The
American Heritage®
Medical Dictionary

The American Heritage® Medical Dictionary

Houghton Mifflin Company
Boston   New York

Visit our website: www.houghtonmifflinbooks.com

Library of Congress Cataloging-in-Publication Data

The American Heritage medical dictionary.
    p. ; cm.
  Rev. ed. of: The American Heritage Stedman's medical dictionary. 2nd ed. c2004.
  Includes index.
  ISBN-13: 978-0-618-82435-9
  ISBN-10: 0-618-82435-9
  1. Medicine--Dictionaries. I. American Heritage Stedman's medical dictionary. II. Title: Medical dictionary.
  [DNLM: 1. Medicine--Dictionary--English. W 13 A5112 2007]
  R121.A4446 2007
  610.3--dc22

               2006028757

Manufactured in the United States of America

QWV 10 9 8 7 6 5 4 3 2 1

EDITORIAL AND PRODUCTION STAFF

Vice President, Publisher of Dictionaries
Margery S. Berube

Vice President, Executive Editor
Joseph P. Pickett

Editorial Project Director
David R. Pritchard

Vice President, Managing Editor
Christopher Leonesio

Project Editor
Susan I. Spitz, MD

Senior Editor
Steven R. Kleinedler

Contributing Editors
Benjamin W. Fortson IV
Hanna Schonthal

Associate Editor
Uchenna C. Ikonné

Assistant Editor
Peter Chipman

Editorial Assistance
Daniel T. Harney
Hiu Ho
Ashley N. O'Bryan

Proofreaders
Kathryn Blatt
Katherine Isaacs
Julia Penelope

Database Production Supervisor
Christopher Granniss

Art and Production Supervisor
Margaret Anne Miles

Manufacturing Supervisor
James W. Mitchell

Production Associate
Katherine M. Getz

Editorial Production Associate
Brianne M. Lutfy

Text Design
Catherine Hawkes, Cat & Mouse

Administrative Coordinators
Darcy Conroy
Kevin McCarthy

Contributors to the First Edition

Lois Principe Borup, James J. Boyle,
Kaethe Ellis, Paul G. Evenson, David A. Jost,
Ann-Marie Imbornoni, Ann Marie Menting,
Joseph M. Patwell, Martha Phelps,
Marion Severynse

TABLE OF CONTENTS

Guide to the Dictionary   ix

Pronunciation Key   xiii

Compound Word Index   xv

The American Heritage Medical Dictionary   1

Appendixes

    Measurements   898

    Metric Conversion Chart   899

    Recommended Daily Allowances   900–901

    Periodic Table of the Elements   902–903

    Skeletal Muscles   904–905

    Skeleton   906

    Vascular System   907

    Nervous System   908

Illustration Credits   909

This Guide explains the conventions used in presenting the array of information contained in the Dictionary, enabling you to find and understand that information quickly and easily.

Guidewords

There are boldface guidewords printed at the top left and top right corners of every two-page spread. The first guideword, at the top left of the two-page spread, shows the first entry on the left page; the second guideword, at the top right of the spread, shows the last entry on the right page. Thus, **alloxuremia** appears at the top left corner of page 30 and **alveolar artery** at the top right corner of page 31. All the entries that fall alphabetically between them are entered and defined on these two pages.

The Entry Words: Alphabetical Order

Each entry word, printed in boldface type, is set slightly to the left of the text column. All entries—including biographical names, abbreviations, symbols, and compounds of two or more words—are listed in strict alphabetical order:

> **denial**
> **denidation**
> **Denis Browne splint**
> **Dennie's line**
> **dens**

Superscript numbers. Words with identical spellings but different etymologies are entered separately and have superscript, or raised, numbers:

> **mole¹** (mōl) *n.* A small congenital growth on the skin
> ...
> **mole²** (mōl) *n.* **1.** A fleshy abnormal mass formed in the uterus ...
> **mole³** *or* **mol** (mōl) *n.* **1.** The amount of a substance that contains as many atoms ...

Syllabification

An entry word and its inflected and derived forms are divided into syllables by means of centered dots:

> **ol·i·go·nu·cle·o·tide** (ŏl′ĭ-gō-no͞o′klē-ə-tīd) *n.*

In compound entries composed of two or more words separated either by a hyphen or by a space, individual words within the compound may not be syllabicated if they are entered separately in the Dictionary with syllabication or if they are common English words that can be found in any general dictionary:

> **digital subtraction angiography** (səb-trăk′shən) *n.*
> **ethyl alcohol** *n.*
> **growth-onset diabetes** *n.*

Pronunciation

Pronunciations, enclosed by parentheses, are given immediately after the boldface entry word. Variant pronunciations are given wherever necessary and follow the form to which they apply. When more than one pronunciation is given, all are acceptable in spite of the fact that there may be differences between them in frequency of occurrence. A full pronunciation key is given on page *xiii.*

Pronunciations are syllabified for the sake of clarity. The syllabication of the pronunciation may not match the syllabification of the entry word because the division of the pronunciation follows phonological rules, while the division of the entry word reflects the long-established practices of printers and editors of breaking words at the end of a line.

Stress. There are three relative degrees of stress or emphasis with which the syllables of a word are spoken. A syllable with primary, or strongest, stress is signaled by a boldface mark (′) after it. A syllable with secondary, or weaker, stress has a lighter mark (′) after it. A syllable with no mark after it has the weakest stress in a multisyllabic word. Monosyllabic words have no stress mark because there is no other level of stress within the word to which the syllable can be compared. (For a full explanation of the pronunciation symbols, see the Pronunciation Key on page xiii.)

Variants

All spelling variants in this Dictionary are set in boldface type with the word *or* between the main entry term and its variant:

ba·be·si·o·sis (bə-bē′zē-ō′sĭs) or **bab·e·si·a·sis** (băb′ĭ-zī′ə-sĭs) *n.*

Variants that occur more than a few entries away from the main entry word in alphabetical order are entered as separate cross-references at the appropriate places in the alphabetical word list:

a·me·ba or **am·oe·ba** (ə-mē′bə) *n.*
am·oe·ba (ə-mē′bə) *n.* Variant of **ameba.**

Part-of-speech Labels

The following italicized labels indicate parts of speech:

adj.	adjective
adv.	adverb
n.	noun
v.	verb

Irregular plurals are indicated with the label *pl.*

Entries that are abbreviations, such as *DDI* and *IVP*, are labeled *abbr.*

Some entries are unlabeled; these include symbols (such as *I*, the symbol for iodine), trademarks (such as *Wellbutrin*), and Greek letters (α).

The labels for word elements are:

pref.	prefix
suff.	suffix

Inflected Forms

An inflected form of a word differs from the main entry form by the addition of a suffix or by a change in its base form to indicate grammatical features such as number, person, mood, or tense. The following inflected forms are given in the main entries in this Dictionary: (1) principal parts of all irregular and regular verbs, (2) all comparative and superlative degrees of adjectives and adverbs formed by inflection, and (3) irregular plurals of nouns.

Inflected forms follow the part-of-speech label. They are set in boldface type, divided into syllables, and given pronunciations as necessary. Inflected forms are usually shortened to the last syllable of the entry word plus the inflectional ending. Irregular inflected forms are spelled out to the extent required for clarity. When inflected forms are shortened, each shortened inflected form is preceded by a boldface hyphen:

ge·la·tin·ize (jə-lăt′n-īz′, jĕl′ə-tn-īz′) *v.* **-nized,** **-niz·ing, -niz·es.**

Principal parts of verbs. The principal parts of verbs are entered in this order: *past tense, past participle, present participle,* and *third person singular present tense.* When the past tense and the past participle are identical, one form represents both:

di·vide (dĭ-vīd′) *v.* **-vid·ed, -vid·ing, -vides.**

Comparison of adjectives and adverbs. Adjectives and adverbs whose comparative and superlative degrees can be formed by adding *–er* and *–est* to the unchanged word show these comparative and superlative suffixes immediately after the part-of-speech label:

sick (sĭk) *adj.* **sick·er, sick·est.**

Irregular comparative and superlative forms are given in full.

Plurals of nouns. Plurals of nouns other than those formed regularly by adding the suffixes *–s* or *–es* are shown and labeled *pl.*:

louse (lous) *n., pl.* **lice** (līs).

When a noun has a regular and an irregular plural form, both forms appear, with the most common shown first:

a·me·ba or **am·oe·ba** (ə-mē′bə) *n., pl.* **–bas** or **–bae** (-bē).

A noun that is chiefly or exclusively plural in both form and meaning is labeled *pl.n.*:

abdominal reflexes *pl.n.* Contractions of the muscles of the abdominal wall upon stimulation of the skin or upon the tapping of neighboring bony structures.

The irregular plural forms of certain nouns are often the more recognizable, and more commonly used, form of the word and have therefore been entered separately in the Dictionary. Examples of such entries include *bacteria, protozoa,* and *teeth.*

Cross-references

A cross-reference signals that additional information about one entry can be found at another entry. Cross-references have two main functions: to avoid needless duplication of information and to indicate where further discussion of a word occurs.

Synonymous cross-references. When two terms are synonymous, a full definition appears at the primary term. A list of synonyms follows. The secondary terms are entered at their own places in the alphabet and are defined by the primary term, set in secondary boldface letters and followed if necessary by the appropriate sense number indicating the sense of the main entry at which a full definition can be found. For instance, **lockjaw** is a cross-reference entry referring the reader to sense **1** of **tetanus:**

> **lock·jaw** (lŏk′jô′) *n.* **1.** See **tetanus** (sense 1). **2.** See **trismus.**

At sense **1** of **tetanus,** the full definition is given:

> **tet·a·nus** (tĕt′n-əs) *n.* **1.** An acute, often fatal disease characterized by spasmodic contraction of voluntary muscles, especially those of the neck and jaw, and caused by the neurotoxin of *Clostridium tetani,* which typically infects the body through a deep wound. Also called *lockjaw.*

If, however, a secondary term falls adjacent to the primary term, it is not given a separate entry.

Symbol cross-references. This type of cross-reference refers to the entry represented by the symbol:

> **Ba** The symbol for the element **barium.**

The main entry likewise contains a reference to its symbol:

> **bar·i·um** (bâr′ē-əm, băr′-) *n. Symbol* **Ba**

Order of Senses

Entries containing more than one sense are arranged so that the word and its meanings can be perceived as a structural unit. Sense are listed from the most common, general, and least detailed to the most technical, specific, and detailed. Senses and subsenses are grouped to show their relationships with each other. Senses that are outdated but that remain in some use or are important for their historical usage contain the admonition "No longer in technical use."

Division of senses. Multisense entries have their meanings numbered sequentially in boldface:

> **a·nas·to·mose** (ə-năs′tə-mōz′, -mōs′) *v.* **–mosed, –mos·es, –mos·ing. 1.** To join by anastomosis. **2.** To be connected by anastomosis.

In a combined entry the senses are numbered in separate sequences that begin after each part-of-speech label:

> **de·cay** (dĭ-kā′) *n.* **1.** The destruction or decomposition of organic matter as a result of bacterial or fungal action; rot. **2.** Dental caries. **3.** The loss of information that was registered by the senses and processed into the short-term memory system. **4.** Radioactive decay. *-v.* **–cayed, –cay·ing, –cays. 1.** To break down into component parts; rot. **2.** To disintegrate or diminish by radioactive decay. **3.** To decline in health or vigor; waste away.

Verbal Illustrations

Verbal illustrations are used only at those entries that are affixes for prefixes or suffixes, to show examples of words formed with these elements. The word acanthocyte is a verbal illustration at the entry acantho-:

> **acantho–** or **acanth–** *pref.* Thorn; spine; spinous process: *acanthocyte.*

Undefined Forms

At the end of many entries additional boldface words appear without definitions—words either formed from the entry word by the addition of suffixes or otherwise closely and clearly related to the entry word or the entry word itself with a different part of speech. These *run-on entries* are related in basic meaning to the entry word but may have different grammatical functions, as indicated by their part-of-speech labels. Multisyllabic run-ons are divided into syllables and show primary and secondary stresses as needed. Pronunciations are included as required:

> **cu·ra·rize** (koŏ-rä′riz′, kyoŏ-) *v.* **–rized, –riz·ing, –riz·es. 1.** To poison with curare. **2.** To treat a person with curare so as to relax the skeletal muscles. **—cu·ra′ri·za′tion** (-rĭ-zā′shən) *n.*

Eponymous Terms

Entries that are terms based on or derived from the name of a person are eponymous terms and often have a biographical entry located near them. More than 400 biographical entries are featured throughout the Dictionary and serve to explain the eponym as well as give an idea of the person and the history behind the term, for example:

> **cu·rie** (kyŏŏr′ē, kyŏŏ-rē′) *n. Abbr.* **Ci** A unit of radioactivity, equal to the amount of a radioactive isotope that decays at the rate of 3.7×1010 disintegrations per second.

Cu·rie (kyŏŏr′ē, kyŏŏ-rē′, kü-), **Marie.** Originally Manja Skłodowska. 1867–1934. Polish-born French chemist. She shared a 1903 Nobel Prize with her husband, **Pierre Curie** (1859–1906), and Henri Becquerel (1852–1908) for fundamental research on radioactivity. In 1911 she won a second Nobel Prize for her discovery and study of the elements radium and polonium.

Pronunciations appear in parentheses after bold-face entry words. If an entry word has a variant, and both have the same pronunciation, the pronunciation follows the variant. If the variant does not have the same pronunciation, pronunciations follow the forms to which they apply. If a word has more than one pronunciation, the first pronunciation is usually more common than the other, but often they are equally common. Pronunciations are shown within an entry where necessary.

Stress. Stress is the relative degree of emphasis with which a word's syllables are spoken. An unmarked syllable has the weakest stress in the word. The strongest, or primary, stress is indicated with a bold mark (**′**). A lighter mark (′) indicates a secondary level of stress. Words of one syllable have no stress mark, because there is no other stress level to which the syllable is compared.

Pronunciation Symbols. The pronunciation symbols used in this Dictionary are shown below. To the right of the symbols are words that show how the symbols are pronounced. The letters whose sound corresponds to the symbols are shown in boldface.

The symbol (ə) is called *schwa*. It represents a vowel with the weakest level of stress in a word. The schwa sound varies slightly according to the vowel it represents or the sounds around it:

a·bun·dant (ə-bŭn**′**dənt)
mo·ment (mō**′**mənt)
grate·ful (grāt**′**fəl)
civ·il (sĭv**′**əl)
pro·pose (prə-pōz**′**)

In English, the consonants *l* and *n* can be complete syllables. Examples of words with syllabic *l* and *n* are **needle** (nēd**′**l) and **sudden** (sŭd**′**n).

Foreign Symbols. Some foreign words use sounds that are not found in English. The (œ) sound is made by rounding the lips as though you were going to make the (ō) sound, but instead you make an (ā) sound. The (ü) sound is made by rounding the lips as though you were going to make the (o͞o) sound, but instead you make an (ē) sound. The (KH) sound is like a (k), but the air is forced through continuously, not stopped as with a (k). The (N) sound shows that the vowel before it is nasalized—that is, air escapes through the nose (and the mouth) when you say it.

Pronunciation Key

ă	pat	ī	pie, by	o͝o	took	ûr	urge, term, firm,
ā	pay	îr	dear, deer, pier	o͝or	lure		word, heard
âr	care	j	judge	o͞o	boot	v	valve
ä	father	k	kick, cat, pique	ou	out	w	with
b	bib	l	lid, needle	p	pop	y	yes
ch	church	m	mum	r	roar	z	zebra, xylem
d	deed, milled	n	no, sudden	s	sauce	zh	vision, pleasure,
ě	pet	ng	thing	sh	ship, dish		garage
ē	bee	ŏ	pot	t	tight, stopped	ə	about, item,
f	fife, phase, rough	ō	toe	th	thin		edible, gallop,
g	gag	ô	caught, paw	*th*	this		circus
h	hat	ôr	core	ŭ	cut	ər	butter
ĭ	pit	oi	noise				

COMPOUND WORD INDEX

This index is an alphabetical guide to common compound words that appear as entries in the dictionary. The **boldfaced** terms are followed by every word that precedes them in a given entry; for example, the word **agent** will appear in the entries **alkylating agent, antianxiety agent,** and so on.

A

aberration chromatic; chromosome; coma; curvature; dioptric; distortion; lateral; longitudinal; meridional; monochromatic; optical; spherical

abortion habitual; incomplete; induced; infected; missed; septic; spontaneous; therapeutic

abscess alveolar; amebic; appendiceal; Bezold's; Brodie's; cold; collar-button; crypt; dental; dentoalveolar; diffuse; dry; Dubois; fecal; gas; gummatous; metastatic; migrating; miliary; Munro's; Pautrier's; perforating; periappendiceal; periarticular; peritonsillar; phlegmonous; Pott's; psoas; pyemic; residual; ring; satellite; septicemic; shirt-stud; stellate; stercoral; stitch; syphilitic; thymic; Tornwaldt's; tropical; tuberculous; wandering

acid acetic; acetoacetic; acetohydroxamic; acetylsalicylic; adenylic; agaric; aliphatic; alpha-amino; alpha-aminosuccinic; alpha-hydroxy; aminobenzoic; arachidonic; argininosuccinic; arsenic; ascorbic; aspartic; barbituric; benzoic; bile; boric; bromic; butanoic; butyric; capric; caproic; caprylic; carbamic; carbolic; cerebronic; chloric; chlorous; cholaic; choleic; cholic; cis-aconitic; citric; cysteic; cytidylic; dehydrocholic; delta-aminolevulinic; deoxyadenylic; deoxycholic; deoxycytidylic; deoxyguanylic; deoxyribonucleic; deoxythymidylic; diacetic; dibasic; dicarboxylic; diethylenetriamine pentaacetic; dihydrofolic; dihydropteroic; edetic; ellagic; erythorbic; ethacrynic; ethanoic; ethylenediaminetetraacetic; folic; folinic; formic; formiminoglutamic; 4-pyridoxic; fumaric; gamma-aminobutyric; gluconic; glucuronic; glutamic; glutaminic; glutaric; glyceric; glycocholic; glycolic; guanylic; heptanedioic; hexadecanoic; homogentisic; homovanillic; hyaluronic; hydrochloric; hydrocyanic; hypochlorous; imino; indoleacetic; inorganic; inosinic; iocetamic; iopanoic; iothalamic; isocitric; keto; kynurenic; lactic; lauric; linoleic; linolenic; lipoic; lysergic; maleic; malic; malonic; mandelic; mefenamic; mercapturic; metaphosphoric; methanesulfonic; monobasic; nalidixic; nervonic; neuraminic; nicotinic; nitric; nitrous; nucleic; oleic; organic; orotic; orthophosphoric; osmic; oxalacetic; oxalic; oxaloacetic; oxalosuccinic; oxolinic; palmitic; palmitoleic; pantothenic; para-aminobenzoic; para-aminohippuric; para-aminosalicylic; pentetic; perchloric; periodic; permanganic; phenaceturic; phenic; phenylacetic; phenylaceturic; phenyllactic; phosphoenolpyruvic; phosphoric; phthalic; phytanic; picric; pimelic; polyadenylic; polybasic; polyenoic; propanoic; propionic; prostanoic; prussic; pteroylglutamic; pteroyltriglutamic; pyrogallic; pyrophosphoric; pyruvic; retinoic; ribonucleic; saccharic; salicylic; sarcolactic; sialic; sorbic; stearic; succinic; sulfonic; sulfosalicylic; sulfuric; tannic; taurocholic; teichoic; thiosulfuric; thymidylic; tranexamic; triacetic; trichloroacetic; uric; uridylic; urocanic; uronic; valproic; vanillylmandelic; vitamin A; xanthurenic

adenoma acidophil; ACTH-producing; adnexal; apocrine; basophil; bronchial; carcinoma ex pleomorphic; chromophil; chromophobe; eosinophil; fibroid; growth hormone-producing; papillary cystic; pituitary basophil; prolactin-producing; sebaceous; villous

agent alkylating; antianxiety; antipsychotic; contrast; delta; disclosing; Eaton; initiating; Pittsburgh pneumonia; promoting; reducing

ampulla duodenal; Henle's; membranous; osseous; rectal; Thoma's; Vater's

amputation A-E; A-K; B-E; birth; central; Chopart's; cineplastic; circular; congenital; double-flap; Dupuytren's; elliptical; flap; flapless; Gritti-Stokes; interpelviabdominal; intrauterine; Krukenberg's; Larrey's; mediotarsal; oval; periosteoplastic; pulp; racket; root; spontaneous; Stokes'; subperiosteal; Teale's; transverse; traumatic

anastomosis antiperistaltic; arteriovenous; Billroth I; Billroth II; conjoined; cruciate; heterocladic; H-graft; homocladic; intestinal; isoperistaltic; postcostal; precostal; Riolan's; Roux-en-Y; termino-terminal

anemia achrestic; Addison's; aplastic; autoallergic hemolytic; autoimmune hemolytic; congenital; congenital hemolytic; congenital hypoplastic; Cooley's; crescent cell; drepanocytic; false; Fanconi's;

hemolytic; hyperchromic; hypochromic; hypoplastic; iron deficiency; macrocytic; malignant; Mediterranean; megaloblastic; metaplastic; microangiopathic hemolytic; microcytic; microdrepanocytic; myelophthisic; neonatal; normochromic; normocytic; pernicious; refractory; sickle cell; sideroblastic; spherocytic; splenic; trophoneurotic; tropical

anesthesia balanced; basal; block; caudal; cerebral; circle absorption; closed; conduction; dissociated; dissociative; epidural; general; girdle; glove; infiltration; inhalation; insufflation; intranasal; intraoral; intravenous; local; muscular; nerve block; nonrebreathing; olfactory; open drop; perineural; rebreathing; rectal; refrigeration; regional; retrobulbar; saddle block; segmental; semi-closed; semi-open; spinal; splanchnic; stocking; surgical; tactile; thermal; topical; traumatic; unilateral; visceral

aneurysm arteriosclerotic; arteriovenous; bacterial; berry; cirsoid; compound; dissecting; false; fusiform; mycotic; racemose; saccular; supraclinoid; syphilitic; varicose

antibody acquired; anaphylactic; anti-; antibasement membrane; antinuclear; blocking; complement-fixing; complete; cross-reacting; cytophilic; cytotropic; heterocytotropic; homocytotropic; incomplete; monoclonal; natural; neutralizing; normal; reaginic

antigen Australia; blood group; capsular; carcinoembryonic; common; complete; delta; flagellar; group; H; hepatitis-associated; hepatitis B core; hepatitis B e; hepatitis B surface; heterogenetic; heterogenic enterobacterial; heterophil; histocompatibility; human leukocyte; H-Y; incomplete; Kveim; mumps skin test; O; oncofetal; organ-specific; partial; sensitized; somatic; species-specific; T; tissue-specific; tumor; tumor-specific transplantation; viral

antitoxin botulism; diphtheria; gas gangrene; normal; scarlet fever; staphylococcus; tetanus and gas gangrene; tetanus; toxin-

aphasia acoustic; acquired epileptic; amnestic; anomic; associative; ataxic; auditory; Broca's; conduction; expressive; global; impressive; jargon; mixed; motor; nominal; receptive; sensory; total; visual

arch abdominothoracic; aortic; branchial; Corti's; costal; dental; fallen; gill; hemal; hyoid; mandibular; neural; palatoglossal; palatopharyngeal; palmar; pectoral; pelvic; pharyngeal; plantar; postoral; primitive costal; pubic; superciliary; supraorbital; tendinous; vertebral; visceral; zygomatic

arteritis cranial; giant cell; obliterating; rheumatic; temporal

artery accessory obturator; acromiothoracic; alveolar; angular; anterior malleolar; appendicular; arcuate; ascending; ascending pharyngeal; atrial; auricular; axillary; basilar; brachial; buccal; carotid; cavernous; celiac; cerebellar; cerebral; cervical; choroidal; ciliary; circumflex humeral; circumflex iliac; circumflex scapular; colic; collateral; communicating; conjunctival; coronary; cortical; costocervical; cremasteric; cystic; deep; descending scapular; dolichoectatic; dorsal digital; dorsal scapular; end; epigastric; episcleral; ethmoidal; external spermatic; facial; femoral; fibular; frontal; gastric; gastroduodenal; gastroepiploic; gastro-omental; gluteal; helicine; hepatic; hyaloid; hypogastric; ileal; ileocolic; iliac; iliolumbar; infraorbital; innominate; intercostal; interlobar; interlobular; internal auditory; internal pudendal; internal spermatic; interosseous; intestinal; jejunal; labial; lacrimal; laryngeal; lienal; lingual; lumbar; mammary; masseteric; maxillary; median; meningeal; mental; mesenteric; metacarpal; metatarsal; middle collateral; musculophrenic; nutrient; obturator; occipital; ophthalmic; ovarian; palatine; palmar digital; palpebral; pancreatic; pancreaticoduodenal; perforating; pericardiacophrenic; perineal; peroneal; phrenic; plantar; plantar digital; popliteal; posterior lateral nasal; pudendal; pulmonary; radial; radial collateral; radial index; ranine; rectal; recurrent; renal; sacral; sigmoid; spermatic; sphenopalatine; spinal; splenic; stylomastoid; subclavian; subcostal; sublingual; submental; subscapular; supraorbital; suprarenal; suprascapular; supratrochlear; sural; tarsal; temporal; terminal; testicular; thoracic; thoracoacromial; thoracodorsal; thyroid; tibial; transverse cervical; transverse facial; transverse scapular; tympanic; ulnar; ulnar collateral; umbilical; urethral; uterine; vaginal; ventricular; vertebral; vesical; zygomatico-orbital

arthritis atrophic; chronic absorptive; gouty; hypertrophic; juvenile; juvenile rheumatoid; Lyme; psoriatic; rheumatoid; suppurative

astigmatism compound hyperopic; compound myopic; corneal; hyperopic; irregular; lenticular; mixed; myopic; regular

atrophy familial spinal muscular; infantile muscular; juvenile muscular; Leber's hereditary optic; linear; olivopontocerebellar; peroneal muscular; Pick's; progressive muscular; spinal; Sudeck's

B

bacillus Bang's; Bordet-Gengou; Calmette-Guérin; colon; comma; Ducrey's; Flexner's; Friedländer's; Gärtner's; gas; Hansen's; Klebs-Löffler; Koch's; Koch-Weeks; Morgan's; Pfeiffer's; Shiga-Kruse;

Sonne; timothy hay; tubercle; typhoid

bandage adhesive; Barton's; capeline; cravat; demigauntlet; Desault's; elastic; figure-of-8; gauntlet; many-tailed; plaster; roller; Scultetus; spica; spiral; suspensory; T-bandage; triangular; Velpeau

biopsy aspiration; brush; endoscopic; excision; incision; needle; open; punch; shave

bladder atonic; autonomic; autonomic neurogenic; low-compliance; nervous; neurogenic; neuropathic; pseudo-neurogenic; reflex neurogenic; uninhibited neurogenic; urinary

block anterograde; atrioventricular; bone; bundle-branch; depolarizing; epidural; field; heart; intra-atrial; intraventricular; nerve; nondepolarizing; periinfarction; phase I; phase II; retrograde; sino-atrial; sinoauricular; sinus; spinal; stellate; sun

blocker alpha-; beta-; calcium channel

blocking agent adrenergic; adrenergic neuronal; alpha-adrenergic; beta-adrenergic; ganglionic; neuromuscular; nondepolarizing neuromuscular

body acetone; aortic; asbestos; Aschoff; asteroid; Auer; Babés-Ernst; Barr; basal; Bollinger; Cabot's ring; Call-Exner; carotid; cavernous; cell; chromaffin; chromatin; ciliary; coccygeal; Councilman; cytoplasmic inclusion; Döhle; Donovan; Ehrlich's inner; foreign; geniculate; Heinz-Ehrlich; Highmore's; Howell-Jolly; hyaline; hyaloid; immune; inclusion; intercarotid; ketone; Lafora; lateral geniculate; Leishman-Donovan; Mallory; malpighian; mamillary; medial geniculate; metachromatic; Michaelis-Gutmann; multilamellar; Negri; Nissl; nuclear inclusion; olivary; pacchionian; Pappenheimer; para-aortic; parabasal; Paschen; persistent anterior hyperplastic primary vitreous; persistent posterior hyperplastic primary vitreous; pineal; polar; psammoma; quadrigeminal; restiform; Russell; sclerotic; striate; trachoma; tuffstone; vitreous; wolffian; Wolf-Orton; zebra

bone ankle-; back-; breast-; brittle; calf; cancellous; capitate; cartilage; cheek-; collar-; compact; cortical; cranial; cuneiform; elbow; endochondral; ethmoid; facial; first cuneiform; flat; frontal; funny; heel; hip-; hollow; hyoid; iliac; incisive; innominate; intermaxillary; intermediate cuneiform; irregular; ischial; jaw-; jugal; knuckle-; lacrimal; lamellar; lateral cuneiform; long; lunate; malar; marble; mastoid; medial cuneiform; membrane; middle cuneiform; multangular; nasal; nonlamellar; occipital; palatine; parietal; perichondral; pisiform; pneumatic; premaxillary; pubic; pyramidal; reticulated; rider's; scroll; second cuneiform; semilunar; shin-; short; sphenoid; spongy; sutural; tail-; tarsal; temporal; thigh-; third cuneiform; trabecular; triangular; turbinate; tympanic; unciform; wedge;

wormian; woven; zygomatic

bundle atrioventricular; ground; His; longitudinal pontine; medial forebrain; Vicq d'Azyr's

bursa Achilles; anserine; Boyer's; Calori's; glutefemoral; iliac; infraspinatus; ischial; Luschka's; omental; pharyngeal; retrohyoid; subacromial; subdeltoid; suprapatellar; synovial

bypass aortoiliac; aortorenal; bowel; cardiopulmonary; coronary; gastric; jejunoileal

C

calculus alternating; biliary; bronchial; cerebral; combination; coral; cystine; decubitus; dendritic; dental; encysted; fibrin; gastric; hematogenetic; matrix; oxalate; pharyngeal; pocketed; stag-horn; urinary; uterine; vesical

calorie gram; kilogram; large; mean; nutritionist's; small

canal adductor; Alcock's; alimentary; anal; Arnold's; arterial; atrioventricular; auditory; birth; carotid; cervical; cochlear; condylar; condyloid; Corti's; crural; dentinal; ear; external auditory; facial; femoral; Haversian; Hirschfeld's; Hunter's; hypoglossal; incisive; incisor; infraorbital; inguinal; interdental; interfacial; lacrimal; musculotubal; nasolacrimal; nutrient; obturator; optic; parturient; portal; pterygoid; pterygopalatine; pudendal; pulp; pyloric; root; sacral; Schlemm's; semicircular; spinal; tarsal; tympanic; urogenital; vertebral; vestibular; Volkmann's; Wirsung's

capillary arterial; blood; continuous; fenestrated; lymph; venous

capsule articular; auditory; bacterial; Bowman's; cartilage; external; fibrous; Gerota's; Glisson's; internal; joint; lenticular; malpighian; nasal; optic; otic; perivascular fibrous; Tenon's

carcinoma adenoid cystic; adenoid squamous cell; alveolar cell; apocrine; basal cell; basosquamous; bronchiolar; bronchogenic; colloid; cylindromatous; embryonal; endometrioid; epidermoid; fibrolamellar liver cell; giant cell; hepatocellular; Hürthle cell; inflammatory; large cell; medullary; melanotic; mesometanephric; metaplastic; mucinous; oat cell; oncoplastic; papillary; scar; scirrhous; secretory; signet ring cell; small cell; spindle cell; squamous cell; sweat gland; transitional cell; tubular; verrucous; villous

cartilage alar; arthrodial; articular; arytenoid; auditory; auricular; connecting; corniculate; costal; cricoid; cuneiform; diarthrodial; elastic; ensiform; epiglottic; epiphysial; floating; hyaline; innominate; interarticular; interosseous; intervertebral; investing; mandibular; permanent; precursory; secondary; semilunar; slipping rib; temporary; thyroid; tracheal; vomerine; vomeronasal; xiphoid; Y; yellow

cataract annular; atopic; axillary; black; blue; capsular; capsulolenticular; coronary; cortical; cupuliform; diffuse; fibrinous; fibroid; galactose; glaucomatous; gray; hypermature; immature; juvenile; lamellar; lenticular; mature; membranous; Morgagni's; nuclear; polar; primary; progressive; pyramidal; secondary; senile; siliculose; siliquose; subcapsular; vascular; zonular

catheter balloon-tip; Bozeman-Fritsch; brush; cardiac; Carlens; central venous; double-channel; Fogarty; Foley; Gouley's; indwelling; intra-cardiac; Nélaton; pacing; Phillips; self-retaining; Swan-Ganz; two-way; vertebrated; winged

cavity abdominal; amniotic; axillary; buccal; cleavage; cotyloid; cranial; glenoid; intracranial; lesser peritoneal; Meckel's; medullary; nasal; oral; orbital; pelvic; pericardial; peritoneal; pleural; pulp; segmentation; tension; thoracic; trigeminal; tympanic; uterine

cell A; acid; acinar; acinous; adipose; adventitial; air; alpha; alveolar; ameboid; anaplastic; Anitschkow; antigen-presenting; APUD; argentaffin; auditory receptor; B; band; basal; basket; beaker; beta; Betz; bipolar; blast; blood; branchial; cartilage; centroacinar; chief; chromaffin; chromophobe; clear; cochlear hair; columnar; commissural; cone; Corti's; cytotoxic T; daughter; decidual; Deiters'; delta; dendritic; Downey; dust; enterochromaffin; enteroendocrine; ependymal; epithelioid; ethmoidal; fat; foam; follicular; follicular dendritic; G; ganglion; Gaucher's; germ; germinal; ghost; giant; glia; glomerulosa; goblet; Golgi; granule; granulosa; gustatory; hair; hairy; HeLa; helper; helper T; Hensen's; heteromeric; hilus; hobnail; Hortega; Hürthle; I; inclusion; interdigitating; interstitial; islet; juvenile; juxtaglomerular; killer; killer T; Kupffer; LAK; Langerhans; LE; Leydig; lupus erythematosus; luteal; lutein; mast; mastoid; mesoglial; mirror-image; mitral; mother; mucoserous; mucous; multipolar; myoid; natural killer; nerve; neurilemma; neurolemma; nevus; Niemann-Pick; NK; null; oat; OKT; olfactory receptor; oligodendroglia; Ortho-Kung T; osteoprogenitor; oxyntic; oxyphil; Paget's; Paneth's granular; parafollicular; parietal; peptic; peritubular contractile; phalangeal; photoreceptor; Pick; pigment; plasma; polychromatic; prickle; Purkinje; pyramidal; red; red blood; Reed-Sternberg; resting; reticular; Rieder; rod; Rouget; satellite; Schwann; segmented; sensitized; serous; Sertoli; sex; Sézary; sickle; signet-ring; somatic; spindle; squamous; stab; staff; stellate; stem; Sternberg-Reed; strap; suppressor T; sustentacular; T; target; tart; taste; tendon; T-helper; Touton giant; transducer; tufted; vasoformative; Virchow's; virus-transformed; visual receptor; wandering; white blood; zymogenic

center birthing; Broca's; burn; chondrification; ciliospinal; crisis; epiotic; medullary; motor speech; optic; respiratory; sensory speech; Wernicke's

chromosome acrocentric; bivalent; Christchurch; duplication of; fragile X-; eterotypical; homologous; metacentric; Philadelphia; reduction of; ring; sex; X-; Y-

circulation collateral; compensatory; enterohepatic; extracorporeal; placental; portal; pulmonary; systemic

cirrhosis alcoholic; biliary; cardiac; cholangiolitic; fatty; Laënnec's; necrotic; portal; posthepatitic; postnecrotic; toxic

colitis amebic; collagenous; granulomatous; hemorrhagic; mucous; myxomembranous; pseudomembranous; ulcerative

complex AIDS-related; anomalous; atrial; avian leukosis-sarcoma; B; Cain; castration; Diana; Eisenmenger's; Electra; femininity; Golgi; HLA; immune; inferiority; Jocasta; Lear; major histocompatibility; Oedipus; primary; QRS; sicca; superiority; symptom; synaptinemal; VATER; ventricular; vitamin B

conjunctivitis acute contagious; acute hemorrhagic; allergic; atopic; calcareous; contagious granular; follicular; gonococcal; granular; inclusion; infantile purulent; spring; swimming pool; vernal

contraction Braxton-Hicks; carpopedal; escaped ventricular; fibrillary; hourglass; hunger; idiomuscular; myotatic; paradoxical; postural; premature ventricular; tonic

cord false vocal; genital; gonadal; spermatic; spinal; tendinous; testicular; true vocal; umbilical; vocal

corpuscle articular; bulboid; corneal; genital; ghost; Golgi-Mazzoni; Hassall's concentric; lamellated; lymphatic; lymph; lymphoid; malpighian; Meissner's; Merkel's; pacinian; phantom; Purkinje; red; renal; Ruffini's; tactile; thymic; thymus; white

cortex adrenal; association; auditory; cerebellar; cerebral; frontal; heterotypic; homotypic; motor; renal; sensory; somatic sensory; somatosensory; visual

crest ampullary; anterior lacrimal; ethmoidal; external occipital; frontal; iliac; infratemporal; internal occipital; intertrochanteric; medial; nasal; neural; obturator; palatine; posterior lacrimal; pubic; sacral; sphenoid; spiral; supramastoid; supraventricular; urethral; vestibular

culture cell; organ; plate; pure; slant; slope; smear;

stab; stock; streak; tissue

cycle carbon; carbon dioxide; carbon-nitrogen; cardiac; cell; citric acid; Cori; dicarboxylic acid; estrous; fatty acid oxidation; Krebs; Krebs-Henseleit; Krebs ornithine; Krebs urea; life; menstrual; nitrogen; ovarian; reproductive; tricarboxylic acid; urea; uterine

cyst adventitious; aneurysmal bone; arachnoid; Baker's; Bartholin's; Blessig's; blood; blue dome; Boyer's; bronchogenic; chocolate; choledochal; daughter; dentigerous; dentinal lamina; dermoid; echinococcus; enterogenous; epidermal; epidermoid; exudation; false; follicular; granddaughter; hemorrhagic; hydatid; keratinous; morgagnian; mother; multilocular; myxoid; nabothian; odontogenic; osseous hydatid; ovarian; parasitic; parent; periapical periodontal; pilar; radicular; retention; sebaceous; serous; solitary bone; sterile; sublingual; synovial; tarry; tarsal; tubular; unicameral; unicameral bone; unilocular; vitellointestinal; wolffian

D

deafness acoustic trauma; Alexander's; central; conductive; cortical; functional; psychogenic; sensorineural; word

defect aorticopulmonary septal; aortic septal; atrial septal; birth; congenital ectodermal; fibrous cortical; filling; ventricular septal

deficiency antitrypsin; familial high-density lipoprotein; galactokinase; glucosephosphate isomerase; immune; LCAT; mental; phosphohexose isomerase; pseudocholinesterase; pyruvate kinase

degeneration adipose; albuminoid; amyloid; ascending; atheromatous; calcareous; caseous; colloid; Crooke's hyaline; descending; disciform; elastoid; fascicular; fatty; fibrinoid; fibroid; glassy; gray; hepatolenticular; heredomacular; hyaline; hydropic; macular; mucoid; orthograde; parenchymatous; reticular; secondary; spongy; transsynaptic; vitelliform; wallerian; waxy; Zenker's

dementia Alzheimer's; dialysis; multi-infarct; paralytic; presenile; senile; vascular

dentin hereditary opalescent; irregular; primary; reparative; sclerotic; secondary; tertiary; transparent

dentition deciduous; delayed; mandibular; maxillary; permanent; primary; retarded; secondary

denture complete; fixed partial; full; immediate; implant; interim; overlay; partial; removable partial; temporary; transitional; trial

dermatitis actinic; atopic; berlock; berloque; bubble gum; chemical; contact; contact-type; diaper; exfoliative; infectious eczematoid; livedoid; mead-

ow; occupational; radiation; schistosome; seborrheic; stasis

diabetes adult-onset; brittle; bronze; chemical; growth-onset; insulin-dependent; juvenile; juvenile-onset; latent; late-onset; mature-onset; maturity-onset; non-insulin-dependent; phosphate; subclinical; sugar; type I; type II

diet acid-ash; alkaline-ash; balanced; bland; challenge; diabetic; elimination; high calorie; ketogenic; low calorie; macrobiotic; smooth; soft

digestion gastric; intestinal; pancreatic; peptic; primary; salivary; secondary

disease Acosta's; Addison's; akamushi; Albers-Schönberg; Albright's; Almeida's; Alpers'; Alzheimer's; Andersen's; aortoiliac occlusive; Aran-Duchenne; autoimmune; Ayerza's; Bamberger-Marie; Bang's; Bannister's; Banti's; Barlow's; Barraquer's; Basedow's; Batten-Mayou; Bayle's; Bazin's; Bechterew's; Benson's; Bernhardt's; Besnier-Boeck-Schaumann; Best's; Bielschowsky's; Binswanger's; Blocq's; Blount's; Boeck's; Bornholm; Bourneville-Pringle; Bourneville's; Bowen's; Breda's; Bright's; Brill's; Brill-Symmers; Brill-Zinsser; bronzed; brown lung; Buerger's; Busse-Buschke; Caffey's; caisson; Calvé-Perthes; Canavan's; Carrión's; cat scratch; celiac; Chagas; Charcot-Marie-Tooth; Charcot's; Chédiak-Higashi; Chiari's; Christensen-Krabbe; Christian's; Christmas; chronic active liver; chronic granulomatous; chronic obstructive pulmonary; Coats; collagen; collagen vascular communicable; Concato's; connective-tissue; constitutional; contagious; Cori's; coronary heart; Cowden's; Creutzfeldt-Jakob; Crohn's; Crouzon's; Cruveilhier's; cystine storage; cytomegalic inclusion; cytomegalovirus; Darier's; Darling's; deficiency; degenerative joint; Dejerine's; demyelinating; de Quervain's; Dercum's; Devic's; Duchenne-Aran; Duchenne's; Duhring's; Dukes; Ebstein's; Engelmann's; Erb's; Eulenburg's; extrapyramidal; Fabry's; familial Alzheimer's; Farber's; fifth; fishskin; Flegel's; foot-and-mouth; Forbes; Fordyce's; Forrestier's; Fothergill's; fourth; Fox-Fordyce; Freiberg's; Friedreich's; functional; Gamna's; Garré's; Gaucher's; genetic; Gierke's; Gilbert's; Gilles de la Tourette's; Glanzmann's; glycogen storage; Goldflam; graft-versus-host; Graves'; Greenfield's; Günther's; Hailey and Hailey; Hallopeau's; Hamman's; hand-foot-and-mouth; Hand-Schüller-Christian; H; Hansen's; Hartnup; Hashimoto's; heart; heavy chain; Heerfordt's; Heine-Medin; hemoglobin; hemoglobin C; hemoglobin H; Hers; Hippel's; Hirschsprung's; Hodgkin's; Hodgson's; hoof-and-mouth; hookworm; Huntington's; Hurler's; hyaline membrane; hydatid; Iceland; immune complex; inclusion body; inclusion cell; industrial; infectious; inflammatory bowel; insufficiency; interstitial; iron-storage; Jakob-Creutzfeldt; Jansky-Bielschowsky; Jensen's; Kashin-Bek; Katayama; Kawasaki; Kienböck's; Kimmelstiel-Wilson; kinky-hair; kissing; Klippel's; Köhler's; Krabbe's; Kufs; Kussmaul's; Lafora body; Lafora's; Legg-Calvé-Perthes; Legionnaires'; Leiner's; Letterer-Siwe; Lhermitte-Duclos; Lindau's; Lou Gehrig's; Lutz-Splendore-Almeida; Lyell's; Lyme; lysosomal; Madelung's; Majocchi's; Manson's; maple syrup urine; marble bone; Marburg virus; Marchiafava-Bignami; Marie's; Marie-Strümpell; McArdle's; McArdle-Schmid-Pearson; Mediterranean-hemoglobin E; Ménétrièr's; Ménière's; mental; Merzbacher-Pelizaeus; Mikulicz; Milroy's; Minamata; Mitchell's; mixed connective-tissue; Möbius; molecular; Mondor's; Monge's; Morgagni's; Morquio's; Morquio-Ulrich; Morvan's; motor neuron; Nicolas-Favre; Niemann-Pick; Norrie's; notifiable; occupational; Oguchi's; Ollier's; Oppenheim's; organic; Ormond's; Osgood-Schlatter; Osler's; Osler-Vaquez; Owren's; Paget's; Panner's; paper mill worker's; Parkinson's; Parrot's; Parry's; Pel-Ebstein; Pelizaeus-Merzbacher; Pellegrini's; Pellegrini-Stieda; pelvic inflammatory; periodic; peripheral vascular; Perthes; Peyronie's; Pick's[1]; Pick's[2]; Pick's[3]; pink; Pompe's; Pott's; primary; Pringle's; pulseless; Quincke's; Raynaud's; Recklinghausen's; Refsum's; Reiter's; Rendu-Osler-Weber; reportable; RH; rheumatic heart; Riggs'; Ritter's; Roger's; Rokitansky's; Sandhoff's; Schamberg's; Scheuermann's; Schilder's; Schlatter-Osgood; Schönlein's; Schüller's; secondary; serum; sexually transmitted; sickle cell; sickle cell C; sickle cell-thalassemia; Simmonds; sixth; sixth venereal; slow virus; social; Spielmeyer-Vogt; Steinert's; Still's; Stokes-Adams; storage; Strümpell-Marie; Strümpell's; Strümpell-Westphal; Sturge's; Sturge-Weber; Sutton's; Swift's; Takahara's; Takayasu's; Tangier; Tay-Sachs; Thomsen's; thyrocardiac; tsutsu-gamushi; tunnel; vagabond's; vagrant's; Vaquez; venereal; Vincent's; Vogt-Spielmeyer; von Economo's; von Gierke's; von Hippel-Lindau; von Recklinghausen's; von Willebrand's; Weber-Christian; Weil's; Werlhof's; Wernicke's; Westphal-Strümpell; Whipple's; Wilson's; Winiwarter-Buerger; Wolman's; wool-sorter's

disk articular; blood; choked; ciliary; embryonic; germinal; hair; herniated; intercalated; intervertebral; optic; Placido's; protruded; ruptured; slipped; tactile

disorder acute brain; acute neuropsychologic; adjustment; affective; antisocial personality; anxiety; attention deficit; behavior; binge eating; bipolar; borderline personality; character; conduct; conversion; cyclothymic; dissociative identity; dysthymic; eating; emotional; focal seizure; functional; generalized anxiety; generalized seizure; generalized tonic-clonic seizure; identity; immunoproliferative; impulse control; intermittent explosive; isolated explosive; mental; neuropsychologic; oppositional; organic mental; overanxious; panic; personality; pervasive developmental; posttraumatic stress; psychogenic pain; psychophysiologic; psychosomatic; seasonal affective; seizure; somatization; somatoform; substance abuse

dose absorbed; booster; curative; effective; erythema; L; lethal; maximal; maximal permissible; minimal; minimal infecting; minimal lethal; minimal reacting; optimum; skin; tolerance

duct aberrant; accessory pancreatic; alveolar; anal; arterial; Bartholin's; Bellini's; bile; biliary; Botallo's; branchial; cochlear; common bile; common hepatic; cystic; deferent; efferent; ejaculatory; endolymphatic; excretory; galactophorous; gall; hepatic; intercalated; interlobar; interlobular; intralobular; lacrimal; lacteriferous; left hepatic; left lymphatic; Luschka's; lymphatic; major sublingual; mamillary; mammary; mesonephric; metanephric; milk; minor sublingual; müllerian; Müller's; nasolacrimal; omphalomesenteric; pancreatic; papillary; paramesonephric; paraurethral; parotid; perilymphatic; prostatic; right hepatic; right lymphatic; right thoracic; Rivinus; salivary; Santorini's; secretory; semicircular; seminal; spermatic; Steno's; Stensen's; sublingual; submandibular; submaxillary; thoracic; Wharton's; wolffian

dwarfism achondroplastic; camptomelic; chondrodystrophic; Laron type; mesomelic; metatropic; micromelic; pituitary; Seckel

dye acid; basic; natural; nitro; Sudan; synthetic; triphenylmethane; xanthene

dysmenorrhea essential; mechanical; membranous; obstructive; primary; secondary; spasmodic

dysplasia anhidrotic ectodermal; anterofacial; bronchopulmonary; cerebral; chondroectodermal; cleidocranial; clidocranial; congenital ectodermal; cretinoid; dentinal; dentin; diaphysial; diastrophic; ectodermal; enamel; faciodigitogenital; hidrotic ectodermal; mandibuloacral; metaphysial; Mondini; oculoauriculovertebral; oculodentodigital; oculovertebral; ophthalmomandibulomelic; periapical, cemental; septo-optic; spondyloepiphysial

dystrophy adiposogenital; adult pseudohypertrophic muscular; childhood muscular; Duchenne's;

epithelial; facioscapulohumeral muscular; Fuchs epithelial; infantile neuroaxonal; Landouzy-Déjérine; limb-girdle muscular; muscular; myotonic; pseudohypertrophic muscular

E

edema angioneurotic; cardiac; cerebral; dependent; gestational; hereditary angioneurotic; pitting; pulmonary

embolism air; cerebral; cholesterol; cotton-fiber; fat; infective; miliary; obturating; paradoxical; pulmonary; pyemic; retrograde

emphysema centri-acinar; centrilobular; interlobular; interstitial; intestinal; mediastinal; panacinar; panlobular; pulmonary; subcutaneous; surgical

encephalitis acute necrotizing; bunyavirus; Coxsackie; herpes; inclusion body; Japanese B; La Crosse; lead; postvaccinal; Powassan; Saint Louis; secondary; varicella

encephalopathy bilirubin; Binswanger's; hepatic; lead; leukoencephalopathy portal-systemic; spongiform; subacute spongiform; transmissible; Wernicke-Korsakoff; Wernicke's

endocarditis atypical verrucous; bacterial; infectious; infective; Libman-Sacks; Löffler's; mural; nonbacterial verrucous; parietal; rheumatic; subacute bacterial; valvular; vegetative; verrucous

enzyme acyl-activating; angiotensin-converting; autolytic; brancher; deamidizing; deaminating; debranching; extracellular; induced; inducible; 1,4-alpha-glucan branching; phosphorylase-rupturing; PR; repressible; respiratory; restriction; yellow

epilepsy anosognosic; audiogenic; complex precipitated; cortical; eating; focal; generalized; generalized tonic-clonic; grand mal; idiopathic; jacksonian; juvenile myoclonic; major; myoclonic astatic; myoclonus; pattern sensitive; petit mal; photogenic; posttraumatic; procursive; psychomotor; reflex; rolandic; sensory; startle; temporal lobe; tonic; uncinate

epithelioma basal cell; chorionic; Malherbe's calcifying; malignant ciliary; sebaceous

epithelium ciliated; columnar; cuboidal; germinal; glandular; junctional; laminated; olfactory; pseudostratified; seminiferous; simple; simple squamous; stratified; surface; transitional

extrasystole atrial; atrioventricular; atrioventricular nodal; A-V; A-V nodal; infranodal; interpolated; nodal; return; ventricular

eye aphakic; black; crossed-; cross-; dark-adapted; dominant; exciting; glass; heavy; light-adapted; phakic; photopic; pink-; raccoon; scotopic; wall-

F

facies adenoid; Corvisart's; hippocratic; hurloid; Hutchinson's; leonine; myasthenic; Parkinson's; Potter's

factor accelerator; angiogenesis; antihemophilic; antihemorrhagic; antinuclear; antipernicious anemia; atrial natriuretic; capillary permeability; Castle's intrinsic; Christmas; citrovorum; clearing; clotting; coagulation; extrinsic; F; fertility; follicle-stimulating hormone-releasing; glycotropic; gonadotropin-releasing; growth; growth hormone-releasing; Hageman; human antihemophilic; initiation; insulin-antagonizing; insulinlike growth; intrinsic; Laki-Lorand; LE; lethal; luteinizing hormone/follicle-stimulating hormone-releasing; lymph node permeability; myocardial depressant; nerve growth; osteoclast-activating; platelet-activating; platelet-aggregating; platelet-derived growth; platelet tissue; prolactin-inhibiting; prolactin-releasing; R; recognition; releasing; resistance; resistance transfer; Rh; Rhesus; rheumatoid; risk; sigma; somatotropin release-inhibiting; somatotropin-releasing; Stuart; sun protection; transfer; transforming; tumor angiogenic; tumor necrosis

fascia broad; clavipectoral; Colles'; deep; endothoracic; extraperitoneal; pelvic; phrenicopleural; renal; Scarpa's; subperitoneal; superficial; thoracolumbar; transverse

fever blackwater; boutonneuse; brain; breakbone; camp; cat scratch; childbed; Colorado tick; continued; dandy; desert; elephantoid; enteric; entericoid; epidemic hemorrhagic; familial Mediterranean; Far Eastern hemorrhagic; Fort Bragg; Haverhill; hay; hemorrhagic; Japanese river; jungle; Kew garden; Korean hemorrhagic; Lassa; Malta; Manchurian hemorrhagic; Mediterranean exanthematous; Mediterranean; metal fume; miliary; milk; mud; Oroya; paratyphoid; parenteric; parrot; Pel-Ebstein; pharyngoconjunctival; phlebotomus; polymer fume; pretibial; prison; puerperal; Q; rat-bite; recurrent; relapsing; rheumatic; Rock; Rocky Mountain spotted; rose; sandfly; scarlet; septic; Sindbis; South African tick-bite; spotted; swamp; tick; trench; typhoid; undifferentiated type; undulant; urticarial; uveoparotid; valley; Yangtze Valley; yellow

fiber A; accelerator; adrenergic; afferent; alpha; arcuate; association; B; beta; C; cholinergic; collagen; collagenous; commissural; depressor; dietary; elastic; exogenous; gamma; gray; inhibitory; intrafusal; medullated; motor; muscle; myelinated; nerve; nonmedullated; osteogenetic; perforating; periodontal membrane; precollagenous; pressor;

projection; Purkinje; reticular; spindle; sudomotor; tautomeric; unmyelinated; white; yellow

fibroma ameloblastic; aponeurotic; cementifying; central ossifying; chondromyxoid; desmoplastic; giant cell; irritation; nonosteogenic; peripheral ossifying; telangiectatic

fissure abdominal; anal; anterior median; auricular; Bichat's; calcarine; caudal transverse; cerebellar; collateral; glaserian; Henle's; hippocampal; palpebral; paracentral; parieto-occipital; petrotympanic; portal; posterior median; Rolando's; superior orbital; sylvian; tympanomastoid

fistula amphibolic; amphibolous; anal; arteriovenous; blind; carotid-cavernous; complete; Eck; external; fecal; gastric; horseshoe; incomplete; internal; intestinal; parietal; pilonidal; reverse Eck; salivary; stercoral; urethrovaginal; vesicouterine

flap advancement; buried; caterpillar; composite; compound; cross; delayed; direct; distant; Filatov; flat; free; full thickness; hinged; immediate; island; jump; local; open; partial-thickness; pedicle; rotation; sliding; split-thickness; subcutaneous; tubed; turnover; waltzed

flexure basicranial; caudal; cephalic; cervical; cranial; dorsal; duodenojejunal; hepatic; left colic; lumbar; mesencephalic; pontine; right colic; sacral; sigmoid; splenic; telencephalic; transverse rhombencephalic

fluid amniotic; body; cerebrospinal; extracellular; extravascular; interstitial; intracellular; labyrinthine; pleural; prostatic; Scarpa's; seminal; serous; spinal; synovial; transcellular

fold amniotic; aryepiglottic; circular; Dennie's; Douglas's; epicanthic; epiglottic; gastric; gluteal; head; interureteric; lacrimal; lateral; mammary; mesonephric; Mongolian; nail; neural; palmate; palpebronasal; rectouterine; semilunar conjunctival; tail; vestibular; vocal

follicle aggregated lymphatic; dental; gastric; gastric lymphatic; Graafian; hair; intestinal; Lieberkühn's; lingual; lymph; nabothian; ovarian; primary ovarian; primordial ovarian; sebaceous; secondary; solitary; splenic lymph; vesicular ovarian

foramen anterior condyloid; anterior palatine; aortic; apical dental; conjugate; epiploic; ethmoidal; external acoustic; external auditory; great; greater palatine; incisive; infraorbital; internal acoustic; internal auditory; interventricular; intervertebral; jugular; lesser palatine; mastoid; mental; Monro's; nutrient; obturator; olfactory; optic; oval; parietal; posterior condyloid; posterior palatine; quadrate; round; sacral; Scarpa's; sciatic; sphenopalatine; stylomastoid; supraorbital; transverse; vertebral; vertebroarterial; Weitbrecht's; zygomaticofacial; zygo-

matico-orbital; zygomaticotemporal

fossa acetabular; adipose; amygdaloid; axillary; condylar; coronoid; cranial; digastric; duodenal; epigastric; gallbladder; glenoid; hyaloid; hypophysial; incisive; infraclavicular; infratemporal; interpeduncular; infraspinous; jugular; mandibular; oval; ovarian; pituitary; rhomboid; subarcuate; temporal; tonsillar; Waldeyer's; zygomatic

fracture avulsion; Barton's; bending; Bennett's; blow-out; capillary; closed; Colles'; comminuted; compound; compression; craniofacial disjunction; depressed skull; direct; dislocation; double; expressed skull; fatigue; fissured; greenstick; gutter; hairline; hangman's; horizontal maxillary; impacted; incomplete; indirect; intrauterine; LeFort I; LeFort II; LeFort III; linear; longitudinal; march; multiple; oblique; occult; open; pathologic; Pott's; pyramidal; reverse Colles'; silverfork; simple; Smith's; spiral; sprain; stellate; strain; stress; torsion; torus; transverse; transverse facial

G

ganglion Acrel's; autonomic; cardiac; carotid; celiac; cervical; cervicothoracic; ciliary; coccygeal; Corti's; dorsal root; gasserian; geniculate; jugular; Ludwig's; lumbar; mesenteric; otic; parasympathetic; paravertebral; pelvic; petrous; phrenic; pterygopalatine; renal; sacral; semilunar; sensory; solar; sphenopalatine; spinal; splanchnic; stellate; submandibular; submaxillary; thoracic; trigeminal; tympanic; vestibular; visceral

gene allelic; autosomal; dominance of; dominant; histocompatibility; holandric; immune response; lethal; mutant; operator; penetrant; pleiotropic; polyphenic; recessive; regulator; repressor; sex-linked; structural; X-linked; Y-linked

gingivitis acute necrotizing ulcerative; chronic desquamative; fusospirillary; fusospirochetal; hyperplastic; necrotizing ulcerative; pregnancy; proliferative; suppurative; ulceromembranous

gland accessory; acinotubular; acinous; adrenal; aggregate; agminate; alveolar; anterior lingual; apical; apocrine; apocrine sweat; areolar; axillary; Bartholin's; Bowman's; bronchial; Brunner's; buccal; bulbourethral; cardiac; celiac; ceruminous; ciliary; circumanal; compound; Cowper's; digestive; ductless; duodenal; eccrine; eccrine sweat; endocrine; excretory; exocrine; fundus; gastric; genal; greater vestibular; hematopoietic; holocrine; intestinal; jugular; lacrimal; lesser vestibular; lymph; major salivary; mammary; master; maxillary; Meibomian; merocrine; minor salivary; mixed; muciparous;

mucous; oil; olfactory; parathyroid; paraurethral; parotid; Peyer's; pileous; pineal; pituitary; preputial; prostate; pyloric; racemose; Rivinus; saccular; salivary; sebaceous; seminal; sentinel; seromucous; serous; sex; solitary; sublingual; submandibular; submaxillary; sudoriferous; suprarenal; sweat; target; tarsal; thyroid; tubular; tubuloacinar; tubuloalveolar; unicellular; urethral; uterine; vaginal; vestibular; vulvovaginal; Weber's; Zeis

glaucoma absolute; angle-closure; combined; congenital; narrow-angle; open-angle; phacogenic; phacomorphic; secondary; simple

globulin accelerator; alpha; antihemophilic; antihuman; beta; chickenpox immune; corticosteroid-binding; gamma; human gamma; immune serum; measles immune; pertussis immune; plasma accelerator; poliomyelitis immune; rabies immune; serum; serum accelerator; specific immune; tetanus immune; thyroid-binding; zoster immune

goiter aberrant; adenomatous; colloid; cystic; diving; exophthalmic; fibrous; follicular; lingual; lymphadenoid; multinodular; nontoxic; parenchymatous; simple; substernal; suffocative; toxic; wandering

graft accordion; allogeneic; autodermic; autogeneic; autologous; autoplastic; avascular; Blair-Brown; cable; chip; composite; corneal; delayed; dermal; Esser; fascia; fascicular; free; full-thickness; funicular; heterologous; heteroplastic; homologous; homoplastic; inlay; isogeneic; isologous; isoplastic; nerve; Ollier-Thiersch; omental; partial-thickness; periosteal; Phemister; pinch; punch; sieve; splitskin; split-thickness; syngeneic; vascularized; Wolfe; Wolfe-Krause

granule acrosomal; alpha; basal; beta; cone; Crooke's; delta; elementary; glycogen; juxtaglomerular; keratohyalin; Langerhans; membranecoating; Nissl; proacrosomal; rod; Schüffner's; seminal

granuloma actinic; amebic; apical; dental; eosinophilic; foreign body; giant cell; lethal midline; lipoid; lipophagic; malignant; paracoccidioidal; periapical; pyogenic; sarcoidal; swimming pool

granulomatosis bronchocentric; lipid; lymphomatoid; Miescher's; Wegener's

groove atrioventricular; developmental; frontal; Harrison's; medullary; neural; olfactory; pontomedullary; posterolateral; urethral

gyrus angular; annectent; callosal; cingulate; dentate; frontal; fusiform; Heschl's; hippocampal; lingual; marginal; medial occipitotemporal; orbital; parahippocampal; paraterminal; postcentral; precentral; straight; subcallosal; supracallosal; supramarginal; temporal; transition; transverse temporal; uncinate

H

headache cluster; fibrositic; histaminic; sick; spinal; tension

heart armored; artificial; athletic; fatty; hairy; irritable; left; right; soldier's; stone; tobacco

heart failure backward; congestive; coronary; forward

hemianopsia absolute; altitudinal; binasal; bitemporal; color; complete; congruous; crossed; heteronymous; homonymous; lateral; quadrantic; unilateral; uniocular

hemoglobin Bart's; carbon monoxide; F; fetal; glycosylated; mean cell; muscle; oxygenated; reduced; sickle cell

hemorrhage cerebral; concealed; extradural; internal; intracranial; intrapartum; parenchymatous; petechial; postpartum; primary; punctate; secondary; subdural

hepatitis active chronic; anicteric virus; cholangiolitic; delta; infectious; lupoid; NANB; neonatal; non-A, non-B; persistent chronic; serum; viral

hernia abdominal; Barth's; Béclard's; Bochdalek's; cerebral; Cloquet's; complete; congenital diaphragmatic; crural; diaphragmatic; epigastric; extrasaccular; fatty; femoral; gastroesophageal; Hesselbach's; hiatal; hiatus; Holthouse's; incarcerated; incisional; inguinal; interstitial; irreducible; ischiatic; labial; Littre's; lumbar; obturator; pannicular; paraperitoneal; parietal; perineal; reducible; retrograde; Richter's; sciatic; scrotal; sliding; slipped; strangulated; synovial; umbilical; vesical; vitreous

hormone adipokinetic; adrenocortical; adrenocorticotropic; androgenic; anterior pituitarylike; antidiuretic; bovine growth; brain; chorionic gonadotropic; corpus luteum; cortical; corticotropin-releasing; follicle-stimulating; follicle-stimulating hormonereleasing; gonadotropic; gonadotropin-releasing; growth; growth hormone-releasing; human chorionic somatomammotropic; human growth; interstitial cell-stimulating; lactogenic; luteinizing; luteinizing hormone-releasing; luteotropic; melanocyte-stimulating; parathyroid; pituitary gonadotropic; pituitary growth; placental growth; progestational; prolactininhibiting; releasing; sex; somatotropic; steroid; thyroid; thyroid-stimulating; thyrotropic; thyrotropinreleasing

host amplifier; dead-end; definitive; final; intermediate; paratenic; reservoir

hydrocephalus communicating; double compartment; noncommunicating; normal pressure; obstructive; occult

hyperemia active; arterial; collateral; fluxionary; passive; reactive; venous

hyperlipoproteinemia acquired; familial broad-beta; familial; nonfamilial; type I familial; type II familial; type III familial; type IV familial; type V familial

hypertension adrenal; benign; essential; malignant; portal; pulmonary; renal; renovascular; white-coat

hypertrophy adaptive; compensatory; complementary; concentric; eccentric; functional; physiologic; vicarious

hysterectomy abdominal; cesarean; radical; subtotal; supracervical; vaginal

hysteria anxiety; conversion; major; mass; minor

I

immunity acquired; active; cell-mediated; cellular; general; genetic; herd; humoral; infection; inherent; innate; local; native; natural; nonspecific; passive; specific

infarction cardiac; cerebral; myocardial; silent myocardial; watershed

infection cross; droplet; endogenous; focal; multi-; opportunistic; slow; terminal

inflammation acute; catarrhal; chronic; exudative; fibrinous; granulomatous; necrotic; proliferative; pseudo-membranous; purulent; serous; subacute; suppurative

influenza Asian; avian; Hong Kong; Spanish; swine

insufficiency acute adrenocortical; adrenocortical; aortic; cardiac; chronic adrenocortical; convergence; coronary; divergence; mitral; myocardial; primary adrenocortical; pulmonary; secondary adrenocortical; tricuspid; valvular; velopharyngeal; venous

J

jaundice acholuric; cholestatic; chronic acholuric; chronic familial; chronic idiopathic; congenital hemolytic; familial nonhemolytic; hematogenous; hemolytic; hepatocellular; hepatogenous; leptospiral; malignant; mechanical; nonobstructive; nuclear; obstructive; physiologic; regurgitation; retention

joint ankle; arthrodial; ball-and-socket; biaxial; bicondylar; bilocular; carpal; carpometacarpal; cartilaginous; Charcot's; Chopart's; cochlear; compound; condylar; coryloid; cubital; diarthrodial; digital; dry; elbow; ellipsoidal; enarthrodial; false; fibrous; flail; ginglymoid; gliding; hinge; hip; immovable; intercarpal; intermetacarpal; intermetatarsal; interphalangeal; intertarsal; knee; Lisfranc's; mandibular; metacarpophalangeal; metatarsophalangeal; mortise; movable; multiaxial; neuropathic; peg-and-socket; phalangeal; pivot; plane; polyaxial; radiocarpal; rotary; saddle; shoulder; simple; spheroid; spiral; synarthrodial; synchondrodial; syndesmodial; synovial; talocalcaneonavicular; talocrural; tarsal; tarsometatarsal; temporomandibular; transverse tarsal; trochoid; uniaxial; unilocular; wedge-and-groove; wrist

K

keratitis dendriform; dendritic; exposure; herpetic; interstitial; lagophthalmic; metaherpetic; neuroparalytic; parenchymatous; phlyctenular; punctate; sclerosing; trachomatous; vascular

keratoconjunctivitis atopic; blepharokeratoconjunctivitis; epidemic; herpetic; superior limbic; ultraviolet; virus; virus punctate

kidney amyloid; artificial; Ask-Upmark; cake; contracted; duplex; fatty; floating; Formad's; fused; Goldblatt; horseshoe; medullary sponge; pancake; polycystic; wandering; waxy

L

layer ameloblastic; bacillary; basal; choriocapillary; corneal; enamel; external elastic; germ; germinative; granular; horny; internal elastic; Malpighian; odontoblastic; osteogenetic; prickle cell; Purkinje; spinous; still; subendocardial; subendothelial; vascular; visceral

leishmaniasis American; anergic; anthroponotic cutaneous; cutaneous; diffuse cutaneous; disseminated cutaneous; lupoid; mucocutaneous; nasopharyngeal; New World; Old World; rural; visceral; wet; zoonotic cutaneous

leprosy anesthetic; cutaneous; histoid; lepromatous; macular; nodular; trophoneurotic; tuberculoid

leukemia acute promyelocytic; adult T-cell; aleukemic; basophilic; embryonal; eosinophilic; granulocytic; hairy cell; leukopenic; lymphatic; lymphoblastic; lymphocytic; lymphoid; mast cell; megakaryocytic; micromyeloblastic; monocytic; myeloblastic; myelocytic; myelogenic; myelogenous; myeloid; plasma cell; Rieder cell; stem cell; subleukemic

leukocyte basophilic; eosinophilic; granular; mast; multinuclear; neutrophilic; oxyphilic; polymorphonuclear

leukocytosis absolute; eosinophilic; lymphocytic; monocytic; physiologic; relative

ligament accessory; alveolodental; annular; arcuate; arterial; calcaneocuboid; capsular; cardinal; collateral; Cooper's; coracoacromial; coracoclavicular; costoclavicular; costotransverse; cystoduodenal; deltoid; extracapsular; falciform; fissure of round; fissure of venous; glenohumeral; iliofemoral; iliotrochanteric; inguinal; intercarpal; intracapsular; lacunar; longitudinal; lumbocostal; medial; meniscofemoral; nuchal; patellar; pectineal; periodontal; phrenicocolic; popliteal; Poupart's; pulmonary; reflex; rhomboid; serous; splenorenal; spring; stellate; sternocostal; sutural; synovial; trapezoid; umbilical; vesicouterine; vocal; Y-shaped

line absorption; anterior median; arterial; base; Beau's; bismuth; blood-; blue; cell; cement; cervical; Clapton's; cleavage; Dennie's; developmental; epiphysial; Futcher's; germ; growth; gum; hair-; Harris'; Hilton's white; His's; illopectineal; inferior temporal; intertrochanteric; intertubercular; isoelectric; Kerley B; lead; M; mamillary; mammary; median; milk; Muehrcke's; Nélaton's; nipple; pectinate; posterior median; Poupart's; semilunar; Shenton's; Spigelius'; spiral; sternal; superior temporal; terminal; trapezoid; vibrating; Voigt's; white; Z

lung air-conditioner; bird-breeder's; black; cheese worker's; farmer's; honeycomb; hyperlucent; iron; miner's; postperfusion; pump; quiet; shock; wet

lymphoma adult T-cell; Burkitt's; follicular; large cell; lymphoblastic; malignant; nodular; non-Hodgkin's; poorly differentiated lymphocytic; well-differentiated lymphocytic

M

malaria acute; chronic; falciparum; malariae; malignant tertian; quartan; quotidian; tertian; vivax

mastectomy extended radical; modified radical; radical; simple; subcutaneous

measles atypical; black; German; hemorrhagic; three-day

membrane adamantine; allantoid; alveolocapillary; alveolodental; arachnoid; atlanto-occipital; basement; Bichat's; Bowman's; Bruch's; Brunn's; cell; cloacal; Corti's; croupous; deciduous; Descemet's; diphtheritic; drum; egg; elastic; embryonic; enamel; false; fenestrated; fetal; fibrous; germinal; germ; glassy; hyaline; hyaloid; hyoglossal; intercostal; Jackson's; keratogenous; medullary; mucous; nuclear; olfactory; ovular; peridental; periodontal; placental; plasma; postsynaptic; presynaptic; pupillary; Reissner's; reticular; Ruysch's; Scarpa's; secondary tympanic; serous; synovial; thyrohyoid; tympanic; undulating; unit; vestibular; vitelline; vitreous; yolk; Zinn's

meningitis basilar; cerebrospinal; eosinophilic; meningococcal; occlusive; otitic; serous; spinal; tuberculous

milk acidophilus; certified; certified pasteurized; condensed; filled; skim; vitamin D; witch's

molar first; second; sixth-year; third; twelfth-year

murmur anemic; aortic; arterial; Austin Flint; cardiac; cardiopulmonary; Carey Coombs; continuous; crescendo; Cruveilhier-Baumgarten; diastolic; Duroziez; ejection; Flint's; functional; Gibson; Graham Steell's; hemic; hourglass; innocent; inorganic; machinery; mitral; obstructive; organic; pansystolic; pericardial; presystolic; pulmonary; regurgitant; Roger's; stenosal; Still's; systolic; tricuspid; vesicular

muscle abdominal external oblique; abdominal internal oblique; anconeous; antagonistic; anterior scalene; appendicular; articular; aryepiglottic; arytenoid; auricular; axial; Bell's; brachial; bronchoesophageal; Brücke's; cardiac; ceratocricoid; cervical iliocostal; cervical longissimus; cheek; chin; ciliary; coccygeal; coracobrachial; corrugator; cricoarytenoid; cricothyroid; cruciate; cutaneous; deltoid; digastric; epicranial; external intercostal; external obturator; extraocular; facial; fixator; Gavard's; gracilis; great; greater psoas; greater rhomboid; greater zygomatic; hamstring; hyoglossus; iliac; iliococcygeal; iliocostal; iliopsoas; index extensor; inferior gemellus; inferior lingual; inferior oblique; inferior rectus; inferior tarsal; infraspinatus; innermost intercostal; intermediate great; intermediate vastus; internal intercostal; internal obturator; interspinal; intertransverse; involuntary; Kohlrausch's; Landström's; lateral pterygoid; lateral rectus; lesser rhomboid; lesser zygomatic; longissimus capitis; longitudinal; long palmar; lumbar iliocostal; lumbar quadrate; Marcacci's; medial pterygoid; medial rectus; middle scalene; nasal; occipitofrontal; orbital; palatopharyngeal; palmar interosseous; papillary; pectinate; pectineal; pectoral; peroneal; piriform; plantar; plantar interosseous; plantar quadrate; pleuroesophageal; popliteal; posterior scalene; posterior tibial; procerus; puboprostatic; puborectal; pubovaginal; pubovesical; pyramidal; quadrate pronator; rectococcygeal; rectourethral; rectouterine; rectovesical; red; Reisseissen's; risorius; rotator; round pronator; Ruysch's; sacrococcygeal; salpingopharyngeal; sartorius; scalene; semimembranosus; semitendinous; skeletal; smaller psoas; smallest scalene; smooth; sternal; straight; striated; stylopharyngeal; subclavian; subcostal; suboccipital; subscapular; superficial lingual; superior gemellus; superior oblique; superior rectus; superior tarsal; supinator; synergistic; tailor's; temporal; temporoparietal; third fibular; third peroneal; thoracic iliocostal; thoracic longissimus; thyroarytenoid; thyroepiglottic; tracheal; triangular; vocal; voluntary; white

mutation lethal; missense; natural; neutral; point; somatic; spontaneous; suppressor; transition; transversion

N

necrosis aseptic; caseous; central; coagulation; colliquative; epiphysial aseptic; fat; focal; ischemic; liquefactive; Zenker's; zonal

nephritis glomerular; interstitial; lupus; mesangial; salt-losing; serum; suppurative; transfusion; tubulointerstitial

nerve abducent; accelerator; accessory; accessory phrenic; acoustic; afferent; anococcygeal; anterior ampullar; anterior auricular; anterior ethmoidal; anterior interosseous; anterior labial; anterior scrotal; anterior supraclavicular; articular; auditory; auriculotemporal; axillary; buccal; caroticotympanic; centrifugal; centripetal; cervical; coccygeal; cochlear; common palmar digital; common peroneal; common plantar digital; cranial; cubital; deep peroneal; deep petrosal; deep temporal; depressor; dorsal digital; dorsal lateral cutaneous; dorsal medial cutaneous; efferent; eighth cranial; eleventh cranial; excitoreflex; excitor; external carotid; facial; femoral; fibular; fifth cranial; first cranial; fourth cranial; frontal; gangliated; genitofemoral; glossopharyngeal; great auricular; greater occipital; greater palatine; greater petrosal; greater splanchnic; hypogastric; hypoglossal; iliohypogastric; ilioinguinal; inferior alveolar; inferior cervical cardiac; inferior cluneal; inferior gluteal; inferior laryngeal; inferior rectal; infraorbital; infratrochlear; inhibitory; intercostal; intercostobrachial; intermediary; intermediate; intermediate dorsal cutaneous; intermediate supraclavicular; internal carotid; jugular; lacrimal; lateral ampullar; lateral plantar; lateral supraclavicular; lesser occipital; lesser palatine; lesser petrosal; lesser splanchnic; lingual; long ciliary; long thoracic; lowest splanchnic; lumbar; lumbar splanchnic; mandibular; masseteric; maxillary; medial plantar; medial supraclavicular; median; mental; middle cervical cardiac; middle cluneal; middle supraclavicular; mixed; motor; musculocutaneous; mylohyoid; nasociliary; nasopalatine; obturator; oculomotor; olfactory; ophthalmic; optic; parasympathetic; pectoral; pelvic splanchnic; perineal; phrenic; plantar; pneumogastric; posterior ampullar; posterior auricular; posterior ethmoidal; posterior interosseous; posterior labial; posterior scrotal; posterior supraclavicular; pressor; proper palmar digital; proper plantar digital; pterygoid; pterygopalatine; pudendal; radial; recurrent laryngeal; saccular; sacral; sacral splanchnic; saphenous; sciatic; second cranial; secretory; sensory; seventh cranial; short ciliary; sixth cranial; somatic; spinal; subclavian; subcostal; sublingual; suboccipital; subscapular; superficial peroneal; superior alveolar; superior cervical cardiac; superior cluneal; superior gluteal; superior laryngeal; supraorbital; suprascapular; supratrochlear; sural; sympathetic; temporomandibular; tenth cranial; terminal; third cranial; third occipital; thoracic; thoracic cardiac; thoracodorsal; tibial; trigeminal; trochlear; twelfth cranial; tympanic; ulnar; utricular; utriculoampullar; vaginal; vagus; vascular; vasomotor; vertebral; vestibular; vestibulocochlear; zygomatic

neuralgia Fothergill's; geniculate; Hunt's; idiopathic; Morton's; red; trifacial; trigeminal

neuritis adventitial; brachial, endemic; interstitial; multiple; optic; parenchymatous; retrobulbar; segmental; toxic; traumatic

neuron associative; bipolar; final motor; ganglionic motor; Golgi type I; Golgi type II; intercalary; internuncial; lower motor; motor; multipolar; peripheral motor; postganglionic motor; preganglionic motor; somatic motor; unipolar; upper motor

neuropathy brachial plexus; diabetic; entrapment; giant axonal; hereditary hypertrophic; segmental

nevus acquired; basal cell; bathing trunk; blue; blue rubber bleb; collagenous; comedo; congenital; dysplastic; halo; intradermal; Ito's; Jadassohn-Tièche; junction; Ota's; spider; strawberry; verrucous; white sponge; woolly-hair

node atrioventricular; AV; axillary lymph; Bouchard's; central lymph; cystic; delphian; Dürck's; foraminal; Haygarth's; Heberden's; Hensen's; inferior mesenteric lymph; jugulodigastric; jugulo-omohyoid; lymph; mandibular; middle rectal; nasolabial; Osler; parietal; primitive; Ranvier's; S-A; signal; singer's; sinoatrial; sinoauricular; sinus; subdigastric; superior mesenteric lymph; Virchow's; visceral

nodule Albini's; apple jelly; Arantius'; Bianchi's; Gamna-Gandy; Jeanselme's; lymph; Morgagni's; pulp; rheumatoid; siderotic; Sister Joseph's; vocal cord

nucleus ambiguous; amygdaloid; caudate; centromedian; cochlear; cuneate; dorsal; hypoglossal; inferior salivary; intermediolateral; intermediomedial; interpeduncular; lenticular; lentiform; motor; oculomotor; olivary; Onuf's; paraventricular; pulpy; raphe; red; secondary sensory; somatic motor;

subthalamic; superior salivary; tegmental; terminal; thoracic; vestibular

nystagmus caloric; central; congenital; conjugate; dissociated; end-position; fixation; gaze; jerky; labyrinthine; latent; lateral; opticokinetic; pendular; positional; retraction; rotational; rotatory; vertical; vestibular

O

occlusion abnormal; afunctional; balanced; centric; coronary; eccentric; functional; hyperfunctional; mesial; mesio-; normal; pathogenic; physiologic; protrusive; retrusive; traumatic; traumatogenic

operation Abbé; Bassini's; Baudelocque's; Beer's; Belsey; Blalock-Taussig; bloodless; Bricker; Caldwell-Luc; cesarean; Cotte's; Dandy; Daviel's; debulking; Dupuy-Dutemps; Elliot's; Estlander; filtering; flap; Fothergill's; Frazier-Spiller; Fredet-Ramstedt; Frost-Lang; Gifford's; Glenn's; Gonin; Graefe's; Halsted's; Hartmann's; Herbert's; Hill; Hoffa's; Hofmeister's; Kasai; Kelly's; Kondoleon; Kraske's; Lagrange's; Lambrinudi; Manchester; Matas; Mayo's; McVay's; Mikulicz; Miles'; morcellation; Motais; Mustard; Naffziger; Pancoast's; Payne; Pomeroy's; Potts'; Putti-Platt; Ramstedt; Saemisch's; Scott; Smith's; Soave; stapes-mobilization; Stookey-Scarff; subcutaneous; Wertheim's; Whipple's; Whitehead's; Ziegler's

organ circumventricular; critical; enamel; end; genital; Golgi tendon; sense; spiral; target; vestibular; vestigial

P

papilla circumvallate; conical; dentinal; dermal; filiform; foliate; fungiform; hair; incisive; interdental; lacrimal; lingual; major duodenal; minor duodenal; optic; parotid; renal; retrocuspid; tactile; urethral; vallate

paralysis acute ascending; Brown-Séquard's; bulbar; central; compression; conjugate; decubitus; Duchenne-Erb; facial; familial periodic; hyperkalemic periodic; hypokalemic periodic; immunological; infantile; Klumpke's; Landry's; mixed; motor; musculospiral; normokalemic periodic; obstetrical; periodic; pressure; progressive bulbar; pseudobulbar; pseudohypertrophic muscular; sensory; sleep; spastic; spinal; supranuclear; tick; Todd's; vasomotor

parasite facultative; heterogenetic; heteroxenous; incidental; obligate; specific; temporary

peduncle cerebral; inferior cerebellar; inferior thalamic; lateral thalamic; middle cerebellar; superior cerebellar; ventral thalamic

pelvis android; anthropoid; assimilation; beaked; brachypellic; contracted; cordate; cordiform; dolichopellic; false; flat; frozen; funnel-shaped; gynecoid; juvenile; kyphotic; large; masculine; mesatipellic; Nägele's; osteomalacic; Otto; platypellic; Prague; rachitic; renal; Robert's; Rokitansky's; scoliotic; small; split; spondylolisthetic; true

peritonitis adhesive; chemical; gas; meconium; pelvic

personality antisocial; authoritarian; avoidant; compulsive; cyclothymic; dependent; hysterical; inadequate; masochistic; multiple; paranoid; passive-aggressive; schizoid; schizotypical; split; type A; type B

phenomenon Anrep; Arias-Stella; dawn; declamping; déjà vu; diaphragm; Donath-Landsteiner; gap; gestalt; Goldblatt; Jod-Basedow; Köbner's; Litten's; Marcus Gunn; on-off; paradoxical diaphragm; psi; quellung; Raynaud's; rebound; Somogyi; staircase; Tyndall

pit anal; arm-; auditory; central; iris; lens; Mantoux; nail; nasal; olfactory; sublingual

placenta battledore; bidiscoidal; fetal; hemochorial; hemoendothelial; maternal; uterine

plaque bacterial; dental; Hollenhorst; neuritic; senile

plasma antihemophilic human; blood; fresh frozen; muscle; normal human

plasmid bacteriocinogenic; conjugative; F; nonconjugative; R; resistance

plate anal; axial; base-; bite-; buttress; cloacal; cutis; dental; end; epiphysial; equatorial; flat; floor; foot-; lateral; medullary; metaphase; motor; muscle; neural; neutralization; roof; tarsal; tympanic; ventral

pleurisy adhesive; diaphragmatic; dry; fibrinous; interlobular; plastic; purulent; serofibrinous; serous; wet

plexus aortic; autonomic; brachial; cardiac; celiac; cervical; choroid; coccygeal; common carotid; external carotid; inferior dental; inferior mesenteric; internal carotid; intraparotid; lumbar; lymphatic; myenteric; nerve; pampiniform; periarterial; pulmonary; sacral; solar; submucosal; subserous; superior dental; superior mesenteric; tympanic

pneumonia apex; apical; aspiration; atypical; bronchial; double; eosinophilic; Friedländer's; giant cell; Hecht's; hypostatic; influenzal; interstitial giant cell; interstitial plasma cell; lipid; lobar; mycoplasmal; Pittsburgh; Pittsburgh pneumonia agent; primary atypical; rheumatic

poisoning bacterial food; blood; carbon monoxide; food; lead; mercury; ptomaine; Salmonella; sausage; scombroid

polyp adenomatous; dental; fibrinous; hyperplastic; juvenile; metaplastic; regenerative; vascular

porphyria acute intermittent; congenital erythropoietic; erythropoietic; hepatic; intermittent acute; symptomatic; variegate

pouch branchial; Douglas; Kock; pharyngeal; rectouterine; rectovesical; vesicouterine

pregnancy abdominal; ampullar; cervical; combined; ectopic; false; interstitial; intraligamentary; intramural; multiple; ovarian; secondary abdominal; tubal; tuboabdominal; tubo-ovarian

presentation breech; brow; cephalic; face; foot; footling; incomplete foot; knee; placental; shoulder; sincipital; transverse; vertex

pressure abdominal; back; blood; central venous; cerebrospinal; continuous positive airway; diastolic; effective osmotic; high blood; intracranial; intraocular; negative; negative end-expiratory; osmotic; partial; positive end-expiratory; pulmonary capillary wedge; pulse; systolic; wedge

process acromial; alveolar; caudate; ciliary; clinoid; condylar; coracoid; coronoid; dendritic; ensiform; falciform; foot; funicular; malar; mandibular; mastoid; maxillary; odontoid; orbital; palatal; palatine; primary; pterygoid; secondary; spinous; temporal; transverse; xiphoid; zygomatic

protein antiviral; Bence-Jones; beta-amyloid; catabolite gene activator; complement; conjugated; C-reactive; M; nonspecific; plasma; receptor; silver; simple

psychosis affective; alcoholic; circular; drug; exhaustion; gestational; hysterical; ICU; infection-exhaustion; involutional; Korsakoff's; polyneuritic; postpartum; schizoaffective; senile; situational

pulse alternating; anacrotic; bigeminal; bisferious; cannonball; Corrigan's; coupled; dicrotic; hard; jugular; nerve impulse paradoxical; plateau; Quincke's; Riegel's; thready; trigeminal; undulating; vagus; venous; vermicular; water-hammer; wiry

pupil Adie's; amaurotic; Argyll Robertson; fixed; Holmes-Adie; Horner's; Hutchinson's; neurotonic; pinhole; tonic; Westphal-Piltz

purpura allergic; anaphylactoid; fibrinolytic; Henoch-Schönlein; idiopathic thrombocytopenic; immune thrombocytopenic; nonthrombocytopenic; psychogenic; Schönlein-Henoch; thrombocytopenic; thrombotic thrombocytopenic

R

reaction acute situational; adverse; alarm; allergic; anamnestic; antigen-antibody; anxiety; Arias-Stella; Bence Jones; bi-bi; biuret; catastrophic; cell-mediated; chain; complement; constitutional; conversion; cross-; cutaneous; cytotoxic; delayed; dissociative; dystonic; false-negative; false-positive; fight-or-flight; flocculation; focal; graft versus host, hemiopic pupillary; Herxheimer's; immediate; immune; intracutaneous; intradermal; Jarisch-Herxheimer; leukemoid; local; mixed agglutination; Neufeld; ninhydrin; Prausnitz-Küstner; precipitin; primary; quellung; reversed Prausnitz-Küstner; Schultz-Charlton; serum; specific; stress; symptomatic; Wassermann; Weil-Felix; Wernicke's; wheal-and-erythema; wheal-and-flare

receptor adrenergic; alpha-adrenergic; beta-adrenergic; cholinergic; NMDA; opiate; stretch

reflex abdominal; accommodation; Achilles; Achilles tendon; anal; ankle; auditory; Babinski's; basal joint; Bechterew-Mendel; biceps; Brain's; celiac plexus; Chaddock; chain; ciliary; ciliospinal; cochleopalpebral; conditioned; conjunctival; corneal; cough; cremasteric; crossed; darwinian; deep; digital; diving; enterogastric; finger-thumb; gag; gastrocolic; gastroileac; grasp; grasping; Hoffmann's; intrinsic; jaw; knee; knee-jerk; latent; light; lip; Mayer's; Mendel-Bechterew; Moro's; myotatic; nasal; nociceptive; orienting; palatal; palatine; parachute; paradoxical; patellar; pharyngeal; pilomotor; plantar; proprioceptive; protective laryngeal; pupillary; pupillary-skin; quadriceps; quadripedal extensor; red; righting; rooting; Rossolimo's; snout; spinal; startle; static; statokinetic; statotonic; stretch; sucking; superficial; swallowing; tendon; toe; triceps; triceps surae; unconditioned; vestibulospinal; vomiting; wink

respiration abdominal; aerobic; anaerobic; artificial; assisted; Biot's; cellular; Cheyne-Stokes; cogwheel; controlled; diffusion; electrophrenic; external; internal; Kussmaul-Kien; Kussmaul; mouth-to-mouth; paradoxical; tissue; vesicular

reticulum agranular endoplasmic; endoplasmic; granular endoplasmic; sarcoplasmic; stellate; trabecular

retinopathy circinate; diabetic; hypertensive; leukemic; pigmentary; proliferative; sickle cell; tapetoretinal

rhinitis acute; allergic; atrophic; caseous; eosinophilic nonallergic; fibrinous; hypertrophic; membranous; purulent; vasomotor

rhythm alpha; atrioventricular nodal; AV nodal; beta; bigeminal; cantering; circadian; coupled; delta; escape; fast; gallop; idioventricular; nodal; quadrigeminal; sinus; theta; trigeminal; ventricular

ridge dental; epidermal; genital; gonadal; mammary; mesonephric; palatine; rete; skin; supraorbital; teeth-; temporal; trapezoid; urogenital; Wolffian

ring abdominal; annular; anterior limiting; Bandl's; benzene; Cannon's; ciliary; conjunctival; constriction; deep inguinal; Kayser-Fleischer; pathologic retraction; physiologic retraction; pleural; posterior limiting; Schwalbe's; subcutaneous; superficial inguinal; tracheal; tympanic; umbilical; vascular

S

sac air; allantoic; alveolar; amniotic; conjunctival; dental; heart; hernial; lacrimal; tear; yolk

sarcoma alveolar soft part; ameloblastic; botryoid; endometrial stromal; giant cell; granulocytic; Kaposi's; myeloid; osteogenic; reticulum cell; telangiectatic osteogenic

schizophrenia catatonic; disorganized; hebephrenic; latent; paranoid; process; reactive; residual

sclerosis amyotrophic lateral; arterial; lateral spinal; Mönckeberg's; multiple; progressive systemic; tuberous

seizure absence; complex partial; disorder; focal; generalized tonic-clonic; grand mal; partial; psychomotor

septum atrioventricular; interalveolar; interatrial; interdental; intermuscular; interventricular; nasal; rectovaginal; rectovesical; scrotal

shock anaphylactic; anaphylactoid; cardiogenic; chronic; culture; declamping; hemorrhagic; hypovolemic; insulin; osmotic; septic; serum; shell; toxic

sickness acute African sleeping; African sleeping; air-; altitude; car-; chronic mountain; chronic sleeping; decompression; milk; morning; motion; mountain; radiation; sea-; serum; sleeping; space

sign Allis's; Amoss'; Baastrup's; Babinski's; Bamberger's; Bárány's; Barré's; Beevor's; Biernacki's; Blumberg's; Boston's; Braxton Hicks; Broadbent's; Brudzinski's; Chaddock; Chvostek's; clenched fist; Comby's; Comolli's; conventional; Cruveilhier-Baumgarten; Cruveilhier's; Cullen's; Dalrymple's; Delbet's; doll's eye; drawer; Ebstein's; Erb's; Erb-Westphal; Ewart's; eyelash; Friedreich's; Goldstein's toe; Goodell's; Graefe's; Gunn's; halo; Higoumenakia; Hill's; Hoffmann's; Homans'; Hoover's; Joffroy's; Kernig's; Kussmaul's; Lasègue's; Leri's; Lhermitte's; Macewen's; Marañon's; Marcus Gunn's; Möbius'; Musset's; Nikolsky's; Osler's; Payr's; physical; Piltz; Porter's; pyramid; Quincke's; Remak's; Romberg's; Rossolimo's; Russell's; Saenger's; scimitar; Steinberg thumb; Stellwag's; Stewart-Holmes; Tinel's; Trendelenburg's; Trousseau's; Uhthoff; vital; von Graefe's; Wernicke's; Westphal-Erb; Westphal's; wrist

sinus anal; aortic; carotid; cavernous; cerebral; circular; coccygeal; coronary; dermal; dural; ethmoidal; frontal; inferior petrosal; inferior sagittal; intercavernous; lactiferous; lymphatic; mastoid; maxillary; occipital; paranasal; parasinoidal; pilonidal; prostatic; rectal; renal; rhomboidal; sigmoid; sphenoidal; sphenoparietal; splenic; straight; superior petrosal; superior sagittal; tarsal; tentorial; transverse; tympanic; urogenital; uterine; uteroplacental; venous

space alveolar dead; anatomical dead; apical; Bowman's; capsular; cartilage; corneal; dead; deep perineal; epidural; episcleral; haversian; intercostal; interpleural; interproximal; interradicular; intervillous; Kiernan's; mediastinal; medullary; perforated; perilymphatic; perineal; personal; physiological dead; pleural; Poiseuille's; retroperitoneal; retropubic; subarachnoid; subchorial; subdural; subgingival; superficial perineal; Tenon's; zonular

spasm canine; carpopedal; clonic; cynic; facial; habit; infantile; intention; muscle; nodding; retrocollic; saltatory; tonic; tonoclonic; torsion

splint active; airplane; air; anchor; Anderson; backboard; Balkan; coaptation; contact; Denis Browne; dynamic; Frejka pillow; functional; interdental; labial; ladder; pillow; shin splints surgical; Thomas

spot Bitot's; blind; blue; café au lait; cherry-red; cotton-wool; Fordyce's; hot; hypnogenic; Koplik's; liver; milk; mongolian; rose; Roth's; Soemmering's; soft; yellow

stain acid; basic fuchsin-methylene blue; basic; C-banding; centromere banding; contrast; differential; double; G-banding; Giemsa; Giemsa chromosome banding; Golgi's; Gram's; hematoxylin-eosin; immunofluorescent; intravital; iodine; Mallory's triple; metachromatic; multiple; negative; neutral; nuclear; Papanicolaou; picrocarmine; port-wine; positive; Q-banding; R-banding; selective; silver protein; supravital; trichrome; vital; Wright's

stenosis aortic; congenital pyloric; hypertrophic pyloric; idiopathic hypertrophic subaortic; laryngeal; mitral; pulmonary; pyloric; subaortic; supravalvar; tricuspid

stomatitis angular; aphthous; gangrenous; primary herpetic; recurrent herpetic; recurrent ulcerative; ulcerative

sulcus calcarine; central; cingulate; collateral; coronary; frontal; gingival; hippocampal; inferior temporal; intraparietal; lateral cerebral; middle temporal; olfactory; parieto-occipital; postcentral; posterior median; precentral; rhinal; superior temporal; terminal

suture absorbable; apposition; approximation; atraumatic; blanket; bridle; buried; button; coaptation; cobbler's; continuous; coronal; cranial; Czerny; Czerny-Lembert; dentate; doubly armed; Faden; false; far-and-near; figure eight; frontal; Frost; glover's; Halsted's; harmonic; implanted; intermaxillary; internasal; interparietal; interrupted; lambdoid; Lembert; mattress; metopic; nonabsorbable; plane; purse-string; relaxation; retention; sagittal; serrate; sphenoethmoidal; squamous; tension; transfixion; uninterrupted; wedge-and-groove; zygomaticomaxillary

syndrome Aarskog-Scott; abdominal muscle deficiency; acquired Fanconi's; acquired immune deficiency; acquired immunodeficiency; Adams-Stokes; Adie; adrenogenital; adult Fanconi's; adult respiratory distress; afferent-loop; Ahumada-Del Castillo; alcohol amnestic; Aldrich; Alport's; Alström's; amenorrhea-galactorrhea; amnestic; Amsterdam; anterior tibial compartment; aortic arch; Apert-Crouzon; Apert's; Asperger's; autoerythrocyte sensitization; Ayerza's; Banti's; Bardet-Biedl; bare lymphocyte; Barrett's; basal-cell nevus; Bassen-Kornzweig; battered child; battered woman; battering parent; Bauer's; Beckwith-Wiedemann; Behçet's; Besnier-Boeck-Schaumann; Beuren; binge-eating; binge-purge; binge-vomit; Bloch-Sulzberger; Boerhaave's; Bonnevie-Ullrich; Börjeson-Forssman-Lehmann; bowel bypass; Brown-Séquard's; Budd-Chiari; Buschke-Ollendorf; Caffey's; carpal tunnel; Carpenter's; cat-cry; cavernous sinus; Ceelen-Gellerstadt; central cord; cerebrohepatorenal; cervical rib; Cestan-Chenais; Charcot's; Chédiak-Steinbrinck-Higashi; cherry-red spot myoclonus; Chiari's; Chinese restaurant; Chotzen; chromosomal; chromosomal breakage; chromosomal instability; chronic fatigue; chronic fatigue immune dysfunction; Clarke-Hadfield; Cobb; Cockayne's; Coffin-Lowry; Coffin-Siris; Cogan-Reese; compression; Conn's; Cornelia de Lange's; Costen's; CREST; cri-du-chat; Crigler-Najjar; crocodile tears; Cronkhite-Canada; CRST; crush; Cruveilhier-Baumgarten; Cushing's; DaCosta's; de Lange's; Del Castillo; dialysis encephalopathy; disk; Down; dry-eye; Dubin Johnson; dumping; dysplastic nevus; Eaton-Lambert; effort; Ehlers-Danlos; Eisenmenger; EMG; erythrodysesthesia; external carotid steal; Fanconi's; Felty's; fetal alcohol; fetal aspiration; fetal distress; fetal warfarin; folded lung; fragile X; Franceschetti's; Ganser's; Gardner-Diamond; Gardner's; general-adaptation; Goodpasture's; Gorlin-Chaudhry-Moss; Gorlin's; Gorman's; gray-baby; gray; Greig's; Guillain-Barré; Gulf War; Hallervorden; Hallervorden-Spatz; Hamman-Rich; Hamman's; happy-puppet; Harada's; Hartnup; Hayem-Widal; hemolytic uremic; hemopleuropneu-

monia; hepatonephric; hepatorenal; Hirschowitz; Holmes-Adie; Horner's; Hunter's; Hunt's; Hurler's; Hutchinson-Gilford; hypereosinophilic; hyperimmunoglobulin E; hyperkinetic; immotile cilia; immunodeficiency; iridocorneal endothelial; iris-nevus; lrvine-Gass; Jadassohn-Lewandowsky; jaw-winking; Jeghers-Peutz; Job's; Joubert's; Kanner's; Kartagener's; Katayama; Kearns-Sayre; Kimmelstiel-Wilson; Klinefelter's; Klippel-Feil; Klumpke-Déjérine; Kniest; Korsakoff's; LAMB; Lambert-Eaton; Landau-Kleffner; Landry; Landry-Guillain-Barré; Laurence-Moon; Laurence-Moon-Bardet-Biedl; Lejeune; Lenègre's; Lennox; Lennox-Gastaut; Leriche's; Leri-Weill; Lermoyez; Lesch-Nyhan; Lev's; Libman-Sacks; Li-Fraumeni cancer; Lorain-Lévi; Lowe's; Lowe-Terrey-MacLachlan; Lutembacher's; Mad Hatter; malabsorption; male Turner's; Mallory-Weiss; Marchiafava-Micheli; Marcus Gunn; Marfan; Maroteaux-Lamy; Mauriac's; Mayer-Rokitansky-Küster-Hauser; May-White; Meadows's; Meckel; megacystic; Menkes; metabolic; middle lobe; Mikulicz; milk-alkali; Möbius; Morgagni's; Morquio's; Morton's; mucocutaneous lymph node; Muir-Torre; multiple lentigines; multiple mucosal neuroma; Munchausen; myeloproliferative; myofacial pain-dysfunction; Naegeli; Naffziger; nail-patella; NAME; Nelson; nephritic; nephrotic; neural crest; neuroleptic malignant; Noonan's; oculocerebrorenal; Omenn's; Oppenheim's; organic brain; organic mental; orofaciodigital; Paget-von Schrötter; Pancoast; paraneoplastic; Parinaud's; oculoglandular; Parkinson's; Peutz-Jeghers; Pfeiffer; pickwickian; Pierre Robin; Pins'; Plummer-Vinson; POEMS; polycystic ovary; polyendocrine deficiency; poly-glandular deficiency; popliteal entrapment; post-adrenalectomy; postcommissurotomy; postgastrectomy; postpartum pituitary necrosis; postpericardiotomy; post-polio; posttraumatic neck; posttraumatic; posttraumatic stress; Potter's; Prader-Willi; preexcitation; premature-senility; premenstrual; prune-belly; pseudo-Turner's; pulmonary dysmaturity; punch-drunk; Putnam-Dana; Ramsay Hunt's; Raynaud's; Reifenstein's; Reiter's; Rendu-Osler-Weber; respiratory distress; restless legs; Rett's; Reye's; Rh null; Riley-Day; Rokitansky-Küster-Hauser; Rothmund's; Russell's; Sanfilippo's; scalenus anterior; scalenus anticus; scapulocostal; Schaumann's; Scheie's; Schwachman; Seabright bantam; Seckel; Secrétan's; Sertoli cell-only; Sézary; shaken infant; Sheehan's; shoulder-girdle; shoulder-hand; Shy-Drager; sicca; sick building; sickle cell; sick sinus; Sipple's; Sjögren's; Spens'; staphylococcal scalded skin; Stein-Leventhal; Stevens-Johnson; Stewart-Treves; Stickler; stiff-man; Stockholm;

Stokes-Adams; Sturge-Weber; subclavian steal; sudden infant death; sump; Swyer-James; tachycardia-bradycardia; Takayasu's; tarsal tunnel; TAR; Taussig-Bing; tegmental; temporomandibular joint; tendon sheath; Terry's; testicular feminization; tethered cord; thoracic outlet; thrombocytopenia-absent radius; Tietze's; Tolosa-Hunt; TORCH; Torre's; Tourette's; toxic shock; translocation Down; triad; trisomy 21; tropical splenomegaly; Trousseau's; tumor lysis; Turcot; Turner's; Usher's; VACTERL; Van Buchem's; vanishing lung; Vernet's; virus-associated hemophagocytic; vitreoretinal choroidopathy; Vohwinkel; von Hippel-Lindau; Waardenburg; Waterhouse-Friderichsen; Weber's; Wells'; Werner's; Wernicke-Korsakoff; Wernicke's; Wilson-Mikity; Wiskott-Aldrich; Wissler's; Wolff-Parkinson-White; WPW; Wyburn-Mason; XO; XXY; XYY; Zollinger-Ellison

T

tachycardia atrial chaotic; bidirectional ventricular; ectopic; essential; paroxysmal; supraventricular

testis descensus; ectopia; ectopic; gubernaculum; inverted; mediastinum; movable; obstructed; retained; rete; tunica vaginalis; undescended

tissue adenoid; adipose; areolar; cancellous, chondroid; chromaffin; connective; elastic; erectile; fibrous; granulation; indifferent; interstitial; lymphatic; lymphoid; mucous connective; myeloid; nerve; reticular; retiform; scar; subcutaneous

toxin botulinus; diagnostic diphtheria; Dick test; erythrogenic; extracellular; intracellular; Schick test; streptococcus erythrogenic; tetanus

tract alimentary; anterior spinocerebellar; digestive; dorsolateral; gastrointestinal; genital; optic; posterior spinocerebellar; pyramidal; respiratory; reticulospinal; solitary; spinothalamic; urinary

transfusion direct; exchange; immediate; indirect; reciprocal; substitution; total; twin-twin

trunk atrioventricular; brachiocephalic; celiac; costocervical; nerve; pulmonary; sympathetic; thyrocervical; vagal

tuberculosis acute; acute miliary; cutaneous; disseminated; enteric; Mycobacterium; open; primary; pulmonary; secondary

tumor acinar cell; adenomatoid; amyloid; aortic-body; benign; Brenner; Buschke-Löwenstein; carcinoid; carotid-body; chromaffin; connective; dermoid; desmoid; embryonal; endodermal sinus; endometrioid; Ewing's; glomus; glomus jugulare; granular cell; granulosa cell; haarscheibe; heterologous; histoid; homologous; Hürthle cell;

Krukenberg's; malignant; melanotic neuroectodermal; mixed; oncocytic hepatocellular; organoid; papillary; pearl; phantom; pontine angle; Recklinghausen's; sand; Sertoli cell; squamous odontogenic; teratoid; theca-cell; triton; Warthin's; Wilms; yolk-sac

typhus endemic; epidemic; mite; murine; recrudescent; scrub; tick; tropical

U

ulcer anastomotic; chiclero's; chronic; cold; Curling's; decubitus; dendritic corneal; gastric; gravitational; hard; Hunner's; Meleney's; peptic; perforated; phagedenic; recurrent aphthous; rodent; soft; stercoral; steroid; stomal; stress; trophic; undermining; varicose; venereal

uterus bicornate; cordiform; Couvelaire; duplex; gravid; masculine; septate; unicorn

V

vaccine acellular pertussis; autogenous; Bacillus Calmette-Guérin; BCG; diphtheria, tetanus toxoids, and pertussis; DPT; DTP; Haemophilus influenza type b conjugate; hepatitis B; heterogenous; human diploid cell rabies; inactivated poliovirus; influenza virus; live; measles, mumps, rubella; measles virus; multivalent; mumps virus; oral poliovirus; pertussis; plague; pneumococcal; poliovirus; polyvalent; rabies; Rocky Mountain spotted fever; rubella virus; Sabin; Salk; smallpox; stock; subunit; TAB; tetanus-diphtheria toxoids; tetanus toxoids; tetanus; tuberculosis; typhoid-paratyphoid A and B; typhoid; typhus; whole-cell; whooping cough; yellow fever

valve aortic; ball; bicuspid; cardiac; congenital; coronary; Heyer-Pudenz; ileocecal; ileocolic; left atrioventricular; mitral; parachute mitral; pulmonary; pyloric; right atrioventricular; semilunar; spiral; tricuspid; urethral; vesicoureteral

vein accessory cephalic; accessory hemiazygos; accessory saphenous; accessory vertebral; accompanying; angular; anterior auricular; anterior cardiac; anterior cardinal; anterior cerebral; anterior facial; anterior intercostal; anterior jugular; anterior labial; anterior scrotal; anterior tibial; anterior vertebral; appendicular; ascending lumbar; axillary; azygos; basal; basilic; basivertebral; brachial; brachiocephalic; bronchial; capillary; cardinal; cephalic; cerebellar; ciliary; circumflex femoral; circumflex iliac; common basal; common cardinal; common facial; common iliac; companion; condylar emissary; conjunctival; coronary; costoaxillary; cutaneous; cystic; deep cervical; deep facial; deep femoral; deep lingual; deep temporal; diploic; dorsal metacarpal; dorsal metatarsal; dorsal scapular; emissary; episcleral; esophageal; ethmoidal; external iliac; external jugular; external nasal; external pudendal; facial; femoral; fibular; genicular; great cardiac; great cerebral; great saphenous; hemiazygos; hemorrhoidal; hepatic; hepatic portal; highest intercostal; hypogastric; ileal; ileocolic; iliolumbar; inferior anastomotic; inferior basal; inferior cerebral; inferior choroid; inferior epigastric; inferior gluteal; inferior labial; inferior laryngeal; inferior mesenteric; inferior ophthalmic; inferior phrenic; inferior pulmonary; inferior rectal; inferior thalamostriate; inferior thyroid; innominate; intercapitular; intermediate antebrachial; intermediate basilic; intermediate cephalic; intermediate cubital; internal auditory; internal cerebral; internal iliac; internal jugular; internal pudendal; internal thoracic; intervertebral; jejunal and ileal; jugular; labial; labyrinthine; lacrimal; lateral sacral; lateral thoracic; left brachiocephalic; left colic; left gastric; left gastroepiploic; left gastro-omental; left ovarian; left suprarenal; left testicular; left umbilical; lingual; lumbar; mastoid emissary; maxillary; median; median sacral; mediastinal; meningeal; middle cardiac; middle cerebral; middle colic; middle meningeal; middle rectal; middle temporal; middle thyroid; musculophrenic; nasofrontal; obturator; occipital; occipital emissary; palatine; palmar digital; palmar metacarpal; pancreatic; pancreaticoduodenal; paraumbilical; parietal emissary; parotid; pectoral; perforating; pericardiacophrenic; pericardial; peroneal; pharyngeal; plantar digital; plantar metatarsal; popliteal; portal; posterior auricular; posterior cardinal; posterior facial; posterior intercostal; posterior labial; posterior scrotal; posterior tibial; precentral cerebellar; prepyloric; pulmonary; pyloric; radial; renal; retromandibular; right brachiocephalic; right colic; right gastric; right gastroepiploic; right gastro-omental; right ovarian; right suprarenal; right testicular; scleral; short gastric; sigmoid; small cardiac; smallest cardiac; small saphenous; spinal; splenic; stellate; sternocleidomastoid; striate; stylomastoid; subclavian; sublingual; submental; superficial epigastric; superficial temporal; superior anastomotic; superior basal; superior cerebral; superior choroid; superior epigastric; superior gluteal; superior intercostal; superior labial; superior laryngeal; superior mesenteric; superior ophthalmic; superior phrenic; superior pulmonary; superior rectal; superior thalamostri-

ate; superior thalamostriate; superior thyroid; supraorbital; suprascapular; supratrochlear; thoracoacromial; thoracoepigastric; thymic; tracheal; tympanic; ulnar; uterine; varicose; vertebral; vesical; vestibular; vortex; vorticose

vesicle acrosomal; allantoic; auditory; blastodermic; cerebral; encephalic; lens; lenticular; ocular; optic; otic; primary brain; seminal; synaptic; umbilical

vessel absorbent; afferent; blood; chyle; collateral; efferent; lymph; lymphatic; nutrient; vitelline

virus adenoidal-pharyngeal-conjunctival; AIDS-related; amphotropic; A-P-C; attenuated; avian leukosis-sarcoma; bacterial; Bornholm disease; CA; California; chickenpox; Coe; Colorado tick fever; common-cold; Coxsackie; croup-associated; cytopathogenic; defective; dengue; DNA; EB; Ebola; ECHO; ecotropic; encephalomyocarditis; enteric; enteric orphan; epidemic gastroenteritis; epidemic keratoconjunctivitis; epidemic parotitis; epidemic pleurodynia; Epstein-Barr; fixed; foamy; German measles; HA1; HA2; helper; hepatitis A; hepatitis B; hepatitis delta; herpes simplex; herpes zoster; human immunodeficiency; human papilloma; human T-cell leukemia; infectious hepatitis; infectious papilloma; infectious warts; influenza; Japanese B encephalitis; Lassa; lymphadenopathy-associated; lymphocytic choriomeningitis; Marburg; masked; measles; Mokola; mumps; naked; negative-strand; oncogenic; orphan; papilloma; parainfluenza; parainfluenza 1; parainfluenza 2; parainfluenza 3; parainfluenza 4; parainfluenza 5; phlebotomus fever; poliomyelitis; rabies; respiratory syncytial; RNA tumor; RNA; Ross River; Rous-associated; Rous sarcoma; Rs; rubella; rubeola; Sabia; Saint Louis encephalitis; Sendai; serum hepatitis; simian; Sindbis; slow; smallpox; snowshoe hare; street; tick-borne encephalitis; tobacco mosaic; tumor; vaccinia; varicella-zoster; variola; verruca vulgaris; visceral disease; West-Nile; xenotropic; yellow fever

vision achromatic; binocular; central; chromatic; direct; double; indirect; multiple; night; oscillating; peripheral; photopic; scotopic; stereoscopic; triple; tunnel

W

wart anatomical; fig; flat; genital; moist; mosaic; necrogenic; Peruvian; pitch; plantar; pointed; postmortem; soft; telangiectatic; tuberculous; venereal

The
American Heritage®
Medical Dictionary

A

α 1. The Greek letter *alpha*. Entries beginning with this character are alphabetized under **alpha. 2.** The symbol for **Bunsen's solubility coefficient. 3.** The symbol for **specific rotation.**

a *abbr.* area; asymmetrical; specific absorption coefficient; systemic arterial blood (used as a subscript); total acidity

A *abbr.* absorbance; alveolar gas (used as a subscript); adenine; AMP (in polynucleotides); ampere; angstrom; area

a– *or* **an–** *pref.* Without; not: *acellular.*

Å *abbr.* angstrom

AA *abbr.* Alcoholics Anonymous; amino acid; aminoacyl

AAFP *abbr.* American Academy of Family Physicians

Aar·skog-Scott syndrome (är′skŏg-) *n.* See **faciodigitogenital dysplasia.**

Ab *abbr.* antibody

ab–¹ *pref.* Away from: *abaxial.*

ab–² *pref.* Used to indicate an electromagnetic unit in the centimeter-gram-second system: *abcoulomb.*

a·bac·te·ri·al (ā′băk-tîr′ē-əl) *adj.* **1.** Not caused by bacteria. **2.** Free of bacteria.

A·ba·die's sign of exophthalmic goiter (ăb′ə-dēz′, ä-bə-) *n.* Spasm of the elevator muscle of the upper eyelid seen in Graves' disease as well as normally as a result of tension or fatigue.

Abadie's sign of tabes dorsalis *n.* Insensibility to pressure over the Achilles tendon.

ab·am·pere (ăb-ăm′pîr′) *n.* The centimeter-gram-second electromagnetic unit of current equal to ten amperes.

A band *n.* Any of various dark-staining anisotropic cross striations in the myofibrils of muscle fibers.

ab·ap·i·cal (ăb-ăp′ĭ-kəl, -ā′pĭ-) *adj.* Opposite to or directed away from the apex.

a·bar·og·no·sis (ā-băr′ŏg-nō′sĭs) *n.* Loss of the ability to sense weight.

a·ba·sia (ə-bā′zhə) *n.* Inability to walk due to impaired muscular coordination. **—a·ba′sic** (ə-bā′sĭk, -zĭk), **a·bat′ic** (ə-băt′ĭk) *adj.*

abasia-astasia *n.* See **astasia-abasia.**

abasia trep·i·dans (trĕp′ĭ-dănz′) *n.* Abasia due to trembling of the legs.

ab·ax·i·al (ăb-ăk′sē-əl) *or* **ab·ax·ile** (ăb-ăk′sīl) *adj.* Located away from or on the opposite side of an axis. **—ab·ax′i·al·ly** *adv.*

Ab·bé operation (ăb′ē) *n.* The transfer of a flap of the full thickness of the middle portion of the lower lip into the upper lip.

Ab·bott's method (ăb′əts) *n.* A method of treating scoliosis by applying plaster jackets after partial correction of the curvature by external force.

ab·cix·i·mab (ăb-sĭk′sə-măb′) *n.* A monoclonal antibody with anticoagulant properties, used to treat occlusive disorders of the arteries.

ab·do·men (ăb′də-mən, ăb-dō′mən) *n.* The part of the body that lies between the chest and the pelvis and encloses the stomach, intestines, liver, spleen, and pancreas. Also called *belly, venter.*

abdomin– *pref.* Variant of **abdomino–.**

ab·dom·i·nal (ăb-dŏm′ə-nəl) *adj.* Of or relating to the abdomen. **—n.** An abdominal muscle.

abdominal angina *n.* Intermittent abdominal pain, frequently occurring at a fixed time after eating, caused by inadequacy of the mesenteric circulation. Also called *intestinal angina.*

abdominal cavity *n.* The space bounded by the abdominal walls, diaphragm, and pelvis and containing most of the organs of digestion, the spleen, the kidneys, and the adrenal glands.

abdominal external oblique muscle *n.* A muscle with origin from the fifth to twelfth ribs, with insertion into the anterior lateral lip of the iliac crest, the inguinal ligament, and the anterior layer of the sheath of the rectus muscle of the abdomen, with nerve supply from the ventral branches of the lower thoracic nerves, and whose action diminishes the capacity of the abdomen and draws the chest down.

abdominal fissure *n.* Congenital failure of the ventral body wall to close.

abdominal guarding *n.* A spasm of the abdominal wall muscles to protect inflamed abdominal viscera from pressure; it usually results from inflammation of the peritoneal surface as in appendicitis, or generalized peritonitis, and is detectable on palpation.

abdominal hernia *n.* A hernia protruding through or into any part of the abdominal wall. Also called *laparocele.*

abdominal hysterectomy *n.* A hysterectomy made through an incision in the abdominal wall. Also called *abdominohysterectomy.*

abdominal hysterotomy *n.* Hysterotomy performed through the abdominal wall. Also called *abdominohysterotomy.*

abdominal internal oblique muscle *n.* A muscle with origin from the iliac fascia deep to the lateral part of the inguinal ligament, to the anterior half of the crest of the ilium, and to the lumbar fascia, with insertion into the tenth to twelfth ribs and the sheath of the rectus muscle of the abdomen, with nerve supply from the lower thoracic nerve, and whose action diminishes the capacity of the abdomen and bends the chest forward.

abdominal muscle deficiency syndrome *n.* Congenital absence of abdominal muscles, in which the outline of the intestines is visible through the protruding abdominal wall and the skin in the abdominal region is wrinkled. Also called *prune-belly syndrome, triad syndrome.*

abdominal pad *n.* See **laparotomy pad.**

abdominal pregnancy *n.* An ectopic pregnancy developing in the peritoneal cavity, usually secondary to an early rupture of a tubal pregnancy. Also called *ab-dominocyesis.*

abdominal pressure *n.* Pressure surrounding the bladder; it is estimated from rectal, gastric, or intraperitoneal pressure.

abdominal reflexes *pl.n.* Contractions of the muscles of the abdominal wall upon stimulation of the skin or upon the tapping of neighboring bony structures.

abdominal region *n.* Any of the subdivisions of the abdomen, including the right or left hypochondriac, the right or left lateral, the right or left inguinal, and the epigastric, umbilical, or pubic regions.

abdominal respiration *n.* Breathing that occurs primarily by the action of the diaphragm.

abdominal ring *n.* See **deep inguinal ring.**

abdominal section *n.* See **celiotomy.**

abdomino– *or* **abdomin–** *pref.* Abdomen: *abdominothoracic.*

ab·dom·i·no·cen·te·sis (ăb-dŏm′ə-nō-sĕn-tē′sĭs) *n.* Surgical puncture of the abdomen by a needle to withdraw fluid; abdominal paracentesis. Also called *celiocentesis, celioparacentesis.*

ab·dom·i·no·cy·e·sis (ăb-dŏm′ə-nō-sī-ē′sĭs) *n.* **1.** See **abdominal pregnancy. 2.** See **secondary abdominal pregnancy.**

ab·dom·i·no·cys·tic (ăb-dŏm′ə-nō-sĭs′tĭk) *adj.* Abdominovesical.

ab·dom·i·no·gen·i·tal (ăb-dŏm′ə-nō-gĕn′ĭ-tl) *adj.* Of or relating to the abdomen and the genital organs.

ab·dom·i·no·hys·ter·ec·to·my (ăb-dŏm′ə-nō-hĭs′tə-rĕk′tə-mē) *n.* See **abdominal hysterectomy.**

ab·dom·i·no·hys·ter·ot·o·my (ăb-dŏm′ə-nō-hĭs′tə-rŏt′ə-mē) *n.* See **abdominal hysterotomy.**

ab·dom·i·no·per·i·ne·al (ăb-dŏm′ə-nō-pĕr′ə-nē′əl) *adj.* Relating to the abdomen and the perineum.

ab·dom·i·no·plas·ty (ăb-dŏm′ə-nō-plăs′tē) *n.* Plastic surgery of the abdomen in which excess fatty tissue and skin are removed, usually for cosmetic purposes.

ab·dom·i·nos·co·py (ăb-dŏm′ə-nŏs′kə-pē) *n.* Internal examination of the abdomen through the use of an endoscope; peritoneoscopy.

ab·dom·i·no·scro·tal (ăb-dŏm′ə-nō-skrōt′l) *adj.* Of or relating to the abdomen and the scrotum.

ab·dom·i·no·tho·rac·ic (ăb-dŏm′ə-nō-thə-răs′ĭk) *adj.* Of or relating to the abdomen and the thorax.

abdominothoracic arch *n.* A bell-shaped line along the lowest of the false ribs and the lower end of the sternum, making a rough boundary line between the abdomen and thorax.

ab·dom·i·no·vag·i·nal (ăb-dŏm′ə-nō-văj′ə-nəl) *adj.* Of or relating to the abdomen and the vagina.

ab·dom·i·no·ves·i·cal (ăb-dŏm′ə-nō-vĕs′ĭ-kəl) *adj.* Of or relating to the abdomen and the urinary bladder or the gallbladder.

ab·duce (ăb-dōōs′) *v.* To abduct.

ab·du·cens oc·u·li (ăb-dōō′sənz ŏk′yə-lī′) *n.* The lateral rectus muscle.

ab·du·cent (ăb-dōō′sənt) *adj.* Abducting; drawing away.

abducent nerve *n.* The small motor nerve supplying the lateral rectus muscle of the eye, originating in the dorsal part of the tegmentum of the pons, passing through

the cavernous sinus, and entering the orbit through the superior orbital fissure. Also called *sixth cranial nerve.*

ab·duct (ăb-dŭkt′) *v.* To draw away from the midline of the body or from an adjacent part or limb. —**ab·duc′tion** *n.*

ab·duc·tor (ăb-dŭk′tər) *n.* A muscle that draws a body part, such as a finger, arm, or toe, away from the midline of the body or of an extremity.

abductor muscle of big toe *n.* A muscle with origin from the medial process of the calcaneal tuberosity, and the plantar aponeurosis, with insertion into the medial side of the proximal phalanx of the big toe, with nerve supply from the medial plantar nerve, and whose action abducts the big toe.

abductor muscle of little finger *n.* A muscle with origin from the pisiform bone and pisohamate ligament, with insertion into the medial side of the base of the proximal phalanx of the little finger, with nerve supply from the ulnar nerve, and whose action abducts and flexes the little finger.

abductor muscle of little toe *n.* A muscle with origin from the lateral and the medial processes of the calcanean tuberosity, with insertion to the lateral side of the proximal phalanx of the fifth toe, with nerve supply from the lateral plantar nerve, and whose action abducts and flexes the little toe.

A·bell-Ken·dall method (ā′bəl-kĕn′dl) *n.* A method for estimating total serum cholesterol without interference from bilirubin, protein, and hemoglobin.

ab·er·rant (ă-bĕr′ənt, ăb′ər-) *adj.* **1.** Deviating from the usual course, as certain ducts, vessels, or nerves. **2.** Deviating from the normal; untrue to type. **3.** Out of place; ectopic. —**ab·er′ran·cy** *n.*

aberrant ductule *n.* Any of the diverticula of the epididymis. Also called *aberrant duct.*

aberrant goiter *n.* Enlargement of a supernumerary or ectopic thyroid gland.

aberrant regeneration *n.* Misdirected regrowth of nerve fibers, commonly seen after oculomotor nerve injury.

ab·er·rat·ed (ăb′ə-rā′tĭd) *adj.* Characterized by defects, abnormality, or deviation from the usual, typical, or expected course.

ab·er·ra·tion (ăb′ə-rā′shən) *n.* **1.** A departure from the normal or typical. **2.** A psychological disorder or abnormal alteration in one's mental state. **3.** A defect of focus, such as blurring in an image. **4.** An imperfect image caused by a physical defect in an optical element, as in a lens. **5.** A deviation in the normal genetic structure or number of chromosomes in an organism.

a·be·ta·lip·o·pro·tein·e·mi·a (ā-bā′tə-lĭp′ō-prō′tē-nē′mē-ə, -tē-ə-nē′-) *n.* An inherited disorder characterized by the absence of low-density lipoproteins in the plasma, the presence of acanthocytes in the blood, retinal pigmentary degeneration, malabsorption of fats, and neuromuscular abnormalities. Also called *Bassen-Kornzweig syndrome.*

ABFP *abbr.* American Board of Family Practice

ABG *abbr.* arterial blood gas

A·bil·i·fy (ə-bĭl′ə-fī′) A trademark for the drug aripiprazole.

a·bi·o·sis (ā′bī-ō′sĭs) *n.* **1.** Absence of life. **2.** See abiotrophy. —**a′bi·ot′ic** (-ŏt′ĭk) *adj.*

a·bi·ot·ro·phy (ā′bī-ŏt′rə-fē) *n.* **1.** Premature loss of vitality or degeneration of cells or tissues, especially when due to genetic causes. **2.** A hereditary degenerative disease. Also called *abiosis.*

ab·ir·ri·tant (ăb-ĭr′ĭ-tənt) *adj.* Relieving irritation; soothing. —**ab·ir′ri·tant** *n.*

ab·ir·ri·ta·tion (ăb-ĭr′ĭ-tā′shən) *n.* The diminution of a reflex or other irritability in a body part.

ab·ir·ri·ta·tive (ăb-ĭr′ĭ-tā′tĭv) *adj.* Abirritant. —**ab·ir′·ri·ta′tive·ly** *adv.*

abl (ā′bəl) *n.* An oncogene found in the Abelson strain of mouse leukemia virus and involved in the Philadelphia chromosome translocation in chronic granulocytic leukemia.

ab·late (ă-blāt′) *v.* To remove or destroy the function of.

ab·la·tion (ă-blā′shən) *n.* Removal of a body part or the destruction of its function, as by a surgery, disease, or noxious substance.

a·ble·phar·i·a (ā′blĕ-fâr′ē-ə) *n.* Congenital absence of the eyelids.

a·blep·si·a (ə-blĕp′sē-ə) *or* **a·blep·sy** (ə-blĕp′sē) *n.* Lack of sight; blindness.

ab·ner·val (ăb-nûr′vəl) *adj.* Flowing away from a nerve. Used of an electric current passing through a muscle.

ab·neu·ral (ăb-nŏŏr′əl) *adj.* Away from the neural axis. —**ab·neur′al·ly** *adv.*

ab·nor·mal·i·ty (ăb′nôr-măl′ĭ-tē) *n.* An anomaly, malformation, or difference from the normal.

ab·nor·mal occlusion (ăb-nôr′məl) *n.* An alignment of the teeth not considered to be within the normal range of variation.

abnormal psychology *n.* Psychopathology.

ABO hemolytic disease of newborn *n.* See erythroblastosis fetalis.

ab·o·rad (ăb-ôr′ăd) *or* **ab·o·ral** (ăb-ôr′əl) *adj.* In a direction away from the mouth.

a·bort (ə-bôrt′) *v.* **1.** To expel or cause to expel an embryo or fetus before it is viable. **2.** To arrest a disease in its earliest stages. **3.** To arrest in growth or development; to cause to remain rudimentary.

a·bort·ed systole (ə-bôr′tĭd) *n.* A loss of the systolic beat in the radial pulse through weakness of the ventricular contraction.

a·bor·tient (ə-bôr′shənt) *adj.* Abortifacient.

a·bor·ti·fa·cient (ə-bôr′tə-fā′shənt) *adj.* Causing or inducing abortion. —**a·bor′ti·fa′cient** *n.*

a·bor·ti·gen·ic (ə-bôr′tə-jĕn′ĭk) *adj.* Abortifacient.

a·bor·tion (ə-bôr′shən) *n.* **1.** Induced termination of pregnancy with destruction of the embryo or fetus; therapeutic abortion. **2.** Any of various procedures that result in such a termination of pregnancy. **3.** Spontaneous abortion. **4.** Cessation of a normal or abnormal process before completion.

a·bor·tive (ə-bôr′tĭv) *adj.* **1.** Not reaching completion, as of a disease subsiding before it has finished its course. **2.** Partially or imperfectly developed; rudimentary. **3.** Abortifacient. —**a·bor′tive·ly** *adv.* —**a·bor′tive·ness** *n.*

abortive transduction *n.* Transduction in which the genetic fragment from the donor bacterium is not integrated in the genome of the recipient bacterium. When the recipient bacterium divides, the genetic fragment from the donor bacterium is transmitted to only one of the daughter cells.

a·bor·tus (ə-bôr′təs) *n.* The product or products of an abortion.

abortus Bang ring test *n.* An agglutination test done on the mixed milk of many cows, usually of entire herds, for the detection of bovine brucellosis. Also called *milk ring test.*

ABO system *n.* A classification system for human blood that identifies four major blood types based on the presence or absence of two antigens, A and B, on red blood cells. The four blood types (A, B, AB, and O, in which O designates blood that lacks both antigens) are important in determining the compatability of blood for transfusion.

a·bou·li·a (ə-bŏŏ′lē-ə, ə-byŏŏ′-) *n.* Variant of **abulia.**

ABR *abbr.* auditory brainstem response (see under **auditory brainstem response audiometry**)

a·bra·chi·a (ə-brā′kē-ə, ā-brā′-) *n.* Congenital absence of the arms.

a·bra·chi·o·ce·pha·li·a (ə-brā′kē-ō-sə-fā′lē-ə,-ā-brā′-) *or* **a·bra·chi·o·ceph·a·ly** (ə-brā′kē-ō-sĕf′ə-lē) *n.* Congenital absence of the arms and head. Also called *acephalobrachia.*

a·brade (ə-brād′) *v.* **1.** To wear away by mechanical action. **2.** To scrape away the surface layer from a part.

a·bra·sion (ə-brā′zhən) *n.* **1.** A scraping away of a portion of a surface. **2.** The wearing down or rubbing away or removal of the superficial layers of skin or mucous membrane in a limited area. **3.** The pathological wearing away of tooth substance by mechanical means; grinding.

a·bra·sive (ə-brā′sĭv) *adj.* Causing abrasion. —*n.* A material used to produce abrasion.

a·bra·sive·ness (ə-brā′sĭv-nĭs) *n.* **1.** The property of a substance that causes surface wear by friction. **2.** The quality of being able to scratch or abrade another material.

ab·re·act (ăb′rē-ăkt′) *v.* To release repressed emotions by acting out the situation causing the conflict, as in words, behavior, or the imagination. —**ab′re·ac′tion** *n.*

ab·rup·ti·o pla·cen·tae (ə-brŭp′shē-ō′ plə-sĕn′tē′) *n.* The premature detachment of a normally situated placenta.

ab·scess (ăb′sĕs′) *n.* **1.** A collection of pus formed by tissue destruction in an inflamed area of a localized infection. **2.** A cavity that is formed by liquefactive necrosis within solid tissue. —*v.* To form an abscess.

ab·scis·sion (ăb-sĭzh′ən) *n.* The act of cutting off or away.

ab·sco·pal (ăb-skō′pəl, -skŏp′əl) *adj.* Of or relating to the remote effect that irradiation of tissue has on nonirradiated tissue.

abscopal effect *n.* A reaction produced following irradiation but occurring outside the zone of actual radiation absorption.

ab·sence (ăb′səns) *n.* See **petit mal.**

absence seizure *n.* A brief, sudden loss of consciousness symptomatic of petit mal epilepsy.

abs feb. *abbr. Latin* absente febre (when fever is absent)

Ab·sid·i·a (ăb-sĭd′ē-ə) *n.* A genus of fungi that may cause phycomycosis in humans.

ab·so·lute accommodation (ăb′sə-lo͞ot′, ăb′sə-lo͞ot′) *n.* Accommodation of one eye independent of the other eye.

absolute alcohol *n.* Ethyl alcohol containing no more than 1 percent water.

absolute glaucoma *n.* The final stage of blindness in glaucoma.

absolute hemianopsia *n.* Hemianopsia in which the affected half of the visual field is insensitive to all visual stimuli.

absolute humidity *n.* The weight of water vapor present per unit volume of a gas or a mixture of gases.

absolute hyperopia *n.* Manifest hyperopia that cannot be overcome by accommodation.

absolute leukocytosis *n.* An increase in the total number of white blood cells in the blood.

absolute scale *n.* See **Kelvin scale.**

absolute temperature *n. Abbr.* **T** Temperature measured in kelvin from absolute zero.

absolute unit *n.* A unit whose value is constant regardless of place or time.

absolute zero *n.* The temperature at which substances possess no thermal energy, equal to −273.15°C, −459.67°F, or 0 K.

ab·sorb (əb-zôrb′) *v.* **1.** To take in by absorption. **2.** To reduce the intensity of transmitted light.

ab·sorb·a·ble gelatin film (əb-zôr′bə-bəl) *n.* A sterile, nonantigenic, absorbable, water-insoluble film, used in the closure and repair of defects in membranes.

absorbable suture *n.* A surgical suture that is composed of a material that is digestible by tissues of the body.

ab·sorb·ance (əb-zôr′bəns) *or* **ab·sorb·an·cy** *or* **ab·sorb·en·cy** (əb-zôr′bən-sē) *n. Abbr.* **A** In spectrophotometry, equal to 2 minus the log of the percentage transmittance of light. Also called *extinction, optical density.*

absorbed dose (əb-zôrbd′) *n.* The quantity of radiation energy, expressed in rads, that is administered or absorbed per unit mass of target.

ab·sor·be·fa·cient (əb-zôr′bə-fā′shənt) *adj.* Causing absorption. —**ab·sor′be·fa′cient** *n.*

ab·sorb·ent (əb-zôr′bənt) *adj.* Capable of absorption; able to absorb. —**ab·sorb′ent** *n.*

absorbent vessel *n.* See **lymphatic vessel.**

ab·sorp·ti·om·e·try (ăb-zôrp′shē-ŏm′ĭ-trē) *n.* A diagnostic technique for measuring bone mineral density in which an image of bone is produced from computerized analysis of absorption rates of photons directed in a focused beam at a body part. —**ab·sorp′ti·om′e·ter** *n.*

ab·sorp·tion (əb-zôrp′shən) *n.* The taking in or incorporation of something, such as a gas, a liquid, light, or heat.

absorption chromatography *n.* See **chromatography.**

absorption coefficient *n.* **1.** The milliliters of a gas at standard temperature and pressure that will saturate 100 milliters of liquid. **2.** The amount of light absorbed in 1 atom or in 1 unit of thickness or mass of a given substance.

absorption spectrum *n.* The electromagnetic spectrum, broken by a specific pattern of dark lines or bands, observed when radiation traverses a particular absorbing medium.

ab·sorp·tive (əb-zôrp′tĭv) *adj.* Absorbent.

ab·sti·nence (ăb′stə-nəns) *n.* The act or practice of refraining from indulgence in an appetite, as for certain foods, drink, alcoholic beverages, drugs, or sex. —**ab′sti·nent** *adj.*

ab·stract (ăb-străkt′, ăb′străkt′) *adj.* **1.** Considered apart from concrete existence. **2.** Not applied or practical; theoretical.

ab·strac·tion (ăb-străk′shən, əb-) *n.* **1.** Distillation or separation of the volatile constituents of a substance. **2.** Exclusive mental concentration; absent-mindedness. **3.** A malocclusion in which the teeth or associated structures are lower than their normal occlusal plane. **4.** The selection of a certain aspect of a concept from the whole.

abstract thinking *n.* Thinking characterized by the ability to use concepts and to make and understand generalizations, such as of the properties or pattern shared by a variety of specific items or events.

ab·ter·mi·nal (ăb-tûr′mə-nəl) *adj.* Flowing away from the end and toward the center of a nerve. Used of an electric current passing through a muscle.

a·bu·li·a *or* **a·bou·li·a** (ə-bo͞o′lē-ə, ə-byo͞o′-) *n.* Loss or impairment of the ability to make decisions or act independently. —**a·bu′lic** (-lĭk) *adj.*

a·buse (ə-byo͞oz′) *v.* **1.** To use wrongly or improperly; misuse. **2.** To hurt or injure physically by maltreatment. **3.** To force sexual activity on; rape or molest. **4.** To assail with contemptuous, coarse, or insulting words; revile. —*n.* (ə-byo͞os′) **1.** Improper use or handling, as of a drug; misuse. **2.** Physical maltreatment, as of a spouse or child. **3.** The forcing of unwanted sexual activity by one person on another. **4.** Sexual activity that is deemed improper or harmful, as between an adult and a minor or with a person of diminished mental capacity. **5.** Insulting or coarse language. —**a·bus′er** *n.*

a·but·ment (ə-bŭt′mənt) *n.* A natural tooth or implanted tooth substitute used to support or anchor a dental prosthesis.

ABVD *abbr.* adriamycin, bleomycin, vinblastine, and dacarbazine (chemotherapy regimen used to treat neoplastic diseases, such as Hodgkin's disease)

ac *abbr. Latin* ante cibum (before a meal)

Ac The symbol for the element **actinium.**

ac– *pref.* Variant of **ad–** (sense 1).

a·cal·cu·li·a (ā′kăl-kyo͞o′lē-ə) *n.* A form of aphasia characterized by the inability to perform mathematical calculations.

a·camp·si·a (ə-kămp′sē-ə, ā-kămp′-) *n.* Stiffening or rigidity of a joint.

a·can·tha (ə-kăn′thə) *n., pl.* **–thae** (-thē) A sharp spiny part or structure, such as the spinous process of a vertebra.

a·can·tha·me·bi·a·sis (ə-kăn′thə-mē-bī′ə-sĭs) *n.* Infection with amebas of the genus *Acanthamoeba* that may result in a necrotizing dermal or tissue infection or in meningoencephalitis.

A·can·tha·moe·ba (ə-kăn′thə-mē′bə) *n.* A free-living ameba found in soil, sewage, and water, several species of which cause acanthamebiasis.

a·can·thes·the·sia (ə-kăn′thĕs-thē′zhə) *n.* An abnormal sensation as of a pinprick.

acan·thi·on (ə-kăn′thē-ŏn′, -thē-ən) *n.* The tip of the anterior nasal spine.

acantho– *or* **acanth–** *pref.* Thorn; spine; spinous process: *acanthocyte.*

A·can·tho·ceph·a·la (ə-kăn′thə-sĕf′ə-lə) *n.* Any of various worms of the phylum Acanthocephala that live parasitically in the intestines of vertebrates and are characterized by a cylindrical, retractile proboscis that bears many rows of hooked spines. Also called *spiny-headed worm.* —**a·can′tho·ceph′a·lan** (-lən), **a·can′-tho·ceph′a·lid** (-lĭd) *adj.*

a·can·tho·ceph·a·li·a·sis (ə-kăn′thə-sĕf′ə-lī′ə-sĭs) *n.* Infection with a species of Acanthocephala.

A·can·tho·chei·lo·ne·ma (ə-kăn′thə-kī′lə-nē′mə) *n.* A genus of filarial worms that are parasitic in humans, now part of the genus *Dipetalonema.* No longer in technical use.

a·can·tho·cyte (ə-kăn′thə-sīt′) *n.* A red blood cell characterized by multiple spiny cytoplasmic projections and found in acanthocytosis. Also called *acanthrocyte.*

a·can·tho·cy·to·sis (ə-kăn′thə-sī-tō′sĭs) *n.* A rare condition in which the majority of the red blood cells are acanthocytes. Also called *acanthrocytosis.*

a·can·thoid (ə-kăn′thoid′) *adj.* Shaped like a thorn or spine.

ac·an·thol·y·sis (ăk′ăn-thŏl′ĭ-sĭs, ăk′ən-) *n., pl.* **–ses** (-sēz′) Separation of individual prickle cells from their neighbors, as in keratosis follicularis.

ac·an·tho·ma (ăk′ăn-thō′mə, ăk′ən-) *n., pl.* **–mas** *or* **–ma·ta** (-mə-tə) A tumor composed of epidermal squamous cells.

a·can·thor·rhex·is (ə-kăn′thə-rĕk′sĭs) *n.* Rupture of the intercellular bridges of the prickle cell layer of the epidermis, as in contact dermatitis.

ac·an·tho·sis (ăk′ăn-thō′sĭs, ăk′ən-) *n., pl.* **–ses** (-sēz′) An increase in the thickness of the prickle cell layer of the epidermis; hyperacanthosis. —**ac′an·thot′ic** (-thŏt′ĭk) *adj.*

acanthosis ni·gri·cans (nī′grĭ-kănz′, nĭg′rĭ-) *n.* An eruption of velvety wartlike growths accompanied by hyperpigmentation in the skin of the armpits, neck, anogenital area, and groin, occurring in a benign form in children, but associated with internal malignancy or reticulosis in adults.

a·can·thro·cyte (ə-kăn′thrə-sīt′) *n.* See **acanthocyte.**

a·can·thro·cy·to·sis (ə-kăn′thrə-sī-tō′sĭs) *n.* See **acanthocytosis.**

a·cap·ni·a (ā-kăp′nē-ə) *n.* A condition marked by the presence of less than the normal amount of carbon dioxide in the blood and tissues.

a·car·di·a (ā-kär′dē-ə) *n.* Congenital absence of the heart, sometimes occurring in the smaller parasitic member of conjoined twins when its partner monopolizes the placental blood supply.

ac·a·ri·a·sis (ăk′ə-rī′ə-sĭs) *n., pl.* **–ses** (-sēz′) A disease, usually of the skin, caused by infestation with mites. Also called *acaridiasis, acarinosis.*

a·car·i·cide (ə-kăr′ĭ-sīd′) *adj.* Destructive to acarids. —*n.* An agent that destroys acarids. —**acaricidal** *adj.*

ac·a·rid (ăk′ə-rĭd) *n.* An arachnid of the order Acarina, which includes the mites and ticks. —**ac′a·rid** *adj.*

A·car·i·dae (ə-kăr′ĭ-dē) *n.* A family of exceptionally small mites, usually 0.5 millimeter or less in length, abundant in dried fruits and meats, grain, meal, and flour, and frequently causing severe dermatitis in persons hypersensitized by frequent handling of infested products.

Ac·a·ri·na (ăk′ə-rī′nə, -rē′-) *n.* An order of Arachnida comprising the mites and ticks and including several species that are parasitic to humans and animals.

ac·a·rine (ăk′ə-rīn′, -rēn′) *adj.* Relating to or caused by an acarid. —*n.* An acarid.

ac·a·ro·der·ma·ti·tis (ăk′ə-rō-dûr′mə-tī′tĭs) *n.* A skin inflammation or eruption produced by an acarid.

ac·a·roid (ăk′ə-roid′) *adj.* Resembling a mite.

ac·a·ro·pho·bi·a (ăk′ə-rə-fō′bē-ə) *n.* **1.** An abnormal fear of mites, small insects, or worms. **2.** An abnormal fear of small particles, or of itching.

Ac·a·rus (ăk′ə-rəs) *n.* A genus of mites.

Acarus fol·lic·u·lo·rum (fə-lĭk′yə-lôr′əm) *n.* Demodex folliculorum.

Acarus sca·bi·e·i (skā′bē-ē′ī) *n. Sarcoptes scabiei.*

Acarus trit·i·ci (trĭt′ĭ-sī′) *n. Pyemotes tritici.*

a·car·y·ote (ā-kăr′ē-ōt′, ə-kăr′-) *n.* See **akaryocyte.**

a·cat·a·la·se·mi·a (ā-kăt′ə-lā-sē′mē-ə) *n.* Hereditary deficiency of catalase in the blood, often manifested by recurrent infection or ulceration of the gums and related oral structures. Also called *acatalasia, Takahara's disease.*

a·cat·a·ma·the·sia (ā-kăt′ə-mə-thē′zhə) *n.* Loss of the faculty of understanding.

a·cat·a·pha·sia (ā-kăt′ə-fā′zhə) *n.* Loss of the power to formulate a statement correctly.

ac·a·thex·i·a (ăk′ə-thĕk′sē-ə) *n.* An abnormal loss of bodily secretions. —**ac′a·thec′tic** (-thĕk′tĭk) *adj.*

ac·a·thex·is (ăk′ə-thĕk′sĭs) *n.* A mental disorder in which certain objects or ideas fail to elicit an emotional response in the individual.

ac·a·this·i·a (ăk′ə-thĭz′ē-ə) *n.* Variant of **akathisia.**

ac·cel·er·ant (ăk-sĕl′ər-ənt) *n.* Accelerator.

ac·cel·er·a·tor (ăk-sĕl′ə-rā′tər) *n.* **1.** One that increases rapidity of action or function. **2.** A nerve, muscle, or substance that quickens movement or response. **3.** A catalyst.

accelerator factor *n.* See **factor V.**

accelerator fiber *n.* Any of the postganglionic sympathetic nerve fibers that originate in the superior middle and inferior cervical ganglia of the sympathetic trunk and convey impulses to the heart that tend to increase the rapidity and force of the cardiac pulsations.

accelerator globulin *n.* Variant of **serum accelerator globulin.**

accelerator nerve *n.* Any of the slender unmyelinated nerves establishing the sympathetic innervation of the heart, and originating from the ganglion cells of the superior, middle, and inferior cervical ganglion of the sympathetic trunk.

ac·cen·tu·a·tor (ăk-sĕn′chŏŏ-ā′tər) *n.* A substance, such as aniline, that allows an otherwise impossible combination between a histologic element and a stain.

ac·cep·tor *or* **ac·cept·er** (ăk-sĕp′tər) *n.* **1.** The reactant in an induced reaction that has an increased rate of reaction in the presence of the inductor. **2.** The atom that contributes no electrons to a covalent bond.

ac·cess (ăk′sĕs) *n.* **1.** A means of approaching, entering, exiting, or making use of; passage. **2.** The space required to view a tooth and manipulate dental instruments to remove decay and prepare the tooth for restoration. **3.** The opening in the crown of a tooth necessary to allow adequate admittance to the pulp space to clean, shape, and seal the root canal.

ac·ces·so·ry (ăk-sĕs′ə-rē) *adj.* Having a secondary, supplementary, or subordinate function.

accessory adrenal *n.* An island of cortical tissue separate from the adrenal gland, usually found in the retroperitoneal tissues, kidneys, or genitals. Also called *adrenal rest.*

accessory cephalic vein *n.* A variable vein that passes along the radial border of the forearm to join the cephalic vein near the elbow.

accessory gland *n.* A small mass of glandular tissue detached from, but lying near, another gland of similar structure.

accessory hemiazygos vein *n.* A vein that is formed by the union of the fourth to seventh left posterior intercostal veins, passes along the fifth, sixth, and seventh thoracic vertebrae, crosses the midline behind the aorta, esophagus, and thoracic duct, and empties into the azygos vein.

accessory ligament *n.* A ligament around a joint that supports or supplements another.

accessory nerve *n.* A nerve that arises by two sets of roots: the cranial set, arising from the side of the medulla, and the spinal set, arising from the ventrolateral part of the first five cervical segments of the spinal cord. These two roots form the accessory nerve trunk, which divides into two branches: the internal, which unites with the vagus nerve in the jugular foramen and supplies the muscles of the pharynx, larynx, and soft palate; and the external, which continues through the jugular foramen to supply the sternocleidomastoid and trapezius muscles. Also called *eleventh cranial nerve.*

accessory obturator artery *n.* An artery that is the pubic branch of the inferior epigastric artery when it contributes a significant supply through the obturator canal.

accessory pancreatic duct *n.* The excretory duct of the head of the pancreas, one branch of which joins the pancreatic duct, the other opening into the duodenum. Also called *Santorini's duct.*

accessory phrenic nerve *n.* Any of the accessory nerve strands that arise from the fifth cervical nerve, often as branches of the nerve to the subclavius, and pass downward to join the phrenic nerve.

accessory saphenous vein *n.* An occasional vein running in the thigh parallel to the great saphenous vein, which it joins just before the latter empties into the femoral vein.

accessory spleen *n.* Any of the small globular masses of splenic tissue occasionally found in the area of the spleen, or in one of the peritoneal folds.

accessory symptom *n.* A symptom that usually but not always accompanies a certain disease. Also called *concomitant symptom.*

accessory vertebral vein *n.* A vein that accompanies the vertebral vein but passes through the foramen of the transverse process of the seventh cervical vertebra and opens independently into the brachiocephalic vein.

ac·ci·den·tal hypothermia (ăk′sĭ-dĕn′tl) *n.* Unintentional decrease in body temperature from exposure to a cold environment.

ac·cli·ma·tion (ăk′lə-mā′shən) *n.* **1.** The process of becoming adjusted to a new environment or situation. **2.** Acclimatization.

Ac·co·late (ăk′ə-lāt′) A trademark for the drug zafirkulast.

ac·com·mo·date (ə-kŏm′ə-dāt′) *v.* To become adjusted, as the eye to focusing on objects at a distance.

ac·com·mo·da·tion (ə-kŏm′ə-dā′shən) *n.* **1.** The act or state of adjustment or adaptation. **2.** The automatic adjustment in the focal length of the lens of the eye to permit retinal focus of images of objects at varying distances.

accommodation reflex *n.* The coordinated changes that occur in the eye when viewing a near object, including constriction of the pupil, convergence of the eyes, and increased convexity of the lens.

ac·com·mo·da·tive (ə-kŏm′ə-dā′tĭv) *adj.* Of or relating to accommodation.

accommodative asthenopia *n.* Asthenopia due to errors of refraction and excessive contraction of the ciliary muscle.

ac·com·pa·ny·ing vein (ə-kŭm′pə-nē-ĭng, ə-kŭmp′nē-ĭng) *n.* **1.** A vein accompanying another structure. **2.** Either of a pair of veins, occasionally more, that closely accompany an artery in such a manner that the pulsations of the artery aid venous return.

ac·cor·di·on graft (ə-kôr′dē-ən) *n.* A skin graft in which multiple slits have been made so that it can be stretched to cover a large area.

ac·cou·cheur's hand (ăk′ŏŏ-shûrz′, ä′kŏŏ-) *n.* The position of the hand in tetany or in muscular dystrophy, in which the fingers are flexed at the metacarpophalangeal joints and extended at the phalangeal joints, with the thumb flexed and drawn into the palm. Also called *obstetrical hand.*

ac·cre·men·ti·tion (ăk′rə-mən-tĭsh′ən) *n.* **1.** Reproduction by budding or germination. **2.** See **accretion** (sense 2).

ac·cre·ti·o cor·dis (ə-krē′shē-ō kôr′dĭs) *n.* Adhesion of the pericardium to adjacent structures outside the heart.

ac·cre·tion (ə-krē′shən) *n.* **1.** Growth or increase in size by gradual external addition, fusion, or inclusion. **2.** Increase by addition to the periphery of material of the same nature as that already present, as in the growth of crystals. Also called *accrementition.* **3.** Foreign material, such as plaque or calculus, collecting on the surface of a tooth or in a cavity. **4.** The growing together or adherence of body parts that are normally separate.

ac·cre·tion·ar·y growth (ə-krē′shə-nĕr′ē) *n.* Growth resulting from an increase of intercellular material.

Ac·cu·pril (ăk′yə-prĭl′) A trademark for the drug quinapril hydrochloride.

Ac·cu·tane (ăk′yoō-tān′) A trademark for the drug isotretinoin.

Ace (ās) A trademark for an elastic bandage.

ACE inhibitor (ās) *n.* Angiotensin-converting enzyme inhibitor; any of a class of drugs that reduce peripheral arterial resistance by inactivating an enzyme that converts angiotensin I to the vasoconstrictor angiotensin II, used in the treatment of hypertension, congestive heart failure, and other cardiovascular disorders.

A cell *n.* See **alpha cell**.

a·cel·lu·lar (ā-sĕl′yə-lər) *adj.* 1. Containing no cells; not made of cells. 2. Devoid of cells; noncellular. 3. Of or relating to unicellular organisms that do not become multicellular and are complete within a single cell unit.

acellular pertussis vaccine *n. Abbr.* **DTaP** A diphtheria, tetanus, pertussis vaccine containing two or more antigens but no whole cells.

a·ce·lo·mate (ā-sē′lə-māt′) *adj.* Lacking a true celom or body cavity lined with mesothelium, as in flatworms. —**a·ce′lo·mate′, a′ce·lom′a·tous** (-lŏm′ə-təs, -lō′mə-) *adj.*

a·ce·nes·the·sia (ā-sē′nĭs-thē′zhə, ā-sĕn′ĭs-) *n.* Absence of the sensation of physical existence and well-being or of the consciousness of normal bodily functioning.

a·cen·tric (ā-sĕn′trĭk) *adj.* 1. Having no center. 2. Not located in the center. 3. Of or relating to a chromosome fragment lacking a centromere.

a·ceph·a·lo·bra·chi·a (ā-sĕf′ə-lō-brā′kē-ə, ə-sĕf′-) *n.* See **abrachiocephalia**.

a·ceph·a·lo·car·di·a (ā-sĕf′ə-lō-kär′dē-ə, ə-sĕf′-) *n.* Absence of the head and heart in the parasitic member of conjoined twins.

a·ceph·a·lo·chei·ri·a *or* **a·ceph·a·lo·chi·ri·a** (ā-sĕf′ə-lō-kī′rē-ə, ə-sĕf′-) *n.* Congenital absence of the head and hands.

a·ceph·a·lo·cyst (ā-sĕf′ə-lō-sĭst, ə-sĕf′-) *n.* A hydatid cyst with no daughter cyst; a sterile hydatid.

a·ceph·a·lo·gas·te·ri·a (ā-sĕf′ə-lō-gă-stîr′ē-ə, ə-sĕf′-) *n.* Congenital absence of the head, chest, and abdomen in the parasitic member of conjoined twins.

a·ceph·a·lor·rha·chi·a (ā-sĕf′ə-lō-rā′kē-ə, ə-sĕf′-) *n.* Congenital absence of the head and spinal column.

a·ceph·a·lo·sto·mi·a (ā-sĕf′ə-lō-stō′mē-ə, ə-sĕf′-) *n.* Congenital absence of most of the head, with the presence of a mouthlike opening.

a·ceph·a·lo·tho·ra·ci·a (ā-sĕf′ə-lō-thə-rā′sē-ə, ə-sĕf′-) *n.* Congenital absence of the head and chest.

a·ceph·a·ly (ā-sĕf′ə-lē, ə-sĕf′-) *or* **a·ce·pha·li·a** (ā′sə-fā′lē-ə, ăs′ə-) *or* **a·ceph·a·lism** (ā-sĕf′ə-lĭz′əm, ə-sĕf′-) *n.* Congenital absence of the head.

a·cer·vu·line (ə-sûr′vyə-lĭn′, -lēn′) *adj.* Occurring in clusters; aggregated.

a·cer·vu·lus (ə-sûr′vyə-ləs) *n., pl.* **-li** (-lī′) See **brain sand**.

acet– *pref.* Variant of **aceto–**.

acetabular fossa *n.* A depressed area in the floor of the acetabulum above the acetabular notch.

ac·e·tab·u·lec·to·my (ăs′ĭ-tăb′yə-lĕk′tə-mē) *n.* Excision of the acetabulum.

ac·e·tab·u·lo·plas·ty (ăs′ĭ-tăb′yə-lō-plăs′tē) *n.* Surgical repair of the acetabulum.

ac·e·tab·u·lum (ăs′ĭ-tăb′yə-ləm) *n., pl.* **-la** (-lə) The cup-shaped cavity at the base of the hipbone into which the ball-shaped head of the femur fits. Also called *cotyloid cavity.* —**ac′e·tab′u·lar** *adj.*

ac·e·tal (ăs′ĭ-tăl′) *n.* 1. A colorless, flammable, volatile liquid used as a solvent. 2. Any of the compounds formed from aldehydes combined with alcohol.

ac·et·al·de·hyde (ăs′ĭ-tăl′də-hīd′) *n.* A colorless, flammable liquid formed during ethanol metabolism and yeast fermentation of organic compounds and used to manufacture acetic acid and drugs. Also called *aldehyde, ethaldehyde.*

a·cet·a·min·o·phen (ə-sē′tə-mĭn′ə-fən, ăs′ə-) *n.* A crystalline compound used in chemical synthesis and in medicine to relieve pain and reduce fevers.

ac·et·an·i·lide (ăs′ĭt-ăn′l-īd′) *or* **ac·et·an·i·lid** (-ăn′l-ĭd) *n.* A white crystalline compound used to relieve pain and reduce fever.

ac·e·tate (ăs′ĭ-tāt′) *n.* A salt or ester of acetic acid containing the radical group CH_3COO.

acetate-CoA ligase *n.* See **acetyl-CoA synthetase**.

a·ce·ta·zo·la·mide (ăs′ĭ-tə-zō′lə-mīd′) *n.* An anticonvulsant drug used in the treatment of altitude sickness, glaucoma, and epilepsy.

a·ce·tic acid (ə-sē′tĭk) *n.* A clear, colorless organic acid with a distinctive pungent odor, the chief acid of vinegar, also used as a solvent. Also called *ethanoic acid.*

aceto– *or* **acet–** *pref.* 1. Acetic acid: *acetaldehyde.* 2. Acetyl: *acetanilide.*

ac·e·to·ac·e·tate (ăs′ĭ-tō-ăs′ĭ-tāt′, ə-sē′tō-) *n.* A salt of acetoacetic acid.

ac·e·to·a·ce·tic acid (ăs′ĭ-tō-ə-sē′tĭk, ə-sē′tō-) *n.* A ketone body that is formed in excessive amounts and excreted in the urine of individuals suffering from starvation or diabetes. Also called *diacetic acid.*

ac·e·to·a·ce·tyl-CoA (ăs′ĭ-tō-ə-sēt′l-kō′ā′, -ăs′ĭ-tl-, ə-sē′tō-) *n.* An intermediate in the oxidation of fatty acids. Also called *acetoacetyl coenzyme A.*

ac·e·to·hy·drox·a·mic acid (ăs′ĭ-tō-hī′drŏk-săm′ĭk, ə-sē′to-) *n.* An inhibitor of urease, used to treat a chronic urinary infection.

ac·e·to·me·naph·thane (ăs′ĭ-tō-mə-năf′thān′, ə-sē′tō-) *n.* A vitamin K analog used to treat and prevent hypoprothrombinemia caused by vitamin K deficiency. Also called *menadiol diacetate.*

ac·e·tone (ăs′ĭ-tōn′) *n.* 1. A colorless, volatile, extremely flammable liquid ketone widely used as an organic solvent. 2. An organic compound produced in excessive amounts in diabetic acidosis.

acetone body *n.* See **ketone body**.

ac·e·ton·e·mi·a (ăs′ĭ-tō-nē′mē-ə) *n.* The presence of acetone or ketone bodies in relatively large amounts in the blood.

ac·e·ton·u·ri·a (ăs′ĭ-tōn-yoōr′ē-ə) *n.* The excretion in the urine of excessive amounts of acetone, an indication of incomplete oxidation of large amounts of fat, and common in diabetic acidosis.

a·ce·tyl (ə-sēt′l, ăs′ĭ-tl) *n.* The acetic acid radical CH_3CO. —**ac′e·tyl′ic** (ăs′ĭ-tĭl′ĭk) *adj.*

a·cet·y·la·tion (ə-sĕt′l-ā′shən) *n.* A reaction, usually with acetic acid, that introduces an acetyl radical into an organic compound.

a·ce·tyl·cho·line (ə-sĕt′l-kō′lēn′) *n. Abbr.* **Ach** A white crystalline derivative of choline that is released at the ends of nerve fibers in the somatic and parasympathetic nervous systems and is involved in the transmission of nerve impulses in the body.

a·ce·tyl·cho·lin·es·ter·ase (ə-sĕt′l-kō′lə-nĕs′tə-rās′, -rāz′) *n.* See **cholinesterase**.

acetylcholinesterase inhibitor *n.* See **cholinesterase inhibitor**.

acetyl CoA *abbr.* acetyl coenzyme A

acetyl-CoA synthetase *n.* A ligase that catalyzes the formation of acetyl CoA from acetate and CoA. Also called *acetate-CoA ligase*.

acetyl coenzyme A *n. Abbr.* **acetyl CoA 1.** An organic compound in which an acetyl group is attached to CoA. **2.** A compound that functions as a coenzyme in many biological acetylation reactions and is formed as an intermediate in the oxidation of carbohydrates, fats, and proteins.

a·cet·y·lene (ə-sĕt′l-ēn′, -ən) *n.* A colorless, highly flammable, and explosive gas used for metal welding and cutting and as an illuminant.

a·ce·tyl·sal·i·cyl·ic acid (ə-sĕt′l-săl′ĭ-sĭl′ĭk) *n. Abbr.* **ASA** See **aspirin**.

a·ce·tyl·trans·fer·ase (ə-sĕt′l-trăns′fə-rās′, -rāz′, ăs′ĭ-tl-) *n.* An enzyme that catalyzes the transfer of acetyl groups from one compound to another. Also called *acetylase, transacetylase*.

Ach *abbr.* acetylcholine

A chain *n.* A polypeptide component of insulin containing 21 amino acids, the composition of which is species-specific.

ach·a·la·sia (ăk′ə-lā′zhə) *n.* The failure of a ring of muscle fibers, such as a sphincter, to relax.

ache (āk) *n.* A dull persistent pain. —*v.* To suffer a dull, sustained pain.

a·chei·li·a *or* **a·chi·li·a** (ə-kī′lē-ə) *n.* Congenital absence of the lips. —**a·chei′lous** *adj.*

a·chei·ri·a *or* **a·chi·ri·a** (ə-kī′rē-ə) *n.* **1.** Congenital absence of the hands. **2.** A condition sometimes occurring in hysteria in which there is a loss of the sense of possession of one or both hands.

a·chei·rop·o·dy *or* **a·chi·rop·o·dy** (ə-kī-rŏp′ə-dē) *n.* Congenital absence of the hands and the feet.

a·chieve·ment age (ə-chēv′mənt) *n.* The level of an individual's educational accomplishment as measured by standard achievement tests and expressed as the age in years of a child for whom the total score would be an average score.

achievement quotient *n.* The ratio of actual performance to expected performance or to the norm achieved by individuals of a particular age, usually on a standard achievement test.

achievement test *n.* A standardized test used to measure acquired learning.

A·chil·les bursa (ə-kĭl′ēz) *n.* The bursa between the Achilles tendon and the upper part of the posterior surface of the calcaneus.

Achilles reflex *n.* A reflex bending of the foot resulting from contraction of the calf muscles when the Achilles tendon is sharply struck. Also called *Achilles jerk, Achilles tendon reflex, ankle reflex, triceps surae reflex*.

Achilles tendon *n.* The large tendon connecting the heel bone to the calf muscle of the leg. Also called *calcanean tendon, heel tendon*.

Achilles tendon reflex *n.* See **Achilles reflex**.

a·chil·lo·bur·si·tis (ə-kĭl′ō-bər-sī′tĭs) *n.* Inflammation of a bursa beneath the Achilles tendon. Also called *retrocalcaneobursitis*.

a·chil·lo·dyn·i·a (ə-kĭl′ō-dĭn′ē-ə) *n.* Pain due to achilloburitis.

ach·il·lot·o·my (ăk′ĭl-ŏt′ə-mē) *n.* Surgical division of the Achilles tendon. Also called *achillotenotomy*.

a·chlor·hy·dri·a (ā′klôr-hī′drē-ə) *n.* Absence of hydrochloric acid from the gastric juice.

a·chlo·ro·phyl·lous (ā-klôr′ə-fĭl′əs) *adj.* Having no chlorophyll.

a·cho·li·a (ā-kō′lē-ə) *n.* Suppression or absence of secretion of bile. —**a·chol′ic** (ā-kŏl′ĭk) *adj.*

a·cho·lu·ri·a (ā′kō-lŏŏr′ē-ə) *n.* Absence of bile pigments from the urine in some forms of jaundice. —**a′cho·lu′ric** *adj.*

acholuric jaundice *n.* Jaundice in which the circulating blood has excessive amounts of unconjugated bilirubin and no bile pigments.

a·chon·dro·gen·e·sis (ā-kŏn′drō-jĕn′ĭ-sĭs, ə-kŏn′-) *n.* Dwarfism characterized by various bone aplasias and hypoplasias of the extremities and a short trunk with delayed ossification of the lower spine.

a·chon·dro·pla·sia (ā-kŏn′drō-plā′zhə, ə-kŏn′-) *or* **a·chon·dro·plas·ty** (ā-kŏn′drō-plăs′tē, ə-kŏn′-) *n.* Improper development of cartilage at the ends of the long bones, resulting in a form of congenital dwarfism. Also called *osteosclerosis congenita*. —**a·chon′dro·plas′tic** (-plăs′tĭk) *adj.*

achondroplastic dwarfism *n.* A congenital dwarfism resulting from a failure of cartilage to normally develop into bone, especially cartilage on the ends of long bones.

a·chres·tic anemia (ə-krĕs′tĭk) *n.* A macrocytic anemia in which the changes in bone marrow and circulating blood resemble those of pernicious anemia.

a·chro·ma·cyte (ā-krō′mə-sīt′, ə-krō′-) *n.* Variant of **achromocyte**.

ach·ro·ma·sia (ăk′rō-mā′zhə) *n.* **1.** Pallor associated with the hippocratic facies of extremely severe and chronic illness. **2.** See **achromia** (sense 2).

ach·ro·mat·ic (ăk′rə-măt′ĭk) *adj.* **1.** Of or relating to color perceived to have zero saturation and therefore no hue, such as neutral grays, white, or black. **2.** Refracting light without spectral color separation. **3.** Of or relating to cells or tissues difficult to stain with standard dyes.

achromatic lens *n.* A combination of lenses made of different glass, used to produce images free of chromatic aberrations.

achromatic objective *n.* An objective that is corrected for two colors chromatically and for one color spherically.

achromatic vision *n.* See **achromatopsia.**

a·chro·ma·tin (ā-krō′mə-tĭn) *n.* The part of a cell nucleus that remains less colored than the rest of the nucleus when stained or dyed. —**a·chro′ma·tin′ic** *adj.*

a·chro·ma·tism (ā-krō′mə-tĭz′əm, ə-krō′-) *n.* **1.** The quality of being achromatic. **2.** The correction of chromatic aberration by combining lenses of different refractive indexes and different dispersion.

a·chro·ma·tol·y·sis (ā-krō′mə-tŏl′ĭ-sĭs, ə-krō′-) *n., pl.* **-ses** (-sēz′) Dissolution of the achromatin of a cell or of its nucleus.

a·chro·mat·o·phil (ā′krō-măt′ə-fĭl, ăk′rō-, ā-krō′mə-tə-, ə-krō′-) *or* **a·chro·mo·phil** (ā-krō′mə-fĭl, ə-krō′-) *adj.* Not able to be colored by histological or bacteriological stains. —*n.* A cell or tissue that cannot be stained in the usual way. —**a′chro·mo·phil′ic** (-fĭl′ĭk), **a′chro·moph′i·lous** (āk′rō-mŏf′ə-ləs, ăk′rō-) *adj.*

a·chro·ma·top·si·a (ā-krō′mə-tŏp′sē-ə, ə-krō′-) *or* **a·chro·ma·top·sy** (ā-krō′mə-tŏp′sē, ə-krō′-) *n.* A severe congenital deficiency in color perception, often associated with nystagmus and reduced visual acuity. Also called *achromatic vision, monochromatism.*

a·chro·ma·to·sis (ā-krō′mə-tō′sĭs, ə-krō′-) *n., pl.* **-ses** (-sēz′) See **achromia** (sense 2).

a·chro·ma·tous (ā-krō′mə-təs, ə-krō′-) *adj.* Having no color; colorless.

a·chro·ma·tu·ri·a (ā-krō′mə-tŏŏr′ē-ə, ə-krō′-) *n.* Passage of colorless or very pale urine.

a·chro·mi·a (ā-krō′mē-ə, ə-krō′-) *n.* **1.** Congenital or acquired deficiency of natural pigmentation. **2.** Lack of capacity to accept stains in cells or tissue. Also called *achromasia, achromatosis.*

a·chro·mic (ā-krō′mĭk, ə-krō′-) *adj.* Having no color; colorless.

a·chro·mo·cyte *or* **a·chro·ma·cyte** (ā-krō′mə-sīt′, ə-krō′-) *or* **a·chro·mat·o·cyte** (ā′krō-măt′ə-sīt′, ăk′rō-, ā-krō′mə-tə-, ə-krō′-) *n.* A decolorized crescent-shaped red blood cell. Also called *ghost corpuscle, phantom corpuscle.*

a·chy·li·a (ā-kī′lē-ə, ə-kī′-) *n.* **1.** Absence of gastric juice or other digestive secretions. **2.** Absence of chyle. —**a·chy′lous** *adj.*

ac·id (ăs′ĭd) *n.* **1.** Any of a large class of sour-tasting substances whose aqueous solutions are capable of turning blue litmus indicators red, of reacting with and dissolving certain metals to form salts, and of reacting with bases or alkalis to form salts. **2.** A substance that ionizes in solution to give the positive ion of the solvent. **3.** A substance capable of yielding hydrogen ions. **4.** A proton donor. **5.** An electron acceptor. **6.** A molecule or ion that can combine with another by forming a covalent bond with two electrons of the other. **7.** A substance having a sour taste. **8.** See **LSD.** —*adj.* **1.** Of or relating to an acid. **2.** Having a high concentration of acid. **3.** Having a sour taste.

ac·id·am·i·nu·ri·a (ăs′ĭd-ăm′ə-nŏŏr′ē-ə) *n.* See **aminoaciduria.**

acid-ash diet *n.* A diet consisting largely of meat or fish, eggs, and cereals with a minimal quantity of milk, fruit,

and vegetables, that when catabolized leaves an acid residue to be excreted in the urine.

acid-base balance *n.* The state that exists when acidic and basic ions in solution neutralize each other.

acid-base indicator *n.* A substance that indicates the degree of acidity or basicity of a solution through characteristic color changes.

acid cell *n.* See **parietal cell.**

acid dye *n.* Any of a class of dyes that contain acidic groups, usually in the form of sodium or potassium salts, and are used in staining cytoplasm and various acidophilic structures of cells or tissues. Also called *acid stain.*

ac·i·de·mi·a (ăs′ĭ-dē′mē-ə) *n.* An increase in the hydrogen ion concentration of the blood.

acid-fast *adj.* Of or relating to bacteria that are not decolorized by an acidic alcohol solution after they have been stained. —**ac′id-fast′ness** *n.*

acid fuchsin *n.* An acid dye used as an indicator and as a stain for cytoplasm and collagen.

acidified serum test *n.* A test for paroxysmal nocturnal hemoglobinuria, in which red blood cells are lysed in acidified fresh serum. Also called *Ham's test.*

a·cid·i·fy (ə-sĭd′ə-fī′) *v.* To make or become acid.

acid indigestion *n.* **1.** Indigestion that results from an excess of hydrochloric acid in the stomach. **2.** Heartburn.

a·cid·i·ty (ə-sĭd′ĭ-tē) *n.* The state, quality, or degree of being acid.

acid maltase *n.* An enzyme found in lysosomes that catalyzes the hydrolysis of maltose and other oligosaccharides to yield glucose; alpha-1,4-glucosidase.

a·cid·o·phil (ə-sĭd′ə-fĭl, ăs′ĭ-də-) *or* **a·cid·o·phile** (-fĭl′) *n.* **1.** A cell that stains readily with acid dyes. **2.** A microorganism that grows well in an acid medium. —**a·cid′o·phil′ic** (-fĭl′ĭk) *adj.*

acidophil adenoma *n.* See **growth hormone-producing adenoma.**

ac·i·doph·i·lus milk (ăs′ĭ-dŏf′ə-ləs) *n.* Milk fermented by bacterial cultures that thrive in dilute acid, often used to alter the bacterial flora of the gastrointestinal tract in the treatment of certain digestive disorders.

ac·i·do·sis (ăs′ĭ-dō′sĭs) *n., pl.* **-ses** (-sēz′) An abnormal increase in the acidity of body fluids, caused either by accumulation of acids or by depletion of bicarbonates. —**ac′i·dot′ic** (-dŏt′ĭk) *adj.*

acid perfusion test *n.* See **Bernstein test.**

acid phosphatase *n.* A phosphatase with optimum functioning at pH 5.4 and present in the prostate gland.

acid-phosphatase test for semen *n.* A screening test for detecting the presence of semen by determining acid phosphatase content.

acid reflux *n.* See **heartburn.**

acid-reflux test *n.* A test to detect esophageal reflux by monitoring esophageal pH, performed either basally or after acid is instilled into the stomach.

acid stain *n.* See **acid dye.**

acid sulfate *n.* See **bisulfate.**

acid tide *n.* A temporary increase in the acidity of the urine, occurring during fasting.

a·cid·u·lous (ə-sĭj′ə-ləs) *adj.* Slightly acid or sour.

ac·i·du·ri·a (ăs′ĭ-dŏŏr′ē-ə) *n.* **1.** Excretion of a specific acid in an abnormal amount. **2.** Excretion of an abnormal amount of any specified acid.

ac·i·du·ric (ăs′ĭ-dŏŏr′ĭk) *adj.* Of or relating to bacteria that tolerate an acid environment.

ac·i·nar (ăs′ĭ-nər, -när′) *adj.* Relating to an acinus.

acinar cell *n.* A secreting cell lining an acinus, especially one of the cells of the pancreas that furnish pancreatic juice. Also called *acinous cell.*

acinar cell tumor *n.* A solid, cystic tumor of the pancreas, occurring in young women.

acinic cell adenocarcinoma *n.* An adenocarcinoma arising from the secreting cells of a racemose gland, particularly the salivary glands.

a·cin·i·form (ə-sĭn′ə-fôrm′) *adj.* Acinar.

ac·i·ni·tis (ăs′ə-nī′tĭs) *n.* Inflammation of an acinus.

ac·i·no·tu·bu·lar gland (ăs′ə-nō-tŏŏ′byə-lər) *n.* See **tubuloacinar gland.**

acinous cell *n.* See **acinar cell.**

acinous gland *n.* A gland in which the secretory unit has a grapelike shape and a very small lumen.

ac·i·nus (ăs′ə-nəs) *n.,* pl. **-ni** (-nī′) Any of several minute grape-shaped secretory portions of an acinous gland. —**a·cin′ic** (ə-sĭn′ĭk) **ac′i·nose′** (ăs′ə-nōs′), **ac′-i·nous** (-nəs) *adj.*

ACL *abbr.* anterior cruciate ligament

ac·la·sis (ăk′lə-sĭs) *n.,* pl. **-ses** (-sēz′) Pathological continuity between normal and abnormal tissue.

a·clas·tic (ə-klăs′tĭk) *adj.* **1.** Not refracting light rays; nonrefractive. **2.** Relating to or exhibiting aclasis.

a·cleis·to·car·di·a (ə-klī′stō-kär′dē-ə) *n.* An opening in the oval foramen of the heart.

ACLS *abbr.* advanced cardiac life support

ac·mes·the·sia (ăk′mĕs-thē′zhə) *n.* **1.** Sensitivity to pinprick. **2.** A sensation of a sharp point on the skin.

ac·ne (ăk′nē) *n.* An inflammatory disease of the sebaceous glands and hair follicles of the skin that is marked by the eruption of pimples or pustules, especially on the face. —**ac′ned** *adj.*

acne con·glo·ba·ta (kŏn′glō-bā′tə) *n.* Severe cystic acne characterized by cystic lesions, abscesses, communicating sinuses, and thickened, nodular scars.

acne cos·met·i·ca (kŏz-mĕt′ĭ-kə) *n.* Mild noninflammatory acne lesions from repeated application of cosmetics.

acne er·y·the·ma·to·sa (ĕr′ə-thē′mə-tō′sə, -thĕm′ə-) *n.* See **rosacea.**

ac·ne·form (ăk′nē-fôrm′) *or* **ac·ne·i·form** (ăk-nē′ə-) *adj.* Resembling acne.

ac·ne·gen·ic (ăk′nĭ-jĕn′ĭk) *n.* Causing or exacerbating lesions of acne.

acne in·du·ra·ta (ĭn′də-rā′tə) *n.* Deeply seated acne with large papules and pustules that can cause severe scarring.

acne keloid *n.* A chronic eruption of fibrous papules that develop at the site of follicular lesions, usually on the back of the neck at the hairline, seen most commonly in Black men. Also called *dermatitis papillaris capillitii, folliculitis keloidalis.*

acne ker·a·to·sa (kĕr′ə-tō′sə) *n.* An inflammatory eruption of papules consisting of horny plugs projecting from the hair follicles.

acne med·i·ca·men·to·sa (mĕd′ĭ-kə-mən-tō′sə) *n.* Acne caused or exacerbated by several types of drugs, such as antiepileptics, halogens, and steroids.

acne pap·u·lo·sa (păp′yə-lō′sə) *n.* Acne vulgaris in which papular lesions predominate.

acne punc·ta·ta (pŭngk-tā′tə) *n.* A condition resembling chloracne in that central blackheads are present in all the lesions.

acne pus·tu·lo·sa (pŭs′tyə-lō′sə) *n.* Acne vulgaris in which pustular lesions predominate.

acne rosacea *n.* See **rosacea.**

acne var·i·o·li·for·mis (văr′ē-ō′lə-fôr′mĭs) *n.* A pyogenic infection of the hair follicles occurring chiefly on the forehead and temples.

acne vul·gar·is (vŭl-gâr′ĭs) *n.* An inflammatory eruption affecting the face, upper back, and chest, consisting of blackheads, cysts, papules, and pustules, and occurring primarily during puberty and adolescence.

ac·o·nite (ăk′ə-nīt′) *n.* The dried leaves and roots of various herbs of the genus *Aconitum,* especially *Aconitum napellus,* containing aconitine. It is used externally as an analgesic and was formerly used internally as a sedative. Also called *monkshood.*

a·con·i·tine (ə-kŏn′ĭ-tēn′, -tĭn) *n.* A poisonous alkaloid found in aconite.

ac·o·re·a (ăk′ə-rē′ə) *n.* The congenital absence of the pupil.

A·cos·ta's disease (ə-kŏs′təz) *n.* See **altitude sickness.**

a·cous·tic (ə-kŏŏ′stĭk) *or* **a·cous·ti·cal** (-stĭ-kəl) *adj.* Of or relating to sound, the sense of hearing, or the perception of sound.

acoustic aphasia *n.* See **auditory aphasia.**

acoustic maculae *pl.n.* The macula sacculi and macula utriculi.

acoustic meatus *n.* **1.** The passage leading inward through the tympanic portion of the temporal bone, from the auricle to the tympanic membrane; external acoustic meatus. **2.** A canal running through the petrous portion of the temporal bone, giving passage to the facial and vestibulocochlear nerves and to the labyrinthine artery and veins; internal acoustic meatus.

acoustic nerve *n.* See **vestibulocochlear nerve.**

acoustic neuroma *n.* A nonmalignant but life-threatening tumor of the vestibular nerve, originating from Schwann cells, that can cause tinnitus, hearing loss, and disturbance of balance.

acoustic radiation *n.* The radiation of fibers that pass from the medial geniculate body to the transverse temporal gyri of the cerebral cortex and form part of the sublentiform part of the internal capsule.

a·cous·tics (ə-kŏŏ′stĭks) *n.* The scientific study of sound, especially of its generation, transmission, and reception.

acoustic stria *n.* See **medullary stria of fourth ventricle.**

acoustic trauma deafness *n.* The impairment or loss of hearing caused by injury to the inner ear after exposure to extremely loud or prolonged sounds.

ACP *abbr.* American College of Physicians

ac·quired (ə-kwīrd′) *adj.* **1.** Of or relating to a disease, condition, or characteristic that is not congenital but develops after birth. **2.** Developed in response to an antigen, as resistance to a disease by vaccination or previous infection.

acquired antibody *n.* An antibody produced by an immune response, in contrast to one occurring naturally in an individual.

acquired character *n.* A nonhereditary change of function or structure in a plant or animal made in response to the environment.

acquired drive *n.* See **secondary drive.**

acquired epileptic aphasia *n.* See **Landau-Kleffner syndrome.**

acquired Fanconi's syndrome *n.* A complex of defects in the functioning of renal tubules associated with multiple myeloma or trauma.

acquired hyperlipoproteinemia *n.* Hyperlipoproteinemia that develops as a consequence of some primary disease, such as thyroid deficiency. Also called *nonfamilial hyperlipoproteinemia.*

acquired immune deficiency syndrome *n.* AIDS.

acquired immunity *n.* Immunity obtained either from the development of antibodies in response to exposure to an antigen, as from vaccination or an attack of an infectious disease, or from the transmission of antibodies, as from mother to fetus through the placenta or the injection of antiserum.

acquired immunodeficiency syndrome *n.* AIDS.

acquired nevus *n.* A melanocytic nevus not visible at birth but appearing in childhood or adult life.

ac·qui·si·tion (ăk′wĭ-zĭsh′ən) *n.* The empirical demonstration in psychology of an increase in the strength of the conditioned response in successive trials in which the conditioned and unconditioned stimuli are paired.

acr– *pref.* Variant of **acro–.**

ac·ral (ăk′rəl) *adj.* Of, relating to, or affecting peripheral parts, such as limbs, fingers, or ears.

a·cra·ni·a (ā-krā′nē-ə, ə-krā′-) *n.* Congenital absence of all or a part of the skull. —**a·cra′ni·al** *adj.*

Ac·rel's ganglion (ăk′rəlz) *n.* **1.** A pseudoganglion on the posterior interosseous nerve on the dorsal aspect of the wrist joint. **2.** A cyst on a tendon of an extensor muscle at the level of the wrist.

Ac·re·mo·ni·um (ăk′rə-mō′nē-əm) *n.* A genus of fungi that cause certain forms of mycetoma.

ac·rid (ăk′rĭd) *adj.* Unpleasantly sharp, pungent, or bitter to the taste or smell. —**a·crid′i·ty** (ə-krĭd′ĭ-tē), **ac′rid·ness** *n.*

ac·ri·dine (ăk′rĭ-dēn′) *n.* A coal tar derivative that has an irritating odor and is used in the manufacture of dyes and synthetics.

acridine orange *n.* A basic fluorescent dye used as a metachromatic stain for nucleic acids and in screening cervical smears for abnormal cells.

acridine yellow *n.* A faintly yellow solution with strong bluish-violet fluorescence used as a topical antiseptic and as a fluorescent stain in histology.

ac·ri·fla·vine (ăk′rə-flā′vēn′, -vĭn) *n.* A brown or orange powder derived from acridine and used as a topical antiseptic.

a·crit·i·cal (ā-krĭt′ĭ-kəl, ə-krĭt′-) *adj.* **1.** Not critical; not marked by crisis. **2.** Indeterminate, especially concerning prognosis.

acro– *or* **acr–** *pref.* **1.** Top; summit; height: *acrophobia.* **2.** Tip; beginning: *acrosome.* **3.** Extremity of the body: *acroparalysis.*

ac·ro·ag·no·sis (ăk′rō-ăg-nō′sĭs) *n.* Absence of sensory perception of the limbs.

ac·ro·an·es·the·sia (ăk′rō-ăn′ĭs-thē′zhə) *n.* Loss of sensation in one or more of the extremities.

ac·ro·a·tax·i·a (ăk′rō-ə-tăk′sē-ə) *n.* Ataxia affecting the hands, fingers, feet, and toes.

ac·ro·blast (ăk′rə-blăst′) *n.* A component of the developing spermatid, composed of numerous Golgi elements and containing the proacrosomal granules.

ac·ro·brach·y·ceph·a·ly (ăk′rə-brăk′ĭ-sĕf′ə-lē) *n.* A type of craniosynostosis in which there is premature closure of the coronal suture, resulting in an abnormally short anteroposterior diameter of the skull.

ac·ro·cen·tric (ăk′rō-sĕn′trĭk) *adj.* Having the centromere located near one end of the chromosome so that one chromosomal arm is long and the other is short. —**ac′ro·cen′tric** *n.*

acrocentric chromosome *n.* A chromosome with the centromere located very close to one end so that the shorter arm is very small.

ac·ro·ceph·a·lo·pol·y·syn·dac·ty·ly (ăk′rə-sĕf′ə-lō-pŏl′ē-sĭn-dăk′tə-lē) *n.* A congenital syndrome characterized by oxycephaly and brachysyndactyly of the hands, polydactyly of the feet, and mental retardation. Also called *Carpenter's syndrome.*

ac·ro·ceph·a·lo·syn·dac·ty·ly (ăk′rə-sĕf′ə-lō-sĭn-dăk′tə-lē) *or* **ac·ro·ceph·a·lo·syn·dac·tyl·i·a** (-sĭn′-dăk-tĭl′ē-ə) *or* **ac·ro·ceph·a·lo·syn·dac·tyl·ism** (-sĭn-dăk′tə-lĭz′əm) *n.* A congenital syndrome characterized by a peaked head due to premature closure of the skull sutures and associated with fusion or webbing of the fingers or toes. Also called *acrodysplasia.*

ac·ro·ceph·a·ly (ăk′rə-sĕf′ə-lē) *or* **ac·ro·ce·pha·li·a** (ăk′rō-sə-fā′lē-ə) *n.* See **oxycephaly.** —**ac′ro·ce·phal′-ic** (-sə-făl′ĭk) *adj.*

ac·ro·chor·don (ăk′rə-kôr′dŏn′) *n.* See **skin tag.**

ac·ro·cy·a·no·sis (ăk′rō-sī′ə-nō′sĭs) *n.* A circulatory disorder in which the hands, and less commonly the feet, are persistently cold, blue, and sweaty. —**ac′ro·cy′a·not′ic** (-nŏt′ĭk) *adj.*

ac·ro·der·ma·ti·tis (ăk′rō-dûr′mə-tī′tĭs) *n.* Inflammation of the skin of the extremities.

acrodermatitis chron·i·ca a·troph·i·cans (krŏn′ĭ-kə ə-trŏf′ĭ-kănz′) *n.* A progressive dermatitis appearing first on the feet, hands, elbows, or knees, composed of hardened erythematous plaques that become atrophic, giving a tissue-paper appearance to the affected areas.

acrodermatitis con·tin·u·a (kən-tĭn′yoō-ə) *n.* A pustular eruption of the fingers and toes, variously attributed to dyshidrosis, pustular psoriasis, and bacterial infection. Also called *acrodermatitis perstans, dermatitis repens, Hallopeau's disease, pustulosis palmaris et plantaris.*

acrodermatitis en·ter·o·path·i·ca (ĕn′tə-rō-păth′ĭ-kə) *n.* A genetic defect in the malabsorption of zinc, beginning as a skin eruption on an extremity or around a body orifice, followed by hair loss and diarrhea or other gastrointestinal disturbances.

acrodermatitis per·stans (pûr′stănz′) *n.* See **acrodermatitis continua.**

ac·ro·der·ma·to·sis (ăk′rō-dûr′mə-tō′sĭs) *n.* Any of several cutaneous diseases affecting the distal portions of the extremities.

ac·ro·dol·i·cho·me·li·a (ăk′rō-dŏl′ĭ-kō-mē′lē-ə, -mēl′-yə) *n.* Abnormal growth of the hands and feet.

ac·ro·dont (ăk′rə-dŏnt′) *adj.* Having teeth attached to the edge of the jawbone without sockets.

ac·ro·dyn·ia (ăk′rō-dĭn′ē-ə) *n.* **1.** A syndrome in children and infants caused by mercury poisoning, characterized by erythema of the extremities, chest, and nose, polyneuritis, and gastrointestinal disorders. Also called *dermatopolyneuritis, erythredema, pink disease, Swift's disease.* **2.** A syndrome associated with ingestion of mercury by adults, characterized by photophobia, sweating, and tachycardia.

ac·ro·dys·os·to·sis (ăk′rō-dĭs′ŏs-tō′sĭs) *n.* A disorder marked by abnormally small hands and feet, facial changes, and mental retardation.

ac·ro·dys·pla·sia (ăk′rō-dĭs-plā′zhə) *n.* See **acrocephalosyndactyly.**

ac·ro·es·the·sia (ăk′rō-ĕs-thē′zhə) *n.* **1.** Extreme hyperesthesia. **2.** Hyperesthesia of one or more of the extremities.

ac·ro·ger·i·a (ăk′rō-jĕr′ē-ə, -gîr′-) *n.* Congenital reduction or loss of subcutaneous fat and collagen of the hands and feet.

ac·ro·ker·a·to·e·las·toi·do·sis (ăk′rō-kĕr′ə-tō-ĭ-lăs′-toi-dō′sĭs) *n.* An inherited disorder marked by hyperkeratotic yellow nodules on the palms and soles with disorganization of the dermal elastic fibers.

ac·ro·ker·a·to·sis (ăk′rō-kĕr′ə-tō′sĭs) *n.* Overgrowth of the horny layer of the skin, characterized usually by nodular configurations of the backs of the fingers and toes.

acrokeratosis ver·ru·ci·for·mis (və-rōō′sə-fôr′mĭs) *n.* A dermatitis of genetic origin, characterized by warty outgrowths of the hands and feet.

ac·ro·meg·a·ly (ăk′rō-mĕg′ə-lē) *n.* A disorder marked by progressive enlargement of the head, face, hands, feet, and chest due to excessive secretion of growth hormone by the anterior lobe of the pituitary gland. Also called *Marie's disease.*

ac·ro·me·lal·gia (ăk′rō-mə-lăl′jə) *n.* A form of erythromelalgia characterized by redness, pain, and swelling of the fingers and toes, headache, and vomiting.

ac·ro·me·li·a (ăk′rō-mē′lē-ə, -mēl′yə) *n.* A form of dwarfism in which shortening is most evident in the most distal segment of the limbs.

ac·ro·mel·ic (ăk′rō-mĕl′ĭk) *adj.* Of or affecting the terminal part of a limb.

ac·ro·met·a·gen·e·sis (ăk′rō-mĕt′ə-jĕn′ĭ-sĭs) *n.* Abnormal development of the extremities resulting in deformity.

a·cro·mi·al angle (ə-krō′mē-əl) *n.* The prominent bony point at the junction of the lateral border of the acromion and the spine of the shoulder blade.

acromial process *n.* See **acromion.**

a·cro·mi·o·cla·vic·u·lar (ə-krō′mē-ō-klə-vĭk′yə-lər) *adj.* **1.** Of or relating to the acromion and the clavicle.

2. Of or relating to the articulation between the clavicle and the scapula and its ligaments.

a·cro·mi·o·cor·a·coid (ə-krō′mē-ō-kôr′ə-koid′) *adj.* Relating to the acromion and the coracoid process.

a·cro·mi·o·hu·mer·al (ə-krō′mē-ō-hyōō′mər-əl) *adj.* Of or relating to the acromion and the humerus.

a·cro·mi·on (ə-krō′mē-ŏn′, -ən) *n.* The outer end of the scapula, extending over the shoulder joint and forming the highest point of the shoulder, to which the collarbone is attached. Also called *acromial process.* —**a·cro′mi·al** *adj.*

a·cro·mi·o·scap·u·lar (ə-krō′mē-ō-skăp′yə-lər) *adj.* Of or relating to both the acromion and the scapula.

a·cro·mi·o·tho·rac·ic (ə-krō′mē-ō-thə-răs′ĭk) *adj.* Of or relating to the acromion and the chest.

acromiothoracic artery *n.* See **thoracoacromial artery.**

a·crom·pha·lus (ə-krŏm′fə-ləs) *n.* Abnormal projection of the umbilicus.

ac·ro·my·o·to·ni·a (ăk′rō-mī′ō-tō′nē-ə) *or* **ac·ro·my·ot·o·nus** (-mī-ŏt′n-əs) *n.* Myotonia affecting only the extremities, resulting in spasmodic deformity of the hand or foot.

ac·ro·neu·ro·sis (ăk′rō-nŏŏ-rō′sĭs) *n.* A vasomotor neuropathy affecting the extremities.

ac·ro·os·te·ol·y·sis (ăk′rō-ŏs′tē-ŏl′ĭ-sĭs) *n.* A disorder that is usually congenital but may also be acquired by exposure to vinyl chloride, marked by ulcers on the palms of the hands and the soles of the feet.

ac·ro·pach·y·der·ma (ăk′rō-păk′ĭ-dûr′mə) *n.* Thickening of the skin of the face, scalp, and extremities with clubbing of the fingers and deformities in the limb bones.

ac·ro·par·es·the·sia (ăk′rō-păr′ĭs-thē′zhə) *n.* Numbness, tingling, or other abnormal sensations in one or more of the extremities.

a·crop·a·thy (ə-krŏp′ə-thē) *n.* Hereditary clubbing of the fingers and toes without an associated progressive disease.

ac·ro·pho·bi·a (ăk′rə-fō′bē-ə) *n.* An abnormal fear of heights.

ac·ro·pus·tu·lo·sis (ăk′rō-pŭs′tyə-lō′sĭs) *n.* Recurring pustular eruptions on the hands and feet.

ac·ro·scle·ro·sis (ăk′rō-sklə-rō′sĭs) *n.* A form of progressive systemic sclerosis occurring with Raynaud's phenomenon, marked by stiffness of the skin of the fingers, atrophy of the soft tissue of the hands and feet, and osteoporosis of the distal phalanges. Also called *acroscleroderma, sclerodactyly.*

ac·ro·sin (ăk′rə-sĭn) *n.* A proteinase that is contained in spermatozoa.

acrosomal cap *n.* A caplike structure at the anterior end of a spermatozoon that produces enzymes aiding in egg penetration. Also called *acrosome, head cap.*

acrosomal granule *n.* A large granule that is formed by the coalescing of proacrosomal granules within the acrosomal vesicle and adheres to the nuclear envelope of a developing spermatozoon.

acrosomal vesicle *n.* A vesicle derived from the Golgi apparatus during spermiogenesis; its membrane adheres to the nuclear envelope of the sperm and, together with the acrosomal granule within the vesicle, spreads in a thin layer over the pole of the nucleus to form the acrosomal cap.

ac·ro·some (ăk′rə-sōm′) *n.* See **acrosomal cap. —ac′ro·so′mal** (-sō′məl) *adj.*

ac·ro·tism (ăk′rə-tĭz′əm) *n.* Absent or imperceptible pulse. **—a·crot′ic** (ə-krŏt′ĭk) *adj.*

ac·ro·tro·pho·neu·ro·sis (ăk′rō-trō′fō-nŏo-rō′sĭs, -trŏf′ō-) *n.* A trophoneurosis of one or more of the extremities.

ACTH (ā′sē′tē-āch′) *n.* Adrenocorticotropic hormone; a hormone that is produced by the anterior lobe of the pituitary gland and that stimulates the secretion of cortisone, aldosterone, and other hormones by the adrenal cortex. Also called *adrenocorticotropin, adrenotropin, corticotropin.*

Ac·thar (ăk′thär′) A trademark for the drug preparation of ACTH.

ACTH-producing adenoma *n.* A pituitary tumor causing Cushing's syndrome, composed of basophilic, densely granulated corticotrophs. Also called *basophil adenoma.*

ac·tin (ăk′tĭn) *n.* One of the protein components found in muscle, existing as F-actin or G-actin, into which actomyosin can be split and which acts with myosin in muscle contraction.

actin filament *n.* One of the contractile elements in skeletal, cardiac, and smooth muscle fibers.

ac·tin·ic (ăk-tĭn′ĭk) *adj.* Of or relating to the chemically active rays of the electromagnetic spectrum.

actinic cheilitis *n.* See **solar cheilitis.**

actinic dermatitis *n.* Dermatitis caused by exposure to actinic radiation, such as sunlight or x-rays.

actinic elastosis *n.* See **colloid acne.**

actinic granuloma *n.* An annular eruption on sun-exposed skin that microscopically shows phagocytosis of dermal elastic fibers by giant cells and histiocytes.

actinic keratosis *n.* A warty lesion, often premalignant, occurring on the sun-exposed skin of the face or hands, especially of light-skinned persons. Also called *senile keratosis.*

ac·ti·nide (ăk′tə-nīd′) *n.* Any of a series of chemically similar radioactive elements with atomic numbers ranging from 89 (actinium) through 103 (lawrencium).

ac·tin·i·um (ăk-tĭn′ē-əm) *n. Symbol* **Ac** A radioactive element found in uranium ores. Its longest lived isotope is Ac 227 with a half-life of 21.6 years. Atomic number 89.

actino– *or* **actin–** *pref.* Actinic radiation: *actinotherapy.*

ac·ti·no·der·ma·ti·tis (ăk′tə-nō-dûr′mə-tī′tĭs) *n.* 1. Inflammation of the skin produced by exposure to sunlight. 2. Adverse reaction of skin to radiation therapy.

Ac·ti·no·mad·u·ra (ăk′tə-nō-măj′ə-rə) *n.* A genus of aerobic, gram-positive, non-acid-fast fungi forming filaments that fragment into spores.

Ac·ti·no·my·ces (ăk′tə-nō-mī′sēz) *n.* A genus of nonmotile, non-spore-producing, anaerobic to facultatively anaerobic bacteria pathogenic to humans.

Actinomyces bo·vis (bō′vĭs) *n.* A species of *Actinomyces* causing actinomycosis in cattle.

Actinomyces is·ra·e·li·i (ĭz′rā-ē′lē-ī) *n.* A species of *Actinomyces* causing human actinomycosis.

Ac·ti·no·my·ce·ta·ce·ae (ăk′tə-nō-mī′sĭ-tā′sē-ē′) *n.* A family of non-spore-producing, nonmotile, mostly facultatively anaerobic bacteria containing gram-positive, non-acid-fast, predominantly diphtheroid cells that tend to form branched filaments.

Ac·ti·no·my·ce·ta·les (ăk′tə-nō-mī′sĭ-tā′lēz) *n.* An order of bacteria consisting of moldlike, rod-shaped, clubbed or filamentous forms that tend to form branching filaments.

ac·ti·no·my·cete (ăk′tə-nō-mī′sēt′, -mĭ-sēt′) *n.* 1. Any of various filamentous or rod-shaped, often pathogenic microorganisms of the genus *Actinomyces.* 2. A member of the family Actinomycetaceae. 3. A member of the order Actinomycetales. **—ac′ti·no·my·ce′tous** *adj.*

ac·ti·no·my·cin (ăk′tə-nō-mī′sĭn) *n.* Any of a large group of red, often toxic, polypeptide antibiotics isolated from soil bacteria of several species of *Streptomyces* (originally *Actinomyces*) that are active against gram-positive bacteria and fungi.

ac·ti·no·my·co·ma (ăk′tə-nō-mī-kō′mə) *n.* A swelling caused by an infection with an actinomycete.

ac·ti·no·my·co·sis (ăk′tə-nō-mī-kō′sĭs) *n.* An inflammatory disease of cattle, hogs, and sometimes humans, caused by microorganisms of the genus *Actinomyces* and characterized by lumpy tumors of the mouth, neck, chest, and abdomen. **—ac′ti·no·my·cot′ic** (-kŏt′ĭk) *adj.*

ac·ti·no·ther·a·py (ăk′tə-nō-thĕr′ə-pē) *n.* The therapeutic use of ultraviolet light.

ac·tion (ăk′shən) *n.* 1. The state or process of acting or doing. 2. A deed. 3. A change that occurs in the body or in a bodily organ as a result of its functioning. 4. Exertion of force or power.

action current *n.* An electrical current generated in a cell such as a neuron or muscle cell during the action potential.

action potential *n.* The change in membrane potential occurring in nerve, muscle, or other excitable tissue when excitation occurs.

ac·ti·vat·ed charcoal (ăk′tə-vā′tĭd) *n.* Finely powdered charcoal treated to increase its adsorptive power; it is used in treating diarrhea, as an antidote, and in purification processes in industry.

activated resin *n.* See **autopolymer resin.**

ac·ti·va·tor (ăk′tə-vā′tər) *n.* 1. An agent that renders another substance active or accelerates a process or reaction. 2. The fragment produced by chemical cleavage of a proactivator that induces the enzymatic activity of another substance.

ac·tive anaphylaxis (ăk′tĭv) *n.* The anaphylactic response produced in an individual following inoculation with an antigen to which the person is sensitized.

active chronic hepatitis *n.* Hepatitis with chronic portal inflammation that extends into the liver parenchyma. Also called *posthepatitic cirrhosis.*

active congestion *n.* Congestion caused by an increased flow of arterial blood to a part of the body.

active hyperemia *n.* Hyperemia due to increased flow of arterial blood in dilated capillaries. Also called *arterial hyperemia, fluxionary hyperemia.*

active immunity *n.* Immunity resulting from the development of antibodies in response to the presence of an antigen, as from vaccination or exposure to an infectious disease.

active methyl *n.* A methyl group, bound to a quaternary ammonium ion or a tertiary sulfonium ion, that can take part in transmethylation reactions.

active principle *n.* A constituent of a drug, usually an alkaloid or glycoside, on which the characteristic therapeutic action of the substance largely depends.

active repressor *n.* A repressor that binds directly with an operator gene to block it and its structural genes from synthesizing enzymes; it is a homeostatic mechanism for the regulation of inducible enzyme systems.

active site *n.* The part of an enzyme molecule at which catalysis of the substrate occurs.

active splint *n.* See **dynamic splint.**

active transport *n.* The passage of ions or molecules across a cell membrane against an electrochemical or concentration gradient, or against the normal direction of diffusion.

ac·ti·vin (ăk′tə-vĭn, ăk-tĭv′ĭn) *n.* A polypeptide growth factor that is synthesized in the pituitary gland and the gonads and stimulates the secretion of follicle-stimulating hormone.

ac·tiv·i·ty (ăk-tĭv′ĭ-tē) *n.* **1.** A physiological process. **2.** The presence of neurogenic electrical energy in electroencephalography. **3.** An ideal concentration for which the law of mass action will apply perfectly. **4.** The intensity of a radioactive source. **5.** The ability to take part in a chemical reaction.

ac·to·my·o·sin (ăk′tə-mī′ə-sĭn) *n.* A protein complex that is the essential contractile substance of muscle, composed of the globulin myosin and actin.

ac·tu·al cautery (ăk′chōō-əl) *n.* An agent or process, such as electrocautery or a hot iron, that cauterizes tissue using heat and not a chemical means.

a·cu·i·ty (ə-kyōō′ĭ-tē) *n.* Sharpness, clearness, and distinctness of perception or vision.

a·cu·le·ate (ə-kyōō′lē-ĭt, -āt′) *adj.* Covered with sharp spines; pointed.

a·cu·mi·nate (ə-kyōō′mə-nĭt, -nāt′) *adj.* Tapering to a point; pointed.

ac·u·pres·sure (ăk′yə-prĕsh′ər) *n.* See **shiatsu.**

ac·u·punc·ture (ăk′yə-pŭngk′chər) *n.* A procedure used in or adapted from Chinese medical practice in which specific body areas are pierced with fine needles for therapeutic purposes or to relieve pain or produce regional anesthesia.

a·cute (ə-kyōōt′) *adj.* **1.** Pointed at the end; sharp. **2.** Of or relating to a disease or a condition with a rapid onset and a short, severe course. **3.** Of or relating to a patient afflicted with such a disease.

acute abdomen *n.* A serious condition within the abdomen characterized by sudden onset, pain, tenderness, and muscular rigidity, and usually requiring emergency surgery. Also called *surgical abdomen.*

acute adrenocortical insufficiency *n.* A severe phase or attack of a chronic adrenocortical disorder such as Addison's disease, characterized by insufficient amounts of the adrenocortical hormones and resulting in nausea, vomiting, low blood pressure, and life-threatening imbalances in electrolytes. Also called *addisonian crisis, adrenal crisis.*

acute African sleeping sickness *n.* See **Rhodesian trypanosomiasis.**

acute alcoholism *n.* See **alcoholism** (sense 3).

acute anterior poliomyelitis *n.* An acute infectious inflammation of the anterior cornua of the spinal cord caused by the poliomyelitis virus and marked by fever, pains, and gastroenteric disturbances, flaccid paralysis, and atrophy of muscular groups. Also called *Heine-Medin disease.*

acute ascending paralysis *n.* Paralysis having a rapid course, beginning in the legs and progressively involving the trunk, arms, and neck. Also called *Landry's paralysis.*

acute brachial radiculitis *n.* See **brachial plexus neuropathy.**

acute brain disorder *n.* An organic brain syndrome that is caused by temporary reversible impairment of brain functioning and is characterized by mood changes that range from mild disorientation to delirium and can include more serious personality and behavior disturbances. Also called *acute neuropsychologic disorder.*

acute bulbar poliomyelitis *n.* A poliomyelitis virus infection affecting nerve cells in the medulla oblongata and causing paralysis of certain motor nerves.

acute care *n.* Short-term medical treatment, usually in a hospital, for patients having an acute illness or injury or recovering from surgery.

acute compression triad *n.* The rising venous pressure, falling arterial pressure, and decreased heart sounds of pericardial tamponade. Also called *Beck's triad.*

acute contagious conjunctivitis *n.* An acute, contagious form of conjunctivitis, caused by the bacterium *Hemophilus aegyptius* and characterized by inflammation of the eyelids and eyeballs and a mucopurulent discharge. Also called *pinkeye.*

acute coronary syndrome *n.* A sudden, severe coronary event that mimics a heart attack, such as unstable angina.

acute disseminated encephalomyelitis *n.* A diffuse inflammation of the brain and spinal cord usually caused by a perivascular hypersensitivity response.

acute epidemic leukoencephalitis *n.* A usually fatal form of leukoencephalitis that is characterized by acute onset of fever, followed by convulsions, delirium, and coma, and is associated with localized hemorrhaging in the central nervous system. Also called *Strümpell's disease.*

acute hemorrhagic conjunctivitis *n.* An acute, endemic form of conjunctivitis usually caused by an enterovirus and characterized by eyelid swelling, tearing, and conjunctival hemorrhages.

acute hemorrhagic pancreatitis *n.* Acute inflammation of the pancreas accompanied by the formation of necrotic areas on the surface of the pancreas and in the omentum and, frequently, also accompanied by hemorrhages into the substance of the gland.

acute idiopathic polyneuritis *n.* A neurologic syndrome, usually following certain virus infections, marked by paresthesia of the limbs and by muscular weakness or a flaccid paralysis. Also called *Guillain-Barré syndrome, infectious polyneuritis, Landry-*

Guillain-Barré syndrome, Landry syndrome, polyradiculoneuropathy, radiculoganglionitis.

acute infectious nonbacterial gastroenteritis *n.* See **epidemic nonbacterial gastroenteritis.**

acute inflammation *n.* Inflammation having a rapid onset and coming to a crisis relatively quickly, with a clear and distinct termination.

acute intermittent porphyria *n.* See **intermittent acute porphyria.**

acute isolated myocarditis *n.* An acute interstitial carditis of unknown etiology and that does not affect the endocardium and pericardium.

acute lymphoblastic leukemia *n. Abbr.* **ALL** Lymphoblastic leukemia occurring mainly in older adults, characterized by rapid onset and progression of symptoms. Also called *acute lymphocytic leukemia.*

acute lymphocytic leukemia *n.* See **acute lymphoblastic leukemia.**

acute malaria *n.* Any of various forms of malaria that may be intermittent or remittent, consisting of a chill accompanied by fever with its attendant general symptoms and terminating in a sweating stage.

acute miliary tuberculosis *n.* See **acute tuberculosis.**

acute myelogenous leukemia *n. Abbr.* **AML** Myelogenous leukemia characterized by rapid abnormal increase in the number of myeloblasts and progression of symptoms. Also called *acute myelocytic leukemia, acute myeloid leukemia, acute nonlymphocytic leukemia.*

acute necrotizing encephalitis *n.* An acute form of encephalitis, caused by herpes simplex virus and affecting the temporal lobes and the limbic system.

acute necrotizing ulcerative gingivitis *n. Abbr.* **ANUG** See **trench mouth.**

acute neuropsychologic disorder *n.* See **acute brain disorder.**

acute non·lym·pho·cyt·ic leukemia (nŏn-lĭm′fə-sĭt′-ĭk) *n.* See **acute myelogenous leukemia.**

acute phase response *n.* A group of physiologic changes that occur shortly after the onset of an infection or other inflammatory process and include an increase in the blood level of various proteins, especially C-reactive protein, fever, and other metabolic changes.

acute pro·my·e·lo·cyt·ic leukemia (prō-mī′ə-lō-sĭt′-ĭk) *n.* A severe bleeding disorder that is a form of leukemia and is characterized by low concentrations of plasma fibrigen, defective coagulation, and infiltration of the bone marrow with abnormal promyelocytes and myelocytes.

acute pulmonary alveolitis *n.* Acute inflammation of the pulmonary alveoli resulting in necrosis and hemorrhage into the lungs.

acute respiratory distress syndrome *n.* See **adult respiratory distress syndrome.**

acute rhinitis *n.* See **cold.**

acute situational reaction *n.* See **stress reaction.**

acute trypanosomiasis *n.* See **Rhodesian trypanosomiasis.**

acute tuberculosis *n.* A rapidly fatal disease in which tubercle bacilli are disseminated by the blood, resulting in the formation of miliary tubercles in various organs and tissues and in profound toxemia. Also called *acute miliary tuberculosis, disseminated tuberculosis.*

acute yellow atrophy of liver *or* **yellow atrophy of liver** *n.* Extensive and rapid death of the parenchymal cells of the liver, sometimes accompanied by fatty degeneration. Also called *Rokitansky's disease.*

a·cy·a·not·ic (ā-sī′ə-nŏt′ĭk) *adj.* Characterized by the absence of cyanosis.

a·cy·clic compound (ā-sī′klĭk, ā-sĭk′lĭk) *n.* An organic compound that has an open chain structure and does not form a ring. Also called *open chain compound.*

a·cy·clo·gua·no·sine (ā-sī′klō-gwä′nə-sēn′, -sĭn) *n.* See **acyclovir.**

a·cy·clo·vir (ā-sī′klō-vîr, -klə-) *n.* A synthetic purine nucleoside analog that is derived from guanine and is used in the treatment of herpes simplex, herpes zoster, and varicella zoster viral infections. Also called *acycloguanosine.*

ac·yl (ăs′əl) *n.* A organic radical having the general formula RCO, derived from the removal of a hydroxyl group from an organic acid.

acyl-activating enzyme *n.* See **acetyl-CoA synthetase.**

ac·yl·am·i·dase (ăs′ə-lăm′ĭ-dās′, -dāz′) *n.* See **amidase.**

ac·yl·ase (ăs′ə-lās′, -lāz′) *n.* See **amidase.**

acyl CoA *abbr.* acyl coenzyme A

acyl-CoA synthetase *n.* Any of various ligases that catalyze the formation of acyl CoA from corresponding fatty acids and CoA. Also called *thiokinase.*

acyl coenzyme A *n. Abbr.* **acyl CoA** A compound that functions as a coenzyme in acylation reactions and is formed as an intermediate in the oxidation of fats. Also called *acyl-CoA synthetase.*

ac·yl·trans·fer·ase (ăs′əl-trăns′fə-rās′, -rāz′) *n.* An enzyme that catalyzes the transfer of an acyl group from an acyl CoA to various acceptors. Also called *transacylase.*

a·cys·ti·a (ā-sĭs′tē-ə, ə-sĭs′-) *n.* Congenital absence of the urinary bladder.

AD *abbr. Latin* auris dextra (right ear)

ad– *pref.* **1.** Toward; to. Before *c, f, g, k, l, p, q, s,* and *t, ad-* is usually assimilated to *ac-, af-, ag-, ac-, al-, ap-, ac-, as-,* and *at-,* respectively: *adductor, acclimation, agglutinant.* **2.** Near; at: *adrenal.*

–ad *suff.* In the direction of; toward: *cephalad.*

a·dac·ty·ly (ā-dăk′tə-lē) *or* **a·dac·tyl·i·a** (ā′dăk-tĭl′ē-ə, ə-dăk-)*or* **a·dac·tyl·ism** (ā-dăk′tə-lĭz′əm) *n.* Congenital absence of fingers or toes. —**a·dac′ty·lous** *adj.*

Ad·a·lat (ăd′ə-lăt′) A trademark for the drug nifedipine.

ad·a·man·tine membrane (ăd′ə-măn′tēn′, -tīn′, -tĭn) *n.* See **dental cuticle.**

ad·a·man·ti·no·ma (ăd′ə-măn′tə-nō′mə) *n., pl.* **–mas** *or* **–ma·ta** (-mə-tə) See **ameloblastoma.**

Ad·am's apple (ăd′əmz) *n.* The slight projection at the front of the throat formed by the largest cartilage of the larynx, usually more prominent in men than in women. Also called *laryngeal prominence.*

Adams-Stokes syndrome *n.* An occasional temporary stoppage or extreme slowing of the pulse as a result of heart block, causing dizziness, fainting, and sometimes convulsions. Also called *Morgagni's disease, Spens' syndrome, Stokes-Adams disease, Stokes-Adams syndrome.*

ad·an·so·ni·an classification (ăd′n-sō′nē-ən) *n*. The classification of organisms based on giving equal weight to every character of the organism.

ad·ap·ta·tion (ăd′ăp-tā′shən) *n*. **1.** The acquisition of modifications in an organism that enable it to adjust to life in a new environment. **2.** An advantageous change in the function or constitution of an organ or tissue to meet new physiological conditions. **3.** Adjustment of the pupil and retina to varying degrees of illumination. **4.** A property of certain receptors through which they become less responsive or cease to respond to repeated or continued stimuli of constant intensity. **5.** The fitting, condensing, or contouring of a restorative dental material to a tooth or cast. **6.** The dynamic process in which the behavior and physiological mechanisms of an individual continually change to adjust to variations in living conditions.

a·dapt·er *or* **a·dap·tor** (ə-dăp′tər) *n*. **1.** One that adapts. **2.** A connecting part that joins two pieces of apparatus. **3.** A converter of electric current to a desired form.

a·dap·tive behavior scale (ə-dăp′tĭv) *n*. A series of tests used to quantify the ability of mentally retarded and developmentally delayed individuals to live independently. The tests assess personal self-sufficiency, as in eating and dressing, community self-sufficiency, as in shopping and communicating, and personal and social responsibility, as in job performance and the use of leisure time.

adaptive hypertrophy *n*. Hypertrophic enlargement in response to a condition, such as the thickening of the walls of a hollow organ when there is obstruction to outflow.

ad·ap·tom·e·ter (ăd′ăp-tŏm′ĭ-tər) *n*. A device for determining the course of ocular dark adaptation and for measuring the minimum light threshold.

ADD *abbr.* attention deficit disorder

add. *abbr. Latin* adde (add)

ad·dict (ăd′ĭkt) *n*. One who is addicted, as to narcotics or a compulsive activity.

ad·dict·ed (ə-dĭk′tĭd) *adj*. **1.** Physiologically or psychologically dependent on a habit-forming substance. **2.** Compulsively or habitually involved in a practice or behavior, such as gambling.

ad·dic·tion (ə-dĭk′shən) *n*. Habitual psychological or physiological dependence on a substance or practice beyond one's voluntary control.

ad·dic·tive (ə-dĭk′tĭv) *adj*. **1.** Causing or tending to cause addiction. **2.** Characterized by or susceptible to addiction.

Ad·dis count (ăd′ĭs) *n*. The number of red blood cells, white blood cells, and casts in a twelve-hour urine specimen, used to follow the progress of kidney disease.

Ad·di·son (ăd′ĭ-sən), **Thomas** 1793–1860. English physician who first described (1849) Addison's disease and Addison's anemia.

ad·di·so·ni·an crisis (ăd′ĭ-sō′nē-ən) *n*. See **acute adrenocortical insufficiency.**

Ad·di·son's anemia (ăd′ĭ-sənz) *or* **addisonian anemia** *n*. See **pernicious anemia.**

Addison's clinical plane *n*. Any of a series of planes used in thoracoabdominal topography. See under **interspinal plane, intertubercular plane, lateral plane,** median plane, transpyloric plane, and transthoracic plane.

Addison's disease *n*. A disease caused by partial or total failure of adrenocortical function, characterized by a bronzelike pigmentation of the skin and mucous membranes, anemia, weakness, nausea, and low blood pressure. Also called *bronzed disease, chronic adrenocortical insufficiency*.

ad·di·tive (ăd′ĭ-tĭv) *n*. A substance added in small amounts to something else to improve, strengthen, or otherwise alter it. —**ad′di·tive** *adj*.

additive effect *n*. An effect in which two substances or actions used in combination produce a total effect the same as the sum of the individual effects.

ad·duct (ə-dŭkt′, ă-dŭkt′) *v*. To draw inward toward the median axis of the body or toward an adjacent part or limb. —**ad·duc′tion** *n*. —**ad·duc′tive** *adj*.

ad·duc·tor (ə-dŭk′tər) *n*. A muscle that draws a body part, such as a finger, an arm, or a toe, inward toward the median axis of the body or of an extremity.

adductor brev·is (brĕv′ĭs) *n*. A muscle with origin in the superior ramus of the pubis, with insertion to the linea aspera, with nerve supply from the obturator nerve, and whose action adducts the thigh.

adductor canal *n*. The space in the thigh between the medial vastus and the adductor muscles through which the femoral vessels pass. Also called *Hunter's canal*.

adductor lon·gus (lŏn′gəs) *n*. A muscle with origin in the symphysis and crest of the pubis, with insertion to a ridge on the shaft of the femur, with nerve supply from the obturator nerve, and whose action adducts the thigh.

adductor mag·nus (măg′nəs) *n*. A muscle with origin in the ischial tuberosity and ischiopubic ramus, with insertion to the linea aspera and femur, with nerve supply from the obturator and sciatic nerves, and whose action adducts and extends the thigh.

adductor muscle of big toe *n*. A muscle with origin from the transverse head from the capsules of the lateral four metatarsophalangeal joints, and from the oblique head from the lateral cuneiform bone and the bases of the third and fourth metatarsal bones, with insertion into the lateral side of the base of the proximal phalanx of the big toe, with nerve supply from the lateral plantar nerve, and whose action adducts the big toe.

adductor muscle of thumb *n*. A muscle with origin from the transverse head from the shaft of the third metacarpal bone and from the oblique head from the front of the base of the second metacarpal, trapezoid, and capitate bones; with insertion to the medial side of the base of the proximal phalanx of the thumb, with nerve supply from the ulnar nerve, and whose action adducts the thumb.

a·del·o·mor·phous (ə-dĕl′ə-môr′fəs, ə-dē′lə-) *adj*. Lacking a clearly defined form.

aden– *pref*. Variant of **adeno–.**

ad·e·nal·gia (ăd′n-ăl′jə) *n*. Pain in a gland. Also called *adenodynia*.

a·den·dric (ā-dĕn′drĭk, ə-dĕn′-) *or* **a·den·drit·ic** (ā′-dĕn-drĭt′ĭk) *adj*. Lacking dendrites.

ad·e·nec·to·my (ăd′n-ĕk′tə-mē) *n.* Surgical excision of a gland.

ad·e·nec·to·pi·a (ăd′n-ĕk-tō′pē-ə) *n.* Presence of a gland in a position other than in its normal anatomical position.

ad·e·nem·phrax·is (ăd′n-ĕm-frăk′sĭs) *n.* The obstruction of the discharge of a glandular secretion.

a·den·i·form (ə-dĕn′ə-fôrm′) *adj.* Having a glandular appearance; glandlike.

ad·e·nine (ăd′n-ēn′, -ĭn) *n. Abbr.* **A** A purine base that is a constituent of DNA and RNA and an important energy transport and storage component in cellular metabolism.

adenine deoxyribonucleotide *n.* See **deoxyadenylic acid.**

adenine nucleotide *n.* See **AMP.**

ad·e·ni·tis (ăd′n-ī′tĭs) *n.* Inflammation of a lymph node or gland.

ad·e·ni·za·tion (ăd′n-ĭ-zā′shən) *n.* Conversion into a glandlike structure.

adeno– or **aden–** *pref.* Gland: *adenectomy.*

ad·e·no·ac·an·tho·ma (ăd′n-ō-ăk′ăn-thō′mə) *n.* A malignant neoplasm consisting chiefly of usually well-differentiated glandular epithelium with foci of metaplasia to squamous neoplastic cells. Also called *adenoid squamous cell carcinoma.*

ad·e·no·am·e·lo·blas·to·ma (ăd′n-ō-ăm′ə-lō-blă-stō′mə, -ə-mĕl′ō-) *n.* A benign tumor, usually in the maxilla of young people, composed of ducts lined by cuboidal or columnar cells.

ad·e·no·blast (ăd′n-ō-blăst′) *n.* A proliferating embryonic cell with the potential to form glandular parenchyma.

ad·e·no·car·ci·no·ma (ăd′n-ō-kär′sə-nō′mə) *n.* A malignant tumor originating in the epithelial cells of glandular tissue and forming glandular structures.

ad·e·no·cel·lu·li·tis (ăd′n-ō-sĕl′yə-lī′tĭs) *n.* Inflammation of a gland and adjacent cellular tissue.

ad·e·no·chon·dro·ma (ăd′n-ō-kŏn-drō′mə) *n.* See **pulmonary hamartoma.**

ad·e·no·cys·to·ma (ăd′n-ō-sĭ-stō′mə) *n.* A glandular cancer in which the neoplastic glandular epithelium forms cysts.

ad·e·no·dyn·i·a (ăd′n-ō-dĭn′ē-ə) *n.* See **adenalgia.**

ad·e·no·fi·bro·ma (ăd′n-ō-fī-brō′mə) *n.* A benign neoplasm composed of glandular and fibrous tissues.

ad·e·no·fi·bro·my·o·ma (ăd′n-ō-fī′brō-mī-ō′mə) *n.* See **adenomatoid tumor.**

ad·e·no·fi·bro·sis (ăd′n-ō-fī-brō′sĭs) *n.* See **sclerosing adenosis.**

ad·e·nog·e·nous (ăd′n-ŏj′ə-nəs) *adj.* Originating in glandular tissue.

ad·e·no·hy·poph·y·sis (ăd′n-ō-hī-pŏf′ĭ-sĭs) *n.* The anterior glandular lobe of the pituitary gland, consisting of distal, intermediate, and infundibular parts, and secreting many hormones, including gonadotropin, prolactin, and somatotropin. Also called *anterior lobe of hypophysis.* —**ad′e·no·hy′po·phy′si·al** (-hī′pə-fĭz′ē-əl, -hī-pŏf′ĭ-sē′əl) *adj.*

ad·e·no·hy·poph·y·si·tis (ăd′n-ō-hī-pŏf′ĭ-sī′tĭs) *n.* Inflammation of the anterior pituitary gland, often related to pregnancy.

ad·e·noid (ăd′n-oid′) *n.* **1.** A lymphoid tissue growth located at the back of the nose in the upper part of the throat that when swollen may obstruct normal breathing and make speech difficult. **2. adenoids** Hypertrophy of the pharyngeal tonsil resulting from chronic inflammation. —*adj.* Of, relating to, or resembling lymphatic glands or lymphatic tissue. —**ad′e·noi′dal** (ăd′n-oid′l) *adj.*

adenoidal-pharyngeal-conjunctival virus *n. Abbr.* **A-P-C virus** See **adenovirus.**

adenoid cystic carcinoma *n.* A carcinoma characterized by large epithelial masses containing round glandlike spaces or cysts, frequently containing mucus, that are bordered by layers of epithelial cells. Also called *cylindromatous carcinoma.*

ad·e·noid·ec·to·my (ăd′n-oi-dĕk′tə-mē) *n.* Surgical removal of adenoid growths in the nasopharynx.

adenoid facies *n.* The appearance in children with adenoid hypertrophy, associated with a pinched nose and an open mouth.

ad·e·noid·i·tis (ăd′n-oi-dī′tĭs) *n.* Inflammation of the adenoids.

adenoid squamous cell carcinoma *n.* See **adenoacanthoma.**

adenoid tissue *n.* See **lymphatic tissue.**

ad·e·no·li·po·ma (ăd′n-ō-lĭ-pō′mə, -lī-) *n.* A benign neoplasm composed of both glandular and adipose tissues.

ad·e·no·li·po·ma·to·sis (ăd′n-ō-lĭ-pō′mə-tō′sĭs) *n.* A condition marked by the development of multiple adenolipomas.

ad·e·no·lym·pho·cele (ăd′n-ō-lĭm′fə-sēl′) *n.* Cystic dilation of a lymph node following obstruction of the efferent lymphatic vessels.

ad·e·no·lym·pho·ma (ăd′n-ō-lĭm-fō′mə) *n.* A benign glandular tumor usually arising in the parotid gland and composed of two rows of eosinophilic epithelial cells with a lymphoid stroma. Also called *papillary cystadenoma lymphomatosum, Warthin's tumor.*

ad·e·nol·y·sis (ăd′n-ŏl′ĭ-sĭs) *n.* Destruction or dissolution of glandular tissue by enzymes.

ad·e·no·ma (ăd′n-ō′mə) *n., pl.* **–mas** or **–ma·ta** (-mə-tə) A benign epithelial tumor having a glandular origin and structure.

adenoma se·ba·ce·um (sĭ-bā′sē-əm) *n.* A hamartoma on the face, composed of fibrovascular tissue and appearing as an aggregation of red or yellow papules that may be associated with tuberous sclerosis. Also called *Pringle's disease.*

ad·e·no·ma·toid (ăd′n-ō′mə-toid′) *adj.* Resembling an adenoma.

adenomatoid tumor *n.* A small benign tumor of the male epididymis or the female genital tract, consisting of fibrous tissue or smooth muscle enclosing spaces lined by flattened cells. Also called *adenofibromyoma, Recklinghausen's tumor.*

ad·e·no·ma·to·sis (ăd′n-ō′mə-tō′sĭs) *n.* Development of multiple glandular overgrowths.

ad·e·nom·a·tous (ăd′n-ŏm′ə-təs, -ō′mə-təs) *adj.* **1.** Of or relating to adenoma. **2.** Of or relating to various types of glandular hyperplasia.

adenomatous goiter *n.* Goiter due to the growth of multiple encapsulated adenomas or multiple nonencapsulated colloid nodules within its substance.

adenomatous polyp *n.* A polyp that consists of benign neoplastic tissue derived from glandular epithelium.

ad·e·no·mere (ăd′n-ō-mîr′) *n.* A structural unit in the parenchyma of a developing gland.

ad·e·no·my·o·ma (ăd′n-ō-mī-ō′mə) *n.* A benign tumor of smooth muscle containing glandular elements, occurring most frequently in the uterus and in the uterine ligaments.

ad·e·no·my·o·sar·co·ma (ăd′n-ō-mī′ō-sär-kō′mə) *n.* See **Wilms′ tumor.**

ad·e·no·my·o·sis (ăd′n-ō-mī-ō′sĭs) *n.* A form of endometriosis characterized by the invasive, usually benign growth of tissue into smooth muscle such as the uterus.

ad·e·nop·a·thy (ăd′n-ŏp′ə-thē) *n.* Swelling or abnormal enlargement of the lymph nodes.

ad·e·no·phar·yn·gi·tis (ăd′n-ō-făr′ĭn-jī′tĭs) *n.* Inflammation of the adenoids and the pharyngeal lymphoid tissue.

ad·e·no·phleg·mon (ăd′n-ō-flĕg′mŏn′) *n.* Acute inflammation of a gland and the adjacent connective tissue.

ad·e·no·sal·pin·gi·tis (ăd′n-ō-săl′pĭn-jī′tĭs) *n.* Nodular thickening of the tunica muscularis of the isthmic portion of the fallopian tube enclosing glandlike or cystic duplications of the lumen. Also called *salpingitis isthmica nodosa.*

ad·e·no·sar·co·ma (ăd′n-ō-sär-kō′mə) *n.* A malignant tumor arising simultaneously or consecutively in mesodermal tissue and glandular epithelium.

a·den·o·sine (ə-dĕn′ə-sēn′) *n.* A nucleoside that is a structural component of nucleic acids and the major molecular component of ADP, AMP, and ATP.

adenosine 3′,5′-cyclic phosphate *n.* Cyclic AMP.

adenosine 3′,5′-monophosphate *n.* Cyclic AMP.

adenosine 5′-diphosphate *n.* ADP.

adenosine 5′-triphosphate *n.* ATP.

adenosine diphosphate *n.* ADP.

adenosine monophosphate *n.* **1.** AMP. **2.** Cyclic AMP.

adenosine phosphate *n.* AMP.

adenosine tri·phos·pha·tase (trī-fŏs′fə-tās′, -tāz′) *n.* ATPase.

adenosine triphosphate *n.* ATP.

ad·e·no·sis (ăd′n-ō′sĭs) *n., pl.* **-ses** (-sēz′) A disease of a gland, especially one marked by the abnormal formation or enlargement of glandular tissue.

ad·e·not·o·my (ăd′n-ŏt′ə-mē) *n.* Surgical incision of a gland.

ad·e·no·ton·sil·lec·to·my (ăd′n-ō-tŏn′sə-lĕk′tə-mē) *n.* Surgical removal of the tonsils and adenoids.

Ad·e·no·vir·i·dae (ăd′n-ō-vîr′ĭ-dē) *n.* A family of double-stranded DNA-containing viruses, of which there are more than 80 antigenic species that cause diseases of the respiratory tract and conjunctiva.

ad·e·no·vi·rus (ăd′n-ō-vī′rəs) *n.* Any of the viruses of the family Adenoviridae. Also called *adenoidal-pharyngeal-conjunctival virus.*

ad·e·nyl (ăd′n-ĭl′) *n.* The univalent radical $C_5H_4N_5$ in adenine.

a·den·yl·ate (ə-dĕn′l-ĭt, ăd′n-ĭl′ĭt) *n.* A salt or ester of AMP.

adenylate cyclase *n.* An enzyme that catalyzes the formation of cyclic AMP from ATP. Also called *3′,5′-cyclic AMP synthetase.*

adenylate kinase *n.* An enzyme that catalyzes the phosphorylation of one molecule of ADP by another, yielding ATP and AMP.

ad·e·nyl·ic acid (ăd′n-ĭl′ĭk) *n.* See **AMP.**

ad·e·quate stimulus (ăd′ĭ-kwĭt) *n.* A stimulus to which a particular receptor responds effectively and that gives rise to a characteristic sensation.

a·der·mi·a (ā-dûr′mē-ə, ə-dûr′-) *n.* Congenital absence of skin.

a·der·mo·gen·e·sis (ā-dûr′mō-jĕn′ĭ-sĭs, ə-dûr′-) *n.* Failure of or imperfection in the regeneration of the skin, especially in the repair of a cutaneous defect.

ADH *abbr.* antidiuretic hormone

ADHD *abbr.* attention deficit hyperactivity disorder

ad·her·ence (ăd-hîr′əns) *n.* The extent to which the patient continues the agreed-upon mode of treatment under limited supervision when faced with conflicting demands, as distinguished from compliance or maintenance.

ad·he·sion (ăd-hē′zhən) *n.* **1.** A condition in which body tissues that are normally separate grow together. **2.** A fibrous band of scar tissue that binds together normally separate anatomical structures. **3.** The union of opposing surfaces of a wound, especially in healing. Also called *conglutination.*

ad·he·si·ot·o·my (ăd-hē′zē-ŏt′ə-mē) *n.* Surgical division or separation of adhesions.

ad·he·sive (ăd-hē′sĭv) *adj.* **1.** Tending to adhere; sticky. **2.** Of, relating to, or having the characteristics of an adhesion. —*n.* A substance that adheres to a surface or causes adherence between surfaces.

adhesive absorbent dressing *n.* A sterile dressing consisting of a plain absorbent gauze or compress affixed to a film of fabric coated on one side with a pressure-sensitive adhesive.

adhesive bandage *n.* A dressing of absorbent gauze affixed to plastic or fabric coated with a pressure-sensitive adhesive.

adhesive capsulitis *n.* See **frozen shoulder.**

adhesive pericarditis *n.* Pericarditis with adhesions between the two pericardial layers, between the pericardium and heart, or between the pericardium and neighboring structures.

adhesive peritonitis *n.* Peritonitis characterized by a fibrinous exudate that mats together the intestines and various other organs.

adhesive pleurisy *n.* See **dry pleurisy.**

adhesive vaginitis *n.* Inflammation of vaginal mucosa accompanied by adhesion of the vagina walls to each other.

adhib. *abbr. Latin* adhibendus (to be administered)

a·di·a·do·cho·ki·ne·sis (ə-dī′ə-dō′kō-kĭ-nē′sĭs, -kī-, ăd′ē-ăd′ə-kō-) *n.* Inability to perform rapid alternating movements.

a·di·a·pho·re·sis (ā-dī′ə-fə-rē′sĭs) *n.* See **anhidrosis.** —**a·di·a·pho·ret·ic** (-rĕt′ĭk) *adj.*

a·di·a·pho·ri·a (ə-dī′ə-fôr′ē-ə) *n.* Failure to respond to a stimulus after a series of stimuli.

A·die's pupil (ā′dēz) *n.* See **Holmes-Adie syndrome.**

Adie syndrome *n.* See **Holmes-Adie syndrome.**

adipo– *or* **adip–** *pref.* Fat: *adipocyte.*

ad·i·po·cele (ăd′ə-pō-sēl′) *n.* See **lipocele.**

ad·i·po·cel·lu·lar (ăd′ə-pō-sĕl′yə-lər) *adj.* Relating to or composed of fatty tissue and connective tissue.

ad·i·po·cere (ăd′ə-pō-sîr′) *n.* A brown, fatty, waxlike substance that forms on dead animal tissue in response to moisture. Also called *lipocere.* —**ad′i·po·cer′a·tous** (-sĕr′ə-təs) *adj.*

ad·i·po·cyte (ăd′ə-pō-sīt′) *n.* See **fat cell.**

ad·i·po·gen·e·sis (ăd′ə-pō-jĕn′ĭ-sĭs) *n.* See **lipogenesis** (sense 1). —**ad′i·po·gen′ic, ad′i·pog′e·nous** (-pŏj′ə-nəs) *adj.*

ad·i·poid (ăd′ə-poid′) *adj.* Lipoid.

ad·i·po·ki·net·ic (ăd′ə-pō-kĭ-nĕt′ĭk, -kī-) *adj.* Of or relating to an agent that mobilizes stored lipids.

ad·i·po·ki·nin (ăd′ə-pō-kī′nĭn) *n.* An anterior pituitary hormone that mobilizes fat from adipose tissue. Also called *adipokinetic hormone.*

ad·i·po·ne·cro·sis (ăd′ə-pō-nə-krō′sĭs) *n.* Necrosis of fat, as occurs in hemorrhagic pancreatitis.

adiponecrosis ne·o·na·to·rum (nē′ō-nā-tôr′əm) *n.* See **sclerema neonatorum.**

ad·i·pose (ăd′ə-pōs′) *adj.* Of, relating to, or composed of animal fat; fatty. —*n.* The fat found in adipose tissue. —**ad′i·pose′ness, ad′i·pos′i·ty** (-pŏs′ĭ-tē) *n.*

adipose cell *n.* See **fat cell.**

adipose degeneration *n.* See **fatty degeneration.**

adipose fossa *n.* Any of the subcutaneous spaces in the breast containing accumulations of fat.

adipose infiltration *n.* The growth of normal adult fat cells in sites where they are not usually present.

adipose tissue *n.* A connective tissue consisting chiefly of fat cells surrounded by reticular fibers and arranged in lobular groups or along the course of one of the smaller blood vessels.

ad·i·po·sis (ăd′ə-pō′sĭs) *n.* Excessive accumulation of fat in the body. Also called *lipomatosis, liposis.*

adiposis car·di·a·ca (kär′dē-ā′kə) *n.* See **fatty heart** (sense 2).

adiposis do·lo·ro·sa (dō′lə-rō′sə) *n.* Uncomfortable or painful deposits of pendulous or symmetrical nodular masses of adipose tissue in various regions of the body. Also called *Dercum's disease.*

adiposis tu·be·ro·sa sim·plex (tōō′bə-rō′sə sĭm′-plĕks′) *n.* Small sensitive or painful masses of fat that occur on the abdomen or the extremities.

ad·i·po·so·gen·i·tal dystrophy (ăd′ə-pō′sō-jĕn′ĭ-tl) *n.* A disorder characterized primarily by obesity and genital hypoplasia either of which may be caused by a tumor of the adenohypophysis or lesions of the hypothalamus.

ad·i·po·su·ri·a (ăd′ə-pō-sōōr′ē-ə) *n.* See **lipuria.**

ad·i·tus (ăd′ĭ-təs) *n., pl.* **aditus** An entrance to a cavity or channel.

ad·just (ə-jŭst′) *v.* **1.** To bring into proper relationship. **2.** To treat disorders of the spine by correcting slight dislocations between vertebrae using chiropractic techniques. **3.** To achieve a psychological balance with re-gard to one's external environment, one's needs, and the demands of others.

ad·just·ed (ə-jŭs′tĭd) *adj.* Having achieved psychological balance, especially regarding others or the demands of everyday life.

ad·just·ment disorder (ə-jŭst′mənt) *n.* Any of a class of disorders that result from an individual's failure to adapt to identifiable stresses in the environment such as divorce, natural disaster, family discord, or retirement, characterized by an impaired ability to function socially or occupationally.

ad·ju·vant (ăj′ə-vənt) *n.* **1.** A pharmacological agent added to a drug, predictably affecting the action of the drug's active ingredient. **2.** An immunological vehicle for enhancing antigenicity, such as a water-in-oil emulsion in which antigen solution is emulsified in mineral oil. Also called *immunoadjuvant.*

ADL *abbr.* activities of daily living

Ad·ler (ăd′lər, äd′-), **Alfred** 1870–1937. Austrian psychiatrist. He rejected Sigmund Freud's emphasis on sexuality and theorized that neurotic behavior is an over-compensation for feelings of inferiority.

ad lib. *abbr. Latin* ad libitum (freely, as desired)

admov. *abbr. Latin* admove (apply)

ad·ner·val (ăd-nûr′vəl) *adj.* **1.** Lying near a nerve. **2.** Flowing toward a nerve. Used of an electric current passing through a muscle.

ad·neu·ral (ăd-nōōr′əl) *adj.* Adnerval.

ad·nex·a (ăd-nĕk′sə) *or* **an·nex·a** (ă-nĕk′sə) *pl.n.* Accessory or adjoining anatomical parts, such as ovaries and oviducts in relation to the uterus. —**ad·nex′al, an·nex′al** *adj.*

adnexal adenoma *n.* A tumor arising in or forming structures resembling skin appendages.

ad·nex·um (ăd-nĕk′-səm) *or* **an·nex·um** (ă-nĕk′-) *n.* Singular of **adnexa.**

ad·o·les·cence (ăd′l-ĕs′əns) *n.* The period of physical and psychological development from the onset of puberty to complete growth and maturity.

ad·o·les·cent (ăd′l-ĕs′ənt) *adj.* Of, relating to, or undergoing adolescence. —*n.* A young person who has undergone puberty but who has not reached full maturity; a teenager.

adolescent medicine *n.* The branch of medicine that is concerned with the treatment of youth between 13 and 21 years of age. Also called *ephebiatrics, hebiatrics.*

a·dop·tive immunotherapy (ə-dŏp′tĭv) *n.* The passive transfer of immunity from an immune donor through inoculation with sensitized white blood cells, transfer factor, immune RNA, or antibodies in serum or gamma globulin.

ad·o·ral (ăd-ôr′əl) *adj.* At, near, or toward the mouth.

ADP (ā′dē′pē′) *n.* Adenosine diphosphate; an ester of adenosine that is converted to ATP for the storage of energy.

adren– *pref.* Variant of **adreno–.**

ad·re·nal (ə-drē′nəl) *adj.* **1.** At, near, or on the kidneys. **2.** Of or relating to the adrenal glands or their secretions. —*n.* An adrenal gland or tissue.

adrenal cortex *n.* The outer part of the adrenal gland, consisting of the zona glomerulosa, the zona fasciculata, and the zona reticularis and yielding various steroid hormones.

adrenal crisis *n.* See **acute adrenocortical insufficiency.**

ad·re·nal·ec·to·my (ə-drē′nə-lĕk′tə-mē) *n.* The surgical excision of one or both of the adrenal glands. Also called *suprarenalectomy.*

adrenal gland *n.* Either of two small, dissimilarly shaped endocrine glands, one located above each kidney, consisting of the cortex, which secretes several steroid hormones, and the medulla, which secretes epinephrine. Also called *epinephros, paranephros, suprarenal gland.*

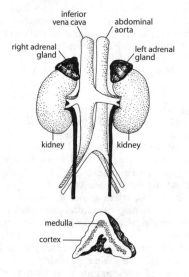

inferior
vena cava

abdominal
aorta

right adrenal
gland

left adrenal
gland

kidney   kidney

medulla

cortex

adrenal gland
Top: *position of adrenal glands in relation to kidneys*
Bottom: *cross section of right adrenal gland*

adrenal hypertension *n.* Hypertension due to pheochromocytoma.

A·dren·a·lin (ə-drĕn′ə-lĭn) A trademark for a preparation of epinephrine.

a·dren·a·line (ə-drĕn′ə-lĭn) *n.* See **epinephrine** (sense 1).

ad·re·nal·i·tis (ə-drē′nə-lī′tĭs) *n.* Inflammation of one or both of the adrenal glands.

adrenal medulla *n.* Medulla of the adrenal gland.

ad·re·na·lop·a·thy (ə-drē′nə-lŏp′ə-thē) *or* **ad·re·nop·a·thy** (ăd′rə-nŏp′ə-thē) *n.* Disease of the adrenal glands.

adrenal rest *n.* See **accessory adrenal.**

ad·re·ner·gic (ăd′rə-nûr′jĭk) *adj.* **1.** Activated by or capable of releasing epinephrine or an epinephrinelike substance, especially in the sympathetic nervous system. **2.** Having physiological effects similar to those of epinephrine.

adrenergic amine *n.* See **sympathomimetic amine.**

adrenergic blockade *n.* Selective inhibition by a drug of the responses of effector cells to adrenergic sympathetic nerve impulses and to adrenergic amines.

adrenergic blocking agent *n.* A compound that selectively inhibits responses to sympathetic adrenergic nerve impulses and to adrenergic amines.

adrenergic fiber *n.* Any of the fibers that transmit impulses to other nerve cells, smooth muscle, or gland cells by norepinephrine.

adrenergic neuronal blocking agent *n.* A drug that blocks sympathetic nerve impulses but does not inhibit the responses of adrenergic receptors to epinephrine and other adrenergic amines.

adrenergic receptor *n.* Any of several reactive components of effector tissues most of which are innervated by adrenergic postganglionic fibers of the sympathetic nervous system and are activated by norepinephrine, epinephrine, and various adrenergic drugs. They are classified as alpha-adrenergic receptors and beta-adrenergic receptors according to their response to various adreneregic activating and blocking agents. Also called *adrenoreceptor.*

adreno– *or* **adren–** *pref.* Adrenal gland; adrenal: *adrenomegaly.*

ad·re·no·cep·tive (ə-drē′nō-sĕp′tĭv) *adj.* Of or relating to chemical sites in effector cells with which the adrenergic mediator unites.

a·dre·no·chrome (ə-drē′nō-krōm′, -nə-) *n.* A naturally occurring chemical formed during the oxidation of epinephrine.

ad·re·no·cor·ti·cal (ə-drē′nō-kôr′tĭ-kəl) *adj.* Of, relating to, or derived from the adrenal cortex.

adrenocortical hormone *n.* Any of the various hormones secreted by the adrenal cortex, especially cortisol, aldosterone, and corticosterone. Also called *cortical hormone.*

adrenocortical insufficiency *n.* Loss or diminution of adrenocortical function, as in Addison's disease. Also called *hypocorticoidism.*

ad·re·no·cor·ti·co·mi·met·ic (ə-drē′nō-kôr′tĭ-kō-mĭ-mĕt′ĭk, -mī-) *adj.* Mimicking the function of the adrenal cortex.

ad·re·no·cor·ti·co·trop·ic (ə-drē′nō-kôr′tĭ-kō-trŏp′-ĭk, -trō′pĭk) *or* **ad·re·no·cor·ti·co·troph·ic** (-trŏf′ĭk, -trō′fĭk) *adj.* Stimulating or otherwise acting on the adrenal cortex.

adrenocorticotropic hormone *or* **adrenocorticotrophic hormone** *n.* ACTH.

ad·re·no·cor·ti·co·trop·in (ə-drē′nō-kôr′tĭ-kō-trŏp′-ĭn, -trō′pĭn) *or* **ad·re·no·cor·ti·co·troph·in** (-trŏf′ĭn, -trō′fĭn) *n.* See **ACTH.**

ad·re·no·gen·ic (ə-drē′nə-jĕn′ĭk) *or* **ad·re·nog·e·nous** (ăd′rə-nŏj′ə-nəs) *adj.* Of adrenal origin.

a·dre·no·gen·i·tal syndrome (ə-drē′nō-jĕn′ĭ-tl) *n.* A group of disorders caused by adrenocortical hyperplasia or malignant tumors, resulting in abnormal secretion of adrenocortical hormones and characterized by masculinization of women, feminization of men, or precocious sexual development in children.

ad·re·no·leu·ko·dys·tro·phy (ə-drē′nō-lōō′kō-dĭs′-trə-fē) *n. Abbr.* **ALD** A genetic disorder affecting boys, characterized by adrenocortical insufficiency, hyperpigmentation, and leukodystrophy.

ad·re·no·lyt·ic (ə-drē′nə-lĭt′ĭk) *adj.* Inhibiting or preventing the action of epinephrine, norepinephrine, and related sympathomimetics. —**ad·re′no·lyt′ic** *n.*

ad·re·no·meg·a·ly (ə-drē′nō-mĕg′ə-lē) *n.* Enlargement of the adrenal glands.

ad·re·no·mi·met·ic (ə-drē′nō-mĭ-mĕt′ĭk, -mī-) *adj.* Having an action similar to that of epinephrine and norepinephrine.

adrenomimetic amine *n.* See **sympathomimetic amine.**

ad·re·nop·a·thy (ăd′rə-nŏp′ə-thē) *n.* Variant of **adrenalopathy.**

ad·re·no·re·cep·tor (ə-drē′nō-rĭ-sĕp′tər) *n.* See **adrenergic receptor.**

ad·re·no·tox·in (ə-drē′nō-tŏk′sĭn) *n.* A substance toxic to the adrenal glands.

ad·re·no·trop·ic (ə-drē′nō-trŏp′ĭk, -trō′pĭk) *or* **ad·re·no·troph·ic** (ə-drē′nō-trŏf′ĭk, -trō′fĭk) *adj.* Adrenocorticotropic.

ad·re·no·trop·in (ə-drē′nō-trŏp′ĭn, -trō′pĭn) *n.* See **ACTH.**

A·dri·a·my·cin (ā′drē-ə-mī′sən) A trademark for the drug doxorubicin.

A·dri·an (ā′drē-ən), **Edgar Douglas** First Baron Adrian. 1889–1977. British physiologist. He shared a 1932 Nobel Prize for major advances in the understanding of the nervous and muscular systems and was one of the first to study electrical activity in the brain and nervous system.

ad sat. *abbr. Latin* ad saturatum (to saturation)

Ad·son's test (ăd′sənz) *n.* A test for thoracic outlet syndrome in which the patient is seated and, with the head extended and turned to the side of the lesion, breathes deeply; a diminution or loss of radial pulse on the affected side is indicative of the syndrome.

ad·sorb (ăd-zôrb′) *v.* To take up by adsorption.

ad·sor·bent (ăd-zôr′bənt) *adj.* Capable of adsorption. —*n.* **1.** An adsorptive substance. **2.** A pharmacological substance capable of attaching other substances to its surface without any chemical action. **3.** An antigen or antibody used in immune adsorption.

ad·sorp·tion (ăd-zôrp′shən) *n.* The property of a solid or liquid to attract and hold to its surface a gas, liquid, solute, or suspension.

adsorption theory of narcosis *n.* The theory that a drug becomes concentrated at the surface of the cell as a result of adsorption and thus alters the cell wall permeability and the cell's metabolism.

adst. feb. *abbr. Latin* adstante febre (when fever is present)

ad·ter·mi·nal (ăd-tûr′mə-nəl) *adj.* At, near, or toward the nerve endings, muscular insertions, or the extremity of any structure.

a·dult (ə-dŭlt′, ăd′ŭlt) *n.* **1.** One who has attained maturity or legal age. **2.** A fully grown, mature organism. —*adj.* Fully developed and mature.

a·dul·ter·ant (ə-dŭl′tər-ənt) *n.* An additive causing an undesirable effect; impurity. —**a·dul·ter·ant** *adj.*

a·dul·ter·a·tion (ə-dŭl′tə-rā′shən) *n.* The alteration, especially the debasement, of a substance by deliberately adding something not ordinarily a part of it.

adult Fanconi's syndrome *n.* A rare hereditary disease characterized by a softening of bone tissue and a malfunctioning of the renal tubules that causes cystine to be excreted in the urine.

adult medulloepithelioma *n.* See **malignant ciliary epithelioma.**

adult-onset diabetes mellitus *n. Abbr.* **AODM** Non-insulin-dependent diabetes.

adult pseudohypertrophic muscular dystrophy *n.* An inherited, relatively mild form of muscular dystrophy that manifests its first symptoms when individuals are in their 20s or 30s.

adult respiratory distress syndrome *n. Abbr.* **ARDS** Interstitial and alveolar edema and hemorrhage of the lungs following injury and associated with hyaline membrane, proliferation of collagen fibers, and swollen epithelium. Also called *acute respiratory distress syndrome.*

adult rickets *n.* See **osteomalacia.**

adult T-cell lymphoma *n. Abbr.* **ATL** An acute or subacute disease associated with a human T-cell virus and characterized by lymphadenopathy, enlargement of the liver and spleen, skin lesions, peripheral blood involvement, and hypercalcemia. Also called *adult T-cell leukemia.*

ad us. ext. *abbr. Latin* ad usum externum (for external use)

adv. *abbr. Latin* adversum (against)

ad·vanced life support (ăd-vănst′) *n.* Emergency medical care for sustaining life, including defibrillation, airway management, and drugs and medications.

advanced practice nurse *n. Abbr.* **APN** A licensed registered nurse who has completed graduate training as a clinical nurse specialist, nurse anesthetist, nurse-midwife, or nurse practitioner.

ad·vance·ment (ăd-văns′mənt) *n.* A surgical procedure in which a tendinous insertion or a skin flap is severed from its attachment and is sutured to a further point on the body.

advancement flap *n.* See **sliding flap.**

ad·ven·ti·tia (ăd′vĕn-tĭsh′ə) *n.* The outermost membranous covering of an organ or structure, especially the outer coat of an artery.

ad·ven·ti·tial (ăd′vĕn-tĭsh′əl) *adj.* **1.** Of or relating to the adventitia of an organ or blood vessel. **2.** Adventitious.

adventitial cell *n.* See **pericyte.**

adventitial neuritis *n.* Inflammation of the sheath of a nerve.

ad·ven·ti·tious (ăd′vĕn-tĭsh′əs) *adj.* **1.** Arising from an external source or occurring in an unusual place or manner; extrinsic. **2.** Occurring accidentally or spontaneously, not caused by heredity. **3.** Adventitial.

adventitious cyst *n.* See **pseudocyst** (sense 1).

ad·verse reaction (ăd-vûrs′, ăd′vûrs′) *n.* A result of drug therapy that is neither intended nor expected in normal therapeutic use and that causes significant, sometimes life-threatening conditions.

Ad·vil (ăd′vĭl) A trademark for the drug ibuprofen.

a·dy·nam·i·a (ā′dī-năm′ēə, ăd′ə-nā′mē-ə) *n.* Loss of strength or vigor, usually because of disease.

a·dy·nam·ic ileus (ā′dī-năm′ĭk, ăd′ə-) *n.* See **paralytic ileus.**

ae– For words beginning with *ae–* that are not found here, see under *e–*.

A-E amputation *n.* Amputation of the limb from above the elbow.

A·e·des (ā-ē′dēz′) *n.* A genus of mosquitoes frequently found in tropical and subtropical regions that includes *Aedes aegypti,* which transmits diseases such as yellow fever and dengue.

–aemia *suff.* Variant of **–emia.**

aer·a·tion (âr′ā′shən) *n.* **1.** Exposure to air. **2.** Saturation of a fluid with air or a gas. **3.** The exchange of carbon dioxide and oxygen in the lungs.

aero– or **aer–** *pref.* **1.** Air; atmosphere: *aerobic.* **2.** Gas: *aerosol.*

aer·o·al·ler·gen (âr′ō-ăl′ər-jən) *n.* Any of various airborne substances, such as pollen or spores, that can cause an allergic response.

aer·obe (âr′ōb′) *n.* An organism, such as a bacterium, requiring oxygen to live.

aer·o·bic (â-rō′bĭk) *adj.* **1.** Living or occurring only in the presence of oxygen, as certain microorganisms. **2.** Of or relating to aerobes. **3.** Relating to or used in aerobics.

aer·o·bi·cize (â-rō′bĭ-sīz′) *v.* To perform vigorous exercise as part of a program to improve physical fitness.

aerobic respiration *n.* Respiration in which molecular oxygen is consumed and carbon dioxide and water are produced.

aer·o·bics (â-rō′bĭks) *n.* **1.** A system of physical conditioning to enhance circulatory and respiratory efficiency that involves vigorous, sustained exercise, such as jogging, swimming, or cycling, thereby improving the body's use of oxygen. **2.** A program of physical fitness that involves such exercise.

Aer·o·bid (âr′ō-bĭd′) A trademark for the drug flunisolide in an inhaler form.

aer·o·bi·ol·o·gy (âr′ō-bī-ŏl′ə-jē) *n.* The study of the sources, dispersion, and effects of airborne biological materials, such as pollen, spores, and microorganisms.

aer·o·bi·o·sis (âr′ō-bī-ō′sĭs) *n.* Life sustained by an organism in the presence of air or oxygen.

aer·o·cele (âr′ō-sēl′) *n.* A cavity or pouch filled with air or gas, especially one connected to the trachea or larynx.

aer·o·col·pos (âr′ō-kŏl′pəs) *n.* Distention of the vagina with air or gas.

aer·o·der·mec·ta·sia (âr′ō-dûr′mĭk-tā′zhə) *n.* See **subcutaneous emphysema.**

aer·o·don·tal·gia (âr′ō-dŏn-tăl′jə) *n.* Toothache that is caused by decreased atmospheric pressure.

aer·o·em·phy·se·ma (âr′ō-ĕm′fĭ-sē′mə, -zē′-) *n.* **1.** See **decompression sickness. 2.** A form of chronic pulmonary emphysema resulting from rapid decompression, as may occur in an inadequately pressurized aircraft.

aer·o·gen (âr′ə-jən, -jĕn′) *n.* A gas-producing microorganism.

aer·o·gen·e·sis (âr′ō-jĕn′ĭ-sĭs) *n.* The formation of gas. —**aer′o·gen′ic** *adj.*

aer·o·med·i·cine (âr′ō-mĕd′ĭ-sĭn) *n.* The medical study and treatment of physiological and psychological disorders associated with atmospheric or space flight.

ae·ro·o·ti·tis me·di·a (âr′ō-ō-tī′tĭs mē′dē-ə) *n.* See **barotitis media.**

aer·op·a·thy (â-rŏp′ə-thē) *n.* A pathological condition induced by a change in the atmospheric pressure.

aer·o·pha·gia (âr′ə-fā′jə) or **aer·oph·a·gy** (-ŏf′ə-jē) *n.* The excessive swallowing of air or gas.

aer·o·phil (âr′ə-fĭl)or **aer·o·phile** (-fīl′) *adj.* Thriving in the presence of air; air-loving. —*n.* An aerobic organism, especially an obligate aerobe.

aer·o·pho·bi·a (âr′ə-fō′bē-ə) *n.* An abnormal fear of air, especially drafts.

aer·o·pi·e·so·ther·a·py (âr′ō-pī-ē′sō-thĕr′ə-pē) *n.* The treatment of disease using compressed air or rarified air.

aer·o·si·nus·i·tis (âr′ō-sī′nə-sī′tĭs) *n.* Inflammation of the paranasal sinuses caused by a difference between the pressure within the sinus cavities and the ambient pressure. Also called *barosinusitis.*

aer·o·sol (âr′ə-sôl′) *n.* **1.** A gaseous suspension of fine solid or liquid particles. **2.** A substance, such as a drug containing therapeutically active ingredients, packaged under pressure with a gaseous propellant for release as a spray of fine particles.

aerosol generator *n.* A device that produces aerosol suspensions, as for inhalation therapy.

aer·o·ti·tis me·di·a (âr′ə-tī′tĭs mē′dē-ə) *n.* See **barotitis media.**

aes·cu·la·pi·an (ĕs′kyə-lā′pē-ən) *adj.* Relating to the art of medicine; medical.

aes·the·sia or **es·the·sia** (ĕs-thē′zhə) *n.* The ability to feel or perceive.

aesthesio– *pref.* Variant of **esthesio–.**

aes·the·si·od·ic or **es·the·si·od·ic** (ĕs-thē′zē-ŏd′ĭk) *adj.* Conveying sensory impressions.

aes·the·si·o·gen·e·sis or **es·the·si·o·gen·e·sis** (ĕs-thē′zē-ō-jĕn′ĭ-sĭs) *n.* The production of sensation, especially of nervous erethism.

aes·the·si·o·gen·ic or **es·the·si·o·gen·ic** (ĕs-thē′zē-ō-jĕn′ĭk) *adj.* Producing a sensation.

aes·the·si·om·e·ter or **es·the·si·om·e·ter** (ĕs-thē′zē-ŏm′ĭ-tər) *n.* An instrument used to measure tactile sensitivity. Also called *tactometer.*

aes·the·si·om·e·try or **es·the·si·om·e·try** (ĕs-thē′zē-ŏm′ĭ-trē) *n.* The measurement of the degree of tactile or other sensibility.

aes·the·si·o·phys·i·ol·o·gy or **es·the·si·o·phys·i·ol·o·gy** (ĕs-thē′zē-ō-fĭz′ē-ŏl′ə-jē) *n.* The physiology of sensation and the sense organs.

aes·thet·ic or **es·thet·ic** (ĕs-thĕt′ĭk) *adj.* **1.** Relating to the sensations. **2.** Relating to esthetics.

aes·thet·ics or **es·thet·ics** (ĕs-thĕt′ĭks) *n.* The study of psychological aspects of beauty, especially with the components thereof as they relate to appearance.

aesthetic surgery *n.* Plastic or cosmetic surgery.

af– *pref.* Variant of **ad–** (sense 1).

AFB *abbr.* acid-fast bacillus

a·feb·rile (ā-fĕb′rəl, ā-fē′brəl) *adj.* Apyretic.

a·fe·tal (ā-fēt′l, ə-fēt′l) *adj.* Lacking a fetus or intrauterine life.

af·fect (ə-fĕkt′) *v.* **1.** To have an influence on or affect a change in. **2.** To attack or infect, as a disease. —*n.*

(ăf**/**ĕkt**/**) Feeling or emotion, especially as manifested by facial expression or body language.

af·fec·tion (ə-fĕk**/**shən) *n.* **1.** A tender feeling toward another; fondness. **2.** A bodily condition; disease.

af·fec·tive (ə-fĕk**/**tĭv) *adj.* **1.** Concerned with or arousing feelings or emotions; emotional. **2.** Influenced by or resulting from the emotions, as of a psychological disorder.

affective disorder *n.* See **mood disorder.**

affective psychosis *n.* Psychosis characterized chiefly by emotional disturbance.

af·fer·ent (ăf**/**ər-ənt) *adj.* Carrying inward to a central organ or section, as nerves that conduct impulses from the periphery of the body to the brain or spinal cord. —*n.* An afferent organ or body part, such as a blood vessel.

afferent fiber *n.* Any of the nerve fibers that convey impulses to a ganglion or to a nerve center in the brain or spinal cord.

afferent glomerular arteriole *n.* A branch of an interlobular artery of the kidney that conveys blood to the glomerule.

afferent-loop syndrome *n.* Chronic obstruction of the duodenum and jejunum after gastrojejunostomy, resulting in abdominal distention and pain.

afferent nerve *n.* A nerve conveying impulses from the periphery to the central nervous system. Also called *centripetal nerve.*

afferent vessel *n.* **1.** An artery conveying blood to a part. **2.** A lymphatic vessel entering a lymph node. **3.** The arteriole that enters a renal glomerulus.

af·fin·i·ty (ə-fĭn**/**ĭ-tē) *n.* **1.** An attraction or a force between particles that causes them to combine. **2.** The attraction between an antigen and an antibody. **3.** A relationship or resemblance in structure between species that suggests a common origin. **4.** The selective staining of a tissue by a dye. **5.** The selective uptake of a dye, chemical, or other substance by a tissue.

af·flux (ăf**/**lŭks**/**) *n.* A flow to or toward an area, especially of blood or other fluid toward a body part.

a-fib (ā**/**fĭb**/**) *n.* See **atrial fibrillation.**

A fiber *n.* Any of the myelinated nerve fibers in somatic nerves, measuring 1 to 22 microns in diameter, conducting nerve impulses at a rate of 6 to 120 meters per second.

a·fi·bril·lar (ā-fī**/**brə-lər, ā-fĭb**/**-) *adj.* Not containing fibrils.

a·fi·brin·o·ge·ne·mi·a (ā**/**fī-brĭn**/**ə-jə-nē**/**mē-ə, ā-fī**/**-brə-nō-) *n.* The absence of fibrinogen in the blood plasma.

af·la·tox·i·co·sis (ăf**/**lə-tŏk**/**sĭ-kō**/**sĭs) *n.* Poisoning that is caused by the consumption of substances or foods contaminated with aflatoxin.

af·la·tox·in (ăf**/**lə-tŏk**/**sĭn) *n.* Any of a group of toxic compounds produced by certain molds, especially *Aspergillus flavus,* that contaminate stored food supplies such as animal feed and peanuts.

AFP *abbr.* alpha-fetoprotein

Af·ri·can sleeping sickness (ăf**/**rĭ-kən) *n.* African trypanosomiasis.

African trypanosomiasis *n.* Either of two types of an often fatal, endemic infectious disease of humans and animals in tropical Africa: Gambian trypanosomiasis or Rhodesian trypanosomiasis.

Af·rin (ăf**/**rĭn) A trademark for the hydrochloride form of the drug oxymetazoline.

af·ter·birth (ăf**/**tər-bûrth**/**) *n.* The placenta and fetal membranes expelled from the uterus following childbirth. Also called *secundines.*

af·ter·care (ăf**/**tər-kâr**/**) *n.* Follow-up care provided after a medical procedure or treatment program.

af·ter·hear·ing (ăf**/**tər-hîr**/**ĭng) *n.* See **aftersound.**

af·ter·im·age (ăf**/**tər-ĭm**/**ĭj) *n.* A visual image that persists after the visual stimulus causing it has ceased to act. Also called *photogene.*

af·ter·im·pres·sion (ăf**/**tər-ĭm-prĕsh**/**ən) *n.* See **aftersensation.**

af·ter·load (ăf**/**tər-lōd**/**) *n.* **1.** The arrangement of a muscle so that it lifts a weight from an adjustable support or works against a constant opposing force to which it is not exposed when at rest. **2.** The load or force thus encountered.

af·ter·pains (ăf**/**tər-pānz**/**) *pl.n.* Cramps or pains following childbirth, caused by contractions of the uterus.

af·ter·per·cep·tion (ăf**/**tər-pər-sĕp**/**shən) *n.* Perception of a sensation after the stimulus that produced it has ceased to act.

af·ter·po·ten·tial (ăf**/**tər-pə-tĕn**/**shəl) *n.* A small negative or positive change in electrical potential in a stimulated nerve that follows and is dependent on the main potential.

af·ter·sen·sa·tion (ăf**/**tər-sĕn-sā**/**shən) *n.* A sensory impression, such as an afterimage or aftertaste, that persists after the stimulus has ceased. Also called *afterimpression.*

af·ter·sound (ăf**/**tər-sound**/**) *n.* The sensation of hearing a sound after the cause of the sound has ceased. Also called *afterhearing.*

af·ter·taste (ăf**/**tər-tāst**/**) *n.* A taste persisting in the mouth after the substance that caused it is no longer present.

a·func·tion·al occlusion (ā-fŭngk**/**shə-nəl) *n.* A malocclusion that does not permit normal biting and chewing function of the teeth.

Ag The symbol for the element **silver.**

ag– *pref.* Variant of **ad–** (sense 1).

AGA *abbr.* appropriate for gestational age

a·ga·lac·ti·a (ā**/**gə-lăk**/**tē-ə, -shē-ə, ăg**/**ə-) *n.* Absence of or faulty secretion of milk following childbirth. Also called *agalactosis.* —**a**'**ga·lac**'**tous** (-təs) *adj.*

a·ga·lac·tor·rhe·a (ā**/**gə-lăk**/**tə-rē**/**ə) *n.* Cessation of the flow of milk.

a·gal·ac·to·sis (ā-găl**/**ək-tō**/**sĭs, ə-găl**/**-) *n.* See **agalactia.**

a·gam·ic (ā-găm**/**ĭk) *or* **ag·a·mous** (ăg**/**ə-məs) *adj.* Occurring or reproducing without the union of male and female cells; asexual or parthenogenetic.

a·gam·ma·glob·u·lin·e·mi·a (ā-găm**/**ə-glŏb**/**yə-lə-nē**/**-mē-ə) *n.* Congenital or acquired absence of, or extremely low levels of, gamma globulins in the blood.

a·gan·gli·on·ic (ā-găng**/**glē-ŏn**/**ĭk) *adj.* Lacking the presence of ganglia.

a·gan·gli·o·no·sis (ā-găng′glē-ə-nō′sĭs) *n.* **1.** Absence of ganglion cells. **2.** Congenital absence of the myenteric plexus ganglion cells.

a·gar (ā′gär′, ä′gär′) *or* **a·gar-a·gar** (ā′gär-ā′gär′, ä′gär-ä′-) *n.* **1.** A gelatinous material derived from marine algae, used as a base for bacterial culture media and as a stabilizer and thickener in food. **2.** A culture medium containing this material.

ag·ar·ic (ăg′ər-ĭk, ə-găr′ĭk) *n.* **1.** Any of various mushrooms of the genera *Agaricus, Fomes,* or related genera, having large umbrellalike caps with numerous gills beneath. **2.** The dried fruiting body of certain fungi of the genus *Fomes,* formerly used to inhibit the production of sweat.

agaric acid *or* **ag·a·ric·ic acid** (ăg′ə-rĭs′ĭk) *or* **a·gar·i·cin·ic acid** (ə-găr′ə-sĭn′ĭk) *n.* An acid obtained from agaric and responsible for the anhidrotic action of the fungus.

a·gas·tric (ā-găs′trĭk, ə-găs′-) *adj.* Lacking a stomach or digestive tract.

age (āj) *n.* The length of time that one has existed; duration of life. —*v.* **1.** To become old. **2.** To manifest traits associated with old age.

a·gen·e·sis (ā-jĕn′ĭ-sĭs) *n.* Absence or incomplete development of an organ or body part.

a·gen·i·tal·ism (ā-jĕn′ĭ-tl-ĭz′əm) *n.* Congenital absence of genitals.

a·gen·o·so·mi·a (ā-jĕn′ə-sō′mē-ə, ə-jĕn′-) *n.* Defective formation or absence of the genitalia in a fetus.

a·gent (ā′jənt) *n.* A force or substance, such as a chemical, that causes a change.

Agent Orange *n.* A herbicide that contains trace amounts of the toxic contaminant dioxin, used in the Vietnam War to defoliate areas of forest.

age spot *n.* A benign, localized brownish patch on the skin, often occurring in old age and most often in people with pale, sun-damaged skin. Also called *liver spot, senile lentigo.*

a·geu·sia (ə-gyōō′zhə, -jōō′-) *n.* Loss of the sense of taste.

ag·glu·ti·nant (ə-glōōt′n-ənt) *n.* A substance that holds parts together or causes agglutination.

ag·glu·ti·nate (ə-glōōt′n-āt′) *v.* **1.** To clump together; undergo agglutination. **2.** To cause substances, such as bacteria, to clump together. —*n.* See **agglutination** (sense 3).

ag·glu·ti·na·tion (ə-glōōt′n-ā′shən) *n.* **1.** The act or process of agglutinating. **2.** The clumping together of red blood cells or bacteria, usually in response to a particular antibody. **3.** A clumped mass of material formed by agglutination. Also called *agglutinate.* **4.** Adhesion of wound surfaces in healing.

agglutination test *n.* Any of various tests in which blood serum causes agglutination of bacteria or blood cells of a foreign type, used to determine infection and to identify pathogens and blood types.

ag·glu·ti·na·tive (ə-glōōt′n-ā′tĭv, -ə-tĭv) *adj.* Concerning or characteristic of agglutination.

ag·glu·ti·nin (ə-glōōt′n-ĭn) *n.* **1.** A substance, such as an antibody, that is capable of causing agglutination of a particular antigen, especially red blood cells or bacteria. **2.** A substance, other than a specific agglutinating antibody, that causes organic particles to agglutinate.

ag·glu·tin·o·gen (ăg′lōō-tĭn′ə-jən, ə-glōōt′n-) *n.* An antigen that stimulates the production of a particular agglutinin, such as an antibody. Also called *agglutogen.* —**ag′glu·tin′o·gen′ic** (ăg′lōō-tĭn′ə-gĕn′ĭk, ə-glōōt′n-) *adj.*

ag·glu·ti·no·phil·ic (ə-glōōt′n-ə-fĭl′ĭk) *adj.* Readily undergoing agglutination.

ag·glu·to·gen (ə-glōō′tə-jən) *n.* See **agglutinogen.**

ag·gre·gate (ăg′rĭ-gĭt) *adj.* Crowded or massed into a dense cluster. —*n.* A total considered with reference to its constituent parts; a gross amount in a mass or cluster. —*v.* (-gāt′) To gather into a mass, sum, or whole.

ag·gre·gat·ed lymphatic follicles (ăg′rĭ-gā′tĭd) *pl.n.* Collections of many lymphoid follicles closely packed together, forming oblong elevations on the mucous membrane of the small intestine. Also called *aggregate glands, agminate glands, Peyer's patches.*

aggregate glands *pl.n.* See **aggregated lymphatic follicles.**

ag·gre·ga·tion (ăg′rĭ-gā′shən) *n.* A massing together or clustering of independent but similar units, such as particles, parts, or bodies.

ag·gres·sion (ə-grĕsh′ən) *n.* Hostile or destructive behavior or actions.

ag·gres·sive (ə-grĕs′ĭv) *adj.* **1.** Characterized by aggression. **2.** Inclined to behave in a hostile fashion. **3.** Tending to spread quickly, as a tumor; fast-growing. **4.** Characterized by or inclined toward vigorous or intensive medical treatment.

aggressive infantile fibromatosis *n.* A childhood counterpart of abdominal or extra-abdominal desmoid tumors, characterized by firm subcutaneous nodules that grow rapidly in any part of the body but do not metastasize.

ag·ing (ā′jĭng) *n.* **1.** The process of growing old or maturing. **2.** The gradual changes in the structure of a mature organism that occur normally over time and increase the probability of death.

agit. ante us. *abbr. Latin* agita ante usum (shake before using)

ag·i·tat·ed depression (ăj′ĭ-tā′tĭd) *n.* A form of depression characterized by restlessness and nervous activity.

agit. bene *abbr. Latin* agita bene (shake well)

a·glos·so·sto·mi·a (ā-glŏs′ə-stō′mē-ə, ə-glŏs′-) *n.* Congenital absence of a tongue and a mouth.

ag·lu·ti·tion (ăg′lōō-tĭsh′ən) *n.* See **dysphagia.**

a·gly·co·su·ri·a (ā-glī′kə-sŏŏr′ē-ə, -shŏŏr′-, ə-glī′-) *n.* Absence of sugar in the urine. —**a·gly′co·su′ric** *adj.*

ag·mi·nate glands (ăg′mə-nāt′, -nĭt) *pl.n.* See **aggregated lymphatic follicles.**

ag·nail (ăg′nāl′) *n.* **1.** A hangnail. **2.** A painful sore or swelling around a fingernail or toenail.

ag·na·thi·a (ăg-nā′thē-ə) *n.* Congenital absence or partial absence of the lower jaw.

ag·no·gen·ic (ăg′nə-jĕn′ĭk) *adj.* Idiopathic.

ag·no·sia (ăg-nō′zhə) *n.* Loss of the ability to interpret sensory stimuli, such as sounds or images.

–agogue *or* **–agog** *suff.* A substance that stimulates the flow of: *hemagogue.*

ag·om·pho·sis (ăg′ŏm-fō′sĭs) *or* **ag·om·phi·a·sis** (-fī′-ə-sĭs) *n.* See **anodontia.**

a·go·nad·al (ā′gō-năd′l, ə-gō′năd′l) *adj.* Congenital or acquired absence of ovaries or testes.

ag·o·nist (ăg′ə-nĭst) *n.* **1.** A contracting muscle that is resisted or counteracted by an antagonistic muscle. **2.** A substance that can combine with a cell receptor to produce a reaction typical for that substance.

ag·o·ra·pho·bi·a (ăg′ər-ə-fō′bē-ə) *n.* Phobia of open or public places. —**ag′o·ra·pho′bic** *adj.*

–agra *suff.* Sudden acute pain: *podagra.*

a·gram·ma·tism (ā-grăm′ə-tĭz′əm, ə-grăm′-) *n.* A form of aphasia characterized by the inability to produce a grammatical or intelligible sentence.

a·gran·u·lar endoplasmic reticulum (ā-grăn′yə-lər) *n.* Endoplasmic reticulum lacking in ribosomal granules, usually a characteristic of cells that secrete steroid hormones.

a·gran·u·lo·cyte (ā-grăn′yə-lō-sīt′, ə-grăn′-) *n.* A nongranular white blood cell.

a·gran·u·lo·cy·to·sis (ā-grăn′yə-lō-sī-tō′sĭs, ə-grăn′-yə-) *n.* An acute disease characterized by high fever, lesions of the mucous membranes and skin, and a sharp drop in circulating granular white blood cells.

a·gran·u·lo·plas·tic (ā-grăn′yə-lō-plăs′tĭk, ə-grăn′yə-) *adj.* **1.** Incapable of forming granular cells. **2.** Forming only nongranular cells.

a·graph·i·a (ā-grăf′ē-ə) *n.* A form of aphasia characterized by loss of the ability to write. Also called *anorthography.* —**a·graph′ic** *adj.*

ag·ri·a (ăg′rē-ə) *n.* An extensive pustular eruption.

a·gue (ā′gyōō) *n.* **1.** A febrile condition, especially associated with malaria, characterized by alternating periods of chills, fever, and sweating. **2.** A chill or fit of shivering.

a·gy·ri·a (ə-jī′rē-ə) *n.* Congenital malformation or absence of the convolutions of the cerebral cortex. Also called *lissencephalia.*

AHF *abbr.* antihemophilic factor

AHG *abbr.* antihemophilic globulin

A·hu·ma·da-Del Castillo syndrome (ä′ōō-mä′də-) *n.* Galactorrhea and amenorrhea when unrelated to the termination of a pregnancy.

AI *abbr.* artificial insemination

AID *abbr.* artificial insemination donor

aid·man (ād′măn′) *n.* A member of an army medical corps attached to a field unit.

AIDS (ādz) *n.* A severe immunological disorder caused by the retrovirus HIV, resulting in a defect in cell-mediated immune response that is manifested by increased susceptibility to opportunistic infections and to certain rare cancers, especially Kaposi's sarcoma. It is transmitted primarily by exposure to contaminated body fluids, especially blood and semen.

AIDS dementia complex *n.* The neurological disease complex that is sometimes experienced by AIDS patients, caused by neuron injury and death and characterized by cognitive impairment.

AIDS-related complex *n. Abbr.* **ARC** A combination of symptoms, including fever, lymphadenopathy, blood abnormalities, and susceptibility to opportunistic infections that is a precursor to AIDS in some individuals infected with HIV.

AIDS virus *n.* See **HIV.**

AIH *abbr.* artificial insemination performed by the husband; artificial insemination, homologous (using the husband's semen)

ail·ment (āl′mənt) *n.* A physical or mental disorder, especially a mild illness.

ai·lu·ro·pho·bi·a (ī-lōōr′ə-fō′bē-ə, ā-lōōr′-) *n.* An abnormal fear of or aversion to cats.

air (âr) *n.* **1.** A colorless, odorless, tasteless, gaseous mixture, approximately 78 percent nitrogen and approximately 21 percent oxygen with lesser amounts of argon, carbon dioxide, hydrogen, neon, helium, and other gases. **2.** This mixture, with varying amounts of moisture and particulate matter, enveloping Earth; the atmosphere. **3.** Any of various respiratory gases. No longer in technical use.

air-bone gap *n.* The difference between the threshold for hearing acuity by bone conduction and by air conduction.

air cell *n.* **1.** A terminal dilation of the bronchiole where gas exchange is thought to occur. **2.** Spaces that contain air in the bones of the skull.

air-conditioner lung *n.* Extrinsic allergic alveolitis caused by forced air contaminated by thermophilic actinomycetes and other organisms.

air conduction *n.* The atmospheric transmission of sound to the inner ear through the external auditory canal and via structures of the middle ear.

air embolism *n.* Bubbles of air in the heart or vascular system that create an obstruction and are usually the result of surgery or trauma.

air·plane splint (âr′plān′) *n.* A splint that holds the arm in abduction at about shoulder level with the forearm midway in flexion.

air pollution *n.* Contamination of air by smoke and harmful gases, mainly oxides of carbon, sulfur, and nitrogen.

air sac *n.* A tiny, thin-walled, capillary-rich sac in the lungs where the exchange of oxygen and carbon dioxide takes place. Also called *alveolar sac.*

air·sick·ness (âr′sĭk′nĭs) *n.* A form of motion sickness caused by air flight and characterized by nausea, vomiting, and dizziness.

air splint *n.* A hollow tubular inflatable splint.

air syringe *n.* See **chip syringe.**

air·way (âr′wā′) *n.* **1.** Any of the various parts of the respiratory tract through which air passes during breathing. **2.** A device used to gain an unobstructed route to convey air into and out of the lungs during general anesthesia or when the respiratory passage is blocked.

AKA *abbr.* above-the-knee amputation

A-K amputation *n.* Amputation of the limb from above the knee.

ak·a·mu·shi disease (ăk′ə-mōō′shē, ä′kə-) *n.* See **scrub typhus.**

a·kar·y·o·cyte (ā-kăr′ē-ə-sīt′, ə-kăr′-) *n.* A cell having no nucleus. Also called *acaryote, akaryote.*

a·kar·y·ote (ā-kăr′ē-ōt′, ə-kăr′-) *n.* See **akaryocyte.**

ak·a·this·i·a *or* **ac·a·this·i·a** (ăk′ə-thĭz′ē-ə) *n.* **1.** Motor restlessness characterized by muscular quivering and the inability to sit still, often a result of chronic ingestion of neuroleptic drugs. **2.** Intense anxiety at the thought of sitting down; inability to sit down.

a·ker·a·to·sis (ə-kĕr′ə-tō′sĭs) *n.* Deficiency or absence of horny tissue such as nails.

Å·ker·lund deformity (ĕk′ər-lŏŏnd′, ô′kər-) *n.* A deformity of the duodenal cap as seen in a radiograph of a duodenal ulcer, consisting of an indentation of the cap in addition to the ulcerated area.

a·ki·ne·sia (ā′kĭ-nē′zhə, -kī-) *or* **a·ki·ne·sis** (-sĭs) *n.* A slowness or loss of normal motor function resulting in impaired muscle movement. —**a′ki·ne′sic** (-zĭk, -sĭk), **a′ki·net′ic** (-nĕt′ĭk) *adj.*

a·kin·es·the·sia (ā-kĭn′ĭs-thē′zhə, ā-kī′nĭs-) *n.* Loss of the ability to perceive movement.

akinetic mutism *n.* A syndrome characterized by the inability to speak, loss of voluntary movement, and apparent loss of emotional feeling. It is related to lesions of the upper brainstem.

Al The symbol for the element **aluminum.**

al– *pref.* Variant of **ad–** (sense 1).

–al *suff.* Aldehyde: *butyral.*

a·la (ā′lə) *n., pl.* **a·lae** (ā′lē) A winglike or expanded structure or part, such as the external ear.

Ala *abbr.* alanine

ALA (ā′ĕl-ā′) *n.* Delta-aminolevulinic acid; an intermediate in the biosynthesis of hematin formed from glycine and succinyl-coenzyme A.

a·lac·ri·ma (ā-lăk′rə-mə) *n.* Hereditary or congenital deficiency or absence of tear secretion.

a·la·li·a (ə-lā′lē-ə) *n.* Impairment or loss of the ability to talk.

ala na·si (nā′zī) *n.* The outer wall of each nostril.

al·a·nine (ăl′ə-nēn′) *n. Abbr.* **Ala** A crystalline amino acid that is a constituent of many proteins.

alanine aminotransferase *n. Abbr.* **ALT** See **SGPT.**

al·a·nyl (ăl′ə-nĭl′) *n.* The acyl radical of alanine, $CH_3CH(NH_2)CO.$

a·lar (ā′lər) *adj.* **1.** Resembling, containing, or composed of wings or alae; axillary. **2.** Relating to the ala of such structures as the nose, sphenoid bone, and sacrum.

alar cartilage *n.* **1.** Either of a pair of cartilages that form the tip of the nose; greater alar cartilage. **2.** Any of the cartilaginous plates of the wing of the nose posterior to the greater alar cartilage; lesser alar cartilage.

a·larm reaction (ə-lärm′) *n.* The initial stage in the body's response to stressful stimuli, characterized by adaptive physiological changes, such as increased hormonal activity and increased heart rate.

alar spine *n.* See **sphenoidal spine.**

al·ba (ăl′bə) *n.* See **white matter.**

Al·bers-Schön·berg disease (ăl′bərs-shûrn′bûrg, -shœn′bĕrk′) *n.* See **osteopetrosis.**

al·bi·cans (ăl′bĭ-kănz′) *n., pl.* **al·bi·can·ti·a** (ăl′bĭ-kăn′tē-ə) The white fibrous scar tissue in an ovary that results after the involution and regression of the corpus luteum. Also called *corpus albicans.*

al·bi·du·ri·a (ăl′bĭ-dŏŏr′ē-ə) *or* **al·bi·nu·ri·a** (-nŏŏr′ē-ə) *n.* The passing of pale or white urine having a low specific gravity.

al·bi·nism (ăl′bə-nĭz′əm) *n.* **1.** Congenital absence of normal pigmentation or coloration in the eyes only or

in the skin, hair, and eyes. **2.** The condition of being an albino. —**al′bi·not′ic** (-nŏt′ĭk) *adj.*

Al·bi·ni's nodules (ăl-bē′nēz, äl-) *pl.n.* Minute fibrous nodules on the margins of the mitral and tricuspid valves of the heart, present in the neonate.

al·bi·no (ăl-bī′nō) *n., pl.* **–nos** A person or an animal lacking normal pigmentation, resulting in abnormally pale or white skin and hair and pink or blue eyes with a deep-red pupil.

Al·bi·nus (ăl-bī′nəs), **Bernard Siegfried** 1697–1770. German anatomist who is noted for his study of the connections between the vascular systems of mother and fetus.

Al·bright's disease (ôl′brīts) *n.* Fibrous dysplasia involving multiple bones and characterized by irregular brown spots on the skin, endocrine dysfunction, and precocious puberty, especially in girls.

al·bu·gin·e·a (ăl′bə-jĭn′ē-ə, -byə-) *n.* A tough whitish layer of fibrous tissue, especially the dense white membrane covering the testicle.

al·bu·men (ăl-byŏŏ′mən) *n.* **1.** The white of an egg, which consists mainly of albumin dissolved in water. **2.** Albumin.

al·bu·min (ăl-byŏŏ′mĭn) *n.* A class of simple, water-soluble proteins that can be coagulated by heat and precipitated by strong acids and are found in egg white, blood serum, milk, and many other animal and plant juices and tissues.

albumin-globulin ratio *n.* The ratio of albumin to globulin in the serum or urine in kidney disease.

al·bu·mi·noid (ăl-byŏŏ′mə-noid′) *n.* **1.** A fibrous protein. **2.** See **scleroprotein.** —*adj.* Composed of or resembling albumin.

albuminoid degeneration *or* **albuminous degeneration** *n.* See **cloudy swelling.**

al·bu·mi·nu·ri·a (ăl-byŏŏ′mə-nŏŏr′ē-ə) *n.* The presence of protein, usually albumin but at times globulin, in the urine, indicating either dysfunction or disease. Also called *proteinuria.*

al·bu·mose (ăl′byə-mōs′, -mōz′) *n.* A class of substances derived from albumins and formed by the enzymatic breakdown of proteins during digestion.

al·bu·ter·ol (ăl-byŏŏ′tə-rôl′, -rōl′) *n.* A beta-adrenergic stimulant used as a bronchodilator in the treatment of asthma and other obstructive lung diseases.

al·cap·ton (ăl-kăp′tŏn′, -tən) *n.* Variant of **alkapton.**

al·cap·to·nu·ri·a (ăl-kăp′tə-nŏŏr′ē-ə) *n.* Variant of **alkaptonuria.**

Alc·mae·on (ălk-mē′ən) fl. sixth century BC. Greek physician and philosopher. He was the first known anatomist and probably the first to perform scientific dissections of human bodies.

Al·cock's canal (ăl′kŏks′, ôl′-) *n.* See **pudendal canal.**

al·co·hol (ăl′kə-hôl′) *n.* **1.** Any of a series of hydroxyl compounds derived from saturated hydrocarbons, including ethanol and methanol. **2.** A colorless, volatile, flammable liquid synthesized or obtained by fermentation of sugars and starches and widely used, either pure or denatured, as a solvent and in drugs. Also called *ethanol, ethyl alcohol.* **3.** Intoxicating liquor containing alcohol.

alcohol dehydrogenase *n.* An enzyme that catalyzes the

oxidation of ethanol to acetaldehyde as the first step in its metabolism by the liver.

al·co·hol·ic (ăl′kə-hô′lĭk) *adj.* **1.** Related to or resulting from alcohol. **2.** Containing or preserved in alcohol. **3.** Suffering from alcoholism. —*n.* A person who drinks alcoholic substances habitually and to excess or who suffers from alcoholism.

alcoholic cirrhosis *n.* Cirrhosis that frequently develops in chronic alcoholism, characterized at an early stage by enlargement of the liver due to fatty change with mild fibrosis, and later by Laënnec's cirrhosis with contraction of the liver.

alcoholic psychosis *n.* Any of various psychoses that result from alcoholism and involve organic brain damage.

al·co·hol·ism (ăl′kə-hô-lĭz′əm) *n.* **1.** The compulsive consumption of and psychophysiological dependence on alcoholic beverages. **2.** A chronic, progressive pathological condition, mainly affecting the nervous and digestive systems, caused by the excessive and habitual consumption of alcohol. Also called *chronic alcoholism.* **3.** Temporary mental disturbance and muscular incoordination caused by excessive consumption of alcohol. Also called *acute alcoholism.*

al·co·hol·y·sis (ăl′kə-hô′lĭ-sĭs) *n., pl.* **–ses** (-sēz′) A reaction in which a chemical bond is broken by the addition of alcohol.

ALD *abbr.* adrenoleukodystrophy

Al·dac·tone (ăl-dăk′tōn) A trademark for the drug spironolactone.

al·de·hyde (ăl′də-hīd′) *n.* **1.** Any of a class of reactive organic chemical compounds obtained by oxidation of primary alcohols, characterized by the common group CHO, and used in the manufacture of resins, dyes, and organic acids. **2.** See **acetaldehyde.**

Al·der (ăl′dər), **Kurt** 1902–1958. German chemist. He shared a 1950 Nobel Prize for discoveries concerning the structure of organic matter.

Al·der's anomaly (ăl′dərz) *n.* Coarse azurophilic granulation of white blood cells, especially granulocytes.

al·dol (ăl′dôl, -dōl) *n.* **1.** A thick, colorless to pale yellow liquid obtained from acetaldehyde and used in perfumery and as a solvent. **2.** A similar aldehyde containing the group CH₃OH–CO–CHOH.

al·dol·ase (ăl′də-lās′, lāz′) *n.* An enzyme present in certain living tissues, including skeletal and heart muscle tissues, that catalyzes the breakdown of a fructose ester into triose sugars.

Al·do·met (ăl′də-mĕt′) A trademark for the drug methyldopa.

al·do·pen·tose (ăl′dō-pĕn′tōs′) *n.* A pentose containing an aldehyde group.

al·dose (ăl′dōs′, -dōz′) *n.* Any of a class of monosaccharide sugars containing an aldehyde group.

al·dos·ter·one (ăl-dŏs′tə-rōn′) *n.* A steroid hormone secreted by the adrenal cortex that regulates the salt and water balance in the body.

al·dos·ter·on·ism (ăl-dŏs′tə-rō-nĭz′əm, ăl′dō-stĕr′ə-) *n.* A disorder marked by excessive secretion of the hormone aldosterone, which can cause weakness, cardiac irregularities, and abnormally high blood pressure. Also called *hyperaldosteronism.*

Al·drich syndrome (ôl′drĭch) *n.* See **Wiskott-Aldrich syndrome.**

a·lec·i·thal (ă-lĕs′ə-thəl) *adj.* Relating to an egg that has little or no yolk.

a·len·dro·nate sodium (ə-lĕn′drə-nāt′) *n.* A synthetic drug analog of pyrophosphate that acts primarily on bone to inhibit its resorption and is used to treat and prevent osteoporosis in postmenopausal women.

A·lep·po boil (ə-lĕp′ō) *n.* The lesion found in cutaneous leishmaniasis. Also called *Bagdad boil, date boil.*

A·lesse (ə-lĕs′) A trademark for an oral contraceptive drug containing ethinyl estradiol and levonorgestrel.

a·leu·ke·mi·a (ā′lōō-kē′mē-ə, ăl′ōō-) *n.* **1.** An absence of white blood cells in the blood. Usually used in reference to varieties of leukemic disease in which the blood's white cell count is normal or low but contains a few young white blood cells. **2.** The leukemic changes in bone marrow associated with a subnormal number of white blood cells in the blood. —**a′leu·ke′mic** *adj.*

aleukemic leukemia *n.* Leukemia characterized by a normal or low number of white blood cells in the blood despite leukemic changes in tissues.

a·leu·ke·moid (ā′lōō-kē′moid′) *adj.* Relating to or characteristic of the symptoms of aleukemia.

a·leu·ki·a (ā-lōō′kē-ə, ə-lōō′-) *n.* An absence or extreme reduction in the number of white blood cells in circulating blood.

a·leu·ko·cy·to·sis (ā-lōō′kō-sī-tō′sĭs) *n.* An absence or severe reduction in the number of white blood cells in blood or in a lesion.

A·leve (ə-lēv′) A trademark for the drug naproxen.

Al·ex·an·der's deafness (ăl′ĭg-zăn′dərz) *n.* The inability to hear high frequencies due to the abnormal development of the cochlear duct.

a·lex·i·a (ə-lĕk′sē-ə) *n.* Loss of the ability to comprehend the meaning of written or printed words and sentences, usually caused by brain lesions. Also called *text blindness, visual aphasia, word blindness.* —**a·lex′ic** *adj.*

a·lex·i·thy·mi·a (ə-lĕk′sə-thī′mē-ə) *n.* Inability to describe emotions in a verbal manner.

al·gae (ăl′jē) *pl.n.* Any of various chiefly aquatic, eukaryotic, photosynthetic organisms, ranging in size from single-celled forms to the giant kelp.

al·ge·si·a (ăl-jē′zē-ə, -zhə) *n.* Hypersensitivity to pain. Also called *algesthesia.*

al·ge·sic (ăl-jē′zĭk) *adj.* **1.** Relating to hypersensitivity to pain. **2.** Relating to or causing pain.

al·ge·si·a·dys·tro·phy (ăl-jē′zĭ-dĭs′trə-fē, -sĭ-) *n.* See **algodystrophy.**

al·ge·si·o·gen·ic (ăl-jē′zē-ə-jĕn′ĭk) *adj.* Producing pain. Also called *algogenic.*

al·ge·si·om·e·ter (ăl-jē′zē-ŏm′ĭ-tər) *or* **al·ge·sim·e·ter** (ăl′jĭ-sĭm′ĭ-tər) *n.* An instrument for measuring sensitivity to a painful stimulus. Also called *algometer, odynometer.*

al·ges·the·sia (ăl′jĕs-thē′zhə) *n.* **1.** The ability to sense pain. **2.** See **algesia.**

al·ges·the·sis (ăl′jĕs-thē′sĭs) *n.* The perception of pain.

–algia *suff.* Pain: *neuralgia.*

al·gi·cide (ăl′jĭ-sīd′) *n.* A substance that kills or inhibits the growth of algae.

al·gid stage (ăl′jĭd) *n.* The stage of collapse in cholera.

algo– *pref.* Pain: *algophobia.*

al·go·dys·tro·phy (ăl′gō-dĭs′trə-fē) *n.* A local disturbance of growth, particularly in bone and cartilage, that causes pain. Also called *algesidystrophy.*

al·go·gen·ic (ăl′gō-jĕn′ĭk) *adj.* See **algesiogenic.**

al·go·lag·ni·a (ăl′gō-lăg′nē-ə) *n.* Sexual gratification derived from inflicting or experiencing pain.

al·gom·e·ter (ăl-gŏm′ĭ-tər) *n.* See **algesiometer.**

al·go·phil·i·a (ăl′gə-fĭl′ē-ə) *n.* Abnormal pleasure in receiving or inflicting pain.

al·go·pho·bi·a (ăl′gə-fō′bē-ə) *n.* An abnormal fear of pain.

al·go·rithm (ăl′gə-rĭth′əm) *n.* A step-by-step protocol, as for management of health care problems.

al·gor mor·tis (ăl′gər môr′tĭs) *n.* The cooling of the body that follows death.

al·go·vas·cu·lar (ăl′gō-văs′kyə-lər) *or* **an·gi·o·vas·cu·lar** (ăn′jē-ō-) *adj.* Relating to the changes in the lumen of blood vessels in response to pain.

al·i·ble (ăl′ə-bəl) *adj.* Having nutrients; nourishing.

al·i·cy·clic (ăl′ĭ-sī′klĭk, -sĭk′lĭk) *adj.* Of or relating to organic compounds having both aliphatic and cyclic characteristics or structures.

al·ien·a·tion (āl′yə-nā′shən, ā′lē-ə-) *n.* A state of estrangement between the self and the objective world or between different parts of the personality.

a·li·e·ni·a (ā′lī-ē′nē-ə) *n.* Absence of the spleen.

al·ien·ist (āl′yə-nĭst, ā′lē-ə-) *n.* A physician accepted by a court of law as an expert on the mental competence of principals or witnesses.

a·li·form (ā′lə-fôrm′, ăl′ə-) *adj.* Shaped like a wing; alar.

a·lign·ment curve (ə-līn′mənt) *n.* The line passing through the center of the teeth lateral to the curve of the dental arch.

al·i·ment (ăl′ə-mənt) *n.* **1.** Something that nourishes; food. **2.** Something that supports or sustains. —*v.* To supply with sustenance, such as food.

al·i·men·ta·ry (ăl′ə-mĕn′tə-rē, -trē) *adj.* **1.** Concerned with food, nutrition, or digestion. **2.** Providing nourishment.

alimentary canal *n.* The mucous membrane-lined tube of the digestive system that extends from the mouth to the anus and through which food passes, digestion takes place, and wastes are eliminated; it includes the pharynx, esophagus, stomach, and intestines. Also called *alimentary tract, digestive tract.*

alimentary glycosuria *n.* Glycosuria developing after the ingestion of a moderate amount of sugar or starch, which normally is metabolized without appearing in the urine.

alimentary lipemia *n.* Transient lipemia occurring after the ingestion of foods with a large content of fat. Also called *postprandial lipemia.*

alimentary pentosuria *n.* The urinary excretion of arabinose and xylose as the result of the excessive ingestion of fruits containing these pentoses.

alimentary system *n.* See **digestive system.**

alimentary tract *n.* See **alimentary canal.**

al·i·men·ta·tion (ăl′ə-mĕn-tā′shən) *n.* **1.** The act or process of giving or receiving nourishment. **2.** Support; sustenance.

al·i·na·sal (ăl′ə-nā′zəl, ā′lə-) *adj.* Relating to the flaring portions of the nostrils.

al·i·phat·ic (ăl′ə-făt′ĭk) *adj.* Of, relating to, or being a group of organic chemical compounds in which the carbon atoms are linked in open chains.

aliphatic acids *n.* The acids of nonaromatic hydrocarbons, such as acetic, propionic, and butyric acids.

al·i·quant (ăl′ĭ-kwŏnt′) *n.* A portion that results from dividing the whole in such a manner that some is left after aliquots have been apportioned.

al·i·quot (ăl′ĭ-kwŏt′, -kwət) *n.* A portion of the whole, especially one of two or more samples of something that have the same volume or weight.

al·i·sphe·noid (ăl′ĭ-sfē′noid, ā′lĭ-) *adj.* Relating to the greater wing of the sphenoid bone.

a·liz·a·rin (ə-lĭz′ər-ĭn) *n.* An orange-red crystalline compound used in making dyes and as an indicator.

al·ka·le·mi·a (ăl′kə-lē′mē-ə) *n.* A decrease in hydrogen-ion concentration of the blood or a rise in pH.

al·ka·les·cent (ăl′kə-lĕs′ənt) *adj.* Becoming alkaline; slightly alkaline.

al·ka·li (ăl′kə-lī′) *n.*, *pl.* **-lis** **1.** A carbonate or hydroxide of an alkali metal, the aqueous solution of which is bitter, slippery, caustic, and characteristically basic in reactions. **2.** Any of various soluble mineral salts found in natural water and arid soils. **3.** Alkali metal.

alkali denaturation test *n.* A test for hemoglobin F, based on the fact that hemoglobin F, unlike other hemoglobins, is not denatured by alkali to alkaline hematin.

alkali metal *n.* Any of a group of soft, white, low-density, low-melting, highly reactive metallic elements, including lithium, sodium, potassium, rubidium, cesium, and francium.

al·ka·line (ăl′kə-lĭn, -līn′) *adj.* **1.** Of, relating to, or containing an alkali. **2.** Having a pH greater than 7.

alkaline-ash diet *n.* A diet consisting mainly of fruits, vegetables, and milk with little meat, fish, eggs, cheese, and cereals, that when catabolized leaves an alkaline residue to be excreted in the urine.

alkaline earth *n.* The oxides of calcium, strontium, radium, and barium, and sometimes magnesium.

alkaline-earth metal *n.* Any of a group of metallic elements including calcium, strontium, magnesium, barium, beryllium, and radium.

alkaline phosphatase *n.* A phosphatase with an optimum functioning at pH 8.6; it is present throughout the body.

alkaline tide *n.* A period of urinary neutrality or alkalinity after meals.

al·ka·lin·i·ty (ăl′kə-lĭn′ĭ-tē) *n.* The alkali concentration or alkaline quality of a substance that contains alkali.

al·ka·li·nu·ri·a (ăl′kə-lə-nŏŏr′ē-ə) *n.* A condition characterized by alkalinity of the urine. Also called *alkaluria.*

alkali reserve *n.* The sum total of the basic ions of the blood and other body fluids that act as buffers and maintain the normal pH of the blood.

al·ka·loid (ăl′kə-loid′) *n.* Any of various organic compounds, such as nicotine and morphine, that have basic chemical properties and that usually contain at least one nitrogen atom in a heterocyclic ring.

al·ka·lo·sis (ăl′kə-lō′sĭs) *n.* Abnormally high alkalinity of the blood and body fluids. —**al′ka·lot′ic** (-lŏt′ĭk) *adj.*

al·ka·lu·ri·a (ăl′kə-lŏŏr′ē-ə) *n.* See **alkalinuria.**

al·kane (ăl′kān′) *n.* Any of various saturated open-chain hydrocarbons having the general formula C_nH_{2n+2}, the most abundant of which is methane.

al·kap·ton *or* **al·cap·ton** (ăl-kăp′tŏn′, -tən) *n.* See **homogentisic acid.**

al·kap·to·nu·ri·a *or* **al·cap·to·nu·ri·a** (ăl-kăp′tə-nŏŏr′-ē-ə) *n.* An inherited disorder that affects phenylalanine and tyrosine metabolism and leads to the excretion of homogentisic acid in the urine. Also called *homogentisuria.*

Al·ka-Selt·zer (ăl′kə-sĕlt′zər) A trademark for an over-the-counter preparation containing aspirin and citric acid.

al·kene (ăl′kēn′) *n.* Any of a series of unsaturated, open chain hydrocarbons with one or more carbon-carbon double bonds, having the general formula C_nH_{2n}.

al·kide (ăl′kīd) *n.* A compound in which a metal is combined with alkyl radicals.

al·kyl (ăl′kəl) *n.* A monovalent radical, such as ethyl or propyl, having the general formula C_nH_{2n+1}.

al·kyl·at·ing agent (ăl′kə-lā′tĭng) *n.* Any of various highly reactive chemical compounds that bond with various nucleophilic groups in nucleic acids and proteins and cause mutagenic, carcinogenic, or cytotoxic effects.

al·kyl·a·tion (ăl′kə-lā′shən) *n.* A process in which one or more alkyl groups are substituted for hydrogen atoms in an organic compound.

ALL *abbr.* acute lymphoblastic leukemia

all– *pref.* Variant of **allo–.**

al·la·ches·the·sia (ăl′ə-kĕs-thē′zhə) *n.* See **allesthesia.**

al·lan·ti·a·sis (ăl′ən-tī′ə-sĭs) *n.* Poisoning due to the ingestion of sausages, usually the result of consuming sausages containing the toxins of *Clostridium botulium.* Also called *sausage poisoning.*

allanto– *or* **allant–** *pref.* Sausage-shaped: *allantoid.*

al·lan·to·cho·ri·on (ə-lăn′tō-kôr′ē-ŏn′) *n.* The extraembryonic membrane formed by the fusion of the allantois and the chorion.

al·lan·to·ic sac (ăl′ən-tō′ĭk, -ăn-) *n.* The dilated distal portion of the allantois.

allantoic stalk *n.* The narrow connection between the intraembryonic portion of the allantois and the extraembryonic allantoic vesicle.

allantoic vesicle *n.* The hollow part of the allantois.

al·lan·toid (ə-lăn′toid′) *or* **al·lan·toid·al** (ăl′ən-toid′l) *adj.* **1.** Of or having an allantois. **2.** Shaped like a sausage. —*n.* See **allantois.**

allantoid membrane *n.* Allantois.

al·lan·toi·do·an·gi·op·a·gous twins (ăl′ən-toi′dō-ăn′jē-ŏp′ə-gəs) *pl.n.* Unequal monozygotic twins with fusion of their allantoic vessels within the placenta. Also called *omphaloangiopagous twins.*

al·lan·to·in (ə-lăn′tō-ĭn) *n.* **1.** A substance present in allantoic fluid, amniotic fluid, and fetal urine. **2.** A crystalline oxidation product of uric acid produced in vertebrate purine metabolism and used medicinally to promote tissue growth.

al·lan·to·i·nu·ri·a (ə-lăn′tō-ə-noor′ē-ə) *n.* The excretion of allantoin in the urine.

al·lan·to·is (ə-lăn′tō-ĭs) *n., pl.* **al·lan·to·i·des** (ăl′ən-tō′ĭ-dēz′) A membranous sac that develops from the posterior part of the alimentary canal in the embryos of mammals, birds, and reptiles, and is important in the formation of the umbilical cord and placenta in mammals. Also called *allantoid.* —**al′lan·to′ic** (ăl′ən-tō′ĭk) *adj.*

Al·leg·ra (ə-lĕg′rə) A trademark for the drug fexofenadine hydrochloride.

al·lele (ə-lēl′) *n.* One member of a pair or series of genes that occupies a specific position on a specific chromosome. Also called *allelomorph.* —**al·le′lic** (ə-lē′lĭk, ə-lĕl′ĭk) *adj.*

allelic gene *n.* Allele.

al·le·lo·morph (ə-lē′lə-môrf′, ə-lĕl′ə-) *n.* See **allele.**

al·le·lo·tax·is (ə-lē′lə-tăk′sĭs, ə-lĕl′ə-) *or* **al·le·lo·tax·y** (ə-lē′lə-tăk′sē, ə-lĕl′ə-) *n.* Development of an organ or part from several different embryonic structures or tissues.

Al·len (ăl′ən), **Edgar** 1892–1943. American anatomist who is noted for his studies of hormones and for the discovery (1923) of estrogen.

Al·len's law (ăl′ənz) *n.* The principle that, in contrast to a normal physiology, the more carbohydrate taken by a diabetic, the less carbohydrate is utilized.

Allen test *n.* A test for occlusion of the radial or ulnar artery, in which one of these arteries is compressed after blood has been forced out of the hand by clenching it into a fist; failure of the blood to diffuse into the hand when opened indicates that the artery not compressed is occluded.

al·ler·gen (ăl′ər-jən) *n.* **1.** A substance, such as pollen, that causes an allergy. **2.** See **antigen.** —**al′ler·gen′ic** (-jĕn′ĭk) *adj.*

allergenic extract *or* **allergic extract** *n.* An extract of allergenic components that usually contains protein, is prepared from various sources, and is used to test for an allergy or for desensitization.

al·ler·gic (ə-lûr′jĭk) *adj.* **1.** Of, caused, or characterized by an allergy. **2.** Having an allergy or exhibiting an allergic reaction to a substance.

allergic conjunctivitis *n.* Conjunctivitis caused by an allergic reaction to a substance. Also called *atopic conjunctivitis.*

allergic purpura *n.* **1.** Nonthrombocytopenic purpura due to sensitization to foods, drugs, or insect bites. Also called *anaphylactoid purpura.* **2.** See **Henoch-Schönlein purpura.**

allergic reaction *n.* A local or generalized reaction of an organism to internal or external contact with a specific allergen to which the organism has been previously sensitized.

allergic rhinitis *n.* Rhinitis associated with hay fever.

allergic sa·lute (sə-lŏŏt′) *n.* A wiping or rubbing of the nose with a transverse or upward movement of the hand.

al·ler·gist (ăl′ər-jĭst) *n.* A physician specializing in the diagnosis and treatment of allergies.

al·ler·gy (ăl**′**ər-jē) *n.* An abnormally high acquired sensitivity to certain substances, such as drugs, pollens, or microorganisms, that may include such symptoms as sneezing, itching, and skin rashes.

al·les·the·sia (ăl**′**ĭs-thē**′**zhə) *n.* A condition in which a sensation or stimulus is perceived at a point on the body that is remote from the point that was stimulated. Also called *allachesthesia, allocheiria.*

al·lied health (ăl**′**īd**′**) *n.* A group of medically prescribed health-care services, such as occupational therapy, speech pathology, and physical therapy, provided by licensed professionals.

al·li·ga·tor forceps (ăl**′**ĭ-gā**′**tər) *n.* Long forceps with a small hinged jaw on the end.

alligator skin *n.* See **ichthyosis.**

Al·lis's sign (ăl**′**ĭ-sĭz) *n.* An indication of fracture in the neck of the femur in which a finger easily sinks into the relaxed fascia between the great trochanter and the iliac crest.

allo– *or* **all–** *pref.* **1.** Other; different: *allotransplantation.* **2.** Isomeric: *allomorphism.*

al·lo·an·ti·bod·y (ăl**′**ō-ăn**′**tĭ-bŏd**′**ē) *n.* See **isoantibody.**

al·lo·an·ti·gen (ăl**′**ō-ăn**′**tĭ-jən) *n.* See **isoantigen.**

al·lo·bar·bi·tal (ăl**′**ō-bär**′**bĭ-tôl**′**, -tăl**′**) *n.* A white, crystalline powder used as a sedative and hypnotic.

al·lo·chei·ri·a (ăl**′**ō-kī**′**rē-ə) *n.* See **allesthesia.**

al·lo·chro·ma·sia (ăl**′**ō-krō-mā**′**zhə) *n.* Change in color of the skin or hair.

al·lo·cor·tex (ăl**′**ō-kôr**′**tĕks**′**) *n.* Any of the regions of the cerebral cortex that have fewer cell layers than the isocortex, especially the olfactory cortex and the hippocampus. Also called *heterotypic cortex.*

al·lo·dyn·i·a (ăl**′**ō-dĭn**′**ē-ə) *n.* Pain that results from a noninjurious stimulus to the skin.

al·lo·er·o·tism (ăl**′**ō-ĕr**′**ə-tĭz**′**əm) *or* **al·lo·e·rot·i·cism** (ăl**′**ō-ĭ-rŏt**′**ĭ-sĭz**′**əm) *n.* Sexual attraction toward another person. Also called *heteroerotism.*

al·lo·ge·ne·ic (ăl**′**ō-jə-nē**′**ĭk) *or* **al·lo·gen·ic** (-jĕn**′**ĭk) *adj.* Being genetically different although belonging to or obtained from the same species, as in tissue grafts.

allogeneic graft *n.* See **allograft.**

allogeneic homograft *n.* See **allograft.**

al·lo·graft (ăl**′**ə-grăft**′**) *n.* A graft of tissue obtained from a donor genetically different from, though of the same species as the recipient. Also called *allogeneic graft, allogeneic homograft, homograft, homologous graft, homoplastic graft.*

al·lo·ker·a·to·plas·ty (ăl**′**ō-kĕr**′**ə-tō-plăs**′**tē) *n.* The replacement of opaque corneal tissue with a transparent prosthesis usually made of acrylic.

al·lo·la·li·a (ăl**′**ō-lā**′**lē-ə) *n.* A speech defect that results from a disorder of the speech center.

al·lom·er·ism (ə-lŏm**′**ə-rĭz**′**əm) *n.* Consistency in crystalline form with variation in chemical composition.

al·lom·e·try (ə-lŏm**′**ĭ-trē) *n.* The study of the change in proportion of various parts of an organism as a consequence of growth.

al·lo·mor·phism (ăl**′**ə-môr**′**fĭz**′**əm) *n.* A change in crystalline form that occurs without a change in chemical composition.

al·lop·a·thy (ə-lŏp**′**ə-thē) *n.* A method of treating disease with remedies that produce effects antagonistic to those caused by the disease itself. —**al′lo·path′ic** (ăl**′**ə-păth**′**ĭk) *adj.*

al·lo·plast (ăl**′**ə-plăst**′**) *n.* **1.** A graft of an inert metal or plastic material. **2.** An inert foreign body used for transplantation into tissues.

al·lo·plas·ty (ăl**′**ə-plăs**′**tē) *n.* **1.** The repair of defects by allotransplantation. **2.** A surgical operation in which a synthetic material, such as stainless steel, replaces a body part or tissue.

al·lo·ploi·dy (ăl**′**ə-ploi**′**dē) *n.* A hybrid individual or cell having two or more sets of chromosomes derived from two different species. —**al′lo·ploid′** *adj.*

al·lo·pol·y·ploid (ăl**′**ə-pŏl**′**ē-ploid**′**) *adj.* Having two or more complete sets of chromosomes derived from different species. —*n.* An allopolyploid organism. —**al′-lo·pol′y·ploi′dy** *n.*

al·lo·psy·chic (ăl**′**ō-sī**′**kĭk) *adj.* Of or relating to the mind in its relation to the outside world.

al·lo·pu·ri·nol (ăl**′**ō-pyoŏr**′**ə-nôl**′**, -nōl**′**) *n.* A drug that inhibits the synthesis of uric acid and is used to treat gout and other hyperuricemic conditions.

al·lo·rhyth·mi·a (ăl**′**ō-rĭth**′**mē-ə) *n.* An irregularity in the rhythm of the heartbeat or pulse that recurs in a regular fashion. —**al′lo·rhyth′mic** (-mĭk) *adj.*

all-or-none law *n.* The principle that the strength by which a nerve or muscle fiber responds to a stimulus is not dependent on the strength of the stimulus. If the stimulus is any strength above threshold, the nerve or muscle fiber will either give a complete response or no response at all. —**all′-or-none′** *adj.*

al·lo·some (ăl**′**ə-sōm**′**) *n.* A chromosome that differs from an ordinary autosome in form, size, or behavior; a sex chromosome. Also called *heterochromosome, heterotypical chromosome.*

allosteric site *n.* The place on an enzyme where a molecule that is not a substrate may bind, thus changing the shape of the enzyme and influencing its ability to be active.

al·lo·ster·ism (ăl**′**ō-stĕr**′**ĭz**′**əm) *or* **al·los·ter·y** (ə-lŏs**′**tə-rē) *n.* A change in the activity and conformation of an enzyme resulting from the binding of a compound at a site on the enzyme other than the active binding site. —**al′lo·ster′ic** (ăl**′**ō-stĕr**′**ĭk) *adj.*

al·lo·trans·plant (ăl**′**ō-trăns**′**plănt**′**) *v.* To transfer an organ or tissue between genetically different individuals of the same species. —*n.* An organ or tissue transferred between genetically different individuals of the same species.

al·lo·trans·plan·ta·tion (ăl**′**ō-trăns**′**plăn-tā**′**shən) *n.* The transfer of an organ or tissue between genetically different individuals of the same species.

al·lo·trich·i·a cir·cum·scrip·ta (ăl**′**ō-trĭk**′**ē-ə sûr**′**kəm-skrĭp**′**tə) *n.* See **woolly-hair nevus.**

al·lo·trope (ăl**′**ə-trōp**′**) *n.* A structurally differentiated form of an element that exhibits allotropism.

al·lo·troph·ic (ăl**′**ə-trŏf**′**ĭk, -trō**′**fĭk) *adj.* Having an altered nutritive value.

al·lo·trop·ic (ăl**′**ə-trŏp**′**ĭk) *adj.* **1.** Relating to allotropism. **2.** Characterizing one who is preoccupied with the reactions of others.

al·lot·ro·pism (ə-lŏt**′**rə-pĭz**′**əm) *or* **al·lot·ro·py** (-rə-pē) *n.* The existence of two or more forms of an element that differ from one another in crystalline or molecular structure.

al·lo·type (ăl′ə-tīp′) *n.* Any of the genetically determined variants in the constant region of a given subclass of immunoglobulin that is detectable as an antigen by members of the same species having a different constant region. —**al′lo·typ′ic** (-tĭp′ĭk) *adj.*

al·lox·u·re·mi·a (ăl′ŏks-yŏo-rē′mē-ə) *n.* The presence of purine bases in the blood.

al·lox·u·ri·a (ăl′ŏks-yŏor′ē-ə) *n.* The presence of purine bases in the urine.

al·loy (ăl′oi′, ə-loi′) *n.* A homogeneous mixture or solid solution of two or more metals, the atoms of one replacing or occupying interstitial positions between the atoms of the other.

al·lyl (ăl′əl) *n.* The univalent, unsaturated organic radical C₃H₅.

Al·mei·da′s disease (ăl-mā′dəz) *n.* See **paracoccidioidomycosis.**

al·oe (ăl′ō) *n.* **1.** Any of various chiefly African plants of the genus *Aloe,* having rosettes of succulent, often spiny-margined leaves and long stalks bearing yellow, orange, or red tubular flowers. **2.** Aloe vera. **3.** Any of various laxative drugs obtained from the processed juice of a certain species of aloe.

aloe vera (vĕr′ə, vîr′ə) *n.* **1.** A species of aloe (*Aloe vera*) native to the Mediterranean region. **2.** The mucilaginous juice or gel obtained from the leaves of this plant, used in pharmaceutical preparations for its soothing and healing properties.

a·lo·gi·a (ə-lō′jē-ə) *n.* The inability to speak because of mental deficiency, mental confusion, or aphasia.

al·o·in (ăl′ō-ĭn) *n.* A bitter, yellow crystalline compound obtained from aloe and used as a laxative.

al·o·pe·cia (ăl′ə-pē′shə) *n.* Loss of hair; baldness. —**al′o·pe′cic** (-pē′sĭk) *adj.*

alopecia ar·e·a·ta (âr′ē-ā′tə) *n.* Hair loss in circumscribed, noninflamed areas of the scalp, eyebrows and beard. Also called *alopecia circumscripta.*

alopecia cap·i·tis to·ta·lis (căp′ĭ-tĭs tō-tā′lĭs) *n.* Progressive loss of scalp hair.

alopecia cir·cum·scrip·ta (sûr′kəm-skrĭp′tə) *n.* See **alopecia areata.**

alopecia he·red·i·tar·i·a (hə-rĕd′ĭ-târ′ē-ə) *n.* See **male pattern baldness.**

alopecia lim·i·nar·is fron·ta·lis (lĭm′ə-nâr′ĭs frŭn-tā′lĭs) *n.* Hair loss occurring at the hair line, usually resulting from friction or trauma but occasionally from seborrheic dermatitis.

alopecia med·i·ca·men·to·sa (mĕd′ĭ-kə-mən-tō′sə) *n.* Diffuse hair loss, most notably of the scalp, caused by administration of various drugs.

alopecia pit·y·ro·des (pĭt′ə-rō′dēz) *n.* Loss of hair on the body and scalp, accompanied by desquamation.

alopecia symp·to·mat·i·ca (sĭm′tə-măt′ĭ-kə, sĭmp′-) *n.* Loss of hair occurring in the course of various diseases or following prolonged febrile illness.

alopecia to·ta·lis (tō-tā′lĭs) *n.* Complete loss of scalp hair occurring either all at one time or within a short period of time.

alopecia u·ni·ver·sa·lis (yŏo′nə-vər-sā′lĭs) *n.* Total hair loss on all parts of the body.

Al·pers′ disease (ăl′pərz) *n.* See **progressive cerebral poliodystrophy.**

al·pha (ăl′fə) *n.* **1.** *Symbol* α The first letter of the Greek alphabet. **2.** The first one in a series; the beginning. **3.** The first position from a designated carbon atom in an organic molecule at which an atom or radical group may be substituted. —*adj.* **1.** Characterizing the atom or radical group that is closest to the functional group of atoms in an organic molecule. **2.** Relating to one of two or more closely related substances, as in stereoisomers. **3.** Relating to or characterizing a polypeptide chain that is one of five types of heavy chains present in immunoglobins.

alpha-adrenergic blocking agent *n.* See **alpha-blocker.**

alpha-adrenergic receptor *n.* Any of various cell membrane receptors that can bind with norepinephrine and related substances that activate or block the actions of the cells containing such receptors; these cells initiate physiological responses such as vasoconstriction, pupil dilation, and contraction of pilomotor muscles. Also called *alpha-receptor.*

alpha-amino acid *n.* Any of the 20 or so amino acids that has the amino and carboxyl groups attached to the same carbon atom, usually has an L-configuration, and is the chemical constituent of a protein.

al·pha-a·mi·no·suc·cin·ic acid (ăl′fə-ə-mē′nō-sək-sĭn′ĭk, -ăm′ə-nō-) *n.* See **aspartic acid.**

alpha angle *n.* **1.** The angle between the visual and the optic axes as they cross at the nodal point of the eye. **2.** The angle between the visual line and the major axis of the corneal ellipse.

alpha-blocker *n.* A drug that opposes the excitatory effects of norepinephrine released from sympathetic nerve endings at alpha-adrenergic receptors and causes vasodilation and a decrease in blood pressure. Also called *alpha-adrenergic blocking agent.*

alpha carotene *n.* An isomer of carotene.

alpha cell *n.* **1.** Cells situated on the periphery of the islets of Langerhans. **2.** Cells containing acidophil granules in the anterior lobe of the pituitary gland. Also called *A cell.*

alpha-fetoprotein *n. Abbr.* **AFP** An antigen produced in the fetal liver that can appear in certain diseases of adults, such as liver cancer, and whose level in amniotic fluid can be used to detect certain fetal abnormalities, including Down syndrome and spina bifida.

alpha fiber *n.* Any of the large somatic motor or proprioceptive nerve fibers conducting impulses at rates near 100 meters per second.

al·pha-fu·co·si·dase (ăl′fə-fyŏo-kō′sĭ-dās′, -dāz′) *n.* An enzyme that catalyzes the metabolism of fucose and fucose-containing compounds.

alpha globulin *n.* A type of globulin in blood plasma that exhibits great colloidal mobility in electrically charged neutral or alkaline solutions.

alpha granule *n.* A granule of an alpha cell.

alpha helix *n.* The helical form, turned in a right-handed direction, of many proteins.

alpha-hemolytic streptococci *pl.n.* Streptococci that partially lyse red blood cells cultured on a blood agar medium, producing a green color around the cell colonies.

al·pha-hy·drox·y acid (ăl′fə-hī-drŏk′sē) *n.* Any of various fruit acids with the capacity to trap moisture in the skin and initiate formation of collagen.

alpha-interferon *n.* A family of glycoproteins that are produced endogenously and prepared commercially for their pharmacologic effects, which include antiviral and antineoplastic activity and immune system regulation.

alpha-lipoprotein *n.* See **high-density lipoprotein.**

alpha particle *n.* A positively charged nuclear particle, indistinguishable from a helium atom nucleus and consisting of two protons and two neutrons.

alpha ray *n.* A stream of alpha particles or a single high-speed alpha particle.

alpha-receptor *n.* See **alpha-adrenergic receptor.**

alpha rhythm *n.* See **alpha wave.**

alpha-tocopherol *n.* A substance that is obtained from wheat germ oil or by synthesis, biologically exhibits the most vitamin E activity of the tocopherols, and is an antioxidant.

al·pha·vi·rus (ăl′fə-vī′rəs) *n.* A member of the genus *Alphavirus.*

Alphavirus *n.* A genus of viruses of the Togaviridae family.

alpha wave *n.* A pattern of smooth, regular electrical oscillations, as recorded by an electroencephalograph, that occur in the human brain when a person is awake and relaxed. Also called *alpha rhythm.*

Al·port's syndrome (ăl′pôrts′) *n.* An inherited syndrome marked by progressive nephropathy and nerve deafness and sometimes ocular defects.

al·pra·zo·lam (ăl-prā′zə-lăm′) *n.* A benzodiazepine tranquilizer that is used in the management of anxiety disorders.

al·pros·ta·dil (ăl-prŏs′tə-dĭl) *n.* A prostaglandin drug that acts as a vasodilator and is used to treat erectile dysfunction.

ALS *abbr.* amyotrophic lateral sclerosis; antilymphocyte serum

Al·ström's syndrome (ăl′strəm, ăl′strœmz) *n.* An inherited syndrome marked by retinal degeneration with nystagmus and loss of central vision, nerve deafness, and diabetes. It is associated with childhood obesity.

ALT (ā′ĕl-tē′) *n.* alanine aminotransferase

al·ter ego (ôl′tər) *n.* Another side of oneself; a second self.

al·ter·nans (ôl-tûr′nănz′) *adj.* Alternating, as in heart contractions. —*n.* Alternation in the contractions of the heart.

al·ter·nate binaural loudness balance test (ôl′tər-nĭt, ăl′-) *n.* Variant of **binaural alternate loudness balance test.**

alternate cover test *n.* A test for detecting phoria or strabismus in which one eye is covered for several seconds, and then the other eye is immediately covered while the person's attention is directed to a small fixation picture.

alternate hemianesthesia *n.* The loss of tactile sensibility on one side of the head as well as on the opposite side of the rest of the body. Also called *crossed hemianesthesia.*

al·ter·nat·ing calculus (ôl′tər-nā′tĭng, ăl′-) *n.* A urinary calculus having successive layers of different composition. Also called *combination calculus.*

alternating hemiplegia *n.* Hemiplegia caused by a lesion on the opposite side of the brainstem, accompanied by an additional paralysis of a motor cranial nerve on the same side as the lesion. Also called *crossed hemiplegia, stauroplegia.*

alternating pulse *n.* A pulse pattern that occurs at regular intervals but alternates between weak and strong beats; usually indicates myocardial disease. Also called *pulsus alternans.*

alternating tremor *n.* Hyperkinesia characterized by regular, symmetrical, to-and-fro movements produced by patterned, alternating contraction of muscles and their antagonists.

al·ter·na·tion (ôl′tər-nā′shən, ăl′-) *n.* Successive change from one thing or state to another and back again.

alternation of generations *n.* The regular alternation of forms or of mode of reproduction in the life cycle of an organism, such as between diploid and haploid phases, or between sexual and asexual reproductive cycles. Also called *metagenesis, xenogenesis.*

alternation of heart *n.* See **mechanical alternation.**

al·ter·na·tive medicine (ôl-tûr′nə-tĭv, ăl-) *n.* A variety of therapeutic or preventive health care practices, such as homeopathy, naturopathy, and herbal medicine, that are not typically taught or practiced in traditional medical communities and offer treatments that differ from standard medical practice.

alt. hor. *abbr. Latin* alternis horis (every other hour)

al·ti·tude sickness (ăl′tĭ-tōōd′) *n.* A collection of symptoms, including shortness of breath, nausea, and nosebleed, brought on by decreased oxygen in the atmosphere, such as that encountered at high altitudes. Also called *Acosta's disease.*

al·ti·tu·di·nal hemianopsia (ăl′tĭ-tōōd′n-əl) *n.* Hemianopsia affecting the upper or lower half of the visual field.

Al·to·cor (ăl′tō-kôr′) A trademark for the drug lovastatin.

al·um (ăl′əm) *n.* Any of various double sulfates of a trivalent metal such as aluminum or iron and a univalent metal such as potassium or sodium that are used as topical astringents and styptics.

a·lu·mi·nat·ed (ə-lōō′mə-nā′tĭd) *adj.* Containing alum.

a·lu·mi·no·sis (ə-lōō′mə-nō′sĭs) *n.* A form of pneumoconiosis caused by exposure to alum-bearing dust.

a·lu·mi·num (ə-lōō′mə-nəm) *n. Symbol* **Al** A silvery-white, ductile metallic element used in making dental alloys and forming compounds with pharmaceutical uses, especially as astringents and antiseptics. Atomic number 13.

Al·u·pent (ăl′yə-pĕnt′) A trademark for the drug metaproterenol sulfate.

al·ve·o·al·gia (ăl′vē-ō-ăl′jə) *or* **al·ve·o·lal·gia** (-lăl′jə) *n.* Pain following a tooth extraction caused by blood clot disintegration and subsequent infection of the empty socket.

al·ve·o·lar (ăl-vē′ə-lər) *adj.* Relating to an alveolus.

alveolar abscess *n*. An abscess in the alveolar ridge of the jaw, usually caused by the spread of infection from an adjacent nonvital tooth. Also called *dental abscess*.

alveolar air *n*. See **alveolar gas**.

alveolar-arterial oxygen difference *n*. The difference or gradient between the partial pressure of oxygen in the alveolar spaces and the arterial blood.

alveolar artery *n*. **1.** An artery that has its origin in the maxillary artery, is distributed through the mandibular canal to the lower teeth, and branches into the mylohyoid, mental, and dental arteries; inferior alveolar artery. **2.** An artery that has its origin in the infraorbital artery and is distributed through the upper incisors, canines, and maxillary sinus. **3.** An artery that has its origin in the maxillary artery and is distributed through the molars, premolars, and gingiva.

alveolar cell *n*. A cell lining the alveoli of the lung.

alveolar cell carcinoma *n*. See **bronchiolar carcinoma**.

alveolar dead space *n*. The difference between physiological dead space and anatomical dead space, representing that part of the physiological dead space resulting from ventilation of relatively underperfused or nonperfused alveoli.

alveolar duct *n*. **1.** The part of the respiratory passages beyond the respiratory bronchioles, from which the alveolar sacs and alveoli arise. **2.** The smallest of the intralobular ducts in the mammary gland, into which the secretory alveoli open.

alveolar gas *n. Abbr.* **A,** The gas in the pulmonary alveoli and alveolar sacs, where the oxygen–carbon dioxide exchange with pulmonary capillary blood occurs. Also called *alveolar air*.

alveolar gingiva *n*. Gum tissue enveloping the alveolar bone.

alveolar gland *n*. A gland having a saclike secretory unit and an obvious lumen.

alveolar macrophage *n*. A vigorously phagocytic macrophage on the epithelial surface of lung alveoli that ingests carbon and other inhaled particulate matter. Also called *coniophage, dust cell*.

alveolar point *n*. See **prosthion**.

alveolar process *n*. The ridge on the surfaces of the upper and lower jaws containing the tooth sockets.

alveolar sac *n*. See **air sac**.

alveolar soft part sarcoma *n*. A malignant tumor formed of a reticular stroma of connective tissue enclosing aggregates of large round or polygonal cells.

alveolar ventilation *n*. The volume of gas expired from alveoli to the outside of the body per minute.

al·ve·o·lec·to·my (ăl′vē-ə-lĕk′tə-mē) *n*. Surgical removal of a portion of the aveolar process to facilitate the fitting of a dental prosthesis.

al·ve·o·li·tis (ăl′vē-ə-lī′tĭs) *n*. **1.** Inflammation of alveoli. **2.** Inflammation of a tooth socket.

alveolo– *pref*. Alveolus; alveolar: *alveoloclasia*.

al·ve·o·lo·cap·il·lar·y membrane (ăl-vē′ə-lō-kăp′ə-lĕr′ē) *n*. A thin layer of tissue that mediates the exchange of gases between the alveoli and the blood in the pulmonary capillaries.

al·ve·o·lo·cla·sia (ăl-vē′ə-lō-klā′zhə) *n*. Destruction of an alveolus.

alveolodental ligament *n*. See **periodontal ligament**.

alveolodental membrane *n*. See **periodontium**.

al·ve·o·lo·lin·gual (ăl-vē′ə-lō-lĭng′gwəl) *or* **al·ve·o·lin·gual** (ăl′vē-ō-) *adj*. Relating to the alveolar processes and the tongue.

al·ve·o·lo·pal·a·tal (ăl-vē′ə-lō-păl′ə-təl) *adj*. Relating to the palatal surface of the alveolar process of the mandible and maxilla.

al·ve·o·lo·plas·ty (ăl-vē′ə-lō-plăs′tē) *or* **al·ve·o·plas·ty** (ăl′vē-ō-plăs′tē) *n*. Surgical preparation of the alveolar ridges for the reception of dentures.

al·ve·o·lot·o·my (ăl′vē-ō-lŏt′ə-mē) *n*. Incision of the alveolar process to drain pus from an abscess.

al·ve·o·lus (ăl-vē′ə-ləs) *n., pl.* **–li** (-lī′) A small angular cavity or pit, such as a tooth socket or an air sac.

al·ve·us (ăl′vē-əs) *n., pl.* **–ve·i** (-vē-ī′) A channel or trough.

a·lym·phi·a (ā-lĭm′fē-ə, ə-lĭm′-) *n*. Absence or deficiency of lymph.

a·lym·pho·cy·to·sis (ā-lĭm′fō-sī-tō′sĭs, ə-lĭm′-) *n*. Total or nearly total absence of lymphocytes.

a·lym·pho·pla·sia (ā-lĭm′fō-plā′zhə, ə-lĭm′-) *n*. Aplasia or hypoplasia of lymphoid tissue.

Alz·hei·mer's disease (älts′hī-mərz, älts′-, ôlts′-) *n*. A degenerative disease of the brain, associated with the development of abnormal tissues and protein deposits in the cerebral cortex and characterized by confusion, disorientation, memory failure, speech disturbances, and the progressive loss of mental capacity.

Am The symbol for the element **americium**.

AMA *abbr*. against medical advice; American Medical Association

am·a·crine (ăm′ə-krĭn, -krīn′) *n*. A cell or structure lacking a long fibrous process. —*adj*. Of, relating to, or being a cell that lacks long processes.

a·mal·gam (ə-măl′gəm) *n*. Any of various alloys of mercury with other metals, as with tin or silver, used for filling teeth.

amalgam tattoo *n*. A bluish-black or gray lesion of the oral mucous membrane caused by accidental implantation of silver amalgam into the tissue during tooth restoration or extraction.

Am·a·ni·ta (ăm′ə-nī′tə, -nē′-) *n*. A genus of mushrooms with many highly poisonous species.

Amanita mus·car·i·a (mŭs-kâr′ē-ə) *n*. A toxic mushroom that contains muscarine.

Amanita phal·loi·des (fə-loi′dēz′) *n*. A mushroom containing toxins such as phalloidine and amanitin that cause gastroenteritis and necrosis of the liver and kidneys.

a·man·ta·dine hydrochloride (ə-măn′tə-dēn′) *n*. An antiviral drug used also in the treatment of Parkinson's disease.

am·a·rine (ăm′ə-rĭn, -rīn′) *n*. Any of various bitter substances derived from plants, especially from the oil of bitter almond.

a·mas·ti·a (ā-măs′tē-ə, ə-măs′-) *n*. Congenital absence of one or both breasts. Also called *amazia*.

a·mas·ti·gote (ə-măs′tĭ-gōt′) *n*. See **Leishman-Donovan body**.

am·au·ro·sis (ăm′ô-rō′sĭs) *n*. Blindness, especially without apparent change in the eye, as from a cortical lesion. —**am′au·rot′ic** (-rŏt′ĭk) *adj*.

amaurosis con·gen·i·ta of Le·ber (kən-jĕn′ĭ-tə, lā′-bər) *n.* A cone-rod abiotrophy that causes blindness or severely reduces vision at birth.

amaurosis fu·gax (fōo′găks′) *n.* A temporary blindness that may result from transient ischemia caused by an insufficiency of the carotid artery or exposure to centrifugal force.

amaurotic pupil *n.* A pupil in an eye that is blind because of ocular or optic nerve disease, and that contracts in response to light only when the normal eye is stimulated with light.

a·ma·zi·a (ə-mā′zē-ə) *n.* See **amastia**.

am·ba·geu·sia (ăm′bə-gyōo′zhə, -jōo′-) *n.* Loss of taste on both sides of the tongue.

am·be·no·ni·um chloride (ăm′bə-nō′nē-əm) *n.* A cholinesterase inhibitor used primarily in the management of myasthenia gravis and occasionally to treat intestinal and urinary tract obstruction.

ambi– *or* **ambo–** *pref.* Both: *ambilateral.*

am·bi·dex·ter·i·ty (ăm′bĭ-dĕk-stĕr′ĭ-tē) *or* **am·bi·dex·trism** (-dĕk′strĭz′əm) *n.* The state or quality of being ambidextrous.

am·bi·dex·trous (ăm′bĭ-dĕk′strəs) *adj.* Able to use both hands with equal facility.

Am·bi·en (ăm′bē-ən) A trademark for the drug zolpidem tartrate.

am·bi·ent (ăm′bē-ənt) *adj.* Surrounding; encircling.

am·big·u·ous external genitalia (ăm-bĭg′yōo-əs) *n.* External genitalia that physically do not appear to be either male or female in form.

ambiguous nucleus *n.* A slender longitudinal column of motor neurons in the ventrolateral region of the medulla oblongata, whose efferent fibers leave with the vagus and glossopharyngeal nerves and innervate the striated muscle fibers of the pharynx and the vocal cord muscles of the larynx.

am·bi·lat·er·al (ăm′bĭ-lăt′ər-əl) *adj.* Relating to both sides.

am·bi·le·vous (ăm′bĭ-lē′vəs) *adj.* Having the ability to perform manual skill tasks with both hands.

am·bi·sex·u·al (ăm′bĭ-sĕk′shōo-əl) *adj.* Sexually attracted to either sex indiscriminately. —*n.* An ambisexual person or organism. —**am′bi·sex′u·al′i·ty** (-ăl′ĭ-tē) *n.*

am·biv·a·lence (ăm-bĭv′ə-ləns) *n.* The coexistence of opposing attitudes or feelings toward a person, an object, or an idea. —**am·biv′a·lent** *adj.*

am·bi·ver·sion (ăm′bĭ-vûr′zhən) *n.* A personality trait including the qualities of both introversion and extroversion.

ambly– *pref.* Dull; dim: *amblyopia.*

am·bly·a·phi·a (ăm′blē-ā′fē-ə) *n.* Reduced sensitivity or dullness of the sense of touch.

am·bly·geu·sti·a (ăm′blĭ-gyōo′stē-ə, -jōo′-) *n.* A dulled sense of taste.

Am·bly·om·ma (ăm′blē-ŏm′ə) *n.* A genus of ticks of the Ixodidae family, certain species of which are vectors of Rocky Mountain spotted fever.

am·bly·o·pi·a (ăm′blē-ō′pē-ə) *n.* Dimness of vision, especially when occurring in one eye without apparent physical defect or disease. Also called *lazy eye.* —**am′bly·o′pic** (-ō′pĭk, -ŏp′ĭk) *adj.*

am·bly·o·scope (ăm′blē-ə-skōp′) *n.* A reflecting stereoscope used for measuring or training binocular vision and for stimulating vision in an amblyopic eye.

ambo– *pref.* Variant of **ambi–**.

am·bo·cep·tor (ăm′bō-sĕp′tər) *n.* The antibody to sheep red blood cells used in complement-fixation tests.

Am·bu bag (ăm′byōo) A trademark for a self-reinflating bag used during resuscitation.

am·bu·lance (ăm′byə-ləns) *n.* A specially equipped vehicle used to transport the sick or injured.

am·bu·lant (ăm′byə-lənt) *adj.* Moving or walking about.

am·bu·la·to·ry (ăm′byə-lə-tôr′ē) *adj.* **1.** Of, relating to, or adapted for walking. **2.** Capable of walking; not bedridden. **3.** Moving about. **4.** Of or relating to medical care or services provided on an outpatient basis.

ambulatory care *n.* Medical care provided to outpatients.

ambulatory surgery *n.* Surgery performed on a person who is admitted to and discharged from a hospital on the same day.

a·me·ba *or* **amoeba** (ə-mē′bə) *n.,* *pl.* **-bas** *or* **-bae** (-bē) A protozoa of the genus *Amoeba* and of related genera, occurring in soil and water and parasitic in animals.

am·e·bi·a·sis *or* **am·oe·bi·a·sis** (ăm′ə-bī′ə-sĭs) *n.* An infection or disease caused by pathogenic amebas, especially *Entamoeba histolytica.* Also called *amebiosis, amebism.*

a·me·bic *or* **a·moe·bic** (ə-mē′bĭk) *adj.* Relating to, resembling, or caused by amebas.

amebic abscess *n.* An abscess in the liver or other organ, containing amebas and usually following amebic dysentery. Also called *tropical abscess.*

amebic colitis *n.* Inflammation of the colon in amebiasis.

amebic dysentery *n.* Severe intestinal infection of humans caused by the ameba *Entamoeba histolytica* and resulting in diarrhea, cramping, fever, and ulceration of the colon.

amebic granuloma *n.* See **ameboma**.

a·me·bi·cide (ə-mē′bĭ-sīd′) *n.* Any of various agents that destroy amebas. —**a·me′bi·cid′al** (-cīd′l) *adj.*

a·me·bi·form (ə-mē′bə-fôrm′) *adj.* Resembling an ameba in shape or appearance.

am·e·bi·o·sis (ăm′ə-bī-ō′sĭs) *n.* See **amebiasis**.

a·me·bism (ə-mē′bĭz′əm) *n.* See **amebiasis**.

a·me·bo·cyte *or* **a·moe·bo·cyte** (ə-mē′bə-sīt′) *n.* **1.** An ameboid cell, such as a white blood cell. **2.** A blood cell in an in vitro tissue culture.

a·me·boid *or* **a·moe·boid** (ə-mē′boid′) *adj.* **1.** Of or resembling an ameba, especially in changeability of form and means of locomotion. **2.** Having an irregular or asymmetric outline with peripheral projections, as the outline of a group of cells growing in a nutrient culture.

ameboid cell *n.* A cell, such as a leukocyte, that is able to change its form and move about like an ameba. Also called *wandering cell.*

am·e·bo·ma (ăm′ə-bō′mə) *n.* An inflamed, tumorlike, spreading nodule that occasionally develops in chronic amebiasis, often in the wall of the colon. Also called *amebic granuloma.*

a·me·bu·la (ə-mē′byə-lə) *n.*, *pl.* **-las** *or* **-lae** (-lē′) **1.** Any of the young amebas of *Entamoeba* species and their immediate progeny that emerge from the cyst in the human gut before localizing in the large intestine. **2.** The ameboid spores of protozoa and other organisms.

a·me·bu·ri·a (ăm′ə-byŏŏr′ē-ə) *n.* The presence of amebas in the urine.

a·mel·i·a (ə-mĕl′ē-ə, ə-mē′lē-ə) *n.* Congenital absence of one or more limbs.

am·e·lo·blast (ăm′ə-lō-blăst′) *n.* A cell of the inner layer of the enamel organ of a developing tooth that is involved in enamel formation.

am·e·lo·blas·tic fibroma (ăm′ə-lō-blăs′tĭk) *n.* A benign mixed tumor of odontogenic origin, distinguished by a simultaneous neoplastic proliferation of both epithelial and mesenchymal components of the tooth bud without the production of hard tissue.

ameloblastic fibrosarcoma *n.* A rapidly growing, painful, destructive tumor of the jaw that usually arises through a malignant change in a benign fibroma. Also called *ameloblastic sarcoma.*

ameloblastic layer *n.* The internal layer of the enamel organ. Also called *enamel layer.*

ameloblastic odontoma *n.* A benign mixed odontogenic tumor having histological characteristics of both an odontoma and an ameloblastoma.

ameloblastic sarcoma *n.* See **ameloblastic fibrosarcoma.**

am·e·lo·blas·to·ma (ăm′ə-lō-blă-stō′mə) *n.* A benign tumor, usually of the posterior regions of the mandible, composed of epithelial cells that resemble enamel-producing cells but do not form enamel. Also called *adamantinoma.*

am·e·lo·den·tal junction (ăm′ə-lō-dĕn′tl) *n.* See **dentinoenamel junction.**

am·e·lo·den·tin·al (ăm′ə-lō-dĕn′tə-nəl, -dĕn-tē′-) *adj.* Dentinoenamel.

amelodentinal junction *n.* See **dentinoenamel junction.**

am·e·lo·gen·e·sis (ăm′ə-lō-jĕn′ĭ-sĭs) *n.* The formation and development of dental enamel. Also called *enamelogenesis.*

amelogenesis im·per·fec·ta (ĭm′pər-fĕk′tə) *n.* A hereditary condition in which the dental enamel does not develop properly, often because of insufficient calcification. Also called *enamel dysplasia.*

a·men·or·rhe·a *or* **a·men·or·rhoe·a** (ā-mĕn′ə-rē′ə) *n.* Abnormal suppression or absence of menstruation. Also called *menostasis.* —**a·men′or·rhe′al** *adj.* —**a·men′or·rhe′ic** *adj.*

amenorrhea-galactorrhea syndrome *n.* Lactation and amenorrhea resulting from endocrinological causes or from a pituitary tumor.

a·ment (ā′mĕnt′, ā′mənt) *n.* A person whose intellectual capacity remains undeveloped.

a·men·tia (ā-mĕn′shə, ə-mĕn′-) *n.* Insufficient mental development or functioning.

American Law Institute Rule *n.* A 1962 US rule used as a test of criminal responsibility and stating that an individual accused of a crime is not criminally responsible if at the time of such conduct as a result of mental disease or defect the person lacks substantial capacity either to appreciate the wrongfulness of the conduct or to conform such conduct to the requirements of law.

American leishmaniasis *n.* See **mucocutaneous leishmaniasis.**

American Sign Language *n.* The primary sign language used by deaf and hearing-impaired people in the United States and Canada.

am·er·i·ci·um (ăm′ə-rĭsh′ē-əm) *n.* *Symbol* **Am** A white metallic synthetic element of the actinide series whose longest-lived isotopes, Am 241 and Am 243, are used as radiation sources for bone mineral analysis and in treating cancer. Atomic number 95.

Ames (āmz), **Bruce Nathan** Born 1928. American biochemist noted for his studies of environmental mutagens and carcinogens. He developed the Ames test.

Ames test *n.* A test in which strains of *Salmonella* that are unable to synthesize histidine are introduced into a test substance lacking in histidine. If the strains then regain the ability to synthesize histidine, the substance is considered mutagenic and thus carcinogenic.

am·e·thop·ter·in (ăm′ə-thŏp′tər-ĭn) *n.* See **methotrexate.**

a·me·tri·a (ā-mē′trē-ə) *n.* Congenital absence of the uterus.

am·e·trom·e·ter (ăm′ĭ-trŏm′ĭ-tər) *n.* An instrument for measuring the degree of ametropia.

am·e·tro·pi·a (ăm′ĭ-trō′pē-ə) *n.* An eye abnormality, such as nearsightedness, farsightedness, or astigmatism, resulting from faulty refractive ability of the eye. —**am′e·trop′ic** (-trŏp′ĭk, -trō′pĭk) *adj.*

AMI *abbr.* acute myocardial infarction

am·i·an·thoid (ăm′ē-ăn′thoid′) *adj.* Having a crystalline appearance like asbestos.

−amic *suff.* Relating to or derived from an amide: *carbamic acid.*

a·mi·cro·bic (ā′mī-krō′bĭk) *adj.* Not relating to or caused by microorganisms.

am·i·dase (ăm′ĭ-dās′, -dāz′) *n.* An enzyme that catalyzes the hydrolysis of monocarboxylic amides, thus freeing ammonia. Also called *acylamidase, acylase.*

am·ide (ăm′īd′, -ĭd) *n.* An organic compound, such as acetamide, containing the acyl radical. —**a·mid′ic** (ə-mĭd′ĭk)

am·i·dine (ăm′ĭ-dēn′, -dĭn) *n.* The monovalent radical having the general formula $RCNHNH_2$.

a·mi·do (ə-mē′dō′, ăm′ĭ-dō′) *n.* A chemical group having a NH_2 radical as well as a CO radical.

am·i·do·hy·dro·lase (ăm′ĭ-dō-hī′drə-lās′, -drə-lāz′, ə-mē′-) *n.* An enzyme that catalyzes the hydrolysis of the C−N bond in an amide. Also called *deamidase, deamidizing enzyme.*

a·mim·i·a (ā-mĭm′ē-ə, ə-mĭm′-) *n.* Loss of the ability to imitate or to communicate by gestures or signs.

am·i·nate (ăm′ə-nāt′) *v.* **1.** To form or convert to an amine. **2.** To add an amino group to a compound.

a·mine (ə-mēn′, ăm′ēn) *n.* Any of a group of organic compounds of nitrogen that may be considered ammonia derivatives in which one or more hydrogen atoms have been replaced by one or more hydrocarbon radicals.

−amine *suff.* Amine: *phenylamine.*

a·mi·no (ə-mē′nō, ăm′ə-nō′) *adj.* Relating to an amine or other compound containing an NH₂ group combined with a nonacid organic radical.

amino– *pref.* Containing the radical NH₂ combined with a nonacid organic radical: *aminobenzoic acid.*

amino acid *n. Abbr.* **AA** Any of various organic acids containing both an amino group and a carboxyl group, especially any of the 20 or more compounds that link together to form proteins.

amino acid dehydrogenase *n.* Any of various enzymes that catalyze the deamination of amino acids to keto acids.

a·mi·no·ac·i·de·mi·a (ə-mē′nō-ăs′ĭ-dē′mē-ə, ăm′ə-nō-) *n.* An excess of specific amino acids in the blood.

amino acid oxidase *n.* An enzyme that catalyzes the oxidative deamination of an amino acid to a keto acid.

a·mi·no·ac·i·du·ri·a (ə-mē′nō-ăs′ĭ-do͝or′ē-ə, ăm′ə-nō-) *n.* A disorder of protein metabolism in which excessive amounts of amino acids are excreted in the urine. Also called *acidaminuria.*

a·mi·no·ac·yl (ə-mē′nō-ăs′əl) *n. Abbr.* **AA** The radical formed when the carboxyl group of an amino acid loses a hydroxyl group.

a·mi·no·ben·zo·ic acid (ə-mē′nō-běn-zō′ĭk, ăm′ə-nō-) *n.* Any of three benzoic acid derivatives, especially the yellowish para form, which is part of the vitamin B complex.

a·mi·no·gly·co·side (ə-mē′nō-glī′kə-sīd′, ăm′ə-nō-) *n.* Any of a group of bacteriocidal antibiotics derived from species of *Streptomyces* or *Micromonosporum* that are effective against aerobic gram-negative bacilli and *Mycobacterium tuberculosis.*

am·i·nol·y·sis (ăm′ə-nŏl′ĭ′-sĭs) *n.* The replacement of a halogen in an alkyl or aryl group by an amine radical and the elimination of hydrogen halide.

a·mi·no·pep·ti·dase (ə-mē′nō-pĕp′tĭ-dās′, -dāz′, ăm′-ə-nō-) *n.* Any of various enzymes that catalyze the hydrolysis of the terminal peptide bond at the amino end of a polypeptide.

am·i·noph·er·ase (ăm′ə-nŏf′ə-rās′, -rāz′) *n.* See **aminotransferase.**

am·i·noph·yl·line (ăm′ə-nŏf′ə-lĭn) *n.* A theophylline derivative, used as a bronchodilator in the treatment of bronchial asthma, emphysema, and bronchitis.

a·mi·no·py·rine (ə-mē′nō-pī′rēn′, ăm′ə-nō-) *n.* A colorless crystalline compound used to reduce fever and relieve pain.

a·mi·no·trans·fer·ase (ə-mē′nō-trăns′fə-rās′, -rāz′, ăm′ə-nō-) *n.* Any of various enzymes that catalyze the transfer of an amino group between an alpha-amino acid and usually a specific carbon on a keto acid. Also called *aminopherase, transaminase.*

am·i·nu·ri·a (ăm′ə-no͝or′ē-ə) *n.* Excretion of an excessive amount of amines in the urine.

a·mi·o·da·rone hydrochloride (ə-mē′ō-də-rōn′) *n.* A vasodilator for the heart used to control ventricular and supraventricular arrhythmias and to manage stenocardia.

am·i·to·sis (ăm′ĭ-tō′sĭs, ā′mī-) *n.* Direct cell division by simple cleavage of the nucleus, without spindle formation or the appearance of chromosomes. Also called *direct nuclear division.* **—am′i·tot′ic** (-tŏt′ĭk) *adj.*

am·i·trip·tyl·ine (ăm′ĭ-trĭp′tə-lēn′) *n.* A tricyclic antidepressant drug.

AML *abbr.* acute myelogenous leukemia

am·mo·ne·mi·a (ăm′ə-nē′mē-ə) *or* **am·mo·ni·e·mi·a** (ə-mō′nē-ē′mē-ə) *n.* Excessive amounts of ammonia or its compounds in the blood.

am·mo·nia (ə-mōn′yə) *n.* A colorless, pungent gas used to manufacture a wide variety of nitrogen-containing organic and inorganic chemicals.

am·mo·ni·ac (ə-mō′nē-ăk′) *n.* A strong-smelling gum resin from the stems of a plant of western Asia, formerly used in perfumery and in medicine as an expectorant and a stimulant.

ammonia-lyase *n.* Any of various enzymes that remove ammonia or an amino compound by breaking the C–N bond, leaving a CC.

am·mo·ni·at·ed (ə-mō′nē-ā′tĭd) *adj.* Containing or combining with ammonia.

ammonio– *pref.* Containing an ammonium group: *ammoniocupric sulfate.*

am·mo·ni·um (ə-mō′nē-əm) *n.* The univalent radical NH₄⁺, that is derived from ammonia and that reacts as a univalent metal in forming ammonium compounds.

ammonium carbonate *n.* **1.** A carbonate of ammonium. **2.** The double salt of ammonium bicarbonate and ammonium carbamate, produced commercially and used in powder form in smelling salts.

am·mo·ni·u·ri·a (ə-mō′nē-yo͝or′ē-ə) *n.* The presence of an excessive amount of ammonia in the urine.

am·mo·nol·y·sis (ăm′ə-nŏl′ĭ-sĭs) *n.* The breaking of a chemical bond by ammonia during which an amino group is added at the point of breakage.

Am·mon's horn (ăm′ənz) *n.* One of the two interlocking gyri composing the hippocampus. Also called *cornu ammonis.*

am·ne·sia (ăm-nē′zhə) *n.* The loss or impairment of memory.

am·ne·si·ac (ăm-nē′zē-ăk′, -zhē-ăk′) *n.* One who is afflicted with amnesia.

am·ne·sic (ăm-nē′zĭk) *adj.* Relating to or affected with amnesia.

am·nes·tic (ăm-nĕs′tĭk) *adj.* Amnesic. **—***n.* An agent that causes amnesia.

amnestic aphasia *or* **amnesic aphasia** *n.* The inability to find specific words or name objects.

amnestic syndrome *n.* An organic brain syndrome marked by short-term memory disturbance.

amnio– *pref.* **1.** Amnion: *amniorrhexis.* **2.** Amniotic fluid: *amniorrhea.*

am·ni·o·cen·te·sis (ăm′nē-ō-sĕn-tē′sĭs) *n., pl.* **–ses** (-sēz′) A procedure in which a small sample of amniotic fluid is drawn out of the uterus through a needle inserted in the abdomen and is then analyzed to detect genetic abnormalities in the fetus or to determine the sex of the fetus.

am·ni·o·cho·ri·al (ăm′nē-ō-kôr′ē-əl) *or* **am·ni·o·cho·ri·on·ic** (-kôr′ē-ŏn′ĭk) *adj.* Of, relating to, or characteristic of the amnion and the chorion.

am·ni·o·gen·e·sis (ăm′nē-ō-jĕn′ĭ-sĭs) *n.* Formation of the amnion.

am·ni·og·ra·phy (ăm′nē-ŏg′rə-fē) *n.* Radiographic examination of the amnion following its injection with a radiopaque substance.

am·ni·o·ma (ăm′nē-ō′mə) *n.* A broad flat skin tumor caused by amnionic adhesion before birth.

am·ni·on (ăm′nē-ən, -ŏn′) *n., pl.* **–ni·ons** *or* **–ni·a** (-nē-ə) The thin, membranous sac filled with a serous fluid in which the embryo or fetus is enclosed and suspended in the uterus. Also called *amniotic sac.* —**am′ni·ot′ic** (-ŏt′ĭk), **am′ni·on′ic** (-ŏn′ĭk) *adj.*

am·ni·o·ni·tis (ăm′nē-ə-nī′tĭs) *n.* Inflammation of the amnion.

amnion no·do·sum (nō-dō′səm) *n.* Nodules in the amnion that consist of stratified squamous epithelium. Also called *squamous metaplasia of amnion.*

am·ni·or·rhe·a (ăm′nē-ə-rē′ə) *n.* The escape of amniotic fluid from the amnion.

am·ni·or·rhex·is (ăm′nē-ə-rĕk′sĭs) *n.* Rupture of the amnion.

am·ni·o·scope (ăm′nē-ə-skōp′) *n.* An endoscope that allows the fetus and amniotic fluid to be observed directly through the intact amniotic sac.

am·ni·os·co·py (ăm′nē-ŏs′kə-pē) *n.* Examination of the amniotic cavity and fetus using an optical instrument that is inserted into the amniotic cavity.

amniotic cavity *n.* The fluid-filled cavity surrounding the developing embryo.

amniotic fluid *n.* The fluid within the amnion that surrounds the fetus and protects it from injury.

amniotic fold *n.* A fold of amniotic membrane enclosing the yolk stalk and extending from the point of insertion of the umbilical cord to the yolk sac.

amniotic sac *n.* See **amnion.**

am·ni·o·tome (ăm′nē-ə-tōm′) *n.* An instrument for puncturing the fetal membranes.

am·ni·ot·o·my (ăm′nē-ŏt′ə-mē) *n.* Surgical rupture of the fetal membranes to induce or expedite labor.

A-mode (ā′mōd′) *n.* A one-dimensional representation of a reflected sound wave in a diagnostic ultrasound.

a·moe·ba (ə-mē′bə) *n.* Variant of **ameba.**

A·moe·ba (ə-mē′bə) *n., pl.* **–bas** *or* **–bae** (-bē) **1.** A genus of protozoa of the class Sarcodina or Rhizopoda. **2.** Any of several genera of protozoa that are parasitic in humans, especially *Entamoeba.*

am·oe·bi·a·sis (ăm′ə-bī′ə-sĭs) *n.* Variant of **amebiasis.**

a·moe·bic (ə-mē′bĭk) *adj.* Variant of **amebic.**

a·moe·bo·cyte (ə-mē′bə-sīt′) *n.* Variant of **amebocyte.**

a·moe·boid (ə-mē′boid′) *adj.* Variant of **ameboid.**

a·morph (ā′môrf′) *n.* A mutant gene that has no phenotypic effect.

a·mor·phi·a (ə-môr′fē-ə) *or* **a·mor·phism** (-fĭz′əm) *n.* The state or quality of being amorphous.

a·mor·phous (ə-môr′fəs) *adj.* **1.** Lacking definite form; shapeless. **2.** Lacking organization; formless. **3.** Lacking distinct crystalline structure.

A·moss′ sign (ā′məs) *n.* An indication of painful flexion of the spine in which it is necessary to support a sitting position by extending the arms behind the torso and placing its weight on the hands.

a·mox·i·cil·lin (ə-mŏk′sĭ-sĭl′ĭn) *n.* A semisynthetic penicillin having an antibacterial spectrum of action similar to that of ampicillin.

A·mox·il (ə-mŏk′sĭl) A trademark for the drug amoxicillin.

AMP (ā′em-pē′) *n.* Adenosine monophosphate; a mononucleotide found in animal cells and reversibly convertible to ADP and ATP. Also called *adenine nucleotide, adenylic acid.*

am·pere (ăm′pîr′) *n. Abbr.* **A 1.** A unit of electric current in the meter-kilogram-second system, equal to the current that, flowing in two parallel wires one meter apart, produces a force of 2×10^{-7} newtons per meter. **2.** A unit in the International System specified as one International coulomb per second and equal to 0.999835 ampere.

am·phet·a·mine (ăm-fĕt′ə-mēn′, -mĭn) *n.* **1.** A colorless, volatile liquid that is used as a central nervous system stimulant in the treatment of certain neurological conditions, such as attention deficit hyperactivity disorder and narcolepsy, and is abused as a stimulant. **2.** A chemical derivative of amphetamine, such as dextroamphetamine sulfate.

amphi– *or* **amph–** *or* **ampho–** *pref.* **1.** Both: *amphibaric.* **2.** On both sides: *amphicentric.*

am·phi·ar·thro·sis (ăm′fē-är-thrō′sĭs) *n.* See **movable joint** (sense 2). —**am′phi·ar·thro′di·al** (-thrō′dē-əl) *adj.*

am·phi·as·ter (ăm′fē-ăs′tər) *n.* A double-star figure present in the cell during mitosis, consisting of two astrospheres connected by a spindle, formed just before the division of the nucleus. Also called *diaster.*

am·phi·bar·ic (ăm′fĭ-băr′ĭk) *adj.* Of, relating to, or characteristic of a drug that can either lower or elevate arterial blood pressure depending on the dose.

am·phi·bol·ic fistula (ăm′fə-bŏl′ĭk) *or* **am·phib·o·lous fistula** (ăm-fĭb′ə-ləs) *n.* A complete anal fistula opening both externally and internally.

am·phi·cen·tric (ăm′fĭ-sĕn′trĭk) *adj.* Centering at both ends. Used of a rete mirabile that begins by the vessel branching out and ends by the branches joining again to form the same vessel.

am·phi·mix·is (ăm′fə-mĭk′sĭs) *n.* The union of the sperm and egg in sexual reproduction.

am·phis·tome (ăm′fĭ-stōm′) *n.* Any trematode of the genus *Paramphistomum.*

am·phit·ri·chate (ăm-fĭt′rĭ-kāt′, -kĭt) *or* **am·phit·ri·chous** (-kəs) *adj.* Of, relating to, or characteristic of a microorganism that has a flagellum or flagella at each end.

am·pho·phil (ăm′fə-fĭl) *or* **am·pho·phile** (-fĭl′) *adj.* Having an affinity for both acid and basic dyes. —*n.* A cell that stains readily with either acid or basic dyes. Also called *amphocyte.*

am·pho·phil·ic (ăm′fə-fĭl′ĭk) *or* **am·phoph·i·lous** (ăm-fŏf′ə-ləs) *adj.* Amphophil.

am·phor·ic (ăm-fôr′ĭk) *adj.* Relating to or characteristic of a sound made by blowing across the mouth of a bottle. Used to describe sounds in percussion and auscultation.

amphoric rale *n.* A sound heard during auscultation and associated with the movement of fluid in a lung cavity communicating with a bronchus.

amphoric resonance *n.* The sound obtained by percussing over a pulmonary cavity when the patient's mouth is open; it is similar to the sound produced by blowing across the neck of an empty bottle.

am·pho·ter·ic (ăm′fə-tĕr′ĭk) *adj.* Having the capacity to react as either an acid or a base.

am·pho·ter·i·cin B (ăm′fə-tĕr′ĭ-sĭn) *n.* An antibiotic derived from strains of the actinomycete *Streptomyces nodosus* and used in treating systemic fungal infections.

am·pho·ter·ism (ăm′fə-tĕr′ĭz′əm, ăm-fŏt′ə-rĭz′əm) *n.* The quality of exhibiting the characteristics of an acid and a base and having the capacity to react either as an acid or a base.

am·pho·trop·ic virus (ăm′fə-trŏp′ĭk, -trō′pĭk) *n.* An oncornavirus that does not produce disease in its natural host, but does replicate in tissue culture cells of the host species and in cells from other species.

am·pi·cil·lin (ăm′pĭ-sĭl′ĭn) *n.* A semisynthetic penicillin having a broader antibacterial spectrum of action than that of penicillin G. It is effective against gram-negative and gram-positive bacteria and used to treat gonorrhea and infections of the intestinal, urinary, and respiratory tracts.

am·pli·fi·ca·tion (ăm′plə-fĭ-kā′shən) *n.* **1.** The process of increasing the magnitude of a variable quantity, especially the magnitude of voltage, power, or current, without altering any other quality. **2.** The result of such a process. **3.** The process by which genes or DNA sequences are copied in an organism or in the laboratory.

am·pli·fi·er host (ăm′plə-fī′ər) *n.* A host in which infectious agents multiply to high concentrations.

am·pli·tude of accommodation (ăm′plĭ-tōōd′) *n.* The difference in refractivity of the eye at rest and when fully accommodated.

am·pule *or* **am·poule** *or* **am·pul** (ăm′pōōl, -pyōōl) *n.* A hermetically sealed vial, usually made of glass, that contains a sterile medicinal solution or a powder to be made into a solution for subcutaneous, intramuscular, or intravenous injection.

am·pul·la (ăm-pōōl′ə, -pŭl′ə) *n., pl.* **–pul·lae** (-pōōl′ē, -pŭl′ē) A dilated portion of a canal or duct, as in the semicircular canal of the ear. **—am·pul′lar** *adj.*

ampulla of uterine tube *n.* The wide portion of the fallopian tube that is situated near the fimbriated extremity.

ampulla of vas deferens *n.* See **Henle's ampulla.**

ampullar pregnancy *n.* A tubal pregnancy situated near the midportion of the oviduct.

am·pul·lar·y crest (ăm′pə-lĕr′ē) *n.* An elevation on the inner surface of the ampulla of each semicircular duct, through which filaments of the vestibular nerve pass to reach hair cells on the surface.

am·pul·li·tis (ăm′pə-lī′tĭs) *n.* Inflammation of an ampulla, especially of the dilated extremity of the vas deferens.

am·pu·tate (ăm′pyōō-tāt′) *v.* To cut off a part of the body, especially by surgery.

am·pu·ta·tion (ăm′pyōō-tā′shən) *n.* **1.** Surgical removal of all or part of a limb, an organ, or projecting part or process of the body. **2.** Traumatic or spontaneous loss of a limb, organ, or part.

amputation in continuity *n.* Amputation through a segment of a limb, not through a joint.

amputation neuroma *n.* See **traumatic neuroma.**

am·pu·tee (ăm′pyōō-tē′) *n.* A person who has had one or more limbs removed by amputation.

am·ri·none lactate (ăm′rə-nōn′) *n.* An inotropic agent that dilates blood vessels, used in treatment of congestive heart failure.

Am·ster·dam syndrome (ăm′stər-dăm′) *n.* See **de Lange's syndrome.**

amu *abbr.* atomic mass unit

a·mu·si·a (ə-myōō′zē-ə, -zhə) *n.* Loss or impairment of the ability to produce or comprehend music or musical tones.

a·my·e·li·a (ā′mī-ē′lē-ə, ăm′ī-) *n.* Congenital absence of the spinal cord. **—a′my·el′ic** (-ĕl′ĭk, -ē′lĭk) *adj.*

a·my·e·li·na·tion (ā-mī′ə-lə-nā′shən, ə-mī′-) *n.* Congenital absence of the myelin sheath on a nerve. **—a·my′e·li·nat′ed** (-nā′tĭd) *adj.*

a·my·e·lin·ic (ā-mī′ə-lĭn′ĭk, ə-mī′-) *adj.* Without myelin; unmyelinated.

a·my·e·lon·ic (ā-mī′ə-lŏn′ĭk, ə-mī′-) *or* **a·my·e·lo·ic** (-lō′ĭk) *adj.* **1.** Amyelous. **2.** Lacking bone marrow or lacking the functional participation of bone marrow in hemopoiesis.

a·my·e·lous (ə-mī′ə-ləs) *adj.* Relating to or characterized by the total or partial absence of a spinal cord.

a·myg·da·la (ə-mĭg′də-lə) *n., pl.* **–lae** (-lē) **1.** One of two almond-shaped masses of gray matter that are part of the limbic system and are located in the temporal lobes of the cerebral hemispheres. Also called *amygdaloid nucleus.* **2.** The cerebellar tonsil. **3.** Any of the lymphatic tonsils.

a·myg·da·lin (ə-mĭg′də-lĭn) *n.* A glycoside found in seeds and other plant parts of many members of the rose family, such as kernels of the apricot, peach, and bitter almond. Also called *amygdaloside.*

a·myg·da·line (ə-mĭg′də-lĭn, -līn′) *adj.* **1.** Relating to or resembling an almond. **2.** Relating to or characteristic of a tonsil or an amygdala. **3.** Tonsillar.

a·myg·da·loid (ə-mĭg′də-loid′) *or* **a·myg·da·loi·dal** (ə-mĭg′də-loid′l) *adj.* **1.** Shaped like an almond. **2.** Of or relating to an amygdala.

amygdaloid fossa *n.* See **tonsillar fossa.**

amygdaloid nucleus *n.* See **amygdala** (sense 1).

a·myg·da·lo·side (ə-mĭg′də-lə-sīd′) *n.* See **amygdalin.**

am·yl (ăm′əl) *n.* The univalent organic radical, C_5H_{11}, occurring in many organic compounds in eight isomeric forms. Also called *pentyl.*

am·y·la·ceous (ăm′ə-lā′shəs) *adj.* Of, relating to, or resembling starch; starchy.

am·y·lase (ăm′ə-lās′, -lāz′) *n.* Any of a group of enzymes that catalyze the hydrolysis of starch to sugar to produce carbohydrate derivatives.

amylase-creatinine clearance ratio *n.* The ratio between amylase and creatinine in serum and urine, used to diagnose acute pancreatitis.

am·y·la·su·ri·a (ăm′ə-lā-sŏor′ē-ə) *n.* The excess of amylase in the urine. Also called *diastasuria.*

am·y·lin (ăm′ə-lĭn) *n.* The insoluble envelope of starch grains; starch cellulose.

amyl nitrite *n.* A volatile yellow liquid formerly used in medicine as a vasodilator, but now replaced by other nitrates, such as nitroglycerin. It is used illicitly to induce euphoria and enhance sexual stimulation.

amylo– *or* **amyl–** *pref.* Starch: *amylose.*

amylo-1,6-glucosidase *n.* An enzyme that catalyzes the

hydrolysis of glycogen at specific branch points in its glucose residue chains; debrancher enzyme.

am·y·lo·gen·e·sis (ăm′ə-lō-jĕn′ĭ-sĭs) *n.* The biosynthesis of starch. —**am′y·lo·gen′ic** *adj.*

am·y·loid (ăm′ə-loid′) *n.* **1.** A starchlike substance. **2.** A hard, waxy deposit consisting of protein and polysaccharides resulting from the degeneration of tissue. —*adj.* Starchlike.

amyloid beta-protein *n.* See **beta-amyloid protein**.

amyloid degeneration *n.* The degeneration of a tissue or an organ characterized by the infiltration of amyloid between cells and fibers. Also called *waxy degeneration.*

amyloid kidney *n.* A kidney in which amyloidosis has occurred, usually in association with a chronic illness. Also called *waxy kidney.*

amyloid nephrosis *n.* The nephrotic syndrome due to deposition of amyloid in the kidney.

am·y·loid·o·sis (ăm′ə-loi-dō′sĭs) *n.* A disorder marked by the deposition of amyloid in various organs and tissues of the body that may be associated with a chronic disease such as rheumatoid arthritis, tuberculosis, or multiple myeloma.

amyloid tumor *n.* See **nodular amyloidosis**.

am·y·lol·y·sis (ăm′ə-lŏl′ĭ-sĭs) *n.* The conversion of starch to sugars by the action of enzymes or acids. —**am′y·lo·lyt′ic** (-lō-lĭt′ĭk) *adj.*

am·y·lo·pec·tin (ăm′ə-lō-pĕk′tĭn) *n.* The highly branched, almost insoluble polysaccharide that is a constituent of starch.

am·y·lo·pec·ti·no·sis (ăm′ə-lō-pĕk′tə-nō′sĭs) *n.* Glycogenosis due to an enzyme deficiency that causes abnormal glycogen to be stored in the liver, kidney, heart, muscle, and recticuloendothelial system.

am·y·lop·sin (ăm′ə-lŏp′sĭn) *n.* The starch-digesting amylase produced by the pancreas and present in pancreatic juice.

am·y·lor·rhe·a (ăm′ə-lō-rē′ə) *n.* The presence of undigested starch in the stool.

am·y·lose (ăm′ə-lōs′, -lōz′) *n.* **1.** The inner portion of a starch granule, consisting of relatively soluble polysaccharides having an unbranched, linear, or spiral structure. **2.** A polysaccharide, such as cellulose.

am·y·lo·su·ri·a (ăm′ə-lō-soŏr′ē-ə, -lōs-yoŏr′ē-ə) *n.* The presence of amylose in the urine. Also called *amyluria.*

am·y·lum (ăm′ə-ləm) *n.* See **starch** (sense 1).

am·y·lu·ri·a (ăm′ə-loŏr′ē-ə) *n.* See **amylosuria**.

a·my·o·es·the·sia (ā-mī′ō-ĭs-thē′zhə, ə-mī′-) *or* **a·my·o·es·the·sis** (-thē′sĭs) *n.* Inability to sense motion, weight, and balance.

a·my·o·pla·sia (ā-mī′ō-plā′zhə, ə-mī′-) *n.* The lack of muscle formation.

amyoplasia con·gen·i·ta (kən-jĕn′ĭ-tə) *n.* See **arthrogryposis** (sense 2).

a·my·o·sta·sia (ā-mī′ō-stā′zhə, ə-mī′-) *n.* A muscular tremor causing difficulty in standing or in coordination. —**a·my′o·stat′ic** (-stăt′ĭk) *adj.*

a·my·os·the·ni·a (ā-mī′əs-thē′nē-ə, ə-mī′-) *n.* Weakness of the muscles. —**a·my′os·then′ic** (-thĕn′ĭk) *adj.*

a·my·o·tax·y (ā-mī′ə-tăk′sē, ə-mī′-) *or* **a·my·o·tax·ia** (ā-mī′ə-tăk′sē-ə, ə-mī′-) *n.* Muscular ataxia or

incoordination due to difficulties in controlling voluntary movements.

a·my·o·to·ni·a (ā′mī-ə-tō′nē-ə) *n.* See **myatonia**.

amyotonia con·gen·i·ta (kən-jĕn′ĭ-tə) *n.* Any of several congenital diseases of children that are marked by general muscle hypotonia, usually in muscles that are functionally connected to the spinal nerves. Also called *myatonia congenita, Oppenheim's disease, Oppenheim's syndrome.*

a·my·o·tro·phi·a (ā-mī′ə-trō′fē-ə, ə-mī′-) *n.* See **amyotrophy**. —**a·my′o·tro′pic** (-trō′pĭk, -trŏp′ĭk) *adj.*

a·my·o·troph·ic lateral sclerosis (ā-mī′ə-trŏf′ĭk, -trō′fĭk) *n.* A disease of the motor tracts of the lateral columns and anterior horns of the spinal cord, causing progressive muscular atrophy, increased reflexes, fibrillary twitching, and spastic irritability of muscles. Also called *Charcot's disease, Lou Gehrig's disease.*

a·my·ot·ro·phy (ā′mī-ŏt′rə-fē, ăm′ī-) *n.* Muscular wasting or atrophy. Also called *amyotrophia.*

am·y·ous (ăm′ē-əs) *adj.* Lacking muscular tissue or muscular strength.

Am·y·tal (ăm′ĭ-tăl′, -tôl′) A trademark for the drug amobarbital.

a·myx·i·a (ā-mĭk′sē-ə, ə-mĭk′-) *n.* Absence of mucus.

a·myx·or·rhe·a (ā-mĭk′sə-rē′ə, ə-mĭk′-) *n.* Absence of mucus secretion.

an– *pref.* Variant of **a–**.

an·a (ăn′ə) *adv.* Both in the same quantity; of each. Used to refer to ingredients in prescriptions.

ANA *abbr.* antinuclear antibody

ana– *pref.* **1.** Upward; up: *anacrotic.* **2.** Backward; back: *anaplasia.* **3.** Again; anew: *anabiosis.*

an·a·bi·o·sis (ăn′ə-bī-ō′sĭs) *n.* A restoring to life from a deathlike condition; resuscitation.

an·a·bi·ot·ic (ăn′ə-bī-ŏt′ĭk) *adj.* Of, relating to, or being restorative; resuscitative. —*n.* A powerful stimulant; a revivifying remedy.

anabolic steroid *n.* A group of synthetic hormones that promote the storage of protein and the growth of tissue.

a·nab·o·lism (ə-năb′ə-lĭz′əm) *n.* The phase of metabolism in which simple substances are synthesized into the complex materials of living tissue. —**an′a·bol′ic** (ăn′ə-bŏl′ĭk) *adj.*

a·nab·o·lite (ə-năb′ə-līt′) *n.* A substance formed as a result of anabolism.

an·a·cid·i·ty (ăn′ə-sĭd′ĭ-tē) *n.* Absence of acidity, especially the absence of hydrochloric acid in the gastric juices.

a·nac·la·sis (ə-năk′lə-sĭs) *n.* **1.** Reflection of light or sound. **2.** Refraction of the ocular media. **3.** Forcible flexion of a joint to break up adhesions associated with fibrous ankylosis.

an·a·cli·sis (ăn′ə-klī′sĭs, ə-năk′lĭ-) *n.* Psychological dependence on others.

an·a·clit·ic (ăn′ə-klĭt′ĭk) *adj.* Having a physical and emotional dependence on another person, especially relating to the dependence of an infant on a mother or surrogate mother.

anaclitic depression *n.* The impairment of an infant's physical, social, and intellectual development following separation from its mother or primary caregiver.

an·a·crot·ic (ăn′ə-krŏt′ĭk) *adj.* Of, relating to, or characteristic of the upstroke or ascending limb of an arterial pulse tracing.

anacrotic pulse *n.* A slow-rising pulse tracing with a notch in the ascending portion.

a·nac·ro·tism (ə-năk′rə-tĭz′əm) *n.* The condition in which one or more notches or waves occur on the ascending limb of an arterial pulse tracing. Also called *anadicrotism.*

an·a·cu·sis *or* **an·a·ku·sis** (ăn′ə-koo′sĭs, -kyoo′-) *n.* Complete deafness.

an·a·di·crot·ic (ăn′ə-dī-krŏt′ĭk) *adj.* Anacrotic.

an·a·di·cro·tism (ăn′ə-dī′krə-tĭz′əm) *n.* See **anacrotism.**

an·ad·re·nal·ism (ăn′ə-drē′nə-lĭz′əm) *n.* Complete absence or failure of adrenal function.

an·aer·obe (ăn′ə-rōb′, ăn-âr′ōb′) *n.* An organism that can live in the absence of atmospheric oxygen.

an·aer·o·bic (ăn′ə-rō′bĭk, -ă-rō′bĭk) *adj.* **1.** Relating to or being an anaerobe. **2.** Living without oxygen.

anaerobic respiration *n.* Respiration in which molecular oxygen is not consumed.

an·aer·o·bi·o·sis (ăn′ə-rō′bī-ō′sĭs, ăn′â-rō′-) *n.* Life sustained by an organism in the absence of oxygen.

an·aer·o·gen·ic (ăn′ə-rō-jĕn′ĭk, ăn′â-rō-) *adj.* Producing no gas.

A·naf·ra·nil (ə-năf′rə-nĭl) A trademark for the drug clomipramine.

an·a·gen (ăn′ə-jĕn′) *n.* The growth phase of the hair cycle during which new hair is formed.

a·nal (ā′nəl) *adj.* **1.** Of, relating to, or near the anus. **2.** Of or relating to the second stage of psychosexual development in psychoanalytic theory, during which gratification is derived from sensations associated with the anus. **3.** Relating to or being personality traits that originated during toilet training and are distinguished as anal-expulsive or anal-retentive.

anal atresia *n.* Congenital absence of an anal opening due to the presence of a membranous septum or to complete absence of the anal canal. Also called *imperforate anus, proctatresia.*

an·al·bu·mi·ne·mi·a (ăn′ăl-byoo′mə-nē′mē-ə) *n.* The absence of albumin from blood serum.

anal canal *n.* The terminal portion of the alimentary canal, extending from the pelvic diaphragm to the anal orifice.

anal column *n.* Any of the vertical ridges in the mucous membrane of the upper half of the anal canal. Also called *rectal column.*

anal duct *n.* One of the short ducts lined with columnar epithelium that extend from the anal valves to the anal sinus.

an·a·lep·tic (ăn′ə-lĕp′tĭk) *adj.* Restorative or stimulating, as a drug or medication. —*n.* A medication used as a central nervous system stimulant.

analeptic enema *n.* An enema of lukewarm water with a small amount of table salt.

anal-expulsive *adj.* Indicating personality traits, such as conceit, ambition, and generosity, originating in habits, attitudes, or values associated with infantile pleasure in the expulsion of feces.

anal fissure *n.* A crack or slit in the mucous membrane of the anus.

anal fistula *n.* A fistula opening at or near the anus, usually into the rectum above the internal sphincter.

an·al·ge·si·a (ăn′əl-jē′zē-ə, -zhə) *n.* A deadening or absence of the sense of pain without loss of consciousness.

analgesia al·ger·a (ăl′jər-ə) *n.* Spontaneous pain in a portion of the body that is not sensitive to painful stimuli. Also called *analgesia dolorosa.*

analgesia do·lo·ro·sa (dō′lə-rō′sə) *n.* See **analgesia algera.**

an·al·ge·sic (ăn′əl-jē′zĭk) *n.* A medication capable of reducing or eliminating pain. Also called *analgetic.* —*adj.* Characterized by analgesia.

an·al·get·ic (ăn′əl-jĕt′ĭk) *n.* See **analgesic.** —*adj.* Having altered pain perception.

a·nal·i·ty (ā-năl′ĭ-tē) *n.* The psychological state derived from and characteristic of the anal period of psychosexual development.

an·al·ler·gic (ăn′ə-lûr′jĭk) *adj.* Not allergic.

a·nal·o·gous (ə-năl′ə-gəs) *adj.* Similar in function but not in structure and evolutionary origin.

an·a·log *or* **an·a·logue** (ăn′ə-lôg′) *n.* **1.** An organ or structure similar in function to one in another species but of dissimilar evolutionary origin. **2.** A structural derivative of a parent chemical compound that often differs from it by a single element.

anal orifice *n.* See **anus.**

anal pecten *n.* The middle third of the anal canal.

anal phase *n.* In psychoanalytic theory, the stage of psychosexual development occurring early in life, usually around the second year, when a child's activities, interests, and concerns are centered around the expulsion and retention of feces.

anal pit *n.* See **proctodeum.**

anal plate *n.* The anal portion of the cloacal plate.

anal reflex *n.* Contraction of the anal sphincter around a finger passed into the rectum.

anal-retentive *adj.* Indicating personality traits, such as meticulousness, avarice, and obstinacy, originating in habits, attitudes, or values associated with infantile pleasure in retention of feces.

anal sinus *n.* Any of the grooves between the anal columns. Also called *Morgagni's crypt, rectal sinus.*

anal sphincter *n.* Either of the two sphincter muscles of the anus. See under **external** and **internal sphincter muscle of anus.**

anal verge *n.* The distal end of the anal canal, forming a transitional zone between the skin of the anal canal and the perianal skin.

a·nal·y·sand (ə-năl′ĭ-sănd′) *n.* An individual who is being psychoanalyzed.

a·nal·y·sis (ə-năl′ĭ-sĭs) *n.,* pl. **–ses** (-sēz′) **1.** The separation of a whole into its constituent parts for individual study. **2.** The separation of a substance into its constituent elements to determine either their nature or proportions. **3.** The stated findings of such a separation or determination. **4.** Psychoanalysis.

an·a·lyst (ăn′ə-lĭst) *n.* **1.** One that analyzes. **2.** A psychoanalyst.

an·a·lyte (ăn′ə-līt′) *n.* A substance or chemical constituent that is undergoing analysis.

an·a·lyt·ic (ăn′ə-lĭt′ĭk) *or* **an·a·lyt·i·cal** (-ĭ-kəl) *adj.* **1.** Of or relating to analysis or analytics. **2.** Expert in or using analysis, especially one who thinks in a logical manner. **3.** Psychoanalytic.

an·a·lyt·ic psychology *n.* The theory of psychoanalysis developed by Carl Jung that focuses on the concept of the collective unconscious and the importance of balancing opposing forces within the personality.

an·a·lyze (ăn′ə-līz′) *v.* **1.** To examine methodically by separating into parts and studying their interrelations. **2.** To separate a chemical substance into its constituent elements to determine their nature or proportions. **3.** To psychoanalyze.

an·a·lyz·er *or* **an·a·ly·zor** (ăn′ə-lī′zər) *n.* **1.** An analyst. **2.** The prism in a polariscope that analyses polarized light. **3.** The neural basis of a conditioned reflex, including the sensory side of the reflex arc and its central connections. **4.** An apparatus attached to electroencephalographic instruments to measure electrical frequency. **5.** Any of various instruments used for performing an analysis.

an·am·ne·sis (ăn′ăm-nē′sĭs) *n.*, *pl.* **–ses** (-sēz) **1.** A recalling to memory; recollection. **2.** The complete case history of a patient.

an·am·nes·tic (ăn′ăm-něs′tĭk) *adj.* **1.** Of or relating to the current or previous medical history of a patient. **2.** Aiding memory; mnemonic.

anamnestic reaction *n.* Augmented production of an antibody due to previous stimulation by the same antigen.

an·an·gi·o·pla·sia (ăn-ăn′jē-ō-plā′zhə) *n.* The imperfect vascularization of a part due to poorly formed or unformed blood vessels. **—an·an′gi·o·plas′tic** (-plăs′tĭk) *adj.*

an·a·phase (ăn′ə-fāz′) *n.* The stage of mitosis and meiosis in which the chromosomes move from the equatorial plate toward opposite ends of the nuclear spindle.

an·a·phi·a (ăn-ā′fē-ə) *n.* Total or partial absence of the sense of touch. **—an·ap′tic** (-ăp′tĭk) *adj.*

an·a·pho·ri·a (ăn′ə-fôr′ē-ə) *n.* A tendency of resting eyes to turn upward. Also called *anatropia*.

an·aph·ro·dis·i·a (ăn-ăf′rə-dĭz′ē-ə, -dĭzh′ə) *n.* A decline or absence of sexual desire.

an·aph·ro·dis·i·ac (ăn-ăf′rə-dĭz′ē-ăk′) *adj.* **1.** Of, relating to, or characteristic of anaphrodisia. **2.** Repressing or destroying sexual desire. **—***n.* An agent that lessens or eliminates sexual desire.

anaphylactic antibody *n.* See **cytotropic antibody.**

anaphylactic shock *n.* A severe, sometimes fatal allergic reaction characterized by a sharp drop in blood pressure, urticaria, and breathing difficulties that is caused by exposure to a foreign substance, such as a drug or bee venom, after preliminary or sensitizing exposure. The reaction may be fatal if emergency treatment, including epinephrine injections, is not given immediately. Also called *anaphylaxis*.

an·a·phy·lac·to·gen (ăn′ə-fə-lăk′tə-jən) *n.* A substance capable of producing anaphylaxis in an individual. **—an′a·phy·lac′to·gen′ic** (-jěn′ĭk) *adj.*

an·a·phy·lac·to·gen·e·sis (ăn′ə-fə-lăk′tə-jěn′ĭ-sĭs) *n.* The production of anaphylaxis.

an·a·phy·lac·toid (ăn′ə-fə-lăk′toid′) *adj.* Of or resembling anaphylaxis.

anaphylactoid purpura *n.* **1.** See **allergic purpura. 2.** See **Henoch-Schönlein purpura.**

anaphylactoid shock *n.* A reaction similar to anaphylactic shock but not requiring the incubation period characteristic of induced sensitivity and unrelated to antibody-antigen reactions.

an·a·phyl·a·tox·in *or* **an·a·phyl·o·tox·in** (ăn′ə-fĭl′ə-tŏk′sĭn) *n.* A substance that may cause the release of histamine and other compounds that cause hypersensitivity, thus triggering some or all of the symptoms of anaphylaxis.

an·a·phy·lax·is (ăn′ə-fə-lăk′sĭs) *n.*, *pl.* **–lax·es** (-lăk′sēz) **1.** Hypersensitivity induced by preliminary exposure to a substance and usually producing a contraction of smooth muscle and a dilation of blood vessels. **2.** See **anaphylactic shock. —an′a·phy·lac′tic** (-lăk′tĭk) *adj.*

an·a·pla·sia (ăn′ə-plā′zhə) *n.* Reversion of cells to an immature or a less differentiated form, as occurs in most malignant tumors.

an·a·plas·tic (ăn′ə-plăs′tĭk) *adj.* **1.** Relating to the surgical restoration of a lost or absent part. **2.** Of, relating to, or characterized by cells that have become less differentiated.

anaplastic cell *n.* **1.** A cell that has reverted to an embryonal state. **2.** An undifferentiated cell, characteristic of a malignant neoplasm.

an·a·poph·y·sis (ăn′ə-pŏf′ĭ-sĭs) *n.* An accessory process of a vertebra, especially in the thoracic or lumbar vertebrae.

An·a·prox (ăn′ə-prŏks′) A trademark for the drug naproxen.

an·a·rith·mi·a (ăn′ə-rĭth′mē-ə, -rĭth′-) *n.* An inability to count or use numbers due to a brain lesion.

an·ar·thri·a (ăn-är′thrē-ə) *n.* Loss of the motor ability that enables speech.

an·a·sar·ca (ăn′ə-sär′kə) *n.* An accumulation of serous fluid in various tissues and cavities of the body. **—an′-a·sar′cous** (-kəs) *adj.*

a·nas·to·mose (ə-năs′tə-mōz′, -mōs′) *v.* **1.** To join by anastomosis. **2.** To be connected by anastomosis.

a·nas·to·mo·sis (ə-năs′tə-mō′sĭs) *n.*, *pl.* **–ses** (-sēz) **1.** The direct or indirect connection of separate parts of a branching system to form a network, especially among blood vessels. **2.** The surgical connection of separate or severed tubular hollow organs to form a continuous channel as between two parts of the intestine. **3.** An opening created by surgery, trauma, or disease between two or more normally separate spaces or organs. **—a·nas′to·mot′ic** (-mŏt′ĭk) *adj.*

anastomotic branch *n.* A blood vessel that connects two neighboring vessels.

anastomotic ulcer *n.* An ulcer of the jejunum occurring after gastroenterostomy.

an·a·tom·i·cal (ăn′ə-tŏm′ĭ-kəl) *or* **an·a·tom·ic** (-tŏm′-ĭk) *adj.* **1.** Concerned with anatomy. **2.** Concerned with dissection. **3.** Related to the structure of an organism.

anatomical dead space *n.* The volume of the conducting airways of the nose, mouth, and trachea down to the level of the alveoli, representing that portion of inspired gas unavailable for exchange of gases with pulmonary capillary blood.

anatomical pathology *n.* The study of the structural and compositional changes that occur in organs and tissues as a result of disease. Also called *pathological anatomy.*

anatomical position *n.* The erect position of the body with the face directed forward, the arms at the side, and the palms of the hands facing forward, used as a reference in describing the relation of body parts to one another.

anatomical sphincter *n.* See **sphincter.**

anatomical wart *n.* See **postmortem wart.**

a·nat·o·mist (ə-năt′ə-mĭst) *n.* An expert in or a student of anatomy.

a·nat·o·mize (ə-năt′ə-mīz′) *v.* To dissect an animal or other organism to study the structure and relation of the parts.

a·nat·o·my (ə-năt′ə-mē) *n.* **1.** The morphological structure of a plant or an animal or of any of its parts. **2.** The science of the shape and structure of organisms and their parts. **3.** Dissection of an animal to study the structure, position, and interrelation of its various parts. **4.** A skeleton. **5.** The human body.

an·a·tri·cro·tism (ăn′ə-trī′krə-tĭz′əm, -trĭk′rə-) *n.* A pulse anomaly manifested by a triple beat on the ascending limb of a sphygmographic tracing. —**an′a·tri·crot′ic** (-trī-krŏt′ĭk) *adj.*

an·a·tro·pi·a (ăn′ə-trō′pē-ə) *n.* See **anaphoria.**

An·be·sol (ăn′bə-sôl′) A trademark for an over-the-counter preparation containing the drug benzocaine.

an·chor·age (ăng′kər-ĭj) *n.* **1.** The surgical fixation of loose or prolapsed abdominal or pelvic organs. **2.** The part to which something is secured or stabilized. **3.** A tooth or an implanted tooth substitute to which a fixed or removable partial denture, crown, or restorative material is fastened. **4.** The resistance to displacement offered by an anatomical structure used to help move a tooth.

an·chor splint (ăng′kər) *n.* A splint used for a fracture of the jaw, with wires around the teeth and a rod to hold it in place.

an·cil·lar·y (ăn′sə-lĕr′ē) *adj.* Relating to or being auxiliary or secondary.

an·cip·i·tal (ăn-sĭp′ĭ-tl) *or* **an·cip·i·tate** (-ĭ-tāt′) *or* **an·cip·i·tous** (-ĭ-təs) *adj.* Of or being two-headed or two-edged.

an·co·nad (ăng′kō-năd′) *adj.* Anatomically located toward the elbow.

an·co·nal (ăng′kə-nəl, ăng-kō′-) *or* **an·co·ne·al** (ăng-kō′nē-əl) *adj.* Relating to the elbow.

an·co·ne·ous muscle (ăng-kō′nē-əs) *n.* A muscle with its origin in the back of the lateral condyle of the humerus, with insertion to the olecranon process and the posterior surface of the ulna, with nerve supply from the radial nerve, and whose action extends the forearm and abducts the ulna in pronation of the wrist.

an·co·ni·tis (ăng′kə-nī′tĭs) *n.* An inflammation of the elbow joint.

an·crod (ăn′krŏd) *n.* A proteinase obtained from the venom of the pit viper, which contains a fibrinogen-splitting enzyme and is used in the treatment of chronic peripheral vascular disease.

ancylo– *pref.* Variant of **ankylo–.**

An·cy·los·to·ma (ăn′sə-lŏs′tə-mə, ăng′kə-) *n.* A genus of hookworms that includes species that are intestinal parasites of humans and other mammals.

Ancylostoma bra·zil·i·en·se (brə-zĭl′ē-ĕn′sē) *n.* A species of hookworm that usually is an intestinal parasite of dogs and cats but can also infest the skin of humans.

Ancylostoma ca·ni·num (kā-nī′nəm) *n.* A species of hookworm that can infest human skin.

Ancylostoma du·o·de·na·le (dōō′ō-də-nā′lē) *n.* A species of hookworm widespread in temperate areas that can infest the small intestine of humans, causing ancylostomiasis.

an·cy·lo·sto·mat·ic (ăn′sə-lō-stō-măt′ĭk, ăng′kə-) *adj.* Of or relating to hookworms of the genus *Ancylostoma.*

an·cy·lo·sto·mi·a·sis (ăn′sə-lō-stō-mī′ə-sĭs, ăng′kə-lō-) *n.* A disease caused by infestation with the hookworm *Ancylostoma duodenale,* characterized by gastrointestinal pain, diarrhea, and progressive anemia. Also called *tunnel disease, uncinariasis.*

an·cy·roid (ăn′sə-roid′) *or* **an·ky·roid** (ăn′kə-) *adj.* Shaped like the fluke of an anchor.

An·der·sen's disease (ăn′dər-sənz) *n.* See **type 4 glycogenosis.**

An·der·son (ăn′dər-sən), **Elizabeth** 1836–1917. British physician. The first licensed British woman doctor (1865), she established medical courses for women at a dispensary in London.

Anderson splint *n.* A skeletal traction splint having pins inserted into the proximal and distal ends of a fracture; reduction is obtained by an external plate attached to the pins.

andro– *or* **andr–** *pref.* Male; masculine: *androgen.*

an·dro·blas·to·ma (ăn′drō-blă-stō′mə) *n.* **1.** A testicular tumor that histologically resembles a fetal testis and contains cells that may produce estrogen. Also called *Sertoli cell tumor.* **2.** Arrhenoblastoma.

an·dro·gen (ăn′drə-jən) *n.* A steroid, such as testosterone or androsterone, that controls the development and maintenance of masculine characteristics. Also called *androgenic hormone.* —**an′dro·gen′ic** (-jĕn′ĭk) *adj.*

an·dro·gen·e·sis (ăn′drō-jĕn′ĭ-sĭs) *n.* The development of an embryo that contains only paternal chromosomes because the egg has been activated by sperm without fusion of the egg and sperm nuclei. —**an·dro·ge·net·ic** (ăn′drō-jə-nĕt′ĭk) *adj.*

androgenetic alopecia *n.* **1.** See **male pattern baldness.** **2.** A condition of hair loss in women similar to male pattern baldness, but beginning later in life and less severe.

androgenic hormone *n.* See **androgen.**

an·drog·e·nize (ăn-drŏj′ə-nīz′) *v.* To treat with male hormones, usually in large doses.

an·drog·y·nism (ăn-drŏj′ə-nĭz′əm) *n.* Female pseudohermaphroditism.

an·drog·y·ny (ăn-drŏj′ə-nē) *n.* **1.** Female pseudohermaphroditism. **2.** The condition of having both masculine and feminine characteristics, as in appearance, attitude, or behavior. —**an·drog′y·nous** (-nəs) *adj.*

an·droid (ăn′droid′) *adj.* Possessing human features and form.

android pelvis *n.* A masculine or funnel-shaped pelvis.

an·dro·pause (ăn′drə-pôz′) *n.* The decrease in function of male reproductive organs that occurs with aging.

an·dro·pho·bi·a (ăn′drə-fō′bē-ə) *n.* An abnormal fear or dislike of men.

an·dro·stane (ăn′drə-stān′) *n.* A steroid hydrocarbon from which androgens are derived.

an·dro·stene (ăn′drə-stēn′) *n.* A unsaturated steroid that exists in two isomeric forms and comprises the basic chemical unit of various androgens.

an·dro·stene·di·ol (ăn′drə-stēn′dī-ôl′, -dē-ôl′) *n.* An unsaturated steroidal derivative of androstane that contains two alcohol groups and exists in three isomeric forms.

an·dro·stene·di·one (ăn′drə-stēn′dī-ōn′, -dē-ōn′) *n.* An unsaturated androgenic steroid existing in three isomeric forms that is secreted by the testis, ovary, and adrenal cortex and has a weaker biological potency than testosterone.

an·dros·ter·one (ăn-drŏs′tə-rōn′) *n.* A steroid hormone excreted in urine that reinforces masculine characteristics.

–ane *suff.* A saturated hydrocarbon: *hexane.*

an·ec·ta·sis (ăn-ĕk′tə-sĭs) *n.* See **primary atelectasis.**

a·ne·mi·a (ə-nē′mē-ə) *n.* A pathological deficiency in the oxygen-carrying component of the blood, measured in unit volume concentrations of hemoglobin, red blood cell volume, or red blood cell number. —**a·ne′mic** (-mĭk) *adj.*

anemic anoxia *n.* See **anemic hypoxia.**

anemic halo *n.* A pale, relatively avascular area in the skin seen around spider nevi, cherry angiomas, and some acute macular eruptions.

anemic hypoxia *n.* Hypoxia resulting from a decreased concentration of functional hemoglobin or a reduced number of erythrocytes. Also called *anemic anoxia.*

anemic infarct *n.* An infarct in which little or no bleeding into tissue occurs when the blood supply is obstructed. Also called *white infarct.*

anemic murmur *n.* A nonvalvular murmur heard on auscultation of the heart and large blood vessels in cases of profound anemia.

an·e·mo·pho·bi·a (ăn′ə-mō-fō′bē-ə, ə-nē′mə-) *n.* An abnormal fear of the wind or drafts.

an·en·ceph·a·ly (ăn′ən-sĕf′ə-lē) *n.* Congenital absence of most of the brain and spinal cord. —**an′en·ce·phal′ic** (-sə-făl′ĭk), **an′en·ceph′a·lous** (-sĕf′ə-ləs) *adj.*

a·neph·ric (ā-nĕf′rĭk, ə-nĕf′-) *adj.* Lacking kidneys.

anergic leishmaniasis *n.* See **diffuse cutaneous leishmaniasis.**

an·er·gy (ăn′ər-jē) *n.* Absence of sensitivity to substances that would normally elicit an antigenic response. —**an·er′gic** (ă-nûr′jĭk, ăn′ər-) *adj.*

an·e·ryth·ro·pla·sia (ăn′ĭ-rĭth′rə-plā′zhə) *n.* A condition in which there is no formation of red blood cells. —**an·e·ryth·ro·plas′tic** (-plăs′tĭk) *adj.*

an·es·the·sia (ăn′ĭs-thē′zhə) *n.* **1.** Total or partial loss of sensation, especially tactile sensibility, induced by disease, injury, acupuncture, or an anesthetic. **2.** Local or general insensibility to pain with or without the loss of consciousness, induced by an anesthetic. **3.** A drug that induces partial or total loss of sensation and may be topical, local, regional, or general, depending on the method of administration and area of the body affected.

anesthesia do·lo·ro·sa (dō′lə-rō′sə) *n.* Severe spontaneous pain occurring in an anesthetic zone.

anesthesia record *n.* A written account of drugs administered, procedures undertaken, and cardiovascular responses observed during the course of surgical or obstetrical anesthesia.

an·es·the·si·ol·o·gy (ăn′ĭs-thē′zē-ŏl′ə-jē) *n.* The medical specialty concerned with the pharmacological, physiological, and clinical basis of anesthesia, including resuscitation, intensive respiratory care, and pain management. —**an·es·the·si·ol·o·gist** (-jĭst) *n.*

an·es·thet·ic (ăn′ĭs-thĕt′ĭk) *n.* An agent that reversibly depresses neuronal function, producing total or partial loss of sensation. —*adj.* **1.** Characterized by the loss of sensation. **2.** Capable of producing a loss of sensation. **3.** Associated with or due to the state of anesthesia. —**an′es·thet′i·cal·ly** *adv.*

anesthetic depth *n.* The degree to which the central nervous system is depressed by a general anesthetic agent, depending on the potency of the anesthetic and the concentration in which it is administered.

anesthetic leprosy *n.* Leprosy chiefly affecting the nerves and marked by heightened then suppressed sensation, and by paralysis, ulceration, and various trophic disturbances, often resulting in gangrene and disfigurement. Also called *trophoneurotic leprosy.*

a·nes·the·tist (ə-nĕs′thĭ-tĭst) *n.* A person trained to administer anesthetics.

a·nes·the·tize (ə-nĕs′thĭ-tīz′) *v.* To induce anesthesia in. —**an·es′the·ti·za′tion** (-tĭ-zā′shən) *n.*

an·es·trous (ăn-ĕs′trəs) *adj.* **1.** Not exhibiting estrus. **2.** Of or relating to anestrus.

an·es·trus (ăn-ĕs′trəs) *n.* An interval of sexual inactivity between two periods of estrus in female mammals that breed cyclically.

an·e·to·der·ma (ăn′ĭ-tō-dûr′mə) *n.* Atrophy of the skin characterized by circumscribed lesions in which the skin becomes baglike and wrinkled.

an·eu·ploid (ăn′yōō-ploid′) *n.* A cell or an organism characterized by aneuploidy.

an·eu·ploi·dy (ăn′yə-ploi′dē) *n.* The state of having a chromosome number that is not a multiple of the haploid number.

an·eu·rysm *or* **an·eu·rism** (ăn′yə-rĭz′əm) *n.* A localized, blood-filled dilation of a blood vessel caused by disease or weakening of the vessel wall. See illustration on page 44. —**an′eu·rys′mal** (-məl), **an′eu·ris·mat′ic** (-măt′ĭk) *adj.*

aneurysmal bone cyst *n.* A solitary benign lesion in a long bone or vertebra, consisting of blood-filled spaces separated by fibrous tissue and causing swelling, pain, and tenderness.

an·eu·rys·mec·to·my (ăn′yə-rĭz-mĕk′tə-mē) *n.* Excision of an aneurysm.

aneurysm of Char·cot (shär-kō′) *n.* A small round nodular aneurysm of a small artery or arteriole of the cerebral cortex or basal ganglia, occurring frequently in hypertensive persons.

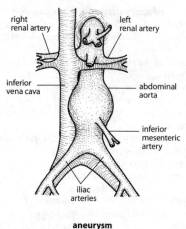

right renal artery

left renal artery

inferior vena cava

abdominal aorta

inferior mesenteric artery

iliac arteries

aneurysm
abdominal aortic aneurysm

an·eu·rys·mo·gram (ăn′yə-rĭz′mə-grăm′) *n.* Demonstration of an aneurysm, usually by means of x-rays and a contrast medium.

an·eu·rys·mo·plas·ty (ăn′yə-rĭz′mə-plăs′tē) *n.* **1.** Treatment of an aneurysm by opening the sac and suturing its walls to reconstruct the artery. Also called *endoaneurysmoplasty, endoaneurysmorrhaphy, Matas operation.* **2.** See **aneurysmorrhaphy.**

an·eu·rys·mor·rha·phy (ăn′yə-rĭz-môr′ə-fē) *n.* The surgical suture of the sac of an aneurysm. Also called *aneurysmoplasty.*

an·eu·rys·mot·o·my (ăn′yə-rĭz-mŏt′ə-mē) *n.* Incision into the sac of an aneurysm.

ANF *abbr.* antinuclear factor

An·fin·sen (ăn′fən-sən), **Christian Boehmer** 1916–1995. American biochemist. He shared a 1972 Nobel Prize for pioneering studies of ribonuclease.

an·gel dust (ān′jəl) *n.* Phencyclidine.

angi– *pref.* Variant of **angio–**.

an·gi·as·the·ni·a (ăn′jē-əs-thē′nē-ə) *n.* Loss of vascular tone.

an·gi·ec·ta·sia (ăn′jē-ĭk-tā′zhə) *or* **an·gi·ec·ta·sis** (-ĕk′tə-sĭs) *n.* Dilation of a lymphatic or blood vessel.

an·gi·ec·tat·ic (ăn′jē-ĭk-tăt′ĭk) *adj.* Marked by the presence of dilated blood vessels.

an·gi·ec·to·my (ăn′jē-ĕk′tə-mē) *n.* Excision of a section of a blood vessel.

an·gi·ec·to·pi·a (ăn′jē-ĕk-tō′pē-ə) *n.* Abnormal location or course of a blood vessel.

an·gi·i·tis (ăn′jē-ī′tĭs) *n.* See **vasculitis.**

an·gi·na (ăn-jī′nə, ăn′jə-) *n.* **1.** A severe constricting pain, especially angina pectoris. **2.** A sore throat. —**an·gi′nal** *adj.* —**an′gi·nose′** (-jə-nōs′) *adj.*

angina cru·ris (krŏŏr′ĭs) *n.* Intermittent claudication.

angina in·ver·sa (ĭn-vûr′sə) *n.* See **Prinzmetal's angina.**

angina pec·to·ris (pĕk′tər-ĭs) *n.* Severe constricting chest pain, often radiating from the precordium to the left shoulder and down the arm, due to insufficient blood supply to the heart that is usually caused by coronary disease. Also called *stenocardia.*

angina pectoris va·so·mo·to·ri·a (vā′zō-mō-tôr′ē-ə) *n.* See **vasomotor angina.**

an·gin·i·form (ăn-jĭn′ə-fôrm′) *adj.* Of or resembling angina.

an·gi·noid (ăn′jə-noid′) *n.* Resembling angina, especially angina pectoris.

anginose scarlatina *n.* A form of scarlatina in which the sore throat is unusually severe. Also called *Fothergill's disease.*

angio– *or* **angi–** *pref.* Blood and lymph vessel: *angiography.*

an·gi·o·blast (ăn′jē-ə-blăst′) *n.* **1.** A cell taking part in blood vessel formation. **2.** The primordial mesenchymal tissue from which embryonic blood cells and vascular endothelium are differentiated. Also called *vasoformative cell.*

an·gi·o·blas·to·ma (ăn′jē-ō-blă-stō′mə) *n.* See **hemangioblastoma.**

an·gi·o·car·di·og·ra·phy (ăn′jē-ō-kär′dē-ŏg′rə-fē) *n.* Examination of the heart and associated blood vessels using x-rays following the injection of a radiopaque substance. —**an′gi·o·car′di·o·graph′ic** (-ə-grăf′ĭk) *adj.*

an·gi·o·car·di·o·ki·net·ic (ăn′jē-ō-kär′dē-ō-kĭ-nĕt′ĭk) *or* **an·gi·o·car·di·o·ci·net·ic** (-sə-nĕt′ĭk) *adj.* Causing dilation or contraction in the heart and the blood vessels.

an·gi·o·car·di·op·a·thy (ăn′jē-ō-kär′dē-ŏp′ə-thē) *n.* A disease affecting the heart and the blood vessels.

an·gi·o·car·di·tis (ăn′jē-ō-kär-dī′tĭs) *n.* Inflammation of the heart and the blood vessels.

an·gi·o·dys·pla·sia (ăn′jē-ō-dĭs-plā′zhə) *n.* Degenerative dilation of the normal vasculature.

an·gi·o·dys·tro·phy (ăn′jē-ō-dĭs′trə-fē) *or* **an·gi·o·dys·tro·phi·a** (-dĭ-strō′fē-ə) *n.* A nutritional disorder affecting the blood vessels.

an·gi·o·e·de·ma (ăn′jē-ō-ĭ-dē′mə) *n.* See **angioneurotic edema.**

an·gi·o·en·do·the·li·o·ma·to·sis (ăn′jē-ō-ĕn′dō-thē′-lē-ō′mə-tō′sĭs) *n.* Proliferation of endothelial cells within blood vessels.

an·gi·o·fi·bro·li·po·ma (ăn′jē-ō-fī′brō-lĭ-pō′mə, -lī-) *n.* A neoplasm composed of fibrocytes, capillaries, and adipose tissue.

an·gi·o·fi·bro·ma (ăn′jē-ō-fī-brō′mə) *n.* See **telangiectatic fibroma.**

an·gi·o·fi·bro·sis (ăn′jē-ō-fī-brō′sĭs) *n.* Fibrosis of the walls of blood vessels.

an·gi·o·gen·e·sis (ăn′jē-ō-jĕn′ĭ-sĭs) *n.* The formation of new blood vessels, especially blood vessels that supply oxygen and nutrients to cancerous tissue. —**an′gi·o·gen′ic** (-jĕn′ĭk) *adj.*

angiogenesis factor *n.* A substance of 2000 to 20,000 molecular weight secreted by macrophages and stimulating neovascularization in healing wounds or in the stroma of tumors.

an·gi·o·gli·o·ma (ăn′jē-ō-glē-ō′mə, -glī-) *n.* A tumor that is a mixed glioma and angioma.

an·gi·o·gram (ăn′jē-ə-grăm′) *n.* An angiographic x-ray of blood vessels used in diagnosing pathological conditions of the cardiovascular system.

an·gi·og·ra·phy (ăn′jē-ŏg′rə-fē) *n.* Examination of the blood vessels using x-rays following the injection of a radiopaque substance. —**an′gi·o·graph′ic** (-ə-grăf′ĭk) *adj.*

an·gi·o·he·mo·phil·i·a (ăn′jē-ō-hē′mə-fĭl′ē-ə, -fēl′yə) *n.* See **von Willebrand's disease.**

an·gi·o·hy·a·li·no·sis (ăn′jē-ō-hī′ə-lə-nō′sĭs) *n.* Hyaline degeneration of the walls of the blood vessels.

an·gi·oid (ăn′jē-oid′) *adj.* Resembling blood vessels.

angioid streak *n.* Any of the breaks in the basal layer of the choroid of the eye occurring in a variety of systemic disorders affecting elastic tissue.

an·gi·o·im·mu·no·blas·tic lymphadenopathy (ăn′jē-ō-ĭm′yə-nō-blăs′tĭc) *n.* Acute or subacute generalized lymphadenopathy in elderly persons associated with polyclonal hypergammaglobulinemia, anemia, and enlargement of the liver and spleen. Also called *immunoblastic lymphadenopathy.*

an·gi·o·ker·a·to·ma (ăn′jē-ō-kĕr′ə-tō′mə) *n.* An intradermal cavernous hemangioma covered by a wartlike thickening of the horny layer of the epidermis. Also called *telangiectatic wart.*

angiokeratoma cor·po·ris dif·fu·sum (kôr′pər-ĭs dĭ-fyoo′səm) *n.* See **Fabry's disease.**

an·gi·o·ker·a·to·sis (ăn′jē-ō-kĕr′ə-tō′sĭs) *n.* A condition characterized by multiple angiokeratomas.

an·gi·o·ki·ne·sis (ăn′jē-ō-kə-nē′sĭs) *n.* See **vasomotion.**

an·gi·o·ki·net·ic (ăn′jē-ō-kə-nĕt′ĭk, -kī-) *n.* See **vasomotor.**

an·gi·o·lei·o·my·o·ma (ăn′jē-ō-lī′ō-mī-ō′mə) *n.* See **vascular leiomyoma.**

an·gi·o·li·po·ma (ăn′jē-ō-lĭ-pō′mə, -lī-) *n.* A benign tumor composed chiefly of fat cells and containing an unusually large number of vascular channels.

an·gi·o·lith (ăn′jē-ə-lĭth′) *n.* A calcareous deposit in the wall of a blood vessel. —**an′gi·o·lith′ic** *adj.*

an·gi·ol·o·gy (ăn′jē-ŏl′ə-jē) *n.* The study of blood vessels and lymphatic vessels.

an·gi·o·lu·poid (ăn′jē-ō-loo′poid′) *n.* An eruption of the skin in which nodular, telangiectatic papules are distributed over the nose and cheeks.

an·gi·ol·y·sis (ăn′jē-ŏl′ĭ-sĭs) *n.* Obliteration of blood vessels, as in the tied umbilical cord of a newborn.

an·gi·o·ma (ăn′jē-ō′mə) *n., pl.* **–mas** *or* **–ma·ta** (-mə-tə) A tumor composed chiefly of lymphatic vessels or blood vessels.

angioma ser·pig·i·no·sum (sər-pĭj′ə-nō′səm) *n.* The presence of rings of red dots on the skin that are due to proliferation and subsequent atrophy of superficial capillaries. Also called *essential telangiectasia.*

an·gi·o·ma·toid (ăn′jē-ō′mə-toid′) *adj.* Resembling a tumor of vascular origin.

an·gi·o·ma·to·sis (ăn′jē-ō-mə-tō′sĭs) *n.* A condition characterized by multiple angiomas.

an·gi·o·ma·tous (ăn′jē-ō′mə-təs, -ŏm′ə-) *adj.* Relating to or resembling an angioma.

an·gi·o·meg·a·ly (ăn′jē-ō-mĕg′ə-lē) *n.* Enlargement of blood vessels, especially in the eyelids.

an·gi·o·my·o·li·po·ma (ăn′jē-ō-mī′ō-lĭ-pō′mə, -lī-) *n.* A benign tumor composed of adipose tissue, muscle cells, and vascular structures.

an·gi·o·my·o·ma (ăn′jē-ō-mī-ō′mə) *n.* See **vascular leiomyoma.**

an·gi·o·my·o·neu·ro·ma (ăn′jē-ō-mī′ō-noo-rō′mə) *n.* See **glomus tumor.**

an·gi·o·my·o·sar·co·ma (ăn′jē-ō-mī′ō-sär-kō′mə) *n.* A myosarcoma that has a large number of proliferated, frequently dilated, vascular channels.

an·gi·o·neu·rec·to·my (ăn′jē-ō-noo-rĕk′tə-mē) *n.* Excision of the vessels and nerves of a part.

an·gi·o·neu·ro·my·o·ma (ăn′jē-ō-noor′ō-mī-ō′mə) *n.* See **glomus tumor.**

an·gi·o·neu·rot·ic edema (ăn′jē-ō-noo-rŏt′ĭk) *n.* Recurring episodes of noninflammatory swelling of the skin, mucous membranes, viscera, and brain, occasionally accompanied by arthralgia, purpura, or fever. Also called *angioedema, atrophedema, Bannister's disease, giant urticaria, Quincke's disease.*

an·gi·o·par·al·y·sis (ăn′jē-ō-pə-răl′ĭ-sĭs) *n.* See **vasoparalysis.**

an·gi·o·pa·re·sis (ăn′jē-ō-pə-rē′sĭs, -păr′ĭ-sĭs) *n.* See **vasoparesis.**

an·gi·o·path·ic (ăn′jē-ō-păth′ĭk) *adj.* Of or relating to angiopathy.

an·gi·op·a·thy (ăn′jē-op′ə-thē) *n.* Any of several diseases of the blood or lymph vessels.

an·gi·o·pha·co·ma·to·sis *or* **an·gi·o·pha·ko·ma·to·sis** (ăn′jē-ō-fə-kō′mə-tō′sĭs, -făk′ō-) *n.* **1.** See **Lindau's disease. 2.** See **Sturge-Weber syndrome.**

an·gi·o·plas·ty (ăn′jē-ə-plăs′tē) *n.* **1.** Surgical reconstruction of a blood vessel. **2.** Balloon angioplasty.

an·gi·o·poi·e·sis (ăn′jē-ō-poi-ē′sĭs) *n.* The formation of blood vessels or lymphatic vessels. Also called *vasifaction, vasoformation.* —**an′gi·o·poi·et′ic** (-ĕt′ĭk) *adj.*

an·gi·o·pres·sure (ăn′jē-ō-prĕsh′ər) *n.* The application of pressure on a blood vessel to arrest bleeding.

an·gi·or·rha·phy (ăn′jē-ôr′ə-fē) *n.* Suture repair of a vessel, especially a blood vessel.

an·gi·o·sar·co·ma (ăn′jē-ō-sär-kō′mə) *n.* A rare malignant tumor occurring most often in the breast and skin and believed to originate from the endothelial cells of blood vessels.

an·gi·os·co·py (ăn′jē-ŏs′kə-pē) *n.* Visualization of the passage of intravenously injected substances, such as radiopaque agents, through the capillaries.

an·gi·o·sco·to·ma (ăn′jē-ō-skō-tō′mə) *n.* A ribbon-shaped defect in the visual field caused by retinal vessels overlying the photoreceptors. Also called *cecocentral scotoma.*

an·gi·o·sco·tom·e·try (ăn′jē-ō-skō-tŏm′ĭ-trē) *n.* Measurement or projection of a pattern resulting from angioscotoma.

an·gi·o·spasm (ăn′jē-ō-spăz′əm) *n.* See **vasospasm.** —**an′gi·o·spas′tic** (-spăs′tĭk) *adj.*

an·gi·o·stax·is (ăn′jē-ō-stăk′sĭs) *n.* **1.** The oozing of blood. No longer in technical use. **2.** Hemophilia. No longer in technical use.

an·gi·o·ste·no·sis (ăn′jē-ō-stə-nō′sĭs) *n.* The narrowing of one or more blood vessels.

an·gi·o·stron·gy·lo·sis (ăn′jē-ō-strŏn′jə-lō′sĭs) *n.* The infection of humans with parasites of the genus *Angiostrongylus.* Also called *eosinophilic meningitis.*

An·gi·o·stron·gy·lus ma·lay·si·en·sis (ăn′jē-ō-strŏn′jə-ləs mə-lā′zē-ĕn′sĭs) *n.* A Malaysian species of the parasitic nematode genus *Angiostrongylus,* an agent of angiostrongylosis.

an·gi·os·tro·phy (ăn′jē-ŏs′trə-fē) *n.* The twisting of the cut end of a blood vessel to arrest bleeding.

an·gi·o·te·lec·ta·sis (ăn′jē-ō-tĕ-lĕk′tə-sĭs) *or* **an·gi·o·tel·ec·ta·sia** (-tĕl′ĭk-tā′zhə) *n.* Dilation of the terminal arterioles, venules, or capillaries.

an·gi·o·ten·sin (ăn′jē-ō-tĕn′sĭn) *n.* Any of a group of peptides with vasoconstrictive activity that function physiologically in controlling arterial pressure.

angiotensin I *n.* A decapeptide that is the precursor to angiotensin II but is itself physiologically inactive.

angiotensin II *n.* An octapeptide that is a potent vasopressor and a powerful stimulus for production and release of aldosterone from the adrenal cortex.

angiotensin III *n.* A heptapeptide derivative of angiotensin II that exhibits some of the vasopressor and aldosterone stimulation effects of its precursor.

angiotensin amide *n.* A peptide analog to angiotensin II that is used as a vasopressor agent in the treatment of certain types of shock and circulatory collapse.

an·gi·o·ten·si·nase (ăn′jē-ō-tĕn′sə-nās′, -nāz′) *n.* **1.** A peptidase in tissues and plasma that degrades angiotensin II. **2.** Any of several enzymes in the blood that hydrolyze angiotensin.

angiotensin-converting enzyme *n.* See **dipeptidyl carboxypeptidase.**

angiotensin-converting enzyme inhibitor *n.* ACE inhibitor.

an·gi·o·ten·sin·o·gen (ăn′jē-ō-tĕn-sĭn′ə-jən) *n.* A serum globulin formed by the liver that is cleaved by renin to form angiotensin I. Also called *angiotensin precursor.*

an·gi·o·ten·sin·o·ge·nase (ăn′jē-ō-tĕn-sĭn′ə-jə-nās′, -nāz′) *n.* See **renin.**

angiotensin precursor *n.* See **angiotensinogen.**

an·gi·ot·o·my (ăn′jē-ŏt′ə-mē) *n.* Incision into a blood vessel.

an·gi·o·to·ni·a (ăn′jē-ō-tō′nē-ə) *n.* See **vasotonia.** —**an′gi·o·ton′ic** (-tŏn′ĭk) *adj.*

an·gi·o·ton·ic (an′jē-ō- tŏn′ik) *adj.* Of or relating to the tone in a blood vessel, especially an arteriole; vasotonic.

an·gi·o·tribe (ăn′jē-ə-trīb′) *n.* A strong forceps used to arrest hemorrhage by crushing the end of a blood vessel and the tissue in which it is embedded.

an·gi·o·trip·sy (ăn′jē-ə-trĭp′sē) *n.* Use of an angiotribe to arrest hemorrhage. Also called *vasotripsy.*

an·gi·o·troph·ic (ăn′jē-ō-trŏf′ĭk) *adj.* Relating to the nutrition of the blood vessels or lymphatics.

an·gle (ăng′gəl) *n.* The figure or space formed by the junction of two lines or planes.

angle-closure glaucoma *n.* Primary glaucoma in which increased pressure occurs because outflow of the aqueous humor is mechanically prevented by contact of the iris with the trabecular drainage meshwork and the peripheral cornea. Also called *narrow-angle glaucoma.*

angle of anomaly *n.* The degree of deviation from parallelism in an eye with strabismus. Also called *angle of abnormality.*

angle of convergence *n.* The angle that the visual axis makes with the medial line when a near object is viewed.

angle of ec·cen·tric·i·ty (ĕk′sĕn-trĭs′ĭ-tē) *n.* The angle between the line of fixation and the line of normal foveal fixation in an eye with strabismus.

angle of iris *n.* See **filtration angle.**

angle of jaw *n.* The angle formed by the junction of the lower edge of the jawbone and the posterior edge of the ramus of the jawbone. Also called *angle of mandible.*

angle of rib *n.* The abrupt change in curvature of the external surface of a rib where the rib is bent in two directions and twisted along its axis. Also called *costal angle.*

angle of torsion *n.* The degree of rotation of a long bone along its axis or between two axes.

An·gle's classification of malocclusion (ăng′gəlz) *n.* A classification of different types of malocclusion, based on the mesiodistal relationship of the permanent molars upon their eruption and locking.

angst[1] (ängkst) *n.* A feeling of anxiety or apprehension often accompanied by depression.

angst[2] *abbr.* angstrom

ang·strom *or* **ång·strom** (ăng′strəm) *n. Abbr.* **A, Å,** angst A unit of length equal to one hundred millionth (10^{-8}) of a centimeter, used especially to specify radiation wavelengths.

Ångstrom unit *n.* An angstrom.

an·gu·lar artery (ăng′gyə-lər) *n.* **1.** An artery that is the terminal branch of the facial artery, distributed through the muscles and skin of the side of the nose, having anastomoses with the lateral nasal and dorsal arteries of the nose and the palpebral arteries from the ophthalmic artery. **2.** See **artery of angular gyrus.**

angular cheilitis *n.* Inflammation and radiating fissures at the corners of the mouth, secondary to predisposing factors such as overclosure of the jaws in denture wearers, nutritional deficiencies, atopic dermatitis, or *Candida albicans* infection. Also called *commissural cheilitis, perlèche.*

angular curvature *n.* Abnormal curvature of the spine caused by tuberculosis of the vertebrae.

angular gyrus *n.* A convolution in the inferior parietal lobe formed by the united posterior ends of the superior and middle temporal gyri and involved in the processing of auditory and visual input and in the comprehension of language.

angular stomatitis *n.* Inflammation at the corners of the mouth, associated with a wrinkled or fissured epithelium that does not involve the mucosa.

angular vein *n.* A short vein at the anterior angle of the eye socket, formed by the supraorbital and supratrochlear veins and continuing as the facial vein.

an·gu·la·tion (ăng′gyə-lā′shən) *n.* The formation of an abnormal angle or bend in an organ. —**an′gu·late′** (-lāt′) *v.*

an·gu·lus (ăng′gyə-ləs) *n., pl.* –**li** (-lī′) An angle or a corner.

an·he·do·ni·a (ăn′hē-dō′nē-ə) *n.* Absence of pleasure from the performance of acts that would normally be pleasurable.

an·hi·dro·sis (ăn′hī-drō′sĭs) *n.* Absence of sweating. Also called *adiaphoresis, ischidrosis.*

an·hi·drot·ic (ăn′hī-drŏt′ĭk) *adj.* Relating to or characterized by anhidrosis. —*n.* An agent that reduces, prevents, or stops sweating.

anhidrotic ectodermal dysplasia *n.* The hereditary absence of sweat glands characterized by heat intolerance, finely wrinkled skin, sunken nose, malformed and missing teeth, and sparse fragile hair.

an·hy·drase (ăn-hīʹdrās′, -drāz′) *n.* An enzyme that catalyzes the removal of water from a compound.

an·hy·dride (ăn-hīʹdrīd′) *n.* A chemical compound formed from another by the removal of water.

anhydro– *pref.* Without water: *anhydride.*

an·hy·drous (ăn-hīʹdrəs) *adj.* Without water, especially water of crystallization.

an·ic·ter·ic virus hepatitis (ăn′ĭk-tĕrʹĭk) *n.* A mild form of viral hepatitis, without jaundice.

an·ile (ănʹīl′, āʹnīl′) *adj.* 1. Of or like an old woman. 2. Senile.

an·i·lide (ănʹə-lĭd, -līd′) *n.* 1. An acyl derivative of aniline. 2. An amide in which a hydrogen in the amido group is replaced by a phenyl group.

a·ni·linc·tion (ā′nə-lĭngkʹshən) *or* **a·ni·linc·tus** (ā′nə-lĭngkʹtəs) *n.* Sexual stimulation by licking or kissing the anus.

an·i·line *or* **an·i·lin** (ănʹə-lĭn) *n.* An oily, poisonous benzene derivative used in the manufacture of dyes and pharmaceuticals. —*adj.* Derived from aniline.

aniline blue *n.* A mixture of sulfonated triphenylmethane dyes used as a connective tissue stain and as a counterstain.

a·ni·lin·gus (ā′nə-lĭngʹgəs) *n.* Anilinction.

an·i·lin·ism (ănʹə-lə-nĭzʹəm) *or* **an·il·ism** (ănʹə-lĭzʹəm) *n.* Chronic aniline poisoning characterized by gastric and cardiac weakness, vertigo, muscular depression, intermittent pulse, and cyanosis.

a·nil·i·ty (ə-nĭlʹĭ-tē) *n.* See **dotage**.

an·i·ma (ănʹə-mə) *n.* 1. The inner self of an individual; the soul. 2. In Jungian psychology, the unconscious or true inner self of an individual, as opposed to the persona, or outer aspect of the personality. 3. In Jungian psychology, the feminine inner personality as present in the unconscious of the male.

an·i·mal (ănʹə-məl) *n.* 1. A multicellular organism with membranous cell walls of the kingdom Animalia, differing from plants in certain typical characteristics such as capacity for locomotion, nonphotosynthetic metabolism, pronounced response to stimuli, restricted growth, and fixed bodily structure. 2. An animal organism other than a human, especially a mammal. 3. A human considered with respect to his or her physical, as opposed to spiritual, nature. —*adj.* 1. Relating to, characteristic of, or derived from an animal or animals. 2. Relating to the physical as distinct from the spiritual nature of humans.

animal pole *n.* The nuclear site in an ovum and the point from which polar bodies are extruded during maturation. Also called *germinal pole*.

animal starch *n.* See **glycogen**.

an·i·ma·tion (ăn′ə-māʹshən) *n.* 1. The state of being alive. 2. Liveliness; high spirits.

an·i·mus (ănʹə-məs) *n.* 1. An animating or energizing spirit. 2. Intention to do something; disposition. 3. A spirit of active hostility; ill will. 4. In Jungian psychology, the masculine inner personality as present in the unconscious of the female.

an·i·on (ănʹīʹən) *n.* A negatively charged ion, especially one that migrates to the anode in electrolysis. —**anʹi·onʹic** (-ŏnʹĭk) *adj.*

anion exchange *n.* The process by which an anion in a liquid phase exchanges with another anion previously bound to a solid, positively charged phase.

anion-exchange resin *n.* An insoluble organic polymer containing cation groups that attract and hold anions present in a surrounding solution in exchange for anions previously held.

anion gap *n.* The difference between the sum of cations and anions found in plasma or serum.

an·i·rid·i·a (ăn′ī-rĭdʹē-ə, ăn′ə-) *n.* Congenital absence of all but the root of the iris.

an·i·sa·ki·a·sis (ăn′ĭ-sə-kīʹə-sĭs) *n.* Infection of the intestinal wall with larvae of the nematode *Anisakis marina,* characterized by symptoms resembling those of septic ulcer or tumor.

An·i·sa·kis (ăn′ĭ-sāʹkĭs) *n.* A genus of nematodes that includes many common parasites of marine mammals and marine fish-eating birds.

an·i·sei·ko·ni·a (ăn-ī′sī-kōʹnē-ə) *n.* A condition in which the shape and size of the ocular image differ in each eye.

aniso– *or* **anis–** *pref.* Unequal; dissimilar: *anisogamy.*

an·i·so·ac·com·mo·da·tion (ăn-ī′sō-ə-kŏm′ə-dāʹshən) *n.* Variation between the two eyes in accommodation capacity.

an·i·so·chro·mat·ic (ăn-ī′sō-krō-mătʹĭk) *adj.* Not uniformly of one color.

an·i·so·co·ri·a (ăn-ī′sō-kôrʹē-ə) *n.* Unequal size of the pupils.

an·i·so·cy·to·sis (ăn-ī′sō-sī-tōʹsĭs) *n.* Considerable variation in the size of cells that are normally uniform, especially such a variation in red blood cells.

an·i·so·dac·ty·ly (ăn-ī′sō-dăkʹtə-lē) *n.* Unequal length in corresponding fingers. —**anʹi·so·dacʹty·lous** (-tə-ləs) *adj.*

an·i·sog·a·my (ăn′ī-sŏgʹə-mē) *n.* A union between two gametes that differ in size or form. —**anʹi·so·gamʹic** (-sə-gămʹĭk) *adj.*

an·i·sog·na·thous (ăn′ī-sŏgʹnə-thəs) *adj.* Having upper and lower jaws of unequal width, especially in the areas of the molars.

an·i·so·kar·y·o·sis (ăn-ī′sō-kăr′ē-ōʹsĭs) *n.* Variation in the size of the nuclei of cells.

an·i·so·mas·ti·a (ăn-ī′sō-măsʹtē-ə) *n.* Asymmetry of the breasts.

an·i·so·me·li·a (ăn-ī′sō-mēʹlē-ə, -mēlʹyə) *n.* Inequality between paired limbs.

an·i·so·me·tro·pi·a (ăn-ī′sə-mĭ-trōʹpē-ə) *n.* A condition in which the refractive power of one eye differs from that of the other. —**anʹi·so·me·tropʹic** (-trŏpʹĭk, -trōʹpĭk) *adj.*

an·i·so·pi·e·sis (ăn-ī′sō-pī-ēʹsĭs) *n.* Unequal arterial blood pressure on the two sides of the body.

an·i·so·sphyg·mi·a (ăn-ī′sō-sfĭgʹmē-ə) *n.* A difference in the volume, force, or time of the pulse in the corresponding arteries on two sides of the body.

an·i·sos·then·ic (ăn-ī′sŏs-thĕnʹĭk) *adj.* Of or relating to two muscles or groups of muscles having unequal strength.

an·i·so·ton·ic (ăn-ī′sə-tŏn′ĭk) *adj.* Having unequal osmotic pressure.

an·i·so·trop·ic (ăn-ī′sə-trŏp′ĭk, -trō′pĭk) *adj.* **1.** Not isotropic. **2.** Having physical properties that differ according to the direction of measurement. —**an·i′so·trop′i·cal·ly** *adv.* —**an′i·sot′ro·pism** (-sŏt′rə-pĭz′əm), **an′i·sot′ro·py** (-sŏt′rə-pē) *n.*

an·i·so·tro·pine meth·yl·bro·mide (ăn-ī′sə-trō′pēn′-mĕth′əl-brō′mīd′) *n.* An anticholinergic agent and intestinal antispasmodic.

A·nitsch·kow cell (ə-nĭch′kôf′, ə-nēch′-) *n.* See **cardiac histiocyte.**

Anitschkow myocyte *n.* See **cardiac histiocyte.**

an·kle (ăng′kəl) *n.* **1.** The joint between the leg and foot in which the tibia and fibula articulate with the talus. **2.** The region of the ankle joint. **3.** The anklebone.

an·kle·bone (ăng′kəl-bōn′) *n.* See **talus** (sense 1).

ankle joint *n.* A hinge joint formed by the articulating of the tibia and the fibula with the talus below. Also called *mortise joint, talocrural joint.*

ankle reflex *n.* See **Achilles reflex.**

ankylo– *or* **ancylo–** *pref.* Stiff; stuck together: *ankyloblepharon.*

an·ky·lo·bleph·a·ron (ăng′kə-lō-blĕf′ə-rŏn′) *n.* See **blepharosynechia.**

an·ky·lo·glos·si·a (ăng′kə-lō-glô′sē-ə) *n.* See **tongue-tie.**

an·ky·lo·poi·et·ic (ăng′kə-lō-poi-ĕt′ĭk) *adj.* Forming or characterized by ankylosis.

an·ky·lo·proc·ti·a (ăng′kə-lō-prŏk′shē-ə) *n.* Imperforation or stricture of the anus.

an·ky·losed (ăng′kə-lōst′, -lōzd′) *adj.* **1.** Stiffened or bound by adhesions. **2.** Of or relating to a joint in a state of ankylosis.

an·ky·los·ing hyperostosis (ăng′kə-lō′sĭng, -lō′zĭng) *n.* See **diffuse idiopathic skeletal hyperostosis.**

ankylosing spondylitis *n.* Arthritis of the spine, resembling rheumatoid arthritis and leading to lipping or fusion of the vertebrae. Also called *Strümpell-Marie disease, Marie-Strümpell disease, rheumatoid spondylitis, Strümpell-Marie disease.*

an·ky·lo·sis (ăng′kə-lō′sĭs) *n.* The stiffening or immobility of a joint resulting from disease, trauma, surgery, or bone fusion. —**an′ky·lot′ic** (-lŏt′ĭk) *adj.*

an·ky·roid (ăng′kə-roid′) *adj.* Variant of **ancyroid.**

an·la·ge *or* **An·la·ge** (än′lä-gə) *n., pl.* **–ges** *or* **–gen** (-gən) **1.** The initial clustering of embryonic cells from which a part or an organ develops; primordium. **2.** A genetic predisposition to a given trait or personality characteristic.

an·nec·tent (ə-nĕk′tənt) *adj.* Connected with; joined.

annectent gyrus *n.* See **transition gyrus.**

an·nex·a (ə-nĕk′sə) *n.* Variant of **adnexa.**

an·nu·lar (ăn′yə-lər) *adj.* Shaped like or forming a ring.

annular cataract *n.* A congenital cataract in which a central white membrane replaces the nucleus.

annular ligament *n.* Any of various ligaments encircling parts such as the stapes, radius, and trachea.

annular ring *n.* An opaque area appearing in radiographs of the lung and indicating a cavity of tuberculosis. Also called *pleural ring.*

annular scotoma *n.* A circular scotoma surrounding the center of the field of vision.

an·nu·lo·plas·ty (ăn′yə-lə-plăs′tē) *n.* Surgical reconstruction of an incompetent cardiac valve.

an·nu·lor·rha·phy (ăn′yə-lôr′ə-fē) *n.* The closure of a hernial ring by suture.

an·nu·lus *or* **an·u·lus** (ăn′yə-ləs) *n., pl.* **–lus·es** *or* **–li** (-lī′) A circular or ring-shaped structure.

annulus hem·or·rhoi·da·lis (hĕm′ə-roi-dā′lĭs) *n.* See **zona hemorrhoidalis.**

annulus u·re·thra·lis (yŏŏr′ĭ-thrā′lĭs) *n.* See **sphincter muscle of urinary bladder.**

a·no·coc·cyg·e·al (ā′nō-kŏk-sĭj′ē-əl) *adj.* Relating to the anus and the coccyx.

anococcygeal nerve *n.* Any of several small nerves arising from the coccygeal plexus, supplying the skin over the coccyx.

a·no·cu·ta·ne·ous line (ā′nō-kyōō-tā′nē-əs) *n.* The line between the simple columnar epithelium of the rectum and the stratified epithelium of the anal canal. Also called *pectinate line.*

an·o·don·tia (ăn′ō-dŏn′shə) *n.* Congenital absence of teeth. Also called *agomphosis.*

an·o·dyne (ăn′ə-dīn′) *n.* An agent that relieves pain.

a·no·gen·i·tal (ā′nō-jĕn′ĭ-tl) *adj.* Relating to the anus and the genitals.

anogenital raphe *n.* In the male embryo, the line of closure of the genital folds and swellings, extending from the anus to the tip of the penis.

a·nom·a·lad (ə-nŏm′ə-lăd′) *n.* A malformation together with its derived structural changes.

a·nom·a·lous complex (ə-nŏm′ə-ləs) *n.* An electrocardiographic reading that differs significantly from the normal reading for that physiological type.

anomalous correspondence *n.* A condition common in strabismus in which light from a viewed object does not strike the same point on each retina.

a·nom·a·ly (ə-nŏm′ə-lē) *n.* A deviation from the average or norm.

an·o·mer (ăn′ə-mər) *n.* A cyclic stereoisomer, such as a sugar, whose sole conformational difference involves the arrangement of atoms or groups in the aldehyde or ketone group.

a·no·mi·a (ə-nō′mē-ə) *n.* See **nominal aphasia.**

a·no·mic (ə-nŏm′ĭk, ə-nō′mĭk) *adj.* Socially unstable, alienated, and disorganized. —*n.* A socially unstable, alienated person.

anomic aphasia *n.* See **nominal aphasia.**

an·o·nych·i·a (ăn′ə-nĭk′ē-ə) *or* **an·o·ny·cho·sis** (ăn′ə-nĭ-kō′sĭs) *n.* Congenital absence of the nails.

A·noph·e·les (ə-nŏf′ə-lēz′) *n.* A genus of mosquitoes containing over 90 species, many of which are vectors of malaria. —**a·noph·e·line** (-līn′) *adj.*

an·oph·thal·mi·a (ăn′ŏf-thăl′mē-ə, -ŏp-) *n.* Complete absence of tissues of the eyes.

a·no·plas·ty (ā′nə-plăs′tē) *n.* Reconstructive surgery on the anus.

an·or·chi·a (ă-nôr′kē-ə) *or* **an·or·chism** (ă-nôr′kĭz′əm) *n.* Congenital absence of the testes.

a·no·rec·tal (ā′nō-rĕk′təl) *adj.* Relating to the anus and the rectum.

an·o·rec·tic (ăn′ə-rĕk′tĭk) *or* **an·o·ret·ic** (-rĕt′ĭk) *adj.* **1.** Marked by loss of appetite. **2.** Suppressing or causing loss of appetite. **3.** Of or affected with anorexia nervosa. —*n.* **1.** An agent that causes loss of appetite. **2.** One affected with anorexia nervosa.

an·o·rex·i·a (ăn′ə-rĕk′sē-ə) *n.* **1.** Loss of appetite, especially as a result of disease. **2.** Anorexia nervosa.

anorexia nerv·o·sa (nûr-vō′sə) *n.* An eating disorder usually occurring in young women, characterized by fear of becoming obese, a persistent aversion to food, and severe weight loss and often causing amenorrhea and other physiological changes.

an·o·rex·i·ant (ăn′ə-rĕk′sē-ənt) *n.* A drug, process, or event that leads to anorexia.

an·o·rex·ic (ăn′ə-rĕk′sĭk) *adj.* Relating to or suffering from anorexia nervosa. —**an′o·rex′ic** *n.*

an·o·rex·i·gen·ic (ăn′ə-rĕk′sə-jĕn′ĭk) *adj.* Promoting or causing anorexia.

an·or·gas·my (ăn′ôr-găz′mē) *or* **an·or·gas·mi·a** (-găz′-mē-ə) *n.* Failure to experience an orgasm. —**an′or·gas′mic** *adj.*

an·or·thog·ra·phy (ăn′ôr-thŏg′rə-fē) *n.* See **agraphia**.

a·no·scope (ā′nə-skōp′) *n.* A short speculum that is used for examining the anal canal and the lower rectum.

a·no·sig·moid·os·co·py (ā′nō-sĭg′moi-dŏs′kə-pē) *n.* Endoscopy of the anus, rectum, and sigmoid colon.

an·os·mi·a (ăn-ŏz′mē-ə) *n.* Loss of the sense of smell. Also called *olfactory anesthesia.* —**an·os′mic** *adj.*

a·no·sog·no·si·a (ə-nō′sŏg-nō′zē-ə, -zhə) *n.* Real or feigned ignorance of the presence of disease, especially of paralysis. —**a·no′sog·no′sic** (-nō′zĭk) *adj.*

anosognosic epilepsy *n.* Epilepsy in which the individual is unaware of, or denies, the occurrence of seizures.

a·no·spi·nal (ā′nō-spī′nəl) *adj.* Relating to the anus and the spinal cord.

an·os·to·sis (ăn′ŏs-tō′sĭs) *n.* Failure of ossification.

an·o·ti·a (ă-nō′shē-ə, -shə) *n.* Congenital absence of one or both ears.

a·no·ves·i·cal (ā′nō-vĕs′ĭ-kəl) *adj.* Relating to the anus and the urinary bladder.

an·ov·u·lant (ăn′ŏv′yə-lənt) *n.* A drug that suppresses ovulation.

an·o·vu·lar (ăn-ō′vyə-lər, -ŏv′yə-) *or* **an·o·vu·la·to·ry** (-ō′vyə-lə-tôr′ē, -ŏv′yə-) *adj.* Not related to or coincident with ovulation.

anovular menstruation *n.* Menstrual bleeding without the discharge of an ovum.

an·o·vu·la·tion (ăn-ō′vyə-lā′shən, -ŏv′yə-) *n.* Suspension or cessation of ovulation.

an·ox·e·mi·a (ăn′ŏk-sē′mē-ə) *n.* An absence of oxygen in arterial blood.

an·ox·i·a (ăn-ŏk′sē-ə, ə-nŏk′-) *n.* The absence or reduced supply of oxygen in inspired gases, arterial blood, or tissues. —**an·ox′ic** *adj.*

anoxic anoxia *n.* See **hypoxic hypoxia**.

An·rep phenomenon (ăn′rĕp, än′-) *n.* Homeometric autoregulation of the heart in which cardiac performance improves as aortic pressure increases.

an·sa (ăn′sə) *n.*, *pl.* **–sae** (-sē) An anatomical structure shaped like a loop or an arc.

An·said (ăn′sād′, -sĕd′) A trademark for the drug flurbiprofen.

an·sate (ăn′sāt′) *adj.* Ansiform.

an·ser·ine bursa (ăn′sə-rīn′, -rĭn) *n.* The bursa between the tibial collateral ligament of the knee joint and the tendons of the sartorius, gracilis, and semitendinosus muscles.

an·si·form (ăn′sə-fôrm′) *adj.* Having a handle or a part resembling a handle.

ant– *pref.* Variant of **anti–**.

An·ta·buse (ăn′tə-byōōs′) A trademark for the drug disulfiram.

ant·ac·id (ănt-ăs′ĭd) *or* **an·ti·ac·id** (ăn′tē-ăs′ĭd, ăn′tī-) *adj.* Counteracting or neutralizing acidity, especially of the stomach. —*n.* A substance, such as sodium bicarbonate, that neutralizes acid.

an·tag·o·nism (ăn-tăg′ə-nĭz′əm) *n.* Mutual opposition in action between structures, agents, diseases, or physiological processes. Also called *mutual resistance.*

an·tag·o·nist (ăn-tăg′ə-nĭst) *n.* Something, such as a muscle, disease, or physiological process, that neutralizes or impedes the action or effect of another.

an·tag·o·nis·tic muscles (ăn-tăg′ə-nĭs′tĭk) *pl.n.* Muscles having opposite functions, the contraction of one neutralizing the contraction of the other.

ant·al·gic (ănt-ăl′jĭk) *adj.* Analgesic.

antalgic gait *n.* A limp in which a phase of the gait is shortened on the injured side to alleviate the pain experienced when bearing weight on that side.

ante– *pref.* **1.** Prior to; earlier: *antenatal.* **2.** In front of; before: *antebrachium.*

an·te·ce·dent (ăn′tĭ-sēd′nt) *n.* A precursor.

an·te·cu·bi·tal (ăn′tē-kyōō′bĭ-tl) *adj.* In front of the elbow.

an·te·feb·rile (ăn′tē-fĕb′rəl, -fē′brəl) *adj.* See **antepyretic**.

an·te·flex·ion (ăn′tē-flĕk′shən) *n.* A sharp forward curve or angulation, especially a forward bend in the uterus at the junction of the corpus and cervix.

an·te·grade (ăn′tĭ-grād′) *adj.* Moving or extending forward.

antegrade urography *n.* X-ray examination of the urinary tract utilizing percutaneous injection of a contrast agent into the renal calices or pelvis, or into the urinary bladder.

an·te·mor·tem (ăn′tē-môr′təm) *adj.* Before death.

an·te·na·tal (ăn′tē-nāt′l) *adj.* See **prenatal**.

an·te·par·tum (ăn′tē-pär′təm) *adj.* Of or occurring in the period before childbirth.

an·te·py·ret·ic (ăn′tē-pī-rĕt′ĭk) *adj.* Before the onset of fever. Also called *antefebrile.*

an·te·ri·or (ăn-tîr′ē-ər) *adj.* **1.** Placed before or in front. **2.** Occurring before in time; earlier. **3.** Of or relating to the front surface of the body, especially of the position of one structure relative to another; ventral. **4.** Near the head or rostral end of certain embryos. —*n.* The front surface of the body.

anterior ampullar nerve *n.* A branch of the utriculoampullar nerve that supplies the ampullary crest of the anterior semicircular duct of the ear.

anterior asynclitism *n.* See **Nägele obliquity**.

anterior auricular nerve *n.* Any of branches of the auriculotemporal nerve that supply the tragus and the upper part of the auricle of the ear.

anterior auricular vein *n.* Any of of several veins emptying into the retromandibular vein.

anterior cardiac vein *n.* One of two or three small veins in the anterior wall of the right ventricle that open into the right atrium independently of the coronary sinus.

anterior cardinal vein *n.* Any of the major drainage channels from the cephalic region of most vertebrate embryos.

anterior cerebral vein *n.* A vein that parallels the anterior cerebral artery and drains into the basal vein.

anterior chamber of eye *n.* The space between the cornea and the iris, filled with the aqueous humor and communicating through the pupil with the posterior chamber.

anterior column of spinal cord *n.* The ventral ridge of gray matter in each half of the spinal cord, containing the motor neurons innervating the skeletal musculature of the trunk, neck, and extremities. Also called *ventral column of spinal cord.*

anterior condyloid foramen *n.* See **hypoglossal canal.**

anterior cruciate ligament *n. Abbr.* **ACL** The cruciate ligament of the knee that crosses from the anterior intercondylar area of the tibia to the posterior part of the lateral condyle of the femur.

anterior embryotoxon *n.* See **arcus cornealis.**

anterior ethmoidal nerve *n.* The anterior branch of the nasociliary nerve.

anterior facial vein *n.* A continuation of the angular vein, uniting with the retromandibular vein below the border of the lower jaw before emptying into the internal jugular vein.

anterior focal point *n.* The point where light rays starting parallel from the retina become focused.

anterior funiculus *n.* A column or bundle of white matter on either side of the anterior median fissure.

anterior horn *n.* **1.** The front section of the lateral ventricle of the brain, extending forward from Monro's foramen. Also called *ventral horn.* **2.** The front or ventral gray column of the spinal cord in cross section. Also called *ventral horn.*

anterior intercostal vein *n.* Any of the tributaries to the musculophrenic or internal thoracic veins from the intercostal spaces.

anterior interosseous nerve *n.* A branch of the median nerve supplying the long flexor muscle of the thumb, part of the deep flexor muscle of the fingers, and the quadrate pronator muscles.

anterior jugular vein *n.* A vein that arises below the chin from the veins draining the chin and lower lip, passes down the front of the neck superficially, and terminates in the external jugular vein at the lateral border of the anterior scalene muscle.

anterior labial nerve *n.* Any of the branches of the ilioinguinal nerve distributed to the labia majora.

anterior labial vein *n.* Any of the veins that pass from the labia majora to the external pudendal veins.

anterior lacrimal crest *n.* A vertical ridge on the frontal process of the upper jaw that forms part of the medial margin of the eye socket.

anterior limiting ring *n.* The periphery of the cornea thickened by a bundle of circular connective and elastic fibers, in front or in the termination of the limiting layer of cornea. Also called *Schwalbe's ring.*

anterior lingual gland *n.* One of the tubuloacinar mixed glands situated behind the tip of the tongue on each side of the frenulum. Also called *apical gland.*

anterior lobe of hypophysis *n.* See **adenohypophysis.**

anterior malleolar artery *n.* **1.** An artery with its origin in the anterior tibial artery, with distribution to the ankle joint, and with anastomoses to the peroneal and lateral tarsal arteries; lateral anterior malleolar artery. **2.** An artery with its origin in the anterior tibial artery, with distribution to the ankle joint and the neighboring integument, and with anastomoses to the branches of the posterior tibial artery; medial anterior artery.

anterior median fissure *n.* The longitudinal groove in the midline of the anterior aspect of the medulla oblongata, continuous with the anterior median fissure of the spinal cord and ending at the foramen cecum medullae oblongatae.

anterior median line *n.* The line of intersection of the midsagittal plane with the anterior surface of the body.

anterior megalophthalmus *n.* Megalophthalmus affecting the anterior segment of the eyeball and causing associated changes in the zonular ligament and the lens. Also called *keratoglobus.*

anterior nasal spine *n.* A pointed projection at the front extremity of the intermaxillary suture.

anterior ocular segment *n.* The portion of the eye made up of the cornea, the iris, and the lens, and their associated chambers and adnexa.

anterior palatine foramen *n.* See **lesser palatine foramen.**

anterior perforated substance *n.* A region at the base of the brain through which numerous small branches of the anterior and middle cerebral arteries enter deep into the cerebral hemisphere.

anterior pituitary gonadotropin *n.* Any of several polypeptide or protein hormones secreted by the anterior lobe of the pituitary gland. Also called *pituitary gonadotropic hormone.*

anterior pituitarylike hormone *n.* See **chorionic gonadotropin.**

anterior pyramid *n.* See **pyramid of medulla oblongata.**

anterior rectus muscle of head *n.* A muscle with origin from the transverse process and the lateral mass of the atlas, with insertion into the basilar process of the occipital bone, with nerve supply from the first and second cervical nerve, and whose action turns and inclines the head forward.

anterior rhinoscopy *n.* Examination of the anterior portion of the nasal cavity.

anterior scalene muscle *n.* A muscle with origin from the anterior tubercles of the transverse processes of the third to the sixth cervical vertebrae, with insertion into the scalene tubercle of the first rib, with nerve supply from the cervical plexus, and whose action raises the first rib.

anterior scleritis *n.* Inflammation of the sclera adjoining the limbus of the cornea and appearing as a dark red or bluish swelling.

anterior scrotal nerve *n.* Any of the branches of the ilioinguinal nerve distributed to the skin of the root of the penis and to the front surface of the scrotum.

anterior scrotal vein *n.* Any of the veins passing from the scrotum to the external pudendal veins.

anterior ser·ra·tus (sə-rā′təs) *n.* A muscle with origin from the center of the lateral aspect of the first eight to nine ribs, with insertion to the superior and inferior angles and the intervening medial margin of the scapula, with nerve supply from the long thoracic nerve from the brachial plexus, and whose action rotates the scapula and pulls it forward, and elevates the ribs.

anterior spinocerebellar tract *n.* A bundle of fibers that originates in the posterior horn along the spinal cord, crosses to the opposite side, ascends peripherally in the ventral half of the lateral funiculus through the rhombencephalon, terminates in the cerebellar vermis, and conveys exteroceptive information from the opposite half of the body.

anterior staphyloma *n.* Bulging near the anterior pole of the eyeball. Also called *corneal staphyloma*.

anterior supraclavicular nerve *n.* See **medial supraclavicular nerve.**

anterior synechia *n.* Adhesion of the iris to the cornea.

anterior tibial compartment syndrome *n.* Swelling, pain, and necrosis of the muscles of the anterior tibial compartment of the leg, usually following unaccustomed exertion.

anterior ti·bi·al·is (tĭb′ē-ăl′ĭs) *n.* A muscle with origin from the lateral surface of the tibia, the interosseous membrane, and the intermuscular septum, with insertion into the medial cuneiform bone and the base of the first metatarsal, with nerve supply from the deep peroneal nerve, and whose action causes the dorsiflexion and inversion of the foot.

anterior tibial vein *n.* One of usually two veins that accompany the anterior tibial artery and empty into the popliteal vein.

anterior vein of septum pel·lu·ci·dum (pə-lōō′sĭ-dəm) *n.* A vein that drains the front part of the septum pellucidum and empties into the superior thalamostriate vein.

anterior vertebral vein *n.* A vein that accompanies the ascending cervical artery and opens below into the vertebral vein.

antero– *pref.* Anterior; in front: *anteroposterior.*

an·ter·o·fa·cial dysplasia (ăn′tə-rō-fā′shəl) *n.* The abnormal growth in an anteroposterior direction of the face or cranium.

an·ter·o·grade (ăn′tə-rō-grād′) *adj.* Moving forward.

anterograde amnesia *n.* A condition in which events that occurred after the onset of amnesia cannot be recalled and new memories cannot be formed.

anterograde block *n.* Block of the conduction of an impulse traveling in its ordinary direction, from the sinoatrial node toward the ventricular myocardium.

an·ter·o·in·fe·ri·or (ăn′tə-rō-ĭn-fēr′ĭ-ər) *adj.* In front and below.

an·ter·o·lat·er·al (ăn′tə-rō-lăt′ər-əl) *adj.* In front and away from the middle line.

an·ter·o·me·di·al (ăn′tə-rō-mē′dē-əl) *adj.* In front and toward the middle line.

an·ter·o·me·di·an (ăn′tə-rō-mē′dē-ən) *adj.* In front and in the central line.

an·ter·o·pos·te·ri·or (ăn′tə-rō-pŏ-stîr′ē-ər, -pō-) *adj.* *Abbr.* **AP 1.** Relating to both front and back. **2.** In x-ray imaging, taken or viewed from front to back through the body.

anteroposterior diameter *n.* See **conjugate.**

an·ter·o·su·pe·ri·or (ăn′tə-rō-sōō-pîr′ē-ər) *adj.* In front and above.

an·te·sys·to·le (ăn′tē-sĭs′tə-lē) *n.* The premature activation of the ventricle of the heart.

an·te·ver·sion (ăn′tē-vûr′zhən) *n.* A turning forward as a whole without bending. —**an′te·vert′ed** (ăn′tē-vûr′tĭd) *adj.*

ant·he·lix (ănt-hē′lĭks) *or* **an·ti·he·lix** (ăn′tē-, ăn′tī-) *n.* Ridge of cartilage anterior and roughly parallel to the posterior portion of the auricle helix.

ant·hel·min·tic (ănt′hĕl-mĭn′tĭk, ăn′thĕl-) *or* **ant·hel·min·thic** (-thĭk) *n.* An agent that destroys or causes the expulsion of parasitic intestinal worms. Also called *helminthagogue, helminthic, vermifuge.* —*adj.* Acting to expel or destroy parasitic intestinal worms.

an·thra·coid (ăn′thrə-koid′) *adj.* **1.** Characteristic of or resembling a carbuncle or cutaneous anthrax. **2.** Resembling anthrax.

an·thra·co·sil·i·co·sis (ăn′thrə-kō-sĭl′ĭ-kō′sĭs) *n.* Accumulation of carbon and silica in the lungs from inhaled coal dust.

an·thra·co·sis (ăn′thrə-kō′sĭs) *n.* Accumulation of carbon in the lungs from inhaled smoke or coal dust. Also called *miner's lung.*

an·thrax (ăn′thrăks′) *n.* **1.** An infectious, usually fatal disease of warm-blooded animals that is characterized by ulcerative skin lesions, can be transmitted to humans, and is caused by the bacterium *Bacillus anthracis.* Also called *carbuncle.* **2.** *pl.* **–thra·ces** (-thrə-sēz′) A lesion that is caused by anthrax. —**an·thrac·ic** (ăn-thrăs′ĭk) *adj.*

anthropo– *pref.* Human: *anthropometry.*

an·thro·po·cen·tric (ăn′thrə-pə-sĕn′trĭk) *adj.* **1.** Regarding humans as the central element of the universe. **2.** Interpreting reality exclusively in terms of human values and experience.

an·thro·poid (ăn′thrə-poid′) *adj.* **1.** Resembling human beings in structure and form. **2.** Of or belonging to the family of great apes including the gorilla, chimpanzee, and orangutan. **3.** Resembling or characteristic of an ape; apelike.

anthropoid pelvis *n.* An apelike pelvis with a long anteroposterior diameter and a narrow transverse diameter.

an·thro·pol·o·gy (ăn′thrə-pŏl′ə-jē) *n.* The scientific study of the origin, the behavior, and the physical, social, and cultural development of humans. —**an′thro·pol′o·gist** *n.*

an·thro·pom·e·try (ăn′thrə-pŏm′ĭ-trē) *n.* The branch of anthropology concerned with comparative measurements of the human body and its parts. —**an′thro·po·met′ric** (-pə-mĕt′rĭk), **an′thro·po·met′ri·cal** (-rĭ-kəl) *adj.* —**an′thro·po·met′ri·cal·ly** *adv.*

an·thro·po·mor·phism (ăn′thrə-pə-môr′fĭz′əm) *n.* The attribution of human motivation, characteristics, or behavior to nonhuman organisms or inanimate objects. —**an′thro·po·mor′phic** *adj.* —**an′thro·po·mor′phi·cal·ly** *adv.*

an·thro·po·not·ic cutaneous leishmaniasis (ăn′thrə-pə-nŏt′ĭk) *n.* A form of cutaneous leishmaniasis occurring in urban areas in western and central Asia and characterized by a painless, chronic, dry ulceration that develops from two to eight months after the bite from the transmitting sandfly bite and heals in about a year, often leaving a scar.

an·thro·po·phil·ic (ăn′thrə-pō-fĭl′ĭk) *adj.* Seeking or preferring a human over another animal. Used of a parasite.

an·thro·po·zo·o·no·sis (ăn′thrə-pō-zō′ə-nō′sĭs) *n.* A zoonosis maintained in nature by animals and transmissible to humans.

anti– *or* **ant–** *pref.* **1.** Opposite: *antimere.* **2.** Opposing; against: *antisocial.* **3.** Counteracting; neutralizing: *antibody.*

an·ti·ac·id (ăn′tē-ăs′ĭd, ăn′tī-) *adj.* Variant of **antacid.**

an·ti·ad·re·ner·gic (ăn′tē-ăd′rə-nûr′jĭk, ăn′tī-) *adj.* Of or relating to an agent that annuls or antagonizes the effects of the sympathetic nervous system.

an·ti·ag·glu·ti·nin (ăn′tē-ə-glōōt′n-ĭn, ăn′tī-) *n.* A specific antibody that inhibits or destroys the action of an agglutinin.

an·ti·ag·ing (ăn′tē-ā′jĭng, ăn′tī-) *adj.* Used to delay or lessen the effects of aging, especially on the skin.

an·ti·al·ler·gic (ăn′tē-ə-lûr′jĭk, ăn′tī-) *adj.* Preventing or relieving allergies.

an·ti·an·a·phy·lax·is (ăn′tē-ăn′ə-fə-lăk′sĭs, ăn′tī-) *n.* See **desensitization** (sense 1).

an·ti·an·dro·gen (ăn′tē-ăn′drə-jən, ăn′tī-) *n.* A substance that prevents expression of biological effects of androgenic hormones on responsive tissues.

an·ti·a·ne·mic (ăn′tē-ə-nē′mĭk, ăn′tī-) *adj.* Relating to factors or substances that prevent or correct anemic conditions.

an·ti·an·gi·o·gen·ic (ăn′tē-ăn′jē-ō-jĕn′ĭk, ăn′tī-) *adj.* Inhibiting the growth of blood vessels.

an·ti·an·ti·bod·y *or* **an·ti·an·ti·bod·y** (ăn′tē-ăn′tĭ-bŏd′ē, ăn′tī-) *n.* An antibody that is specifically directed against another antibody.

an·ti·an·ti·tox·in (ăn′tē-ăn′tē-tŏk′sĭn, ăn′tī-) *n.* An antiantibody that is directed against an antitoxin and counteracts its effects.

an·ti·anx·i·e·ty (ăn′tē-ăng-zī′ĭ-tē, ăn′tī-) *adj.* Preventing or reducing anxiety.

antianxiety agent *n.* Any of a group of drugs used to treat anxiety without causing excessive sedation.

an·ti·ar·rhyth·mic (ăn′tē-ə-rĭth′mĭk, ăn′tī-) *adj.* Preventing or alleviating irregularities in the force or the rhythm of the heart. —*n.* An antiarrythmic drug.

an·ti·bac·te·ri·al (ăn′tē-băk-tîr′ē-əl, ăn′tī-) *adj.* Destroying or inhibiting the growth of bacteria. —**an′ti·bac·te′ri·al** *n.*

anti-basement membrane antibody *n.* Autoantibody to a renal glomerular basement membrane antigen.

anti-basement membrane glomerulonephritis *n.* Glomerulonephritis resulting from anti-basement membrane antibodies.

an·ti·bi·o·sis (ăn′tē-bī-ō′sĭs, ăn′tī-) *n.* **1.** An association between two or more organisms that is detrimental to at least one of them. **2.** The antagonistic association between an organism and the metabolic substances produced by another.

an·ti·bi·ot·ic (ăn′tī-bī-ŏt′ĭk, ăn′tī-) *n.* A substance, such as penicillin or streptomycin, produced by or derived from certain fungi, bacteria, and other organisms, that can destroy or inhibit the growth of other microorganisms. —*adj.* **1.** Of or relating to antibiotics. **2.** Of or relating to antibiosis.

antibiotic enterocolitis *n.* Enterocolitis caused by oral administration of broad-spectrum antibiotics, resulting from antibiotic-resistant staphylococci or the overgrowth of yeasts and fungi when the normal fecal gram-negative organisms are absent.

an·ti·bod·y (ăn′tĭ-bŏd′ē) *n.* **1.** *Abbr.* **Ab** A protein substance produced in the blood or tissues in response to a specific antigen, such as a bacterium or a toxin, that destroys or weakens bacteria and neutralizes organic poisons, thus forming the basis of immunity. **2.** An immunoglobulin present in the blood serum or body fluids as a result of antigenic stimulus and interacting only with the antigen that induced it or with an antigen closely related to it.

antibody excess *n.* In a precipitation test, the presence of antibody in an amount greater than that required to combine with all of the antigen present.

an·ti·cho·lin·er·gic (ăn′tē-kō′lə-nûr′jĭk, ăn′tī-) *n.* An agent that is antagonistic to the action of parasympathetic or other cholinergic nerve fibers.

an·ti·cho·lin·es·ter·ase (ăn′tē-kō′lə-nĕs′tə-rās′, -rāz′, ăn′tī-) *n.* A substance that inhibits the activity of cholinesterases, including acetylcholinesterase.

an·ti·cli·nal (ăn′tē-klī′nəl, ăn′tī-) *adj.* Inclined in opposite directions, as two sides of a pyramid.

an·ti·co·ag·u·lant (ăn′tē-kō-ăg′yə-lənt, ăn′tī-) *n.* A substance that prevents the clotting of blood. —*adj.* Acting as an anticoagulant. —**an′ti·co·ag′u·la′tive** (-lā′tĭv, -lə-tĭv) *adj.*

an·ti·co·don (ăn′tē-kō′dŏn, ăn′tī-) *n.* A sequence of three adjacent nucleotides in tRNA designating a specific amino acid that binds to a corresponding codon in mRNA during protein synthesis.

an·ti·com·ple·ment (ăn′tē-kŏm′plə-mənt, ăn′tī-) *n.* A substance that neutralizes the action of a complement by combining with it and preventing its union with an antibody.

an·ti·con·vul·sant (ăn′tē-kən-vŭl′sənt, ăn′tī-) *n.* A drug that prevents or relieves convulsions. —**an′ti·con·vul′sive** (-sĭv) *adj.*

an·ti·de·pres·sant (ăn′tē-dĭ-prĕs′ənt, ăn′tī-) *n.* A drug used to prevent or treat clinical depression. —**an′ti·de·pres′sant, an′ti·de·pres′sive** (-prĕs′ĭv) *adj.*

an·ti·di·ar·rhe·al (ăn′tē-dī′ə-rē′əl, ăn′tī-) *n.* A substance used to prevent or treat diarrhea.

an·ti·di·u·re·sis (ăn′tē-dī′ə-rē′sĭs, ăn′tī-) *n.* The reduction of urinary volume.

an·ti·di·u·ret·ic (ăn′tē-dī′ə-rĕt′ĭk, ăn′tī-) *n.* An agent that reduces the output of urine.

antidiuretic hormone *n.* *Abbr.* **ADH** See **vasopressin.**

an·ti·dote (ăn′tĭ-dōt′) *n.* An agent used to neutralize or counteract the effects of a poison. —**an′ti·dot′al** (ăn′-tĭ-dōt′l) *adj.*

an·ti·drom·ic (ăn′tĭ-drŏm′ĭk) *adj.* Relating to the propagation of an impulse along an axon in a direction that is the reverse of normal.

an·ti·drug (ăn′tē-drŭg′, ăn′tī-) *adj.* Directed against the production, distribution, and consumption of illegal drugs.

an·ti·e·lec·tron (ăn′tē-ĭ-lĕk′trŏn′) *n.* See **positron.**

an·ti·e·met·ic (ăn′tē-ĭ-mĕt′ĭk, ăn′tī-) *adj.* Preventing or arresting vomiting. —*n.* An agent that prevents or arrests vomiting.

an·ti·en·zyme (ăn′tē-ĕn′zīm′, ăn′tī-) *n.* An agent or principle, especially an inhibitory enzyme or an antibody to an enzyme, that retards, inhibits, or destroys enzymic activity. —**an′ti·en′zy·mat′ic** (-zĭ-măt′ĭk, -zī-), **an′ti·en·zy′mic** (-zī′mĭk) *adj.*

an·ti·es·tro·gen (ăn′tē-ĕs′trə-jən, ăn′tī-) *n.* A substance capable of preventing full expression of the biological effects of an estrogen.

an·ti·feb·rile (ăn′tē-fĕb′rəl, -fē′brəl, -brĭl′, ăn′tī-) *n.* See **antipyretic.**

an·ti·fer·til·i·ty (ăn′tē-fər-tĭl′ĭ-tē, ăn′tī-) *adj.* Capable of reducing or eliminating fertility; contraceptive.

an·ti·fi·bri·nol·y·sin (ăn′tē-fī′brə-nŏl′ĭ-sĭn, ăn′tī-) *n.* See **antiplasmin.**

an·ti·fi·bri·no·lyt·ic (ăn′tē-fī′brə-nə-lĭt′ĭk, ăn′tī-) *adj.* Of or relating to a substance, such as aminocaproic acid, that decreases the breakdown of fibrin.

an·ti·flat·u·lent (ăn′tē-flăch′ə-lənt, ăn′tī-) *adj.* Preventing and treating excessive gas in the gastrointestinal tract. —*n.* An antiflatulent drug.

an·ti·fun·gal (ăn′tē-fŭng′gəl, ăn′tī-) *adj.* Destroying or inhibiting the growth of fungi. —*n.* An antifungal drug.

an·ti·gen (ăn′tĭ-jən) *n.* Any of various substances, including toxins, bacteria, and the cells of transplanted organs, that when introduced into the body stimulate the production of antibodies. Also called *allergen, immunogen.* —**an′ti·gen′ic** (-jĕn′ĭk) *adj.*

antigen-antibody reaction *n.* The binding of an antibody with an antigen of the type that stimulated the formation of the antibody, resulting in agglutination, precipitation, complement fixation, greater susceptibility to ingestion and destruction by phagocytes, or neutralization of an exotoxin.

an·ti·gen·e·mi·a (ăn′tə-jə-nē′mē-ə) *n.* The presence of an antigen in circulating blood.

antigen excess *n.* In a precipitation test, the presence of uncombined antigen above that required to combine with all of the antibody.

antigenic determinant *n.* Epitope.

an·ti·ge·nic·i·ty (ăn′tĭ-jə-nĭs′ĭ-tē) *n.* **1.** The capacity to induce an immune response. **2.** The degree to which a substance induces an immune response. Also called *immunogenicity.*

antigenic shift *n.* A sudden, major change in the antigenic structure of a virus, usually the result of genetic mutation.

antigen-presenting cell *n.* A cell, originating in the bone marrow and subsequently found as a dendritic cell in various locations, that facilitates the immune response by holding antigens on its surface and presenting them to lymphocytes.

antigen unit *n.* The smallest amount of antigen that, in the presence of specific antiserum, will bind to one complement unit.

an·ti·glob·u·lin test (ăn′tē-glŏb′yə-lĭn, ăn′tī-) *n.* See **Coombs′ test.**

an·ti-HB$_c$ (ăn′tē-āch′bē-sē′, ăn′tī-) *n. Abbr.* **HB$_c$Ab** The antibody to the hepatitis B core antigen.

an·ti-HB$_s$ (ăn′tē-āch′bē-ĕs′, ăn′tī-) *n. Abbr.* **HB$_s$Ab** The antibody to the hepatitis B surface antigen.

an·ti-HB$_e$ (ăn′tē-āch′bē-ē′, ăn′tī-) *n. Abbr.* **HB$_e$Ab** The antibody to the hepatitis B e antigen.

an·ti·he·lix (ăn′tē-hē′lĭks, ăn′tī-) *n.* Variant of **anthelix.**

an·ti·he·mag·glu·ti·nin (ăn′tē-hē′mə-glōōt′n-ĭn, ăn′tī-) *n.* A substance that inhibits or prevents the effects of hemagglutinin.

an·ti·he·mol·y·sin (ăn′tē-hĭ-mŏl′ĭ-sĭn,-hē′mə-lī′-, ăn′tī-) *n.* A substance that inhibits or prevents the effects of hemolysin.

an·ti·he·mo·lyt·ic (ăn′tē-hē′mə-lĭt′ĭk, ăn′tī-) *adj.* Preventing hemolysis.

an·ti·he·mo·phil·ic factor (ăn′tē-hē′mə-fĭl′ĭk, ăn′tī-) *n. Abbr.* **AHF** See **factor VIII.**

antihemophilic globulin *n. Abbr.* **AHG 1.** See **factor VIII. 2.** See **human antihemophilic factor.**

antihemophilic globulin A *n.* See **factor VIII.**

antihemophilic globulin B *n.* See **factor IX.**

antihemophilic human plasma *n.* Normal human plasma in which the labile antihemophilic globulin component has been preserved, used to temporarily relieve dysfunction of the hemostatic mechanism in hemophilia.

an·ti·hem·or·rhag·ic (ăn′tē-hĕm′ə-răj′ĭk, ăn′tī-) *adj.* Arresting or reducing hemorrhage.

antihemorrhagic factor *n.* See **vitamin K.**

an·ti·hi·drot·ic (ăn′tē-hī-drŏt′ĭk, ăn′tī-) *adj.* Acting to reduce or prevent sweating; anhidrotic.

an·ti·his·ta·mine (ăn′tē-hĭs′tə-mēn′, -mĭn) *n.* Any of several drugs used to counteract the physiological effects of histamine. —**an′ti·his′ta·mine′** *adj.*

an·ti·his·ta·min·ic (ăn′tē-hĭs′tə-mĭn′ĭk) *adj.* Tending to neutralize or antagonize the action of histamine or inhibit its production in the body. —*n.* An antihistaminic drug.

an·ti·hor·mone (ăn′tē-hôr′mōn′, ăn′tī-) *n.* A substance that inhibits or that prevents the effects of a hormone.

an·ti·hu·man globulin (ăn′tē-hyōō′mən, ăn′tī-) *n.* See **Coombs′ serum.**

an·ti·hy·per·ten·sive (ăn′tē-hī′pər-tĕn′sĭv, an′tī-) *adj.* Reducing high blood pressure. —*n.* A drug or treatment that reduces high blood pressure.

an·ti·in·fec·tive (ăn′tē-ĭn-fĕk′tĭv, ăn′tī-) *adj.* Capable of preventing or counteracting infection. —*n.* An anti-infective agent or drug.

an·ti·in·flam·ma·to·ry *or* **an·ti·in·flam·ma·to·ry** (ăn′-tē-ĭn-flăm′ə-tôr′ē, ăn′tī-) *adj.* Reducing inflammation by acting on body mechanisms. —**an′ti·in·flam′ma·to′ry** *n.*

an·ti·lew·is·ite (ăn′tē-lōō′ĭ-sīt′, ăn′tī-) *n.* See **dimercaprol.**

an·ti·lith·ic (ăn′tē-lĭth′ĭk, ăn′tī-) *adj.* Preventing the formation of calculi or promoting their dissolution.

an·ti·lym·pho·cyte serum (ăn′tē-lĭm′fə-sīt′, ăn′tī-) *n. Abbr.* **ALS** The globulin fraction of serum from a horse or another animal, usually used in conjunction with other immunosuppressive agents to suppress rejection of grafts or organ transplants.

an·ti·ly·sin (ăn′tē-lī′sĭn, ăn′tī-) *n.* An antibody that inhibits or prevents the effects of lysin.

an·ti·ma·lar·i·al (ăn′tē-mə-lâr′ē-əl, ăn′tī-) *adj.* Preventing or relieving the symptoms of malaria.

an·ti·mere (ăn′tĭ-mîr′) *n.* **1.** A segment of an animal body formed by planes cutting the axis of the body at right angles. **2.** One of the corresponding parts of a bilaterally symmetrical organism. **3.** The right or left half of the body. —**an′ti·mer′ic** (-mĕr′ĭk) *adj.*

an·ti·me·tab·o·lite (ăn′tē-mĭ-tăb′ə-līt′, ăn′tī-) *n.* A substance that closely resembles an essential metabolite and competes with, interferes with, or replaces the metabolite in physiological reactions.

an·ti·mi·cro·bi·al (ăn′tē-mī-krō′bē-əl, ăn′tī-) *or* **an·ti·mi·cro·bic** (-bĭk) *adj.* Tending to destroy microbes, prevent their development, or inhibit their pathogenic action.

an·ti·mo·ny (ăn′tə-mō′nē) *n. Symbol* **Sb** A toxic metallic element, compounds of which are used as anthelmintics, especially in the treatment of schistosomiasis. Atomic number 51.

an·ti·mu·ta·gen (ăn′tē-myōō′tə-jən, -jĕn′, ăn′tī-) *n.* A substance that reduces or interferes with the mutagenic effects of another substance. —**an′ti·mu′ta·gen′ic** *adj.*

an·ti·my·cot·ic (ăn′tē-mī-kŏt′ĭk, ăn′tī-) *adj.* Inhibiting the growth of fungi; antifungal.

an·ti·ne·o·plas·tic (ăn′tē-nē′ə-plăs′tĭk, ăn′tī-) *adj.* Preventing the development, maturation, or spread of neoplastic cells. —**an′ti·ne′o·plas′tic** *n.*

an·tin·i·on (ăn-tĭn′ē-ən) *n.* The space between the eyebrows.

an·ti·nu·cle·ar antibody (ăn′tē-nōō′klē-ər, ăn′tī-) *n. Abbr.* **ANA** An antibody that attacks cell nuclei.

antinuclear factor *n. Abbr.* **ANF** A factor present in serum having a strong affinity for nuclei and present in lupus erythematosus and rheumatic arthritis.

an·ti·on·co·gene (ăn′tē-ŏng′kə-jēn, ăn′tī-) *n.* See **tumor suppressor gene.**

an·ti·ox·i·dant (ăn′tē-ŏk′sĭ-dənt, ăn′tī-) *n.* **1.** A chemical compound or substance that inhibits oxidation. **2.** A substance, such as vitamin E, vitamin C, or beta–carotene, thought to protect body cells from the damaging effects of oxidation.

an·ti·par·a·sit·ic (ăn′tē-păr′ə-sĭt′ĭk, ăn′tī-) *adj.* Destroying or inhibiting the growth and reproduction of parasites. —**an′ti·par′a·sit′ic** *n.*

an·ti·pe·dic·u·lot·ic (ăn′tē-pə-dĭk′yə-lŏt′ĭk, ăn′tī-) *adj.* Destructive to lice. —**an′ti·pe·dic′u·lot′ic** *n.*

an·ti·pep·tic (ăn′tē-pĕp′tĭk, ăn′tī-) *adj.* Inhibiting the action of pepsin.

an·ti·per·i·stal·sis (ăn′tē-pĕr′ĭ-stôl′sĭs, -stăl′-, ăn′tī-) *n.* See **reversed peristalsis.**

an·ti·per·i·stal·tic (ăn′tē-pĕr′ĭ-stôl′tĭk, -stăl′-, ăn′tī-) *adj.* **1.** Of or relating to antiperistalsis. **2.** Impeding or arresting peristalsis.

antiperistaltic anastomosis *n.* A surgical connection of intestinal segments to divert the normal flow of the intestinal contents.

an·ti·per·ni·cious anemia factor (ăn′tē-pər-nĭsh′əs, ăn′tī-) *n. Abbr.* **APA** See **vitamin B₁₂.**

an·ti·per·spi·rant (ăn′tē-pûr′spər-ənt, ăn′tī-) *n.* An astringent preparation applied to the skin to decrease perspiration.

an·ti·phlo·gis·tic (ăn′tē-flə-jĭs′tĭk, ăn′tī-) *adj.* Reducing inflammation or fever; anti-inflammatory.

an·ti·plas·min (ăn′tē-plăz′mĭn, ăn′tī-) *n.* A substance that inhibits or prevents the effects of plasmin. Also called *antifibrinolysin.*

an·ti·plate·let (ăn′tē-plāt′lĭt, ăn′tī-) *adj.* Acting against or destroying blood platelets.

an·ti·port (ăn′tē-pôrt′) *n.* A mechanism for the coupled transport of two different molecules or ions through a membrane in opposite directions.

an·ti·pro·throm·bin (ăn′tē-prō-thrŏm′bĭn, ăn′tī-) *n.* An anticoagulant that inhibits or prevents the conversion of prothrombin into thrombin.

an·ti·pru·rit·ic (ăn′tē-prōō-rĭt′ĭk, ăn′tī-) *adj.* Preventing or relieving itching. —**an′ti·pru·rit′ic** *n.*

an·ti·psy·chot·ic (ăn′tē-sī-kŏt′ĭk, ăn′tī-) *adj.* Counteracting or diminishing the symptoms of a psychotic disorder such as schizophrenia, paranoia, or bipolar disorder. —**an′ti·psy·chot′ic** *n.*

an·ti·py·ret·ic (ăn′tē-pī-rĕt′ĭk, ăn′tī-) *n.* An agent that reduces or prevents fever. Also called *antifebrile, antithermic.* —*adj.* Reducing or preventing fever. —**an′ti·py·re′sis** (-rē′sĭs) *n.*

an·ti·py·rot·ic (ăn′tē-pī-rŏt′ĭk, ăn′tī-) *adj.* Relieving the pain and promoting the healing of superficial burns. —**an′ti·py·rot′ic** *n.*

an·ti·ra·chit·ic (ăn′tē-rə-kĭt′ĭk, ăn′tī-) *adj.* Curing or preventing rickets.

an·ti·re·jec·tion (ăn′tē-rĭ-jĕk′shən, ăn′tī-) *adj.* Preventing rejection of a transplanted tissue or organ.

an·ti·ret·ro·vi·ral (ăn′tē-rĕt′rō-vī′rəs, ăn′tī-) *adj.* Destroying or inhibiting the replication of retroviruses.

an·ti·scor·bu·tic (ăn′tē-skôr-byōō′tĭk, ăn′tī-) *adj.* Preventing or relieving scurvy.

an·ti·se·cre·to·ry (ăn′tē-sĭ-krē′tə-rē, ăn′tī-) *adj.* Inhibiting or decreasing secretion, especially gastric secretion.

an·ti·sense (ăn′tē-sĕns′, ăn′tī-) *adj.* Of or relating to a nucleotide sequence that is complementary to a sequence of messenger RNA. When antisense DNA or RNA is added to a cell, it binds to a specific messenger RNA molecule and inactivates it.

an·ti·sep·sis (ăn′tĭ-sĕp′sĭs) *n.* Destruction of pathogenic organisms to prevent infection.

an·ti·sep·tic (ăn′tĭ-sĕp′tĭk) *adj.* **1.** Of, relating to, or producing antisepsis. **2.** Capable of preventing infection by inhibiting the growth of infectious agents. —*n.* A substance that inhibits the proliferation of infectious agents.

antiseptic dressing *n.* A sterile dressing of gauze impregnated with an antiseptic.

an·ti·se·rum (ăn′tĭ-sîr′əm) *n.* A serum containing antibodies that are specific for one or more antigens. Also called *immune serum.*

antiserum anaphylaxis *n.* See **passive anaphylaxis**.

an·ti·si·al·a·gogue (ăn′tē-sī-ăl′ə-gôg′, ăn′tī-) *n.* An agent that diminishes or arrests the flow of saliva.

an·ti·si·al·ic (ăn′tē-sī-ăl′ĭk, ăn′tī-) *adj.* Reducing the flow of saliva.

an·ti·so·cial (ăn′tē-sō′shəl, ăn′tī-) *adj.* Behaving in a manner that violates the social or legal norms of society. —**an′ti·so′cial·ly** *adv.*

antisocial personality disorder *n.* A personality disorder characterized by chronic antisocial behavior and violation of the law and the rights of others.

an·ti·spas·mod·ic (ăn′tē-spăz-mŏd′ĭk, ăn′tī-) *adj.* Preventing or relieving convulsions or spasms. —*n.* An antispasmodic agent.

an·ti·strep·to·coc·cic (ăn′tē-strĕp′tə-kŏk′sĭk, ăn′tī-) *adj.* Destructive to streptococci or antagonistic to their toxins.

an·ti·su·dor·if·ic (ăn′tē-soo′də-rĭf′ĭk, ăn′tī-) *adj.* Capable of inhibiting the secretion of sweat.

an·ti·the·nar (ăn′tĭ-thē′när′, -nər, ăn-tĭth′ə-) *n.* See **hypothenar**.

an·ti·ther·mic (ăn′tē-thûr′mĭk, ăn′tī-) *n.* See **antipyretic**.

an·ti·throm·bin (ăn′tē-thrŏm′bĭn, ăn′tī-) *n.* An anticoagulant that inhibits or prevents the effects of thrombin.

an·ti·tox·ic (ăn′tē-tŏk′sĭk) *adj.* 1. Neutralizing the action of a toxin or poison. 2. Of, relating to, or containing an antitoxin.

an·ti·tox·in (ăn′tē-tŏk′sĭn) *n.* 1. An antibody formed in response to and capable of neutralizing a specific biological toxin. 2. Serum containing antitoxins that is used to prevent or treat diseases caused by biological toxins, such as tetanus and diphtheria.

antitoxin unit *n.* A unit expressing the strength or activity of an antitoxin.

an·ti·tra·gus (ăn′tĭ-trā′gəs) *n.* A projection of the auricle of the ear posterior to the tragus.

an·ti·trep·o·ne·mal (ăn′tē-trĕp′ə-nē′məl, ăn′tī-) *n.* See **treponemicidal**.

an·ti·tro·pic (ăn′tĭ-trō′pĭk) *adj.* Bilaterally symmetrical but in an opposite direction, as the right thumb to the left thumb.

an·ti·tryp·sin (ăn′tē-trĭp′sĭn, ăn′tī-) *n.* A serum protein that inhibits the activity of trypsin and other proteolytic enzymes.

antitrypsin deficiency *n.* An inherited deficiency of a trypsin-inhibiting serum protein that may increase one's susceptibility to emphysema and cirrhosis.

an·ti·tryp·tic (ăn′tē-trĭp′tĭk, ăn′tī-) *or* **an·ti·tryp·sic** (-trĭp′sĭk) *adj.* Having the properties of antitrypsin.

an·ti·tus·sive (ăn′tē-tŭs′ĭv, ăn′tī-) *adj.* Capable of relieving or suppressing coughing. —**an′ti·tus′sive** *n.*

an·ti·ven·in (ăn′tē-vĕn′ĭn, ăn′tī-) *n.* An antitoxin active against venom.

An·ti·vert (ăn′tĭ-vûrt′) A trademark for the drug meclizine hydrochloride.

an·ti·vi·ral (ăn′tē-vī′rəl, ăn′tī-) *adj.* Destroying or inhibiting the growth and reproduction of viruses. —**an′ti·vi′ral** *n.*

antiviral protein *n.* A human or animal factor that is induced by interferon in virus-infected cells and mediates interferon inhibition of virus replication.

an·ti·vi·ta·min (ăn′tē-vī′tə-mĭn, ăn′tī-) *n.* A substance that prevents a vitamin from exerting its typical metabolic effects.

an·trec·to·my (ăn-trĕk′tə-mē) *n.* Excision of an antrum, such as removing the pyloric antrum of the stomach.

antro– *pref.* Antrum: *antroscope.*

an·tro·du·o·de·nec·to·my (ăn′trō-doo′ō-d-n-ĕk′tə-mē, -doo-ŏd′n-ĕk′tə-mē) *n.* Surgical removal of the antrum of the stomach and the ulcer-bearing part of the duodenum.

an·tro·na·sal (ăn′trō-nā′zəl) *adj.* Relating to a maxillary sinus and the corresponding nasal cavity.

an·tro·scope (ăn′trə-skōp′) *n.* An instrument for examining a cavity or an antrum.

an·tros·co·py (ăn-trŏs′kə-pē) *n.* Examination by means of an antroscope.

an·tros·to·my (ăn-trŏs′tə-mē) *n.* The surgical formation of an opening into an antrum.

an·trot·o·my (ăn-trŏt′ə-mē) *n.* Incision through the wall of an antrum.

an·tro·tym·pan·ic (ăn′trō-tĭm-păn′ĭk) *adj.* Relating to the mastoid antrum and the tympanic cavity.

an·trum (ăn′trəm) *n., pl.* **–tra** (-trə) 1. A nearly closed cavity or chamber, especially in a bone. 2. The pyloric end of the stomach, partially shut off during digestion from the cardiac end by sphincter muscles in the stomach wall. —**an′tral** (-trəl) *adj.*

antrum of Highmore *n.* See **maxillary sinus**.

ANUG *abbr.* acute necrotizing ulcerative gingivitis

an·u·lus (ăn′yə-ləs) *n.* Variant of **annulus**.

an·u·re·sis (ăn′yə-rē′sĭs) *n.* The inability to pass urine. —**an′u·ret′ic** (-rĕt′ĭk) *adj.*

a·nu·ri·a (ə-noor′ē-ə) *n.* The absence of urine formation. —**a·nu′ric** (ə-noor′ĭk) *adj.*

a·nus (ā′nəs) *n., pl.* **a·nus·es** The opening at the lower end of the alimentary canal through which solid waste is eliminated from the body. Also called *anal orifice, fundament.*

an·vil (ăn′vĭl) *n.* See **incus**.

anx·i·e·ty (ăng-zī′ĭ-tē) *n.* 1. A state of uneasiness and apprehension, as about future uncertainties. 2. A cause of anxiety. 3. A state of intense apprehension, uncertainty, and fear resulting from the anticipation of a threatening event or situation, often to a degree that normal physical and psychological functioning is disrupted.

anxiety attack *n.* See **panic attack**.

anxiety disorder *n.* Any of various psychiatric disorders in which anxiety is either the primary disturbance or is the result of confronting a feared situation or object.

anxiety hysteria *n.* Hysteria characterized by manifest anxiety.

anxiety reaction *n.* A psychological state or experience involving the apprehension of danger, accompanied by a feeling of dread and such physical symptoms as restlessness and rapid heartbeat, occurring in the absence of any clearly identifiable fear stimulus. Also called *anxiety state.*

anxiety state *n.* See **anxiety reaction**.

anx·i·o·lyt·ic (ăng′zē-ō-lĭt′ĭk, -sē-, ăngk′sē-) *n.* A drug that relieves anxiety. —**anx′i·o·lyt′ic** *adj.*

AODM *abbr.* adult-onset diabetes mellitus

a·or·ta (ā-ôr**′**tə) *n., pl.* **–tas** *or* **–tae** (-tē) The large artery that is the main trunk of the systemic arterial system, arising from the base of the left ventricle, ending at the left side of the body of the fourth lumbar vertebra, dividing to form the right and left common iliac arteries, and whose parts are the ascending aorta, the aortic arch, and the descending aorta. —**a·or′tal, a·or′tic** *adj.*

a·or·tal·gia (ā**′**ôr-tăl**′**jə) *n.* Pain attributed to aneurysm or another pathologic condition of the aorta.

aortic arch *n.* **1.** The curved portion between the ascending and descending portions of the aorta, lying behind the manubrium and giving rise to the brachiocephalic trunk, the left common carotid, and the left subclavian arteries. Also called *arch of aorta.* **2.** Any of several pairs of arterial channels encircling the embryonic pharynx in the mesenchyme of the branchial arches.

aortic arch syndrome *n.* Obstruction of the branches of the aortic arch caused by thrombosis.

aortic atresia *n.* The congenital absence of the normal valvular orifice into the aorta.

aortic body *n.* One of the small bilateral structures, attached to a small branch of the aorta near its arch, and containing chemoreceptors that respond primarily to decreases in blood oxygen concentration.

aortic-body tumor *n.* See **chemodectoma.**

aortic bulb *n.* The dilated first part of the aorta containing the aortic semilunar valves and the aortic sinuses.

aortic dissection *n.* A dissecting aneurysm of the aorta.

aortic foramen *n.* The opening in the diaphragm through which the aorta and thoracic duct pass.

aortic insufficiency *n.* See **aortic regurgitation.**

aortic murmur *n.* An obstructive or regurgitant murmur produced at the aortic orifice.

aortic notch *n.* A slight notch in a sphygmographic tracing caused by rebound from the closure of the aortic valves.

aorticopulmonary septal defect *n.* See **aortic septal defect.**

aortic ostium *n.* The opening from the left ventricle of the heart into the ascending aorta, guarded by the aortic valve.

aortic plexus *n.* **1.** A plexus of lymph nodes and connecting vessels lying along the lower portion of the abdominal aorta. **2.** An autonomic plexus surrounding the abdominal aorta and continuous with the thoracic aortic plexus; abdominal aortic plexus. **3.** An autonomic plexus surrounding the thoracic aorta and passing with it through the aortic opening in the diaphragm to become continuous with the abdominal aortic plexus; thoracic aortic plexus.

aortic regurgitation *n.* Incompetence of the aortic valve of the heart, resulting in backward flow of blood. Also called *aortic insufficiency.*

aortic septal defect *n.* A small congenital opening between the aorta and pulmonary artery just above the semilunar valves. Also called *aorticopulmonary septal defect.*

aortic sinus *n.* The space between each semilunar valve and the wall of the aorta.

aortic stenosis *n. Abbr.* **AS** Pathological narrowing of the orifice of the aortic valve.

aortic valve *n.* The valve between the left ventricle of the heart and the ascending aorta, consisting of three semilunar cusps.

aortic vestibule *n.* The part of the left ventricle of the heart below the aortic orifice that allows room for segments of the closed aortic valve.

aortic window *n.* A radiolucent region, located below the aortic arch, formed by the bifurcation of the trachea, and traversed by the left pulmonary artery.

a·or·ti·tis (ā**′**ôr-tī**′**tĭs) *n.* Inflammation of the aorta.

a·or·to·cor·o·nar·y (ā-ôr**′**tə-kôr**′**ə-nĕr**′**ē) *adj.* Relating to the aorta and the coronary arteries.

a·or·to·gram (ā-ôr**′**tə-grăm**′**) *n.* An image or set of images of the aorta made after the injection of a radiopaque substance.

a·or·tog·ra·phy (ā**′**ôr-tŏg**′**rə-fē) *n.* The radiographic visualization of the aorta and its branches by injection of a radiopaque substance.

a·or·to·il·i·ac bypass (ā-ôr**′**tō-ĭl**′**ē-ăk**′**) *n.* A shunt uniting the aorta and iliac artery to relieve obstruction of the lower abdominal aorta.

aortoiliac occlusive disease *n.* Obstruction of the abdominal aorta and its main branches by atherosclerosis. Also called *Leriche's syndrome.*

a·or·top·a·thy (ā**′**ôr-tŏp**′**ə-thē) *n.* Disease of the aorta.

a·or·to·plas·ty (ā-ôr**′**tə-plăs**′**tē) *n.* Surgical repair of the aorta.

a·or·to·re·nal bypass (ā-ôr**′**tō-rē**′**nəl) *n.* A shunt between the aorta and the distal renal artery to circumvent an obstruction of the renal artery.

a·or·tor·rha·phy (ā**′**ôr-tôr**′**ə-fē) *n.* Suture of the aorta.

a·or·to·scle·ro·sis (ā-ôr**′**tō-sklə-rō**′**sĭs) *n.* Arteriosclerosis of the aorta.

a·or·tot·o·my (ā**′**ôr-tŏt**′**ə-mē) *n.* Incision into the aorta.

AP *abbr.* anteroposterior

ap. *abbr.* apothecary

ap–[1] *pref.* Variant of **ad–** (sense 1).

ap–[2] *pref.* Variant of **apo–.**

APA *abbr.* antipernicious anemia factor

a·pal·les·the·sia (ə-păl**′**ĭs-thē**′**zhə) *n.* See **pallanesthesia.**

a·par·a·lyt·ic (ā-păr**′**ə-lĭt**′**ĭk) *adj.* Not paralyzed; without paralysis.

ap·a·thet·ic (ăp**′**ə-thĕt**′**ĭk) *adj.* Lacking interest or concern; indifferent. —**ap′a·thet′i·cal·ly** *adv.*

ap·a·thism (ăp**′**ə-thĭz**′**əm) *n.* Sluggishness in reacting to stimuli.

ap·a·thy (ăp**′**ə-thē) *n.* Lack of interest, concern, or emotion; indifference.

APC *abbr.* acetylsalicylic acid, phenacetin, and caffeine (combined as an antipyretic and analgesic); antigen-presenting cell

A-P-C virus *abbr.* adenoidal-pharyngeal-conjunctival virus

a·pel·lous (ə-pĕl**′**əs) *adj.* **1.** Not covered by skin. **2.** Having no foreskin; circumcised.

a·pe·ri·od·ic (ā**′**pîr-ē-ŏd**′**ĭk) *adj.* Not occurring periodically. —**a′pe·ri·od′i·cal·ly** *adv.* —**a·pe′ri·o·dic′i·ty** (-ə-dĭs**′**ĭ-tē) *n.*

a·per·i·stal·sis (ā-pĕr**′**ĭ-stôl**′**sĭs, -stăl**′**-) *n.* The absence of peristalsis.

A·pert-Crouzon syndrome (ə-pĕr′-) *n.* See **type II acrocephalosyndactyly.**

a·per·tog·na·thi·a (ə-pûr′tŏg-nā′thē-ə, -tō-nǎth′ē-ə) *n.* A type of malocclusion characterized by the premature occlusion of posterior teeth and the absence of anterior occlusion. Also called *open bite.*

A·pert's syndrome (ə-pĕrz′) *n.* See **type I acrocephalosyndactyly.**

ap·er·ture (ăp′ər-chər) *n.* **1.** An opening, such as a hole, gap, or slit. **2.** A usually adjustable opening in an optical instrument, such as a microscope, a camera, or a telescope, that limits the amount of light passing through a lens or onto a mirror. **3.** The diameter of such an opening. **4.** The diameter of the objective of a telescope or microscope. —**ap′er·tur′al** *adj.*

a·pex (ā′pĕks) *n., pl.* **a·pex·es** *or* **a·pi·ces** (ā′pĭ-sēz′, ăp′ĭ-) The pointed end of a conical or pyramidal structure.

apex beat *n.* A pulsation, either visible or palpable or both, made by the apex of the left ventricle of the heart as it strikes the chest wall in systole.

apex pneumonia *or* **apical pneumonia** *n.* Pneumonia of the apex of the lung.

Ap·gar score (ăp′gär) *n.* A system of evaluating a newborn's physical condition by assigning a value (0, 1, or 2) to each of five criteria: heart rate, respiratory effort, muscle tone, response to stimuli, and skin color.

a·pha·gia (ə-fā′jə) *n.* See **dysphagia.**

a·pha·ki·a (ə-fā′kē-ə) *n.* Absence of the crystalline lens of the eye. —**a·pha′ki·al, a·pha′kic** (ə-fā′kĭk) *adj.*

aph·a·lan·gia (ăf′ə-lăn′jə, ā′fə-) *n.* Absence of a digit or of one or more phalanges of a finger or toe.

a·pha·sia (ə-fā′zhə) *n.* Partial or total loss of the ability to articulate ideas or comprehend spoken or written language, resulting from brain damage due to injury or disease. Also called *logagnosia, logamnesia, logasthenia.* —**a·pha·si·ac′** (-zē-ăk′) *n.* —**a·pha′sic** (-zĭk, -sĭk) *adj. & n.*

a·pha·si·ol·o·gy (ə-fā′zē-ŏl′ə-jē) *n.* The study of aphasia. —**a·pha′si·ol′o·gist** *n.*

a·phe·mi·a (ə-fē′mē-ə) *n.* A form of motor aphasia in which the ability to express ideas verbally is lost.

aph·e·re·sis (ăf′ə-rē′sĭs) *n.* A procedure in which blood is drawn from a donor and separated into its components, some of which are retained, such as plasma or platelets, and the remainder returned by transfusion to the donor. Also called *hemapheresis.*

a·pho·ni·a (ā-fō′nē-ə) *n.* Loss of the voice resulting from disease, injury to the vocal cords, or psychological causes, such as hysteria. —**a·phon′ic** (ā-fŏn′ĭk, ā-fō′nĭk) *adj.*

a·phra·sia (ə-frā′zhə) *n.* The inability to speak.

aph·ro·dis·i·ac (ăf′rə-dĭz′ē-ăk′, -dē′zē-) *adj.* Arousing, increasing, or intensifying sexual desire. —*n.* An aphrodisiac drug or food. —**aph′ro·di·si′a·cal** (-dĭ-zī′ĭ-kəl) *adj.*

aph·tha (ăf′thə) *n., pl.* **–thae** (-thē′) A minute painful ulcer on a mucous membrane of the mouth, often covered by a gray or white exudate.

aph·thae (ăf′thē′) *pl.n.* Canker sores.

aphthae ma·jo·res (mə-jôr′ēz) *n.* A severe form of aphthae characterized by large numerous, frequently occurring ulcers that may take up to six weeks to heal. Also called *Mikulicz' aphthae.*

aphthae mi·no·res (mə-nôr′ēz) *n.* Aphthae.

aph·thoid (ăf′thoid′) *adj.* Relating to or resembling aphthae.

aph·tho·sis (ăf-thō′sĭs) *n.* A condition characterized by the presence of aphthae.

aph·thous (ăf′thəs) *adj.* Of or relating to aphthae or aphthosis.

aphthous stomatitis *n.* See **canker sore.**

a·phy·lax·is (ā′fə-lăk′sĭs, ăf′ə-) *n.* Lack of protection against disease. Also called *nonimmunity.* —**a′phy·lac′tic** (-lăk′tĭk) *adj.*

a·pi·cal (ā′pĭ-kəl, ăp′ĭ-) *adj.* **1.** Relating to the apex of a pyramidal or pointed structure. **2.** Situated nearer to the apex of a structure in relation to a specific reference point. —**a′pi·cal·ly** *adv.*

apical dental foramen *n.* The opening at the apex of the root of a tooth through which the nerves and blood vessels pass.

apical gland *n.* See **anterior lingual gland.**

apical granuloma *n.* See **periapical granuloma.**

apical pneumonia *n.* Variant of **apex pneumonia.**

apical space *n.* The space between the alveolar wall and the apex of the root of a tooth, where an alveolar abscess usually has its origin.

a·pi·cec·to·my (ā′pĭ-sĕk′tə-mē, ăp′ĭ-) *n.* The surgical removal of the apex of the petrous part of the temporal bone.

ap·i·ci·tis (ăp′ĭ-sī′tĭs, ā′pĭ-) *n.* Inflammation of the apex of a structure or organ.

apico– *pref.* Apex: *apicotomy.*

ap·i·co·ec·to·my (ăp′ĭ-kō-ĕk′tə-mē, ā′pĭ-) *n.* Surgical removal of a dental root apex. Also called *root resection.*

ap·i·col·y·sis (ăp′ĭ-kŏl′ĭ-sĭs) *n.* Surgical collapse of the apex of the lung.

ap·i·cot·o·my (ăp′ĭ-kŏt′ə-mē, ā′pĭ-) *n.* Incision into an apical structure.

a·pla·cen·tal (ā′plə-sĕn′tl) *adj.* Having no placenta.

ap·la·nat·ic (ăp′lə-năt′ĭk) *adj.* Of or relating to an optical lens that is free from chromatic or spherical aberration.

aplanatic lens *n.* A lens designed to correct spherical and coma aberration.

a·pla·sia (ə-plā′zhə) *n.* **1.** Congenital absence of an organ or tissue. **2.** Incomplete, retarded, or defective development of an organ or tissue. **3.** Cessation of the usual regenerative process in an organ or tissue.

aplasia ax·i·a·lis ex·tra·cor·ti·ca·lis (ăk′sē-ā′lĭs ĕk′strə-kôr′tĭ-kā′lĭs) *n.* See **Merzbacher-Pelizaeus disease.**

aplasia cu·tis con·gen·i·ta (kyoō′tĭs kən-jĕn′ĭ-tə) *n.* The congenital absence or deficiency of a localized area of skin, usually on the scalp, with the base of the defect covered by a thin translucent membrane.

a·plas·tic (ā-plăs′tĭk, ə-plăs′-) *adj.* **1.** Unable to form or regenerate tissue. **2.** Of, relating to, or characterized by aplasia.

aplastic anemia *n.* A form of anemia in which the capacity of the bone marrow to generate red blood cells is defective, caused by bone marrow disease or exposure to toxic agents, such as radiation, chemicals, or drugs.

aplastic lymph *n.* Lymph containing a relatively large number of leukocytes but comparatively little fibrinogen and manifesting only a slight tendency to become organized. Also called *corpuscular lymph*.

APN *abbr.* advanced practice nurse

ap·ne·a (ăp′nē-ə, ăp-nē′ə) *n.* Temporary absence or cessation of breathing. —**ap·ne′ic** *adj. & n.*

apneic pause *n.* Cessation of air flow in respiration for more than ten seconds.

ap·neu·mi·a (ăp-nŏŏ′mē-ə) *n.* Congenital absence of the lungs.

ap·neus·tic breathing (ăp-nŏŏ′stĭk) *n.* A series of slow, deep inspirations, each one held for 30 to 90 seconds, after which the air is suddenly expelled by the elastic recoil of the lung.

apo– *or* **ap–** *pref.* **1.** Away from; off: *aponeurosis*. **2.** Separate: *apocrine*. **3.** Without; lacking; not: *apoferritin*. **4.** Related to; derived from: *apomorphine*.

ap·o·chro·mat·ic objective (ăp′ə-krō-măt′ĭk) *n.* An objective in which chromatic aberration is corrected for three colors and spherical aberration is corrected for two.

ap·o·crine (ăp′ə-krĭn, -krīn′, -krēn′) *adj.* Of or relating to an apocrine gland or its secretions. —*n.* The apocrine gland.

apocrine adenoma *n.* See **papillary hidradenoma**.

apocrine carcinoma *n.* **1.** A carcinoma composed predominantly of anaplastic cells resembling those of apocrine epithelium, often found in the breast. **2.** A carcinoma of the apocrine glands.

apocrine chromesthesia *n.* The excretion of colored sweat, usually black, from apocrine glands of the face.

apocrine gland *n.* **1.** A coiled, tubular gland whose secretory cells accumulate their products on their apical surfaces that are then pinched off to become the secretion, as in the mammary glands. **2.** Apocrine sweat gland.

apocrine metaplasia *n.* Transformation of acinar epithelium of breast tissue to resemble apocrine sweat glands, as in fibrocystic disease of the breast.

apocrine sweat gland *n.* Any of numerous sweat glands found primarily in the skin of the armpit, pubic region, and areolae of the breasts that produce a secretion that is more viscous than that formed by the eccrine glands. Secretions from these glands occur most frequently during periods of emotional stress or sexual excitement.

ap·o·dal (ăp′ə-dl) *or* **ap·o·dous** (-dəs) *adj.* Having no feet or footlike appendages.

a·po·di·a (ā-pō′dē-ə, ə-pō′-) *or* **ap·o·dy** (ăp′ə-dē) *n.* Congenital absence of feet.

ap·o·en·zyme (ăp′ō-ĕn′zīm) *n.* The protein component of an enzyme that combines with the coenzyme to form the active enzyme.

ap·o·fer·ri·tin (ăp′ə-fĕr′ĭ-tĭn) *n.* A protein present in the intestinal mucosa that binds and stores iron by combining with a ferric hydroxide-phosphate compound to form ferritin.

ap·o·lip·o·pro·tein (ăp′ə-lĭp′ō-prō′tēn′, -lī′pō-) *n.* The protein component that combines with a lipid to form a lipoprotein.

ap·o·mor·phine (ăp′ə-môr′fēn′) *n.* A poisonous, white, crystalline alkaloid derived from morphine and used medicinally to induce vomiting.

ap·o·neu·rec·to·my (ăp′ə-nŏŏ-rĕk′tə-mē) *n.* Excision of an aponeurosis.

ap·o·neu·ror·rha·phy (ăp′ə-nŏŏ-rôr′ə-fē) *n.* See **fasciorrhaphy**.

ap·o·neu·ro·sis (ăp′ə-nŏŏ-rō′sĭs) *n.* A sheetlike fibrous membrane resembling a flattened tendon that serves as a fascia to bind muscles together or to connect muscle to bone. —**ap′o·neu·rot′ic** (-rŏt′ĭk) *adj.*

ap·o·neu·ro·si·tis (ăp′ə-nŏŏr′ə-sī′tĭs) *n.* Inflammation of an aponeurosis.

aponeurotic fibroma *n.* A calcifying, recurrent but infiltrating nonmetastasizing fibromatosis appearing as small nodules that are unattached to the overlying skin and seen most frequently on the palms of children.

ap·o·neu·rot·o·my (ăp′ə-nŏŏ-rŏt′ə-mē) *n.* Incision into an aponeurosis.

a·poph·y·sis (ə-pŏf′ĭ-sĭs) *n., pl.* **–ses** (-sēz′) An outgrowth or projection of an organ or part, especially an outgrowth from a bone that lacks an independent center of ossification. —**ap′o·phys′i·al** (ăp′ə-fĭz′ē-əl), **a·poph′y·se′al** (-sē′əl) *adj.*

a·poph·y·si·tis (ə-pŏf′ĭ-sī′tĭs) *n.* Inflammation of an apophysis.

ap·o·plec·tic (ăp′ə-plĕk′tĭk) *adj.* Relating to, having, or predisposed to apoplexy. —**ap′o·plec′ti·cal·ly** *adv.*

ap·o·plex·y (ăp′ə-plĕk′sē) *n.* **1.** Sudden impairment of neurological function, especially from a cerebral hemorrhage; a stroke. **2.** An effusion of blood into a tissue or organ.

ap·o·pro·tein (ăp′ə-prō′tēn′) *n.* A polypeptide that combines with a prosthetic group to form a conjugated protein.

ap·op·to·sis (ăp′əp-tō′sĭs, ăp′ə-tō′-) *n.* A natural process of self-destruction in certain cells that is determined by the genes and can be initiated by a stimulus or by removal of a repressor agent. Also called *programmed cell death*.

ap·o·re·pres·sor (ăp′ə-rĭ-prĕs′ər) *n.* A repressor that combines with a specific corepressor to inhibit transcription of certain genes; it is a homeostatic mechanism for the regulation of repressible enzyme systems. Also called *inactive repressor*.

ap·o·stax·is (ăp′ə-stăk′sĭs) *n.* Slight bleeding; bleeding by drops.

a·pos·thi·a (ə-pŏs′thē-ə) *n.* Congenital absence of the prepuce.

a·poth·e·car·ies′ measure (ə-pŏth′ĭ-kĕr′ēz) *n.* A system of liquid volume measure used in pharmacy.

apothecaries′ weight *n.* A system of weights used in compounding prescriptions and in which an ounce equals 480 grains and a pound equals 12 ounces.

a·poth·e·car·y (ə-pŏth′ĭ-kĕr′ē) *n., pl.* **–ies** *Abbr.* **ap.** **1.** One that prepares and sells drugs and other medicines; a pharmacist. **2.** See **pharmacy** (sense 2).

ap·pa·ra·tus (ăp′ə-rā′təs, -răt′əs) *n., pl.* **apparatus** *or* **–tus·es 1.** An integrated group of materials or devices used for a particular purpose. **2.** A group or system of organs that collectively performs a specific function or process.

ap·pend·age (ə-pĕn′dĭj) *n.* A part or organ attached to a main structure and subordinate in function or size.

appendages of eye *pl.n.* The eyelids, lashes, eyebrows, lacrimal apparatus, and conjunctiva.

appendages of skin *pl.n.* The hairs and nails and the sweat, sebaceous, and mammary glands.

ap·pen·dec·to·my (ăp′ən-dĕk′tə-mē) *n.* Surgical removal of the vermiform appendix. Also called *appendicectomy.*

ap·pen·di·ce·al (ə-pĕn′dĭ-sē′əl, ăp′ən-dĭs′ē-əl, -dĭsh′-) *or* **ap·pen·di·cal** (ə-pĕn′dĭ-kəl) *adj.* Relating to an appendix.

appendiceal abscess *n.* An abscess in the peritoneal cavity resulting from the spread of infection in acute appendicitis, especially with perforation of the appendix. Also called *periappendiceal abscess.*

ap·pen·di·cec·to·my (ə-pĕn′dĭ-sĕk′tə-mē) *n.* See **appendectomy.**

ap·pen·di·ci·tis (ə-pĕn′dĭ-sī′tĭs) *n.* Inflammation of the vermiform appendix.

appendico– *pref.* Vermiform appendix: *appendicolithiasis.*

ap·pen·di·co·li·thi·a·sis (ə-pĕn′dĭ-kō-lĭ-thī′ə-sĭs) *n.* Concretions in the vermiform appendix.

ap·pen·di·col·y·sis (ə-pĕn′dĭ-kŏl′ĭ-sĭs) *n.* Surgical freeing of the appendix from adhesions.

ap·pen·di·cos·to·my (ə-pĕn′dĭ-kŏs′tə-mē) *n.* Surgical opening of the tip of the veriform appendix to irrigate the bowel.

ap·pen·dic·u·lar (ăp′ən-dĭk′yə-lər) *adj.* 1. Relating to an appendix. 2. Relating to the limbs.

appendicular artery *n.* The branch of the ileocolic artery that supplies the vermiform appendix.

appendicular muscle *n.* Any of of the skeletal muscles of the limbs.

appendicular skeleton *n.* The bones of the limbs, including the bones of the pectoral and pelvic girdles.

appendicular vein *n.* A tributary of the ileocolic vein that accompanies the appendicular artery.

ap·pen·dix (ə-pĕn′dĭks) *n., pl.* **–dix·es** *or* **–di·ces** (-dĭ-sēz′) 1. A supplementary or an accessory part of an organ or a structure of the body. 2. The vermiform appendix.

ap·per·cep·tion (ăp′ər-sĕp′shən) *n.* 1. Conscious perception with full awareness. Also called *comprehension.* 2. The process of understanding by which newly observed qualities of an object are related to past experience. —**ap′per·cep′tive** (-sĕp′tĭv) *adj.*

ap·pe·stat (ăp′ĭ-stăt′) *n.* The area in the brain that is believed to regulate appetite and food intake.

ap·pe·tite (ăp′ĭ-tīt′) *n.* An instinctive physical desire, as for food or sex.

ap·pla·na·tion (ăp′lə-nā′shən) *n.* 1. The flattening of the cornea by pressure, as with an applanation tonometer. 2. Undue flatness, as of the cornea.

applanation tonometer *n.* An instrument for determining intraocular tension by measuring the pressure required to flatten a small area of the cornea.

ap·pla·nom·e·try (ăp′lə-nŏm′ĭ-trē) *n.* The use of an applanation tonometer to measure the pressure within the eye.

ap·ple jelly nodules (ăp′əl) *n.* The papular lesions of lupus vulgaris as they appear on diascopy.

ap·pli·ance (ə-plī′əns) *n.* A dental or surgical device designed to perform a therapeutic or corrective function.

ap·pli·ca·tor (ăp′lĭ-kā′tər) *n.* An instrument for applying something, such as a medication.

ap·plied anatomy (ə-plīd′) *n.* The application of anatomical knowledge to the diagnosis and treatment of disease.

ap·po·si·tion (ăp′ə-zĭsh′ən) *n.* 1. The putting in contact of two parts or substances. 2. The condition of being placed or fitted together. 3. The growth of successive layers of a cell wall. —**ap′po·si′tion·al** *adj.* —**ap′po·si′tion·al·ly** *adv.*

appositional growth *n.* Growth by the addition of new layers on those previously formed, characteristic of tissues formed of rigid materials.

apposition suture *n.* A superficial suture of the skin only. Also called *coaptation suture.*

ap·prox·i·mate (ə-prŏk′sə-māt′) *v.* To bring together, as cut edges of tissue. —*adj.* (-mĭt) 1. Relating to the contact surfaces, either proximal or distal, of two adjacent teeth; proximate. 2. Close together. Used of the teeth in the human jaw.

ap·prox·i·ma·tion (ə-prŏk′sə-mā′shən) *n.* Bringing tissue edges into desired apposition for suturing.

approximation suture *n.* A suture that pulls together the deep tissues of a wound.

a·prag·ma·tism (ā-prăg′mə-tĭz′əm) *n.* An interest in theory or dogma rather than practical results. —**ap′rag·mat′ic** (ăp′răg-măt′ĭk) *adj.*

a·prax·i·a (ā-prăk′sē-ə) *n.* 1. A disorder of voluntary movement consisting of the partial or complete inability to execute purposeful movements without the impairment of muscular power and coordination. 2. A psychomotor defect characterized by the inability to make proper use of a known object.

a·proc·ti·a (ā-prŏk′shē-ə, ə-prŏk′-) *n.* The congenital absence or imperforation of the anus.

a·pro·so·pi·a (ā′prə-sō′pē-ə, ăp′rə-) *n.* The congenital absence of part or all of the face, usually associated with other malformations.

a·pro·ti·nin (ā-prōt′n-ĭn, ă-prōt′-) *n.* A natural polypeptide and protease inhibitor that affects blood clotting and is used during high-risk surgery, such as cardiopulmonary bypass, to reduce bleeding.

ap·ti·tude test (ăp′tĭ-tōōd′) *n.* An occupation-oriented test for evaluating intelligence, achievement, and interest.

ap·ty·a·li·a (ăp′tī-ā′lē-ə, ăp′tĭ-) *or* **ap·ty·a·lism** (ăp-tī′-ə-lĭz′əm, ā-tī′-) *n.* See **asialism.**

APUD cell (ā′pəd) *n.* A cell capable of amine precursor uptake and decarboxylation and of synthesizing and secreting polypeptide hormones.

ap·y·rase (ăp′ə-rās′, -rāz′) *n.* Any of various enzymes that catalyze the hydrolysis of ATP, causing the release of phosphate and energy.

a·py·ret·ic (ā′pī-rĕt′ĭk, ăp′ə-) *adj.* Having no fever.

a·py·rex·i·a (ā′pī-rĕk′sē-ə, ăp′ə-) *n.* The absence of fever.

aq·ua·gen·ic pruritus (ăk′wə-jĕn′ĭk) *n.* Intense itching that is the result of brief contact with water of any temperature but that does not produce visible changes in the skin, associated with local release of acetylcholine, mast-cell degranulation, and increased histamine concentrations.

aq·ua·pho·bi·a (ăk′wə-fō′bē-ə) *n.* An abnormal fear of water.

aq·ue·duct (ăk′wĭ-dŭkt′) *n.* A channel or passage in a body part or an organ.

aq·ue·duc·tus (ăk′wĭ-dŭk′təs) *n., pl.* **aqueductus** Aqueduct.

a·que·ous (ā′kwē-əs, ăk′wē-) *adj.* Relating to, similar to, containing, or dissolved in water; watery.

aqueous chamber *n.* Either of the anterior or posterior chambers of the eye, containing the aqueous humor.

aqueous humor *n.* The clear, watery fluid circulating in the chamber of the eye between the cornea and the lens.

aqueous phase *n.* The water portion of a system consisting of two liquid phases, one that is primarily water and a second that is a liquid immiscible with water.

Ar The symbol for the element **argon.**

ar·a·chi·don·ic acid (ăr′ə-kĭ-dŏn′ĭk) *n.* An unsaturated fatty acid found in animal fats that is essential in human nutrition and is a precursor in the biosynthesis of some prostaglandins.

A·rach·ni·da (ə-răk′nĭ-də) *n.* A class of arthropods that includes spiders, scorpions, mites, and ticks.

a·rach·nid·ism (ə-răk′nĭ-dĭz′əm) *n.* Systemic poisoning following the bite of a spider.

a·rach·no·dac·ty·ly (ə-răk′nō-dăk′tə-lē) *n.* A condition in which the hands and fingers, and often the feet and toes, are abnormally long and slender, characteristic of Marfan syndrome.

a·rach·noid (ə-răk′noid′) *adj.* Resembling a cobweb. Used of the arachnoid membrane covering the brain and spinal cord.

arachnoid cyst *n.* A fluid-filled cyst lined with arachnoid membrane, frequently situated in the sylvian fissure of the brain.

arachnoid granulation *n.* Any of numerous villuslike projections of the cranial arachnoid through the dura into the superior sagittal sinus or into its lateral venous lacunae. Also called *arachnoid villus, pacchionian body.*

a·rach·noid·i·tis (ə-răk′noi-dī′tĭs) *n.* Inflammation of the arachnoid membrane and subarachnoid space.

arachnoid membrane *n.* A delicate fibrous membrane forming the middle of the three coverings of the brain and spinal cord, closely attached to the dura mater, from which it is separated only by the subdural cleft, but separated from the pia mater by the subarachnoid space.

arachnoid villus *n.* See **arachnoid granulation.**

a·rach·no·pho·bi·a (ə-răk′nə-fō′bē-ə, -nō-) *or* **a·rach·ne·pho·bi·a** (ə-răk′nə-) *n.* An abnormal fear of spiders.

Ar·a·len (âr′ə-lĕn′) A trademark for the drug chloroquine phosphate.

A·ran-Duchenne disease (ə-răn′-, ä-räN′-) *n.* See **progressive muscular atrophy.**

A·ran·ti·us′ nodule (ə-răn′shē-ə-sĭz) *n.* See **nodule of semilunar valve.**

Arantius′ ventricle *n.* See **calamus scriptorius.**

Ar·ber (är′bər), **Werner** Born 1929. Swiss microbiologist. He shared a 1978 Nobel Prize for the discovery of restriction enzymes, an important step in the development of genetic engineering.

ar·bor (är′bər) *n., pl.* **ar·bo·res** (är′bə-rēz′) A treelike anatomical structure.

ar·bo·res·cent (är′bə-rĕs′ənt) *adj.* Dendriform.

ar·bo·ri·za·tion (är′bər-ĭ-zā′shən) *n.* **1.** The treelike terminal branching of nerve fibers or blood vessels. **2.** The leaflike pattern formed under certain conditions by a dried smear of cervical mucus.

ar·bo·rize (är′bə-rīz′) *v.* To ramify.

ar·bo·vi·rus (är′bə-vī′rəs) *or* **ar·bor·vi·rus** (är′bər-) *n.* Any of a large group of viruses transmitted by arthropods, such as mosquitoes and ticks, that include the causative agents of encephalitis, yellow fever, and dengue.

arc (ärk) *n.* A curved line or segment of a circle.

ARC *abbr.* AIDS-related complex

arch (ärch) *n.* An organ or structure having a curved or bowlike appearance, especially either of two arched sections of the bony structure of the foot.

ar·chen·ter·on (är-kĕn′tə-rŏn′, -tər-ən) *n.* See **gastrocele** (sense 1).

ar·che·o·ki·net·ic (är′kē-ō-kĭ-nĕt′ĭk, -kī-) *adj.* Of or relating to a primitive type of motor nerve mechanism, as in the peripheral and the ganglionic nervous systems.

ar·che·type (är′kĭ-tīp′) *n.* **1.** An original model or type after which other similar things are patterned. **2.** In Jungian psychology, an inherited pattern of thought or symbolic image that is derived from the past collective experience of humanity and is present in the unconscious of the individual. Also called *imago.* —**ar′che·typ′al** (-tī′pəl) **ar′che·typ′ic** (-tĭp′ĭk), **ar′che·typ′i·cal** *adj.* —**ar′che·typ′i·cal·ly** *adv.*

archi– *or* **arch–** *or* **arche–** *pref.* Earlier; primitive: *archenteron.*

arch of aorta *n.* See **aortic arch** (sense 1).

arch of foot *n.* **1.** The longitudinal arch consisting of a medial arch, comprised of the calcaneus, talus, navicular, three cuneiform bones, and the three medial metatarsals, and a lateral arch formed by the calcaneus, cuboid, and the two lateral metatarsals. **2.** The transverse arch formed by the proximal parts of the metatarsal bones, the three cuneiform bones, and the cuboid.

arch of palate *n.* The vaulted roof of the mouth.

ar·ci·form (är′sə-fôrm′) *adj.* Arcuate.

arc·ta·tion (ärk-tā′shən) *n.* A narrowing, contraction, or stricture of a canal or opening.

ar·cu·ate (är′kyōō-ĭt, -āt′) *adj.* Formed in the shape of an arc. —**ar′cu·ate·ly** *adv.*

arcuate artery *n.* An artery with its origin in the dorsal artery of the foot, with deep plantar, dorsal metatarsal, and dorsal digital branches.

arcuate artery of kidney *n.* Any of the branches of the interlobar arteries of the kidney that turn at the junction of the cortex and medulla and proceed at right angles to the parent stem and approximately parallel to the surface of the kidney.

arcuate fiber *n.* Any of the nervous or tendinous fibers forming an arch between parts, such as those connecting adjacent gyri in the cerebral cortex.

arcuate ligament *n.* **1.** A thickening of the fascia of the lumbar quadrate muscle, between the transverse process of the first lumbar vertebra and the twelfth rib on either side, that gives attachment to a portion of the diaphragm; lateral arcuate ligament. **2.** A tendinous thickening of the fascia of the greater psoas muscle that extends from the body of the first lumbar vertebra to its transverse process on either side and from which a portion of the diaphragm arises; medial arcuate ligament. **3.** A tendinous connection between the crura of the diaphragm that arches in front on the aorta; median arcuate ligament.

arcuate nuclei *pl.n.* A variable assembly of small-cell groups on the ventral and medial aspects of the pyramid in the medulla oblongata.

arcuate veins of kidney *pl.n.* The veins that parallel the arcuate arteries, receive blood from the interlobular veins and the rectal venules, and terminate in the interlobar veins.

arcuate zone *n.* The inner third of the basilar membrane of the cochlear duct, from the tympanic lip of the osseous spiral lamina to the outer pillar cell of the spiral organ. Also called *zona tecta*.

ar·cu·a·tion (är′kyōō-ā′shən) *n.* A curvature.

ar·cus (är′kəs) *n., pl.* **arcus** A structure resembling a bent bow or an arch.

arcus cor·ne·a·lis (kôr′nē-ā′lĭs) *n.* An opaque, grayish ring at the periphery of the cornea just within the sclerocorneal junction, common among the elderly and resulting from a deposit of fatty granules in, or hyaline degeneration of, the lamellae and cells of the cornea. Also called *anterior embryotoxon, arcus adiposus, arcus juvenilis, arcus senilis, gerontoxon*.

ARDS *abbr.* adult respiratory distress syndrome

ar·e·a (âr′ē-ə) *n., pl.* **–as** *or* **–ae** (-ē-ē′) **1.** A circumscribed surface or space. **2.** All of a part that is supplied by a given artery or nerve. **3.** A part of an organ having a special function.

area of cardiac dullness *n.* A triangular area determined by percussion of the front of the chest that corresponds to the part of the heart that is not covered by lung tissue.

a·re·flex·i·a (ā′rĭ-flĕk′sē-ə) *n.* The absence of reflexes.

Ar·e·na·vir·i·dae (ăr′ə-nə-vîr′ĭ-dē) *n.* A family of RNA viruses comprising the genus *Arenavirus*.

Ar·e·na·vi·rus (ăr′ə-nə-vī′rəs, ə-rē′nə-) *n.* The single genus of viruses in the family Arenaviridae that includes the viruses that cause lymphocytic choriomeningitis and Lassa fever.

a·re·o·la (ə-rē′ə-lə) *n., pl.* **–las** *or* **–lae** (-lē′) **1.** A small area. **2.** Any of numerous spaces or interstices in areolar tissue. **3.** Areola mammae. **4.** A pigmented, depigmented, or erythematous zone surrounding a papule, pustule, wheal, or cutaneous neoplasm. **—a·re′o·lar, a·re′o·late** (-lĭt) *adj.*

areola mam·mae (măm′ē) *n.* The circular pigmented area surrounding the nipple of the breast, dotted with small projections from the glands beneath.

areolar gland *n.* Any of several cutaneous glands forming small, rounded projections from the surface of the areola of the breast.

areolar tissue *n.* Loose, irregularly arranged connective tissue that consists of collagenous and elastic fibers, a protein polysaccharide ground substance, and connective tissue cells.

areola umbilicus *n.* A pigmented ring surrounding the umbilicus of a pregnant woman.

Arg *abbr.* arginine

Ar·gas (är′gəs, -găs′) *n.* A genus of ticks that includes some species that usually infest birds but that may infect humans.

ar·gas·id (är-găs′ĭd) *n.* A member of Argasidae.

Ar·gas·i·dae (är-găs′ĭ-dē) *n.* A family of soft-bodied ticks.

ar·gen·taf·fin (är-jĕn′tə-fĭn) *adj.* Of or relating to cells or tissue elements that reduce silver ions in solution, thereby staining brown or black.

argentaffin cell *n.* See enteroendocrine cell.

ar·gen·taf·fi·no·ma (är-jĕn′tə-fə-nō′mə, är′jən-tăf′ə-) *n.* See carcinoid.

ar·gen·to·phil (är-jĕn′tə-fĭl) *or* **ar·gen·to·phile** (-fīl′) *adj.* Argyrophil.

ar·gi·nase (är′jə-nās′, -nāz′) *n.* An enzyme found primarily in the liver that catalyzes the hydrolysis of arginine to urea and ornithine.

ar·gi·nine (är′jə-nēn′) *n. Abbr.* **Arg** An amino acid obtained from the hydrolysis or digestion of plant and animal protein.

ar·gi·ni·no·suc·cin·ic acid (är′jə-nĭ-nō-sək-sĭn′ĭk, är′-jə-nē′-) *n.* An acid formed as an intermediate during the urea cycle in a reaction involving aspartic acid and adenosine triphosphate.

ar·gi·ni·no·suc·cin·ic·ac·i·du·ri·a (är′jə-nĭ-nō-sək-sĭn′ĭk-ăs′ĭ-dōŏr′ē-ə, är′jə-nē′-) *n.* A disorder characterized by excessive excretion of argininosuccinic acid in the urine, epilepsy, ataxia, mental retardation, liver disease, and friable, tufted hair.

ar·gon (är′gŏn′) *n. Symbol* **Ar** A colorless, inert gaseous element constituting approx. one percent of the earth's atmosphere, used in electric bulbs and fluorescent tubes and in lasers used for opthalmic procedures. Atomic number 18.

Ar·gyll Rob·ert·son pupil (är-gīl′ rŏb′ərt-sən) *n.* A pupil that contracts or expands to accommodate changes in focal length but that does not respond to light.

ar·gyr·i·a (är-jîr′ē-ə, -jī′rē-ə) *n.* A slate-gray or bluish discoloration of the skin and deep tissues due to the deposit of insoluble albuminate of silver. Also called *argyrism.* **—ar·gyr′ic** *adj.*

Ar·gy·rol (är′jə-rôl′, -rōl′) A trademark for a silver-protein compound used as a local antiseptic.

ar·gy·ro·phil (är-jī′rə-fĭl, är′jə-rō-fĭl′) *or* **ar·gy·ro·phile** (-fīl′) *adj.* Of or relating to tissue elements capable of impregnation with silver salts and of being made visible through the use of a reducing agent.

a·rhin·i·a (ə-rĭn′ē-ə, ə-rī′nē-ə) *n.* See arrhinia.

A·ri·as-Stel·la phenomenon (ä′rē-ä-stĕl′ə, är′yä-stĕ′yä) *n.* Focal, unusual, decidual changes in endometrial epithelium that consist of intraluminal budding, nuclear enlargement, and hyperchromatism with cytoplastic swelling and vacuolation. Also called *Arias-Stella reaction.*

Arias-Stella reaction *n.* See **Arias-Stella phenomenon.**

a·ri·bo·fla·vin·o·sis (ā-rī′bō-flā′və-nō′sĭs) *n.* A condition caused by a riboflavin deficiency, characterized by chilosis or angular stomatitis and a magenta-colored tongue. Also called *hyporiboflavinosis.*

Ar·i·cept (âr′ə-sĕpt′) A trademark for the drug donepezil hydrochloride.

a·ri·pip·ra·zole (ā′rə-pĭp′rə-zōl′) *n.* An antipsychotic drug that functions as a partial dopamine receptor agonist and is used in the treatment of schizophrenia and other psychoses.

A·ris·to·cort (ə-rĭs′tə-kôrt′) A trademark for the drug triamcinolone.

Ar·is·to·te·li·an method (ăr′ĭ-stə-tē′lē-ən, -tēl′yən, ə-rĭs′tə-) *n.* A method of study that emphasizes the relation between a general category and a specific object.

Ar·is·tot·le (ăr′ĭ-stŏt′l) 384–322 BC. Greek philosopher. A pupil of Plato, the tutor of Alexander the Great, and the author of works on logic, metaphysics, ethics, natural sciences, politics, and poetics, he profoundly influenced Western intellectual and scientific thought. In his works on science he emphasized the direct observation of nature and the philosophy that theory follows empirical observation.

a·rith·me·tic mean (ə-rĭth′mĭ-tĭk) *n.* The value obtained by calculating the sum of a set of quantities and then dividing that sum by the number of quantities in the set. Also called *average.*

arm (ärm) *n.* An upper limb of the human body, connecting the hand and wrist to the shoulder.

ar·ma·men·tar·i·um (är′mə-mĕn-târ′ē-əm) *n.,* *pl.* **–i·ums** or **–i·a** (-ē-ə) The complete equipment of a physician or medical institution, including drugs, books, supplies, and instruments.

Ar·mil·li·fer (är-mĭl′ə-fər) *n.* A genus of parasitic organisms, including the tongue worms, whose adult members are found in the lungs of reptiles and whose larvae or nymphs are sometimes found in humans.

ar·mored heart (är′mərd) *n.* A heart condition characterized by calcareous deposits in the pericardium.

arm·pit (ärm′pĭt′) *n.* The hollow under the upper part of the arm below the shoulder joint, bounded by the pectoralis major, the latissimus dorsi, the anterior serratus muscles, and the humerus, and containing the axillary artery and vein, the infraclavicular part of the brachial plexus, lymph nodes and vessels, and areolar tissue. Also called *axilla, axillary fossa.*

Arndt's law (ärnts) *n.* The principle stating that weak stimuli excite physiological activity, moderately strong stimuli favor it, strong stimuli retard it, and very strong stimuli arrest it.

Ar·neth count (är′nĕt′) *n.* The analysis by percentage of the distribution of neutrophils based on the number of lobes in the nuclei, ranging from 1 to 5 lobes. Also called *Arneth index.*

Ar·nold-Chiari deformity (är′nəld-, -nōlt′-) *n.* A congenital deformity at the base of the brain, often associated with spina bifida, in which the cerebellar tissue is elongated and extends into the fourth ventricle.

Ar·nold's canal (är′nəldz, -nôlts) *n.* A bony canal in the petrous portion of the temporal bone through which the lesser petrosal nerve passes.

a·roma·tase (ə-rō′mə-tāz′, -tāz′) *n.* An enzyme that catalyzes the conversion of androgens to estrogens.

aromatase inhibitor *n.* A drug that inhibits tumor growth, especially breast cancer, by inhibiting the enzyme aromatase and thereby lowering estrogen levels in the blood or in tumor tissues.

a·ro·ma·ther·a·py (ə-rō′mə-thĕr′ə-pē) *n.* The use of selected fragrant substances in lotions and inhalants in an effort to affect mood and promote health.

ar·o·mat·ic (ăr′ə-măt′ĭk) *adj.* **1.** Having an agreeable, somewhat pungent, spicy odor. **2.** Of, relating to, or containing one or more six-carbon rings characteristic of the benzene series and related organic groups. —*n.* **1.** Any of a group of vegetable-derived drugs having a fragrant odor and slight stimulative properties. **2.** An aromatic organic compound. —**ar′o·mat′i·cal·ly** *adv.*

aromatic compound *n.* A cyclic compound containing at least one benzene ring and characterized by the presence of alternating double bonds within the ring.

aromatic series *n.* Chemical compounds derived from benzene or similar closed-chain hydrocarbon compounds containing conjugated double bonds.

ar·rec·tor (ə-rĕk′tər, ă-rĕk′-) *n.,* *pl.* **ar·rec·to·res** (ăr′-ĕk-tôr′ēz) See **erector.**

ar·rest (ə-rĕst′) *v.* **1.** To stop; check. **2.** To undergo cardiac arrest. —*n.* **1.** An interference with or a checking of the regular course of a disease or symptom, a stoppage. **2.** Interference with the performance of a function. **3.** The inhibition of a developmental process, usually the ultimate stage of development.

Ar·rhe·ni·us-Mad·sen theory (ə-rē′nē-əs-măd′sən, ə-rā′-) *n.* The theory that the reaction of an antigen with its antibody is a reversible reaction.

ar·rhe·no·blas·to·ma (ăr′ə-nō-blă-stō′mə, ə-rē′nō-) *n.* An ovarian tumor that contains luteinized cells and immature testicular tubules and that may result in masculinization.

ar·rhin·i·a (ə-rĭn′ē-ə, ə-rī′nē-ə) *n.* The congenital absence of the nose. Also called *arhinia.*

ar·rhyth·mi·a (ə-rĭth′mē-ə) *n.* An irregularity in the force or rhythm of the heartbeat.

ar·rhyth·mic (ə-rĭth′mĭk) *adj.* Lacking rhythm or regularity of rhythm.

ar·rhyth·mo·gen·ic (ə-rĭth′mō-jĕn′ĭk) *adj.* Capable of inducing arrhythmias.

ar·se·nate (är′sə-nĭt, -nāt′) *n.* A salt of arsenic acid.

ar·se·ni·a·sis (är′sə-nī′ə-sĭs) *n.* Chronic arsenical poisoning. Also called *arsenicalism.*

ar·se·nic (är′sə-nĭk) *n.* *Symbol* **As** A poisonous metallic element, compounds of which are used as antamebics. Atomic number 33. —*adj.* **ar·sen·ic** (är-sĕn′ĭk) Of or containing arsenic, especially with valence 5.

ar·sen·ic acid (är-sĕn′ĭk) *n.* A poisonous, white, translucent crystalline compound used to manufacture medical arsenates.

ar·sen·i·cal (är-sĕn′ĭ-kəl) *n.* An agent containing arsenic. —*adj.* Of, relating to, or containing arsenic.

ar·sen·i·cal·ism (är-sĕn′ĭ-kə-lĭz′əm) *n.* See **arseniasis.**

ars·phen·a·mine (ärs-fĕn′ə-mēn′) *n.* A drug formerly used in the treatment of syphilis, yaws, and other protozoal diseases.

ar·te·fact (är′tə-făkt′) *n.* Variant of **artifact.**

ar·te·ri·a (är-tîr′ē-ə) *n., pl.* **–te·ri·ae** (-tîr′ē-ē′) Artery.

ar·te·ri·al (är-tîr′ē-əl) *adj.* **1.** Of or relating to one or more arteries or to the entire system of arteries. **2.** Of, relating to, or being the bright red oxygenated blood in the arteries. **—ar·te′ri·al·ly** *adv.*

arterial blood *n.* Blood that is oxygenated in the lungs, is found in the left chambers of the heart and in the arteries, and is relatively bright red.

arterial canal *n.* See **ductus arteriosus.**

arterial capillary *n.* A capillary opening from an arteriole or metarteriole.

arterial cone *n.* See **conus arteriosus.**

arterial duct *n.* See **ductus arteriosus.**

arterial forceps *n.* Locking forceps with sloping blades for grasping the end of a blood vessel until a ligature is applied.

arterial hyperemia *n.* See **active hyperemia.**

arterial ligament *n.* The fibrous cord that develops from the embryonic arterial duct.

arterial line *n.* An intra-arterial catheter.

arterial murmur *n.* A murmur heard during auscultation of an artery.

arterial nephrosclerosis *or* **ar·te·ri·o·neph·ro·scle·ro·sis** (är-tîr′ē-ō-nĕf′rō-sklə-rō′sĭs) *n.* Patchy atrophic scarring of the kidney due to arteriosclerotic narrowing of the lumens of large branches of the renal artery; it occurs in the aged or in hypertensive persons and occasionally causes hypertension.

arterial sclerosis *n.* See **arteriosclerosis.**

arterial spider *n.* A telangiectatic arteriole in the skin having capillary branches that radiate from a central area in a manner similar to legs from the body of a spider. Also called *spider nevus, spider telangiectasia, vascular spider.*

arteria lu·so·ri·a (lōō-sôr′ē-ə) *n.* An abnormally placed artery or vascular ring causing pressure on the esophagus and producing dysphagia.

ar·te·ri·arc·ti·a (är-tîr′ē-ärk′shē-ə, -tē-ə) *n.* Vasoconstriction of the arteries.

ar·te·ri·ec·ta·sis (är-tîr′ē-ĕk′tə-sĭs) *or* **ar·te·ri·ec·ta·sia** (-ĕk-tā′zhə) *n.* The vasodilation of the arteries.

ar·te·ri·ec·to·my (är-tîr′ē-ĕk′tə-mē) *n.* Excision of part of an artery.

arterio– *or* **arteri–** *pref.* Artery: *arteriovenous.*

ar·te·ri·o·at·o·ny (är-tîr′ē-ō-ăt′ə-nē) *n.* A relaxed state of the arterial walls.

ar·te·ri·o·cap·il·lar·y (är-tîr′ē-ō-kăp′ə-lĕr′ē) *adj.* Of or relating to the arteries and the capillaries.

ar·te·ri·og·ra·phy (är-tîr′ē-ŏg′rə-fē) *n.* Examination of the arteries using x-rays following injection of a radiopaque substance. **—ar·te′ri·o·gram′** (-ə-grăm′) *n.* **—ar·te′ri·o·graph′ic** (-ə-grăf′ĭk) *adj.*

ar·te·ri·o·la (är-tîr′ē-ō′lə) *n., pl.* **–lae** (-lē′) Arteriole.

arteriolae rec·tae (rĕk′tē′) *pl.n.* Branches of the arcuate arteries of the kidney, arising at the bases of the pyramids, running through the renal medulla toward the apex of each pyramid, then reversing direction back toward the base of each pyramid. Also called *vasa recta.*

arteriolar nephrosclerosis *n.* Scarring of the kidney due to arteriolar sclerosis resulting from chronic hypertension. Also called *arteriolonephrosclerosis.*

ar·te·ri·ole (är-tîr′ē-ōl′) *n.* A minute artery, especially a terminal artery continuous with the capillary network. **—ar·te′ri·o′lar** (-ō′lər, -ə-lər) *adj.*

ar·te·ri·o·lith (är-tîr′ē-ō-lĭth′) *n.* A calcareous deposit in an arterial wall or thrombus.

ar·te·ri·o·li·tis (är-tîr′ē-ō-lī′tĭs) *n.* Inflammation of the arterioles.

arteriolo– *pref.* Arteriole: *arteriolosclerosis.*

ar·te·ri·o·lo·ne·cro·sis (är-tîr′ē-ō′lō-nə-krō′sĭs) *n.* Necrosis of the arterioles.

ar·te·ri·o·lo·neph·ro·scle·ro·sis (är-tîr′ē-ō′lō-nĕf′rō-sklə-rō′sĭs) *n.* See **arteriolar nephrosclerosis.**

ar·te·ri·o·lo·scle·ro·sis (är-tîr′ē-ō′lō-sklə-rō′sĭs) *n.* Arteriosclerosis mainly affecting the arterioles.

ar·te·ri·o·mo·tor (är-tîr′ē-ō-mō′tər) *adj.* Relating to or causing changes in the caliber of an artery.

ar·te·ri·o·my·o·ma·to·sis (är-tîr′ē-ō-mī′ō-mə-tō′sĭs) *n.* An overgrowth of irregular muscular fibers causing a thickening of the walls of an artery.

ar·te·ri·o·neph·ro·scle·ro·sis (är-tîr′ē-ō-nĕf′rō-sklə-rō′sĭs) *n.* Variant of **arterial nephrosclerosis.**

ar·te·ri·op·a·thy (är-tîr′ē-ŏp′ə-thē) *n.* A disease of the arteries.

ar·te·ri·o·plas·ty (är-tîr′ē-ə-plăs′tē) *n.* Surgical reconstruction of the wall of an artery.

ar·te·ri·o·pres·sor (är-tîr′ē-ō-prĕs′ər) *adj.* Causing increased arterial blood pressure.

ar·te·ri·or·rha·phy (är-tîr′ē-ôr′ə-fē) *n.* Suture of an artery.

ar·te·ri·or·rhex·is (är-tîr′ē-ō-rĕk′sĭs) *n.* Rupture of an artery.

ar·te·ri·o·scle·ro·sis (är-tîr′ē-ō-sklə-rō′sĭs) *n.* Any of a group of chronic diseases in which thickening, hardening, and loss of elasticity of the arterial walls result in impaired blood circulation. Also called *arterial sclerosis.* **—ar·te′ri·o·scle·rot′ic** (-rŏt′ĭk) *adj.*

arteriosclerosis o·blit·er·ans (ə-blĭt′ə-rănz′) *n.* Arteriosclerosis producing narrowing and occlusion of the arterial lumen.

arteriosclerotic aneurysm *n.* The most common type of aneurysm, occurring in the abdominal aorta and other large arteries primarily in the older persons, due to weakening of the tunica media by severe atherosclerosis.

ar·te·ri·o·spasm (är-tîr′ē-ō-spăz′əm) *n.* Spasm of one or more arteries.

ar·te·ri·o·ste·no·sis (är-tîr′ē-ō-stə-nō′sĭs) *n.* A temporary or permanent narrowing of the caliber of an artery, as, for example, by vasoconstriction or arteriosclerosis.

ar·te·ri·ot·o·my (är-tîr′ē-ŏt′ə-mē) *n.* Incision into the lumen of an artery.

ar·te·ri·ot·o·ny (är-tîr′ē-ŏt′n-ē) *n.* See **blood pressure.**

ar·te·ri·o·ve·nous (är-tĕr′ĭ-ō-vē′nəs) *adj. Abbr.* **AV** Of, relating to, or connecting arteries and veins.

arteriovenous anastomosis *n.* A vessel that shunts blood from an artery to a vein in order to bypass a capillary.

arteriovenous aneurysm *n.* A dilated connection between an artery and a vein that allows blood to flow from the artery into the vein.

arteriovenous carbon dioxide difference *n.* The difference in carbon dioxide content, in milliliters per 100 milliliters blood, between the arterial and venous bloods.

arteriovenous fistula *n.* An abnormal communication between an artery and a vein, usually resulting in the formation of an arteriovenous aneurysm.

arteriovenous nicking *n.* A constriction of a vein in the retina of the eye at an artery-vein crossing.

arteriovenous oxygen difference *n.* The difference in the oxygen content, in milliliters per 100 milliliters blood, between arterial and venous blood.

arteriovenous shunt *n.* The passage of blood directly from arteries to veins, without going through the capillary network.

ar·te·ri·tis (är′tə-rī′tĭs) *n.* Inflammation of an artery or arteries.

ar·ter·y (är′tə-rē) *n.* Any of a branching system of muscular, elastic blood vessels that, except for the pulmonary and umbilical arteries, carry aerated blood away from the heart to the cells, tissues, and organs of the body.

artery of angular gyrus *n.* An artery that is the last branch of the terminal part of the middle cerebral artery, distributed to parts of the temporal parietal and occipital lobes. Also called *angular artery.*

artery of bulb of penis *n.* A branch of the internal pudendal artery that supplies the bulb of the penis.

artery of bulb of vestibule *n.* A branch of the internal pudendal artery in the female that supplies the bulb of the vestibule.

artery of ductus deferens *n.* An artery with its origin in the anterior division of the internal iliac or sometimes in the superior vesical artery, with distribution to the ductus deferens, seminal vesicles, testicles, and ureter, and with anastomoses to the testicular artery and the cremasteric branch of the inferior epigastric artery.

artery of kidney *n.* Any of the usually five branches of the renal artery that supply the kidney and give off the interlobar, arcuate, and interlobular arteries in sequence.

artery of labyrinth *n.* The branch of the basilar artery that enters the labyrinth through the internal acoustic meatus. Also called *internal auditory artery.*

artery of pterygoid canal *n.* A tiny artery in the pterygoid canal connecting the maxillary and internal carotid arteries.

artery of round ligament of uterus *n.* An artery with its origin in the inferior epigastric artery and with distribution to the round ligament.

ar·thral·gia (är-thrăl′jə) *n.* Severe pain in a joint. Also called *arthrodynia.* —**ar·thral′gic** (-jĭk) *adj.*

ar·threc·to·my (är-thrĕk′tə-mē) *n.* The surgical excision of a joint.

arthritic general pseudoparalysis *n.* A disease, occurring in arthritis, having symptoms resembling those of general paresis and associated with intracranial atheroma. Also called *Klippel's disease.*

ar·thri·tide (är′thrĭ-tīd′, -tēd′) *n.* A skin eruption possibly of gouty or rheumatic origin.

ar·thri·tis (är-thrī′tĭs) *n., pl.* **–thrit·i·des** (-thrĭt′ĭ-dēz′) Inflammation of a joint, usually accompanied by pain, swelling, and stiffness, resulting from infection, trauma, degenerative changes, metabolic disturbances, or other causes. —**ar·thrit′ic** (-thrĭt′ĭk) *adj. & n.* —**ar·thrit′i·cal·ly** *adv.*

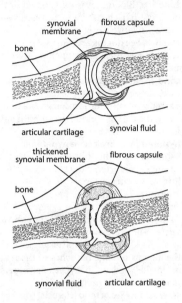

arthritis
Top: *normal finger joint*
Bottom: *arthritic finger joint*

arthritis de·for·mans (dē-fôr′mănz′) *n.* See **rheumatoid arthritis.**

arthritis mu·ti·lans (myōōt′l-ănz′) *n.* Rheumatoid arthritis accompanied by osteoporosis and destruction of the joint cartilages that results in severe deformities, chiefly of the hands and feet.

arthro– *or* **arthr–** *pref.* Joint: *arthropathy.*

ar·thro·cele (är′thrə-sēl′) *n.* **1.** Hernia of the synovial membrane through the capsule of a joint. **2.** Swelling of a joint.

ar·thro·cen·te·sis (är′thrō-sĕn-tē′sĭs) *n.* The surgical puncture and aspiration of a joint.

ar·thro·chon·dri·tis (är′thrō-kŏn-drī′tĭs) *n.* Inflammation of an articular cartilage.

ar·thro·cla·sia (är′thrō-klā′zhə) *n.* A forcible breaking up of the adhesions in an ankylosis to allow more mobility in the joint.

ar·throd·e·sis (är-thrŏd′ĭ-sĭs, är′thrə-dē′sĭs) *n.* The surgical fixation of a joint to promote bone fusion. Also called *artificial ankylosis, syndesis.*

ar·thro·di·a (är-thrō′dē-ə) *n.* See **plane joint.** —**ar·thro′di·al** *adj.*

arthrodial cartilage *n.* See **articular cartilage.**

arthrodial joint *n.* See **plane joint.**

ar·thro·dyn·i·a (är'thrō-dĭn'ē-ə) *n.* See **arthralgia.** —**ar'thro·dyn'ic** (-dĭn'ĭk) *adj.*

ar·thro·dys·pla·sia (är'thrō-dĭs-plā'zhə) *n.* Abnormal joint development.

ar·thro·en·dos·co·py (är'thrō-ĕn-dŏs'kə-pē) *n.* See **arthroscopy.**

ar·throg·ra·phy (är-thrŏg'rə-fē) *n.* Examination of the interior of a joint using x-rays following the injection of a radiopaque substance. —**ar'thro·gram'** (är'thrə-grăm') *n.*

ar·thro·gry·po·sis (är'thrə-grə-pō'sĭs) *n.* **1.** The permanent fixation of a joint in a contracted position. **2.** A congenital disorder marked by generalized stiffness of the joints, often accompanied by muscle and nerve degeneration, resulting in severely impaired mobility of the limbs. Also called *amyoplasia congenita, arthrogryposis multiplex congenita.*

ar·thro·lith (är'thrə-lĭth') *n.* A concretion within a joint.

ar·throl·y·sis (är-thrŏl'ĭ-sĭs) *n.* The surgical restoration of mobility in ankylosed joints.

ar·throm·e·ter (är-thrŏm'ĭ-tər) *n.* A calibrated device for measuring the arc or range of mobility of a joint. Also called *goniometer.*

ar·throm·e·try (är-thrŏm'ĭ-trē) *n.* The measurement of the range of movement in a joint.

ar·thro·oph·thal·mop·a·thy (är'thrō-ŏf'thəl-mŏp'ə-thē, -thăl-, -ŏp'-) *n.* Disease affecting the joints and eyes.

ar·throp·a·thy (är-thrŏp'ə-thē) *n.* A disease or an abnormality of a joint.

ar·thro·phy·ma (är'thrō-fī'mə) *n.* A tumor or swelling of a joint.

ar·thro·plas·ty (är'thrə-plăs'tē) *n.* **1.** The creation of an artificial joint. **2.** The surgical restoration of the integrity and functional power of a joint.

ar·thro·pod (är'thrə-pŏd') *n.* Any of numerous invertebrate animals of the phylum Arthropoda, including insects, crustaceans, arachnids, and myriapods.

Ar·throp·o·da (är-thrŏp'ə-də) *n.* A phylum of the Metazoa that includes crustaceans, insects, arachnids, centipedes, millipedes, and horseshoe crabs.

ar·thro·po·di·a·sis (är'thrō-pə-dī'ə-sĭs) *n.* A pathological disorder caused by an arthropod, as acariasis, allergy, dermatosis, or entomophobia.

ar·thro·py·o·sis (är'thrō-pī-ō'sĭs) *n.* The formation of pus in a joint.

ar·thro·scle·ro·sis (är'thrō-sklə-rō'sĭs) *n.* Stiffness or hardening of the joints.

ar·thros·co·py (är-thrŏs'kə-pē) *n.* Examination of the interior of a joint using an endoscope that is inserted into the joint through a small incision. Also called *arthroendoscopy.* —**ar'thro·scope'** (är'thrə-skōp') *n.* —**ar'thro·scop'ic** (-skŏp'ĭk) *adj.*

ar·thro·sis (är-thrō'sĭs) *n., pl.* **-ses** (-sēz) **1.** An articulation between bones. **2.** A degenerative disease of a joint.

ar·thros·to·my (är-thrŏs'tə-mē) *n.* Surgical construction of a temporary opening into a joint cavity.

ar·thro·syn·o·vi·tis (är'thrō-sĭn'ə-vī'tĭs, -sī'nə-) *n.* Inflammation of the synovial membrane of a joint.

ar·throt·o·my (är-thrŏt'ə-mē) *n.* Incision into a joint. Also called *synosteotomy.*

ar·throx·e·sis (är-thrŏk'sĭ-sĭs) *n.* The surgical removal of diseased tissue from a joint by scraping.

ar·tic·u·lar (är-tĭk'yə-lər) *adj.* Of or relating to a joint or joints.

articular capsule *n.* A sac enclosing a joint, formed by an outer fibrous membrane and an inner synovial membrane. Also called *joint capsule.*

articular cartilage *n.* The cartilage covering the articular surfaces of the bones forming a synovial joint. Also called *arthrodial cartilage, diarthrodial cartilage, investing cartilage.*

articular chondrocalcinosis *n.* A disease that is characterized by deposits of calcium hypophosphate crystals in synovial fluid, articular cartilage, and adjacent soft tissue and that produces goutlike attacks of pain and swelling of the involved joints. Also called *pseudogout.*

articular corpuscle *n.* Any of the encapsulated nerve endings in a joint capsule.

articular disk *n.* A plate or ring of fibrocartilage attached to the joint capsule and separating the articular surfaces of the bones. Also called *interarticular cartilage, interarticular fibrocartilage.*

articular lamella *n.* The compact layer of bone on its articular surface that is firmly attached to the overlying articular cartilage.

articular muscle *n.* A muscle that inserts directly into the capsule of a joint, acting to retract the capsule in certain movements.

articular muscle of elbow *n.* A small portion of the medial head of the triceps that inserts into the capsule of the elbow joint.

articular muscle of knee *n.* A muscle with origin from the lower anterior surface of the shaft of the femur, with insertion into the capsule of the knee joint, with nerve supply from the femoral nerve, and whose action retracts the suprapatellar bursa.

articular nerve *n.* Nerve branch supplying a joint.

ar·tic·u·late (är-tĭk'yə-lĭt) *adj.* **1.** Capable of speaking distinctly and connectedly. **2.** Consisting of sections united by joints; jointed. —*v.* (-lāt') **1.** To speak distinctly and connectedly. **2.** To join or connect together loosely to allow motion between the parts. **3.** To unite by forming a joint or joints. **4.** To form a joint; be jointed.

ar·tic·u·la·ted (är-tĭk'yə-lā-tĭd) *adj.* Characterized by or having articulations; jointed.

ar·tic·u·la·ti·o (är-tĭk'yə-lā'shē-ō') *n., pl.* **-la·ti·o·nes** (-lā'shē-ō'nēz) Articulation.

ar·tic·u·la·tion (är-tĭk'yə-lā'shən) *n.* **1.** The place of anatomical union, usually movable, between two or more bones. **2.** A joining or connecting together loosely so as to allow motion between the parts. **3.** Distinct connected speech or enunciation. **4.** The contact relationship of the occlusal surfaces of the teeth during jaw movement. **5.** Placement of artificial teeth on a denture base so that the teeth approximate normal position and contact.

ar·tic·u·la·tor (är-tĭk'yə-lā'tər) *n.* A mechanical device representing the temporomandibular joints and the jaw bones, used in dentistry to obtain proper articulation of artificial teeth.

ar·ti·fact *or* **ar·te·fact** (är′tə-făkt′) *n.* **1.** A structure or substance not normally present but produced by an external agent or action, such as a structure seen in a microscopic specimen after fixation that is not present in the living tissue. **2.** A skin lesion produced or perpetuated by self-inflicted action. —**ar′ti·fac·ti′tious** (-făk-tĭsh′əs), **ar′ti·fac′tu·al** (-făk′chŏo-əl) *adj.*

ar·ti·fi·cial ankylosis (är′tə-fĭsh′əl) *n.* See **arthrodesis.**

artificial heart *n.* A mechanical pump used to replace the function of a damaged heart, either temporarily or as a permanent internal prosthesis.

artificial insemination *n. Abbr.* **AI** The introduction of semen into the vagina or uterus without sexual contact.

artificial kidney *n.* See **hemodialyzer.**

artificial pacemaker *n.* An electronic device that substitutes for the natural pacemaker of the heart. It may be surgically implanted or placed externally on the chest.

artificial radioactivity *n.* The radioactivity of isotopes that have been artificially produced through the bombardment of naturally occurring isotopes by subatomic particles or by high levels of x-rays or gamma rays. Also called *induced radioactivity.*

artificial respiration *n.* A procedure to mechanically or manually force air into and out of the lungs in a rhythmic manner to restore or maintain respiration in a person who has stopped breathing. Also called *artificial ventilation.*

artificial selection *n.* Human intervention in animal or plant reproduction to ensure certain characteristics are represented in successive generations.

artificial ventilation *n.* See **artificial respiration.**

arts medicine *n.* A branch of medicine dealing with the special health needs of artists, such as the injuries and disorders suffered by musicians that result from playing a musical instrument.

art therapy *n.* Psychotherapy that incorporates the production of visual art, such as painting or sculpture, in order to understand and express one's feelings.

ar·y·ep·i·glot·tic fold (är′y-ĕp′ĭ-glŏt′ĭk) *n.* A prominent fold of mucous membrane stretching between the lateral margin of the epiglottis and the arytenoid cartilage on either side to enclose the aryepiglottic muscle.

aryepiglottic muscle *n.* A band of muscular fibers of the oblique arytenoid muscle that extends from the summit of the arytenoid cartilage to the side of the epiglottis and whose action constricts the laryngeal aperture.

ar·yl (ăr′əl) *n.* An organic radical derived from an aromatic compound by the removal of one hydrogen atom.

ar·y·te·noid (är′ĭ-tē′noid′, ə-rĭt′n-oid′) *n.* **1.** Either of two small pitcher-shaped cartilages at the back of the larynx to which the vocal cords are attached. **2.** A muscle that is connected to either of these cartilages. **3.** Any of several small mucous glands located in front of these cartilages. —*adj.* Of or relating to these cartilages or an associated muscle or gland. —**ar′y·te·noid′al** *adj.*

arytenoid cartilage *n.* Either of a pair of small pyramidal laryngeal cartilages that articulate with the lamina

of the cricoid cartilage and give attachment to the posterior part of the corresponding vocal ligament and to several muscles.

ar·y·te·noi·dec·to·my (är′ĭ-tē′noi-děk′tə-mē, ə-rĭt′n-oi-) *n.* Excision of an arytenoid cartilage.

ar·y·te·noi·di·tis (är′ĭ-tē′noi-dī′tĭs, ə-rĭt′n-oi-) *n.* Inflammation of an arytenoid cartilage.

arytenoid muscle *n.* **1.** A muscle with its origin in the muscular process of the arytenoid cartilage, with insertion to the summit of the arytenoid cartilage of the opposite side and the aryepiglottic fold as far as the epiglottis, with nerve supply from the recurrent laryngeal nerve, and whose action narrows the rima glottidis; oblique arytenoid muscle. **2.** A band of muscular fibers passing between the two arytenoid cartilages posteriorly, with nerve supply from the recurrent laryngeal nerve, and whose action narrows the rima glottidis; transverse arytenoid muscle.

ar·y·te·noi·do·pexy (är′ĭ-tə-noi′də-pěk′sē,ə-rĭt′n-oi′-) *n.* Surgical fixation of the arytenoid cartilages or muscles.

As The symbol for the element **arsenic.**

AS *abbr.* aortic stenosis; *Latin* auris sinistra (left ear)

as– *pref.* Variant of **ad–** (sense 1).

ASA *abbr.* acetylsalicylic acid

A·sa·col (ā-sə-kôl′) A trademark for the drug mesalamine.

as·bes·toid (ăs-běs′toid′, ăz-) *adj.* Amianthoid.

as·bes·tos (ăs-běs′təs, ăz-) *n.* Either of two incombustible, chemical-resistant, fibrous mineral forms of impure magnesium silicate, formerly used for fireproofing, electrical insulation, brake linings, and chemical filters but now banned because it causes pleural mesothelioma and asbestosis. —*adj.* Of, made of, or containing one or the other of these two mineral forms.

asbestos body *n.* A ferruginous body containing asbestos fibers as a core and a histologic indication of exposure to asbestos.

as·bes·to·sis (ăs′běs-tō′sĭs, ăz′-) *n.* Pneumoconiosis due to prolonged inhalation of asbestos particles.

as·ca·ri·a·sis (ăs′kə-rī′ə-sĭs) *n.* A disease caused by infestation with worms of the genus *Ascaris.*

as·car·i·cide (ə-skăr′ĭ-sīd′) *n.* An agent or substance that kills ascarids.

as·ca·rid (ăs′kə-rĭd) *n.* A worm of the family Ascarididae. —**as′ca·rid** *adj.*

As·ca·rid·i·dae (ăs′kə-rĭd′ĭ-dē) *n.* A family of large intestinal roundworms including the genus *Ascaris.*

As·ca·ris (ăs′kə-rĭs) *n.* A genus of large roundworms parasitic in the small intestine of humans and other vertebrates.

Ascaris lum·bri·coi·des (lŭm′brĭ-koi′dēz) *n.* A common roundworm that is parasitic in the intestines of humans and that causes restlessness, fever, and sometimes diarrhea.

as·cend·ing artery (ə-sĕn′dĭng) *n.* The branch of the ileocolic artery that communicates with a branch of the colic artery and supplies the ascending colon.

ascending colon *n.* The part of the colon between the ileocecal orifice and the right colic flexure.

ascending degeneration *n.* The degeneration of nerve

fibers progressing toward the spinal cord or brain from the point of injury.

ascending lumbar vein *n.* A vein that arises from the sacral and lumbar veins and at the diaphragm becomes the azygos vein on the right side and the hemiazygos vein on the left.

ascending pharyngeal artery *n.* An artery with its origin in the external carotid artery and with distribution to both the wall of the pharynx and the soft palate.

Asc·hel·min·thes (ăsk'hĕl-mĭn'thēz') *n.* A phylum of the Metazoa that includes nematodes and other round-worms that are nonsegmented, bilaterally symmetrical, and cylindrical in form, with a pseudocele body cavity and rounded or pointed ends.

Asch·off body (ăsh'ôf', ä'shôf') *n.* A granulomatous inflammation characteristic of acute rheumatic carditis, consisting of fibrinoid changes in connective tissue and lymphocytes.

as·ci·tes (ə-sī'tēz) *n., pl.* **ascites** The accumulation of serous fluid in the peritoneal cavity. Also called *hydroperitoneum.* —**as·cit'ic** (-sĭt'ĭk) *adj.*

As·cle·pi·a·des (ăs'klə-pī'ə-dēz') fl. first century BC. Greek physician born in Bithynia who theorized that disease is caused by an inharmonious flow of the corpuscles of the body. His methods for restoring harmony in the body included diet, exercise, and bathing. Asclepiades also advocated humane treatment of the mentally ill.

as·co·my·cete (ăs'kō-mī'sēt', -mī-sēt') *n.* A member of the class Ascomycetes.

As·co·my·ce·tes (ăs'kō-mī-sē'tēz') *n.* A class of fungi characterized by the presence of asci and spores, and having two distinct reproductive phases, a perfect stage and an imperfect stage.

a·scor·base (ə-skôr'bās) *n.* A copper-containing enzyme that catalyzes the oxidation of ascorbic acid.

a·scor·bate (ə-skôr'bāt, -bĭt) *n.* A salt of ascorbic acid.

a·scor·bic acid (ə-skôr'bĭk) *n.* A white, crystalline vitamin found in citrus fruits, tomatoes, potatoes, and leafy green vegetables and used to prevent scurvy. Also called *vitamin C.*

as·cus (ăs'kəs) *n., pl.* **as·ci** (ăs'ī', -kī') A membranous, often club-shaped structure in which typically eight spores are formed through sexual reproduction of ascomycetes.

ASCVD *abbr.* arteriosclerotic cardiovascular disease

ASD *abbr.* atrial septal defect

-ase *suff.* Enzyme: *amylase.*

A·sel·li (ə-sĕl'ē, ä-sĕl'ē), **Gasparo** *Latin* **Gaspar A·sel·i·us** (ə-sĕl'ē-əs) 1581–1626. Italian anatomist who discovered the lacteal vessels of the intestine.

as·e·ma·sia (ăs'ə-mā'zhə) *or* **a·se·mi·a** (ə-sē'mē-ə) *n.* See **asymbolia** (sense 2).

a·sep·sis (ə-sĕp'sĭs, ā-) *n.* **1.** The state of being free of living pathogenic microorganisms. **2.** The process of removing pathogenic microorganisms or protecting against infection by such organisms.

a·sep·tic (ə-sĕp'tĭk, ā-) *adj.* Of, relating to, or characterized by asepsis.

aseptic necrosis *n.* Necrosis occurring in the absence of infection.

aseptic surgery *n.* Surgery performed under sterilized conditions to prevent the introduction of infectious microorganisms.

a·sex·u·al (ā-sĕk'shoo-əl) *adj.* **1.** Having no evident sex or sex organs; sexless. **2.** Relating to, produced by, or involving reproduction that occurs without the union of male and female gametes, as in binary fission or budding. **3.** Lacking interest in or desire for sex. —**a·sex'u·al'i·ty** (-ăl'ĭ-tē) *n.* —**a·sex'u·al·ly** *adv.*

asexual dwarf *n.* A dwarf who is not developed sexually yet is beyond the age of puberty.

asexual generation *n.* **1.** A generation that reproduces by asexual means only. **2.** Reproduction without the union of individuals or of the male and female germ cells; asexual reproduction. Also called *nonsexual generation.*

asexual reproduction *n.* Reproduction occurring without the sexual union of male and female gametes.

ASHD *abbr.* arteriosclerotic heart disease

a·si·a·lism (ə-sī'ə-lĭz'əm) *or* **a·si·a·li·a** (ā'sī-ā'lē-ə, -ăl'ē-ə) *n.* Diminished or arrested secretion of saliva. Also called *aptyalia.*

Asian influenza *n.* Influenza that is caused by a strain of influenza virus type A, which was first isolated in China during the 1957 epidemic.

A·si·at·ic schistosomiasis (ā'zhē-ăt'ĭk, -shē-, -zē-) *n.* See **schistosomiasis japonicum.**

Ask-Up·mark kidney (ăsk'ŭp'märk) *n.* A kidney disorder characterized by renal hypoplasia with decreased lobules and deep transverse grooving of the cortical surfaces of the organ.

a·sleep (ə-slēp') *adj.* **1.** In a state of sleep; sleeping. **2.** Numb, as of a limb. **3.** Dead. —*adv.* **1.** In or into a state of sleep. **2.** In or into a state of apathy or indifference. **3.** Into the sleep of the dead.

Asn *abbr.* asparagine

a·so·cial (ā-sō'shəl) *adj.* **1.** Avoiding or averse to the society of others; not sociable. **2.** Unable or unwilling to conform to normal standards of social behavior; antisocial.

Asp *abbr.* aspartic acid

as·par·a·gin·ase (ə-spăr'ə-jə-nās', -năz') *n.* A bacterial enzyme that catalyzes the hydrolysis of asparagine and is used in the treatment of leukemia.

as·par·a·gine (ə-spăr'ə-jēn') *n. Abbr.* **Asn** An amino acid found in proteins that is the beta-amide of aspartic acid. Also called *asparamide.*

as·par·tame (ăs'pər-tām', ə-spär'-) *n.* A low-calorie, artificial sweetening agent derived from aspartic acid.

a·spar·tase (ə-spär'tās', -tāz') *n.* An enzyme found in various bacteria, yeasts, and plants that catalyzes the conversion of aspartic acid to fumaric acid by removing ammonia and catalyzes the reverse reaction by adding ammonia. Also called *aspartate ammonialyase.*

a·spar·tate (ə-spär'tāt) *n.* **1.** A salt of aspartic acid. **2.** An ester of aspartic acid.

aspartate aminotransferase *n. Abbr.* **AST** See **SGOT.**

as·par·tic ac·id (ə-spär'tĭk) *n. Abbr.* **Asp** One of the nonessential amino acids that occur in proteins. Also called *alpha-aminosuccinic acid.*

as·pect (ăs'pĕkt) *n.* **1.** An appearance or look. **2.** The side of an object that faces in a particular direction.

As·per·ger's syndrome (ăs′pər-gərz) *n.* A pervasive developmental disorder, usually of childhood, characterized by impairments in social interactions and repetitive behavior patterns.

as·per·gil·lo·ma (ăs′pər-jə-lō′mə) *n.* **1.** An infectious granuloma caused by fungi of the genus *Aspergillus.* **2.** A variety of bronchopulmonary aspergillosis characterized by a ball-like mass of the fungus *Aspergillus fumigatus* in an existing cavity in the lung. Also called *fungus ball.*

as·per·gil·lo·sis (ăs′pər-jə-lō′sĭs) *n.* An infection or a disease caused by fungi of the genus *Aspergillus.*

As·per·gil·lus (ăs′pər-jĭl′əs) *n.* A genus of fungi that includes many common molds.

a·sper·ma·tism (ā-spûr′mə-tĭz′əm, ə-spûr′-) *or* **a·sper·mi·a** (ā-spûr′mē-ə, ă-spûr′-) *n.* The inability to secrete or ejaculate semen.

as·phyx·i·a (ăs-fĭk′sē-ə) *n.* A condition in which an extreme decrease in the amount of oxygen in the body accompanied by an increase of carbon dioxide leads to loss of consciousness or death.

asphyxia liv·i·da (lĭv′ĭ-də) *n.* Asphyxia in which the skin is cyanotic, but the heart is strong and the reflexes are preserved.

asphyxia ne·o·na·to·rum (nē′ō-nā-tôr′əm) *n.* Asphyxia occurring in a newborn.

as·phyx·i·ant (ăs-fĭk′sē-ənt) *adj.* Inducing or tending to induce asphyxia. —*n.* A substance, such as a toxic gas, or an event, such as drowning, that induces asphyxia.

as·phyx·i·ate (ăs-fĭk′sē-āt′) *v.* To induce asphyxia. —**as·phyx′i·a′tion** *n.*

as·pi·rate (ăs′pə-rāt′) *v.* To take in or remove by aspiration. —*n.* (-pər-ĭt) A substance removed by aspiration.

as·pi·ra·tion (ăs′pə-rā′shən) *n.* **1.** The removal of a gas or fluid by suction. **2.** The sucking of fluid or a foreign body into the airway when drawing breath. **3.** A surgical technique used in the treatment of cataracts of the eye, in which an incision is made into the cornea, the lens capsule is severed, and the material of the lens is fragmented and aspirated by a needle.

aspiration biopsy *n.* See **needle biopsy.**

aspiration pneumonia *n.* Bronchopneumonia resulting from the entrance of foreign material, usually food particles or vomit, into the bronchi.

as·pi·ra·tor (ăs′pə-rā′tər) *n.* An apparatus for removing fluid from a body cavity, consisting usually of a hollow needle and a cannula, connected by tubing to a container in which a vacuum is created by a syringe or a suction pump.

as·pi·rin (ăs′pər-ĭn, -prĭn) *n.* A white, crystalline compound derived from salicylic acid and commonly used to relieve pain and reduce fever and inflammation. It is also used as an antiplatelet agent. Also called *acetylsalicylic acid.*

a·sple·ni·a (ə-splē′nē-ə) *n.* Congenital absence of the spleen. —**a·sple′nic** (ə-splē′nĭk, -splĕn′ĭk) *adj.*

as·sas·sin bug (ə-săs′ĭn) *n.* A predatory bug of the family Reduviidae having powerful piercing mouthparts that inflict irritating, painful bites on humans.

as·say (ăs′ā′, ă-sā′) *n.* **1.** Qualitative or quantitative analysis of a substance, especially of an ore or a drug, to determine its components. **2.** A substance to be so analyzed. **3.** The result of such an analysis. **4.** An analysis or examination. —*v.* (ă-sā′, ăs′ā′) **1.** To subject a substance to chemical analysis. **2.** To examine a person's capability by trial or experiment; put to a test. **3.** To evaluate a situation; assess. **4.** To attempt; try. **5.** To be shown by analysis to contain a certain proportion of atoms, molecules, compounds, or precious metal.

as·sim·i·late (ə-sĭm′ə-lāt′) *v.* **1.** To consume and incorporate nutrients into the body after digestion. **2.** To transform food into living tissue by the process of anabolism.

as·sim·i·la·tion (ə-sĭm′ə-lā′shən) *n.* **1.** The incorporation of digested substances from food into the tissues of an organism. **2.** The amalgamation and modification of newly perceived information and experiences into the existing cognitive structure.

as·sist-con·trol ventilation (ə-sĭst′kən-trōl′) *n.* A method of artificial respiration in which inspiration is produced automatically after a set interval if the person has not begun to inspire earlier.

as·sist·ed living (ə-sĭs′tĭd) *n.* A living arrangement in which people with special needs, especially older people with disabilities, reside in a facility that provides help with everyday tasks such as bathing, dressing, and taking medication.

assisted reproduction *n.* The use of medical techniques, such as drug therapy, artificial insemination, or in vitro fertilization, to enhance fertility.

assisted respiration *n.* A procedure for applying mechanically or manually generated positive pressure to gases in or surrounding the airway during inhalation to augment movement of gases into the lungs. Also called *assisted ventilation.*

assisted suicide *n.* Suicide accomplished with the aid of another person, especially a physician.

as·so·ci·at·ed movement (ə-sō′shē-ā′tĭd, -sē-) *n.* Involuntary movement in one limb corresponding to a voluntary movement in the opposite limb.

as·so·ci·a·tion (ə-sō′sē-ā′shən, -shē-) *n.* **1.** A connection of persons, things, or ideas by some common factor; union. **2.** A functional connection of two ideas, events, or psychological phenomena established through learning or experience.

association area *n.* See **association cortex.**

association constant *n.* A mathematical constant describing the bonding affinity of two molecules at equilibrium, especially the bonding affinity of an antibody and an antigen.

association cortex *n.* Any of the expanses of the cerebral cortex that are not sensory or motor in the customary sense, but instead are associated with advanced stages of sensory information processing, multisensory integration, or sensorimotor integration. Also called *association area.*

association fiber *n.* Any of the nerve fibers connecting individual subdivisions of a brain structure or different segments of the spinal cord.

association test *n.* A word association test used diagnostically in psychiatry and psychology in which a word is spoken to an individual who responds with whatever word comes to mind as a result of hearing the first word.

as·so·ci·a·tive aphasia (ə-sō′shē-ā′tĭv, -sē-, -shə-tĭv) *n.* See **conduction aphasia.**

associative learning *n.* A learning principle based on the belief that ideas and experiences reinforce one another and can be mentally linked to enhance the learning process.

associative neuron *n.* A nerve cell within the central nervous system that links sensory and motor neurons.

as·sor·ta·tive mating (ə-sôr′tə-tĭv) *n.* Nonrandom mating in which individuals mate preferentially according to phenotype.

as·sort·ment (ə-sôrt′mənt) *n.* The relationship between non-allelic genetic traits that are transmitted from parent to child independently and according to the degree of linkage between the respective loci.

AST *abbr.* aspartate aminotransferase

a·sta·sia (ə-stā′zhə) *n.* The inability to stand due to muscular incoordination.

astasia-abasia *n.* Inability to stand or walk normally as a symptom of conversion hysteria. Also called *abasia-astasia, Blocq's disease.*

a·stat·ic (ə-stăt′ĭk) *adj.* **1.** Relating to astasia. **2.** Unsteady; unstable.

as·ta·tine (ăs′tə-tēn′, -tĭn) *n.* *Symbol* **At** A radioactive halogen element. Its longest lived isotope has a mass number of 210 and a half-life of 8.1 hours. Atomic number 85.

a·ste·a·to·sis (ə-stē′ə-tō′sĭs, ăs′tē-) *n.* Diminished or arrested action of the sebaceous glands.

as·ter (ăs′tər) *n.* See **astrosphere.**

a·ster·e·og·no·sis (ə-stĕr′ē-ŏg-nō′sĭs) *n.* The inability to determine the form of an object by touch.

as·te·ri·on (ăs-tîr′ē-ŏn′, -ən) *n.* The junction of the lambdoid, occipitomastoid, and parietomastoid sutures on the skull.

as·ter·ix·is (ăs′tə-rĭk′sĭs) *n.* An abnormal tremor consisting of involuntary jerking movements, especially in the hands, frequently occurring with impending hepatic coma and other forms of metabolic encephalopathy. Also called *flapping tremor.*

a·ster·nal (ā-stûr′nəl, ə-stûr′-) *adj.* **1.** Not related to or connected with the sternum, as a rib. **2.** Lacking a sternum.

a·ster·ni·a (ā-stûr′nē-ə, ə-stûr′-) *n.* The congenital absence of the sternum.

as·ter·oid body (ăs′tə-roid′) *n.* **1.** An eosinophilic inclusion body having radiating lines, found in a vacuolated area of cytoplasm of a multinucleated giant cell, especially seen in sarcoidosis but occurring also in other granulomas. **2.** A structure characteristic of sporotrichosis when found in the skin or in secondary lesions of sporotrichosis.

asteroid hyalosis *n.* A form of hyalosis in which numerous small spherical bodies form in the vitreous humor but do not affect vision, associated with increasing age. Also called *Benson's disease.*

as·the·ni·a (ăs-thē′nē-ə) *n.* Loss or lack of bodily strength; weakness. —**as·then′ic** (-thĕn′ĭk) *adj.*

as·the·no·pi·a (ăs′thə-nō′pē-ə) *n.* See **eyestrain.** —**as′-the·nop′ic** (-nŏp′ĭk) *adj.*

as·the·no·sper·mi·a (ăs′thə-nō-spûr′mē-ə) *n.* The loss or reduction of spermatozoan motility.

asth·ma (ăz′mə, ăs′-) *n.* Bronchial asthma. —**asth·mat′ic** (-măt′ĭk) *adj. & n.*

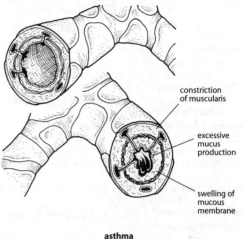

asthma
Top: *normal bronchiole*
Bottom: *asthmatic bronchiole*

constriction of muscularis

excessive mucus production

swelling of mucous membrane

astigmatic lens *n.* See **cylindrical lens.**

a·stig·ma·tism (ə-stĭg′mə-tĭz′əm) *n.* A visual defect in which the unequal curvature of one or more refractive surfaces of the eye, usually the cornea, prevents light rays from focusing clearly at one point on the retina, resulting in blurred vision. Also called *astigmia.* —**as′-tig·mat′ic** (ăs′tĭg-măt′ĭk) *adj. & n.*

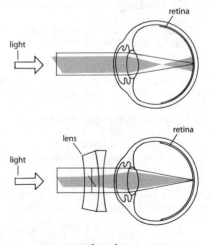

retina

light

lens

light

retina

astigmatism
Top: *astigmatic vision*
Bottom: *corrected vision*

a·stig·ma·tom·e·ter (ə-stĭg′mə-tŏm′ĭ-tər) *or* **as·tig·mom·e·ter** (ăs′tĭg-mŏm′ĭ-tər) *n.* An instrument for measuring the degree of and determining the variety of astigmatism. —**a·stig′ma·tom′e·try** (-trē), **as′tig·mom′e·try** *n.*

as·tig·mat·o·scope (ăs′tĭg-măt′ə-skōp′) *or* **a·stig·mo·scope** (ə-stĭg′mə-skōp′) *n.* An instrument for detecting and measuring the degree of astigmatism. —**a·stig·ma·tos′co·py** (-tŏs′kə-pē), **as′tig·mos′co·py** (-mŏs′kə-pē) *n.*

a·stig·mi·a (ə-stĭg′mē-ə) *n.* See **astigmatism.**

a·sto·mi·a (ə-stō′mē-ə) *n.* Congenital absence of a mouth.

A-strabismus *n.* **1.** Strabismus in which esotropia is more marked in looking upward than downward. **2.** Strabismus in which exotropia is more marked on looking downward than upward.

as·trag·a·lec·to·my (ə-străg′ə-lĕk′tə-mē) *n.* Surgical removal of the ankle bone.

as·trag·a·lus (ə-străg′ə-ləs) *n.* See **talus** (sense 1).

as·tral (ăs′trəl) *adj.* **1.** Of, relating to, emanating from, or resembling the stars. **2.** Of, relating to, or shaped like the mitotic aster; having the shape of an astrosphere; star-shaped.

as·tra·pho·bi·a (ăs′trə-fō′bē-ə) *n.* An abnormal fear of lightning and thunder.

as·tric·tion (ə-strĭk′shən) *n.* **1.** Astringent action. **2.** Compression to arrest hemorrhage.

as·trin·gent (ə-strĭn′jənt) *adj.* Causing the contraction of tissues, arrest of secretion, or control of bleeding. —*n.* A substance or preparation, such as alum, that draws together or constricts body tissues and is effective in stopping the flow of blood or other secretions. —**as·trin′gen·cy** *n.*

as·tro·blast (ăs′trə-blăst′) *n.* A primitive cell that develops into an astrocyte.

as·tro·blas·to·ma (ăs′trō-blă-stō′mə) *n.* A poorly differentiated tumor composed of astrocytes and arranged radially with short fibrils terminating on small blood vessels. Also called *grade II astrocytoma, grade III astrocytoma.*

as·tro·cyte (ăs′trə-sīt′) *n.* One of the large neuroglia cells of nervous tissue. Also called *astroglia, Deiters' cell, macroglia.*

as·tro·cy·to·ma (ăs′trō-sī-tō′mə) *n.*, *pl.* **-mas** *or* **-ma·ta** (-mə-tə) A malignant tumor of nervous tissue composed of well-differentiated astrocytes. Also called *grade I astrocytoma.*

as·trog·li·a (ăs-trŏg′lē-ə) *n.* See **astrocyte.**

as·tro·sphere (ăs′trō-sfîr′) *n.* A set of radiating fibrils extending outward from the centrosome and centrosphere of a dividing cell. Also called *aster, attraction sphere.*

a·sy·lum (ə-sī′ləm) *n.* An institution for the care of people, especially individuals with physical or mental impairments, who require organized supervision or assistance.

a·sym·bo·li·a (ā′sĭm-bō′lē-ə) *n.* **1.** A loss of the ability to comprehend by touch the form and nature of an object. **2.** A form of aphasia in which the significance of signs cannot be comprehended. Also called *asemasia.*

a·sym·met·ri·cal (ā′sĭ-mĕt′rĭ-kəl) *or* **a·sym·met·ric** (-rĭk) *adj. Abbr.* **a** Lacking symmetry between two or more like parts; not symmetrical.

a·sym·me·try (ā-sĭm′ĭ-trē) *n.* Disproportion between two or more like parts; lack of symmetry.

a·symp·to·mat·ic (ā′sĭmp-tə-măt′ĭk) *adj.* Exhibiting or producing no symptoms.

a·syn·cli·tism (ā-sĭn′klĭ-tĭz′əm, ə-sĭn′-) *n.* Absence of synclitism or parallelism between the axis of the presenting part of the fetus and the pelvic planes during childbirth. Also called *obliquity.*

a·syn·de·sis (ə-sĭn′dĭ-sĭs) *n.* A disorder in which separate ideas or thoughts cannot be joined into a coherent concept.

a·syn·ech·i·a (ā′sə-nĕk′ē-ə, ăs′ə-) *n.* A discontinuity of structure.

a·sy·ner·gia (ā′sə-nûr′jə) *or* **a·syn·er·gy** (ā-sĭn′ər-jē) *n.* The lack of cooperation or working together of parts that normally act in unison. —**a′sy·ner′gic** *adj.*

a·sys·tem·at·ic (ā-sĭs′tə-măt′ĭk) *or* **a·sys·tem·ic** (ā′sĭ-stĕm′ĭk) *adj.* Not specific to one system or set of organs; not systematic.

a·sys·to·le (ā-sĭs′tə-lē, ə-sĭs′-) *n.* The absence of contractions of the heart. —**a′sys·tol′ic** (ā′sĭ-stŏl′ĭk) *adj.*

At The symbol for the element **astatine.**

at– *pref.* Variant of **ad–** (sense 1).

At·a·brine (ăt′ə-brĭn, -brēn′) A trademark for the drug quinacrine hydrochloride.

At·a·cand (ăt′ə-kănd′) A trademark for the drug candesartan cilexetil.

At·a·rax (ăt′ə-răks′) A trademark for the hydrochloride salt of the drug hydroxyzine.

at·a·vism (ăt′ə-vĭz′əm) *n.* The appearance of characteristics that are presumed to have been present in some remote ancestor; reversion to an earlier biological type. —**at′a·vist** *n.* —**at′a·vis′tic** *adj.*

a·tax·i·a (ə-tăk′sē-ə) *or* **a·tax·y** (ə-tăk′sē) *n.* Loss of the ability to coordinate muscular movement. Also called *dyssynergia, incoordination.*

a·tax·i·a·pha·sia (ə-tăk′sē-ə-fā′zhə) *n.* Inability to form connected sentences.

ataxia telangiectasia *n.* A disease characterized by progressive ataxia due to disease in the cerebellum, oculocutaneous telangiectases, proneness to pulmonary infections, and immunodeficiency.

a·tax·ic (ə-tăk′sĭk) *or* **a·tac·tic** (ə-tăk′tĭk) *adj.* Of, relating to, or characterized by ataxia.

ataxic abasia *or* **atactic abasia** *n.* Abasia due to ataxia of the legs.

ataxic aphasia *n.* See **motor aphasia.**

ataxic gait *n.* An unsteady, staggering, or irregular gait.

a·tax·i·o·phe·mi·a (ə-tăk′sē-ō-fē′mē-ə) *n.* Incoordination of the speech muscles.

–ate *suff.* **1.** A derivative of a specified chemical compound or element: *aluminate.* **2.** A salt or ester of a specified acid whose name ends in *-ic: acetate.*

at·e·lec·ta·sis (ăt′l-ĕk′tə-sĭs) *n.* **1.** The absence of gas from all or a part of the lungs, due to failure of expansion or resorption of gas from the alveoli. **2.** A congenital condition characterized by the incomplete expansion of the lungs at birth. —**at′e·lec·tat′ic** (-ĕk-tăt′ĭk) *adj.*

a·te·li·o·sis (ə-tē′lē-ō′sĭs, ə-tĕl′ē-) *n.* Incomplete development of the body or any of its parts, as in infantilism and dwarfism. Also called *atelia.* —**a·te′li·ot′ic** (-ŏt′ĭk) *adj.*

ateliotic dwarf *n.* A normally proportioned individual of unusually short stature.

atelo– *or* **atel–** *pref.* Incomplete; imperfect: *atelectasis.*

a·ten·o·lol (ə-tĕn′ə-lôl′, -lŏl′) *n.* A beta-blocking agent used primarily in the treatment of angina pectoris and hypertension.

a·the·li·a (ə-thē′lē-ə) *n.* The congenital absence of the nipples.

athero– *pref.* Soft gruel-like deposit; atheroma: *atherogenesis.*

ath·er·o·em·bo·lism (ăth′ə-rō-ĕm′bə-lĭz′əm) *n.* See **cholesterol embolism.**

ath·er·o·gen·e·sis (ăth′ə-rō-jĕn′ĭ-sĭs) *n.* Formation of atheromatous deposits, especially on the innermost layer of arterial walls.

ath·er·o·gen·ic (ăth′ə-rō-jĕn′ĭk) *adj.* Initiating, increasing, or accelerating atherogenesis.

ath·er·o·ma (ăth′ə-rō′mə) *n., pl.* **–mas** *or* **–ma·ta** (-mə-tə) A deposit or degenerative accumulation of lipid-containing plaques on the innermost layer of the wall of an artery. —**ath′er·o·ma·to′sis** (-tō′sĭs) *n.* —**ath′er·om·a′tous** (-rŏm′ə-təs, -rō′mə-) *adj.*

atheromatous degeneration *n.* The accumulation of lipid deposits on the inner surface of the arteries, eventually resulting in fibrous thickening or calcification of the arteries.

ath·er·o·scle·ro·sis (ăth′ə-rō-sklə-rō′sĭs) *n.* A form of arteriosclerosis characterized by the deposition of atheromatous plaques containing cholesterol and lipids on the innermost layer of the walls of large and medium-sized arteries. —**ath′er·o·scle·rot′ic** (-rŏt′ĭk) *adj.*

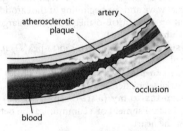

atherosclerosis

ath·e·to·sis (ăth′ĭ-tō′sĭs) *n.* A constant succession of slow, writhing, involuntary movements of flexion, extension, pronation, and supination of fingers and hands, and sometimes of toes and feet. —**ath′e·toid′ ath′e·to′sic, ath′e·tot′ic** (-tŏt′ĭk) *adj.*

ath·lete's foot (ăth′lēts) *n.* A contagious fungal skin infection caused by a species of *Trichophyton* or *Epidermophyton* that usually affects the feet, especially the skin between the toes, and is characterized by itching, blisters, cracking, and scaling; ringworm of the foot. Also called *tinea pedis.*

ath·let·ic heart (ăth-lĕt′ĭk) *n.* Enlargement of the heart observed in some athletes.

a·threp·si·a (ə-thrĕp′sē-ə) *or* **ath·rep·sy** (ăth′rəp-sē) *n.* See **marasmus.** —**a·threp′tic** (-tĭk) *adj.*

a·thy·mi·a (ə-thī′mē-ə) *n.* **1.** The absence of emotion; morbid impassivity. **2.** The absence of the thymus

gland or the suppression of its secretion. Also called *athymism.*

a·thy·mism (ə-thī′mĭz′əm) *n.* See **athymia** (sense 2).

a·thy·roid·ism (ā-thī′roi-dĭz′əm, ə-thī′-) *or* **a·thy·re·a** (ā-thī′rē-ə, ə-thī′-) *or* **a·thy·ro·sis** (ā′thī-rō′sĭs, ăth′ī-) *n.* The absence of the thyroid gland or the suppression of its secretion. —**a′thy·rot′ic** (ā′thī-rŏt′ĭk, ăth′ī-) *adj.*

At·i·van (ăt′ə-văn′) A trademark for the drug lorazepam.

ATL *abbr.* adult T-cell lymphoma

at·lan·tad (ăt-lăn′tăd′, ət-) *adv.* Toward the atlas.

at·lan·tal (ăt-lăn′təl, ət-) *adj.* Characteristic of or relating to the atlas.

atlanto– *pref.* Atlas: *atlantoaxial.*

at·lan·to·ax·i·al (ăt-lăn′tō-ăk′sē-əl) *adj.* Relating to the atlas and the axis or to the joint between the two vertebrae.

at·lan·to·oc·cip·i·tal membrane (ăt-lăn′tō-ŏk-sĭp′ĭ-tl) *n.* **1.** The fibrous layer extending from the anterior arch of the atlas to the anterior margin of the great foramen. **2.** The fibrous membrane that attaches between the posterior arch of the atlas and the posterior margin of the great foramen.

at·las (ăt′ləs) *n.* The top or first cervical vertebra of the neck, supporting the skull and articulating with the occipital bone and rotating around the dens of the axis.

atlo– *pref.* Atlas: *atloaxoid.*

at·lo·ax·oid (ăt′lō-ăk′soid′) *adj.* Atlantoaxial.

atm *or* **atm.** *abbr.* atmosphere

atmo– *pref.* Steam; vapor: *atmosphere.*

at·mos·phere (ăt′mə-sfîr′) *n.* **1.** A gas surrounding a given body; a gaseous medium. **2.** *Abbr.* **atm, atm.** A unit of pressure equal to the air pressure at sea level, approximately equal to 1.01325×10^5 newtons per square meter.

at. no. *or* **at no** *abbr.* atomic number

at·om (ăt′əm) *n.* **1.** A unit of matter, the smallest unit of an element, having all the characteristics of that element and consisting of a dense, central, positively charged nucleus surrounded by a system of electrons. The entire structure has an approximate diameter of 10^{-8} centimeter and characteristically remains undivided in chemical reactions except for limited removal, transfer, or exchange of certain electrons. **2.** This unit regarded as a source of nuclear energy. **3.** A part or particle considered to be an irreducible constituent of a specified system. **4.** The irreducible, indestructible material unit postulated by ancient atomism. **5.** An extremely small part, quantity, or amount. —**a·tom′ic** (ə-tŏm′ĭk) *adj.*

atomic mass *n.* The mass of an atom, usually expressed in atomic mass units.

atomic mass unit *n. Abbr.* **amu** A unit of mass equal to $\frac{1}{12}$ the mass of an atom of carbon 12, which is assigned a mass of 12. Also called *dalton.*

atomic number *n. Abbr.* **at. no., at no** The number of protons in an atomic nucleus; it indicates the position of an element in the periodic table.

atomic weight *n. Abbr.* **at wt, AW** The average mass of an atom of an element, usually expressed relative to the atomic mass of carbon 12.

at·om·iz·er (ăt′ə-mī′zər) *n.* A device used to reduce liquid medication to a fine spray or aerosol.

a·ton·ic (ā-tŏn′ĭk) *adj.* Relating to, caused by, or exhibiting lack of muscle tone. —**at′o·nic′i·ty** (ăt′ə-nĭs′ĭ-tē, ăt′n-ĭs′-) *n.*

atonic bladder *n.* A large dilated urinary bladder that does not empty, usually due to disturbance of innervation or to chronic obstruction.

at·o·ny (ăt′ə-nē, ăt′n-ē) *or* **a·to·ni·a** (ā-tō′nē-ə) *n.* Lack of normal tone or tension; flaccidity.

at·o·pen (ăt′ə-pən, -pĕn′) *n.* An agent that causes an atopic reaction.

atopic allergy *n.* See **atopy**.

atopic cataract *n.* A cataract associated with atopic dermatitis.

atopic conjunctivitis *n.* See **allergic conjunctivitis**.

atopic dermatitis *n.* Dermatitis characterized by intense itching, occurring in individuals predisposed to developing certain hypersensitivity reactions.

atopic keratoconjunctivitis *n.* Inflammation of the cornea and conjunctiva occurring as a consequence of atopic eczema.

a·top·og·no·si·a (ā-tŏp′ŏg-nō′zē-ə, -zhə, ə-tŏp′-) *or* **a·top·og·no·sis** (-nō′sĭs) *n.* The inability to discern the origin of a sensation.

at·o·py (ăt′ə-pē) *n.* A hereditary disorder marked by the tendency to develop immediate allergic reactions to substances such as pollen, food, dander, and insect venoms and manifested by hay fever, asthma, or similar allergic conditions. Also called *atopic allergy.* —**a·top′ic** (ā-tŏp′ĭk) *adj.*

a·tor·va·stat·in calcium (ə-tôr′və-stăt′n) *n.* A statin drug used to treat hyperlipidemia.

a·tox·ic (ā-tŏk′sĭk) *n.* Not toxic.

ATP (ā′tē′pē′) *n.* Adenosine triphosphate; an adenosine-derived nucleotide that supplies large amounts of energy to cells for various biochemical processes, including muscle contraction and sugar metabolism, through its hydrolysis to ADP.

ATP·ase (ā′tē-pē′ās, -āz) *n.* Adenosine triphosphatase; an enzyme that catalyzes the hydrolysis of ATP.

at·ra·cu·ri·um be·syl·ate (ăt′rə-kyoor′ē-əm bĕs′ə-lāt′) *n.* A nondepolarizing neuromuscular relaxant used as an adjunct to general anesthesia.

a·trau·mat·ic suture (ā′trô-măt′ĭk, -trou-, -trə-) *n.* A suture affixed to the end of a small eyeless needle.

a·tre·sia (ə-trē′zhə, -zhē-ə) *n.* **1.** The congenital absence or closure of a normal body orifice or tubular passage such as the anus, intestine, or external ear canal. **2.** The degeneration and resorption of one or more ovarian follicles before maturation.

a·tret·ic (ə-trĕt′ĭk) *or* **a·tre·sic** (ə-trē′zĭk) *adj.* Relating to atresia.

a·tri·al (ā′trē-əl) *adj.* Of or relating to an atrium.

atrial artery *n.* Any of the branches of the right and left coronary arteries distributed to the muscle of the atria.

atrial auricle *n.* A small conical pouch projecting from the upper anterior portion of each atrium of the heart. Also called *auricula atrii, auricular appendage, auricular appendix.*

atrial chaotic tachycardia *n.* Tachycardia originating

from several foci within the atrium, often confused with atrial fibrillation.

atrial complex *n.* The P wave in an electrocardiogram.

atrial conduction *n.* See **intra-atrial conduction**.

atrial dissociation *n.* Independent beating of the two atria or of parts of the atria.

atrial extrasystole *n.* A premature contraction of the heart arising from an ectopic atrial focus.

atrial fibrillation *n. Abbr.* **AF** Fibrillation in which the normal rhythmical contractions of the cardiac atria are replaced by rapid irregular twitchings of the muscular wall that cause the ventricles to respond irregularly. Also called *a-fib, auricular fibrillation.*

atrial flutter *n.* Rapid regular atrial contractions occurring usually at rates between 250 and 400 per minute and often producing saw-tooth waves in an electrocardiogram. Also called *auricular flutter.*

atrial fusion beat *n.* A pulsation occurring when the atria of the heart are activated partly by a sinus impulse and partly by a retrograde impulse from the atrioventricular node or ventricle.

atrial natriuretic factor *n.* A peptide hormone released from cardiac atrial tissue that causes increased elimination of sodium by the kidney.

atrial septal defect *n. Abbr.* **ASD** A defect in the interatrial septum of the heart, due to failure of the embryonic foramen to close normally.

a·trich·i·a (ā-trĭk′ē-ə, ə-trĭk′-) *n.* The congenital or acquired absence of hair. Also called *atrichosis.*

at·ri·chous (ăt′rĭ-kəs) *adj.* Having no hair.

atrio– *pref.* Atrium: *atrioventricular.*

a·tri·o·ca·rot·id interval (ā′trē-ō-kə-rŏt′ĭd) *n.* In a venous pulse tracing, the time between the beginning of the atrial wave and the beginning of the carotid wave.

a·tri·o·meg·a·ly (ā′trē-ō-mĕg′ə-lē) *n.* Enlargement of the atrium of the heart.

a·tri·o·sep·to·pex·y (ā′trē-ō-sĕp′tə-pĕk′sē) *n.* Surgical repair of an atrial septal defect.

a·tri·o·sep·to·plas·ty (ā′trē-ō-sĕp′tə-plăs′tē) *n.* Repair of an atrial septal defect by plastic surgery.

a·tri·o·sep·tos·to·my (ā′trē-ō-sĕp-tŏs′tə-mē) *n.* The surgical establishment of a communication between the atria of the heart.

a·tri·o·ven·tric·u·lar (ā′trē-ō-vĕn-trĭk′yə-lər) *adj. Abbr.* **A-V** Of or relating to the atria and the ventricles of the heart.

atrioventricular block *n.* Impairment of the normal conduction of impulses between the atria and the ventricles.

atrioventricular bundle *n.* See **bundle of His**.

atrioventricular canal *n.* The canal in the embryonic heart joining the atrium to the ventricle.

atrioventricular canal cushion *n.* Either of a pair of mounds of embryonic connective tissue covered by endothelium, bulging dorsally and ventrally into the embryonic atrioventricular canal, eventually growing together and dividing the canal into right and left atria. Also called *endocardial cushion.*

atrioventricular conduction *n.* Forward conduction of the cardiac impulse from the atria to ventricles via the atrioventricular node, represented in an electrocardiogram by the P-R interval.

atrioventricular dissociation *n.* A condition in which the atria and ventricles contract independently, especially as resulting from the slowing of an atrial pacemaker or the acceleration of a ventricular pacemaker.

atrioventricular extrasystole *n.* A premature contraction of the heart in which the stimulus arises from either the A-V node or A-V bundle. Also called *A-V extrasystole.*

atrioventricular groove *n.* See **coronary sulcus.**

atrioventricular interval *n.* The time from the beginning of atrial systole to the beginning of ventricular systole as measured on an electrocardiogram.

atrioventricular nodal extrasystole *n.* A premature beat arising from the A-V node and leading to a simultaneous or almost simultaneous contraction of atria and ventricles. Also called *A-V nodal extrasystole, nodal extrasystole.*

atrioventricular nodal rhythm *n.* The cardiac rhythm that results when the heart is controlled by the atrioventricular node in which the impulse arises in the atrioventricular node, ascends to the atria, and descends to the ventricles more or less simultaneously. Also called *A-V nodal rhythm, nodal bradycardia, nodal rhythm.*

atrioventricular node *n.* A small mass of specialized cardiac muscle fibers, located near the ostium of the coronary sinus and giving rise to the atrioventricular bundle of the conduction system of the heart. Also called *A-V node.*

atrioventricular septum *n.* The small part of the membranous septum of the heart just above the septal cusp of the tricuspid valve, separating the right atrium from the left ventricle.

a·tri·um (ā′trē-əm) *n.,* *pl.* **–ums** or **a·tri·a** (ā′trē-ə) **1.** A chamber or cavity to which several chambers or passageways are connected. **2.** Either the right or the left upper chamber of the heart that receives blood from the veins and forces it into a ventricle. **3.** That part of the tympanic cavity that lies below the eardrum. **4.** A subdivision of the alveolar duct in the lung from which the alveolar sacs open.

a·troph·e·de·ma (ə-trŏf′ĭ-dē′mə) *n.* See **angioneurotic edema.**

a·tro·phi·a (ə-trō′fē-ə) *n.* See **atrophy.**

atrophic arthritis *n.* Arthritis, usually rheumatoid arthritis, occurring without formation of new bone.

atrophic excavation *n.* An exaggeration of the normal or physiological cupping of the optic disk caused by atrophy of the optic nerve.

atrophic gastritis *n.* Chronic gastritis with atrophy of the mucous membrane and destruction of the peptic glands.

atrophic rhinitis *n.* Chronic rhinitis with thinning of the mucous membrane, often associated with crust formation and foul-smelling discharge.

atrophic vaginitis *n.* Thinning and atrophy of the vaginal epithelium usually resulting from diminished endocrine stimulation and seen most commonly in postmenopausal women.

at·ro·phied (ăt′rə-fēd) *adj.* Characterized by atrophy.

at·ro·pho·der·ma (ăt′rə-fō-dûr′mə) *n.* Atrophy of the skin occurring in localized or widespread areas.

at·ro·pho·der·ma·to·sis (ăt′rə-fō-dûr′mə-tō′sĭs) *n.* A cutaneous disorder characterized by skin atrophy.

at·ro·phy (ăt′rə-fē) *n.* A wasting or decrease in the size of an organ or tissue, as from death and reabsorption of cells, diminished cellular proliferation, pressure, ischemia, malnutrition, decreased function, or hormonal changes. Also called *atrophia.* —*v.* To undergo atrophy. —**a·troph·ic** (ā-trŏf′ĭk) *adj.*

at·ro·pine (ăt′rə-pēn′, -pĭn) or **at·ro·pin** (-pĭn) *n.* An alkaloid obtained from belladonna and related plants, used to dilate the pupils of the eyes and as an antispasmodic, antisudorific, and anticholinergic.

At·ro·vent (ăt′rə-věnt′) A trademark for the drug ipratropium bromide.

at·tached gingiva (ə-tăcht′) *n.* The portion of the oral mucous membrane bound to the tooth and to the alveolar arches of the jaw.

at·tach·ment disorder (ə-tăch′mənt) *n.* A behavioral disorder caused by the lack of an emotionally secure attachment to a caregiver in the first two years of life, characterized by an inability to form healthy relationships. Other common symptoms, especially in children, are poor impulse control, chronic anger, and antisocial tendencies.

at·tack (ə-tăk′) *n.* An episode or onset of a disease, often sudden in nature. —**at·tack′** *v.*

attack rate *n.* A cumulative incidence rate used for particular groups observed for limited periods under special circumstances, such as during an epidemic.

at·tend·ing physician (ə-těn′dĭng) *n.* A physician who, as a member of a hospital staff, admits and treats patients and may supervise or teach house staff, fellows, and students.

at·ten·tion deficit disorder (ə-těn′shən) *n. Abbr.* **ADD** A syndrome, usually diagnosed in childhood, characterized by a persistent pattern of impulsiveness, a short attention span, and sometimes hyperactivity, and interfering especially with academic, occupational, and social performance.

attention deficit hyperactivity disorder *n. Abbr.* **ADHD** Attention deficit disorder in which hyperactivity is present.

at·ten·u·ate (ə-těn′yoō-āt′) *v.* **1.** To reduce in force, value, amount, or degree; weaken; diminish. **2.** To make bacteria or viruses less virulent. —*adj.* Reduced or weakened, as in strength, value, or virulence.

at·ten·u·at·ed virus (ə-těn′yoō-ā′tĭd) *n.* A strain of a virus whose pathogenicity has been reduced so that it will initiate the immune response without producing the specific disease. Attenuated viruses are used in some vaccines.

at·ten·u·a·tion (ə-těn′yoō-ā′shən) *n.* **1.** A dilution, thinning, or weakening of a substance, especially a reduction in the virulence of a pathogen through repeated inoculation, growth in a different culture medium, or exposure to heat, light, air, or other weakening agents. **2.** The energy loss of an ultrasonic beam as it passes through a material.

at·tic (ăt′ĭk) *n.* The upper portion of the tympanic cavity above the tympanic membrane that contains the head of the malleus and the body of the incus. Also called *epitympanum.*

at·ti·cot·o·my (ăt′ĭ-kŏt′ə-mē) *n*. Incision into the tympanic attic.

at·ti·tude (ăt′ĭ-tōōd′) *n*. **1.** The position of the body and limbs; posture. **2.** A manner of acting. **3.** A relatively stable and enduring predisposition to behave or react in a characteristic way.

atto– *pref*. One quintillionth (10^{-18}): *attometer.*

at·trac·tion (ə-trăk′shən) *n*. A force acting mutually between particles of matter to draw them together and to resist their separation.

attraction sphere *n*. See **astrosphere.**

at·tri·tion (ə-trĭsh′ən) *n*. A wearing away by friction or rubbing, such as the loss of tooth structure caused by abrasive foods or grinding of the teeth.

at wt *abbr*. atomic weight

a·typ·i·cal (ā-tĭp′ĭ-kəl) *adj*. Not corresponding to the normal form or type; not typical. —**a·typ′i·cal·ly** *adv*.

atypical lipoma *n*. A benign lipoma occurring primarily in older men on the posterior neck, shoulders, and back, and containing multinucleated giant cells. Also called *pleomorphic lipoma.*

atypical measles *n*. A severe form of measles caused by natural infection with the measles virus in persons whose immunity by vaccination is diminished; it is characterized by high fever, atypical rash, and pneumonia.

atypical pneumonia *n*. See **primary atypical pneumonia.**

atypical verrucous endocarditis *n*. See **Libman-Sacks endocarditis.**

Au The symbol for the element **gold.**

AU *abbr*. *Latin* auris utraque (each ear)

au·dile (ô′dĭl′) *adj*. Relating to hearing; auditory.

audio– *pref*. **1.** Hearing: *audiology.* **2.** Sound: *audiogenic.*

au·di·o·an·al·ge·si·a (ô′dē-ō-ăn′əl-jē′zē-ə, -zhə) *n*. A deadening of pain produced by listening to a sound or sounds.

au·di·o·gen·ic (ô′dē-ō-jěn′ĭk) *adj*. Caused by sound, especially a loud sound.

audiogenic epilepsy *n*. A form of reflex epilepsy induced by sound, usually a sudden loud noise.

au·di·o·gram (ô′dē-ə-grăm′) *n*. A graphic record of hearing ability for various sound frequencies.

au·di·ol·o·gy (ô′dē-ŏl′ə-jē) *n*. The study of hearing disorders and the rehabilitation of people with hearing impairments. —**au′di·ol′o·gist** *n*.

au·di·om·e·ter (ô′dē-ŏm′ĭ-tər) *n*. An electrical instrument for measuring the threshold of hearing for pure tones of normally audible frequencies generally varying from 200 to 8000 hertz and recorded in decibels. —**au′di·o·met′ric** (-ō-mět′rĭk) *adj*. —**au′di·o·me·tri′cian** (-ō-mə-trĭsh′ən) *n*. —**au′di·om′e·try** *n*.

au·di·o·vis·u·al or **au·di·o·vis·u·al** (ô′dē-ō-vĭzh′ōō-əl) *adj*. **1.** Both audible and visible. **2.** Of or relating to materials, such as films and videotapes, that present information in audible and pictorial form.

au·di·tion (ô-dĭsh′ən) *n*. The sense, ability, or power of hearing.

au·di·to·ry (ô′dĭ-tôr′ē) *adj*. Of or relating to hearing, the organs of hearing, or the sense of hearing.

auditory aphasia *n*. Impairment of the ability to comprehend spoken language even though hearing is normal. Also called *acoustic aphasia.*

auditory area *n*. See **auditory cortex.**

auditory brainstem response audiometry *n*. *Abbr*. **ABR audiometry** An electronic measure of auditory function using responses produced by the auditory nerve and the brainstem. Also called *brainstem evoked response audiometry.*

auditory canal *n*. Either of two passages of the ear, the internal or the external acoustic meatus. See under *acoustic meatus.*

auditory cartilage *n*. The embryonic tissue that surrounds the developing auditory vesicle. Also called *auditory capsule.*

auditory cortex *n*. The region of the cerebral cortex that receives auditory data from the medial geniculate body. Also called *auditory area.*

auditory field *n*. The space or range within which a specified sound can be heard.

auditory hair *n*. Any of the cilia on the free surface of the auditory cells.

auditory nerve *n*. See **cochlear nerve.**

auditory pit *n*. One of a pair of depressions, one on either side of the head of an embryo, marking the location of the future auditory vesicles.

auditory receptor cell *n*. A columnar cell in the epithelium of the organ of Corti having hairs. Also called *Corti's cell.*

auditory reflex *n*. A reflex in response to a sound.

auditory tube *n*. See **eustachian tube.**

auditory vertigo *n*. See **Ménière's disease.**

auditory vesicle *n*. Either of the paired sacs of invaginated ectoderm in the embryo that develop into the membranous labyrinth of the internal ear. Also called *otic vesicle.*

Au·en·brug·ger (ou′ən-brŏŏg′ər), **Leopold** 1722–1809. Austrian physician who in 1761 developed the technique of using percussion to diagnose diseases of the thorax and lungs.

Au·er body (ou′ər) *n*. A rod-shaped structure of uncertain nature in the cytoplasm of immature myeloid cells, especially myeloblasts, in cases of acute myelocytic leukemia. Also called *Auer rod.*

aug·men·ta·tion mammaplasty (ôg′měn-tā′shən) *n*. Plastic surgery to enlarge the breast, often by insertion of an implant.

Aug·men·tin (ôg-měn′tĭn) A trademark for a preparation of amoxicillin and clavulanic acid.

au·ra (ôr′ə) *n.*, *pl*. **–ras** or **au·rae** (ôr′ē) A sensation, as of a cold breeze or a bright light, that precedes the onset of certain disorders, such as an epileptic seizure or an attack of migraine.

au·ral¹ (ôr′əl) *adj*. Relating to or perceived by the ear.

au·ral² (ôr′əl) *adj*. Characterized by or relating to an aura.

au·ran·o·fin (ô-răn′ə-fĭn) *n*. A compound of radiogold colloid used to treat rheumatoid arthritis.

au·ran·ti·a·sis cu·tis (ôr′ăn-tī′ə-sĭs kyōō′tĭs) *n*. See **carotenosis cutis.**

auri– *pref*. Ear: *auriscope.*

au·ric (ôr′ĭk) *adj*. Of, relating to, derived from, or containing gold, especially with valence 3.

au·ri·cle (ôr′ĭ-kəl) *n*. **1**. Atrial auricle. **2**. The projecting shell-like structure on the side of the head constituting, with the external acoustic meatus, the external ear. Also called *pinna*.

auricle a·tri·a·lis (ā′trē-ā′lĭs) *n*. Atrial auricle.

au·ric·u·la (ô-rĭk′yə-lə) *n*., *pl*. **-lae** (-lē′) Auricle.

auricula a·tri·i (ā′trē-ī′) *n*. See **atrial auricle**.

au·ric·u·lar (ô-rĭk′yə-lər) *adj*. **1**. Of or relating to the sense of hearing or the organs of hearing. **2**. Perceived by or spoken into the ear, as when testing hearing. **3**. Shaped like an ear or an earlobe; having earlike parts or extensions. **4**. Of or relating to an auricle of the heart.

auricular appendage *n*. See **atrial auricle**.

auricular appendix *n*. See **atrial auricle**.

auricular artery *n*. **1**. An artery with origin in the external carotid artery, with muscular, posterior tympanic, auricular, occipital, and stylomastoid branches; posterior auricular artery. **2**. An artery with origin in the maxillary artery, with distribution to the articulation of the jaw, parotid gland, and external acoustic meatus, and with anastomoses to the branches of the superficial temporal and the posterior auricular arteries; deep auricular artery.

auricular cartilage *n*. The cartilage of the auricle of the ear.

auricular fibrillation *n*. See **atrial fibrillation**.

auricular fissure *n*. See **tympanomastoid fissure**.

auricular flutter *n*. See **atrial flutter**.

auricular muscle *n*. **1**. A muscle with origin in the galea, with insertion to the auricular cartilage, with nerve supply from the facial nerve, and whose action draws the pinna of the ear upward and forward; anterior auricular muscle. **2**. A muscle with origin in the mastoid process, with insertion to the root of the auricle, with nerve supply from the facial nerve, and whose action draws back the pinna; posterior auricular muscle. **3**. A muscle with origin in the galea, with insertion to the auricular cartilage, with nerve supply from the facial nerve, and whose action draws the pinna of the ear upward and backward; superior auricular muscle.

auricular point *n*. A craniometric point usually located at the center of the opening of the external acoustic meatus.

auricular tubercle *n*. See **Darwinian tubercle**.

au·ric·u·lo·tem·po·ral (ô-rĭk′yə-lō-tĕm′pər-əl, -tĕm′-prəl) *adj*. Of or relating to the auricle of the ear and the temple.

auriculotemporal nerve *n*. A branch of the mandibular nerve that passes through the parotid gland, terminates in the skin of the temple and the scalp, sends branches to the external acoustic meatus, tympanic membrane, parotid gland, and auricle, and also sends a communicating branch to the facial nerve.

au·ris (ôr′ĭs) *n*. Ear.

au·ri·scope (ôr′ĭ-skōp′) *n*. See **otoscope**.

au·rum (ôr′əm) *n*. Gold.

aus·cul·tate (ô′skəl-tāt′) *or* **aus·cult** (ô′skəlt) *v*. To examine by auscultation. —**aus′cul·ta·tive** *adj*. —**aus·cul′ta·to·ry** (ô-skŭl′tə-tôr′ē) *adj*.

aus·cul·ta·tion (ô′skəl-tā′shən) *n*. The act of listening for sounds made by internal organs, such as the heart and lungs, to aid in the diagnosis of certain disorders.

auscultatory alternans *n*. Alternation in the intensity of heart sounds or murmurs in the presence of regular cardiac rhythm.

auscultatory gap *n*. In measuring blood pressure by the auscultatory method, the period during which sounds indicating true systolic pressure fade away and reappear at a lower pressure point.

auscultatory percussion *n*. Auscultation performed at the same time that percussion is made.

Aus·tin Flint murmur (ô′stən flĭnt′) *n*. See **Flint's murmur**.

Aus·tra·lia antigen (ô-strāl′yə) *n*. See **hepatitis B surface antigen**.

au·ta·coid *or* **au·to·coid** (ô′tə-koid′) *n*. An organic substance, such as a hormone, produced in one part of an organism and transported by the blood or lymph to another part of the organism where it exerts a physiologic effect on that part.

au·te·cic (ô-tē′sĭk) *or* **au·te·cious** (-shəs) *adj*. Relating to or being a parasite that infects the same host throughout its entire lifecycle.

au·thor·i·tar·i·an personality (ə-thôr′ĭ-târ′ē-ən) *n*. A personality pattern reflecting a desire for security, order, power, and status, with a desire for structured lines of authority, a conventional set of values or outlook, a demand for unquestioning obedience, and a tendency to be hostile toward or use as scapegoats individuals of minority or nontraditional groups.

au·thor·i·ty figure (ə-thôr′ĭ-tē) *n*. A real or projected person in a position of power.

au·tism (ô′tĭz′əm) *n*. A pervasive developmental disorder characterized by severe deficits in social interaction and communication, by an extremely limited range of activities and interests, and often by the presence of repetitive, stereotyped behaviors. It is evident in the first years of life and is usually associated with some degree of mental retardation. Also called *infantile autism*, *Kanner's syndrome*. —**au·tis′tic** (ô-tĭs′tĭk) *adj*.

auto– *or* **aut–** *pref*. Self; same: *autogamy*.

au·to·ag·glu·ti·na·tion (ô′tō-ə-glōōt′n-ā′shən) *n*. **1**. The nonspecific agglutination or clumping together of cells (bacteria or erythrocytes, for example) as the result of physical-chemical factors. **2**. The agglutination of a person's red blood cells in his or her own serum as a consequence of a specific autoantibody.

au·to·ag·glu·ti·nin (ô′tō-ə-glōōt′n-ĭn) *n*. An agglutinating autoantibody.

autoallergic hemolytic anemia *n*. See **autoimmune hemolytic anemia**.

au·to·al·ler·gy (ô′tō-ăl′ər-jē) *n*. An altered reactivity in which autoantibodies are produced against one's own tissues, causing a destructive rather than a protective effect. —**au′to·al·ler′gic** (ə-lûr′jĭk) *adj*.

au·to·an·ti·bod·y (ô′tō-ăn′tĭ-bŏd′ē) *n*. An antibody that attacks the cells, tissues, or native proteins of the organism in which it was formed.

au·to·an·ti·gen (ô′tō-ăn′tĭ-jən) *n*. An endogenous antigen that stimulates the production of autoantibodies.

au·to·ca·tal·y·sis (ô′tō-kə-tăl′ĭ-sĭs) *n*. Catalysis of a chemical reaction by one of the products of the reaction. —**au′to·cat′a·lyt′ic** (-kăt′l-ĭt′ĭk) *adj*.

au·toch·tho·nous (ô-tŏk′thə-nəs) *adj.* **1.** Native to the place inhabited; indigenous. **2.** Originating in the place where found. Used of a disease originating in the part of the body where found, or of a disease acquired in the place where the patient is.

autochthonous idea *n.* A thought that suddenly bursts into the consciousness and is often believed to have come from an outside source.

au·toc·la·sis (ô-tŏk′lə-sĭs) *or* **au·to·cla·sia** (ô′tō-klā′-zhə) *n.* **1.** A breaking up or rupturing from intrinsic or internal causes. **2.** Progressive, immunologically induced tissue destruction.

au·to·clave (ô′tō-klāv′) *n.* A pressurized, steam-heated vessel used for sterilization. —*v.* To treat in an autoclave.

au·to·coid (ô′tə-koid′) *n.* Variant of **autacoid**.

au·to·crine (ô′tə-krĭn, -krēn′) *adj.* Of or relating to self-stimulation through cellular production of a factor and a specific receptor for it.

autocrine hypothesis *n.* The hypothesis that tumor cells containing viral oncogenes may have encoded a growth factor normally produced by other cell types and thereby produce the factor autonomously, leading to uncontrolled proliferation.

au·to·cy·tol·y·sin (ô′tō-sī-tŏl′ĭ-sĭn) *n.* See **autolysin**.

au·to·cy·tol·y·sis (ô′tō-sī-tŏl′ĭ-sĭs) *n.* See **autolysis** (sense 2).

au·to·cy·to·tox·in (ô′tō-sī′tə-tŏk′sĭn) *n.* A cytotoxic autoantibody.

au·to·der·mic graft (ô′tō-dûr′mĭk) *n.* A skin graft taken from the body receiving it.

au·to·di·ges·tion (ô′tō-dī-jĕs′chən, -dĭ-) *n.* See **autolysis** (sense 1).

au·to·ech·o·la·li·a (ô′tō-ĕk′ō-lā′lē-ə) *n.* The repetition of some or all words in one's statements.

autoerotic asphyxia *n.* A form of sexual masochism in which oxygen flow to the brain is reduced, as by controlled strangulation or suffocation, in order to enhance the pleasure of masturbation.

au·to·er·o·tism (ô′tō-ĕr′ə-tĭz′əm) *or* **au·to·e·rot·i·cism** (-ĭ-rŏt′ĭ-sĭz′əm) *n.* **1.** Self-satisfaction of sexual desire, as by masturbation. **2.** The arousal of sexual feeling without an external stimulus. —**au′to·e·rot′ic** (-ĭ-rŏt′-ĭk) *adj.*

au·to·e·ryth·ro·cyte sensitization syndrome (ô′tō-ĭ-rĭth′rə-sīt′) *n.* A condition, usually occurring in women, in which bruising occurs easily, with the resulting ecchymoses tending to enlarge and involve adjacent tissues, causing pain in the affected parts; it may be a form of autosensitization or may be due to psychogenic causes. Also called *autoerythrocyte sensitization, Gardner-Diamond syndrome, psychogenic purpura*.

au·tog·a·my (ô-tŏg′ə-mē) *n.* Self-fertilization in which fission of the cell nucleus occurs without complete cellular division, forming two pronuclei that reunite to form the synkaryon. —**au·tog′a·mous** *adj.*

au·to·gen·e·sis (ô′tō-jĕn′ĭ-sĭs) *n.* **1.** The supposed development of living organisms from nonliving matter. **2.** The process by which a vaccine is made from bacteria obtained from the patient's own body. —**au′to·ge·net′ic** (-jə-nĕt′ĭk) *adj.* —**au′to·ge·net′i·cal·ly** *adv.*

au·tog·e·nous (ô-tŏj′ə-nəs) *or* **au·to·gen·ic** (ô′tə-jĕn′-ĭk) *adj.* **1.** Of or relating to autogenesis; self-generating. **2.** Of or relating to vaccines prepared from bacteria obtained from the infected person. —**au·tog′e·nous·ly** *adv.*

autogenous vaccine *n.* A vaccine made from a culture of bacteria taken from the person to be vaccinated.

au·to·graft (ô′tō-grăft′) *n.* A tissue or an organ grafted into a new position in or on the body of the same individual. Also called *autologous graft, autotransplant*.

au·to·hem·ag·glu·ti·na·tion (ô′tō-hē′mə-glōōt′n-ā′-shən) *n.* Clumping of an individual's red blood cells by his or her own plasma.

au·to·he·mol·y·sin (ô′tō-hĭ-mŏl′ĭ-sĭn, -hē′mə-lĭ′-) *n.* An autoantibody that acts on the red blood cells in the same person in whose body it is formed.

au·to·he·mol·y·sis (ô′tō-hĭ-mŏl′ĭ-sĭs, -hē′mə-lī′sĭs) *n.* Hemolysis occurring in certain diseases through the action of an autohemolysin.

au·to·he·mo·ther·a·py (ô′tō-hē′mō-thĕr′ə-pē) *n.* Treatment of disease by the withdrawal and reinjection of the patient's own blood.

au·to·im·mune (ô′tō-ĭ-myōōn′) *adj.* Of or relating to an immune response by the body against one of its own tissues, cells, or molecules. —**au′to·im·mu′ni·ty** *n.* —**au′to·im′mu·ni·za′tion** (ô′tō-ĭm′yə-nə-zā′shən) *n.*

autoimmune disease *n.* A disease resulting from an immune reaction produced by an individual's white blood cells or antibodies acting on the body's own tissues or extracellular proteins.

autoimmune hemolytic anemia *n.* Either of two forms of hemolytic anemia involving autoantibodies against red cell antigens; a cold-antibody type, caused by hemagglutinating cold antibody; and a warm-antibody type, due to serum autoantibodies that react with the patient's red blood cells, with antigenic specificity being chiefly in the Rh complex. Also called *autoallergic hemolytic anemia*.

au·to·im·mu·no·cy·to·pe·ni·a (ô′tō-ĭm′yə-nō-sī′tō-pē′nē-ə) *n.* Anemia, thrombocytopenia, and leukopenia resulting from cytotoxic autoimmune reactions.

au·to·in·fec·tion (ô′tō-ĭn-fĕk′shən) *n.* **1.** Reinfection by microbes or parasitic organisms that are present on or within the body. **2.** Self-infection by direct contact with a contagious agent, as with parasite eggs in the infectious state transmitted by fingernails. Also called *autoreinfection*.

au·to·in·fu·sion (ô′tō-ĭn-fyōō′zhən) *n.* Forcing the blood from the extremities, as by the application of a bandage or pressure device, to raise the blood pressure and fill vessels in the vital organs.

au·to·in·oc·u·la·tion (ô′tō-ĭ-nŏk′yə-lā′shən) *n.* A secondary infection originating from the site of an infection already present in the body.

au·to·in·tox·i·ca·tion (ô′tō-ĭn-tŏk′sĭ-kā′shən) *n.* Self-poisoning resulting from the absorption of waste products of metabolism, decomposed intestinal matter, or other toxins produced within the body. Also called *endogenic toxicosis*.

au·to·i·sol·y·sin (ô′tō-ī-sŏl′ĭ-sĭn, -ī′sō-lĭ′-) *n.* An antibody that with complement causes lysis of cells in the organism in whose body the lysin is formed, as well as in others of the same species.

au·to·ker·a·to·plas·ty (ô′tō-kĕr′ə-tō-plăs′tē) *n.* The grafting of corneal tissue from one eye to the other eye.

au·to·ki·ne·sia (ô′tō-kĭ-nē′zhə, -kī-) *or* **au·to·ki·ne·sis** (-nē′sĭs) *n.* Voluntary movement. —**au′to·ki·net′ic** (-nĕt′ĭk) *adj.*

au·tol·o·gous (ô-tŏl′ə-gəs) *adj.* **1.** Of or relating to a natural, normal occurrence in a certain type of tissue or in a specific structure of the body. **2.** Of or relating to a graft in which the donor and recipient areas are in the same individual.

autologous graft *n.* See **autograft.**

au·tol·y·sate (ô-tŏl′ĭ-sāt′, -zāt′) *n.* An end product of autolysis.

au·tol·y·sin (ô-tŏl′ĭ-sĭn, ô′tə-lī′sĭn) *n.* A substance, such as an enzyme, that is capable of destroying the cells or tissues of an organism within which it is produced. Also called *autocytolysin.*

au·tol·y·sis (ô-tŏl′ĭ-sĭs) *n.* **1.** The destruction of tissues or cells of an organism by the action of substances, such as enzymes, that are produced within the organism. **2.** Self-destruction of tissues within the living body. Also called *autodigestion.* **3.** The hemolytic action of blood serum or plasma upon its own cells. Also called *autocytolysis.* —**au′to·lyt′ic** (ô′tə-lĭt′ĭk) *adj.*

autolytic enzyme *n.* An enzyme that digests the cell in which it is produced, usually marking the death of the cell.

au·to·mat·ic beat (ô′tə-măt′ĭk) *n.* An ectopic beat that arises anew and is not precipitated by the preceding beat.

au·tom·a·tism (ô-tŏm′ə-tĭz′əm) *n.* **1.** The involuntary functioning of an organ or other body structure that is not under conscious control, such as the beating of the heart or the dilation of the pupil of the eye. **2.** The reflexive action of a body part. **3.** An act performed without intent or conscious exercise of the will, often without realization of its occurrence, as for certain types of epilepsy. **4.** A condition in which one is consciously or unconsciously, but involuntarily, compelled to the performance of certain acts. Also called *telergy.*

au·to·nom·ic (ô′tə-nŏm′ĭk) *adj.* **1.** Functionally independent; not under voluntary control. **2.** Relating to the autonomic nervous system. —**au′to·nom′i·cal·ly** *adv.*

autonomic bladder *n.* Involuntary, spontaneous, or induced reflex emptying of the urinary bladder.

autonomic dysreflexia *n.* See **dysreflexia.**

autonomic ganglion *n.* Any of the various ganglia that are part of the autonomic nervous system and are located along the sympathetic trunks, on the peripheral plexuses, and within the walls of organs. Also called *visceral ganglion.*

autonomic imbalance *n.* A lack of balance between the sympathetic and parasympathetic nervous systems, especially when manifested by vasomotor disturbances. Also called *vasomotor imbalance.*

autonomic nervous system *n.* The part of the nervous system that regulates involuntary action, as of the intestines, smooth muscle, heart, and glands, and that is divided into two physiologically and anatomically distinct, mutually antagonistic systems, the sympathetic nervous system and the parasympathetic nervous system.

autonomic neurogenic bladder *n.* A malfunctioning urinary bladder secondary to low spinal cord lesions. Also called *neuropathic bladder.*

autonomic plexus *n.* Any of the plexuses of nerves in relation to blood vessels and viscera, whose component fibers are sympathetic, parasympathetic, and sensory.

au·to·nom·o·tro·pic (ô′tə-nŏm′ə-trŏp′ĭk) *adj.* Acting on the autonomic nervous system.

au·to·ox·i·da·tion (ô′tō-ŏk′sĭ-dā′shən) *n.* The combination of a substance with molecular oxygen at ordinary temperatures. Also called *autoxidation.*

au·to·pha·gia (ô′tə-fā′jə) *n.* **1.** The biting of one's own flesh. **2.** *or* **au·toph·a·gy** (ô-tŏf′ə-jē) The segregation and disposal of damaged organelles within a cell. **3.** *or* **autophagy** The maintenance of the nutrition of the whole body by metabolic consumption of some of the body tissues. —**au′to·phag′ic** (-făj′ĭk) *adj.*

au·to·plas·ty (ô′tō-plăs′tē) *n.* Surgical repair or reconstruction of a body part using tissue taken from another part of the body. —**au′to·plas′tic** *adj.* —**au′to·plas′ti·cal·ly** *adv.*

au·to·pol·y·mer resin (ô′tō-pŏl′ə-mər) *n.* A resin that can be polymerized by chemical catalysis rather than by the application of heat, as of dental restoration material. Also called *activated resin, cold-cure resin, quick-cure resin, self-curing resin.*

au·top·sy (ô′tŏp′sē) *n.* An examination of a cadaver in order to determine the cause of death or to study pathologic changes. Also called *necropsy, postmortem, postmortem examination.*

au·to·ra·di·o·graph (ô′tō-rā′dē-ō-grăf′) *n.* An image recorded on a photographic film or plate produced by the radiation emitted from a specimen, such as a section of tissue, that has been treated or injected with a radioactively labeled isotope or that has absorbed or ingested such an isotope. Also called *radioautograph.* —**au′to·ra′di·o·graph′ic** *adj.* —**au′to·ra′di·og′ra·phy** (-ŏg′rə-fē) *n.*

au·to·reg·u·la·tion (ô′tō-rĕg′yə-lā′shən) *n.* **1.** The tendency of the blood flow toward an organ or part to remain at or return to the same level despite changes in arterial pressure. **2.** A biological system equipped with inhibitory feedback systems such that a given change tends to be largely or completely counteracted.

au·to·re·in·fec·tion (ô′tō-rē′ĭn-fĕk′shən) *n.* See **autoinfection** (sense 2).

au·to·re·pro·duc·tion (ô′tō-rē′prə-dŭk′shən) *n.* The capability of a gene, virus, or nucleoprotein molecule to bring about the synthesis of another molecule like itself from smaller molecules within the cell; replication.

au·to·sep·ti·ce·mi·a (ô′tō-sĕp′tĭ-sē′mē-ə) *n.* Septicemia originating with microorganisms existing within the individual and not introduced from outside the person.

au·to·se·rum (ô′tō-sîr′əm) *n.* Serum derived from an individual's own blood.

au·to·site (ô′tō-sīt′) *n.* The usually larger component of abnormal, unequally conjoined twins that is able to live independently and nourish the other parasitic component.

autosomal gene *n.* A gene located on an autosome.

au·to·some (ô′tə-sōm′) *n.* A chromosome other than a sex chromosome, normally occurring in pairs in somatic cells and singly in gametes. —**au·to·so′mal** (-sō′məl) *adj.* —**au′to·so′mal·ly** *adv.*

au·to·sug·ges·tion (ô′tō-səg-jĕs′chən) *n.* **1.** The dwelling upon an idea, thought, or concept, thereby inducing some change in the mental or bodily functions. **2.** The process by which a person induces self-acceptance of an opinion, belief, or plan of action.

au·tot·o·my (ô-tŏt′ə-mē) *n.* The spontaneous casting off of a body part, especially of an invertebrate, when injured or under attack.

au·to·top·ag·no·si·a (ô′tō-tŏp′ăg-nō′zē-ə, -zhə) *n.* The inability to recognize or correctly orient the parts of one's own body.

au·to·tox·in (ô′tō-tŏk′sĭn) *n.* A poison that acts on the organism in which it is generated. —**au′to·tox′ic** *adj.*

au·to·trans·fu·sion (ô′tō-trăns-fyoō′zhən) *n.* Infusion of blood or blood products into the individual from whom they were originally withdrawn.

au·to·trans·plant (ô′tō-trăns′plănt′) *n.* See **autograft.**

au·to·trans·plan·ta·tion (ô′tō-trăns′plăn-tā′shən) *n.* The transplantation of a tissue or an organ from one site onto another on or in the body of the same individual.

au·to·troph (ô′tə-trŏf′, -trōf′) *n.* An organism that is capable of synthesizing its own food from inorganic substances using light or chemical energy. Green plants, algae, and certain bacteria are autotrophs. —**au′to·troph′ic** (-trŏf′ĭk, -trō′fĭk) *adj.*

au·to·vac·ci·na·tion (ô′tō-văk′sə-nā′shən) *n.* Revaccination of an individual using vaccine obtained from that individual.

au·tox·i·da·tion (ô-tŏk′sĭ-dā′shən) *n.* See **autooxidation.**

aux·an·o·gram (awk-săn′ō-gram) *n.* A plate culture of microorganisms that is exposed to a variety of conditions in order to determine the effect these conditions have on the microorganisms' growth.

aux·a·nog·ra·phy (ôk′sə-nŏg′rə-fē) *n.* A method, using auxanograms, for determining the appropriate culture medium for growing a particular strain of microorganism. —**aux′a·no·graph′ic** (-nə-grăf′ĭk) *adj.*

aux·e·sis (ôg-zē′sĭs, ôk-sē′-) *n.* Growth resulting from increase in cell size without cell division. —**aux·et′ic** (ôg-zĕt′ĭk) *adj.*

aux·il·ia·ry (ôg-zĭl′yə-rē, -zĭl′ə-rē) *adj.* **1.** Functioning in an augmenting capacity; supplementary. **2.** Functioning as a subordinate; secondary.

aux·i·lyt·ic (ôk′sə-lĭt′ĭk) *adj.* Increasing the effectiveness of a lysin; favoring lysis.

auxo– *or* **aux–** *pref.* Increase: *auxotroph.*

aux·o·ton·ic (ôk′sə-tŏn′ĭk) *adj.* Relating to a muscle contracting to accommodate an increasing load.

aux·o·troph (ôk′sə-trŏf′, -trōf′) *n.* A mutated microorganism having nutritional requirements that differ from those of unmutated microorganisms from the same strain.

aux·o·troph·ic (awk-sō-trŏf′ĭk) *adj.* Requiring one or more specific substances for growth and metabolism that the parent organism was able to synthesize on its own. Used with respect to organisms, such as strains of bacteria, algae, or fungi, that can no longer synthesize certain growth factors because of mutational changes.

A-V *abbr.* arteriovenous; atrioventricular

Av·a·pro (ăv′ə-prō′) A trademark for the drug irbesartan.

a·vas·cu·lar (ā-văs′kyə-lər) *adj.* Not associated with or supplied by blood vessels. —**a·vas′cu·lar′i·ty** (-lăr′ĭ-tē) *n.*

avascular graft *n.* A skin allograft that does not become vascularized.

a·vas·cu·lar·i·za·tion (ā-văs′kyə-lər-ĭ-zā′shən) *n.* **1.** The exclusion of blood from a part or a tissue. **2.** A loss of blood vessels, as in the tissue that forms in scarring.

A·ven·tyl (ə-vĕn′tl) A trademark for the drug nortriptyline hydrochloride.

Av·en·zo·ar (ăv′ən-zō′ər) 1090?–1162. Spanish-Arab physician whose *Practical Manual of Treatments and Diet* showed an understanding of the human body based on science rather than speculation.

av·er·age (ăv′ər-ĭj, ăv′rĭj) *n.* **1.** A number that typifies a set of numbers of which it is a function. **2.** See **arithmetic mean. 3.** An intermediate level or degree. —*adj.* **1.** Of, relating to, or constituting an average. **2.** Being intermediate between extremes, as on a scale. —*v.* **1.** To calculate the average of. **2.** To do or have an average of. **3.** To distribute proportionately, as over a period of time.

A·ver·ro·ës *or* **A·ver·rho·ës** (ə-vĕr′ō-ēz′, ăv′ə-rō′ēz) 1126–1198. Arab physician and philosopher, born in Spain. He is best known for his commentaries on Aristotle.

a·ver·sion (ə-vûr′zhən) *n.* **1.** A fixed, intense dislike; repugnance, as of crowds. **2.** A feeling of extreme repugnance accompanied by avoidance or rejection.

aversion therapy *n.* A type of behavior therapy designed to modify antisocial habits or addictions by creating a strong association with a disagreeable or painful stimulus.

a·ver·sive (ə-vûr′sĭv, -zĭv) *adj.* Causing avoidance of a thing, situation, or behavior by using an unpleasant or punishing stimulus, as in techniques of behavior modification.

A·ver·y (ā′və-rē), Oswald 1877–1955. American bacteriologist noted for establishing (1944) that DNA is responsible for the transmission of heritable characteristics.

A-V extrasystole *n.* See **atrioventricular extrasystole.**

a·vi·an (ā′vē-ən) *adj.* Of, relating to, or characteristic of birds.

avian influenza *n.* A potentially fatal infection in birds caused by any of various subtypes of the influenza type A virus, especially the H5N1 virus, which is highly contagious among birds and can be transmitted to humans who have been in direct contact with infected birds.

avian leukosis-sarcoma complex *n.* **1.** A division of the RNA tumor viruses that causes a group of transmissable diseases of poultry. Also called *avian leukosis-sarcoma virus.* **2.** The group of diseases caused by this division of viruses.

Av·i·cen·na (ăv′ĭ-sĕn′ə) 980–1037. Persian physician and philosopher noted for his *Canon of Medicine,* a standard medical textbook used in Europe until the 17th century.

av·i·din (ăv′ĭ-dĭn) *n.* A protein, found in uncooked egg white, that binds to and inactivates biotin and which, when present in abundance, can result in a deficiency of biotin.

a·vir·u·lent (ā-vîr′yə-lənt, ā-vîr′ə-) *adj.* Not virulent.

A·vi·ta (ə-vē′tə) A trademark for the drug tretinoin.

a·vi·ta·min·o·sis (ā-vī′tə-mĭ-nō′sĭs) *n.* A disease, such as scurvy, beriberi, or pellagra, caused by deficiency of one or more essential vitamins.

A-V nodal extrasystole *n.* See **atrioventricular nodal extrasystole.**

A-V nodal rhythm (ā′vē′) *n.* See **atrioventricular nodal rhythm.**

A-V node *n.* See **atrioventricular node.**

A·vo·ga·dro's constant (ä′və-gä′drōz, ä′vō-) *n.* See **Avogadro's number.**

Avogadro's law *n.* The principle that equal volumes of all gases under identical conditions of pressure and temperature contain the same number of molecules.

Avogadro's number *n.* The number of molecules in a mole of a substance, approximately 6.0225×10^{23}. Also called *Avogadro's constant.*

a·void·ant personality (ə-void′nt) *n.* A personality disorder characterized by hypersensitivity to potential or actual rejection and criticism, a strong need for uncritical acceptance, social withdrawal in spite of a desire for affection and acceptance, and low self-esteem.

av·oir·du·pois (ăv′ər-də-poiz′) *n.* Avoirdupois weight.

avoirdupois weight *n.* A system of weights and measures based on a pound containing 16 ounces or 7,000 grains and equal to 453.59 grams.

a·vulsed wound (ə-vŭlst) *n.* A wound that is caused by avulsion.

a·vul·sion (ə-vŭl′shən) *n.* The forcible tearing away of a body part by trauma or surgery.

avulsion fracture *n.* A fracture occurring when a joint capsule, ligament, tendon, or muscle is pulled from a bone, taking with it a fragment of the bone to which it was attached.

AW *abbr.* atomic weight

ax *abbr.* axis

Ax·el·rod (ăk′səl-rŏd′), **Julius** 1912–2004. American biochemist and pharmacologist. He shared a 1970 Nobel Prize for studies of the ways in which different substances affect neural impulses.

a·xen·ic (ā-zĕn′ĭk, ā-zē′nĭk) *adj.* Not contaminated by or associated with any other living organisms; sterile. Used especially in reference to pure cultures of microorganisms.

axi– *pref.* Variant of **axio–.**

ax·i·al (ăk′sē-əl) *adj.* **1.** Relating to or characterized by an axis; axile. **2.** Relating to or situated in the head and trunk region of the body. **3.** Relating to or parallel with the long axis of a tooth.

axial angle *n.* The angle formed by two surfaces of a structure, as of a tooth, in which the line of union is parallel with its axis.

axial current *n.* The central, rapidly moving portion of the bloodstream in an artery.

axial filament *n.* The central filament of a flagellum or cilium. Also called *axoneme.*

axial hyperopia *n.* Hyperopia due to shortening of the anteroposterior diameter of the globe of the eye.

axial muscle *n.* Any of the skeletal muscles of the trunk or head.

axial plate *n.* The primitive streak of an embryo.

axial point *n.* See **nodal point.**

axial skeleton *n.* The bones of the head and trunk, excluding the pectoral and pelvic girdles.

Ax·id (ăk′sĭd) A trademark for the drug nizatidine.

ax·if·u·gal (ăk-sĭf′yə-gəl, -sĭf′ə-) *or* **ax·of·u·gal** (-sŏf′-yə-gəl, -sŏf′ə-, ăk′sə-fyoo′gəl) *adj.* **1.** Directed away from an axon or axis. **2.** Relating to nerve impulses that move from the body of a nerve cell.

ax·ile (ăk′sīl) *adj.* Axial.

ax·il·la (ăk-sĭl′ə) *n.,* pl. **–il·lae** (-sĭl′ē) See **armpit.**

ax·il·lar·y (ăk′sə-lĕr′ē) *n.* Relating to the axilla.

axillary artery *n.* A continuation of the subclavian artery in the armpit, becoming the brachial artery in the arm, with superior thoracic, thoracoacromial, lateral thoracic, subscapular, and posterior and superior circumflex humeral branches.

axillary cataract *n.* A type of hereditary cataract in which the opacity of the lens or capsule is deep and central.

axillary cavity *n.* Axilla.

axillary fossa *n.* See **armpit.**

axillary gland *n.* Any of numerous nodes situated around axillary veins that receive lymphatic drainage from the upper limb, pectoral girdle, and mammary gland. Also called *axillary lymph node.*

axillary nerve *n.* A nerve that arises from the posterior cord of the brachial plexus in the axilla and supplies the deltoid and teres minor muscles.

axillary vein *n.* The continuation of the basilic and brachial veins that runs from the lower border of the teres major muscle to the outer border of the first rib where it becomes the subclavian vein.

axio– *or* **axi–** *pref.* Axis: *axioversion.*

ax·i·o·plasm (ăk′sē-ə-plăz′əm) *n.* Variant of **axoplasm.**

ax·i·o·ver·sion (ăk′sē-ō-vûr′zhən, -shən) *n.* An abnormal inclination of the long axis of a tooth.

ax·ip·e·tal (ăk-sĭp′ĭ-tl) *adj.* Centripetal.

ax·is (ăk′sĭs) *n.,* pl. **ax·es** (ăk′sēz′) **1.** A real or imaginary straight line about which a body or geometric object rotates or may be conceived to rotate. **2.** A center line to which parts of a structure or body may be referred. **3.** The second cervical vertebra. Also called *epistropheus, vertebra dentata.* **4.** An artery that divides into many branches at its origin.

axis deviation *n.* The deflection of the electrical axis of the heart to the right or left of its normal position. Also called *axis shift.*

axis traction *n.* Traction upon the fetal head in the line of the birth canal by means of forceps.

axis-trac·tion forceps *n.* Obstetrical forceps provided with a second handle so attached that traction can be made in the line in which the head must move along the axis of the pelvis.

axo– *pref.* **1.** Axis: *axoneme.* **2.** Axon: *axodentritic.*

ax·o·ax·on·ic (ăk′sō-ăk-sŏn′ĭk) *adj.* Relating to or being a synapse between the axon of one nerve cell and the axon of another such cell.

ax·o·den·drit·ic (ăk′sō-dĕn-drĭt′ĭk) *adj.* Relating to or being a synapse between the axon of one nerve cell and the dendrite of another.

ax·of·u·gal (ăk-sŏf′yə-gəl, -sŏf′ə-, ăk′sə-fyoō′gəl) *adj.* Variant of **axifugal.**

ax·o·lem·ma (ăk′sō-lĕm′ə) *n.* The plasma membrane of an axon. Also called *Mauthner's sheath.*

ax·ol·y·sis (ăk-sŏl′ĭ-sĭs) *n.* Degeneration and destruction of the axon of a nerve cell.

ax·om·e·ter (ăk-sŏm′ĭ-tər) *n.* An instrument used in the determination of the position of the optical axes, especially for adjustment of eyeglasses. Also called *axonometer.*

ax·on (ăk′sŏn′) *or* **ax·one** (-sōn′) *n.* The usually long process of a nerve fiber that generally conducts impulses away from the body of the nerve cell. —**ax′on·al** (ăk′sə-nəl, ăk-sŏn′əl) *adj.*

ax·o·neme (ăk′sə-nēm′) *n.* **1.** The axial thread of a chromosome. **2.** See **axial filament.**

axon hillock *n.* The conical area of origin of the axon from the nerve cell body.

ax·o·nog·ra·phy (ăk′sə-nŏg′rə-fē) *n.* A procedure for recording electrical changes in axons.

ax·o·nom·e·ter (ăk′sə-nŏm′ĭ-tər) *n.* See **axometer.**

ax·on·ot·me·sis (ăk′sə-nŏt-mē′sĭs) *n.* Damage to nerve cells that destroys the axons but that does not destroy the supporting structures of the cells, making regeneration possible.

axon terminals *pl.n.* The somewhat enlarged, often club-shaped endings by which axons make synaptic contacts with other nerve cells or with effector cells. Also called *end-feet, neuropodia, terminal boutons.*

ax·op·e·tal (ăk-sŏp′ĭ-tl) *adj.* Relating to nerve impulses transmitted along an axon toward the body of a nerve cell.

ax·o·plasm (ăk′sə-plăz′əm) *or* **ax·i·o·plasm** (ăk′sē-ə-) *n.* The cytoplasm of an axon.

ax·o·plas·mic transport (ăk′sə-plăz′mĭk) *n.* Transport, by way of flow of axoplasm, toward a cell body or toward an axon terminal.

ax·o·so·mat·ic (ăk′sō-sō-măt′ĭk) *adj.* Relating to or being the synapse between an axon of one nerve cell and the body of another nerve cell.

A·yer·za's disease (ə-yûr′səz, ä-yĕr′-) *n.* A condition resembling erythremia but resulting from primary pulmonary arteriosclerosis or primary pulmonary hypertension and is characterized by chronic cyanosis, chronic dyspnea, and enlargement of the liver and spleen.

Ayerza's syndrome *n.* Sclerosis of the pulmonary arteries in chronic cor pulmonale, caused by primary pulmonary arteriosclerosis or primary pulmonary hypertension. It is associated with severe cyanosis. Also called *cardiopathia nigra.*

A·yur·ve·da (ī′yər-vā′də, -vē′-) *n.* The ancient Hindu science of health and medicine.

A·yur·ve·dic medicine (ī′yər-vā′dĭk, -vē′-) *n.* A holistic approach to health care that is based on principles of Ayurveda and designed to maintain or improve health through the use of dietary modification, massage, yoga, herbal preparations, and other measures.

A·zac·tam (ə-zăk′təm) A trademark for the drug aztreonam.

az·a·gua·nine (ăz′ə-gwä′nēn′) *n.* Nitrogen-containing form of guanine believed to block the growth of certain tumors in mice. Also called *guanazolo.*

a·za·spi·ro·dec·ane·di·one (ā′zə-spī′rō-dĕk′ān-dī′ōn′) *n.* A class of antianxiety agents that are chemically and pharmacologically unrelated to other classes of sedative and anxiolytic drugs.

a·zat·a·dine ma·le·ate (ə-zăt′ə-dēn′ mā′lē-āt′, mə-lē′ət) *n.* An antihistaminic that has anticholinergic and antiserotonin properties.

az·a·thi·o·prine (ăz′ə-thī′ə-prēn′) *n.* An immunosuppressive agent used especially to prevent organ rejection in kidney transplant recipients.

a·ze·o·trope (ə-zē′ə-trōp′, ā′zē-) *n.* A liquid mixture of two or more substances that retains the same composition in the vapor state as in the liquid state when distilled or partially evaporated under a certain pressure. —**a′ze·o·trop′ic** (a′zē-ə-trŏp′ĭk, -trō′pĭk) *adj.*

az·i·do·thy·mi·dine (ăz′ĭ-dō-thī′mĭ-dēn′) *n.* AZT.

a·zith·ro·my·cin dihydrate (ə-zĭth′rō-mī′sĭn) *n.* An antibiotic of the macrolide class used primarily to treat respiratory tract and skin infections.

az·lo·cil·lin sodium (ăz′lō-sĭl′ĭn) *n.* A derivative of penicillin used in treating infections caused by *Pseudomonas aeruginosa, Escherichia coli,* and *Haemophilus influenzae.*

Az·ma·cort (ăz′mə-kôrt′) A trademark for the drug triamcinolone acetonide.

azo– *or* **az–** *pref.* Containing a nitrogen group, especially one attached at both ends in a covalent bond to other groups: *azole.*

a·zo·ic (ā-zō′ĭk) *adj.* Containing no living things; lacking organic life.

az·ole (ăz′ōl′, ā′zōl′) *n.* A class of organic compounds having a five-membered heterocyclic ring with two double bonds; pyrrole.

a·zo·o·sper·mi·a (ā-zō′ə-spûr′mē-ə, ə-zō′-) *n.* **1.** Absence of live spermatozoa in the semen. **2.** Failure to form live spermatozoa.

az·o·pro·tein (ăz′ō-prō′tēn′, ā′zō-) *n.* Any of various compounds formed by coupling proteins with diazonium compounds, often used as synthetic antigens.

az·o·te·mi·a (ăz′ə-tē′mē-ə, ā′zə-) *n.* See **uremia** (sense 1). —**az′o·te′mic** (-mĭk) *adj.*

az·o·tu·ri·a (ăz′ə-toōr′ē-ə) *n.* Increase of nitrogenous substances, especially urea, in the urine.

AZT (ā′zē-tē′) *n.* Azidothymidine; a nucleoside analog antiviral drug that inhibits the replication of retroviruses such as HIV by interfering with the enzyme reverse transcriptase.

az·tre·o·nam (ăz-trē′ə-năm′) *n.* A synthetic bactericidal antibiotic that acts against a wide spectrum of gram-negative aerobic pathogens.

az·ure (ăzh′ər) *n.* Any of various dyes used in biological stains, especially for blood and nuclear staining.

az·u·res·in (ăzh′ə-rĕz′ĭn) *n.* A complex of an azure dye and a carbacrylic resin that is used to detect gastric achlorhydria without intubation.

a·zu·ro·phil (ă-zhŏŏr′ə-fĭl′, ăzh′ə-rō-fĭl′) *or* **a·zu·ro·phile** (-fĭl′, -fĭl′) *adj.* Staining readily with an azure dye. Used especially in reference to certain cytoplasmic granules in white blood cells.

az·y·go·gram (ăz′ĭ-gə-grăm′) *n.* The radiographic image obtained by azygography.

az·y·gog·ra·phy (ăz′ĭ-gŏg′rə-fē) *n.* The radiographic visualization of the azygos venous system following the injection of a radiopaque contrast medium.

az·y·gos (ăz′ĭ-gŏs′, ā-zī′gŏs′) *n.* An unpaired anatomical structure. —*adj. or* **a·zy·gous** (ā-zī′gəs) Not one of a pair, as a vein or muscle; occurring singly.

azygos vein *n.* A vein that arises from the right ascending lumbar vein or the inferior vena cava, ascends through the aortic orifice of the diaphragm, lies in the posterior mediastinum, and terminates in the superior vena cava.

B

β The Greek letter *beta*. Entries beginning with this character are alphabetized under **beta**.

b *or* **B** *abbr.* blood (used as a subscript)

B The symbol for the element **boron**.

Ba The symbol for the element **barium**.

Baas·trup's sign (bä′strŭps) An indication on x-ray of bridging of the spinous processes in adjacent lumbar vertebrae, associated with back pain and degenerative diseases of the spine. Also called *Baastrup's syndrome*.

Ba·bès-Ernst body (bä′bāz-ûrnst′, -ĕrnst′, bä′bäsh-) *n.* An intracellular granule present in many species of bacteria, possessing a strong affinity for nuclear stains.

Ba·be·si·a (bə-bē′zē-ə, -zhə) *n.* A genus of parasitic sporozoans of the family Babesiidae that infect the red blood cells of humans and of animals such as dogs, cattle, and sheep.

Babesia mi·cro·ti (mī-krō′tī) *n.* A species of *Babesia* that causes babesiosis in humans, usually transmitted by the northern deer tick.

ba·be·si·o·sis (bə-bē′zē-ō′sĭs) *or* **bab·e·si·a·sis** (băb′ĭ-zī′ə-sĭs) *n.* A human protozoan disease of the red blood cells that is caused by infection with a species of *Babesia* that is transmitted by ticks. Babesiosis is characterized by fever, malaise, and hemolytic anemia. Also called *piroplasmosis*.

Ba·bin·ski (bə-bĭn′skē), **Joseph François Felix** 1857–1932. French neurologist who described the diagnostic relevance of Babinski's reflex.

Ba·bin·ski's reflex (bə-bĭn′skēz) *n.* An extension of the great toe, sometimes with fanning of the other toes, in response to stroking of the sole of the foot. It is a normal reflex in infants, but is associated with a disturbance of the pyramidal tract in children and adults. Also called *Babinski's sign, toe reflex*.

Babinski's sign *n.* **1.** See **Babinski's reflex**. **2.** Weakness of the platysma muscle on the affected side in hemiplegia, evident in such actions as blowing or opening the mouth. **3.** A sign of hemiplegia in which the thigh on the paralyzed side flexes and the heel is raised when a person attempts to sit up while lying supine with legs extended and arms crossed upon the chest. **4.** A sign of hemiplegia in which the forearm on the affected side, when placed in a position of supination, turns into the pronated position.

ba·by (bā′bē) *n.* A very young child; an infant.

baby tooth *n.* See **deciduous tooth**.

bac·cate (băk′āt′) *adj.* Resembling a berry in texture or form; berrylike.

Bac·il·la·ce·ae (băs′ə-lā′sē-ē′) *n.* A family of bacteria including the genera *Bacillus* and *Clostridium* that are generally rod-shaped, gram-negative, and spore-producing.

bac·il·lar·y (băs′ə-lĕr′ē, bə-sĭl′ə-rē) *or* **ba·cil·lar** (bə-sĭl′ər, băs′ə-lər) *adj.* **1.** Shaped like a rod. **2.** Consisting of small rods or rodlike structures. **3.** Caused by, relating to, or resembling bacilli.

bacillary angiomatosis *n.* A skin disease characterized by raised, red lesions, caused by bacterial infection in individuals with weakened immune systems, and treatable with antibiotics, although potentially fatal if untreated.

bacillary dysentery *n.* Any of various severe infections of the colon caused by microorganisms, especially of the genus *Shigella*, that result in abdominal cramping, fever, and passage of blood-stained stools or of material consisting of blood and mucus.

bacillary layer *n.* See **layer of rods and cones**.

ba·cil·le Cal·mette-Gué·rin (bă-sĕl′ kăl-mĕt′gā-răn′, kăl-mĕt′gā-răn′) *n.* See **bacillus Calmette-Guérin**.

bac·il·le·mi·a (băs′ə-lē′mē-ə) *n.* The presence of bacilli in the blood.

ba·cil·li·form (bə-sĭl′ə-fôrm′) *adj.* Having a rodlike shape.

ba·cil·lin (bə-sĭl′ĭn) *n.* An antibiotic substance produced by a species of *Bacillus*.

bac·il·lo·sis (băs′ə-lō′sĭs) *n.* An infection caused by bacilli.

bac·il·lu·ri·a (băs′ə-lŏŏr′ē-ə) *n.* The presence of bacilli in the urine.

ba·cil·lus (bə-sĭl′əs) *n.*, *pl.* **–cil·li** (-sĭl′ī′) **1.** Any of various rod-shaped, usually gram-positive aerobic bacteria of the genus *Bacillus* that often occur in chains and include *Bacillus anthracis*, the causative agent of anthrax. **2.** Any of various bacteria, especially a rod-shaped bacterium.

Bacillus *n.* A genus of rod-shaped gram-positive bacteria capable of producing endospores.

bacillus Cal·mette-Gué·rin (kăl-mĕt′gā-răn′, kăl-mĕt′-gā-răn′) *n. Abbr.* **BCG** An attenuated strain of tubercle bacillus grown in repeated cultures on medium containing bile and used in tuberculosis vaccines. Also called *bacille Calmette-Guérin*.

Bacillus ce·re·us (sîr′ē-əs) *n.* A species of *Bacillus* that causes an emetic type and a diarrheal type of food poisoning in humans.

Bacillus sphae·ri·cus (sfîr′ĭ-kəs) *n.* A species of *Bacillus* associated with infections in humans.

bac·i·tra·cin (băs′ĭ-trā′sĭn) *n.* A polypeptide antibiotic obtained from a strain of the bacterium *Bacillus subtilis* and used as a topical treatment for certain bacterial infections, especially those caused by cocci.

back (băk) *n.* **1.** The posterior portion of the trunk of the human body between the neck and the pelvis; the dorsum. **2.** The backbone or spine.

back·ache (băk′āk′) *n.* Discomfort or a pain in the region of the back or spine.

back·board (băk′bôrd′) *n.* **1.** A board placed under or behind something to provide firmness or support. **2.** A board placed beneath the body of a person with an injury to the neck or back, used especially in transporting the person in such a way as to avoid further injury.

backboard splint *n.* A board splint with slots for fixation by straps; shorter ones are used for neck injuries, longer ones for back injuries.

back·bone (băk′bōn′) *n.* See **spinal column.**

back·ground radiation (băk′ground′) *n.* Relatively constant low-level radiation from environmental sources such as building materials, cosmic rays, and ingested radionucleides in the body.

back pressure *n.* Pressure exerted upstream in the circulation as a result of obstruction to forward flow, as when congestion in the pulmonary circulation results from failure of the left ventricle.

back·ward heart failure (băk′wərd) *n.* Congestive heart failure resulting from passive engorgement of the veins caused by a rise in pressure near the failing cardiac chambers.

bac·lo·fen (băk′lə-fĕn) *n.* A gamma-aminobutyric acid receptor agonist used as a muscle relaxant, especially in patients with multiple sclerosis and spinal cord injuries.

bacter– *pref.* Variant of **bacterio–.**

bac·te·re·mi·a (băk′tə-rē′mē-ə) *n.* The presence of bacteria in the blood. —**bac′te·re′mic** (-mĭk) *adj.*

bac·te·ri·a (băk-tîr′ē-ə) *n.* Plural of **bacterium.**

bacterial capsule *n.* A mucopolysaccharide outer shell enveloping certain bacteria.

bacterial endocarditis *n.* Infectious endocarditis caused by the direct invasion of bacteria and leading to deformity of the heart valves.

bacterial plaque *n.* See **dental plaque.**

bacterial vaginosis *n.* Overgrowth of anaerobic vaginal flora (especially species of *Bacteroides* and *Gardnerella*) and loss of normal lactobacilli, often causing irritation and a discharge with a "fishy" odor, and increasing the risk of pelvic inflammatory disease and adverse pregnancy outcomes.

bacterial virus *n.* A virus that injects its genome into a host bacteria, initiating production of new viruses and viral DNA; a bacteriophage.

bac·te·ri·cide (băk-tēr′ĭ-sīd′) *or* **bac·te·ri·o·cide** (-tēr′ē-ə-sīd′) *n.* An agent that destroys bacteria. —**bac′te′·ri·cid′al, bac·te′ri·cid′al** (-sīd′l) *adj.*

bac·ter·id (băk′tər-ĭd) *n.* A recurrent or persistent eruption of pustules on the palms and soles that is associated with a bacterial infection.

bac·ter·in (băk′tər-ĭn) *n.* A suspension of killed or weakened bacteria used as a vaccine.

bacterio– *or* **bacteri–** *or* **bacter–** *pref.* Bacteria; bacterial: *bacteriology.*

bac·te·ri·o·cide (băk-tîr′ē-ə-sīd′) *n.* Variant of **bactericide.**

bac·te·ri·o·cid·in (băk-tîr′ē-ə-sīd′n) *n.* An antibody capable of destroying bacteria.

bac·te·ri·o·cin (băk-tîr′ē-ə-sĭn′) *n.* An antibacterial substance, such as colicin, produced by a strain of bacteria and harmful to another strain within the same family.

bac·te·ri·o·gen·ic (băk-tîr′ē-ə-jĕn′ĭk) *or* **bac·te·ri·og·e·nous** (-ŏj′ə-nəs) *adj.* Caused by bacteria.

bacteriogenic agglutination *n.* The clumping of red blood cells due to the action of bacteria.

bac·te·ri·o·cin·o·gen·ic plasmid (băk-tîr′ē-ə-sĭn′ə-jĕn′ĭk) *n.* A bacterial plasmid that controls the synthesis of bacteriocin.

bac·te·ri·ol·o·gy (băk-tîr′ē-ŏl′ə-jē) *n.* The study of bacteria, especially in relation to medicine and agriculture. —**bac′te′ri·o·log′ic** (-ə-lŏj′ĭk) *adj.* —**bac·te′ri·ol′o·gist** *n.*

bac·te·ri·ol·y·sin (băk-tîr′ē-ŏl′ĭ-sĭn, -ə-lī′sĭn) *n.* An antibody that, together with other substances, destroys a bacterium.

bac·te·ri·ol·y·sis (băk-tîr′ē-ŏl′ĭ-sĭs) *n., pl.* **–ses** (-sēz′) Dissolution or destruction of bacteria. —**bac′te′ri·o·lyt′ic** (-ə-lĭt′ĭk) *adj.*

bac·te·ri·o·pex·y (băk-tîr′ē-ə-pĕk′sē) *n.* Immobilization of bacteria by phagocytic cells.

bac·te·ri·o·phage (băk-tîr′ē-ə-fāj′) *n.* A virus capable of infecting and lysing bacterial cells. Also called *phage.*

bac·te·ri·op·so·nin (băk-tîr′ē-ŏp′sə-nĭn) *n.* An opsonin that acts on bacteria.

bac·te·ri·o·sis (băk-tîr′ē-ō′sĭs) *n.* An infection caused by bacteria.

bac·te·ri·o·stat (băk-tîr′ē-ə-stăt′) *n.* An agent, such as a chemical, that inhibits bacterial growth. —**bac·te′ri·o·stat′ic** (-stăt′ĭk) *adj.*

bac·te·ri·um (băk-tîr′ē-əm) *n., pl.* **–te·ri·a** (-tîr′ē-ə) Any of the unicellular, prokaryotic microorganisms of the class Schizomycetes, which vary in terms of morphology, of oxygen and nutritional requirements, and of motility, and may be free-living, saprophytic, or pathogenic, the latter causing disease in plants or in animals.

Bac·te·roi·des (băk′tə-roi′dēz) *n.* A genus of gram-negative, anaerobic, rod-shaped, non-spore-forming bacteria that occur in the respiratory, intestinal, and urogenital tracts of warm-blooded animals and include some pathogenic species.

Bacteroides cap·il·lo·sus (kăp′ə-lō′səs) *n.* A species of bacterium found in human cysts and wounds, the mouth, and feces.

Bacteroides di·si·ens (dī′sē-ənz) *n.* A bacterium found in abdominal and urogenital infections and in the mouth.

Bacteroides frag·i·lis (frăj′ə-lĭs) *n.* A bacterium that is one of the predominant microorganisms in the lower intestinal tract of humans.

Bacteroides me·lan·i·no·gen·i·cus (mə-lăn′ə-nō-jĕn′ĭ-kəs) *n.* A bacterium found in the mouth, in feces, and in infections of the respiratory, urogenital, or intestinal tracts, pathogenic only in association with other microorganisms.

Bacteroides o·ris (ôr′ĭs) *n.* A bacterium found in the gingival crevice and in abscesses of the face, neck, or chest.

bac·te·roi·do·sis (băk′tə-roi-dō′sĭs) *n.* An infection caused by a species of *Bacteroides.*

Bac·trim (băk′trĭm) A trademark for a mixture of sulfamethoxazole and trimethoprim.

Bac·tro·ban (băk′trə-băn′) A trademark for the drug mupirocin calcium.

Baer (bâr), **Karl Ernst von** 1792–1876. Estonian-born German naturalist and pioneer embryologist who discovered (1827) the mammalian egg in the ovary. He later described the process by which the fertilized egg develops first into germ layers and then into different organs and tissues.

BAER *abbr.* brainstem auditory evoked response

bag (băg) *n.* An anatomical sac or pouch, such as the udder of a cow.

bag·as·so·sis (băg′ə-sō′sĭs) *n.* A respiratory disorder caused by dust from waste sugar cane fiber.

Bag·dad boil (băg′dăd′) *n.* See **Aleppo boil.**

Ba·ker's cyst (bā′kərz) *n.* A collection of synovial fluid that has escaped from the knee joint or from a bursa and has formed a synovial-lined sac behind the knee.

bak·ing soda (bā′kĭng) *n.* A white crystalline compound, used as a gastric and systemic antacid, to alkalize urine, and for washes of body cavities. Also called *sodium bicarbonate.*

BAL *abbr.* British anti-Lewisite

bal·ance (băl′əns) *n.* **1.** A weighing device, especially one consisting of a rigid beam horizontally suspended by a low-friction support at its center, with identical weighing pans hung at either end, one of which holds an unknown weight while the effective weight in the other is increased by known amounts until the beam is level and motionless. **2.** A state of bodily equilibrium. **3.** The difference in magnitude between opposing forces or influences, such as for bodily parts or organs. **4.** Equality of mass and net electric charge of reacting species on each side of a chemical equation.

bal·anced anesthesia (băl′ənst) *n.* A technique of general anesthesia based on the concept that administration of a mixture of small amounts of several neuronal depressants summates the advantages but not the disadvantages of the individual components of the mixture.

balanced diet *n.* A diet that furnishes in proper proportions all of the nutrients necessary for adequate nutrition.

balanced occlusion *n.* The even alignment of upper and lower teeth on the right and left and in front and back within the functional range.

balanced polymorphism *n.* A system of genes in which two alleles are maintained in stable equilibrium because the heterozygote is more fit than either of the homozygotes.

balanced translocation *n.* Translocation of the long arm of an acrocentric chromosome to another chromosome, accompanied by loss of the small fragment containing the centromere.

ba·lan·ic (bə-lăn′ĭk) *adj.* Of or relating to the glans penis or the glans clitoridis.

bal·a·ni·tis (băl′ə-nī′tĭs) *n.* Inflammation of the glans penis or glans clitoridis.

balano– *or* **balan–** *pref.* Glans penis or glans clitoridis: *balanitis.*

bal·a·no·plas·ty (băl′ə-nō-plăs′tē) *n.* Surgical repair of the glans penis.

bal·a·no·pos·thi·tis (băl′ə-nō-pŏs-thī′tĭs) *n.* Inflammation of the glans penis and the prepuce.

bal·a·no·pre·pu·tial (băl′ə-nō-prē-pyōō′shəl) *adj.* Relating to the glans penis and the prepuce.

bal·a·nor·rha·gia (băl′ə-nō-rā′jə) *n.* A continual discharge from the glans penis.

bal·an·ti·di·a·sis (băl′ən-tĭ-dī′ə-sĭs) *n.* An intestinal disease caused by a species of *Balantidium* and characterized by diarrhea, dysentery, and occasionally ulceration.

Bal·an·tid·i·um (băl′ən-tĭd′ē-əm) *n.* A genus of ciliates found in the digestive tract of vertebrates and invertebrates.

bald (bôld) *adj.* Lacking hair on the head.

bald·ness (bôld′nĭs) *n.* The lack of all or a significant part of the hair on the head and sometimes on other parts of the body.

Bal·four (băl′fŏŏr′, -fôr′), **Francis Maitland** 1851–1882. Scottish embryologist and zoologist noted for his studies of the development of the urogenital and nervous systems in vertebrates.

Bal·kan frame (bôl′kən) *n.* An over-the-bed or free-standing horizontal pole, supported by uprights, from which a splinted limb can be suspended. Also called *Balkan splint.*

ball (bôl) *n.* **1.** A spherical object or mass. **2.** A bezoar. **3.** A large pill or bolus.

ball-and-socket joint *n.* A multiaxial joint in which a sphere on the head of one bone fits into a rounded cavity in the other bone, as in the hip joint. Also called *cotyloid joint, enarthrosis.*

bal·lis·mus (bə-lĭz′məs) *n.* Jerky or shaking movements of the arms or legs, especially such movements occurring in chorea.

bal·lis·to·car·di·o·gram (bə-lĭs′tō-kär′dē-ə-grăm′) *n. Abbr.* **BCG** A recording of the body's recoil as measured by a ballistocardiograph.

bal·lis·to·car·di·o·graph (bə-lĭs′tō-kär′dē-ə-grăf′) *n.* A device used to determine the volume of blood passing through the heart in a specific period of time and the force of cardiac contraction by measuring the body's recoil as blood is ejected from the ventricles with each heartbeat. —**bal·lis′to·car′di·og′ra·phy** (-ŏg′rə-fē) *n.*

ball of foot *n.* The padded portion of the sole of the human foot between the toes and the arch, on which the weight of the body rests when the heel is raised.

bal·loon (bə-lōōn′) *n.* An inflatable spherical device that is inserted into a body cavity or structure and distended with air or gas for therapeutic purposes.

balloon angioplasty *n.* A procedure in which a catheter equipped with a tiny balloon at the tip is inserted into an artery that has been narrowed by the accumulation of fatty deposits. The balloon is then inflated to clear the blockage and widen the artery.

balloon catheter *n.* A catheter with an inflatable balloon at its tip, used especially to expand a partially obstructed blood vessel or bodily passage and to measure blood pressure in a blood vessel. Also called *balloon-tip catheter.*

bal·loon·sep·tos·to·my (bə-lōōn′sĕp-tŏs′tə-mē) *n.* The surgical creation of an artificial interatrial septal defect by cardiac catheterization during which an inflated balloon is pulled across the interatrial septum through the oval foramen.

balloon-tip catheter *n.* See **balloon catheter.**

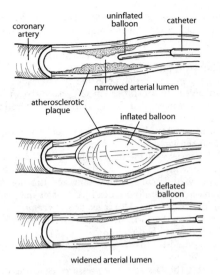

balloon angioplasty
Top: *uninflated balloon approaching obstructed artery*
Center: *inflated balloon clearing atherosclerotic plaque*
Bottom: *withdrawal of deflated balloon*

bal·lotte·ment (bə-lŏt′mənt) *n.* **1.** A palpatory technique for detecting or examining an organ not near the surface of the body. **2.** The use of a finger to push sharply against the uterus and detect the presence or position of a fetus by its return impact.

ball thrombus *n.* An antemortem thrombus sometimes found in the left atrium in mitral stenosis.

ball valve *n.* A valve regulated by the position of a free-floating ball that moves in response to fluid or mechanical pressure.

ball-valve thrombus *n.* A ball thrombus intermittently occluding the mitral orifice.

balm (bäm) *n.* **1.** An aromatic salve or oil. **2.** A soothing, healing, or comforting agent.

Bal·ti·more (bôl′tə-môr′), **David** Born 1938. American microbiologist. He shared a 1975 Nobel Prize for research on the interaction of tumor viruses and genetic material.

Bam·ber·ger-Marie disease (băm′bər-gər-, bäm′-) *n.* See **hypertrophic pulmonary osteoarthropathy.**

Bam·ber·ger's sign (băm′bər-gərz, bäm′-) *n.* **1.** The jugular pulse occurring in tricuspid insufficiency of the heart. **2.** An indication of pericarditis with effusion in which the dullness of sound generated upon percussion at the angle of the scapula disappears as the patient leans forward.

bam·boo hair (băm-bōō′) *n.* Hair having nodules along the shaft caused by intermittent fracturing. Also called *trichorrhexis invaginata.*

band (bănd) *n.* **1.** An appliance or a part of an apparatus that encircles or binds a part of the body. **2.** A cordlike tissue that connects or that holds bodily structures together. **3.** A chromatically, structurally, or functionally differentiated strip or stripe in or on an organism.

band·age (băn′dĭj) *n.* A strip of material such as gauze used to protect, immobilize, compress, or support a wound or injured body part. —*v.* To apply a bandage to.

Band-Aid (bănd′ād′) A trademark for an adhesive bandage with a gauze pad in the center, employed to protect minor wounds.

band cell *n.* Any of the blood granulocytic cells that have a densely staining unsegmented nucleus. Also called *stab cell, staff cell.*

band·ing (băn′dĭng) *n.* The differential staining of metaphase chromosomes in cultured cells to reveal their characteristic patterns of stripes in order to identify individual chromosome pairs.

Bandl's ring (băn′dlz) *n.* See **pathologic retraction ring.**

band-shaped keratopathy *n.* A horizontal, gray, inter-palpebral opacity of the cornea that progresses from the limbus.

Bang (băng, bäng), **Bernhard Lauritz Frederik** 1848–1932. Danish veterinarian who discovered *Brucella abortus,* the agent of brucellosis in cattle and of undulant fever in humans.

Bang's bacillus (băngz) *n.* A gram-negative bacterium, *Brucella abortus,* that causes abortion in cows, mares, and sheep, and undulant fever in humans.

Bang's disease *n.* See **brucellosis.**

Ban·nis·ter's disease (băn′ĭ-stərz) *n.* See **angioneurotic edema.**

Ban·ting (băn′tĭng), Sir **Frederick Grant** 1891–1941. Canadian physiologist. He shared a 1923 Nobel Prize for the discovery and successful clinical application of insulin.

Ban·ti's syndrome (băn′tēz, bän′-) *n.* Chronic congestive enlargement of the spleen that occurs primarily in children following hypertension in the portal or splenic veins and is characterized by anemia, splenomegaly, ascites, jaundice, leukopenia, thrombocytopenia, and gastrointestinal bleeding. Also called *Banti's disease, splenic anemia.*

bar (bär) *n.* **1.** The international unit of pressure equal to 1 megadyne (10^6 dyne) per square centimeter or 0.987 atmosphere. **2.** A metal segment of greater length than width which serves to connect two or more parts of a removable partial denture. **3.** A segment of tissue or a tight cellular junction that serves to constrict the passage of fluid, usually urine.

bar– *pref.* Variant of **baro–.**

bar·ag·no·sis (băr′ăg-nō′sĭs) *n.* Loss or impairment of the ability to differentiate varying weights or pressures, sometimes the result of a brain lesion.

Bá·rá·ny (bä′rän′yə), **Robert** 1876–1936. Austrian physician and otologist. He won a 1914 Nobel Prize for research on the balancing system of the inner ear.

Bá·rá·ny's caloric test (bä′rän′yəz) *n.* A test for assessing vestibular function in which the ear is irrigated with either hot or cold water, normally stimulating the vestibular apparatus, resulting in nystagmus; a lack of nystagmus indicates impaired vestibular functioning.

Bárány's sign *n.* An indication of ear disease despite a healthy vestibule in which injection into the external auditory canal of water below the body temperature causes rotary nystagmus toward the opposite side while injection of water above the body temperature causes nystagmus toward the injected side.

bar·ber's itch (bär′bərz) *n.* Any of various skin eruptions on the face and neck, especially ringworm of the beard. Also called *folliculitis barbae, tinea barbae, tinea sycosis.*

bar·bi·tal (bär′bĭ-tôl′, -tăl′) *n.* A white crystalline barbiturate used as a sedative and hypnotic, especially in the form of its soluble salt, sodium barbital.

bar·bi·tu·rate (bär-bĭch′ər-ĭt, -ə-rāt′, bär′bĭ-tŏŏr′ĭt, -āt′) *n.* **1.** A salt or ester of barbituric acid. **2.** Any of a group of barbituric acid derivatives that act as central nervous system depressants and are used as sedatives or hypnotics.

bar·bi·tu·ric acid (bär′bĭ-tŏŏr′ĭk) *n.* An organic acid used in the manufacture of barbiturates.

bar·bi·tu·rism (bär-bĭch′ə-rĭz′əm, bär′bĭ-tŏŏr′ĭz′əm) *n.* Chronic poisoning caused by any of the derivatives of barbituric acid.

bar·bo·tage (bär′bə-täzh′) *n.* The production of spinal anesthesia in which a portion of the anesthetic solution is injected into the cerebral spinal fluid, which is then aspirated into the syringe and a second portion of the contents of the syringe is injected. The partial reinjections and aspirations are repeated until the contents of the syringe are used.

Bar·det-Biedl syndrome (bär-dā′bēd′l) *n.* An inherited disorder characterized by mental retardation, pigmentary retinopathy, polydactyly, obesity, and hypogenitalism.

bare·foot doctor (bâr′fŏŏt′) *n.* A lay health care worker, especially in rural China, trained in such activities as first aid, childbirth assistance, the dispensing of drugs, and preventive medicine.

bare lymphocyte syndrome (bâr) *n.* The absence of human leukocyte antigens on peripheral mononuclear cells, which may result in immunodeficiency.

bar·es·the·si·om·e·ter (bär′ĕs-thē′zē-ŏm′ĭ-tər) *n.* An instrument for measuring an individual's sense of pressure.

barf bag (bärf) *n.* A disposable plastic or paper bag provided to a passenger by an airline for use in case of airsickness.

bar·i·at·rics (bär′ē-ăt′rĭks) *n.* The branch of medicine that deals with the causes, prevention, and treatment of obesity. —**bar′i·at′ric** *adj.*

bar·i·um (bâr′ē-əm, băr′-) *n. Symbol* **Ba** A soft alkaline-earth metal that is a component in compounds used in radiography and as radiopaque media. Atomic number 56.

barium enema *n.* The administration of barium in enema form for radiographic study of the lower intestinal tract. Also called *contrast enema.*

barium hydroxide *n.* A water soluble base used as a chemical reagent.

barium sulfate *n.* A fine white powder used as a pigment and as a contrast medium in x-ray photography of the digestive tract.

barium swallow *n.* See **upper GI series.**

Bar·low's disease (bär′lōz′) *n.* See **infantile scurvy.**

Bar·nard (bär′nərd, bär-närd′), **Christiaan Neethling** 1923–2001. South African surgeon who performed the first human heart transplant (1967).

Barnes curve (bärnz) *n.* The segment of a circle whose center is the promontory of the sacrum.

baro– *or* **bar–** *pref.* Weight; pressure: *baroreceptor.*

bar·o·phil·ic (bär′ō-fĭl′ĭk) *adj.* Of, relating to, or being a microorganism that thrives under high environmental pressure.

bar·o·re·cep·tor (băr′ō-rĭ-sĕp′tər) *or* **bar·o·cep·tor** (băr′ō-sĕp′tər) *n.* A sensory nerve ending in the walls of the auricles of the heart, vena cava, carotid sinus, and aortic arch, sensitive to stretching of the wall due to increased pressure from within, and functioning as the receptor of central reflex mechanisms that tend to reduce that pressure. Also called *pressoreceptor.*

bar·o·re·flex (bär′ō-rē′flĕks′) *n.* A reflex triggered by stimulation of a baroreceptor.

bar·o·si·nus·i·tis (băr′ō-sī′nə-sī′tĭs) *n.* See **aerosinusitis.**

bar·o·stat (băr′ə-stăt′) *n.* A pressure-regulating device or structure, such as a baroreceptor.

bar·o·ti·tis me·di·a (băr′ō-tī′tĭs mē′dē-ə) *n.* An acute or chronic traumatic inflammation of the middle ear caused by differences between the pressure in the tympanic cavity and the ambient pressure. Also called *aero-otitis media.*

bar·o·trau·ma (băr′ō-trô′mə, -trou′-) *n.* Injury caused by pressure, especially to the middle ear or paranasal sinuses due to an imbalance between the ambient pressure and pressure within the cavity.

Bar·ra·quer's disease (băr′ə-kârz′, bä-rä-kĕrz′) *n.* See **progressive lipodystrophy.**

Barr body (bär) *n.* The condensed, inactive, single X-chromosome found in the nuclei of somatic cells of most female mammals and whose presence is the basis of sex determination tests that are performed, for example, on athletes. Also called *sex chromatin.*

bar·rel chest (băr′əl) *n.* A large chest with increased anteroposterior diameter and usually some degree of kyphosis, sometimes seen in cases of emphysema.

bar·ren (băr′ən) *adj.* **1.** Not producing offspring. **2.** Incapable of producing offspring.

Bar·ré's sign (bă-rāz′) *n.* An indication of disease of the corticospinal tracts in which an individual, when placed in a prone position with the legs flexed at the knees, is unable to maintain a flexed position on the side of the lesion but can extend the leg.

Bar·rett's esophagus (băr′ĭts) *n.* Chronic peptic ulcer of the lower esophagus due to the presence of columnar epithelium resembling the mucosa of the gastric cardia.

bar·ri·er (băr′ē-ər) *n.* **1.** A boundary or limit. **2.** An obstacle or impediment. **3.** Something that separates or holds apart. **4.** Something immaterial that obstructs or impedes behavior. **5.** A physical or biological factor that limits the migration, interbreeding, or free movement of individuals or populations.

Bar·tho·lin (bär′tl-ĭn, -thə-lĭn), **Caspar** 1585–1629. Danish anatomist and physician who was the first to describe Bartholin's glands of the vagina.

bar·tho·lin·i·tis (bär′tə-lə-nī′tĭs) *n.* Inflammation of Bartholin's gland.

Bar·tho·lin's cyst (bär′tl-ĭnz, -thə-lĭnz) *n.* A vaginal cyst arising from Bartholin's gland or from its ducts.

Bartholin's duct *n.* The duct that drains the anterior portion of the sublingual salivary glands. Also called *major sublingual duct.*

Bartholin's gland *n.* Either of two compound tubuloalveolar mucus-secreting glands situated in the lateral walls on each side of the vestibule of the vagina. Also called *greater vestibular gland.*

Bar·thol·o·mew's rule of fourths (bär-thŏl′ə-myōoz′) *n.* A rule for determining the duration of pregnancy by measuring the height of the fundus of the uterus above the pubic symphysis.

Barth's hernia (bärths, bärts) *n.* A hernia of a loop of intestine between a persistent vitelline duct and the abdominal wall.

Bar·ton (bär′tn), **Clara** Full name **Clarissa Harlowe Barton.** 1821–1912. American administrator who did battlefield relief work during the Civil War and organized the American Red Cross (1881).

Bar·ton·el·la (bär′tn-ĕl′ə) *n.* A genus of bacteria found in humans and arthropods that multiply in red blood cells and reproduce by binary fission.

Bartonella ba·cil·li·for·mis (bə-sĭl′ə-fôr′mĭs) *n.* An aerobic coccobacilli of the genus *Bartonella* that causes Oroya fever in humans.

bar·ton·el·lo·sis (bär′tn-ĕl-ō′sĭs) *n.* A disease caused by *Bartonella bacilliformis* and transmitted by the bite of the sandfly.

Bar·ton's bandage (bär′tnz) *n.* A figure-of-8 bandage for support of a fractured mandible.

Barton's fracture *n.* A dislocation fracture of the radiocarpal joint.

Bart's hemoglobin (bärts) *n. Abbr.* **Hb Bart's** An abnormal hemoglobin that is not effective in oxygen transport, found in beta-thalassemia.

ba·sad (bā′săd′) *adj.* Having a direction toward the base of an object or structure.

ba·sal (bā′səl, -zəl) *adj.* **1.** Of, relating to, located at, or forming a base, usually of an organ or a tooth. **2.** Of, relating to, of situated at the lowest level, as of an organ.

basal anesthesia *n.* Parenteral administration of one or more sedatives to produce a state of depressed consciousness short of a general anesthesia.

basal body *n.* A cellular organelle associated with the formation of cilia and flagella and resembling the centriole in structure. Also called *basal granule.*

basal cell *n.* A type of cell found in the deepest layer of the epithelium.

basal cell carcinoma *n.* A slow-growing, locally invasive, but rarely metastasizing neoplasm of the skin derived from basal cells of the epidermis or hair follicles. Also called *basal cell epithelioma.*

basal cell nevus *n.* A hereditary disease characterized by lesions of the eyelids, nose, cheeks, neck, and axillae that are usually benign and that appear as uneroded papules histologically indistinguishable from basal cell epithelioma.

basal-cell nevus syndrome *n.* An inherited syndrome marked by the presence of numerous basal-cell carcinomas of the skin, cysts of the jawbones, erythema-

tous pitting of the palms and soles, and often skeletal anomalies. Also called *Gorlin's syndrome.*

basal ganglia *pl.n.* **1.** The caudate and lentiform nuclei of the brain and the cell groups associated with them, considered as a group. **2.** All of the large masses of gray matter at the base of the cerebral hemisphere. No longer in technical use.

basal granule *n.* See **basal body.**

basal joint reflex *n.* A reflex of the thumb in which the metacarpophalangeal joint flexes and the interphalangeal joint extends in response to firm passive flexion of the third, fourth, or fifth finger. Also called *finger-thumb reflex, Mayer's reflex.*

basal lamina *n.* The ventral division of the lateral walls of the neural tube in the embryo, containing the neuroblasts that give rise to the somatic and visceral motor neurons. Also called *ventral plate of neural tube.*

basal layer *n.* **1.** The outermost layer of the endometrium, which undergoes only minimal changes during the menstrual cycle. **2.** The inner layer of the choroid in contact with the pigmented layer of the retina. Also called *Bruch's membrane, vitreous membrane.* **3.** The inner layer of the ciliary body of the eye, continuous with the basal layer of the choroid. **4.** The deepest layer of the epidermis.

basal metabolic rate *n. Abbr.* **BMR** The rate at which energy is used by an organism at complete rest, measured in humans by the heat given off per unit time, and expressed as the calories released per kilogram of body weight or per square meter of body surface per hour.

basal metabolism *n.* The minimum amount of energy required to maintain vital functions in an organism at complete rest, measured by the basal metabolic rate in a fasting individual.

basal rod *n.* See **costa** (sense 2).

basal vein *n.* A large vein passing caudally and dorsally along the medial surface of the temporal lobe and emptying into the great cerebral vein from the lateral side.

base (bās) *n.* **1.** The part of an organ nearest its point of attachment. **2.** A fundamental ingredient; a chief constituent of a mixture. **3.** Any of a large class of compounds, including the hydroxides and oxides of metals, having a bitter taste, a slippery solution, the capacity to turn litmus blue, and to react with acids to form salts. **4.** A molecular or ionic substance capable of combining with a proton to form a new substance. Also called *Brønsted base.* **5.** A nitrogen-containing organic compound that combines in such a manner. **6.** A substance that provides a pair of electrons for a covalent bond with an acid.

base·ball finger (bās′bôl′) *n.* Permanent flexion of the terminal phalanx of a finger due to a break in the extensor tendon resulting from a blow from a ball or other object. Also called *hammer finger, mallet finger.*

base deficit *n.* A decrease in the total concentration of bicarbonate indicative of metabolic acidosis or of compensated respiratory alkalosis.

Ba·se·dow's disease (băz′ĭ-dōz′, bä′zĭ-) *n.* See **Graves' disease.**

base excess *n.* A measure of metabolic alkalosis based on the amount of strong acid that would have to be added per unit volume of whole blood to titrate it to pH 7.4 while at a specified temperature and carbon dioxide pressure.

base line *n.* **1.** A line corresponding to the base of the skull, passing from the infraorbital ridge to the midline of the occiput, through the ear canal. **2.** A line serving as a basis, as for measurement or calculation.

base·ment membrane (bās′mənt) *n.* A thin, delicate layer of connective tissue underlying the epithelium of many organs. Also called *basilemma.*

base of heart *n.* The part of the heart formed mainly by the left atrium and to a lesser extent by the posterior part of the right atrium, directed backward and to the right, and separated from the vertebral column by the esophagus and aorta.

base of lung *n.* The lower concave part of the lung that rests upon the convex part of the diaphragm.

base of skull *n.* **1.** The interior aspect of the skull, on which the brain rests. **2.** The inferior or external aspect of the skull.

base of stapes *n.* The flat portion of the stirrup of the ear that fits in the oval window between the middle and inner ear. Also called *footplate.*

base pair *n.* The pair of nitrogenous bases that connects the complementary strands of DNA or of double-stranded RNA and consists of a purine linked by hydrogen bonds to a pyrimidine: adenine-thymine and guanine-cytosine in DNA, and adenine-uracil and guanine-cytosine in RNA.

base·plate (bās′plāt′) *n.* **1.** The portion of an artificial denture in contact with the jaw. **2.** A temporary form representing the base of a denture and used to help establish jaw relationships and the arrangement of teeth.

base unit *n.* Any of the fundamental units of length, mass, time, electric current, thermodynamic temperature, amount of substance, or luminous intensity in the International System of Units, consisting respectively of the meter, kilogram, second, ampere, kelvin, mole, and candela.

basi– *or* **baso–** *pref.* **1.** Base; lower part: *basifacial.* **2.** Chemical base; chemically basic: *basophil.*

ba·si·breg·mat·ic axis (bā′sə-brĕg-măt′ĭk) *n.* A vertical line connecting the basion to the bregma; the maximum height of the cranium.

ba·sic (bā′sĭk) *adj.* **1.** Of, being, or serving as a starting point or basis. **2.** Producing, resulting from, or relating to a base. **3.** Containing a base, especially in excess of acid. **4.** Containing oxide or hydroxide anions.

basic cardiac life support *n. Abbr.* **BCLS** Emergency procedures performed to sustain life that include cardiopulmonary resuscitation, control of bleeding, treatment of shock, stabilization of injuries and wounds, and first aid.

basic dye *n.* Any of various usually synthetic dyes that produce brilliant colors, react as bases, and are usually used as stains. Also called *basic stain.*

basic fuchsin *n.* A mixture of rosanilin and pararosanilin chlorides used to stain cellular elements, certain tissues, and bacteria, especially tubercle bacilli.

basic fuchsin-methylene blue stain *n.* A stain that produces differential staining in which nuclei stain purple; collagen and connective tissue stain blue; mitochondria, myelin, and lipid droplets stain red; and cytoplasm, smooth muscle cells, and chrondroblasts stain pink.

ba·si·chro·mat·ic (bā′sĭ-krō-măt′ĭk) *adj.* Easily stained with basic dye.

ba·sic·i·ty (bā-sĭs′ĭ-tē) *n.* **1.** The ability of an acid to react based on the number of replaceable hydrogen atoms it contains. **2.** The quality of being basic.

basic personality type *n.* **1.** An individual's unique, covert, or underlying personality characteristics. **2.** The shared behavioral traits of individuals raised in the same culture and experiencing similar child-rearing practices.

ba·si·cra·ni·al axis (bā′sĭ-krā′nē-əl) *n.* A line connecting the basion to the midpoint of the sphenoethmoidal suture of the cranium.

basicranial flexure *n.* See **pontine flexure.**

basic stain *n.* See **basic dye.**

Ba·sid·i·o·my·ce·tes (bə-sĭd′ē-ō-mī-sē′tēz′) *n.* A large group of fungi including puffballs, shelf fungi, rusts, smuts, and mushrooms that bear sexually produced spores on a basidium.

ba·sid·i·um (bə-sĭd′ē-əm) *n., pl.* **–i·a** (-ē-ə) A small club-shaped structure that typically bears four spores at the tips of minute projections, is unique to Basidiomycetes, and is used as a distinguishing characteristic.

ba·si·fa·cial (bā′sə-fā′shəl) *adj.* Of or relating to the lower portion of the face.

basifacial axis *n.* A line connecting the subnasal point of the cranium to the midpoint of the sphenoethmoidal suture. Also called *facial axis.*

ba·si·hy·al (bā′sə-hī′əl) *adj.* Of or relating to the base or body of the hyoid bone.

ba·si·hy·oid (bā′sə-hī′oid′) *adj.* Basihyal.

bas·i·lar (băs′ə-lər) *adj.* Of, relating to, or located at or near the base, especially the base of the skull.

basilar artery *n.* The union of the two vertebral arteries, running from the lower to the upper border of the pons, with anterior spinal, the two inferior cerebellar, the labyrinthine, pontine, and superior cerebellar branches.

basilar membrane *n.* The membrane that extends from the margin of the bony shelf of the cochlea to its outer wall and on which the sensory cells of the organ of Corti rest.

basilar meningitis *n.* Meningitis at the base of the brain, usually caused by tuberculosis, syphilis, or a low-grade chronic granulomatous condition.

basilar vertebra *n.* The lowest lumbar vertebra.

ba·si·lat·er·al (bā′sə-lăt′ər-əl) *adj.* Variant of **basolateral.**

ba·si·lem·ma (bā′sə-lĕm′ə) *n.* See **basement membrane.**

ba·sil·ic vein (bə-sĭl′ĭk) *n.* A vein that arises on the back of the hand, curves around the medial side of the forearm, and passes up the medial side of the arm to join the axillary vein.

ba·si·on (bā′sē-ŏn′, -zē-) *n.* The middle point on the anterior margin of the great foramen opposite the opisthion.

ba·sip·e·tal (bā-sĭp′ĭ-tl, -zĭp′-) *adj.* Of or relating to the development or maturation of tissues or organs or the movement of substances, such as hormones, from the apex downward toward the base.

ba·si·pho·bi·a (bā′sə-fō′bē-ə) *n.* An abnormal fear of walking or standing erect.

ba·sis (bā′sĭs) *n., pl.* **–ses** (-sēz′) The foundation upon which something, such as an anatomical part, rests.

ba·si·sphe·noid (bā′sĭ-sfē′noid′) *adj.* **1.** Of or relating to the base or body of the sphenoid bone. **2.** Relating to or being the independent center of ossification in the embryo that forms the posterior portion of the body of the sphenoid bone.

ba·si·ver·te·bral vein (bā′sə-vûr′tə-brəl, -vər-tē′brəl) *n.* Any of a number of veins in the spongy substance of the verterbral bodies, emptying into the venous plexus running along the anterior of the vertebral canal to the dura.

bas·ket cell (băs′kĭt) *n.* **1.** Any of the neurons in the cerebellum whose terminal axons form a basketlike network around another cell. **2.** A myoepithelial cell with branching processes that occurs basal to the secretory cells of certain salivary and lacrimal gland alveoli.

baso– *pref.* Variant of **basi–**.

ba·so·e·ryth·ro·cyte (bā′sō-ĭ-rĭth′rə-sīt′) *n.* A red blood cell that shows stippling associated with basic staining granules, representing a condition such as severe anemia, leukemia, or lead poisoning.

ba·so·e·ryth·ro·cy·to·sis (bā′sō-ĭ-rĭth′rə-sī-tō′sĭs) *n.* An increase of red blood cells that show stippling resulting from the presence of basic staining granules and frequently observed in diseases characterized by prolonged hypochromic anemia.

ba·so·lat·er·al *or* **ba·si·lat·er·al** (bā′sə-lăt′ər-əl) *adj.* Of or relating to the base and one or more sides of a part.

ba·so·phil (bā′sə-fĭl) *or* **ba·so·phile** (-fĭl′) *n.* A cell, especially a white blood cell, having granules that stain readily with basic dyes.

basophil adenoma *n.* See **ACTH-producing adenoma**.

ba·so·phil·i·a (bā′sə-fĭl′ē-ə) *n.* **1.** The affinity of cellular structures for basic dyes, such as methylene blue. **2.** An increase in the number of basophils in the circulating blood. Also called *basophilism*. **3.** An abnormal stippling of red blood cells with basic staining granules. —**ba·so·phil′ic** (-fĭl′ĭk) *adj.*

basophilic leukemia *n.* A form of granulocytic leukemia characterized by abnormally large numbers of basophilic granulocytes in the tissues and blood. Also called *mast cell leukemia*.

basophilic leukocyte *n.* A white blood cell having granules that contain histamine and heparin and stain deeply with basic dye. Also called *mast leukocyte*.

basophilic leukopenia *n.* A condition characterized by a decrease in the number of basophilic granulocytes normally present in the blood.

ba·soph·i·lism (bā-sŏf′ə-lĭz′əm) *n.* See **basophilia** (sense 2).

ba·so·squa·mous carcinoma (bā′sə-skwā′məs, -skwä′-) *n.* Carcinoma of the skin that is considered transitional between basal cell and squamous cell carcinoma.

Bas·sen-Korn·zweig syndrome (băs′ən-kôrn′zwīg) *n.* See **abetalipoproteinemia**.

Bas·si·ni's operation (bə-sē′nēz, bä-) *n.* An operation for the radical correction of inguinal hernia.

Bate·son (bāt′sən), **William** 1861–1926. British biologist who was one of the founders of the science of genetics. He experimentally proved Gregor Mendel's theories on heredity and published the first English translation of Mendel's work in 1900.

bath (băth) *n., pl.* **baths** (bă*thz*, băths) **1.** The act of soaking or cleansing the body or any of its parts, as in water. **2.** The apparatus used in giving a bath. **3.** The fluid used to maintain the metabolic activities of an organism.

bath·ing trunk nevus (bā′thĭng) *n.* A congenital nevus that is large, hairy, and pigmented and that usually occurs on the lower trunk of the body. Also called *tierfellnaevus*.

bath itch *n.* See **bath pruritus**.

bath·mo·trop·ic (băth′mə-trŏp′ĭk) *adj.* Influencing the excitability of muscular tissue, especially cardiac muscle.

bath·o·pho·bi·a (băth′ə-fō′bē-ə) *n.* An abnormal fear of depths.

bath pruritus *n.* Itching caused by inadequate rinsing off of soap or by overdrying of skin as a result of excessive bathing. Also called *bath itch*.

bathy– *or* **batho–** *pref.* Deep; depth: *bathophobia*.

bat·o·pho·bi·a (băt′ə-fō′bē-ə) *n.* An abnormal fear of being near an object of great height, such as a skyscraper or mountain.

Bat·ten-May·ou disease (băt′n-mā′ōō) *n.* See **Spielmeyer-Vogt disease**.

bat·tered child (băt′ərd) *n.* A child upon whom multiple, continuing, often serious nonaccidental injuries have been inflicted.

battered child syndrome *n.* A combination of continuing, often serious physical injuries, such as bruises, scratches, hematomas, burns, or malnutrition, inflicted on a child through gross abuse usually by parents, guardians, or other individuals.

battered woman syndrome *n.* A pattern of signs and symptoms, such as fear and a perceived inability to escape, appearing in women who are physically and mentally abused over an extended period by a husband or other dominant individual.

bat·ter·y (băt′ə-rē) *n.* **1.** The act of beating or pounding. **2.** An array of similar things intended for use together, such as achievement tests.

bat·tle·dore placenta (băt′l-dôr′) *n.* A placenta in which the umbilical cord is attached at the border.

bat·tle fatigue *or* **bat·tle neurosis** (băt′l) *n.* See **combat fatigue**.

Baude·locque's operation (bōd-lôks′) *n.* In extrauterine pregnancy, an incision through the posterior culde-sac of the vagina to remove the embryo.

Bau·er's syndrome (bou′ərz) *n.* Aortitis and aortic endocarditis due to rheumatoid arthritis.

Bau·mé (bō-mā′), **Antoine** 1728–1804. French pharmacist who invented a process for making sal ammonia and in 1768 devised an improved hydrometer using the scale that now bears his name.

Baumé scale *n.* A hydrometer scale used to measure the specific gravity of liquids.

Bayle's disease (bālz) *n.* See **general paresis.**

Bay·ley Scales of Infant Development (bā′lē) *pl.n.* Standardized tests used to assess the mental, motor, and behavioral progress of children during the first two and one-half years of life.

Bay·liss (bā′lĭs), Sir **William Maddock** 1860–1924. British physiologist. With Ernest Starling he discovered (1902) secretin. He also developed a treatment for surgical or wound shock in which saline injections replaced lost blood, a technique credited with saving many lives in World War I.

bay·o·net hair (bā′ə-nĭt, -nĕt′, bā′ə-nĕt′) *n.* Hair that is spindle-shaped at its tapered ends because of a developmental defect.

Ba·zin's disease (bə-zănz′, bä-zănz′) *n.* See **erythema induratum.**

BBB *abbr.* blood-brain barrier; bundle-branch block

B cell *n.* 1. See **beta cell.** 2. A type of lymphocyte that, when stimulated by a particular antigen, differentiates into plasma cells that synthesize the antibodies that circulate in the blood and react with the specific antigens. Also called *B lymphocyte.*

BCG *abbr.* bacillus Calmette-Guérin; ballistocardiogram

BCG vaccine *n.* A vaccine containing attenuated human tubercle bacilli that is used for immunization against tuberculosis. Also called *tuberculosis vaccine.*

B chain *n.* A polypeptide component of insulin containing 30 amino acids, the composition of which is species-specific.

BCL2 (bē′sē-ĕl-tōō′) *n.* A gene associated with non-Hodgkin's lymphoma that normally helps regulate the life span of a white blood cell but when mutated prevents such cells from dying, allowing possible further mutations and the development of cancer.

BCLS *abbr.* basic cardiac life support

BCNU (bē′sē′ĕn′yōō′) *n.* See **carmustine.**

B complex *n.* See **vitamin B complex.**

B-DNA (bē′-dē′ĕn-ā′) *n.* The most common form of DNA in living organisms, in which the double helix twists in a right-hand direction.

Be The symbol for the element **beryllium.**

bead·ed (bē′dĭd) *adj.* 1. Having numerous small rounded projections often in a row. 2. Relating to, or being a series of noncontinuous bacterial colonies along the line of inoculation in a stab culture. 3. Of, relating to, or being stained bacteria that have more deeply stained granules occurring at regular intervals.

beaded hair *n.* See **monilethrix.**

bead·ing of ribs (bē′dĭng) *n.* See **rachitic rosary.**

Bea·dle (bēd′l), **George Wells** 1903–1989. American biologist. He shared a 1958 Nobel Prize for discovering how genes transmit hereditary characteristics.

beaked pelvis (bēkt) *n.* See **osteomalacic pelvis.**

beak·er cell (bē′kər) *n.* See **goblet cell.**

B-E amputation *n.* Amputation of arm from below the elbow.

bear·ing down (bâr′ĭng) *n.* Forceful contraction of the abdominal muscles and diaphragm during the second stage of labor, either as a reflex or as a conscious effort.

bearing-down pain *n.* A uterine contraction accompanied by straining and tenesmus, usually appearing in the second stage of labor.

beat (bēt) *v.* 1. To strike repeatedly. 2. To pulsate; throb. —*n.* A stroke, impulse, or pulsation, especially one that produces a sound as of the heart or pulse.

Beau's line (bōz) *n.* Transverse depressions on the fingernails occurring after trauma such as severe febrile disease, malnutrition, or coronary occlusion.

Bech·te·rew-Mendel reflex (bĕk′tə-rĕf-, -rĕv-) *n.* The flexion of the toes caused by percussion of the upper surface of the foot, indicative of lesions of the pyramidal tract. Also called *Mendel-Bechterew reflex.*

Bech·te·rew's disease (bĕk′tə-rĕfs′, -rĕvz′) *n.* See **spondylitis deformans.**

Beck Depression Inventory (bĕk) A trademark for a standardized questionnaire used to diagnose depression.

Beck·er muscular dystrophy (bĕk′ər) *n.* A form of pseudohypertrophic muscular dystrophy that is less severe than Duchenne's muscular dystrophy, in which patients remain ambulatory and usually live until the third or fourth decade.

Beck·er's test (bĕk′ərz) *n.* A test for astigmatism that uses diagrams of sets of three lines radiating in different meridians.

Beck's triad (bĕks) *n.* See **acute compression triad.**

Beck·with-Wie·de·mann syndrome (bĕk′wĭth-wē′də-mən, -vē′də-män′) *n.* See **EMG syndrome.**

Bé·clard's hernia (bā-klärz′) *n.* A femoral hernia through the opening for the great saphenous vein.

bec·lo·meth·a·sone di·pro·pi·o·nate (bĕk′lə-mĕth′ə-sōn′ dī-prō′pē-ə-nāt′, -zōn′) *n.* A corticosteroid usually used as an inhalant to treat asthma.

Bec·o·nase (bĕk′ə-nāz′) A trademark for the drug beclomethasone dipropionate.

bec·que·rel (bĕ-krĕl′, bĕk′ə-rĕl′) *n.* A unit of measurement of radioactivity, equal to one disintegration per second.

bed (bĕd) *n.* 1. A piece of furniture for reclining and sleeping, typically consisting of a flat, rectangular frame and a mattress resting on springs. 2. Such a piece of furniture used for rest, recuperation, or treatment. 3. A supporting, underlying, or securing base or structure, especially an anatomical one.

BED *abbr.* binge eating disorder

bed·bug (bĕd′bŭg′) *n.* A wingless, odorous insect with a flat, reddish body that infests dwellings and bedding and feeds on human blood.

Bed·nar's aphthae (bĕd′närz) *n.* Aphthae affecting the newborn, consisting of two patches, one on either side of the median raphe of the palate.

bed·pan (bĕd′păn′) *n.* A metal, glass, or plastic receptacle for the urinary and fecal discharges of persons confined to bed.

bed·rid·den (bĕd′rĭd′n) *or* **bed·rid** (-rĭd′) *adj.* Confined to bed because of illness or infirmity.

bed·side manner (bĕd′sīd′) *n.* The attitude and conduct of a physician in the presence of a patient.

Bed·so·ni·a (bĕd-sō′nē-ə) *n.* See **Chlamydia.**

bed·sore (bĕd′sôr′) *n.* A pressure-induced ulceration of the skin occurring in persons confined to bed for long periods of time. Also called *decubitus ulcer, pressure sore.*

bed-wet·ting (bĕd′wĕt′ĭng) *n.* Involuntary discharge of urine, especially when occurring nocturnally during sleep. Also called *nocturnal enuresis.*

Beer's operation (bārz) *n.* A flap amputation for treatment of a cataract.

Bee·vor's sign (bē′vərz) *n.* An indication of paralysis of the lower portions of the straight muscles of the abdomen in which the navel moves upward.

be·hav·ior (bĭ-hāv′yər) *n.* **1.** The actions or reactions of persons or things in response to external or internal stimuli. **2.** The manner in which one behaves. —**be·hav′ior·al** *adj.*

behavioral genetics *n.* The study of the genetic underpinnings of behavioral phenotypes such as eating or mating activity, substance abuse, social attitudes, violence, and mental abilities.

behavioral immunogen *n.* A lifestyle or pattern of behavior associated with greater longevity and decreased risk for illness.

behavioral medicine *n.* The application of behavior therapy techniques, such as biofeedback and relaxation training, to the prevention and treatment of medical and psychosomatic disorders and to the treatment of undesirable behaviors, such as overeating. Also called *behavior medicine.*

behavioral pathogen *n.* The lifestyle and pattern of behavior associated with an increased risk of physical illness and dysfunction.

behavioral psychology *n.* See **behaviorism.**

behavior disorder *n.* **1.** Any of various forms of behavior that are considered inappropriate by members of the social group to which an individual belongs. **2.** A functional disorder or abnormality.

be·hav·ior·ism (bĭ-hāv′yə-rĭz′əm) *n.* A school of psychology that confines itself to the study of observable and quantifiable aspects of behavior and excludes subjective phenomena, such as emotions or motives. Also called *behavioral psychology.*

behavior medicine *n.* See **behavioral medicine.**

behavior modification *n.* **1.** The use of basic learning techniques, such as conditioning, biofeedback, reinforcement, or aversion therapy, in order to teach simple skills or alter undesirable behavior. **2.** See **behavior therapy.**

behavior therapy *n.* A form of psychotherapy that uses basic learning techniques to modify maladaptive behavior patterns by substituting new responses to given stimuli for undesirable ones. Also called *behavior modification.* —**behavior therapist** *n.*

Beh·çet's syndrome (bĕch′ĕts′, bĕ-chĕts′) *n.* Recurrent attacks of genital and oral ulcerations and uveitis or iridocyclitis with hypopyon, often accompanied by arthritis.

Beh·ring (bâr′ĭng, bĕr′-), **Emil Von** 1854–1917. German physiologist. He won a 1901 Nobel Prize for work on serum immunization against diphtheria and tetanus.

Beh·ring's law (bâr′ĭngz, bĕr′-) *n.* The principle stating that parenteral administration of serum from a person immunized to a particular disease provides the recipient with passive immunity.

Bé·ké·sy (bā′kā-shē), **Georg von** 1899–1972. Hungarian-born American physiologist. He won a 1961 No-

bel Prize for discoveries concerning the mechanisms of stimulation that occur within the cochlea of the ear.

Bekh·te·rev (bĕk′tə-rĕf, -rĕv), **Vladimir Mikhailovich** 1857–1927. Russian neuropathologist noted for his studies of the pathology and anatomy of the nervous system. His applications of the principles of conditioned responses influenced the development of behaviorism in the United States.

bel (bĕl) *n.* A unit expressing the relative intensity of a sound, equal to ten decibels.

belch (bĕlch) *v.* To expel stomach gas noisily through the mouth; burp.

Bell (bĕl), Sir **Charles** 1774–1842. British anatomist and surgeon who published detailed anatomies of the nervous system and the brain. He was the first to distinguish between sensory and motor nerves. Bell's Law and Bell's palsy are named for him.

bel·la·don·na (bĕl′ə-dŏn′ə) *n.* **1.** A poisonous Eurasian perennial herb having usually solitary, purplish-brown, bell-shaped flowers and glossy black berries. Also called *deadly nightshade.* **2.** An alkaloidal extract or tincture derived from this plant.

belladonna alkaloids *pl.n.* A group of alkaloids, including atropine and scopolamine, found in plants such as belladonna, used to dilate the pupils, dry respiratory passages, prevent motion sickness, and relieve cramping of the intestines and bladder.

belle in·dif·fér·ence (bĕl′ ăɴ-dē-fâ-räɴs′) *n.* See **la belle indifference.**

Bel·li·ni (bə-lē′nē), **Lorenzo** 1643–1704. Italian anatomist known for his description of the anatomy of the kidney and his investigation into the sense of taste. Bellini's duct is named for him.

Bel·li·ni's duct (bə-lē′nēz) *n.* One of the straight collecting tubules of the kidney.

Bell's Law (bĕlz) *n.* A law stating that the anterior or ventral roots of the spinal nerves are motor and the posterior or dorsal roots are sensory.

Bell's muscle *n.* A band of muscular fibers forming a slight fold in the wall of the bladder, running from the uvula vesicae to the opening of the ureter on either side, and bounding the trigonum.

Bell's palsy *n.* See **facial palsy.**

bel·ly (bĕl′ē) *n.* **1.** See **abdomen. 2.** The stomach. **3.** The womb; the uterus. **4.** The bulging, central part of a muscle. Also called *venter.*

bel·ly·ache (bĕl′ē-āk′) *n.* Pain in the stomach or abdomen; colic.

bel·ly·but·ton (bĕl′ē-bŭt′n) *n.* See **navel.**

bel·o·ne·pho·bi·a (bĕl′ə-nə-fō′bē-ə) *n.* An abnormal fear of sharply pointed objects, especially needles.

Bel·sey operation (bĕl′sē) *n.* A transthoracic procedure for the treatment of sliding hiatal hernia.

Ben·a·cer·raf (bĕn-ăs′ər-əf), **Baruj** Born 1920. Venezuelan-born American immunologist. He shared a 1980 Nobel Prize for discoveries concerning cell structure that enhanced understanding of the immunological system, resulting in higher success rates in organ transplantation.

Ben·a·dryl (bĕn′ə-drĭl) A trademark for a hydrochloride of diphenhydramine.

be·na·ze·pril hydrochloride (bə-nā′zə-prĭl′) *n.* An ACE inhibitor drug used in the treatment of hypertension, congestive failure, and other cardiovascular disorders.

Bence-Jones protein (bĕns′jōnz′) *n.* A protein with high thermosolubility occurring in the serum and urine of patients with certain diseases, especially multiple myeloma.

Bence-Jones proteinuria *n.* The presence of Bence-Jones proteins in the urine, usually indicative of multiple myeloma, amyloidosis, or Waldenström's macroglobulinemia.

Bence-Jones reaction *n.* The test used to determine the presence of Bence-Jones proteins in the urine.

bend (bĕnd) *v.* To incline the body; stoop.

Ben·der gestalt test (bĕn′dər) *n.* A test of visuospatial and visuomotor coordination used to detect brain damage by measuring a person's ability to copy a set of geometric designs.

bend·ing fracture (bĕn′dĭng) *n.* A curving of a long bone due to multiple minute fractures.

bends (bĕndz) *n.* See **decompression sickness.**

Ben·e·dict's test (bĕn′ĭ-dĭkts′) *n.* A test for detecting glucose in urine in which urine is heated with a blue solution containing sodium carbonate, sodium citrate, and copper sulfate, producing a red, yellow, or orange precipitate in the presence of glucose.

Ben·Gay (bĕn′gā′) An over-the-counter preparation containing menthol and methyl salicylate.

be·nign (bĭ-nīn′) *adj.* Of no danger to health, especially relating to a tumorous growth; not malignant.

benign hypertension *n.* Essential hypertension that runs a relatively long and symptomless course.

benign inoculation lymphoreticulosis *n.* See **cat scratch disease.**

benign juvenile melanoma *n.* A benign, slightly pigmented or red superficial skin tumor composed of spindle-shaped, epithelioid, and multinucleated cells and seen usually in children.

benign migratory glossitis *n.* See **geographical tongue.**

benign mucosal pemphigoid *n.* A chronic disease that produces progressive scarring and shrinkage of the conjunctivae and denuded areas in the mucous membrane of the mouth.

benign myalgic encephalomyelitis *n.* See **epidemic neuromyasthenia.**

benign prostatic hyperplasia *n. Abbr.* **BPH** A nonmalignant enlargement of the prostate gland commonly occurring in men after the age of 50, and sometimes leading to compression of the urethra and obstruction of the flow of urine.

benign tumor *n.* A tumor that does not metastasize or invade and destroy adjacent normal tissue.

Ben·nett's fracture (bĕn′ĭt) *n.* A dislocation fracture of the first metacarpal bone at the carpal-metacarpal joint.

ben·ox·a·pro·fen (bĕ-nŏk′sə-prō′fən) *n.* A nonsteroidal, anti-inflammatory, analgesic agent.

Ben·son's disease (bĕn′sənz) *n.* See **asteroid hyalosis.**

ben·tir·o·mide (bĕn-tîr′ə-mīd′) *n.* A peptide used as a screening test for exocrine pancreatic insufficiency and to monitor the adequacy of supplemental pancreatic therapy.

bentiromide test *n.* A test of pancreatic exocrine function in which orally administered bentiromide is cleaved by chymotrypsin within the lumen of the small intestine, releasing *p*-aminobenzoic acid. Diminished urinary excretion of *p*-aminobenzoic acid may indicate pancreatic insufficiency.

ben·ton·ite flocculation test (bĕn′tə-nīt′) *n.* A flocculation test for rheumatoid arthritis in which sensitized bentonite particles are added to inactivated serum; if half of the particles are clumped while the other half remain in suspension, the test is positive.

Ben·tyl (bĕn′tĭl) A trademark for the drug dicyclomine hydrochloride.

benz·al·ko·ni·um chloride (bĕn′zăl-kō′nē-əm) *n.* A powder prepared in an aqueous solution and used as a fungicide, bactericide, and spermicide.

benz·an·thra·cene (bĕn-zăn′thrə-sēn′) *or* **benz·an·threne** (-thrēn′) *n.* A crystalline, weakly carcinogenic cyclic hydrocarbon.

ben·zene (bĕn′zēn′, bĕn-zēn′) *n.* A clear, colorless, highly refractive flammable liquid derived from petroleum and used in or to manufacture a wide variety of chemical products, including DDT, insecticides, and motor fuels. Also called *benzine.*

benzene ring *n.* The hexagonal ring structure in the benzene molecule and its substitutional derivatives, each vertex of which is occupied and distinguished by a carbon atom.

ben·ze·tho·ni·um chloride (bĕn′zə-thō′nē-əm) *n.* A synthetic quaternary ammonium compound used as a germicide and bacteriostat.

ben·zi·dine (bĕn′zĭ-dēn′) *n.* A yellowish, white, or reddish-gray crystalline powder used in dyes and to detect blood.

ben·zim·id·az·ole (bĕn′zə-mĭ-dăz′ō′, -mĭd′ə-zōl′) *n.* A crystalline compound that is used in organic synthesis and that inhibits the growth of certain microorganisms and parasitic worms.

ben·zine (bĕn′zēn′, bĕn-zēn′) *or* **ben·zin** (bĕn′zĭn) *n.* **1.** A colorless, flammable, liquid mixture of hydrocarbons obtained in distilling petroleum, used in cleaning and dyeing and as a motor fuel; naphtha. Also called *petroleum benzin.* **2.** See **benzene.**

benzo– *or* **benz–** *pref.* Benzene; benzoic acid: *benzodiazepine.*

ben·zo·ate (bĕn′zō-āt′) *n.* A salt or ester of benzoic acid.

ben·zo·caine (bĕn′zə-kān′) *n.* The white, odorless, tasteless crystalline ester of *para*-aminobenzoate, used as a local anesthetic.

ben·zo·di·az·e·pine (bĕn′zō-dī-ăz′ə-pēn′, -pĭn) *n.* Any of a group of psychotropic agents used as antianxiety agents, muscle relaxants, sedatives, and hypnotics.

ben·zo·ic acid (bĕn-zō′ĭk) *n.* An aromatic white crystalline acid used to season tobacco and in perfumes, dentifrices, and germicides.

ben·zo·na·tate (bĕn-zō′nə-tāt′) *n.* A colorless to faintly yellow oil that is soluble in most organic solvents and is used as an antitussive drug.

ben·zo·py·rene (bĕn′zō-pī′rēn′, -pī-rēn′) *n.* A yellow, crystalline, aromatic hydrocarbon that is a carcinogen found in coal tar and cigarette smoke.

ben·zo·sul·fi·mide (bĕn′zō-sŭl′fə-mīd′, -mĭd) *n.* See saccharin.

ben·zo·thi·a·di·a·zide (bĕn′zō-thī′ə-dī′ə-zīd′) *n.* Any of a group of diuretics that increase both sodium and chloride excretion and the volume of water excreted. Also called *thiazide.*

ben·zo·yl (bĕn′zō-ĭl′, -zoil′) *n.* The univalent radical $C_6H_5ICO^-$ derived from benzoic acid.

benzoyl peroxide *n.* A flammable white granular solid used as a bleaching agent for flour, fats, waxes, and oils, and in pharmaceuticals.

ben·zyl (bĕn′zĭl, -zēl′) *n.* The univalent radical $C_6H_5CH_2^-$ that is derived from toluene. —**ben·zyl′·ic** (-zĭl′ĭk) *adj.*

ben·zyl·i·dene (bĕn-zĭl′ĭ-dēn′) *n.* The divalent hydrocarbon radical $C_6H_5CH.$

ben·zyl·pen·i·cil·lin (bĕn′zĭl-pĕn′ĭ-sĭl′ĭn) *n.* See penicillin G.

ber·ber·ine (bûr′bə-rēn′) *n.* A bitter-tasting yellow plant alkaloid used as an antipyretic and antibacterial agent.

Berg (bûrg), **Paul** Born 1926. American chemist. He shared a 1980 Nobel Prize for developing recombinant methods of inserting genes from simple organisms into the genetic material of similar organisms.

Ber·gey (bûr′gē), **David Hendricks** 1860–1937. American bacteriologist noted for his study of hygiene and classifications of bacteria.

Berg·strom (bĕrg′strəm), **Sune Karl** 1916–2004. Swedish biochemist and physician. He shared a 1982 Nobel Prize for research into the chemical structure of prostaglandins.

ber·i·ber·i (bĕr′ē-bĕr′ē) *n.* A disease caused by a deficiency of thiamine, endemic in eastern and southern Asia, and characterized by neurological symptoms, cardiovascular abnormalities, and edema. Also called *endemic neuritis.*

ber·ke·li·um (bər-kē′lē-əm, bûrk′lē-əm) *n. Symbol* **Bk** A synthetic radioactive element. Its most stable isotope, Bk 247, has a half-life of 1,380 years. Atomic number 97.

Ber·lin blue (bûr-lĭn′) *n.* An insoluble dark blue pigment and dye, ferric ferrocyanide or one of its modifications. Also called *Prussian blue.*

ber·loque dermatitis (bər-lŏk′) *or* **ber·lock dermatitis** (bûr′lŏk′) *n.* A skin disorder characterized by brown pigmented patches that appear after an individual has been exposed to certain essential oils in perfume and then to sunlight.

Ber·nard (bĕr-när′), **Claude** 1813–1878. French physiologist noted for his study of the digestive and nervous systems.

Ber·nard-Cannon homeostasis (bĕr-när′-) *n.* The set of mechanisms by which cybernetic adjustment of physiological and biochemical states is made in postnatal life.

Bern·hardt's disease (bûrn′härts′, bĕrn′-) *n.* See meralgia paraesthetica.

Ber·noul·li's law (bər-nōō′lēz) *n.* **1.** An expression of the conservation of energy for any incompressible flowing fluid in terms of its pressure, velocity, density, acceleration, and vertical height. **2.** See **law of large numbers.**

Bern·stein test (bûrn′stīn′, -stēn′) *n.* A test to establish that substernal pain is due to reflux esophagitis, performed by instillation of a weak solution of hydrochloric acid directly into the lower esophagus. The symptoms disappear when the acid solution is replaced by normal saline solution. Also called *acid perfusion test.*

ber·ry aneurysm (bĕr′ē) *n.* A small saccular aneurysm of a cerebral artery that resembles a berry.

Ber·ti·el·la (bûr′tē-ĕl′ə) *n.* A genus of tapeworm parasitic in humans and higher primates.

ber·ti·el·lo·sis (bûr′tē-ə-lō′sĭs) *n.* The infection of primates, including humans, with tapeworms of the genus *Bertiella.*

be·ryl·li·o·sis (bə-rĭl′ē-ō′sĭs) *n.* Beryllium poisoning characterized by the occurrence of granulomatous fibrosis, especially of the lungs, due to inhalation of beryllium salts.

be·ryl·li·um (bə-rĭl′ē-əm) *n. Symbol* **Be** A lightweight, corrosion-resistant, toxic and possibly carcinogenic metallic element used in making precision instruments. Atomic number 4.

Bes·nier-Boeck-Schaumann disease *or* **Bes·nier-Boeck-Schaumann syndrome** (bĕ-nyā′-) *n.* See **sarcoidosis.**

Best (bĕst), **Charles Herbert** 1899–1978. American-born Canadian physiologist noted for the discovery and successful clinical application of insulin.

bes·ti·al·i·ty (bĕs′chē-ăl′ĭ-tē, bēs′-) *n.* **1.** The quality or condition of being an animal or like an animal. **2.** Conduct or an action marked by depravity or brutality. **3.** Sexual relations between a human and an animal.

Best's disease (bĕsts) *n.* Congenital degeneration of the macula of the retina occurring during the first few years of life.

be·ta (bā′tə, bē′-) *n.* **1.** *Symbol* **β** The second letter of the Greek alphabet. **2.** The second item in a series or system of classification. **3.** A beta particle. **4.** A beta ray. —*adj.* **1.** Of or relating to the second position from a designated carbon atom in an organic molecule at which an atom or a radical may be substituted. **2.** Of or relating to an isomeric variation of a chemical compound, such as a stereoisomer.

beta-adrenergic *adj.* Of, relating to, or being a beta-adrenergic receptor.

beta-adrenergic blocking agent *n.* See **beta-blocker.**

beta-adrenergic receptor *n.* Any of various cell membrane receptors that can bind with epinephrine and related substances that activate or block the actions of cells containing such receptors. These cells initiate physiological responses such as increasing the rate and force of contraction of the heart as well as relaxing bronchial and vascular smooth muscle. Also called *beta-receptor.*

beta-agonist *n.* An agent, such as albuterol, that stimulates beta-receptors in the autonomic nervous system.

beta-amyloid protein *n.* An amyloid that circulates in human blood and in cerebrospinal fluid and is deposited into plaques that are found in the brains of patients with Alzheimer's disease. Also called *amyloid beta-protein.*

beta-blocker *n.* A drug that opposes the excitatory effects of norepinephrine released from sympathetic nerve endings at beta-adrenergic receptors and is used for the treatment of angina, hypertension, arrhythmia, and migraine. Also called *beta-adrenergic blocking agent.*

beta–carotene *n.* An isomer of carotene.

beta cell *n.* 1. Any of the basophilic chromophil cells located in the anterior lobe of the pituitary gland. 2. Any of the insulin-producing cells of the islets of Langerhans in the pancreas. Also called *B cell.*

be·ta·cism (bā′tə-sĭz′əm, bē′-) *n.* A defect in speech in which the sound of *b* is given to other consonants.

Be·ta·dine (bā′tə-dīn′) An trademark for an over-the-counter preparation of povidone iodine.

beta-endorphin *n.* An endorphin produced by the pituitary gland that is a potent pain suppressant.

beta fiber *n.* A nerve fiber having a conduction velocity of about 40 meters per second.

be·ta·fruc·to·fu·ran·o·sid·ase (bā′tə-frŭk′tō-fyə-răn′ō-sī′dās′, -dāz′) *n.* See **invertase.**

beta globulin *n.* A type of globulin in blood plasma that in electrically charged solutions exhibits colloidal mobility between that of the alpha and gamma globulins.

beta-glucuronidase *n.* An enzyme the catalyzes the hydrolysis of various proteoglycans.

beta granule *n.* A granule of a beta cell.

beta-hemolytic streptococci *pl.n.* Streptococci that lyse red blood cells cultured on blood agar medium, producing a clear area around the cell colonies.

be·ta·ine (bē′tə-ēn′, -ĭn) *n.* A sweet crystalline alkaloid occurring in sugar beets and other plants and used in the treatment of muscular degeneration.

betaine hydrochloride *n.* An acidifying agent used in the treatment of achlorhydria and hypochlorhydria.

beta-interferon *n.* A family of glycoproteins that are produced by fibroblasts, have antiviral properties, and are used in the treatment of multiple sclerosis.

beta-lactam *n.* Any of a class of broad-spectrum antibiotics that are structurally and pharmacologically related to the penicillins and cephalosporins.

be·ta·lac·ta·mase (bā′tə-lăk′tə-mās′, -māz′) *n.* Any of various enzymes that are produced by gram-negative bacteria and hydrolyze lactam rings, thereby inactivating penicillin and cephalosporin antibiotics. Also called *cephalosporinase, penicillinase.*

beta-lipoprotein *n.* See **low-density lipoprotein.**

be·ta·meth·a·sone (bā′tə-mĕth′ə-sōn′, bē′-) *n.* A synthetic crystalline glucocorticoid powder used as a topical anti-inflammatory agent for the treatment of dermatological conditions.

beta particle *n.* A high-speed electron or positron, especially one emitted from the nucleus of an atom in radioactive decay.

beta ray *n.* A stream of beta particles, especially of electrons.

beta-receptor *n.* See **beta-adrenergic receptor.**

beta rhythm *n.* The second most common waveform occurring in electroencephalograms of the adult brain, characteristically having a frequency from 13 to 30 hertz. It is associated with an alert waking state but can also occur as a sign of anxiety or apprehension. Also called *beta wave.*

be·ta·tron (bā′tə-trŏn′, bē′-) *n.* A magnetic induction device capable of accelerating electrons to energies of several hundred million electron volts.

beta wave *n.* See **beta rhythm.**

be·tax·o·lol hydrochloride (bā-tăk′sə-lôl, bē-) *n.* A beta-adrenergic blocking agent used to treat ocular hypertension and chronic open-angle glaucoma.

be·than·e·chol (bĕ-thăn′ĭ-kôl′) *n.* A cholinergic drug that stimulates the parasympathetic nervous system and is used in the form of its chloride to treat abdominal distention and urinary retention.

Be·thes·da unit (bə-thĕz′də) *n.* A measure of inhibitor activity expressed as the amount of inhibitor that will inactivate 50 percent or 0.5 unit of a coagulation factor during a given incubation period.

Be·top·tic S (bā-tŏp′tĭk ĕs′) A trademark for the drug betaxolol hydrochloride.

be·tween·brain (bĭ-twēn′brān′) *n.* See **diencephalon.**

Betz cell (bĕts) *n.* Any of the large pyramidal cells in the motor area of the cerebral cortex.

Beu·ren syndrome (byoor′ən) *n.* Supravalvular aortic stenosis with multiple areas of peripheral pulmonary arterial stenosis accompanied by mental retardation and dental anomalies.

be·zoar (bē′zôr′) *n.* A hard indigestible mass of material, such as hair, vegetable fibers, or the seeds and skins of fruits, formed in the alimentary canal.

Be·zold's abscess (bā′zōlts) *n.* An abscess deep in the neck associated with suppuration in the mastoid cells.

B fiber *n.* Any of the myelinated nerve fibers in autonomic nerves, having a diameter of 2 microns or less, conducting nerve impulses at a rate of 3 to 15 meters per second.

BGH *abbr.* bovine growth hormone

Bh The symbol for the element **bohrium.**

BHA (bē′ăch-ā′) *n.* A white, waxy phenolic antioxidant used to preserve fats and oils, especially in foods.

BHT (bē′ăch-tē′) *n.* A crystalline phenolic antioxidant used to preserve fats and oils, especially in foods.

Bi The symbol for the element **bismuth.**

bi–[1] *or* **bin–** *pref.* 1. Two: *bilateral.* 2. Both: *binaural.* 3. Both sides, parts, or directions: *biconcave.* 4. Containing twice the proportion of a specified chemical element or group necessary for stability: *bicarbonate.* 5. Containing two chemical atoms, radicals, or groups: *biphenyl.*

bi–[2] *pref.* Variant of **bio–.**

Bi·an·chi's nodule (bē-ăng′kēz, byäng′kēz) *n.* See **nodule of semilunar valve.**

bi·ar·tic·u·lar (bī′är-tĭk′yə-lər) *adj.* Relating to two joints; diarthric.

bi·au·ric·u·lar axis (bī′ô-rĭk′yə-lər) *n.* A straight line connecting the auricles of the ears.

bi·ax·i·al joint (bī-ăk′sē-əl) *n.* A joint in which there are two principal axes of movement situated at right angles to each other.

Bi·ax·in (bī-ăk′sĭn) A trademark for the drug clarithromycin.

bib. *abbr. Latin* bibe (drink)

bi-bi reaction (bī′bī′) *n.* A reaction catalyzed by a single enzyme and involving two substrates and two products.

bib·li·o·ther·a·py (bĭb′lē-ō-thĕr′ə-pē) *n.* A form of psychotherapy in which selected reading materials are used to assist a person in solving personal problems or for other therapeutic purposes.

bi·cam·er·al (bī-kăm′ər-əl) *adj.* Composed of or having two chambers, especially an abscess divided by a septum.

bi·cap·su·lar (bī-kăp′sə-lər) *adj.* Having a double capsule.

bi·car·bon·ate (bī-kär′bə-nāt′, -nĭt) *n.* The radical group HCO₃ or a compound, such as sodium bicarbonate, containing it.

bi·cel·lu·lar (bī-sĕl′yə-lər) *adj.* Having two cells or subdivisions.

bi·ceps (bī′sĕps′) *n., pl.* **biceps** *or* **–ceps·es** (-sĕp′sĭz) **1.** A muscle with two heads or points of origin. **2.** The biceps brachii. **3.** The biceps femoris. —**bi·cip′i·tal** (-sĭp′ĭ-tl) *adj.*

biceps bra·chi·i (brā′kē-ī′, -kē-ē′, brăk′ē-ī′, -ē-ē′) *n.* A muscle whose long head has origin from the supraglenoidal tuberosity of the scapula and whose short head has origin from the coracoid process, with insertion into the tuberosity of the radius, with nerve supply from the musculocutaneous nerve, and whose action flexes and supinates the forearm.

biceps fem·or·is (fĕm′ər-ĭs) *n.* A muscle whose long head has origin from the tuberosity of the ischium and whose short head has origin from the lower half of the lateral lip of the linea aspera, with insertion into the head of the fibula, with nerve supply from the tibial nerve for the long head and from the peroneal nerve for the short head, and whose action flexes the knee and rotates the leg laterally.

biceps reflex *n.* Contraction of the biceps muscle when its tendon is struck.

Bi·chat (bē-shä′), **Marie François Xavier** 1771–1802. French physiologist and anatomist who pioneered the histological study of organs.

Bi·chat's fissure (bē-shäz′) *n.* The nearly circular fissure corresponding to the medial margin of the pallium, marking the hilum of the cerebral hemisphere.

Bichat's membrane *n.* The inner elastic membrane of arteries.

bi·chro·mate (bī-krō′māt′, -mĭt) *n.* See **dichromate**.

bi·cip·i·tal rib (bī-sĭp′ĭ-tl) *n.* Fusion of the first thoracic rib with the corresponding cervical vertebra.

bi·clo·nal·i·ty (bī′klō-năl′ĭ-tē) *n.* A condition in which some cells have markers of one cell line and other cells have markers of another cell line, as in biclonal leukemias. —**bi·clon′al** (-klō′nəl) *adj.*

bi·con·cave (bī′kŏn-kāv′, bī-kŏn′kāv′) *adj.* Concave on both sides or surfaces.

biconcave lens *n.* A lens that is concave on two opposing surfaces. Also called *concavo-concave lens.*

bi·con·dy·lar joint (bī-kŏn′də-lər) *n.* A joint in which two rounded surfaces of one bone articulate with shallow depressions on another bone.

bi·con·vex (bī′kŏn-vĕks′, bī-kŏn′vĕks′) *adj.* Convex on both sides or surfaces.

biconvex lens *n.* A lens with both surfaces convex. Also called *convexo-convex lens.*

bi·cor·nate uterus (bī-kôr′nāt′, -nĭt) *n.* A uterus that is divided into two lateral horns as a result of imperfect fusion of the paramesonephric ducts.

bi·cor·nu·ate (bī-kôr′nyo͞o-ĭt, -āt′) *adj.* **1.** Having two horns or horn-shaped parts. **2.** Shaped like a crescent. —**bi·cor′nu·ous** (-əs) *adj.*

bi·cus·pid (bī-kŭs′pĭd) *adj.* Having two points or cusps. —*n.* See **premolar**.

bicuspid valve *n.* See **mitral valve**.

b.i.d. *abbr. Latin* bis in die (twice a day)

bi·dac·ty·ly (bī-dăk′tə-lē) *n.* Congenital absence of all fingers or toes except the first and fifth digits.

bi·di·rec·tion·al ventricular tachycardia (bī′dĭ-rĕk′-shə-nəl, -dī-) *n.* Ventricular tachycardia in which the QRS complexes in the electrocardiogram are alternately positive and negative.

bi·dis·coi·dal placenta (bī′dĭ-skoid′l) *n.* A placenta with two separate disc-shaped portions attached to opposite walls of the uterus, occasionally found in humans.

BIDS (bĭdz) *n.* A congenital condition resulting from a deficiency of high-sulfur protein and characterized by brittle hair, impaired intelligence, decreased fertility, and short stature.

Biel·schow·sky's disease (bē′ĕl-shō′skēz, bēl-shôv′-skēz) *n.* See **Jansky-Bielschowsky disease**.

Bier·nac·ki's sign (byĕr-nät′skēz) *n.* Analgesia of the ulnar nerve occurring in cases of tabes dorsalis and general paresis.

Bier's method (bîrz) *n.* A method for administering anesthesia to a part through intravenous injections of anesthesia after the part has been constricted and elevated so as to be exsanguinated.

bi·fid (bī′fĭd) *adj.* Forked or split into two parts.

bifid cranium *n.* See **encephalocele**.

bifid tongue *n.* A tongue whose tip is divided longitudinally for a certain distance. Also called *cleft tongue, diglossia.*

bi·fo·cal (bī-fō′kəl, bī′fō′-) *adj.* **1.** Having two focal lengths. **2.** Having one section that corrects for distant vision and another that corrects for near vision.

bifocal lens *n.* A lens having one section that corrects for distant vision and another section that corrects for near vision.

bi·fo·rate (bī-fôr′āt′) *adj.* Having two openings.

bi·fur·cate (bī′fər-kāt′, bī-fûr′-) *v.* To divide into two parts or branches. —*adj.* (-kāt′, -kĭt) Forked or divided into two parts or branches.

bi·fur·ca·tion (bī′fər-kā′shən) *n.* A division into two branches; a forking.

bi·gem·i·nal (bī-jĕm′ə-nəl) *adj.* Occurring in pairs; doubled or twinned.

bigeminal pulse *n.* A pulse in which the beats occur in pairs followed by a pause. Also called *coupled pulse.*

bigeminal rhythm *n.* Cardiac rhythm in which a normal heartbeat is followed by a premature beat, so that the heartbeats occur in pairs. Also called *coupled rhythm, coupling.*

bi·gem·i·ny (bī-jĕm′ə-nē) *n.* **1.** An association in pairs. **2.** A bigeminal pulse.

big toe *n.* The largest and innermost toe of the human foot.

bi·lat·er·al (bī-lăt′ər-əl) *adj.* **1.** Having or formed of two sides; two-sided. **2.** Having or marked by bilateral symmetry.

bilateral hermaphroditism *n.* Hermaphroditism with testicular and ovarian tissue occurring on both sides of the body.

bilateral symmetry *n.* Symmetrical arrangement, as of an organism or a body part, along a central axis, so that the body is divided into equivalent right and left halves by only one plane.

bi·lay·er (bī′lā′ər) *n.* A structure, such as a film or membrane, consisting of two molecular layers.

bile (bīl) *n.* **1.** A bitter, alkaline, brownish-yellow or greenish-yellow fluid that is secreted by the liver, stored in the gallbladder, and discharged into the duodenum and aids in the emulsification, digestion, and absorption of fats. Also called *gall.* **2.** Either of two bodily humors, black bile or yellow bile, in ancient and medieval physiology.

bile acid *n.* Any of several acids formed in the liver that commonly occur in the bile in combination with glycine or taurine as sodium salts.

bile canaliculus *n.* See **biliary canaliculus.**

bile duct *or* **biliary duct** *n.* Any of the excretory ducts in the liver that convey bile between the liver and the intestine, including the hepatic, cystic, and common bile ducts. Also called *gall duct.*

bile pigment *n.* Any of the coloring materials in the bile derived from porphyrins, such as bilirubin.

bile salt *n.* **1.** Any of the sodium salts of the bile acids, such as taurocholate and glycocholate, occurring in bile. **2.** A mixture, such as a commercial preparation derived from the bile of the ox, that is used medicinally as a hepatic stimulant or laxative.

Bil·har·zi·a (bĭl-här′zē-ə) *n.* See **Schistosoma.**

bil·har·zi·al dysentery (bĭl-här′zē-əl) *n.* Intestinal damage or hemorrhage that is caused by passage of the spined eggs of certain trematode worms of the genus *Schistosoma.*

bil·har·zi·a·sis (bĭl′här-zī′ə-sĭs) *n.* See **schistosomiasis.**

bili– *pref.* Bile: *biliuria.*

bil·i·ar·y (bĭl′ē-ĕr′ē) *adj.* **1.** Of or relating to bile, the bile ducts, or the gallbladder. **2.** Transporting bile.

biliary atresia *n.* Atresia of the major bile ducts resulting in cholestasis and jaundice.

biliary calculus *n.* See **gallstone.**

biliary canaliculus *n.* Any of the intercellular channels between liver cells. Also called *bile canaliculus.*

biliary cirrhosis *n.* Cirrhosis due to obstruction or infection of the bile ducts.

biliary duct *n.* Variant of **bile duct.**

biliary ductule *n.* Any of the excretory ducts of the liver that connect the interlobular ductules to the right or left hepatic duct.

biliary dyskinesia *n.* Spasms of the gallbladder or its ducts that impair filling or emptying and are caused by intrinsic or extrinsic disease.

biliary xanthomatosis *n.* Xanthomatosis with hypercholesterolemia caused by biliary cirrhosis.

bil·i·gen·e·sis (bĭl′ĭ-jĕn′ĭ-sĭs) *n.* The production of bile. —**bil′i·gen′ic** (-ĭk) *adj.*

bil·ious (bĭl′yəs) *adj.* **1.** Of, relating to, or containing bile; biliary. **2.** Characterized by an excess secretion of bile. **3.** Relating to, characterized by, or experiencing gastric distress caused by a disorder of the liver or gallbladder.

bil·i·ra·chi·a (bĭl′ĭ-rā′kē-ə) *n.* The presence of bile in the spinal fluid.

bil·i·ru·bin (bĭl′ĭ-roō′bĭn, bĭl′ĭ-roō′-) *n.* A red bile pigment derived from the degradation of hemoglobin during the normal and abnormal destruction of red blood cells.

bil·i·ru·bi·ne·mi·a (bĭl′ĭ-roō′bə-nē′mē-ə) *n.* The presence of excess bilirubin in the blood.

bilirubin encephalopathy *n.* Encephalopathy due to the toxic effects of bilirubin, as in kernicterus.

bil·i·ru·bin·oid (bĭl′ĭ-roō′bə-noid′) *n.* Any of various intermediate chemical substances, usually found in urine and feces, produced during the conversion of bilirubin to stercobilin through the action of reductive enzymes in intestinal bacteria.

bil·i·ru·bi·nu·ri·a (bĭl′ĭ-roō′bə-noōr′ē-ə) *n.* The presence of bilirubin in the urine.

bil·i·u·ri·a (bĭl′ĭ-yoŏr′ē-ə) *n.* The presence of various bile salts, or bile, in the urine. Also called *choluria.*

bil·i·ver·din (bĭl′ĭ-vûr′dĭn, bĭl′ĭ-vûr′-) *n.* A green pigment occurring in bile.

bill of health *n.* **1.** A certificate stating whether there is infectious disease aboard a ship or in a port of departure, given to the ship's master to present at the next port of arrival. **2.** An attestation as to condition, especially a favorable one.

Bill·roth (bĭl′rōt), **(Christian Albert) Theodor** 1829–1894. Austrian surgeon who was a pioneer of modern abdominal surgery. He performed the first successful excision of the larynx in 1874, and the first resection of the intestine in 1881.

Bill·roth's operation I (bĭl′rōts) *n.* Excision of the pylorus with end-to-end anastomosis of the upper portion of the stomach and the duodenum. Also called *Billroth I anastomosis.*

Billroth's operation II *n.* The surgical resection of the pylorus to the stomach, followed by closure of the cut ends of the duodenum and gastrojejunostomy. Also called *Billroth II anastomosis.*

bi·lo·bate (bī-lō′bāt′) *or* **bi·lo·bat·ed** (-bā′tĭd) *or* **bi·lobed** (bī′lōbd′) *adj.* Divided into or having two lobes.

bi·lob·u·lar (bī-lŏb′yə-lər, -lō′byə-) *adj.* Having two lobules.

bi·loc·u·lar (bī-lŏk′yə-lər) *or* **bi·loc·u·late** (-lĭt, -lāt′) *adj.* Divided into or containing two chambers.

bilocular joint *n.* A joint in which the intra-articular disk is complete, dividing the joint into two distinct cavities.

Bil·tri·cide (bĭl′trĭ-sīd′) A trademark for the drug praziquantel.

bi·man·u·al (bī-măn′yōō-əl) *adj.* Using or requiring the use of both hands.

bimanual version *n.* A turning of the fetus in utero, performed by both internal and external manipulation with the hands. Also called *bipolar version, combined version.*

bi·mas·toid (bī-măs′toid′) *adj.* Relating to both mastoid processes.

bi·max·il·lar·y (bī-măk′sə-lĕr′ē) *adj.* Relating to or affecting both jaws.

bin– *pref.* Variant of **bi–**[1].

bi·na·ry (bī′nə-rē) *adj.* **1.** Characterized by or consisting of two parts or components; twofold. **2.** Consisting of or containing only molecules having two kinds of atoms.

binary fission *n.* A method of asexual reproduction that involves the splitting of a parent cell into two daughter cells.

bi·na·sal hemianopsia (bī-nā′zəl) *n.* Blindness in the nasal field of vision of both eyes.

bin·au·ral (bī-nôr′əl, bĭn-ôr′-) *adj.* Having or relating to both ears.

binaural alternate loudness balance test *or* **alternate binaural loudness balance test** *n.* A test for recruitment in one ear that compares the relative loudness of a series of intensities presented alternately to each ear.

binaural diplacusis *n.* A form of diplacusis in which the same sound is heard differently by the two ears.

bind·er (bīn′dər) *n.* A broad bandage, especially one encircling the abdomen.

Bi·net (bĭ-nā′), **Alfred** 1857–1911. French psychologist. With French physician Théodore Simon (1873–1961), he developed (1905) the first widely accepted test for measuring intelligence.

Binet-Simon scale *n.* An evaluation of the relative mental development of children by a series of psychological tests of intellectual ability. Also called *Binet scale, Binet-Simon test, Binet test.*

binge eating disorder *n. Abbr.* **BED** A recurrent eating disorder characterized by the uncontrolled, excessive intake of any available food and often occurring following stressful events.

binge-purge syndrome *n.* See bulimarexia.

bin·oc·u·lar (bə-nŏk′yə-lər, bī-) *adj.* Adapted to the use of both eyes. Used of an optical instrument.

binocular microscope *n.* A microscope having two eyepieces, one for each eye, so that the object can be viewed with both eyes.

binocular vision *n.* Vision in which both eyes are used synchronously to produce a single image.

bi·no·mi·al (bī-nō′mē-əl) *adj.* Consisting of two terms or names, such as the genus and species names of organisms. —*n.* A taxonomic name used in binomial nomenclature.

binomial nomenclature *n.* The scientific naming of species whereby each species receives a Latin or Lat-inized name of two parts, the first indicating the genus and the second being the specific name.

bin·o·tic (bĭn-ō′tĭk, -ŏt′ĭk) *adj.* Binaural.

bin·o·vu·lar (bĭn-ō′vyə-lər, -ŏv′yə-) *adj.* Relating to or derived from two ova.

Bins·wang·er's disease (bĭn′swăng′ərz, bĭns′văng′ərz) *n.* Organically caused dementia that is associated with chronic high blood pressure and that is characterized by recurrent edema of cerebral white matter with secondary demyelination. Also called *Binswanger's encephalopathy.*

bi·nu·cle·ate (bī-nōō′klē-ĭt, -āt′) *or* **bi·nu·cle·ar** (-ər) *adj.* Having two nuclei.

bi·nu·cle·o·late (bī-nōō′klē-ə-lāt′) *adj.* Having two nucleoli.

bio– *or* **bi–** *pref.* **1.** Life; living organism: *biology.* **2.** Biology; biological: *biophysics.*

bi·o·ac·cu·mu·la·tion (bī′ō-ə-kyōōm′yə-lā′shən) *n.* The increase in the concentration of a substance, especially a contaminant, in an organism or in the food chain over time.

bi·o·a·cous·tics (bī′ō-ə-kōō′stĭks) *n.* The study of sounds produced by or affecting living organisms, especially those sounds involved in communication.

bi·o·ac·tive (bī′ō-ăk′tĭv) *adj.* Of or relating to a substance that has an effect on living tissue.

bi·o·ac·tiv·i·ty (bī′ō-ăk-tĭv′ĭ-tē) *n.* The effect of a given agent, such as a vaccine, upon a living organism or on living tissue.

bi·o·as·say (bī′ō-ăs′ā′, -ă-sā′) *n.* **1.** Determination of the strength or biological activity of a substance, such as a drug or hormone, by comparing its effects with those of a standard preparation on a test organism. **2.** A test that is used to determine such strength or activity. —*v.* To cause to undergo a bioassay. Also called *biologic assay.*

bi·o·a·vail·a·bil·i·ty (bī′ō-ə-vā′lə-bĭl′ĭ-tē) *n.* The physiological availability of a given amount of a drug, as distinct from its chemical potency.

bi·o·be·hav·ior·al (bī′ō-bĭ-hāv′yə-rəl) *adj.* Of or relating to the interrelationships among psychosocial, behavioral, and biological processes, as in the progression or treatment of a disease.

biochemical oxygen demand *n.* The amount of oxygen required by aerobic microorganisms to decompose the organic matter in a sample of water and used as a measure of the degree of water pollution. Also called *biological oxygen demand.*

biochemical profile *n.* An array of biochemical tests, usually involving the use of automated instrumentation, performed on individuals admitted to a hospital or clinic.

bi·o·chem·is·try (bī′ō-kĕm′ĭ-strē) *n.* **1.** The study of the chemical substances and vital processes occurring in living organisms. **2.** The chemical composition of a particular living system or biological substance. —**bi′·o·chem′i·cal** (-ĭ-kəl) *adj.*

bi·o·cid·al (bī′ə-sīd′l) *adj.* Of or relating to an agent that is destructive to living organisms.

bi·o·cy·tin (bī′ō-sīt′n) *n.* A colorless crystalline peptide occurring naturally, as in yeast, and yielding biotin and lysine when hydrolyzed.

bi·o·de·grad·a·ble (bī′ō-dĭ-grā′də-bəl) *adj.* Capable of being decomposed by biological agents, especially bacteria.

bi·o·deg·ra·da·tion (bī′ō-dĕg′rə-dā′shən) *n.* See **biotransformation.**

bi·o·en·gi·neer·ing (bī′ō-ĕn′jə-nîr′ĭng) *n.* **1.** The application of engineering principles to the fields of biology and medicine, as in the development of aids or replacements for defective or missing body organs. **2.** Genetic engineering.

bi·o·e·quiv·a·lent (bī′ō-ĭ-kwĭv′ə-lənt) *n.* A value indicating the rate at which a substance enters the bloodstream and becomes available to the body. —**bi′o·e·quiv′a·lence** *n.*

bi·o·eth·ics (bī′ō-ĕth′ĭks) *n.* The study of the ethical and moral implications of new biological discoveries and biomedical advances, as in the fields of genetic engineering and drug research. —**bi′o·eth′i·cal** (-ĭ-kəl) *adj.*

bi·o·feed·back (bī′ō-fēd′băk′) *n.* A training technique that enables a person to gain some element of voluntary control over autonomic body functions. It is based on the principle that a desired response is learned when received information indicates that a specific thought or action has produced the desired response.

bi·o·fla·vo·noid (bī′ō-flā′və-noid′) *n.* See **flavonoid.**

bi·o·gen·e·sis (bī′ō-jĕn′ĭ-sĭs) *n.* **1.** The principle that life originates from preexisting life and not from nonliving material. **2.** See **biosynthesis.** —**bi′o·ge·net′ic** (-jə-nĕt′ĭk), **bi′o·ge·net′i·cal** (-ĭ-kəl) *adj.*

biogenetic law *n.* The theory that the stages in an organism's embryonic development and differentiation correspond to the stages of evolutionary development characteristic of the species. Also called *Haeckel's law, law of recapitulation, recapitulation theory.*

bi·o·gen·ic amine (bī′ō-jĕn′ĭk) *n.* Any of a group of naturally occurring, biologically active amines, such as serotonin, that act primarily as neurotransmitters and are capable of affecting mental functioning.

bi·o·haz·ard (bī′ō-hăz′ərd) *n.* **1.** A biological agent, such as a virus or a condition that constitutes a threat to humans, especially in biological research or experimentation. **2.** The potential danger or harm from exposure to such an agent or condition.

bi·o·in·for·mat·ics (bī′ō-ĭn′fər-măt′ĭks) *n.* Information technology as applied to the life sciences, especially the technology used for the collection, storage, and retrieval of genomic data.

bi·o·in·stru·ment (bī′ō-ĭn′strə-mənt) *n.* A sensor or device attached to or embedded in body tissue to record and transmit physiological data to a receiving and monitoring station.

bi·o·ki·net·ics (bī′ō-kĭ-nĕt′ĭks, kī-) *n.* The study of the growth changes and movements that developing organisms undergo.

bi·o·log·ic (bī′ə-lŏj′ĭk) *or* **bi·o·log·i·cal** (-ĭ-kəl) *n.* A preparation, such as a drug, a vaccine, or an antitoxin, that is synthesized from living organisms or their products and used as a diagnostic, preventive, or therapeutic agent.

bi·o·log·i·cal (bī′ə-lŏj′ĭ-kəl) *adj.* **1.** Of, relating to, caused by, or affecting life or living organisms. **2.** Having to do with biology. **3.** Related by blood, as in a child's biological parents.

biological clock *n.* An innate mechanism in living organisms that controls the periodicity or rhythm of various physiological functions or activities.

biological half-life *n.* See **half-life** (sense 2).

biological oxygen demand *n.* See **biochemical oxygen demand.**

biological response modifier *n.* A substance, such as interferon, that is produced naturally or manufactured as a drug designed to strengthen, direct, or restore the body's immune response against infection or cancer.

biological vector *n.* A vector that is essential in the life cycle of a pathogenic organism.

biological warfare *n.* The use of disease-producing microorganisms, toxic biological products, or organic biocides to cause death or injury to humans, animals, or plants.

biologic assay *n.* See **bioassay.**

biologic evolution *n.* The doctrine that all forms of life have been derived by gradual changes from simpler forms or from a single cell. Also called *organic evolution.*

bi·ol·o·gy (bī-ŏl′ə-jē) *n.* **1.** The science of life and of living organisms, including their structure, function, growth, origin, evolution, and distribution. It includes botany and zoology. **2.** The life processes or characteristic phenomena of a group or category of living organisms. —**bi·ol′o·gist** *n.*

bi·ol·y·sis (bī-ŏl′ĭ-sĭs) *n.* **1.** Death of a living organism or tissue caused or accompanied by lysis. **2.** The decomposition of organic material by living organisms, such as microorganisms.

bi·o·mark·er (bī′ō-mär′kər) *n.* **1.** See **marker** (sense 2). **2.** A specific physical trait used to measure or indicate the effects or progress of a disease, illness, or condition.

bi·o·mass (bī′ō-măs′) *n.* The total mass of all living things within a given area, biotic community, species population, or habitat; a measure of total biotic productivity.

bi·o·ma·te·ri·al (bī′ō-mə-tîr′ē-əl) *n.* Material used to construct artificial organs, rehabilitation devices, or prostheses and replace natural body tissues.

bi·ome (bī′ōm′) *n.* The total complex of biotic communities occupying and characterizing a particular area or zone, such as a desert or deciduous forest.

bi·o·me·chan·ics (bī′ō-mĭ-kăn′ĭks) *n.* **1.** The study of the mechanics of a living body, especially of the forces exerted by muscles and gravity on the skeletal structure. **2.** The mechanics of a part or function of a living body, such as of the heart or of locomotion.

bi·o·med·i·cal (bī′ō-mĕd′ĭ-kəl) *adj.* **1.** Of or relating to biomedicine. **2.** Of, relating to, or involving biological, medical, and physical sciences.

bi·o·med·i·cine (bī′ō-mĕd′ĭ-sĭn) *n.* **1.** The branch of medical science that deals with the ability of humans to tolerate environmental stresses and variations, as in space travel. **2.** The application of the principles of the natural sciences, especially biology and physiology, to clinical medicine.

bi·o·me·tri·cian (bī′ō-mĭ-trĭsh′ən) *n.* One who specializes in the science of biometry.

bi·om·e·try (bī-ŏm′ĭ-trē) *n.* The statistical analysis of biological data. Also called *biometrics.*

bi·o·mi·cro·scope (bī′ō-mī′krə-skōp′) *n.* An instrument consisting of a microscope combined with a rectangular light source, used for examination of the cornea, aqueous humor, and retina of the eye. Also called *slitlamp.*

bi·o·mi·cros·co·py (bī′ō-mī-krŏs′kə-pē) *n.* **1.** The microscopic examination of living tissue in the body. **2.** The examination of structures of the eye with a biomicroscope.

bi·o·ne·cro·sis (bī′ō-nə-krō′sĭs) *n.* See **necrobiosis** (sense 2).

bi·on·ic (bī-ŏn′ĭk) *adj.* **1.** Of, relating to, or developed from bionics. **2.** Having anatomical structures or physiological processes that are replaced or enhanced by electronic or mechanical components. **3.** Having extraordinary strength, powers, or capabilities; superhuman.

bi·on·ics (bī-ŏn′ĭks) *n.* The science of biological functions and mechanisms as analogous to electronics, using knowledge of human and other animal systems to devise improvements in various machines, especially computers.

bi·o·phar·ma·ceu·ti·cal (bī′ō-fär′mə-sōō′tĭ-kəl) *n.* A drug created by means of biotechnology, especially genetic engineering.

bi·o·phar·ma·ceu·tics (bī′ō-fär′mə-sōō′tĭks) *n.* The study of the physical and chemical properties of drugs and their proper dosage as related to the onset, duration, and intensity of drug action.

bi·o·phys·ics (bī′ō-fĭz′ĭks) *n.* **1.** The study of biological processes using the theories and tools of physics. **2.** The study of physical processes occurring in living organisms. —**bi′o·phys′i·cal** *adj.* —**bi′o·phys′i·cal·ly** *adv.* —**bi′o·phys′i·cist** *n.*

bi·o·pol·y·mer (bī′ō-pŏl′ə-mər) *n.* A macromolecule, such as a protein or nucleic acid, that is formed in a living organism.

bi·op·sy (bī′ŏp′sē) *n. Abbr.* **bx 1.** The removal and examination of a sample of tissue from a living body for diagnostic purposes. **2.** A specimen so obtained.

bi·o·psy·chol·o·gy (bī′ō-sī-kŏl′ə-jē) *n.* See **psychobiology.**

bi·o·rhythm (bī′ō-rĭth′əm) *n.* A biologically inherent cyclic variation or recurrence of an event or state, such as sleep cycles, circadian rhythms, and periodic diseases. —**bi′o·rhyth′mic** (-rĭth′mĭk) *adj.*

bi·o·sci·ence (bī′ō-sī′əns) *n.* See **life science.** —**bi′o·sci′en·tif′ic** (-sī′ən-tĭf′ĭk) *adj.* —**bi′o·sci′en·tist** *n.*

bi·os·co·py (bī-ŏs′kə-pē) *n.* Medical examination of a body to determine the presence or absence of life.

bi·o·sen·sor (bī′ō-sĕn′sər, -sôr) *n.* **1.** A device that detects, records, and transmits information regarding a physiological change or process. **2.** A device that uses biological materials to monitor the presence of various chemicals in a substance.

–biosis *suff.* A way of living: *parabiosis.*

bi·o·spec·trom·e·try (bī′ō-spĕk-trŏm′ĭ-trē) *n.* The spectroscopic determination of the types and amounts

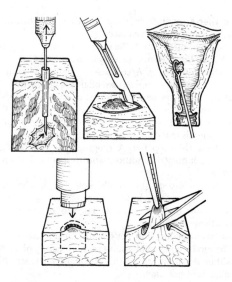

biopsy
Top left to right: *needle, excisional, and curettage biopsy procedures*
Bottom: *punch excisional biopsy procedure*

of various substances in living tissue or body fluids. Also called *clinical spectrometry.*

bi·o·spec·tros·co·py (bī′ō-spĕk-trŏs′kə-pē) *n.* Spectroscopic examination of specimens of living tissue or body fluids. Also called *clinical spectroscopy.*

bi·o·sphere (bī′ə-sfîr′) *n.* **1.** All the regions of the earth and its atmosphere in which living organisms are found or can live. **2.** The living organisms and their environment composing the biosphere. —**bi′o·spher′ic** (-sfîr′ĭk, -sfĕr′-) *adj.*

bi·o·sta·tis·tics (bī′ō-stə-tĭs′tĭks) *n.* The science of statistics applied to the analysis of biological or medical data.

bi·o·syn·the·sis (bī′ō-sĭn′thĭ-sĭs) *n.* Formation of a chemical compound by a living organism. Also called *biogenesis.* —**bi′o·syn·thet′ic** (-thĕt′ĭk) *adj.*

bi·o·sys·tem (bī′ō-sĭs′təm) *n.* A living organism or a system of living organisms that can directly or indirectly interact with others.

bi·o·ta (bī-ō′tə) *n.* The flora and fauna of a region.

bi·o·tech·nol·o·gy (bī′ō-tĕk-nŏl′ə-jē) *n.* **1.** The use of microorganisms, such as bacteria or yeasts, or biological substances, such as enzymes, to perform specific industrial or manufacturing processes. Applications include production of certain drugs, synthetic hormones, and bulk foodstuffs. **2.** The application of the principles of engineering and technology to the life sciences.

bi·o·te·lem·e·try (bī′ō-tə-lĕm′ĭ-trē) *n.* The monitoring, recording, and measuring of a living organism's basic physiological functions, such as heart rate, muscle activity, and body temperature, by the use of telemetry techniques.

bi·o·ter·ror·ism (bī′ō-tĕr′ə-rĭz′əm) *n.* The use of biological agents, such as pathogenic organisms or agricultural pests, for terrorist purposes.

bi·o·ther·a·py (bī′ō-thĕr′ə-pē) *n.* Treatment of disease with biologicals, such as vaccines.

bi·ot·ic (bī-ŏt′ĭk) *adj.* **1.** Relating to life or living organisms. **2.** Produced or caused by living organisms.

bi·o·tin (bī′ə-tĭn) *n.* A colorless crystalline vitamin of the vitamin B complex, essential for the activity of many enzyme systems and found in large quantities in liver, egg yolk, milk, and yeast.

bi·o·tin·ide (bī′ə-tə-nīd′) *n.* Any of various chemical compounds that contain biotin, such as biocytin.

bi·o·tope (bī′ə-tōp′) *n.* A geographical area uniform in environmental conditions and in its distribution of biota.

bi·o·tox·i·col·o·gy (bī′ō-tŏk′sĭ-kŏl′ə-jē) *n.* The study of poisons produced by living organisms.

bi·o·tox·in (bī′ō-tŏk′sĭn) *n.* A toxic substance produced by a living organism.

bi·o·trans·for·ma·tion (bī′ō-trăns′fər-mā′shən) *n.* Chemical alteration of a substance, especially of a drug, within the body, as by the action of enzymes. Also called *biodegradation.*

Bi·ot's respiration (bē-ōz′, byōz) *n.* Abrupt and irregularly alternating periods of apnea with periods of breathing that are consistent in rate and depth, often the result of increased intracranial pressure.

bi·o·type (bī′ə-tīp′) *n.* A population or group of individuals having the same genotype. —**bi′o·typ′ic** (-tĭp′ĭk) *adj.*

bi·o·var (bī′ō-vâr′, -văr′) *n.* A group of bacterial strains that are distinguishable from other strains of the same species on the basis of their physiological characteristics.

bi·o·vu·lar (bī-ō′vyə-lər, -ŏv′yə-) *adj.* Diovular.

bi·pa·ren·tal (bī′-pə-rĕn′tl) *adj.* **1.** Having two parents, male and female. **2.** Of or derived from two parents.

bi·pa·ri·e·tal diameter (bī′pə-rī′ĭ-tl) *n.* The diameter of the fetal head as measured from one parietal eminence to the other.

bip·a·rous (bĭp′ər-əs) *adj.* Bearing two offspring from the same pregnancy.

bi·par·tite (bī-pär′tīt′) *adj.* Consisting of two parts or divisions.

bi·pen·nate (bī-pĕn′āt′) *adj.* Of or relating to a muscle with a central tendon toward which the fibers converge on either side like the barbs of a feather.

bi·pen·ni·form (bī-pĕn′ə-fôrm′) *adj.* Bipennate.

bi·pha·sic pill (bī′fā′zĭk) *adj.* A drug, such as an oral contraceptive, in which the dosage level changes during the number of days it is taken.

bi·phe·no·typ·y (bī-fē′nə-tīp′ē) *n.* The appearance in one cell type of distinguishing characteristics of other cell types, as in certain leukemias. —**bi·phe′no·typ′ic** *adj.*

bi·phen·yl (bī-fĕn′əl, -fē′nəl) *n.* A colorless crystalline aromatic hydrocarbon used in fungicides and in organic synthesis. Also called *diphenyl.*

bi·po·lar (bī-pō′lər) *adj.* **1.** Having two poles; used especially of nerve cells in which the branches project from two usually opposite points. **2.** Of or relating to both ends or poles of a bacterial or other cell. **3.** Of or relating to a major mood disorder that is characterized by episodes of mania and depression. —**bi′po·lar′i·ty** (-lăr′ĭ-tē) *n.*

bipolar II *n.* See **dysphoric hypomania.**

bipolar cautery *n.* Cauterization using a high frequency electrical current passed through tissue from one electrode to another.

bipolar cell *n.* A neuron having two processes.

bipolar disorder *n.* Any of several mood disorders usually characterized by alternating periods of depression with mania or hypomania. Also called *manic-depressive illness.*

bipolar lead (lēd) *n.* **1.** The electrical connection of two electrodes to a recording instrument and to two different places on the body, such as the chest and a limb. **2.** A record obtained from the combined input of the two electrodes.

bipolar neuron *n.* A neuron that has two processes arising from opposite poles of the cell body.

bipolar version *n.* See **bimanual version.**

bi·po·ten·ti·al·i·ty (bī′pə-tĕn′shē-ăl′ĭ-tē) *n.* **1.** The capability of differentiating along two developmental pathways, as of a gonad. **2.** The capacity to function either as a male or a female. **3.** The condition of having both male and female reproductive organs; hermaphroditism.

bi·ra·mous (bī-rā′məs) *adj.* Consisting of or having two branches, as the appendages of an arthropod.

birch tar oil (bûrch) *n.* An oil obtained by the dry distillation of the wood of the white birch and used externally in the treatment of skin diseases.

bird-breeder's lung *n.* Extrinsic allergic alveolitis that is caused by an acquired sensitivity to inhaled particles from bird excreta.

bird face *n.* See **brachygnathia.**

bi·re·frin·gence (bī′rĭ-frĭn′jəns) *n.* The resolution or splitting of a light wave into two unequally reflected waves by an optically anisotropic medium such as calcite or quartz. —**bi′re·frin′gent** *adj.*

birth (bûrth) *n.* **1.** The emergence and separation of offspring from the body of the mother. **2.** The act or process of bearing young; parturition. **3.** The circumstances or conditions relating to this event, as its time or location. **4.** The set of characteristics or circumstances received from one's ancestors; inheritance. **5.** Origin; extraction.

birth canal *n.* The passage through which the fetus is expelled during parturition, leading from the uterus through the cervix, vagina, and vulva. Also called *parturient canal.*

birth control *n.* Voluntary limitation or control of the number of children conceived, especially by planned use of contraceptive techniques.

birth control pill *n.* See **oral contraceptive.**

birth defect *n.* A physiological or structural abnormality that develops at or before birth and is present at the time of birth, especially as a result of faulty development, infection, heredity, or injury. Also called *congenital anomaly.*

birth family *n.* A family consisting of one's biological as opposed to adoptive parents and their offspring.

birth father *or* **birthfather** *n.* A biological father.

birth·ing (bûr′thĭng) *adj.* Having to do with or used during birth. —*n.* The act of giving birth.

birthing center *n.* A medical facility, often associated with a hospital, that is designed to provide a comfortable, homelike setting during childbirth and that is generally less restrictive than a hospital in its regulations, as in permitting midwifery or allowing family members or friends to attend the delivery.

birthing room *n.* An area of a hospital or outpatient medical facility equipped for labor, delivery, and recovery and designed as a homelike environment.

birth·mark (bûrth′märk′) *n.* A mole or blemish present on the skin from birth; a nevus.

birth mother *or* **birthmother** *n.* A biological mother.

birth palsy *n.* Paralysis due to cerebral hemorrhage occurring at birth or to anoxic injury to the fetal brain. Also called *obstetrical paralysis.*

birth pang *n.* One of the repetitive pains occurring in childbirth.

birth parent *or* **birthparent** *n.* A biological parent.

birth·rate *or* **birth rate** (bûrth′rāt′) *n.* The ratio of total live births to total population in a specified community or area over a specified period of time, often expressed as the number of live births per 1,000 of the population per year.

birth trauma *n.* **1.** A physical injury sustained by an infant during birth. **2.** The psychological shock said to be experienced by an infant during birth.

birth weight *n.* In humans, the first weight of an infant, obtained within the first hour after birth. An infant of birth weight $5\frac{1}{2}$ pounds or more is considered to be full-sized.

bis– *pref.* **1.** Two; twice: *bisalbuminemia.* **2.** Having two identical but separated complex chemical groups in one molecule: *1,4-bis(5-phenyloxazol-2-yl)-benzene.*

bis·ac·o·dyl (bĭs-ăk′ə-dĭl, bĭs′ə-kō′dĭl) *n.* An over-the-counter laxative taken by mouth or per rectum to treat constipation.

bis·al·bu·mi·ne·mi·a (bĭs′ăl-byōō′mə-nē′mē-ə) *n.* The condition of having two kinds of serum albumin that differ in mobility on electrophoresis.

bi·sex·u·al (bī-sĕk′shōō-əl) *adj.* **1.** Relating to both sexes. **2.** Having both male and female reproductive organs; hermaphroditic. **3.** Relating to or having a sexual orientation to persons of either sex. —*n.* **1.** A bisexual organism; a hermaphrodite. **2.** A bisexual person. —**bi′sex·u·al′i·ty** (-ăl′ĭ-tē) *n.*

bis·fer·i·ous pulse (bĭs-fĕr′ē-əs, -fîr′-) *n.* An arterial pulse with two palpable peaks, with the second stronger than the first.

Bish·op (bĭsh′əp), **J. Michael** Born 1936. American microbiologist. He shared a 1989 Nobel Prize for discovering a sequence of genes that can cause cancer when mutated.

bis·hy·drox·y·cou·ma·rin (bĭs′hī-drŏk′sē-kōō′mər-ĭn) *n.* See **dicumarol.**

bis·muth (bĭz′məth) *n. Symbol* **Bi** A metallic element used in various low-melting alloys and having many medical applications, including as an x-ray contrast medium and in compounds that are used as astringents, antiseptics, treatments of gastrointestinal disturbances, and suppressants of lupus erythematosus. Atomic number 83.

bismuth line *n.* A black zone on the gingiva, often the first sign of bismuth poisoning.

bis·muth·o·sis (bĭz′mə-thō′sĭs) *n.* Chronic bismuth poisoning.

bismuth sub·sa·lic·y·late (sŭb-sə-lĭs′ə-lāt′, -lĭt, -săl′ĭ-sĭl′ĭt) *n.* A salicylate used to treat nausea, indigestion, and diarrhea.

bis·muth·yl (bĭz′mə-thĭl, -thēl′) *n.* The univalent radical BiO.

bis·tou·ry (bĭs′tə-rē) *n.* A long, narrow-bladed knife used for opening abscesses or for slitting sinuses and fistulas.

bi·sul·fate (bī-sŭl′fāt′) *n.* **1.** The univalent inorganic acid group HSO$_4$. **2.** A salt of sulfuric acid containing this group. Also called *acid sulfate.*

bi·sul·fide (bī-sŭl′fīd′) *n.* See **disulfide.**

bi·sul·fite (bī-sŭl′fīt′) *n.* **1.** The univalent inorganic acid group HSO$_3$. **2.** A salt of sulfurous acid containing this group.

bi·tar·trate (bī-tär′trāt′) *n.* **1.** The group $C_4H_5O_6$. **2.** A salt of tartaric acid containing this group.

bite (bīt) *v.* **1.** To cut, grip, or tear with the teeth. **2.** To pierce the skin of with the teeth, fangs, or mouthparts. —*n.* **1.** The act of biting. **2.** A puncture or laceration of the skin by the teeth of an animal or the mouthparts of an insect or similar organism.

bite analysis *n.* See **occlusal analysis.**

bite gauge *n.* See **gnathodynamometer.**

bi·tem·po·ral hemianopsia (bī-tĕm′pər-əl, -tĕm′prəl) *n.* Blindness in the temporal field of vision of both eyes.

bite·plate *or* **bite plate** (bīt′plāt′) *n.* A removable dental appliance, made of wire and plastic, worn in the palate and used as a diagnostic or therapeutic aid in orthodontics or prosthodontics. Also called *bite plane.*

bite·wing (bīt′wĭng′) *n.* A dental x-ray film having a central projection on which the teeth can close, holding it in position for the radiographic imagery of several upper and lower teeth simultaneously.

bit·ing stage (bīt′ĭng) *n.* In psychoanalytic theory, the second stage of the oral phase of psychosexual development, from approximately 8 to 18 months of age, during which a child may express hostility by biting, spitting, or chewing on objects.

Bi·tot's spots (bē-tōz′) *pl.n.* Small grayish foamy triangular deposits on the conjunctiva adjacent to the cornea in the area of the palpebral fissure, associated with vitamin A deficiency.

bi·tro·chan·ter·ic (bī′trō-kən-tĕr′ĭk, -kăn-) *adj.* Of or relating to two trochanters, either to the trochanters of one femur, or to both greater trochanters.

bi·u·ret (bī′yə-rĕt′, bī′yə-rĕt′) *n.* A derivative of urea obtained by heating. Also called *carbamylurea.*

biuret reaction *n.* A test to determine the concentration in biological fluids of biuret, peptides that contain more than three amino acids or that contain amido groups in which such compounds react with copper sulfate in highly alkaline solutions to produce a violet color. Also called *biuret test.*

bi·va·lent (bī-vā′lənt) *adj.* **1.** Having a valence of 2; divalent. **2.** Consisting of a pair of homologous, synapsed chromosomes, as occurs during meiosis. —*n.* A pair of homologous, synapsed chromosomes associated together during meiosis. —**bi·va′lence, bi·va′len·cy** *n.*

bivalent chromosome *n.* A pair of chromosomes temporarily united.

bi·ven·tral (bī-vĕn′trəl) *adj.* Digastric.

Bk The symbol for the element **berkelium**.

BKA *abbr.* below-the-knee amputation

Black (blăk), Sir **James Whyte** Born 1924. British pharmacologist. He shared a 1988 Nobel Prize for developing drugs to treat heart disease and stomach and duodenal ulcers.

black bile *n.* One of the four humors of ancient and medieval physiology, supposed to cause melancholy when present in excess.

black cataract *n.* A cataract in which the lens is hardened and dark brown.

Black Death *n.* A form of bubonic plague, caused by *Yersinia pestis*, that was pandemic throughout Europe and much of Asia in the 14th century.

black eye *n.* A bruised discoloration of the flesh surrounding the eye.

black fly *n.* Any of various small dark humpbacked flies of whom the females are aggressive biters and serve as vectors in the transmission of onchocerciasis.

black·head (blăk′hĕd′) *n.* A plug of keratin and sebum within a hair follicle that is blackened at the surface. Also called *open comedo.*

black lung *n.* A form of pneumoconiosis common in coal miners, characterized by the deposit of carbon particles in the lungs.

black measles *n.* A severe form of measles characterized by dark, hemorrhagic skin eruptions. Also called *hemorrhagic measles.*

black·out (blăk′out′) *n.* **1.** Temporary loss of consciousness due to decreased blood flow to the brain. **2.** Temporary loss of memory.

black tongue *n.* The presence of a blackish- to yellowish-brown patch or patches on the tongue, accompanied by elongation of the papillae. Also called *melanoglossia.*

black vomit *n.* **1.** Dark vomit consisting of digested blood and gastric contents. **2.** Severe yellow fever marked by regurgitation of dark vomited matter.

black·wa·ter fever (blăk′wô′tər) *n.* A serious, often fatal complication of falciparum malaria, characterized by the passage of bloody, dark red, or black urine.

Black·well (blăk′wĕl′, blăk′wəl), **Elizabeth** 1821–1910. British-born American physician who was the first woman to be awarded a medical doctorate in modern times (1849). In 1853 she founded an infirmary for women and children in New York City that her sister **Emily Blackwell** (1826–1910), also a physician, directed (1869–1910) and built into an accredited medical school.

blad·der (blăd′ər) *n.* **1.** Any of various distensible membranous sacs, such as the urinary bladder, that serve as receptacles for fluid or gas. **2.** A blister, pustule, or cyst filled with fluid or air; vesicle.

bladder worm *n.* The bladderlike, encysted larva of a tapeworm that is characteristic of the cysticercus stage.

blain (blān) *n.* A skin swelling or sore; a blister; a blotch.

Blair-Brown graft (blâr′broun′) *n.* A split-skin graft of intermediate thickness.

Bla·lock (blā′lŏk′), **Alfred** 1899–1964. American surgeon who developed surgical techniques for repairing congenital defects of the heart and associated blood vessels. With pediatrician Helen Taussig he developed the pulmonary bypass operation for the treatment of blue babies.

Blalock-Taussig operation *n.* Surgical anastomosis of a subclavian artery to a pulmonary artery in order to direct blood from the systemic circulation to the lungs in cases of congenital malformations of the heart in which an abnormally small volume of blood passes through the pulmonary circuit.

bland diet (blănd) *n.* A regular diet omitting foods that may irritate the gastrointestinal tract.

blan·ket suture (blăng′kĭt) *n.* A continuous lock-stitch suture used to pull together the skin of a wound.

–blast *suff.* An immature, embryonic stage in the development of cells or tissues: *erythroblast.*

blast cell (blăst) *n.* An immature precursor of a blood cell.

blas·te·ma (blă-stē′mə) *n.* **1.** The formative, undifferentiated material from which cells are formed. **2.** A mass of embryonic cells from which an organ or a body part develops, either in normal development or in regeneration of a lost body part. —**blas·te′mal blas′te·mat′ic** (blăs′tə-măt′ĭk), **blas·te′mic** (blă-stē′mĭk) *adj.*

–blastic *suff.* Having a specified number or kind of formative elements such as buds, germs, cells, or cell layers: *epiblastic.*

blast injury *n.* The tearing of lung tissue or rupture of abdominal viscera without external injury, as by the force of an explosion.

blasto– *or* **blast–** *pref.* Bud; germ; budding; germination: *blastocyst.*

blas·to·coel *or* **blas·to·cele** *or* **blas·to·coele** (blăs′tə-sēl′) *n.* The fluid-filled cavity in the blastula of a developing embryo. Also called *cleavage cavity, segmentation cavity.* —**blas′to·coe′lic** *adj.*

blas·to·cyst (blăs′tə-sĭst′) *n.* The modified blastula stage of mammalian embryos, consisting of the inner cell mass and a thin trophoblast layer enclosing the blastocoel. Also called *blastodermic vesicle.* —**blas′to·cys′tic** *adj.*

blas·to·cyte (blăs′tə-sīt′) *n.* An undifferentiated blastomere of the morula or the blastula stage of an embryo.

blas·to·cy·to·ma (blăs′tō-sī-tō′mə) *n.* See **blastoma**.

blas·to·derm (blăs′tə-dûrm′) *or* **blas·to·der·ma** (blăs′-tə-dûr′mə) *n.* The layer of cells formed by the cleavage of a fertilized mammalian egg, which later divides into the three germ layers from which the embryo develops. Also called *germinal membrane, germ membrane.* —**blas′to·der′mal, blas′to·der′mic** *or* **blas′to·der·mat′ic** (-dər-măt′ĭk) *adj.*

blastodermic vesicle *n.* See **blastocyst**.

blas·to·disk *or* **blas·to·disc** (blăs′tə-dĭsk′) *n.* **1.** The disk of active cytoplasm at the animal pole of a telolecithal egg. **2.** The blastoderm, especially in very early stages when its extent is small.

blas·to·gen·e·sis (blăs′tə-jĕn′ĭ-sĭs) *n.* **1.** Reproduction of unicellular organisms by budding. **2.** Development of an embryo during cleavage and germ layer formation. **3.** Transformation of small lymphocytes of human peripheral blood into large, undifferentiated cells capable of undergoing mitosis. —**blas′to·ge·net′ic** (-jə-nĕt′ĭk), **blas′to·gen′ic** (-jĕn′ĭk) *adj.*

blas·to·ma (blă-stō′mə) *n., pl.* **-mas** *or* **-ma·ta** (-mə-tə) A neoplasm composed of immature, undifferentiated cells. Also called *blastocytoma, embryonal carcinosarcoma.*

blas·to·mere (blăs′tə-mîr′) *n.* Any of the cells resulting from the cleavage of a fertilized ovum during early embryonic development. —**blas′to·mer′ic** (-mîr′ĭk, -mĕr′-) *adj.*

blas·to·my·co·sis (blăs′tō-mī-kō′sĭs) *n.* A chronic granulomatous and suppurative disease caused by the dimorphic fungus *Blastomyces dermatitidis,* originating as a respiratory infection, and usually spreading to the lungs, bones, and skin.

blas·to·pore (blăs′tə-pôr′) *n.* The opening into the archenteron formed by the invagination of the blastula to form a gastrula. —**blas′to·por′ic, blas′to·por′al** (-pôr′əl) *adj.*

blas·to·spore (blăs′tə-spôr′) *n.* An asexual reproductive sphore formed by budding, as in yeasts.

blas·tu·la (blăs′chə-lə) *n., pl.* **-las** *or* **-lae** (-lē′) An early embryonic form produced by cleavage of a fertilized ovum and consisting of a spherical layer of cells surrounding a fluid-filled cavity. —**blas′tu·lar** *adj.* —**blas′tu·la′tion** (-lā′shən) *n.*

bleb (blĕb) *n.* A large flaccid vesicle.

bleed (blēd) *v.* **1.** To lose blood as a result of rupture or severance of blood vessels. **2.** To take or remove blood from.

bleed·er (blē′dər) *n.* **1.** A person, such as a hemophiliac, who bleeds freely or is subject to frequent hemorrhages. **2.** A blood vessel from which there is uncontrolled bleeding. **3.** A blood vessel severed by trauma or surgery that requires cautery or ligature to arrest the flow of blood. **4.** A person who draws blood from another; a phlebotomist.

blem·ish (blĕm′ĭsh) *n.* A small circumscribed alteration of the skin considered to be unesthetic but insignificant.

blenno– *or* **blenn–** *pref.* Mucus: *blennuria.*

blen·no·gen·ic (blĕn′ə-jĕn′ĭk) *or* **blen·nog·e·nous** (blĕ-nŏj′ə-nəs) *adj.* Producing mucus; muciparous.

blen·noid (blĕn′oid′) *adj.* Resembling mucus; muciform.

blen·nor·rhe·a (blĕn′ə-rē′ə) *n.* **1.** A mucous discharge, especially from the urethra or the vagina. Also called *myxorrhea.* **2.** Gonorrhea. This term is no longer in technical use. —**blen′nor·rhe′al, blen′nor·rhag′ic** (-răj′ĭk) *adj.*

blen·nos·ta·sis (blĕ-nŏs′tə-sĭs) *n.* The reduction or suppression of secretion from the mucous membranes. —**blen′no·stat′ic** (blĕn′ə-stăt′ĭk) *adj.*

blen·nu·ri·a (blĕ-nŏŏr′ē-ə) *n.* The presence of mucus in the urine.

Ble·nox·ane (blə-nŏk′sān′) A trademark for the drug bleomycin.

ble·o·my·cin (blē′ə-mī′sĭn) *n.* Any of several glycopeptide antibiotics obtained from the bacterium *Streptomyces verticillus.* Their sulfates were once used as antineoplastic agents.

bleph·a·rec·to·my (blĕf′ə-rĕk′tə-mē) *n.* Excision of all or part of an eyelid.

bleph·ar·e·de·ma (blĕf′ər-ĭ-dē′mə) *n.* Edema of the

eyelids, that produces swelling and often a baggy appearance.

bleph·a·ri·tis (blĕf′ə-rī′tĭs) *n.* Inflammation of the eyelids.

blepharo– *or* **blephar–** *pref.* Eyelid; eyelids: *blepharospasm.*

bleph·a·ro·ad·e·no·ma (blĕf′ə-rō-ăd′n-ō′mə) *n.* A glandular tumor of the eyelid.

bleph·a·ro·chal·a·sis (blĕf′ə-rō-kăl′ə-sĭs) *n.* Hypertrophy of the upper eyelids so that a fold of skin hangs down, often concealing the tarsal margin when the eye is open.

bleph·a·ro·con·junc·ti·vi·tis (blĕf′ə-rō-kən-jŭngk′tə-vī′tĭs) *n.* A condition in which the eyelids and conjunctiva become inflamed.

bleph·a·ro·ker·a·to·con·junc·ti·vi·tis (blĕf′ə-rō-kĕr′-ə-tō-kən-jŭngk′tə-vī′tĭs) *n.* Inflammation of the margins of the eyelids, cornea, and conjunctiva.

bleph·a·ro·phi·mo·sis (blĕf′ə-rō-fə-mō′sĭs, -fī-) *n.* Decrease in the size of the fissure between the eyelids without fusion of the eyelid margins. Also called *blepharostenosis.*

bleph·a·ro·plas·ty (blĕf′ər-ə-plăs′tē) *n.* Plastic surgery of the eyelids. Also called *tarsoplasty.* —**bleph′a·ro·plas′tic** (-plăs′tĭk) *adj.*

bleph·a·ro·ple·gia (blĕf′ə-rō-plē′jə) *n.* Paralysis of an eyelid.

bleph·a·rop·to·sis (blĕf′ə-rŏp-tō′-sĭs, -rō-tō′-) *n.* Drooping of the upper eyelid.

blepharoptosis ad·i·po·sa (ăd′ə-pō′sə) *n.* Excessive elasticity of skin so that it hangs over the free border of the eyelid.

bleph·a·ror·rha·phy (blĕf′ə-rôr′ə-fē) *n.* See **tarsorrhaphy.**

bleph·a·ro·spasm (blĕf′ə-rō-spăz′əm) *n.* Spasmodic winking caused by the involuntary contraction of an eyelid muscle.

bleph·a·ro·stat (blĕf′ə-rō-stăt′) *n.* An instrument used to hold the eyelids apart.

bleph·a·ro·ste·no·sis (blĕf′ə-rō-stə-nō′sĭs) *n.* See **blepharophimosis.**

bleph·a·ro·syn·ech·i·a (blĕf′ə-rō-sə-nĕk′ē-ə, -nē′kē-ə) *n.* Adhesion of the eyelids to each other or to the eyeball. Also called *ankyloblepharon.*

bleph·a·rot·o·my (blĕf′ə-rŏt′ə-mē) *n.* Incision of an eyelid.

Bles·sig's cysts (blĕs′ĭgz) *pl.n.* Cystic spaces caused by tissue degeneration on the periphery of the sensory retina.

blind (blīnd) *adj.* **1.** Unable to see; without useful sight. **2.** Having a maximal visual acuity of the better eye, after correction by refractive lenses, of one-tenth normal vision or less (20/200 or less on the Snellen test). **3.** Of, relating to, or for sightless persons. **4.** Closed at one end, as a tube or sac. —**blind′ness** *n.*

blind fistula *n.* A fistula that is open at one end only. Also called *incomplete fistula.*

blind gut *n.* See **cecum** (sense 1).

blind spot *n.* **1.** See **optic disk. 2.** The area of blindness in the visual field corresponding to the optic disk. Also called *physiologic scotoma, punctum cecum.* **3.** An area or facet of one's personality of which one remains ignorant or fails to gain understanding. Also called *mental scotoma, scotoma.*

blis·ter (blĭs′tər) *n.* A local swelling of the skin that contains watery fluid and is caused by burning, infection, or irritation.

blis·ter·ing (blĭs′tər-ĭng) *n.* See **vesiculation** (sense 1).

bloat (blōt) *n.* Abdominal distention due to swallowed air or intestinal gas production. —**bloat′ed** (blō′tĭd) *adj.*

Blo·ca·dren (blō′kə-drĕn′) A trademark for the drug timolol maleate.

Bloch (blŏk, blôкн), **Konrad Emil** 1912–2000. German-born American biochemist. He shared a 1964 Nobel Prize for research on cholesterol and fatty acid metabolism.

Bloch-Sulz·ber·ger syndrome (-sŭlz′bûr′gər) *n.* See **incontinentia pigmenti.**

block (blŏk) *n.* **1.** Interruption, especially obstruction, of a normal physiological function. **2.** Interruption, complete or partial, permanent or temporary, of the passage of a nervous impulse. **3.** Atrioventricular block. **4.** Sudden cessation of speech or a thought process without an immediate observable cause, sometimes considered a consequence of repression. —*v.* To arrest passage through; obstruct. —**block′age** (blŏk′ĭj) *n.*

block·ade (blŏ-kād′) *n.* **1.** Intravenous injection of large amounts of colloidal dyes in which the reaction of the reticuloendothelial cells to other influences is temporarily prevented. **2.** Arrest of nerve impulse transmission at autonomic synaptic junctions, autonomic receptor sites, or myoneural junctions through the action of a drug.

block anesthesia *n.* See **conduction anesthesia.**

block·ing activity (blŏk′ĭng) *n.* The repression or elimination of electrical activity in the brain because of the arrival of a sensory stimulus.

blocking agent *n.* A drug that blocks transmission of nerve impulses at an autonomic receptor site, autonomic synapse, or neuromuscular junction.

blocking antibody *n.* **1.** An antibody that combines with an antigen without a reaction but that blocks another antibody from later combining with that antigen. **2.** An immunoglobulin that combines specifically with an atopic allergen but does not elicit an allergic reaction.

Blocq's disease (blŏks) *n.* See **astasia-abasia.**

blood (blŭd) *n.* **1.** The fluid consisting of plasma, red blood cells, white blood cells, and platelets that is circulated by the heart through the arteries and veins, carrying oxygen and nutrients to and waste materials away from all body tissues. **2.** One of the four humors of ancient and medieval physiology, identified with the blood found in the blood vessels, and believed to cause cheerfulness. **3.** Descent from a common ancestor; parental lineage.

blood agar *n.* A nutrient culture medium that is enriched with whole blood and used for the growth of certain strains of bacteria.

blood-air barrier *n.* The material intervening between alveolar air and the blood that consists of a nonstructural film or surfactant, alveolar epithelium, basement membrane, and endothelium.

blood albumin *n.* See **seralbumin.**

blood alcohol concentration *n.* The concentration of alcohol in the blood, expressed as the weight of alcohol in a fixed volume of blood and used as a measure of the degree of intoxication in an individual. The concentration depends on body weight, the quantity and rate of alcohol ingestion, and the rates of alcohol absorption and metabolism.

blood-aqueous barrier *n.* A membrane of the capillary bed of the ciliary body of the eye that permits two-way transfer of fluids between the aqueous chamber of the eye and the blood.

blood bank *n.* **1.** A place, usually a separate division of a hospital laboratory, in which blood is collected from donors, typed, and often separated into several components for future transfusion to recipients. **2.** Blood or plasma stored in such a place.

blood blister *n.* A blister containing blood, resulting from a pinch or a crushing injury.

blood-brain barrier *n. Abbr.* **BBB** A physiological mechanism that alters the permeability of brain capillaries so that some substances, such as certain drugs, are prevented from entering brain tissue, while other substances are allowed to enter freely.

blood capillary *n. Abbr.* **c** One of the minute blood vessels that connect arterioles and venules and are a part of an intricate network throughout the body for the interchange of oxygen, carbon dioxide, and other substances between blood and tissue cells.

blood cell *n.* Any of the cells contained in blood; an erythrocyte or leukocyte; a blood corpuscle.

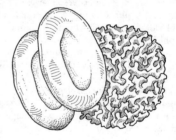

blood cell
Red blood cells (left) *and a white blood cell*

blood-cerebrospinal fluid barrier *n.* A barrier located at the tight junctions that surround and connect the cuboidal epithelial cells on the surface of the choroid plexus.

blood clot *n.* A semisolid, gelatinous mass of coagulated blood that consists of red blood cells, white blood cells, and platelets in a fibrin network.

blood count *n.* **1.** Calculation of the number of red blood cells, white blood cells, and platelets in a cubic millimeter of blood by counting the cells in an accurate volume of diluted blood. **2.** The determination of the percentages of various types of white blood cells observed in a stained film of blood. **3.** Complete blood count.

blood crystal *n.* A crystal of hematoidin in the blood.

blood cyst *n.* See **hemorrhagic cyst.**

blood disk *n.* A platelet.

blood dyscrasia *n.* A diseased state of the blood, usually one in which the blood contains permanent abnormal cellular elements.

blood fluke *n.* See **schistosome**.

blood gas *n.* Any of the gases that become dissolved in blood plasma, including oxygen, nitrogen, and carbon dioxide.

blood gas analysis *n.* The measurement of the partial pressure of oxygen and carbon dioxide concentrations in blood.

blood group *n.* **1.** Any of several immunologically distinct, genetically determined classes of human blood that are based on the presence or absence of certain antigens, are clinically identified by characteristic agglutination reactions, and are important with respect to blood transfusions and organ transplantation. **2.** Blood type.

blood group antigen *n.* Any of various inherited antigens found on the surface of red blood cells that determine a blood grouping reaction with a specific antiserum.

blood grouping *n.* The process of identifying an individual's blood group by serologic testing of a sample of blood. Also called *blood typing*.

blood group-specific substances A and B *n.* A solution of complexes of polysaccharides and amino acids that is used to render group O blood reasonably safe for transfusion into persons of group A, B, or AB.

blood heat *n.* The normal temperature (about 37.0°C or 98.6°F) of human blood.

blood·less operation (blŭd′lĭs) *n.* An operation performed with negligible loss of blood.

blood·let·ting (blŭd′lĕt′ĭng) *n.* The therapeutic removal of blood, usually from a vein. —**blood′let′ter** *n.*

blood·line (blŭd′līn′) *n.* The direct line of descent; a pedigree.

blood·mo·bile (blŭd′mə-bēl′) *n.* A motor vehicle that is equipped for collecting blood from donors.

blood plasma *n.* The yellow or gray-yellow, protein-containing fluid portion of blood in which the blood cells and platelets are normally suspended.

blood plasma fraction *n.* The components of blood plasma that are separated by electrophoresis or a similar analytical technique.

blood platelet *n.* See **platelet**.

blood poisoning *n.* **1.** See **septicemia**. **2.** See **toxemia**.

blood pressure *n. Abbr.* **BP** The pressure exerted by the blood against the walls of the arteries, maintained by the contraction of the left ventricle, the resistance of the arterioles and capillaries, the elasticity of the arterial walls, and by the viscosity and volume of the blood. Also called *arteriotony*.

blood profile *n.* See **complete blood count**.

blood relation *n.* A person who is related to another by birth rather than by marriage.

blood relationship *n.* Relationship by blood or by a common ancestor.

blood·shot (blŭd′shŏt′) *adj.* Red and inflamed as a result of locally congested blood vessels, as of the eyes.

blood·stream (blŭd′strēm′) *n.* The flow of blood through the circulatory system of an organism.

blood sugar *n.* **1.** See **glucose**. **2.** The concentration of glucose in the blood, measured in milligrams of glucose per 100 milliliters of blood.

blood test *n.* **1.** An examination of a sample of blood to determine its chemical, physical, or serologic characteristics. **2.** A serologic test for certain diseases, such as syphilis or AIDS.

blood thinner *n.* A drug used to prevent the formation of blood clots.

blood type *n.* **1.** The specific reaction pattern of red blood cells of an individual to the antisera of one blood group as, for example, of the ABO blood group, which consists of four major blood types, O, A, B, and AB. **2.** Blood group.

blood typing *n.* See **blood grouping**.

blood urea nitrogen *n. Abbr.* **BUN** Nitrogen in the form of urea in the blood or serum, used as a indicator of kidney function.

blood vessel *n.* An elastic tubular channel, such as an artery, a vein, a sinus, or a capillary, through which the blood circulates.

blood·y (blŭd′ē) *adj.* **1.** Stained with blood. **2.** Of, characteristic of, or containing blood. **3.** Suggesting the color of blood; blood-red. —*v.* **1.** To stain, spot, or color with or as if with blood. **2.** To make bleed, as by injuring or wounding.

Bloom's syndrome (bloomz) *n.* A rare genetic disease that is carried by an autosomal recessive gene and results in small stature, photosensitive skin, and a predisposition to various cancers.

blot (blŏt) *n.* The Northern, Southern, or Western blot analyses.

Blount's disease (blŭnts) *n.* Bowing of the legs in children due to a growth disturbance in the proximal tibial epiphysis.

blow·ing wound (blō′ĭng) *n.* See **open pneumothorax**.

blow-out fracture *n.* A fracture of the bone at the floor of the eye socket caused by a blow to the eye.

blue baby (bloo) *n.* An infant born with cyanosis as a result of a congenital cardiac or pulmonary defect that causes incomplete oxygenation of the blood.

blue·ber·ry muf·fin baby (bloo′bĕr·ē mŭf′ĭn) *n.* An infant that has jaundice and purpura, especially of the face, which may result from intrauterine viral infection.

blue cataract *n.* A coronary cataract of bluish color.

blue devil *n.* **1.** A blue capsule or tablet containing barbiturate amobarbital or its sodium derivative. **2.** A feeling of depression; despondency.

blue dome cyst *n.* **1.** A benign retention cyst of the mammary gland in fibrocystic disease, containing a light yellow fluid that gives the cyst a blue color when seen through the surrounding tissue. **2.** One of a number of small dark-blue nodules or cysts in the vaginal fornix caused by retained menstrual blood in endometriosis affecting this region.

blue line *n.* A bluish line along a border of the gums resulting from chronic lead poisoning.

blue nevus *n.* A dark-blue or blue-black smooth nevus that is formed by melanin-pigmented spindle cells situated in the lower dermis. Also called *Jadassohn-Tièche nevus*.

blue pus *n.* Pus that is tinged with blue because of the presence of pyocyanin, a product of the bacterium *Pseudomonas aeruginosa.*

blue rubber bleb nevus *n.* A skin disorder characterized by erectile, easily compressible, thin-walled, hemangiomatous nodules that occur in association with similar nodules in the alimentary canal and, sometimes, in other tissues.

blue spot *n.* 1. See **macula cerulea.** 2. See **mongolian spot.**

Blum·berg (blŭm′bərg, bloom′-), **Baruch Samuel** Born 1925. American virologist noted for research on the origin and spread of infectious diseases. He shared a 1976 Nobel Prize for discovering the antigen that led to a vaccine against hepatitis B.

Blum·berg's sign (blŭm′bərgz, bloom′-) *n.* An indication of peritonitis in which pain is felt upon sudden release of steadily applied pressure on a suspected area of the abdomen.

blunt duct adenosis (blŭnt) *n.* A glandular disease of the breast in which the ducts are enlarged.

blush (blŭsh) *n.* A sudden and brief redness of the face and neck due to emotion; flush. —**blush** *v.*

B lymphocyte *or* **B-lymphocyte** *n.* See **B cell.**

BM *abbr.* bowel movement

BMI *abbr.* body mass index

B-mode *n.* A two-dimensional diagnostic ultrasound presentation of echo-producing interfaces in a single plane.

BMR *abbr.* basal metabolic rate

board certification (bôrd) *n.* The process by which a person is tested and approved to practice in a specialty field, especially medicine, after successfully completing the requirements of a board of specialists in that field. For a physician, board certification is required in order to practice in a hospital. —**board-certified** *adj.*

board·er baby (bôr′dər) *n.* An infant, often the offspring of drug addicts or AIDS victims, who remains for months, sometimes up to a year, at the hospital where he or she was born, waiting for placement in a home.

Boch·da·lek's hernia (bŏk′də-lĕks′) *n.* A diaphragmatic hernia associated with a developmental defect in the pleuroperitoneal membrane.

Bo·dan·sky unit (bō-dăn′skē) *n.* A unit used as a measure of phosphatase concentration in the blood and based on the activity of phosphatase incubated for a given period in a particular buffered substrate.

bod·y (bŏd′ē) *n.* 1. The entire material or physical structure of an organism, especially of a human. 2. The physical part of a person. 3. A corpse or carcass. 4. The trunk or torso of a human, as distinguished from the head, neck, and extremities. 5. The largest or principal part, as of an organ; corpus. 6. A physical thing or kind of substance.

body clock *n.* An internal mechanism of the body that is thought to regulate physical and mental functions in rhythm with normal daily activities.

body fluid *n.* 1. A natural bodily fluid or secretion of fluid such as blood, semen, or saliva. 2. Total body water, contained principally in blood plasma and in intracellular and interstitial fluids.

body image *n.* 1. The cerebral representation of all body sensation organized in the parietal cortex. 2. The subjective concept of one's physical appearance based on self-observation and reactions of others.

body louse *n.* A parasitic louse that infests the body and clothes of humans.

body mass index *n. Abbr.* **BMI** A measurement of the relative percentages of fat and muscle mass in the human body, in which mass in kilograms is divided by height in meters squared and the result used as an index of obesity.

body mechanics *n.* The application of kinesiology to the use of proper body movement in daily activities, to the prevention and correction of problems associated with posture, and to the enhancement of coordination and endurance.

body of stomach *n.* The part of the stomach that lies between the fundus and the pyloric antrum.

Boeck's disease *or* **Boeck's sarcoid** (bĕks) *n.* See **sarcoidosis.**

Boer·haa·ve (bôr′hä′və, boor′-), **Hermann** 1668–1738. Dutch physician and educator noted for developing the modern technique of clinical medical instruction.

Boer·haa·ve's syndrome (bôr′hä′vəz, boor′-) *n.* Complete and spontaneous rupture of the lower esophagus, often causing painful swallowing.

Bohr (bôr), **Niels Henrik David** 1885–1962. Danish physicist. He won a 1922 Nobel Prize for his investigation of atomic structure and radiations. His son **Aage Niels Bohr** (born 1922), also a physicist, shared a 1975 Nobel Prize for discovering the asymmetry of atomic nuclei.

Bohr effect *n.* The influence of carbon dioxide on the oxygen dissociation curve of blood. The shift of the curve to the right means a reduction in the affinity of hemoglobin for oxygen.

bohr·i·um (bôr′ē-əm) *n. Symbol* **Bh** A radioactive synthetic element whose most long-lived isotopes have mass numbers of 261, 262, and 264 with half-lives of 11.8 milliseconds, 0.1 seconds, and 0.44 seconds. Atomic number 107.

boil (boil) *n.* A painful, circumscribed pus-filled inflammation of the skin and subcutaneous tissue usually caused by a local staphylococcal infection. Also called *furuncle.*

Bol·ling·er body (bŏl′ĭng-ər) *n.* A relatively large, somewhat granular, acidophilic, intracytoplasmic inclusion body observed in the infected tissues of birds with avian pox.

bo·lus (bō′ləs) *n., pl.* **-lus·es 1.** A round mass. **2.** A single, relatively large dose of a drug that is administered for therapeutic purposes and taken orally. **3.** A concentrated mass of a pharmaceutical substance administered intravenously for therapeutic or diagnostic purposes. **4.** A soft mass of chewed food within the mouth or alimentary canal.

bom·be·sin (bŏm′bĭ-sĭn) *n.* A neuropeptide found in brain tissue and at vagal nerve endings in the gastrointestinal mucosa.

bond (bŏnd) *n.* The linkage or force holding two neighboring atoms of a molecule in place and resisting their separation, usually accomplished by the transfer or sharing of one or more electrons or pairs of electrons between the atoms.

bond·ing (bŏn′dĭng) *n.* The emotional and physical attachment occurring between a parent or parent figure, especially a mother, and offspring, that usually begins at birth and is the basis for further emotional affiliation.

bone (bōn) *n.* **1.** The dense, semirigid, porous, calcified connective tissue forming the major portion of the skeleton of most vertebrates, consisting of a dense organic matrix and an inorganic, mineral component. **2.** Any of the more than 200 anatomically distinct structures making up the human skeleton. **3.** A piece of bone.

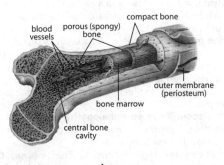

bone
cross section of an adult femur

bone block *n.* A surgical procedure in which the bone next to the joint is modified to limit the motion of the joint.

bone canaliculus *n.* Any of various channels interconnecting bone lacunae or connecting them with a haversian canal.

bone conduction *n.* The process by which sound waves are transmitted to the inner ear by the cranial bones without traveling through the air in the ear canal.

bone density *n.* A measurement corresponding to the mineral density of bone and used to diagnose osteopenia and osteoporosis. Also called *bone mineral density.*

bone forceps *n.* Strong forceps used for seizing or removing fragments of bone.

bone grafting *n.* See **osteoplasty** (sense 1).

bone·let (bōn′lĭt) *n.* See **ossicle.**

bone marrow *n.* The soft, fatty, vascular tissue filling the cavities of bones, having a stroma of reticular fibers and cells.

bone marrow transplantation *n.* A technique used to enhance or restore a person's immune response or supply of blood cells or to replace diseased or destroyed bone marrow with normally functioning bone marrow. The technique involves the removal of bone marrow from a donor and transplantation of it to a patient.

bone mass *n.* The mineral content of bone.

bone matrix *n.* The intercellular substance of bone tissue consisting of collagen fibers, ground substance, and inorganic bone salts.

bone mineral density *n.* See **bone density.**

bones of digits *pl.n.* The phalanges and sesamoid bones of the fingers or toes.

Bo·nine (bō′nēn′) A trademark for the drug meclizine.

Bo·ni·va (bō-nē′və) A trademark for the drug ibandronate sodium.

Bon·ne·vie-Ull·rich syndrome (bôn′ə-vē-ōol′rĭk, -rĭкн) *n.* See **pseudo-Turner's syndrome.**

bon·y *or* **bon·ey** (bō′nē) *adj.* **1.** Of, relating to, resembling, or consisting of bone. **2.** Having an internal skeleton of bones. **3.** Having prominent or protruding bones. **4.** Lean; scrawny.

bony ankylosis *n.* See **synostosis.**

bony labyrinth *n.* See **osseous labyrinth.**

bony palate *n.* A concave elliptical bony plate, constituting the roof of the oral cavity.

boost·er (bōo′stər) *n.* An additional dose of an immunizing agent, such as a vaccine or toxoid, given at a time after the initial dose to sustain the immune response elicited by the previous dose of the same agent. Also called *booster dose, booster shot.*

bo·rate (bôr′āt′) *n.* A salt or ester of boric acid.

bo·rax (bôr′ăks′, -əks) *n.* Sodium borate.

bor·bo·ryg·mus (bôr′bə-rĭg′məs) *n., pl.* **-mi′** (-mī′) A rumbling noise that is produced by the movement of gas through the intestines.

bor·der·line personality disorder (bôr′dər-līn′) *n.* A personality disorder marked by instability in interpersonal relationships, behavior, mood, and self-image that can interfere with social or occupational functioning or cause extreme emotional distress.

Bor·det (bôr-dā′), **Jules Jean Baptiste Vincent** 1870–1961. Belgian bacteriologist. With French bacteriologist Octave Gengou (1875–1957), he developed (1900) the technique of complement fixation testing and discovered (1906) the agent of whooping cough. Bordet won a 1919 Nobel Prize for advances in immunology.

Bor·de·tel·la (bôr′dĭ-tĕl′ə) *n.* A genus of aerobic bacteria that contain minute gram-negative coccobacilli and are parasites and pathogens of the mammalian respiratory tract.

Bordet-Gen·gou bacillus (-zhän-gōo′) *n.* An aerobic gram-negative bacterium *Bordetella pertussis* that causes whooping cough in humans.

bo·ric acid (bôr′ĭk) *n.* A water-soluble white or colorless crystalline compound used as an antiseptic and preservative.

bo·rism (bôr′ĭz′əm) *n.* The symptoms that result from the ingestion of borax or of another compound of boron.

Bör·je·son-Forssman-Leh·mann syndrome (bôr′yə-sən-, bœr′yĕ-sōon-; -lā′mən, -män′) *n.* An inherited disorder that is marked by mental retardation, epilepsy, hypogonadism, hypometabolism, obesity, and narrow palpebral fissures.

Born·holm disease (bôrn′hōm′, -hōlm′, -hôlm′) *n.* See **epidemic pleurodynia.**

Bornholm disease virus *n.* See **epidemic pleurodynia virus.**

bo·ron (bôr′ŏn′) *n. Symbol* **B** A soft, nonmetallic element found in compounds used in treating cancer and as astringents and antiseptics. Atomic number 5.

boron neutron capture therapy *n.* A treatment for cancers, especially virulent ones of the brain, in which a person who has been injected with a boron compound that concentrates in cancerous cells is exposed to neutron irradiation causing the boron compound to emit alpha particles that destroy the cancer cells.

Bor·re·li·a (bə-rē′lē-ə, -rĕl′ē-ə) *n.* A genus of parasitic irregularly coiled helical spirochetes, some species of which cause relapsing fever in humans.

Borrelia burg·dor·fe·ri (bərg-dôr′fə-rī) *n.* A spirochete causing Lyme disease in humans.

bor·re·li·o·sis (bə-rē′lē-ō′sĭs, -rĕl′ē-) *n.* Disease caused by bacteria of the genus *Borrelia.*

bos·om (bŏŏz′əm, bōō′zəm) *n.* **1.** The chest of a human. **2.** A woman's breast or breasts.

boss (bôs) *n.* **1.** A circumscribed rounded swelling; a protuberance. **2.** The prominence of a kyphosis.

Bos·ton's sign (bô′stənz) *n.* An indication of Graves' disease in which the lowering of the upper eyelid is jerky during the downward rotation of the eye.

bot (bŏt) *n.* **1.** The parasitic larva of a botfly. **2. bots** A disease of mammals, especially cattle and horses, caused by infestation of the stomach or intestines with botfly larvae.

Bo·tal·lo's duct (bə-tăl′ōz, -tä′lōz) *n.* See **ductus arteriosus.**

bot·fly (bŏt′flī′) *n.* A robust hairy fly of the order Diptera whose larvae produce a variety of myiasis conditions in humans and various domestic animals.

Both·ri·o·ceph·a·lus (bŏth′rē-ō-sĕf′ə-ləs) *n.* A genus of tapeworms with both plerocercoid and adult stages in fishes.

Bo·tox (bō′tŏks′) A trademark for a preparation of botulinum toxin, used to treat blepharospasms, strabismus, and muscle dystonias and to smooth facial wrinkles.

bot·ry·oid (bŏt′rē-oid′) *adj.* Having numerous rounded protuberances resembling a bunch of grapes.

botryoid sarcoma *n.* A polypoid form of rhabdomyosarcoma occurring in children, most frequently in the urogenital tract, and characterized by the formation of grapelike clusters of neoplastic tissue.

bot·u·lin (bŏch′ə-lĭn) *n.* See **botulinus toxin.**

bot·u·li·num (bŏch′ə-lī′nəm) *or* **bot·u·li·nus** (-nəs) *n.* An anaerobic, rod-shaped bacterium (*Clostridium botulinum*) that secretes botulin and inhabits soils.

botulinus toxin *n.* Any of several potent neurotoxins produced by the bacterium *Clostridium botulinum* and resistant to proteolytic digestion. Also called *botulin.*

bot·u·lism (bŏch′ə-lĭz′əm) *n.* A severe, sometimes fatal food poisoning caused by ingestion of a toxin produced by the bacterium *Clostridium botulinum* in improperly canned or preserved food and characterized by nausea, vomiting, disturbed vision, and paralysis.

botulism antitoxin *n.* The antitoxin to the toxins of the various strains of *Clostridium botulinum.*

bou·bas (bōō′bəz) *n.* See **yaws.**

Bou·chard's node (bōō-shärdz′) *n.* A bony outgrowth on the dorsal aspect of a proximal interphalangeal joint, characteristic of osteoarthritis.

bou·gie (bōō′zhē, -jē) *n.* A cylindrical instrument, usually somewhat flexible and yielding, used for calibrating or dilating constricted areas in tubular organs, such as the urethra or rectum.

bou·gie·nage (bōō′zhē-näzh′) *n.* The examination or treatment of the interior of a canal by the passage of a bougie or cannula.

Bour·ne·ville-Pringle disease (bōōr′nə-vēl′-) *n.* Tuberous sclerosis occurring in association with adenoma sebaceum.

Bour·ne·ville's disease (bōōr′nə-vēlz′) *n.* See **tuberous sclerosis.**

bou·ton (bōō-tôn′) *n.* A button, pustule, or knoblike swelling.

bou·ton·neuse fever (bōō′tə-nœz′) *n.* A tick-borne disease seen primarily in the Mediterranean and South Africa, caused by *Rickettsia conori,* and characterized by rash, fever, headache, and muscle and joint pain.

Bo·vet (bō-vā′, -vĕt′), **Daniel** 1907–1992. Swiss-born Italian physiologist. He won a Nobel Prize 1957 for the development of muscle relaxants and the first synthetic antihistamine.

bovine growth hormone *n.* A naturally occurring hormone of cattle that regulates growth and milk production. It may also be produced artificially by genetic engineering techniques and administered to cows to increase milk production. Also called *bovine somatotropin.*

bovine spongiform encephalopathy *n. Abbr.* **BSE** An infectious degenerative brain disease occurring in cattle. Also called *mad cow disease.*

Bow·ditch's law (bou′dĭch′ĭz) *n.* The principle that heart muscle, regardless of the strength of the stimulus it receives, will contract to its fullest extent or will not contract at all.

bow·el (bou′əl, boul) *n.* The intestine. Often used in the plural.

bowel bypass *n.* See **jejunoileal bypass.**

bowel bypass syndrome *n.* A syndrome following and resulting from bowel bypass surgery whose symptoms include fever, chills, malaise, and inflammatory cutaneous papules and pustules on the extremities and upper trunk.

bowel movement *n. Abbr.* **BM 1.** The discharge of waste matter from the large intestine; defecation. **2.** The waste matter discharged from the large intestine; feces.

bowel sounds *pl.n.* Abdominal sounds caused by the products of digestion as they move through the lower gastrointestinal tract, usually heard on auscultation.

Bow·en's disease (bō′ənz) *n.* A dermatosis or form of intraepidermal carcinoma characterized by the development of pinkish or brownish skin papules covered with a thickened horny layer.

bow·leg (bō′lĕg′) *n.* A leg having an outward curvature in the region of the knee.

Bow·man (bō′mən), Sir **William** 1816–1892. British histologist, ophthalmologist, and surgeon who is noted for his studies of the eye, the kidney, and striated muscle.

Bow·man's capsule (bō′mənz) *n.* A double-walled, cup-shaped structure around the glomerulus of each nephron of the vertebrate kidney. It serves as a filter to remove organic wastes, excess inorganic salts, and water. Also called *malpighian capsule.*

Bowman's gland *n.* See **olfactory gland.**

Bowman's membrane *n.* See **limiting layer of cornea** (sense 1).

Bowman's space *n.* See **capsular space.**

Boy·den meal (boid′n) *n.* A meal consisting of three or four egg yolks, beaten up in milk and sweetened, used to test the evacuation time of the gallbladder.

Boy·er's bursa (bwä-yāz′) *n.* See **retrohyoid bursa.**

Boyer's cyst *n.* A cyst of the subhyoid bursa.

Boyle's law (boilz) *n.* The principle that at a constant temperature the volume of a confined ideal gas varies inversely with its pressure.

Boze·man-Fritsch catheter (bōz′mən-frĭch′) *n.* A slightly curved double-channel uterine catheter with several openings at the tip.

Boze·man's position (bōz′mənz) *n.* A knee-elbow position in which the patient is strapped to supports.

BP *abbr.* blood pressure; boiling point; British Pharmacopoeia

BPH *abbr.* benign prostatic hyperplasia

Br The symbol for the element **bromine.**

brace (brās) *n.* **1.** An orthopedic appliance that supports or holds a movable part of the body in correct position while allowing motion of the part. **2.** *Often* **braces** A dental appliance, constructed of bands and wires that is fixed to the teeth to correct irregular alignment.

bra·chi·al (brā′kē-əl) *adj.* Relating to the arm.

brachial artery *n.* **1.** An artery that is a continuation of the axillary artery, with branches to the deep brachial, superior and inferior ulnar collateral, muscular, and nutrient arteries, and with bifurcations at the elbow into the radial and the ulnar arteries. **2.** An artery that is an occasional variation of the brachial artery and in which the brachial artery lies superficial to the median nerve in the arm; superficial brachial artery. **3.** An artery with origin in the brachial artery, with distribution to the shoulder and to the muscles and integument of the arm, and with anastomoses to the radial recurrent, recurrent interosseous, ulnar collateral, and posterior circumflex humeral arteries; deep brachial artery.

bra·chi·al·gia (brā′kē-ăl′jə) *n.* Pain in the arm.

brachial muscle *n.* A muscle with its origin in the anterior two thirds of the humerus, with insertion to the coronoid process of the ulna, with nerve supply from the musculocutaneous and radial nerves, and whose action flexes the forearm.

brachial neuritis *n.* See **brachial plexus neuropathy.**

brachial plexus *n.* A network of nerves located in the neck and axilla, composed of the anterior branches of the lower four cervical and first two thoracic spinal nerves and supplying the chest, shoulder, and arm.

brachial plexus neuropathy *n.* An acute syndrome of unknown cause marked by pain in the shoulder girdle, flaccid weakness of the muscles innervated by the brachial plexus, and mild sensory loss in the affected dermatomes, usually of limited duration with spontaneous recovery. Also called *acute brachial radiculitis, brachial neuritis, shoulder-girdle syndrome, shoulder-hand syndrome.*

brachial vein *n.* Either of two veins in either arm accompanying the brachial artery and emptying into the axillary vein.

brachio– *pref.* Arm: *brachiocephalic.*

bra·chi·o·ce·phal·ic (brā′kē-ō-sə-făl′ĭk, brăk′ē-) *adj.* Relating to the arm and the head.

brachiocephalic trunk *n.* See **innominate artery.**

brachiocephalic vein *n.* Either of two veins formed by the union of the internal jugular and subclavian veins. See under **left brachiocephalic vein** and **right brachiocephalic vein.** Also called *innominate vein.*

bra·chi·o·cru·ral (brā′kē-ō-krŏŏr′əl, brăk′ē-) *adj.* Relating to the arm and the thigh.

bra·chi·o·cu·bi·tal (brā′kē-ō-kyōō′bĭ-tl, brăk′ē-) *adj.* **1.** Relating to the arm and the elbow. **2.** Relating to the arm and the forearm.

bra·chi·o·ra·di·al·is (brā′kē-ō-rā′dē-əl, brăk′ē-) *n.* A muscle with its origin in the lateral supracondylar ridge of the humerus, with insertion to the front of the base of the styloid process of the radius, with nerve supply from the radial nerve, and whose action flexes the forearm.

bra·chi·um (brā′kē-əm, brăk′ē-) *n., pl.* **bra·chi·a** (brā′-kē-ə, brăk′ē-ə) **1.** The arm, especially between the shoulder and the elbow. **2.** An armlike structure.

Bracht maneuver (bräkt, bräкнт) *n.* Delivery of a fetus in breech position by extending the legs and trunk of the fetus over the pubic symphysis and abdomen of the mother, which leads to spontaneous delivery of the fetal head.

brachy– *pref.* Short: *brachydactyly.*

brach·y·ba·sia (brăk′ē-bā′zhə) *n.* The shuffling gait characteristic of partial paraplegia.

brach·y·ba·so·camp·to·dac·ty·ly (brăk′ē-bā′sō-kămp′tō-dăk′tə-lē) *n.* A condition marked by abnormally short and crooked fingers.

brach·y·ba·so·pha·lan·gia (brăk′ē-bā′sō-fə-lăn′jə) *n.* Abnormally short proximal phalanges.

brach·y·car·di·a (brăk′ē-kär′dē-ə) *n.* See **bradycardia.**

brach·y·chei·li·a *or* **brach·y·chi·li·a** (brăk′ē-kī′lē-ə) *n.* Abnormally short lips.

brach·y·dac·ty·ly (brăk′ē-dăk′tə-lē) *n.* An abnormal shortness of the fingers.

brach·yg·na·thi·a (brăk′ĭg-nā′thē-ə) *n.* An abnormal shortness or recession of the mandible. Also called *bird face.*

brach·y·mel·i·a (brăk′ē-mĕl′ē-ə, -mē′lē-ə) *n.* Disproportionate shortness of the limbs.

brach·y·mes·o·pha·lan·gia (brăk′ē-mĕz′ō-fə-lăn′jə) *n.* Abnormal shortness of the middle phalanxes of the digits.

brach·y·met·a·car·pi·a (brăk′ē-mĕt′ə-kär′pē-ə) *n.* Abnormal shortness of the metacarpal bones.

brach·y·met·a·tar·si·a (brăk′ē-mĕt′ə-tär′sē-ə) *n.* Abnormal shortness of the metatarsal bones.

brach·y·pel·lic pelvis (brăk′ē-pĕl′ĭk) *n.* A pelvis in which the transverse diameter is longer than the anteroposterior diameter.

brach·y·pha·lan·gia (brăk′ē-fə-lăn′jə) *n.* Brachybasophalangia.

brach·y·syn·dac·ty·ly (brăk′ē-sĭn-dăk′tə-lē) *n.* Abnormal shortness of fingers or toes combined with a webbing between the adjacent digits.

brach·y·tel·e·pha·lan·gia (brăk′ē-tĕl′ə-fə-lăn′jə) *n.* Abnormal shortness of the distal phalanges.

brach·y·ther·a·py (brăk′ē-thĕr′ə-pē) *n.* Radiotherapy in which the source of irradiation is placed close to the surface of the body or within a body cavity.

Brad·ford frame (brăd′fərd) *n.* A rectangular metal frame having canvas or webbing straps and used to support individuals with diseases or fractures of the spine, hip, or pelvis.

brady– *pref.* Slow: *bradycardia.*

brad·y·ar·rhyth·mi·a (brăd′ē-ə-rĭth′mē-ə) *n.* A disturbance of the heart's rhythm resulting in a rate under 60 beats per minute.

brad·y·ar·thri·a (brăd′ē-är′thrē-ə) *n.* A form of dysarthria that is characterized by an abnormal slowness or deliberation in speech. Also called *bradyglossia, bradylalia.*

brad·y·car·di·a (brăd′ĭ-kär′dē-ə) *n.* A slowness of the heartbeat, usually under 60 beats per minute in adults. Also called *brachycardia.* —**brad′y·car′dic** (-dĭk), **brad′y·car′di·ac′** (-dē-ăk′) *adj.*

bra·dy·di·as·to·le (brăd′ē-dī-ăs′tə-lē) *n.* The prolongation of the diastole of the heart.

brad·y·es·the·sia (brăd′ē-ĕs-thē′zhə) *n.* Retardation in the rate of transmission of sensory impressions.

brad·y·glos·si·a (brăd′ē-glô′sē-ə) *n.* **1.** Slow or difficult tongue movement. **2.** See **bradyarthria.**

brad·y·ki·ne·sia (brăd′ē-kĭ-nē′zhə, -kī-) *n.* Extreme slowness in movement. —**brad′y·ki·net′ic** (-nĕt′ĭk) *adj.*

brad·y·ki·nin (brăd′ĭ-kī′nĭn, -kĭn′ĭn) *n.* A biologically active polypeptide that forms from a blood plasma globulin and mediates the inflammatory response, increases vasodilation, and causes contraction of smooth muscle. Also called *kallidin I.*

brad·y·ki·nin·o·gen (brăd′ē-kə-nĭn′ə-jən, -jĕn′, -kī-) *n.* A plasma alpha globulin that is the precursor to bradykinin. Also called *kallidin II.*

brad·y·la·li·a (brăd′ē-lā′lē-ə) *n.* See **bradyarthria.**

brad·y·lex·i·a (brăd′ē-lĕk′sē-ə) *n.* Abnormal slowness in reading.

brad·y·pha·sia (brăd′ə-fā′zhə) *n.* Abnormal slowness in speech.

brad·yp·ne·a (brăd′ĭp-nē′ə, brăd′ē-nē′ə) *n.* Abnormal slowness of respiration.

brad·y·sper·ma·tism (brăd′ē-spûr′mə-tĭz′əm) *n.* Absence of ejaculatory force.

brad·y·sphyg·mi·a (brăd′ē-sfĭg′mē-ə) *n.* Slowness of the pulse, as in bradycardia.

brad·y·stal·sis (brăd′ē-stăl′sĭs) *n.* Slow bowel motion.

brad·y·to·ci·a (brăd′ē-tō′sē-ə) *n.* Slow childbirth.

brad·y·u·ri·a (brăd′ē-yŏŏr′ē-ə) *n.* Slow passage of urine.

brain (brān) *n.* The portion of the central nervous system that is enclosed within the cranium, continuous with the spinal cord, and composed of gray matter and white matter. It is the primary center for the regulation and control of bodily activities, receiving and interpreting sensory impulses, and transmitting information to the muscles and body organs. It is also the seat of consciousness, thought, memory, and emotion. Also called *encephalon.*

brain·case (brān′kās′) *n.* The part of the skull that encloses the brain; the cranium.

brain concussion *n.* A clinical syndrome occurring as the result of trauma to the head and characterized by immediate and transient impairment of neural function, such as loss of consciousness.

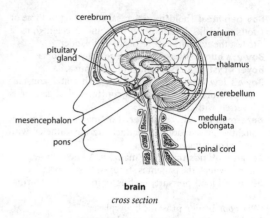

brain
cross section

brain damage *n.* Injury to the brain that is caused by various conditions, such as head trauma, inadequate oxygen supply, infection, or intracranial hemorrhage, and that may be associated with a behavioral or functional abnormality.

brain death *n.* Irreversible brain damage and loss of brain function, as evidenced by cessation of breathing and other vital reflexes, unresponsiveness to stimuli, absence of muscle activity, and a flat electroencephalogram for a specific length of time. Also called *cerebral death.* —**brain′-dead′** *adj.*

brain fever *n.* Inflammation of the brain or meninges.

brain hormone *n.* Any of various hormones produced in the hypothalamic region of the brain, especially those acting on the pituitary gland to release other hormones.

brain mantle *n.* See **pallium.**

brain sand *n.* A gritty substance present in central nervous tissue or in the pineal gland. Also called *acervulus, psammoma body.*

Brain's reflex (brānz) *n.* See **quadripedal extensor reflex.**

brain·stem *or* **brain stem** (brān′stĕm′) *n.* The portion of the brain, consisting of the medulla oblongata, pons Varolii, and mesencephalon, that connects the spinal cord to the forebrain and cerebrum.

brainstem evoked response audiometry *n.* See **auditory brainstem response audiometry.**

brain sugar *n.* See **galactose.**

brain swelling *n.* A localized or generalized increase in the bulk of brain tissue due to congestion or edema.

brain·wash·ing (brān′wŏsh′ĭng) *n.* Inducing a person to modify his or her beliefs, attitudes, or behavior by conditioning through various forms of pressure or torture.

brain wave *n.* A rhythmic fluctuation of electric potential between parts of the brain, as seen on an electroencephalogram.

bran (brăn) *n.* The outer layers of a cereal grain such as wheat, approximately 20 percent of which is indigestible cellulose, used as a source of dietary fiber.

branch (brănch) *n.* An offshoot or a division of the main portion of a structure, especially that of a nerve, blood vessel, or lymphatic vessel; a ramus.

branched chain ketoaciduria (brăncht) *n.* See **maple syrup urine disease.**

bran·cher deficiency amylopectinosis (brăn′chər) *n.* See **type 4 glycogenosis.**

brancher enzyme *n.* **1.** 1,4-alpha-glucan branching enzyme. **2.** An enzyme that catalyzes the conversion of amylose to glycogen.

bran·chi·al (brăng′kē-əl) *adj.* Of, relating to, or resembling the gills of a fish, their homologous embryonic structures, or the derivatives of their homologous parts in higher animals.

branchial arch *n.* Any of usually six embryonic arches that give rise to specialized structures in the head and neck in the higher vertebrates. Also called *gill arch, pharyngeal arch, visceral arch.*

branchial cell *n.* Any of various cartilage cells forming the embryonic aggregate of pharyngeal arches, pouches, and membranes.

branchial cleft *n.* **1.** One of a bilateral series of slit-like openings into the pharynx through which water is drawn by aquatic animals. **2.** Any of the homologous branchialectodermal grooves of the mammalian embryo.

branchial duct *n.* The lumen of one of the embryonic pharyngeal pouches that has elongated and narrowed as a result of differentiation.

branchial pouch *n.* See **pharyngeal pouch.**

bran·chi·o·mo·tor nuclei (brăng′ē-ō-mō′tər) *pl.n.* Motoneuronal nuclei of the brainstem that develop from the branchiomotor column of the embryo and innervate striated muscle fibers developed from the mesenchyme of the branchial arches.

Brandt-An·drews maneuver (brănt′ăn′drōōz) *n.* A method of expressing the placenta by grasping the umbilical cord with one hand and placing the other hand on the abdomen.

Bran·ha·mel·la (brăn′hə-měl′ə) *n.* A genus of aerobic, nonmotile, asporogenic bacteria containing gram-negative cocci and occurring in the mucous membranes of the upper respiratory tract.

bran·ny (brăn′ē) *adj.* Resembling broken layers of small husklike scales.

brawn·y (brô′nē) *adj.* **1.** Strong and muscular. **2.** Hardened; calloused.

Brax·ton-Hicks contraction *or* **Brax·ton Hicks contraction** (brăk′stən hĭks′) *n.* One of a series of usually painless uterine contractions that occur with increasing frequency during pregnancy.

Braxton Hicks sign *n.* Irregular uterine contractions occurring after the third month of pregnancy.

BRCA1 (bē′är-sē′ā-wŭn′) *n.* A tumor suppressor gene that, when inherited in a mutated state, is associated with the development of various cancers, especially breast and ovarian cancer.

BRCA2 (bē′är-sē′ā-tōō′) *n.* A tumor suppressor gene that, when inherited in a mutated state, is associated with the development of various cancers, especially breast and ovarian cancer.

break·bone fever (brāk′bōn′) *n.* See **dengue.**

break·down (brāk′doun′) *n.* **1.** The act or process of failing to function or continue. **2.** A typically sudden collapse in physical or mental health. **3.** Disintegration or decomposition into parts or elements.

break·ing point (brā′kĭng) *n.* **1.** The point at which physical, mental, or emotional strength gives way under stress. **2.** The point at which a condition or situation becomes critical.

breast (brĕst) *n.* **1.** Either of two milk-secreting, glandular organs on the chest of a woman; mammary gland; mamma. **2.** A corresponding rudimentary gland in the male. **3.** The superior ventral surface of the human body, extending from the neck to the abdomen.

breast·bone (brĕst′bōn′) *n.* See **sternum.**

breast-feed (brĕst′fēd) *v.* To feed a baby mother's milk from the breast; suckle.

breast pump *n.* A suction device for withdrawing milk from the breast.

breath (brĕth) *n.* **1.** The air inhaled and exhaled in respiration. **2.** A single respiration.

breath-holding test *n.* A test used as a rough index of cardiopulmonary reserve, measured by the length of time a person can hold his or her breath. Diminished cardiac or pulmonary reserve is indicated if one's breath is held for less than 20 seconds.

breath·ing (brē′thĭng) *n.* The alternate inhalation and exhalation of air in respiration.

breathing bag *n.* A collapsible reservoir from which gases are inhaled and into which gases may be exhaled during general anesthesia or artificial ventilation. Also called *reservoir bag.*

breathing reserve *n.* The difference between the volume of air breathed under ordinary resting conditions and the maximum breathing capacity.

breath sounds *pl.n.* Sounds, such as rales or rhonchi, that are heard upon auscultation of the lungs or associated parts of the respiratory system.

Bre·da's disease (brā′dəz, brĕ′däz) *n.* See **espundia.**

breech (brēch) *n.* The lower rear portion of the human trunk; the buttocks.

breech delivery *n.* Delivery of a fetus with the buttocks or feet appearing first. Also called *breech birth.*

breech presentation *n.* Presentation of the fetus during birth with the buttocks or less commonly the knees or feet first.

breg·ma (brĕg′mə) *n., pl.* **–ma·ta** (-mə-tə) The junction of the sagittal and coronal sutures at the top of the skull. **—breg·mat·ic** (-măt′ĭk) *adj.*

Bren·ner tumor (brĕn′ər) *n.* A rare benign neoplasm of the ovary consisting primarily of fibrous tissue with nests of cells resembling transitional type epithelium and glandlike structures containing mucin.

Bres·low's thickness (brĕs′lōz) *n.* The greatest thickness of a primary cutaneous melanoma, measured in tissue sections from the top of the epidermal granular layer, or from the ulcer base if the tumor is ulcerated, to the bottom of the tumor, and used to estimate the rate of metastasis.

Bre·ton·neau (brĭ-tô-nō′), **Pierre** 1778–1862. French surgeon who described typhoid and diphtheria and performed the first tracheotomy (1825).

Breus mole (brois) *n.* An aborted ovum in which the fetal surface of the placenta contains numerous hematomas, the chorion has no blood vessels, and the ovum is much smaller than normal for its given point in the pregnancy.

brev·i·col·lis (brĕv′ĭ-kŏl′ĭs) *n.* Shortness of the neck.

brew·er's yeast (broō′ərz) *n.* A yeast (genus *Saccharomyces*) used as a source of B-complex vitamins.

Brick·er operation (brĭk′ər) *n.* An operation utilizing an isolated segment of ileum to collect urine from both ureters and conduct it to the skin surface.

Brick·ner's position (brĭk′nərz) *n.* A position in which the wrist is tied to the elevated head of the bed, used to obtain traction in abduction and external rotation.

bridge (brĭj) *n.* **1.** An anatomical structure resembling a bridge or span. **2.** The upper part of the ridge of the nose formed by the nasal bones. **3.** A fixed or removable replacement for one or several but not all of the natural teeth, usually anchored at each end to a natural tooth. **4.** One of the threads of protoplasm that appears to pass from one cell to another.

Bridg·es (brĭj′ĭz), Calvin Blackman 1889–1938. American geneticist noted for his work on the chromosome theory of heredity and the mapping of chromosomes.

bridge·work (brĭj′wûrk′) *n.* See **partial denture.**

bri·dle suture (brīd′l) *n.* A suture passed through the superior rectus muscle to rotate the globe downward in eye surgery.

Bright's disease (brīts) *n.* Any of several diseases of the kidney marked especially by edema and the presence of albumin in the urine.

bril·liant cre·syl blue (brĭl′yənt krē′sĭl) *n.* A basic dye used for reticulocytes.

brilliant green *n.* An indicator dye that changes from yellow to green at pH 0.0 to 2.6 and is also used as a topical antiseptic and as a selective bacteriostatic agent in culture media.

Brill's disease (brĭlz) *n.* See **Brill-Zinsser disease.**

Brill-Sym·mers disease (-sĭm′ərz) *n.* See **nodular lymphoma.**

Brill-Zins·ser disease (-zĭn′sər) *n.* A relatively mild recurrence of epidemic typhus in persons previously infected with the *Rickettsia prowazekii* bacterium. Also called *Brill's disease, recrudescent typhus.*

brim (brĭm) *n.* The rim of the upper opening of the pelvis.

brise·ment for·cé (brēz-mäN′ fôr-sā′) *n.* The forcible manipulation of an ankylosed joint or joints.

Brit·ish anti-lewisite (brĭt′ĭsh) *n.* See **dimercaprol.**

British thermal unit *n. Abbr.* **Btu 1.** The quantity of heat required to raise the temperature of one pound of water from 60° to 61°F at a constant pressure of one atmosphere. **2.** The quantity of heat equal to $\frac{1}{180}$ of the heat required to raise the temperature of one pound of water from 32° to 212°F at a constant pressure of one atmosphere.

brit·tle bones (brĭt′l) *n.* See **osteogenesis imperfecta.**

brittle diabetes *n.* Insulin-dependent diabetes in which there are wide unpredictable fluctuations in blood glucose concentrations.

broach (brōch) *n.* A dental instrument for removing the pulp of a tooth or exploring its canal.

Broad·bent's sign (brôd′bĕnts′) *n.* An indication of adherent pericardium in which the retraction of the thoracic wall is synchronous with cardiac systole and is visible in the left posterior axillary line.

broad fascia (brôd) *n.* The strong fascia enveloping the muscles of the thigh.

broad ligament of uterus *n.* The peritoneal fold passing from the lateral margin of the uterus to the wall of the pelvis on either side.

broad-spectrum *adj.* Effective against a wide range of organisms, especially gram-positive and gram-negative bacteria.

Bro·ca (brō′kə, brō-kä′), Paul 1824–1880. French anthropologist and surgeon. He became the first to offer anatomical proof of the localization of brain functions when he discovered (1861) the center of articulate speech in the brain.

Bro·ca's aphasia (brō′kəz) *n.* See **motor aphasia.**

Broca's area *n.* A small posterior part of the inferior frontal gyrus of the left cerebral hemisphere, identified as an essential component of the motor mechanisms governing articulated speech. Also called *Broca's center, motor speech center.*

Bro·die's abscess (brō′dēz) *n.* A chronic abscess of bone surrounded by dense fibrous tissue and sclerotic bone.

Brod·mann's area (brŏd′mənz) *n.* Any of the areas of the cerebral cortex mapped out on the basis of the cortical cytoarchitectural patterns.

bro·mate (brō′māt′) *n.* **1.** A salt of bromic acid. **2.** An ion of bromic acid. —*v.* To treat a substance chemically with a bromate.

bro·me·lain (brō′mə-lān′) *or* **bro·me·lin** (-lĭn) *n.* A peptide hydrolase obtained from pineapple used in treating inflammation and edema of soft tissues associated with traumatic injury.

bro·mic acid (brō′mĭk) *n.* A corrosive, colorless bromine-containing liquid used in making dyes and pharmaceuticals.

bro·mide (brō′mīd′) *n.* **1.** A binary compound of bromine with another element, especially a salt containing monovalent negatively charged bromine. **2.** Potassium bromide.

bro·mi·dro·sis (brō′mĭ-drō′sĭs) *or* **brom·hi·dro·sis** (brō′mĭ-drō′sĭs, brōm′hĭ-) *n.* Fetid or foul-smelling perspiration. Also called *osmidrosis.*

bro·mi·nate (brō′mə-nāt′) *v.* To combine with bromine or with a compound containing bromine.

bro·mine (brō′mēn) *n. Symbol* **Br** A volatile nonmetallic liquid element having a highly irritating vapor and used in disinfecting water and in various pharmaceuticals. Atomic number 35.

bro·mism (brō′mĭz′əm) *or* **bro·min·ism** (brō′mə-nĭz′-əm) *n.* Chronic bromide poisoning, characterized by headache, drowsiness, confusion, occasionally violent delirium, muscular weakness, cardiac depression, acneform eruption, foul breath, anorexia, and gastric distress.

bromo– *or* **brom–** *pref.* Bromine: *bromide.*

bro·mo·crip·tine (brō′mō-krĭp′tēn′) *n.* An ergot alkaloid that slows dopamine turnover and inhibits prolactin secretion and thus is used in the treatment of Parkinson's disease and to retard the growth of various pituitary tumors.

bro·mo·der·ma (brō′mə-dûr′mə) *n.* An acneform or granulomatous eruption due to hypersensitivity to bromide.

brom·phen·ir·a·mine maleate (brōm′fĕn-ĭr′ə-mēn′) *n.* A white, soluble, crystalline powder that is used as an antihistamine.

brom·phe·nol test (brōm-fē′nôl′, -nōl′) *n.* A colorimetric test that measures amounts of protein, albumin, and globulin in urine by the use of reagent strips.

Bromp·ton cocktail (brŏmp′tən, brŏm′-) *n.* A mixture of morphine and cocaine usually used for analgesia in terminal cancer patients.

bronch– *pref.* Variant of **broncho–**.

bronchi– *pref.* Variant of **broncho–**.

bron·chi·al (brŏng′kē-əl) *adj.* Relating to the bronchi, the bronchial tubes, or the bronchioles.

bronchial adenoma *n.* A slow-growing benign or malignant polypoid epithelial tumor of the bronchial mucosa.

bronchial asthma *n.* A condition of the lungs characterized by widespread narrowing of the airways due to spasm of the smooth muscle, edema of the mucosa, and the presence of mucus in the lumen of the bronchi and bronchioles. It is caused by the local release of spasmogens and vasoactive substances in the course of an allergic reaction.

bronchial calculus *n.* See **broncholith**.

bronchial gland *n.* Any of the mucous and seromucous glands having secretory units outside the muscle of the bronchi.

bronchial pneumonia *n.* See **bronchopneumonia**.

bronchial tube *n.* Any of the smaller divisions of the bronchi of the lung.

bronchial vein *n.* Any of the veins that run in front of and behind the bronchi and unite into two main trunks emptying on the right into the azygos vein and on the left into the accessory hemiazygos vein or the left superior intercostal vein.

bron·chi·ec·ta·sis (brŏng′kē-ĕk′tə-sĭs) *n.* Chronic dilation of bronchi or bronchioles, often due to inflammatory disease or obstruction. —**bron′chi·ec·tat′ic** (-ĕk-tăt′ĭk), **bron′chi·ec·ta′sic** (-tā′zĭk) *adj.*

bron·chil·o·quy (brŏng-kĭl′ə-kwē) *n.* See **bronchophony**.

bron·chi·o·cele (brŏng′kē-ə-sēl′) *n.* Variant of **bronchocele**.

bron·chi·o·gen·ic (brŏng′kē-ə-jĕn′ĭk) *or* **bron·cho·gen·ic** (brŏng′kə-jĕn′ĭk) *adj.* Of bronchial origin; emanating from the bronchi.

bron·chi·o·lar carcinoma (brŏng′kē-ō′lər) *n.* Carcinoma of the lung that includes symptoms of severe coughing and expectoration. Also called *alveolar cell carcinoma*.

bron·chi·ole (brŏng′kē-ōl′) *n.* Any of the fine, thin-walled, tubular extensions of a bronchus.

bron·chi·o·lec·ta·sis (brŏng′kē-ō-lĕk′tə-sĭs) *n.* Chronic dilation of the bronchioles.

bron·chi·o·li·tis (brŏng′kē-ō-lī′tĭs) *n.* Inflammation of the bronchioles, often associated with bronchopneumonia.

bron·chi·o·lus (brŏng-kī′ə-ləs) *n.,* pl. **–li** (-lī′) A respiratory bronchiole.

bron·chi·o·ste·no·sis (brŏng′kē-ō-stə-nō′sĭs) *n.* Variant of **bronchostenosis**.

bron·chi·tis (brŏn-kī′tĭs, brŏng-) *n.* Inflammation of the mucous membrane of the bronchial tubes. —**bron·chit′ic** (-kĭt′ĭk) *adj.*

broncho– *or* **bronch–** *or* **bronchi–** *pref.* Bronchus; bronchial: *bronchoscope*.

bron·cho·al·ve·o·lar (brŏng′kō-ăl-vē′ə-lər) *adj.* Bronchovesicular.

bron·cho·cav·ern·ous (brŏng′kō-kăv′ər-nəs) *adj.* Relating to a bronchus or bronchial tube and a pulmonary cavity.

bron·cho·cele (brŏng′kə-sēl′) *or* **bron·chi·o·cele** (-kē-ə-sēl′) *n.* Circumscribed dilation of a bronchus.

bron·cho·cen·tric granulomatosis (brŏng′kō-sĕn′trĭk) *n.* A severe form of allergic bronchopulmonary aspergillosis.

bron·cho·con·stric·tor (brŏng′kō-kən-strĭk′tər) *n.* An agent that causes a reduction in the caliber of a bronchus or bronchial tube. —**bron·cho·con·stric·tion** (-shən) *n.*

bron·cho·di·la·tion (brŏng′kō-dī-lā′shən) *or* **bron·cho·dil·a·ta·tion** (-dĭl′ə-tā′shən, -dī′lə-) *n.* An increase in the caliber of a bronchus or bronchial tube.

bron·cho·di·la·tor (brŏng′kō-dī-lā′tər, -dī′lā′-, -dī-lā′-) *n.* An agent that causes an increase in the caliber of a bronchus or bronchial tube and eases breathing by relaxing bronchial smooth muscle.

bron·cho·e·soph·a·ge·al muscle (brŏng′kō-ĭ-sŏf′ə-jē′əl) *n.* Any of the muscular fascicles that arise from the wall of the left bronchus and reinforce the musculature of the esophagus.

bron·cho·e·soph·a·gol·o·gy (brŏng′kō-ĭ-sŏf′ə-gŏl′ə-jē) *n.* The medical specialty concerned with peroral endoscopic examination of the esophagus and tracheobronchial tree.

bron·cho·e·soph·a·gos·co·py (brŏng′kō-ĭ-sŏf′ə-gŏs′kə-pē) *n.* Examination of the tracheobronchial tree or esophagus through the use of an endoscope.

bron·cho·fi·ber·scope (brŏng′kō-fī′bər-skōp′) *n.* A fiberoptic endoscope specialized for viewing the trachea and bronchi.

bron·cho·gen·ic (brŏng′kə-jĕn′ĭk) *adj.* Variant of **bronchiogenic**.

bronchogenic carcinoma *n.* Squamous cell or oat cell carcinoma that develops in the mucosa of the large bronchi and produces a persistent productive cough or hemoptysis.

bronchogenic cyst *n.* A cyst lined with bronchial epithelium and sometimes containing mucous glands, usually found in the mediastinum.

bron·chog·ra·phy (brŏng-kŏg′rə-fē) *n.* The radiographic examination of the tracheobronchial tree following the injection of a radiopaque material. —**bron·cho·gram** (brŏng′kə-grăm) *n.*

bron·cho·lith (brŏng′kə-lĭth′) *n.* A hard concretion in a bronchus or bronchial tube. Also called *bronchial calculus*.

bron·cho·li·thi·a·sis (brŏng′kō-lĭ-thī′ə-sĭs) *n.* Bronchial inflammation or obstruction caused by the presence of broncholiths.

bron·cho·ma·la·cia (brŏng′kō-mə-lā′shə) *n.* Degeneration of the elastic and connective tissue of the bronchi and trachea.

bron·cho·mo·tor (brŏng′kō-mō′tər) *adj.* Causing a change in the caliber, dilation, or contraction of a bronchus or bronchiole.

bron·cho·my·co·sis (brŏng′kō-mī-kō′sĭs) *n.* A disease of the bronchial tubes or of the bronchi that is caused by a fungus.

bron·choph·o·ny (brŏng-kŏf′ə-nē) *n.* An exaggerated vocal resonance that can be heard over a bronchus that is surrounded by consolidated lung tissue. Also called *bronchiloquy.*

bron·cho·plas·ty (brŏng′kə-plăs′tē) *n.* Surgical repair of a defect in the bronchus.

bron·cho·pleu·ral (brŏng′kō-plŏŏr′əl) *adj.* **1.** Of or relating to a bronchus and the pleura. **2.** Joining a bronchus and the pleural cavity.

bron·cho·pneu·mon·ia (brŏng′kō-nŏŏ-mōn′yə) *n.* Acute inflammation of the walls of the smaller bronchial tubes, with irregular areas of consolidation due to spread of the inflammation into the peribronchiolar alveoli and the alveolar ducts of the lungs. Also called *bronchial pneumonia.*

bron·cho·pul·mo·nary (brŏng′kō-pŏŏl′mə-něr′ē, -pŭl′-) *adj.* Of or relating to the bronchial tubes and to the lungs.

bronchopulmonary dysplasia *n.* A chronic pulmonary insufficiency resulting from long-term artificial pulmonary ventilation, more common in premature infants than in mature infants.

bronchopulmonary segment *n.* The largest subdivision of a lobe of the lung, supplied by a direct branch of a lobar bronchus and separated from adjacent segments by connective tissue septa.

bronchopulmonary sequestration *n.* A congenital anomaly in which a mass of embryonic lung tissue becomes isolated from the rest of the lung with the bronchi in the mass usually being dilated or cystic and unconnected to the bronchial tree.

bron·chor·rha·phy (brŏng-kôr′ə-fē) *n.* The suture of a wound of the bronchus.

bron·chor·rhe·a (brŏng′kə-rē′ə) *n.* Excessive mucal secretion from bronchial mucous membranes.

bron·cho·scope (brŏng′kə-skōp′) *n.* An endoscope for inspecting the interior of the tracheobronchial tree. —**bron′cho·scop′ic** (-skŏp′ĭk) *adj.* —**bron·chos′co·py** (-kŏs′kə-pē) *n.*

bron·cho·spasm (brŏng′kə-spăz′əm) *n.* A contraction of smooth muscle in the walls of the bronchi and bronchioles, causing narrowing of the lumen.

bron·cho·spi·rog·ra·phy (brŏng′kō-spī-rŏg′rə-fē) *n.* The use of a single-lumen endobronchial tube for measuring the ventilatory function of one lung.

bron·cho·spi·rom·e·ter (brŏng′kō-spī-rŏm′ĭ-tər) *n.* A device for measuring rates and volumes of air flow into each lung separately. —**bron′cho·spi·rom′e·try** (-ĭ-trē) *n.*

bron·cho·stax·is (brŏng′kō-stăk′sĭs) *n.* Hemorrhage from the bronchi.

bron·cho·ste·no·sis (brŏng′kō-stə-nō′sĭs) *or* **bron·chi·o·ste·no·sis** (brŏng′kē-ō-) *n.* Chronic narrowing of a bronchus.

bron·chos·to·my (brŏng-kŏs′tə-mē) *n.* The surgical formation of a new opening into a bronchus.

bron·chot·o·my (brŏng-kŏt′ə-mē) *n.* Incision into a bronchus.

bron·cho·tra·che·al (brŏng′kō-trā′kē-əl) *adj.* Relating to the bronchi and the trachea.

bron·cho·ve·sic·u·lar (brŏng′kō-vě-sĭk′yə-lər, -və-) *adj.* Relating to the bronchial tubes and alveoli.

bron·chus (brŏng′kəs) *n., pl.* **–chi** (-kī′, -kē′) Either of two main branches of the trachea, leading directly to the lungs.

Brøn·sted base (brŏn′stĕd, broen′stĕth′) *n.* See **base** (sense 4).

Brønsted theory *n.* The theory that an acid is a substance that liberates hydrogen ions in solution and that a base is a substance that removes hydrogen ions from solution.

bronzed disease (brŏnzd) *n.* **1.** See **Addison's disease. 2.** See **hemochromatosis.**

bronze diabetes (brŏnz) *n.* A type of diabetes associated with hemochromatosis.

brood (brŏŏd) *n.* See **litter.**

brow (brou) *n.* **1.** The eyebrow. **2.** See **forehead.**

brow·lift (brou′lĭft′) *n.* Plastic surgery to elevate the eyebrows and thereby remove excess skin folds or fullness in the upper eyelids.

Brown (broun), **Michael** Born 1941. American geneticist. He shared a 1985 Nobel Prize for discoveries related to cholesterol metabolism.

Brownian movement (brŏu′nē-ən) *n.* The random movement of microscopic particles suspended in a liquid or gas, caused by collisions with molecules of the surrounding medium. Also called *Brownian motion, molecular movement, pedesis.*

brown induration of the lung *n.* A lung condition characterized by tissue firmness and brown pigmentation associated with hemosiderin-pigmented macrophages in the alveoli, resulting from prolonged congestion caused by heart disease.

brown lung disease *n.* See **byssinosis.**

Brown-Sé·quard's syndrome (broun′sā-kärz′) *n.* A syndrome caused by damage to one side of the spinal cord and resulting in ipsilateral hemiparaplegia and loss of muscle and joint sensation and contralateral hemianesthesia. Also called *Brown-Séquard's paralysis.*

brow presentation *n.* Presentation of the fetus during birth in which the brow is the presenting part.

Bruce (brŏŏs), Sir **David** 1855–1931. Australian physician and bacteriologist known for his description (1887) of the bacterium that causes brucellosis.

Bru·cel·la (brŏŏ-sĕl′ə) *n.* A genus of encapsulated, nonmotile bacteria containing short, rod-shaped to coccoid gram-negative cells that are parasites in and pathogens for humans.

Brucella a·bor·tus (ə-bôr′təs) *n.* Bang's bacillus.

Bru·cel·la·ce·ae (brŏŏ′sə-lā′sē-ē′) *n.* A family of bacteria containing small, coccoid to rod-shaped, gram-negative cells that are parasites in and pathogens for warm-blooded animals, including humans.

Brucella mel·i·ten·sis (mĕl′ĭ-tĕn′sĭs) *n.* A bacterium causing brucellosis in humans, abortion in goats, and a wasting disease in chickens.

Brucella su·is (sŏŏ′ĭs) *n.* A bacterium that causes abortion in swine and brucellosis in humans.

bru·cel·lo·sis (brŏŏ′sə-lō′sĭs) *n.* An infectious disease caused by any of several species of *Brucella* and marked by fever, sweating, weakness, and headache. It is transmitted to humans by direct contact with diseased animals or through ingestion of infected meat, milk, or cheese. Also called *Bang's disease, Malta fever, Mediterranean fever, Rock fever, undulant fever.*

Bruch's membrane (brŏŏks, brŏŏкнs) *n.* See **basal layer** (sense 2).

Brück·e's muscle (brŏō′kəz, brü′-) *n.* The part of the ciliary muscle formed by the radiating fibers.

Bru·dzin·ski's sign (brŏō-jĭn′skēz) *n.* **1.** An indication of meningitis in which passive flexion of the leg on one side causes a similar movement in the opposite leg. **2.** Such an indication in which passive flexion of the neck causes flexion of the legs.

Bru·gi·a (brŏō′jē-ə) *n.* A genus of filarial worms transmitted by mosquitoes to humans and including a species that is an important agent of filariasis and elephantiasis in Southeast Asia and Indonesia.

bruise (brŏōz) *n.* An injury to underlying tissues or bone in which the skin is unbroken, often characterized by ruptured blood vessels and discolorations; a contusion.

bru·it (brŏō′ē) *n.* A sound, especially an abnormal one, heard in auscultation.

Brun·ner's gland (brŏŏn′ərz) *n.* See **duodenal gland.**

Brunn's membrane (brŏŏnz) *n.* The epithelium of the olfactory region of the nose.

brush biopsy (brŭsh) *n.* A biopsy obtained by passing a bristled catheter into suspected areas of disease and removing cells that are entrapped in the bristles.

brush border *n.* An epithelial cell surface consisting of microvilli, as on the cells of the proximal tubule of the kidney.

brush catheter *n.* A catheter with a finely bristled brush tip that is endoscopically passed into the ureter or renal pelvis to obtain a brush biopsy.

brux·ism (brŭk′sĭz′əm) *n.* The habitual involuntary grinding or clenching of the teeth, usually during sleep, as from anger, tension, fear, or frustration.

Bry·ant's triangle (brī′ənts) *n.* A triangle drawn in order to determine the upward displacement of the trochanter in fracture of the neck of the femur. A line is drawn around the body at the level of the anterior superior iliac spines, another line is drawn perpendicular to it as far as the great trochanter of the femur, and the third line is drawn from the trochanter to the iliac spine. Also called *iliofemoral triangle.*

BSE *abbr.* bovine spongiform encephalopathy

Btu *abbr.* British thermal unit

bu·ba ma·dre (brŏō′bə mä′drā) *n.* See **mother yaw.**

bu·bas (brŏō′bəz) *n.* See **yaws.**

bub·ble gum dermatitis (bŭb′əl gŭm′) *n.* Allergic contact dermatitis that develops about the lips of some children who chew bubble gum.

bu·bo (brŏō′bō) *n.,* *pl.* **–boes** Inflammatory swelling of one or more lymph nodes, especially in the groin.

bu·bon·al·gia (brŏō′bə-năl′jə) *n.* Pain in the groin.

bu·bon·ic (brŏō-bŏn′ĭk) *adj.* Of or relating to a bubo.

bubonic plague *n.* A contagious, often fatal epidemic disease caused by the bacterium *Yersinia pestis,* transmitted from person to person or by the bite of fleas from an infected host, especially a rat, and characterized by chills, fever, vomiting, diarrhea, and the formation of buboes.

bu·bon·o·cele (brŏō-bŏn′ə-sēl′) *n.* An inguinal hernia,

especially one in which the knuckle of intestine has not yet emerged from the external abdominal ring.

bu·car·di·a (brŏō-kär′dē-ə, byŏō-) *n.* Extreme hypertrophy of the heart. Also called *cor bovinum.*

buc·ca (bŭk′ə) *n.* The cheek.

buc·cal (bŭk′əl) *adj.* **1.** Of, relating to, adjacent to, or in the direction of the cheek. **2.** Of or relating to the mouth cavity.

buccal artery *n.* An artery with its origin in the maxillary artery, with distribution to the buccinator muscle, skin, and mucous membrane of the cheek, and with anastomoses to the buccal branch of the facial artery.

buccal cavity *n.* The portion of the oral cavity bounded by the lips, cheeks, and gums. Also called *vestibule of mouth.*

buccal gland *n.* Any of the mixed glands situated in the mucous membrane of the cheeks. Also called *genal gland.*

buccal nerve *n.* A sensory branch of the mandibular division of the trigeminal nerve, supplying the buccal mucous membrane and the skin of the cheek near the angle of the mouth.

buc·ci·na·tor (bŭk′sə-nā′tər) *n.* A muscle with origin from the alveolar portion of the maxilla, mandible, and pterygomandibular ligament, with insertion into the orbicular muscle of the mouth, with nerve supply from the facial nerve, and whose action flattens the cheek and retracts the angle of the mouth. Also called *cheek muscle.*

bucco– *pref.* Cheek: *buccogingival.*

buc·co·gin·gi·val (bŭk′ō-jĭn′jə-vəl, -jĭn-jī′-) *adj.* Relating to the cheek and the gums.

buc·co·la·bi·al (bŭk′ō-lā′bē-əl) *adj.* **1.** Relating to the cheek and the lip. **2.** Relating to the aspect of the dental arch or the surfaces of the teeth that are in contact with the mucosa of the lip and cheek.

buc·co·lin·gual (bŭk′ō-lĭng′gwəl) *adj.* Relating to the cheek and the tongue.

buc·co·pha·ryn·geal (bŭk′ō-fə-rĭn′jəl, -făr′ĭn-jē′əl) *adj.* Relating to the cheek or mouth and the pharynx.

buc·co·ver·sion (bŭk′ō-vûr′zhən) *n.* Malposition of a posterior tooth from its normal line of occlusion in the direction of the cheek.

Buck's extension (bŭks) *n.* An apparatus for applying skin traction on the leg in which adhesive tape is connected to the skin and to a suspended weight.

buck·tooth (bŭk′tŏōth′) *n.* A prominent, projecting upper front tooth. —**buck′toothed′** (-tŏŏtht′) *adj.*

bud (bŭd) *n.* **1.** A small, rounded anatomical structure or organic part, such as a taste bud. **2.** An asexual reproductive structure, as in yeast or a hydra, that consists of an outgrowth capable of developing into a new individual. —*v.* **1.** To put forth or cause to put forth buds. **2.** To reproduce asexually by forming a bud.

Budd-Chiari syndrome (bŭd′-) *n.* See **Chiari's syndrome.**

bud·ding (bŭd′ĭng) *n.* See **gemmation.**

bu·des·o·nide (byŏō-dĕs′ə-nīd′) *n.* A corticosteroid used in inhalant form to treat asthma.

bud fission *n.* See **gemmation.**

Buer·ger's disease (bûr′gərz, bŏōr′-) *n.* See **thromboangiitis obliterans.**

buf·fa·lo neck (bŭf'ə-lō') *n.* Moderate kyphosis accompanied by a thick heavy fat pad on the neck.

buff·er (bŭf'ər) *n.* A substance that minimizes change in the acidity of a solution when an acid or base is added to the solution. —*v.* To treat a solution with a buffer.

buffer value *n.* The value indicating the capability of a substance in solution to absorb acid or alkali without changing the pH.

buf·fy coat (bŭf'ē) *n.* The upper, lighter portion of the blood clot occurring when coagulation is delayed or when blood has been centrifuged.

bu·fo·ten·ine (byōō'fə-tĕn'ēn, -ĭn) *n.* A poisonous hallucinogenic alkaloid that is obtained from the skin glands of toads of the genus *Bufo* or from some mushrooms.

bug (bŭg) *n.* **1.** A true bug, specifically one having a beaklike structure that allows piercing and sucking. **2.** An insect or similar organism, such as a centipede or an earwig. **3.** A disease-producing microorganism, such as a flu bug. **4.** The illness or disease so produced. **5.** A defect or difficulty, as in a system or design.

bulb (bŭlb) *n.* A globular or fusiform anatomical structure or enlargement.

bul·bar (bŭl'bər, -bär') *adj.* **1.** Resembling or relating to a bulb. **2.** Relating to the rhombencephalon.

bulbar myelitis *n.* Inflammation of the medulla oblongata of the brain.

bulbar paralysis *n.* See **progressive bulbar paralysis**.

bul·bi·tis (bŭl-bī'tĭs) *n.* Inflammation of the bulbous portion of the urethra.

bulbo– *pref.* Bulb; bulbus: *bulbospinal.*

bul·bo·cav·er·no·sus (bŭl'bō-kăv'ər-nəs) *n.* See **bulbospongiosus**.

bulb of corpus spongiosum *n.* See **bulb of penis**.

bulb of eye *n.* See **eyeball** (sense 1).

bulb of penis *n.* The expanded posterior part of the corpus spongiosum of the penis lying in the interval between the crura of the penis. Also called *bulb of corpus spongiosum, bulb of urethra.*

bulb of vestibule *n.* A mass of erectile tissue on either side of the vagina.

bul·boid (bŭl'boid') *adj.* Bulb-shaped.

bulboid corpuscle *n.* Any of the nerve terminals in the skin, mouth, and conjunctiva, consisting of a laminated capsule of connective tissue enclosing the terminal ending of an afferent nerve fiber.

bul·bo·spi·nal (bŭl'bō-spī'nəl) *adj.* Relating to the medulla oblongata and spinal cord, particularly to the nerve fibers interconnecting the two.

bul·bo·spon·gi·o·sus (bŭl'bō-spŏn'jē-ō'səs, -spŭn'-) *n.* A muscle with origin in the inferior fascia of the urogenital diaphragm, the corpus cavernosum of the clitoris or the penis, and in the dorsum of the clitoris or the bulb of the penis; with insertion to the central tendon of the perineum and in the male also to the median raphe on the bulb of the penis; and whose action controls the weak sphincter of the vagina or constricts the bulbous urethra. Also called *bulbocavernosus.*

bul·bo·u·re·thral (bŭl'bō-yōō-rē'thrəl) *adj.* Relating to the bulbus penis and the urethra.

bulbourethral gland *n.* Either of two small racemose glands in the male that are located below the prostate

and discharge a component of the seminal fluid into the urethra. Also called *Cowper's gland.*

bul·bous bougie (bŭl'bəs) *n.* A bougie with a bulb-shaped tip, sometimes shaped like an olive.

bul·bus (bŭl'bəs) *n., pl.* **-bi** (-bī') A bulb.

bu·li·ma·rex·i·a (bōō-lē'mə-rĕk'sē-ə, -lĭm'ə-, byōō-) *n.* An eating disorder marked by an alternation between abnormal craving for and aversion to food. It is manifested by episodes of excessive food intake followed by periods of fasting and self-induced vomiting or diarrhea. Also called *binge-purge syndrome.*

bu·li·mi·a (bōō-lē'mē-ə, -lĭm'ē-ə, byōō-) *n.* A chronic eating disorder involving repeated and secretive episodes of eating, characterized by uncontrolled rapid ingestion of large quantities of food over a short period of time, followed by self-induced vomiting, purging, and anorexia and accompanied by feelings of guilt, depression, or self-disgust. Also called *bulimia nervosa, hyperorexia.* —**bu·lim'ic** *adj. & n.*

bul·la (bōōl'ə) *n., pl.* **bul·lae** (bōōl'ē) **1.** A large blister or vesicle of pathological origin. **2.** A bubblelike structure.

bull·dog forceps (bōōl'dôg') *n.* A short spring forceps for grasping and occluding a blood vessel.

bul·let forceps (bōōl'ĭt) *n.* A forceps having thin curved blades with serrated grasping surfaces for extracting a bullet from tissues.

bull neck *n.* A heavy, thick neck caused by hypertrophied muscles or enlarged cervical lymph nodes.

bul·lous (bōōl'əs) *adj.* Relating to or characterized by bullae.

bullous keratopathy *n.* Corneal edema characterized by the formation of large subepithelial bullae that cause intense pain when they rupture and expose corneal nerves.

bullous pemphigoid *n.* A chronic generally benign skin disease, usually of old age, characterized by subepidermal blisters that cause detachment of the epidermis but that tend to heal without scarring.

bullous urticaria *n.* Urticaria marked by the eruption of wheals capped with subepidermal vesicles.

bu·met·a·nide (byōō-mĕt'ə-nīd') *n.* A diuretic used in the treatment of edema associated with congestive heart failure, hepatic cirrhosis, and renal disease.

Bu·mex (byōō'mĕks') A trademark for the drug bumetanide.

BUN *abbr.* blood urea nitrogen

bun·dle (bŭn'dl) *n.* A structure composed of a group of fibers, such as a fasciculus.

bundle-branch block *n. Abbr.* **BBB** Intraventricular block due to interruption of conduction in one of the two main branches of the bundle of His and manifested in the electrocardiogram by marked prolongation of the QRS complex.

bundle of His (hĭs) *n.* The bundle of cardiac muscle fibers that begins at the atrioventricular node and passes through the right atrioventricular fibrous ring to the membranous part of the interventricular septum. It conducts the electrical impulse that regulates the heartbeat from the right atrium to the ventricles. Also called *atrioventricular bundle, His bundle.*

bun·ion (bŭn'yən) *n.* A localized swelling at either the medial or dorsal aspect of the first joint of the big toe, caused by an inflamed bursa.

bun·ion·ec·to·my (bŭn′yə-nĕk′tə-mē) *n.* Excision of a bunion.

Bun·sen burner (bŭn′sən) *n.* A small laboratory burner consisting of a vertical metal tube connected to a gas source and producing a very hot flame from a mixture of gas and air let in through adjustable holes at the base.

Bun·sen's solubility coefficient (bŭn′sənz) *n. Symbol* α The milliliters of gas dissolved per milliliter of liquid that is maintained at atmospheric pressure and at a given temperature.

Bun·ya·vi·rus (bŭn′yə-vī′rəs) *n.* A large genus of arboviruses that carry single-strand RNA.

bunyavirus encephalitis *n.* A form of encephalitis having an abrupt onset, with severe frontal headache and low-grade to moderate fever, caused by a virus of the genus *Bunyavirus.*

buph·thal·mi·a (boof-thăl′mē-ə) *or* **buph·thal·mos** (-məs, -mŏs′) *or* **buph·thal·mus** (-məs) *n.* A disease of infancy marked by an increase of intraocular fluid and consequent enlargement of the eyeball. Also called *congenital glaucoma.*

bu·piv·a·caine (byoo-pĭv′ə-kān′) *n.* A potent, long-acting local anesthetic used in regional anesthesia.

bu·pre·nor·phine hydrochloride (byoo′prə-nôr′fēn′) *n.* A semisynthetic opioid analgesic used for the relief of moderate to severe pain.

Bu·pren·ex (byoo′prĕ-nĕks′) A trademark for the drug buprenorphine hydrochloride.

bu·pro·pi·on hydrochloride (byoo-prō′pē-ŏn′) *n.* A drug used to treat depression and nicotine dependence.

bur *or* **burr** (bûr) *n.* **1.** A rotary cutting instrument used in dentistry for excavating decay, shaping cavity forms, and reducing tooth structure. **2.** A drilling tool for enlarging a trephine hole in the cranium.

bu·rette *or* **bu·ret** (byoo-rĕt′) *n.* A uniform-bore tube with fine gradations and a stopcock at the bottom, used especially in laboratory procedures for accurate fluid dispensing and measurement.

bur·ied flap (bĕr′ēd) *n.* A surgical flap denuded of both surface epithelium and superficial dermis and transferred into the subcutaneous tissues.

buried suture *n.* A suture placed entirely below the surface of the skin.

Bur·kitt (bûr′kĭt), **Denis Parsons** 1911–1993. British surgeon who first described the cancer now known as Burkitt's lymphoma. He is also noted for his work in Africa in geographical pathology.

Bur·kitt's lymphoma (bûr′kĭts) *n.* An undifferentiated malignant lymphoma usually occurring among children in central Africa, characterized by a large osteolytic lesion in the mandible or by a mass in the retroperitoneal area and associated with the Epstein-Barr virus.

burn (bûrn) *v.* **1.** To undergo or cause to undergo combustion. **2.** To consume or use as fuel or energy. **3.** To damage or injure by fire, heat, radiation, electricity, or a caustic agent. **4.** To irritate or inflame, as by chafing or sunburn. **5.** To become sunburned or windburned. **6.** To metabolize a substance, such as glucose, in the body.

7. To impart a sensation of intense heat to. **8.** To feel or look hot. —*n.* **1.** An injury produced by fire, heat, radiation, electricity, or a caustic agent. **2.** A burned place or area. **3.** The process or result of burning. **4.** A stinging sensation. **5.** A sunburn or windburn.

burn center *n.* A multidisciplinary health care facility in which victims of burns are treated.

Bur·net (bər-nĕt′, bûr′nĭt), Sir **(Frank) Macfarlane** 1899–1985. Australian virologist. He shared a 1960 Nobel Prize for his work on acquired immunological tolerance.

bur·nish·er (bûr′nə-shər) *n.* An instrument for smoothing and polishing the surface or edge of a dental restoration.

burp (bûrp) *n.* Noisy expulsion of gas from the stomach through the mouth. —*v.* **1.** To expel gas from the stomach through the mouth. **2.** To cause a baby to expel gas from the stomach, as by patting the back after feeding.

burr (bûr) *n.* Variant of **bur.**

bur·sa (bûr′sə) *n., pl.* **–sas** *or* **–sae** (-sē) A sac or saclike bodily cavity, especially one containing a viscous lubricating fluid and located between a tendon and a bone or at points of friction between moving structures. —**bur′sal** *adj.*

bursal synovitis *n.* See **bursitis.**

bursa of gastrocnemius *n.* A subtendinous bursa consisting of a lateral and a medial bursa between the heads of the gastrocnemius and the capsule of the knee joint.

bursa of semimembranosus *n.* The bursa between the semimembranous muscle, the head of the gastrocnemius, and the knee joint.

bur·sec·to·my (bər-sĕk′tə-mē) *n.* Surgical removal of a bursa.

bur·si·tis (bər-sī′tĭs) *n.* Inflammation of a bursa, especially in the shoulder, elbow, or knee joint. Also called *bursal synovitis.*

bur·so·lith (bûr′sə-lĭth′) *n.* A calculus formed in a bursa.

bur·sop·a·thy (bər-sŏp′ə-thē) *n.* A disease of a bursa.

bur·sot·o·my (bər-sŏt′ə-mē) *n.* Incision through the wall of a bursa.

Busch·ke-Lö·wen·stein tumor (boosh′kə-lō′wən-stīn′, -lœ′vən-) *n.* See **giant condyloma.**

Buschke-Ol·len·dorf syndrome (-ô′lən-dôrf′) *n.* See **osteodermatopoikilosis.**

Bu·spar (byoo′spär′) A trademark for the drug buspirone hydrochloride.

bu·spi·rone hydrochloride (byoo-spī′rōn′) *n.* An agent used in the management of anxiety disorders or for short-term relief of the symptoms of anxiety.

Bus·se-Buschke disease (boos′ə-) *n.* See **cryptococcosis.**

bu·sul·fan (byoo-sŭl′fən) *n.* An alkylating agent that is used as an antineoplastic drug in the treatment of chronic myelocytic leukemia.

bu·tam·ben (byoo-tăm′bən) *n.* See **butyl aminobenzoate.**

bu·tane (byoo′tān′) *n.* Either of two isomers of a gaseous hydrocarbon produced synthetically from petroleum and used as a refrigerant, as a aerosol propellant, and in the manufacture of synthetic rubber.

bu·ta·no·ic acid (byoo′tə-nō′ĭk) *n.* See **butyric acid.**

Bu·ta·zol·i·din (byōō′tə-zŏl′ĭ-dĭn) A trademark for the drug phenylbutazone.

Bu·te·nandt (bōōt′n-änt′), **Adolf Friedrich** 1903–1995. German chemist. He shared a 1939 Nobel Prize for his work on sexual hormones but declined the honor following a Nazi edict prohibiting acceptance of such prizes.

bu·to·con·a·zole nitrate (byōō′tə-kŏn′ə-zōl′) *n.* An antifungal agent used primarily in the treatment of vulvovaginal candidiasis.

but·ter (bŭt′ər) *n.* **1.** A soft yellowish or whitish emulsion of butterfat, water, air, and sometimes salt, churned from milk or cream and processed for use in cooking and as a food. **2.** A soft solid having at room temperature a consistency like that of butter.

but·ter·fly rash (bŭt′ər-flī′) *n.* A scaling lesion that appears on each cheek and is joined by a narrow band across the nose, seen in lupus erythematosus and seborrheic dermatitis.

but·tock (bŭt′ək) *n.* **1.** Either of the two rounded prominences on the human torso that are posterior to the hips and formed by the gluteal muscles and underlying structures. **2. buttocks** The rear pelvic area of the human body.

but·ton (bŭt′n) *n.* A knoblike structure, device, or lesion.

but·ton·hole (bŭt′n-hōl′) *n.* **1.** A short straight surgical cut made through the wall of a cavity or canal. **2.** The contraction of an orifice down to a narrow slit, as in mitral stenosis.

button suture *n.* A suture that is passed through a button, to prevent the threads from cutting through the flesh, and then tied.

but·tress plate (bŭt′rĭs) *n.* A metal plate used to support the internal fixation of a fracture.

bu·tyl (byōōt′l) *n.* A hydrocarbon radical, C_4H_9.

butyl a·mi·no·ben·zo·ate (ə-mē′nō-bĕn′zō-āt′, ăm′ə-nō-) *n.* A local anesthetic that is very insoluble and only slightly absorbed. Also called *butamben.*

bu·ty·ra·ceous (byōō′tə-rā′shəs) *or* **bu·ty·rous** (byōō′-tə-rəs) *adj.* Buttery in consistency.

bu·ty·rate (byōō′tə-rāt′) *n.* A salt or ester of butyric acid.

bu·tyr·ic acid (byōō-tîr′ĭk) *n.* Either of two colorless isomeric acids occurring in animal milk fats and used in disinfectants, emulsifying agents, and pharmaceuticals. Also called *butanoic acid.*

bu·ty·roid (byōō′tə-roid′) *adj.* Resembling or having the consistency of butter.

bu·ty·ro·phe·none (byōō-tîr′ō-fə-nōn′, byōō′tə-rō-) *n.* Any of a group of neuroleptic drugs, such as haloperidol, that are administered in the treatment of acute psychotic episodes, schizophrenia, and other psychiatric disorders.

bu·ty·ryl (byōō′tə-rĭl′) *n.* The radical C_3H_7COO of butyric acid.

bx *abbr.* biopsy

by·pass (bī′păs′) *n.* **1.** A passage created surgically to divert the flow of blood or other bodily fluid or to circumvent an obstructed or diseased organ. **2.** A surgical procedure to create such a channel.

bys·si·no·sis (bĭs′ĭ-nō′sĭs) *n.* A form of pneumoconiosis that affects cotton, flax, and hemp workers and is characterized by symptoms, such as wheezing, that are most severe at the beginning of each work week. Also called *brown lung disease.*

C

χ The Greek letter *chi.* Entries beginning with this letter are alphabetized under **chi.**

c *abbr.* blood capillary; small calorie

C¹ The symbol for the element **carbon.**

C² *abbr.* Celsius; centigrade; coulomb; cytosine; large calorie

ca *abbr.* circa

Ca The symbol for the element **calcium.**

CA *abbr.* cancer; carcinoma; chronologic age; cytosine arabinoside

CABG *abbr.* coronary artery bypass graft

ca·ble graft (kā′bəl) *n.* A multiple-strand nerve graft that is arranged as a pathway for the regeneration of axons.

Cab·ot's ring body (kăb′əts) *n.* A ring-shaped or figure-8 structure, staining red with Wright's stain, found in red blood cells in severe anemias.

ca·chec·tic (kə-kĕk′tĭk) *adj.* Affected by or relating to cachexia.

ca·chec·tin (kə-kĕk′tĭn) *n.* A polypeptide hormone produced by macrophages that releases fat and reduces the concentration of enzymes needed to produce and store fat.

ca·chet (kă-shā′) *n.* An edible wafer capsule used for enclosing an unpleasant-tasting drug.

ca·chex·i·a (kə-kĕk′sē-ə) *n.* Weight loss, wasting of muscle, loss of appetite, and general debility that can occur during a chronic disease.

cachexia hy·po·phys·i·o·pri·va (hī′pō-fĭz′ē-ō-prī′və) *n.* A condition following removal of the pituitary gland, marked by a fall in body temperature, electrolyte imbalance, hypoglycemia, and ultimately resulting in coma and death.

cachexia stru·mi·pri·va (strōō′mə-prī′və) *n.* A condition having the signs and symptoms of hypothyroidism, resulting from the loss of thyroid tissue, either from surgery or radiation.

cach·in·na·tion (kăk′ə-nā′shən) *n.* Loud, hard, or compulsive laughter without apparent cause.

caco– *or* **cac–** *pref.* Bad: *cacogeusia.*

cac·o·geu·sia (kăk′ə-gyōō′zhə, -jōō′-) *n.* A bad taste not due to food, drugs, or other ingested matter.

cac·o·me·li·a (kăk′ə–mē′lē-ə, -mēl′yə) *n.* Congenital deformity of one or more limbs.

ca·cos·mi·a (kă-kŏs′mē-ə, -kŏz′-) *n.* The imagining of unpleasant odors, particularly odors that are putrefactive.

ca·cu·men (kə-kyōō′mən) *n., pl.* **-mi·na** (-mə-nə) The top or apex, as of an anatomical structure. —**ca·cu′mi·nal** (-mə-nəl) *adj.*

CAD *abbr.* coronary artery disease

ca·dav·er (kə-dăv′ər) *n.* A dead body, especially one intended for dissection. —**ca·dav′er·ic** (-ər-ĭk) *adj.*

ca·dav·er·ine (kə-dăv′ə-rēn′) *n.* A syrupy, colorless, fuming ptomaine formed by the carboxylation of lysine by bacteria in decaying animal flesh.

ca·dav·er·ous (kə-dăv′ər-əs) *adj.* **1.** Suggestive of death; corpselike. **2.** Having a corpselike pallor.

cad·mi·um (kăd′mē-əm) *n. Symbol* **Cd** A soft metallic element occurring primarily in zinc, copper, and lead ores that is used in low-friction fatigue-resistant alloys, solders, batteries, nuclear reactor shields, and electroplating. Atomic number 48.

ca·du·ce·us (kə-dōō′sē-əs, -shəs) *n., pl.* **-ce·i** (-sē-ī′) **1.** A winged staff with two serpents twined around it, carried by Hermes. **2.** An insignia modeled on Hermes' staff and used as the symbol of the medical profession.

cae– For words beginning with *cae-* that are not found here, see under *ce-.*

cae·cum (sē′kəm) *n.* Variant of **cecum.**

caesarean *n.* Variant of **cesarean.**

caesarean hysterectomy *n.* Variant of **cesarean hysterectomy.**

caesarean section *n.* Variant of **cesarean section.**

caesarian *n.* Variant of **cesarean.**

ca·fé au lait spots (kă-fā′ ō lā′) *pl.n.* Uniformly light brown, sharply defined, and usually oval-shaped patches of the skin characteristic of neurofibromatosis, though also found in healthy individuals.

caf·feine *or* **caf·fein** (kă-fēn′, kăf′ēn′) *n.* A bitter white alkaloid often derived from tea or coffee and used chiefly as a mild stimulant and in the treatment of certain kinds of headache.

caf·fein·ism (kă-fē′nĭz′əm, kăf′ē-) *n.* A toxic condition marked by diarrhea, elevated blood pressure, rapid breathing, heart palpitations, and insomnia, caused by excessive ingestion of coffee and other caffeine-containing substances.

Caf·fey's disease (kăf′ēz) *n.* See **infantile cortical hyperostosis.**

Caffey's syndrome *n.* See **infantile cortical hyperostosis.**

Ca·got ear (kă-gō′) *n.* An ear having no lower lobe.

Cain complex (kān) *n.* A complex characterized by rivalry, competition, and extreme envy or jealousy of a brother, leading to hatred.

–caine *suff.* A synthetic alkaloid anesthetic: *dibucaine.*

cai·no·to·pho·bi·a (kā-nō-tə-fō′bē-ə) *n.* An abnormal fear of newness.

cais·son disease (kā′sŏn′, -sən) *n.* See **decompression sickness.**

cake kidney (kāk) *n.* A solid irregularly shaped lobed mass, usually situated in the pelvis toward the midline, that is produced by congenital fusion of the embryonic kidneys.

cal *abbr.* mean calorie; small calorie

Cal *abbr.* large calorie

Cal·a·dryl (kăl′ə-drĭl′) A trademark for an over-the counter-preparation containing calamine.

cal·a·mine (kăl′ə-mīn′, -mĭn) *n.* A pink, odorless, tasteless powder of zinc oxide with a small amount of ferric oxide, dissolved in mineral oils and used in skin lotions.

cal·a·mus scrip·to·ri·us (kăl′ə-məs skrĭp-tôr′ē-əs) *n.* The inferior reedlike part of the rhomboid fossa of the fourth ventricle of the brain. Also called *Arantius' ventricle.*

Cal·an (kăl′ăn′) A trademark for the drug verapamil.

cal·ca·ne·an tendon (kal-kā′nē-ən) *n.* See **Achilles tendon.**

calcaneo– *pref.* Calcaneus: *calcaneotibial.*

cal·ca·ne·o·a·poph·y·si·tis (kăl-kā′nē-ō-ə-pŏf′ĭ-sī′tĭs) *n.* Inflammation at the posterior part of the calcaneus, at the insertion of the Achilles' tendon.

cal·ca·ne·o·as·trag·a·loid (kăl-kā′nē-ō-ə-străg′ə-loid′) *adj.* Relating to the calcaneus and the talus.

cal·ca·ne·o·cu·boid (kăl-kā′nē-ō-kyōō′boid′) *adj.* Relating to the calcaneus and the cuboid bone.

calcaneocuboid ligament *n.* The ligament that connects the calcaneus and the cuboid bones.

cal·ca·ne·o·dyn·i·a (kal-kā′nē-ō-dĭn′ē-ə) *n.* Variant of calcodynia.

cal·ca·ne·o·na·vic·u·lar (kăl-kā′nē-ō-nə-vĭk′yə-lər) *adj.* Relating to the calcaneus and the navicular bones.

cal·ca·ne·o·tib·i·al (kăl-kā′nē-ō-tĭb′ē-əl) *adj.* Relating to the calcaneus and the tibia.

cal·ca·ne·us (kăl-kā′nē-əs) *or* **cal·ca·ne·um** (-nē-əm) *n., pl.* **–ne·i** (-nē-ī′) *or* **–ne·a** (-nē-ə) The quadrangular bone at the back of the tarsus, the largest of the tarsal bones. Also called *heel bone.* **—cal·ca′ne·al** *adj.*

cal·car (kăl′kär′) *n., pl.* **cal·car·i·a** (kăl-kâr′ē-ə) **1.** A small spurlike projection from a structure. **2.** An internal septum at the level of division of arteries and confluence of veins when branches or roots form an acute angle. **3.** A dull spine or projection from a bone. **4.** A horny outgrowth from the skin.

cal·car·e·ous (kăl-kâr′ē-əs) *adj.* Composed of, containing, or characteristic of calcium carbonate, calcium, or limestone; chalky.

calcareous conjunctivitis *n.* A form of conjuctivitis characterized by the appearance of minute calcareous concretions on the conjunctiva of the eyelids.

calcareous degeneration *n.* The deposition of insoluble calcium salts in degenerated tissue that has become necrotic, as in dystrophic calcification.

calcareous infiltration *n.* See **calcification** (sense 1).

cal·car·ine (kăl′kə-rīn′, -rēn′) *adj.* **1.** Relating to or having a calcar. **2.** Having the shape of a spur.

calcarine sulcus *n.* A deep fissure on the medial aspect of the cerebral cortex, marking the border between the lingual gyrus below and the cuneus above. Also called *calcarine fissure.*

cal·car·i·u·ri·a (kăl-kâr′ē-yōor′ē-ə) *n.* Excretion of calcium salts in the urine.

cal·cic (kăl′sĭk) *adj.* Composed of, containing, derived from, or relating to calcium or lime.

cal·ci·co·sis (kăl′sĭ-kō′sĭs) *n.* Pneumoconiosis resulting from the inhalation of limestone dust.

cal·cif·er·ol (kăl-sĭf′ə-rôl′, -rōl′) *n.* See **vitamin D₂.**

cal·ci·fi·ca·tion (kăl′sə-fĭ-kā′shən) *n.* **1.** Impregnation with calcium or calcium salts. Also called *calcareous infiltration.* **2.** Hardening, as of tissue, by such impregnation. **3.** A calcified substance or part.

cal·ci·fy (kăl′sə-fī′) *v.* To make or become stony or chalky by deposition of calcium salts.

cal·cine (kăl-sīn, kăl′sīn) *v.* To heat a substance to a high temperature but below the melting or fusing point, causing loss of moisture, reduction, or oxidation and the decomposition of carbonates and other compounds.

cal·ci·no·sis (kăl′sə-nō′sĭs) *n.* The abnormal deposition of calcium salts in a part or tissue of the body.

calcinosis cir·cum·scrip·ta (sûr′kəm-skrĭp′tə) *n.* Localized deposits of calcium salts in the skin and subcutaneous tissues, usually surrounded by granulomatous inflammation.

calcinosis u·ni·ver·sa·lis (yōō′nə-vər-sā′lĭs) *n.* Diffuse deposits of calcium salts in the skin and subcutaneous tissues, connective tissues, and other bodily sites.

cal·ci·pex·is (kăl′sə-pěk′sĭs) *or* **cal·ci·pex·y** (kăl′sə-pěk′sē) *n.* Fixation of calcium in the tissues. **—cal′ci·pex′ic** *adj.*

cal·ci·phil·i·a (căl′sə-fĭl′ē-ə) *n.* A condition in which the tissues show an unusual affinity for, and fixation of, calcium salts circulating in the blood.

cal·ci·phy·lax·is (kăl′sə-fə-lăk′sĭs,) *n.* An adaptive response following induced systemic hypersensitivity to a calcifying factor such as vitamin D and an agent such as a metallic salt, usually resulting in localized inflammation and calcification of tissues.

cal·ci·priv·ic (kăl′sə-prĭv′ĭk) *adj.* Deprived of calcium.

cal·ci·to·nin (kăl′sĭ-tō′nĭn) *n.* A peptide hormone, produced by the thyroid gland in humans, that acts to lower plasma calcium and phosphate levels without augmenting calcium accretion. Also called *thyrocalcitonin.*

cal·ci·um (kăl′sē-əm) *n. Symbol* **Ca** A soft metallic element that is a basic component of animals and plants and constitutes approx. 3 percent of Earth's crust. It occurs naturally in limestone, gypsum, and fluorite. Atomic number 20.

calcium carbonate *n.* A calcium salt used as a dietary supplement and as an antacid.

calcium channel blocker *n.* Any of a class of drugs that inhibit movement of calcium ions across a cell membrane, used in the treatment of cardiovascular disorders.

calcium cyclamate *n.* An artificially prepared salt of cyclamic acid formerly used as a nonnutritive low-calorie sweetener but now banned because of possible carcinogenic effects of its metabolic products.

calcium hypochlorite *n.* A white crystalline solid used as a bactericide, fungicide, and bleaching agent.

calcium oxide *n.* A white, caustic, lumpy powder used in analytical and manufacturing procedures, in glassmaking, in waste treatment, in insecticides, and as an industrial alkali. Also called *lime.*

cal·ci·u·ri·a (kăl′sē-yōor′ē-ə) *n.* The presence of calcium in the urine.

cal·co·dyn·i·a (kăl′kō-dĭn′ē-ə) *or* **cal·ca·ne·o·dyn·i·a** (kăl-kā′nē-ō-) *n.* A condition in which bearing weight on the heel causes pain of varying severity.

cal·co·sphe·rite (kăl′kō-sfîr′īt′, -sfěr′-) *n.* A tiny round laminated body containing calcium salts. Also called *psammoma body.*

cal·cu·lo·sis (kăl′kyə-lō′sĭs) *n.* The formation of or the condition of having calculi.

cal·cu·lus (kăl′kyə-ləs) *n.*, *pl.* **-lus·es** *or* **-li** (-lī′) **1.** An abnormal concretion in the body, usually formed of mineral salts and most commonly found in the gallbladder, kidney, or urinary bladder. Also called *stone.* **2.** Dental tartar.

Cald·well-Luc operation (kôld′wěl′look′, -lük′) *n.* An intraoral surgical opening into the maxillary antrum through the fossa above the maxillary premolar teeth.

Caldwell-Mo·loy classification (-mə-loi′) *n.* A system of classification of variations in the female pelvis, based on the type of posterior and anterior segments of the inlet.

cal·e·fa·cient (kăl′ə-fā′shənt) *adj.* Causing a sense of warmth. —*n.* An agent that produces a sense of warmth in the part to which it is applied.

calf (kăf) *n.*, *pl.* **calves** (kăvz) The fleshy, muscular back part of the human leg between the knee and ankle, formed chiefly by the bellies of the gastrocnemius and soleus muscles.

calf bone *n.* See **fibula.**

cal·i·ber (kăl′ə-bər) *n.* The diameter of the inside of a round cylinder, such as a tube.

cal·i·brate (kăl′ə-brāt′) *v.* **1.** To check, adjust, or determine the graduations of a quantitative measuring instrument by comparison with a standard. **2.** To determine the caliber of a tube. **3.** To make corrections in or adjust a procedure or process. —**cal′i·bra′tor** *n.*

cal·i·ce·al (kăl′ĭ-sē′əl) *adj.* Of or relating to a calix.

cal·i·cec·ta·sis (kăl′ĭ-sěk′tə-sĭs, kā′lĭ-) *or* **cal·i·ec·ta·sis** (kăl′ē-ěk′tə-sĭs, kā′lē-) *n.* Dilation of the calices, usually due to obstruction or infection. Also called *pyelocaliectasis.*

cal·i·cec·to·my (kăl′ĭ-sěk′tə-mē, kā′lĭ-) *or* **cal·i·ec·to·my** (kăl′ē-ěk′tə-mē, kā′lē-) *n.* Excision of a calix.

cal·i·ci·vi·rus (kăl′ĭ-sĭ-vī′rəs) *n.* Any of a group of single-stranded RNA viruses, including the Norwalk virus, that cause acute gastroenteritis and some kinds of hepatitis.

ca·li·co·plas·ty (kā′lĭ-kō-plăs′tē) *n.* Plastic surgery of a calix, usually designed to increase its lumen at the infundibulum.

ca·li·cot·o·my (kā′lĭ-kŏt′ə-mē) *n.* Incision into a calix, usually to remove a calculus.

ca·lic·u·lus (kə-lĭk′yə-ləs) *n.*, *pl.* **-li** (-lī′) A bud-shaped or cup-shaped structure.

Cal·i·for·nia virus (kăl′ĭ-fôr′nyə) *n.* A strain of *Bunyavirus* that causes encephalitis.

cal·i·for·ni·um (kăl′ə-fôr′nē-əm) *n.* Symbol **Cf** A synthetic radioactive element produced in trace quantities by neutron bombardment of curium. Its most stable isotope, Cf 251, has a half-life of 790 years. Atomic number 98.

ca·li·or·rha·phy (kā′lē-ôr′ə-fē) *n.* **1.** The suturing of a calix. **2.** Reconstructive surgery on a dilated or obstructed calix to improve urinary drainage.

cal·i·per *or* **cal·li·per** (kăl′ə-pər) *n.* An instrument consisting essentially of two curved hinged legs, used to measure thickness and distances.

cal·is·then·ics (kăl′ĭs-thĕn′ĭks) *pl.n.* Gymnastic exercises, such as sit-ups, designed to develop muscular tone and promote physical fitness.

ca·lix *or* **ca·lyx** (kā′lĭks, kăl′ĭks) *n.*, *pl.* **ca·li·ces** *or* **ca·ly·ces** (kā′lĭ-sēz′, kăl′ĭ-) **1.** A flower-shaped or funnel-shaped structure. **2.** Any of the branches or recesses of the pelvis of the kidney into which the orifices of the malpighian renal pyramids project.

Call-Ex·ner body (kôl′ěks′nər) *n.* A small fluid-filled space between granulosal cells in ovarian follicles and in ovarian tumors of granulosal origin.

Cal·liph·o·ra (kə-lĭf′ər-ə) *n.* A genus of blowfies whose larvae feed on dead flesh.

cal·lo·sal (kə-lō′səl) *adj.* Of or relating to the corpus callosum.

callosal gyrus *n.* See **cingulate gyrus.**

cal·los·i·ty (kə-lŏs′ĭ-tē) *n.* A localized thickening and enlargement of the horny layer of the skin. Also called *callus, keratoma, poroma, tyloma.*

cal·lous (kăl′əs) *adj.* Of, relating to, or characteristic of a callus or callosity.

cal·lus (kăl′əs) *n.*, *pl.* **-lus·es 1.** See **callosity. 2.** The hard bony tissue that develops around the ends of a fractured bone during healing.

calm·a·tive (kä′mə-tĭv, kăl′mə-) *adj.* Having relaxing or pacifying properties. —*n.* A sedative.

Cal·mette (kăl-mět′), **Albert Léon Charles** 1863–1933. French bacteriologist. With Camille Guérin he developed (c. 1921) the Bacillus Calmette-Guérin vaccine for immunization against tuberculosis.

cal·mod·u·lin (kăl-mŏj′ə-lĭn) *n.* A ubiquitous, eukaryotic calcium-binding protein that regulates cellular processes by modifying the activity of specific calcium-sensitive enzymes.

cal·o·mel (kăl′ə-měl′, -məl) *n.* A colorless, white or brown tasteless compound used as a purgative and an insecticide. Also called *mercurous chloride.*

cal·or (kăl′ôr, -ər, kā′lôr) *n.* The bodily heat indicating an inflammation.

ca·lor·ic (kə-lôr′ĭk) *adj.* **1.** Of or relating to calories. **2.** Of or relating to heat.

caloric nystagmus *n.* A jerky nystagmus as part of Bárány's sign.

caloric test *n.* Bárány's caloric test.

cal·o·rie (kăl′ə-rē) *n.* **1.** A unit of energy-producing potential that is supplied by food and is released upon oxidation by the body, equal to the amount of energy required to raise the temperature of 1 kilogram of water by 1°C at one atmosphere pressure. Also called *nutritionist's calorie.* **2.** The unit of heat equal to the amount of heat that is required to raise the temperature of 1 kilogram of water by 1°C at 1 atmosphere pressure. Also called *kilocalorie, kilogram calorie, large calorie.* **3.** Any of several approximately equal units of heat, each measured as the quantity of heat that is required to raise the temperature of 1 gram of water by 1°C from a standard initial temperature at 1 atmosphere pressure. Also called *gram calorie, small calorie.* **4.** The unit of heat equal to $\frac{1}{100}$ the quantity of heat that is required to raise the temperature of 1 gram of water from 0 to 100°C at 1 atmosphere pressure. Also called *mean calorie.*

ca·lor·i·gen·ic (kə-lôr′ə-jěn′ĭk, kăl′ər-ə-) *adj.* Heat-producing, especially with regard to food or certain hormones.

cal·o·rim·e·ter (kăl′ə-rĭm′ĭ-tər) *n.* An apparatus for measuring the heat generated by a chemical reaction, change of state, or formation of a solution. —**ca·lor′i·met′ric** (kə-lôr′ə-mĕt′rĭk) *adj.*

cal·o·rim·e·try (kăl′ə-rĭm′ĭ-trē) *n.* Measurement of the amount of heat evolved or absorbed in a chemical reaction, change of state, or formation of a solution.

Ca·lo·ri's bursa (kə-lôr′ēz, kä-) *n.* The bursa between the arch of the aorta and the trachea.

Ca·lot's triangle (kă-lōz′) *n.* A triangle that is bounded by the cystic artery, the cystic duct, and the hepatic duct.

cal·var·i·a (kăl-vâr′ē-ə) *n., pl.* –**i·ae** (-ē-ē′) Roof of the skull; the upper domelike portion of the skull without the lower jaw or the lower jaw and facial parts. Also called *calvarium, skullcap.*

Cal·vé-Perthes disease (kăl-vā′-) *n.* See **osteochondritis deformans juvenilis.**

calx (kălks) *n., pl.* **calx·es** *or* **cal·ces** (kăl′sēz′) **1.** The crumbly residue left after a mineral or metal has been calcined or roasted. **2.** The posterior rounded extremity of the foot; the heel.

Ca·lym·ma·to·bac·te·ri·um (kə-lĭm′ə-tō-băk-tîr′ē-əm) *n.* A genus of nonmotile bacteria containing gram-negative, pleomorphic rods that cause granulomatous lesions in humans, especially in the inguinal region.

ca·lyx (kā′lĭks, kăl′ĭks) *n.* Variant of **calix.**

cam·er·a (kăm′ər-ə, kăm′rə) *n., pl.* –**er·ae** (-ə-rē) A chamber or cavity, such as one of the chambers of the heart or eye.

cAMP *abbr.* cyclic AMP

camp fever *n.* See **typhus.**

cam·phor (kăm′fər) *n.* An aromatic crystalline compound obtained from the wood or leaves of the camphor tree or synthesized and used as an insect repellent and in external preparations to relieve mild pain and itching.

cam·pim·e·ter (kăm-pĭm′ĭ-tər) *n.* A portable, hand-held device used to measure the visual field.

camp·to·cor·mi·a (kămp′tə-kôr′mē-ə) *n.* A hysterical condition in which the body is bent completely forward at the trunk and is unable to be straightened. Also called *camptospasm.*

camp·to·me·li·a (kămp′tō-mē′lē-ə, mēl′yə) *n.* A bending of the limbs that produces a permanent curving or bowing. —**camp′to·mel′ic** *adj.*

camptomelic dwarfism *n.* Dwarfism that is caused by the shortening of the lower limbs as a result of the femur and tibia bending anteriorly.

camp·to·spasm (kămp′tə-spăz′əm) *n.* See **camptocormia.**

Cam·py·lo·bac·ter (kăm′pə-lō-băk′tər) *n.* A genus of motile bacteria containing gram-negative, nonspore-forming, spirally curved rods with a single polar flagellum at one or both ends of the cell; certain species can cause illness in humans.

cam·py·lo·bac·ter·o·sis (kăm′pə-lō-băk′tə-rō′sĭs) *n.* A gastrointestinal condition characterized by diarrhea, abdominal cramps, and fever, caused by eating raw meat or unpasteurized milk contaminated with *Campylobacter jejuni,* a bacterium that infects poultry, cattle, and sheep.

cam·py·lo·dac·ty·ly (kăm′pə-lō-dăk′tə-lē) *n.* Permanent flexion of one or more of the finger joints. Also called *camptodactyly.*

ca·nal (kə-năl′) *n.* A duct, a channel, or a tubular structure.

can·a·lic·u·li·tis (kăn′ə-lĭk′yə-lī′tĭs) *n.* Inflammation of the lacrimal duct. —**can′a·lic′u·lar** (-lĭk′yə-lər) *adj.*

can·a·lic·u·li·za·tion (kăn′ə-lĭk′yə-lĭ-zā′shən) *n.* The formation of small canals or channels in tissue.

can·a·lic·u·lus (kăn′ə-lĭk′yə-ləs) *n., pl.* –**li** (-lī′) A small canal or duct in the body, as one of the minute channels in compact bone.

ca·na·lis (kə-nā′lĭs) *n., pl.* –**les** (-lēz′) A canal.

can·a·li·za·tion (kăn′ə-lĭ-zā′shən) *n.* The formation of canals or channels in tissue.

Ca·nas·a (kə-năs′ə) A trademark for the drug mesalamine.

Can·a·van's disease (kăn′ə-vănz′, -vənz) *n.* See **spongy degeneration.**

can·cel·lat·ed (kăn′sə-lā′tĭd) *adj.* Having an open, latticed, or porous structure, as in a bone.

can·cel·lous (kăn-sĕl′əs, kăn′sə-ləs) *adj.* Cancellated.

cancellous bone *n.* See **spongy bone** (sense 1).

cancellous tissue *n.* Lattice-like or spongy bone tissue.

can·cel·lus (kăn-sĕl′əs) *n., pl.* –**li** (-lī′) A latticelike structure, such as spongy bone.

can·cer (kăn′sər) *n.* **1.** *Abbr.* **CA** Any of various malignant neoplasms characterized by the proliferation of anaplastic cells that tend to invade surrounding tissue and metastasize to new body sites. **2.** The pathological condition characterized by such growths. —**can′cer·ous** (kăn′sər-əs) *adj.*

cancer á deux (ä′ dœ′) *n.* Carcinomas occurring at approximately the same time, or in fairly close succession, in two persons who live together.

cancer family *n.* A group of blood relatives in which cancer has been reported. The mode of aggregation may be genetic, as in familial cancer, or due to common exposure to a carcinogenic or oncogenic agent.

can·cer·o·pho·bi·a (kăn′sə-rō-fō′bē-ə) *or* **car·ci·no·pho·bi·a** (kär′sə-nō-) *n.* An abnormal fear of developing a malignant growth.

can·cri·form (kăng′krə-fôrm′) *adj.* Of or resembling a cancer.

can·croid (kăng′kroid′) *adj.* **1.** Of or relating to squamous cell carcinoma. **2.** Of or resembling a cancer. —*n.* See **squamous cell carcinoma.**

can·crum (kăng′krəm) *n., pl.* –**cra** (-krə) A gangrenous, ulcerative, inflammatory lesion.

can·del·a (kăn-dĕl′ə) *n. Abbr.* **cd** A unit of measurement of luminous flux, equal to the amount of light given out through a solid angle by a source of one candela radiating equally in all directions. Also called *candle.*

can·de·sar·tan ci·lex·e·til (kăn′də-sär′tn sĭ-lĕk′sə-tĭl) *n.* An angiotensin II receptor antagonist drug used primarily to treat hypertension.

can·di·ci·din (kăn′dĭ-sīd′n) *n.* An antibiotic agent derived from a soil actinomycete and active against some fungi of the genus *Candida.*

Can·di·da (kăn′dĭ-də) *n.* A genus of the pathogenic yeastlike fungi.

can·di·de·mi·a (kăn′dĭ-dē′mē-ə) *n.* The presence of any fungus of the genus *Candida* in the blood.

can·di·di·a·sis (kăn′dĭ-dī′ə-sĭs) *or* **can·di·do·sis** (-dō′-sĭs) *n.* A fungous infection caused by a species of *Candida*, especially *Candida albicans,* that can involve various parts of the body, such as the skin and mucous membranes. Also called *moniliasis.*

can·dle (kăn′dl) *n.* See **candela.**

can·dle-me·ter (kăn′dl-mē′tər) *n.* See **lux.**

can·dy strip·er (kăn′dē strī′pər) *n.* A volunteer worker in a hospital.

Can·i·dae (kăn′ĭ-dē′) *n.* A family of carnivorous mammals that includes dogs, wolves, jackals, and foxes.

ca·nine (kā′nīn) *adj.* **1.** Of, relating to, or characteristic of members of the family Canidae. **2.** Of, relating to, or being one of the pointed conical teeth that is located between the incisors and the first bicuspids. —*n.* **1.** An animal of the family Canidae, especially a dog. **2.** A canine tooth.

canine spasm *n.* See **risus caninus.**

canine tooth *n.* Any of four teeth having a thick conical crown and a long conical root, adjacent to the distal surface of the lateral incisors, in both deciduous and permanent dentition. Also called *cuspid.*

ca·ni·ti·es (kə-nĭsh′ē-ēz′) *n.* The diminishing of pigment in hair producing a range of colors from normal to white that is perceived as gray.

can·ker (kăng′kər) *n.* **1.** Ulceration of the mouth and lips. **2.** An acute inflammation or infection of the ear and auditory canal, especially in dogs and cats. **3.** Cancrum.

canker sore *n.* A small painful ulcer of the mucous membrane of the mouth; an aphtha. Also called *aphthous stomatitis, recurrent aphthous ulcers, ulcerative stomatitis.*

can·nab·i·noid (kə-năb′ə-noid′) *n.* Any of various organic substances, such as THC, found in cannabis.

can·na·bis (kăn′ə-bĭs) *n.* Any of several mildly euphoriant, intoxicating hallucinogenic drugs, such as hashish or marijuana, prepared from various parts of the hemp plant.

can·na·bism (kăn′ə-bĭz′əm) *n.* Poisoning by preparations of cannabis.

Can·non (kăn′ən), **Walter Bradford** 1871–1945. American physiologist noted for his research on the autonomic nervous system, including the "fight or flight" response that is induced by stressful stimuli and the effects of hormones on nerve conduction. He also invented the use of barium in x-ray studies of the gastrointestinal tract.

can·non·ball pulse (kăn′ən-bôl′) *n.* See **water-hammer pulse.**

Can·non's ring (kăn′ənz) *n.* A tonically contracted muscular band in the transverse colon close to the hepatic flexure.

can·nu·la *or* **can·u·la** (kăn′yə-lə) *n., pl.* **–las** *or* **–lae** (-lē′) A flexible tube, usually containing a trocar at one end, that is inserted into a bodily cavity, duct, or vessel to drain fluid or administer a substance such as a medication.

can·nu·la·tion (kăn′yə-lā′shən) *or* **can·nu·li·za·tion** (-yə-lĭ-zā′shən) *n.* Insertion of a cannula.

can·thec·to·my (kăn-thĕk′tə-mē) *n.* An excision of a canthus.

can·thi·tis (kăn-thī′tĭs) *n.* Inflammation of a canthus.

can·thol·y·sis (kăn-thŏl′ĭ-sĭs) *n.* See **canthoplasty** (sense 2).

can·tho·me·a·tal plane (kăn′thō-mē-āt′l) *n.* A plane passing through the junction of the upper and lower eyelids and the center of the ear canal.

can·tho·plas·ty (kăn′thə-plăs′tē) *n.* **1.** The lengthening of the palpebral fissure by cutting through the external canthus. Also called *cantholysis.* **2.** Surgical restoration of the canthus.

can·thor·rha·phy (kăn-thôr′ə-fē) *n.* The surgical shortening of the palpebral fissure of the eyelids by suturing the canthus.

can·thot·o·my (kăn-thŏt′ə-mē) *n.* An incision of the canthus.

can·thus (kăn′thəs) *n., pl.* **–thi** (-thī′) The angle formed by the meeting of the upper and lower eyelids at either side of the eye. —**can′thal** (-thəl) *adj.*

can·u·la (kăn′yə-lə) *n.* Variant of **cannula.**

cap (kăp) *n.* A protective cover or seal, especially one that closes off an end or a tip and that resembles a close-fitting head covering.

CAP *abbr.* catabolite gene activator protein

ca·pac·i·ta·tion (kə-păs′ĭ-tā′shən) *n.* The change undergone by spermatozoa in the female genital tract that enables them to penetrate and fertilize an egg.

ca·pac·i·ty (kə-păs′ĭ-tē) *n.* **1.** The measure of potential cubic contents of a cavity or receptacle; volume. **2.** Ability to perform or produce; capability.

cap·ac·tin (kă-păk′tĭn) *n.* Any of a class of proteins capping the ends of actin filaments.

cap·e·line bandage (kăp′ə-lēn′, -lĭn) *n.* A caplike bandage covering the head or the stump from an amputation.

cap·il·lar·ec·ta·sia (kăp′ə-lĕr′ĭk-tā′zhə) *n.* Dilation of the capillary blood vessels.

cap·il·lar·i·o·mo·tor (kăp′ə-lĕr′ē-ō-mō′tər) *adj.* Relating to the functional activity of the capillaries.

cap·il·la·ri·tis (kăp′ə-lə-rī′tĭs) *n.* Inflammation of a capillary or capillaries.

cap·il·lar·i·ty (kăp′ə-lăr′ĭ-tē) *n.* The interaction between contacting surfaces of a liquid and a solid that distorts the liquid surface from a planar shape.

cap·il·la·rop·a·thy (kăp′ə-lə-rŏp′ə-thē) *n.* A disease of the capillaries. Also called *microangiopathy.*

cap·il·lary (kăp′ə-lĕr′ē) *adj.* **1.** Of or relating to the capillaries. **2.** Relating to or resembling a hair; fine and slender. —*n.* Blood capillary.

capillary arteriole *n.* A minute artery that terminates in a capillary.

capillary attraction *n.* A surface force of adhesion that causes fluids to rise along or into solid materials.

capillary bed *n.* The capillaries of the blood system considered collectively with their volume capacity.

capillary drainage *n.* The use of a wick of gauze or other material to drain a cavity or wound.

capillary fracture *n.* See **hairline fracture.**

capillary hemangioma *n.* A congenital lesion consisting of numerous, closely packed capillaries usually separated only by a thin network of reticulin.

capillary lake *n.* The total mass of blood contained in capillary vessels.

capillary loop *n.* Any of the small blood vessels that carry blood in the papillae of the skin.

capillary permeability factor *n.* See **vitamin P**.

capillary vein *n.* See **venule**.

ca·pil·lus (kə-pĭl′əs) *n.*, *pl.* **–li** (-lī′) A hair on the head.

cap·i·stra·tion (kăp′ĭ-strā′shən) *n.* See **paraphimosis** (sense 1).

cap·i·tate (kăp′ĭ-tāt′) *adj.* Enlarged and globular at the tip, as a bone of the wrist having a rounded, knoblike end.

capitate bone *n.* The largest of the carpal bones, located in the distal row of the carpus.

cap·i·ta·tion (kăp′ĭ-tā′shən) *n.* A fixed payment remitted at regular intervals to a medical provider by a managed care organization for an enrolled patient.

cap·i·tel·lum (kăp′ĭ-tĕl′əm) *n.*, *pl.* **–tel·la** (-tĕl′ə) **1.** Capitulum. **2.** The rounded protuberance at the lower end of the humerus that articulates with the radius.

ca·pit·i·um (kă-pĭt′ē-əm) *n.* A bandage for the head.

cap·i·ton·nage (kăp′ĭ-tə-näzh′) *n.* Surgical closure of a cyst cavity.

ca·pit·u·lum (kə-pĭch′ə-ləm) *n.*, *pl.* **–la** (-lə) A small head or rounded articular extremity of a bone. —**ca·pit′u·lar** *adj.*

cap·let (kăp′lĭt) *n.* A smooth, coated, oval-shaped medicine tablet intended to be tamper-resistant.

Cap·o·ten (kăp′ə-tn) A trademark for the drug captopril.

capped elbow (kăpt) *n.* A swelling of the bursa on the point of the elbow of a horse.

cap·rate (kăp′rāt′) *n.* A salt or ester of capric acid.

cap·re·o·my·cin (kăp′rē-ō-mī′sĭn) *n.* An antibiotic derived from *Streptomyces capreolus* and effective against the microorganism responsible for tuberculosis in humans.

cap·ric acid (kăp′rĭk) *n.* A fatty acid obtained from animal fats and oils and used in the manufacture of perfumes and fruit flavorings.

cap·rine (kăp′rēn′) *n.* See **norleucine**.

cap·ro·ate (kăp′rō-āt′) *n.* A salt or ester of caproic acid.

ca·pro·ic acid (kə-prō′ĭk, kă-) *n.* A liquid fatty acid found in animal fats and oils or synthesized and used in the manufacture of pharmaceuticals.

cap·ro·yl (kăp′rō-ĭl, kə-prō′ĭl, kă-) *n.* The radical $C_5H_{11}CO$ of caproic acid.

cap·ry·late (kăp′rə-lāt′) *n.* A salt or ester of caprylic acid.

ca·pryl·ic acid (kə-prĭl′ĭk, kă-) *n.* A liquid fatty acid found in butter and other fats and oils and having a rancid taste; used in the manufacture of dyes.

cap·sa·i·cin (kăp-sā′ĭ-sĭn) *n.* A colorless, pungent, crystalline compound that is derived from the capsicum pepper and is a strong irritant to skin and mucous membranes.

cap·sid (kăp′sĭd) *n.* The protein shell that surrounds a virus particle.

cap·so·mere (kăp′sə-mîr′) *or* **cap·so·mer** (-mər) *n.* A subunit of a viral capsid.

cap·su·la (kăp′sə-lə) *n.*, *pl.* **–lae** (-lē′) **1.** A membranous structure, usually dense collagenous connective tissue, that envelops an organ, joint, or other part. **2.** An anatomical structure resembling a capsule or envelope.

capsula fi·bro·sa (fī-brō′sə) *n.*, *pl.* **capsulae fi·bro·sae** (-sē′) Fibrous capsule.

capsular antigen *n.* An antigen found only in the capsules of certain microorganisms.

capsular cataract *n.* A cataract in which the opacity affects the capsule only.

capsular ligament *n.* The thickened portions of the fibrous membrane of an articular capsule.

capsular space *n.* The slitlike space between the visceral and parietal layers of the capsule of the renal corpuscle. Also called *Bowman's space*.

cap·sule (kăp′səl, -sool) *n.* **1.** A fibrous, membranous, or fatty sheath that encloses an organ or part, such as the sac surrounding the kidney or the fibrous tissues that surround a joint. **2.** A small soluble container, usually made of gelatin, that encloses a dose of an oral medicine or a vitamin. **3.** The thin-walled, spore-containing structure of mosses and related plants. —**cap′su·lar** (kăp′sə-lər) *adj.*

capsule forceps *n.* A fine strong forceps for removing the capsule of the lens in extracapsular extraction of cataract.

cap·su·li·tis (kăp′sə-lī′tĭs) *n.* Inflammation of the capsule of an organ or part.

cap·su·lo·len·tic·u·lar (kăp′sə-lō-lĕn-tĭk′yə-lər) *adj.* Relating to the lens of the eye and its capsule.

capsulolenticular cataract *n.* A cataract involving both the lens of the eye and its capsule.

cap·su·lo·plas·ty (kăp′sə-lə-plăs′tē) *n.* The surgical repair of a capsule, especially a joint capsule.

cap·su·lor·rha·phy (kăp′sə-lôr′ə-fē) *n.* Suture of a tear in a capsule, especially of a joint capsule to prevent recurring dislocation.

cap·su·lot·o·my (kăp′sə-lŏt′ə-mē) *n.* Incision into a capsule, especially that of the crystalline lens of the eye, as to remove cataracts.

cap·to·pril (kăp′tə-prĭl′) *n.* An ACE inhibitor drug that is used in the treament of hypertension, congestive heart failure, and other cardiovascular disorders.

cap·ture (kăp′chər) *n.* The act of catching, taking, or holding a particle or impulse.

capture beat *n.* The cardiac cycle resulting when, after atrioventricular dissociation, the atria regain control of the ventricles.

cap·ut (kăp′oot, -ət) *n.*, *pl.* **cap·i·ta** (kăp′ĭ-tə) The head.

caput me·du·sae (mĭ-doo′sē′) *n.* **1.** See **Medusa head**. **2.** Dilated ciliary arteries surrounding the corneoscleral limbus in absolute glaucoma.

caput suc·ce·da·ne·um (sŭk′sē-dā′nē-əm) *n.* A swelling formed on the presenting part of the head of a fetus during labor, resulting in edema and varying degrees of scalp hemorrhage.

Car·a·fate (kâr′ə-fāt′) A trademark for the drug sucralfate.

carb– *pref.* Variant of **carbo–**.

car·ba·mate (kär′bə-māt′, kär-băm′āt′) *n.* A salt or ester of carbamic acid.

car·ba·maz·e·pine (kär′bə-măz′ə-pēn′) *n.* An anticonvulsant and analgesic drug used in the treatment of certain forms of epilepsy and to relieve pain associated with trigeminal neuralgia.

car·bam·ic acid (kär-băm′ĭk) *n.* A hypothetical acid that exists only in the form of its esters and salts.

car·ba·mide (kär′bə-mīd′, kär-băm′ĭd) *n.* See **urea.**

carb·a·mi·no compound (kär′bə-mē′nō, kär-băm′ə-nō) *n.* Any of various carbamic acid derivatives formed by the combination of carbon dioxide with an amino acid or a protein, such as hemoglobin forming carbaminohemoglobin.

carb·a·mi·no·he·mo·glo·bin (kär′bə-mē′nō-hē′mə-glō′bĭn, kär-băm′ə-nō-) *n.* A compound of carbon dioxide and hemoglobin, which is one of the forms in which carbon dioxide exists in the blood.

car·ba·myl (kär′bə-mĭl) *or* **car·bam·o·yl** (kär-băm′ō-ĭl′) *n.* The radical NH_2CO from carbamic acid.

car·ba·myl·trans·fer·ase (kär′bə-mĭl-trăns′fə-rās′, -răz′) *n.* See **transcarbamylase.**

car·ba·myl·u·re·a (kär′bə-mĭl-yŏŏ-rē′ə) *n.* See **biuret.**

car·ben·i·cil·lin (kär-bĕn′ĭ-sĭl′ĭn) *n.* A semisynthetic derivative of penicillin that is effective in the treatment of infections caused by certain susceptible strains of gram-negative bacteria.

carbenicillin disodium *n.* The disodium salt of a semisynthetic derivative of penicillin used in the treatment of severe systemic infections, septicemia, and urinary, genitourinary, respiratory, and soft-tissue infections.

car·bi·do·pa (kär′bĭ-dō′pə) *n.* A drug that increases the availability of L-dopa to the brain and is administered with it in the treatment of Parkinson's disease

car·bi·nol (kär′bə-nôl′, -nōl′) *n.* See **methanol.**

carbo– *or* **carb–** *pref.* Carbon: *carbohydrate.*

car·bo·ben·zox·y (kär′bō-bĕn-zŏk′sē) *adj.* Relating to or containing the radical $COOCH_2C_6H_5$.

car·bo·hy·drase (kär′bō-hī′drās′, -drāz′) *n.* Any of various enzymes, such as amylase, that catalyze the hydrolysis of a carbohydrate.

car·bo·hy·drate (kär′bō-hī′drāt′) *n.* Any of a group of organic compounds that includes sugars, starches, celluloses, and gums and serves as a major energy source in the diet of animals; they are produced by photosynthetic plants and contain only carbon, hydrogen, and oxygen, usually in the ratio 1:2:1.

carbohydrate-induced hyperlipemia *n.* **1.** See **type III familial hyperlipoproteinemia. 2.** See **type IV familial hyperlipoproteinemia.**

carbohydrate loading *n.* A dietary practice that increases carbohydrate reserves in muscle tissue through the consumption of extra quantities of high-starch foods and is often followed by some endurance athletes prior to competition.

car·bo·hy·dra·tu·ri·a (kär′bō-hī′drā-tŏŏr′ē-ə) *n.* The presence of an abnormally large concentration of carbohydrates in the urine.

car·bol·fuch·sin (kär′bôl-fyŏŏk′sĭn) *n.* A mixture of an aqueous solution of phenol and an alcoholic solution of fuchsin used as a stain in microscopy, especially to stain bacteria.

car·bol·ic acid (kär-bŏl′ĭk) *n.* See **phenol** (sense 1).

car·bo·lu·ri·a (kär′bə-lŏŏr′ē-ə) *n.* The presence of phenol in the urine.

car·bon (kär′bən) *n. Symbol* **C** A nonmetallic element occurring in many inorganic and in all organic compounds, existing as graphite and diamond and as a constituent of coal, limestone, and petroleum, and capable of chemical self-bonding to form a number of important molecules. Atomic number 6.

car·bon·ate (kär′bə-nāt′) *n.* A salt or ester of carbonic acid.

carbon cycle *n.* **1.** The combined processes, including photosynthesis, decomposition, and respiration, by which carbon as a component of various compounds cycles between its major reservoirs—the atmosphere, oceans, and living organisms. Also called *carbon dioxide cycle.* **2.** See **carbon-nitrogen cycle.**

carbon dioxide *n.* A colorless, odorless, incombustible gas formed during respiration, combustion, and organic decomposition and used in inert atmospheres, fire extinguishers, and aerosols.

carbon dioxide cycle *n.* See **carbon cycle.**

car·bo·ni·um (kär-bō′nē-əm) *n.* An organic cation having one less electron than a corresponding free radical and with positive charge localized on the carbon atom.

carbon monoxide *n.* A colorless, odorless, highly poisonous gas that is formed by the incomplete combustion of carbon or of a carbonaceous material, such as gasoline.

carbon monoxide hemoglobin *n.* See **carboxyhemoglobin.**

carbon monoxide poisoning *n.* A potentially fatal condition caused by inhalation of carbon monoxide gas which competes favorably with oxygen for binding with hemoglobin and thus interferes with the transportation of oxygen and carbon dioxide by the blood. Also called *carboxyhemoglobinemia.*

carbon-nitrogen cycle *n.* A chain of thermonuclear reactions in which nitrogen isotopes are formed in intermediate stages and carbon acts essentially as a catalyst to convert four hydrogen atoms into one helium atom with the emission of two positrons. The entire sequence is thought to generate significant amounts of energy in the sun and certain other stars. Also called *carbon cycle, nitrogen cycle.*

carbon tetrachloride *n.* A poisonous, nonflammable, colorless liquid used in fire extinguishers and as a dry-cleaning fluid. Also called *tetrachloromethane.*

car·bon·yl (kär′bə-nĭl′) *n.* The bivalent radical CO.

car·bo·prost tromethamine (kär′bō-prŏst′) *n.* A prostaglandin used as an abortifacient and in the treatment of refractory postpartum bleeding.

car·box·y·he·mo·glo·bin (kär-bŏk′sē-hē′mə-glō′bĭn) *n.* The compound that is formed when inhaled carbon monoxide combines with hemoglobin in the blood. Also called *carbon monoxide hemoglobin.*

car·box·y·he·mo·glo·bi·ne·mi·a (kär-bŏk′sē-hē′mə-glō′bə-nē′mē-ə) *n.* See **carbon monoxide poisoning.**

car·box·yl (kär-bŏk′səl) *n.* The univalent radical, COOH, characteristic of all organic acids.

car·box·yl·ase (kär-bŏk′sə-lās′, -lāz′) *n.* An enzyme that catalyzes a carboxylation or decarboxylation reaction.

car·box·yl·a·tion (kär-bŏk′sə-lā′shən) *n.* The introduction of a carboxyl group into a compound or molecule.

car·box·yl·trans·fer·ase (kär-bŏk′səl-trăns′fə-rās′, -rāz′) *n.* Any of various enzymes that catalyze the transfer of carboxyl groups from one compound to another. Also called *transcarboxylase*.

car·box·y·pep·ti·dase (kär-bŏk′sē-pĕp′tĭ-dās′, -dāz′) *n.* An enzyme that catalyzes the hydrolysis of a terminal amino acid from the end of a peptide or polypeptide that contains a free carboxyl group.

car·bun·cle (kär′bŭng′kəl) *n.* **1.** A deep-seated pyogenic infection of several contiguous hair follicles, with formation of connecting sinuses, often preceded or accompanied by fever, malaise, and prostration. **2.** See **anthrax** (sense 1). —**car·bun′cu·lar** (-kyə-lər) *adj.*

car·bun·cu·lo·sis (kär-bŭng′kyə-lō′sĭs) *n.* The occurrence of several carbuncles simultaneously or within a short period of time.

carcino– or **carcin–** *pref.* Cancer; cancerous: *carcinogenesis.*

car·ci·no·em·bry·on·ic antigen (kär′sə-nō-ĕm′brē-ŏn′ĭk) *n. Abbr.* **CEA** A glycoprotein that is present in fetal gastrointestinal tissue and is generally absent from adult cells, with the exception of some kinds of carcinomas.

car·cin·o·gen (kär-sĭn′ə-jən, kär′sə-nə-jĕn′) *n.* A substance or agent that causes cancer. —**car′cin·o·gen′ic** (kär′sə-nə-jĕn′ĭk) *adj.*

car·ci·no·gen·e·sis (kär′sə-nə-jĕn′ĭ-sĭs) *n.* The production of cancer.

car·ci·noid (kär′sə-noid′) *n.* A small, slow-growing, benign or malignant tumor, usually in the gastrointestinal tract, that is composed of islands of rounded cells with small vesicular nuclei and secretes serotonin. Also called *argentaffinoma.*

carcinoid syndrome *n.* A group of signs and symptoms including diarrhea, bronchospasm, skin flushing, and valvular heart disease caused primarily by serotonin secreted by carcinoid tumors that have metastasized to the liver.

car·ci·no·lyt·ic (kär′sə-nō-lĭt′ĭk) *adj.* Destructive to the cancer cells.

car·ci·no·ma (kär′sə-nō′mə) *n., pl.* **–mas** or **–ma·ta** (-mə-tə) *Abbr.* **CA** An invasive malignant tumor derived from epithelial tissue that tends to metastasize to other areas of the body.

carcinoma ex pleomorphic adenoma *n.* A carcinoma developing in a benign mixed tumor of a salivary gland and characterized by rapid growth and pain.

carcinoma in situ *n.* A neoplasm whose cells are localized in the epithelium and show no tendency to invade or metastasize to other tissues.

carcinoma sim·plex (sĭm′plĕks′) *n.* A carcinoma that is poorly differentiated or lacks differentiation.

car·ci·no·ma·to·sis (kär′sə-nō′mə-tō′sĭs) *n.* A pathological condition characterized by the presence of carcinomas that have metastasized to many parts of the body.

car·ci·no·ma·tous (kär′sə-nō′mə-təs, -nŏm′ə-) *adj.* Relating to or manifesting the characteristic properties of carcinoma.

carcinomatous myopathy *n.* See **Lambert-Eaton syndrome.**

car·ci·no·pho·bi·a (kär′sə-nō-fō′bē-ə) *n.* Variant of **cancerophobia.**

car·ci·no·sar·co·ma (kär′sə-nō-sär-kō′mə) *n.* A malignant neoplasm that contains elements of carcinoma and sarcoma. Also called *sarcocarcinoma.*

car·ci·no·sis (kär′sə-nō′sĭs) *n.* Carcinomatosis.

Car·dene (kär′dēn′) A trademark for the drug nicardipine.

cardi– *pref.* Variant of **cardio–.**

car·di·a (kär′dē-ə) *n., pl.* **–di·as** or **–di·ae** (-dē-ē′) **1.** The opening of the esophagus into the stomach. **2.** The upper portion of the stomach that adjoins this opening.

car·di·ac (kär′dē-ăk′) *adj.* **1.** Of, near, or relating to the heart. **2.** Of, near, or relating to the cardia. —*n.* A person with a heart disorder.

cardiac arrest *n. Abbr.* **CA** A sudden cessation of cardiac function, resulting in loss of effective circulation.

cardiac arrhythmia *n.* See **cardiac dysrhythmia.**

cardiac asthma *n.* An asthmatic attack due to bronchoconstriction caused by pulmonary congestion and failure of the left ventricle.

cardiac catheter *n.* A long, fine catheter that can be passed into the chambers of the heart via a vein or artery as a means of withdrawing samples of blood, measuring pressures within the heart's chambers or great vessels, or injecting contrast media. Also called *intracardiac catheter.*

cardiac cirrhosis *n.* An extensive fibrotic reaction occurring within the liver as a result of prolonged congestive heart failure. Also called *pseudocirrhosis.*

cardiac cycle *n.* A complete beat of the heart, including systole and diastole and the intervals between, beginning with any event in the heart's action to the moment when that same event is repeated.

cardiac decompression *n.* The relief of pressure on the heart caused by blood or fluid in the pericardial sac by means of an incision in the pericardium. Also called *pericardial decompression.*

cardiac dysrhythmia *n.* Any abnormality in the rate, regularity, or sequence of cardiac activation. Also called *cardiac arrhythmia.*

cardiac edema *n.* Edema resulting from congestive heart failure.

cardiac ganglion *n.* Any of the parasympathetic ganglia of the cardiac plexus between the arch of the aorta and the bifurcation of the pulmonary artery.

cardiac gland *n.* A coiled tubular gland situated in the cardiac region of the stomach.

cardiac glycoside *n.* Any of several glycosides obtained chiefly from plant sources such as the foxglove, used medicinally to increase the force of contraction of heart muscle and to regulate heartbeats.

cardiac histiocyte *n.* A large mononuclear cell found in connective tissue of the heart wall in inflammatory conditions, especially in the Aschoff body. Also called *Anitschkow cell, Anitschkow myocyte.*

cardiac index *n.* The volume of blood pumped by the heart in a unit of time divided by the body surface area, usually expressed in liters per minute per square meter.

cardiac infarction *n.* See **myocardial infarction.**

cardiac insufficiency *n.* See **heart failure** (sense 1).

cardiac jelly *n.* The gelatinous noncellular material between the endothelial lining and the myocardial layer of the heart in very young embryos, later serving as a substratum for cardiac mesenchyme.

cardiac massage *n.* A resuscitative procedure that employs the rhythmic compression of the chest and heart in an effort to restore and maintain the circulation after cardiac arrest or ventricular fibrillation. Also called *heart massage.*

cardiac murmur *n.* A murmur that is produced within the heart.

cardiac muscle *n.* The muscle of the heart, consisting of anastomosing transversely striated muscle fibers formed of cells united at intercalated disks; the myocardium. Also called *muscle of heart.*

cardiac notch *n.* A deep notch in the alimentary canal at the junction of the esophagus and the stomach.

cardiac opening *n.* The opening of the esophagus into the stomach.

cardiac output *n. Abbr.* **CO** The volume of blood pumped from the right or left ventricle in one minute. It is equal to the stroke volume multiplied by the heart rate.

cardiac plexus *n.* A wide-meshed network of anastomosing cords from the sympathetic and vagus nerves that surrounds the arch of the aorta and the pulmonary artery and continues to the atria, ventricles, and coronary vessels.

cardiac reserve *n.* The work that the heart is able to perform beyond that required of it under ordinary circumstances.

cardiac souffle *n.* A soft puffing heart murmur.

cardiac sound *n.* See **heart sound.**

cardiac sphincter *n.* See **lower esophageal sphincter.**

cardiac tamponade *n.* Compression of venous return to the heart because of increased volume of fluid in the pericardium.

cardiac valve *n.* Any of the valves regulating the flow of blood through and from the heart, consisting of the aortic valve, the left and right atrioventricular valves, and the pulmonary valve.

car·di·al·gia (kär′dē-ăl′jə) *n.* **1.** See **heartburn. 2.** Cardiodynia.

car·di·ec·ta·sia (kär′dē-ĭk-tā′zhə) *n.* Dilation of the heart.

car·di·nal ligament (kär′dn-əl, kärd′nəl) *n.* See **cervical ligament of uterus.**

cardinal point *n.* **1.** One of four points in the pelvic inlet toward which the occiput of the fetus is usually directed in cases of head presentation. **2.** Any of six reference points in the eye: the anterior focal point, posterior focal point, two principal points, and two nodal points.

cardinal symptom *n.* The primary or major symptom by which a diagnosis is made.

cardinal veins *pl.n.* Any of three major systemic venous channels in certain adult vertebrates and in the embryos of other vertebrates, such as humans.

cardio– *or* **cardi–** *pref.* **1.** Heart: *cardiovascular.* **2.** Cardia: *cardiodiosis.*

car·di·o·ac·cel·er·a·tor (kär′dē-ō′ăk-sĕl′ə-rā′tər) *n.* An agent that increases the heart rate.

car·di·o·ac·tive (kär′dē-ō-ăk′tĭv) *adj.* Affecting the heart.

car·di·o·a·or·tic (kär′dē-ō-ā-ôr′tĭk) *adj.* Relating to the heart and the aorta.

car·di·o·ar·te·ri·al (kär′dē-ō-är-tîr′ē-əl) *adj.* Relating to the heart and the arteries.

cardioarterial interval *n.* The time between the apex beat of the heart and the radial pulse beat.

car·di·o·cele (kär′dē-ə-sēl′) *n.* Herniation or protrusion of the heart through an opening in the diaphragm or through a wound.

car·di·o·cen·te·sis (kär′dē-ō-sĕn-tē′sĭs) *n.* Puncture of a chamber of the heart for diagnosis or therapy.

car·di·o·cha·la·sia (kär′dē-ō-kə-lā′zhə) *n.* Relaxation or incompetence of sphincter action of the cardiac orifice of the stomach.

car·di·o·di·o·sis (kär′dē-ō-dē-ō′sĭs, -dī-ō′sĭs) *n.* Dilation of the cardiac end of the stomach by passing an instrument through the esophagus.

car·di·o·dy·nam·ics (kär′dē-ō-dī-năm′ĭks) *n.* The mechanics of the heart's action in pumping blood.

car·di·o·dyn·i·a (kär′dē-ō-dĭn′ē-ə) *n.* Localized pain in the region of the heart.

car·di·o·e·soph·a·ge·al (kär′dē-ō-ĭ-sŏf′ə-jē′əl) *adj.* Relating to the junction of the esophagus and the cardiac part of the stomach.

car·di·o·gen·ic (kär′dē-ō-jĕn′ĭk) *adj.* **1.** Having origin in the heart. **2.** Resulting from a disease or disorder of the heart.

cardiogenic shock *n.* Shock that results from a decline in cardiac output that occurs as a result of serious heart disease, especially myocardial infarction.

car·di·o·gram (kär′dē-ə-grăm′) *n.* **1.** The curve traced by a cardiograph, used in the diagnosis of heart disorders. **2.** See **electrocardiogram.**

car·di·o·graph (kär′dē-ə-grăf′) *n.* **1.** An instrument used to record the mechanical movements of the heart. **2.** See **electrocardiograph.** —**car′di·og′ra·phy** (-ŏg′rə-fē) *n.*

car·di·o·he·pat·ic (kär′dē-ō-hĭ-păt′ĭk) *adj.* Relating to the heart and the liver.

car·di·o·in·hib·i·to·ry (kär′dē-ō-ĭn-hĭb′ĭ-tôr′ē) *adj.* Arresting or slowing the action of the heart.

car·di·o·ki·net·ic (kär′dē-ō-kĭ-nĕt′ĭk, -kī-) *adj.* Influencing the action of the heart.

car·di·o·ky·mo·gram (kär′dē-ō-kī′mə-grăm′) *n.* A tracing of the changes in the size of the heart made by a cardiokymograph.

car·di·o·ky·mo·graph (kär′dē-ō-kī′mə-grăf′) *n.* A noninvasive device, placed on the chest, capable of recording motion made by the anterior left ventricle segmental wall of the heart.

car·di·o·lip·in (kär′dē-ō-lĭp′ĭn) *n.* A phospholipid usually obtained from beef heart, used in combination with lecithin and cholesterol as an antigen to diagnose syphilis.

car·di·o·lith (kär′dē-ə-lĭth′) *n.* A concretion in the heart, or an area of calcareous degeneration in its walls or valves.

car·di·ol·o·gy (kär′dē-ŏl′ə-jē) *n.* The medical study of the structure, function, and disorders of the heart.

car·di·ol·y·sis (kär′dē-ŏl′ĭ-sĭs) *n.* Surgery to break up adhesions in chronic mediastinopericarditis.

car·di·o·ma·la·cia (kär′dē-ō-mə-lā′shə) *n.* Pathological softening of the walls of the heart.

car·di·o·meg·a·ly (kär′dē-ō-měg′ə-lē) *n.* Enlargement of the heart. Also called *macrocardia, megalocardia.*

car·di·o·mo·til·i·ty (kär′dē-ō-mō-tĭl′ĭ-tē) *n.* The movements of the heart.

car·di·o·mus·cu·lar (kär′dē-ō-mŭs′kyə-lər) *adj.* Relating to the musculature of the heart.

car·di·o·my·o·li·po·sis (kär′dē-ō-mī′ō-lĭ-pō′sĭs) *n.* Fatty degeneration of the myocardium.

car·di·o·my·op·a·thy (kär′dē-ō-mī-ŏp′ə-thē) *n.* A disease or disorder of the heart muscle, especially of unknown cause. Also called *myocardiopathy.*

car·di·o·neph·ric (kär′dē-ō-něf′rĭk) *adj.* Cardiorenal.

car·di·o·neu·ral (kär′dē-ō-nŏŏr′əl) *adj.* Relating to the innervation of the heart.

car·di·o·o·men·to·pexy (kär′dē-ō-ō-měn′tə-pěk′sē) *n.* Surgical attachment of the omentum to the heart to improve its blood supply.

car·di·o·path·i·a ni·gra (kär′dē-ō-păth′ē-ənī′grə, nĭg′-rə) *n.* See **Ayerza's syndrome.**

car·di·op·a·thy (kär′dē-ŏp′ə-thē) *n.* A disease or disorder of the heart.

car·di·o·per·i·car·di·o·pex·y (kär′dē-ō-pěr′ĭ-kär′dē-ə-pěk′sē) *n.* Surgery to increase the blood supply to the myocardium.

car·di·o·pho·bi·a (kär′dē-ə-fō′bē-ə) *n.* An abnormal fear of heart disease.

car·di·o·plas·ty (kär′dē-ə-plăs′tē) *n.* See **esophagogastroplasty.**

car·di·o·ple·gia (kär′dē-ō-plē′jə) *n.* **1.** Paralysis of the heart, or cardiac arrest, as from direct blow or trauma. **2.** Elective, temporary stopping of cardiac activity, usually by using drugs.

car·di·op·to·si·a (kär′dē-ŏp-tō′sē-ə, -shə) *n.* Downward displacement or prolapse of the heart.

car·di·o·pul·mo·nar·y (kär′dē-ō-pŏŏl′mə-něr′ē, -pŭl′-) *adj.* Of, relating to, or involving both the heart and the lungs.

cardiopulmonary bypass *n.* A procedure to circulate and oxygenate the blood during heart surgery involving the diversion of blood from the heart and lungs through a heart-lung machine and the return of oxygenated blood to the aorta.

cardiopulmonary murmur *n.* A murmur, synchronous with the heart's beat but disappearing when the breath is held, due to movement of the air in a segment of lung compressed by the contracting heart.

cardiopulmonary resuscitation *n. Abbr.* **CPR** Restoration of cardiac output and pulmonary ventilation by artificial respiration and closed-chest massage after cardiac arrest and apnea.

car·di·o·py·lo·ric (kär′dē-ō-pī-lôr′ĭk, -pĭ-) *adj.* Of, relating to, or involving the cardiac and the pyloric portions of the stomach.

car·di·o·re·nal (kär′dē-ō-rē′nəl) *adj.* Of, relating to, or involving the heart and the kidney.

car·di·or·rha·phy (kär′dē-ôr′ə-fē) *n.* The suturing of the heart wall.

car·di·or·rhex·is (kär′dē-ə-rěk′sĭs) *n.* A rupture of the heart wall.

car·di·os·chi·sis (kär′dē-ŏs′kĭ-sĭs) *n.* Surgical division of adhesions between the heart and the pericardium or the chest wall.

car·di·o·se·lec·tiv·i·ty (kär′dē-ō-sĭ-lěk′tĭv′ĭ-tē, -sē′-lěk-) *n.* The relatively predominant cardiovascular effect of a drug that has many pharmacologic effects. —**car′di·o·se·lec′tive** (-sĭ-lěk′tĭv) *adj.*

car·di·o·spasm (kär′dē-ə-spăz′əm) *n.* See **esophageal achalasia.**

car·di·o·sphyg·mo·graph (kär′dē-ō-sfĭg′mə-grăf′) *n.* An instrument for recording graphically the movements of the heart and the radial pulse.

car·di·o·ta·chom·e·ter (kär′dē-ō-tă-kŏm′ĭ-tər, -tə-) *n.* An instrument for measuring the rapidity of the heartbeat.

car·di·o·tho·rac·ic (kär′dē-ō-thə-răs′ĭk) *n.* Of or relating to the heart and the chest.

cardiothoracic ratio *n.* The transverse diameter of the heart, as determined by x-ray examination, compared with that of the thoracic cage, used to help determine enlargement of the heart.

car·di·ot·o·my (kär′dē-ŏt′ə-mē) *n.* **1.** Incision of the heart wall. **2.** Incision of the cardiac end of the stomach.

car·di·o·ton·ic (kär′dē-ō-tŏn′ĭk) *adj.* Relating to or having a favorable effect upon the action of the heart. —**car′di·o·ton′ic** *n.*

car·di·o·val·vot·o·my (kär′dē-ō-văl-vŏt′ə-mē) *n.* See **cardiovalvulotomy.**

car·di·o·val·vu·li·tis (kär′dē-ō-văl′vyə-lī′tĭs) *n.* Inflammation of the heart valves.

car·di·o·val·vu·lot·o·my (kär′dē-ō-văl′vyə-lŏt′ə-mē) *n.* Surgical correction of valvular stenosis by cutting or excising a part of a heart valve. Also called *cardiovalvotomy.*

car·di·o·vas·cu·lar (kär′dē-ō-văs′kyə-lər) *adj. Abbr.* **CV** Of, relating to, or involving the heart and the blood vessels.

cardiovascular system *n.* The heart and blood vessels considered as a whole.

car·di·o·ver·sion (kär′dē-ō-vûr′zhən) *n.* Restoration of the heartbeat to normal by electrical countershock or by use of medication.

car·di·o·ver·ter (kär′dē-ō-vûr′tər) *n.* A device for administering an electric shock in cardioversion.

car·di·tis (kär-dī′tĭs) *n.* Inflammation of the muscle tissue of the heart. Also called *myocarditis.*

Car·di·zem (kär′dĭ-zěm′) A trademark for the drug diltiazem hydrochloride.

Car·dur·a (kär-dŏŏr′ə) A trademark for the drug doxazosin mesylate.

care·giv·er (kâr′gĭv′ər) *n.* **1.** An individual, such as a physician, nurse, or social worker, who assists in the identification, prevention, or treatment of an illness or disability. **2.** An individual, such as a parent, foster parent, or head of a household, who attends to the needs of a child or dependent adult.

Car·ey Coombs murmur (kâr′ē kŏŏmz′) *n.* An apical mid-diastolic murmur occurring in the acute stage of rheumatic mitral valvulitis and disappearing as the valvulitis subsides.

car·ies (kâr′ēz) *n., pl.* **caries** Decay of a bone or tooth, especially dental caries.

ca·ri·na (kə-rī′nə, kə-rē′nə) *n., pl.* **-nae** (-nē) A keel-shaped ridge or structure, such as the ridge on the under surface of the fornix of the brain.

car·i·nate (kăr′ə-nāt′, -nĭt) *adj.* Shaped like or having a carina or keel; ridged.

carinate abdomen *n.* A sloping of the sides of the abdomen with a prominence of the central line.

car·i·nat·ed (kăr′ə-nā′tĭd) *adj.* Carinate.

cario– *pref.* Caries: *cariology.*

car·i·o·gen·e·sis (kâr′ē-ō-jĕn′ĭ-sĭs) *n.* The production of dental caries. —**car′i·o·gen′ic** (-jĕn′ĭk) *adj.*

car·i·o·ge·nic·i·ty (kâr′ē-ō-jə-nĭs′ĭ-tē) *n.* The quality of being conducive to cariogenesis.

car·i·ol·o·gy (kâr′ē-ŏl′ə-jē) *n.* The study of dental caries and cariogenesis.

car·i·ous (kâr′ē-əs) *adj.* Having caries; decayed.

Car·len's catheter (kär′lənz) *n.* A double lumen, flexible catheter for bronchospirometry and for isolation of a portion of the lung to control secretions into the remainder of the tracheobronchial tree during general anesthesia. Also called *endobronchial tube.*

car·min·a·tive (kär-mĭn′ə-tĭv, kär′mə-nā′-) *adj.* Inducing the expulsion of gas from the stomach and intestines. —*n.* A drug or agent that induces the expulsion of gas from the stomach or intestines.

car·mine (kär′mĭn, -mīn′) *n.* A crimson pigment derived from cochineal.

car·min·o·phil (kär-mĭn′ə-fĭl) *adj.* Staining readily with carmine dyes.

car·mus·tine (kär′mŭs-tēn′) *n.* An alkylating agent used to treat various cancers, including brain tumors, non-Hodgkin's lymphoma, melanoma, and multiple myeloma. Also called *BCNU.*

car·ni·tine (kär′nĭ-tēn′) *n.* A betaine commonly occurring in the liver and in skeletal muscle that functions in the transport of fatty acids across mitochondrial membranes.

car·o·ten·ase (kăr′ə-tē-nās′, kə-rŏt′n-ās′) *n.* An enzyme that catalyzes the conversion of beta-carotene to retinaldehyde by adding molecular oxygen.

car·o·tene (kăr′ə-tēn′) *or* **car·o·tin** (-tĭn) *n.* An orange-yellow to red crystalline pigment that exists in three isomeric forms designated alpha, beta, and gamma; it is converted to vitamin A in the liver and is found in animal tissue and certain plants, such as carrots and squash.

car·o·te·ne·mi·a (kăr′ə-tən-ē′mē-ə) *n.* The presence of excess carotene in the blood, often resulting in yellowing of the skin. Also called *xanthemia.*

ca·rot·e·noid (kə-rŏt′n-oid′) *n.* Any of a class of yellow to red pigments, including the carotenes and the xanthophylls. —*adj.* Of, relating to, or characterizing such a pigment.

car·o·te·no·sis cu·tis (kăr′ə-tən-ō′sĭs kyōō′tĭs) *n.* A yellow or golden coloration of the skin that is caused by an excessive intake of carotene. Also called *aurantiasis cutis.*

ca·rot·i·co·tym·pan·ic (kə-rŏt′ĭ-kō-tĭm-păn′ĭk) *adj.* Of, relating to, or involving the carotid canal and the tympanum.

caroticotympanic nerve *n.* Either of the two sympathetic branches from the internal carotid plexus to the tympanic plexus.

ca·rot·id (kə-rŏt′ĭd) *n.* Either of two major arteries, one on each side of the neck, that carry blood to the head. —*adj.* Relating to either of these arteries.

carotid artery *n.* **1.** An artery that originates on the right from the brachiocephalic artery and on the left from the aortic arch, runs upward into the neck and divides opposite the upper border of the thyroid cartilage, with the external and internal carotid arteries as its terminal branches; common carotid artery. **2.** An artery with its origin in the common carotid artery, with branches to the superior thyroid, lingual, facial, occipital, posterior auricular, and ascending pharyngeal arteries, and with the maxillary and superficial temporal arteries as its terminal branches; external carotid artery. **3.** An artery that arises from the common carotid artery opposite the upper border of the thyroid cartilage and terminates in the middle cranial fossa by dividing into the anterior and the middle cerebral arteries; internal carotid artery.

carotid body *n.* A small epithelioid structure, located just above the bifurcation of the common carotid artery on each side that serves as a chemoreceptor organ responsive to lack of oxygen, excess of carbon dioxide, and increased concentration of hydrogen ions. Also called *intercarotid body.*

carotid-body tumor *n.* See **chemodectoma.**

carotid bruit *n.* A bruit produced by blood flow in a carotid artery.

carotid canal *n.* A passage through the petrous part of the temporal bone that transmits the internal carotid artery.

carotid-cavernous fistula *n.* An arteriovenous communication due to rupture of the intracavernous portion of the carotid artery.

carotid ganglion *n.* A small ganglionic swelling on the filaments from the internal carotid plexus, lying on the undersurface of the carotid artery in the cavernous sinus.

carotid sheath *n.* The dense fibrous tissue enveloping the carotid artery, internal jugular vein, and vagus nerve on either side.

carotid sinus *n.* A dilation of the common carotid artery at its bifurcation into the internal and external carotids, containing baroreceptors that when stimulated cause slowing of the heart, vasodilation, and a fall in blood pressure.

carotid sinus syncope *n.* Syncope resulting from overactivity of the carotid sinus and occurring either spontaneously or in reaction to pressure on a sensitive carotid sinus.

carotid triangle *n.* A space bounded by the superior belly of the omohyoid muscle, by the anterior border of the sternocleidomastoid muscle, and by the posterior belly of the digastric muscle, containing the bifurcation of the common carotid artery.

ca·rot·o·dyn·i·a (kə-rŏt′ə-dĭn′ē-ə) *n.* Pain caused by pressure on the carotid artery.

car·pal (kär′pəl) *adj.* Of, relating to, or near the carpus. —*n.* Any of the bones of the carpus, including the scaphoid, lunate, triquetrum, pisiform, trapezium, trapezoid, capitate, and hamate bones.

carpal joint *n.* Any of the joints between the carpal bones. Also called *intercarpal joint.*

carpal tunnel *n.* The space between the flexor retinaculum of the wrist and the carpal bones, through which the median nerve and the flexor tendons of the fingers and thumb pass.

carpal tunnel syndrome *n. Abbr.* **CTS** Chronic pain and paresthesia in the hand in the area of distribution of the median nerve, caused by compression of the median nerve by fibers of the flexor retinaculum and associated with repetitive motion, as in typing or playing a musical instrument.

car·pec·to·my (kär-pĕk′tə-mē) *n.* Surgical removal of all or part of the carpus.

Car·pen·ter's syndrome (kär′pən-tərz) *n.* See **acrocephalopolysyndactyly.**

car·phen·a·zine maleate (kär-fĕn′ə-zēn′) *n.* A yellow, powdered, phenothiazine antipsychotic agent used in the treatment of acute or chronic schizophrenia.

car·po·car·pal (kär′pō-kär′pəl) *adj.* Mediocarpal.

car·po·met·a·car·pal (kär′pō-mĕt′ə-kär′pəl) *adj.* Of, relating to, or involving the carpus and metacarpus.

carpometacarpal joint *n.* Any of the joints between the carpal and the metacarpal bones.

car·po·ped·al (kär′pə-pĕd′l) *adj.* Of, relating to, or involving the wrists and feet or the fingers and toes.

carpopedal spasm *n.* A spasm of the feet and hands observed in hyperventilation, calcium deprivation, and tetany. Also called *carpopedal contraction.*

car·pop·to·sis (kär′pŏp-tō′sĭs) *or* **car·pop·to·sia** (-tō′zhə) *n.* See **wrist-drop.**

car·pus (kär′pəs) *n., pl.* **–pi** (-pī′) **1.** The group of eight carpal bones and associated soft parts forming the joint between the forearm and the hand, articulating with the radius and indirectly with the ulna, and with the five metacarpal bones. Also called *wrist.* **2.** The carpal bones considered as a group.

car·ra·geen·an *or* **car·ra·geen·in** (kär′ə-gē′nən) *n.* Any of a group of closely related colloids derived from several red algae, widely used as a thickening, stabilizing, emulsifying, or suspending agent in pharmaceuticals.

Car·rel (kə-rĕl′, kär′əl), **Alexis** 1873–1944. French-born American surgeon and biologist. He won a 1912 Nobel Prize for his work on vascular ligature and grafting of blood vessels and organs.

car·ri·er (kär′ē-ər) *n.* **1.** A person or an animal that shows no symptoms of a disease but harbors the infectious agent of that disease and is capable of transmitting it to others. **2.** A compound that is capable of transferring a hydrogen atom from one compound to another. **3.** A quantity of naturally occurring element that is added to a minute amount of pure isotope, especially a radioactive one, to facilitate the chemical handling of the isotope. **4.** An individual that carries, but does not express, a gene for a particular recessive trait, yet when mated with another carrier, can produce offspring that do.

carrier screening *n.* Indiscriminate examination of members of a population to detect heterozygotes for serious disorders and to discourage sexual union and marriage with other carriers. Prenatal diagnosis is used for a married couple who are both carriers.

Car·rión's disease (kăr′ē-ōnz′, kä-ryônz′) *n.* See **Oroya fever.**

Car·roll (kăr′əl), **James** 1854–1907. British-born American physician noted for his research on yellow fever. In 1900 he deliberately infected himself with the disease for experimental purposes.

car·sick (kär′sĭk′) *adj.* Suffering from motion sickness caused by travel in a motor vehicle.

car·sick·ness (kär′sĭk′nĭs) *n.* A form of motion sickness caused by travel in a motor vehicle.

car·ti·lage (kär′tl-ĭj) *n.* A tough, elastic, fibrous connective tissue that is a major constituent of embryonic and young vertebrate skeletons, is converted largely to bone with maturation, and is found in various parts of the adult body, such as the joints, outer ear, and larynx.

cartilage bone *n.* A bone that develops in the region of a cartilage after the cartilage is partially or completely destroyed. Also called *endochondral bone.*

cartilage capsule *n.* The basophilic matrix in hyaline cartilage surrounding a lacuna and its enclosed chondrocyte.

cartilage cell *n.* See **chondrocyte.**

cartilage lacuna *n.* A cavity within the matrix of cartilage, occupied by a chondrocyte. Also called *cartilage space.*

cartilage matrix *n.* The intercellular substance of cartilage consisting of fibers and ground substance.

cartilage of nasal septum *n.* A thin cartilaginous plate located between the vomer, the perpendicular plate of the ethmoid, and the nasal bones.

cartilage space *n.* See **cartilage lacuna.**

car·ti·lag·i·noid (kär′tl-ăj′ə-noid′) *adj.* Chondroid.

car·ti·lag·i·nous (kär′tl-ăj′ə-nəs) *adj.* **1.** Chondral. **2.** Having a skeleton consisting primarily of cartilage. **3.** Having the texture of cartilage.

cartilaginous joint *n.* See **movable joint** (sense 2).

ca·run·cle (kə-rŭng′kəl, kăr′ŭng′-) *n.* A fleshy, naked outgrowth.

Ca·rus curve (kä′rōōs, -rəs) *n.* A curved line representing the outlet of the pelvic canal.

caryo– *pref.* Variant of **karyo–.**

cas·cade (kă-skād′) *n.* A succession of actions, processes, or operations, as of a physiological process.

cascade stomach *n.* A stomach in which the upper posterior wall is pushed forward, creating an upper portion that fills until sufficient volume is present to spill into the antrum.

case (kās) *n.* An occurrence of a disease or disorder.

ca·se·a·tion (kā′sē-ā′shən) *n.* Necrotic degeneration of bodily tissue into a soft, cheeselike substance.

case fatality rate *n.* The proportion of individuals contracting a disease who die of that disease.

case history *n.* A detailed account of the facts affecting the development or condition of a person or group under treatment or study, especially in medicine, psychiatry, or psychology.

ca·sein (kā′sēn′, -sē-ĭn) *n.* A white, tasteless, odorless protein precipitated from cow's milk by rennin that is the basis of cheese and is used to make plastics, adhesives, paints, and foods.

ca·se·ous (kā′sē-əs) *adj.* Of, relating to, or having the gross and microscopic features of tissue affected by caseation.

caseous necrosis *n.* A type of tissue death in which all cellular outline is lost and tissue appears crumbly and cheeselike, usually seen in tuberculosis. Also called *caseous degeneration.*

caseous osteitis *n.* Osteitis characterized by tuberculous caries.

caseous rhinitis *n.* Chronic rhinitis in which the nasal cavities are more or less completely filled with an ill-smelling cheesy material.

case study *n.* **1.** A detailed analysis of a person or group, especially as a model of medical, psychiatric, psychological, or social phenomena. **2.** An exemplary or cautionary model; an instructive example.

cast (kăst) *n.* **1.** An object formed by the solidification of molten liquid poured into an impression or mold, as in a dental cast of the maxillary or mandibular arch. **2.** A rigid dressing, usually made of gauze and plaster of Paris, used to immobilize an injured, fractured, or dislocated body part, as in a fracture or dislocation. Also called *plaster cast.* **3.** A mass of fibrous material, coagulated protein, or exudate that has taken the form of the cavity in which it has been molded, such as the bronchial, renal, intestinal, or vaginal cavity, and that is found histologically as well as in urine or sputum samples.

cast brace *n.* A specially designed plaster cast incorporating hinges and other brace components and used in the treatment of fractures to promote activity and joint motion.

Cas·tle's intrinsic factor (kăs'əlz) *n.* See **intrinsic factor.**

cas·tor oil (kăs'tər) *n.* A colorless or pale yellowish oil extracted from the seeds of the castor-oil plant, used pharmaceutically as a laxative and skin softener and industrially as a lubricant.

cas·trate (kăs'trāt') *v.* **1.** To remove the testicles of a male; emasculate. **2.** To remove the ovaries of a female; spay.

cas·tra·tion (kă-strā'shən) *n.* **1.** Removal of the testicles or ovaries; sterilization. **2.** A psychological disorder that is manifested in the female as the fantasized loss of the penis or in the male as fear of its actual loss.

castration complex *n.* **1.** In psychoanalytic theory, a child's fear of injury to the genitals by the parent of the same sex as punishment for unconscious guilt over oedipal feelings. **2.** An unconscious fear of injury from those in authority.

CAT *abbr.* computerized axial tomography

cata– *pref.* **1.** Down: *catabolism.* **2.** Reverse; backward; degenerative: *cataplasia.*

cat·a·bi·ot·ic (kăt'ə-bī-ŏt'ĭk) *adj.* Relating to the dissipation or using up of energy derived from food in the performance of bodily functions.

ca·tab·o·lism (kə-tăb'ə-lĭz'əm) *n.* The metabolic breakdown of complex molecules into simpler ones, often resulting in a release of energy. —**cat'a·bol'ic** (kăt'ə-bŏl'ĭk) *adj.*

ca·tab·o·lite (kə-tăb'ə-līt') *n.* A substance produced by the process of catabolism.

catabolite gene activator protein *n. Abbr.* **CAP** A protein that can be activated by cyclic AMP, whereupon it

affects the action of RNA polymerase by binding the polymerase with or near itself on the DNA to be transcribed. Also called *catabolite gene activator.*

cat·a·chron·o·bi·ol·o·gy (kăt'ə-krŏn'ə-bī-ŏl'ə-jē) *n.* The study of the deleterious effects of time on a living system.

ca·tac·ro·tism (kə-tăk'rə-tĭz'əm) *n.* A condition of the pulse in which there are one or more secondary expansions of the artery following the main beat, producing upward notches or waves on the downstroke of the pulse tracing. —**cat'a·crot'ic** (kăt'ə-krŏt'ĭk) *adj.*

cat·a·di·cro·tism (kăt'ə-dī'krə-tĭz'əm) *n.* A condition of the pulse marked by two expansions of the artery following the main beat, producing two upward notches on the downstroke of the pulse tracing. —**cat'a·dicrot'ic** (-krŏt'ĭk) *adj.*

cat·a·gen (kăt'ə-jən, -jĕn') *n.* A transitional phase of the hair cycle between growth and resting of the hair follicle.

cat·a·gen·e·sis (kăt'ə-jĕn'ĭ-sĭs) *n.* See **involution** (sense 3).

cat·a·lase (kăt'l-ās', -āz') *n.* An enzyme found in most living cells that catalyzes the decomposition of hydrogen peroxide to water and oxygen.

cat·a·lep·sy (kăt'l-ĕp'sē) *n.* A condition that occurs in a variety of physical and psychological disorders and is characterized by lack of response to external stimuli and by muscular rigidity, so that the limbs remain in whatever position they are placed. —**cat'a·lep'tic** (kăt'l-ĕp'tĭk) *adj.* —**cat'a·lep'toid'** *adj.*

ca·tal·y·sis (kə-tăl'ĭ-sĭs) *n., pl.* **-ses** (-sēz') The action of a catalyst, especially an increase in the rate of a chemical reaction.

cat·a·lyst (kăt'l-ĭst) *n.* A substance, usually used in small amounts relative to the reactants, that modifies and increases the rate of a reaction without being consumed in the process. —**cat'a·lyt'ic** (kăt'l-ĭt'ĭk) *adj.*

cat·a·lyze (kăt'l-īz') *v.* To modify, especially to increase, the rate of a chemical reaction by catalysis.

cat·a·me·nia (kăt'ə-mē'nē-ə) *n.* See **menses.** —**cat'a·me'ni·al** *adj.*

cat·am·ne·sis (kăt'ăm-nē'sĭs) *n.* The medical history of a patient following an illness; the follow-up history. —**cat'am·nes'tic** (-nĕs'tĭk) *adj.*

cat·a·pha·sia (kăt'ə-fā'zhə) *n.* A speech disorder in which the same word or series of words is repeated involuntarily.

ca·taph·o·ra (kə-tăf'ə-rə) *n.* **1.** Semicoma. **2.** Somnolence marked by periods of partial consciousness.

cat·a·phy·lax·is (kăt'ə-fə-lăk'sĭs) *n.* **1.** Movement or transportation of white blood cells and antibodies to the site of infection. **2.** A deterioration or breakdown in the natural mechanisms by which the body resists infectious disease.

cat·a·pla·sia (kăt'ə-plā'zhə) *or* **cat·a·pla·sis** (-plā'sĭs) *n.* Degenerative reversion of cells or tissue to a less differentiated form.

cat·a·plasm (kăt'ə-plăz'əm) *n.* See **poultice.**

cat·a·plex·y (kăt'ə-plĕk'sē) *n.* A sudden loss of muscle tone and strength, usually caused by an intense emotional stimulus. —**cat'a·plec'tic** (-plĕk'tĭk) *adj.*

cat·a·ract (kăt′ə-răkt′) *n.* Opacity of the lens or capsule of the eye, causing impairment of vision or blindness. —**cat′a·rac′tous** (-răk′təs) *adj.*

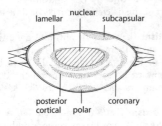

lamellar / nuclear / subcapsular

posterior cortical / polar / coronary

cataract
location in the lens of different types of cataracts

cat·a·rac·to·gen·ic (kăt′ə-răk′tə-jĕn′ĭk) *adj.* Relating to or having the ability to produce a cataract.

ca·tarrh (kə-tär′) *n.* Inflammation of mucous membranes, especially of the nose and throat. —**ca·tarrh′al** *adj.*

catarrhal gastritis *n.* Gastritis with excessive secretion of mucus.

catarrhal inflammation *n.* An inflammatory process that occurs in mucous membranes and is characterized by increased blood flow to the mucosal vessels, edema of the interstitial tissue, enlargement of the secretory epithelial cells, and profuse discharge of mucus and epithelial debris.

cat·a·stal·sis (kăt′ə-stôl′sĭs, -stăl′-) *n.* A downward wave of contraction occurring in the gastrointestinal tract during digestion.

cat·a·stal·tic (kăt′ə-stôl′tĭk, -stăl′-) *adj.* Restricting or inhibitory; restraining.

cat·a·stroph·ic reaction (kăt′ə-strŏf′ĭk) *n.* Disorganized behavior due to a severe shock or threatening situation with which the person cannot cope.

cat·a·to·ni·a (kăt′ə-tō′nē-ə) *n.* An abnormal condition often associated with schizophrenia and variously characterized by stupor, stereotypy, mania, and either rigidity or extreme flexibility of the limbs. —**cat′a·ton′ic** (-tŏn′ĭk) *adj.*

catatonic rigidity *n.* Rigidity associated with catatonic psychotic states in which muscles exhibit flexibilitas cerea.

catatonic schizophrenia *n.* A type of schizophrenia characterized by marked disturbances in activity resulting in either generalized inhibition or excessive activity.

cat·a·tri·cro·tism (kăt′ə-trī′krə-tĭz′əm) *n.* A condition of the pulse marked by three expansions of the artery following the main beat and producing three upward notches on the downstroke of a pulse tracing. —**cat′a·tri·crot′ic** (-trī-krŏt′ĭk) *adj.*

cat-cry syndrome *n.* See **cri-du-chat syndrome.**

cat·e·chol (kăt′ĭ-kôl′, -kōl′) *n.* See **pyrocatechol.**

cat·e·cho·la·mine (kăt′ĭ-kō′lə-mēn′, -kô′-) *n.* Any of a group of amines composed of a pyrocatechol molecule and the aliphatic portion of an amine that have important physiological effects as neurotransmitters and hormones, such as epinephrine, norepinephrine, and L-dopa.

cat·er·pil·lar flap (kăt′ər-pĭl′ər, kăt′ə-) *n.* A tubed flap that is transferred end-over-end in stages from the donor area to a distant recipient area. Also called *waltzed flap.*

cat·gut (kăt′gŭt′) *n.* A tough, thin cord made from the treated and stretched intestines of certain animals, especially sheep, and used for surgical ligatures.

ca·thar·sis (kə-thär′sĭs) *n., pl.* **-ses** (-sēz) **1.** Purgation. **2.** A psychological technique used to relieve tension and anxiety by bringing repressed feelings and fears to consciousness. **3.** The therapeutic result of this process; abreaction.

ca·thar·tic (kə-thär′tĭk) *adj.* Inducing catharsis; purgative. —*n.* An agent for purging the bowels, especially a laxative.

ca·thec·tic (kə-thĕk′tĭk) *adj.* Of or relating to cathexis.

cath·e·ter (kăth′ĭ-tər) *n.* A hollow, flexible tube inserted into a body cavity, duct, or vessel to allow the passage of fluids or distend a passageway; its many uses include the diagnosis of heart disorders when inserted through a blood vessel into the heart.

catheter embolus *n.* A coiled worm-shaped aggregate of platelets and fibrin that develops on the catheter or the guide wire used in vascular catheterization.

cath·e·ter·ize (kăth′ĭ-tə-rīz′) *v.* To introduce a catheter into. —**cath′e·ter·i·za′tion** (-rĭ-zā′shən) *n.*

ca·thex·is (kə-thĕk′sĭs) *n., pl.* **-thex·es** (-thĕk′sēz) Concentration of emotional energy on an object or on an idea.

cath·ode ray (kăth′ōd′) *n.* **1.** A stream of electrons emitted by the cathode in electrical discharge tubes. **2.** One of the electrons that is emitted in a stream from a cathode-ray tube.

cat·i·on (kăt′ī′ən) *n.* An ion or group of ions having a positive charge and characteristically moving toward the negative electrode in electrolysis.

cation exchange *n.* A chemical process in which cations of like charge are exchanged equally between a solid, such as zeolite, and a solution, such as water.

cation-exchange resin *n.* An insoluble organic polymer having negatively charged radicals attached to it that can attract and hold cations in a surrounding solution.

CAT scan (kăt) *n.* An image produced by a CAT scanner. Also called *CT scan.*

CAT scanner *n.* A device that uses computerized axial tomography to produce cross-sectional views of an internal body structure. Also called *CT scanner.*

cat scratch disease *n.* An infectious disease that may follow the scratch or bite of a cat, producing localized inflammation of lymph nodes and a low-grade fever. Also called *benign inoculation lymphoreticulosis, cat scratch fever.*

cau·da (kô′də) *n., pl.* **-dae** (-dē′) A tail or taillike structure, or a tapering or elongated extremity of an organ or other part.

cau·dad (kô′dăd′) *adv.* Toward the tail or posterior end of the body; caudally.

cauda e·qui·na (ĭ-kwī′nə) *n.* The bundle of spinal nerve roots running through the lower part of the subarachnoid space within the vertebral canal below the first lumbar vertebra.

cau·dal (kôd′l) *adj.* **1.** Of, at, or near the tail or hind parts; posterior. **2.** Situated beneath or on the underside; inferior. **3.** Taillike.

caudal anesthesia *n.* Regional anesthesia by injection of a local anesthetic into the epidural space via the sacral hiatus.

caudal flexure *n.* The bend in the lumbosacral region of the embryo. Also called *sacral flexure.*

caudal transverse fissure *n.* See **portal fissure.**

cauda pan·cre·a·tis (păng-krē′ə-tĭs) *n.* The left extremity of the pancreas within the splenorenal ligament; tail of the pancreas.

cau·date lobe (kô′dāt′) *n.* A small lobe of the liver situated posteriorly between the sulcus for the vena cava and the fissure for the venous ligament. Also called *Spigelius' lobe.*

caudate nucleus *n.* An elongated, curved mass of gray matter consisting of three portions: an anterior, thick portion that projects into the anterior horn of the lateral ventricle; a portion extending along the floor of the body of the lateral ventricle; and an elongated, thin portion that curves downward and backward in the temporal lobes to the wall of the lateral ventricle. Also called *caudatum.*

caudate process *n.* A narrow band of hepatic tissue connecting the caudate and right lobes of the liver behind the portal fissure.

cau·da·tum (kô-dā′təm) *n.,* *pl.* **-ta** (-tə) See **caudate nucleus.**

caul (kôl) *n.* **1.** A portion of the amnion, especially when it covers the head of a fetus at birth. Also called *veil.* **2.** See **greater omentum.**

cau·li·flow·er ear (kô′lĭ-flou′ər) *n.* An ear that is swollen, hardened, and deformed from extravasation of blood following repeated blows.

cau·mes·the·sia (kô′mĭs-thē′zhə) *n.* A sensation of burning heat irrespective of the temperature of the air.

cau·sal·gia (kô-săl′jē-ə, -zăl′-) *n.* A persistent, severe burning sensation of the skin, usually following injury to a peripheral nerve.

caus·tic (kô′stĭk) *n.* **1.** A hydroxide of a light metal. **2.** A caustic material or substance. —*adj.* **1.** Capable of burning, corroding, dissolving, or eating away by chemical action. **2.** Of or relating to light emitted from a point source and reflected or refracted from a curved surface. **3.** Causing a burning or stinging sensation.

caustic soda *n.* See **sodium hydroxide.**

cau·ter·ant (kô′tər-ənt) *n.* A cauterizing substance.

cau·ter·ize (kô′tə-rīz′) *v.* To burn or sear with a cautery. —**cau′ter·i·za′tion** (-tər-ĭ-zā′shən) *n.*

cau·ter·y (kô′tə-rē) *n.* **1.** An agent or instrument used to destroy tissue by burning, searing, cutting, or scarring, including caustic substances, electric currents, and lasers. **2.** The act or process of cauterizing.

ca·va (kā′və) *n.* See **vena cava.**

ca·va·gram (kā′və-grăm′) *n.* Variant of **cavogram.**

ca·val (kā′vəl) *adj.* Of, relating to, or having the characteristics of a vena cava.

ca·ve·o·la (kă-vē′ə-lə) *n.,* *pl.* **-lae** (-lē′) A small vesicle or recess, especially one communicating with the outside of a cell and extending inward, indenting the cytoplasm and the cell membrane.

Cav·er·ject (kăv′ûr-jĕkt′) A trademark for the drug alprostadil.

ca·ver·na (kə-vûr′nə, kă-) *n.,* *pl.* **-nae** (-nē′) An anatomical cavity or hollow space.

cav·er·nil·o·quy (kăv′ər-nĭl′ə-kwē) *n.* A low-pitched, resonant pectoriloquy detected over a lung cavity.

cav·er·ni·tis (kăv′ər-nī′tĭs) *n.* Inflammation of the cavernous body of the penis.

cav·er·nos·to·my (kăv′ər-nŏs′tə-mē) *n.* Surgical opening and drainage of a cavity.

cav·ern·ous (kăv′ər-nəs) *adj.* Filled with cavities or hollow areas; porous.

cavernous angioma *n.* See **cavernous hemangioma.**

cavernous artery *n.* Any of several small branches of the internal carotid artery that supply the trigeminal ganglion and the walls of the cavernous and petrosal sinuses.

cavernous hemangioma *n.* A vascular tumor composed of large dilated blood vessels and containing large blood-filled spaces, due to dilation and thickening of the walls of the capillary loops. Also called *cavernous angioma.*

cavernous lymphangioma *n.* Conspicuous dilation of lymphatic vessels in a circumscribed region, frequently with the formation of lymph-filled cavities.

cavernous nerve of clitoris *n.* Either of two nerves, designated major and minor, that are derived from the inferior hypogastric plexus, supply the sympathetic and the parasympathetic fibers to the corpus cavernosum, and correspond to the cavernous nerves of the penis.

cavernous nerve of penis *n.* Either of two nerves, designated major and minor, that are derived from the inferior hypogastric plexus, supply the sympathetic and the parasympathetic fibers to the corpus cavernosum, and correspond to the cavernous nerves of the clitoris.

cavernous rale *n.* A hollow bubbling sound heard on auscultation, caused by air entering a cavity partly filled with fluid.

cavernous sinus *n.* Either of a pair of dural sinuses on either side of the sella turcica, connected by anastomoses in front of and behind the pituitary gland.

cavernous sinus syndrome *n.* A syndrome caused by thrombosis of the cavernous intracranial sinus and characterized by edema of the eyelids and conjunctivae and by paralysis of the third, fourth, and sixth nerves.

CA virus (sē-ā) *n.* Variant of **croup-associated virus.**

cav·i·tar·y (kăv′ĭ-tĕr′ē) *adj.* **1.** Relating to or having a cavity or cavities. **2.** Of, relating to, or being an animal parasite that has a body cavity and lives within the host's body.

cav·i·ta·tion (kăv′ĭ-tā′shən) *n.* The formation of cavities in a body tissue or an organ, especially those cavities that form in the lung as a result of tuberculosis.

cav·i·tis (kă-vī′tĭs) *n.* Inflammation of a vena cava. Also called *celophlebitis.*

cav·i·ty (kăv′ĭ-tē) *n.* **1.** A hollow area within the body, such as a sinus cavity. **2.** A pitted area in a tooth caused by caries.

ca·vo·gram *or* **ca·va·gram** (kā′və-grăm′) *n.* A radiographic depiction of a vena cava.

ca·vog·ra·phy (kā-vŏg′rə-fē) *n.* Angiography of a vena cava.

ca·vo·sur·face (kā′vō-sûr′fəs) *adj.* Of or relating to the wall of a cavity and the surface of a tooth.

cavosurface angle *n.* The angle formed by the junction of a cavity wall and the surface of a tooth.

ca·vum (kā′vəm) *n., pl.* **-va** (-və) A hollow space, hole, or cavity.

CB (sē-bē′) *n.* A bipolar lead of an electrocardiograph that has electrodes that are attached to the chest and back.

C-banding stain *n.* A selective chromosome stain in which Giemsa stain is used to stain heterochromatic regions close to the centromeres except for the Y-chromosome, which shows a light diffuse stain throughout. Also called *centromere banding stain.*

CBC *abbr.* complete blood count

cc *abbr.* chief complaint (as recorded on a patient's medical history); cubic centimeter

CCK *abbr.* cholecystokinin

CCU *abbr.* coronary care unit; critical care unit

cd *abbr.* candela

Cd The symbol for the element **cadmium.**

CD4 (sē′dē-fôr′) *n.* A glycoprotein on the surface of helper T cells that serves as a receptor for HIV.

CD4 count *n.* A measure of the number of helper T cells per cubic millimeter of blood, used to analyze the prognosis of patients infected with HIV.

CD8 (sē′dē-āt′) *n.* A glycoprotein on the surface of killer cells that enhances binding with major histocompatibility complex molecules.

CDC *abbr.* Centers for Disease Control and Prevention

cDNA (sē′dē′ĕn-ā′) *n.* Complementary DNA; single-stranded DNA that is complementary to mRNA in the presence of reverse transcriptase.

Ce The symbol for the element **cerium.**

CEA *abbr.* carcinoembryonic antigen

ce·cal (sē′kəl) *adj.* Of, relating to, or having the characteristics of the cecum.

ce·cec·to·my (sē-sĕk′tə-mē) *n.* Excision of all or part of the cecum. Also called *typhlectomy.*

ce·ci·tis (sē-sī′tĭs) *n.* Inflammation of the cecum. Also called *typhlenteritis, typhlitis.*

ceco- *or* **cec-** *pref.* Cecum: *cecotomy.*

ce·co·cen·tral scotoma (sē′kō-sĕn′trəl) *n.* Any of three forms of scotoma involving the optic disk and papillomacular fibers. Also called *angioscotoma.*

ce·co·co·los·to·my (sē′kō-kə-lŏs′tə-mē) *n.* Surgical formation of an anastomosis between the cecum and the colon.

ce·co·il·e·os·to·my (sē′kō-ĭl′ē-ŏs′tə-mē) *n.* See **ileocecostomy.**

ce·co·pex·y (sē′kə-pĕk′sē) *n.* Surgical operation for anchoring the cecum to the abdominal wall. Also called *typhlopexy.*

ce·co·pli·ca·tion (sē′kə-plĭ-kā′shən) *n.* Surgical reduction in size of a dilated cecum by making folds or tucks in its wall.

ce·cor·rha·phy (sē-kôr′ə-fē) *n.* Suture of the cecum. Also called *typhlorrhaphy.*

ce·co·sig·moid·os·to·my (sē′kō-sĭg′moi-dŏs′tə-mē) *n.* Surgical formation of an anastomosis between the cecum and the sigmoid colon.

ce·cos·to·my (sē-kŏs′tə-mē) *n.* Surgical formation of a permanent artificial opening into the cecum. Also called *typhlostomy.*

ce·cot·o·my (sē-kŏt′ə-mē) *n.* Incision into the cecum. Also called *typhlotomy.*

ce·cum *or* **cae·cum** (sē′kəm) *n., pl.* **-ca** (-kə) **1.** The large blind pouch forming the beginning of the large intestine. Also called *blind gut.* **2.** A saclike cavity with only one opening.

Ce·dax (sē′dăks′) A trademark for the drug ceftibuten.

Cee·len-Gel·ler·stadt syndrome (sē′lən-gĕl′ər-stät′) *n.* See **idiopathic pulmonary hemosiderosis.**

cef·a·clor (sĕf′ə-klôr′) *n.* A semisynthetic analog of cephalosporin that has a broad spectrum of antibiotic activity.

cef·a·drox·il (sĕf′ə-drŏk′səl) *n.* A semisynthetic, broad-spectrum antibiotic derived from cephalosporin with action similar to the penicillins.

ce·faz·o·lin (sə-făz′ə-lĭn) *n.* A broad-spectrum cephalosporin antibiotic that is given intravenously in its salt form.

cef·di·nir (sĕf′dĭ-nîr′) *n.* A broad-spectrum cephalosporin antibiotic given orally to treat respiratory, ear, and skin infections.

cef·di·tor·en pi·vox·il (sĕf′dĭ-tôr′ən pĭ-vŏk′sĭl) *n.* A broad-spectrum oral cephalosporin antibiotic used to treat respiratory and skin infections.

cef·e·pime hydrochloride (sĕf′ə-pēm′) *n.* A broad-spectrum parenteral cephalosporin antibiotic.

Cef·i·zox (sĕf′ĭ-zŏks′) A trademark for the drug ceftizoxime sodium.

Cef·o·bid (sĕf′ə-bĭd′) A trademark for the drug cefoperazone sodium.

cef·o·per·a·zone sodium (sĕf′ō-pĕr′ə-zōn′) *n.* A semisynthetic, parenteral cephalosporin antibiotic effective against a wide range of aerobic and anaerobic, gram-positive and gram-negative pathogens.

Cef·o·tan (sĕf′ə-tăn′) A trademark for the drug cefotetan.

cef·o·tax·ime sodium (sĕf′ō-tăk′sēm′) *n.* A semisynthetic, parenteral cephalosporin antibiotic that inhibits cell-wall synthesis and is effective against a wide range of infections.

cef·o·te·tan (sĕf′ō-tēt′n) *n.* A semisynthetic cephalosporin antibiotic that is stable in the presence of beta-lactamases that are produced by gram-negative bacteria.

ce·fox·i·tin sodium (sə-fŏk′sĭ-tĭn) *n.* A semisynthetic, broad-spectrum antibiotic that acts by inhibiting bacterial cell-wall synthesis; used for lower respiratory, genitourinary, intra-abdominal, gynecological, skin and joint infections, and septicemia.

cef·po·dox·ime prox·e·til (sĕf′pə-dŏk′sēm′ prŏk′sə-tĭl) *n.* A broad-spectrum oral cephalosporin antibiotic.

cef·pro·zil (sĕf-prō′zĭl) *n.* A broad-spectrum oral cephalosporin antibiotic used to treat respiratory and skin infections.

cef·taz·i·dime (sĕf-tăz′ĭ-dēm′) *n.* A cephalosporin antibiotic especially effective against enterobacteria and species of *Pseudomonas.*

cef·ti·bu·ten (sĕf-tī′byoo-tn) *n.* A broad-spectrum cephalosporin antibiotic that is given orally to treat ear and respiratory infections.

Cef·tin (sĕf′tn) A trademark for an ester of the drug cefuroxime.

cef·ti·zox·ime sodium (sĕf′tĭ-zŏk′sēm′) *n.* A broad-spectrum, semisynthetic cephalosporin antibiotic effective against a range of infections including gonorrhea and septicemia.

cef·tri·ax·one (sĕf′trī-ăk′sōn′) *n.* A semisynthetic, broad-spectrum cephalosporin antibiotic.

cef·u·rox·ime (sĕf′yə-rŏk′sēm′) *n.* A broad-spectrum cephalosporin antibiotic given orally and parenterally for respiratory, skin, and other infections.

Cef·zil (sĕf′zĭl) A trademark for the drug cefprozil.

–cele[1] *suff.* Tumor; hernia: *cystocele.*

–cele[2] *suff.* Variant of **–coel**.

Cel·e·brex (sĕl′ə-brĕks′) A trademark for the drug celecoxib.

cel·e·cox·ib (sĕl′ə-cŏk′sĭb) *n.* A nonsteroidal anti-inflammatory drug that selectively inhibits the formation of prostaglandins and is used primarily to treat pain and other symptoms of osteoarthritis, rheumatoid arthritis, and other musculoskeletal conditions.

Ce·lex·a (sə-lĕk′sə) A trademark for the drug citalopram hydrobromide.

ce·li·ac *or* **coe·li·ac** (sē′lē-ăk′) *adj.* Of or relating to the abdomen or abdominal cavity.

celiac artery *n.* See **celiac trunk**.

celiac disease *n.* A gastrointestinal disease that is characterized by sensitivity to gluten with malabsorption and mucosal atrophy, resulting in diarrhea, steatorrhea, and nutritional and vitamin deficiencies. Also called *gluten enteropathy, gluten-sensitive enteropathy, nontropical sprue.*

celiac ganglion *n.* Any of the largest and highest group of sympathetic prevertebral ganglia, on the upper part of the abdominal aorta on either side of the celiac artery, containing the sympathetic neurons whose unmyelinated postganglionic axons innervate the stomach, liver, gallbladder, spleen, kidney, small intestine, and the ascending and transverse colon. Also called *semilunar ganglion, solar ganglion.*

celiac gland *n.* Any of the various nodes situated along the celiac trunk that receive lymphatic drainage from the stomach, duodenum, pancreas, spleen, and biliary tract.

celiac plexus *n.* **1.** The largest of the autonomic plexuses, lying in front of the aorta at the level of the origin of the celiac artery and behind the stomach, formed by the splanchnic and the vagus nerves and by cords from the celiac and superior mesenteric ganglia, and branching to all the abdominal viscera through its connections with the other abdominal plexuses. Also called *solar plexus.* **2.** A lymphatic plexus formed of the superior mesenteric lymph nodes and of the nodes behind the stomach, duodenum, and pancreas, with the connecting vessels.

celiac plexus reflex *n.* A fall in arterial blood pressure coincident with surgical manipulations in the upper abdomen during general anesthesia.

celiac trunk *n.* An artery that has its origin in the abdominal aorta just below the diaphragm, with branches to the left gastric, common hepatic, and splenic arteries. Also called *celiac artery.*

celio– *pref.* Variant of **celo–**[1].

ce·li·o·cen·te·sis (sē′lē-ō-sĕn-tē′sĭs) *n.* See **abdominocentesis**.

ce·li·o·en·ter·ot·o·my (sē′lē-ō-ĕn′tə-rŏt′ə-mē) *n.* An incision into the intestine through the wall of the abdomen.

ce·li·o·gas·trot·o·my (sē′lē-ō-gă-strŏt′ə-mē) *n.* An incision into the stomach through the abdomen.

ce·li·o·my·o·si·tis (sē′lē-ō-mī′ə-sī′tĭs) *n.* Inflammation of the abdominal muscles.

ce·li·o·par·a·cen·te·sis (sē′lē-ō-păr′ə-sĕn-tē′sĭs) *n.* See **abdominocentesis**.

ce·li·op·a·thy (sē′lē-ŏp′ə-thē) *n.* A disease affecting the abdominal region.

ce·li·or·rha·phy (sē′lē-ôr′ə-fē) *n.* Suture of the abdominal wall. Also called *laparorrhaphy.*

ce·li·os·co·py (sē′lē-ŏs′kə-pē) *n.* See **peritoneoscopy**.

ce·li·ot·o·my (sē′lē-ŏt′ə-mē) *n.* Incision of the abdomen. Also called *abdominal section, laparotomy, ventrotomy.*

ce·li·tis (sē-lī′tĭs) *n.* Inflammation of the abdomen.

cell (sĕl) *n.* **1.** The smallest structural unit of an organism that is capable of independent functioning, consisting of one or more nuclei, cytoplasm, and various organelles, all surrounded by a semipermeable cell membrane. **2.** A small enclosed cavity or space.

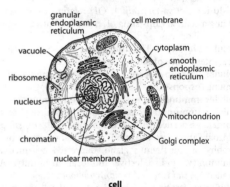

cell
human cell sectioned for electron microscopy

cell body *n.* The part of a neuron containing the nucleus but not incorporating the axon and dendrites. Also called *soma.*

cell bridge *n.* See **intercellular bridge**.

cell culture *n.* **1.** The maintenance or growth of dispersed cells in a medium after removal from the body. **2.** A culture of such cells.

cell cycle *n.* The series of biochemical and structural events involving the growth, replication, and division of a eukaryotic cell.

cell division *n.* The process by which a cell divides to form two daughter cells, each of which contains the same genetic material as the original cell and roughly half of its cytoplasm.

cell fusion *n.* The nondestructive merging of the contents of two cells by artificial means, resulting in a heterokaryon that will reproduce genetically alike, multinucleated progeny for a few generations.

cell inclusion *n.* **1.** Nonliving material in the protoplasm of a cell, such as pigment granules, fat droplets, or nutritive substances. Also called *metaplasm.* **2.** A storage material such as glycogen or fat.

cell line *n.* Cells grown in tissue culture and representing generations of a primary culture.

cell-mediated immune response *n.* The immune response produced when sensitized T cells attack foreign antigens and secrete lymphokines that initiate the body's humoral immune response. Also called *cell-mediated reaction, cellular immune response.*

cell-mediated immunity *n.* *Abbr.* **CMI** Immunity resulting from a cell-mediated immune response. Also called *cellular immunity.*

cell-mediated reaction *n.* See **cell-mediated immune response.**

cell membrane *n.* The semipermeable membrane that encloses the cytoplasm of a cell. Also called *cytomembrane, plasmalemma, plasma membrane.*

cell-transfer therapy *n.* A therapeutic technique in which cells from an individual with a disease, usually cancer, are removed and genetically modified to make the cells cytotoxic or to improve their cytotoxic abilities before they are returned to the donor.

cel·lu·la (sĕl′yə-lə) *n., pl.* **cel·lu·lae** (-lē′) **1.** A small anatomical compartment that is still visible to the eye. **2.** A small cell.

cel·lu·lar (sĕl′yə-lər) *adj.* **1.** Of, relating to, or resembling a cell. **2.** Consisting of, composed of, or containing a cell or cells.

cellular biology *n.* The study of the molecular or chemical interactions of biological phenomena.

cellular immune response *n.* See **cell-mediated immune response.**

cellular immunity *n.* See **cell-mediated immunity.**

cellular immunodeficiency *n.* Any of a group of disorders associated with recurrent bacterial, fungal, protozoal, and viral infections and characterized by atrophy of the thymus gland, depressed cell-mediated immunity, and defective humoral immunity. Also called *Nezelof type of thymic alymphoplasia.*

cellular infiltration *n.* The migration of cells from their sources of origin, or the direct extension of cells as a result of unusual growth and multiplication, into organs or tissues.

cel·lu·lar·i·ty (sĕl′yə-lăr′ĭ-tē) *n.* The state of a tissue or other mass with regard to the degree, quality, or condition of cells present in it.

cellular pathology *n.* **1.** The interpretation of disease origins in terms of cellular alterations or the failure of cells to maintain homeostasis. **2.** Cytopathology.

cellular respiration *n.* The series of metabolic processes by which living cells produce energy through the oxidation of organic substances.

cel·lu·lase (sĕl′yə-lās′, -lāz′) *n.* Any of several enzymes produced chiefly by fungi, bacteria, and protozoans that catalyze the hydrolysis of cellulose.

cel·lule (sĕl′yool) *n.* A small cell.

cel·lu·li·cid·al (sĕl′yə-lĭ-sīd′l) *adj.* Destructive to cells.

cel·lu·lif·u·gal (sĕl′yə-lĭf′yə-gəl, -lĭf′ə-) *adj.* Moving from, repelling, or extending away from a cell or cell body.

cel·lu·lip·e·tal (sĕl′yə-lĭp′ĭ-tl) *adj.* Moving or extending toward a cell or cell body.

cel·lu·lite (sĕl′yə-līt′) *n.* A fatty deposit causing a dimpled or uneven appearance, as around the thighs.

cel·lu·li·tis (sĕl′yə-lī′tĭs) *n.* A spreading inflammation of subcutaneous or connective tissue.

cel·lu·lose (sĕl′yə-lōs′, -lōz′) *n.* A complex carbohydrate that is composed of glucose units, forms the main constituent of the cell wall in most plants, and is important in the manufacture of numerous products, such as pharmaceuticals.

cellulose nitrate *n.* A pulpy or cottonlike polymer derived from cellulose treated with sulfuric and nitric acids and used in the manufacture of explosives and plastics. Also called *nitrocellulose.*

cell wall *n.* The rigid outermost cell layer found in plants and certain algae, bacteria, and fungi but characteristically absent from animal cells.

celo–¹ or **celio–** *pref.* Abdomen: *celoschisis.*

celo–² *pref.* Any body cavity: *celoscope.*

celo–³ *pref.* Hernia: *celotomy.*

ce·lom (sē′ləm) *n.* Variant of **coelom.** —**ce·lom′ic** (sē′lŏm′ĭk) *adj.*

ce·lo·nych·i·a (sē′lō-nĭk′ē-ə) *n.* See **koilonychia.**

ce·lo·phle·bi·tis (sē′lō-flĭ-bī′tĭs) *n.* See **cavitis.**

ce·los·chi·sis (sē-lŏs′kĭ-sĭs) *n.* See **gastroschisis.**

ce·lo·scope (sē′lə-skōp′) *n.* An optical device for examining the interior of a body cavity.

ce·los·co·py (sē-lŏs′kə-pē) *n.* The examination of a body cavity with a celoscope.

ce·lo·so·mi·a (sē′lō-sō′mē-ə) *n.* A congenital protrusion of the abdomen or thorax, usually accompanied by defects of the sternum and ribs as well as of the abdominal walls.

ce·lot·o·my (sē-lŏt′ə-mē) *n.* See **herniotomy.**

ce·lo·zo·ic (sē′lō-zō′ĭk) *adj.* Of, relating to, or being within any of the cavities of the body.

Cel·si·us (sĕl′sē-əs, -shəs) *adj. Abbr.* **C** Of or relating to a temperature scale that registers the freezing point of water as 0° and the boiling point as 100° under normal atmospheric pressure.

Cel·sus (sĕl′səs), **Aulus Cornelius** 1st century AD. Roman writer and physician who compiled *De medicina,* an eight-volume encyclopedia of medicine that is the only surviving portion of a larger work and describes symptoms and treatments of diseases, surgical methods, and medical history.

ce·ment (sĭ-mĕnt′) *n.* **1.** A substance that is used for filling dental cavities or anchoring crowns, inlays, or other restorations. **2.** See **cementum.** **3.** A substance that hardens to act as an adhesive; glue.

ce·ment·i·cle (sĭ-mĕn′tĭ-kəl) *n.* A spherical calcified body lying free within the periodontal membrane or fused with the cementum of the tooth.

ce·men·ti·fy·ing fibroma (sĭ-mĕn′tə-fī′ĭng) *n.* A form of cementoma occurring in the mandible of the elderly and consisting of cellular fibrous tissue containing round or lobulated masses of cementum.

cement line *n.* The refractile boundary of an osteon in compact bone.

ce·men·to·blast (sĭ-mĕn′tə-blăst′) *n.* One of the cells that takes part in the formation of the cementum.

ce·men·to·blas·to·ma (sĭ-mĕn′tō-blă-stō′mə) *n*. A benign tumor in which cells are developing into cementoblasts and there is a small amount of cementum or cementumlike material at the tooth root.

ce·men·to·cla·sia (sĭ-mĕn′tō-klā′zhə) *n*. The destruction of cementum by cementoclasts.

ce·men·to·clast (sĭ-mĕn′tə-klăst′) *n*. One of the multinucleated giant cells, similar to osteoclasts, that destroy cementum.

ce·men·to·cyte (sĭ-mĕn′tə-sīt′) *n*. A cell with multiple processes present in the cavities of the cementum.

ce·men·to·den·tin·al junction (sĭ-mĕn′tō-dĕn′tə-nəl, -dĕn-tē′-) *n*. The surface at which the cementum and dentin of the root of a tooth are joined. Also called *dentinocemental junction*.

ce·men·to·e·nam·el junction (sĭ-mĕn′tō-ĭ-năm′əl) *n*. The surface at which the enamel of the crown and the cementum of the root of a tooth are joined.

ce·men·to·ma (sē′mĕn-tō′mə, sĭ-mĕn′-) *n*. A tumor composed of tissue resembling cementum.

ce·men·tum (sĭ-mĕn′təm) *n*. A bonelike substance covering the root of a tooth. Also called *cement*.

ce·nes·the·sia (sē′nĭs-thē′zhə) *n*. The sensation that is caused by the normal functioning of the internal organs; a sense of conscious existence. —**ce′nes·the′sic** (-zĭk) *adj*.

ceno– or **cen–** or **coeno–** or **coen–** *pref*. Common: *cenesthesia*.

ce·no·site (sē′nə-sīt′, sĕn′ə-) *n*. An animal parasite that can live independently of its usual host. Also called *coinosite*.

cen·sor (sĕn′sər) *n*. The hypothetical agent in the unconscious mind that is responsible for suppressing unconscious thoughts and wishes.

cen·ter (sĕn′tər) *n*. **1.** A point or place in the body that is equally distant from its sides or outer boundaries; the middle. **2.** A group of neurons in the central nervous system that control a particular function.

center of ossification *n*. **1.** The site where bone begins to form in a specific bone or part of bone as a result of the accumulation of osteoblasts in the connective tissue. **2.** The site where bone begins to form in the shaft of a long bone or the body of an irregular bone; primary ossification center. **3.** The site where bone formation continues after beginning in the long shaft or body of the bone, usually in an epiphysis; secondary ossification center. **4.** The site of earliest destruction of cartilage prior to bone formation; ossific center.

cen·te·sis (sĕn-tē′sĭs) *n*., *pl.* **-ses** (-sēz′) See **puncture**.

centi– *pref*. **1.** One-hundredth part (10^{-2}): *centiliter*. **2.** One hundred (10^2): *centigrade*.

cen·ti·grade (sĕn′tĭ-grād′) *adj*. Celsius.

cen·ti·gram (sĕn′tĭ-grăm′) *n*. A metric unit of mass equal to one hundredth (10^{-2}) of a gram.

cen·ti·li·ter (sĕn′tə-lē′tər) *n*. A unit of volume equal to one hundredth (10^{-2}) of a liter or ten milliliters.

cen·ti·me·ter (sĕn′tə-mē′tər) *n*. *Abbr*. **cm** A unit of length equal to one hundredth (10^{-2}) of a meter.

centimeter-gram-second system *n*. *Abbr*. **CGS system, cgs system** The scientific system of expressing the fundamental physical units of length, mass, and time, as well as units derived from them, in centimeters, grams, and seconds.

cen·ti·mor·gan (sĕn′tə-môr′gən) *n*. *Abbr*. **cM** A unit of crossover frequency in linkage maps of chromosomes equal to one hundredth of a morgan.

cen·ti·nor·mal (sĕn′tə-nôr′məl) *n*. A unit of concentration of a solution that is equal to one hundredth of normal.

cen·ti·poise (sĕn′tə-poiz′) *n*. A unit in the centimeter-gram-second system that is of dynamic viscosity equal to one hundredth (10^{-2}) of a poise.

cen·ti·stoke (sĕn′tĭ-stōk′) *n*. A unit of kinematic viscosity that equals one hundredth of a stoke.

centr– *pref*. Variant of **centro–**.

cen·trad (sĕn′trăd′) *adv*. Toward the center.

cen·tral amputation (sĕn′trəl) *n*. An amputation in which the scar runs at or near the center of the stump.

central apnea *n*. Apnea resulting from medullary depression that inhibits respiratory movement.

central artery of retina *n*. The branch of the ophthalmic artery that penetrates the optic nerve behind the eye, enters the eye at the optic papilla in the retina, and divides into superior and inferior temporal and nasal branches.

central cord syndrome *n*. A syndrome characterized by paraplegia most severely involving the upper extremities, which may be accompanied by sensory loss and bladder dysfunction and is caused by injury to the central part of the cervical spinal cord.

central deafness *n*. The loss or impairment of hearing caused by disease or a defect in the auditory system of the brain.

central fovea *n*. See **fovea centralis**.

central ganglioneuroma *n*. A rare form of glioma composed of nearly mature, slowly growing, neuronlike cells, found in the optic chiasm or cerebral white matter. Also called *ganglioglioma*.

central gyri *pl.n.* The postcentral gyrus and the precentral gyrus considered together.

central lymph node *n*. Any of the lymph nodes located around the midportion of the axillary artery.

central necrosis *n*. Necrosis involving the inner portions of a tissue or organ.

central nervous system *n*. *Abbr*. **CNS** The portion of the vertebrate nervous system consisting of the brain and spinal cord. Also called *cerebrospinal axis*.

central nystagmus *n*. Nystagmus that is a reflex from stimulation arising in the central nervous system.

central ossifying fibroma *n*. A painless, slow-growing, sharply circumscribed benign fibro-osseous tumor of the jaws that is derived from cells of the periodontal ligament.

central osteitis *n*. **1.** See **osteomyelitis**. **2.** See **endosteitis**.

central paralysis *n*. Paralysis due to a lesion in the brain or spinal cord.

central pit *n*. See **fovea centralis**.

central scotoma *n*. A scotoma involving the fixation point.

central spindle *n*. A central group of microtubules that extend uninterrupted between the asters.

central sulcus *n.* See **fissure of Rolando**.

central vein of retina *n.* The vein formed by union of the retinal veins and accompanying the central artery of the retina in the optic nerve.

central vein of suprarenal gland *n.* The single vein draining the adrenal gland that receives a number of medullary veins and empties on the right directly into the inferior vena cava and on the left into the left renal vein.

central veins of liver *pl.n.* The terminal branches of the hepatic veins, lying centrally in the hepatic lobules and receiving blood from the liver sinusoids.

central venous catheter *n.* A catheter passed through a peripheral vein and ending in the thoracic vena cava; it is used to measure venous pressure or to infuse concentrated solutions.

central venous pressure *n. Abbr.* **CVP** The pressure of the blood within the superior and inferior vena cava, depressed in circulatory shock and deficiencies of circulating blood volume, and increased with cardiac failure and congestion of circulation.

central vision *n.* Vision produced by light rays falling directly on the fovea centralis of the eye. Also called *direct vision*.

cen·tren·ce·phal·ic (sĕn′trĕn-sə-făl′ĭk) *adj.* Of or relating to the center of the brain.

centri– *pref.* Variant of **centro–**.

cen·tri·ac·i·nar emphysema (sĕn′trē-ăs′ĭ-nər, -när′) *n.* See **centrilobular emphysema**.

cen·tric (sĕn′trĭk) *or* **cen·tri·cal** (-trĭ-kəl) *adj.* Situated at or near the center; central.

–centric *suff.* **1.** Having a specified kind or number of centers: *polycentric* **2.** Having a specified object as the center: *egocentric*.

centric fusion *n.* See **robertsonian translocation**.

cen·tric·i·put (sĕn-trĭs′ə-pŭt′, -pət) *n.* The central portion of the upper surface of the skull, between the occiput and the sinciput.

centric occlusion *n.* **1.** The relation of opposing occlusal surfaces of the teeth providing the maximal intercuspation. **2.** The occlusion of the teeth when the lower jaw is in centric relation to the upper jaw.

cen·trif·u·gal (sĕn-trĭf′yə-gəl, -trĭf′ə-) *adj.* **1.** Moving or directed away from a center or axis. **2.** Transmitting nerve impulses away from the central nervous system; efferent.

centrifugal nerve *n.* See **efferent nerve**.

cen·tri·fuge (sĕn′trə-fyōōj′) *n.* An apparatus consisting essentially of a compartment spun about a central axis to separate contained materials of different densities, or to separate colloidal particles that are suspended in a liquid. —*v.* To rotate something in a centrifuge or to separate, dehydrate, or test by means of this apparatus.

cen·tri·lob·u·lar (sĕn′trə-lŏb′yə-lər) *adj.* Relating to or being at or near the center of a lobule, as of an internal organ.

centrilobular emphysema *n.* Emphysema that primarily affects the lobules around their central bronchioles and that is causally related to bronchiolitis. Also called *centri-acinar emphysema*.

cen·tri·ole (sĕn′trē-ōl′) *n.* One of two cylindrical cel-

lular structures composed of nine triplet microtubules and forming the mitotic astrospheres.

cen·trip·e·tal (sĕn-trĭp′ĭ-tl) *adj.* **1.** Moving or directed toward a center or axis. **2.** Transmitting nerve impulses toward the central nervous system; afferent.

centripetal nerve *n.* See **afferent nerve**.

centro– *or* **centr–** *or* **centri–** *pref.* Center: *centrostaltic*.

cen·tro·ac·i·nar cell (sĕn′trō-ăs′ĭ-nər, -när′) *n.* A nonsecretory cell of a pancreatic ductule occupying the lumen of an acinus. Also called *Langerhans cell*.

cen·tro·ki·ne·sia (sĕn′trō-kĭ-nē′zhə, -kī-) *n.* A movement occurring as a result of a stimulus of central origin. —**cen′tro·ki·net′ic** (-nĕt′ĭk) *adj.*

cen·tro·me·di·an nucleus (sĕn′trō-mē′dē-ən) *n.* The largest and most caudal of the intralaminar nuclei, receiving numerous fibers from the internal segment of the globus pallidus and from one area of the motor cortex, and whose major efferent connection is with the putamen.

cen·tro·mere (sĕn′trə-mîr′) *n.* The most condensed and constricted region of a chromosome to which the spindle fiber is attached during mitosis. Also called *kinetochore*.

centromere banding stain *n.* See **C-banding stain**.

cen·tro·nu·cle·ar myopathy (sĕn′trō-nōō′klē-ər) *n.* Slowly progressing generalized muscle weakness and atrophy, beginning in childhood, in which the nuclei of most muscle fibers are located near the center rather than at the periphery of the fiber. Also called *myotubular myopathy*.

cen·tro·some (sĕn′trə-sōm′) *n.* A small region of cytoplasm adjacent to the nucleus that contains the centrioles and serves to organize microtubules. Also called *cytocentrum, microcentrum*.

cen·tro·sphere (sĕn′trə-sfîr′) *n.* The mass of cytoplasm surrounding the centriole in a centrosome.

cen·tro·stal·tic (sĕn′trō-stôl′tĭk, -stăl′-) *adj.* Relating to or being the center of motion.

cen·trum (sĕn′trəm) *n., pl.* **–trums** *or* **–tra** (-trə) **1.** A center of any kind, especially an anatomical center. **2.** The major part of a vertebra, exclusive of the bases of the neural arch.

CEP *abbr.* congenital erythropoietic porphyria

cephal– *pref.* Variant of **cephalo–**.

ceph·a·lad (sĕf′ə-lăd′) *adv.* Toward the head or anterior section.

ceph·al·al·gia (sĕf′ə-lăl′jə) *n.* Pain in the head. Also called *headache*.

ceph·al·e·de·ma (sĕf′ə-lĭ-dē′mə) *n.* Edema of the head.

ceph·a·lex·in (sĕf′ə-lĕk′sĭn) *n.* A semisynthetic cephalosporin antibiotic used especially in the treatment of respiratory and urinary tract infections.

ceph·al·he·ma·to·cele (sĕf′əl-hē′mə-tə-sēl′, -hĭ-măt′ə-) *or* **ceph·a·lo·he·ma·to·cele** (sĕf′ə-lō-) *n.* A cephalhematoma that communicates with the cerebral sinuses.

ceph·al·he·ma·to·ma (sĕf′əl-hē′mə-tō′mə) *or* **ceph·a·lo·he·ma·to·ma** (sĕf′ə-lō-) *n.* A blood cyst, tumor, or swelling of the scalp in a newborn due to an effusion of blood beneath the pericranium, often resulting from birth trauma.

ceph·al·hy·dro·cele (sĕf′əl-hī′drə-sēl′) *n.* Effusion of cerebrospinal fluid beneath the scalp in fractures of the skull.

ce·phal·ic (sə-făl′ĭk) *adj.* 1. Of or relating to the head. 2. Located on, in, or near the head.

–cephalic *suff.* Having a specified kind or number of heads: *dolichocephalic.*

cephalic flexure *n.* The sharp, ventrally concave bend in the developing midbrain of the embryo. Also called *cranial flexure, mesencephalic flexure.*

cephalic index *n.* The ratio of the maximum width of the head to its maximum length, multiplied by 100.

cephalic pole *n.* The head end of the fetus.

cephalic presentation *n.* Presentation of the fetus head-first during birth.

cephalic tetanus *n.* A condition caused by trauma to the head, especially to the facial nerve, characterized by tonic spasms in the face and throat. Also called *cerebral tetanus.*

cephalic vein *n.* A vein that arises at the radial border of the dorsal venous rete of the hand, passes upward in front of the elbow and along the lateral side of the arm, and empties into the upper part of the axillary vein.

cephalic version *n.* Version in which the fetus is turned so that the head presents.

ceph·a·lin (sĕf′ə-lĭn) *or* **keph·a·lin** (kĕf′-) *n.* Any of a group of phospholipids having hemostatic properties and found especially in the nervous tissue of the brain and spinal cord.

ceph·a·li·tis (sĕf′ə-lī′tĭs) *n.* See **encephalitis**.

cephalo– *or* **cephal–** *pref.* Head: *cephalometry.*

ceph·a·lo·cau·dal axis (sĕf′ə-lō-kôd′l) *n.* The long axis of the body.

ceph·a·lo·cele (sĕf′ə-lō-sēl′) *n.* See **encephalocele**.

ceph·a·lo·cen·te·sis (sĕf′ə-lō-sĕn-tē′sĭs) *n.* The passage of a hollow needle or a trocar and cannula into the brain to allow drainage.

ceph·a·lo·dyn·i·a (sĕf′ə-lō-dĭn′ē-ə) *n.* Pain in the head; headache.

ceph·a·lo·gy·ric (sĕf′ə-lō-jī′rĭk) *adj.* Of or relating to circular movements of the head.

ceph·a·lo·he·ma·to·cele (sĕf′ə-lō-hē′mə-tə-sēl′, -hĭ-măt′ə-) *n.* Variant of **cephalhematocele**.

ceph·a·lo·he·ma·to·ma (sĕf′ə-lō-hē′mə-tō′mə) *n.* Variant of **cephalhematoma**.

ceph·a·lo·meg·a·ly (sĕf′ə-lō-mĕg′ə-lē) *n.* Enlargement of the head.

ceph·a·lo·men·in·gi·tis (sĕf′ə-lō-mĕn′ĭn-jī′tĭs) *n.* Inflammation of the membranes of the brain.

ceph·a·lom·e·ter (sĕf′ə-lŏm′ĭ-tər) *n.* An instrument used to position the head for measurement and radiographic examination. Also called *cephalostat.*

ceph·a·lom·e·try (sĕf′ə-lŏm′ĭ-trē) *n.* 1. The scientific measurement of the bones of the cranium and the face. 2. A scientific study of the measurement of the head with relation to specific reference points to assess facial growth and development. —**ceph′a·lo·met′ric** (-lō-mĕt′rĭk) *adj.* —**ceph′a·lo·met′rics** (-rĭks) *n.*

ceph·a·lo·mo·tor (sĕf′ə-lō-mō′tər) *adj.* Relating to movements of the head.

ceph·a·lop·a·thy (sĕf′ə-lŏp′ə-thē) *n.* See **encephalopathy**.

ceph·a·lo·pel·vic (sĕf′ə-lō-pĕl′vĭk) *adj.* Relating to the size of the fetal head, especially in relation to the maternal pelvis.

ceph·a·lo·spo·rin (sĕf-ə-lə-spôr′ĭn) *n.* Any of various broad-spectrum antibiotics, closely related to the penicillins, that were originally derived from the fungus *Cephalosporium acremonium* and are used to treat bacterial infections.

ceph·a·lo·spor·i·nase (sĕf-ə-lə-spôr′ə-nās′, -năz′) *n.* See **beta-lactamase**.

ceph·a·lo·stat (sĕf′ə-lō-stăt′) *n.* See **cephalometer**.

ceph·a·lo·tho·rac·ic (sĕf′ə-lō-thə-răs′ĭk) *adj.* Relating to the head and the chest.

–cephalous *suff.* Having a specified kind of head or number of heads: *nanocephalous.*

–cephaly *suff.* A specified condition affecting the head: *microcephaly.*

–ceptor *suff.* Taker, receiver: *nociceptor.*

cer·am·i·dase (sə-răm′ĭ-dās′, -dāz′) *n.* An enzyme that catalyzes the breakdown of ceramides into sphingosine and fatty acids.

cer·am·ide (sə-răm′īd′, sûr′ə-mīd′) *n.* Any of a group of amides formed by linking a fatty acid to sphingosine and found in plant and animal tissue.

cerat– *pref.* Variant of **kerato–**.

cerato– *pref.* Variant of **kerato–**.

cer·a·to·cri·coid muscle (sĕr′ə-tō-krī′koid′) *n.* A fasciculus from the cricoarytenoid muscle, inserted into the inferior cornu of the thyroid cartilage.

Cer·a·to·phyl·lus (sĕr′ə-tō-fĭl′əs, -tŏf′ə-ləs) *n.* A genus of fleas found in temperate climates, including species parasitic to birds and small mammals.

cer·car·i·a (sər-kâr′ē-ə) *n.*, *pl.* **–i·as** *or* **–i·ae** (-ē-ē′) The parasitic larva of a trematode worm, having a tail that disappears in the adult stage.

cer·clage (sär-kläzh′, sər-) *n.* 1. The use of an encircling wire loop or ring to bring together the ends of an obliquely fractured bone or the fragments of a broken patella. Also called *tiring.* 2. The use of an encircling silicone band around the sclera of the eye to correct detachment of the retina. 3. The placement of a non-absorbable suture around a functionally incompetent uterine cervix.

cer·co·cys·tis (sûr′kō-sĭs′tĭs) *n.* A cysticercoid larva of a tapeworm that develops within a vertebrate host.

cer·cus (sûr′kəs) *n.*, *pl.* **cer·ci** (sûr′sī, -kī) 1. A stiff hairlike structure. 2. Either of a pair of terminal, dorsolateral sensory appendages of certain insects, such as the female mosquito.

ce·re·a flex·i·bil·i·tas (sîr′ē-ə flĕk′sə-bĭl′ĭ-təs) *n.* The capacity to maintain the limbs or other bodily parts in the position they are placed, as in catalepsy.

cerebellar artery *n.* 1. An artery with origin in the basilar artery, with distribution to the lateral lobes of the cerebellum, and with anastomosis to the posterior inferior cerebellar artery; anterior inferior cerebellar artery. 2. An artery with origin in the vertebral artery, with distribution to the medulla, choroid plexus, and cerebellum, and with anastomoses to the superior cerebellar and the anterior inferior cerebellar arteries; posterior inferior cerebellar artery. 3. An artery with origin in the basilar artery, with distribution to the cerebellum and colliculi, and with anastomoses to the posterior inferior cerebellar artery; superior cerebellar artery.

cerebellar cortex *n.* The thin gray surface layer of the cerebellum, consisting of an outer molecular layer and an inner granular layer.

cerebellar fissure *n.* Any of the deep furrows between the lobules of the cerebellum.

cerebellar gait *n.* A staggering gait, often with a tendency to fall.

cerebellar hemisphere *n.* Either of the two lobes of the cerebellum lateral to the vermis cerebelli.

cerebellar pyramid *n.* A subdivision of the inferior vermis of the cerebellum between the tuber and the uvula.

cerebellar tonsil *n.* A rounded lobule on the undersurface of each cerebellar hemisphere, continuous medially with the uvula of the vermis.

cerebellar vein *n.* The veins draining the cerebellum, including the inferior and the superior veins of the cerebellar hemisphere, the petrosal vein, the precentral cerebellar vein, and the inferior and the superior veins of the vermis.

cer·e·bel·li·tis (sĕr′ə-bĕ-lī′tĭs) *n.* Inflammation of the cerebellum.

cer·e·bell·o·med·ull·ar·y cistern (sĕr′ə-bĕl′ō-mĕd′l-ĕr′ē, -mə-dŭl′ə-rē) *n.* The largest of the subarachnoid cisterns between the undersurface of the cerebellum and the dorsal surface of the medulla oblongata.

cer·e·bel·lum (sĕr′ə-bĕl′əm) *n.*, *pl.* **–bel·lums** *or* **–bel·la** (-bĕl′ə) The trilobed structure of the brain, lying posterior to the pons and medulla oblongata and inferior to the occipital lobes of the cerebral hemispheres, responsible for the regulation and coordination of complex voluntary muscular movement and the maintenance of posture and balance. —**cer′e·bel′lar** (-bĕl′ər) *adj.*

cerebr– *pref.* Variant of **cerebro–**.

cer·e·bral (sĕr′ə-brəl, sə-rē′-) *adj.* Of or relating to the brain or cerebrum.

cerebral accident *n.* See **stroke** (sense 2).

cerebral amyloid angiopathy *n.* A pathological condition of small cerebral vessels characterized by deposits of amyloid in the vessel walls which may lead to infarcts or hemorrhage.

cerebral anesthesia *n.* Loss of sensation due to a lesion in the cerebrum.

cerebral aqueduct *n.* A short canal in the cerebrum, lined with ependymal cells and leading downward through the mesencephalon from the third to the fourth ventricle. Also called *sylvian aqueduct.*

cerebral artery *n.* **1.** An artery that is one of two terminal branches of the internal carotid artery, divided into two parts and supplying the branches to the thalamus and corpus striatum and to the cortex of the medial parts of the frontal and parietal lobes. **2.** An artery that is one of two terminal branches of the internal carotid artery, divided into three parts and supplying the perforating branches to the internal capsule, thalamus, and corpus striatum, the insula and adjacent cortical areas, and a large part of the central cortical convexity. **3.** An artery that is formed by a bifurcation of the basilar artery and is divided into three parts supplying part of the thalamus and hypothalamus, the thalamus,

cerebral peduncles, and choroid plexuses of the lateral and third ventricles, and the cortex of the temporal and occipital lobes.

cerebral calculus *n.* See **encephalolith**.

cerebral death *n.* See **brain death**.

cerebral decompression *n.* The relief of intracranial pressure by surgical removal of a piece of the cranium, usually in the subtemporal region, and incision of the dura mater.

cerebral dysplasia *n.* An abnormal development of the telencephalon portion of the brain.

cerebral edema *n.* Brain swelling due to increased volume of the extravascular compartment from the uptake of water in the gray and white matter.

cerebral embolism *n.* An obstruction in a cerebral artery by an embolus, usually resulting in transient or permanent impairment of cognitive, motor, or sensory function.

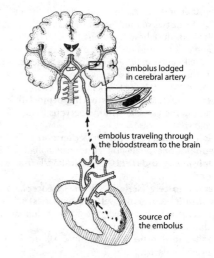

embolus lodged in cerebral artery

embolus traveling through the bloodstream to the brain

source of the embolus

cerebral embolism
An embolus arising from a mural thrombus of the left ventricle of the heart, traveling to an artery in the brain.

cerebral gigantism *n.* A syndrome of unknown cause characterized by large size at birth and an accelerated growth rate in infancy and early childhood without a like increase in serum growth hormone levels, acromegalic features, moderate mental retardation, and impaired coordination.

cerebral hemisphere *n.* Either of the two symmetrical halves of the cerebrum, as divided by the longitudinal cerebral fissure.

cerebral hemorrhage *n.* Bleeding into the substance of the cerebrum, usually in the internal capsule. Also called *encephalorrhagia, hematencephalon.*

cerebral hernia *n.* The protrusion of brain substance through a defect in the skull.

cerebral infarction *n.* See **stroke** (sense 2).

cerebral lipidosis *n.* See **cerebral sphingolipidosis**.

cerebral localization *n.* **1.** The mapping of the cerebral cortex into areas, and the correlation of these areas with cerebral function. **2.** The diagnosis of the location in the cerebrum of a brain lesion, made either from the signs and symptoms manifested by the patient or from an electroencephalogram.

cerebral palsy *n. Abbr.* **CP** A disorder usually caused by brain damage occurring at or before birth and marked by muscular impairment. Often accompanied by poor coordination, it sometimes involves speech and learning difficulties. —**cer′e·bral-pal′sied** (sĕr′ə-brəl-pôl′-zēd, sə-rē′-) *adj.*

cerebral peduncle *n.* **1.** The massive bundle of corticofugal nerve fibers passing longitudinally over the ventral surface of the midbrain on each side of the midline. **2.** Either of the two halves of the midbrain connecting the forebrain to the hindbrain.

cerebral sinus *n.* See **sinus of dura mater.**

cerebral sphingolipidosis *n.* Any of a group of inherited diseases characterized by progressive spastic paralysis, blindness, convulsions, mental retardation, and, ultimately, death, and caused by abnormal phospholipid metabolism. The disease occurs almost exclusively in individuals of eastern European Jewish descent in four enzymatically distinct forms: infantile (Tay-Sachs disease); early juvenile (Jansky-Bielschowsky disease); late juvenile (Spielmeyer-Vogt disease); and adult (Kufs disease). Also called *cerebral lipidosis.*

cerebral tetanus *n.* See **cephalic tetanus.**

cerebral vesicle *n.* Any of the three divisions of the early embryonic brain: prosencephalon, mesencephalon, and rhombencephalon. Also called *encephalic vesicle, primary brain vesicle.*

cer·e·bra·tion (sĕr′ə-brā′shən) *n.* Activity of the mental processes; thinking.

ce·re·bri·form (sə-rē′brə-fôrm′) *adj.* Resembling the external fissures and convolutions of the brain.

cer·e·bri·tis (sĕr′ə-brī′tĭs) *n.* Nonlocalized inflammation of the cerebrum.

cerebro– or **cerebr–** or **cerebri–** *pref.* Brain; cerebrum: *cerebrospinal.*

cer·e·bro·hep·a·to·re·nal syndrome (sĕr′ə-brō-hĕp′-ə-tō-rē′nəl, sə-rē′brō-) *n.* An inherited syndrome marked by hypotonia, incomplete myelinization of nervous tissue, craniofacial malformations, hepatomegaly, and small glomerular kidney cysts.

cer·e·bro·ma (sĕr′ə-brō′mə) *n.* See **encephaloma.**

cer·e·bro·ma·la·cia (sĕr′ə-brō-mə-lā′shə) *n.* See **encephalomalacia.**

cer·e·bro·men·in·gi·tis (sĕr′ə-brō-mĕn′ĭn-jī′tĭs) *n.* See **meningoencephalitis.**

cer·e·bron·ic acid (sĕr′ə-brŏn′ĭk) *n.* A constituent of phrenosin.

cer·e·brop·a·thy (sĕr′ə-brŏp′ə-thē) *n.* See **encephalopathy.**

cer·e·bro·scle·ro·sis (sĕr′ə-brō-sklə-rō′sĭs) *n.* Hardening of the substance of the cerebral hemispheres.

cer·e·bro·side (sĕr′ə-brə-sīd′, sə-rē′-) *n.* Any of various lipid compounds containing glucose or galactose and glucose, and found in the brain and other nerve tissue, especially the myelin sheath. Also called *galactolipid, galactolipin.*

cerebroside lipidosis *n.* See **Gaucher's disease.**

cer·e·bro·si·do·sis (sĕr′ə-brō-sī-dō′sĭs) *n.* See **Gaucher's disease.**

cer·e·bro·sis (sĕr′ə-brō′sĭs) *n.* See **encephalosis.**

cer·e·bro·spi·nal (sĕr′ə-brō-spī′nəl, sə-rē′brō-) *adj.* Relating to the brain and the spinal cord.

cerebrospinal axis *n.* See **central nervous system.**

cerebrospinal fluid *n. Abbr.* **CSF** The serumlike fluid that circulates through the ventricles of the brain, the cavity of the spinal cord, and the subarachnoid space, functioning as a shock absorber. Also called *spinal fluid.*

cerebrospinal fluid rhinorrhea *n.* A discharge of cerebrospinal fluid from the nose.

cerebrospinal meningitis *n.* See **meningococcal meningitis.**

cerebrospinal pressure *n.* Tension of the cerebrospinal fluid, normally 100 to 150 millimeters when measured by an instrument such as a manometer.

cer·e·bro·spi·nant (sĕr′ə-brō-spī′nənt) *adj.* Acting upon the brain and spinal cord.

cer·e·bro·ten·di·nous xanthomatosis (sĕr′ə-brō-tĕn′-də-nəs, sə-rē′brō-) *n.* An inherited disorder associated with the deposition of a form of cholesterol in the brain and other tissues and with elevated levels of cholesterol in plasma but with normal total cholesterol level; it is characterized by progressive cerebellar ataxia beginning after puberty and by juvenile cataracts, and tendinous or tuberous xanthomas.

cer·e·brot·o·my (sĕr′ə-brŏt′ə-mē) *n.* Incision of the brain substance.

cer·e·bro·vas·cu·lar (sĕr′ə-brō-văs′kyə-lər, sə-rē′brō-) *adj.* Relating to the blood supply to the brain, particularly with reference to pathological changes.

cerebrovascular accident *n. Abbr.* **CVA** See **stroke** (sense 2).

cer·e·brum (sĕr′ə-brəm, sə-rē′-) *n., pl.* **–brums** or **–bra** (-brə) The largest portion of the brain, including practically all the parts within the skull except the medulla, pons, and cerebellum and now usually referring only to the parts derived from the telencephalon and including mainly the cerebral hemispheres that are joined at the bottom by the corpus callosum. It controls and integrates motor, sensory, and higher mental functions, such as thought, reason, emotion, and memory.

ce·ri·um (sîr′ē-əm) *n. Symbol* **Ce** A lustrous, malleable metallic rare-earth element that occurs chiefly in the minerals monazite and bastnaesite, exists in four allotropic states, and is used in lighter flint alloys. Atomic number 58.

ce·roid lipofuscinosis (sîr′oid′) *n.* See **Spielmeyer-Vogt disease.**

cer·ti·fi·a·ble (sûr′tə-fī′ə-bəl) *adj.* **1.** That can or must be certified. Used of infectious, industrial, and other diseases that are required by law to be reported to health authorities. **2.** Relating to or being a person showing disordered behavior of sufficient gravity to justify involuntary mental hospitalization.

cer·ti·fi·ca·tion (sûr′tə-fĭ-kā′shən) *n.* **1.** The reporting to health authorities of those diseases legally required to be reported. **2.** The attainment of board certification in a specialty. **3.** The court procedure by which a patient is committed to a mental institution. **4.** Involuntary mental hospitalization.

cer·ti·fied milk (sûr′tə-fīd′) *n.* Pasteurized or unpasteurized cow's milk having no more than 10,000 bacteria per milliliter at any time prior to delivery, and maintained at 50° F or less prior to delivery.

certified pas·teur·ized milk (păs′chə-rīzd′, păs′tə-) *n.* Pasteurized cow's milk having no more than 10,000 bacteria per milliliter prior to pasteurization and no more than 500 bacteria per milliliter following pasteurization, and maintained at 45°F or less prior to delivery.

ce·ru·le·in (sə-rōō′lē-ən) *n.* A decapeptide that stimulates smooth muscle, especially gallbladder contraction, and increases digestive secretions.

ce·ru·lo·plas·min (sə-rōō′lō-plăz′mĭn) *n.* A blue, copper-containing globulin that may play a part in erythropoiesis and oxygen reduction.

ce·ru·men (sə-rōō′mən) *n.* The brownish yellow, waxy secretion of the ceruminous glands of the external auditory meatus; earwax. —**ce·ru′mi·nal** (-mə-nəl), **ce·ru′mi·nous** (-mə-nəs) *adj.*

ce·ru·mi·no·lyt·ic (sə-rōō′mə-nō-lĭt′ĭk) *n.* A substance instilled into the external auditory canal to soften earwax.

ce·ru·mi·no·sis (sə-rōō′mə-nō′sĭs) *n.* Excessive formation of cerumen.

ce·ru·mi·nous gland (sə-rōō′mə-nəs) *n.* Any of the modified sudiferous glands producing a waxy secretion and situated in the external auditory canal.

cer·vi·cal (sûr′vĭ-kəl) *adj.* Relating to a neck or a cervix.

cervical ansa *n.* A loop in the cervical plexus consisting of fibers from the first three cervical nerves. Also called *cervical loop.*

cervical artery *n.* **1.** An artery with origin in the inferior thyroid artery, with distribution to muscles of the neck, and spinal cord, and with anastomoses to the branches of the vertebral, occipital, ascending pharyngeal, and deep cervical arteries; ascending cervical artery. **2.** An artery with origin in the costocervical trunk, with distribution to the posterior deep muscles of the neck, and with anastomoses to the branches of the occipital, ascending cervical, and vertebral arteries; superior cervical ganglion.

cervical canal *n.* A spindle-shaped canal extending from the isthmus of the uterus to the opening of the uterus into the vagina.

cervical cap *n.* A small, rubber, cup-shaped contraceptive device that fits over the uterine cervix to prevent the entry of sperm.

cervical flexure *n.* The ventrally concave bend at the juncture of the brainstem and spinal cord in the embryo.

cervical ganglion *n.* **1.** The cervicothoracic ganglion. **2.** A small sympathetic ganglion at the level of the cricoid cartilage. **3.** The uppermost and largest of the ganglia of the sympathetic trunk, near the base of the skull between the internal carotid artery and the internal jugular vein.

cervical gland of uterus *n.* Any of the branched mucus-secreting glands in the uterine cervical mucosa.

cervical iliocostal muscle *n.* A muscle with its origin from the angles of the upper six ribs, with insertion to the transverse processes of the middle cervical vertebrae, with nerve supply from the upper thoracic nerves, and whose action extends, abducts, and rotates the cervical vertebrae.

cervical in·tra·ep·i·the·li·al neoplasia (ĭn′trə-ĕp′ə-thē′lē-əl) *n.* Dysplastic changes beginning at the squamocolumnar junction in the uterine cervix that may be precursor to squamous cell carcinoma.

cervical ligament of uterus *n.* A fibrous band attached to the uterine cervix and to the vault of the lateral fornix of the vagina and continuous with the tissue sheathing the pelvic vessels. Also called *cardinal ligament.*

cervical line *n.* A continuous anatomical, irregularly curved line marking the cervical end of the crown of a tooth.

cervical longissimus muscle *n.* A muscle with origin from the transverse processes of the upper thoracic vertebrae, with insertion into the transverse processes of the middle and upper cervical vertebrae, with nerve supply from the dorsal branches of the lower cervical and the upper thoracic nerves, and whose action extends the cervical vertebrae.

cervical loop *n.* See **cervical ansa.**

cervical nerve *n.* Any of the nerves whose nuclei of origin are in the cervical spinal cord.

cervical plexus *n.* A plexus that lies beneath the sternocleidomastoid muscle, is formed by loops joining the anterior branches of the first four cervical nerves, receives communicating branches from the superior cervical ganglion, and sends out many cutaneous, muscular, and communicating branches.

cervical pregnancy *n.* An ectopic pregnancy developing in the cervical canal.

cervical rib *n.* A supernumerary rib articulating with a cervical vertebra, usually the seventh, but not reaching the sternum in front.

cervical rib syndrome *n.* A syndrome caused by pressure from the cervical rib on the nerves of the brachial plexus and manifested by pain and tingling along the forearm and hand that may develop into anesthesia with cyanosis.

cer·vi·cec·to·my (sûr′vĭ-sĕk′tə-mē) *n.* Excision of the cervix of the uterus. Also called *trachelectomy.*

cer·vi·ci·tis (sûr′vĭ-sī′tĭs) *n.* Inflammation of the mucous membrane of the uterine cervix, frequently affecting the deeper structures. Also called *trachelitis.*

cervico– *pref.* Cervix: *cervicoplasty.*

cer·vi·co·bra·chi·al (sûr′vĭ-kō-brā′kē-əl, -brăk′ē-) *adj.* Relating to the neck and the arm.

cer·vi·co·dyn·ia (sûr′vĭ-kō-dĭn′ē-ə) *n.* Neck pain. Also called *trachelodynia.*

cer·vi·co·fa·cial (sûr′vĭ-kō-fā′shəl) *adj.* Relating to the neck and the face.

cer·vi·cog·ra·phy (sûr′vĭ-kŏg′rə-fē) *n.* A technique, equivalent to colposcopy, for photographing part or all of the uterine cervix.

cer·vi·co·oc·cip·i·tal (sûr′vĭ-kō-ŏk-sĭp′ĭ-tl) *adj.* Relating to the neck and the back part of the skull.

cer·vi·co·plas·ty (sûr′vĭ-kə-plăs′tē) *n.* Plastic surgery on the neck or on the cervix of the uterus.

cer·vi·co·tho·rac·ic (sûr′vĭ-kō-thə-răs′ĭk) *adj.* **1.** Relating to the neck and thorax. **2.** Relating to the disk between the seventh cervical vertebra and first thoracic vertebra, or to the fusion of these vertebrae.

cervicothoracic ganglion *n.* A sympathetic trunk ganglion behind the subclavian artery near the origin of the vertebral artery, at the level of the seventh cervical vertebra, and close to the first thoracic ganglion, with which it is usually fused. Also called *stellate ganglion*.

cer·vi·cot·o·my (sûr′vĭ-kŏt′ə-mē) *n.* Incision into the cervix of the uterus. Also called *trachelotomy*.

cer·vi·co·ves·i·cal (sûr′vĭ-kō-věs′ĭ-kəl) *adj.* Relating to the cervix of the uterus and the bladder.

cer·vix (sûr′vĭks) *n.*, *pl.* **cer·vix·es** *or* **cer·vi·ces** (sûr′vĭ-sēz′, sər-vī′sēz) **1.** The neck. **2.** See **collum. 3.** A neck-shaped anatomical structure, such as the narrow outer end of the uterus.

cervix u·ter·i (yo͞o′tə-rī′) *n.* The lower part of the uterus extending from the isthmus of the uterus into the vagina; neck of uterus; neck of womb.

cervix ve·si·cae u·ri·nar·i·ae (vĭ-sī′kē′ yo͝or′ə-nâr′ē-ē′, vĭ-sē′kē′) *n.* The lowest part of the bladder, formed by the junction of the fundus and the inferolateral surfaces; neck of urinary bladder.

ce·sar·e·an *or* **cae·sar·e·an** *or* **cae·sar·i·an** *or* **ce·sar·i·an** (sĭ-zâr′ē-ən) *adj.* Of or relating to a cesarean section. —*n.* A cesarean section.

cesarean hysterectomy *or* **caesarean hysterectomy** *n.* A cesarean section followed by removal of the uterus.

cesarean section *or* **caesarean section** *n.* An incision through the abdominal wall and uterus, so as to deliver a fetus. Also called *cesarean operation*.

ce·si·um *or* **cae·si·um** (sē′zē-əm) *n. Symbol* **Cs** A soft ductile metal, liquid at room temperature, the most electropositive and alkaline of the elements, used in photoelectric cells. Atomic number 55.

Ces·tan-Che·nais syndrome (sĕ-stän′shə-nā′, sĕ-stän′-) *n.* A syndrome caused by lesions of the brainstem and resulting in contralateral hemiplegia, hemianesthesia, paralysis of the larynx and soft palate, enophthalmos, miosis, and ptosis.

Ces·to·da (sĕs-tō′də) *n.* A subclass of parasitic flatworms including the segmented tapeworms that parasitize humans and domestic animals.

ces·tode (sĕs′tōd′) *or* **ces·toid** (-toid′) *n.* Any of various parasitic flatworms of the class Cestoidea, including the tapeworms, having a long, flat body equipped with a specialized organ of attachment at one end. —**ces′-tode, ces′toid′** *adj.*

Ces·toi·de·a (sĕs-toi′dē-ə) *n.* A class of flatworms characterized by lack of an alimentary canal and, in typical forms, by a segmented body with a scolex at one end; adult worms are vertebrate parasites, usually found in the small intestine.

Ce·ta·caine (sē′tə-kān′) A trademark for a combination of the drugs tetracaine hydrochloride, butyl aminobenzoate, and benzocaine.

ce·tir·i·zine hydrochloride (sə-tîr′ə-zēn′) *n.* A nonsedating antihistamine used to treat allergic rhinitis and other allergic disorders.

ce·tyl (sēt′l) *n.* The univalent radical $C_{16}H_{33}$ occurring in compounds found in waxes.

Cf The symbol for the element **californium.**

CF[1] *abbr.* cystic fibrosis

CF[2] (sē-ĕf′) *n.* A bipolar lead of an electrocardiograph that has electrodes attached to the chest and the left leg.

C fiber *n.* Any of the unmyelinated fibers, 0.4 to 1.2 micrometers in diameter, conducting nerve impulses at a velocity of 0.7 to 2.3 meters per second.

CFIDS *abbr.* chronic fatigue and immune dysfunction syndrome

CFS *abbr.* chronic fatigue syndrome

CG *abbr.* chorionic gonadotropin

CGS *or* **cgs** *abbr.* centimeter-gram-second system.

Chad·dock sign (chăd′ək) *n.* Extension of the big toe in response to irritation of the skin covering the malleolus of the ankle joint, observed in organic disease of the corticospinal reflex paths. Also called *Chaddock reflex*.

chafe (chāf) *v.* To cause irritation of the skin by friction.

Cha·gas disease *or* **Cha·gas-Cruz disease** (shä′gəs-) *n.* See **South American trypanosomiasis.**

cha·go·ma (shə-gō′mə) *n.* The skin lesion in acute Chagas disease.

chain (chān) *n.* **1.** A group of atoms that are covalently bonded in a spatial configuration like links in a chain. **2.** A linear arrangement of living things such as cells or bacteria.

Chain (chān), **Ernst Boris** 1906–1979. German-born British biochemist. He shared a 1945 Nobel Prize for isolating and purifying penicillin, discovered in 1928 by Sir Alexander Fleming.

chain reaction *n.* **1.** A series of events in which each induces or influences the next. **2.** A series of chemical reactions in which one product of a reacting set is a reactant in the following set. **3.** A multistage nuclear reaction, especially a self-sustaining series of fissions in which the release of neutrons from the splitting of one atom leads to the splitting of others.

chain reflex *n.* A series of reflexes, each serving as a stimulus for the next.

cha·la·sia (kə-lā′zhə) *or* **cha·la·sis** (-lā′sĭs) *n.* The inhibition and relaxation of a previously sustained contraction of a muscle or synergistic group of muscles, such as the cardiac sphincter.

cha·la·zi·on (kə-lā′zē-ən, -ŏn′) *n.* A cyst of a tarsal gland.

chal·co·sis (kăl-kō′sĭs) *n.* **1.** Chronic copper poisoning. **2.** A deposit of fine particles of copper in the lungs or other tissues.

chal·i·co·sis (kăl′ĭ-kō′sĭs) *n.* Pneumoconiosis caused by the inhalation of dust, occurring especially in stone cutters.

chal·lenge diet (chăl′ənj) *n.* A diet in which specific substances are included for the purpose of determining whether an abnormal reaction occurs.

cha·lone (kā′lōn′, kăl′ōn′) *n.* **1.** A hormone that inhibits rather than stimulates. **2.** Any of several polypeptides produced by a tissue and causing the reversible inhibition of mitosis in cells of that tissue.

cha·lyb·e·ate (kə-lĭb′ē-ĭt) *adj.* Impregnated with or containing iron salts.

cham·ber (chām′bər) *n.* A compartment or enclosed space.

Cham·ber·land (chām′bər-lənd, shäɴ-běr-läɴ′), **Charles Édouard** 1851–1908. French bacteriologist. A colleague of Louis Pasteur, he contributed to the development of sterilization techniques.

chan·cre (shăng′kər) *n.* The primary lesion of syphilis; a hard, nonsensitive, dull red papule or area of infiltration that begins at the site of infection after an interval of 10 to 30 days. Also called *hard chancre, hard ulcer*. —**chan′crous** (-krəs) *adj.*

chan·cri·form (shăng′krə-fôrm′) *adj.* Resembling chancre.

chan·croid (shăng′kroid′) *n.* An infectious venereal ulcer located at the site of infection by *Haemophilus ducreyi* beginning after an incubation period of 3 to 5 days. Also called *soft ulcer, venereal ulcer.* —**chan′croi′dal** (-kroid′l) *adj.*

Chang (chăng), **Chueh** 1908–1991. American Chinese-born who helped develop (1954) the first effective oral contraceptive.

change of life (chānj) *n.* Menopause.

chan·nel (chăn′əl) *n.* **1.** A furrow, a tube, or another groovelike passageway through which something flows. **2.** An aqueous pathway through a protein molecule in a cell membrane that modulates the electrical potential across the membrane by controlling the passage of small inorganic ions into and out of the cell. Also called *ion channel, protein channel.*

chapped (chăpt) *adj.* Having or relating to skin that is dry, scaly, and fissured, owing to excessive evaporation of moisture from the skin surface.

char·ac·ter (kăr′ək-tər) *n.* **1.** A distinguishing feature or attribute, as of an individual, group, or category. **2.** A structure, function, or attribute determined by a gene or group of genes. **3.** In psychoanalysis, an individual's personality or temperament.

char·ac·ter·is·tic (kăr′ək-tə-rĭs′tĭk) *n.* **1.** A distinguishing feature or attribute; character. **2.** A structure or function determined by a gene or genes; trait. —**char′ac·ter·is′tic** *adj.*

char·coal (chär′kōl′) *n.* **1.** Carbon obtained by heating or burning organic material with restricted access of air. **2.** Activated charcoal.

Char·cot (shär-kō′), **Jean Martin** 1825–1893. French neurologist. A teacher of Sigmund Freud and Alfred Binet, he is known for his investigations of nervous diseases, his work on hysteria, and his studies of hypnotism.

Charcot-Ley·den crystals (-līd′n) *pl.n.* Crystals in the shape of elongated double pyramids, formed from eosinophils, found in the sputum in bronchial asthma and in the feces in some intestinal infections.

Charcot-Marie-Tooth disease (-tōōth′) *n.* See **peroneal muscular atrophy.**

Char·cot's disease (shär-kōz′) *n.* See **amyotrophic lateral sclerosis.**

Charcot's joint *n.* See **tabetic arthropathy.**

Charcot's syndrome *n.* See **intermittent claudication.**

Charcot's triad *n.* The symptoms of nystagmus, tremor, and scanning speech as manifested in multiple sclerosis.

char·la·tan (shär′lə-tən) *n.* A person fraudulently claiming knowledge and skills not possessed.

Charles's law (chärl′zĭz) *n.* The physical law that the volume of a fixed mass of gas that is held at a constant pressure will vary directly with the absolute temperature.

char·ley horse (chär′lē hôrs′) *n.* Localized pain or stiffness in a muscle following excessive muscular exertion or the contusion of a muscle.

Charn·ley (chärn′lē), **Sir John** 1911–1982. British orthopedic surgeon who pioneered total hip replacement surgery. He also developed the technique of arthrodesis for the treatment of rheumatoid arthritis in the knee and hip.

Char·riè·re scale (shär-yâr′) *n.* See **French scale.**

chart (chärt) *n.* **1.** A recording, in tabular form, of clinical data relating to a case. **2.** A group of symbols of graduated size for measuring visual acuity.

Chaus·sier's areola (shō-syāz′, -sē-āz′) *n.* A ring of indurated tissue that forms around a lesion of cutaneous anthrax.

ChB *abbr. Latin* Chirurgiae Baccalaureus (Bachelor of Surgery)

ChD *abbr. Latin* Chirurgiae Doctor (Doctor of Surgery)

check ligament of eyeball (chĕk) *n.* Either of two expansions of the sheaths of the medial and lateral rectus muscles of the eyeball that act to restrain the activity of these muscles.

check·up (chĕk′ŭp′) *n.* **1.** An examination or inspection. **2.** A general physical examination.

Chédiak-Steinbrinck-Higashi syndrome (shäd′yäk-stīn′brĭngk-hĭ-gä′shē, -shtīn-) *n.* An inherited syndrome marked by abnormalities of granulation and nuclear structure of all types of white blood cells; it is often accompanied by hepatosplenomegaly, lymphadenopathy, anemia, thrombocytopenia, radiologic changes of bones, lungs, and heart, skin and psychomotor abnormalities, and susceptibility to infection. Also called *Chédiak-Higashi disease, Chédiak-Steinbrinck-Higashi anomaly.*

cheek (chēk) *n.* **1.** The fleshy part of either side of the face below the eye and between the nose and ear. **2.** Either of the buttocks.

cheek·bone (chēk′bōn′) *n.* See **zygomatic bone.**

cheek muscle *n.* See **buccinator.**

cheese worker's lung (chēz) *n.* Extrinsic allergic alveolitis caused by the inhalation of spores of *Penicillium casei* from moldy cheese.

chei·lal·gia *or* **chi·lal·gia** (kī-lăl′jə) *n.* Pain in the lip.

chei·lec·to·my *or* **chi·lec·to·my** (kī-lĕk′tə-mē) *n.* **1.** Excision of a portion of the lip. **2.** The chiseling away of bony irregularities on the lips of a joint cavity that interfere with movements of the joint.

chei·lec·tro·pi·on *or* **chi·lec·tro·pi·on** (kī′lĭk-trō′pē-ŏn′, -ən) *n.* Eversion of the lips or a lip.

chei·li·tis *or* **chi·li·tis** (kī-lī′tĭs) *n.* Inflammation of the lips or of a lip, including redness and the production of fissures radiating from the angles of the mouth.

cheilo– *or* **cheil–** *or* **chilo–** *or* **chil–** *pref.* Lip: *cheilotomy.*

chei·lo·plas·ty *or* **chi·lo·plas·ty** (kī′lə-plăs′tē) *n.* Plastic surgery of the lips.

chei·lor·rha·phy *or* **chi·lor·rha·phy** (kī-lôr′ə-fē) *n.* Suturing of the lip.

chei·los·chi·sis *or* **chi·los·chi·sis** (kī-lŏs′kĭ-sĭs) *n.* See **cleft lip.**

chei·lo·sis *or* **chi·lo·sis** (kī-lō′sĭs) *n.* A disorder of the lips often due to riboflavin deficiency and other B-complex vitamin deficiencies and characterized by fissures, especially in the corners of the mouth.

chei·lo·sto·ma·to·plas·ty *or* **chi·lo·sto·ma·to·plas·ty** (kī′lō-stō′mə-tə-plăs′tē) *n.* Plastic surgery of the lips and mouth.

chei·lot·o·my *or* **chi·lot·o·my** (kī-lŏt′ə-mē) *n.* Incision into the lip.

cheiro– or **cheir–** or **chiro–** or **chir–** pref. Hand: *cheirospasm.*

chei·rog·nos·tic or **chi·rog·nos·tic** (kī'rəg-nŏs'tĭk) n. Able to recognize the hand, or to distinguish between right and left.

chei·ro·kin·es·the·sia or **chi·ro·kin·es·the·sia** (kī'rō-kĭn'ĭs-thē'zhə, -kī'nĭs-) n. The subjective sensation of movement of the hands. —**chei'ro·kin'es·thet'ic** (-thĕt'ĭk) adj.

chei·ro·meg·a·ly or **chi·ro·meg·a·ly** (kī'rō-mĕg'ə-lē) n. See **macrocheiria.**

chei·ro·plas·ty or **chi·ro·plas·ty** (kī'rə-plăs'tē) n. Plastic surgery on the hand.

chei·ro·po·dal·gia or **chi·ro·po·dal·gia** (kī'rō-pō-dăl'-jə) n. Pain in the hands and the feet.

chei·ro·pom·pho·lyx or **chi·ro·pom·pho·lyx** (kī'rō-pŏm'fə-lĭks) n. See **dyshidrosis.**

chei·ro·spasm or **chi·ro·spasm** (kī'rə-spăz'əm) n. Spasm of the muscles of the hand, as in writers' cramp.

che·late (kē'lāt') n. A chemical compound in the form of a heterocyclic ring, containing a metal ion attached by coordinate bonds to at least two nonmetal ions. —v. 1. To combine a metal ion with a chemical compound to form a ring. 2. To remove a heavy metal, such as lead or mercury, from the bloodstream by means of a chelate. —**che'late'** adj. —**che·la'tion** n.

chem. abbr. chemical; chemist; chemistry

chem– pref. Variant of **chemo–.**

chem·ex·fo·li·a·tion (kĕm'ĕks-fō'lē-ā'shən) n. A chemosurgical technique designed to remove acne scars or treat chronic skin defects caused by exposure to sunlight.

chemi– pref. Variant of **chemo–.**

chem·i·cal (kĕm'ĭ-kəl) adj. Abbr. **chem.** 1. Of or relating to chemistry. 2. Of or relating to the properties or actions of chemicals. —n. 1. A substance with a distinct molecular composition that is produced by or used in a chemical process. 2. A drug, especially an illicit or addictive one. —**chem'i·cal·ly** adv.

chemical abuse n. See **substance abuse.**

chemical antidote n. A substance that unites with a poison to form an innocuous chemical compound.

chemical attraction n. The force of attraction between atoms that causes them to form and maintain certain combinations.

chemical dependency n. A physical and psychological habituation to a mood- or mind-altering drug, such as alcohol or cocaine.

chemical dermatitis n. Contact dermatitis due to exposure of the skin to a chemical, usually characterized by erythema, edema, and vesiculation of the exposed or contacted site.

chemical diabetes n. See **latent diabetes.**

chemical energy n. Energy liberated by a chemical reaction or absorbed in the formation of a chemical compound.

Chemical Mace A trademark for a temporarily disabling liquid packed in aerosol form and sprayed in self-defense into the face of an attacker, thereby causing dizziness, irritation of the eyes, and immobilization for a short period.

chemical peritonitis n. Peritonitis resulting from the escape of bile, pancreatic juice, or the contents of the gastrointestinal tract into the peritoneal cavity; infection may be preceded by symptoms such as shock and peritoneal exudation.

chemical repair n. Conversion of a free radical to a stable molecule.

chemical sensitivity n. See **multiple chemical sensitivity.**

chem·ist (kĕm'ĭst) n. Abbr. **chem.** 1. A scientist specializing in chemistry. 2. A pharmacist.

chem·is·try (kĕm'ĭ-strē) n. Abbr. **chem.** 1. The science of the composition, structure, properties, and reactions of matter, especially of atomic and molecular systems. 2. The composition, structure, properties, and reactions of a substance.

che·mo (kē'mō) n. Chemotherapy or a chemotherapeutic treatment.

chemo– or **chemi–** or **chem–** pref. Chemicals; chemical: *chemotherapy.*

che·mo·au·to·troph (kē'mō-ô'tə-trōf', -trŏf') n. An organism that depends on inorganic chemicals for its energy and principally on carbon dioxide for its carbon. Also called *chemolithotroph.* —**che'mo·au'to·tro'-phic** (-trō'fĭk, -trŏf'ĭk) adj.

che·mo·bi·ot·ic (kē'mō-bī-ŏt'ĭk) n. A combination of an antibiotic with a chemotherapeutic agent.

che·mo·cau·ter·y (kē'mō-kô'tə-rē) n. A chemical substance that destroys tissue to which it is applied.

che·mo·dec·to·ma (kē'mō-dĕk-tō'mə) n. A relatively rare, usually benign tumor originating in chemoreceptor tissue. Also called *aortic-body tumor, carotid-body tumor, glomus jugulare tumor, nonchromaffin paraganglioma.*

che·mo·dec·to·ma·to·sis (kē'mō-dĕk-tō'mə-tō'sĭs) n. A condition that is characterized by multiple tumors of perivascular tissue of the carotid body or of other chemoreceptor tissue.

che·mo·kine (kē'mō-kīn', kĕm'mō-) n. Any of various cytokines produced in acute and chronic inflammation that mobilize and activate white blood cells.

che·mo·ki·ne·sis (kē'mō-kə-nē'sĭs, -kī-) n. Stimulation of an organism by a chemical. —**che'mo·ki·net'ic** (-kĭ-nĕt'ĭk, -kī-) adj.

che·mo·lith·o·troph (kē'mō-lĭth'ə-trōf', -trŏf') n. See **chemoautotroph.** —**che'mo·lith'o·tro'phic** (-trō'fĭk, -trŏf'ĭk) adj.

che·mo·lu·mi·nes·cence (kē'mō-lōō'mə-nĕs'əns) n. Emission of light as a result of a chemical reaction.

che·mo·nu·cle·ol·y·sis (kē'mō-nōō'klē-ŏl'ĭ-sĭs) n. The enzymatic dissolution of the pulpy nucleus by injection of chymopapain, used in the treatment of intervertebral disk lesions.

che·mo·or·ga·no·troph (kē'mō-ôr'gə-nō-trōf', -trŏf') n. An organism that depends on organic chemicals for its energy and carbon.

che·mo·pre·ven·tion (kē'mō-prĭ-vĕn'shən) n. The use of chemical agents, drugs, or food supplements to prevent disease.

che·mo·pro·phy·lax·is (kē'mō-prō'fə-lăk'sĭs) n. Disease prevention by use of chemicals or drugs. —**che'-mo·pro'phy·lac'tic** (-lăk'tĭk) n. & adj.

che·mo·pro·tec·tion (kē'mō-prə-tĕk'shən) n. A therapeutic technique in which bone marrow cells are removed from an individual with cancer and are genetically modified to withstand higher doses of chemotherapy before being returned to the donor.

che·mo·re·cep·tion (kē′mō-rĭ-sĕp′shən) *n.* The physiological response of a sense organ to a chemical stimulus. —**che′mo·re·cep′tive** *adj.*

che·mo·re·cep·tor (kē′mō-rĭ-sĕp′tər) *n.* A sensory nerve cell or sense organ, as of smell or taste, that responds to chemical stimuli.

che·mo·sen·si·tive (kē′mō-sĕn′sĭ-tĭv) *adj.* Capable of perceiving changes in the chemical composition of the environment.

che·mo·sen·si·tiz·er (kē′mō-sĕn′sĭ-tī′zər) *n.* Any of several compounds that inhibit the functioning of a particular cellular glycoprotein and make cells, especially tumor cells, sensitive to chemotherapeutic agents.

che·mo·se·ro·ther·a·py (kē′mō-sîr′ō-thĕr′ə-pē) *n.* The combination of serum and drugs to treat disease.

che·mo·sis (kē-mō′sĭs) *n.* Edema of the bulbar conjunctiva, forming a swelling around the cornea. —**che·mot′ic** (-mŏt′ĭk) *adj.*

che·mo·sur·ger·y (kē′mō-sûr′jə-rē) *n.* Selective destruction of tissue by use of chemicals.

che·mo·tac·tic (kē′mō-tăk′tĭk) *adj.* Of or relating to chemotaxis.

che·mo·tax·is (kē′mō-tăk′sĭs) *n.* The characteristic movement or orientation of an organism or cell along a chemical concentration gradient either toward or away from the chemical stimulus. Also called *chemotropism.*

che·mo·ther·a·py (kē′mō-thĕr′ə-pē) *n.* **1.** The treatment of cancer using specific chemical agents or drugs that are selectively destructive to malignant cells and tissues. **2.** The treatment of disease using chemical agents or drugs that are selectively toxic to the causative agent of the disease, such as a virus or other microorganism. —**che′mo·ther′a·peu′tic** (-pyōō′tĭk) *adj.* —**che′mo·ther′a·pist** *n.*

che·mot·ro·pism (kĭ-mŏt′rə-pĭz′əm) *n.* See **chemotaxis.**

cher·ry angioma (chĕr′ē) *n.* See **senile hemangioma.**

cherry-red spot *n.* The choroid appearing as a red spot through the fovea centralis surrounded by a contrasting white edema; it is noted in cases of infantile cerebral sphingolipidosis.

cherry-red spot myoclonus syndrome *n.* Either of two types of neuronal storage disorders in children characterized by a cherry-red spot at the macula, progressive myoclonus, and easily controlled seizures, and resulting from a deficiency of sialidase. Also called *sialidosis.*

cher·ub·ism (chĕr′ə-bĭz′əm) *n.* A hereditary disease marked by an enlargement of the jawbones in young children, producing a cherublike facial appearance.

chest (chĕst) *n.* The part of the body between the neck and the abdomen, enclosed by the ribs and the breastbone; thorax.

chest lead (lēd) *n.* See **precordial lead.**

chest wall *n.* The system of structures outside the lungs that move as a part of breathing, including the rib cage, diaphragm, and abdomen. Also called *thoracic wall.*

Cheyne (chān, chā′nē), **John** 1777–1836. Scottish physician who described (1818) the breathing irregularity now known as Cheyne-Stokes respiration.

Cheyne-Stokes respiration *n.* An abnormal pattern of breathing marked by a gradual increase in depth and sometimes in rate to a maximum depth, followed by a decrease resulting in apnea, usually seen in comatose people with diseased nervous centers of respiration.

CHF *abbr.* congestive heart failure

chi[1] or **khi** (kī) *n. Symbol* χ The 22nd letter of the Greek alphabet.

chi[2] or **ch'i** or **Qi** or **qi** (chē) *n.* In traditional Chinese thought, the vital force believed to be inherent in all things. Unimpeded circulation of chi and a balance of its negative and positive forms in the body are held to be essential to good health.

Chi·a·ri's syndrome (kē-ä′rēz) *n.* Thrombosis of the hepatic vein with enlargement of the liver and extensive development of collateral vessels, intractable ascites, and severe portal hypertension. Also called *Budd-Chiari syndrome, Chiari's disease, Rokitansky's disease.*

chi·as·ma (kī-ăz′mə) or **chi·asm** (kī′ăz′əm) *n., pl.* −**mas** or −**ma·ta** (-mə-tə) or −**asms 1.** A crossing or intersection of two tracts, as of nerves or ligaments. **2.** The point of contact between paired chromatids during meiosis, resulting in a cross-shaped configuration, representing the cytological manifestation of crossing over. —**chi·as′mal chi·as′mic, chi·as·mat′ic** (-măt′ĭk) *adj.*

chick·en breast (chĭk′ən) *n.* See **pigeon breast.** —**chick′en-breast′ed** (-brĕs′tĭd) *adj.*

chicken fat clot *n.* A clot formed in vitro or postmortem from leukocytes and plasma of sedimented blood.

chick·en·pox or **chicken pox** (chĭk′ən-pŏks′) *n.* An acute contagious disease, primarily of children, that is caused by the varicella-zoster virus and characterized by skin eruptions, slight fever, and malaise. Also called *varicella.*

chickenpox immune globulin (human) *n.* Globulin fraction of serum from persons recently recovered from herpes zoster infection, used to inoculate high-risk children to prevent infection.

chickenpox virus *n.* See **varicella-zoster virus.**

chi·cler·o's ulcer (chĭ-klĕr′ōz) *n.* A form of cutaneous leishmaniasis found among forest workers in Mexico and Central America that commonly erodes the pinna of the ear over a long course of infection, and transmitted by the bite of a sandfly.

chief agglutinin *n.* See **major agglutinin.**

chief cell (chēf) *n.* **1.** The principle cell of the parathyroid gland, often divided into dark chief cells and light chief cells. **2.** See **zymogenic cell.**

chig·ger (chĭg′ər) *n.* **1.** The six-legged larva of mites of the family Trombiculidae, parasitic on humans and other vertebrates and inflicting a bite that produces a wheal accompanied by intense itching. Also called *harvest bug, harvest mite, jigger, red bug.* **2.** Chigoe.

chig·oe (chĭg′ō) *n.* A small tropical flea (*Tunga penetrans*) the fertilized female of which burrows under the skin, frequently under the toenails, causing intense irritation and sores that may become severely infected. Also called *jigger, sand flea.*

chil– *pref.* Variant of **cheilo–.**

chi·lal·gia (kī-lăl′jə) *n.* Variant of **cheilalgia.**

chil·blain (chĭl′blān′) *n.* Erythema, itching, and burning, especially of the dorsa of the fingers and toes, and of the heels, nose, and ears, resulting from exposure to moist cold. Also called *erythema pernio*.

child (chīld) *n*. **1.** A person who has not yet reached puberty. **2.** A son or daughter; an offspring. **3.** A person who is not of legal age; a minor.

child·bear·ing (chīld'bâr'ĭng) *n*. Pregnancy and parturition. —**child'bear'ing** *adj*.

child·bed fever (chīld'bĕd') *n*. See **puerperal fever**.

child·birth (chīld'bûrth') *n*. Parturition.

child·hood (chīld'hŏŏd') *n*. The period of life between infancy and puberty.

childhood muscular dystrophy *n*. See **pseudohypertrophic muscular dystrophy**.

child psychiatry *n*. The branch of psychiatry that deals with the diagnosis, treatment, and prevention of mental and emotional disorders in children.

chi·lec·to·my (kī-lĕk'tə-mē) *n*. Variant of **cheilectomy**.

chi·lec·tro·pi·on (kī'lĭk-trō'pē-ŏn', -ən) *n*. Variant of **cheilectropion**.

chi·li·tis (kī-lī'tĭs) *n*. Variant of **cheilitis**.

chill (chĭl) *n*. A feeling of cold, with shivering and pallor, sometimes accompanied by an elevation of temperature in the interior of the body.

chilo– *pref*. Variant of **cheilo–**.

chi·lo·plas·ty (kī'lə-plăs'tē) *n*. Variant of **cheiloplasty**.

chi·lor·rha·phy (kī-lôr'ə-fē) *n*. Variant of **cheilorrhaphy**.

chi·los·chi·sis (kī-lŏs'kĭ-sĭs) *n*. Variant of **cheiloschisis**.

chi·lo·sis (kī-lō'sĭs) *n*. Variant of **cheilosis**.

chi·lo·sto·ma·to·plas·ty (kī'lō-stō'mə-tə-plăs'tē) *n*. Variant of **cheilostomatoplasty**.

chi·lot·o·my (kī-lŏt'ə-mē) *n*. Variant of **cheilotomy**.

chi·me·ra (kī-mîr'ə, kĭ-) *n*. **1.** One who has received a transplant of genetically and immunologically different tissue. **2.** Twins with two immunologically different types of red blood cells.

chi·mer·ic (kī-mĕr'ĭk, -mîr'-) *adj*. **1.** Of, relating to, or being a chimera. **2.** Composed of parts of different origin.

chin (chĭn) *n*. The prominence formed by the anterior projection of the lower jaw.

Chi·nese restaurant syndrome (chī-nēz', -nēs') *n*. A group of symptoms, including dizziness and headache, that may occur after the ingestion of food containing large amounts of monosodium glutamate.

chin muscle *n*. A muscle with origin from the incisor fossa of the mandible, with insertion into the skin of the chin, with nerve supply from the facial nerve, and whose action raises and wrinkles the skin of the chin and pushes up the lower lip.

chip graft (chĭp) *n*. A graft in which small pieces of cartilage or bone are packed into a bone defect.

chip syringe *n*. A tube, usually made of metal, through which air is blown to dry or to remove debris from a cavity in preparing teeth for restoration. Also called *air syringe*.

chir– *pref*. Variant of **cheiro–**.

chi·ral (kī'rəl) *adj*. Of or relating to the structural characteristic of a molecule that makes it impossible to superimpose it on its mirror image. —**chi·ral'i·ty** (kī-răl'ĭ-tē) *n*.

chiro– *pref*. Variant of **cheiro–**.

chi·rog·nos·tic (kī'rəg-nŏs'tĭk) *n*. Variant of **cheirognostic**.

chi·ro·kin·es·the·sia (kī'rō-kĭn'ĭs-thē'zhə, -kī'nĭs-) *n*. Variant of **cheirokinesthesia**.

chi·ro·meg·a·ly (kī'rō-mĕg'ə-lē) *n*. Variant of **cheiromegaly**.

chi·ro·plas·ty (kī'rə-plăs'tē) *n*. Variant of **cheiroplasty**.

chi·ro·po·dal·gia (kī'rō-pō-dăl'jə) *n*. Variant of **cheiropodalgia**.

chi·rop·o·dy (kĭ-rŏp'ə-dē, shĭ-) *n*. See **podiatry**.

chi·ro·prac·tic (kī'rə-prăk'tĭk) *n*. A system of therapy that utilizes the recuperative powers of the body and the relationship between the musculoskeletal structures and the functions of the body, particularly of the spinal column and the nervous system, in the restoration and maintenance of health. —**chi'ro·prac'tor** *n*.

chi·ro·spasm (kī'rə-spăz'əm) *n*. Variant of **cheirospasm**.

chi·rur·gi·cal (kī-rûr'jĭ-kəl) *adj*. Surgical. No longer in technical use.

chi-square *n*. A test statistic that is calculated as the sum of the squares of observed values minus expected values divided by the expected values.

chi-square test *n*. A test that uses the chi-square statistic to test the fit between a theoretical frequency distribution and a frequency distribution of observed data for which each observation may fall into one of several classes.

chi·tin (kīt'n) *n*. A tough, protective, semitransparent polysaccharide forming the principal component of arthropod exoskeletons and the cell walls of certain fungi. —**chi'tin·ous** *adj*.

chla·myd·i·a (klə-mĭd'ē-ə) *n*., *pl*. **–i·ae** (-ē-ē') Any of several common, often asymptomatic, sexually transmitted diseases that are caused by the microorganism *Chlamydia trachomatis*. —**chla·myd'i·al** *adj*.

Chla·myd·i·a (klə-mĭd'ē-ə) *n*. A genus of coccoid, gram-negative microorganisms that are pathogenic to humans and animals, causing diseases such as conjunctivitis in cattle and sheep, and trachoma, nonspecific urethritis, and proctitis in humans. Also called *Bedsonia, Miyagawanella*.

Chlamydia psit·ta·ci (sĭt'ə-sī') *n*. A species of *Chlamydia* that causes psittacosis in humans and ornithosis, pneumonitis, abortion, encephalomyelitis, and enteritis in various animals.

Chlamydia tra·cho·ma·tis (trə-kō'mə-tĭs) *n*. A species of *Chlamydia* that causes trachoma, inclusion conjunctivitis, lymphogranuloma venereum, nonspecific urethritis, and proctitis in humans.

chla·myd·i·o·sis (klə-mĭd'ē-ō'sĭs) *n*. Any of the diseases that are caused by *Chlamydia psittaci* and *C. trachomatis*.

chlo·as·ma (klō-ăz'mə) *n*., *pl*. **–ma·ta** (-mə-tə) A patchy brown or dark brown skin discoloration that usually occurs on a woman's face and may result from hormonal changes, as in pregnancy. Also called *mask of pregnancy, melasma*.

chlor– *pref*. Variant of **chloro–**.

chlor·ac·ne (klôr-ăk'nē) *n*. An acnelike skin disorder caused by prolonged exposure to chlorinated hydrocarbons. Also called *chlorine acne*.

chlo·ral hydrate (klôr′əl) *n.* A crystalline compound used medicinally as a sedative and hypnotic.

chlor·am·bu·cil (klôr-ăm′byə-sĭl) *n.* An anticancer drug that is a deriritive of nitrogen mustard and is used to depress the proliferation and maturation of lymphocytes in such diseases as leukemia and Hodgkin's disease.

chlor·am·phen·i·col (klôr′ăm-fĕn′ĭ-kôl′, -kōl′) *n.* A broad-spectrum antibiotic derived from the soil bacterium *Streptomyces venezuelae* or produced synthetically.

chlo·rate (klôr′āt′) *n.* **1.** A salt of chloric acid containing the chlorate ion. **2.** The inorganic ion $ClO_3{}^-$.

chlor·dane (klôr′dān′) *n.* A chlorinated hydrocarbon used as an insecticide that may be absorbed through the skin with resultant severe toxic effects.

chlor·di·az·e·pox·ide (klôr′dī-ăz′ə-pŏk′sīd′) *n.* A benzodiazepine drug whose hydrochloride is used primarily to treat anxiety and alcohol withdrawal.

chlo·re·mi·a (klôr-ē′mē-ə) *n.* **1.** See **chlorosis**. **2.** See **hyperchloremia**.

chlor·hy·dri·a (klôr-hī′drē-ə) *n.* See **hyperchlorhydria**.

chlo·ric acid (klôr′ĭk) *n.* A strongly oxidizing unstable chlorine acid that exists only in solution and as chlorates.

chlo·ride (klôr′īd′) *n.* A binary compound of chlorine. —**chlo·rid′ic** (klə-rĭd′ĭk) *adj.*

chloride shift *n.* The movement of chloride ions from the plasma into red blood cells as a result of the transfer of carbon dioxide from tissues to the plasma, a process that serves to maintain blood pH.

chlo·ri·du·ri·a (klôr′ĭ-dŏŏr′ē-ə) *n.* See **chloruresis**.

chlo·ri·nate (klôr′ə-nāt′) *v.* To treat or combine with chlorine or a chlorine compound. —**chlo′ri·na′tion** *n.*

chlo·rine (klôr′ēn′, -ĭn) *n. Symbol* **Cl** A highly irritating poisonous halogen, capable of combining with nearly all other elements, produced principally by electrolysis of sodium chloride and used widely to purify water, as a disinfectant and bleaching agent, and in the manufacture of many important compounds. Atomic number 17.

chlorine acne *n.* See **chloracne**.

chlo·rite (klôr′īt′) *n.* **1.** A salt of chlorous acid. **2.** The inorganic group ClO_2 or a salt containing it.

chloro– or **chlor–** *pref.* **1.** Green: *chlorosis*. **2.** Chlorine: *chloroform*.

chlo·ro·form (klôr′ə-fôrm′) *n.* A clear, colorless, heavy, sweet-smelling liquid used sometimes as a general anesthetic; it has generally been replaced by less toxic, more easily controlled agents.

chlo·ro·form·ism (klôr′ə-fôr′mĭz′əm) *n.* **1.** Habituation to chloroform inhalation. **2.** The symptoms caused by chloroform.

chlo·ro·i·o·do·quin (klôr′ō-ī-ō′də-kwĭn) *n.* See **iodochlorhydroxyquin**.

chlo·ro·ma (klə-rō′mə) *n.* The development of multiple, malignant, localized green masses of abnormal cells, usually myeloblasts, especially beneath the periosteum of the skull, spine, and ribs. Also called *chloroleukemia, chloromyeloma*.

Chlo·ro·my·ce·tin (klôr′ō-mī-sēt′n) A trademark for an antibiotic preparation of chloramphenicol.

chlo·ro·my·e·lo·ma (klôr′ō-mī′ə-lō′mə) *n.* See **chloroma**.

chlo·ro·phe·nol (klôr′ō-fē′nôl′, -nōl′) *n.* One of several substitution products obtained by the action of chlorine on phenol and used as an antiseptic.

chlo·ro·phyll or **chlo·ro·phyl** (klôr′ə-fĭl) *n.* Any of a group of related green pigments found in photosynthetic cells that converts light energy into ATP and other forms of energy needed for biochemical processes; it is found in green plants, brown and red algae, and certain aerobic and anaerobic bacteria.

chlo·ro·pro·caine hydrochloride (klôr′ō-prō′kān′) *n.* An anesthetic drug given locally by infiltration or by caudal or epidural nerve block.

chlo·rop·si·a (klə-rŏp′sē-ə) *n.* A condition in which all objects appear to be colored green, as may occur in digitalis intoxication.

Chlo·rop·tic (klə-rŏp′tĭk) A trademark for the drug chloramphenicol.

chlo·ro·quine phosphate (klôr′ə-kwīn′, -kwĕn′) *n.* An antimalarial drug also used in the treatment of hepatic amebiasis and certain skin diseases.

chlo·ro·sis (klə-rō′sĭs) *n.* A form of chronic anemia, primarily of young women, that is characterized by a greenish-yellow discoloration of the skin and is usually associated with deficiency in iron and protein. Also called *chloremia*. —**chlo·rot′ic** (-rŏt′ĭk) *adj.*

chlo·rous acid (klôr′əs) *n.* An acid that has not been isolated but whose chlorite salts are known.

chlor·phen·ir·a·mine maleate (klôr′fĕn-ĭr′ə-mēn′) *n.* An antihistamine usually used in the treatment of respiratory infections and allergic conditions.

chlor·prom·a·zine (klôr-prŏm′ə-zēn′, -prō′mə-) *n.* A phenothiazine antipsychotic agent with antiemetic, antiadrenergic, and anticholinergic actions.

chlor·pro·pa·mide (klôr-prō′pə-mīd′) *n.* An orally effective hypoglycemic agent, related chemically and pharmacologically to tolbutamide and used in controlling hyperglycemia in certain cases of diabetes mellitus.

chlor·thi·a·zide (klôr-thī′ə-zīd′, -zĭd) *n.* A diuretic drug of the thiazide class.

Chlor-Trim·e·ton (klôr-trĭm′ə-tŏn′) A trademark for the drug chlorpheniramine maleate.

chlor·u·re·sis (klôr′yə-rē′sĭs) *n.* Excretion of chloride in the urine. Also called *chloriduria, chloruria*.

chlor·u·ret·ic (klôr′yə-rĕt′ĭk) *n.* An agent that increases the excretion of chloride in urine. —**chlor′u·ret′ic** *adj.*

chlor·u·ri·a (klôr-yŏŏr′ē-ə) *n.* See **chloruresis**.

cho·a·na (kō′ə-nə) *n., pl.* **–nae** (-nē′) The opening into the nasopharynx of the nasal cavity on either side; posterior naris.

choc·o·late cyst (chô′kə-lĭt, chôk′lĭt, chŏk′-) *n.* A cyst of the ovary containing old brown blood.

choke (chōk) *v.* **1.** To interfere with the respiration of by compression or obstruction of the larynx or trachea. **2.** To have difficulty in breathing, swallowing, or speaking.

choked disk (chōkt) *n.* See **papilledema**.

chokes (chōks) *n.* A manifestation of caisson disease or altitude sickness characterized by dyspnea, coughing, and choking.

chol– *pref.* Variant of **chole–**.

cho·la·gogue (kō′lə-gôg′) *n.* An agent that promotes the flow of bile into the intestine, especially as a result of contraction of the gallbladder. —**cho′la·gog′ic** (-gŏj′ĭk) *adj. & n.*

cho·la·ic acid (kō-lā′ĭk) *n.* See **taurocholic acid.**

cho·lan·gei·tis (kō′lăn-jī′tĭs) *n.* Variant of **cholangitis.**

cho·lan·gi·ec·ta·sis (kō-lăn′jē-ĕk′tə-sĭs) *n.* Dilation of a bile duct.

cho·lan·gi·o·car·ci·no·ma (kō-lăn′jē-ō-kär′sə-nō′mə) *n.* An adenocarcinoma of the intrahepatic bile ducts.

cho·lan·gi·o·en·ter·os·to·my (kō-lăn′jē-ō-ĕn′tə-rŏs′-tə-mē) *n.* The surgical connection of a bile duct to the intestine.

cho·lan·gi·o·fi·bro·sis (kō-lăn′jē-ō-fī-brō′sĭs) *n.* Fibrosis of the bile ducts.

cho·lan·gi·o·gas·tros·to·my (kō-lăn′jē-ō-gă-strŏs′tə-mē) *n.* The surgical formation of a communication between a bile duct and the stomach.

cho·lan·gi·o·gram (kō-lăn′jē-ə-grăm′) *n.* A radiographic image of the bile ducts that is obtained by cholangiography.

cho·lan·gi·og·ra·phy (kō-lăn′jē-ŏg′rə-fē) *n.* A radiographic examination of the bile ducts following administration of a radiopaque contrast medium.

cho·lan·gi·ole (kō-lăn′jē-ōl′) *n.* A ductule that occurs between a bile canaliculus and an interlobular bile duct.

cho·lan·gi·o·lit·ic cirrhosis (kō-lăn′jē-ō-lĭt′ĭk) *n.* Chronic cirrhosis in which there is diffuse inflammation of the cholangioles, with inflammation, fibrosis, and regeneration; it is characterized by relapses and febrile episodes.

cholangiolitic hepatitis *n.* Hepatitis with inflammatory changes around the small bile ducts, producing obstructive jaundice.

cho·lan·gi·o·li·tis (kō-lăn′jē-ə-lī′tĭs) *n.* Inflammation of the small bile radicles or cholangioles.

cho·lan·gi·o·ma (kō-lăn′jē-ō′mə) *n.* A neoplasm of bile duct origin, especially within the liver.

cho·lan·gi·o·pan·cre·a·tog·ra·phy (kō-lăn′jē-ō-păng′krē-ə-tŏg′rə-fē) *n.* Radiographic examination of the bile ducts and pancreas following administration of a radiopaque contrast medium.

cho·lan·gi·os·co·py (kō-lăn′jē-ŏs′kə-pē) *n.* The examination of bile ducts utilizing a cystoscope or fiberoptic endoscope.

cho·lan·gi·os·to·my (kō-lăn′jē-ŏs′tə-mē) *n.* The surgical formation of a fistula into a bile duct.

cho·lan·gi·ot·o·my (kō-lăn′jē-ŏt′ə-mē) *n.* Incision into a bile duct.

cho·lan·gi·tis *or* **cho·lan·gei·tis** (kō′lăn-jī′tĭs) *n.* Inflammation of a bile duct.

cho·lan·o·poi·e·sis (kō-lăn′ō-poi-ē′sĭs) *n.* Synthesis of cholic acid or its conjugates and natural bile salts by the liver. —**cho·lan′o·poi·et′ic** (-ĕt′ĭk) *adj.*

cho·late (kō′lāt′) *n.* A salt or ester of cholic acid.

chole– *or* **chol–** *or* **cholo–** *pref.* Bile: *choleperitoneum.*

cho·le·cal·cif·er·ol (kō′lĭ-kăl-sĭf′ə-rôl′, -rōl′) *n.* See **vitamin D₃.**

cho·le·cyst (kō′lĭ-sĭst′) *n.* See **gallbladder.**

cho·le·cys·ta·gog·ic (kō′lĭ-sĭs′tə-gŏj′ĭk) *adj.* Stimulating activity of the gallbladder.

cho·le·cys·ta·gogue (kō′lĭ-sĭs′tə-gôg′) *n.* A substance that stimulates the activity of the gallbladder.

cho·le·cys·tec·ta·sia (kō′lĭ-sĭs′tĭk-tā′zhə) *n.* Dilation of the gallbladder.

cho·le·cys·tec·to·my (kō′lĭ-sĭ-stĕk′tə-mē) *n.* Surgical removal of the gallbladder.

cho·le·cyst·en·ter·os·to·my (kō′lĭ-sĭ-stĕn′tə-rŏs′tə-mē) *n.* The surgical formation of a direct communication between the gallbladder and the intestine.

cho·le·cys·tic (kō′lĭ-sĭs′tĭk) *adj.* Relating to the gallbladder.

cho·le·cys·tis (kō′lĭ-sĭs′tĭs) *n.* See **gallbladder.**

cho·le·cys·ti·tis (kō′lĭ-sĭ-stī′tĭs) *n.* Inflammation of the gallbladder.

cho·le·cys·to·co·los·to·my (kō′lĭ-sĭs′tō-kə-lŏs′tə-mē) *or* **co·lo·cho·le·cys·tos·to·my** (kō′lō-kō′lĭ-sĭ-stŏs′tə-mē) *n.* The surgical formation of a communication between the gallbladder and the colon.

cho·le·cys·to·du·o·de·nos·to·my (kō′lĭ-sĭs′tō-dōō′ə-dn-ŏs′tə-mē, -dōō-ŏd′n-ŏs′-) *n.* The surgical formation of a communication between the gallbladder and the duodenum.

cho·le·cys·to·gas·tros·to·my (kō′lĭ-sĭs′tō-gă-strŏs′tə-mē) *n.* The surgical formation of a communication between the gallbladder and the stomach.

cho·le·cys·to·gram (kō′lĭ-sĭs′tə-grăm′) *n.* A radiographic image of the gallbladder that is obtained by cholecystography.

cho·le·cys·tog·ra·phy (kō′lĭ-sĭ-stŏg′rə-fē) *n.* Visualization of the gallbladder by x-rays after the administration of a radiopaque substance.

cho·le·cys·to·il·e·os·to·my (kō′lĭ-sĭs′tō-ĭl′ē-ŏs′tə-mē) *n.* The surgical formation of a communication between the gallbladder and the ileum.

cho·le·cys·to·je·ju·nos·to·my (kō′lĭ-sĭs′tō-jə-jōō′-nŏs′tə-mē, -jē′jōō-, -jĕj′ōō-) *n.* The surgical formation of a communication between the gallbladder and the jejunum.

cho·le·cys·to·ki·net·ic (kō′lĭ-sĭs′tō-kĭ-nĕt′ĭk, -kī-) *adj.* Promoting emptying of the gallbladder.

cho·le·cys·to·ki·nin (kō′lĭ-sĭs′tə-kī′nĭn) *n. Abbr.* **CCK** A polypeptide hormone produced principally by the small intestine in response to the presence of fats, causing contraction of the gallbladder, release of bile, and secretion of pancreatic digestive enzymes. Also called *pancreozymin.*

cho·le·cys·to·li·thi·a·sis (kō′lĭ-sĭs′tō-lĭ-thī′ə-sĭs) *n.* The presence of one or more gallstones in the gallbladder.

cho·le·cys·top·a·thy (kō′lĭ-sĭ-stŏp′ə-thē) *n.* Disease of the gallbladder.

cho·le·cys·to·pex·y (kō′lĭ-sĭs′tə-pĕk′sē) *n.* Suture of the gallbladder to the abdominal wall.

cho·le·cys·tor·rha·phy (kō′lĭ-sĭ-stôr′ə-fē) *n.* Suture of an incised or ruptured gallbladder.

cho·le·cys·to·so·nog·ra·phy (kō′lĭ-sĭs′tō-sə-nŏg′rə-fē) *n.* Ultrasonic examination of the gallbladder.

cho·le·cys·tos·to·my (kō′lĭ-sĭ-stŏs′tə-mē) *n.* The establishment of a fistula into the gallbladder.

cho·le·cys·tot·o·my (kō′lĭ-sĭ-stŏt′ə-mē) *n.* Incision into the gallbladder.

cho·led·o·chal (kə-lĕd′ə-kəl, kō′lĭ-dŏk′əl) *adj.* Relating to the common bile duct.

choledochal cyst *n.* A cyst originating in the common bile duct, usually apparent early in life as a right upper abdominal mass in association with jaundice.

cho·led·o·chec·to·my (kə-lĕd′ə-kĕk′tə-mē, kō′lĭ-dō-) *n.* Surgical removal of a portion of the common bile duct.

cho·led·o·chi·tis (kə-lĕd′ə-kī′tĭs, kō′lĭ-dō-) *n.* Inflammation of the common bile duct.

choledocho– *or* **choledoch–** *pref.* Common bile duct: *choledochectomy.*

cho·led·o·cho·du·o·de·nos·to·my (kə-lĕd′ə-kō-dōō′-ō-dn-ŏs′tə-mē, dōō-ŏd′n-ŏs′-) *n.* The surgical formation of a communication between the common bile duct and the duodenum.

cho·led·o·cho·en·ter·os·tomy (kə-lĕd′ə-kō-ĕn′tə-rŏs′tə-mē) *n.* The surgical formation of a communication between the common bile duct and any part of the intestine.

cho·led·o·cho·je·ju·nos·to·my (kə-lĕd′ə-kō-jə-jōō′-nŏs′tə-mē, -jē′jōō-) *n.* The surgical formation of a communication between the common bile duct and the jejunum.

cho·led·o·cho·li·thi·a·sis (kə-lĕd′ə-kō-lĭ-thī′ə-sĭs) *n.* The presence of a gallstone in the common bile duct.

cho·led·o·cho·li·thot·o·my (kə-lĕd′ə-kō-lĭ-thŏt′ə-mē) *n.* Incision of the common bile duct for the extraction of an impacted gallstone.

cho·led·o·cho·plas·ty (kə-lĕd′ə-kō-plăs′tē) *n.* Plastic surgery on the common bile duct.

cho·led·o·chor·rha·phy (kə-lĕd′ə-kôr′ə-fē) *n.* The suturing together of the divided ends of the common bile duct.

cho·led·o·chos·to·my (kə-lĕd′ə-kŏs′tə-mē) *n.* The establishment of a fistula into the common bile duct.

cho·led·o·chot·o·my (kə-lĕd′ə-kŏt′ə-mē) *n.* Incision into the common bile duct.

cho·led·o·chous (kə-lĕd′ə-kəs) *adj.* Containing or conveying bile.

cho·le·ic (kō-lē′ĭk) *adj.* Variant of **cholic.**

choleic acid *n.* Any of several compounds formed of bile acids and sterols.

cho·le·lith (kō′lə-lĭth′) *n.* See **gallstone.**

cho·le·li·thi·a·sis (kō′lə-lĭ-thī′ə-sĭs) *n.* The presence or formation of gallstones in the gallbladder or bile ducts.

cho·le·li·thot·o·my (kō′lə-lĭ-thŏt′ə-mē) *n.* Surgical removal of a gallstone.

cho·le·lith·o·trip·sy (kō′lə-lĭth′ə-trĭp′sē) *n.* The crushing of a gallstone.

cho·lem·e·sis (kō-lĕm′ĭ-sĭs) *n.* The vomiting of bile.

cho·le·mi·a (kō-lē′mē-ə) *n.* The presence of bile salts in the circulating blood. —**cho·le′mic** (-mĭk) *adj.*

cho·le·per·i·to·ne·um (kō′lə-pĕr′ĭ-tn-ē′əm) *n.* The presence of bile in the peritoneum.

cho·le·poi·e·sis (kō′lə-poi-ē′sĭs) *n.* Formation of bile.

choler *n.* 1. Anger; irritability. 2. One of the four humors of ancient and medieval physiology, thought to cause anger and bad temper when present in excess. Also called *yellow bile.*

chol·er·a (kŏl′ər-ə) *n.* 1. An acute epidemic infectious disease caused by *Vibrio cholerae,* characterized by profuse watery diarrhea, extreme loss of fluid and electrolytes, and prostration. 2. Any of various diseases of domesticated animals marked by severe gastroenteritis. —**chol′e·ra′ic** (-ə-rā′ĭk) *adj.*

choleraic diarrhea *n.* See **summer diarrhea.**

cholera mor·bus (môr′bəs) *n.* Acute gastroenteritis occurring seasonally and marked by cramps, diarrhea, and vomiting. No longer in scientific use.

cho·le·re·sis (kō′lə-rē′sĭs) *n.* The secretion of bile by the liver into the gallbladder.

cho·le·ret·ic (kō′lə-rĕt′ĭk) *adj.* Relating to choleresis. —*n.* An agent, usually a drug, that stimulates the liver to increase output of bile.

chol·er·ic (kŏl′ə-rĭk, kə-lĕr′ĭk) *adj.* 1. Easily angered; bad-tempered. 2. Showing or expressing anger.

chol·er·i·form (kŏl′ər-ə-fôrm′) *adj.* Of or resembling cholera.

chol·er·ine (kŏl′ər-ĭn, -ə-rēn′) *n.* A mild form of diarrhea occurring during epidemics of cholera.

chol·er·oid (kŏl′ə-roid′) *adj.* Choleriform.

chol·er·rha·gia (kō′lə-rā′jə) *n.* Excessive flow of bile.

chol·er·rhag·ic (kō′lə-răj′ĭk) *adj.* Relating to the flow of bile.

cho·le·sta·sis (kō′lĭ-stā′sĭs) *n.* An arrest in the flow of bile. —**cho′le·stat′ic** (-stăt′ĭk) *adj.*

cholestatic jaundice *n.* Jaundice caused by thickened bile or bile plugs in the small biliary passages of the liver.

cho·les·te·a·to·ma (kə-lĕs′tē-ə-tō′mə, kō′lĭ-stē′ə-) *n.,* *pl.* **–mas** *or* **–ma·ta** (-mə-tə) A tumorlike mass of keratinizing squamous epithelium and cholesterol, usually occurring in the middle ear and mastoid region. Also called *pearl tumor.*

cho·les·ter·in (kə-lĕs′tər-ĭn) *n.* Cholesterol.

cho·les·ter·ol (kə-lĕs′tə-rôl′, -rōl′) *n.* A white crystalline substance found in animal tissues and various foods, normally synthesized by the liver and important as a constituent of cell membranes and a precursor to steroid hormones. Its level in the bloodstream can influence the pathogenesis of certain conditions, such as the development of atherosclerotic plaque and coronary artery disease.

cholesterol embolism *n.* An embolism of lipid debris from an ulcerated atheromatous deposit, generally from a large artery to small arterial branches. Also called *atheroembolism.*

cho·les·ter·ol·e·mi·a (kə-lĕs′tər-ə-lē′mē-ə) *or* **cho·les·ter·e·mi·a** (kə-lĕs′tə-rē′mē-ə) *n.* The presence of elevated levels of cholesterol in the blood.

cho·les·ter·ol·o·sis (kə-lĕs′tər-ə-lō′sĭs) *or* **cho·les·ter·o·sis** (kə-lĕs′tə-rō′sĭs) *n.* A condition marked by abnormal deposition of cholesterol, as in tissues or blood vessels.

cho·les·ter·ol·u·ri·a (kə-lĕs′tər-ə-lōōr′ē-ə) *n.* Excretion of cholesterol in the urine.

cho·le·styr·a·mine (kō′lĭ-stîr′ə-mēn′, kō-lĕs′tə-răm′-ēn) *n.* A drug used to lower serum cholesterol levels and treat itching associated with jaundice through its ability to promote excretion of bile acids.

cho·le·u·ri·a (kō′lə-yŏŏr′ē-ə) *n.* Variant of **choluria.**

cho·lic (kō′lĭk) *or* **cho·le·ic** (kō-lē′ĭk) *adj.* Of or relating to bile.

cholic acid *n.* An abundant crystalline bile acid derived from cholesterol.

cho·line (kō′lēn′) *n.* A natural amine often classed in the vitamin B complex and a constituent of many other biologically important molecules, such as acetylcholine and lecithin.

choline acetyltransferase *n.* An enzyme, present at the presynaptic ends of axons, that catalyzes the transfer of the acetyl group of acetyl CoA to choline, forming acetylcholine.

choline kinase *n.* An enzyme that catalyzes the reaction between choline and ATP, forming ADP and phosphocholine.

cho·lin·er·gic (kō′lə-nûr′jĭk) *adj.* **1.** Relating to nerve cells or fibers that employ acetylcholine as their neurotransmitter. **2.** Relating to an agent that mimics the action of acetylcholine.

cholinergic blockade *n.* **1.** Inhibition by a drug of nerve impulse transmission at autonomic ganglionic synapses, postganglionic parasympathetic effector cells, and myoneural junctions. **2.** Inhibition of a cholinergic agent.

cholinergic fiber *n.* Any of the nerve fibers that transmit impulses to other nerve cells or to muscle fibers or gland cells by acetylcholine.

cholinergic receptor *n.* Any of the sites in effector cells or at synapses through which acetylcholine exerts its action. Also called *cholinoreceptor.*

cholinergic urticaria *n.* A form of nonallergic or physical urticaria initiated by heat or by excitement, consisting of pruritic areas surrounded by bright red macules. Also called *heat urticaria.*

cho·lin·es·ter·ase (kō′lə-nĕs′tə-rās′, -rāz′) *n.* An enzyme that catalyzes the hydrolysis of choline esters chiefly at nerve terminals, where it hydrolyzes and inactivates acetylcholine. Also called *acetylcholinesterase.*

cholinesterase inhibitor *n.* A drug, such as neostigmine, that restores myoneural function by inhibiting the biodegradation of acetylcholine. Also called *acetylcholinesterase inhibitor.*

cho·li·no·cep·tive (kō′lə-nō-sĕp′tĭv) *adj.* Of or relating to chemical sites in effector cells with which acetylcholine unites to exert its actions.

cho·li·no·lyt·ic (kō′lə-nō-lĭt′ĭk) *adj.* Preventing the action of acetylcholine.

cho·li·no·mi·met·ic (kō′lə-nō-mĭ-mĕt′ĭk, -mī-) *adj.* Having an action similar to that of acetylcholine.

cho·li·no·re·ac·tive (kō′lə-nō-rē-ăk′tĭv) *adj.* Responding to acetylcholine and related compounds.

cho·li·no·re·cep·tor (kō′lə-nō-rĭ-sĕp′tər) *n.* See **cholinergic receptor.**

cholo– *pref.* Variant of **chole–.**

cho·lo·yl (kō′lō-ĭl′) *n.* The radical, $C_{23}H_{41}COO$, present in cholic acid.

chol·u·ri·a (kō-loŏr′ē-ə) or **cho·le·u·ri·a** (kō′lə-yoŏr′ē-ə) *n.* See **biliuria.**

chon·dral (kŏn′drəl) *adj.* Of, relating to, or consisting of cartilage; cartilaginous.

chon·dral·gia (kŏn-drăl′jə) *n.* See **chondrodynia.**

chon·drec·to·my (kŏn-drĕk′tə-mē) *n.* The excision of cartilage.

chon·dri·fi·ca·tion center (kŏn′drə-fĭ-kā′shən) *n.* Any of the various aggregations of embryonic mesenchymal cells at sites of future cartilage formation.

chon·dri·fy (kŏn′drə-fī′) *v.* To change into or become cartilage.

chon·dri·tis (kŏn-drī′tĭs) *n.* Inflammation of cartilage.

chon·dro·blast (kŏn′drə-blăst′) *n.* A cell of growing cartilage tissue. Also called *chondroplast.*

chon·dro·blas·to·ma (kŏn′drō-blă-stō′mə) *n.* A tumor arising in the epiphyses of long bones in young males, consisting of tissue resembling fetal cartilage.

chon·dro·cal·ci·no·sis (kŏn′drō-kăl′sə-nō′sĭs) *n.* The calcification of cartilage.

chon·dro·clast (kŏn′drə-klăst′) *n.* A multinucleated cell involved in the reabsorption of cartilage.

chon·dro·cos·tal (kŏn′drō-kŏs′təl) *adj.* Relating to the costal cartilages.

chon·dro·cra·ni·um (kŏn′drō-krā′nē-əm) *n.* The cartilaginous parts of the developing skull.

chon·dro·cyte (kŏn′drə-sīt′) *n.* A connective tissue cell that occupies a lacuna within the cartilage matrix. Also called *cartilage cell.*

chon·dro·dyn·i·a (kŏn′drō-dĭn′ē-ə) *n.* Pain in cartilage. Also called *chondralgia.*

chon·dro·dys·pla·sia (kŏn′drō-dĭs-plā′zhə) *n.* See **chondrodystrophy.**

chon·dro·dys·tro·phi·a (kŏn′drō-dĭ-strō′fē-ə) *n.* See **chondrodystrophy.**

chon·dro·dys·troph·ic dwarfism (kŏn′drō-dĭ-strŏf′ĭk, -strō′fĭk) *n.* A congenital dwarfism in which the disturbed development of the cartilage of the long bones arrests the growth of long bones, resulting in extremely shortened extremities.

chon·dro·dys·tro·phy (kŏn′drə-dĭs′trə-fē) *n.* A disturbance that affects the development of the cartilage of the long bones and that especially involves the region of the epiphysial plates, resulting in arrested growth of the long bones. Also called *chondrodysplasia, chondrodystrophia.*

chon·dro·ec·to·der·mal dysplasia (kŏn′drō-ĕk′tə-dûr′məl) *n.* An inherited complex characterized by chondrodystrophy, ectodermal dysplasia, and polydactyly, and often congenital heart defects.

chon·dro·fi·bro·ma (kŏn′drō-fī-brō′mə) *n.* See **chondromyxoid fibroma.**

chon·dro·gen·e·sis (kŏn′drō-jĕn′ĭ-sĭs) *n.* The formation of cartilage. Also called *chondrosis.*

chon·droid (kŏn′droid′) *adj.* Resembling cartilage; cartilaginoid.

chondroid tissue *n.* **1.** Tissue resembling cartilage and occurring in adults. Also called *pseudocartilage.* **2.** An early form of cartilage occurring in an embryo.

chon·dro·i·tin sulfate (kŏn-drō′ĭ-tĭn) *n.* A component of proteoglycan, thought by some to bring relief to osteoarthritis pain when taken as a dietary supplement.

chon·drol·y·sis (kŏn-drŏl′ĭ-sĭs) *n.* The disappearance of articular cartilage as the result of lysis or dissolution of the cartilage matrix and cells.

chon·dro·ma (kŏn-drō′mə) *n., pl.* **–mas** *or* **–ma·ta** (-mə-tə) A benign neoplasm derived from mesodermal cells that form cartilage.

chon·dro·ma·la·cia (kŏn′drō-mə-lā′shə) *n.* Abnormal softening or degeneration of cartilage of the joints, especially of the knee.

chon·dro·ma·to·sis (kŏn′drō-mə-tō′sĭs) *n.* The presence of multiple chondromas.

chon·dro·ma·tous (kŏn-drō′mə-təs, -drŏm′ə-) *adj.* Relating to or having the features of a chondroma.

chon·dro·mere (kŏn′drə-mîr′) *n.* A cartilage unit of the embryonic vertebral column.

chon·dro·myx·oid fibroma (kŏn′drō-mĭk′soid′) *n.* An uncommon benign bone tumor usually affecting the long bones of the leg, composed of lobulated myxoid tissue with few chondroid foci. Also called *chondrofibroma, chondromyxoma.*

chon·dro·os·se·ous (kŏn′drō-ŏs′ē-əs) *adj.* Relating to cartilage and bone, either as a mixture of the two tissues or as a junction between the two.

chon·dro·os·te·o·dys·tro·phy (kŏn′drō-ŏs′tē-ō-dĭs′trə-fē) *n.* A group of disorders of bone and cartilage, including Morquio's syndrome and similar conditions. Also called *osteochondrodystrophy.*

chon·drop·a·thy (kŏn-drŏp′ə-thē) *n.* A disease involving cartilage.

chon·dro·phyte (kŏn′drə-fīt′) *n.* An abnormal cartilaginous mass that develops at the articular surface of a bone.

chon·dro·plast (kŏn′drə-plăst′) *n.* See **chondroblast.**

chon·dro·plas·ty (kŏn′drə-plăs′tē) *n.* Reparative or plastic surgery of cartilage.

chon·dro·po·ro·sis (kŏn′drō-pə-rō′sĭs) *n.* A state of cartilage in which spaces appear during normal ossification or in pathological conditions.

chon·dro·sar·co·ma (kŏn′drō-sär-kō′mə) *n.* A malignant neoplasm derived from cartilage cells and occurring most frequently in pelvic bones or near the ends of long bones.

chon·dro·sis (kŏn-drō′sĭs) *n.* See **chondrogenesis.**

chon·dro·ster·nal (kŏn′drō-stûr′nəl) *adj.* Relating to the costal cartilages and the sternum.

chon·dro·ster·no·plas·ty (kŏn′drō-stûr′nə-plăs′tē) *n.* Surgical correction of malformations of the sternum.

chon·drot·o·my (kŏn-drŏt′ə-mē) *n.* The surgical division of a cartilage.

chon·dro·xiph·oid (kŏn′drō-zĭf′oid′) *adj.* Relating to the xiphoid cartilage.

Cho·part's amputation (shō-pärz′) *n.* Surgical removal of the foot through the midtarsal joint but retaining the calcaneus, talus, and other parts of the tarsus. Also called *mediotarsal amputation.*

Chopart's joint *n.* See **transverse tarsal joint.**

chord (kôrd) *n.* Variant of **cord.**

chord– *pref.* Variant of **cordo–.**

chor·da (kôr′də) *n., pl.* **-dae** (-dē′) **1.** A tendon. **2.** A tendinous or cordlike structure.

chord·al (kôr′dl) *adj.* Of or relating to a chorda or cord.

Chor·da·ta (kôr-dā′tə) *n.* The phylum of animals whose members have a single dorsal nerve cord and a notochord and gill slits during some stage in their development.

chor·date (kôr′dāt′, -dĭt) *n.* An animal of the phylum Chordata, which includes all vertebrates.

chor·dee (kôr′dē′, -dā′, kôr-dā′) *n.* **1.** Painful erection and curvature of the penis in gonorrhea or Peyronie's disease. **2.** Ventral curvature of the penis, most apparent on erection, as seen in hypospadias due to congenital shortness of the urethra.

chor·di·tis (kôr-dī′tĭs) *n.* Inflammation of a cord, usually a vocal cord.

chordo– *pref.* Variant of **cordo–.**

chor·do·ma (kôr-dō′mə) *n.* A rare solitary neoplasm of skeletal tissue in adults.

chor·do·skel·e·ton (kôr′dō-skĕl′ĭ-tn) *n.* The part of the skeleton in the embryo that develops in relation with the notochord.

chor·dot·o·my (kôr-dŏt′ə-mē) *n.* Variant of **cordotomy.**

cho·re·a (kô-rē′ə, kə-) *n.* Irregular, spasmodic, involuntary movements of the limbs or facial muscles. **—cho·re′al, cho·re′ic** *adj.*

choreic abasia *n.* Abasia due to abnormal movements of the legs.

choreic movement *n.* An involuntary spasmodic twitching or jerking in muscle groups that is not associated with the production of definite purposeful movements.

cho·re·o·ath·e·to·sis (kôr′ē-ō-ăth′ĭ-tō′sĭs) *n.* A condition marked by abnormal movements of the body that have a combined choreic and athetoid pattern. **—cho′re·o·ath′e·toid′** (-toid′) **—cho′re·o·ath′e·tot′-ic** (-tŏt′ĭk) *adj.*

cho·re·oid (kôr′ē-oid′) *or* **cho·re·i·form** (kô-rē′ə-fôrm′, kə-) *adj.* Resembling chorea.

cho·re·o·phra·sia (kôr′ē-ō-frā′zhə) *n.* The continual repetition of meaningless phrases.

chorio– *pref.* **1.** Chorion: *chorioadenoma.* **2.** Choroid coat: *chorioretinitis.*

cho·ri·o·ad·e·no·ma (kôr′ē-ō-ăd′n-ō′mə) *n.* A benign neoplasm of the chorion, especially one having early hydatidiform mole formation. Also called *deciduoma malignum.*

chorioadenoma des·tru·ens (dĕ-strōo′ənz) *n.* A hydatidiform mole in which there is an unusual degree of invasion of the myometrium or its blood vessels, causing hemorrhage, necrosis, and occasionally rupture of the uterus.

cho·ri·o·al·lan·to·is (kôr′ē-ō′ə-lăn′tō-ĭs) *n.* The highly vascular extraembryonic membrane formed by the fusion of the allantois with the chorion that constitutes the placenta in most mammals. **—cho′ri·o·al′lan·to′ic** (-ō-ăl′ən-tō′ĭk) *adj.*

cho·ri·o·am·ni·o·ni·tis (kôr′ē-ō-ăm′nē-ə-nī′tĭs) *n.* Inflammation of the amniotic membranes caused by infection.

cho·ri·o·an·gi·o·ma (kôr′ē-ō-ăn′jē-ō′mə) *n.* A benign tumor of placental blood vessels usually of no clinical significance.

cho·ri·o·an·gi·o·sis (kôr′ē-ō-ăn′jē-ō′sĭs) *n.* An abnormal increase in the number of vascular channels that are present in the villi of the placenta; severe chorioangiosis is associated with a high incidence of neonatal death and major congenital malformations. Also called *chorioangiomatosis.*

cho·ri·o·cap·il·lar·is (kôr′ē-ō-kăp′ə-lăr′ĭs) *n.* The capillaries forming the inner vascular layer of the choroid of the eye.

cho·ri·o·cap·il·lar·y layer (kôr′ē-ō-kăp′ə-lĕr′ē) *n.* The internal layer of the choroid of the eye, composed of a very close capillary network. Also called *entochoroidea, Ruysch's membrane.*

cho·ri·o·car·ci·no·ma (kôr′ē-ō-kär′sə-nō′mə) *n.* A malignant tumor of syncytial trophoblasts and cytotrophoblasts, almost always occurring in the uterus. Also called *chorioepithelioma, chorionic epithelioma, trophoblastoma.*

cho·ri·o·cele (kôr′ē-ə-sēl′) *n.* A hernia of the choroid coat of the eye through a defect in the sclera.

cho·ri·o·ep·i·the·li·o·ma (kôr′ē-ō-ĕp′ə-thē′lē-ō′mə) *n.* See **choriocarcinoma.**

chorioid– *pref.* Variant of **choroido–.**

chorioido– *pref.* Variant of **choroido–.**

cho·ri·o·ma (kôr′ē-ō′mə) *n.* A benign or malignant tumor of chorionic tissue.

cho·ri·o·men·in·gi·tis (kôr′ē-ō-mĕn′ĭn-jī′tĭs) *n.* Cerebral meningitis in which there is marked cellular infiltration of the meninges, often with a lymphocytic infiltration of the choroid plexuses.

cho·ri·on (kôr′ē-ŏn′) *n.* The outer membrane enclosing the embryo in reptiles, birds, and mammals. In placental mammals it contributes to the development of the placenta. —**cho′ri·on′ic** (-ŏn′ĭk) *adj.*

chorionic epithelioma *n.* See **choriocarcinoma.**

chorionic gonadotropin *n. Abbr.* **CG** A glycoprotein that is produced by the placenta and is excreted in the urine of pregnant women, and that acts to stimulate ovarian secretion of the estrogen and progesterone that are required to maintain the conceptus; it is used as an aid for conception and in the treatment of cryptorchidism. Also called *anterior pituitary-like hormone, chorionic gonadotropic hormone, human chorionic gonadotropin.*

chorionic growth hormone-prolactin *n.* See **human placental lactogen.**

chorionic villus *n.* Any of the various fingerlike projections of the chorion of the embryo that contain fetal blood vessels and grow into the intervillous lacuna of the placenta.

chorionic villus sampling *n. Abbr.* **CVS** A prenatal test to detect birth defects that is performed at an early stage of pregnancy and involves retrieval and examination of tissue from the chorionic villi.

cho·ri·o·ret·i·nal (kôr′ē-ō-rĕt′n-əl) *adj.* Relating to the choroid coat of the eye and to the retina.

cho·ri·o·ret·i·ni·tis (kôr′ē-ō-rĕt′n-ī′tĭs) *n.* Inflammation of the choroid and retina. Also called *choroidoretinitis, retinochoroiditis.*

cho·ri·o·ret·i·nop·a·thy (kôr′ē-ō-rĕt′n-ŏp′ə-thē) *n.* A noninflammatory abnormality of the choroid with extension to the retina.

cho·ris·ta (kə-rĭs′tə, kô-) *n.* A focus of tissue that is histologically normal, but is not normally found in the organ or structure in which it is located.

cho·ris·to·ma (kôr′ĭ-stō′mə) *n.* A mass formed by the faulty development of tissue of a type not normally found at that site.

cho·roid (kôr′oid′) *or* **cho·ri·oid** (kôr′ē-oid′) *n.* The dark-brown vascular coat of the eye between the sclera and the retina. —*adj.* Of or relating to the chorion or corium.

cho·roi·dal (kə-roid′l, kô-) *adj.* Of or relating to the choroid.

choroidal artery *n.* **1.** An artery with origin in the internal carotid or middle cerebral artery, with distribution to the optic tract, cerebral peduncle, uncus, hippocampus, pallidum, posterior part of the internal capsule, the geniculate bodies of thalamus, and the choroid plexus in the inferior horn of the lateral ventricle; anterior choroidal artery. **2.** An artery that is one of several branches of the posterior cerebral artery supplying the choroid plexus of the body of the lateral and third ventricles; posterior choroidal artery.

cho·roi·de·a (kə-roi′dē-ə, kô-) *n.* The choroid.

cho·roid·e·re·mi·a (kôr′oi-də-rē′mē-ə, kô-) *n.* **1.** The congenital absence of the choroid of the eye. **2.** The progressive degeneration of the choroid in males, beginning with peripheral pigmentary retinopathy, followed by atrophy of the retinal pigment epithelium and of the choriocapillaris, night blindness, progressive constriction of visual fields, and finally complete blindness.

cho·roid·i·tis (kôr′oi-dī′tĭs) *n.* Inflammation of the choroid.

choroido– *or* **choroid–** *or* **chorioido–** *or* **chorioid–** *pref.* Choroid coat: *choroidoiritis.*

cho·roi·do·cy·cli·tis (kə-roi′dō-sĭ-klī′tĭs, -sī-, kô-) *n.* Inflammation of the choroid and the ciliary body.

cho·roi·dop·a·thy (kôr′oi-dŏp′ə-thē) *n.* Noninflammatory degeneration of the choroid.

cho·roi·do·ret·i·ni·tis (kə-roi′dō-rĕt′n-ī′tĭs, kô-) *n.* See **chorioretinitis.**

choroid plexus *n.* A vascular proliferation of the cerebral ventricles that serves to regulate intraventricular pressure by secretion or absorption of cerebrospinal fluid.

choroid tela of fourth ventricle *n.* The sheet of pia mater covering the lower part of the ependymal roof of the fourth ventricle of the brain.

choroid tela of third ventricle *n.* A double fold of pia mater, enclosing the subarachnoid trabeculae and located between the fornix above and the epithelial roof of the third ventricle and the thalami below.

Chot·zen syndrome (kŏt′zən, ĸнôt′-) *n.* See **type III acrocephalosyndactyly.**

Christ·church chromosome (krĭst′chûrch′) *n.* An abnormal small acrocentric chromosome with complete or almost complete deletion of the short arm; it is found in the white blood cells in some cases of chronic lymphocytic leukemia.

Chris·ten·sen-Krabbe disease (krĭs′tən-sən-) *n.* See **progressive cerebral poliodystrophy.**

Chris·tian's disease (krĭs′chənz) *n.* **1.** See **Hand-Schüller-Christian disease. 2.** See **nodular nonsuppurative panniculitis.**

Christ·mas disease (krĭs′məs) *n.* See **hemophilia B.**

Christmas factor *n.* See **factor IX.**

chrom– *pref.* Variant of **chromo–.**

chro·maf·fin (krō′mə-fĭn) *adj.* Staining a brownish yellow upon reaction with chromic salts. Used of certain cells in the medulla of the adrenal glands and in paraganglia.

chromaffin body *n.* See **paraganglion.**

chromaffin cell *n.* A cell that stains readily with chromium salts, especially a cell of the adrenal medulla.

chro·maf·fin·o·ma (krō′mə-fə-nō′mə, krō-măf′ə-) *n.* A tumor composed of chromaffin cells. Also called *chromaffin tumor.*

chro·maf·fi·nop·a·thy (krō-măf′ə-nŏp′ə-thē) *n.* A pathological condition of chromaffin tissue.

chromaffin tissue *n.* A cellular tissue, vascular and well supplied with nerves, made up chiefly of chromaffin cells and found in the medulla of the adrenal glands and in the paraganglia.

chromaffin tumor *n.* See **chromaffinoma.**

chro·mate (krō′māt′) *n.* A salt of chromic acid.

chro·mat·ic (krō-măt′ĭk) *adj.* **1.** Relating to color or colors. **2.** Produced by or made in a color or colors.

chromatic aberration *n.* Color distortion in an image produced by a lens, caused by the inability of the lens to bring the various colors of light to focus at a single point. Also called *chromatism.*

chromatic vision *n.* See **chromatopsia.**

chro·ma·tid (krō′mə-tĭd) *n.* Either of the two daughter strands of a duplicated chromosome that are joined by a single centromere and separate during cell division to become individual chromosomes.

chro·ma·tin (krō′mə-tĭn) *n.* A complex of nucleic acids and proteins in the cell nucleus that stains readily with basic dyes and condenses to form chromosomes during cell division.

chromatin body *n.* The genetic material of bacteria.

chro·ma·tism (krō′mə-tĭz′əm) *n.* **1.** Abnormal pigmentation. **2.** See **chromatic aberration.**

chromato– *or* **chromat–** *pref.* **1.** Color: *chromatophore.* **2.** Chromatin: *chromatolysis.*

chro·ma·tog·e·nous (krō′mə-tŏj′ə-nəs) *adj.* Producing color; causing pigmentation.

chro·mat·o·gram (krō-măt′ə-grăm′) *n.* The pattern of separated substances obtained by chromatography.

chro·ma·tog·ra·phy (krō′mə-tŏg′rə-fē) *n.* Any of various techniques for the separation of complex mixtures that rely on the differential affinities of substances for a gas or liquid mobile medium and for a stationary adsorbing medium through which they pass, such as paper, gelatin, or magnesia. Also called *absorption chromatography.* —**chro′ma·tog′ra·pher** *n.*

chro·ma·tol·y·sis (krō′mə-tŏl′ĭ-sĭs) *n.* The disintegration of chromophil substance in a nerve cell body; it may occur after exhaustion of the cell or after damage to its peripheral process. Also called *chromolysis.* —**chro·mat′o·lyt′ic** (-măt′l-ĭt′ĭk) *adj.*

chro·mat·o·phil (krō-măt′ə-fĭl′, krō′mə-tō-) *or* **chro·mat·o·phile** (-fĭl′) *n.* Variant of **chromophil.**

chro·mat·o·phil·i·a (krō-măt′ə-fĭl′ē-ə, -fēl′yə, krō′mə-tō-) *n.* Variant of **chromophilia.**

chro·mat·o·pho·bi·a (krō-măt′ə-fō′bē-ə, krō′mə-tō-) *n.* Variant of **chromophobia.**

chro·mat·o·phore (krō-măt′ə-fôr′) *n.* **1.** A specialized pigment-bearing organelle in certain photosynthetic bacteria and cyanobacteria. **2.** A pigment-bearing phagocyte found chiefly in the skin, mucous membrane, and choroid coat of the eye, as well as in melanomas. Also called *pigment cell.* **3.** Variant of **chromophore.** —**chro·mat′o·phor′ic** (-fôr′ĭk) *adj.*

chro·ma·top·si·a (krō′mə-tŏp′sē-ə) *n.* A condition in which objects appear to be abnormally colored or tinged with color. Also called *chromatic vision.*

chro·ma·tu·ri·a (krō′mə-tŏor′ē-ə) *n.* Abnormal coloration of the urine.

chrome (krōm) *n.* Chromium, especially as a source of pigment.

chro·mes·the·sia (krō′mĕs-thē′zhə) *n.* A condition in which another sensation, such as taste or smell, is stimulated by the perception of color.

chro·mi·dro·sis (krō′mĭ-drō′sĭs) *or* **chrom·hi·dro·sis** (krōm′hĭ-drō′sĭs, -hī-) *n.* The excretion of sweat containing pigment.

chro·mi·um (krō′mē-əm) *n. Symbol* **Cr** A lustrous hard metallic element, resistant to tarnish and corrosion and found primarily in chromite. It is used to harden steel alloys, in decorative platings, and as a pigment in glass. Atomic number 24.

chromo– *or* **chrom–** *pref.* Color: *chromogenesis.*

chro·mo·blast (krō′mə-blăst′) *n.* An embryonic cell having the potential to develop into a pigment cell.

chro·mo·blas·to·my·co·sis (krō′mō-blăs′tō-mī-kō′sĭs) *n.* See **chromomycosis.**

chro·mo·cys·tos·co·py (krō′mō-sĭ-stŏs′kə-pē) *n.* See **cystochromoscopy.**

chro·mo·cyte (krō′mə-sīt′) *n.* A pigmented cell, such as a red blood corpuscle.

chro·mo·gen (krō′mə-jən) *n.* **1.** A substance that lacks definite color but may be transformed into a pigment. **2.** A strongly pigment-generating or pigmented organelle, organ, or microorganism.

chro·mo·gen·e·sis (krō′mə-jĕn′ĭ-sĭs) *n.* Production of coloring matter or pigment.

chro·mo·gen·ic (krō′mə-jĕn′ĭk) *adj.* Of or relating to a chromogen or to chromogenesis.

chro·mol·y·sis (krō-mŏl′ĭ-sĭs) *n.* See **chromatolysis.**

chro·mo·mere (krō′mə-mîr′) *n.* **1.** A condensed segment of a chromonema. **2.** See **granulomere.**

chro·mo·my·co·sis (krō′mō-mī-kō′sĭs) *n.* A localized chronic mycosis of skin, characterized by rough, irregular lesions and caused by several dark-colored fungi. Also called *chromoblastomycosis, dermatitis verrucosa.*

chro·mo·ne·ma (krō′mə-nē′mə) *n., pl.* **–ma·ta** (-mə-tə) The coiled filament that extends the entire length of a chromosome and on which the genes are located.

chro·mo·phil (krō′mə-fĭl′) *or* **chro·mat·o·phil** (krō-măt′ə-fĭl′, krō′mə-tō-) *or* **chro·mo·phile** (-fĭl′) *n.* A cell or other histologic element that stains readily. —*adj.* Staining readily. Used of a cell or cell structure. —**chro′mo·phil′ic** (krō′mə-fĭl′ĭk) *adj.*

chromophil adenoma *n.* An adenoma composed of cells that stain readily.

chro·mo·phil·i·a (krō′mə-fĭl′ē-ə, -fēl′yə) *or* **chro·mat·o·phil·i·a** (krō-măt′ə-, krō′mə-tō-) *n.* The property possessed by most cells of staining readily with appropriate dyes.

chro·mo·phobe (krō'mə-fōb') *or* **chro·mo·pho·bic** (krō'mə-fō'bĭk) *adj.* Resistant to stains; staining with difficulty or not staining at all. —*n.* A cell that is resistant to stains.

chromophobe adenoma *n.* An adenoma of the chromophobe cells of the anterior pituitary gland.

chromophobe cell *n.* Any of the faintly staining cells of the anterior lobe of the pituitary gland.

chro·mo·pho·bi·a (krō'mə-fō'bē-ə) *or* **chro·mat·o·pho·bi·a** (krō-măt'ə-, krō'mə-tō-) *n.* **1.** Resistance to stains. Used of certain cells and histologic structures. **2.** An abnormal fear of colors or a color.

chro·mo·phore (krō'mə-fôr') *or* **chro·mat·o·phore** (krō-măt'ə-) *n.* A chemical group capable of selective light absorption resulting in coloration of certain organic compounds. Also called *color radical*.

chro·mo·phor·ic (krō'mə-fôr'ĭk) *n.* **1.** Of or relating to a chromophore. **2.** Of or relating to microorganisms that produce or carry color.

chromosomal instability syndrome *n.* Any of a group of Mendelian inheritance conditions associated with chromosomal instability and breakage in vitro and often leading to an increased tendency to develop certain types of malignancies. Also called *chromosomal breakage syndrome*.

chromosomal map *n.* A representation of the karyotype and of the positioning and ordering on it of those loci that have been localized by any of several mapping methods.

chromosomal region *n.* The part of a chromosome defined either by anatomical details, especially by banding, or by its linkage groups.

chromosomal syndrome *n.* Any of a number of syndromes attributable to a chromosomal aberration and typically associated with mental retardation and multiple congenital anomalies.

chromosomal trait *n.* A trait dependent on a chromosomal aberration.

chro·mo·some (krō'mə-sōm') *n.* **1.** A threadlike linear strand of DNA and associated proteins in the nucleus of animal and plant cells that carries the genes and functions in the transmission of hereditary information. **2.** A circular strand of DNA in bacteria and cyanobacteria that contains the hereditary information necessary for cell life. —**chro·mo·so·mal** (-sō'məl), **chro·mo·so'mic** (-sō'mĭk) *adj.*

chromosome aberration *n.* A deviation in the normal number of chromosomes or in their morphology.

chromosome band *n.* An area across the width of a chromosome that stains darkly or in a contrasting manner.

chromosome mapping *n.* The process of determining the position of specific genes on specific chromosomes and constructing a diagram of each chromosome showing the relative positions of the genes.

chron– *pref.* Variant of **chrono–**.

chro·nax·ie *or* **chro·nax·y** (krō'năk'sē, krŏn'ăk'-) *n., pl.* **–ies** The minimum interval of time necessary to electrically stimulate a muscle or nerve fiber, using twice the minimum current needed to elicit a threshold response.

chron·ic (krŏn'ĭk) *adj.* Of long duration. Used of a disease of slow progress and long continuance.

chronic absorptive arthritis *n.* Arthritis, especially of the hands, accompanied by pronounced resorption of bone with shortening and deformity.

chronic acholuric jaundice *n.* See **hereditary spherocytosis**.

chronic active liver disease *n.* Any of several types of hepatitis that persist for more than six months and often progress to cirrhosis.

chronic adrenocortical insufficiency *n.* See **Addison's disease**.

chronic alcoholism *n.* See **alcoholism** (sense 2).

chronic atrophic thyroiditis *n.* Replacement of the thyroid gland by fibrous tissue.

chronic bronchitis *n.* Inflammation of the bronchial mucous membrane, characterized by cough, hypersecretion of mucus, and expectoration of sputum over a long period of time and associated with increased vulnerability to bronchial infection.

chronic desquamative gingivitis *n.* A diffuse or patchy, often painful inflamed area of the gum that is caused by changes to the connective tissue as a result of the atrophy of epithelial cells. Also called *gingivosis*.

chronic familial jaundice *n.* See **hereditary spherocytosis**.

chronic fatigue and immune dysfunction syndrome *n. Abbr.* **CFIDS** Chronic fatigue syndrome.

chronic fatigue syndrome *n. Abbr.* **CFS** A syndrome of unknown origin characterized by persistent or relapsing debilitating fatigue of definite onset that is not alleviated by sleep, combined with other symptoms such as headache, sore throat, impaired short-term memory or concentration, immunologic abnormalities, muscle and joint pain, and lengthy malaise following exertion.

chronic granulomatous disease *n.* A congenital defect in the ability of polymorphonuclear leukocytes to kill phagocytized bacteria, resulting in increased susceptibility to severe infections. Also called *congenital dysphagocytosis*.

chronic idiopathic jaundice *n.* See **Dubin Johnson syndrome**.

chronic inflammation *n.* Inflammation that may have a rapid or slow onset but is characterized primarily by its persistence and lack of clear resolution; it occurs when the tissues are unable to overcome the effects of the injuring agent.

chronic interstitial salpingitis *n.* Salpingitis in which fibrosis or mononuclear cell infiltration involves all layers of the fallopian tube or eustachian tube. Also called *pachysalpingitis*.

chronic lymphocytic leukemia *n. Abbr.* **CLL** Lymphocytic leukemia occurring mainly in older adults, characterized by slow onset and gradual progression of symptoms.

chronic malaria *n.* Malaria that develops after repeated attacks of one of the acute forms, usually falciparum malaria, and is characterized by profound anemia, enlargement of the spleen, emaciation, mental depression, sallow complexion, edema of the ankles, and muscular weakness.

chronic mountain sickness *n.* Altitude sickness that occurs despite acclimatization to high altitudes, characterized by high levels of circulating red blood cells, hypoxemia, and reduced mental and physical capacity. Also called *Monge's disease.*

chronic obstructive pulmonary disease *n.* *Abbr.* **COPD** A chronic lung disease, such as asthma or emphysema, in which breathing becomes slowed or forced.

chronic shock *n.* The state of subnormal blood volume that develops in an individual with a debilitating disease, especially in the elderly, and that makes the person susceptible to hemorrhagic shock if moderate blood loss occurs, as that which may occur during an operation.

chronic sleeping sickness *n.* See **Gambian trypanosomiasis.**

chronic trypanosomiasis *n.* See **Gambian trypanosomiasis.**

chronic ulcer *n.* A long-standing ulcer with fibrous scar tissue at its base.

chrono– *or* **chron–** *pref.* Time: *chronobiology.*

chron·o·bi·ol·o·gy (krŏn′ō-bī-ŏl′ə-jē) *n.* The study of the effect of time on biological events, especially repetitive or cyclic phenomena in individuals.

chron·o·log·i·cal age (krŏn′ə-lŏj′ĭ-kəl) *n.* *Abbr.* **CA** The number of years a person has lived, used especially in psychometrics as a standard against which certain variables, such as behavior and intelligence, are measured.

chron·o·on·col·o·gy (krŏn′ō-ŏng-kŏl′ə-jē) *n.* **1.** The study of the influence of biological rhythms on neoplastic growth. **2.** Anticancer treatment based on the timing of drug administration.

chron·o·ther·a·py (krŏn′ō-thĕr′ə-pē′, krō′nə-) *n.* **1.** Medical treatment that is administered according to a schedule that corresponds to a person's daily, monthly, seasonal, or yearly biological clock. **2.** Treatment of a sleep disorder by altering an individual's sleeping and waking times and resetting his or her biological clock.

chron·o·trop·ic (krŏn′ə-trŏp′ĭk, -trō′pĭk) *adj.* Affecting the rate of rhythmic movements, such as the heartbeat.

chro·not·ro·pism (krə-nŏt′rə-pĭz′əm) *n.* The modification of the rate of a periodic movement, such as the heartbeat, through some external influence.

chry·si·a·sis (krĭ-sī′ə-sĭs) *n.* A permanent slate-gray discoloration of the skin and sclera resulting from deposition of gold in the connective tissue of the skin and eye after the therapeutic administration of gold salts. Also called *chrysoderma.*

chryso– *or* **chrys–** *pref.* Gold; golden: *chrysotherapy.*

chrys·o·der·ma (krĭs′ō-dûr′mə) *n.* See **chrysiasis.**

Chrys·o·my·ia (krĭs′ə-mī′ə, -yə) *n.* A genus of flies that includes species that cause myiasis in humans.

Chry·sops (krī′sŏps′, krĭs′ŏps′) *n.* A genus of biting flies, including the deer fly species and others that transmit diseases to humans and animals.

chrys·o·ther·a·py (krĭs′ə-thĕr′ə-pē) *n.* The treatment of disease by the administration of gold salts.

Chvos·tek's sign (vô′stĕks, кнvô′-) *n.* An indication of tetany in which a unilateral spasm of the oris muscle is initiated by a slight tap over the facial nerve anterior to the external auditory canal.

chyl·an·gi·o·ma (kī-lăn′jē-ō′mə) *n.* A tumor composed of prominent, dilated lacteals and larger intestinal lymphatic vessels.

chyle (kīl) *n.* A turbid, white or pale yellow fluid taken up by the lacteals from the intestine during digestion and carried by the lymphatic system via the thoracic duct into the circulation. —**chy·la′ceous** (kī-lā′shəs), **chy′lous** (kī′ləs) *adj.*

chy·le·mi·a (kī-lē′mē-ə) *n.* The presence of chyle in the blood.

chyle vessel *n.* See **lacteal.**

chy·li·fac·tion (kī′lə-făk′shən) *n.* See **chylopoiesis.** —**chy′li·fac′tive** (-făk′tĭv) *adj.*

chy·lif·er·ous (kī-lĭf′ə-rəs) *adj.* Conveying chyle.

chy·li·fi·ca·tion (kī′lə-fĭ-kā′shən) *n.* See **chylopoiesis.**

chy·li·form (kī′lə-fôrm′) *adj.* Resembling chyle.

chylo– *or* **chyli–** *or* **chyl–** *pref.* Chyle: *chyluria.*

chy·lo·cele (kī′lə-sēl′) *n.* A cystlike lesion resulting from the effusion of chyle into the tunica propria of the vagina or into the cavity of the serous sheath of the testis.

chy·lo·der·ma (kī′lō-dûr′mə) *n.* Swelling of the scrotum as a result of chronic lymphatic obstruction. Also called *elephantiasis scroti.*

chy·lo·me·di·as·ti·num (kī′lō-mē′dē-ə-stī′nəm) *n.* An abnormal presence of chyle in the mediastinum.

chy·lo·mi·cron (kī′lō-mī′krŏn′) *n.* One of the microscopic particles of fat occurring in chyle and in the blood, especially after a meal high in fat.

chy·lo·mi·cro·ne·mi·a (kī′lō-mī′krə-nē′mē-ə) *n.* The presence of chylomicrons, especially an increased number, in the circulating blood.

chy·lo·per·i·car·di·um (kī′lō-pĕr′ĭ-kär′dē-əm) *n.* A milky pericardial effusion resulting from obstruction of the thoracic duct or from trauma.

chy·lo·per·i·to·ne·um (kī′lō-pĕr′ĭ-tn-ē′əm) *n.* See **chylous ascites.**

chy·lo·phor·ic (kī′lə-fôr′ĭk) *adj.* Conveying chyle.

chy·lo·pneu·mo·tho·rax (kī′lō-nōō′mō-thôr′ăks′) *n.* The presence of chyle and air in the pleural space.

chy·lo·poi·e·sis (kī′lō-poi-ē′sĭs) *n.* The formation of chyle in the intestine and its absorption by the lacteals. Also called *chylifaction, chylification.* —**chi′lo·poi·et′ic** (-poi-ĕt′ĭk) *adj.*

chy·lo·sis (kī-lō′sĭs) *n.* The formation of chyle from the food in the intestine, its absorption by the lacteals, and its mixture with the blood and conveyance to the tissues.

chy·lo·tho·rax (kī′lō-thôr′ăks′) *n.* An accumulation of chyle in the thoracic cavity.

chylous ascites *n.* The presence of a milky fluid containing suspended fat in the peritoneal cavity. Also called *chyloperitoneum.*

chy·lu·ri·a (kī-lŏŏr′ē-ə) *n.* The presence of chyle in the urine.

chyme (kīm) *n.* The thick semifluid mass of partly digested food that is passed from the stomach to the duodenum. —**chy′mous** (kī′məs) *adj.*

chy·mi·fi·ca·tion (kī′mə-fĭ-kā′shən) *n.* See **chymo-poiesis.**

chy·mo·pa·pa·in (kī′mō-pə-pā′ĭn, -pī′ĭn) *n.* A prote-olytic enzyme obtained from the fruit of a tropical tree resembling papain; it is used in the treatment of herni-ated intervertebral disks.

chy·mo·poi·e·sis (kī′mō-poi-ē′sĭs) *n.* The conversion of food to chyme, brought about by digestion in the stomach. Also called *chymification.*

chy·mo·sin (kī′mə-sĭn) *n.* See **rennin.**

chy·mo·tryp·sin (kī′mə-trĭp′sĭn) *n.* A pancreatic diges-tive enzyme that catalyzes the hydrolysis of certain pro-teins in the small intestine into polypeptides and amino acids. —**chy′mo·tryp′tic** (-tĭk) *adj.*

chy·mo·tryp·sin·o·gen (kī′mō-trĭp-sĭn′ə-jən, -jĕn′) *n.* A precursor of chymotrypsin in the pancreas.

Ci *abbr.* curie

CI *abbr.* color index

Ci·al·is (sē-ăl′ĭs) A trademark for the drug tadalafil.

CIB *abbr. Latin* cibus (food)

cic·a·trec·to·my (sĭk′ə-trĕk′tə-mē) *n.* The excision of a scar.

cicatricial alopecia *n.* Loss of hair resulting from scar formation that occurs in certain dermatoses.

cicatricial horn *n.* A keratinous growth projecting out-ward from a scar.

cic·a·trix (sĭk′ə-trĭks′, sĭ-kā′trĭks) *n., pl.* **cic·a·tri·ces** (sĭk′ə-trī′sēz, sĭ-kā′trĭ-sēz′) A scar left by the forma-tion of new connective tissue over a healing sore or wound. —**cic′a·tri′cial** (sĭk′ə-trĭsh′əl), **ci·cat′ri·cose′** (sĭ-kăt′rĭ-kōs′) *adj.*

cic·a·tri·zant (sĭk′ə-trī′zənt, sĭ-kăt′rĭ-zənt) *adj.* Causing or promoting cicatrization.

cic·a·tri·za·tion (sĭk′ə-trĭ-zā′shən) *n.* The process of scar formation.

cic·a·trize (sĭk′ə-trīz′) *v.* To heal by forming scar tissue.

ci·clo·pir·ox ol·a·mine (sī′klō-pîr′ŏks′ ô′lə-mēn′, sĭk′-lō-) *n.* A broad-spectrum antifungal agent used in the treatment of a variety of fungal and yeast infections of the skin.

–cide *suff.* **1.** Killer: *bactericide.* **2.** Act of killing: *suicide.*

cig·a·rette drain (sĭg′ə-rĕt′, sĭg′ə-rĕt′) *n.* A drain made of gauze surrounded by a rubber tissue, rubber dam, or rubber tubing.

ci·gua·ter·a (sē′gwə-tĕr′ə) *n.* Poisoning caused by in-gesting fish contaminated with ciguatoxin, character-ized by gastrointestinal and neurological symptoms such as diarrhea, vomiting, tingling, itchiness, and re-versal of temperature perception.

ci·gua·tox·in (sē′gwə-tŏk′sĭn) *n.* A potent neurotoxin that is secreted by various dinoflagellates, especially *Gambierdiscus toxicus,* and can accumulate in the flesh of tropical reef fish, causing ciguatera poisoning if they are eaten.

cili– *pref.* Variant of **cilio–.**

cil·i·a·rot·o·my (sĭl′ē-ə-rŏt′ə-mē) *n.* Surgical division of the ciliary zone of the iris.

cil·i·ar·y (sĭl′ē-ĕr′ē) *adj.* **1.** Of, relating to, or resembling cilia. **2.** Of or relating to the ciliary body and associated structures of the eye.

ciliary artery *n.* **1.** Any of the arteries derived from the muscular branches of the ophthalmic artery, which perforate the anterior part of the sclera and have anas-tomoses with the posterior ciliary arteries; anterior cil-iary artery. **2.** Any of several branches of the oph-thalmic artery distributed to the choroid coat of the eye; short posterior artery. **3.** Either of two branches of the ophthalmic artery to the iris that have anastomoses at the inner and outer margins of the iris; long posterior artery.

ciliary body *n.* A thickened portion of the vascular tunic of the eye located between the choroid and the iris.

ciliary disk *n.* The dark pigmented posterior zone of the ciliary body continuous with the retina at the ora ser-rata. Also called *ciliary ring, pars plana.*

ciliary ganglion *n.* A small parasympathetic ganglion in the orbit behind the eye that receives preganglionic in-nervation through the oculomotor nerve and gives rise to the postganglionic fibers that innervate the ciliary and sphincter muscles of the pupil.

ciliary gland *n.* Any of several modified sudoriferous glands in the margins of the eyelids producing secre-tions that lubricate the eyeball and having ducts that open into the follicles of the eyelashes. Also called *gland of Moll.*

ciliary margin *n.* **1.** The border of the iris that is attached to the ciliary body. **2.** The border of the tarsus of an eyelid.

ciliary movement *n.* The rhythmic sweeping movement characteristic of epithelial cell cilia or ciliate proto-zoans.

ciliary muscle *n.* A smooth muscle of the ciliary body of the eye, consisting of circular fibers and radiating fibers, and whose action changes the shape of the lens in the process of accommodation.

ciliary process *n.* Any of the radiating pigmented ridges on the inner surface of the ciliary body that, with the folds in the furrows between them, constitute the ante-rior portion of the ciliary body.

ciliary reflex *n.* Contraction of the pupil in the accom-modation reflex.

ciliary ring *n.* See **ciliary disk.**

ciliary vein *n.* Any of several small veins, designated an-terior and posterior, coming from the ciliary body of the eye.

ciliary zone *n.* The outer area of the anterior surface of the iris, adjacent to the pupillary zone.

ciliary zonule *n.* Any of a series of delicate meridional fibers arising from the inner surface of the ciliary disk and diverging into two groups that attach to the cap-sule of the eye on the anterior and posterior surfaces of the lens. Also called *suspensory ligament of lens, Zinn's zonule.*

Cil·i·a·ta (sĭl′ē-ā′tə) *n.* A class of protozoans whose members bear cilia or structures derived from them.

cil·i·ate (sĭl′ē-ĭt, -āt′) *n.* Any of various protozoans of the class Ciliata. —*adj.* Ciliated.

cil·i·at·ed (sĭl′ē-ā′tĭd) *adj.* Having cilia.

ciliated epithelium *n.* Epithelium having cilia on the surface not attached to another cell or structure.

cil·i·ec·to·my (sĭl′ē-ĕk′tə-mē) *n.* See **cyclectomy.**

cilio– *or* **cili–** *pref.* Cilia; ciliary: *ciliospinal.*

cil·i·o·ret·i·nal (sĭl′ē-ō-rĕt′n-əl) *adj.* Relating to the cil-iary body and the retina.

cil·i·o·scle·ral (sĭl′ē-ō-sklîr′əl) *adj.* Relating to the ciliary body and the sclera.

cil·i·o·spi·nal (sĭl′ē-ō-spī′nəl) *adj.* Relating to the ciliary body and the spinal cord.

ciliospinal center *n.* The group of preganglionic motor neurons in the first thoracic segment of the spinal cord that become the sympathetic innervation of the dilator muscle of the eye's pupil.

ciliospinal reflex *n.* See **pupillary-skin reflex.**

cil·i·um (sĭl′ē-əm) *n., pl.* **-i·a** (-ē-ə) **1.** See **eyelash** (sense 1). **2.** A microscopic hairlike process extending from the surface of a cell or unicellular organism, capable of rhythmical motion, and acting with other such structures to cause the movement of the cell or of the surrounding medium.

cil·lo·sis (sĭ-lō′sĭs) *n.* Spasmodic twitching of an eyelid.

ci·met·i·dine (sĭ-mĕt′ĭ-dēn′, -dĭn′) *n.* A histamine antagonist used to treat peptic ulcer and hypersecretory conditions by inhibiting gastric acid secretion.

cin·cho·na (sĭng-kō′nə, sĭn-chō′-) *n.* **1.** Any of several trees and shrubs of the genus *Cinchona,* native chiefly to the Andes and cultivated for bark that yields the medicinal alkaloids quinine and quinidine. **2.** The dried bark of any of these plants.

cin·cho·nine (sĭng′kə-nēn′, sĭn′chə-) *n.* An alkaloid derived from the bark of various cinchona trees and used as an antimalarial agent.

cine– *or* **cin–** *pref.* Motion picture: *cineangiography.*

cin·e·an·gio·car·di·og·ra·phy (sĭn′ē-ăn′jē-ō-kär′dē-ŏg′rə-fē) *n.* The use of a movie camera to film the passage of a contrast medium through chambers of the heart and great vessels for diagnostic purposes.

cin·e·an·gi·og·ra·phy (sĭn′ē-ăn′jē-ŏg′rə-fē) *n.* The use of a movie camera to film the passage of a contrast medium through blood vessels for diagnostic purposes.

cin·e·fluo·rog·ra·phy (sĭn′ē-flŏŏ-rŏg′rə-fē, -flô-) *n.* The use of a movie camera to obtain fluoroscopic views, especially of the heart and great vessels or gastrointestinal tract, after the administration of a contrast medium.

ci·ne·plas·tic amputation (sĭn′ə-plăs′tĭk) *n.* Surgical removal of an extremity in which the muscles and tendons in the stump are arranged so that they can perform independent movements and communicate motion to a specially constructed prosthetic apparatus. Also called *cineplastics.*

cin·e·ra·di·og·ra·phy (sĭn′ē-ā′dē-ŏg′rə-fē) *n.* The use of a movie camera to film an organ in motion.

ci·ne·re·a (sĭ-nîr′ē-ə) *n.* The gray matter of the brain and other parts of nervous system. —**ci·ne′re·al** *adj.*

cin·gu·late (sĭng′gyə-lāt′, -lĭt) *adj.* Of or relating to a cingulum.

cingulate gyrus *n.* A long curved convolution of the medial surface of the cortical hemisphere, arched over the corpus callosum from which it is separated by the deep sulcus of the corpus callosum. Also called *callosal gyrus.*

cingulate sulcus *n.* A fissure on the mesial surface of the cerebral hemisphere, bounding the upper surface of the cingulate gyrus, curving up to the superomedial margin of the hemisphere, and bordering the paracentral lobule posteriorly.

cin·gu·lec·to·my (sĭng′gyə-lĕk′tə-mē) *n.* Surgical removal of a portion of the cingulate gyrus.

cin·gu·lot·o·my (sĭng′gyə-lŏt′ə-mē) *n.* Electrolytic destruction of the cortex and white matter of the cingulate gyrus and the anterior corpus callosum.

cin·gu·lum (sĭng′gyə-ləm) *n., pl.* **-la** (-lə) **1.** A structure that has the form of a belt or girdle. **2.** A well-marked fiber bundle passing longitudinally in the white matter of the cingulate gyrus, composed largely of fibers from the anterior thalamic nucleus to the cingulate and parahippocampal gyri.

Cip·ro (sĭp′rō) A trademark for ciprofloxacin and its hydrochloride derivative.

Cip·ro·dex (sĭp′rō-dĕks′) A trademark for a combination of the drugs ciprofloxacin and dexamethasone.

cip·ro·flox·a·cin (sĭp′rō-flŏk′sə-sĭn) *n.* A synthetic broad-spectrum antibiotic of the fluoroquinolone class, used also in its hydrochloride form.

circa (sûr′kə) *prep. Abbr.* **ca** In approximately; about.

cir·ca·di·an (sər-kā′dē-ən, -kăd′ē-, sûr′kə-dī′ən, -dē′-) *adj.* Relating to biological variations or rhythms with a cycle of about 24 hours.

circadian rhythm *n.* A daily rhythmic activity cycle, based on 24-hour intervals, that is exhibited by many organisms.

cir·ci·nate (sûr′sə-nāt′) *adj.* Circular; ring-shaped.

circinate retinopathy *n.* Retinal degeneration, usually bilateral, characterized by sharply defined white exudates encircling a grayish macula. Also called *circinate retinitis.*

cir·cle (sûr′kəl) *n.* **1.** A ring-shaped structure or group of structures. **2.** A line or process with every point equidistant from the center.

circle absorption anesthesia *n.* Inhalation anesthesia in which a circuit with carbon dioxide absorbent is used for the complete or partial rebreathing of exhaled gases.

circle of Wil·lis (wĭl′ĭs) *n.* A roughly circular anastomosis that is located at the base of the brain and formed by the anterior communicating artery, the two anterior cerebral, the two internal carotid, the two posterior communicating, and the two posterior cerebral arteries.

cir·cu·lar amputation (sûr′kyə-lər) *n.* Amputation performed by making a circular incision through the skin, higher up through the muscles, and continuing even higher through the bone but staying vertical to the long axis of the limb.

circular fold *n.* Any of the numerous folds of the mucous membrane of the small intestine, running transversely for about two thirds of the circumference of the gut.

circular sinus *n.* **1.** A venous sinus at the periphery of the placenta. **2.** See **venous sinus of sclera.**

cir·cu·la·tion (sûr′kyə-lā′shən) *n.* Movement in a circle or circuit, especially the movement of blood through bodily vessels as a result of the heart's pumping action.

cir·cu·la·to·ry (sûr′kyə-lə-tôr′ē) *n.* **1.** Relating to circulation. **2.** Relating to the circulatory system.

circulatory system *n.* The system of structures, consisting of the heart, blood vessels, and lymphatics, by which blood and lymph are circulated throughout the body. Also called *vascular system.*

cir·cu·lus (sûr′kyə-ləs) *n.*, *pl.* **–li** (-lī′) **1.** A ringlike or circular structure. **2.** A circle formed by connecting arteries, veins, or nerves.

circum– *pref.* Around; about: *circumduction.*

cir·cum·a·nal gland (sûr′kəm-ā′nəl) *n.* Any of several sebaceous and apocrine sweat glands situated in the skin surrounding the anus.

cir·cum·cise (sûr′kəm-sīz′) *v.* To perform a circumcision.

cir·cum·ci·sion (sûr′kəm-sĭzh′ən) *n.* **1.** The surgical removal of part or all of the prepuce. Also called *peritomy.* **2.** The cutting around an anatomical part.

cir·cum·duc·tion (sûr′kəm-dŭk′shən) *n.* Movement of a part in a circular direction.

cir·cum·fer·en·tial fibrocartilage (sər-kŭm′fə-rĕn′-shəl) *n.* A ring of fibrocartilage surrounding the articular end of a bone and serving to deepen the joint cavity.

circumferential lamella *n.* A bony layer that underlies the periosteum or endosteum.

cir·cum·flex (sûr′kəm-flĕks′) *adj.* **1.** Curving or bending around. **2.** Bowed.

circumflex artery of thigh *n.* **1.** An artery with origin in the deep artery of the thigh, with distribution to the hip joint and thigh muscles, and with anastomoses to the medial circumflex femoral, inferior gluteal, superior gluteal, and popliteal arteries; lateral circumflex artery of the thigh. **2.** An artery with origin in the deep artery of the thigh, with distribution to the hip joint and muscles of the thigh, and with anastomoses to the inferior gluteal, superior gluteal, and lateral circumflex femoral arteries; medial circumflex artery of the thigh.

circumflex femoral vein *n.* **1.** Any of the veins that accompany the lateral circumflex femoral artery; lateral circumflex femoral vein. **2.** Any of the veins that parallel the medial circumflex femoral artery; medial circumflex femoral vein.

circumflex humeral artery *n.* **1.** An artery with origin in the axillary artery, with distribution to the shoulder joint and biceps muscle, and with anastomoses to the posterior circumflex humeral artery; anterior circumflex humeral artery. **2.** An artery with origin in the axillary artery, with distribution to the shoulder joint and muscles and with anastomoses to the anterior circumflex humeral, suprascapular, thoracoacromials, and deep brachial arteries; posterior circumflex humeral artery.

circumflex iliac artery *n.* **1.** An artery with origin in the external iliac artery, with distribution to the muscles and skin of the lower abdomen, the sartorius muscle, and the tensor muscle of the broad fascia; and with anastomoses to the lumbar, epigastric, gluteal, iliolumbar, and superficial circumflex iliac arteries; deep circumflex iliac arterty. **2.** An artery with origin in the femoral artery, with distribution to inguinal lymph nodes and integument, to the sartorius muscle and the tensor muscle of the broad fascia, and with anastomoses to the deep circumflex iliac artery; superficial circumflex iliac artery.

circumflex iliac vein *n.* **1.** A vein that corresponds to the deep circumflex iliac artery and empties near or in a common trunk with the inferior epigastric vein into the external iliac vein; deep circumflex iliac vein. **2.** A vein that corresponds to the superficial circumflex iliac artery and empties usually into the greater saphenous vein; superficial circumflex iliac vein.

circumflex scapular artery *n.* An artery with its origin in the subscapular artery, with distribution to the muscles of the shoulder and shoulder blade, and with anastomoses to the branches of the suprascapular and transverse cervical arteries.

cir·cum·scribed (sûr′kəm-skrībd′) *adj.* Bounded by a line; limited or confined.

circumscribed myxedema *n.* Nodules and plaques of mucoid edema of the skin, usually in the pretibial region, occurring in some patients with hyperthyroidism. Also called *pretibial myxedema.*

circumscribed scleroderma *n.* See **morphea.**

cir·cum·stan·ti·al·i·ty (sûr′kəm-stăn′shē-ăl′ĭ-tē) *n.* A disturbance in the thought process by detail that is often tangential and irrelevant.

cir·cum·val·late (sûr′kəm-văl′āt′) *adj.* Surrounded by a ridge or wall-like structure.

circumvallate papilla *n.* See **vallate papilla.**

cir·cum·ven·tric·u·lar organ (sûr′kəm-vĕn-trĭk′yə-lər) *n.* Any of the structures in or near the base of the brain that differ from normal brain tissue in having capillaries that lack the usual blood-brain barrier and thus are not isolated from certain compounds in the blood.

cir·cum·vo·lute (sûr′kəm-vō′lōot′) *adj.* Rolled about; twisted around.

cir·rhog·e·nous (sĭ-rŏj′ə-nəs) *or* **cir·rho·gen·ic** (sĭr′ə-jĕn′ĭk) *adj.* Tending to produce cirrhosis.

cir·rho·sis (sĭ-rō′sĭs) *n.* **1.** A chronic disease of the liver characterized by the replacement of normal tissue with fibrous tissue and the loss of functional liver cells. It can result from alcohol abuse, nutritional deprivation, or infection, especially by the hepatitis virus. **2.** Chronic interstitial inflammation of any tissue or organ. Also called *fibroid induration.* **—cir·rhot′ic** (-rŏt′-ĭk) *adj.*

cir·sec·to·my (sər-sĕk′tə-mē) *n.* Excision of a section of a varicose vein.

cir·soid (sûr′soid′) *adj.* Resembling a dilated vein.

cirsoid aneurysm *n.* Dilation of a group of blood vessels due to congenital malformation with arteriovenous shunting. Also called *racemose aneurysm.*

cis (sĭs) *adj.* Having two mutations on two genes on the same chromosome of a homologous pair.

cis– *pref.* Having a pair of identical atoms or groups on the same side of a plane that passes through two carbon atoms linked by a double bond: cis-*butene.*

cis-ac·o·nit·ic acid (sĭs′ăk′ə-nĭt′ĭk) *n.* An intermediate in the tricarboxylic acid cycle produced by the dehydration of citric acid.

cis·plat·in (sĭs-plăt′n) *n.* A platinum-containing chemotherapeutic drug used to treat metastatic ovarian or testicular cancers and advanced bladder cancer. Also called *cisplatinum.*

cis·plat·i·num (sĭs-plăt′n-əm) *n.* See **cisplatin.**

cis·tern (sĭs′tərn) *n.* A cisterna.

cis·ter·na (sĭ-stûr′nə) *n.*, *pl.* **–nae** (-nē′) **1.** A cavity or enclosed space serving as a reservoir, especially for chyle, lymph, or cerebrospinal fluid. **2.** An ultramicroscopic space or channel occurring between the membranes of the flattened sacs of the endoplasmic reticulum, the Golgi complex, or the two membranes of the nuclear envelope. —**cis·ter′nal** *adj.*

cisternal puncture *n.* Passage of a hollow needle through the posterior atlanto-occipital membrane into the cerebellomedullary cistern.

cis·ter·nog·ra·phy (sĭs′tər-nŏg′rə-fē) *n.* The radiographic study of the basal cisterns of the brain after the introduction of an opaque contrast medium.

cis·tron (sĭs′trŏn′) *n.* The smallest functional unit of heredity; a length of chromosomal DNA associated with a single biochemical function and essentially equivalent to a gene. —**cis·tron′ic** *adj.*

ci·tal·o·pram hy·dro·bro·mide (sĭ-tăl′ō-prăm′ hī′drō-brō′mīd′) *n.* A drug of the SSRI class that is used primarily to treat depression.

cit·rate (sĭt′rāt′) *n.* A salt or ester of citric acid.

cit·ric acid (sĭt′rĭk) *n.* A colorless translucent crystalline acid principally derived by fermentation of carbohydrates; an intermediate in metabolism.

citric acid cycle *n.* See **Krebs cycle.**

citrovorum factor *n.* See **folinic acid.**

cit·rul·line (sĭt′rə-lēn′) *n.* An amino acid produced as an intermediate in the conversion of ornithine to arginine during urea formation in the liver.

cit·rul·li·ne·mi·a (sĭt′rə-lə-nē′mē-ə, sĭ-trŭl′ə-) *n.* A disease of amino acid metabolism in which there are elevated levels of citrulline in the blood, urine, and cerebrospinal fluid; it is manifested clinically by vomiting, ammonia intoxication, and mental retardation beginning in infancy.

cit·rul·li·nu·ri·a (sĭt′rə-lə-no͞or′ē-ə, sĭ-trŭl′ə-) *n.* Enhanced urinary excretion of citrulline; a manifestation of citrullinemia.

CJD *abbr.* Creutzfeldt-Jakob disease

Cl The symbol for the element **chlorine.**

CL (sē-ĕl) *n.* A bipolar lead of an electrocardiograph that has electrodes attached to chest and left arm.

clad·o·spo·ri·o·sis (klăd′ə-spôr′ē-ō′sĭs) *n.* Infection with a fungus of the genus *Cladosporium.*

Clad·o·spo·ri·um (klăd′ə-spôr′ē-əm) *n.* A genus of fungi commonly isolated in soil or plant residues including some species that cause abscesses of the brain or lungs or lesions on the skin.

Claf·o·ran (klăf′ər-ĭn) A trademark for the drug cefotaxime sodium.

clair·voy·ance (klâr-voi′əns) *n.* The perception of objects or events that cannot be perceived by the senses.

clamp (klămp) *n.* An instrument for the compression or grasping of a structure.

clamp forceps *n.* A forceps with pronged jaws designed to engage the jaws of a rubber dam clamp so that they may be separated to pass over the widest buccolingual contour of a tooth.

clang association (klăng) *n.* Psychic associations resulting from sounds, often observed in the manic phase of manic-depressive psychosis.

clap (klăp) *n.* Gonorrhea. Often used with *the.*

Clap·ton's line (klăp′tənz) *n.* A greenish discoloration of the dental margin of the gums occurring in chronic copper poisoning.

cla·rif·i·cant (klə-rĭf′ĭ-kənt) *n.* An agent that clears a turbid liquid.

cla·rith·ro·my·cin (klə-rĭth′rə-mī′sĭn) *n.* A macrolide antibiotic used primarily to treat bacterial respiratory infections.

Clar·i·tin (klâr′ĭ-tn) A trademark for the drug loratadine.

Clarke-Had·field syndrome (klärk′hăd′fēld′) *n.* See **cystic fibrosis.**

Clark's level (klärks) *n.* Any of four levels that mark the invasion of malignant melanoma through the skin layers to the subcutaneous fat layer, each successive level indicating a worsening prognosis.

Clark's weight rule *n.* A rule for determining the approximate dose of medicine appropriate for a child two years of age or older by dividing the child's weight in pounds by 150 and multiplying the result by the adult dose.

clasp (klăsp) *n.* A part of a removable partial denture that directly retains or stabilizes a denture.

clasp-knife spasticity *n.* Rigidity of the extensor muscles of a joint that gives resistance to passive flexion but gives way abruptly to allow easy flexion, resulting from an exaggeration of the stretch reflex. Also called *clasp-knife rigidity.*

class (klăs) *n.* A taxonomic category ranking below a phylum or division and above an order.

clas·si·fi·ca·tion (klăs′ə-fĭ-kā′shən) *n.* **1.** A systematic arrangement into classes or groups. **2.** The systematic grouping of organisms into categories on the basis of evolutionary or structural relationships between them; taxonomy.

clas·tic (klăs′tĭk) *adj.* **1.** Breaking up into pieces or exhibiting a tendency to break or divide. **2.** Separable into parts or having removable sections, as an anatomical model.

clas·to·gen·ic (klăs′tə-jĕn′ĭk) *adj.* Capable of causing breakage of chromosomes.

clas·to·thrix (klăs′tə-thrĭks′) *n.* See **trichorrhexis nodosa.**

clath·rate (klăth′rāt′) *adj.* **1.** Having a latticelike structure or appearance. **2.** Of or relating to inclusion complexes in a chemical compound in which molecules of one substance are completely enclosed within the crystal structure of another. —*n.* A clathrate compound, such as urea.

Claude (klōd), **Albert** 1899–1983. Belgian-born American biologist who was among the first to use the electron microscope for biological research. He shared a 1974 Nobel Prize for developing methods of separating and analyzing cell components.

clau·di·ca·tion (klô′dĭ-kā′shən) *n.* **1.** A halt or lameness in a person's walk; a limp. **2.** See **intermittent claudication.**

clau·di·ca·to·ry (klô′dĭ-kə-tôr′ē) *adj.* Relating to claudication, especially intermittent claudication.

claus·tro·pho·bi·a (klô′strə-fō′bē-ə) *n.* An abnormal fear of being in narrow or enclosed spaces. —**claus′tro·phobe′** *n.* —**claus′tro·pho′bic** *adj.*

claus·trum (klô′strəm) *n.*, *pl.* **–tra** (-trə) Any of several anatomical structures resembling a barrier, especially a thin vertical lamina of gray matter of the brain lying close to the outer portion of the lenticular nucleus, from which it is separated by the external capsule. —**claus′tral** *adj.*

clav·i·cle (klăv′ĭ-kəl) *n*. Either of two slender bones that extend from the manubrium of the sternum to the acromion of the scapula. Also called *collarbone*. —**cla·vic′u·lar** (klə-vĭk′yə-lər) *adj*. —**cla·vic·u·late′** (-lāt′) *adj*.

clav·i·cot·o·my (klăv′ĭ-kŏt′ə-mē) *n*. Surgical division of the clavicle.

clav·i·pec·to·ral fascia (klăv′ə-pĕk′tər-əl) *n*. A fascia that extends between the coracoid process, the clavicle, and the thoracic wall, envelops the subclavian and the smaller pectoral mucles, and forms a strong membrane in the interval between them.

clav·u·lan·ic acid (klăv′yo͞o-lăn′ĭk) *n*. A drug that inhibits the action of beta-lactamase produced by bacteria, thereby counteracting bacterial resistance to beta-lactam antibiotics.

cla·vus (klā′vəs, klä′-) *n*., *pl*. **–vi** (-vī′) **1.** See **corn. 2.** A condition resulting from healing of a granuloma of the foot in yaws, in which a core falls out, leaving an erosion.

claw foot (klô) *n*. A deformity of the foot marked by an exaggerated arch and downward flexion of the toes.

claw·hand *or* **claw hand** *n*. Atrophy of the interosseous muscles of the hand with hyperextension of the joints of the metacarpus and flexion of the fingers.

clear·ance (klîr′əns) *n*. The removal of a substance from the blood, expressed as the volume of blood or plasma cleared of the substance per unit time.

clear cell (klîr) *n*. A cell, especially a neoplastic one, containing abundant glycogen or other material that is not stained by hematoxylin or eosin, so that the cytoplasm appears clear histologically.

clear·ing factor (klîr′ĭng) *n*. Any of the lipoprotein lipases that appear in plasma during lipemia and catalyze the hydrolysis of triglycerides bound to protein when an acceptor such as serum albumin is present.

clear layer of epidermis *n*. The layer of the epidermis just beneath the stratum corneum, consisting of two or three layers of flat clear cells with atrophied nuclei. Also called *stratum lucidum.*

cleav·age (klē′vĭj) *n*. **1.** A series of cell divisions in the ovum immediately following fertilization. Also called *segmentation.* **2.** The splitting of a complex molecule into two or more simpler molecules. Also called *scission.* **3.** The linear clefts in the skin, indicating the general direction of the fibers in the dermis.

cleavage cavity *n*. See **blastocoel.**

cleavage division *n*. The rapid mitotic division of a zygote with decrease in size of individual cells or blastomeres and the formation of a morula.

cleavage line *n*. Any of the various linear openings that occur when a pin is driven into the skin of a cadaver, whose appearance depends on the axis of orientation of the subcutaneous connective tissue fibers and whose direction varies with the region of the body surface.

cleavage product *n*. Any of the various substances resulting from the splitting of a complex molecule into two or more simpler molecules.

cleavage site *n*. See **restriction site.**

cleavage spindle *n*. The spindle formed during the cleavage of a zygote or its blastomeres.

cleft (klĕft) *n*. A split or fissure between two parts.

cleft hand *n*. A congenital deformity in which the division between the fingers, especially between the third and fourth fingers, extends into the metacarpal region. Also called *split hand.*

cleft lip *n*. A congenital facial deformity of the lip, usually the upper lip, due to a mesodermal deficiency or to a failure of merging in one or more of the embryologic processes that form the lip; it is frequently associated with cleft tooth socket and cleft palate. Also called *cheiloschisis, harelip.*

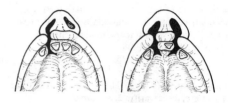

cleft lip
Left: *unilateral cleft lip*
Right: *bilateral cleft lip*

cleft palate *n*. A congenital fissure in the roof of the mouth, resulting from incomplete fusion of the palate during embryonic development. It may involve only the uvula or extend through the entire palate. Also called *palatoschisis.*

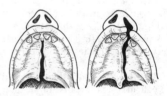

cleft palate
Left: *cleft palate*
Right: *unilateral cleft palate and lip*

cleft spine *n*. See **spondyloschisis.**

cleft tongue *n*. See **bifid tongue.**

clei·dal *or* **cli·dal** (klīd′l) *adj*. Relating to the clavicle.

cleido– *or* **cleid–** *or* **clido–** *or* **clid–** *pref*. Clavicle; clavicular: *cleidocranial.*

clei·do·cos·tal *or* **cli·do·cos·tal** (klī′dō-kŏs′təl) *adj*. Relating to the clavicle and a rib.

clei·do·cra·ni·al *or* **cli·do·cra·ni·al** (klī′dō-krā′nē-əl) *adj*. Relating to the clavicle and the cranium.

cleidocranial dysostosis *or* **clidocranial dysostosis** *n*. A congenital complex that may be hereditary and is characterized by absent or rudimentary development of the clavicles, an enlarged incompletely ossified skull with frontal protuberances, and poor tooth formation. Also called *cleidocranial dysplasia, craniocleidodysostosis.*

–cleisis *or* **–clisis** *suff*. Closure; occlusion: *corecleisis.*

clem·a·stine fumarate (klĕm′ə-stēn′) *n*. An antihistamine used primarily to treat allergic rhinitis and allergic skin disorders.

clenched fist sign (klĕncht) *n*. An indication of the pain of angina pectoris in which an individual presses a clenched fist against the chest as a means of showing its constricting, pressing quality.

Cle·o·cin (klē′ə-sĭn) A trademark for the drug clindamycin.

click (klĭk) *n.* A slight sharp sound, such as that heard from the heart during systole.

cli·ent-cen·tered therapy (klī′ənt-sĕn′tərd) *n.* A system of psychotherapy based on the assumption that the patient has the internal resources to improve and is in the best position to resolve his or her own personality dysfunction.

cli·mac·ter·ic (klī-măk′tər-ĭk, klī′măk-tĕr′ĭk) *n.* **1.** See **menopause. 2.** See **perimenopause. 3.** The period in a man's life corresponding to female menopause, characterized by decreased libido.

cli·mat·ic bubo (klī-măt′ĭk) *n.* See **venereal lymphogranuloma.**

cli·max (klī′măks′) *n.* **1.** The height of a disease; the stage of greatest severity. **2.** See **orgasm.**

clin– *pref.* Variant of **clino–.**

clin·da·my·cin (klĭn′də-mī′sĭn) *n.* A semisynthetic antibiotic derived from lincomycin, active against gram-positive bacteria.

clin·ic (klĭn′ĭk) *n.* **1.** A facility, often associated with a hospital or medical school, that is devoted to the diagnosis and care of outpatients. **2.** A medical establishment that is run by several specialists working in cooperation and sharing the same facilities. **3.** A group session offering counsel or instruction in a particular field or activity. **4.** A seminar or meeting of physicians and medical students in which medical instruction is conducted in the presence of the patient, as at the bedside. **5.** A place where such instruction occurs. **6.** A class or lecture of medical instruction conducted in this manner.

clin·i·cal (klĭn′ĭ-kəl) *adj.* **1.** Relating to the bedside treatment of a patient or to the course of the disease. **2.** Relating to the observed symptoms and course of a disease.

clinical depression *n.* See **depression** (sense 7).

clinical diagnosis *n.* Diagnosis based on a study of the signs and symptoms of a disease.

clinical genetics *n.* The study of the possible genetic determinants affecting the occurrence of diseases and disorders.

clinical medicine *n.* The study and practice of medicine based on direct observation of patients.

clinical nurse specialist *n.* A nurse who has advanced knowledge and competence in a particular area of nursing practice, such as in cardiology, oncology, or psychiatry.

clinical pathology *n.* **1.** The practice of pathology as it pertains to the care of patients. **2.** The subspecialty in pathology concerned with the theoretical and technical aspects of laboratory technology that pertain to the diagnosis and prevention of disease.

clinical psychology *n.* The branch of psychology that studies and treats emotional or behavioral disorders.

clinical spectrometry *n.* See **biospectrometry.**

clinical spectroscopy *n.* See **biospectroscopy.**

clinical thermometer *n.* A thermometer having a graduated glass tube with a bulb containing a liquid, typically mercury or colored alcohol, that expands and rises in the tube as the temperature increases.

clinical trial *n.* A research study using consenting human subjects that tests the effectiveness and safety of a treatment, a diagnostic tool, or a prophylactic intervention.

cli·ni·cian (klĭ-nĭsh′ən) *n.* A physician, psychologist, or psychiatrist specializing in the treatment of patients, not in other areas such as research.

clin·i·co·path·o·log·ic (klĭn′ĭ-kō-păth′ə-lŏj′ĭk) *adj.* Relating to the signs and symptoms that are observed in a patient, in conjunction with the results of laboratory examination.

clino– *or* **clin–** *pref.* Slope; slant: *clinocephaly.*

cli·no·ceph·a·ly (klī′nō-sĕf′ə-lē) *n.* Concavity of the upper surface of the skull, causing a saddle-shaped appearance in profile. Also called *saddle head.*

cli·no·dac·ty·ly (klī′nō-dăk′tə-lē) *n.* Permanent deflection of one or more fingers.

cli·noid process (klī′noid′) *n.* Any of three pairs of bony projections, designated anterior, middle, and superior, from the sphenoid bone.

Clin·o·ril (klĭn′ə-rĭl) A trademark for the drug sulindac.

cli·no·scope (klī′nə-skōp′) *n.* An instrument for measuring cyclophoria in the eyes.

clip (klĭp) *n.* A fastener used in surgery to hold skin or other tissue in position or to control hemorrhage.

clip forceps *n.* A small forceps with a spring catch to hold a bleeding vessel.

–clisis *suff.* Variant of **–cleisis.**

clith·ro·pho·bi·a (klĭth′rə-fō′bē-ə) *n.* An abnormal fear of being locked in.

clit·o·ri·dec·to·my (klĭt′ər-ĭ-dĕk′tə-mē, klī′tər-) *n.* Excision of the clitoris.

clit·o·ri·di·tis (klĭt′ər-ĭ-dī′tĭs, klī′tər-) *or* **clit·o·ri·tis** (klĭt′ə-rī′tĭs, klī′tə-) *n.* Inflammation of the clitoris.

clit·o·ris (klĭt′ər-ĭs, klī′tər-) *n., pl.* **cli·to·ri·des** (klĭ-tôr′ĭ-dēz′) A small erectile body situated at the anterior portion of the vulva and projecting between the branched extremities of the labia minora forming its prepuce and frenulum.

clit·o·rism (klĭt′ə-rĭz′əm, klī′tə-) *n.* Prolonged and usually painful erection of the clitoris.

clit·o·ro·meg·a·ly (klĭt′ə-rō-mĕg′ə-lē) *n.* An enlarged clitoris.

cli·vus (klī′vəs) *n., pl.* **–vi** (-vī′) A downward-sloping surface.

CLL *abbr.* chronic lymphocytic leukemia

clo·a·ca (klō-ā′kə) *n.* **1.** In early embryos, the entodermally lined chamber into which the hindgut and allantois empty. **2.** The common cavity into which the intestinal, genital, and urinary tracts open in vertebrates such as fish, reptiles, birds, and some mammals. **3.** An opening in a diseased bone containing a fragment of dead bone. **—clo·a′cal** (-kəl) *adj.*

cloacal membrane *n.* A transitory membrane in the caudal area of the ventral wall of the embryo, forming a temporary barrier between the hindgut and the exterior.

cloacal plate *n.* A structure in the embryo composed of endoderm and ectoderm that ruptures and forms the anal and urogenital openings.

clo·fi·brate (klō-fī′brāt, -fíb′rāt) *n.* A synthetic drug formerly prescribed to reduce abnormally elevated levels of plasma cholesterol and triglyceride.

Clo·mid (klō′mĭd) A trademark for the drug clomiphene.

clom·i·phene (klŏm′ə-fēn, klō′mə-) *n.* A synthetic drug that is used to stimulate ovulation.

clo·mip·ra·mine (klō-mĭp′rə-mēn′) *n.* A tricyclic antidepressant drug, used in the form of its hydrochloride to treat anxiety and obsessive-compulsive disorder.

clonal selection theory *n.* The theory that the mutation of stem cells produces all possible templates for antibody production and that exposure to a specific antigen selectively stimulates the proliferation of the cell with the appropriate template to form a clone or colony of specific antibody-forming cells.

clo·naz·e·pam (klō-năz′ə-păm′) *n.* A benzodiazepine used as an anticonvulsant for epilepsy and as a sedative for sleep disorders.

clone (klōn) *n.* **1.** A cell, group of cells, or organism descended from and genetically identical to a single common ancestor, such as a bacterial colony whose members arose from a single original cell. **2.** An organism descended asexually from a single ancestor, such as a plant produced by layering or a polyp produced by budding. **3.** A DNA sequence, such as a gene, that is transferred from one organism to another and replicated by genetic engineering techniques. —*v.* **1.** To make multiple identical copies of a DNA sequence. **2.** To create or propagate an organism from a clone cell: **3.** To establish and maintain pure lineages of a cell under laboratory conditions. **4.** To reproduce or propagate asexually. —**clon′al** (klō′nəl) *adj.*

clon·ic (klŏn′ĭk, klō′nĭk) *adj.* Of the nature of clonus, marked by contraction and relaxation of muscle.

clonic convulsion *n.* A convulsion in which the muscles alternately contract and relax.

clo·nic·i·ty (klō-nĭs′ĭ-tē, klŏ-) *n.* The state of being clonic.

clon·i·co·ton·ic (klŏn′ĭ-kō-tŏn′ĭk) *adj.* Both clonic and tonic. Used of certain forms of muscular spasm.

clonic spasm *n.* Alternate involuntary contraction and relaxation of a muscle.

clon·i·dine (klŏn′ĭ-dēn′, klō′nĭ-) *n.* A synthetic drug used in the treatment of hypertension and for the prevention of migraine headaches.

clon·ing (klō′nĭng) *n.* The transplantation of a nucleus from a somatic cell into an ovum, which then develops into an embryo.

cloning vector *n.* An autonomously replicating plasmid having regions into which foreign DNA can be inserted.

clo·nism (klō′nĭz′əm, klŏn′ĭz′-) *n.* A succession of clonic spasms.

clo·no·gen·ic (klō′nə-jĕn′ĭk) *adj.* Arising from or consisting of a clone.

clo·nor·chi·a·sis (klō′nôr-kī′ə-sĭs) *n.* A disease caused by infestation with *Clonorchis sinensis* that affects the distal bile ducts after transmission by ingestion of raw, smoked, or undercooked fish.

Clo·nor·chis si·nen·sis (klō-nôr′kĭs sə-nĕn′sĭs) *n.* A trematode worm that causes clonorchiasis in humans; the Oriental liver fluke.

clo·nus (klō′nəs) *n.,* *pl.* **–nus·es** A form of movement marked by contractions and relaxations of a muscle, occurring in rapid succession, after forcible extension or flexion of a part. Also called *clonospasm.*

Clo·quet's hernia (klō-kāz′, klô-) *n.* A femoral hernia perforating the aponeurosis of the pectineus muscle.

closed anesthesia (klōzd) *n.* Inhalation anesthesia in which there is complete rebreathing of all exhaled gases, except for carbon dioxide, which is removed by the anesthetic apparatus.

closed chain compound *n.* See cyclic compound.

closed chest massage *n.* Cardiac massage in which pressure is applied over the sternum.

closed circuit method *n.* A method for measuring oxygen consumption in which an initial quantity of oxygen is rebreathed through a carbon dioxide absorber and any decrease in the volume of oxygen taken in is noted.

closed comedo *n.* See whitehead (sense 1).

closed dislocation *n.* A dislocation not complicated by an external wound. Also called *simple dislocation.*

closed drainage *n.* The use of a water- or air-tight system to drain a body cavity.

closed fracture *n.* A bone fracture that causes little or no damage to the surrounding soft tissues. Also called *simple fracture.*

closed head injury *n.* A head injury in which the scalp and mucous membranes remain unbroken.

closed hospital *n.* A hospital in which only physicians who are members of the attending and consulting staff may admit and treat patients.

closed reduction *n.* Reduction of a fractured bone by manipulation without incision into the skin.

closed surgery *n.* Surgery performed without an incision into skin, as in a closed reduction.

clos·ing snap (klō′zĭng) *n.* The accentuated first heart sound of mitral stenosis, related to closure of the abnormal valve.

closing volume *n.* The amount of air in the lungs at which the flow from the lower sections of the lungs becomes severely reduced or halts altogether during expiration.

clos·trid·i·al (klŏ-strĭd′ē-əl) *adj.* Relating to a bacterium of the genus *Clostridium.*

Clos·trid·i·um (klŏ-strĭd′ē-əm) *n.* A genus of rod-shaped, spore-forming, chiefly anaerobic bacteria including the nitrogen-fixing bacteria found in soil and those causing botulism and tetanus.

Clostridium bi·fer·men·tans (bī′fər-mĕn′tănz′) *n.* A bacterium found in putrid meat and gaseous gangrene, and in soil, feces, and sewage.

Clostridium bot·u·li·num (bŏch′ə-lī′nəm) *n.* A bacterium that occurs widely in nature and is a cause of botulism; its six main types, A to F, are characterized by antigenically distinct but pharmacologically similar, very potent neurotoxins.

Clostridium his·to·lyt·i·cum (hĭs′tə-lĭt′ĭ-kəm) *n.* A bacterium found in wounds, where it induces necrosis of tissue by producing a cytolytic exotoxin.

Clostridium no·vy·i (nō'vē-ī') *n.* A bacterium consisting of three types: A, B, and C; type A causes gaseous gangrene and necrotic hepatitis.

Clostridium par·a·bot·u·li·num (păr'ə-bŏch'ə-lī'nəm) *n.* A bacterium that produces a powerful exotoxin and is pathogenic to humans; it was formerly classified as *Clostridium botulinum* types A and B.

Clostridium per·frin·gens (pər-frĭn'jənz) *or* **Clostridium welchii** (wĕl'chē-ī') *n.* Gas bacillus.

Clostridium tet·a·ni (tĕt'ə-nī') *n.* A bacterium that causes tetanus.

clo·sure principle (klō'zhər) *n.* In psychology, the principle that, when one views fragmentary stimuli forming a nearly complete figure, one tends to ignore the missing parts and perceive the figure as whole.

clot (klŏt) *n.* A soft, nonrigid, insoluble mass formed when blood or lymph gels. —*v.* To coagulate.

clo·trim·a·zole (klō-trĭm'ə-zōl') *n.* A broad-spectrum antifungal drug that is used topically to treat a variety of superficial fungal infections, including candidiasis and tinea.

clot·tage (klŏt'ĭj) *n.* The blocking of a canal or duct by a blood clot.

clot·ting factor (klŏt'ĭng) *n.* Any of various plasma components involved in the clotting of blood, including fibrinogen, prothrombin, thromboplastin, and calcium ion. Also called *coagulation factor.*

cloud·y swelling (klou'dē) *n.* A degenerative change in cells, in which the cells swell due to injury to the membranes affecting ionic transfer, causing the cytoplasm to appear cloudy and water to accumulate between cells, with resultant swelling of tissues. Also called *albuminoid degeneration, hydropic degeneration, parenchymatous degeneration.*

clove oil (klōv) *n.* An aromatic oil obtained from the buds, stems, or leaves of the clove tree, used as a temporary anesthetic for toothaches.

clo·za·pine (klō'zə-pēn', -pĭn) *n.* An antipsychotic drug used as a sedative and in treating of schizophrenia.

Clo·za·ril (klō'zə-rĭl') A trademark for the drug clozapine.

clubbed digit (klŭbd) *n.* A finger or toe affected with clubbing.

clubbed finger *n.* A finger affected with clubbing. Also called *drumstick finger, hippocratic finger.*

club·bing (klŭb'ĭng) *n.* A condition affecting the fingers and toes in which the extremities are broadened and the nails are shiny and abnormally curved.

club·foot (klŭb'fŏŏt') *n.* A congenital deformity of the foot that is usually characterized by a curled shape or a twisted position of the ankle, heel, and toes. Also called *talipes.*

club hair (klŭb) *n.* A hair before normal shedding, in which the bulb has become a club-shaped mass.

club·hand (klŭb'hănd') *or* **club hand** *n.* See **talipomanus.**

clump·ing (klŭm'pĭng) *n.* The massing together of bacteria or other cells suspended in a fluid.

clu·nes (klōō'nēz) *pl.n.* The buttocks.

clus·ter headache (klŭs'tər) *n.* A recurring headache that is marked by severe pain in the eye or temple on one side of the head, usually occurring in males. Also called *erythroprosopalgia, histaminic headache.*

cly·sis (klī'sĭs) *n., pl.* **–ses** (-sēz') An infusion of fluid, usually subcutaneously, for therapeutic purposes.

clys·ter (klĭs'tər) *n.* An enema.

cm *abbr.* centimeter

cM *abbr.* centimorgan

Cm The symbol for the element **curium.**

CM *abbr. Latin* Chirurgiae Magister (Master in Surgery)

CMA *abbr.* Certified Medical Assistant

CMI *abbr.* cell-mediated immunity

CMT *abbr.* Certified Medical Transcriptionist

CMV *abbr.* controlled mechanical ventilation; cytomegalovirus

CNA *abbr.* certified nursing assistant

CNM *abbr.* Certified Nurse Midwife

CNS *abbr.* central nervous system

Co The symbol for the element **cobalt.**

CO *abbr.* cardiac output

co– *pref.* **1.** Together; joint; jointly; mutually: *coaptation.* **2.** Subordinate or auxiliary: *coenzyme.* **3.** To the same extent or degree: *codominant.*

Co·A (kō'ā') *abbr.* coenzyme A

co·ac·er·vate (kō-ăs'ər-vāt') *n.* **1.** A cluster of molecules. **2.** A cluster of droplets that is separated out of a lyophilic colloid. —**co·ac·er·vate'** *v. & adj.* —**co·ac'er·va'tion** *n.*

co·ad·ap·ta·tion (kō'ăd-ăp-tā'shən) *n.* The joint correlated changes in two or more interdependent organs.

co·ag·glu·ti·nin (kō'ə-glōōt'n-ĭn) *n.* A substance that does not agglutinate an antigen, but induces the agglutination of an antigen that is appropriately coated with a univalent antibody.

co·ag·u·la·ble (kō-ăg'yə-lə-bəl) *adj.* Capable of being coagulated or clotted.

co·ag·u·lant (kō-ăg'yə-lənt) *n.* An agent that causes a sol or liquid, especially blood, to coagulate. —**co·ag'u·lant** *adj.*

co·ag·u·lase (kō-ăg'yə-lās', -lāz') *n.* An enzyme, such as rennin or thrombin, that induces coagulation.

co·ag·u·late (kō-ăg'yə-lāt') *v.* To change from the liquid state to a solid or a gel; clot. —**co·ag'u·la·bil'i·ty** *n.* —**co·ag'u·la'tor** *n.*

co·ag·u·la·tion (kō-ăg'yə-lā'shən) *n.* **1.** The change, especially of blood, from liquid to solid; clotting. **2.** A clot; coagulum.

coagulation factor *n.* See **clotting factor.**

coagulation necrosis *n.* Necrosis in which the affected cells or tissue are converted into a dry, dull, fairly homogeneous eosinophilic mass as a result of the coagulation of protein.

co·ag·u·la·tive (kō-ăg'yə-lā'tĭv, -lə-tĭv) *adj.* Of or being a coagulant.

co·ag·u·lop·a·thy (kō-ăg'yə-lŏp'ə-thē) *n.* A disease affecting the coagulability of the blood.

co·ag·u·lum (kō-ăg'yə-ləm) *n., pl.* **–la** (-lə) **1.** A clot; a curd. **2.** A soft insoluble mass formed when a sol or liquid is coagulated.

co·a·les·cence (kō'ə-lĕs'əns) *n.* See **concrescence.**

coal tar (kōl) *n.* A viscous black liquid containing numerous organic compounds that is obtained by the destructive distillation of coal and that has many uses including as raw material for many dyes, drugs, and paints.

co·ap·ta·tion (kō′ăp-tā′shən) *n.* The joining together or fitting of two surfaces, such as the edges of a wound or the ends of a broken bone.

coaptation splint *n.* A short splint that is designed to prevent overriding of the ends of a fractured bone and that is often supplemented by a longer splint to fix the entire limb.

coaptation suture *n.* See **apposition suture.**

co·arct (kō-ärkt′) *v.* To restrict or press together, as a blood vessel.

co·arc·tate (kō-ärk′tāt′) *adj.* Constricted, narrowed, or compressed, as a segment of a blood vessel.

co·arc·ta·tion (kō′ärk-tā′shən) *n.* A constriction, stricture, or stenosis.

coat (kōt) *n.* The outer covering or enveloping layer or layers of an organ or part.

coat·ed tongue (kō′tĭd) *n.* The presence of a whitish layer on the upper surface of the tongue, composed of epithelial debris, food particles, and bacteria.

Coats disease (kōts) *n.* See **exudative retinitis.**

co·bal·a·min (kō-băl′ə-mĭn) or **co·bal·a·mine** (-mēn′) *n.* See **vitamin B₁₂.**

co·balt (kō′bôlt′) *n. Symbol* **Co** A metallic element, used chiefly for magnetic and high-temperature alloys and in the form of its salts for blue glass and ceramic pigments. Atomic number 27.

cob·bler's suture (kŏb′lərz) *n.* See **doubly armed suture.**

Cobb syndrome (kŏb) *n.* A syndrome caused by vascular abnormality of the spinal cord and resulting in neurologic symptoms and cutaneous angiomas. Also called *cutaneomeningospinal angiomatosis.*

co·caine (kō-kān′, kō′kān′) *n.* A colorless or white crystalline alkaloid extracted from coca leaves, sometimes used as a local anesthetic, especially for the eyes, nose, or throat, and widely used as an illicit drug for its euphoric and stimulating effects.

co·car·cin·o·gen (kō′kär-sĭn′ə-jən, kō-kär′sə-nə-jĕn′) *n.* A substance that works in combination with a carcinogen in the production of cancer.

Coc·cid·i·a (kŏk-sĭd′ē-ə) *n.* An order of protozoans that are intracellular parasites in many vertebrates.

coc·cid·i·oi·dal (kŏk-sĭd′ē-oid′l) *adj.* Of or relating to coccidioidomycosis or its causative agent.

Coc·cid·i·oi·des (kŏk-sĭd′ē-oi′dēz) *n.* A genus of fungi, a single species of which, *Coccidiodes immitis,* causes coccidioidomycosis.

coc·cid·i·oi·din (kŏk-sĭd′ē-oid′n) *n.* A sterile solution containing the byproducts of growth of *Coccidioides immitis;* it is used as an intracutaneous skin test for coccidioidomycosis.

coc·cid·i·oi·do·ma (kŏk-sĭd′ē-oi-dō′mə) *n.* A benign localized residual granulomatous lesion or scar in a lung following primary coccidioidomycosis.

coc·cid·i·oi·do·my·co·sis (kŏk-sĭd′ē-oi′dō-mī-kō′sĭs) *n.* An infectious respiratory disease of humans and other animals caused by inhaling the fungus *Coccidioides immitis;* it is characterized by fever and various respiratory symptoms. Also called *valley fever.*

coc·cid·i·o·sis (kŏk-sĭd′ē-ō′sĭs) *n.* An intestinal disease caused by a coccidium.

coc·cid·i·um (kŏk-sĭd′ē-əm) *n., pl.* **–i·a** (-ē-ə) Any of various protozoan parasites belonging to the order Coccidia. —**coc·cid′i·al** *adj.*

coc·co·bac·il·lar·y (kŏk′ō-băs′ə-lĕr′ē, -bə-sĭl′ə-rē) *adj.* Relating to a coccobacillus.

coc·co·ba·cil·lus (kŏk′ō-bə-sĭl′əs) *n., pl.* **–cil·li** (-sĭl′ī) A short, thick bacterial rod having the shape of an oval or slightly elongated coccus.

coc·cus (kŏk′əs) *n., pl.* **coc·ci** (kŏk′sī, kŏk′ī) A bacterium of round, spheroidal, or ovoid form. —**coc′-coid′** (kŏk′oid′), **coc′cal** (kŏk′əl) *adj.*

–coccus *suff.* A microorganism that is of spherical or spheroidal shape: *streptococcus.*

coc·cy·al·gia (kŏk′sē-ăl′jə) *n.* See **coccygodynia.**

coc·cy·dyn·i·a (kŏk′sĭ-dĭn′ē-ə) *n.* See **coccygodynia.**

coc·cyg·e·al (kŏk-sĭj′ē-əl) *adj.* Relating to the coccyx.

coccygeal body *n.* An arteriovenous anastomosis supplied by the middle sacral artery and located on the pelvic surface of the coccyx.

coccygeal ganglion *n.* The lowest unpaired ganglion of the sympathetic nerve trunk. Also called *ganglion impar.*

coccygeal muscle *n.* A muscle with origin in the spine of the ischium and sacrospinous ligament, with insertion to the sides of the lower part of the sacrum and the upper part of the coccyx, with nerve supply from the third and fourth sacral nerves, and whose action assists in raising and supporting the pelvic floor.

coccygeal nerve *n.* The lowest of the spinal nerves, entering into the formation of the coccygeal plexus.

coccygeal plexus *n.* A small plexus formed by the fifth sacral and the coccygeal nerves and giving origin to the anococcygeal nerves.

coccygeal sinus *n.* A fistula opening in the region of the coccyx due to incomplete closure of the caudal end of the neural tube.

coc·cy·gec·to·my (kŏk′sə-jĕk′tə-mē) *n.* Surgical removal of the coccyx.

coc·cy·go·dyn·i·a (kŏk′sĭ-gō-dĭn′ē-ə) *n.* Pain in the region of the coccyx. Also called *coccyalgia, coccydynia, coccyodynia.*

coc·cy·got·o·my (kŏk′sĭ-gŏt′ə-mē) *n.* An operation for freeing the coccyx from its attachments.

coc·cy·o·dyn·i·a (kŏk′sē-ō-dĭn′ē-ə) *n.* See **coccygodynia.**

coc·cyx (kŏk′sĭks) *n., pl.* **coc·cy·ges** (kŏk-sī′jēz, kŏk′-sĭ-jēz′) The small triangular bone located at the base of the spinal column, formed by the fusion of four rudimentary vertebrae, and articulating above with the sacrum. Also called *tailbone.*

coch·i·neal (kŏch′ə-nēl′, kŏch′ə-nēl′, kō′chə-nēl′, kō′-chə-nēl′) *n.* A red dye made of dried, pulverized female cochineal insects and used as a biological stain and as an indicator in acid-base titrations.

coch·le·a (kŏk′lē-ə, kō′klē-ə) *n., pl.* **–le·as** or **–le·ae** (-lē-ē′) A spiral-shaped cavity in the petrous portion of the temporal bone of the inner ear, containing the nerve endings essential for hearing and forming one of the divisions of the labyrinth. —**coch′le·ar** (-ər) *adj.*

cochlear aqueduct *n.* See **perilymphatic duct.**

cochlear canal *n.* **1.** A minute canal in the temporal bone that passes from the cochlea inferiorly to open in front of the medial side of the jugular fossa. **2.** See **spiral canal of cochlea.**

cochlear duct *n.* A spiral membranous tube suspended within the cochlea, occupying the lower portion of the vestibular canal.

cochlear hair cell *n.* A sensory cell in the spiral organ in synaptic contact with sensory as well as efferent fibers of the auditory nerve. Also called *Corti's cell.*

cochlear implant *n.* An electronic device that stimulates auditory nerve fibers in the inner ear in individuals who have severe or profound bilateral hearing loss, allowing them to recognize some sounds, especially speech sounds.

cochlear joint *n.* A form of hinge joint in which the opposing articular surfaces form part of a spiral and flexion is accompanied by a certain amount of lateral movement. Also called *spiral joint.*

cochlear labyrinth *n.* The part of the inner ear containing the spiral organ.

cochlear nerve *n.* The cochlear part of the vestibulocochlear nerve peripheral to the cochlear root, composed of nerve processes with terminals on the four rows of hair cells and the bipolar neurons of the spiral ganglion. Also called *auditory nerve.*

cochlear nucleus *n.* Any of the nuclei that are located on the dorsal and lateral surface of the inferior cerebellar peduncle in the floor of the lateral recess of the rhomboid fossa, receive the incoming fibers of the cochlear part of the vestibulocochlear nerve, and are the major source of the lateral lemniscus or central auditory pathway.

coch·le·o·pal·pe·bral reflex (kŏk′lē-ō-păl′pə-brə, -păl-pē′-) *n.* A form of the wink reflex in which the palpebral part of the orbicular muscle of the eye contracts when a sudden noise is made close to the ear; it is absent in labyrinthine disease involving total deafness. Also called *startle reflex.*

coch·le·o·ves·tib·u·lar (kŏk′lē-ō-vĕ-stĭb′yə-lər, kō′-klē-) *adj.* Relating to the cochlea and the vestibule of the ear.

Coch·li·o·my·ia (kŏk′lē-ō-mī′yə) *n.* A genus of fleshflies whose larvae develop in decaying flesh or carrion or in wounds or sores.

coch·li·tis (kŏk-lī′tĭs) *or* **coch·le·i·tis** (kŏk′lē-ī′tĭs) *n.* Inflammation of the cochlea.

Cock·ayne's syndrome (kŏ-kānz′) *n.* A hereditary syndrome characterized by dwarfism, a precociously senile appearance, pigmentary degeneration of the retina, optic atrophy, deafness, sensitivity to sunlight, and mental retardation.

cock·tail (kŏk′tāl) *n.* **1.** A mixture of drugs, usually in solution, for the diagnosis or treatment of a condition. **2.** A treatment regimen that includes a combination of several drugs that enhances their individual potency.

code blue (kōd) *n.* A medical emergency in which a team of medical personnel work to revive an individual in cardiac arrest.

co·deine (kō′dēn′) *n.* An alkaloid narcotic derived from opium or morphine and used as a cough suppressant, analgesic, and hypnotic. Also called *methylmorphine.*

co·de·pen·dent *or* **co-de·pen·dent** (kō′dĭ-pĕn′dənt) *adj.* Of or relating to a relationship in which one person is psychologically dependent in an unhealthy way on someone who is addicted to a drug or self-destructive behavior, such as chronic gambling.

cod·ing sequence (kō′dĭng) *n.* See **exon.**

cod-liv·er oil (kŏd′lĭv′ər) *n.* An oil obtained from the liver of cod and related fishes and used as a dietary source of vitamins A and D.

Cod·man's triangle (kŏd′mənz) *n.* The interface between a growing bone tumor and normal bone, appearing in an x-ray as an incomplete triangle formed by the periosteum.

co·dom·i·nant (kō-dŏm′ə-nənt) *adj.* Of or relating to an equal degree of dominance of two genes, both being expressed in the phenotype of the individual.

codominant inheritance *n.* Inheritance in which two alleles of a gene pair in a heterozygote both have full phenotypic expression.

co·don (kō′dŏn′) *n.* A sequence of three adjacent nucleotides constituting the genetic code that specifies the insertion of an amino acid in a specific structural position in a polypeptide chain during the synthesis of proteins.

coe– *pref.* For words beginning with *coe-* that are not found here, see under *ce-.*

co·ef·fi·cient (kō′ə-fĭsh′ənt) *n.* The mathematical expression of the amount or degree of any quality possessed by a substance, or of the degree of physical or chemical change normally occurring in that substance under stated conditions.

–coel *or* **–coele** *or* **–cele** *suff.* Chamber; cavity: *blastocoel.*

Coe·len·ter·a·ta (sĭ-lĕn′tə-rā′tə) *n.* A phylum of invertebrate animals including the jellyfishes, hydras, sea anemones, and corals.

coe·li·ac (sē′lē-ăk′) *adj.* Variant of **celiac.**

coe·lom *or* **ce·lom** *or* **coe·lome** (sē′ləm) *n.* The cavity formed by the splitting of the embryonic mesoderm into two layers; in mammals it then forms into the peritoneal, pleural, and pericardial cavities.

coen– *pref.* Variant of **ceno–.**

coeno– *pref.* Variant of **ceno–.**

co·en·zyme (kō-ĕn′zīm′) *n.* A thermostable nonprotein organic substance that usually contains a vitamin or mineral and combines with a specific apoenzyme to form an active enzyme system.

coenzyme A *n. Abbr.* **CoA** A coenzyme present in all living cells that functions as an acyl group carrier and is necessary for fatty acid synthesis and oxidation, pyruvate oxidation, and other acetylation.

coenzyme Q *n.* Ubiquinone.

coeur en sa·bot (kûr′ ŏn sə-bō′, kœr än sä-bō′) *n.* A heart that is visible radiographically as having an elevated apex combined with a transverse rectangular enlargement, thereby giving it the appearance of a wooden shoe.

Coe virus (kō) *n.* A virus serologically identical to a strain of coxsackievirus that causes a disease similar to the common cold.

co·fac·tor (kō′făk′tər) *n.* A substance, such as a metallic iron or coenzyme, that must be associated with an enzyme for the substance to function.

Cof·fin-Sir·is syndrome (kŏfin-sĭr′ĭs) *n.* An inherited syndrome that in males causes mental retardation with a wide bulbous nose and low nasal bridge, moderate hirsutism, and digital anomalies with nail hypoplasia. In females the syndrome may cause digital abnormalities and mild mental retardation. Also called *Coffin-Lowry syndrome.*

Co·gan-Reese syndrome (kō′gən-rēs′) *n.* See **iridocorneal endothelial syndrome.**

Cog·nex (kŏg′něks′) A trademark for the drug tacrine hydrochloride.

cog·ni·tion (kŏg-nĭsh′ən) *n.* The mental faculty of knowing, which includes perceiving, recognizing, conceiving, judging, reasoning, and imagining.

cog·ni·tive (kŏg′nĭ-tĭv) *adj.* **1.** Of, characterized by, involving, or relating to cognition. **2.** Having a basis in or reducible to empirical factual knowledge.

cognitive behavioral therapy *n.* A highly structured psychotherapeutic method that is used to alter distorted attitudes and problem behavior by identifying and replacing negative inaccurate thoughts and changing the rewards for behaviors.

cognitive laterality quotient *n.* A test that is designed to measure the difference in cognitive performance of left and right sides of the brain.

cognitive therapy *n.* Any of a variety of techniques in psychotherapy that utilize guided self-discovery, imaging, self-instruction, and related forms of elicited cognitions as the principal mode of treatment.

cog·wheel respiration (kŏg′wēl′) *n.* Respiration in which the inspiratory sound is punctuated by two or three silent intervals.

cogwheel rigidity *n.* Rigidity in which the muscles respond with cogwheel-like jerks to the use of force in bending the limb, as occurs in Parkinson's disease.

Co·hen (kō′ən), **Stanley** Born 1922. American biochemist. He shared a 1986 Nobel Prize for the discovery of the epidermal growth factor.

co·he·sion (kō-hē′zhən) *n.* The intermolecular attraction that holds molecules and masses together.

Cohn (kōn), **Ferdinand Julius** 1828–1898. German botanist considered the founder of bacteriology. The first to recognize bacteria as plants, he proposed a classification system for bacteria based on genus and species.

Cohn·heim (kōn′hīm′), **Julius Friedrich** 1839–1884. German pathologist noted for his microscopic investigations into inflammation and pus formation and for his development of the technique of freezing a tissue sample before cutting it into thin slices for microscopic examination.

co·hort (kō′hôrt′) *n.* A defined population group followed prospectively in an epidemiological study.

coin lesion of lungs (koin) *n.* Any of various solitary, round, circumscribed shadows appearing in radiographic examinations of the lungs that are believed to be caused by tuberculosis, carcinoma, cysts, infarcts, or vascular anomalies.

coi·no·site (koi′nə-sīt′) *n.* See **cenosite.**

co·i·tus (kō′ĭ-təs, kō-ē′-) *n.* Sexual union between a male and a female involving insertion of the penis into the vagina. Also called *coition, copulation.* —**co′i·tal** *adj.*

coitus in·ter·rup·tus (ĭn′tə-rŭp′təs) *n.* Sexual intercourse deliberately interrupted by withdrawal of the penis from the vagina prior to ejaculation. Also called *onanism.*

coitus res·er·va·tus (rĕz′ər-vā′təs) *n.* Coitus in which ejaculation is delayed or suppressed.

coke (kōk) *n.* Cocaine.

col (kŏl) *n.* A craterlike area of the interproximal oral mucosa joining the lingual and buccal interdental papillae.

col–[1] *pref.* Variant of **com–.**

col–[2] *pref.* Variant of **colo–.**

Co·lace (kō′lās′) A trademark for a preparation containing docusate sodium.

cold (kōld) *n.* A viral infection characterized by inflammation of the mucous membranes lining the upper respiratory passages and usually accompanied by malaise, fever, chills, coughing, and sneezing. Also called *coryza, acute rhinitis, common cold, coryza.*

cold abscess *n.* An abscess not accompanied by heat or other usual signs of inflammation.

cold agglutination *n.* The clumping of red blood cells by their own serum or by any other serum when the blood is cooled below body temperature.

cold agglutinin *n.* An agglutinin associated with cold agglutination.

cold-blooded *adj.* Ectothermic.

cold-cure resin *n.* See **autopolymer resin.**

cold pack *n.* A compress of gauze, cloth, or plastic filled or moistened with a cold fluid and applied externally to swollen or injured body parts to relieve pain and swelling.

cold sore *n.* A small blister occurring on the lips and face and caused by a herpes simplex virus.

cold stage *n.* The stage of chill in a malarial paroxysm.

cold sweat *n.* A reaction to nervousness, fear, pain, or shock, characterized by simultaneous perspiration and chill and cold moist skin.

cold ulcer *n.* A small gangrenous ulcer on the extremities, due to defective circulation.

co·lec·to·my (kə-lĕk′tə-mē) *n.* Surgical removal of part or all of the colon.

coli– *pref.* Variant of **colo–.**

co·li·bac·il·le·mi·a (kō′lə-băs′ə-lē′mē-ə, kō′lē-) *n.* The presence of *Escherichia coli* in the blood.

co·li·bac·il·lo·sis (kō′lə-băs′ə-lō′sĭs, kō′lē-) *n.* A diarrheal disease caused by *Escherichia coli.*

co·li·ba·cil·lu·ri·a (kō′lə-băs′ə-lŏor′ē-ə, kō′lē-) *n.* The presence of *Escherichia coli* in aseptically voided urine. Also called *coliuria.*

co·li·ba·cil·lus (kō′lə-bə-sĭl′əs, kō′lē-) *n.* The colon bacillus *Escherichia coli.*

col·ic (kŏl′ĭk) *n.* **1.** Spasmodic pains in the abdomen. **2.** Paroxysms of pain with crying and irritability in young infants, due to a variety of causes, such as swallowing air, emotional upset, or overfeeding. —*adj.* (kō′lĭk) Of or relating to the colon.

colic artery *n.* **1.** An artery with origin in the superior mesenteric artery, sometimes by a common trunk with the ileocolic artery, with distribution to the ascending colon, and with anastomoses to the middle colic and ileocolic arteries; right colic artery. **2.** An artery with origin in the superior mesenteric artery, with distribution to the transverse colon, and with anastomoses to the right and left colic arteries; middle colic artery. **3.** An artery with origin in the inferior mesenteric artery, with distribution to the descending colon and splenic flexure, and with anastomoses to the middle colic and sigmoid arteries; left colic artery.

col·i·cin (kŏl′ĭ-sĭn, kō′lĭ-) *n.* Any of various antibacterial proteins produced by certain strains of the colon bacillus that are lethal to other closely related strains of bacteria.

col·ick·y (kŏl′ĭ-kē) *adj.* Relating to or affected by colic.

co·li·form (kō′lĭ-fôrm′, kŏl′ə-) *adj.* Of or relating to the bacilli that commonly inhabit the intestines of humans and other vertebrates, especially the colon bacillus. —**co′li·form′** *n.*

co·lip·ase (kō-lĭp′ās′, -lī′pās′) *n.* A small protein in pancreatic juice that is essential for the action of pancreatic lipase.

co·li·phage (kō′lə-fāj′) *n.* A bacteriophage with an affinity for a strain of *Escherichia coli.*

co·lis·tin (kə-lĭs′tĭn, kō-) *n.* An antibiotic produced by the bacterium *Bacillus polymyxa* or *B. colistinus* that is effective against a range of gram-negative bacteria and is used especially in the treatment of infections of the gastrointestinal tract.

co·li·tis (kə-lī′tĭs) *n.* Inflammation of the colon.

co·li·tox·e·mi·a (kō′lĭ-tŏk-sē′mē-ə) *n.* A condition resulting from the toxic effects of *Escherichia coli* in the blood.

co·li·u·ri·a (kō′lĭ-yŏŏr′ē-ə) *n.* See **colibacilluria.**

col·la·gen (kŏl′ə-jən) *n.* The fibrous protein constituent of bone, cartilage, tendon, and other connective tissue that converts into gelatin by boiling.

col·lag·e·nase (kə-lăj′ə-nās′, -nāz′, kŏl′ə-jə-) *n.* Any of various enzymes that catalyze the hydrolysis of collagen and gelatin.

col·lag·e·na·tion (kə-lăj′ə-nā′shən, kŏl′ə-jə-) *n.* **1.** The replacement of normal tissue by collagenous connective tissue. **2.** The production of collagen by fibroblasts.

collagen disease *n.* Any of a group of inflammatory, often autoimmune diseases affecting connective tissue, including lupus erythematosus, rheumatoid arthritis, polyarteritis nodosa, scleroderma and dermatomyositis. Also called *collagenosis, collagen vascular disease.*

collagen fiber *or* **collagenous fiber** *n.* An individual scleroprotein fiber composed of fibrils and usually arranged in branching bundles of indefinite length. Also called *white fiber.*

col·la·gen·ic (kŏl′ə-jĕn′ĭk) *adj.* Collagenous.

col·lag·e·no·lyt·ic (kə-lăj′ə-nə-lĭt′ĭk, kŏl′ə-jə-nə-) *adj.* Relating to or having the capacity to lyse collagen, gelatin, and other proteins containing proline.

col·lag·e·no·sis (kə-lăj′ə-nō′sĭs, kŏl′ə-jə-) *n.* See **collagen disease.**

col·lag·e·nous (kə-lăj′ə-nəs) *adj.* Producing or containing collagen.

collagenous colitis *n.* Colitis that occurs mostly in middle-aged women and is characterized by persistent watery diarrhea and a deposit of a band of collagen beneath the basement membrane of the colon surface epithelium.

collagenous nevus *n.* A skin condition characterized by plaques of smooth or nodular papules occurring symmetrically on the trunk or extremities.

collagen vascular disease *n.* See **collagen disease.**

col·lapse (kə-lăps′) *v.* **1.** To break down suddenly in strength or health and thereby fall into a condition of extreme prostration. **2.** To fall together or inward suddenly. —*n.* **1.** A condition of extreme prostration. **2.** A falling together of the walls of a structure. **3.** The failure of a physical system.

collapse therapy *n.* Surgical treatment of pulmonary tuberculosis in which the diseased lung is caused to collapse and is then immobilized.

col·lar·bone (kŏl′ər-bōn′) *n.* See **clavicle.**

col·lar-but·ton abscess (kŏl′ər-bŭt′n) *n.* See **shirt-stud abscess.**

col·lat·er·al (kə-lăt′ər-əl) *adj.* **1.** Indirect, subsidiary, or accessory to the main thing. **2.** Having an ancestor in common but descended from a different line. —*n.* **1.** A branch of a nerve axon or blood vessel. **2.** A collateral relative. —**col·lat′er·al·ly** *adv.*

collateral artery *n.* **1.** An artery that runs parallel with a nerve or other structure. **2.** An artery through which a collateral circulation is established.

collateral circulation *n.* Circulation that is maintained in small anastomosing vessels when the main artery is obstructed.

collateral fissure *n.* See **collateral sulcus.**

collateral hyperemia *n.* Hyperemia resulting from increased blood flow through collateral channels when the flow through the main artery is arrested.

collateral inheritance *n.* The appearance of traits in collateral members of a family group, as when an uncle and a niece show the same trait inherited from a common ancestor.

collateral ligament *n.* A ligament located on either side of a hinge joint such as the knee or wrist that acts as a radius of movement for the joint.

collateral sulcus *n.* A long, deep sagittal fissure on the undersurface of the temporal lobe of the brain, marking the border between the fusiform gyrus on its lateral side and the hippocampal and lingual gyri on its medial side. Also called *collateral fissure.*

collateral vessel *n.* A branch of an artery running parallel with the parent trunk.

col·lect·ing tubule (kə-lĕk′tĭng) *n.* Any of the various straight tubules of the kidney, present in the medulla and the medullary ray of the cortex.

col·lec·tive unconscious (kə-lĕk′tĭv) *n.* In Jungian psychology, a part of the unconscious mind that is shared by a society, a people, or all humankind. The product of ancestral experience, it contains such concepts as science, religion, and morality.

Col·les (kŏl′ĭs, kŏl′ēz), **Abraham** 1773–1843. Irish surgeon who first described Colles' fracture of the wrist.

Col·les′ fascia (kŏl′ēz, -ĭs) *n.* See **superficial fascia of perineum.**

Colles' fracture *n.* A bone fracture of the radius of the wrist in which the lower fragment becomes displaced dorsally.

col·lic·u·lec·to·my (kə-lĭk′yə-lĕk′tə-mē) *n.* Excision of the seminal colliculus.

col·lic·u·li·tis (kə-lĭk′yə-lī′tĭs) *n.* Inflammation of the urethra in the region of the seminal colliculus.

col·lic·u·lus (kə-lĭk′yə-ləs) *n., pl.* **-li** (-lī′) A small elevation above the surrounding parts of a structure.

col·li·ma·tion (kŏl′ə-mā′shən) *n.* **1.** The process of restricting and confining an x-ray beam to a given area. **2.** In nuclear medicine, the process of restricting the detection of emitted radiations to a given area of interest.

Col·lip (kŏl′ĭp), **James Bertram** 1892–1965. American biochemist who, together with Frederick Banting and John Macleod, developed insulin.

col·li·qua·tion (kŏl′ĭ-kwā′shən) *n.* **1.** Excessive discharge of fluid. **2.** Softening of tissue. **3.** Degeneration of tissue to a liquid state.

col·liq·ua·tive (kə-lĭk′wə-tĭv, kŏl′ĭ-kwā′tĭv) *adj.* Relating to or producing colliquation.

colliquative necrosis *n.* See **liquefactive necrosis**.

col·lo·di·on (kə-lō′dē-ən) *n.* A highly flammable, colorless or yellowish syrupy solution of pyroxylin, ether, and alcohol, used as an adhesive to close small wounds and hold surgical dressings, in topical medications, and for making photographic plates.

collodion baby *n.* An infant born with skin that is bright red, shiny, translucent, and drawn tight, giving the appearance the face is immobilized.

col·loid (kŏl′oid′) *n.* **1.** A suspension of finely divided particles in a continuous medium from which the particles do not settle out rapidly and are not readily filtered. **2.** The particulate matter so suspended. **3.** The gelatinous stored secretion of the thyroid gland, consisting mainly of thyroglobulin. **4.** Gelatinous material resulting from colloid degeneration in diseased tissue. Also called *colloidin.* —*adj.* Of, relating to, containing, or having the nature of a colloid. —**col·loi′dal** (kə-loid′l, kŏ-) *adj.*

colloid acne *n.* Colloid degeneration of the elastic tissue of the dermis due to repeated exposure to sunlight over a period of many years. Also called *actinic elastosis, elastosis colloidalis conglomerata.*

colloidal gel *n.* A colloid that has developed resistance to flow because of chemical or thermal change.

colloidal solution *n.* See **disperse system**.

colloid bath *n.* A bath prepared by adding soothing agents to the water.

colloid carcinoma *n.* See **mucinous carcinoma**.

colloid degeneration *n.* A form of degeneration similar to mucoid degeneration in which the gelatinous material is generally thicker.

colloid goiter *n.* Goiter in which the contents of the follicles increase greatly, thereby causing pressure atrophy of the epithelium so that the gelatinous matter predominates.

col·loi·din (kə-loid′n) *n.* See **colloid** (sense 4).

colloid theory of narcosis *n.* The theory that coagulation or flocculation of protein causes dehydration and reduction of metabolism.

col·lum (kŏl′əm) *n., pl.* **col·la** (kŏl′ə) **1.** The part of the

body between the shoulders or thorax and the head; neck. **2.** The constricted or necklike portion of an anatomical structure. Also called *cervix.*

col·lu·to·ry (kŏl′yə-tôr′ē) *n.* See **mouthwash**.

col·lyr·i·um (kə-lîr′ē-əm) *n., pl.* **-i·ums** *or* **-i·a** (-ē-ə) **1.** A medicinal lotion applied to the eye. **2.** Any preparation for the eye.

colo– *or* **coli–** *or* **col–** *pref.* Colon: *colostomy.*

col·o·bo·ma (kŏl′ə-bō′mə) *n., pl.* **-mas** *or* **-ma·ta** (-mə-tə) An anomaly of the eye, usually a developmental defect, often resulting in some vision loss.

co·lo·cen·te·sis (kō′lə-sĕn-tē′sĭs) *n.* Surgical puncture of the colon to relieve distention. Also called *colopuncture.*

co·lo·cho·le·cys·tos·to·my (kō′lō-kō′lĭ-sĭ-stŏs′tə-mē) *n.* Variant of **cholecystocolostomy**.

co·lo·co·los·to·my (kō′lə-kə-lŏs′tə-mē) *n.* The surgical formation of a communication between two noncontinuous segments of the colon.

co·lo·en·ter·i·tis (kō′lō-ĕn′tə-rī′tĭs) *n.* See **enterocolitis**.

co·lon (kō′lən) *n., pl.* **-lons** *or* **-la** (-lə) The division of the large intestine extending from the cecum to the rectum. —**co·lon′ic** (kə-lŏn′ĭk) *adj.*

co·lon·al·gia (kō′lə-năl′jə) *n.* Pain in the colon.

colon bacillus *n.* A rod-shaped bacterium, especially *Escherichia coli,* a generally nonpathogenic commensal found in all vertebrate intestinal tracts, but which can be virulent, causing diarrhea and other dysenteric symptoms. Its presence in water is an indicator of fecal contamination.

co·lon·op·a·thy (kō′lə-nŏp′ə-thē) *or* **co·lop·a·thy** (kə-lŏp′ə-thē) *n.* Disease of the colon.

co·lon·or·rha·gia (kō′lə-nō-rā′jə) *n.* Variant of **colorrhagia**.

co·lon·or·rhe·a (kō′lə-nō-rē′ə) *n.* Variant of **colorrhea**.

co·lon·o·scope (kō-lŏn′ə-skōp′, kə-) *n.* A long flexible endoscope, often equipped with a device for obtaining tissue samples, that is used for visual examination of the colon. Also called *coloscope.*

co·lon·os·co·py (kō′lə-nŏs′kə-pē) *n.* Examination of the inner surface of the colon by means of a colonoscope. Also called *coloscopy.*

col·o·ny (kŏl′ə-nē) *n.* A discrete group of organisms, such as a group of cells growing on a solid nutrient surface.

colony stimulating factor *n.* A hormone produced in the cells lining the blood vessels that stimulates the bone marrow to synthesize white blood cells.

co·lo·pex·os·to·my (kō′lə-pĕk-sŏs′tə-mē) *n.* The surgical formation of an artificial anus by creation of an opening into the colon after its fixation to the abdominal wall.

col·o·pex·y (kŏl′ə-pĕk′sē, kō′lə-) *n.* The attachment of a portion of the colon to the abdominal wall.

co·lo·pli·ca·tion (kō′lə-plĭ-kā′shən) *n.* The surgical reduction of the lumen of a dilated colon by making folds or tucks in its walls.

co·lo·proc·ti·tis (kō′lə-prŏk-tī′tĭs) *n.* Inflammation of the colon and the rectum. Also called *colorectitis.*

co·lo·proc·tos·to·my (kō′lə-prŏk-tŏs′tə-mē) *n.* The surgical formation of a communication between the rectum and a discontinuous segment of the colon. Also called *colorectostomy*.

co·lop·to·sis (kō′lŏp-tō′sĭs) *or* **co·lop·to·si·a** (-tō′sē-ə, -zē-ə) *n.* Downward displacement or prolapse of the colon, especially of the transverse portion.

co·lo·punc·ture (kō′lə-pŭngk′chər) *n.* See **colocentesis**.

col·or (kŭl′ər) *n.* **1.** That aspect of the appearance of objects and light sources that may be specified in terms of hue, lightness, and saturation. **2.** That portion of the visible electromagnetic spectrum specified in terms of wavelength, luminosity, and purity. **3.** The general appearance of the skin. **4.** The skin pigmentation of a person not classified as white.

Col·o·ra·do tick fever (kŏl′ə-răd′ō, -rä′dō) *n.* A viral infection transmitted to humans by the tick *Dermacentor andersoni* and characterized by mild symptoms and intermittent fever.

Colorado tick fever virus *n.* An *Orbivirus* transmitted by a tick and causing Colorado tick fever.

col·or·blind *or* **col·or-blind** (kŭl′ər-blīnd′) *adj.* Partially or totally unable to distinguish certain colors.

color blindness *n.* Deficiency of color perception, whether hereditary or acquired, partial or complete.

color chart *n.* An assembly of chromatic samples used in checking color vision.

co·lo·rec·tal (kō′lə-rĕk′təl) *adj.* Relating to the colon and the rectum, or to the entire large bowel.

co·lo·rec·ti·tis (kō′lə-rĕk-tī′tĭs) *n.* See **coloproctitis**.

co·lo·rec·tos·to·my (kō′lə-rĕk-tŏs′tə-mē) *n.* See **coloproctostomy**.

color hearing *n.* The imaginary perception of colors in response to the actual perception of sounds. Also called *pseudochromesthesia*.

color hemianopsia *n.* Loss of the ability to perceive colors in one half of the visual field.

col·or·im·e·try (kŭl′ə-rĭm′ĭ-trē) *n.* A technique for measuring the concentration of a known constituent of a solution by comparison of colors of standard solutions of that constituent. —**col′or·i·met′ric** (-ər-ə-mĕt′rĭk) *adj.*

color radical *n.* See **chromophore**.

co·lor·rha·gia (kŭl′ə-rā′jə) *or* **co·lon·or·rha·gia** (kō′-lə-nō-rā′jə) *n.* An abnormal discharge from the colon.

co·lor·rha·phy (kə-lôr′ə-fē) *n.* Suture of the colon.

co·lor·rhe·a (kō′lə-rē′ə) *or* **co·lon·or·rhe·a** (kō′lə-nō-rē′ə) *n.* Diarrhea thought to originate from a process confined to or affecting chiefly the colon.

color scotoma *n.* An area of depressed color vision in the visual field.

color taste *n.* A form of synesthesia in which taste and color sense are associated and stimulation of either also induces a subjective sensation on the part of the other. Also called *pseudogeusesthesia*.

co·lo·scope (kō′lə-skōp′) *n.* See **colonoscope**.

co·los·co·py (kə-lŏs′kə-pē) *n.* See **colonoscopy**.

co·lo·sig·moid·os·to·my (kō′lə-sĭg′moi-dŏs′tə-mē) *n.* The surgical formation of an anastomosis between the sigmoid colon and another part of the colon.

co·los·to·my (kə-lŏs′tə-mē) *n.* **1.** Surgical construction of an artificial excretory opening from the colon. **2.** The opening created by such a surgical procedure.

colostomy bag *n.* A receptacle worn over the stoma to collect feces following a colostomy.

co·los·tror·rhe·a (kə-lŏs′trə-rē′ə) *n.* An abnormally profuse secretion of colostrum.

co·los·trum (kə-lŏs′trəm) *n.* The first milk secreted at the time of parturition, differing from the milk secreted later by containing more lactalbumin and lactoprotein, and also being rich in antibodies that confer passive immunity to the newborn. Also called *foremilk*. —**co·los′tral** (-trəl) *adj.*

co·lot·o·my (kə-lŏt′ə-mē) *n.* Incision into the colon.

col·pal·gia (kŏl-păl′jə) *n.* See **vaginodynia**.

col·pa·tre·sia (kŏl′pə-trē′zhə) *n.* See **vaginal atresia**.

col·pec·ta·sis (kŏl-pĕk′tə-sĭs) *or* **col·pec·ta·sia** (kŏl′-pĕk-tā′zhə) *n.* Distention of the vagina.

col·pec·to·my (kŏl-pĕk′tə-mē) *n.* See **vaginectomy**.

col·pi·tis (kŏl-pī′tĭs) *n.* See **vaginitis**.

colpo– *or* **colp–** *pref.* Vagina: *colpospasm*.

col·po·cele (kŏl′pə-sēl′) *n.* **1.** A hernia projecting into the vagina. Also called *vaginocele*. **2.** See **colpoptosis**.

col·po·clei·sis (kŏl′pō-klī′sĭs) *n.* Surgical obliteration of the lumen of the vagina.

col·po·cys·ti·tis (kŏl′pō-sĭ-stī′tĭs) *n.* Inflammation of the vagina and the bladder.

col·po·cys·to·cele (kŏl′pō-sĭs′tə-sēl′) *n.* See **cystocele**.

col·po·cys·to·plas·ty (kŏl′pō-sĭs′tə-plăs′tē) *n.* Plastic surgery to repair the vesicovaginal wall.

col·po·dyn·i·a (kŏl′pō-dĭn′ē-ə) *n.* See **vaginodynia**.

col·po·hy·per·pla·sia (kŏl′pō-hī′pər-plā′zhə) *n.* A thickening of the vaginal mucous membrane.

col·po·mi·cros·co·py (kŏl′pō-mī-krŏs′kə-pē) *n.* Direct observation and study of cells within the vagina and cervix by means of a special microscope.

col·po·per·i·ne·o·plas·ty (kŏl′pō-pĕr′ə-nē′ə-plăs′tē) *n.* See **vaginoperineoplasty**.

col·po·per·i·ne·or·rha·phy (kŏl′pō-pĕr′ə-nē-ôr′ə-fē) *n.* See **vaginoperineorrhaphy**.

col·po·pex·y (kŏl′pə-pĕk′sē) *n.* See **vaginofixation**.

col·po·plas·ty (kŏl′pə-plăs′tē) *n.* See **vaginoplasty**.

col·po·poi·e·sis (kŏl′pə-poi-ē′sĭs) *n.* Surgical construction of an artificial vagina.

col·po·pto·sis (kŏl′pō-tō′sĭs, -pŏp-tō′-) *or* **col·po·pto·si·a** (-tō′sē-ə, -zē-ə) *n.* Prolapse of the vaginal walls. Also called *colpocele*.

col·por·rha·gia (kŏl′pō-rā′jə) *n.* A hemorrhage of the vagina.

col·por·rha·phy (kŏl-pôr′ə-fē) *n.* Repair of a rupture of the vagina by suturing the edges of the tear.

col·por·rhex·is (kŏl′pō-rĕk′sĭs) *n.* A tearing of the vaginal wall; vaginal laceration.

col·po·scope (kŏl′pə-skōp′) *n.* An endoscopic instrument that magnifies the epithelia of the vagina and cervix in vivo to allow direct observation and study of these tissues. —**col′po·scop′ic** (-skŏp′ĭk) *adj.*

col·pos·co·py (kŏl-pŏs′kə-pē) *n.* Coldoscopic examination of the vaginal and cervical epithelia.

col·po·spasm (kŏl′pə-spăz′əm) *n.* A spasmodic contraction of the vagina.

col·po·ste·no·sis (kŏl′pō-stə-nō′sĭs) *n.* A narrowing of the lumen of the vagina.

col·po·ste·not·o·my (kŏl′pō-stə-nŏt′ə-mē) *n.* Surgical correction of colpostenosis.

col·pot·o·my (kŏl-pŏt′ə-mē) *n.* See **vaginotomy**.

col·po·xe·ro·sis (kŏl′pō-zĭ-rō′sĭs) *n.* Abnormal dryness of the vaginal mucous membrane.

Co·lum·bi·a Mental Maturity scale (kə-lŭm′bē-ə) *n.* An individually administered test for assessing the intellectual ability of children ranging from 3 to 12 years old.

col·u·mel·la (kŏl′yə-mĕl′ə) *or* **col·um·nel·la** (kŏl′əm-nĕl′ə) *n., pl.* **–mel·lae** (-mĕl′ē) *or* **–nel·lae** (-nĕl′ē) A column-shaped anatomical structure. **—col′u·mel′lar** (-mĕl′ər) *adj.* **—col′u·mel′late′** (-mĕl′āt′) *adj.*

col·umn (kŏl′əm) *n.* Any of various tubular or pillarlike supporting structures in the body, such as the spinal column, each generally having a single tissue origin and function.

co·lum·na (kə-lŭm′nə) *n., pl.* **–nae** (-nē) Column.

co·lum·nar cell (kə-lŭm′nər) *n.* A cell, usually epithelial, that is tall, narrow, and somewhat cylindrical.

columnar epithelium *n.* Epithelium made up of cells that are taller than they are wide and that form a single layer.

column chromatography *n.* A form of partition chromatography in which a liquid phase flows down a column packed with a solid phase.

column of fornix *n.* The part of the fornix, consisting primarily of fibers originating in the hippocampus, that is the direct continuation of the body of the fornix.

com– or col– or con– *pref.* Together; with; joint; jointly: *commensalism.*

co·ma (kō′mə) *n.* A state of profound unconsciousness in which an individual is incapable of sensing or responding to external stimuli.

coma aberration *n.* The distortion in image formation occurring when a bundle of light rays enters an optical system that is not parallel to the optic axis.

coma scale *n.* A clinical test for assessing impaired consciousness in which motor responsiveness, verbal performance, eye opening, and sometimes the function of cranial nerves are assessed.

co·ma·tose (kō′mə-tōs′, kŏm′ə-) *adj.* **1.** Of, relating to, or affected with coma. **2.** Marked by lethargy; torpid.

com·bat fatigue (kŏm′băt′) *n.* Posttraumatic stress disorder resulting from wartime combat or similar experiences. No longer in scientific use. Also called *battle fatigue, shell shock.*

com·bi·na·tion calculus (kŏm′bə-nā′shən) *n.* See **alternating calculus**.

combination therapy *n.* Method of treating disease through the simultaneous use of a variety of drugs to eliminate or control the biochemical cause of the disease.

com·bined fat and carbohydrate-induced hyperlipemia (kəm-bīnd′) *n.* See **type V familial hyperlipoproteinemia**.

combined glaucoma *n.* Glaucoma with angle-closure and open-angle mechanisms in the same eye.

combined immunodeficiency *n.* Immunodeficiency of both the B-cells and T-cells.

combined pregnancy *n.* Coexisting uterine and ectopic pregnancy.

combined version *n.* See **bimanual version**.

com·bus·ti·ble (kəm-bŭs′tə-bəl) *adj.* Capable of igniting and burning. **—n.** A substance that ignites and burns readily.

com·bus·tion (kəm-bŭs′chən) *n.* **1.** The process of burning. **2.** A chemical change, especially oxidation, accompanied by the production of heat and light.

Com·by's sign (kŏm-bēz′, kôɴ-) *n.* An early indication of measles in which thin whitish patches appear on the gums and buccal mucous membrane.

com·e·do (kŏm′ĭ-dō′) *n., pl.* **–dos** *or* **–do·nes** (-dō′nēz) A blackhead and the primary lesion of acne vulgaris.

com·e·do·car·ci·no·ma (kŏm′ĭ-dō-kär′sə-nō′mə) *n.* A form of breast carcinoma in which plugs of necrotic malignant cells may be expressed from the ducts.

com·e·do·gen·ic (kŏm′ĭ-dō-jĕn′ĭk) *adj.* Tending to produce or aggravate acne.

comedo nevus *n.* A congenital skin condition characterized by linear keratinous cystic invaginations of the epidermis and a failure to develop normal pilosebaceous follicles.

co·mes (kō′mēz) *n., pl.* **com·i·tes** (kŏm′ĭ-tēz′) A blood vessel accompanying another vessel or a nerve.

com·fort zone (kŭm′fərt) *n.* The temperature range between 28° and 30°C or 82.5° and 86°F at which the naked body maintains heat balance without shivering or sweating; in the clothed body, the range is between 13° and 21°C or 55.5° and 70°F.

com·ma bacillus (kŏm′ə) *n.* See **Koch's bacillus**.

com·man·do procedure (kə-măn′dō) *n.* A surgical operation for malignant tumors of the floor of the oral cavity, involving resection of portions of the mandible in continuity with the oral lesion and radical neck dissection.

com·men·sal (kə-mĕn′səl) *adj.* Of, relating to, or characterized by a symbiotic relationship in which one species is benefited while the other is unaffected. **—n.** An organism participating in a symbiotic relationship in which one species derives some benefit while the other is unaffected.

com·men·sal·ism (kə-mĕn′sə-lĭz′əm) *n.* A symbiotic relationship in which one organism derives benefit and the other is unharmed.

com·mi·nute (kŏm′ə-nōōt′) *v.* To reduce to powder; to pulverize. **—com′mi·nu′tion** *n.*

com·mi·nut·ed (kŏm′ə-nōō′tĭd) *adj.* Broken into fragments. Used of a fractured bone.

comminuted fracture *n.* A fracture in which the bone is splintered, crushed, or broken into pieces.

commissural cell *n.* A nerve cell of the gray matter of the spinal cord, the axon of which passes through a commissure and enters the white matter of the other side of the cord. Also called *heteromeric cell.*

commissural cheilitis *n.* See **angular cheilitis**.

commissural fiber *n.* Any of the nerve fibers crossing the midline and connecting the symmetrical halves of the nervous system.

com·mis·sure (kŏm′ə-shōōr′) *n.* **1.** A line or place at which two things are joined. **2.** A tract of nerve fibers passing from one side to the other of the spinal cord or brain. **3.** The point, angle, or surface where two parts, such as the eyelids, lips, or cardiac valves, join or connect. **—com′mis·su′ral** *adj.*

commissure of cerebral hemispheres *n.* See **corpus callosum.**

com·mis·sur·ot·o·my (kŏm′ə-shoo-rŏt′ə-mē, -soo-) *n.* **1.** Surgical division of a commissure, fibrous band, or ring. **2.** See **midline myelotomy.**

com·mit (kə-mĭt′) *v.* To place officially in confinement or custody, as in a mental health facility.

com·mon antigen (kŏm′ən) *n.* A hapten that occurs in the bacterial cell wall and is shared by most gram-negative bacteria. Also called *heterogenic enterobacterial antigen.*

common basal vein *n.* A tributary to the inferior pulmonary veins that receives blood from the superior and inferior basal veins.

common bile duct *n.* The duct that is formed by the union of the hepatic and cystic ducts and discharges into the duodenum. Also called *gall duct.*

common cardinal vein *n.* Any of the major drainage channels that are formed by anastomosis of the anterior and posterior cardinal veins and are the main systemic return channels to the heart in the embryos of humans and other vertebrates.

common carotid plexus *n.* An autonomic plexus accompanying the common carotid artery and formed by fibers from the middle cervical ganglion.

common cold *n.* See **cold.**

common-cold virus *n.* Any of numerous strains of viruses associated with the common cold, especially the rhinoviruses, and also including strains of adenovirus, ECHO virus, and parainfluenza virus.

common facial vein *n.* A short vein formed by the union of the facial and the retromandibular veins, emptying into the jugular vein.

common hepatic duct *n.* The part of the biliary duct system that is formed by the confluence of the right and left hepatic ducts and is joined by the cystic duct to become the common bile duct.

common iliac vein *n.* A vein that is formed by union of the external and internal iliac veins at the brim of the pelvis and passes upward to the right of the fifth lumbar vertebra where it unites with its fellow of the opposite side to form the inferior vena cava.

common palmar digital nerve *n.* Any of four nerves in the palm of the hand that send branches to the adjacent sides of two digits. Three of these nerves are branches of the median nerve; the fourth is from the ulnar nerve.

common peroneal nerve *n.* A terminal division of the sciatic nerve, passing through the lateral portion of the popliteal space to opposite the head of the fibula where it divides into the superficial and the deep peroneal nerves.

common plantar digital nerve *n.* Any of three nerves derived from the medial plantar nerve and one from the lateral plantar nerve that supply the skin of the ball of the foot and terminate as the proper plantar digital nerves to the side of each toe.

common variable immunodeficiency *n.* Immunodeficiency of unknown cause characterized chiefly by abnormally low levels of immunoglobulin; it is associated with increased susceptibility to pyogenic infections and with autoimmune disease.

com·mu·ni·ca·ble (kə-myoo′nĭ-kə-bəl) *adj.* Transmittable between persons or species; contagious.

communicable disease *n.* A disease that is transmitted through direct contact with an infected individual or indirectly through a vector. Also called *contagious disease.*

com·mu·ni·cat·ing artery (kə-myoo′nĭ-kā′tĭng) *n.* **1.** An artery that connects two larger arteries. **2.** A short artery joining the two anterior cerebral arteries and completing anteriorly the circle of Willis; anterior communicating artery. **3.** An artery with origin in the internal carotid artery, with distribution to the optic tract, cerebral peduncle, and hippocampal gyrus; and with anastomoses with the posterior cerebral artery to form the circle of Willis; posterior communicating artery.

communicating branch *n.* A bundle of nerve fibers passing from one nerve to join another.

communicating hydrocephalus *n.* A form of hydrocephalus in which there is a connection between the ventricles and the spinal subarachnoid space, thus allowing cerebrospinal fluid to pass easily from the brain to the spinal cord.

com·mu·ni·ca·tion (kə-myoo′nĭ-kā′shən) *n.* **1.** The exchange of thoughts, messages, or information, as by speech, signals, writing, or behavior. **2.** An opening or a connecting passage between two structures. **3.** A joining or connecting of solid fibrous structures, such as tendons and nerves.

communication disorder *n.* Any of various disorders, such as stuttering or perseveration, characterized by impaired written or verbal expression.

com·mu·ni·ty medicine (kə-myoo′nĭ-tē) *n.* Public health services emphasizing preventive medicine and epidemiology for members of a given community or region.

community psychiatry *n.* Psychiatry focusing on detection, prevention, early treatment, and rehabilitation of emotional and behavioral disorders as they develop in a community.

community psychology *n.* The application of psychology to community programs for the prevention of mental disorders and the promotion of mental health.

Co·mol·li's sign (kə-mō′lēz) *n.* An indication of fracture of the scapula in which a triangular cushionlike swelling appears that corresponds to the outline of that bone.

co·mor·bid (kō-môr′bĭd) *adj.* Coexisting or concomitant with an unrelated pathological or disease process.

co·mor·bid·i·ty (kō′môr-bĭd′ĭ-tē) *n.* A concomitant but unrelated pathological or disease process.

com·pact bone (kəm-păkt′, kŏm-, kŏm′păkt′) *n.* The compact noncancellous portion of bone that consists largely of concentric lamellar osteons and interstitial lamellae. Also called *compact substance.*

com·pan·ion artery to sciatic nerve (kəm-păn′yən) *n.* An artery with its origin in the inferior gluteal artery, with distribution to the sciatic nerve, and with anastomoses to the branches of the deep artery of the thigh.

companion vein *n.* An accompanying vein.

com·par·a·tive anatomy (kəm-păr′ə-tĭv) *n.* The investigation and comparison of the structures of different animals.

comparative pathology *n.* The pathology of animal diseases, especially in relation to human pathology.

com·pat·i·ble (kəm-păt′ə-bəl) *adj.* **1.** Capable of existing or performing in harmonious or agreeable combination. **2.** Capable of being grafted, transfused, or transplanted from one individual to another without reaction or rejection. **3.** Capable of forming a chemically or biochemically stable system.

Com·pa·zine (kŏm′pə-zēn′) A trademark for the drug prochlorperazine.

com·pen·sat·ed acidosis (kŏm′pən-sā′tĭd) *n.* Acidosis in which the pH of body fluids is normal due to compensation by respiratory or renal mechanisms.

compensated alkalosis *n.* A rise in alkalinity that is compensated for by physiological changes to the pH of body fluids.

com·pen·sa·tion (kŏm′pən-sā′shən) *n.* **1.** A process in which a tendency for a change in a given direction is counteracted by another change so that the original change is not evident. **2.** An unconscious psychological mechanism by which one tries to make up for imagined or real deficiencies in personality or physical ability.

com·pen·sa·to·ry (kəm-pĕn′sə-tôr′ē) *adj.* Relating to or characterized by compensation.

compensatory circulation *n.* Circulation established in dilated collateral vessels when the main artery of the part is obstructed.

compensatory hypertrophy *n.* Increase in size of an organ or tissue when called upon to do additional work or to perform the work of destroyed tissue or of a paired organ.

compensatory pause *n.* A pause in the heartbeat following an extrasystole that is long enough to compensate for the prematurity of the extrasystole.

compensatory polycythemia *n.* Polycythemia resulting from anoxia, as in congenital heart disease, pulmonary emphysema, or prolonged residence at a high altitude.

com·pe·tence (kŏm′pĭ-təns) *n.* **1.** The quality of being competent or capable of performing an allotted function. **2.** The quality or condition of being legally qualified to perform an act. **3.** The mental ability to distinguish right from wrong and to manage one's own affairs. **4.** The ability of a cell, especially a bacterial cell, to be genetically transformable. **5.** The ability to respond immunologically to viruses or other antigenic agents. **6.** Integrity, especially the normal tight closure of a cardiac valve.

com·pe·tent (kŏm′pĭ-tənt) *adj.* **1.** Properly or sufficiently qualified; capable. **2.** Capable of performing an allotted or required function. **3.** Legally qualified or fit to perform an act. **4.** Able to distinguish right from wrong and to manage one's affairs.

com·pe·ti·tion (kŏm′pĭ-tĭsh′ən) *n.* **1.** The process by which the activity or presence of one substance interferes with or suppresses the activity of another substance with similar affinities, as of antigens. **2.** The simultaneous demand by two or more organisms for limited environmental resources.

com·pet·i·tive binding assay (kəm-pĕt′ĭ-tĭv) *n.* An assay in which a biologically specific binding agent competes for radioactively labeled or unlabeled compounds, used especially to measure the concentration of hormone receptors in a sample by introducing a radioactively labeled hormone.

competitive inhibition *n.* Blockage of the action of an enzyme on its substrate by replacement of the substrate with a similar but inactive compound that can combine with the active site of the enzyme but that is not acted upon or split by the enzyme. Also called *selective inhibition.*

com·ple·ment (kŏm′plə-mənt) *n.* A group of proteins found in normal blood serum and plasma that are activated sequentially in a cascadelike mechanism that allows them to combine with antibodies and destroy pathogenic bacteria and other foreign cells.

com·ple·men·tal air (kŏm′plə-mĕn′tl) *n.* See **inspiratory reserve volume.**

com·ple·men·tar·i·ty (kŏm′plə-mĕn-tăr′ĭ-tē) *n.* **1.** The correspondence or similarity between nucleotides or strands of nucleotides of DNA and RNA molecules that allows precise pairing. **2.** The affinity that an antigen and an antibody have for each other as a result of the chemical arrangement of their combining sites.

com·ple·men·ta·ry air (kŏm′plə-mĕn′tə-rē, -trē) *n.* See **inspiratory capacity.**

complementary DNA *n.* cDNA.

complementary hypertrophy *n.* Increase in size or expansion of part of an organ or tissue to fill the space left by the destruction of another portion of the same organ or tissue.

complementary medicine *n.* A method of health care that combines the therapies and philosophies of conventional medicine with those of alternative medicines, such as acupuncture and herbal medicine.

com·ple·men·ta·tion (kŏm′plə-mən-tā′shən, -mĕn-) *n.* **1.** Functional interaction between two defective viruses permitting replication under conditions that are inhibitory to the single virus. **2.** Interaction between two genetic units, one or both of which are defective, permitting the organism containing these units to function normally, whereas it could not do so if one unit were absent.

complement binding assay *n.* An assay for detecting immune complexes.

complement fixation *n.* The binding of active complement to a specific antigen-antibody pair used in diagnostic tests, such as the Wasserman test, to detect the presence of a specific antigen or antibody.

complement-fixation test *n.* An immunological test for determining the presence of a particular antibody in which serum is treated in a manner that allows existing antibodies to accept and bind to a known amount of antigen. If binding occurs the presence of the antibody is verified and its concentration in the serum can be calculated based on the amount of antigen added to the system.

complement-fixing antibody *n.* An antibody that combines with and sensitizes an antigen, leading to activation of complement and sometimes lysis.

complement protein *n.* A substance that is produced by a predecessor protein or in response to the presence of foreign material in the body and that triggers or participates in a complement reaction.

complement reaction *n.* A physiological reaction to the presence of a foreign microorganism in which a cascade of enzymatic reactions, triggered by molecular features of the microorganism, result in lysis or phagocytosis of the foreign material.

complement unit *n.* The smallest amount of complement that will activate a hemolysin unit, causing lysis of a given quantity of red blood cells.

com·plete antibody (kəm-plēt′) *n.* See **saline agglutinin.**

complete antigen *n.* An antigen capable of stimulating formation of an antibody with which it reacts.

complete blood count *n. Abbr.* **CBC** A combination of totals from the red blood cell count, white blood cell count, erythrocyte indices, hematocrit, and differential blood count. Also called *blood profile.*

complete carcinogen *n.* A chemical that is able to induce cancer without inducement by an agent that promotes tumor growth or development.

complete denture *n.* A dental prosthesis that replaces all the natural teeth and their associated maxillary and mandibular structures. Also called *full denture.*

complete fistula *n.* A fistula that is open at both ends.

complete hemianopsia *n.* Hemianopsia affecting a full half of the visual field of each eye.

complete hernia *n.* An inguinal hernia in which the hernial sac and its contents extend through the opening.

complete transduction *n.* Transduction in which the transferred genetic fragment is fully integrated in the genome of the recipient bacterium.

com·plex (kŏm′plĕks′) *n.* **1.** A group of related, often repressed memories, thoughts, and impulses that compel characteristic or habitual patterns of feelings, thought, and behavior. **2.** The relatively stable combination of two or more ions or compounds into a larger structure without covalent binding. **3.** A composite of chemical or immunological structures. **4.** An entity made up of three or more interrelated components. **5.** A group of individual structures known or believed to be anatomically, embryologically, or physiologically related. **6.** The combination of factors, symptoms, or signs that forms a syndrome. —*adj.* (kəm-plĕks′, kŏm′plĕks′) **1.** Consisting of interconnected or interwoven parts; composite. **2.** Composed of two or more units. **3.** Relating to a group of individual structures known or considered to be anatomically, embryologically, or physiologically related.

complex absence *n.* Paroxysmal impairment of consciousness that may be accompanied by other abnormalities such as atonia, automatisms, hypertonicity, myoclonus, episodes of coughing or sneezing, and vasomotor changes.

complex carbohydrate *n.* A polysaccharide consisting of a chain of glucose molecules; starch.

com·plex·ion (kəm-plĕk′shən) *n.* The natural color, texture, and appearance of the skin, especially of the face.

complex odontoma *n.* An odontoma in which the various odontogenic tissues appear in a haphazard arrangement that bears no resemblence to teeth.

complex partial seizure *n.* Psychomotor epilepsy.

complex precipitated epilepsy *n.* A form of reflex epilepsy initiated by particular sensory stimuli, such as certain visual patterns.

com·pli·ance (kəm-plī′əns) *n.* **1.** A measure of the ease with which a structure or substance may be deformed, especially a measure of the ease with which a hollow organ may be distended. **2.** The degree of constancy and accuracy with which a patient follows a prescribed regimen, as distinguished from adherence or maintenance.

com·pli·ca·tion (kŏm′plĭ-kā′shən) *n.* A pathological process or event occurring during a disease that is not an essential part of the disease; it may result from the disease or from independent causes.

com·po·nent of complement (kəm-pō′nənt) *n.* Any one of the nine distinct protein units (designated C1 through C9) that are responsible for the immunological activities associated with complement.

com·pos·ite flap (kəm-pŏz′ĭt) *n.* A skin flap incorporating underlying muscle, bone, or cartilage. Also called *compound flap.*

composite graft *n.* A graft composed of multiple structures, such as skin and cartilage.

com·pos men·tis (kŏm′pəs mĕn′tĭs) *adj.* Of sound mind; sane.

com·pound (kŏm′pound′) *n.* **1.** A combination of two or more elements or parts. **2.** A pure, macroscopically homogeneous substance that consists of atoms or ions of different elements in definite proportions that cannot be separated by physical means, and that have properties unlike those of its constituent elements. —*adj.* (kŏm′pound′, kŏm-pound′, kəm-) Consisting of two or more substances, ingredients, elements, or parts. —*v.* (kŏm-pound′, kəm-, kŏm′pound′) **1.** To combine so as to form a whole; mix. **2.** To produce or create by combining two or more ingredients or parts.

compound aneurysm *n.* An aneurysm in which some of the coats of the artery are ruptured, while others remain intact.

compound dislocation *n.* See **open dislocation.**

compound flap *n.* See **composite flap.**

compound fracture *n.* See **open fracture.**

compound gland *n.* A gland composed of a branching system of ducts that combine, eventually opening into a secretory duct.

compound heterozygote *n.* An organism that has two different, harmful, mutant alleles at the same loci.

compound hyperopic astigmatism *n.* Astigmatism in which all meridians are hyperopic but to different degrees.

compound joint *n.* A joint composed of three or more skeletal elements.

compound microscope *n.* A microscope consisting of an objective and an eyepiece at opposite ends of an adjustable tube.

compound myopic astigmatism *n.* Astigmatism in which all meridians are myopic to different degrees.

compound odontoma *n.* An odontoma in which the odontogenic tissues are organized and bear a superficial resemblence to teeth.

com·pre·hen·sion (kŏm′prĭ-hĕn′shən) *n.* See **apperception** (sense 1).

com·press (kŏm′prĕs′) *n.* A soft pad of gauze or other material applied with pressure to a part of the body to control hemorrhage or to supply heat, cold, moisture, or medication in order to alleviate pain or reduce infection. —*v.* (kəm-prĕs′) To press or squeeze together.

com·pres·sion (kəm-prĕsh′ən) *n.* **1.** See **condensation**. **2.** The state of being compressed.

compression cyanosis *n.* Cyanosis accompanied by petechial hemorrhages of the head, neck, and upper chest, caused by severe or prolonged compression of the chest or abdomen.

compression fracture *n.* A fracture caused by the compression of one bone, especially a vertebra, against another.

compression paralysis *n.* Paralysis due to compression of a nerve, as by prolonged pressure.

compression syndrome *n.* See **crush syndrome**.

com·pres·sor (kəm-prĕs′ər) *n.* A muscle that causes compression of a structure upon contraction.

com·pro·mise (kŏm′prə-mīz′) *v.* To impair by disease, toxicity, or injury. —**com′pro·mised′** *adj.*

com·pul·sion (kəm-pŭl′shən) *n.* An uncontrollable impulse to perform an act, often repetitively, as an unconscious mechanism to avoid unacceptable ideas and desires which, by themselves, arouse anxiety.

com·pul·sive (kəm-pŭl′sĭv) *adj.* Caused or conditioned by compulsion or obsession. —*n.* A person with behavior patterns governed by a compulsion.

compulsive personality *n.* A personality pattern characterized by rigidity, perfectionistic standards, meticulous attention to order and detail, and excessive concern with conformity, duty, and adherence to standards of conscience.

com·put·er·ized axial tomography (kəm-pyōo′tə-rīzd′) *n. Abbr.* **CAT** Tomography used in diagnostic studies of internal bodily structures, in which computer analysis of a series of cross-sectional scans made along a single axis of a bodily structure or tissue is used to construct a three-dimensional image of that structure. Also called *computed tomography*.

con– *pref.* Variant of **com–**.

conA *or* **con A** *abbr.* concanavalin A

co·nar·i·um (kō-nâr′ē-əm) *n.* See **pineal body**.

co·na·tion (kō-nā′shən) *n.* The aspect of mental processes or behavior directed toward action or change and including impulse, desire, volition, and striving. —**co′na·tive** (kō′nə-tĭv, kŏn′ə-) *adj.*

con·ca·nav·a·lin A (kŏn′kə-năv′ə-lĭn) *n. Abbr.* **conA** A glycoprotein extracted from the jack bean that promotes mitosis and stimulates T lymphocytes.

Con·ca·to's disease (kən-kä′tōz, kŏn-) *n.* See **polyserositis**.

con·cave (kŏn-kāv′, kŏn′kāv′) *adj.* Curved like the inner surface of a sphere. —*n.* A concave surface, structure, or line.

concave lens *n.* A lens having at least one surface curved like the inner surface of a sphere.

con·cav·i·ty (kŏn-kăv′ĭ-tē) *n.* A hollow or depression that is curved like the inner surface of a sphere.

con·ca·vo-con·cave (kŏn-kā′vō-kŏn-kāv′) *adj.* Of or being biconcave.

concavo-concave lens *n.* See **biconcave lens**.

con·ca·vo-con·vex (kŏn-kā′vō-kŏn-vĕks′) *adj.* Of or being concave on one surface and convex on the opposite surface.

concavo-convex lens *n.* A lens that is concave on one surface and convex on the opposite surface.

con·cealed hemorrhage (kən-sēld′) *n.* See **internal hemorrhage**.

con·ceive (kən-sēv′) *v.* **1.** To become pregnant. **2.** To apprehend mentally; to understand.

con·cen·tra·tion (kŏn′sən-trā′shən) *n.* **1.** An increase of the strength of a pharmaceutical preparation by the extraction, precipitation, and drying of its crude active agent. **2.** An increase in the strength of a fluid or gas in a mixture by purification, evaporation, or diffusion. **3.** The amount of a specified substance in a unit amount of another substance.

con·cen·tric (kən-sĕn′trĭk) *adj.* Having a common center or center point, as of circles.

concentric hypertrophy *n.* Hypertrophic growth of a hollow organ without overall enlargement, in which the walls of the organ are thickened and its capacity or volume is diminished.

concentric lamella *n.* One of the tubular layers of bone surrounding the central canal in an osteon. Also called *haversian lamella*.

con·cept (kŏn′sĕpt′) *n.* **1.** An abstract idea or notion. **2.** An explanatory principle in a scientific system. Also called *conception*.

concept formation *n.* In psychology, the development of ideas based on the common properties of objects, events, or qualities using the processes of abstraction and generalization.

con·cep·tion (kən-sĕp′shən) *n.* **1.** The act of forming a general idea or notion. **2.** The formation of a viable zygote by the union of a spermatozoon and an ovum; fertilization. **3.** See **concept** (sense 2).

con·cep·tu·al (kən-sĕp′chōo-əl) *adj.* Relating to concepts or the formation of concepts.

con·cep·tus (kən-sĕp′təs) *n., pl.* **–tus·es** The products of conception; that is, the embryo, chorionic sac, placenta, and fetal membranes.

con·cha (kŏng′kə) *n., pl.* **–chae** (-kē′) Any of various structures, such as the external ear, that resemble a shell in shape. —**con′chal** (-kəl) *adj.*

concha au·ric·u·lae (ô-rĭk′yə-lē′) *n.* The large hollow or floor of the external ear, between the front part of the helix and the antihelix.

concha sphe·noi·da·lis (sfē′noi-dā′lĭs) *n.* Either of a pair of pyramid-shaped ossicles whose bases form the roof of the nasal cavity.

con·chi·tis (kŏng-kī′tĭs) *n.* Inflammation of a concha.

con·cli·na·tion (kŏn′klə-nā′shən) *n.* See **intorsion** (sense ?).

con·com·i·tant strabismus (kən-kŏm′ĭ-tənt) *n.* Strabismus in which the degree of imbalance is the same regardless of which direction the eyes are looking.

concomitant symptom *n.* See **accessory symptom**.

con·cor·dance (kən-kôr′dns) *n.* The presence of a given trait in both members of a pair of twins. —**con·cor′dant** *adj.*

concordance rate *n.* A quantitative statistical expression for the concordance of a given genetic trait, especially in pairs of twins in genetic studies.

concordant alternation *n.* An alternation in either the mechanical or electrical activity of the heart, occurring in both systemic and pulmonary circuits. Also called *concordant alternans.*

con·cres·cence (kən-krĕs′əns) *n.* The growing together of separate parts. Also called *coalescence.*

con·crete (kŏn-krēt′, kŏn′krēt′) *adj.* **1.** Relating to an actual, specific thing or instance; particular. **2.** Existing in reality or in real experience; perceptible by the senses; real. **3.** Relating to a material thing or group of things as opposed to an abstraction. **4.** Formed by the coalescence of separate particles or parts into one mass; solid.

concrete thinking *n.* Thinking characterized by a predominance of actual objects and events and the absence of concepts and generalizations.

con·cre·ti·o cor·dis (kən-krē′shē-ō kôr′dĭs) *n.* Extensive adhesion between parietal and visceral layers of the pericardium with partial or complete obliteration of the pericardial cavity. Also called *internal adhesive pericarditis.*

con·cre·tion (kən-krē′shən) *n.* A solid mass, usually composed of inorganic material, formed in a cavity or tissue of the body; a calculus.

con·cus·sion (kən-kŭsh′ən) *n.* **1.** A violent shaking or jarring. **2.** An injury to a soft structure, especially the brain, produced by a violent blow and followed by a temporary or prolonged loss of function.

con·den·sa·tion (kŏn′dĕn-sā′shən, -dən-) *n.* **1.** The act of making more solid or dense. Also called *compression.* **2.** The process by which a gas or vapor changes to a liquid. **3.** The liquid formed when a gas is condensed. **4.** The psychological process by which a single symbol or word is associated with the emotional content of a group of ideas, feelings, memories, or impulses, especially as expressed in dreams. **5.** The dental process of packing a filling material into a cavity.

con·dens·er (kən-dĕn′sər) *n.* **1.** An apparatus for cooling a gas in order to convert it to to a liquid. **2.** An instrument for packing a material into a cavity of a tooth. **3.** The simple or compound lens on a microscope that is used to focus light on the specimen under observation.

con·dens·ing osteitis (kən-dĕn′sĭng) *n.* See **sclerosing osteitis.**

con·di·tion (kən-dĭsh′ən) *n.* **1.** A disease or physical ailment. **2.** A state of health or physical fitness. —*v.* To cause an organism to respond in a specific manner to a conditioned stimulus in the absence of an unconditioned stimulus.

con·di·tioned (kən-dĭsh′ənd) *adj.* **1.** Exhibiting or trained to exhibit a conditioned response. **2.** Physically fit.

conditioned response *n. Abbr.* **CR** A new or modified response elicited by a stimulus after conditioning. Also called *conditioned reflex.*

conditioned stimulus *n.* A previously neutral stimulus that, after repeated association with an unconditioned stimulus, elicits the response produced by the unconditioned stimulus itself.

con·di·tion·ing (kən-dĭsh′ə-nĭng) *n.* A process of behavior modification by which a subject comes to associate a desired behavior with a previously unrelated stimulus.

con·dom (kŏn′dəm) *n.* **1.** A flexible sheath, usually made of thin rubber or latex, designed to cover the penis or vagina during sexual intercourse for contraceptive purposes or as a means of preventing sexually transmitted diseases. **2.** A similar device, consisting of a loose-fitting polyurethane sheath closed at one end, that is inserted into the vagina before sexual intercourse. Also called *female condom.*

con·duct (kən-dŭkt′) *v.* To act as a medium for conveying something such as heat or electricity. —*n.* (kŏn′dŭkt′) The way a person acts, especially from the standpoint of morality. —**con·duc·tive** *adj.*

con·duc·tance (kən-dŭk′təns) *n.* **1.** A measure of a material's ability to conduct electric charge; the reciprocal of the resistance. **2.** The ease with which a fluid or gas enters and flows through a conduit, air passage, or respiratory tract.

con·duct disorder (kŏn′dŭkt′) *n.* A behavior disorder of childhood or adolescence characterized by a pattern of conduct in which either the basic rights of others or the societal norms or rules appropriate for a certain age are violated.

con·duc·tion (kən-dŭk′shən) *n.* The transmission or conveying of something through a medium or passage, especially the transmission of electric charge or heat through a conducting medium without perceptible motion of the medium itself.

conduction analgesia *n.* The pharmacological deactivation of sensory nerves in a portion of the body.

conduction anesthesia *n.* Regional anesthesia in which a local anesthetic solution is injected about the nerves to inhibit nerve transmission. Also called *block anesthesia.*

conduction aphasia *n.* A form of aphasia in which there is ability to speak and write but words are skipped, repeated, or substituted for one another. Also called *associative aphasia.*

con·duc·tive deafness (kn-dŭk′tĭv) *n.* Hearing loss or impairment caused by a defect in part of the ear that conducts sound, specifically the external canal or middle ear.

conductive hearing impairment *n.* Hearing impairment caused by an interference with the apparatus conducting sound to the inner ear.

conductive heat *n.* Heat transmitted to the body by direct contact, as by an electric pad.

con·duc·tiv·i·ty (kŏn′dŭk-tĭv′ĭ-tē) *n.* **1.** The ability or power to conduct or transmit heat, electricity, or sound. **2.** The ability of a body structure to transmit an electric impulse, especially the ability of a nerve to transmit a wave of excitation.

con·duc·tor (kən-dŭk′tər) *n.* **1.** A substance or medium that conducts heat, light, sound, or especially an electric charge. **2.** An instrument or probe having a groove along which a knife is passed in slitting open a sinus or fistula; a grooved director.

con·duit (kŏn′dōo-ĭt) *n.* A channel for the passage of fluids.

con·du·pli·cate (kŏn-doo′plĭ-kĭt) *adj.* Folded upon itself lengthwise.

con·dy·lar (kŏn′də-lər) *adj.* Relating to a condyle.

condylar canal *n.* The opening through the occipital bone posterior to the condyle on each side, transmitting the occipital emissary vein. Also called *condyloid canal, posterior condyloid foramen.*

condylar emissary vein *n.* A vein that connects the sigmoid sinus and the venous plexuses surrounding the vertebral processes and vertebral bodies through the condylar canal of the occipital bone.

condylar fossa *n.* A depression behind the condyle of the occipital bone in which the posterior margin of the superior facet of the atlas lies in extension.

condylar joint *n.* See **ellipsoidal joint.**

condylar process *n.* The articular process of the ramus of the mandible.

con·dy·lar·thro·sis (kŏn′dl-är-thrō′sĭs) *n.* A joint that is formed by condylar surfaces, such as the knee.

con·dyle (kŏn′dīl′, -dl) *n.* A rounded prominence at the end of a bone, most often for articulation with another bone.

con·dy·lec·to·my (kŏn′dl-ĕk′tə-mē) *n.* Excision of a condyle.

con·dy·loid (kŏn′dl-oid′) *adj.* Relating to or resembling a condyle.

condyloid canal *n.* See **condylar canal.**

con·dy·lo·ma (kŏn′dl-ō′mə) *n.,* *pl.* **-mas** *or* **-ma·ta** (-mə-tə) A wartlike growth on the skin or mucous membrane, usually in the area of the anus or external genitalia. —**con′dy·lo′ma·tous** (-mə-təs) *adj.*

condyloma a·cu·mi·na·tum (ə-kyoo′mə-nā′təm) *n.* See **genital wart.**

condyloma la·tum (lā′təm) *n.* See **flat condyloma.**

con·dy·lot·o·my (kŏn′dl-ŏt′ə-mē) *n.* Incision or surgical division of a condyle.

con·dy·lus (kŏn′dl-əs) *n.,* *pl.* **-dy·li** (-dl-ī′) Condyle.

cone (kōn) *n.* **1.** A solid body having a circle for its base and sides inclined so as to meet at a point above the base. **2.** See **cone cell.**

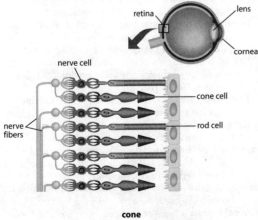

cone
detail of a retina showing cone and rod cells

cone cell *n.* One of the photoreceptors in the retina of the eye that is responsible for daylight and color vision;

they are densely concentrated in the fovea centralis, creating the area of greatest visual acuity. Also called *cone, retinal cone.*

cone granule *n.* The nucleus of a retinal cell connecting with one of the cones.

cone of light *n.* The bright triangular area of reflected light on the tympanic membrane during examination. Also called *light reflex.*

con·fab·u·la·tion (kən-făb′yə-lā′shən) *n.* The unconscious filling of gaps in one's memory by fabrications that one accepts as facts. —**con·fab′u·late′** *v.*

con·fec·tion (kən-fĕk′shən) *n.* A sweetened medicinal compound. Also called *electuary.*

con·fi·den·ti·al·i·ty (kŏn′fĭ-dĕn′shē-ăl′ĭ-tē) *n.* The ethical principle or legal right that a physician or other health professional will hold secret all information relating to a patient, unless the patient gives consent permitting disclosure.

con·fig·u·ra·tion (kən-fĭg′yə-rā′shən) *n.* **1.** The arrangement of parts or elements of a whole, especially the structural arrangement of atoms in a compound or molecule. **2.** Gestalt.

con·fine·ment (kən-fīn′mənt) *n.* **1.** The act of restricting or the state of being restricted in movement. **2.** Lying-in.

con·flict (kŏn′flĭkt′) *n.* A psychic struggle between opposing or incompatible impulses, desires, or tendencies.

con·flu·ence (kŏn′floo-əns) *n.* A flowing or meeting together; a joining.

confluence of sinuses *n.* The dilated area at the internal occipital protuberance where the superior sagittal, straight, occipital, and transverse sinuses of the dura mater meet.

con·flu·ent (kŏn′floo-ənt) *adj.* **1.** Flowing together; blended into one. **2.** Merging or running together so as to form a mass, as sores in a rash.

confluent and re·tic·u·late papillomatosis (rĭ-tĭk′yə-lĭt, -lāt′) *n.* A genodermatosis occurring predominantly in females at puberty and characterized by gradually spreading discrete and confluent papules of the anterior and posterior mid-chest.

con·for·ma·tion (kŏn′fər-mā′shən) *n.* One of the spatial arrangements of atoms in a molecule that can come about through free rotation of the atoms about a single chemical bond.

con·fu·sion (kən-fyoo′zhən) *n.* Impaired orientation with respect to time, place, or person; a disturbed mental state.

con·ge·ner (kŏn′jə-nər) *n.* **1.** A member of the same kind, class, or group. **2.** An organism of the same taxonomic genus as another organism. **3.** One of two or more muscles having the same function.

con·gen·i·tal (kən-jĕn′ĭ-tl) *adj.* **1.** Existing at or before birth usually through heredity, as a disorder. **2.** Acquired at birth or during uterine development, usually as a result of environmental influences.

congenital afibrinogenemia *n.* A hereditary disorder of blood coagulation in which little or no fibrinogen is present in the plasma.

congenital alopecia *n.* A congenital condition in which all hair is absent.

congenital amputation *n.* Loss of a fetal limb, usually the result of an intrinsic deficiency of embryonic tissue. Also called *birth amputation, intrauterine amputation.*

congenital anemia *n.* See **erythroblastosis fetalis.**

congenital anomaly *n.* See **birth defect.**

congenital diaphragmatic hernia *n.* The absence of the pleuroperitoneal membrane, allowing protrusion of abdominal viscera into the chest.

congenital dysphagocytosis *n.* See **chronic granulomatous disease.**

congenital ectodermal defect *n.* Incomplete development of the epidermis and skin appendages, causing the skin to be hairless and sweating to be deficient. Also called *congenital ectodermal dysplasia.*

congenital erythropoietic porphyria *n. Abbr.* **CEP** Enhanced porphyrin formation by erythroid cells in bone marrow, leading to severe porphyrinuria, often with hemolytic anemia and persistent cutaneous photosensitivity. Also called *Günther's disease.*

congenital generalized fibromatosis *n.* A rare disorder that is often fatal in the first week of life, although sometimes undergoing spontaneous remission, characterized by multiple subcutaneous and visceral fibrous tumors that are present at birth.

congenital glaucoma *n.* See **buphthalmia.**

congenital hemolytic anemia *n.* See **hereditary spherocytosis.**

congenital hemolytic jaundice *n.* See **hereditary spherocytosis.**

congenital hypoplastic anemia *n.* A form of anemia resulting from congenital hypoplasia of the bone marrow. Also called *erythrogenesis imperfecta.*

congenital ichthyosiform erythroderma *or* **ichthyosiform erythroderma** *n.* A hereditary skin disease characterized by diffuse chronic erythema and the formation of thickened, scaly skin on the palms and soles, sometimes associated with ocular and neural changes.

congenital megacolon *n.* Congenital dilation and hypertrophy of a segment of the colon due to an absence or marked reduction in the number of motor neurons innervating its muscular coat, resulting in extreme constipation and, if untreated, growth retardation. Also called *Hirschsprung's disease.*

congenital myxedema *n.* See **cretinism.**

congenital nevus *n.* A melanocytic nevus that is visible at birth, is often larger than an acquired nevus, and usually involves deeper dermal structures than an acquired nevus.

congenital nystagmus *n.* **1.** A congenitally predetermined nystagmus that is caused by lesions sustained in utero or at the time of birth. **2.** An inherited, nonprogressive, usually sex-linked nystagmus without associated neurologic lesions. **3.** The nystagmus associated with albinism, achromatopsia, and hypoplasia of the macula.

congenital pancytopenia *n.* See **Fanconi's anemia.**

congenital paramyotonia *n.* A nonprogressive disease characterized by myotonia induced by exposure to cold, with episodes of intermittent flaccid paralysis but no atrophy or hypertrophy of muscles. Also called *Eulenburg's disease.*

congenital pyloric stenosis *n.* See **hypertrophic pyloric stenosis.**

congenital stridor *n.* Stridor occurring at birth or within the first few months of life. It may be due to abnormal flaccidity of the epiglottis or arytenoids.

congenital syphilis *n.* Syphilis acquired by the fetus in utero.

congenital total lipodystrophy *n.* An inherited disorder characterized by an almost complete lack of subcutaneous fat, accelerated rate of growth and skeletal development during the first 3 to 4 years of life, muscular hypertrophy, cardiac enlargement, hepatosplenomegaly, hypertrichosis, renal enlargement, hyperlipemia, and hypermetabolism.

congenital valve *n.* An abnormal fold in a lining membrane that obstructs a passage, as of mucous membrane in the urethra.

con·gest (kən-jĕst′) *v.* To cause the accumulation of excessive blood or tissue fluid in a vessel or an organ.

con·gest·ed (kən-jĕs′tĭd) *adj.* Affected with or characterized by congestion.

con·ges·tion (kən-jĕs′chən) *n.* The presence of an abnormal amount of fluid in a vessel or organ; especially excessive accumulation of blood, due either to increased afflux or to obstruction of return flow.

con·ges·tive (kən-jĕs′tĭv) *adj.* Of or characterized by congestion.

congestive heart failure *n. Abbr.* **CHF** See **heart failure** (sense 1).

congestive splenomegaly *n.* Enlargement of the spleen due to passive congestion.

con·glo·bate (kŏn-glō′bāt′, kŏng′glō-) *adj.* Formed into a single, rounded mass.

con·glom·er·ate (kən-glŏm′ər-ĭt) *adj.* Gathered or aggregated into a mass. **—con·glom′er·a′tion** (-ə-rā′shən) *n.*

con·glu·ti·nant (kən-glōōt′n-ənt, kŏn-) *adj.* **1.** Promoting union, as of the edges of a wound. **2.** Relating to or characterizing the abnormal adhering of tissues to one another.

con·glu·ti·na·tion (kən-glōōt′n-ā′shən, kŏn-) *n.* **1.** Agglutination of the complex of antigen, antibody, and complement by normal bovine serum and other colloidal materials. **2.** See **adhesion** (sense 3).

con·go·phil·ic angiopathy (kŏng′gō-fĭl′ĭk) *n.* A condition of blood vessels characterized by deposits in the vessel walls of a substance, usually amyloid, that is easily stained by Congo red.

Con·go red (kŏng′gō) *n.* An acid dye used as an indicator in testing for free hydrochloric acid in gastric contents, as a laboratory aid in the diagnosis of amyloidosis, and as a histologic stain for amyloid.

con·gru·ous hemianopsia (kŏng′grōō-əs) *n.* Hemianopsia in which the defects in the visual field of each eye are symmetrical in every respect.

con·i·cal (kŏn′ĭ-kəl) *or* **con·ic** (-ĭk) *adj.* Of, relating to, or shaped like a cone.

conical cornea *n.* See **keratoconus.**

conical papilla *n.* Any of numerous projections on the back of the tongue, scattered among, similar to, but shorter than the filiform papillae.

co·nid·i·o·phore (kə-nĭd′ē-ə-fôr′) *n.* A specialized fungal hypha that produces conidia. —**co·nid'i·oph'or·ous** (kə-nĭd'ē-ŏf'ər-əs) *adj.*

co·nid·i·um (kə-nĭd'ē-əm) *n., pl.* **–i·a** (-ē-ə) An asexually produced fungal spore, formed on a conidiophore. —**co·nid'i·al** *adj.*

co·ni·o·fi·bro·sis (kō'nē-ō-fī-brō'sĭs) *n.* Fibrosis, especially of the lungs, caused by dust.

co·ni·o·phage (kō'nē-ə-fāj') *n.* See **alveolar macrophage.**

co·ni·o·sis (kō'nē-ō'sĭs) *n.* Any of various diseases or pathological conditions caused by dust.

con·i·za·tion (kŏn'ī-zā'shən, kō'nĭ-) *n.* The excision of a cone of tissue, such as the mucosa of the uterine cervix.

con·joined anastomosis (kən-joind') *n.* The side-by-side surgical connection of two small blood vessels to create a stoma.

conjoined twins *pl.n.* Identical twins born with their bodies joined at some point and having varying degrees of residual duplication, a result of the incomplete division of the ovum from which the twins developed. Also called *diplosomia.*

con·ju·gant (kŏn'jə-gənt) *n.* Either of a pair of organisms, cells, or gametes undergoing conjugation.

con·ju·ga·ta (kŏn'jə-gā'tə) *n.* Conjugate.

con·ju·gate (kŏn'jə-gāt') *v.* To undergo conjugation. —*adj.* (-gĭt, -gāt') **1.** Joined together, especially in pairs. **2.** Pertaining to an acid and a base that are related by the difference of a proton. —*n.* (-gĭt, -gāt') A distance between the points on the periphery of the pelvic canal, especially the promontory of the sacrum and the upper edge of the pubic symphysis. Also called *anteroposterior diameter, conjugate diameter, conjugate of inlet, internal conjugate, true conjugate.*

conjugate acid-base pair *n.* Two molecular species that easily transfer a hydrogen ion between them, especially from the acid to the base.

con·ju·gat·ed (kŏn'jə-gā'tĭd) *adj.* Conjugate.

conjugated double bond *n.* Two double bonds in a compound that are separated by a single bond.

conjugate deviation of eyes *n.* **1.** The turning of eyes in parallel and at the same time, as occurs normally. **2.** A pathological condition in which both eyes are turned to the same side as a result of either paralysis or muscular spasms.

conjugate diameter *n.* See **conjugate.**

conjugated protein *n.* A compound, such as hemoglobin, that is made up of a protein molecule and a nonprotein prosthetic group; compound protein.

conjugate foramen *n.* A foramen that is formed by the notches of two bones in apposition.

conjugate nystagmus *n.* A nystagmus in which the eyes move simultaneously in the same direction.

conjugate of inlet *n.* See **conjugate.**

conjugate of outlet *n.* The distance from the tip of the coccyx to the lower edge of the pubic symphysis.

conjugate paralysis *n.* Paralysis of one or more of the external muscles of the eye, resulting in loss of conjugate movement of the eyes.

con·ju·ga·tion (kŏn'jə-gā'shən) *n.* **1.** The temporary union of two bacterial cells during which one cell transfers part or all of its genome to the other. **2.** A process

of sexual reproduction in which ciliate protozoans of the same species temporarily couple and exchange genetic material. **3.** A process of sexual reproduction in certain algae and fungi in which temporary or permanent fusion occurs, resulting in the union of the male and female gametes. **4.** The addition of glucuronic or sulfuric acid to certain toxic substances to terminate their biological activity and prepare them for excretion.

conjugation tube *n.* A slender tube in certain bacteria and algae that connects two individuals during conjugation and through which the transfer of genetic material occurs.

con·ju·ga·tive plasmid (kŏn'jə-gā'tĭv) *n.* A plasmid that can move from one cell to another during the process of conjugation.

con·junc·ti·va (kŏn'jŭngk-tī'və) *n., pl.* **–vas** *or* **–vae** (-vē) The mucous membrane that lines the inner eyelid and the exposed surface of the eyeball.

con·junc·ti·val (kŏn'jŭngk-tī'vəl) *adj.* Relating to the conjunctiva.

conjunctival artery *n.* **1.** Any of various branches of anterior ciliary arteries supplying the conjunctiva; anterior conjunctival artery. **2.** Any of a series of branches from the tarsal arterial arches supplying the conjunctiva; posterior conjunctival artery.

conjunctival reflex *n.* Closing of the eyes in response to irritation of the conjunctiva.

conjunctival ring *n.* A narrow ring at the junction of the cornea and the conjunctiva.

conjunctival sac *n.* The space bound by the conjunctival membrane between the palpebral and bulbar conjunctiva of the eye.

conjunctival test *n.* A test in which an allergen is placed on the conjunctiva.

conjunctival varix *n.* See **varicula.**

conjunctival vein *n.* Any of the various veins that drain the conjunctiva.

con·junc·ti·vi·tis (kən-jŭngk'tə-vī'tĭs) *n.* Inflammation of the conjunctiva, characterized by redness and often accompanied by a discharge.

con·junc·ti·vo·ma (kən-jŭnk'tə-vō'mə) *n.* A tumor of the conjunctiva made up of conjunctival tissue.

con·junc·ti·vo·plas·ty (kŏn'jŭngk-tī'və-plăs'tē) *n.* Plastic surgery of the conjunctiva.

con·nect (kə-nĕkt') *v.* **1.** To join or fasten together. **2.** To become joined or united. —**con·nec'tor** *n.*

connecting cartilage *n.* The cartilage in a cartilaginous joint such as the pubic symphysis. Also called *interosseous cartilage.*

con·nec·tion (kə-nĕk'shən) *n.* **1.** The act of connecting or the state of being connected. **2.** Something that connects.

con·nec·tive tissue (kə-nĕk'tĭv) *n.* The supporting or framework tissue of the body, arising chiefly from the embryonic mesoderm and including collagenous, elastic and reticular fibers, adipose tissue, cartilage, and bone. Also called *interstitial tissue.*

connective-tissue disease *n.* Any of a group of noninheritable diseases that affect the connective tissue, such as rheumatic fever and rheumatoid arthritis, and that are characterized by fever, pain, stiffness, and inflammation.

connective tumor *n.* A tumor formed from connective tissue, such as an osteoma, fibroma, or sarcoma.

Conn's syndrome (kŏnz) *n.* See **primary aldosteronism.**

con·san·guin·e·ous (kŏn'săng-gwĭn'ē-əs) *adj.* Exhibiting consanguinity.

con·san·guin·i·ty (kŏn'săng-gwĭn'ĭ-tē) *n.* Relationship by blood or by a common ancestor.

con·science (kŏn'shəns) *n.* **1.** The awareness of a moral or ethical aspect to one's conduct together with the urge to prefer right over wrong. **2.** The part of the superego that judges the ethical nature of one's actions and thoughts and then transmits such determinations to the ego for consideration.

con·scious (kŏn'shəs) *adj.* **1.** Having an awareness of one's environment and one's own existence, sensations, and thoughts. **2.** Intentionally conceived or done; deliberate. —*n.* In psychoanalysis, the component of waking awareness perceptible by a person at any given instant. —**con'scious·ly** *adv.*

con·scious·ness (kŏn'shəs-nĭs) *n.* **1.** The state or condition of being conscious. **2.** A sense of one's personal or collective identity, especially the complex of attitudes, beliefs, and sensitivities held by or considered characteristic of an individual or a group. **3.** In psychoanalysis, the conscious.

consciousness-raising *n.* A process, as by group therapy, of achieving greater awareness of one's needs in order to fulfill one's potential as a person.

con·sec·u·tive anophthalmia (kən-sĕk'yə-tĭv) *n.* Anopthalmia due to atrophy or degeneration of the optic vesicle.

con·sen·su·al (kən-sĕn'shōō-əl) *adj.* **1.** Of or relating to a reflexive response of one body structure following stimulation of another, such as the concurrent constriction of one pupil in response to light shined in the other. **2.** Of or relating to involuntary movement of a body part accompanying voluntary movement of another. —**con·sen'su·al·ly** *adv.*

con·ser·va·tive (kən-sûr'və-tĭv) *adj.* Of or relating to treatment by gradual, limited, or well-established procedures; not radical. —**con·ser'va·tive·ly** *adv.*

con·sis·ten·cy principle (kən-sĭs'tən-sē) *n.* In psychology, the desire to be consistent, especially in attitudes and beliefs.

con·sol·i·da·tion (kən-sŏl'ĭ-dā'shən) *n.* The process of becoming a firm solid mass, as in an infected lung when the alveoli are filled with exudate.

con·stant (kŏn'stənt) *adj.* **1.** Continually occurring; persistent. **2.** Unchanging in nature, value, or extent; invariable. —*n.* **1.** A quantity assumed to have a fixed value in a specified mathematical context. **2.** An experimental or theoretical condition, factor, or quantity that does not vary or that is regarded as invariant in specified circumstances.

constant positive pressure breathing *n.* *Abbr.* **CPPB** Inhalation and exhalation of respiratory gases that are under a small constant positive pressure relative to the ambient pressure.

constant region *n.* The portion of the carboxyl terminal of an immunoglobulin's heavy and light chains having an amino acid sequence that does not vary within a given class or subclass of immunoglobulin.

con·sti·pate (kŏn'stə-pāt') *v.* To cause constipation in the bowels.

con·sti·pat·ed (kŏn'stə-pā'tĭd) *adj.* Suffering from constipation.

con·sti·pa·tion (kŏn'stə-pā'shən) *n.* Difficult, incomplete, or infrequent evacuation of dry, hardened feces from the bowels.

con·sti·tu·tion (kŏn'stĭ-tōō'shən) *n.* **1.** The physical makeup of the body, including its functions, metabolic processes, reactions to stimuli, and resistance to the attack of pathogenic organisms. **2.** The composition or structure of a molecule.

con·sti·tu·tion·al (kŏn'stĭ-tōō'shə-nəl) *adj.* **1.** Of or relating to one's physical makeup. **2.** Of or proceeding from the basic structure or nature of a person or thing; inherent.

constitutional disease *n.* A disease involving the entire body or having a widespread array of symptoms.

constitutional reaction *n.* **1.** A generalized or systemic reaction to a stimulus. **2.** An allergic or immune response occurring at sites remote from that of the introduction of an antigen.

constitutional symptom *n.* A symptom indicating that a disease or disorder is affecting the whole body.

con·strict (kən-strĭkt') *v.* To make smaller or narrower, especially by binding or squeezing.

con·stric·tion (kən-strĭk'shən) *n.* **1.** The act of constricting or the state of being constricted. **2.** A feeling of tightness or pressure, as in the chest. **3.** A constricted or narrow part.

constriction ring *n.* True spastic stricture of the uterine cavity caused by a zone of muscle undergoing tetanic contraction and forming a tight constriction about some part of the fetus.

con·stric·tive pericarditis (kən-strĭk'tĭv) *n.* Tuberculous or other infection of the pericardium, with thickening of the membrane and constriction of the cardiac chambers.

con·stric·tor (kən-strĭk'tər) *n.* One that constricts, especially a muscle that contracts or compresses a part or organ of the body.

con·sul·tant (kən-sŭl'tənt) *n.* **1.** A physician or surgeon who does not take actual charge of a patient, but acts in an advisory capacity to the patient's primary physician. **2.** Such a member of a hospital staff who may advise the attending physician or surgeon.

con·sul·ta·tion (kŏn'səl-tā'shən) *n.* A meeting of two or more health professionals to discuss the diagnosis, prognosis, and treatment of a particular case.

con·sult·ing staff (kən-sŭl'tĭng) *n.* The body of specialists affiliated with a hospital who serve in an advisory capacity to the attending staff.

con·sump·tion (kən-sŭmp'shən) *n.* **1.** The act or process of using up something. **2.** A progressive wasting of body tissue. **3.** Pulmonary tuberculosis. No longer in technical use.

consumption coagulopathy *n.* See **disseminated intravascular coagulation.**

con·sump·tive (kən-sŭmp'tĭv) *adj.* Of, relating to, or afflicted with consumption.

con·tact (kŏn'tăkt') *n.* **1.** A coming together or touching, as of bodies or surfaces. **2.** A person recently exposed to a contagious disease, usually through close association with an infected individual. —*v.* (kŏn′tăkt′, kən-tăkt′) To bring, be, or come in contact. —*adj.* **1.** Of, sustaining, or making contact. **2.** Caused or transmitted by touching, as a rash.

contact allergy *n.* A cutaneous hypersensitivity caused by direct contact with an antigen.

con·tac·tant (kən-tăk′tənt) *n.* Any of a group of allergens that elicit manifestations of induced sensitivity by direct contact with the skin or mucosa.

contact cheilitis *n.* Inflammation of the lips resulting from contact with a specific allergen.

contact dermatitis *n.* An acute or chronic skin inflammation resulting from contact with an irritating substance or allergen.

contact inhibition *n.* Cessation of replication of dividing cells that come into contact.

contact lens *n.* A thin plastic or glass lens that is fitted over the cornea of the eye to correct various vision defects.

contact splint *n.* A slotted plate, held by screws, used in the treatment of fracture of long bones.

contact-type dermatitis *n.* Dermatitis that resembles contact dermatitis but is caused by an ingested or injected allergen and is more widespread.

contact with reality *n.* The ability to understand or interpret external phenomena in relation to the norms of one's societal or cultural milieu.

con·ta·gion (kən-tā′jən) *n.* **1.** Disease transmission by direct or indirect contact. **2.** A disease that is or may be transmitted by direct or indirect contact; a contagious disease. **3.** The direct cause, such as a bacterium or virus, of a communicable disease. **4.** The spread of a behavior pattern, attitude, or emotion from person to person or group to group through suggestion, propaganda, rumor, or imitation.

con·ta·gious (kən-tā′jəs) *adj.* **1.** Of or relating to contagion. **2.** Transmissible by direct or indirect contact; communicable. **3.** Capable of transmitting disease; carrying a disease. —**con·ta′gious·ness** *n.*

contagious disease *n.* See **communicable disease.**

contagious granular conjunctivitis *n.* See **trachoma.**

con·ta·gium (kən-tā′jəm) *n.,* *pl.* **–gia** (-jə) The causative agent of a communicable disease; contagion.

con·tam·i·nate (kən-tăm′ə-nāt′) *v.* **1.** To make impure or unclean by contact or mixture. **2.** To expose to or permeate with radioactivity. —**con·tam·i·nant** (-nənt) *n.*

con·tam·i·na·tion (kən-tăm′ə-nā′shən) *n.* **1.** The act or process of rendering something harmful or unsuitable. **2.** The presence of extraneous, especially infectious, material that renders a substance or preparation impure or harmful.

con·tent (kŏn′tĕnt′) *n.* **1.** Something contained, as in a receptacle. **2.** The proportion of a specified substance present in something else, as of protein in a food. **3.** The subject matter or essential meaning of something, especially a dream.

content analysis *n.* Any of various techniques for classifying and studying the verbalizations of normal or psychologically impaired individuals.

con·ti·gu·i·ty (kŏn′tĭ-gyōo′ĭ-tē) *n.* The state of being contiguous.

con·tig·u·ous (kən-tĭg′yōo-əs) *adj.* **1.** Sharing a boundary or an edge; touching. **2.** Neighboring; adjacent. —**con·tig′u·ous·ness** *n.*

con·ti·nence (kŏn′tə-nəns) *n.* **1.** Self-restraint; moderation. **2.** Voluntary control over urinary and fecal discharge. **3.** Partial or complete abstention from sexual activity. —**con′ti·nent** *adj.*

con·tin·ued fever (kən-tĭn′yōod) *n.* A fever of some duration in which there are no intermissions or marked remissions in the temperature.

con·ti·nu·i·ty (kŏn′tə-nōo′ĭ-tē) *n.* **1.** The state or quality of being continuous. **2.** An uninterrupted succession or flow; a coherent whole.

con·tin·u·ous (kən-tĭn′yōo-əs) *adj.* **1.** Uninterrupted in time, sequence, substance, or extent. **2.** Attached together in repeated units.

continuous bar retainer *n.* A metal bar, usually resting on lingual surfaces of teeth, to aid in their stabilization and to act as an indirect retainer after orthodontic treatment.

continuous capillary *n.* A blood capillary found in muscle, in which small caveolae are numerous and pores are absent.

continuous murmur *n.* A murmur heard without interruption throughout systole and into diastole.

continuous passive motion *n.* *Abbr.* **CPM** A technique in which a joint, usually the knee, is moved constantly in a mechanical splint to prevent stiffness and to increase the range of motion.

continuous positive airway pressure *n.* *Abbr.* **CPAP** A technique of respiratory therapy for individuals breathing with or without mechanical assistance in which airway pressure is maintained above atmospheric pressure throughout the respiratory cycle by pressurization of the ventilatory circuit.

continuous positive pressure breathing *n.* See **controlled mechanical ventilation.**

continuous positive pressure ventilation *n.* See **controlled mechanical ventilation.**

continuous suture *n.* A suture made from an uninterrupted series of stitches and fastened at each end by a knot. Also called *uninterrupted suture.*

contra– *pref.* Against; opposite; contrasting: *contraindication.*

con·tra·ap·er·ture (kŏn′trə-ăp′ər-chər) *n.* See **counteropening.**

con·tra·cep·tion (kŏn′trə-sĕp′shən) *n.* Intentional prevention of conception or impregnation through the use of various devices, agents, drugs, sexual practices, or surgical procedures.

con·tra·cep·tive (kŏn′trə-sĕp′tĭv) *adj.* Capable of preventing conception. —*n.* A device, drug, or chemical agent that prevents conception.

contraceptive device *n.* Any of various devices used to prevent pregnancy, including the diaphragm, condom, and intrauterine device.

contraceptive sponge *n.* A small absorbent contraceptive pad that contains a spermicide and that is positioned against the cervix of the uterus before sexual intercourse.

con·tract (kən-trăkt′, kŏn′trăkt′) *v.* **1.** To reduce in size by drawing together. **2.** To become reduced in size by or as if by being drawn together, as the pupil of the eye. **3.** To acquire or incur by contagion or infection.

contracted kidney *n.* A diffusely scarred kidney in which the presence of abnormal fibrous tissue and ischemic atrophy leads to a reduction in its size.

contracted pelvis *n.* A pelvis with less than normal measurements in any diameter.

con·trac·tile (kən-trăk′təl, -tīl′) *adj.* Capable of contracting or causing contraction, as a tissue. —**con′-trac·til′i·ty** (kŏn′trăk-tĭl′ĭ-tē) *n.*

con·trac·tion (kən-trăk′shən) *n.* **1.** The act of contracting or the state of being contracted. **2.** The shortening and thickening of functioning muscle or muscle fiber.

con·trac·tu·al psychiatry (kən-trăk′chōō-əl) *n.* An arrangement in which a person undergoing psychiatric treatment retains control over his or her participation with the psychiatrist and decides when to seek help.

con·trac·ture (kən-trăk′chər) *n.* An abnormal, often permanent shortening, as of muscle or scar tissue, that results in distortion or deformity, especially of a joint of the body.

con·tra·fis·su·ra (kŏn′trə-fə-shōōr′ə) *n.* A fracture of a bone opposite to the point where a blow was received. Also called *fracture by contrecoup.*

con·tra·ges·tive (kŏn′trə-jĕs′tĭv) *adj.* Capable of preventing gestation, either by preventing implantation or by causing the uterine lining to shed after implantation. —*n.* A contragestive drug or agent.

con·tra·in·di·cate (kŏn′trə-ĭn′dĭ-kāt′) *v.* To indicate the inadvisability of something, such as a medical treatment.

con·tra·in·di·ca·tion (kŏn′trə-ĭn′dĭ-kā′shən) *n.* A factor that renders the administration of a drug or the carrying out of a medical procedure inadvisable.

con·tra·lat·er·al (kŏn′trə-lăt′ər-əl) *adj.* Taking place or originating in a corresponding part on an opposite side, as pain or paralysis in a part opposite the site of a lesion.

contralateral hemiplegia *n.* Paralysis occurring on the side of the body opposite to the side of the brain in which the causal lesion occurs.

con·trast agent (kŏn′trăst′) *n.* See **contrast medium.**

contrast bath *n.* A bath in which a part of the body is immersed alternately in hot and cold water.

contrast enema *n.* See **barium enema.**

contrast medium *n.* A substance, such as barium or air, used in radiography to increase the contrast of an image. A positive contrast medium absorbs x-rays more strongly than the tissue or structure being examined; a negative contrast medium, less strongly. Also called *contrast agent.*

contrast stain *n.* A dye used to color a portion of a tissue or cell that remained uncolored when the other part was stained by a dye of different color.

con·tre·coup (kŏn′trə-kōō′) *n.* Injury to a part opposite the site of the primary injury, as an injury to the skull opposite the site of a blow.

contrecoup injury of brain *n.* Injury to the brain occurring beneath the skull opposite to the area of impact.

cont. rem. *abbr. Latin* continuetur remedium, continuentur remedia (let the remedy be continued, let the

remedies be continued; continue the remedy, continue the remedies)

con·trol (kən-trōl′) *v.* **1.** To verify or regulate a scientific experiment by conducting a parallel experiment or by comparing with another standard. **2.** To hold in restraint; check. —*n.* **1.** A standard of comparison for checking or verifying the results of an experiment. **2.** An individual or group used as a standard of comparison in a control experiment.

control experiment *n.* An experiment that isolates the effect of one variable on a system by holding constant all variables but the one under observation.

control group *n.* A group used as a standard of comparison in a control experiment.

con·trolled hypotension (kən-trōld′) *n.* See **induced hypotension.**

controlled mechanical ventilation *n. Abbr.* **CMV** A method of artificial ventilation in which all inspirations are provided by positive pressure applied to the airway. Also called *continuous positive pressure breathing, continuous positive pressure ventilation, intermittent positive pressure breathing, intermittent positive pressure ventilation.*

controlled respiration *n.* See **controlled ventilation.**

controlled substance *n.* A drug or chemical substance whose possession and use are regulated under the Controlled Substances Act.

controlled ventilation *n.* Intermittent application of positive pressure to a gas or gases in or about the airway in order to force gas into the lungs in the absence of spontaneous ventilatory efforts. Also called *controlled respiration.*

control syringe *n.* A type of Luer syringe with thumb and finger rings attached to the proximal end of the barrel and to the tip of the plunger, allowing operation with one hand. Also called *ring syringe.*

con·tuse (kən-tōōz′) *v.* To injure without breaking the skin; bruise.

con·tused wound (kən-tōōzd′) *n.* A bruise.

con·tu·sion (kən-tōō′zhən) *n.* An injury in which the skin is not broken, often characterized by ruptured blood vessels and discolorations; a bruise.

co·nus (kō′nəs) *n., pl.* **-ni** (-nī′) **1.** Cone. **2.** Posterior staphyloma in myopic choroidopathy.

conus ar·te·ri·o·sus (är-tîr′ē-ō′səs) *n.* A conical extension of the right ventricle in the heart, from which the pulmonary artery originates. Also called *arterial cone, infundibulum.*

con·va·lesce (kŏn′və-lĕs′) *v.* To return to health and strength after illness; recuperate.

con·va·les·cence (kŏn′və-lĕs′əns) *n.* **1.** Gradual return to health and strength after an illness, an injury, or a surgical operation. **2.** The period needed for returning to health after an illness, an injury, or a surgical operation.

con·va·les·cent (kŏn′və-lĕs′ənt) *adj.* Relating to convalescence. —*n.* A person who is recovering from an illness, an injury, or a surgical operation.

con·vec·tion (kən-vĕk′shən) *n.* **1.** Heat transfer in a gas or liquid by the circulation of currents from one region to another. **2.** Fluid motion caused by an external force such as gravity.

con·vec·tive heat (kən-věk′tĭv) *n.* Heat conveyed to the body by a moving warm medium, such as air or water.

con·ven·tion·al sign (kən-věn′shə-nəl) *n.* Any of various signs, such as words or symbols, that acquire their function through linguistic custom.

conventional thoracoplasty *n.* Surgical removal of part of the ribs to allow inward retraction of the chest wall and collapse of a diseased lung.

con·ver·gence (kən-vûr′jəns) *n.* **1.** The process of coming together or the state of having come together toward a common point. **2.** Such a gathering at a single preganglionic motor neuron of several postganglionic motor neurons. **3.** The coordinated turning of the eyes inward to focus on an object at close range. **4.** The adaptive evolution of superficially similar structures, such as the wings of birds and insects, in unrelated species subjected to similar environments. Also called *convergent evolution.* **5.** The movement of cells from the periphery of the embryo toward the midline during gastrulation. —**con·verge′** *v.* —**con·ver′gent** *adj.*

convergence excess *n.* That condition in which an esophoria or esotropia is greater for near vision than for far vision.

convergence insufficiency *n.* The condition in which an esophoria or esotropia is greater for far vision than for near vision.

convergent evolution *n.* See **convergence** (sense 4).

convergent strabismus *n.* See **esotropia.**

con·ver·sion (kən-vûr′zhən, -shən) *n.* **1.** The acquisition by bacteria of a new property associated with presence of a prophage. **2.** A defense mechanism in which repressed ideas, conflicts, or impulses are manifested by various bodily symptoms, such as paralysis or breathing difficulties, that have no physical cause. —**con·ver′sive** (-sĭv) *adj.*

conversion disorder *n.* A disorder involving the loss or alteration of physical functioning, such as paralysis, voice loss, tunnel vision, or seizures, that is the result of a psychological involvement or need rather than a physical illness or disease. Also called *conversion hysteria, conversion reaction.*

conversive heat *n.* Heat produced in the body by the absorption of waves, such as the sun's rays, which are not in themselves hot.

con·ver·tase (kŏn′vər-tās′, kən-vûr′-) *n.* An enzyme that catalyzes the conversion of a substance, such as complement, to its active state.

con·ver·tin (kən-vûr′tn) *n.* See **factor VII.**

con·vex (kŏn′věks′, kən-věks′) *adj.* Having a surface or boundary that curves or bulges outward, as the exterior of a sphere. —**con·vex′i·ty** *n.*

convex lens *n.* A lens having at least one surface that curves outward like the exterior of a sphere.

con·vex·o-con·cave (kən-věk′sō-kən-kāv′) *adj.* **1.** Being convex on one side and concave on the other. **2.** Having greater curvature on the convex side than on the concave side. Used of a lens.

convexo-concave lens *n.* A lens having one surface convex and the opposite surface concave, with the concave surface having the greater curvature.

con·vex·o-con·vex (kən-věk′sō-kən-věks′) *adj.* Convex on both sides; biconvex. Used of a lens.

convexo-convex lens *n.* See **biconvex lens.**

con·vo·lut·ed tubule (kŏn′və-loo′tĭd) *n.* The highly convoluted segments of nephron in the renal labyrinth of the kidney, made up of the proximal tubule that leads from the Bowman's capsule to the descending limb of Henle's loop and the distal tubule that leads from the ascending limb of Henle's loop to a collecting tubule.

con·vo·lu·tion (kŏn′və-loo′shən) *n.* **1.** A form or part that is folded or coiled. **2.** One of the convex folds of the surface of the brain.

con·vul·sant (kən-vŭl′sənt) *adj.* Causing or producing convulsions. —*n.* An agent, such as a drug, that causes convulsions.

con·vulse (kən-vŭls′) *v.* To affect or be affected with irregular and involuntary muscular contractions; throw or be thrown into convulsions.

con·vul·sion (kən-vŭl′shən) *n.* An intense, paroxysmal, involuntary muscular contraction or a series of such contractions. Also called *seizure.*

con·vul·sive (kən-vŭl′sĭv) *adj.* **1.** Characterized by or having the nature of convulsions. **2.** Having or producing convulsions.

Coo·ley (koo′lē), **Denton Arthur** Born 1920. American surgeon and educator who in 1969 performed the first artificial heart transplant on a human.

Coo·ley's anemia (koo′lēz) *n.* See **thalassemia major.**

Coombs' serum (koomz) *n.* Serum from a rabbit or other animal previously immunized with purified human globulin to prepare antibodies directed against IgG and complement, used in the direct and indirect Coombs' tests. Also called *antihuman globulin.*

Coombs' test *n.* Either of two tests for detecting red blood cell antibodies: the direct test, for detecting sensitized red blood cells in erythroblastosis fetalis and in acquired hemolytic anemia; and the indirect test, for cross-matching blood or investigating transfusion reactions. Also called *antiglobulin test.*

Coo·per's ligament (koo′pərz) *n.* See **transverse ligament of elbow.**

co·or·di·nate bond (kō-ôr′dn-ĭt, -āt′) *n.* A covalent chemical bond between two atoms that is produced when one atom shares a pair of electrons with another atom lacking such a pair. Also called *semipolar bond.*

co·or·di·na·tion (kō-ôr′dn-ā′shən) *n.* **1.** The harmonious adjustment or interaction of parts. **2.** Harmonious functioning of muscles or groups of muscles in the execution of movements.

co·pay·ment (kō′pā′mənt) *n.* A fixed fee that subscribers to a medical plan must pay for their use of specific medical services covered by the plan.

COPD *abbr.* chronic obstructive pulmonary disease

cope (kōp) *v.* To contend with difficulties with the intent to overcome them.

co·pe·pod (kō′pə-pŏd′) *n.* Any of numerous minute marine and freshwater crustaceans of the subclass Copepoda, having an elongated body and a forked tail.

co·pol·y·mer (kō-pŏl′ə-mər) *n.* A polymer of two or more different monomers.

copolymer resin *n.* A synthetic resin produced by joint polymerization of two or more different monomers or polymers.

cop·per (kŏp'ər) *n. Symbol* **Cu** A malleable metallic trace element used in its salt forms as an astringent, deodorant, and antifungal, and whose radioisotope is used in brain scans and for diagnosing Wilson's disease. Atomic number 29.

copper penny *n.* See **sclerotic body.**

copper-sulfate method *n.* A method for determining the specific gravity of blood or plasma in which the test fluid is delivered by drops into solutions of copper sulfate having graduated specific gravities.

cop·rem·e·sis (kŏ-prĕm'ĭ-sĭs) *n.* See **fecal vomiting.**

copro– *pref.* Excrement; dung: *coprostasis.*

cop·ro·an·ti·bod·y (kŏp'rō-ăn'tĭ-bŏd'ē) *n.* Any of various antibodies occurring in the intestinal tract and found in feces that are formed by plasma cells in the intestinal mucosa.

cop·ro·lag·ni·a (kŏp'rə-lăg'nē-ə) *n.* A form of sexual perversion in which pleasure is obtained from the thought, sight, or touching of excrement.

cop·ro·la·li·a (kŏp'rə-lā'lē-ə) *n.* The uncontrolled or involuntary use of obscene or scatological language that may accompany certain mental disorders, such as schizophrenia or Tourette's syndrome.

cop·ro·lith (kŏp'rə-lĭth') *n.* A hard mass of fecal matter in the intestine. Also called *fecalith, stercolith.*

cop·rol·o·gy (kŏ-prŏl'ə-jē) *n.* See **scatology.**

cop·ro·ma (kŏ-prō'mə) *n.* The accumulation of hardened feces in the colon or rectum giving the appearance of an abdominal tumor. Also called *fecaloma, stercoroma.*

cop·roph·a·gy (kŏ-prŏf'ə-jē) *n.* See **scatophagy.** —**cop·roph'a·gous** (-gəs) *adj.*

cop·ro·phil·i·a (kŏp'rə-fĭl'ē-ə) *n.* An abnormal, often obsessive interest in excrement, especially the use of feces for sexual excitement. —**cop'ro·phil'i·ac'** (-ē-ăk') *n.*

cop·ro·phil·ic (kŏp'rə-fĭl'ĭk) *adj.* **1.** Occurring in fecal matter. **2.** Relating to coprophilia.

cop·roph·i·lous (kŏ-prŏf'ə-ləs) *adj.* Living or growing on excrement, as certain fungi.

cop·ro·pho·bi·a (kŏp'rə-fō'bē-ə) *n.* An abnormal abhorrence of defecation and feces.

cop·ro·por·phyr·i·a (kŏp'rə-pôr-fîr'ē-ə) *n.* The presence of coproporphyrins in the urine, as in variegate porphyria.

cop·ro·por·phy·rin (kŏp'rə-pôr'fə-rĭn) *n.* Either of two porphyrin compounds found normally in feces as a decomposition product of bilirubin.

cop·ros·ta·sis (kŏ-prŏs'tə-sĭs, kŏp'rə-stā'-) *n.* The impaction of feces in the intestine.

cop·ro·zo·a (kŏp'rə-zō'ə) *n.* Protozoa that can be cultivated in fecal matter but do not necessarily live in feces within the intestine. —**cop·ro·zo'ic** *adj.*

cop·u·la (kŏp'yə-lə) *n.* A narrow part connecting two structures.

cop·u·late (kŏp'yə-lāt') *v.* To engage in coitus or sexual intercourse.

cop·u·la·tion (kŏp'yə-lā'shən) *n.* **1.** Conjugation between two cells that do not fuse but separate after mutual fertilization. **2.** See **coitus.** —**cop'u·late'** *v.*

cor (kôr) *n., pl.* **cor·da** (kôr'də) Heart.

cor– *pref.* Variant of **core–.**

cor·a·co·a·cro·mi·al (kôr'ə-kō-ə-krō'mē-əl) *adj.* Of or relating to the coracoid and the acromial processes; acromiocoracoid.

coracoacromial ligament *n.* The heavy arched fibrous band that passes between the coracoid process and the acromion above the shoulder joint.

cor·a·co·bra·chi·al muscle (kôr'ə-kō-brā'kē-əl, -brăk'-ē-) *n.* A muscle with its origin in the coracoid process of the scapula, with insertion to the middle of the medial border of the humerus, with nerve supply from the musculocutaneous nerve, and whose action adducts and flexes the arm.

cor·a·co·cla·vic·u·lar (kôr'ə-kō-klə-vĭk'yə-lər) *adj.* Relating to the coracoid process and the clavicle.

coracoclavicular ligament *n.* The strong ligament that unites the clavicle to the coracoid process.

cor·a·co·hu·mer·al (kôr'ə-kō-hyōō'mər-əl) *adj.* Of or relating to the coracoid process and the humerus.

cor·a·coid (kôr'ə-koid') *n.* **1.** A bony process projecting from the scapula toward the sternum in mammals. **2.** A beak-shaped bone articulating with the scapula and sternum in most nonmammalia vertebrates, such as birds and reptiles. —*adj.* Of, relating to, or resembling a coracoid.

coracoid process *n.* A long curved projection from the neck of the scapula, overhanging the glenoid cavity and giving attachment to the short head of the biceps, the coracobrachial muscle, the smaller pectoral muscle, and the coracoacromial ligament.

cor ad·i·po·sum (ăd'ə-pō'səm) *n.* See **fatty heart** (sense 2).

cor·al calculus (kôr'əl) *n.* See **stag-horn calculus.**

cor bi·loc·u·lar·e (bī-lŏk'yə-lâr'ē) *n.* A congenital heart abnormality in which the interatrial and interventricular septa are absent or incomplete.

cor bo·vi·num (bō-vī'nəm) *n.* See **bucardia.**

cord *or* **chord** (kôrd) *n.* A long ropelike bodily structure, such as a nerve or tendon.

Cor·da·rone (kôr'də-rōn') A trademark for the drug amiodarone hydrochloride.

cor·date (kôr'dāt') *adj.* Heart-shaped.

cordate pelvis *n.* A pelvis in which the sacrum projects forward between the iliac bones, giving a heart shape to the brim. Also called *cordiform pelvis.*

cord blood *n.* Blood present in the umbilical vessels at the time of delivery.

cor·dec·to·my (kôr-dĕk'tə-mē) *n.* Excision of all or a part of a cord, as of a vocal cord.

cor·di·form (kôr'də-fôrm') *adj.* Heart-shaped.

cordiform pelvis *n.* See **cordate pelvis.**

cordiform uterus *n.* An incomplete bicornate uterus with a wedge-shaped depression at the fundus.

cordo– *or* **cord–** *or* **chordo–** *or* **chord–** *pref.* Cord: *cordopexy.*

cord of tympanum *n.* A nerve arising from the facial nerve in the facial canal to join the lingual branch of the mandibular nerve and conveying taste sensation from the front two thirds of the tongue.

cor·don sa·ni·taire (kôr-dôn' sä-nē-târ') *n.* A barrier designed to prevent a disease or other undesirable condition from spreading.

cor·do·pex·y (kôr'də-pĕk'sē) *n.* The surgical fixation

of a cord, as of one or both vocal cords for the relief of laryngeal stenosis.

cor·dot·o·my or **chor·dot·o·my** (kôr-dŏt′ə-mē) n. **1.** An operation on the spinal cord. **2.** Surgical division of tracts of the spinal cord, as for the relief of severe pain.

Cor·dran (kôr′drăn′) A trademark for the drug flurandrenolide.

core (kôr) n. **1.** The central or innermost part. **2.** The part of a nuclear reactor where fission occurs.

core– or **cor–** or **coreo–** or **coro–** pref. Pupil: corectopia.

cor·e·clei·sis or **cor·e·cli·sis** (kôr′ĭ-klī′sĭs) n. Occlusion of the pupil of the eye.

cor·ec·ta·sia (kôr′ĭk-tā′zhə) or **cor·ec·ta·sis** (kôr-ĕk′tə-sĭs) n. Pathological dilation of the pupil of the eye.

cor·ec·to·me·di·al·y·sis (kôr-ĕk′tə-mē-dī-ăl′ĭ-sĭs) n. A peripheral iridectomy to form an artificial pupil.

cor·ec·to·pi·a (kôr′ĭk-tō′pē-ə) n. Abnormal location of the pupil so that it is not in the center of the iris.

co·rel·y·sis (kô-rĕl′ĭ-sĭs) n. Surgical detachment of the adhesions between the capsule of the lens and the iris.

cor·e·o·plas·ty (kôr′ē-ə-plăs′tē) n. Plastic surgery to correct a deformed or occluded pupil. Also called coroplasty.

cor·e·prax·y (kôr′ə-prăk′sē) n. An operation to centralize a pupil that is abnormally situated. Also called corepexy.

co·re·pres·sor (kō′rĭ-prĕs′ər) n. A substance that combines with and activates a genetic repressor, thus preventing gene transcription and inhibiting protein synthesis.

Cor·gard (kôr′gärd′) A trademark for the drug nadolol.

Co·ri (kôr′ē), **Gerty Theresa Radnitz** 1896–1957. Czechborn American biochemist. She shared a 1947 Nobel Prize with her husband, **Carl Ferdinand Cori** (1896–1984), and Bernardo A. Houssay for discovering the intermediate steps in glycogen-glucose conversion.

Cori cycle n. The phases in the metabolism of carbohydrates in which muscles convert glycogen to lactic acid, which is carried by the blood to the liver where it is converted to glycogen then broken down to glucose that, in turn, is carried by the blood to muscles, where it is converted to glycogen and used as an energy source for muscular activity.

Co·ri's disease (kôr′ēz) n. See **type 3 glycogenosis**.

co·ri·um (kôr′ē-əm) n., pl. **co·ri·a** (kôr′ē-ə) See **dermis**.

corn (kôrn) n. A small conical callosity caused by pressure over a bony prominence, usually on a toe. Also called clavus, heloma.

cor·ne·a (kôr′nē-ə) n. The transparent, convex, anterior portion of the outer fibrous coat of the eyeball that covers the iris and the pupil and is continuous with the sclera. —**cor′ne·al** adj.

corneal astigmatism n. Astigmatism due to a defect in the curvature of the corneal surface.

corneal corpuscle n. A connective tissue cell found between the layers of fibrous tissue in the cornea. Also called Virchow's cell.

corneal graft n. See **keratoplasty**.

corneal layer n. See **stratum corneum**.

corneal margin n. The margin of the cornea that is overlapped by the sclera. Also called sclerocorneal junction.

corneal reflex n. Contraction of the eyelids when the cornea is lightly touched.

corneal space n. Any of the stellate spaces containing a cell or corneal corpuscle between the lamellae of the cornea. Also called lacuna.

corneal staphyloma n. See **anterior staphyloma**.

Cor·ne·lia de Lang·e's syndrome (kôr-nēl′yə də lăng′-ēz, läng′əz) n. Variant of **de Lange's syndrome**.

cor·ne·o·scle·ra (kôr′nē-ō-sklîr′ə) n. The cornea and sclera considered as the external coat of the eyeball. —**cor′ne·o·scle′ral** adj.

cor·ne·ous (kôr′nē-əs) adj. Made of horn or a hornlike substance; horny.

Corn·forth (kôrn′fərth, -fôrth′), **John Warcup** Born 1917. Australian-born British chemist. He shared a 1975 Nobel Prize for research on the structure of biological molecules.

cor·nic·u·late (kôr-nĭk′yə-lāt′, -lĭt) adj. Having horns or hornlike projections.

corniculate cartilage n. A conical nodule of elastic cartilage surmounting the apex of each arytenoid cartilage.

cor·nic·u·lum (kôr-nĭk′yə-ləm) n., pl. **–la** (-lə) A small cornu or hornlike process.

cor·ni·fi·ca·tion (kôr′nə-fĭ-kā′shən) n. See **keratinization**.

cor·ni·fy (kôr′nə-fī′) v. To undergo cornification.

corn sugar n. Dextrose obtained from cornstarch.

cor·nu (kôr′nōō) n., pl. **–nu·a** (-nōō-ə) **1.** A part or structure, such as a protuberance, that is composed of a horny substance. **2.** See **horn** (sense 4). —**cor′nu·al** adj.

cornu am·mo·nis (ă-mō′nĭs) n. See **Ammon's horn**.

coro– pref. Variant of **core–**.

co·ro·na (kə-rō′nə) n., pl. **–nas** or **–nae** (-nē) The crownlike upper portion of a body part or structure, such as the top of the head.

corona glan·dis (glăn′dĭs) n. The prominent posterior border of the glans penis.

cor·o·nal (kôr′ə-nəl, kə-rō′nəl) adj. **1.** Of or relating to a corona, especially of the head. **2.** Of, relating to, or having the direction of the coronal suture or of the plane dividing the body into front and back portions.

coronal plane n. A vertical plane at right angles to a sagittal plane, dividing the body into anterior and posterior portions. Also called frontal plane.

coronal suture n. The suture extending across the skull between the two parietal bones and the frontal bone.

cor·o·na·rism (kôr′ə-nə-rĭz′əm) n. **1.** Coronary insufficiency. **2.** Angina pectoris.

cor·o·na·ri·tis (kôr′ə-nə-rī′tĭs) n. Inflammation of the coronary arteries.

cor·o·nar·y (kôr′ə-nĕr′ē) adj. **1.** Of, relating to, or being the coronary arteries or coronary veins. **2.** Of or relating to the heart. —n. A coronary thrombosis.

coronary artery n. **1.** An artery with origin in the right aortic sinus; with distribution to the right side of the heart in the coronary sulcus, and with branches to the right atrium and ventricle, including the atrioventricular branches and posterior interventricular branch; right coronary artery. **2.** An artery with its origin in the left aortic sinus; with distribution into two major branches, the anterior interventricular, which descends in the anterior interventricular sulcus, and the circumflex branch, which passes to the diaphragmatic surface of the left ventricle, and with the atrial, ventricular, and atrioventricular branches; left coronary artery.

coronary artery bypass graft *n. Abbr.* **CABG** A surgical procedure in which a section of vein or other conduit is grafted between the aorta and a coronary artery below the region of an obstruction in that artery.

coronary artery disease *n. Abbr.* **CAD** Atherosclerosis of the coronary arteries associated with genetic predisposition or other risk factors, including hyperlipidemia, hypertension, smoking, and diabetes mellitus.

coronary bypass *n.* A surgical procedure performed to improve blood supply to the heart by creating new routes for blood flow when one or more of the coronary arteries become obstructed. The surgery involves removing a healthy blood vessel from another part of the body, such as the leg, and grafting it onto the heart to circumvent the blocked artery. Also called *coronary bypass surgery.*

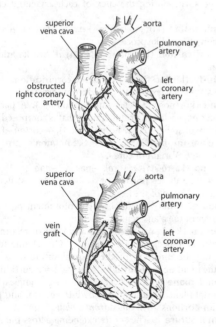

coronary bypass
Top: *a human heart with an obstructed right coronary artery*
Bottom: *the same heart after coronary bypass surgery*

coronary care unit *n. Abbr.* **CCU** A hospital unit that is specially equipped to treat and monitor patients with serious heart conditions, such as coronary thrombosis.

coronary cataract *n.* A cataract believed to be congenital, in which club-shaped opacities develop in the periphery of the cortex near the lens equator.

coronary failure *n.* Acute coronary insufficiency.

coronary heart disease *n.* A disease of the heart and the coronary arteries that is characterized by atherosclerotic arterial deposits that block blood flow to the heart, causing myocardial infarction.

coronary insufficiency *n.* Inadequate coronary circulation leading to anginal pain.

coronary occlusion *n.* Blockage of a coronary vessel, usually by thrombosis or atheroma and often leading to myocardial infarction.

coronary sinus *n.* A short trunk receiving most of the veins of the heart, running in the posterior part of the coronary sulcus and emptying into the right atrium between the inferior vena cava and the atrioventricular orifice.

coronary sulcus *n.* A groove on the outer surface of the heart marking the division between the atria and the ventricles. Also called *atrioventricular groove.*

coronary thrombosis *n.* Obstruction of a coronary artery by a thrombus, often leading to the destruction of heart muscle.

coronary valve *n.* A fold of endocardium at the opening of the coronary sinus into the right atrium.

coronary vein *n.* Any of the veins that drain blood from the muscular tissue of the heart and empty into the coronary sinus.

co·ro·na·vi·rus (kə-rō′nə-vī′rəs) *n.* Any of various single-stranded, RNA-containing viruses that cause respiratory infection in humans and resemble a crown when viewed under an electron microscope because of their petal-shaped projections.

cor·o·ner (kôr′ə-nər) *n.* A public officer whose primary function is to investigate by inquest any death thought to be of other than natural causes.

cor·o·noid·ec·to·my (kôr′ə-noi-děk′tə-mē) *n.* Surgical removal of the coronoid process of the mandible.

cor·o·noid fossa (kôr′ə-noid′) *n.* A hollow on the anterior surface of the distal end of the humerus, just above the trochlea, in which the coronoid process of the ulna rests when the elbow is flexed.

coronoid process *n.* **1.** The triangular anterior process of the mandibular ramus, giving attachment to the temporal muscle. **2.** A bracketlike projection from the anterior portion of the proximal extremity of the ulna, giving attachment to the brachial muscle and entering into formation of the trochlear notch.

cor·o·plas·ty (kôr′ə-plăs′tē) *n.* See **coreoplasty.**

co·rot·o·my (kô-rŏt′ə-mē) *n.* See **iridotomy.**

cor·po·re·al (kôr-pôr′ē-əl) *adj.* Of, relating to, or characteristic of the body.

corpse (kôrps) *n.* **1.** A dead body, especially the dead body of a human. **2.** A cadaver.

cor·pu·lence (kôr′pyə-ləns) *n.* The condition of being excessively fat; obesity.

cor·pu·lent (kôr′pyə-lənt) *adj.* Excessively fat.

cor pul·mo·na·le (pool′mə-nä′lē, pŭl′-) *n.* Acute strain or hypertrophy of the right ventricle caused by a disorder of the lungs or of the pulmonary blood vessels.

cor·pus (kôr′pəs) *n., pl.* **–po·ra** (-pər-ə) **1.** The human body, consisting of the head, neck, trunk, and limbs. **2.** The main part of a bodily structure or organ. **3.** A distinct bodily mass or organ having a specific function.

corpus al·bi·cans (ăl′bĭ-kănz′) *n.* See **albicans.**

corpus am·y·la·ce·um (ăm′ə-lā′sē-əm, -shē-) *n.* One of numerous small ovoid or rounded bodies thought to be derived from degenerated cells or secretions containing protein and found in nervous tissue, in the prostate, and in the pulmonary alveoli.

corpus cal·lo·sum (kə-lō′səm) *n.* The commissural plate of nerve fibers connecting the two cerebral hemispheres except for most of the temporal lobes. Also called *commissure of cerebral hemispheres.*

corpus cav·er·no·sum (kăv′ər-nō′səm) *n.* **1.** Either of two parallel columns of erectile tissue forming the body of the clitoris in women and the dorsal part of the body of the penis in men. **2.** The median column of erectile tissue located between and ventral to these two columns of tissue in the penis, expanding posteriorly into the bulb of the penis and terminating anteriorly as the enlarged glans penis.

cor·pus·cle (kôr′pə-səl, -pŭs′əl) *n.* **1.** An unattached body cell, such as a blood or lymph cell. **2.** A globular mass of cells, such as the pressure receptor on certain nerve endings. —**cor·pus′cu·lar** (-pŭs′kyə-lər) *adj.*

corpuscular lymph *n.* See **aplastic lymph.**

corpuscular radiation *n.* Radiation that consists of streams of subatomic particles such as protons, electrons, and neutrons.

cor·pus·cu·lum (kôr-pŭs′kyə-ləm) *n., pl.* **-la** (-lə) A small mass or body; corpuscle.

corpus fim·bri·a·tum (fĭm′brē-ā′təm) *n.* See **fimbria hippocampi.**

corpus hem·or·rhag·i·cum (hĕm′ə-răj′ĭ-kəm) *n.* A corpus luteum containing a blood clot that is gradually absorbed and replaced by clear fluid.

corpus lu·te·um (lōō′tē-əm) *n.* A yellow, progesterone-secreting mass of cells that forms from a Graafian follicle after the release of a mature egg. Also called *yellow body.*

corpus luteum hormone *n.* See **progesterone** (sense 1).

cor·rect (kə-rĕkt′) *v.* To remove, remedy, or counteract something, such as a malfunction or defect. —*adj.* Free from error or fault; true or accurate.

cor·rec·tive (kə-rĕk′tĭv) *adj.* Counteracting or modifying what is malfunctioning, undesirable, or injurious. —*n.* An agent that corrects.

Cor·rens (kôr′əns), **Karl Erich** 1864–1933. German botanist and geneticist whose research led to the rediscovery (1900) of Mendel's law of inheritance.

cor·re·spon·dence (kôr′ĭ-spŏn′dəns) *n.* A relationship between corresponding points on each retina such that stimulation produces a single image.

Cor·ri·gan's pulse (kôr′ĭ-gəns) *n.* See **water-hammer pulse.**

cor·rin (kôr′ĭn) *n.* The cyclic system of four pyrrole rings forming the central structure of the vitamin B$_{12}$ and related compounds.

cor·ro·sive (kə-rō′sĭv) *adj.* Causing or tending to cause the gradual destruction of a substance by chemical action. —*n.* A substance having the capability or tendency to cause slow destruction.

cor·ru·ga·tor (kôr′ə-gā′tər) *n.* A muscle that draws the skin together, causing it to wrinkle.

corrugator muscle *n.* A muscle with origin from the orbital portion of the orbicular muscle, with insertion to the skin of the eyebrow, with nerve supply from the facial nerve, and whose action draws the medial end of the eyebrow downward and wrinkles the forehead vertically.

Cor·tef (kôr′tĕf′) A trademark for the drug hydrocortisone.

cor·tex (kôr′tĕks′) *n., pl.* **-tex·es** *or* **-ti·ces** (-tĭ-sēz′) **1.** The outer layer of an internal organ or body structure, as of the kidney. **2.** The cerebral cortex.

cortex of ovary *n.* The layer of the ovarian stroma lying immediately beneath the tunica albuginea, composed of connective tissue cells and fibers, among which are scattered primary and secondary follicles in various stages of development.

cortic– *pref.* Variant of **cortico–.**

cor·ti·cal (kôr′tĭ-kəl) *adj.* **1.** Of, relating to, derived from, or consisting of cortex. **2.** Of, relating to, associated with, or depending on the cerebral cortex.

cortical artery *n.* Any of several branches of the anterior, middle, and posterior cerebral arteries that supply the cerebral cortex.

cortical audiometry *n.* Measurement of the electric potentials that arise in the auditory system above the level of the brainstem.

cortical blindness *n.* Loss of sight due to an organic lesion in the visual cortex.

cortical bone *n.* See **cortical substance.**

cortical cataract *n.* A cataract in which the opacity affects the cortex of the lens.

cortical deafness *n.* Deafness resulting from a lesion of the cerebral cortex.

cortical epilepsy *n.* See **focal epilepsy.**

cortical hormone *n.* See **adrenocortical hormone.**

cortical substance *n.* The thin superficial layer of compact bone. Also called *cortical bone.*

cor·ti·cec·to·my (kôr′tĭ-sĕk′tə- mē) *n.* See **topectomy.**

cor·ti·cif·u·gal (kôr′tĭ-sĭf′yə-gəl) *adj.* Passing, conducting, or moving from the cortex, as nerve fibers.

cor·ti·cip·e·tal (kôr′tĭ-sĭp′ĭ-tl) *adj.* Passing, conducting, or moving toward the cortex, as nerve fibers.

cortico– *or* **cortic–** *pref.* Cortex: *corticobulbar.*

cor·ti·co·bul·bar (kôr′tĭ-kō-bŭl′bər, -bär′) *adj.* Of or relating to or connecting the cerebral cortex and the medulla oblongata.

cor·ti·cof·u·gal (kôr′tĭ-kŏf′yə-gəl) *adj.* Corticifugal.

cor·ti·coid (kôr′tĭ-koid′) *n.* A corticosteroid.

cor·ti·co·lib·er·in (kôr′tĭ-kō-lĭb′ər-ĭn) *n.* See **corticotropin-releasing hormone.**

cor·ti·co·spi·nal (kôr′tĭ-kō-spī′nəl) *adj.* Of or relating to the cerebral cortex and the spinal cord.

cor·ti·co·ste·roid (kôr′tĭ-kō-stîr′oid′, -stĕr′-) *n.* Any of the steroid hormones produced by the adrenal cortex or their synthetic equivalents.

corticosteroid-binding globulin *n.* See **transcortin.**

cor·ti·cos·ter·one (kôr′tĭ-kŏs′tə-rōn′) *n.* A corticosteroid produced in the adrenal cortex that functions in the metabolism of carbohydrates and proteins.

cor·ti·co·troph (kôr′tĭ-kō-trŏf′, trōf′) *n.* Any of the cells of the anterior lobe of the pituitary gland that produce adrenocorticotropic hormone.

cor·ti·co·tro·pin (kôr′tĭ-kō-trō′pən) *or* **cor·ti·co·tro·phin** (-trō′fĭn) *n.* See **ACTH.**

corticotropin-releasing hormone *n. Abbr.* **CRH** A hormone produced by the hypothalamus that stimulates the anterior pituitary gland to release adrenocorticotropic hormone. Also called *corticoliberin, corticotropin-releasing factor.*

cor·tin (kôr′tĭn) *n.* An adrenal cortex extract that contains a mixture of hormones including cortisone.

Cor·ti's arch (kôr′tēz) *n.* The arch formed by the junction of the heads of the inner and outer pillar cells in the spinal organ.

Corti's canal *n.* See **Corti's tunnel**.

Corti's cell *n.* **1.** See **cochlear hair cell**. **2.** See **auditory receptor cell**.

Corti's ganglion *n.* See **spiral ganglion of cochlea**.

Corti's membrane *n.* See **tectorial membrane of cochlear duct**.

cor·ti·sol (kôr′tĭ-sôl′, -zôl′, -sōl′, -zōl′) *n.* See **hydrocortisone** (sense **?**).

cor·ti·sone (kôr′tĭ-sōn′, -zōn′) *n.* A naturally occurring corticosteroid that functions primarily in carbohydrate metabolism and is used in the treatment of rheumatoid arthritis, adrenal insufficiency, certain allergies, and gout.

Corti's tunnel *n.* The spiral canal in the ear's spiral organ that is filled with fluid and occasionally crossed by nonmedullated nerve fibers. Also called *Corti's canal*.

cor tri·a·tri·a·tum (trī-ā′trē-ā′təm) *n.* A congenital heart abnormality in which the heart has three atrial chambers, the left atrium being subdivided by a transverse septum with a single small opening that separates the openings of the pulmonary veins from the mitral valve.

cor tri·loc·u·lar·e (trī-lŏk′yə-lâr′ē) *n.* A congenital heart abnormality in which the heart has three chambers due to the absence of the interatrial or interventricular septum.

Cor·tro·syn (kôr′trə-sĭn′) A trademark for the drug cosyntropin.

cor·us·ca·tion (kôr′ə-skā′shən) *n.* A sensation of a flash of light before the eyes.

Cor·vi·sart des Ma·rets (kôr-vē-sär′ dĕ mä-rā′), Baron Jean Nicolas 1755–1821. French physician who developed the technique of percussion to diagnose diseases of the heart and chest.

Cor·vi·sart's facies (kôr′vē-särz′) *n.* The characteristic appearance seen in cardiac insufficiency or aortic regurgitation, consisting of a swollen, purplish, cyanotic face with shiny eyes and puffy eyelids.

co·rym·bi·form (kə-rĭm′bə-fôrm′) *adj.* Relating to or producing the flowerlike clustering of skin lesions seen in granulomatous diseases.

co·ry·ne·bac·te·ri·um (kôr′ə-nē-băk-tîr′ē-əm, kə-rĭn′ə-) *n.* Any of various gram-positive, rod-shaped bacterium of the genus *Corynebacterium*.

Corynebacterium diph·the·ri·ae (dĭf-thēr′ē-ē′, dĭp-) *n.* Klebs-Loeffler bacillus.

co·ry·za (kə-rī′zə) *n.* See **cold**.

co·ry·za·vi·rus (kə-rī′zə-vī′rəs) *n.* See **rhinovirus**.

cos·me·ceu·ti·cal (kŏz′mə-soo′tĭ-kəl) *n.* A cosmetic that has or is purported to have medicinal properties.

Cos·me·gen (kŏs′mə-jən) *n.* A trademark for the drug dactinomycin.

cos·met·ic (kŏz-mĕt′ĭk) *n.* A preparation, such as powder or a skin cream, designed to beautify the body by direct application. —*adj.* **1.** Serving to beautify the body, especially the face and hair. **2.** Serving to improve the appearance of a physical feature or defect.

cosmetic surgery *n.* Surgery that modifies or improves the appearance of a physical feature or defect.

cos·mo·pol·i·tan (kŏz′mə-pŏl′ĭ-tn) *adj.* Growing or occurring in many parts of the world; widely distributed. —*n.* A cosmopolitan organism.

cos·ta (kŏs′tə) *n., pl.* **–tae** (-tē) **1.** Rib. **2.** A rodlike internal supporting organelle that runs along the base of the undulating membrane of certain flagellate parasites. Also called *basal rod*. —**cos′tal** *adj.*

costal angle *n.* See **angle of rib**.

costal arch *n.* The portion of the lower opening of the chest formed by the cartilages of the seventh to tenth ribs.

costal cartilage *n.* The cartilage forming the anterior continuation of a rib.

cos·tal·gia (kŏ-stăl′jə) *n.* Pain in the ribs.

cos·tec·to·my (kŏ-stĕk′tə-mē) *n.* Excision of a rib.

Cos·ten's syndrome (kŏs′tənz) *n.* A complex of symptoms that includes loss of hearing, tinnitus, dizziness, headache, and a burning sensation of the throat, tongue, and side of the nose; its anatomical and physiological causes are uncertain but was originally believed to be the result of temporomandibular joint syndrome.

cos·tive (kŏs′tĭv) *adj.* **1.** Suffering from constipation. **2.** Causing constipation.

costo– *pref.* Rib: *costovertebral*.

cos·to·ax·il·lar·y vein (kŏs′tō-ăk′sə-lĕr′ē) *n.* Any of a number of anastomotic veins connecting the intercostal veins of the first to the seventh intercostal spaces with the lateral thoracic or the thoracoepigastric vein.

cos·to·cer·vi·cal artery (kŏs′tō-sûr′vĭ-kəl) *n.* A short artery that arises from the subclavian artery on each side and divides into deep cervical and highest intercostal branches. Also called *costocervical trunk*.

cos·to·chon·dral (kŏs′tō-kŏn′drəl) *adj.* Relating to the ribs and their cartilages.

cos·to·chon·dri·tis (kŏs′tō-kŏn-drī′tĭs) *n.* The inflammation of the costal cartilages, characterized by pain of the anterior chest wall that may radiate.

cos·to·cla·vic·u·lar (kŏs′tō-klə-vĭk′yə-lər) *adj.* Relating to the ribs and the clavicle.

costoclavicular ligament *n.* The ligament that connects the first rib to the clavicle near its sternal end. Also called *rhomboid ligament*.

cos·to·cor·a·coid (kŏs′tō-kôr′ə-koid′) *adj.* Relating to the ribs and the coracoid process of the scapula.

cos·to·gen·ic (kŏs′tə-jĕn′ĭk) *adj.* Arising from a rib.

cos·to·scap·u·lar (kŏs′tō-skăp′yə-lər) *adj.* Relating to the ribs and the scapula.

cos·to·ster·nal (kŏs′tō-stûr′nəl) *adj.* Relating to the ribs and the sternum.

cos·to·ster·no·plas·ty (kŏs′tō-stûr′nə-plăs′tē) *n.* Surgical correction of a malformation of the anterior chest wall.

cos·tot·o·my (kŏ-stŏt′ə-mē) *n.* Surgical division of a rib.

cos·to·trans·verse (kŏs′tō-trănz-vûrs′, trăns-) *adj.* Relating to the ribs and the transverse processes of the vertebrae articulating with them.

cos·to·trans·ver·sec·to·my (kŏs′tō-trănz′vûr-sĕk′tə-mē, -trăns′-) *n.* Excision of a portion of a rib and the articulating transverse process.

costotransverse ligament *n.* **1.** The ligament that connects the dorsal aspect of the neck of a rib to the ventral aspect of the corresponding transverse process; middle costotransverse ligament. **2.** The short quadrangular ligament that passes across behind the costotransverse joint from the tip of the transverse process to the posterior surface of the neck of the rib; lateral costotransverse ligament. **3.** The fibrous band that extends upward from the neck of a rib to the transverse process of the next higher vertebra; superior costotranverse ligament.

cos·to·ver·te·bral (kŏs′tō-vûr′tə-brəl, -vər-tē′brəl) *adj.* Of or relating to the ribs and the thoracic vertebrae with which they articulate; vertebrocostal.

cos·to·xiph·oid (kŏs′tō-zĭf′oid′) *adj.* Relating to the ribs and the xiphoid cartilage of the sternum.

co·syn·tro·pin (kō′sĭn-trō′pĭn) *n.* A synthetic corticotropin. Also called *tetracosactide.*

co·throm·bo·plas·tin (kō-thrŏm′bō-plăs′tĭn) *n.* See **factor VII.**

Cotte's operation (kŏts, kôts) *n.* See **presacral neurectomy.**

cot·ton-fi·ber embolism (kŏt′n-fī′bər) *n.* An obstruction, often in small pulmonary arteries, produced by cotton fibers derived from sterile gauze used in intravenous medication or transfusion.

cotton-wool patches *pl.n.* Accumulations of cytoplasmic debris in the retina that appear as white opacities and are especially seen in hypertensive retinopathy. Also called *cotton-wool spots.*

cot·y·le·don (kŏt′l-ēd′n) *n.* **1.** One of the lobules constituting the uterine side of the placenta, consisting mainly of a rounded mass of villi. **2.** A leaf of the embryo of a seed plant, which, upon germination, either remains in the seed or emerges, enlarges, and becomes green; a seed leaf.

cot·y·loid (kŏt′l-oid′) *adj.* **1.** Shaped like a cup. **2.** Relating to the acetabulum.

cotyloid cavity *n.* See **acetabulum.**

cotyloid joint *n.* See **ball-and-socket joint.**

cough (kôf) *v.* To expel air from the lungs suddenly and noisily, often to keep the respiratory passages free of irritating material. —*n.* **1.** The act of coughing. **2.** An illness marked by frequent coughing.

cough drop *n.* A small, often medicated and sweetened lozenge taken orally to ease coughing or soothe a sore throat.

cough reflex *n.* The reflex which initiates coughing in response to irritation of the larynx or tracheobronchial tree.

cough syrup *n.* A sweetened medicated liquid taken orally to ease coughing.

cou·lomb (kōō′lŏm′, -lōm′) *n. Abbr.* **C** The unit of electrical charge in the meter-kilogram-second system equal to the quantity of charge transferred in one second by a steady current of one ampere.

Cou·ma·din (kōō′mə-dĭn) A trademark for the drug warfarin sodium.

Coun·cil·man body (koun′səl-mən) *n.* An eosinophilic globule seen in the liver in yellow fever and derived from necrosis of a single hepatic cell.

count (kount) *v.* To name or list the units of a group or collection one by one in order to determine a total. —*n.* **1.** The act of counting or calculating. **2.** The totality of specific items in a particular sample.

count·er (koun′tər) *n.* One that counts, especially an electronic or mechanical device that automatically counts occurrences or repetitions of phenomena or events.

counter– *pref.* **1.** Contrary; opposite; opposing: *countertransport.* **2.** Corresponding; complementary: *counterincision.*

coun·ter·con·di·tion·ing (koun′tər-kən-dĭsh′ə-nĭng) *n.* Any of a group of conditioning techniques used to replace a negative conditioned response to a stimulus with a positive response.

coun·ter·ex·ten·sion (koun′tər-ĭk-stĕn′shən) *n.* See **countertraction.**

coun·ter·im·mu·no·e·lec·tro·pho·re·sis (koun′tər-ĭm′yə-nō-ĭ-lĕk′trə-fə-rē′sĭs, -ĭ-myōō′-) *n.* A modification of immunoelectrophoresis in which antigen and antibody move in opposite directions and form precipitates in the area between the cells where they meet in concentrations of optimal proportions.

coun·ter·in·ci·sion (koun′tər-ĭn-sĭzh′ən) *n.* A second incision made adjacent to a primary incision.

coun·ter·ir·ri·tant (koun′tər-îr′ĭ-tənt) *n.* An agent that induces local inflammation to relieve inflammation in underlying or adjacent tissues. —*adj.* Relating to or producing counterirritation.

coun·ter·ir·ri·ta·tion (koun′tər-îr′ĭ-tā′shən) *n.* Irritation or mild inflammation that is produced in order to relieve inflammation of underlying or adjacent tissues.

coun·ter·o·pen·ing (koun′tər-ō′pə-nĭng) *n.* A second opening made at the lowest part of an abscess or other fluid-containing cavity to assist in drainage. Also called *contra-aperture, counterpuncture.*

coun·ter·shock (koun′tər-shŏk′) *n.* An electric shock that is applied to the chest to restore normal rhythm of the heart.

coun·ter·stain (koun′tər-stān′) *n.* A stain of a contrasting color used to color the components in a microscopic specimen that are not made visible by the principal stain. —**count′er·stain′** *v.*

coun·ter·trac·tion (koun′tər-trăk′shən) *n.* Traction used to offset or oppose another traction in the reduction of fractures. Also called *counterextension.*

coun·ter·trans·fer·ence (koun′tər-trăns-fûr′əns) *n.* The surfacing of a psychotherapist's own repressed feelings through identification with the emotions, experiences, or problems of a person undergoing treatment.

counting chamber *n.* A standardized glass slide used for counting cells, especially red blood cells and white blood cells, and other particulate material in a measured volume of fluid; a hemocytometer.

coup injury of brain (kōō) *n.* Injury to the brain occurring directly beneath the area of impact.

cou·pled pulse (kŭp′əld) *n.* See **bigeminal pulse.**

coupled rhythm *n.* See **bigeminal rhythm.**

cou·pling (kŭp′lĭng) *n.* **1.** The act of uniting sexually. **2.** See **bigeminal rhythm. 3.** The configuration of two different mutant genes on the same chromosome, leading to the likelihood they will both either be inherited or omitted in the next generation.

Cour·nand (kōōr′nänd, -nənd, kōōr-näN′), **André Frédéric** 1895–1988. French-born American physician. He shared a 1956 Nobel Prize for developing cardiac catheterization.

cou·vade (ko͞o-väd′) *n.* A practice in certain non-Western cultures in which the husband of a woman in labor takes to his bed as though he were bearing the child.

Cou·ve·laire uterus (ko͞o-və-lĕr′) *n.* Extravasation of blood into the uterine musculature and beneath the uterine peritoneum in association with premature detachment of the placenta.

co·va·lent (kō-vā′lənt) *adj.* Of or relating to a chemical bond characterized by one or more pairs of shared electrons.

covalent bond *n.* A chemical bond formed by the sharing of one or more electrons, especially pairs of electrons, between atoms.

cov·ert sensitization (kŭv′ərt, kō′vərt, kō-vûrt′) *n.* Aversive conditioning during which an individual is taught to imagine unpleasant or aversive consequences while engaging in an unwanted habit.

cov·er-un·cov·er test (kŭv′ər-ŭn-kŭv′ər) *n.* A test to detect strabismus in which one eye focusing on a given point is covered; if the uncovered eye moves, strabismus is present.

Cow·den's disease (koud′nz) *n.* An inherited condition characterized by benign tissue masses that form on the skin, hair follicles, and gums during infancy, and in the breasts following puberty, and are associated with a higher risk for developing malignancies.

cow·per·i·tis (ko͞o′pə-rī′tĭs, kou′-) *n.* Inflammation of the Cowper's glands.

Cow·per's gland (kou′pərz, ko͞o′-) *n.* See **bulbourethral gland.**

cow·pox (kou′pŏks′) *n.* A mild, contagious skin disease of cattle, usually affecting the udder, that is caused by a virus and characterized by the eruption of a pustular rash. When the virus is transmitted to humans, as by vaccination, it can confer immunity to smallpox. Also called *vaccinia.*

COX-2 inhibitor (kŏks′to͞o′) *n.* Any of a class of nonsteroidal anti-inflammatory drugs thought to have fewer side effects than traditional NSAIDs.

cox·a (kŏk′sə) *n., pl.* **cox·ae** (kŏk′sē′) **1.** See **hipbone. 2.** See **hip joint.**

cox·al·gia (kŏk-săl′jə) *n.* Pain in or disease of the hip or hip joint.

coxa mag·na (măg′nə) *n.* Enlargement and deformation of the head of the femur.

coxa pla·na (plā′nə) *n.* See **osteochondritis deformans juvenilis.**

coxa val·ga (văl′gə) *n.* Deformity of the hip in which the angle made by the femoral neck and the femoral shaft is increased.

coxa var·a (vâr′ə) *n.* Deformity of the hip in which the angle made by the neck and shaft of the femur is decreased.

Cox·i·el·la (kŏk′sē-ĕl′ə) *n.* A genus of filterable parasitic bacteria containing small rod-shaped or coccoid, gram-negative cells; it includes the species that causes Q fever in humans.

cox·i·tis (kŏk-sī′tĭs) *n.* Inflammation of the hip joint.

cox·o·dyn·i·a (kŏk′sə-dĭn′ē-ə) *n.* Pain in the hip joint.

cox·o·fem·o·ral (kŏk′sə-fĕm′ər-əl) *adj.* Relating to the hipbone and the femur.

cox·o·tu·ber·cu·lo·sis (kŏk′sə-to͞o-bûr′kyə-lō′sĭs) *n.* Tuberculous disease of the hip joint.

Cox·sack·ie encephalitis (kŏk-săk′ē, ko͞ok-sä′kē) *n.* An inflammation of the brain, caused by a coxsackie virus and seen mainly in infants, that chiefly involves the gray matter of the medulla and the spinal cord.

coxsackievirus *or* **Coxsackie virus** *n.* Any of various *Enteroviruses* that are associated with a variety of illnesses including herpangina, epidemic pleurodynia, and a disease resembling poliomyelitis but without paralysis.

Co·zaar (kō′zär′) A trademark for the drug losartan potassium.

CP *abbr.* cerebral palsy; chest pain

CPAP *abbr.* continuous positive airway pressure

CPM *abbr.* continuous passive motion

CPPB *abbr.* constant positive pressure breathing

CPR *abbr.* cardiopulmonary resuscitation

cps *abbr.* cycles per second

Cr The symbol for the element **chromium.**

CR[1] *abbr.* conditioned response; crown-rump length

CR[2] *n.* A bipolar lead of an electrocardiograph that has electrodes attached to the chest and right arm.

crab louse (krăb) *n.* A sucking louse that generally infests the pubic region and causes severe itching.

crack cocaine (krăk) *n.* Chemically purified, very potent cocaine in pellet form that is smoked through a glass pipe and is considered highly and rapidly addictive.

cracked heel *n.* See **keratoderma plantare sulcatum.**

cra·dle (krād′l) *n.* **1.** A small low bed for an infant, often furnished with rockers. **2.** A frame that is used to keep the bedclothes from pressing on an injured part.

cradle cap *n.* A form of dermatitis that occurs in infants and is characterized by heavy, yellow, crusted lesions on the scalp.

cramp (krămp) *n.* **1.** A sudden, involuntary, spasmodic muscular contraction causing severe pain, often occurring in the leg or shoulder as the result of strain or chill. **2.** A temporary partial paralysis of habitually or excessively used muscles. **3. cramps** Spasmodic contractions of the uterus, such as those occurring during menstruation or labor, usually causing pain in the abdomen that may radiate to the lower back and thighs. —*v.* To affect with or experience a cramp or cramps.

Cramp·ton test (krămp′tən) *n.* A test for physical condition and resistance in which one's pulse and blood pressure are recorded both in the recumbent and in the standing position, and the difference is graded from theoretical perfection (100) downward. High values indicate a good physical resistance, but low ones may indicate general weakness and a potential for shock after surgery.

crani– *pref.* Variant of **cranio–.**

cra·ni·ad (krā′nē-ăd′) *adv.* Toward the head or anterior end; cephalad.

cra·ni·al (krā′nē-əl) *adj.* Of or relating to the skull or cranium.

cranial arteritis *n.* See **temporal arteritis.**

cranial bone *n.* Any of the bones surrounding the brain, comprising the paired parietal and temporal bones and the unpaired occipital, frontal sphenoid, and ethmoid bones.

cranial cavity *n.* The space or hollow within the skull. Also called *intracranial cavity.*

cranial flexure *n.* See **cephalic flexure.**

cranial fossa *n.* The internal base of the skull in which rest the frontal and temporal lobes of the brain, the pituitary gland, the cerebellum, the pons, and the medulla oblongata.

cranial index *n.* The ratio of the maximum breadth to the maximum length of the skull, multiplied by 100.

cranial nerve *n.* Any of 12 pairs of nerves that emerge from or enter the brain, comprising the olfactory (I), optic (II), oculomotor (III), trochlear (IV), trigeminal (V), abducent (VI), facial (VII), vestibulocochlear (VIII), glossopharyngeal (IX), vagus (X), accessory (XI), and hypoglossal (XII) nerves.

cranial root *n.* Any of the roots of the accessory nerve that arise from the medulla.

cranial suture *n.* Any of the sutures between the bones of the skull.

cranial vertebra *n.* A segment of the skull regarded as homologous with a spinal column segment.

cra·ni·ec·to·my (krā′nē-ĕk′tə-mē) *n.* Surgical removal of a portion of the cranium.

cranio– *or* **crani–** *pref.* Cranium: *craniospinal.*

cra·ni·o·cele (krā′nē-ə-sēl′) *n.* See **encephalocele.**

cra·ni·o·cer·e·bral (krā′nē-ō-sĕr′ə-brəl, -sə-rē′brəl) *adj.* Relating to both cranium and cerebrum.

cra·ni·o·clei·do·dys·os·to·sis (krā′nē-ō-klī′dō-dĭs′ŏs-tō′sĭs) *n.* See **cleidocranial dysostosis.**

cra·ni·o·fa·cial (krā′nē-ō-fā′shəl) *adj.* Of or involving both the cranium and the face.

craniofacial disjunction fracture *n.* A fracture in which the facial bones separate from the cranial bones. Also called *LeFort III fracture, transverse facial fracture.*

craniofacial dysostosis *n.* An inherited cranial deformity characterized by widening of the skull and high forehead, abnormal width between and protrusion of the eyes, a beaked nose, and hypoplasia of the maxilla. Also called *Crouzon's disease.*

cra·ni·o·fe·nes·tri·a (krā′nē-ō-fə-nĕs′trē-ə) *n.* Incomplete formation of the bones of the vault of the fetal skull resulting in nonossified areas in the calvaria. Also called *craniolacunia.*

cra·ni·ol·o·gy (krā′nē-ŏl′ə-jē) *n.* The scientific study of the characteristics of the skull, such as size and shape, especially in humans.

cra·ni·o·ma·la·cia (krā′nē-ō-mə-lā′shə) *n.* Softening of the bones of the skull.

cra·ni·om·e·ter (krā′nē-ŏm′ĭ-tər) *n.* An instrument or device used to measure the skull. —**cra′ni·o·met′ric** (-ə-mĕt′rĭk), **cra′ni·o·met′ri·cal** (-rĭ-kəl) *adj.*

craniometric point *n.* Any of the fixed points on the skull used as reference points in craniometry.

cra·ni·om·e·try (krā′nē-ŏm′ĭ-trē) *n.* Measurement of the skull to determine its characteristics as related to sex, race, or body type.

cra·ni·op·a·thy (krā′nē-ŏp′ə-thē) *n.* Any of various pathological conditions of the cranial bones.

cra·ni·o·pha·ryn·geal (krā′nē-ō-fə-rĭn′jəl, -făr′ĭn-jē′-əl) *adj.* Relating to the cranium and the pharynx.

cra·ni·o·pha·ryn·gi·o·ma (krā′nē-ō-fə-rĭn′jē-ō′mə, -făr′ĭn-jē-) *n.* A tumor of the brain that develops from the epithelium derived from Rathke's pouch and usually affects children.

cra·ni·o·plas·ty (krā′nē-ə-plăs′tē) *n.* Surgical repair of a defect or deformity of the skull.

cra·ni·o·punc·ture (krā′nē-ō-pŭngk′chər) *n.* Surgical puncture of the skull.

cra·ni·or·rha·chis·chi·sis (krā′nē-ō-rə-kĭs′kĭ-sĭs) *n.* Congenital fissure of the skull and spinal column.

cra·ni·o·sa·cral (krā′nē-ō-sā′krəl, -săk′rəl) *adj.* **1.** Associated with both the cranium and the sacrum. **2.** Relating to the parasympathetic nervous system.

craniosacral therapy *n.* A treatment in alternative medicine that identifies and reduces perceived restrictions in movement of the dural sheath and in the flow of cerebrospinal fluid as a means of restoring well-being.

cra·ni·os·chi·sis (krā′nē-ŏs′kĭ-sĭs) *n.* Congenital failure of the skull to close, usually accompanied by defective development of the brain.

cra·ni·o·scle·ro·sis (krā′nē-ō-sklə-rō′sĭs) *n.* Thickening of the skull.

cra·ni·o·spi·nal (krā′nē-ō-spī′nəl) *adj.* Relating to the cranium and the spinal column.

cra·ni·o·ste·no·sis (krā′nē-ō-stə-nō′sĭs) *n.* Premature closure of the cranial sutures, resulting in malformation of the skull.

cra·ni·o·syn·os·to·sis (krā′nē-ō-sĭn′ŏs-tō′sĭs) *n.* Premature ossification of the skull and closure of the sutures.

cra·ni·o·ta·bes (krā′nē-ō-tā′bēz) *n.* An abnormal condition of the skull bones, characterized by thin, soft areas, usually caused by syphilis or rickets.

cra·ni·ot·o·my (krā′nē-ŏt′ə-mē) *n.* Incision into the skull.

cra·ni·o·tym·pan·ic (krā′nē-ō-tĭm-păn′ĭk) *adj.* Relating to the skull and the middle ear.

cra·ni·um (krā′nē-əm) *n., pl.* **–ni·ums** *or* **–ni·a** (-nē-ə) **1.** The bones of the head considered as a group; skull. **2.** The bony case enclosing the brain, excluding the bones of the face; braincase.

crap·u·lence (krăp′yə-ləns) *n.* **1.** Sickness caused by excessive eating or drinking. **2.** Excessive indulgence; intemperance.

cra·ter (krā′tər) *n.* A circular depression or pit in the surface of a tissue or body part.

cra·vat bandage (krə-văt′) *n.* A bandage made by bringing the point of a triangular bandage to the middle of the base and then folding lengthwise to the desired width.

C-reactive protein *n.* An antibody found in the blood in certain acute and chronic conditions including infections and cancers. It is a nonspecific indicator of inflammation and, therefore, not diagnostic of any one disease.

cream (krēm) *n.* **1.** The yellowish fatty component of unhomogenized milk that tends to accumulate at the surface. **2.** A pharmaceutical preparation consisting of a semisolid emulsion of either the oil-in-water or the water-in-oil type and is ordinarily intended for topical use.

crease (krēs) *n.* A line made by folding or wrinkling, as in the skin.

cre·a·ti·nase (krē′ə-tə-nās′, -nāz′) *n.* An enzyme that catalyzes the hydrolysis of creatine to sarcosine and urea.

cre·a·tine (krē′ə-tēn′, -tĭn) *or* **cre·a·tin** (-tĭn) *n.* A nitrogenous organic acid that is found in the muscle tissue of vertebrates mainly in the form of phosphocreatine and supplies energy for muscle contraction.

creatine kinase *n.* An enzyme present in muscle, brain, and other tissues of vertebrates that catalyzes the reversible conversion of ADP and phosphocreatine into ATP and creatine.

cre·a·ti·ne·mi·a (krē′ə-tə-nē′mē-ə) *n.* The presence of excessive creatine in the blood.

creatine phosphate *n.* See **phosphocreatine.**

cre·at·i·nin·ase (krē-ăt′n-ēn-ās′, -āz′, -ə-nās′, -nāz′) *n.* An enzyme that catalyzes the conversion of creatine to creatinine, with participation of ATP.

cre·at·i·nine (krē-ăt′n-ēn′, -ĭn) *n.* A creatine anhydride formed by the metabolism of creatine and found in muscle tissue and blood and normally excreted in the urine as metabolic waste.

creatinine clearance *n.* The volume of serum or plasma that would be cleared of creatinine by one minute's excretion of urine.

cre·a·ti·nu·ri·a (krē′ə-tə-nŏor′ē-ə) *n.* An increase in the amount of creatine in the urine.

Cre·dé's method (krā-dāz′) *n.* **1.** A method for preventing ophthalmia neonatorum by administering one drop of a 2 percent solution of silver nitrate into each eye of a newborn infant. **2.** A method for expelling the afterbirth by resting the hand on the fundus of the uterus after expulsion of the fetus, gently rubbing the fundus with the hand in case of hemorrhage or failing contractions, then, when the afterbirth is loosened, expelling it by firmly squeezing the fundus with the hand. **3.** A method for expressing urine by pressing the hand on the bladder, especially a paralyzed bladder.

creep·ing eruption (krē′pĭng) *n.* A skin disorder characterized by itchiness and a progressive netlike tunneling in the skin caused by the burrowing larvae of various parasites, especially a type of hookworm. Also called *cutaneous larva migrans.*

cre·mas·ter (krə-măs′tər, krē-) *n.* A muscle with origin from the internal oblique and inguinal ligament, enveloping the spermatic cord and the testis and supplied by the genitofemoral nerve, and whose action raises the testicle. —**cre′mas·ter′ic** (krē′mă-stĕr′ĭk) *adj.*

cremasteric artery *n.* An artery with origin in the inferior epigastric artery, with distribution to the coverings of the spermatic cord, and with anastomoses to the external pudendal, spermatic, and perineal arteries. Also called *external spermatic artery.*

cremasteric reflex *n.* A drawing up of the scrotum and the testicle in response to scratching of the skin over Scarpa's triangle or on the inner side of the thigh on the same side of the body.

crem·no·cele (krĕm′nə-sēl′) *n.* A protrusion of the intestine into one of the labia majora. Also called *labial hernia.*

cre·na (krē′nə) *n., pl.* **–nae** (-nē) Any of the notches into which the opposing projections fit in the cranial sutures.

cre·nate (krē′nāt′) *or* **cre·nat·ed** (-nā′tĭd) *adj.* Having a margin with low, rounded or scalloped projections or indentations.

cre·na·tion (krĭ-nā′shən) *n.* **1.** The condition or state of being crenate. **2.** A process resulting from osmosis in which red blood cells, in a hypertonic solution, shrink and acquire a scalloped surface.

cre·no·cyte (krē′nə-sīt′, krĕn′ə-) *n.* A red blood cell with notched edges.

crep·i·tant (krĕp′ĭ-tənt) *adj.* Relating to or characterized by crepitation.

crepitant rale *n.* A fine bubbling or crackling sound that is heard on auscultation, produced by the presence of a very thin secretion in the smaller bronchial tubes.

crep·i·tate (krĕp′ĭ-tāt′) *v.* To make a crackling or popping sound; crackle.

crep·i·ta·tion (krĕp′ĭ-tā′shən) *n.* **1.** A rattling or crackling sound like that made by rubbing hair between the fingers close to the ear. **2.** The sensation felt on placing the hand over the seat of a fracture when the broken ends of the bone are moved, or over tissue in which gas gangrene is present. **3.** The noise produced by rubbing bone or irregular cartilage surfaces together, as in arthritis.

crep·i·tus (krĕp′ĭ-təs) *n.* **1.** Crepitation. **2.** A noisy discharge of gas from the intestine.

cres·cen·do angina (krə-shĕn′dō) *n.* Angina pectoris that occurs with increasing frequency, intensity, or duration.

crescendo murmur *n.* A murmur that increases in intensity and suddenly ceases.

cres·cent (krĕs′ənt) *n.* Something having concave and convex edges terminating in points. —*adj.* Crescent-shaped. —**cres·cen′tic** (krə-sĕn′tĭk) *adj.*

crescent cell anemia *n.* See **sickle cell anemia.**

cre·sol (krē′sôl′, -sōl′) *n.* Any of three isomeric phenols used as a disinfectant.

cresol red *n.* An acid-base indicator with pK value of 8.3; yellow at pH values below 7.4, red above 9.0.

crest (krĕst) *n.* A projection or ridge, especially of bone; cresta.

Cres·tor (krĕs′tôr′) A trademark for the drug rosuvastatin calcium.

CREST syndrome (krĕst) *n.* A form of scleroderma that is a combination of calcinosis, Raynaud's phenomenon, esophageal motility disorders, sclerodactyly, and telangiectasia.

cre·tin (krēt′n) *n.* A person who is afflicted with cretinism. —**cre′tin·oid′** (-oid′) *adj.* —**cre′tin·ous** (-əs) *adj.*

cre·tin·ism (krēt′n-ĭz′əm) *n.* A congenital condition due to thyroid hormone deficiency during fetal development and marked in childhood by dwarfed stature, mental retardation, dystrophy of the bones, and a low basal metabolism. Also called *congenital myxedema, cretinoid dysplasia.*

Creutz·feldt-Jakob disease (kroits′fĕlt-) *n. Abbr.* **CJD** A rare, usually fatal encephalopathy that is likely caused by a prion and is characterized by progressive dementia and gradual loss of muscle control, usually in middle age. Also called *Jakob-Creutzfeldt disease.*

crev·ice (krĕv′ĭs) *n.* A narrow crack, fissure, or cleft.

cre·vic·u·lar (krə-vĭk′yə-lər) *adj.* Of or relating to a crevice, especially the gingival crevice.

CRF *abbr.* chronic renal failure

CRH *abbr.* corticotropin-releasing hormone

crib death (krĭb) *n.* See **sudden infant death syndrome.**

crib·rate (krĭb′rāt′, -rĭt) *adj.* Cribriform.

cri·bra·tion (krə-brā′shən) *n.* The condition of being cribriform.

crib·ri·form (krĭb′rə-fôrm′) *adj.* Perforated like a sieve.

cri·brum (krī′brəm, krĭb′rəm) *n., pl.* **cri·bra** (krī′brə, krĭb′rə) A horizontal lamina that fits into the ethmoidal notch of the frontal bone and supports the olfactory lobes of the cerebrum. Also called *cribriform plate of ethmoid bone.*

crick (krĭk) *n.* A painful cramp or muscle spasm, as in the back or neck. —*v.* To cause a painful cramp or muscle spasm in by turning or wrenching.

Crick (krĭk), **Francis Henry Compton** 1916–2004. British biologist who with James D. Watson proposed a spiral model, the double helix, for the molecular structure of DNA. He shared a 1962 Nobel Prize for advances in the study of genetics.

cri·co·ar·y·te·noid (krī′kō-ăr′ĭ-tē′noid′, -ə-rĭt′n-oid′) *adj.* Relating to the cricoid and arytenoid cartilages.

cricoarytenoid muscle *n.* **1.** A muscle with origin from the upper margin of the arch of the cricoid cartilage, with insertion to the muscular process of the arytenoid, with nerve supply from the recurrent laryngeal nerve, and whose action narrows the rima glottidis; lateral cricoarytenoid muscle. **2.** A muscle with its origin from the depression on the posterior surface of the lamina of the cricoid, with insertion to the muscular process of the arytenoid, with nerve supply from the recurrent laryngeal nerve, and whose action widens the rima glottidis; posterior cricoarytenoid muscle.

cri·coid (krī′koid′) *adj.* Ring-shaped.

cricoid cartilage *n.* The lowermost of the laryngeal cartilages, expanded into a nearly quadrilateral plate. Also called *innominate cartilage.*

cri·coi·dec·to·my (krī′koi-dĕk′tə-mē) *n.* Excision of the cricoid cartilage.

cri·co·pha·ryn·geal (krī′kō-fə-rĭn′jəl, -făr′ĭn-jē′əl) *adj.* Relating to the cricoid cartilage and the pharynx.

cri·co·thy·roid (krī′kō-thī′roid′) *adj.* Relating to the cricoid and the thyroid cartilages.

cricothyroid muscle *n.* A muscle with origin from the anterior surface of the arch of the cricoid, with insertion either upward to the ala of the thyroid or outward to the inferior cornu of the thyroid, with nerve supply from the superior laryngeal nerve, and whose action makes the vocal folds tense.

cri·co·thy·rot·o·my (krī′kō-thī-rŏt′ə-mē) *n.* Incision through the skin and the cricothyroid membrane for emergency relief of upper respiratory obstruction. Also called *intercricothyrotomy.*

cri·cot·o·my (krī-kŏt′ə-mē) *n.* Incision of the cricoid cartilage.

cri-du-chat syndrome (crē-dōō-shä′) *n.* A chromosomal disorder marked by microcephaly, epicanthal folds, micrognathia, strabismus, mental and physical retardation, and a characteristic catlike whine. Also called *cat-cry syndrome, Lejeune syndrome.*

Crig·ler-Naj·jar syndrome (krĭg′lər-nä′jär′) *n.* An inherited defect in the ability to form bilirubin glucuronide, characterized by familial nonhemolytic jaundice and, in its severe form, by irreversible brain damage that resembles kernicterus.

crim·i·nal psychology (krĭm′ə-nəl) *n.* The branch of psychology that studies criminal behavior.

crin·o·gen·ic (krĭn′ə-jĕn′ĭk) *adj.* Stimulating a gland to increased function; causing secretion.

cri·noph·a·gy (krə-nŏf′ə-jē) *n.* The disposal of excess secretory granules by lysosomes.

crip·ple (krĭp′əl) *n.* One that is partially disabled or unable to use a limb or limbs. —*v.* To cause to lose the use of a limb or limbs.

cri·sis (krī′sĭs) *n., pl.* **–ses** (-sēz) **1.** A sudden change in the course of a disease or fever, toward either improvement or deterioration. **2.** An emotionally stressful event or a traumatic change in one's life.

crisis center *n.* A center staffed especially by volunteers who give support and advice to people experiencing personal crises.

cris·pa·tion (krĭs-pā′shən) *n.* A slight involuntary muscular contraction, often producing a crawling sensation of the skin.

cris·ta (krĭs′tə) *n., pl.* **–tae** (-tē) **1.** A ridge, crest, or elevated line projecting from a level or evenly rounded surface. **2.** One of the inward projections or folds of the inner membrane of a mitochondrion.

crista gal·li (găl′ī′) *n.* The triangular midline process of the ethmoid bone extending upward from the cribriform plate and giving attachment to the falx cerebri.

cri·thid·i·a (krə-thĭd′ē-ə) *n.* The stage of development of certain flagellate parasites of vertebrates in the insect host, such as the multiplying form of the agent of African sleeping sickness in the tsetse fly.

crit·i·cal (krĭt′ĭ-kəl) *adj.* **1.** Of or relating to a medical crisis. **2.** Being or relating to a grave physical condition especially of a patient. **3.** Of or relating to the value of a measurement, such as temperature, at which an abrupt change in a chemical of physical quality, property, or state occurs.

critical care unit *n. Abbr.* **CCU** See **intensive care unit.**

critical organ *n.* The organ or physiological system that would first be subjected to radiation in excess of the maximum permissible amount as the dose of a radioactive material is increased.

critical temperature *n.* The temperature above which a gas cannot be liquefied, regardless of the pressure applied.

CRNA *abbr.* Certified Registered Nurse Anesthetist

crocodile tears syndrome (krŏk′ə-dīl′) *n.* A syndrome caused by a lesion of the seventh cranial nerve central to the geniculate ganglion and resulting in residual facial paralysis with profuse lacrimation during eating. Also called *crocodile tears.*

Crohn's disease (krōnz) *n.* Enteritis of unknown cause that is usually limited to the terminal ileum but can progress to other segments of the intestine, characterized by nodule formation and fibrous tissue buildup, abdominal pain, and patchy deep ulceration. Also called *granulomatous enteritis, regional enteritis, regional ileitis, terminal ileitis.*

Cro·lom (krouʹləm) A trademark for the drug cromolyn sodium.

cro·mo·lyn sodium (krōʹmə-lĭn) *n.* A drug usually administered by inhalation and used to prevent certain allergic attacks, especially those associated with asthma or hay fever.

Cron·khite-Can·a·da syndrome (krôngʹkītʹkănʹə-də) *n.* A sporadically occurring syndrome whose symptoms include gastrointestinal polyps, diffuse hair loss, and nail dystrophy.

Crooke's granule (krŏŏks) *n.* One of the lumpy masses of basophilic material in the basophil cells of the anterior lobe of the pituitary gland, associated with Cushing's disease or appearing after the administration of ACTH.

Crooke's hyaline degeneration *n.* A form of degeneration in which the cytoplasmic granules of basophil cells of the pituitary gland are replaced by hyaline, characteristic of Cushing's syndrome.

cross·bite (krôsʹbītʹ) *n.* An abnormal relation of one or more teeth of one arch to the opposing tooth or teeth of the other arch, caused by deviation of tooth position or abnormal jaw position.

crossed diplopia (krŏst) *n.* See **heteronymous diplopia.**

crossed eyes *n.* See **esotropia.**

crossed hemianesthesia *n.* See **alternate hemianesthesia.**

crossed hemianopsia *n.* Altitudinal hemianopsia involving the upper visual field of one eye and the lower visual field of the other. Also called *heteronymous hemianopsia.*

crossed hemiplegia *n.* See **alternating hemiplegia.**

crossed reflex *n.* A reflex movement on one side of the body in response to a stimulus applied to the opposite side.

cross-eye (krôsʹīʹ) *n.* A form of strabismus in which one or both eyes deviate toward the nose. —**crossʹ-eyedʹ** *adj.*

cross flap *n.* A skin flap transferred between corresponding body parts, as from one arm, breast, or eyelid to the other.

cross infection *n.* An infection spread from one organism to another.

cross·ing o·ver *or* **cross·ing-o·ver** (krôʹsĭng-ōʹvər) *n.* The exchange of genetic material between homologous chromosomes that occurs during meiosis and contributes to genetic variability.

cross matching *or* **crossmatching** *n.* **1.** A test for determining the compatibility between the blood of a donor and that of a recipient before transfusion; the clumping of red blood cells indicates incompatibility. **2.** A test for determining tissue compatibility between a transplant donor and the recipient before transplantation, in which the recipient's serum is tested for antibodies that may react with the lymphocytes or other cells of the donor.

cross-reacting agglutinin *n.* See **group agglutinin.**

cross-reacting antibody *n.* An antibody that reacts with an antigen other than the one that induced its production.

cross reaction *n.* A specific reaction between an antiserum and an antigen complex other than the complex that caused the production of the specific antibodies of the antiserum.

cross-sectional study *n.* See **synchronic study.**

cross tolerance *n.* Resistance to an effect or effects of a compound as a result of tolerance previously developed to a pharmacologically similar compound.

cro·ta·mi·ton (krōʹtə-mīʹtŏn) *n.* A topical scabicide.

crotch (krŏch) *n.* The angle or region of the angle formed by the junction of two parts or members, such as two branches, limbs, or legs.

croup (krōōp) *n.* **1.** See **laryngotracheobronchitis.** **2.** A pathological condition of the larynx, especially in infants and children, characterized by respiratory difficulty and a hoarse, brassy cough. —**croupʹous** (krōōʹpəs), **croupʹy** *adj.*

croup-associated virus *or* **CA virus** *n.* See **parainfluenza 2 virus.**

croupous membrane *n.* See **false membrane.**

Crou·zon's disease (krōō-zŏnzʹ, -zônʹ) *n.* See **craniofacial dysostosis.**

crowd·ing (krouʹdĭng) *n.* A condition in which the teeth are crowded in the dental arch, assuming altered positions, as by overlapping and twisting.

crown (kroun) *n.* **1.** The top or highest part of bodily structure, especially the head. **2.** The part of a tooth that is covered by enamel and projects beyond the gum line. **3.** An artificial substitute for the natural crown of a tooth. —*v.* **1.** To put a crown on a tooth. **2.** To reach a stage in labor when a large segment of the fetal scalp is visible at the vaginal orifice. Used of a fetus or the head of a fetus.

crown-heel length *n.* The length of an embryo or fetus measured from the skull vertex to the heel.

crown-rump length *n.* The length of an embryo or fetus measured from the skull vertex to the midpoint between the apices of the buttocks.

CRST syndrome (sēʹär-ĕs-tēʹ) *n.* A scleroderma that is a combination of calcinosis cutis, Raynaud's phenomenon, sclerodactyly, and telangiectasia.

cru·ci·ate (krōōʹshē-ātʹ) *or* **cru·cial** (krōōʹshəl) *adj.* **1.** Having the form of a cross, as in certain ligaments of the knee. **2.** Arranged in or forming a cross, as for a bandage. **3.** Overlapping or crossing, as the wings of some insects when at rest.

cruciate anastomosis *or* **crucial anastomose** *n.* A surgical connection between the branches of the perforating, gluteal, and circumflex femoral arteries that are located behind the upper part of the femur.

cruciate ligament of knee *n.* Either of two ligaments, anterior and posterior, that pass from the intercondylar area of the tibia to the condyles of the femur.

cruciate muscle *n.* A muscle in which the bundles of muscle fibers cross in an x-shaped configuration.

cru·ral (krōōrʹəl) *adj.* **1.** Of or relating to the leg, shank, or thigh. **2.** Of or relating to a body part that resembles a leg.

crural canal *n.* See **femoral canal.**

crural hernia *n.* See **femoral hernia.**

crural sheath *n.* See **femoral sheath.**

crus (krōōs, krŭs) *n., pl.* **cru·ra** (krōŏr**′**ə) **1.** The section of the leg between the knee and foot; lower leg; shank. **2.** A body part consisting of elongated masses or diverging bands that resemble legs or roots. **3.** Either of a pair of diverging bands or elongated masses.

crush syndrome (krŭsh) *n.* A severe shocklike condition that follows release of a limb or other large body part after a prolonged period of compression, characterized by edema, hematuria, and renal failure. Also called *compression syndrome.*

crus of clitoris *n.* The continuation of the clitoris on each side of the corpus cavernosum, diverging from the body posteriorly and attached to the pubic arch.

crus of diaphragm *n.* Any of the muscular origins of the diaphragm from the bodies of the upper lumbar vertebrae that pass the aorta upward to the central tendon.

crus of fornix *n.* The part of the fornix that rises in a forward curve behind the thalamus and continues forward as the body of the fornix below the corpus callosum.

crus of penis *n.* The posterior portion of the corpus cavernosum of the penis attached to the ischiopubic ramus.

crust (krŭst) *n.* **1.** A hard, crisp covering or surface. **2.** An outer layer or coating that is formed by the drying of a bodily exudate such as pus or blood; a scab. —*v.* To cover with, become covered with, or harden into a crust.

crutch (krŭch) *n.* A staff or support used by a physically injured or disabled individual as an aid in walking, usually designed to fit under the armpit and often used in pairs.

Cru·veil·hier (krōō-vāl-yā**′**, krü-vĕ-), Jean 1791–1874. French anatomist who was the first to describe multiple sclerosis.

Cruveilhier-Baumgarten murmur (boum**′**gär**′**tn) *n.* A murmur heard over the collateral veins in the abdominal wall that connect the portal and caval venous systems.

Cruveilhier-Baumgarten sign *n.* An indication of hepatic cirrhosis with portal hypertension in which a murmur, created by recanalization of the umbilical vein and reverse blood flow from the liver into the abdominal veins, is heard over a Medusa head.

Cruveilhier-Baumgarten syndrome *n.* Cirrhosis of the liver associated with patent umbilical or paraumbilical veins and varicose periumbilical veins.

Cru·veil·hier's disease (krōō-vāl-yāz**′**, krü-vĕ-) *n.* See **progressive muscular atrophy.**

Cruveilhier's sign *n.* See **Medusa head.**

crux (krŭks, krōōks) *n., pl.* **crux·es** *or* **cru·ces** (krōō**′**sēz) A cross or a crosslike structure.

crux of heart *n.* The area of the junction of the walls of the four chambers of the heart.

crux pi·lo·rum (pī-lôr**′**əm) *n.* A crosslike figure formed by hairs growing from two directions that meet and then separate in a direction perpendicular to the original orientation.

Cruz trypanosomiasis (krōōz, krōōs) *n.* See **South American trypanosomiasis.**

cry·al·ge·si·a (krī**′**əl-jē**′**zē-ə, -zhə) *n.* Pain caused by cold. Also called *crymodynia.*

cry·an·es·the·sia (krī**′**ăn-ĭs-thē**′**zhə) *n.* The loss of sensation or perception of cold.

cry·es·the·sia (krī**′**ĭs-thē**′**zhə) *n.* **1.** The ability to sense cold. **2.** Extreme sensitivity to cold.

crymo– *pref.* Cold: *crymotherapy.*

cry·mo·dyn·i·a (krī**′**mō-dĭn**′**ē-ə) *n.* See **cryalgesia.**

cry·mo·phil·ic (krī**′**mə-fĭl**′**ĭk) *adj.* Growing best at low temperatures. Used of microorganisms.

cry·mo·phy·lac·tic (krī**′**mō-fə-lăk**′**tĭk) *adj.* Having resistance to cold temperatures. Used of microorganisms.

cry·mo·ther·a·py (krī**′**mō-thĕr**′**ə-pē) *n.* See **cryotherapy.**

cryo– *or* **cry–** *pref.* Cold; freezing: *cryoprotein.*

cry·o·an·es·the·sia (krī**′**ō-ăn**′**ĭs-thē**′**zhə) *n.* Localized application of cold as a means of producing regional anesthesia. Also called *refrigeration anesthesia.*

cry·o·bank (krī**′**ə-bangk**′**) *n.* A place of storage that uses very low temperatures to preserve semen or transplantable tissues.

cry·o·bi·ol·o·gy (krī**′**ō-bī-ŏl**′**ə-jē) *n.* The study of the effects of very low temperatures on living organisms. —**cry′o·bi′o·log′i·cal** (-bī**′**ə-lŏj**′**ĭ-kəl) *adj.* —**cry′o·bi·ol′o·gist** *n.*

cry·o·cau·ter·y (krī**′**ō-kô**′**tə-rē) *n.* A substance or an instrument that destroys tissue by freezing.

cry·o·ex·trac·tion (krī**′**ō-ĭk-străk**′**shən) *n.* The removal of a cataract by the adhesion of a freezing probe to the lens.

cry·o·fi·brin·o·gen (krī**′**ō-fī-brĭn**′**ə-jən) *n.* An abnormal type of fibrinogen that precipitates upon cooling, but redissolves when warmed to room temperature; it is rarely found in human plasma.

cry·o·fi·brin·o·ge·ne·mi·a (krī**′**ō-fī-brĭn**′**ə-jə-nē**′**mē-ə) *n.* The presence of cryofibrinogens in the blood.

cry·o·gen (krī**′**ə-jən) *n.* A liquid, such as liquid nitrogen, that boils at a temperature below about 110 Kelvin (−160°C) and is used to obtain very low temperatures; a refrigerant.

cry·o·gen·ic (krī**′**ə-jĕn**′**ĭk) *adj.* **1.** Relating to or producing low temperatures. **2.** Requiring or suitable for storage at low temperatures. —**cry′o·gen′i·cal·ly** *adv.*

cry·o·glob·u·lin (krī**′**ō-glŏb**′**yə-lĭn) *n.* Any of various abnormal globulins that precipitate from plasma when cooled.

cry·o·glob·u·li·ne·mi·a (krī**′**ō-glŏb**′**yə-lə-nē**′**mē-ə) *n.* The presence of abnormal quantities of cryoglobulin in the blood plasma.

cry·ol·y·sis (krī-ŏl**′**ĭ-sĭs) *n.* Destruction by cold.

cry·om·e·ter (krī-ŏm**′**ĭ-tər) *n.* A thermometer capable of measuring very low temperatures.

cry·op·a·thy (krī-ŏp**′**ə-thē) *n.* Any of various diseased conditions caused by exposure to cold.

cry·o·pex·y (krī**′**ə-pĕk**′**sē) *n.* Surgical attachment of the sensory retina to the pigment epithelium and choroid by applying a cryoprobe to the sclera.

cry·o·phil·ic (krī**′**ə-fĭl**′**ĭk) *or* **cry·oph·i·lous** (krī-ŏf**′**ə-ləs) *adj.* Having an affinity for or thriving at low temperatures. Used of microorganisms.

cry·o·phy·lac·tic (krī**′**ō-fə-lăk**′**tĭk) *adj.* Of or having crymophylactic resistance.

cry·o·pre·cip·i·tate (krī′ō-prĭ-sĭp′ĭ-tāt′, -tĭt) *n.* A precipitate that forms when soluble material is cooled, especially a precipitate rich in factor VIII that is formed when normal blood plasma is cooled.

cry·o·pres·er·va·tion (krī′ō-prĕz′ər-vā′shən) *n.* Maintenance of the viability of excised tissues or organs by freezing at extremely low temperatures. —**cry′o·pre·serve′** (krī′ō-prĭ-zûrv′) *v.*

cry·o·probe (krī′ə-prōb′) *n.* A surgical instrument used to apply extreme cold to tissues during cryosurgery.

cry·o·pro·tec·tant (krī′ō-prə-tək′tənt) *n.* A substance that is used to protect cells or tissues from damage during freezing. —**cry′o·pro·tec′tant** *adj.* —**cry′o·pro·tec′tive** *adj.*

cry·o·pro·tein (krī′ō-prō′tēn′) *n.* A protein, such as cryoglobulin, that precipitates from solution when cooled and redissolves upon warming.

cry·o·scope (krī′ə-skōp′) *n.* An instrument that is used to measure the freezing point, usually of a liquid.

cry·os·co·py (krī-ŏs′kə-pē) *n.* A technique for determining the freezing point of a liquid, such as blood or urine.

cry·o·sur·ger·y (krī′ō-sûr′jə-rē) *n.* The selective exposure of tissues to extreme cold, often by applying a probe containing liquid nitrogen, to bring about the destruction or elimination of abnormal cells.

cry·o·ther·a·py (krī′ō-thĕr′ə-pē) *n.* The local or general use of low temperatures in medical therapy. Also called *crymotherapy.*

cry·o·tol·er·ant (krī′ō-tŏl′ər-ənt) *adj.* Able to withstand very low temperatures.

crypt (krĭpt) *n.* A small pit, recess, or glandular cavity in the body.

crypt abscesses *pl.n.* Abscesses that are characteristic of ulcerative colitis, and are located in the mucosa of the large intestine.

cryp·tec·to·my (krĭp-tĕk′tə-mē) *n.* Excision or obliteration of a crypt, especially a tonsillar crypt.

crypt·es·the·sia *or* **crypt·aes·the·sia** (krĭp′tĭs-thē′zhə) *n.* A mode of paranormal perception, such as clairvoyance.

cryp·tic (krĭp′tĭk) *n.* **1.** Hidden or concealed. **2.** Tending to conceal or camouflage, as the coloring of an animal.

cryp·ti·tis (krĭp-tī′tĭs) *n.* Inflammation of a crypt or crypts, particularly in the rectum.

crypto– *or* **crypt–** *pref.* **1.** Crypt: *cryptectomy.* **2.** Hidden; secret: *cryptogenic.*

cryp·to·coc·co·sis (krĭp′tə-kŏ-kō′sĭs) *n.* A systemic infection caused by *Cryptococcus neoformans* that can affect the lungs, skin, or other body organs but that occurs most often in the brain and meninges. Also called *Busse-Buschke disease.*

Cryp·to·coc·cus (krĭp′tə-kŏk′əs) *n.* Any of a genus of yeastlike fungi commonly occurring in the soil and including certain pathogenic species.

crypt of iris *n.* Any of a group of pits found on the iris close to the pupil.

cryp·to·gen·ic (krĭp′tə-jĕn′ĭk) *adj.* Of obscure or unknown origin. Used of diseases.

cryptogenic septicemia *n.* A form of septicemia in which no primary focus of infection can be found.

cryp·to·lith (krĭp′tə-lĭth′) *n.* A concretion in a crypt.

cryp·to·men·or·rhe·a (krĭp′tō-mĕn′ə-rē′ə) *n.* Occurrence of the menses without any external flow of blood, as in cases of imperforate hymen.

cryp·to·mer·or·rha·chis·chis (krĭp′tō-mĕr′ôr-ə-kĭs′kĭ-sĭs) *n.* See **spina bifida occulta.**

cryp·toph·thal·mi·a (krĭp′tŏf-thăl′mē-ə) *or* **cryp·toph·thal·mus** (-məs) *n.* A congenital abnormality in which the eyelids are absent and skin passes continuously from the forehead to the cheek over rudimentary eyes.

cryp·to·po·di·a (krĭp′tō-pō′dē-ə) *n.* A condition characterized by swelling of the lower part of the leg and the foot so that the sole seems to be a broad flattened pad.

crypt·or·chi·dec·to·my (krĭp-tôr′kĭ-dĕk′tə-mē) *n.* Surgical removal of an undescended testicle.

crypt·or·chi·do·pexy (krĭp-tôr′kĭ-dō-pĕk′sē) *n.* See **orchiopexy.**

crypt·or·chism (krĭp-tôr′kĭz′əm) *or* **crypt·or·chi·dism** (-kĭ-dĭz′əm) *n.* A developmental defect marked by failure of the testes to descend into the scrotum.

cryp·to·spo·rid·i·o·sis (krĭp′tō-spə-rĭd′ē-ō′sĭs) *n.* Infection that is caused by *Cryptosporidium,* characterized by chronic diarrhea.

Cryp·to·spo·rid·i·um (krĭp′tō-spô-rĭd′ē-əm) *n.* A genus of parasitic coccidian protozoans that infect the epithelial cells of the gastrointestinal tract in vertebrates and flourish in humans under conditions of intense immunosuppression.

cryp·to·zo·ite (krĭp′tō-zō′īt′) *n.* A malarial parasite at the stage of development in which it inhabits bodily tissue before invading the red blood cells.

cryp·to·zy·gous (krĭp′tō-zī′gəs, krĭp-tŏz′ĭ-gəs) *adj.* Having a narrow face as compared with the width of the cranium, so that the zygomatic arches are not visible when the skull is viewed from above.

crys·tal (krĭs′təl) *n.* **1.** A homogenous solid formed by a repeating, three-dimensional pattern of atoms, ions, or molecules and having fixed distances between constituent parts. **2.** A mineral, especially a transparent form of quartz that has a crystalline structure and is often characterized by external planar faces.

crys·tal·lin (krĭs′tə-lĭn) *n.* A globulin in the lens of the eye.

crys·tal·line (krĭs′tə-lĭn, -līn′, -lēn′) *adj.* **1.** Being, relating to, or composed of crystal or crystals. **2.** Resembling crystal, as in transparency or distinctness of structure or outline.

crys·tal·li·za·tion (krĭs′tə-lĭ-zā′shən) *n.* The formation of crystals or the assumption of a crystalline form. —**crys′tal·lize′** (-līz′) *v.*

crys·tal·loid (krĭs′tə-loid′) *n.* A substance that in solution can pass through a semipermeable membrane and be crystallized, as distinguished from a colloid. —*adj.* Resembling or having properties of a crystal or crystalloid.

crys·tal·lu·ri·a (krĭs′tə-lŏŏr′ē-ə) *n.* The excretion of crystals in the urine.

crystal violet *n.* A dye derived from gentian violet that is used as a general biological stain, an acid-base indicator, and an agent against infection by bacteria, fungi, pinworms, and other parasites.

Cs The symbol for the element **cesium.**

C-section *n.* A cesarean section.

CSF *abbr.* cerebrospinal fluid

Cten·o·ce·phal·i·des (tĕn'ō-sə-făl'ĭ-dēz') *n.* A genus of fleas that includes species that are parasitic on dogs and cats; the species found on dogs can transmit tapeworm to humans.

CTS *abbr.* carpal tunnel syndrome

CT scan (sē'tē') *n.* See **CAT scan.**

CT scanner *n.* See **CAT scanner.**

Cu The symbol for the element **copper.**

cu·bic centimeter (kyoo'bĭk) *n. Abbr.* **cc** A unit of volume equal to one thousandth (10^{-3}) of a liter or to one milliliter.

cu·bi·tal (kyoo'bĭ-tl) *adj.* Relating to the elbow or the ulna.

cubital joint *n.* See **elbow joint.**

cubital nerve *n.* See **ulnar nerve.**

cu·bi·tus (kyoo'bĭ-təs) *n., pl.* **cubitus 1.** See **elbow** (sense 1). **2.** See **ulna.**

cubitus val·gus (văl'gəs) *n.* A deformity of the elbow in which the forearm deviates away from the midline of the body when extended.

cubitus var·us (vâr'əs) *n.* A deformity of the elbow in which the forearm deviates toward the midline of the body when extended.

cu·boid (kyoo'boid') *adj.* Having the approximate shape of a cube. —*n.* A tarsal bone on the outer side of the foot, articulating in front with the calcaneus and lateral cuneiform, and behind with the fourth and fifth metatarsal bones. —**cu·boi'dal** (kyoo-boid'l) *adj.*

cuboidal epithelium *n.* Epithelium made up of cells that look like cubes in a vertical section but appear to be polyhedral when viewed on their surface.

cuff (kŭf) *n.* **1.** A bandlike structure encircling a part. **2.** An inflatable band, usually wrapped around the upper arm, that is used along with a sphygmomanometer in measuring arterial blood pressure.

cul-de-sac (kŭl'dĭ-săk', kool'-) *n., pl.* **culs-de-sac** (kŭlz'-, koolz'-) *or* **cul-de-sacs** A saclike cavity or tube open only at one end.

cul·do·cen·te·sis (kŭl'dō-sĕn-tē'sĭs, kool'-) *n.* Aspiration of fluid from the rectouterine space by puncture of the vaginal vault near the midline between the uterosacral ligaments.

cul·do·plas·ty (kŭl'də-plăs'tē, kool'-) *n.* A surgical procedure to remedy relaxation of the posterior fornix of the vagina.

cul·do·scope (kŭl'də-skōp', kool'-) *n.* An endoscope used in culdoscopy.

cul·dos·co·py (kŭl-dŏs'kə-pē, kool-) *n.* The visual examination of the rectovaginal pouch and pelvic viscera by the introduction of an endoscope through the posterior vaginal wall.

Cu·lex (kyoo'lĕks') *n.* A genus of mosquitoes that act as vectors for many diseases of humans and domestic and wild animals.

cu·li·cide (kyoo'lĭ-sīd') *n.* An agent that destroys mosquitoes. —**cu'li·cid'al** (kyoo'lĭ-sīd'l) *adj.*

cu·lic·i·fuge (kyoo-lĭs'ə-fyooj') *n.* An agent that repels mosquitoes or gnats.

Cu·li·coi·des (kyoo'lĭ-koi'dēz') *n.* A genus of minute biting gnats or midges.

Cul·len's sign (kŭl'ənz) *n.* An indication of intraperitoneal hemorrhage, especially in ruptured ectopic pregnancy, in which blood causes periumbilical darkening of the skin.

cul·men (kŭl'mən) *n., pl.* **cul·mi·na** (kŭk'mə-nə) The front prominent portion of the monticulus of the vermis of the cerebellum.

cul·ti·va·tion (kŭl'tə-vā'shən) *n.* The process of promoting the growth of a biological culture. —**cul'ti·vate'** *v.*

cul·ture (kŭl'chər) *n.* **1.** The growing of microorganisms, tissue cells, or other living matter in a specially prepared nutrient medium. **2.** Such a growth or colony, as of bacteria. —*v.* **1.** To grow microorganisms or other living matter in a specially prepared nutrient medium. **2.** To use a substance as a medium for culture.

culture medium *n.* A liquid or gelatinous substance containing nutrients in which microorganisms or tissues are cultivated for scientific purposes.

culture shock *n.* A condition of confusion and anxiety affecting a person suddenly exposed to an unfamiliar culture or milieu.

cu·mu·la·tive (kyoom'yə-lā'tĭv, -lə-tĭv) *adj.* **1.** Increasing or enlarging by successive addition. **2.** Acquired by or resulting from accumulation. **3.** Of or relating to the sum of the frequencies of experimentally determined values of a random variable that are less than or equal to a specified value. **4.** Of or relating to experimental error that increases in magnitude with each successive measurement.

cumulative effect *n.* The state at which repeated administration of a drug may produce effects that are more pronounced than those produced by the first dose. Also called *cumulative action.*

cu·ne·ate (kyoo'nē-ĭt, -āt') *adj.* Wedge-shaped.

cuneate fasciculus *n.* The larger lateral subdivision of the posterior funiculus of the spinal cord. Also called *cuneate funiculus.*

cuneate nucleus *n.* One of the three nuclei of the posterior column of the spinal cord, located near the dorsal surface of the medulla oblongata, receiving posterior root fibers corresponding to the sensory innervation of the arm and hand of the same side, and forming with the nucleus gracilis the major source of the origin of the lateral meniscus.

cu·ne·i·form (kyoo'nē-ə-fôrm', kyoo-nē'-) *adj.* **1.** Wedge-shaped. **2.** Of, relating to, or being a wedge-shaped bone or cartilage. —*n.* A wedge-shaped bone, especially one of three such bones of the foot.

cuneiform bone *n.* **1.** A wedge-shaped bone, especially one of three bones in the tarsus of the foot. **2.** See **triquetrum .**

cuneiform cartilage *n.* A small nonarticulating rod of elastic cartilage in the aryepiglottic fold above the corniculate cartilage.

cu·ne·o·cu·boid (kyoo'nē-ō-kyoo'boid') *adj.* Relating to the lateral cuneiform and cuboid bones.

cu·ne·o·na·vic·u·lar (kyoo'nē-ō-nə-vĭk'yə-lər) *adj.* Relating to the cuneiform and navicular bones.

cu·ne·us (kyoo'nē-əs) *n., pl.* **–ne·i** (-nē-ī') The region of the medial aspect of the occipital lobe of each cerebral hemisphere that is bounded by the parieto-occipital sulcus and the calcarine sulcus.

cu·nic·u·lus (kyōo-nĭk′yə-ləs) *n., pl.* **–li** (-lī′) The burrow of the itch mite in the skin.

cun·ni·lin·gus (kŭn′ə-lĭng′gəs) *n.* Oral stimulation of the clitoris or vulva.

cup (kŭp) *n.* **1.** A cup-shaped structure or organ. **2.** See **cupping glass. 3.** A unit of capacity or volume equal to 16 tablespoons or 8 fluid ounces. —*v.* To subject a person or body part to the therapeutic procedure of cupping.

cup biopsy forceps *n.* A slender flexible forceps with movable cup-shaped jaws, used to obtain biopsy specimens by introduction through a specially designed endoscope.

cu·po·la (kyōo′pə-lə) *n.* A cup-shaped or domelike structure.

cup·ping (kŭp′ĭng) *n.* **1.** The formation of a hollow or cup-shaped excavation. **2.** A therapeutic procedure, no longer in use, in which evacuated glass cups are applied to intact or scarified skin in order to draw blood to the surface.

cupping glass *n.* A glass vessel from which the air has been exhausted by heat or suction, applied to the skin to draw blood to the surface for therapeutic purposes. Also called *cup.*

cu·pric (kōo′prĭk) *adj.* Of or containing divalent copper.

Cup·ri·mine (kŭp′rə-mēn′) A trademark for the drug penicillamine.

cu·pu·la (kyōo′pyə-lə) *n., pl.* **–lae** (-lē′) Cupola.

cu·pu·li·form cataract (kyōo′pyə-lə-fôrm′) *n.* A common form of senile cataract often confined to a region within the posterior capsule.

cu·pu·lo·gram (kyōo′pyə-lə-grăm′) *n.* A graphic representation of vestibular function relative to normal performance obtained during cupulometry.

cu·pu·lom·e·try (kyōo′pyə-lŏm′ĭ-trē) *n.* A method for testing vestibular function, in which a person rotates in a chair and the duration of vertigo and nystagmus after the chair has stopped is plotted against angular deceleration.

cur·a·ble (kyōor′ə-bəl) *adj.* Capable of being cured.

cu·ra·re *or* **cu·ra·ri** (kōo-rä′rē, kyōo-) *n.* **1.** An extract obtained from several tropical American woody plants, especially *Chondrodendron tomentosum,* used as an arrow poison by some Indian peoples of South America. **2.** A purified preparation or alkaloid obtained from *Chondrodendron tomentosum,* used to relax skeletal muscles.

cu·ra·ri·form (kōo-rä′rə-fôrm′, kyōo-) *adj.* Having a biochemical action like that of curare.

cu·ra·rize (kōo-rä′rīz′, kyōo-) *v.* **1.** To poison with curare. **2.** To treat a person with curare so as to relax the skeletal muscles. —**cu·ra′ri·za′tion** (-rĭ-zā′shən) *n.*

cu·ra·tive (kyōor′ə-tĭv) *adj.* **1.** Serving or tending to cure. **2.** Relating to the cure of disease. —*n.* Something that cures; a remedy.

curative dose *n.* The dose that is required to eliminate the symptoms of a disease or to correct the manifestations of a deficiency in the diet.

curb tenotomy (kûrb) *n.* Excision of the tendon of the shortened muscle in strabismus, and fixation of it farther back on the aponeurosis of the globe.

cure (kyōor) *n.* **1.** Restoration of health; recovery from disease. **2.** A method or course of treatment used to restore health. **3.** An agent that restores health; a remedy. —*v.* **1.** To restore a person to health. **2.** To effect a recovery from a disease or disorder.

cure-all (kyōor′ôl′) *n.* A remedy that cures all diseases or evils; a panacea.

cu·ret·tage (kyōor′ĭ-täzh′) *n.* The removal of tissue or growths from the interior of a body cavity, such as the uterus, by scraping with a curette. Also called *curettement.*

cu·rette *or* **cu·ret** (kyōo-rĕt′) *n.* A surgical instrument shaped like a scoop or spoon, used to remove tissue or growths from a body cavity. —*v.* To scrape tissue or a body part with a curette.

cu·rette·ment *or* **cu·ret·ment** (kyōo-rĕt′mənt) *n.* See **curettage.**

cu·rie (kyōor′ē, kyōo-rē′) *n. Abbr.* **Ci** A unit of radioactivity, equal to the amount of a radioactive isotope that decays at the rate of 3.7×10^{10} disintegrations per second.

Cu·rie (kyōor′ē, kyōo-rē′, kü-), **Marie** Originally **Manja Skłodowska.** 1867–1934. Polish-born French chemist. She shared a 1903 Nobel Prize with her husband, **Pierre Curie** (1859–1906), and Henri Becquerel (1852–1908) for fundamental research on radioactivity. In 1911 she won a second Nobel Prize for her discovery and study of the elements radium and polonium.

cu·ri·um (kyōor′ē-əm) *n. Symbol* **Cm** A metallic synthetic radioactive transuranic element whose longest-lived isotope is Cm 247, with a half-life of 16.4 million years. Atomic number 96.

Cur·ling's ulcer (kûr′lĭngz) *n.* An ulcer of the duodenum in a patient with extensive superficial burns or severe bodily injury.

cur·rant jelly clot (kûr′ənt) *n.* A jellylike mass of red blood cells and fibrin formed by the in vitro or postmortem clotting of whole or sedimented blood.

cur·rent (kûr′ənt) *n.* **1.** A stream or flow of a liquid or gas. **2.** *Symbol* **I** A flow of electric charge. **3.** *Symbol* **I,** i The amount of electric charge flowing past a specified circuit point per unit time.

Cursch·mann's spirals (kûrsh′mənz, kōorsh′mänz) *n.* Spirally twisted masses of mucus occurring in the sputum in bronchial asthma.

cur·va·ture (kûr′və-chōor′) *n.* A curving or bending, especially an abnormal one.

curvature aberration *n.* A lack of spatial correspondence that causes the visual image of a straight extended object to appear curved.

curvature hyperopia *n.* Hyperopia due to diminution of convexity of the refracting media of the eye.

curvature myopia *n.* Myopia due to refractive errors in the corneal curvature.

curve (kûrv) *n.* **1.** A line or surface that deviates from straightness in a smooth, continuous fashion. **2.** Something characterized by such a line or surface, especially a rounded line or contour of the human body. **3.** A curved line representing variations in data on a graph. —*v*. To move in or take the shape of a curve.

curve of occlusion *n.* **1.** A curved surface that makes simultaneous contact with the major portion of the incisal and occlusal prominences of the existing teeth. **2.** The curve of a dentition on which the occlusal surfaces lie.

Cush·ing (ko͞osh′ĭng), **Harvey Williams** 1869–1939. American surgeon known for his innovations in the field of neurosurgery and for his studies of the pituitary gland.

cush·ing·oid (ko͞osh′ĭng-oid′) *adj.* Resembling the signs and symptoms of Cushing's disease or Cushing's syndrome.

Cush·ing's syndrome (ko͞osh′ĭngz) *n.* A syndrome caused by an increased production of ACTH from a tumor of the adrenal cortex or of the anterior lobe of the pituitary gland. It is characterized by obesity and weakening of the muscles. Also called *Cushing's basophilism, Cushing's disease, pituitary basophilism.*

Cushing's syndrome med·i·ca·men·to·sus (mĕd′ĭ-kə-mən-tō′səs) *n.* A condition that is caused by the chronic administration of large doses of glucocorticoids and that produces the signs and symptoms of Cushing's syndrome.

cush·ion (ko͞osh′ən) *n.* A padlike body part.

cusp (kŭsp) *n.* **1.** A pointed or rounded projection on the chewing surface of a tooth. **2.** A triangular fold or flap of a heart valve.

cusp·al (kŭs′pəl) *adj.* Relating to a cusp.

cus·pate (kŭs′pāt′) *or* **cus·pat·ed** (-pā′tĭd) *adj.* **1.** Having a cusp. **2.** Shaped like a cusp.

cusp height *n.* **1.** The shortest distance between the tip of a cusp of a tooth and its base plane. **2.** The shortest distance between the deepest part of the central fossa of a posterior tooth and a line connecting the points of the cusps of the tooth.

cus·pid (kŭs′pĭd) *n.* See **canine tooth.** —*adj.* Having one cusp; cuspidate.

cut (kŭt) *v.* **1.** To penetrate with a sharp edge; strike a narrow opening in. **2.** To separate into parts with or as if with a sharp-edged instrument; sever. **3.** To make an incision or a separation. **4.** To have a new tooth grow through the gums. **5.** To form or shape by severing or incising. **6.** To separate from a body; detach. **7.** To lessen the strength of; dilute. —*n.* **1.** The act of cutting. **2.** The result of cutting, especially an opening or wound made by a sharp edge.

cu·ta·ne·o·me·nin·go·spi·nal angiomatosis (kyo͞o-tā′nē-ō-mə-nĭng′gō-spī′nəl) *n.* See **Cobb syndrome.**

cu·ta·ne·ous (kyo͞o-tā′nē-əs) *adj.* Of, relating to, or affecting the skin.

cutaneous horn *n.* A protruding keratotic growth of the skin.

cutaneous larva migrans *n.* See **creeping eruption.**

cutaneous leishmaniasis *n.* An endemic disease in northern Africa and western and central Asia that is caused by infection with promastigotes of *Leishmania tropica* and is transmitted by the bite of a sandfly of the genus *Phlebotomus*. It begins as a papule that enlarges to a nodule and then breaks down into an ulcer that leaves

an indented scar. Also called *Old World leishmaniasis.*

cutaneous leprosy *n.* See **tuberculoid leprosy.**

cutaneous muscle *n.* A muscle that lies in the subcutaneous tissue and attaches to the skin, with or without a bony attachment.

cutaneous reaction *n.* See **cutireaction.**

cutaneous tuberculosis *n.* Pathologic skin lesions that are caused by *Mycobacterium tuberculosis.* Also called *scrofuloderma.*

cutaneous vasculitis *n.* A form of vasculitis affecting the skin, often with involvement of other organs, characterized by a polymorphonuclear infiltrate of the small vessels.

cutaneous vein *n.* Any of several veins in the subcutaneous tissue that empty into deep veins.

cut·down (kŭt′doun′) *n.* The incision of a vein to facilitate the insertion of a cannula or needle, as for the administration of intravenous medication. Also called *venostomy.*

cu·ti·cle (kyo͞o′tĭ-kəl) *n.* **1.** The strip of hardened skin at the base and sides of a fingernail or toenail. **2.** The outermost layer of the skin; epidermis. **3.** Dead or cornified epidermis.

cu·ti·re·ac·tion (kyo͞o′tĭ-rē-ăk′shən) *n.* An inflammatory reaction to a skin test. Also called *cutaneous reaction.*

cu·tis (kyo͞o′tĭs) *n.*, *pl.* **–tis·es** *or* **–tes** (-tēz) Dermis.

cutis an·se·ri·na (ăn′sə-rī′nə) *n.* See **goose bumps.**

cu·ti·sec·tor (kyo͞o′tĭ-sĕk′tər) *n.* **1.** An instrument for cutting small pieces of skin for grafting. **2.** An instrument used to remove a section of skin for microscopic examination.

cutis hy·per·e·las·ti·ca (hī′pər-ĭ-lăs′tĭ-kə) *n.* See **Ehlers-Danlos syndrome.**

cutis lax·a (lăk′sə) *n.* A congenital condition characterized by an excessive amount of skin hanging in folds. Also called *pachydermatocele.*

cutis mar·mo·ra·ta (mär′mə-rā′tə) *n.* A pink marble-like mottling of the skin caused by exposure to cold temperature or associated with various debilitating diseases.

cutis plate *n.* See **dermatome** (sense 3).

cutis rhom·boi·da·lis nu·chae (rŏm′boi-dā′lĭs no͞o′kē, nyo͞o′-) *n.* A condition in which the skin on the back of the neck becomes leathery and furrowed and appears to have rhomboid configurations, caused by aging or prolonged exposure to sunlight.

cutis ve·ra (vîr′ə) *n.* See **dermis.**

cutis ver·ti·cis gy·ra·ta (vûr′tĭ-sĭs jī-rā′tə) *n.* A congenital condition in which the skin of the scalp is thickened, forming folds and furrows.

cu·vette (kyo͞o′vĕt) *n.* A small, transparent, often tubular laboratory vessel.

CV *abbr.* cardiovascular

CVA *abbr.* cerebrovascular accident

CVP *abbr.* central venous pressure

CVS *abbr.* chorionic villus sampling

CXR *abbr.* chest x-ray

cy·a·nide (sī′ə-nīd′) *or* **cy·a·nid** (-nĭd) *n.* Any of various salts or esters of hydrogen cyanide containing a CN group, especially the extremely poisonous compounds potassium cyanide and sodium cyanide.

cy·an·met·he·mo·glo·bin (sī′ăn-mĕt′hē′mə-glō′bĭn, sī′ən-) *n.* A relatively nontoxic compound of cyanide with methemoglobin, formed when methylene blue is administered in cases of cyanide poisoning.

cyano– *or* **cyan–** *pref.* **1.** Blue: *cyanosis.* **2.** Cyanide: *cyanocoalbumin.*

Cy·a·no·bac·te·ri·a (sī′ə-nō-băk-tîr′ē-ə) *n.* A group of Procaryotae consisting of unicellular or filamentous gram-negative microorganisms that are either non-motile or possess a gliding motility, may reproduce by binary fission, and photosynthetically produce oxygen; some species are capable of fixing nitrogen. Members of this phylum were formerly called blue-green algae.

cy·a·no·co·bal·a·min (sī′ə-nō′kō-băl′ə-mĭn, sī-ăn′ō-) *n.* See **vitamin B₁₂.**

cy·an·o·phil (sī-ăn′ə-fĭl′, sī′ə-nō-fĭl′) *n.* A cell or tissue element that is capable of being colored by a blue stain.

cy·a·noph·i·lous (sī′ə-nŏf′ə-ləs) *adj.* Readily stainable with a blue dye.

cy·a·nop·si·a (sī′ə-nŏp′sē-ə) *n.* A condition of the eye in which all objects appear blue; it may temporarily follow cataract extraction.

cy·a·nosed (sī′ə-nōzd′, -nōsd′) *adj.* Cyanotic.

cy·a·nose tardive (sī′ə-nōz′, -nōs′) *n.* Cyanosis caused by congenital heart disease in which there is an abnormal communication between systemic and pulmonary circulations; cyanosis appears only when there is a right-to-left shunt, such as that which occurs after exercise or late in the course of the disease. Also called *tardive cyanosis.*

cy·a·no·sis (sī′ə-nō′sĭs) *n.* A bluish discoloration of the skin and mucous membranes resulting from inadequate oxygenation of the blood. —**cy′a·not′ic** (-nŏt′-ĭk) *adj.*

cyanotic induration *n.* Induration related to chronic venous congestion in an organ or tissue, frequently resulting in fibrous thickening of the walls of the veins and eventual fibrosis of adjacent tissues.

cy·ber·net·ics (sī′bər-nĕt′ĭks) *n.* The theoretical study of communication and control processes in biological, mechanical, and electronic systems, especially the comparison of these processes in biological and artificial systems.

cycl– *pref.* Variant of **cyclo–.**

cy·cla·mate (sī′klə-māt′, sĭk′lə-) *n.* A salt or ester of cyclamic acid formerly used as a sweetening agent, especially calcium cyclamate or sodium cyclamate.

cy·clar·thro·di·al (sī′klär-thrō′dē-əl, sĭk′lär-) *adj.* Relating to a cyclarthrosis.

cy·clar·thro·sis (sī′klär-thrō′sĭs, sĭk′lär-) *n.* A joint capable of rotation.

cy·clase (sī′klās′, -klāz′) *n.* An enzyme that acts as a catalyst in the cyclization of a compound.

cy·cle (sī′kəl) *n.* **1.** An interval of time during which a characteristic, often regularly repeated event or sequence of events occurs. **2.** A single complete execution of a periodically repeated phenomenon. **3.** A periodically repeated sequence of events.

cy·clec·to·my (sī-klĕk′tə-mē, sĭ-klĕk′-) *n.* Excision of a portion of the ciliary body. Also called *ciliectomy.*

cy·clen·ceph·a·ly (sī′klən-sĕf′ə-lē, sĭk′lən-) *n.* A fetal condition in which the cerebral hemispheres are fused and underdeveloped. Also called *cyclocephaly.*

cy·clic (sī′klĭk, sĭk′lĭk) *or* **cy·cli·cal** (sī′klĭ-kəl, sĭk′lĭ-kəl) *adj.* **1.** Relating to or characterized by cycles. **2.** Recurring or moving in cycles. **3.** Relating to chemical compounds having atoms arranged in a ring or closed-chain structure. —**cy′cli·cal′i·ty** (sĭk′lə-kăl′ĭ-tē, sī′klə-) *n.* —**cy′cli·cal·ly** *adv.*

cyclic AMP *n. Abbr.* **cAMP** Adenosine 3′,5′-monophosphate; a cyclic nucleotide of adenosine that acts at the cellular level as a regulator of various metabolic processes.

cyclic compound *n.* A compound in which carbon or other atoms are arranged in a ring. Also called *closed chain compound.*

cyclic GMP *n.* Cyclic guanosine monophosphate; a cyclic nucleotide of guanosine that acts at the cellular level as a regulator of various metabolic processes, possibly as an antagonist to cyclic AMP.

cyclic guanosine monophosphate *n.* Cyclic GMP.

cyclic neutropenia *n.* See **periodic neutropenia.**

cy·cli·cot·o·my (sī′klī-kŏt′ə-mē, sĭk′lĭ-) *n.* See **cyclotomy.**

cy·cli·tis (sī-klī′tĭs, sĭ-) *n.* Inflammation of the ciliary body.

cyclo– *or* **cycl–** *pref.* **1.** Circle; cycle: *cyclophoria.* **2.** A cyclic compound: *cyclopeptide.*

cy·clo·ben·za·prine hydrochloride (sī′klō-bĕn′zə-prēn′, sĭk′lō-) *n.* A skeletal muscle relaxant used to relieve acute muscular spasms.

cy·clo·ceph·a·ly (sī′klō-sĕf′ə-lē) *n.* See **cyclencephaly.**

cy·clo·cho·roid·i·tis (sī′klō-kôr′oi-dī′tĭs) *n.* Inflammation of the ciliary body and the choroid coat of the eye.

cy·clo·cry·o·ther·a·py (sī′klō-krī′ō-thĕr′ə-pē) *n.* The application of a freezing probe to the sclera of the eye in the region of the ciliary body in the treatment of glaucoma.

cy·clo·di·al·y·sis (sī′klō-dī-ăl′ĭ-sĭs) *n.* Surgical opening of a passage between the anterior chamber and the suprachoroidal space in order to reduce pressure within the eye in glaucoma.

cy·clo·di·a·ther·my (sī′klō-dī′ə-thûr′mē) *n.* The destruction of part of the ciliary body of the eye by diathermy, performed in the treatment of glaucoma.

cy·clo·pep·tide (sī′klō-pĕp′tīd′) *n.* A polypeptide in which the terminal amine and carboxyl groups form a peptide bond, thus making the compound cyclic.

cy·clo·pho·rase (sī′klō-fôr′ās′, -āz′) *n.* Any of a group of mitochondrial enzymes that catalyze the oxidation of pyruvic acid to carbon dioxide and water; a Krebs-cycle enzyme.

cy·clo·pho·ri·a (sī′klō-fôr′ē-ə) *n.* A strabismus in which the eye or eyes rotate inward or outward.

cy·clo·phos·pha·mide (sī′klə-fŏs′fə-mīd′) *n.* A highly toxic, immunosuppressive, antineoplastic drug, used in the treatment of Hodgkin's disease, lymphoma, and certain other forms of cancer, such as leukemia and breast cancer.

cy·clo·pho·to·co·ag·u·la·tion (sī′klō-fō′tō-kō-ăg′yə-lā′shən) *n.* Photocoagulation by directing a laser through the pupil to destroy individual ciliary processes, used in treating glaucoma.

cy·clo·pi·a (sī-klō′pē-ə) *n.* A congenital defect in which the two orbits merge to form a single cavity containing one eye. Also called *synophthalmia.*

cy·clo·ple·gia (sī′klə-plē′jə) *n.* Paralysis of the ciliary muscles of the eye that results in the loss of visual accommodation.

cy·clo·ple·gic (sī′klə-plē′jĭk) *adj.* Relating to, characterized by, or causing cycloplegia.

cy·clo·sis (sī-klō′sĭs) *n., pl.* **–ses** (-sēz) The streaming rotary motion of protoplasm within certain cells and one-celled organisms.

cy·clo·spor·ine (sī′klə-spôr′ēn, -ĭn) *or* **cy·clo·spor·in A** (-ĭn) *n.* A cyclic oligopeptide immunosuppressant produced by fungus and used to inhibit organ transplant rejection.

cy·clo·thyme (sī′klə-thīm′) *n.* A person afflicted with cyclothymia.

cy·clo·thy·mi·a (sī′klə-thī′mē-ə) *n.* A mild mood disorder characterized by alternating periods of elation and depression.

cy·clo·thy·mic disorder (sī′klə-thī′mĭk) *n.* A chronic mood disturbance generally lasting at least two years and characterized by mood swings including periods of hypomania and depression.

cyclothymic personality *n.* A personality disorder characterized by frequently alternating periods of elation and depression, usually occurring spontaneously and not related to external circumstances.

cy·clot·o·my (sī-klŏt′ə-mē) *n.* Incision of the ciliary muscle. Also called *cyclicotomy.*

cy·clo·tro·pi·a (sī′klə-trō′pē-ə) *n.* An eye disorder in which one eye deviates from the other by turning around its anteroposterior axis.

cy·e·sis (sī-ē′sĭs) *n.* See **pregnancy** (sense 2).

cyl·in·der (sĭl′ən-dər) *n.* **1.** The surface generated by a straight line intersecting and moving along a closed plane curve, the directrix, while remaining parallel to a fixed straight line that is not on or parallel to the plane of the directrix. **2.** A solid bounded by two parallel planes and such a surface, especially such a surface having a circle as its directrix. **3.** A cylindrical or rodlike renal cast. **4.** A cylindrical lens. **5.** A cylindrical metal container for gases stored under high pressure.

cyl·in·dri·cal (sə-lĭn′drĭ-kəl) *adj.* Of, relating to, or having the shape of a cylinder, especially of a circular cylinder.

cylindrical lens *n.* A lens in which one of the surfaces is curved in one meridian and less curved in the opposite meridian. Also called *astigmatic lens.*

cyl·in·dro·ad·e·no·ma (sĭl′ən-drō-ăd′n-ō′mə, sə-lĭn′-) *n.* See **cylindroma.**

cyl·in·droid (sĭl′ən-droid′) *n.* **1.** A cylindrical surface or solid all of whose sections perpendicular to the elements are elliptical. **2.** A mucous thread with pointed or split ends, observed microscopically in the urine, and resembling a urinary cast. —*adj.* Resembling a cylinder.

cyl·in·dro·ma (sĭl′ən-drō′mə) *n.* A type of epithelial tumor characterized by islands of neoplastic cells embedded in a cylindrical hyalinized stroma formed from ducts of glands; it occurs especially in the salivary glands, skin, and bronchi and is frequently malignant. Also called *cylindroadenoma.*

cyl·in·dro·ma·tous carcinoma (sĭl′ĭn-drō′mə-təs, -drŏm′ə) *n.* See **adenoid cystic carcinoma.**

cyl·in·dru·ri·a (sĭl′ən-drŏŏr′ē-ə) *n.* The presence of renal casts in the urine.

cym·bo·ce·phal·ic (sĭm′bō-sə-făl′ĭk) *or* **cym·bo·ceph·a·lous** (-sĕf′ə-ləs) *adj.* Scaphocephalic.

cy·nan·che (sə-năng′kē, sī-) *n.* Severe sore throat.

cyn·ic spasm (sĭn′ĭk) *n.* See **risus caninus.**

cy·no·ceph·a·ly (sī′nə-sĕf′ə-lē) *n.* Craniostenosis in which the skull slopes back from the orbits.

cy·no·pho·bi·a (sī′nə-fō′bē-ə) *n.* An abnormal fear of dogs.

cy·pro·hept·a·dine hydrochloride (sī′prō-hĕp′tə-dēn) *n.* An antihistamine that is used to relieve the symptoms of various allergic reactions, such as itching and skin rash.

cy·prot·er·one (sī-prŏt′ə-rōn′) *n.* A synthetic steroid that inhibits the secretion of androgens.

Cys *abbr.* cysteine

cyst (sĭst) *n.* **1.** An abnormal membranous sac containing a gaseous, liquid, or semisolid substance. **2.** A sac or vesicle in the body. **3.** A small capsulelike sac that encloses certain organisms in their dormant or larval stage.

cyst– *pref.* Variant of **cysto–.**

cyst·ad·e·no·car·ci·no·ma (sĭ-stăd′n-ō-kär′sə-nō′mə) *n.* A malignant tumor derived from glandular tissue, in which secretions are retained and accumulate in cysts.

cyst·ad·e·no·ma (sĭ-stăd′n-ō′mə) *n.* A benign tumor derived from glandular tissue, in which secretions are retained and accumulate in cysts. Also called *cystoadenoma.*

cys·tal·gia (sĭs′tăl′jə) *n.* Pain in the bladder.

cys·ta·thi·o·nase (sĭs′tə-thī′ə-nās′, -nāz′) *n.* A liver enzyme that catalyzes the hydrolysis of cystathionine to cysteine.

cys·ta·thi·o·nine (sĭs′tə-thī′ə-nēn′, -nĭn′) *n.* An intermediate in the conversion of methionine to cysteine.

cystathionine gamma-synthase *n.* An enzyme that catalyzes the reaction between cystathionine and succinate to form cysteine.

cys·ta·thi·o·ni·nu·ri·a (sĭs′tə-thī′ə-nē-nŏŏr′ē-ə) *n.* An inherited disorder of cystathionine metabolism characterized by elevated concentrations of cystathionine in the blood, tissues, and urine, and sometimes mental retardation.

cys·tec·ta·sia (sĭs′tĭk-tā′zhə) *or* **cys·tec·ta·sy** (sĭ-stĕk′tə-sē) *n.* Dilation of the bladder.

cys·tec·to·my (sĭ-stĕk′tə-mē) *n.* **1.** Surgical removal of a cyst. **2.** Surgical removal of all or a part of the gallbladder. **3.** Surgical removal of all or part of the urinary bladder.

cys·te·ic acid (sĭs-stē′ĭk) *n.* A crystalline amino acid formed in the oxidation of cysteine; it is a precursor of taurine.

cys·te·ine (sĭs′tē-ēn′, -ĭn, sĭ-stē′ĭn) *n. Abbr.* **Cys** An alpha-amino acid found in most proteins and especially abundant in keratin.

cysti– *pref.* Variant of **cysto–.**

cys·tic (sĭs′tĭk) *adj.* **1.** Of, relating to, or having the characteristic of a cyst. **2.** Having or containing cysts or a cyst. **3.** Enclosed in a cyst. **4.** Of, relating to, or involving the gallbladder or urinary bladder.

cystic acne *n.* Acne in which the predominant lesions are cysts and deep-seated scars.

cystic artery *n.* An artery with its origin in the right branch of the hepatic artery, with distribution to the gallbladder and visceral surface of the liver.

cystic disease of renal medulla *n.* The presence of small cysts in the medulla of the kidney, associated with anemia, sodium depletion, and chronic renal failure.

cystic disease of breast *n.* See **fibrocystic disease of breast.**

cystic duct *n.* The duct that leads from the gallbladder and joins the hepatic duct to form the common bile duct.

cys·ti·cer·coid (sĭs′tĭ-sûr′koid′) *n.* The larval stage of certain tapeworms, resembling a cysticercus but having the scolex completely filling the enclosing cyst.

cys·ti·cer·co·sis (sĭs′tĭ-sər-kō′sĭs) *n.* Infection with cysticerci in subcutaneous, muscle, or central nervous system tissues.

cys·ti·cer·cus (sĭs′tĭ-sûr′kəs) *n.*, *pl.* **–ci** (-sī′) The larval stage of many tapeworms, consisting of a single invaginated scolex enclosed in a fluid-filled cyst.

cystic fibrosis *n. Abbr.* **CF** A hereditary metabolic disorder of the exocrine glands, usually developing during early childhood and affecting mainly the pancreas, respiratory system, and sweat glands. It is marked by the production of abnormally viscous mucus by the affected glands, usually resulting in chronic respiratory infections and impaired pancreatic function. Also called *Clarke-Hadfield syndrome, fibrocystic disease of pancreas, mucoviscidosis.*

cystic goiter *n.* Goiter due to the presence of one or more cysts within the gland.

cystic lymphangioma *n.* A condition characterized by a fairly circumscribed group of several cystlike dilated vessels or spaces lined with endothelium and filled with lymph.

cystic node *n.* A lymph node at the neck of the gallbladder draining lymph into the hepatic nodes.

cystic vein *n.* A vein that drains the gallbladder and passes along the cystic duct to enter the right branch of the portal vein.

cys·ti·form (sĭs′tə-fôrm′) *adj.* Cystoid.

cys·tine (sĭs′tēn′) *n.* A white crystalline amino acid that is found in many proteins, especially keratin, and is the major source of metabolic sulfur.

cystine calculus *n.* A soft type of urinary calculus composed of cystine.

cys·ti·ne·mi·a (sĭs′tə-nē′mē-ə) *n.* The presence of cystine in blood.

cys·ti·no·sis (sĭs′tə-nō′sĭs) *n.* A hereditary dysfunction of the renal tubules characterized by the presence of carbohydrates and amino acids in the urine, excessive urination, and low blood levels of potassium ions and phosphates, and caused by the abnormal metabolism of cystine and the accumulation of cystine crystals in tissues; it occurs in young children. Also called *cystine storage disease.*

cys·ti·nu·ri·a (sĭs′tə-nōōr′ē-ə) *n.* A hereditary condition characterized by excessive urinary excretion of cystine, lysine, arginine, and ornithine, caused by a defect in the renal tubules that impairs reabsorption of these acids.

cys·ti·stax·is (sĭs′tĭ-stăk′sĭs) *n.* The oozing of blood from the mucous membrane of the bladder. Also called *cystostaxis.*

cys·ti·tis (sĭ-stī′tĭs) *n.* Inflammation of the urinary bladder.

cystitis cys·ti·ca (sĭs′tĭ-kə) *n.* Chronic cystitis glandularis accompanied by the formation of cysts.

cystitis glan·du·lar·is (glăn′jə-lâr′ĭs) *n.* Chronic cystitis with glandlike invaginations of transitional epithelium.

cysto– or **cysti–** or **cyst–** *pref.* Bladder; cyst; sac: *cystocele.*

cys·to·ad·e·no·ma (sĭs′tō-ăd′n-ō′mə) *n.* See **cystadenoma.**

cys·to·car·ci·no·ma (sĭs′tō-kär′sə-nō′mə) *n.* A carcinoma that is accompanied by the formation of cysts. Also called *cystoepithelioma.*

cys·to·cele (sĭs′tə-sēl′) *n.* Herniation of the bladder. Also called *colpocystocele, vesicocele.*

cys·to·chro·mos·co·py (sĭs′tō-krə-mŏs′kə-pē) *n.* Examination of the interior of the bladder after administration of a colored dye to aid in the identification or study of the function of the ureteral orifices. Also called *chromocystoscopy.*

cys·to·du·o·de·nal ligament (sĭs′tō-dōō′ə-dē′nəl, -dōō-ŏd′n-əl) *n.* A peritoneal fold occurring occasionally and passing from the gallbladder to the first part of the duodenum.

cys·to·ep·i·the·li·o·ma (sĭs′tō-ĕp′ə-thē′lē-ō′mə) *n.* See **cystocarcinoma.**

cys·to·fi·bro·ma (sĭs′tō-fī-brō′mə) *n.* A fibroma in which cysts have formed.

cys·to·gram (sĭs′tə-grăm′) *n.* An x-ray image produced by cystography.

cys·tog·ra·phy (sĭ-stŏg′rə-fē) *n.* Radiographic visualization of the bladder following injection of a radiopaque substance.

cys·toid (sĭs′toid′) *adj.* Formed like or resembling a cyst. —*n.* A structure resembling a cyst but having no capsule.

cystoid maculopathy *n.* Cystic degeneration of the central retina; it may occur after cataract extraction, in senile macular degeneration, and in other retinal abnormalities.

cys·to·lith (sĭs′tə-lĭth′) *n.* See **urinary calculus.**

cys·to·li·thec·to·my (sĭs′tō-lĭ-thĕk′tə-mē) *n.* See **cystolithotomy.**

cys·to·li·thi·a·sis (sĭs′tō-lĭ-thī′ə-sĭs) *n.* The presence of a urinary calculus in the bladder.

cys·to·lith·ic (sĭs′tə-lĭth′ĭk) *adj.* Relating to a urinary calculus.

cys·to·li·thot·o·my (sĭs′tō-lĭ-thŏt′ə-mē) *n.* Surgical removal of a urinary calculus from the bladder through an incision in its wall. Also called *cystolithectomy.*

cys·to·ma (sĭ-stō′mə) *n.*, *pl.* **–mas** or **–ma·ta** (-mə-tə) A cystic tumor.

cys·tom·e·ter (sĭ-stŏm′ĭ-tər) *n.* A device for studying bladder function by measuring capacity, sensation, internal pressure, and residual urine.

cys·to·met·ro·gram (sĭs′tō-mĕt′rə-grăm′) *n.* The graphic record produced by a cystometer.

cys·to·me·trog·ra·phy (sĭs′tō-mĭ-trŏg′rə-fē) *n.* Measurement of bladder function, as by a cystometer.

cys·to·mor·phous (sĭs′tə-môr′fəs) *adj.* Cystoid.

cys·to·pan·en·dos·co·py (sĭs′tō-păn′ĕn-dŏs′kə-pē) *n.* Internal examination of the bladder and urethra by an endoscope introduced through the urethra.

cys·to·pa·ral·y·sis (sĭs′tō-pə-răl′ĭ-sĭs) *n.* See **cystoplegia**.

cys·to·pex·y (sĭs′tə-pĕk′sē) *n.* Surgical attachment of the gallbladder or of the urinary bladder to the abdominal wall or to other supporting structures.

cys·to·plas·ty (sĭs′tə-plăs′tē) *n.* Surgical repair of a defect in the urinary bladder.

cys·to·ple·gia (sĭs′tə-plē′jə) *n.* Paralysis of the bladder. Also called *cystoparalysis*.

cys·to·proc·tos·to·my (sĭs′tō-prŏk-tŏs′tə-mē) *n.* See **vesicorectostomy**.

cys·to·pto·sis (sĭs′tō-tō′sĭs, sĭs′tŏp-tō′-) *or* **cys·to·pto·si·a** (-tō-tō′sē-ə, -zē-ə, -tŏp-tō′-) *n.* Prolapse of the mucous membrane of the bladder into the urethra.

cys·to·py·e·li·tis (sĭs′tō-pī′ə-lī′tĭs) *n.* Inflammation of the bladder and the pelvis of the kidney.

cys·to·py·e·lo·ne·phri·tis (sĭs′tō-pī′ə-lō-nĭ-frī′tĭs) *n.* Inflammation of the bladder, the pelvis of the kidney, and the kidney itself.

cys·to·rec·tos·to·my (sĭs′tō-rĕk-tŏs′tə-mē) *n.* See **vesicorectostomy**.

cys·tor·rha·phy (sĭ-stôr′ə-fē) *n.* Suturing of a wound or defect in the urinary bladder.

cys·tor·rhe·a (sĭs′tə-rē′ə) *n.* A mucous discharge from the bladder.

cys·to·sar·co·ma (sĭs′tō-sär-kō′mə) *n.* A sarcoma in which cysts have formed.

cys·to·scope (sĭs′tə-skōp′) *n.* A tubular instrument equipped with a light and used to examine the interior of the urinary bladder and ureter. Also called *lithoscope*. —**cys′to·scop′ic** (-skŏp′ĭk) *adj.*

cystoscopic urography *n.* See **retrograde urography**.

cys·tos·co·py (sĭs-tŏs′kə-pē) *n.* A medical procedure in which a cystoscope is used to examine the bladder.

cys·to·stax·is (sĭs′tə-stăk′sĭs) *n.* See **cystistaxis**.

cys·tos·to·my (sĭ-stŏs′tə-mē) *n.* The surgical formation of an opening into the urinary bladder.

cys·to·tome (sĭs′tə-tōm′) *n.* **1.** An instrument for cutting into the urinary bladder. **2.** An instrument for cutting into the capsule of a lens.

cys·tot·o·my (sĭ-stŏt′ə-mē) *n.* Incision into the bladder. Also called *vesicotomy*.

cys·to·u·re·ter·i·tis (sĭs′tō-yōō-rē′tə-rī′tĭs, -yōōr′ĭ-tə-) *n.* Inflammation of the bladder and of one or both ureters.

cys·to·u·re·ter·og·ra·phy (sĭs′tō-yōō-rē′tə-rŏg′rə-fē, -yōōr′ĭ-tə-) *n.* Radiography of the bladder and the ureter.

cys·to·u·re·thri·tis (sĭs′tō-yōōr′ĭ-thrī′tĭs) *n.* Inflammation of the bladder and urethra.

cys·to·u·re·thro·gram (sĭs′tō-yōō-rē′thrə-grăm′) *n.* A radiograph of the urinary bladder and urethra made after a contrast medium has been introduced. Also called *voiding cystogram*.

cys·to·u·re·throg·ra·phy (sĭs′tō-yōōr′ĭ-thrŏg′rə-fē) *n.* Radiography of the bladder and the urethra after the introduction of a radiopaque substance.

cys·to·u·re·thro·scope (sĭs′tō-yōō-rē′thrə-skōp′) *n.* An instrument for visually examining the bladder and urethra.

cy·ta·phe·re·sis (sī′tə-fə-rē′sĭs) *n.* A procedure in which various cells can be separated from withdrawn blood and retained, with the plasma and other formed elements retransfused into the donor.

cyt·ar·a·bine (sī-tăr′ə-bēn′) *n.* See **cytosine arabinoside**.

–cyte *suff.* Cell: *leukocyte*.

cy·ti·dine (sī′tĭ-dēn′) *n.* A white crystalline nucleoside composed of one molecule each of cytosine and ribose. Also called *cytosine ribonucleoside*.

cytidine 5-triphosphate *n.* A nucleotide necessary to the synthesis of RNA and to the production of choline and ethanolamine.

cytidine diphosphate *n.* A nucleotide that serves an important role in the synthesis of phospholipids, such as those used in cellular membranes.

cy·ti·dyl·ic acid (sī′tĭ-dĭl′ĭk, sĭt′ĭ-) *n.* A component of RNA that hydrolyzes to yield cytosine, D-ribose, and phosphoric acid. Also called *cytidine monophosphate*.

cyto– *or* **cyt–** *pref.* Cell: *cytoplasm*.

cy·to·ar·chi·tec·ture (sī′tō-är′kĭ-tĕk′chər) *n.* The arrangement of cells in a tissue, especially the arrangement of nerve-cell bodies in the cerebral cortex.

cy·to·cen·trum (sī′tō-sĕn′trəm) *n.* See **centrosome**.

cy·to·chal·a·sin (sī′tō-kăl′ə-sĭn, -zĭn, -kə-lā′-) *n.* Any of a group of substances derived from molds that interfere with the division of cytoplasm, inhibit cell movement, and cause extrusion of the nucleus.

cy·to·chem·is·try (sī′tō-kĕm′ĭ-strē) *n.* The branch of biochemistry that deals with the study of the chemical composition and activity of cells.

cy·to·chrome (sī′tə-krōm′) *n.* Any of a class of iron-containing proteins important in cell respiration as catalysts of oxidation-reduction reactions.

cytochrome oxidase *n.* An oxidizing enzyme containing iron and a porphyrin, found in mitochondria and important in cell respiration as an agent of electron transfer from certain cytochrome molecules to oxygen molecules.

cy·to·cide (sī′tə-sīd′) *n.* An agent that is destructive to cells. —**cy·to·cid′al** (-sīd′l) *adj.*

cy·toc·la·sis (sī-tŏk′lə-sĭs) *n.* The destruction of cells by fragmentation.

cy·to·clas·tic (sī′tə-klăs′tĭk) *adj.* Relating to cytoclasis.

cy·to·di·ag·no·sis (sī′tō-dī′əg-nō′sĭs) *n.* Diagnosis of disease through the microscopic study of cells.

cy·to·gen·e·sis (sī′tō-jĕn′ĭ-sĭs) *n.* The formation, development, and variation of cells. Also called *cytogeny*. —**cy′to·gen′ic** *adj.*

cy·to·ge·net·ics (sī′tō-jə-nĕt′ĭks) *n.* The branch of biology that deals with heredity and the cellular components, particularly chromosomes, associated with heredity. —**cy′to·ge·net′i·cist** (-ĭ-sĭst) *n.*

cytogenic reproduction *n.* Reproduction by means of unicellular germ cells, including sexual reproduction and asexual reproduction by means of spores.

cy·tog·e·nous (sī-tŏj′ə-nəs) *adj.* Forming cells.

cy·tog·e·ny (sī-tŏj′ə-nē) *n.* See **cytogenesis.**

cy·to·glu·co·pe·ni·a (sī′tō-glōō′kə-pē′nē-ə) *n.* Deficiency of glucose within cells.

cy·toid (sī′toid′) *adj.* Resembling a cell.

cy·to·kine (sī′tə-kīn′) *n.* Any of several nonantibody proteins, such as lymphokines, that are released by a cell population on contact with a specific antigen and act as intercellular mediators, as in the generation of an immune response.

cy·to·ki·ne·sis (sī′tō-kə-nē′sĭs, -kī-) *n.* The division of the cytoplasm of a cell following the division of the nucleus. —**cy′to·ki·net′ic** (-nĕt′ĭk) *adj.*

cytologic smear *n.* A cytologic specimen made by smearing a sample, then fixing it and staining it, usually with 95% ethyl alcohol and Papanicolaou stain. Also called *cytosmear.*

cy·tol·o·gist (sī-tŏl′ə-jĭst) *n.* A specialist in cytology.

cy·tol·o·gy (sī-tŏl′ə-jē) *n.* The branch of biology that deals with the formation, structure, and function of cells. —**cy′to·log′ic** (-tə-lŏj′ĭk) *adj.*

cy·tol·y·sin (sī-tŏl′ĭ-sĭn) *n.* A substance, such as an antibody, capable of dissolving or destroying cells.

cy·tol·y·sis (sī-tŏl′ĭ-sĭs) *n.* The dissolution or destruction of a cell. —**cy′to·lyt′ic** (sī′tə-lĭt′ĭk) *adj.*

cy·to·ly·so·some (sī′tō-lī′sə-sōm′) *n.* An enlarged vacuole in the cellular cytoplasm containing mitochondria, ribosomes, and other organelles that fuses with cytoplasmic lysosomes and enzymatically digests their contents.

cy·to·me·gal·ic (sī′tō-mĭ-găl′ĭk) *adj.* Of, relating to, or characterized by greatly enlarged cells.

cytomegalic inclusion disease *n.* A disease caused by infection with cytomegalovirus, characterized by the presence of inclusion bodies in infected cells, enlargement of the liver and spleen, jaundice, purpura, thrombocytopenia, and fever; it often occurs in newborn infants, acquired in the womb or when passing through the birth canal of an infected mother, and can also occur in individuals with impaired immune systems. Also called *cytomegalovirus disease, inclusion body disease.*

cy·to·meg·a·lo·vi·rus (sī′tə-mĕg′ə-lō-vī′rəs) *n. Abbr.* **CMV** Any of a group of herpes viruses that attack and enlarge epithelial cells. Such viruses also cause a disease of infants characterized by circulatory dysfunction and microcephaly. Also called *visceral disease virus.*

cytomegalovirus disease *n.* See **cytomegalic inclusion disease.**

cy·to·mem·brane (sī′tə-mĕm′brān) *n.* See **cell membrane.**

cy·to·met·a·pla·sia (sī′tō-mĕt′ə-plā′zhə) *n.* A change in the form or function of a cell other than that related to neoplasia.

cy·tom·e·ter (sī-tŏm′ĭ-tər) *n.* A standardized glass slide or small glass chamber of known volume, used in counting and measuring cells, especially blood cells.

cy·tom·e·try (sī-tŏm′ĭ-trē) *n.* The counting of cells, especially blood cells, using a cytometer or hemocytometer.

cy·to·mor·phol·o·gy (sī′tō-môr-fŏl′ə-jē) *n.* The study of the structure of cells.

cy·to·mor·pho·sis (sī′tō-môr-fō′sĭs) *n.* The series of changes that a cell undergoes during the various stages of its existence.

cy·to·path·ic (sī′tə-păth′ĭk) *adj.* Of or relating to degeneration or disease of cells.

cy·to·path·o·gen·ic (sī′tə-păth′ə-jĕn′ĭk) *adj.* Of, relating to, or producing pathological changes in cells. —**cy′to·path′o·ge·nic′i·ty** (-jə-nĭs′ĭ-tē) *n.*

cytopathogenic virus *n.* A virus whose multiplication leads to degenerative changes in the host cell.

cy·to·path·o·log·ic (sī′tō-păth′ə-lŏj′ĭk) *or* **cy·to·path·o·log·i·cal** (-ĭ-kəl) *adj.* Of, relating to, or characterizing cytopathology.

cy·to·pa·thol·o·gy (sī′tō-pə-thŏl′ə-jē) *n.* **1.** The study of changes caused by disease within cells. **2.** See **exfoliative cytology.** —**cy′to·pa·thol′o·gist** *n.*

cy·top·a·thy (sī-tŏp′ə-thē) *n.* A disorder of a cell.

cy·to·pe·ni·a (sī′tə-pē′nē-ə) *n.* A deficiency or lack of cellular elements in the circulating blood.

cy·to·pha·gic panniculitis (sī′tə-fā′jĭk, -făj′ĭk) *n.* A chronic form of panniculitis marked by the infiltration of histiocytes that have phagocytized red blood cells, white blood cells, and platelets.

cy·toph·a·gous (sī-tŏf′ə-gəs) *adj.* Devouring or destroying cells.

cy·toph·a·gy (sī-tŏf′ə-jē) *n.* The ingestion of cells by phagocytes.

cy·to·phil·ic (sī′tə-fĭl′ĭk) *adj.* Having an affinity for cells.

cytophilic antibody *n.* See **cytotropic antibody.**

cy·to·pho·tom·e·ter (sī′tō-fō-tŏm′ĭ-tər) *n.* An instrument used to determine the identity and location of the chemical compounds within a cell by measuring the intensity of light passing through stained sections of the cytoplasm.

cy·to·pho·tom·e·try (sī′tə-fō-tŏm′ĭ-trē) *n.* The study of cells and chemical compounds within cells by means of a cytophotometer. —**cy′to·pho′to·met′ric** (-tə-mĕt′rĭk) *adj.*

cy·to·phy·lax·is (sī′tō-fə-lăk′sĭs) *n.* The protection of cells against lytic agents. —**cy′to·phy·lac′tic** (-lăk′tĭk) *adj.*

cy·to·plasm (sī′tə-plăz′əm) *n.* The protoplasm outside a cell nucleus. —**cy′to·plas′mic** (-plăz′mĭk) *adj.*

cytoplasmic bridge *n.* See **intercellular bridge.**

cytoplasmic inclusion body *n.* Either of two types of inclusion bodies: acidophilic, as in variola and rabies, or basophilic, as in trachoma and psittacosis.

cytoplasmic inheritance *n.* See **extrachromosomal inheritance.**

cy·to·plast (sī′tə-plăst′) *n.* The living intact cytoplasm that remains after the cell nucleus has been removed. —**cy′to·plas′tic** (-plăs′tĭk) *adj.*

cy·to·re·duc·tive therapy (sī′tō-rĭ-dŭk′tĭv) *n.* Therapy to reduce the number of cells in a lesion, usually a malignancy.

cy·to·sine (sī′tə-sēn′) *n. Abbr.* **C** A pyrimidine base that is an essential constituent of RNA and DNA.

cytosine ar·a·bin·o·side (ăr′ə-bĭn′ə-sīd′, ə-răb′ə-nō-sīd′) *n. Abbr.* **CA** A compound of arabinose and cytosine that inhibits both DNA synthesis and the proliferation of viruses that contain DNA, used as a chemotherapeutic agent. Also called *cytarabine.*

cytosine ribonucleoside *n.* See **cytidine.**

cy·to·sis (sī-tō′sĭs) *n.* A condition in which there is more than the usual number of cells.

cy·to·skel·e·ton (sī′tə-skĕl′ĭ-tn) *n.* The internal framework of a cell, composed largely of actin filaments and microtubules.

cy·to·smear (sī′tō-smîr′) *n.* See **cytologic smear.**

cy·to·sol (sī′tə-sôl′) *n.* The fluid component of cytoplasm, excluding organelles and the insoluble, usually suspended, cytoplasmic components.

cy·to·some (sī′tə-sōm′) *n.* **1.** The cell body exclusive of the nucleus. **2.** Any of the osmiophilic bodies that have concentric lamellae and occur in cells of the lung. Also called *multilamellar body.*

cy·to·sta·sis (sī′tə-stā′sĭs, -stăs′ĭs) *n.* **1.** The slowing of movement and accumulation of blood cells in the capillaries, as in a region of inflammation. **2.** Arrest of cellular growth and multiplication.

cy·to·stat·ic (sī′tə-stăt′ĭk) *adj.* **1.** Obstructing a capillary by the accumulation of blood cells. **2.** Inhibiting or suppressing cellular growth and multiplication. —*n.* A cytostatic agent.

cy·to·tax·is (sī′tə-tăk′sĭs) *n.* The attraction or repulsion of cells for one another. —**cy′to·tac′tic** (-tăk′tĭk) *adj.*

cy·to·tax·on·o·my (sī′tō-tăk-sŏn′ə-mē) *n.* The classification of organisms based on cellular structure and function, especially on the structure and number of chromosomes. —**cy′to·tax′o·nom′ic** (-tăk′sə-nŏm′ĭk) *adj.* —**cy′to·tax·on′o·mist** *n.*

cy·to·tech·nol·o·gist (sī′tō-tĕk-nŏl′ə-jĭst) *n.* A technician trained in medical examination and identification of cellular abnormalities.

cy·toth·e·sis (sī-tŏth′ĭ-sĭs, sī′tə-thē′sĭs) *n.* The repair of injury in a cell.

cy·to·tox·ic (sī′tə-tŏk′sĭk) *adj.* Of, relating to, or producing a toxic effect on cells. —**cy′to·tox·ic′i·ty** (-tŏk-sĭs′ĭ-tē) *n.*

cytotoxic reaction *n.* An immunological reaction in which a noncytotropic antibody combines with a specific antigen on the surface of a cell and forms a complex that initiates the activation of complement, leading to cell lysis or other damage.

cytotoxic T cell *n.* See **killer cell.**

cy·to·tox·in (sī′tə-tŏk′sĭn) *n.* A substance having a specific toxic effect on certain cells.

cy·to·tro·pho·blast (sī′tə-trō′fə-blăst′) *n.* The inner layer of the trophoblast.

cy·to·trop·ic (sī′tə-trŏp′ĭk, -trō′pĭk) *adj.* Having an affinity for cells; cytophilic.

cytotropic antibody *n.* An antibody that has an affinity for additional kinds of cells unrelated to its specific affinity for the antigen that induced it. Also called *anaphylactic antibody, cytophilic antibody.*

cy·tot·ro·pism (sī-tŏt′rə-pĭz′əm) *n.* Affinity for cells, especially the ability of viruses to localize in and damage specific cells.

Cy·to·vene (sī′tə-vēn′) A trademark for the drug ganciclovir.

Cy·tox·an (sī-tŏk′sən) A trademark for the drug cyclophosphamide.

cy·to·zo·ic (sī′tə-zō′ĭk) *adj.* Living in a cell. Used of certain parasitic protozoa.

cy·to·zo·on (sī′tə-zō′ŏn′) *n., pl.* **–zo·a** (-zō′ə) A protozoan cell or organism.

cy·tu·ri·a (sī-tŏor′ē-ə) *n.* The presence of cells in unusual numbers in the urine.

Czer·ny-Lembert suture (chĕr′nē-) *n.* An intestinal suture made up of two rows, the first being the Czerny suture and the second being the Lembert suture.

Czerny suture *n.* A suture of the intestine in which the needle enters the serosa and passes out through the submucosa or muscularis, and then enters the submucosa or muscularis of the opposite side and emerges from the serosa.

D

δ, Δ **1.** The Greek letter *delta*. Entries beginning with this character are alphabetized under **delta**. **2.** *Symbol* Δ The symbol for **double bond**.

D– *pref.* Of or relating to the configuration of D-glyceraldehyde, a compound that is chosen as the basis for stereochemical nomenclature because it is the simplest carbohydrate that can form optical isomers: D-*fructose*.

D¹ The symbol for the isotope deuterium.

D² *abbr.* dexter; diffusing capacity; dead space

D. *abbr.* diopter; dose

d– *pref.* **d–** To the right; dextro: d-*tartaric acid*.

DA *abbr.* developmental age

da·car·ba·zine (dă-kär′bə-zēn′, dā-) *n.* An antineoplastic agent used in the treatment of malignant melanoma and Hodgkin's disease.

Da·Cos·ta's syndrome (də-kŏs′təz) *n.* See **neurocirculatory asthenia**.

dac·ry·a·gogue (dăk′rē-ə-gôg′) *n.* An agent that stimulates a lacrimal gland to secrete, promoting the flow of tears.

dacryo– *or* **dacry–** *pref.* Lacrimal system; tears: *dacryorrhea*.

dac·ry·o·ad·e·nal·gia (dăk′rē-ō-ăd′n-ăl′jə) *n.* Pain in a lacrimal gland.

dac·ry·o·ad·e·ni·tis (dăk′rē-ō-ăd′n-ī′tĭs) *n.* Inflammation of a lacrimal gland.

dac·ry·o·blen·nor·rhe·a (dăk′rē-ō-blĕn′ə-rē′ə) *n.* Chronic discharge of mucus from a lacrimal sac. Also called *dacryocystoblennorrhea*.

dac·ry·o·cele (dăk′rē-ə-sēl′) *n.* See **dacryocystocele**.

dac·ry·o·cyst (dăk′rē-ə-sĭst′) *n.* See **lacrimal sac**.

dac·ry·o·cys·tal·gia (dăk′rē-ō-sĭs′tăl′jə) *n.* Pain in the lacrimal sac.

dac·ry·o·cys·tec·to·my (dăk′rē-ō-sĭ-stĕk′tə-mē) *n.* Surgical removal of the lacrimal sac.

dac·ry·o·cys·ti·tis (dăk′rē-ō-sĭ-stī′tĭs) *n.* Inflammation of the lacrimal sac.

dac·ry·o·cys·to·blen·nor·rhe·a (dăk′rē-ō-sĭs′tə-blĕn′-ə-rē′ə) *n.* See **dacryoblennorrhea**.

dac·ry·o·cys·to·cele (dăk′rē-ō-sĭs′tə-sēl′) *n.* Protrusion of the lacrimal sac. Also called *dacryocele*.

dac·ry·o·cys·top·to·sis (dăk′rē-ō-sĭs′tŏp-tō′sĭs) *n.* Downward displacement of the lacrimal sac.

dac·ry·o·cys·to·rhi·no·ste·no·sis (dăk′rē-ō-sĭs′tō-rī′-nō-stə-nō′sĭs) *n.* Obstruction of the nasolacrimal duct.

dac·ry·o·cys·to·rhi·nos·to·my (dăk′rē-ō-sĭs′tə-rī-nŏs′tə-mē) *n.* The surgical opening of a passage for drainage from the lacrimal sac into the nasal cavity.

dac·ry·o·cys·tot·o·my (dăk′rē-ō-sĭ-stŏt′ə-mē) *n.* Incision of the lacrimal sac.

dac·ry·o·lith (dăk′rē-ə-lĭth′) *n.* A concretion in a lacrimal sac or lacrimal duct. Also called *ophthalmolith*, *tear stone*.

dac·ry·o·li·thi·a·sis (dăk′rē-ō-lĭ-thī′ə-sĭs) *n.* The formation and presence of dacryoliths.

dac·ry·o·ma (dăk′rē-ō′mə) *n.* **1.** A swelling caused by the accumulation of tears in an obstructed lacrimal duct. **2.** A tumor of the lacrimal apparatus.

dac·ry·ops (dăk′rē-ŏps′) *n.* **1.** Excess of tears in the eye. **2.** A swelling of a lacrimal duct caused by excess fluid.

dac·ry·o·py·or·rhe·a (dăk′rē-ō-pī′ə-rē′ə) *n.* The discharge of tears containing pus.

dac·ry·o·py·o·sis (dăk′rē-ō-pī-ō′sĭs) *n.* The formation of pus in a lacrimal sac or duct.

dac·ry·or·rhe·a (dăk′rē-ə-rē′ə) *n.* Excessive flow of tears.

dac·ry·o·scin·tig·ra·phy (dăk′rē-ō-sĭn-tĭg′rə-fē) *n.* Scintigraphy of the lacrimal ducts to determine whether or how much they are blocked.

dac·ry·o·so·le·ni·tis (dăk′rē-ō-sō′lə-nī′tĭs) *n.* Inflammation of a lacrimal or nasal duct.

dac·ry·o·ste·no·sis (dăk′rē-ō-stə-nō′sĭs) *n.* Stricture or narrowing of a lacrimal duct.

dac·ry·o·syr·inx (dăk′rē-ō-sîr′ĭngks) *n.* **1.** An abnormal opening into a tear duct or lacrimal sac. **2.** A syringe for irrigating the lacrimal ducts.

dac·ti·no·my·cin (dăk′tə-nō-mī′sĭn) *n.* An antibiotic isolated from bacteria and used as an antineoplastic agent in the treatment of certain cancers.

dac·tyl (dăk′təl) *n.* A finger or toe; digit.

dac·ty·li·tis (dăk′tə-lī′tĭs) *n.* Inflammation of a finger or toe.

dactylo– *or* **dactyl–** *pref.* Digit: *dactylomegaly*.

dac·tyl·o·gram (dăk-tĭl′ə-grăm′) *n.* A fingerprint.

dac·ty·log·ra·phy (dăk′tə-lŏg′rə-fē) *n.* The study of fingerprints as a method of identification.

dac·ty·lol·o·gy (dăk′tə-lŏl′ə-jē) *n.* The use of the fingers and hands to communicate and convey ideas, as in the manual alphabet used by hearing-impaired and speech-impaired people.

dac·ty·lo·meg·a·ly (dăk′tə-lō-mĕg′ə-lē) *n.* Abnormally large fingers or toes.

Da·kin (dā′kĭn), **Henry Drysdale** 1880–1952. British chemist noted for his study of antiseptics. He developed Dakin's solution, which was widely used in treating wounds during both World Wars and is still used as a disinfectant.

Da·kin's solution (dā′kĭnz) *n.* Buffered sodium hypochlorite solution, used as a bactericidal irrigant of open wounds.

Dale (dāl), Sir **Henry Hallett** 1875–1968. British physiologist. He shared a 1936 Nobel Prize for work on the chemical transmission of nerve impulses, particularly for the isolation and study of acetylcholine (1914).

Dal·mane (dăl′mān) A trademark for the drug flurazepam hydrochloride.

Dal·rym·ple's sign (dăl-rĭm′pəlz, dăl′rĭm-) *n.* An indication of Graves' disease in which there is abnormal wideness of the palpebral fissures with retraction of the upper lid of the eye.

dal·ton (dôl′tən) *n.* See **atomic mass unit**.

dal·ton·ism (dôl′tə-nĭz′əm) *n.* An inherited defect in the perception of red and green; red-green colorblindness.

Dal·ton's law (dôl′tənz) *n.* A principle that each gas in a mixture of gases exerts a pressure proportionately to the percentage of the gas and independently of the presence of the other gases present. Also called *law of partial pressures.*

dam (dăm) *n.* A barrier against the passage of liquid or loose material, especially a rubber sheet used in dentistry to isolate one or more teeth from the rest of the mouth.

Dam (dăm, däm), **(Carl Peter) Henrik** 1895–1976. Danish biochemist. He shared a 1943 Nobel Prize for the discovery of vitamin K.

dance therapy (dăns) *n.* A method of psychological treatment in which movement and dance are used to express and deal with feelings and experiences, both positive and negative.

D & C *abbr.* dilation and curettage

D & E *abbr.* dilation and evacuation

dan·der (dăn′dər) *n.* Small scales from the skin, hair, or feathers of an animal, often causing an allergic reaction in sensitive individuals.

dan·druff (dăn′drəf) *n.* A scaly scurf formed on and shed from the scalp.

dan·dy fever (dăn′dē) *n.* See **dengue.**

Dandy operation *n.* **1.** A suboccipital trigeminal rhizotomy. **2.** See **third ventriculostomy** (sense 2).

Dane particle (dān) *n.* Any of the larger spherical forms of hepatitis-associated antigens comprising the virion of hepatitis B virus.

DANS (dē′ā-ĕn-ĕs′) *n.* 1-dimethylaminonaphthalene-5-sulfonic acid; a green fluorescing compound used in immunohistochemistry to detect antigens.

dap·sone (dăp′sōn′, -zōn′) *n.* An antibacterial drug used primarily to treat leprosy and some forms of dermatitis.

Dar·a·prim (dăr′ə-prĭm′) A trademark for the drug pyrimethamine.

Da·rier's disease (dăr′ē-āz′, dä-ryāz′) *n.* See **keratosis follicularis.**

dark adaptation (därk) *n.* The adjustment of the eye under reduced illumination, in which sensitivity to light is greatly increased. Also called *scotopic adaptation.*

dark-adapted eye *n.* An eye that has been in darkness or semidarkness for some time and has undergone dark adaptation. Also called *scotopic eye.*

dark-field microscope *n.* A microscope in which an object is illuminated only from the sides so that it appears bright against a dark background.

Dar·ling's disease (där′lĭngz) *n.* See **histoplasmosis.**

darm·stadt·i·um (därm-shtät′ē-əm) *n. Symbol* **Ds** A radioactive synthetic element whose longest-lived isotope has a half-life of 0.18 milliseconds. Atomic number 110.

Dar·vo·cet (där′və-sĕt′) A trademark for a drug combination of propoxyphene napsylate and acetaminophen.

Dar·von (där′vŏn) A trademark for the drug propoxyphene hydrochloride.

Dar·win (där′wĭn), **Charles Robert** 1809–1882. British naturalist who revolutionized the study of biology with his theory of evolution based on natural selection. His most famous works include *Origin of Species* (1859) and *The Descent of Man* (1871).

Dar·win·i·an (där-wĭn′ē-ən) *adj.* Relating to, following, or derived from the work or ideas of date rape Charles Darwin.

darwinian reflex *n.* The tendency of young infants to grasp a bar and hang suspended.

Darwinian tubercle *n.* A small projection from the upper end of free margin of the helix of the ear. Also called *auricular tubercle.*

Dar·win·ism (där′wĭ-nĭz′əm) *n.* A theory of biological evolution developed by Charles Darwin and others, stating that all species of organisms arise and develop through the natural selection of small, inherited variations that increase the individual's ability to compete, survive, and reproduce.

date boil (dāt) *n.* See **Aleppo boil.**

date rape *n.* Rape perpetrated by the victim's social escort, sometimes after the surreptitious administration of a sedative or hypnotic drug.

da·tum plane (dā′təm, dăt′əm, dä′təm) *n.* An arbitrary plane used as a base from which to make craniometric measurements.

daugh·ter cell (dô′tər) *n.* Either of the two identical cells that form when a cell divides.

daughter cyst *n.* A small cyst that develops from a mother cyst.

daughter star *n.* One of the figures forming the diaster of a dividing cell. Also called *polar star.*

Daus·set (dō-sā′), **Jean** Born 1916. French physiologist. He shared a 1980 Nobel Prize for discoveries concerning cell structure that enhanced understanding of the immunological system, resulting in higher success rates in organ transplantation.

Da·vaine (dä-vān′, -vĕn′), **Casimir Joseph** 1812–1882. French physician and microbiologist who identified a bacillus as the causative agent of anthrax and advocated the germ theory of disease before Pasteur.

Da·viel's operation (dăv′ē-ĕlz′, dä-vyĕlz′) *n.* An extracapsular cataract extraction.

dawn phenomenon (dôn) *n.* The occurrence of abrupt increases in fasting levels of plasma glucose concentrations between the hours of 5 and 9 a.m., without preceding hypoglycemia, especially in diabetic patients receiving insulin therapy.

day blindness (dā) *n.* See **hemeralopia.**

dB *abbr.* decibel

Db The symbol for the element **dubnium.**

DC *abbr.* Doctor of Chiropractic

DDAVP (dē′dē′ā′vē′pē′) A trademark for the drug desmopressin acetate.

ddC (dē′dē-sē′) *n.* Dideoxycytidine; a nucleoside analog drug similar to AZT. Also called *zalcitabine.*

ddI (dē′dē-ī′) *n.* Dideoxyinosine; a nucleoside analog drug similar to AZT. Also called *didanosine.*

DDS *abbr.* Doctor of Dental Science; Doctor of Dental Surgery

DDT (dē′dē-tē′) *n.* Dichlorodiphenyltrichloroethane; a colorless contact insecticide, toxic to humans and animals when swallowed or absorbed through the skin, that has been banned in the United States for most uses since 1972.

de– *pref.* **1.** Do or make the opposite of; reverse: *decomposition.* **2.** Remove or remove from: *deoxygenation.* **3.** Reduce; degrade: *decholesterolization.*

de·ac·yl·ase (dē-ăs′ə-lās′, -lāz′) *n.* Any of a group of enzymes that catalyze the hydrolysis of an acyl group.

dead (dĕd) *adj.* **1.** Having lost life; no longer alive. **2.** Lacking feeling or sensitivity; unresponsive.

dead-end host *n.* A host from which infectious agents are not transmitted to other susceptible hosts.

dead·ly nightshade (dĕd′lē) *n.* See **belladonna** (sense 1).

dead pulp *n.* See **necrotic pulp.**

dead space *n.* **1.** An actual or potential cavity remaining after the closure of an incision and not obliterated by operative technique. **2.** Anatomical dead space. **3.** Physiological dead space.

deaf (dĕf) *adj.* **1.** Partially or completely lacking in the sense of hearing. **2. Deaf** Of or relating to the Deaf or their culture. —*n.* **1.** Deaf people considered as a group. **2. Deaf** The community of deaf people who use American Sign Language as a primary means of communication.

deaf·en (dĕf′ən) *v.* To make deaf, especially momentarily by a loud noise.

de·af·fer·en·ta·tion (dē-ăf′ər-ən-tā′shən) *n.* The elimination or interruption of sensory nerve impulses by destroying or injuring the sensory nerve fibers.

deaf-mute (dĕf′myo͞ot′) *n.* A person who can neither hear nor speak. No longer in technical use. —*adj.* (dĕf′myo͞ot′) Unable to speak or hear.

deaf·mut·ism (dĕf′myo͞o′tĭz′əm) *n.* Inability to hear and speak. No longer in technical use.

deaf·ness (dĕf′nĭs) *n.* The lack or loss of the ability to hear.

de·al·co·hol·i·za·tion (dē-ăl′kə-hô-lĭ-zā′shən) *n.* The removal of alcohol from a fluid.

de·am·i·dase (dē-ăm′ĭ-dās′, -dāz′) *n.* See **amidohydrolase.**

de·am·i·da·tion (dē-ăm′ĭ-dā′shən) *or* **de·am·i·di·za·tion** (-ĭ-dĭ-zā′shən) *n.* The removal of an amide group, usually by hydrolysis.

de·am·i·diz·ing enzyme (dē-ăm′ĭ-dī′zĭng) *n.* See **amidohydrolase.**

de·am·i·nase (dē-ăm′ĭ-nās′) *n.* Any of a class of enzymes that catalyze the hydrolysis of compounds containing an amino group. Also called *deaminating enzyme.*

de·am·i·na·tion (dē-ăm′i-nā′shŭn) *or* **de·am·i·ni·za·tion** (-ĭ-nĭ-zā′shən) *n.* The removal of an amine group, usually by hydrolysis.

de·ar·te·ri·al·i·za·tion (dē′är-tîr′ē-ə-lĭ-zā′shən) *n.* The deoxygenation of arterial blood to blood resembling venous blood.

death (dĕth) *n.* The end of life; the permanent cessation of vital bodily functions, as manifested in humans by the loss of heartbeat, the absence of spontaneous breathing, and brain death.

death instinct *n.* A primitive impulse for destruction, decay, and death, manifested by a turning away from pleasure, postulated by Sigmund Freud as coexisting with and opposing the life instinct. Also called *Thanatos.*

death rate *n.* The ratio of total deaths to total population in a specified community or area over a specified period of time; often expressed as the number of deaths per 1,000 of the population per year. Also called *fatality rate, mortality rate.*

death rattle *n.* A gurgling or rattling sound sometimes made in the throat of a dying person, caused by loss of the cough reflex and passage of the breath through accumulating mucus.

death wish *n.* **1.** A desire for self-destruction, often accompanied by feelings of depression, hopelessness, and self-reproach. **2.** A suicidal urge that presumably drives certain people to put themselves consistently into dangerous situations.

De Ba·key (də bā′kē), **Michael Ellis** Born 1908. American heart surgeon who implanted the first totally artificial heart in a human (1966).

de·band·ing (dē-băn′dĭng) *n.* The removal of fixed orthodontic appliances.

de·bil·i·tat·ing (dĭ-bĭl′ĭ-tā′tĭng) *adj.* Causing a loss of strength or energy.

de·bil·i·ty (dĭ-bĭl′ĭ-tē) *n.* The state of being weak or feeble; infirmity.

de·branch·er deficiency limit dextrinosis (dē-brăn′-chər) *n.* See **type 3 glycogenosis.**

de·branch·ing enzyme (dē-brăn′chĭng) *n.* **1.** 4-Alpha-D-glucanotransferase. **2.** Amylo-1,6-glucosidase.

dé·bride·ment (dā′brēd-män′, dĭ-brēd′mənt) *n.* The removal of dead or contaminated tissue and foreign matter from a wound, especially by excision.

debt (dĕt) *n.* Something that is deficient or required to restore a normal state.

de·bulk·ing operation (dē-bŭl′kĭng) *n.* The excision of a major part of a malignant tumor that cannot be completely removed surgically, performed to enhance the effectiveness of radiation therapy or chemotherapy.

deca– *or* **dec–** *or* **deka–** *or* **dek–** *pref.* Ten: *decane.*

Dec·a·dron (dĕk′ə-drŏn′) A trademark for the drug dexamethasone.

de·cal·ci·fy (dē-kăl′sə-fī′) *v.* To remove calcium or calcium compounds from a substance. —**de·cal′ci·fi·ca′tion** (-fĭ-kā′shən) *n.*

de·ca·pac·i·ta·tion (dē′kə-păs′ĭ-tā′shən) *n.* The prevention of capacitation by spermatozoa, and thus of their ability to fertilize egg cells.

de·cap·i·ta·tion (dĭ-kăp′ĭ-tā′shən) *n.* The removal of a head, as of an animal, a fetus, or a bone.

de·cap·su·la·tion (dē-kăp′sə-lā′shən) *n.* Surgical removal of a capsule or enveloping membrane, as of the kidney.

de·car·box·yl·ase (dē′kär-bŏk′sə-lās′, -lāz′) *n.* Any of various enzymes that catalyze the hydrolysis of the carboxyl radical.

de·car·box·yl·a·tion (dē′kär-bŏk′sə-lā′shən) *n.* Removal of a carboxyl group from a chemical compound, usually with hydrogen replacing it.

de·cay (dĭ-kā′) *n.* **1.** The destruction or decomposition of organic matter as a result of bacterial or fungal action; rot. **2.** Dental caries. **3.** The loss of information that was registered by the senses and processed into the short-term memory system. **4.** Radioactive decay. —*v.* **1.** To break down into component parts; rot. **2.** To disintegrate or diminish by radioactive decay. **3.** To decline in health or vigor; waste away.

decay constant *n. Symbol* **λ** The constant ratio for the number of atoms of a radionuclide that decay in a given period of time compared with the total number of atoms of the same kind present at the beginning of that period. Also called *disintegration constant, radioactive constant.*

decay theory *n.* The theory of memory loss that holds that an engram deteriorates progressively with time during the interval when it is not activated.

de·cer·e·brate (dē-sĕr′ə-brāt′, -brĭt) *adj.* Of, relating to, or characteristic of an individual who has suffered a brain injury that results in neurological function comparable to that resulting from decerebration of an animal. —*v.* (-brāt′) To eliminate cerebral brain function in an animal by decerebration.

de·cer·e·bra·tion (dē-sĕr′ə-brā′shən) *n.* The elimination of cerebral function in an animal by removing the cerebrum, cutting across the brainstem, or severing certain arteries in the brainstem, as may be done for experimentation.

de·cho·les·ter·ol·i·za·tion (dē′kə-lĕs′tə-rôl′ĭ-zā′shən) *n.* The therapeutic reduction of cholesterol in the blood.

deci– *pref.* One tenth (10^{-1}): *decibel.*

de·ci·bel (dĕs′ə-bəl, -bĕl′) *n. Abbr.* **dB** A unit used to express relative difference in power or intensity, usually between two acoustic or electric signals, equal to ten times the common logarithm of the ratio of the two levels.

de·cid·u·a (dĭ-sĭj′ōō-ə) *n., pl.* **–u·as** *or* **–u·ae** (-ōō-ē′) A mucous membrane lining the uterus, modified during pregnancy and shed at parturition or during menstruation. Also called *deciduous membrane.* —**de·cid′u·al** *adj.*

decidua ba·sa·lis (bə-sā′lĭs) *n.* The area of endometrium between the implanted chorionic vesicle and the myometrium, which becomes the maternal part of the placenta. Also called *decidua serotina.*

decidua cap·su·lar·is (kăp′sə-lâr′ĭs) *n.* The layer of endometrium overlying the implanted chorionic vesicle that progressively diminishes as the chorionic vesicle enlarges. Also called *decidua reflexa, membrana adventitia.*

decidual cell *n.* An enlarged, ovoid, connective tissue cell in the uterine mucous membrane that enlarges and specializes during pregnancy.

decidua men·stru·a·lis (mĕn′strōō-ā′lĭs) *n.* The mucous membrane of the nonpregnant uterus at the menstrual period.

decidua pa·ri·e·ta·lis (pə-rī′ĭ-tā′lĭs) *n.* The mucous membrane lining the main cavity of the pregnant uterus elsewhere than at the site of attachment of the chorionic vesicle. Also called *decidua vera.*

decidua pol·y·po·sa (pŏl′ə-pō′sə, -zə) *n.* Decidua parietalis having polypoid projections of the endometrial surface.

decidua re·flex·a (rĭ-flĕk′sə) *n.* See **decidua capsularis.**

decidua se·rot·i·na (sə-rŏt′ən-ə, sĕr′ə-tī′nə) *n.* See **decidua basalis.**

decidua spon·gi·o·sa (spŏn′jē-ō′sə) *n.* The portion of the decidua basalis attached to the myometrium.

de·cid·u·a·tion (dĭ-sĭj′ōō-ā′shən) *n.* The shedding of endometrial tissue during menstruation.

decidua ve·ra (vîr′ə) *n.* See **decidua parietalis.**

de·cid·u·i·tis (dĭ-sĭj′ōō-ī′tĭs) *n.* Inflammation of the decidua.

de·cid·u·o·ma (dĭ-sĭj′ōō-ō′mə) *n.* An intrauterine mass of decidual tissue, probably the result of hyperplasia of decidual cells retained in the uterus after parturition. Also called *placentoma.*

deciduoma ma·lig·num (mə-lĭg′nəm) *n.* See **chorioadenoma.**

de·cid·u·ous (dĭ-sĭj′ōō-əs) *adj.* **1.** Falling off or shed at a specific stage of growth, as teeth of the first dentition. **2.** Of, relating to, or being the first or primary dentition.

deciduous dentition *n.* See **primary dentition.**

deciduous membrane *n.* See **decidua.**

deciduous tooth *n.* Any of the teeth of the primary dentition. Also called *baby tooth, milk tooth, primary tooth, temporary tooth.*

de·clamp·ing phenomenon (dē-klăm′pĭng) *n.* The occurrence of shock or hypotension following the abrupt release of clamps from a large portion of the vascular bed, such as the aorta, that is believed to be caused by transient pooling of blood in a previously ischemic area. Also called *declamping shock.*

dec·li·na·tion (dĕk′lə-nā′shən) *n.* **1.** A bending, sloping, or other deviation from a normal vertical position. **2.** A deviation of the vertical meridian of the eye to one or the other side due to rotation of the eyeball about its anteroposterior axis.

de·clive (dĭ-klīv′) *n.* The posterior sloping portion of the monticulus of the vermis of the cerebellum.

de·com·pen·sa·tion (dē′kŏm-pən-sā′shən) *n.* **1.** Failure of the heart to maintain adequate blood circulation, characterized by labored breathing, engorged blood vessels, and edema. **2.** The appearance or exacerbation of a mental disorder due to failure of defense mechanisms.

de·com·po·si·tion (dē-kŏm′pə-zĭsh′ən) *n.* **1.** The act or result of decomposing; disintegration. **2.** Separation into constituents by chemical reaction. **3.** The breakdown or decay of organic materials; lysis. —**de·com′po·si′tion·al** *adj.*

de·com·pres·sion (dē′kəm-prĕsh′ən) *n.* **1.** The relief of pressure on a body part by surgery. **2.** The restoration of deep-sea divers and caisson workers to atmospheric pressure by means of a decompression chamber.

decompression chamber *n.* A compartment in which atmospheric pressure can be gradually raised or lowered, used especially in readjusting divers or underwater workers to normal atmospheric pressure or in treating decompression sickness.

decompression sickness *n.* A disorder, seen especially in deep-sea divers or in caisson and tunnel workers, caused by the formation of nitrogen bubbles in the blood following a rapid drop in pressure and characterized by severe pains in the joints and chest, skin irritation, cramps, and paralysis. Also called *aeroemphysema, bends, caisson disease.*

de·con·gest (dē′kən-jĕst′) *v.* To relieve congestion, such as of the sinuses.

de·con·ges·tant (dē′kən-jĕs′tənt) *n.* A medication or treatment that breaks up congestion, as that of the sinuses, by reducing swelling. —*adj.* Capable of relieving congestion.

de·con·tam·i·na·tion (dē′kən-tăm′ə-nā′shən) *n.* The removal or neutralization of a contaminating substance, such as poisonous gas or a radioactive material. —**de′con·tam′i·nate** (-nāt′) *v.*

de·cor·ti·ca·tion (dē-kôr′tĭ-kā′shən) *n.* The removal of the surface layer, membrane, or fibrous cover of an organ or a structure. —**de·cor′ti·cate′** *v.*

de·cru·des·cence (dē′krōō-dĕs′əns) *n.* Abatement of the symptoms of a disease.

de·cu·bi·tal (dĭ-kyōō′bĭ-tl) *adj.* Of or relating to a bedsore.

de·cu·bi·tus (dĭ-kyōō′bĭ-təs) *n.* 1. The position of a patient in bed. 2. A bedsore.

decubitus calculus *n.* A calculus of the urinary tract formed as a result of long immobilization.

decubitus paralysis *n.* A form of compression paralysis due to pressure on a limb during sleep.

decubitus ulcer *n.* See **bedsore**.

de·cus·sate (dĭ-kŭs′āt′, dĕk′ə-sāt′) *v.* To cross or become crossed so as to form an X; intersect. —*adj.* Intersected or crossed in the form of an X.

dec·us·sa·tion (dĕk′ə-sā′shən, dē′kə-) *n.* 1. A crossing in the shape of an X. 2. An X-shaped crossing, especially of homonymous nerves or bands of nerve fibers, connecting corresponding parts on opposite sides of the brain or spinal cord.

decussation of medial lemniscus *n.* Crossing of the fibers of the left and right medial lemniscus in the medulla oblongata.

decussation of superior cerebellar peduncles *n.* Crossing of the left and right superior cerebellar peduncles in the tegmentum of the mesencephalon.

de·dif·fer·en·ti·a·tion (dē′dĭf-ə-rĕn′shē-ā′shən) *n.* Regression of a specialized cell or tissue to a simpler unspecialized form. —**de′dif·fer·en′ti·ate′** *v.*

deep artery of clitoris (dēp) *n.* An artery that is the deep terminal branch of the pudendal artery in the female and supplies the crus of the clitoris.

deep artery of penis *n.* An artery with its origin as the terminal branch of the internal pudendal artery in the male, and with distribution to the corpus cavernosum of the penis.

deep artery of thigh *n.* An artery with its origin in the femoral artery, with branches to the lateral circumflex femoral, medial circumflex femoral, and perforating arteries. Also called *femoral artery.*

deep cervical vein *n.* A vein that accompanies the deep cervical artery between the semispinal muscle of the head and the semispinal muscle of the neck and empties into the brachiocephalic vein or the vertebral vein.

deep dorsal vein of clitoris *n.* A tributary of the vesical venous plexus deep in the fascia on the dorsum of the clitoris.

deep dorsal vein of penis *n.* A tributary of the prostatic plexus deep in the fascia on the dorsum of the penis.

deep facial vein *n.* A valveless communicating vein that passes from the facial vein to the pterygoid plexus in the infratemporal fossa.

deep fascia *n.* A thin fibrous membrane forming an intricate network that envelops and separates muscles, forms sheaths for nerves and vessels, forms or strengthens ligaments around joints, envelops various organs and glands, and binds all structures together into a firm compact mass.

deep femoral vein *n.* A vein that accompanies the deep femoral artery, receives perforating veins from the posterior aspect of the thigh, and joins the femoral vein in the femoral triangle, usually with the medial and lateral circumflex femoral veins.

deep flexor muscle of fingers *n.* A muscle with its origin in the anterior surface of the upper third of the ulna, with insertion to the base of the distal phalanx of each finger, with nerve supply from the ulnar and median nerves, and whose action flexes the distal phalanges of the fingers.

de·ep·i·car·di·al·i·za·tion (dē-ĕp′ĭ-kär′dē-ə-lĭ-zā′shən) *n.* The surgical destruction of the epicardium, usually by the application of phenol, designed to promote collateral circulation to the myocardium.

deep inguinal ring *n.* The opening in the transverse fascia that allows for the passage of the male spermatic cord or the female round ligament. Also called *abdominal ring.*

deep lingual vein *n.* A vein that accompanies the deep lingual artery, drains the body and apex of the tongue, and joins the lingual vein.

deep perineal space *n.* The cleft between the superior and inferior fasciae of the urogenital diaphragm, occupied by the membranous part of the urethra, the bulbourethral gland (male), the deep transverse perineal and sphincter urethrae muscles, and the dorsal nerve and artery of the penis or clitoris.

deep peroneal nerve *n.* A terminal branch of the common peroneal nerve, passing into the anterior compartment of the leg and supplying the anterior tibial muscle, the long extensor muscle of the big toe, the long extensor muscle of the toes, the third peroneal muscle, the skin of the big toe, and the medial surface of the second toe.

deep petrosal nerve *n.* The sympathetic part of the greater petrosal nerve, which arises from the internal carotid plexus and joins the nerve at the entrance of the pterygoid canal.

deep reflex *n.* An involuntary muscular contraction following percussion of a tendon or bone. Also called *jerk.*

deep temporal nerve *n.* Either of two branches from the mandibular nerve, designated anterior and posterior, that supply the temporal muscle.

deep temporal vein *n.* Any of the veins that correspond to the deep temporal arteries and empty into the pterygoid venous plexus.

deep tendon reflex *n. Abbr.* **DTR** Tonic contraction of the muscles in response to a stretching force, due to stimulation of muscle proprioceptors. Also called *myotatic reflex.*

deep transverse muscle of perineum *n.* A muscle with origin from the ramus of the ischium, with insertion with its fellow muscle in a median raphe, with nerve supply from the pudendal nerve, and whose action assists the sphincter urethrae.

deep vein of clitoris *n.* Any of the veins that pass from the dorsum of the clitoris to join the vesical venous plexus.

deep vein of penis *n.* The vein that is deep in the fascia and enters the prostatic plexus.

deep venous thrombosis *n. Abbr.* **DVT** A condition in which one or more thrombi form in a deep vein, especially in the leg or pelvis, resulting in an increased risk of pulmonary embolism.

deer tick (dîr) *n.* Any of several ticks of the genus *Ixodes* that are parasitic on deer and other animals and transmit the infectious agents of febrile diseases, such as Lyme disease.

def *abbr.* decayed, extraction indicated due to caries, or filled (used for deciduous teeth)

DEF *abbr.* decayed, extraction indicated due to caries, or filled (used for permanent teeth)

def·e·cate (dĕf′ĭ-kāt′) *v.* To void feces from the bowels. —**def′e·ca′tion** *n.*

de·fect (dē′fĕkt′, dĭ-fĕkt′) *n.* A lack of or abnormality in something necessary for normal functioning; a deficiency or imperfection.

de·fec·tive (dĭ-fĕk′tĭv) *n.* **1.** Having an imperfection or malformation. **2.** Lacking or deficient in some physical or mental function.

defective bacteriophage *n.* A temperate bacteriophage mutant that cannot fully infect but that can replicate in the bacterial genome as a defective probacteriophage.

defective virus *n.* A virus particle that contains insufficient nucleic acid to provide for production of all essential viral components, thus infection is not produced except under certain conditions.

de·fense (dĭ-fĕns′) *n.* A means or method that helps protect the body or mind, as against disease or anxiety. —**de·fen′sive** (-fĕn′sĭv) *adj.*

defense mechanism *n.* **1.** Any of a variety of usually unconscious mental processes used to protect oneself from shame, anxiety, loss of self-esteem, conflict, or other unacceptable feelings or thoughts, and including behaviors such as repression, projection, denial, and rationalization. **2.** See **immunological mechanism.**

de·fen·sive circle (dĭ-fĕn′sĭv) *n.* The addition of a secondary disease that limits or arrests the progress of the primary disease, the two diseases exerting a reciprocally antagonistic action.

defensive medicine *n.* Diagnostic or therapeutic measures conducted primarily as a safeguard against possible malpractice liability.

def·er·ent (dĕf′ər-ənt, dĕf′rənt) *adj.* Carrying down or away, as a duct or vessel.

deferent duct *n.* See **vas deferens.**

def·er·en·tec·to·my (dĕf′ər-ən-tĕk′tə-mē) *n.* See **vasectomy.**

def·er·en·tial (dĕf′ə-rĕn′shəl) *adj.* Of or relating to the vas deferens.

def·er·en·ti·tis (dĕf′ər-ən-tī′tĭs) *n.* Inflammation of the vas deferens. Also called *vasitis.*

de·fer·ves·cence (dē′fər-vĕs′əns, dĕf′ər-) *n.* The abatement of a fever.

de·fib·ril·la·tion (dē-fĭb′rə-lā′shən, -fī′brə-) *n.* The stopping of fibrillation of the heart muscle and the restoration of normal contractions using drugs or electric shock. —**de·fib′ril·late′** *v.*

de·fib·ril·la·tor (dē-fĭb′rə-lā′tər, -fī′brə-) *n.* An electrical device used to counteract fibrillation of the heart muscle and restore normal heartbeat by applying a brief electric shock.

de·fi·bri·na·tion (dē-fī′brə-nā′shən, -fĭb′rə-) *n.* The removal of fibrin from blood. —**de·fi′bri·nate′** *v.*

de·fi·cien·cy (dĭ-fĭsh′ən-sē) *n.* A lack or shortage of something essential to health; an insufficiency.

deficiency disease *n.* A disease that is caused by a dietary deficiency of specific nutrients, especially a vitamin or mineral, possibly stemming from insufficient intake, digestion, absorption, or utilization of a nutrient. Also called *insufficiency disease.*

deficiency symptom *n.* A symptom caused by the lack of a substance, such as an enzyme or a vitamin, that is necessary for normal structure and function of an organism.

de·fi·cient (dĭ-fĭsh′ənt) *adj.* **1.** Lacking an essential quality or element. **2.** Inadequate in amount or degree; insufficient.

def·i·cit (dĕf′ĭ-sĭt) *n.* **1.** A lack or deficiency of a substance. **2.** A lack or impairment in mental or physical functioning.

de·fin·i·tive host (dĭ-fĭn′ĭ-tĭv) *n.* A host in which a parasite develops to an adult or sexually mature stage. Also called *final host.*

de·flec·tion (dĭ-flĕk′shən) *n.* **1.** A turning aside or deviation. **2.** The deviation of an indicator in a measuring instrument, such as an electrocardiograph, from zero or from its normal position.

de·flu·vi·um (dē-floō′vē-əm) *n.* Defluxion.

de·flux·ion (dē-flŭk′shən) *n.* **1.** A falling down or out, as of the hair. **2.** A flowing down or discharge of fluid.

de·for·ma·tion (dē′fôr-mā′shən, dĕf′ər-) *n.* **1.** An alteration in shape or structure of a previously normally formed part. **2.** A deformity.

de·formed (dĭ-fôrmd′) *adj.* Distorted in form.

de·for·mi·ty (dĭ-fôr′mĭ-tē) *n.* **1.** The state of being deformed. **2.** A deviation from the normal shape or size of a body part, resulting in disfigurement.

deg *or* **deg.** *abbr.* degree

de·gen·er·ate (dĭ-jĕn′ər-ĭt) *adj.* **1.** Characterized by degeneration, as of tissue, a cell, or an organ. **2.** Having lost one or more highly developed functions, characteristics, or structures through evolution. —*v.* (-ə-rāt′) To undergo the process of degeneration.

de·gen·er·a·tion (dĭ-jĕn′ə-rā′shən) *n.* **1.** The gradual deterioration of specific tissues, cells, or organs with impairment or loss of function, caused by injury, disease, or aging. **2.** The evolutionary decline or loss of a function, characteristic, or structure in an organism or a species.

de·gen·er·a·tive (dĭ-jĕn′ər-ə-tĭv) *adj.* Of, relating to, causing, or characterized by degeneration.

degenerative joint disease *n. Abbr.* **DJD** See **osteoarthritis.**

de·glov·ing (dē-glŭv′ĭng) *n.* The surgical exposure of the front part of the mandible while working from within the mouth, as used in plastic surgery.

deglut *abbr. Latin* degluttiatur (let be swallowed; swallow)

de·glu·ti·tion (dē′glo͞o-tĭsh′ən) *n.* The act or process of swallowing.

deg·ra·da·tion (dĕg′rə-dā′shən) *n.* Progressive decomposition of a chemical compound into a less complex compound.

de·gree (dĭ-grē′) *n.* **1.** *Abbr.* **deg, deg.** A unit of measure on a temperature scale. **2.** A division of a circle, equal to $^1/_{360}$ of its circumference. **3.** A position or rank within a graded series.

de·gus·ta·tion (dē′gŭ-stā′shən) *n.* **1.** The act or function of tasting. **2.** The sense of taste.

de·hisce (dĭ-hĭs′) *v.* To rupture or break open, as a surgical wound.

de·his·cence (dĭ-hĭs′əns) *n.* A bursting open or splitting along natural or sutured lines.

de·hy·drase (dē-hī′drās′, -drāz′) *n.* Dehydratase.

de·hy·dra·tase (dē-hī′drə-tās′, -tāz′) *n.* An enzyme that catalyzes the removal of oxygen and hydrogen from organic compounds in the form of water.

de·hy·drate (dē-hī′drāt′) *v.* **1.** To remove water from; make anhydrous. **2.** To preserve by removing water from something, such as vegetables. **3.** To deplete the bodily fluids of an individual.

de·hy·dra·tion (dē′hī-drā′shən) *n.* **1.** Excessive loss of water from the body or from an organ or a body part, as occurs during illness or fluid deprivation. **2.** The process of removing water from a substance or compound.

dehydro– *pref.* Losing one or more hydrogen atoms: *dehydrogenation.*

de·hy·dro·cho·lic acid (dē-hī′drə-kō′lĭk) *n.* A crystalline acid derived from cholic acid and used in its sodium salt form as a choleretic and diuretic.

de·hy·dro·cor·ti·cos·ter·one (dē-hī′drō-kôr′tĭ-kŏs′tə-rōn′) *n.* A steroid occurring in the adrenal cortex or produced synthetically and having biological activity similar to that of corticosterone.

de·hy·dro·ep·i·an·dros·ter·one (dē-hī′drō-ĕp′ē-ăn-drŏs′tə-rōn′) *n. Abbr.* **DHEA 1.** An androgenic steroid that is secreted largely by the adrenal cortex and is found in human urine. **2.** A synthetic preparation of this hormone, used as a dietary supplement.

de·hy·dro·gen·ase (dē′hī-drŏj′ə-nās′, -nāz′, dē-hī′-drə-jə-) *n.* An enzyme that catalyzes the removal and transfer of hydrogen from a substrate in an oxidation-reduction reaction.

de·hy·dro·gen·a·tion (dē′hī-drŏj′ə-nā′shən, dē-hī′drə-jə-) *n.* The removal of hydrogen.

de·hy·dro·ret·i·nal·de·hyde (dē-hī′drō-rĕt′n-ăl′də-hīd′) *n.* An orange-red crystalline aldehyde that is a derivative of vitamin A and acts in the retina to form the visual pigments of the rods and cones. Also called *retinene.*

de·in·sti·tu·tion·al·i·za·tion (dē-ĭn′stĭ-to͞o′shə-nə-lĭ-zā′shən) *n.* The release of institutionalized people, especially mental health patients, from an institution for placement and care in the community. —**de·in′sti·tu′tion·al·ize′** *v.*

Dei·ters′ cell (dī′tərz, -tərs) *n.* **1.** See **phalangeal cell. 2.** See **astrocyte.**

dé·jà vu phenomenon *or* **dé·jà vu** (dā′zhä vü′) *n.* **1.** The illusion of having already experienced something actu-

ally being experienced for the first time. **2.** An impression of having seen or experienced something before.

de·jec·tion (dĭ-jĕk′shən) *n.* **1.** Lowness of spirits; depression; melancholy. **2.** The evacuation of the bowels; defecation. **3.** Feces; excrement.

De·je·rine′s disease (dĕ-zhə-rēnz′) *or* **De·je·rine-Sot·tas disease** (-sŏt′əs, -sô-täs′) *n.* See **hereditary hypertrophic neuropathy.**

deka– *or* **dek–** *pref.* Variants of **deca–.**

de·lac·ri·ma·tion (dē-lăk′rə-mā′shən) *n.* The excessive secretion of tears.

de·lam·i·na·tion (dē-lăm′ə-nā′shən) *n.* **1.** A splitting or separation into layers. **2.** The splitting of the blastoderm into two layers of cells to form a gastrula.

de Lang·e′s syndrome (də lăng′ĕz, läng′əz) *or* **Cor·ne·lia de Lange′s syndrome** (kôr-nēl′yə) *n.* A syndrome of unknown cause characterized by mental retardation, short stature, thick eyebrows and low hairline, and flat, spadelike hands with short tapering fingers. Also called *Amsterdam syndrome.*

del·a·vir·dine (dĕl′ə-vîr′dēn) *n.* A non-nucleoside analog that is used as an antiviral drug in the treatment of HIV infection.

de·layed allergy (dĭ-lād′) *n.* A hypersensitivity that reaches its peak several hours after exposure to an antigen, then recedes.

delayed dentition *n.* The delayed eruption of the first or second set of teeth.

delayed flap *n.* A flap detached from its donor area in two or more stages to increase its chances of survival after transfer.

delayed graft *n.* The application of a skin graft after waiting several days for healthy granulations to form.

delayed reaction *n.* An allergic or immune response that begins 24 to 48 hours after exposure to an antigen to which the individual has been sensitized.

Del·bet′s sign (dĕl-bāz′) *n.* An indication of aneurysm of a main artery in which the pulse disappears although collateral circulation remains efficient and nutrition of the part below the main artery is well maintained.

Del·brück (dĕl′bro͝ok′, -brük′), **Max** 1906–1981. German-born American biologist. He shared a 1969 Nobel Prize for investigating the mechanism of viral infection in living cells.

Del Cas·til·lo syndrome (dĕl kä-stē′yōz, kä-stē′yôz) *n.* See **Sertoli cell-only syndrome.**

de·lead (dē-lĕd′) *v.* To remove lead deposited in the bones and other tissues, as by use of a chelating agent or acid salts.

del·e·te·ri·ous (dĕl′ĭ-tîr′ē-əs) *adj.* Having a harmful effect; injurious.

de·le·tion (dĭ-lē′shən) *n.* Loss, as from mutation, of one or more nucleotides from a chromosome.

de·lim·it·ing keratotomy (dĭ-lĭm′ĭ-tĭng) *n.* Incision in the cornea along the margin of an advancing ulcer. Also called *Gifford′s operation.*

del·i·ques·cence (dĕl′ĭ-kwĕs′əns) *n.* The process of dissolving or of becoming liquid through the absorption of moisture from the atmosphere.

de·lir·i·ous (dĭ-lîr′ē-əs) *adj.* Of, suffering from, or characteristic of delirium.

de·lir·i·um (dĭ-lîr′ē-əm) *n., pl.* **–i·ums** *or* **–i·a** (-ē-ə) A temporary state of mental confusion resulting from high fever, intoxication, shock, or other causes, and characterized by anxiety, disorientation, memory impairment, hallucinations, trembling, and incoherent speech.

delirium tre·mens (trē′mənz) *n. Abbr.* **DT** An acute, sometimes fatal episode of delirium that is usually caused by withdrawal or abstinence from alcohol following habitual excessive drinking and that is characterized by sweating, trembling, anxiety, confusion, and hallucinations.

de·liv·er (dĭ-lĭv′ər) *v.* **1.** To assist a woman in giving birth to a baby. **2.** To extract something from an enclosed place, as a foreign body or a tumor.

de·liv·er·y (dĭ-lĭv′ə-rē, -lĭv′rē) *n.* The expulsion or extraction of a child and the fetal membranes through the birth canal into the external world.

delivery room *n.* A room or an area in a hospital that is equipped for delivering babies.

del·le (dĕl′ə) *n.* The lighter-colored area in the center of a stained red blood cell.

del·len (dĕl′ən) *pl.n.* Shallow excavations along the outer edge of the cornea that are caused by localized dehydration.

del·phi·an node (dĕl′fī-ən, -fē-) *n.* A midline prelaryngeal lymph node, adjacent to the thyroid gland, enlargement of which indicates thyroid disease.

Del·sym (dĕl′sĭm′) A trademark for the drug dextromethorphan.

del·ta (dĕl′tə) *n.* **1.** *Symbol* **δ, Δ** The fourth letter of the Greek alphabet. **2.** The fourth one in a series. **3.** A surface or part that resembles a triangle, such as the terminus of a pattern in a fingerprint or the shape of a muscle. —*adj.* **1.** Of or characterizing the atom or radical group that is fourth in position from the functional group of atoms in an organic molecule. **2.** Of or relating to one of four closely related chemical substances. **3.** Relating to or characterizing a polypeptide chain that is one of five types of heavy chains present in immunoglobins.

delta agent *n.* See **hepatitis delta virus.**

del·ta-a·mi·no·lev·u·lin·ic acid (dĕl′tə-ə-mē′nō-lĕv′-yə-lĭn′ĭk) *n.* ALA.

delta antigen *n.* See **hepatitis delta virus.**

delta cell *n.* **1.** A type of beta cell of the adenohypophysis. **2.** A cell of the islets of Langerhans containing fine granules that stain with aniline blue.

delta granule *n.* A granule of a delta cell.

delta hepatitis *n.* See **hepatitis D.**

delta rhythm *n.* A brain wave pattern originating from the forward portion of the brain and having a frequency of between 1.5 and 4.0 hertz; it is associated with deep sleep in normal adults. Also called *delta wave.*

Del·ta·sone (dĕl′tə-sōn′) A trademark for the drug prednisolone.

delta wave *n.* **1.** A slurring of the R-wave upstroke in an electrocardiogram as seen in Wolff-Parkinson-White syndrome. **2.** See **delta rhythm.**

del·toid (dĕl′toid′) *adj.* **1.** Of or relating to the deltoid muscle. **2.** Triangular in shape or outline. —*n.* The deltoid muscle.

deltoid ligament *n.* A ligament consisting of four parts that pass downward from the medial malleolus of the tibia to the tarsal bones of the foot. Also called *medial ligament.*

deltoid muscle *n.* A muscle with origin from the lateral third of the clavicle, the lateral border of acromion process, and the lower border of spine of scapula, with insertion to the side of the shaft of the humerus, with nerve supply from the axillary nerve from the fifth and sixth cervical nerves through the brachial plexus, and whose action causes the abduction, flexion, extension, and rotation of the arm.

de·lu·sion (dĭ-lōō′zhən) *n.* A false belief strongly held in spite of invalidating evidence, especially as a symptom of mental illness. —**de·lu′sion·al** *adj.*

delusion of gran·deur (grăn′jər, -jōōr′) *n.* A delusion in which one believes oneself possessed of great importance, power, wealth, intellect, or ability.

delusion of negation *n.* A depressive delusion in which one imagines the world no longer exists.

delusion of persecution *n.* A delusion that one is being persecuted or conspired against, characteristic of paranoid schizophrenia.

de·mand pacemaker (dĭ-mănd′) *n.* An artificial pacemaker usually implanted into cardiac tissue because its output of electrical stimuli can be inhibited by endogenous cardiac electrical activity.

de·mat·i·a·ceous (dĭ-măt′ē-ā′shəs) *adj.* Having a dark color, usually olive, gray, or black, as some fungi.

de·ment·ed (dĭ-mĕn′tĭd) *adj.* **1.** Mentally ill; insane. **2.** Suffering from dementia.

de·men·tia (dĭ-mĕn′shə) *n.* Deterioration of intellectual faculties, such as memory, concentration, and judgment, resulting from an organic disease or a disorder of the brain, and often accompanied by emotional disturbance and personality changes.

dementia prae·cox (prē′kŏks′) *n.* Schizophrenia. No longer in technical use.

Dem·er·ol (dĕm′ə-rôl′, -rōl′) A trademark for the drug meperidine hydrochloride.

demi– *pref.* Half: *demilune.*

dem·i·gaunt·let bandage (dĕm′ē-gônt′lĭt, -gänt′-) *n.* A gauntlet bandage that covers the hand but leaves the fingers exposed.

dem·i·lune (dĕm′ē-lōōn′) *n.* A small body shaped like a half-moon or crescent, such as one of the crescent-shaped cells surrounding certain mucous glands.

de·min·er·al·i·za·tion (dē-mĭn′ər-ə-lĭ-zā′shən) *n.* The loss, deprivation, or removal of minerals or mineral salts from the body, especially through disease, as the loss of calcium from bones or teeth.

Dem·o·dex (dĕm′ə-dĕks′, dē′mə-) *n.* A genus of parasitic, usually nonpathogenic mites that invade the skin and are usually found in the sebaceous glands and hair follicles of humans and animals.

Demodex fol·lic·u·lo·rum (fə-lĭk′yə-lôr′əm) *n.* The follicular or mange mite, a very common, universally distributed, probably nonpathogenic species parasitic to human hair follicles and sebaceous glands usually around the nose and scalp margins.

dem·o·graph·ic (dĕm′ə-grăf′ĭk, dē′mə-) *adj.* Of or relating to demography.

de·mog·ra·phy (dĭ-mŏg′rə-fē) *n.* The study of the characteristics of human populations, such as size, growth, density, distribution, and vital statistics. —**de·mog′ra·pher** *n.*

de·mu·co·sa·tion (dē-myōō′kə-sā′shən) *n.* The surgical removal of a mucous membrane from a part of the body.

de·mul·cent (dĭ-mŭl′sənt) *adj.* Relieving irritation; soothing. —*n.* A soothing, usually mucilaginous or oily substance, such as glycerin or lanolin, used especially to relieve pain in inflamed or irritated mucous membranes.

de·my·e·lin·at·ing disease (dē-mī′ə-lə-nā′tĭng) *n.* Any of a group of diseases of unknown cause in which there is extensive loss of the myelin sheaths of nerve fibers, as in multiple sclerosis.

de·my·e·lin·a·tion (dē-mī′ə-lə-nā′shən) *or* **de·my·e·lin·i·za·tion** (-lə-nĭ-zā′shən, -lĭn′ĭ-) *n.* The destruction or removal of the myelin sheath of a nerve fiber, as through disease.

de·na·ture (dē-nā′chər) *v.* **1.** To change the nature or natural qualities of. **2.** To render unfit to eat or drink without destroying usefulness in other applications, especially adding methyl alcohol to ethyl alcohol. **3.** To alter the chemical structure of a protein, as with heat, alkali, or acid, so that some of its original properties, especially its biological activity, are diminished or eliminated. —**de·na′tur·a′tion** *n.*

de·natured alcohol (dē-nā′chərd) *n.* Ethyl alcohol to which a poisonous substance, such as acetone or methanol, has been added to make it unfit for consumption.

den·dri·form (dĕn′drə-fôrm′) *adj.* Being tree-shaped, branching.

den·drite (dĕn′drīt′) *n.* Any of the various branched protoplasmic extensions of a nerve cell that conducts impulses from adjacent cells inward toward the cell body. Also called *dendritic process, dendron, neurodendrite, neurodendron.*

den·drit·ic (dĕn-drĭt′ĭk) *adj.* Relating to the dendrites of nerve cells.

dendritic calculus *n.* See **stag-horn calculus.**

dendritic cell *n.* **1.** A cell that has branching processes. **2.** Any of the cells in the neural crest of the embryonic ectoderm having extensive processes and developing early as producers of melanin. **3.** See **follicular dendritic cell.**

dendritic corneal ulcer *n.* Keratitis caused by herpes simplex virus.

dendritic keratitis *or* **dendriform keratitis** *n.* A form of keratitis associated with herpes simplex virus and characterized by branching ulceration of the corneal tissue.

dendritic process *n.* See **dendrite.**

dendritic spine *n.* Any of various outgrowths of certain nerve-cell dendrites, ranging in shape from small knobs to thornlike or filamentous processes, that are preferential sites of synaptic axodendritic contact.

den·droid (dĕn′droid′) *adj.* Dendriform.

den·dron (dĕn′drŏn′) *n.* See **dendrite.**

de·ner·vate (dē-nûr′vāt) *v.* To deprive an organ or body part of a nerve supply, as by surgically removing or cutting a nerve or by blocking a nerve connection with drugs. —**de′ner·va′tion** *n.*

den·gue (dĕng′gē, -gā) *n.* An acute, infectious tropical disease caused by an arbovirus transmitted by mosquitoes, characterized by high fever, rash, headache, and severe muscle and joint pain. Also called *breakbone fever, dandy fever.*

dengue virus *n.* A virus of the genus *Flavivirus* that is the cause of dengue.

de·ni·al (dĭ-nī′əl) *n.* An unconscious defense mechanism characterized by refusal to acknowledge painful realities, thoughts, or feelings.

den·i·da·tion (dĕn′ĭ-dā′shən) *n.* The detachment and expulsion of the endometrium of the uterus during menstruation.

Den·is Browne splint (dĕn′ĭs broun′) *n.* A light aluminum splint applied to the lateral aspect of the leg and foot, used for clubfoot.

Den·nie's line (dĕn′ēz) *n.* An accentuated line that is located below the margin of the lower eyelid and is characteristic of atopic dermatitis. Also called *Dennie's fold.*

dens (dĕnz) *n., pl.* **den·tes** (dĕn′tēz′) **1.** Tooth. **2.** A toothlike process projecting upward from the body of the axis around which the atlas rotates. Also called *odontoid process of epistropheus.*

den·sim·e·ter (dĕn-sĭm′ĭ-tər) *n.* An instrument used to measure density or specific gravity. Also called *densitometer.* —**den′si·met′ric** (-sə-mĕt′rĭk) *adj.*

dens in den·te (ĭn dĕn′tē) *n.* A developmental disturbance in tooth formation resulting from invagination of the epithelium associated with coronal development into the area that was to be pulp space.

den·si·tom·e·ter (dĕn′sĭ-tŏm′ĭ-tər) *n.* **1.** An apparatus for measuring the optical density of a material, such as a photographic negative. **2.** See **densimeter.** —**den′si·tom′e·try** (-ĭ-trē) *n.*

den·si·ty (dĕn′sĭ-tē) *n.* **1.** The mass per unit volume of a substance at a specified pressure and temperature. **2.** The quantity of something per unit measure, especially per unit length, area, or volume. **3.** The quality or condition of being dense.

dent– *pref.* Variant of **denti–.**

den·tal (dĕn′tl) *adj.* **1.** Of, relating to, or for the teeth. **2.** Of, relating to, or intended for dentistry.

dental abscess *n.* See **alveolar abscess.**

dental anatomy *n.* The study of the morphology of teeth, their location, position, and relationships.

dental arch *n.* **1.** The curved composite structure of natural dentition. **2.** The teeth that are supported by the alveolar part of the mandible; inferior dental arch. Also called *mandibular dentition.* **3.** The teeth that are supported by the alveolar process of the maxillae; superior dental arch. Also called *maxillary dentition.*

dental assistant *n.* A person trained to assist a dentist with clinical and administrative procedures.

dental bulb *n.* The papilla, derived from mesoderm, that forms the part of the tooth primordium that is situated within the cup-shaped enamel organ.

dental calculus *n.* See **tartar.**

dental caries *n.* The formation of cavities in the teeth by the action of bacteria; tooth decay.

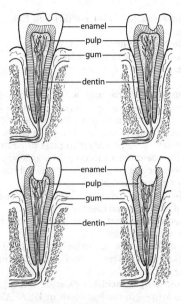

dental caries

Top left: *acid from bacterial action destroys enamel and forms a cavity*
Top right: *unchecked decay spreads to the dentin*
Bottom left: *an enlarged cavity allows bacteria to attack exposed dental pulp*
Bottom right: *untreated and infected dental pulp causes the eventual death of the pulp and tooth*

dental crypt *n.* The space filled by a dental follicle.

dental cuticle *n.* Either of two thin layers, one clear and structureless, one cellular, covering the crown of newly erupted teeth and abraded by mastication. Also called *adamantine membrane.*

dental floss *n.* A waxed or unwaxed thread used to remove food particles and plaque from the teeth.

dental follicle *n.* The dental sac with its enclosed developing tooth.

dental forceps *n.* A forceps used in grasping and extracting teeth. Also called *extracting forceps.*

dental formula *n.* Tabular representation of the number of deciduous and permanent teeth in the jaw.

den·tal·gia (děn-tăl′jə) *n.* See **toothache.**

dental granuloma *n.* See **periapical granuloma.**

dental hygiene *n.* The practice of keeping the mouth, teeth, and gums clean and healthy to prevent disease.

dental hygienist *n.* A person trained and licensed to provide preventive dental services, such as cleaning the teeth, usually in conjunction with a dentist.

dental implant *n.* An artificial tooth that is anchored in the gums or jawbone to replace a missing tooth.

dental lamina *n.* A band of ectodermal cells growing from the epithelium of the embryonic jaws into the underlying mesenchyme and giving rise to the primordia of the enamel organs of the teeth.

dental orthopedics *n.* Orthodontics.

dental plaque *n.* A film of mucus and bacteria on a tooth surface. Also called *bacterial plaque.*

dental plate *n.* See **denture** (sense 1).

dental polyp *n.* Hyperplastic pulpal tissue growing out of a decayed tooth with wide pulpal exposure.

dental pulp *n.* The soft tissue forming the inner structure of a tooth and containing nerves and blood vessels. Also called *tooth pulp.*

dental ridge *n.* The prominent border of a cusp or margin of a tooth.

dental sac *n.* The envelope of connective tissue surrounding a developing tooth.

dental surgeon *n.* A general practitioner of dentistry having a DDS or DMD degree.

dental syringe *n.* A breech-loading syringe fitted with a sealed cartridge containing anesthetic solution.

dental technician *n.* A person who makes dental appliances and restorative devices, such as bridges or dentures, to the specifications of a dentist.

den·tate (děn′tāt′) *adj.* Edged with toothlike projections; toothed.

dentate gyrus *n.* One of the two interlocking gyri composing the hippocampus.

dentate nucleus of cerebellum *n.* The most lateral and largest of the deep cerebellar nuclei, receiving axons of the Purkinje cells of the neocerebellum, and serving as a source of fibers composing the superior cerebellar peduncle.

dentate suture *n.* See **serrate suture.**

denti– *or* **dent–** *or* **dento–** *pref.* **1.** Tooth: *dentalgia.* **2.** Dental: *dentilabial.*

den·ti·cle (děn′tĭ-kəl) *n.* **1.** See **pulp stone.** **2.** A small tooth or toothlike projection.

den·ti·frice (děn′tə-frĭs′) *n.* A substance, such as a paste or powder, for cleaning the teeth.

den·tig·er·ous (děn-tĭj′ər-əs) *adj.* Having or furnished with teeth.

dentigerous cyst *n.* A cyst arising in the odontogenic epithelium after the crown of a developing tooth has been formed.

den·ti·la·bi·al (děn′tə-lā′bē-əl) *adj.* Of or relating to the teeth and lips.

den·ti·lin·gual (děn′tə-lĭng′gwəl) *adj.* Relating to the teeth and tongue.

den·tin (děn′tĭn) *or* **den·tine** (-tēn′) *n.* The main, calcareous part of a tooth, beneath the enamel and surrounding the pulp chamber and root canals.

den·tin·al (děn′tə-nəl, děn-tē′-) *adj.* Relating to dentin.

dentinal canal *n.* Any of the minute, wavy, branching tubes in the dentin that contain dentinal fibers and extend radially from the pulp to the dentoenamel junction. Also called *dentinal tubule.*

dentinal dysplasia *n.* See **dentinogenesis imperfecta.**

den·ti·nal·gia (děn′tə-năl′jə) *n.* Pain in the dentin of a tooth.

dentinal lamina cyst *n.* A small keratin-filled cyst derived from remnants of the dental lamina and usually appearing in groups on newborns' alveolar ridge.

dentinal papilla *n.* A projection of the mesenchymal tissue of the developing jaw into the cup of the enamel organ; its outer layer becomes odontoblasts that form the dentin of the tooth.

dentinal sheath *n.* A relatively acid-resistant layer of tissue that forms the walls of the dentinal tubules.

dentinal tubule *n.* See **dentinal canal.**

dentin dysplasia *n.* A hereditary disorder of both the primary and permanent teeth characterized by short roots, obliteration of the pulp chambers and canals, and mobility and premature loss.

den·ti·no·ce·men·tal (děn′tə-nō-sĭ-měn′tl) *adj.* Of, relating to, or characteristic of the dentin and cementum of teeth.

dentinocemental junction *n.* See **cementodentinal junction**.

den·ti·no·e·nam·el (děn′tə-nō-ĭ-năm′əl) *adj.* Of or relating to or characteristic of the dentin and the enamel of teeth.

dentinoenamel junction *n.* The surface at which the enamel and the dentin of the crown of a tooth are joined. Also called *amelodental junction, amelodentinal junction.*

den·ti·no·gen·e·sis (děn′tə-nō-jěn′ĭ-sĭs) *n.* The formation of dentin.

dentinogenesis im·per·fec·ta (ĭm′pər-fěk′tə) *n.* A hereditary defect of dentin formation characterized by a translucent or opalescent color of the teeth, easy fracturing of the enamel, wearing of occlusal surfaces, and staining of exposed dentin. Also called *dentinal dysplasia, hereditary opalescent dentin.*

den·ti·noid (děn′tə-noid′) *adj.* Resembling dentin. —*n.* See **dentinoma**.

den·ti·no·ma (děn′tə-nō′mə) *n.* A tumor containing dentin, occurring in the tissues that form teeth. Also called *dentinoid.*

den·ti·num (děn′tə-nəm, děn-tī′nəm) *n.* Dentin.

den·tip·a·rous (děn-tĭp′ə-rəs) *adj.* Bearing teeth.

den·tist (děn′tĭst) *n.* A person who is trained and licensed to practice dentistry.

den·tist·ry (děn′tĭ-strē) *n.* The science concerned with the prevention, diagnosis, and treatment of diseases of the teeth, gums, and related structures of the mouth and including the repair or replacement of defective teeth.

den·ti·tion (děn-tĭsh′ən) *n.* **1.** The natural teeth, considered collectively, in the dental arch. **2.** The type, number, and arrangement of a set of teeth. **3.** The process of growing new teeth; teething.

dento– *pref.* Variant of **denti–**.

den·to·al·ve·o·lar (děn′tō-ăl-vē′ə-lər) *adj.* **1.** Relating to a tooth and the part of the alveolar bone that immediately surrounds it. **2.** Relating to the functional unity of the teeth and the alveolar bone.

dentoalveolar abscess *n.* An abscess confined to the dentoalveolar process enclosing a tooth root.

den·tu·lous (děn′chə-ləs) *adj.* Having natural teeth.

den·ture (děn′chər) *n.* **1.** A partial or complete set of artificial teeth for either the upper or lower jaw. Also called *dental plate.* **2. dentures** A complete set of removable artificial teeth for both jaws.

denture base *n.* **1.** The part of a denture that rests on the oral mucus membrane and to which teeth are attached. **2.** The part of a complete or partial denture that rests on the denture foundation and to which teeth are attached.

denture foundation *n.* The portion of the oral structure that can be used to support a denture.

de·nu·cle·at·ed (dē-nōō′klē-ā′tĭd) *adj.* Deprived of a nucleus.

de·nu·da·tion (dē′nōō-dā′shən, děn′yōō-) *n.* The removal of a covering or surface layer.

de·nude (dĭ-nōōd′) *v.* To divest of a covering, as myelin.

de·o·dor·ant (dē-ō′dər-ənt) *n.* An agent that masks, suppresses, or neutralizes odors, especially a cosmetic applied to the skin to mask body odors. —*adj.* Capable of masking, suppressing, or neutralizing odors.

de·o·dor·ize (dē-ō′də-rīz′) *v.* To mask or neutralize the odor of. —**de·o′dor·i·za′tion** (-dər-ĭ-zā′shən) *n.*

de·o·dor·iz·er (dē-ō′də-rī′zər) *n.* A substance that masks or neutralizes odors.

de·os·si·fi·ca·tion (dē-ŏs′ə-fĭ-kā′shən) *n.* The loss or removal of the mineral constituents of bone.

deoxy– *or* **desoxy–** *pref.* Losing one or more atoms of oxygen: *deoxyadenosine.*

de·ox·y·a·den·o·sine (dē-ŏk′sē-ə-děn′ə-sēn′) *n.* One of the four principal nucleosides of DNA, composed of adenine and deoxyribose.

de·ox·y·ad·e·nyl·ic acid (dē-ŏk′sē-ăd′n-ĭl′ĭk) *n.* A nucleotide formed in the hydrolysis of DNA. Also called *adenine deoxyribonucleotide.*

de·ox·y·cho·lic acid (dē-ŏk′sē-kō′lĭk) *n.* A bile acid used as a choleretic and digestant and in the synthesis of adrenocortical hormones such as cortisone.

de·ox·y·cor·ti·cos·ter·one (dē-ŏk′sē-kôr′tĭ-kŏs′tə-rōn′) *n.* A steroid hormone produced synthetically or by the adrenal cortex and used to treat adrenal insufficiency. Also called *21-hydroxyprogesterone.*

de·ox·y·cy·ti·dine (dē-ŏk′sē-sī′tĭ-dēn′) *n.* One of the principal nucleosides of DNA, composed of cytosine and deoxyribose.

de·ox·y·cy·ti·dyl·ic acid (dē-ŏk′sē-sī′tĭ-dĭl′ĭk) *n.* A nucleotide formed in the hydrolysis of DNA.

de·ox·y·gen·a·tion (dē-ŏk′sə-jə-nā′shən) *n.* The process of removing dissolved oxygen from a liquid, such as water.

de·ox·y·gua·no·sine (dē-ŏk′sē-gwä′nə-sēn′, -sĭn) *n.* One of the principal nucleosides of DNA, composed of guanine and deoxyribose.

de·ox·y·gua·nyl·ic acid (dē-ŏk′sē-gwä-nĭl′ĭk) *n.* A nucleotide formed in the hydrolysis of DNA. Also called *guanine deoxyribonucleotide.*

de·ox·y·ri·bo·nu·cle·ase (dē-ok′sē-rī′bō-nōō′klē-ās′, -āz′) *n.* DNase.

de·ox·y·ri·bo·nu·cle·ic acid (dē-ŏk′sē-rī′bō-nōō-klē′ĭk, -klā′-) *n.* DNA.

de·ox·y·ri·bo·nu·cle·o·pro·tein (dē-ŏk′sē-rī′bō-nōō′-klē-ō-prō′tēn′) *n.* DNP.

de·ox·y·ri·bo·nu·cle·o·side (dē-ŏk′sē-rī′bō-nōō′klē-ə-sīd′) *n.* A nucleoside containing deoxyribose that is a constituent of DNA.

de·ox·y·ri·bo·nu·cle·o·tide (dē-ŏk′sē-rī′bō-nōō′klē-ə-tīd′) *n.* A nucleotide containing deoxyribose that is a constituent of DNA.

de·ox·y·ri·bose (dē-ŏk′sē-rī′bōs′) *n.* A sugar that is a constituent of DNA.

de·ox·y sugar (dē-ŏk′sē) *n.* A sugar containing fewer oxygen atoms than carbon atoms, resulting in one or more carbons in the molecule lacking an attached hydroxyl group.

de·ox·y·thy·mi·dyl·ic acid (dē-ŏk′sē-thī′mǐ-dǐl′ĭk) *n.* A nucleotide containing deoxyribose and formed in the hydrolysis of DNA.

Dep·a·kene (dĕp′ə-kēn′) A trademark for valproic acid.

Dep·a·kote (dĕp′ə-kōt′) A trademark for the drug divalproex sodium.

de·pend·ence (dǐ-pĕn′dəns) *n.* **1.** The state of being dependent, as for support. **2.** Subordination to someone or something needed or greatly desired. **3.** A compulsive or chronic need; an addiction. —**de·pend′en·cy** *n.*

de·pend·ent (dǐ-pĕn′dənt) *adj.* **1.** Contingent on or subordinate to another. **2.** Relying on or requiring the aid of another for support. **3.** Hanging down. —*n.* One who relies on another especially for financial support.

dependent drainage *n.* A procedure for draining a cavity or structure from its lowest part into a receptacle positioned at yet a level lower.

dependent edema *n.* A detectable increase in extracellular fluid volume localized in a dependent area such as a limb, characterized by swelling or pitting.

dependent personality *n.* A personality disorder characterized by a long-term pattern of passively allowing others to take responsibility for major areas of life, by a lack of self-confidence and independence, and of subordinating personal needs to the needs of others.

de·per·son·al·i·za·tion (dē-pûr′sə-nə-lǐ-zā′shən) *n.* A state in which the normal sense of personal identity and reality is lost, characterized by feelings that one's actions and speech cannot be controlled.

de·pig·men·ta·tion (dē-pĭg′mən-tā′shən, -mĕn-) *n.* The loss or removal of normal pigmentation.

dep·i·late (dĕp′ə-lāt′) *v.* To remove hair from the body.

dep·i·la·tion (dĕp′ə-lā′shən) *n.* See **epilation**.

de·pil·a·to·ry (dǐ-pĭl′ə-tôr′ē) *adj.* Having the capability to remove hair. —*n.* A preparation in the form of a liquid or cream that is used to remove unwanted hair from the body. Also called *epilatory.*

de·plete (dǐ-plēt′) *v.* **1.** To use up something, such as a nutrient. **2.** To empty something out, as the body of electrolytes.

de·ple·tion (dǐ-plē′shən) *n.* **1.** The act or process of depleting. **2.** The state of being depleted; exhaustion. **3.** Removal of or reduction in a body substance, such as blood, a fluid, or a nutrient.

de·plu·ma·tion (dē′ploo-mā′shən) *n.* The falling out or loss of the eyelashes.

de·po·lar·i·za·tion (dē-pō′lər-ĭ-zā′shən) *n.* Elimination or neutralization of polarity, as in nerve cells.

de·po·lar·iz·ing block (dē-pō′lə-rī′zĭng) *n.* Paralysis of skeletal muscle associated with loss of polarity of the motor end plate, as occurs following administration of succinylcholine.

de·pol·y·mer·ase (dē-pŏl′ə-mə-rās′, -rāz′) *n.* Any of various enzymes that catalyze the decomposition of macromolecules to simpler molecules.

de·pos·it (dǐ-pŏz′ĭt) *v.* **1.** To lay down or leave behind by a natural process. **2.** To become deposited; settle. —*n.* **1.** An accumulation of organic or inorganic material, such as a lipid, in a body tissue, structure, or fluid. **2.** A sediment or precipitate that has settled out of a solution.

de·pot injection (dē′pō, dĕp′ō) *n.* An injection of a substance in a form that tends to keep it at the site of injection so that absorption occurs over a prolonged period.

de·press (dǐ-prĕs′) *v.* **1.** To lower in spirits; deject. **2.** To cause to drop or sink; lower. **3.** To press down. **4.** To lessen the activity or force of something.

de·pres·sant (dǐ-prĕs′ənt) *adj.* Tending to lower the rate of vital physiological activities. —*n.* An agent, especially a drug, that decreases the rate of vital physiological activities.

de·pressed (dǐ-prĕst′) *adj.* **1.** Lower in amount, degree, or position. **2.** Sunk below the surrounding area. **3.** Flattened along the dorsal and ventral surfaces. **4.** Low in spirits; dejected. **5.** Suffering from psychological depression.

depressed skull fracture *n.* A fracture in which bone from part of the skull is pushed inward.

de·pres·sion (dǐ-prĕsh′ən) *n.* **1.** The act of depressing or the state of being depressed. **2.** A reduction in physiological vigor or activity. **3.** A lowering in amount, degree, or position. **4.** An inward displacement of a body part. **5.** A hollow or sunken area. **6.** The condition of feeling sad or despondent. **7.** A psychiatric disorder characterized by an inability to concentrate, insomnia, loss of appetite, anhedonia, feelings of extreme sadness, guilt, helplessness and hopelessness, and thoughts of death. Also called *clinical depression.*

de·pres·sive (dǐ-prĕs′ĭv) *adj.* **1.** Tending to depress or lower. **2.** Depressing; gloomy. **3.** Of or relating to psychological depression. —*n.* A person suffering from psychological depression.

de·pres·so·mo·tor (dǐ-prĕs′ə-mō′tər) *adj.* Retarding motor activity.

de·pres·sor (dǐ-prĕs′ər) *n.* **1.** Any of various muscles that act by drawing down a part of the body. **2.** Something that depresses or retards functional activity. **3.** An instrument used to push certain structures out of the way during an operation or examination. **4.** An agent that lowers blood pressure. Also called *hypotensor.* **5.** A nerve that when stimulated acts to lower arterial blood pressure.

depressor fiber *n.* Any of the sensory nerve fibers having pressure-sensitive nerve endings in the walls of certain arteries and capable of activating blood pressure-lowering brainstem mechanisms when stimulated by an increase in intra-arterial pressure.

depressor muscle of angle of mouth *n.* A muscle with origin from the lower border of the mandible, with insertion near the angle of the mouth, with nerve supply from the facial nerve, and whose action pulls down the corners of the mouth. Also called *triangular muscle.*

depressor muscle of eyebrow *n.* Muscular fibers of the orbital part of the orbicular muscle of the eye that insert in the eyebrow.

depressor muscle of lower lip *n.* A muscle with origin from the lower border of the mandible, with insertion into the skin of the lower lip, with nerve supply from the facial nerve, and whose action depresses the lower lip.

depressor muscle of septum *n.* A vertical fasciculus from the orbicular muscle of the mouth passing upward along the median line of the upper lip and inserted into the cartilaginous septum of the nose.

depressor nerve *n.* A nerve that when stimulated acts to lower arterial blood pressure.

dep·ri·va·tion (děp′rə-vā′shən) *n.* The absence, loss, or withholding of something needed.

de·prive (dĭ-prīv′) *v.* **1.** To take something from someone or something. **2.** To keep from possessing or enjoying something.

de·pro·gram (dē-prō′grăm′, -grəm) *v.* To counteract or try to counteract the effect of an indoctrination, especially a religious or cult indoctrination.

depth (děpth) *n.* The extent, measurement, or dimension downward, backward, or inward.

depth of focus *n.* See **focal depth.**

depth perception *n.* The ability to perceive spatial relationships, especially distances between objects, in three dimensions.

depth psychology *n.* **1.** Psychology of the unconscious mind. **2.** Psychoanalysis.

de Quer·vain's disease (də kâr-vănz′, kĕr-vănz′) *n.* Fibrosis of the sheath of a tendon of the thumb.

de·range·ment (dĭ-rānj′mənt) *n.* **1.** Disturbance of the regular order or arrangement of parts in a system. **2.** Mental disorder; insanity. —**de·range′** *v.*

Der·cum's disease (dûr′kəmz) *n.* See **adiposis dolorosa.**

de·re·al·i·za·tion (dē-rē′ə-lĭ-zā′shən) *n.* The feeling that things in one's surroundings are strange, unreal, or somehow altered, as seen in schizophrenia.

de·re·ism (dē-rē′ĭz′əm, dē′rē-) *n.* Mental activity that is absorbed in fantasy, lacking any connection to the external world or reality. —**de′re·is′tic** *adj.*

der·en·ceph·a·ly (dĕr′ĕn-sĕf′ə-lē) *n.* A malformation in which the skull bones are underdeveloped and the cervical vertebrae are bifurcated, with a rudimentary brain usually resting in the cleft.

de·re·pres·sion (dē′rĭ-prĕsh′ən) *n.* The activation of an operator gene by the deactivation of a repressor gene. —**de′re·press′** (-prĕs′) *v.*

de·riv·a·tive (dĭ-rĭv′ə-tĭv) *n.* **1.** Something obtained or produced by modification of something else. **2.** A chemical compound that may be produced from another compound of similar structure in one or more steps. —*adj.* Resulting from, characterized by, or employing derivation.

de·rive (dĭ-rīv′) *v.* **1.** To obtain or receive from a source. **2.** To produce or obtain a chemical compound from another substance by chemical reaction.

–derm *suff.* Skin; covering: *blastoderm.*

der·ma (dûr′mə) *n.* See **dermis.**

derma– *or* **derm–***or* **dermo–** *pref.* Skin: *dermabrasion.*

–derma *suff.* Skin; skin disease: *scleroderma.*

der·ma·brad·er (dûr′mə-brā′dər) *n.* A motor-driven device used in dermabrasion.

der·ma·bra·sion (dûr′mə-brā′zhən) *n.* A surgical procedure designed to remove skin imperfections, such

as scars, by abrading the surface of the skin with fine sandpaper or wire brushes. Also called *planing.*

Der·ma·cen·tor (dûr′mə-sĕn′tər) *n.* A genus of hard ticks in the family Ixodidae, including certain species that transmit disease.

Dermacentor an·der·so·ni (ăn′dər-sō′nī′) *n.* A tick that is the vector of Rocky Mountain spotted fever in the Rocky Mountains and also transmits tularemia and causes tick paralysis; the Rocky Mountain wood tick.

Dermacentor var·i·a·bi·lis (văr′ē-ā′bə-lĭs) *n.* A tick that transmits tularemia and is the principal vector of Rocky Mountain spotted fever in the central and eastern US; the American dog tick.

der·mal (dûr′məl) *or* **der·mic** (-mĭk) *adj.* Of or relating to the skin or dermis.

dermal graft *n.* A skin graft made with a thin split-thickness graft of dermis.

dermal papilla *n.* Any of the superficial projections of the corium or dermis that interlock with recesses in the overlying epidermis, contain vascular loops and specialized nerve endings, and are arranged in ridgelike lines most prominent in the hand and foot. Also called *papilla of corium.*

dermal sinus *n.* A sinus lined with epidermis and skin appendages extending from the skin to a deeper structure, especially the spinal cord.

dermat– *pref.* Variant of **dermato–.**

der·ma·tan sulfate (dûr′mə-tăn′) *n.* A mucopolysaccharide that is a structural component of certain body tissues, especially the skin.

der·mat·ic (dər-măt′ĭk) *adj.* Dermal.

der·ma·ti·tis (dûr′mə-tī′tĭs) *n.,* pl. **-ti·tis·es** or **-tit·i·des** (-tĭt′ĭ-dēz′) Inflammation of the skin.

dermatitis ex·fo·li·a·ti·va in·fan·tum (ĕks-fō′lē-ə-tī′-və ĭn-făn′təm) *n.* See **impetigo neonatorum.**

dermatitis her·pet·i·for·mis (hər-pĕt′ə-fôr′mĭs) *n.* A chronic disease of the skin marked by severe itching and the extensive eruption of vesicles and groups of papules. Also called *Duhring's disease.*

dermatitis med·i·ca·men·to·sa (mĕd′ĭ-kə-mən-tō′sə) *n.* See **drug eruption.**

dermatitis pap·il·lar·is cap·il·li·ti·i (păp′ə-lâr′ĭs kăp′ə-lĭsh′ē-ī′) *n.* See **acne keloid.**

dermatitis re·pens (rē′pənz) *n.* See **acrodermatitis continua.**

dermatitis ver·ru·co·sa (vĕr′ə-kō′sə) *n.* See **chromomycosis.**

dermato– *or* **dermat–** *pref.* Skin: *dermatophyte.*

der·ma·to·au·to·plas·ty (dûr′mə-tō-ô′tō-plăs′tē) *n.* The grafting of skin from one part of the body to another.

Der·ma·to·bi·a (dûr′mə-tō′bē-ə) *n.* A genus of botflies, one species of which has larvae that develop in boil-like cysts in the skin of humans, many domestic animals, and some fowl.

der·ma·to·bi·a·sis (dûr′mə-tō-bī′ə-sĭs) *n.* The infection of humans and animals with larvae of *Dermatobia hominis.*

der·ma·to·fi·bro·ma (dûr′mə-tō-fī-brō′mə) *n.* A benign skin nodule consisting mostly of fibrous tissue. Also called *sclerosing hemangioma.*

der·ma·to·fi·bro·sar·co·ma (dûr′mə-tō-fī′brō-sär-kō′mə) *n.* A fibrosarcoma of the skin.

dermatofibrosarcoma pro·tu·ber·ans (prō-tōō′bə-rănz′) *n.* A slow-growing dermal neoplasm consisting of one or more purplish nodules that tends to recur but usually does not metastasize.

der·ma·to·glyph·ics (dûr′mə-tō-glĭf′ĭks) *n.* **1.** The patterns of lines and ridges on the skin of the fingertips, palms, and soles, used to establish the identity of individuals or as an indicator of chromosomal abnormalities. **2.** The study of such patterns.

der·ma·tog·ra·phism (dûr′mə-tŏg′rə-fĭz′əm) *n.* A form of urticaria in which skin welts develop along the lines where one has been stroked or scratched. Also called *dermographia, dermographism.*

der·ma·to·het·er·o·plas·ty (dûr′mə-tō-hĕt′ər-ə-plăs′tē) *n.* The grafting of skin obtained from a member of a different species.

der·ma·tol·o·gist (dûr′mə-tŏl′ə-jĭst) *n.* A physician who specializes in the diagnosis and treatment of skin disorders.

der·ma·tol·o·gy (dûr′mə-tŏl′ə-jē) *n.* The branch of medicine that deals with the diagnosis and treatment of skin diseases. —**der′ma·to·log′i·cal** (-tə-lŏj′ĭ-kəl), **der′ma·to·log′ic** *adj.*

der·ma·tol·y·sis (dûr′mə-tŏl′ĭ-sĭs) *n.* Any of various disorders characterized by loosening or hanging of the skin.

der·ma·tome (dûr′mə-tōm′) *n.* **1.** An area of skin innervated by sensory fibers from a single spinal nerve. **2.** An instrument used in cutting thin slices of the skin, as for skin grafts. **3.** The part of a mesodermal somite from which the dermis develops. Also called *cutis plate.*

der·ma·to·meg·a·ly (dûr′mə-tō-mĕg′ə-lē) *n.* A congenital defect in which the skin hangs in folds.

der·ma·to·mere (dûr′mə-tə-mîr′, dər-măt′ə-) *n.* A metameric area of the embryonic integument.

der·ma·to·my·co·sis (dûr′mə-tō-mī-kō′sĭs) *n.* An infection of the skin caused by dermatophytes or other fungi.

der·ma·to·my·o·ma (dûr′mə-tō-mī-ō′mə) *n.* A leiomyoma located in the skin.

der·ma·to·my·o·si·tis (dûr′mə-tō-mī′ə-sī′tĭs) *n.* A progressive inflammatory condition characterized by muscular weakness, a skin rash, and edema of the eyelids and periorbital tissue.

der·ma·to·neu·ro·sis (dûr′mə-tō-nōō-rō′sĭs) *n.* A skin eruption caused by emotional distress.

der·ma·to·path·ic lymphadenopathy (dûr′mə-tō-păth′ĭk) *n.* Enlargement of lymph nodes with proliferation of histiocytes and macrophages containing fat and melanin, secondary to various forms of dermatitis. Also called *dermatopathic lymphadenitis.*

der·ma·to·pa·thol·o·gy (dûr′mə-tō-pă-thŏl′ə-jē) *n.* The histopathology of skin lesions.

der·ma·top·a·thy (dûr′mə-tŏp′ə-thē) *n.* A disease of the skin. Also called *dermopathy.*

Der·ma·toph·a·goi·des pter·o·nys·si·nus (dûr′mə-tŏf′ə-goi′dēz′ tĕr′ə-nĭ-sī′nəs) *n.* A cosmopolitan species of mites that are found in house dust and are a common cause of atopic asthma.

der·mat·o·phyte (dûr-măt′ə-fīt′, dûr′mə-tə-) *n.* Any of various fungi causing parasitic infections of the skin, hair, or nails. —**der·mat′o·phyt′ic** (-fĭt′ĭk) *adj.*

der·ma·to·phy·tid (dûr′mə-tō-fī′tĭd, -tŏf′ĭ-tĭd) *n.* An allergic manifestation of dermatophytosis characterized by lesions that begin as vesicles on the hands and arms and may spread widely but do not contain any of the fungus.

der·ma·to·phy·to·sis (dûr′mə-tō′fī-tō′sĭs) *n.* An infection of the skin, hair, or nails caused by a dermatophyte and characterized by redness of the skin, small papular vesicles, fissures, and scaling.

der·ma·to·plas·ty (dûr′mə-tō-plăs′tē) *n.* The use of skin grafts in plastic surgery to correct defects or replace skin destroyed by injury or disease. Also called *dermoplasty.* —**der′ma·to·plas′tic** (-plăs′tĭk) *adj.*

der·ma·to·pol·y·neu·ri·tis (dûr′mə-tō-pŏl′ē-nōō-rī′tĭs) *n.* See **acrodynia** (sense 1).

der·ma·to·scle·ro·sis (dûr′mə-tō-sklə-rō′sĭs) *n.* See **scleroderma.**

der·ma·to·sis (dûr′mə-tō′sĭs) *n., pl.* **-ses** (-sēz) A skin disease, especially one that is not accompanied by inflammation.

dermatosis med·i·ca·men·to·sa (mĕd′ĭ-kə-mən-tō′-sə) *n.* See **drug eruption.**

dermatosis pap·u·lo·sa ni·gra (păp′yə-lō′sə nī′grə, nĭg′rə) *n.* A skin disorder seen in Blacks, similar to seborrheic keratosis and characterized by dark-brown papular lesions on the face and upper body.

der·ma·to·ther·a·py (dûr′mə-tō-thĕr′ə-pē) *n.* The treatment of skin diseases.

der·ma·to·trop·ic (dûr′mə-tō-trŏp′ĭk, -trō′pĭk) *n.* Having an affinity for the skin.

–dermatous *suff.* Having a specified kind of skin: *sclerodermatous.*

der·mic (dûr′mĭk) *adj.* Variant of **dermal.**

der·mis (dûr′mĭs) *n.* The sensitive connective tissue layer of the skin located below the epidermis, containing nerve endings, sweat and sebaceous glands, and blood and lymph vessels. Also called *corium, cutis vera, derma.*

dermo– *pref.* Variant of **derma–.**

der·mo·blast (dûr′mə-blăst′) *n.* The part of the mesoderm that develops into the dermis.

der·mo·graph·i·a (dûr′mə-grăf′ē-ə) *n.* See **dermatographism.**

der·mog·ra·phism (dər-mŏg′rə-fĭz′əm) *n.* See **dermatographism.**

der·moid (dûr′moid′) *adj.* Resembling skin; skinlike. —*n.* See **dermoid cyst.**

dermoid cyst *n.* A benign tumor resulting from abnormal embryonic development, occurring in the skin or ovary, and consisting of displaced ectodermal structures along the lines of embryonic fusion. Also called *dermoid, dermoid tumor.*

der·moid·ec·to·my (dûr′moi-dĕk′tə-mē) *n.* Surgical removal of a dermoid cyst.

dermoid tumor *n.* See **dermoid cyst.**

der·mop·a·thy (dər-mŏp′ə-thē) *n.* See **dermatopathy.**

der·mo·plas·ty (dûr′mə-plăs′tē) *n.* See **dermatoplasty.**

der·mo·trop·ic (dûr′mə-trŏp′ĭk, -trō′pĭk) *adj.* Having an affinity for the skin.

der·mo·vas·cu·lar (dûr′mō-văs′kyə-lər) *adj.* Of or relating to the blood vessels of the skin.

DES (dē′ē-ĕs′) *n.* Diethylstilbestrol; a synthetic nonsteroidal substance having estrogenic properties and once used to treat menstrual disorders. It is no longer used due to the incidence of certain vaginal cancers in the daughters of women so treated.

de·sat·u·ra·tion (dē-săch′ə-rā′shən) *n.* Conversion of a saturated compound to an unsaturated compound by the removal of hydrogen.

De·sault's bandage (də-sōz′) *n.* A bandage that binds the elbow to a person's side and is used for fractures of the clavicle.

des·ce·me·ti·tis (dĕs′ə-mĭ-tī′tĭs) *n.* Inflammation of Descemet's membrane on the posterior surface of the cornea.

des·ce·met·o·cele (dĕs′ə-mĕt′ə-sēl′) *n.* A hernia of Descemet's membrane.

Des·ce·met's membrane (dĕs′ə-māz′) *n.* See **limiting layer of cornea** (sense 2).

de·scend·ing artery of knee (dĭ-sĕn′dĭng) *n.* An artery with origin in the femoral artery, with distribution to the knee joint and adjacent parts, and with anastomoses to the several genicula arteries, and the lateral circumflex femoral and the anterior tibial recurrent arteries.

descending colon *n.* The part of the colon extending from the left colic flexure to the pelvic brim.

descending degeneration *n.* The degeneration of nerve fibers starting at the point of injury and progressing away from the brain or spinal cord.

descending scapular artery *n.* See **dorsal scapular artery.**

de·scen·sus (dĭ-sĕn′səs) *n.* The process of descending or falling from a higher position.

descensus testis *n.* The descent of the testis from the abdomen into the scrotum, normally occurring during the seventh and eighth months of fetal life.

de·scent (dĭ-sĕnt′) *n.* **1.** The process of descending or falling down from a higher position. **2.** The passage of the presenting part of the fetus into and through the birth canal.

de·sen·si·ti·za·tion (dē-sĕn′sĭ-tĭ-zā′shən) *n.* **1.** The reduction or abolition of allergic sensitivity or reactions to a specific allergen. Also called *antianaphylaxis.* **2.** The mitigation of an individual's emotional response to a distressing stimulus by repeated exposure to or imagination of that stimulus.

de·sen·si·tize (dē-sĕn′sĭ-tīz′) *v.* **1.** To render insensitive or less sensitive, as a nerve or tooth. **2.** To make an individual nonreactive or insensitive to an antigen. **3.** To make a person emotionally insensitive or unresponsive, as by long exposure or repeated shocks.

des·ert fever (dĕz′ərt) *n.* See **primary coccidioidomycosis.**

de·sex (dē-sĕks′) *v.* To remove part or all of the reproductive organs of.

des·ic·cant (dĕs′ĭ-kənt) *n.* A substance, such as calcium oxide or silica gel, that has a high affinity for water and is used as a drying agent. —*adj.* Causing or promoting dryness.

des·ic·cate (dĕs′ĭ-kāt′) *v.* To dry thoroughly; render free from moisture.

des·ic·ca·tion (dĕs′ĭ-kā′shən) *n.* The process of being desiccated. —**des′ic·ca·tive** (-tĭv) *adj.*

de·sign·er drug (dĭ-zī′nər) *n.* A drug with properties and effects similar to a known hallucinogen or narcotic but having a slightly altered chemical structure, especially such a drug created in order to evade restrictions against illegal substances.

de·sip·ra·mine hydrochloride (dĭ-zĭp′rə-mēn, dĕz′ə-prăm′ĭn) *n.* A tricyclic antidepressant that selectively blocks reuptake of norepinephrine.

Des·i·tin (dĕs′ĭ-tn) An over-the-counter ointment containing zinc oxide.

des·mi·tis (dĕz-mī′tĭs) *n.* The inflammation of a ligament.

desmo– *or* **desm–** *pref.* **1.** Bond; adhesion: *desmosome.* **2.** Ligament; connective tissue: *desmogenous.*

des·mo·cra·ni·um (dĕz′mō-krā′nē-əm) *n.* The mass of embryonic mesenchymal cells that develop into the cranium.

des·mog·e·nous (dĕz-mŏj′ə-nəs) *adj.* Originating from or caused by connective tissue or ligament, as a deformity.

des·moid (dĕz′moid′) *adj.* Fibrous or ligamentous. —*n.* A benign tumor of firm scarlike connective tissue resulting from the proliferation of fibroblasts and occurring most frequently in the abdominal muscles of women who have borne children. Also called *desmoid tumor.*

des·mo·lase (dĕz′mə-lās′, -lāz′) *n.* Any of various enzymes that break or form carbon-to-carbon bonds in a molecule and that play a role in respiration and fermentation.

des·mop·a·thy (dĕz-mŏp′ə-thē) *n.* A disease of the ligaments.

des·mo·pla·sia (dĕz′mə-plā′zhə) *n.* The formation and proliferation of fibroblasts and fibrous connective tissue, especially in tumors.

des·mo·plas·tic (dĕz′mə-plăs′tĭk) *adj.* **1.** Producing or forming adhesions. **2.** Causing fibrosis in the vascular stroma of a neoplasm.

desmoplastic fibroma *n.* A benign fibrous tumor of bone affecting children and young adults.

desmoplastic trichoepithelioma *n.* A solitary, hard, annular, centrally depressed papule, occurring usually in women on the face, consisting of dermal strands of basaloid cells and small keratinous cysts within desmoplastic stroma.

des·mo·pres·sin acetate (dĕs′mə-prĕs′ĭn) *n.* An analog of vasopressin, used as an antidiuretic and to manage bleeding in some forms of hemophilia and in von Willebrand's disease.

des·mo·some (dĕz′mə-sōm′) *n.* A structure that forms the site of adhesion between two cells, consisting of a dense plate in each adjacent cell separated by a thin layer of extracellular material. Also called *macula adherens.*

Des·o·gen (dĕs′ə-jən) A trademark for an oral contraceptive containing ethinyl estradiol and desogestrel.

des·o·ges·trel (dĕs′ə-jĕs′trəl) A synthetic progestin used with ethinyl estradiol in birth control pills.

des·o·nide (dĕs′ə-nīd′) *n.* An anti-inflammatory corticosteroid used in topical preparations.

des·ox·i·met·a·sone (dĕs-ŏk′sē-mĕt′ə-sōn′) *n.* An anti-inflammatory corticosteroid containing fluorine and used in topical preparations.

desoxy– *pref.* Variant of **deoxy–**.

de·spe·ci·a·tion (dē-spē′shē-ā′shən, -sē-) *n.* **1.** The alteration or loss of species characteristics. **2.** The removal of species-specific antigenic properties from a foreign protein.

des·qua·mate (dĕs′kwə-māt′) *v.* To shed, peel, or come off in scales. Used of skin.

des·qua·ma·tion (dĕs′kwə-mā′shən) *n.* **1.** The shedding or peeling of the epidermis in scales. **2.** The shedding of the outer layer of a surface.

des·quam·a·tive (dĕs-kwăm′ə-tĭv, dĕs′kwə-mā′tĭv) *adj.* Relating to or marked by desquamation.

desquamative inflammatory vaginitis *n.* Acute inflammation of the vagina having no known cause and characterized by a grayish pseudomembrane, a purulent discharge, and easy bleeding on trauma.

de·sul·fur·ase (dē-sŭl′fə-rās′, -rāz′) *n.* An enzyme that catalyzes the removal of sulfur, usually as hydrogen sulfide, from organic compounds. Also called *desulfhydrase.*

Des·y·rel (dĕs′ûr-əl) A trademark for the drug trazodone hydrochloride.

DET (dē′ē-tē′) *n.* Diethyltryptamine; a hallucinogenic agent similar to DMT.

det. *abbr. Latin* detur (let there be given; give)

de·tach (dĭ-tăch′) *v.* **1.** To separate or unfasten; disconnect. **2.** To remove from association or union with something.

de·tached (dĭ-tăcht′) *adj.* **1.** Separated; disconnected. **2.** Standing apart from others; separate.

detached retina *n.* See **detachment of retina**.

de·tach·ment (dĭ-tăch′mənt) *n.* **1.** The act or process of disconnecting or detaching; separation. **2.** The state of being separate or detached. **3.** Indifference to or remoteness from the concerns of others; aloofness. **4.** Absence of prejudice or bias; disinterest.

detachment of retina *n.* The separation of the sensory layer of the retina from the pigment layer. Also called *detached retina, retinal detachment.*

de·ter·gent (dĭ-tûr′jənt) *n.* A cleansing substance that acts similarly to soap but is made from chemical compounds rather than fats and lye. —*adj.* Having cleansing power.

de·te·ri·o·rate (dĭ-tîr′ē-ə-rāt′) *v.* **1.** To grow worse in function or condition. **2.** To weaken or disintegrate.

de·te·ri·o·ra·tion (dĭ-tîr′ē-ə-rā′shən) *n.* The process or condition of becoming worse.

de·ter·mi·nant (dĭ-tûr′mə-nənt) *n.* **1.** An influencing or determining element or factor. **2.** Antigenic determinant. —*adj.* Tending or serving to determine.

de·ter·mi·na·tion (dĭ-tûr′mə-nā′shən) *n.* **1.** A change for the better or for the worse in the course of a disease. **2.** A fixed movement or tendency toward an object or end. **3.** The ascertaining of the quantity, quality, position, or character of something.

de·ter·min·ism (dĭ-tûr′mə-nĭz′əm) *n.* The philosophical doctrine that every event, act, and decision is the inevitable consequence of antecedents, such as genetic and environmental influences, that are independent of the human will.

de·tox (dē-tŏks′) *v.* To subject to detoxification. —*n.* (dē′tŏks′) A section of a hospital or clinic in which patients are detoxified.

de·tox·i·cate (dē-tŏk′sĭ-kāt′) *v.* To detoxify. —**de·tox′·i·ca′tion** *n.*

de·tox·i·fi·ca·tion (dē-tŏk′sə-fĭ-kā′shən) *n.* **1.** The process of detoxifying. **2.** The state or condition of being detoxified. **3.** The metabolic process by which the toxic qualities of a poison or toxin are reduced by the body. **4.** A medically supervised treatment program for alcohol or drug addiction designed to purge the body of intoxicating or addictive substances and used as a first step in overcoming physiological or psychological addiction.

de·tox·i·fy (dē-tŏk′sə-fī′) *v.* **1.** To counteract or destroy the toxic properties of a substance. **2.** To remove the effects of poison from something, such as the blood. **3.** To treat a person for alcohol or drug dependence, usually under a medically supervised program designed to rid the body of intoxicating or addictive substances.

de·tri·tion (dĭ-trĭsh′ən) *n.* The act of wearing away by friction.

de·tri·tus (dĭ-trī′təs) *n., pl.* **detritus** Loose matter resulting from the wearing away or disintegration of tissue or other material.

de·tru·sor (dĭ-trōō′zər) *n.* A muscle that pushes down, such as the muscle that expels urine from the bladder.

de·tu·mes·cence (dē′tōō-mĕs′əns) *n.* Reduction, subsidence, or lessening of a swelling, especially the restoration of a swollen organ or part to normal size.

deu·ter·a·no·pi·a (dōō′tər-ə-nō′pē-ə) *n.* A form of colorblindness characterized by insensitivity to green. —**deu′ter·a·nop′ic** (-nŏp′ĭk, -nō′pĭk) *adj.*

deu·te·ri·um (dōō-tîr′ē-əm) *n.* An isotope of hydrogen with one proton and one neutron in the nucleus having an atomic weight of 2.014. Also called *heavy hydrogen, hydrogen-2.*

deutero– or **deuter–** *pref.* Second; secondary: *deuteropathy.*

Deu·ter·o·my·ce·tes (dōō′tə-rō-mī-sē′tēz′) *n.* See **Fungi Imperfecti**.

deu·te·rop·a·thy (dōō′tə-rŏp′ə-thē) *n.* A disease that occurs secondary to another. —**deu′ter·o·path′ic** (-ə-păth′ĭk) *adj.*

deu·ter·o·plasm (dōō′tə-rō-plăz′əm) *n.* See **deutoplasm**.

deuto– or **deut–** *pref.* Second; secondary: *deutoplasm.*

deu·to·plasm (dōō′tə-plăz′əm) *n.* The nutritive substances in the cytoplasm, especially the yolk of an ovum. Also called *deuteroplasm.*

de·vas·cu·lar·i·za·tion (dē-văs′kyə-lər-ĭ-zā′shən) *n.* The interruption of the blood supply to a part of the body by the blocking or destroying of blood vessels.

de·vel·op (dĭ-vĕl′əp) *v.* **1.** To progress from earlier to later stages of a life cycle. **2.** To progress from earlier to later or from simpler to more complex stages of evolution. **3.** To aid in the growth of; strengthen. **4.** To grow by degrees into a more advanced or mature state. **5.** To become affected with a disease; contract.

de·vel·op·ment (dǐ-vĕl′əp-mənt) *n*. **1**. The act of developing. **2**. The state of being developed. **3**. A significant event, occurrence, or change. **4**. The natural progression from a previous, simpler, or embryonic stage to a later, more complex, or adult stage. —**de·vel′op·men′-tal** (-mĕn′tl) *adj*.

developmental age *n*. **1**. The age of a fetus from conception to any point in time prior to birth. Also called *fetal age*. **2**. *Abbr*. **DA** An index of development stated as the age in years of an individual and determined by specified standardized measurements such as motor and mental tests and body measurements.

developmental anatomy *n*. The study of the structural changes of an individual from fertilization to adulthood.

developmental anomaly *n*. An anomaly that is established during intrauterine life.

developmental delay *n*. A chronological delay in the appearance of normal developmental milestones achieved during infancy and early childhood, caused by organic, psychological, or environmental factors.

developmental disability *n*. A cognitive, emotional, or physical impairment, especially one related to abnormal sensory or motor development, that appears in infancy or childhood and involves a failure or delay in progressing through the normal developmental stages of childhood.

developmental groove *n*. One of the fine lines found in the enamel of a tooth that mark the junction of the lobes of the crown in its development. Also called *developmental line*.

developmental psychology *n*. The branch of psychology concerned with the study of behavioral changes in an individual from birth until death.

de·vi·ant (dē′vē-ənt) *adj*. Differing from a norm or from the accepted standards of a society. —*n*. One that differs from a norm, especially a person whose behavior and attitudes differ from accepted social standards. —**de′vi·ance, de′vi·an·cy** *n*.

de·vi·a·tion (dē′vē-ā′shən) *n*. **1**. A turning away or aside from a normal course. **2**. An abnormality. **3**. Deviant behavior or attitudes. **4**. The difference, especially the absolute difference, between one number in a set and the mean of the set.

de·vice (dǐ-vīs′) *n*. A contrivance or an invention serving a particular purpose, especially a machine used to perform one or more relatively simple tasks.

De·vic's disease (də-vēks′, dĕ-) *n*. See **neuromyelitis optica**.

dev·il's grip (dĕv′əlz) *n*. See **epidemic pleurodynia**.

de·vi·om·e·ter (dē′vē-ŏm′ĭ-tər) *n*. A type of strabismometer.

de·vi·tal·ized (dē-vīt′l-īzd′) *adj*. Devoid of vitality or life, as a tooth with destroyed pulp.

devitalized pulp *n*. See **necrotic pulp**.

De Vries (də vrēs′), **Hugo Marie** 1848–1935. Dutch botanist who studied evolution by observing mutations rather than natural selection. He was an early proponent of the works of Gregor Mendel.

dex·a·meth·a·sone (dĕk′sə-mĕth′ə-sōn′, -zōn′) *n*. A synthetic glucocorticoid used primarily in the treatment of inflammatory disorders.

dex·am·phet·a·mine sulfate (dĕk′săm-fĕt′ə-mēn′, -mĭn) *n*. See **dextroamphetamine sulfate**.

Dex·e·drine (dĕk′sĭ-drĭn, -drēn′) A trademark for the drug dextroamphetamine sulfate.

dex·pan·the·nol (dĕks-păn′thə-nôl′, -nōl′) *n*. A bitter, viscous liquid that is synthetically derived and used therapeutically as a cholinergic agent and as a supplemental source of pantothetic acid.

dex·ter (dĕk′stər) *adj*. Of or located on the right side.

dextr– *pref*. Variant of **dextro–**.

dex·trad (dĕk′străd′) *adj*. Toward the right side.

dex·tral (dĕk′strəl) *adj*. **1**. Of, facing, or located on the right side; right. **2**. Right-handed.

dex·tral·i·ty (dĕk-străl′ĭ-tē) *n*. Preference for the right hand in performing manual tasks; right-handedness.

dex·tran (dĕk′străn′, -strən) *n*. Any of a group of long-chain polymers of glucose with various molecular weights that are used in isotonic sodium chloride solution for the treatment of shock, in distilled water for the relief of the edema of nephrosis, and as plasma volume expanders.

dex·tran·ase (dĕk′strə-nās′, -nāz′) *n*. An enzyme that catalyzes the hydrolysis of dextran.

dex·trase (dĕk′strās′, -strāz′) *n*. A complex of enzymes that catalyze the conversion of dextrose to lactic acid.

dex·trin (dĕk′strĭn) *or* **dex·trine** (dĕk′strĭn, -strēn′) *n*. Any of various soluble polysaccharides obtained from starch by the application of heat or acids and used mainly as adhesives and thickening agents.

dextrin 6-alpha-glucosidase *n*. Amylo-1,6-glucosidase.

dex·trin·ase (dĕk′strə-nās′, -nāz′) *n*. An enzyme that catalyzes the hydrolysis of dextrins.

dextrin dextranase *n*. A transferase enzyme that catalyzes the synthesis of dextran from dextrin.

dex·tri·no·sis (dĕk′strə-nō′sĭs) *n*. See **glycogenosis**.

dex·tri·nu·ri·a (dĕk′strə-nŏŏr′ē-ə) *n*. The presence of dextrin in the urine.

dextro– *or* **dextr–** *pref*. **1**. On or to the right; right: *dextroposition*. **2**. Dextrorotatory: *dextrose*.

dex·tro·am·phet·a·mine sulfate (dĕk′strō-ăm-fĕt′ə-mēn′, -mĭn) *n*. A white crystalline isomer of amphetamine that acts as a central nervous stimulant and is used to treat narcolepsy and attention deficit hyperactivity disorder. Also called *dexamphetamine sulfate*.

dex·tro·car·di·a (dĕk′strō-kär′dē-ə) *n*. The displacement of the heart to the right, either as dextroposition of a normal heart, or as cardiac heterotaxia, in which the left and right chambers are transposed.

dex·tro·cer·e·bral (dĕk′strō-sĕr′ə-brəl, -sə-rē′-) *adj*. Relating to the right cerebral hemisphere.

dex·tro·cli·na·tion (dĕk′strō-klə-nā′shən) *n*. See **dextrotorsion** (sense 2).

dex·troc·u·lar (dĕk-strŏk′yə-lər) *adj*. Right-eyed.

dex·tro·gas·tri·a (dĕk′strō-găs′trē-ə) *n*. The displacement of the stomach to the right.

dex·tro·gy·ra·tion (dĕk′strō-jī-rā′shən) *n*. A twisting to the right, as of a plane of polarized light.

dex·tro·man·u·al (dĕk′strō-măn′yōō-əl) *adj*. Being or tending to be right-handed.

dex·tro·me·thor·phan (dĕk′strō-mə-thôr′făn) *n*. A drug that is used in its hydrobromide form as a cough suppressant and that is less addictive and has fewer side effects than codeine.

dex·trop·e·dal (děk-strŏp′ĭ-dl, děk′strō-pěd′l, -pēd′l) *adj.* Being or tending to be right-footed.

dex·tro·po·si·tion (děk′strō-pə-zĭsh′ən) *n.* The displacement of a body part to the right.

dex·tro·ro·ta·to·ry (děk′strə-rō′tə-tôr′ē) *or* **dex·tro·ro·ta·ry** (-rō′tə-rē) *adj.* Turning or rotating the plane of polarization of light to the right or clockwise, as for solutions or isomers, usually designated as *d-* in chemical names.

dex·trose (děk′strōs′) *n.* The dextrorotatory form of glucose found naturally in animal and plant tissue and derived synthetically from starch.

dex·tro·sin·is·tral (děk′strō-sĭn′ĭ-strəl, -sĭ-nĭs′trəl) *adj.* Extending from right to left.

dex·tro·tor·sion (děk′strō-tôr′shən) *n.* **1.** A twisting to the right. **2.** Rotation of the upper poles of both corneas to the right. Also called *dextroclination.*

dex·tro·trop·ic (děk′strō-trŏp′ĭk, -trō′pĭk) *adj.* Turning to the right.

dex·tro·ver·sion (děk′strə-vûr′zhən) *n.* **1.** A turning to the right, as of the eyes. **2.** Rotation of both eyes to the right.

df *abbr.* decayed and filled (deciduous teeth)

DF *abbr.* decayed and filled (permanent teeth)

DHEA *abbr.* dehydroepiandrosterone

DHT *abbr.* dihydrotachysterol; dihydrotestosterone

di– *pref.* **1.** Two; twice; double: *dichromatic.* **2.** Containing two atoms, radicals, or groups: *diiodide.*

dia– *or* **di–** *pref.* **1.** Through: *diapedesis.* **2.** Across: *diameter.*

Di·a·be·ta (dī′ə-bā′tə) A trademark for the drug glyburide.

di·a·be·tes (dī′ə-bē′tĭs, -tēz) *n.* Any of several metabolic disorders marked by excessive discharge of urine and persistent thirst, especially one of the two types of diabetes mellitus.

diabetes in·sip·i·dus (ĭn-sĭp′ĭ-dəs) *n.* A chronic metabolic disorder characterized by intense thirst and excessive urination, caused by a deficiency of the pituitary hormone vasopressin.

diabetes in·ter·mit·tens (ĭn′tər-mĭt′ənz) *n.* Diabetes mellitus in which there are periods of relatively normal carbohydrate metabolism followed by relapses to a diabetic state.

diabetes mel·li·tus (mə-lī′təs, měl′ĭ-) *n. Abbr.* **DM** **1.** A severe, chronic form of diabetes caused by insufficient production of insulin and resulting in abnormal metabolism of carbohydrates, fats, and proteins. The disease typically appears in childhood or adolescence and is characterized by increased sugar levels in the blood and urine, excessive thirst, frequent urination, acidosis, and wasting. Also called *insulin-dependent diabetes, type 1 diabetes.* **2.** A mild form of diabetes that typically appears first in adulthood and is exacerbated by obesity and an inactive lifestyle. This disease often has no symptoms, is usually diagnosed by tests that indicate glucose intolerance, and is treated with changes in diet and an exercise regimen. Also called *adult-onset diabetes, late-onset diabetes, non-insulin-dependent diabetes mellitus, type 2 diabetes.*

di·a·bet·ic (dī′ə-bět′ĭk) *adj.* **1.** Relating to, having, or resulting from diabetes. **2.** Intended for use by a person with diabetes. —*n.* One who has diabetes.

diabetic acidosis *n.* See **diabetic ketoacidosis.**

diabetic coma *n.* A coma that develops in severe and inadequately treated cases of diabetes mellitus. Also called *Kussmaul's coma.*

diabetic dermopathy *n.* A skin disorder most commonly occurring on the shins of people with diabetes mellitus, characterized by discolored patches and small papules that often become pigmented and ulcerated and result in scars.

diabetic diet *n.* A diet for a diabetic person, with the aim of maintaining normal blood sugar levels.

diabetic glomerulosclerosis *n.* Rounded hyaline or laminated nodules in the periphery of the renal glomeruli with capillary basement membrane thickening and increased mesangial matrix. Also called *intercapillary glomerulosclerosis.*

diabetic ketoacidosis *n. Abbr.* **DKA** Decreased pH and bicarbonate concentration in the body fluids caused by accumulation of ketone bodies in uncontrolled diabetes mellitus. Also called *diabetic acidosis.*

diabetic neuropathy *n.* A combined sensory and motor neuropathy, usual symmetric and segmental and involving autonomic neurons, seen frequently in older diabetic patients.

diabetic retinopathy *n.* Retinal changes occurring in long-term diabetes and characterized by punctate hemorrhages, microaneurysms, and sharply defined waxy exudates.

di·a·be·to·gen·ic (dī′ə-bē′tə-jěn′ĭk, -bět′ə-) *adj.* Causing diabetes.

di·a·be·tog·en·ous (dī′ə-bĭ-tŏj′ə-nəs) *adj.* Caused by diabetes.

Di·ab·i·nese (dī-ăb′ə-nēz′) A trademark for the drug chlorpropamide.

di·ac·e·tate (dī-ăs′ĭ-tāt′) *n.* A salt or ester containing two acetate groups.

di·a·ce·tic acid (dī′ə-sē′tĭk) *n.* See **acetoacetic acid.**

di·a·ce·tyl·mor·phine (dī′ə-sēt′l-môr′fēn′, dī-ăs′ĭ-tl-) *n.* See **heroin.**

di·a·chron·ic (dī′ə-krŏn′ĭk) *adj.* Of or concerned with phenomena as they change through time.

di·ac·la·sis (dī-ăk′lə-sĭs, dī′ə-klā′sĭs) *n.* See **osteoclasis.**

di·a·crit·ic (dī′ə-krĭt′ĭk) *or* **di·a·crit·i·cal** (-ĭ-kəl) *adj.* Diagnostic or distinctive.

di·ad·o·cho·ki·ne·sia (dī-ăd′ə-kō-kĭ-nē′zhə, -kī-) *or* **di·ad·o·cho·ki·ne·sis** (-sĭs) *n.* The normal power of alternately bringing a limb into opposite positions, as flexion and extension or pronation and supination. —**di·ad·o·cho·ki·net·ic** (-nět′ĭk) *adj.*

di·ag·nose (dī′əg-nōs′, -nōz′) *v.* **1.** To distinguish or identify a disease by diagnosis. **2.** To identify a person as having a particular disease or condition by diagnosis.

di·ag·no·sis (dī′əg-nō′sĭs) *n., pl.* **-ses** (-sēz) *Abbr.* **dx** **1.** The act or process of identifying or determining the nature and cause of a disease or injury through evaluation of patient history, examination, and review of laboratory data. **2.** The opinion derived from such an evaluation. **3.** A brief description of the distinguishing characteristics of an organism, as for taxonomic classification.

diagnosis by exclusion *n.* Diagnosis made by excluding all other known diseases.

di·ag·nos·tic (dī′əg-nŏs′tĭk) *adj.* **1.** Of, relating to, or used in a diagnosis. **2.** Serving to identify a particular disease; characteristic. —*n.* **1. diagnostics** The art or practice of medical diagnosis. **2.** A symptom or a distinguishing feature serving as supporting evidence in a diagnosis. **3.** An instrument or a technique used in medical diagnosis.

diagnostic diphtheria toxin *n.* See **Schick test toxin.**

di·ag·nos·ti·cian (dī′əg-nŏ-stĭsh′ən) *n.* A person who diagnoses, especially a physician specializing in medical diagnostics.

diagnostic specificity *n.* The probability that, given the absence of disease, a normal test result will exclude the disease.

diagnostic ultrasound *n.* Use of ultrasound to obtain images for medical diagnostic purposes.

di·ag·o·nal conjugate (dī-ăg′ə-nəl) *n.* The distance from the promontory of the sacrum to the lower margin of the pubic symphysis. Also called *false conjugate.*

di·a·ki·ne·sis (dī′ə-kə-nē′sĭs, -kī-) *n.* The final stage of the prophase in meiosis, characterized by shortening and thickening of the paired chromosomes, formation of the spindle fibers, disappearance of the nucleolus, and degeneration of the nuclear membrane.

di·al·y·sance (dī-ăl′ĭ-səns) *n.* The number of milliliters of blood completely cleared of any substance by an artificial kidney or by peritoneal dialysis in a unit of time, usually a minute.

di·al·y·sate (dī-ăl′ĭ-sāt′) *n.* The material that passes through the membrane in dialysis and usually contains substances that diffuse easily in solution. Also called *diffusate.*

di·al·y·sis (dī-ăl′ĭ-sĭs) *n.,* *pl.* **–ses** (-sēz′) **1.** The separation of smaller molecules from larger molecules or of dissolved substances from colloidal particles in a solution by selective diffusion through a semipermeable membrane. Also called *diffusion.* **2.** Hemodialysis. —**di′a·lyt′ic** (-ə-lĭt′ĭk) *adj.*

dialysis encephalopathy syndrome *n.* A degenerative brain disease that occurs in some individuals on chronic hemodialysis and is marked by the loss of intellectual abilities, involuntary muscular jerks, and personality changes. Also called *dialysis dementia.*

di·a·lyze (dī′ə-līz′) *v.* To subject to or undergo dialysis or hemodialysis. —**di′a·lyz′a·bil′i·ty** *n.* —**di′a·lyz′a·ble** *adj.*

di·a·lyz·er (dī′ə-lī′zər) *n.* **1.** A machine equipped with a semipermeable membrane and used for performing dialysis. **2.** A hemodialyzer.

di·a·mel·i·a (dī′ə-mĕl′ē-ə, -mē′lē-ə) *n.* Absence of two limbs.

di·am·e·ter (dī-ăm′ĭ-tər) *n.* **1.** A straight line connecting two opposite points on the surface of a spherical or cylindrical body, or at the boundary of an opening or foramen, passing through the center of such body or opening. **2.** The distance measured along such a line.

Di·a·mox (dī′ə-mŏks′) A trademark for the drug acetazolamide.

Di·an·a complex (dī-ăn′ə) *n.* In psychoanalytic theory, the adoption of perceived masculine traits and behavior in a female.

di·a·pause (dī′ə-pôz′) *n.* A period during which growth or development is suspended and physiological activity is diminished, as in certain insects in response to adverse environmental conditions.

di·a·pe·de·sis (dī′ə-pĭ-dē′sĭs) *n.* The movement or passage of blood cells, especially white blood cells, through intact capillary walls into surrounding body tissue. Also called *migration.*

di·a·per dermatitis (dī′ə-pər, dī′pər) *n.* A form of dermatitis occurring where a diaper makes contact with the skin and caused by exposure to feces and urine and possibly by the ammonia produced by decomposing urine; diaper rash. Also called *diaper rash.*

di·aph·a·no·scope (dī-ăf′ə-nə-skōp′) *n.* An instrument for illuminating the interior of a body cavity to determine the translucency of its walls.

di·aph·a·nos·co·py (dī-ăf′ə-nŏs′kə-pē) *n.* Examination of a body part with a diaphanoscope.

di·aph·e·met·ric (dī-ăf′ə-mĕt′rĭk) *adj.* Relating to the measurement of tactile sensibility.

di·a·pho·re·sis (dī′ə-fə-rē′sĭs, dī-ăf′ə-) *n.* Perspiration, especially when copious and medically induced.

di·a·pho·ret·ic (dī′ə-fə-rĕt′ĭk, dī-ăf′ə-) *adj.* Producing or increasing perspiration. —*n.* A medicine or other agent that produces perspiration.

di·a·phragm (dī′ə-frăm′) *n.* **1.** A musculomembranous partition separating the abdominal and thoracic cavities and functioning in respiration. Also called *midriff.* **2.** A membranous part that divides or separates. **3.** A contraceptive device consisting of a thin flexible disk, usually made of rubber, that is designed to cover the uterine cervix to prevent the entry of sperm during sexual intercourse. **4.** A disk having a fixed or variable opening used to restrict the amount of light traversing a lens or optical system. —**di′a·phrag·mat′ic** (-frăg-măt′ĭk) *adj.*

diaphragmatic flutter *n.* Rapid rhythmical contractions of the diaphragm, averaging around 150 per minute, that resemble atrial flutter clinically and sometimes electrocardiographically.

diaphragmatic hernia *n.* The protrusion of abdominal parts, such as the stomach and small intestine, into the chest through a weakness in the diaphragm. Also called *diaphragmatocele.*

diaphragmatic ligament of mesonephros *n.* The segment of the embryonic urogenital ridge extending from the mesonephros to the diaphragm. Also called *urogenital mesentery.*

diaphragmatic pleurisy *n.* See **epidemic pleurodynia.**

di·a·phrag·mat·o·cele (dī′ə-frăg-măt′ə-sēl′) *n.* See **diaphragmatic hernia.**

diaphragm phenomenon *n.* A lowering of the line of retraction on the side of the chest that marks the insertion of the diaphragm during inspiration followed by an elevation during expiration. This phenomenon does not occur when the pleural sac is distended. Also called *Litten's phenomenon.*

di·aph·y·sec·to·my (dī-ăf′ĭ-sĕk′tə-mē, dī′ə-fĭ-) *n.* The partial or complete removal of the shaft of a long bone.

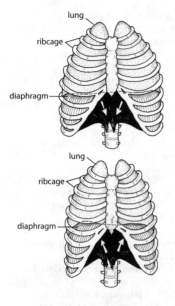

diaphragm
Top: *during inhalation the diaphragm contracts downward,*
forcing air into the lungs
Bottom: *during exhalation the diaphragm relaxes upward,*
forcing air out of the lungs

diaphysial aclasis *n.* See **hereditary multiple exostoses.**

diaphysial dysplasia *n.* Symmetrical thickening of the shafts of long bones, progressing from the middle toward the ends. Also called *Engelmann's disease.*

di·aph·y·sis (dī-ăf′ĭ-sĭs) *n., pl.* **–ses** (-sēz′) The shaft of a long bone. —**di′a·phys′i·al** (dī′ə-fĭz′ē-əl), **di·aph′y·se′al** (dī-ăf′ĭ-sē′əl, dī′ə-fĭz′ē-əl) *adj.*

di·aph·y·si·tis (dī-ăf′ĭ-sī′tĭs) *n.* Inflammation of the shaft of a long bone.

di·a·poph·y·sis (dī′ə-pŏf′ĭ-sĭs) *n., pl.* **–ses** (-sēz′) The superior or articular surface of the transverse process of a vertebra.

di·ar·rhe·a *or* **di·ar·rhoe·a** (dī′ə-rē′ə) *n.* Excessive and frequent evacuation of watery feces. —**di′ar·rhe′al, di′ar·rhe′ic** (-ĭk), **di′ar·rhet′ic** (-rĕt′ĭk) *adj.*

di·ar·thric (dī-är′thrĭk) *adj.* Of or relating to two different joints.

di·ar·thro·di·al cartilage (dī′är-thrō′dē-əl) *n.* See **articular cartilage.**

diarthrodial joint *n.* See **movable joint** (sense 1).

di·ar·thro·sis (dī′är-thrō′sĭs) *n.* See **movable joint** (sense 1).

di·ar·tic·u·lar (dī′är-tĭk′yə-lər) *adj.* Diarthric.

di·as·chi·sis (dī-ăs′kĭ-sĭs) *n.* A sudden loss of function in a portion of the brain that is at a distance from the site of injury, but is connected to it by neurons.

di·a·scope (dī′ə-skōp′) *n.* A flat glass plate through which one can examine superficial skin lesions by means of pressure. —**di′as·co·py** (-ăs′kə-pē) *n.*

di·a·stal·sis (dī′ə-stôl′sĭs, -stăl′-) *n.* Peristalsis in which a region of inhibition precedes the wave of contraction, as in the intestinal tract. —**di′a·stal′tic** (-stôl′tĭk, -stăl′-) *adj.*

di·a·stase (dī′ə-stās′, -stāz′) *n.* An amylase or a mixture of amylases that converts starch to dextrin and maltose, is found in certain germinating grains such as malt, and is used to make soluble starches, to aid the digestion of starches, and to digest glycogen in histological sections.

di·as·ta·sis (dī-ăs′tə-sĭs) *n.* **1.** Separation of normally joined parts, such as the separation of certain abdominal muscles during pregnancy. Also called *divarication.* **2.** The last stage of diastole in the heart, occurring just before contraction and during which little additional blood enters the ventricle.

di·a·sta·su·ri·a (dī′ə-stā-soŏr′ē-ə) *n.* See **amylasuria.**

di·a·stat·ic (dī′ə-stăt′ĭk) *adj.* **1.** Relating to diastasis. **2.** Relating to a diastase.

di·a·ste·ma (dī′ə-stē′mə) *n., pl.* **–ma·ta** (-mə-tə) **1.** A fissure or abnormal opening in a part, especially when congenital. **2.** A gap or space that is between two adjacent teeth in the same dental arch.

di·a·ste·ma·to·cra·ni·a (dī′ə-stē′mə-tō-krā′nē-ə) *n.* A congenital fissure of the skull along the sagittal plane.

di·a·ste·ma·to·my·e·li·a (dī′ə-stē′mə-tō-mī-ē′lē-ə) *n.* A congenital defect in which the spinal cord is divided into halves by a bony or cartilaginous septum, often seen in spina bifida.

di·as·ter (dī-ăs′tər) *n.* See **amphiaster.**

di·as·to·le (dī-ăs′tə-lē) *n.* The normal rhythmically occurring relaxation and dilatation of the heart chambers, especially the ventricles, during which they fill with blood. —**di′a·stol′ic** (dī′ə-stŏl′ĭk) *adj.*

diastolic murmur *n.* A murmur heard during diastole.

diastolic pressure *n.* The lowest arterial blood pressure reached during any given ventricular cycle.

diastolic thrill *n.* A thrill felt during ventricular diastole on palpation over the precordium or over a blood vessel.

di·as·troph·ic dysplasia (dī′ə-strŏf′ĭk) *n. Abbr.* **DTD** A type of dwarfism characterized by clubfoot, deformed spine, incomplete bone growth, stubby fingers, and, often, cleft palate.

di·a·tax·i·a (dī′ə-tăk′sē-ə) *n.* Ataxia affecting both sides of the body.

di·a·ther·mal (dī′ə-thûr′məl) *adj.* Diathermic.

di·a·ther·ma·nous (dī′ə-thûr′mə-nəs) *adj.* Permeable by heat rays.

di·a·ther·mic (dī′ə-thûr′mĭk) *adj.* Relating to or affected by diathermy.

di·a·ther·my (dī′ə-thûr′mē) *n.* The therapeutic generation of local heat in body tissues by high-frequency electromagnetic radiation, electric currents, or ultrasonic waves.

di·ath·e·sis (dī-ăth′ĭ-sĭs) *n., pl.* **–ses** (-sēz′) A hereditary predisposition of the body to a disease, a group of diseases, an allergy, or another disorder. —**di′a·thet′ic** (dī′ə-thĕt′ĭk) *adj.*

di·a·to·ma·ceous earth (dī′ə-tə-mā′shəs, dī-ăt′ə-) *n.* A powder made of the desiccated shells of diatoms, used as a filtering agent, adsorbent, and abrasive in many chemical operations.

di·a·tom·ic (dī′ə-tŏm′ĭk) *adj.* Made up of two atoms.

di·az·e·pam (dī-ăz′ə-păm′) *n.* A tranquilizer used in the treatment of anxiety and tension and as a sedative, a muscle relaxant, and an anticonvulsant.

di·a·zine (dī′ə-zēn′, dī-ăz′ĭn) *n.* Any of a group of chemical compounds containing a benzene ring in which two of the carbon atoms have been replaced by nitrogen atoms.

di·ba·sic (dī-bā′sĭk) *adj.* **1.** Containing two hydrogen atoms that are replaceable by bases. **2.** Of or relating to salts or acids forming salts with two atoms of a univalent metal.

dibasic acid *n.* An acid containing two replaceable hydrogen atoms.

Di·ben·zy·line (dī-běn′zĭ-lēn′) A trademark for the drug phenoxybenzamine.

di·bu·caine (dī-byōō′kān′) *n.* A local anesthetic used topically on the skin and mucous membranes or administered by injection into the subarachnoid space to produce spinal anesthesia.

dibucaine number *n. Abbr.* **DN** A number indicating the percentage by which cholinesterase activity in a serum sample is inhibited by dibucaine.

DIC *abbr.* disseminated intravascular coagulation

di·car·box·yl·ic acid cycle (dī′kär-bŏk-sĭl′ĭk) *n.* The final portion of the Krebs cycle involving the reactions of dicarboxylic acids, specifically succinic, fumaric, malic, and oxaloacetic acid.

di·cen·tric (dī-sĕn′trĭk) *adj.* Having two centromeres.

di·ceph·a·lous (dī-sĕf′ə-ləs) *adj.* Having two heads.

di·chlo·ro·di·phen·yl·tri·chlo·ro·eth·ane (dī-klôr′ō-dī-fĕn′əl-trī-klôr′ō-ĕth′ān′, -fē′nəl-) *n.* DDT.

di·chlor·vos (dī-klôr′vōs′, -vəs) *n.* A nonpersistent organophosphorous pesticide that is of low toxicity to humans.

di·cho·ri·al (dī-kôr′ē-əl) *or* **di·cho·ri·on·ic** (-kôr′ē-ŏn′-ĭk) *adj.* Having two chorions, as the placenta of dizygotic twins.

di·chro·ism (dī′krō-ĭz′əm) *n.* **1.** The property of some solutions of showing different colors at different concentrations. **2.** The property of some crystals of exhibiting two different colors when viewed along different axes. —**di·chro′ic** *adj.*

di·chro·mate (dī-krō′māt′, dī′krō-) *n.* A compound containing the divalent negative ion, Cr_2O_7, usually having a characteristic orange-red color. Also called *bichromate.*

di·chro·mat·ic (dī′krō-măt′ĭk) *adj.* **1.** Having or exhibiting two colors. **2.** Of, relating to, or characterized by dichromatism.

di·chro·ma·tism (dī-krō′mə-tĭz′əm) *n.* **1.** The state of being dichromatic. **2.** A form of colorblindness in which only two of the three fundamental colors can be distinguished due to a lack of one of the retinal cone pigments. Also called *dichromatopsia, dyschromatopsia, parachromatopsia.*

Dick·ens shunt (dĭk′ĭnz) *n.* See **pentose phosphate pathway.**

Dick test (dĭk) *n.* A skin test used to determine immunity or susceptibility to scarlet fever.

Dick test toxin *n.* See **streptococcus erythrogenic toxin.**

di·clo·fen·ac potassium (dī′klō-fĕn′ăk) *n.* A nonsteroidal anti-inflammatory drug used to treat pain.

di·clox·a·cil·lin sodium (dī-klŏk′sə-sĭl′ĭn) *n.* An oral antibiotic derived from penicillin and used to treat infections caused by staphylococcal bacteria that produce beta-lactamase.

di·co·ri·a (dī-kôr′ē-ə) *n.* See **diplocoria.**

dicrotic notch *n.* The notch in a pulse tracing that precedes the dicrotic wave.

dicrotic pulse *n.* A pulse marked by a double beat, with the second beat weaker than the first.

dicrotic wave *n.* The second rise in the tracing of a dicrotic pulse.

di·cro·tism (dī′krə-tĭz′əm) *n.* A condition in which the pulse is felt as two beats per single heartbeat. —**di·crot′ic** (-krŏt′ĭk) *adj.*

dic·ty·o·ma (dĭk′tē-ō′mə) *n.* A benign tumor of the nonpigmented layer of the ciliary epithelium that has a netlike structure.

dic·ty·o·tene (dĭk′tē-ə-tēn′) *n.* The stage of meiosis at which the primary oocyte is arrested in the female fetus during the period from late fetal life through birth and childhood until ovulation occurs.

di·cu·ma·rol (dī-kōō′mə-rôl′, -rōl′) *n.* An anticoagulant that inhibits the formation of prothrombin in the liver. Also called *bishydroxycoumarin.*

di·cy·clo·mine hydrochloride (dī-sī′klə-mēn′) *n.* An anticholinergic drug that is used as an antispasmodic in the treatment of gastrointestinal disorders.

di·dac·tic (dī-dăk′tĭk) *adj.* Of or relating to medical teaching by lectures or textbooks as distinguished from clinical demonstration with patients.

di·dac·tyl·ism (dī-dăk′tə-lĭz′əm) *n.* A congenital defect in which there are only two digits on a hand or a foot.

di·dan·o·sine (dī-dăn′ə-sĭn, -sēn′) *n.* See **ddI.**

di·del·phic (dī-dĕl′fĭk) *adj.* Having or relating to a double uterus.

di·de·ox·y·cy·ti·dine (dī′dē-ŏk′sē-sī′tĭ-dēn′) *n.* ddC.

di·de·ox·y·in·o·sine (dī′dē-ŏk′sē-ĭn′ə-sēn, -sĭn, -ī′nə-) *n.* ddI.

Di·dro·nel (dī-drō′nəl) A trademark for the drug etidronate disodium.

did·y·mal·gia (dĭd′ə-măl′jə) *n.* See **orchialgia.**

did·y·mi·tis (dĭd′ə-mī′tĭs) *n.* See **orchitis.**

did·y·mus (dĭd′ə-məs) *n.* See **testis.**

die (dī) *v.* **1.** To cease living; become dead; expire. **2.** To cease existing, especially by degrees; fade.

dieb. alt. *abbr. Latin* diebus alternis (every other day)

di·e·cious (dī-ē′shəs) *adj.* Variant of **dioecious.**

di·el·drin (dī-ĕl′drĭn, dēl′-) *n.* A chlorinated hydrocarbon used as an insecticide and in mothproofing.

di·en·ceph·a·lon (dī′ĕn-sĕf′ə-lŏn′, -lən) *n.* The posterior part of the prosencephalon, composed of the epithalamus, the dorsal thalamus, the subthalamus, and the hypothalamus. Also called *betweenbrain, interbrain.*

Di·ent·a·moe·ba frag·i·lis (dī-ĕn′tə-mē′bə frăj′ə-lĭs) *n.* A small amoeba that is parasitic in the large intestine and is capable of causing low-grade inflammation coupled with mucous diarrhea and gastrointestinal disturbance.

di·er·e·sis (dī-ĕr′ĭ-sĭs) *n.* See **solution of continuity.**

di·e·ret·ic (dī′ə-rĕt′ĭk) *adj.* **1.** Of or relating to dieresis. **2.** Dividing; ulcerating; corroding.

di·es·trus (dī-ĕs′trəs) *or* **di·es·trum** (-trəm) *n.* The period of sexual quiescence intervening between two periods of estrus. —**di·es′trous** (-trəs) *adj.*

di·et (dī′ĭt) *n.* **1.** Food and drink in general. **2.** A prescribed course of eating and drinking in which the amount and kind of food, as well as the times at which it is to be taken, are regulated for therapeutic purposes. 3. Reduction of caloric intake so as to lose weight. —*v.* To eat and drink according to a regulated system, especially so as to lose weight or control a medical condition.

di·e·tar·y (dī′ĭ-tĕr′ē) *adj.* Of or relating to diet.

dietary amenorrhea *n.* Cessation of menstruation because of rapid weight loss.

dietary fiber *n.* Coarse, indigestible plant matter, consisting primarily of polysaccharides, that when eaten stimulates intestinal peristalsis.

di·e·tet·ic (dī′ĭ-tĕt′ĭk) *adj.* 1. Of or relating to diet. 2. Of or being a food that, naturally or through processing, has a low caloric content.

di·e·tet·ics (dī′ĭ-tĕt′ĭks) *n.* The branch of therapeutics concerned with the practical application of diet in relation to health and disease.

di·eth·yl·ene·tri·a·mine pen·ta·a·ce·tic acid (dī-ĕth′-ə-lēn-trī′ə-mēn′ pĕn′tə-ə-sē′tĭk) *n.* Pentetic acid.

di·eth·yl ether (dī-ĕth′əl) *n.* A pungent, volatile, highly flammable liquid derived from the distillation of ethyl alcohol with sulfuric acid and widely used as an inhalation anesthetic. Also called *ethyl ether, ethyl oxide, sulfuric ether.*

di·eth·yl·stil·bes·trol (dī-ĕth′əl-stĭl-bĕs′trôl, -trōl) *n.* DES.

di·eth·yl·tryp·ta·mine (dī-ĕth′əl-trĭp′tə-mēn′) *n.* DET.

di·e·ti·tian *or* **di·e·ti·cian** (dī′ĭ-tĭsh′ən) *n.* A person specializing in dietetics.

Dietl's crisis (dēt′lz) *n.* A sudden attack of acute lumbar and abdominal pain accompanied by nausea and vomiting, caused by kinking of the ureter in persons with wandering kidney.

dif·fer·ence (dĭf′ər-əns, dĭf′rəns) *n.* The magnitude or degree by which one quantity differs from another of the same kind.

dif·fer·en·tial blood count (dĭf′ə-rĕn′shəl) *n.* An estimate, based on cell counts in a representative sample, of the percentage of white blood cell types that make up the total white blood cell count.

differential diagnosis *n.* Determination of which one of two or more diseases with similar symptoms is the one from which the patient is suffering. Also called *differentiation.*

differential stain *n.* A stain that facilitates the differentiation of the elements of a cell or specimen

differential u·re·ter·al·cath·e·ter·i·za·tion test (yŏŏ-rē′tər-əl-kăth′ĭ-tər-ĭ-zā′shən) *n.* A test that is used to determine various functional parameters of one kidney compared with the other kidney. Also called *split renal-function test.*

dif·fer·en·ti·a·tion (dĭf′ə-rĕn′shē-ā′shən) *n.* 1. The acquisition or possession of a character or function different from that of the original type. Also called *specialization.* 2. See **differential diagnosis.**

dif·frac·tion (dĭ-frăk′shən) *n.* Change in the directions and intensities of a group of waves after passing by an obstacle or through an aperture.

diffraction halo *n.* The hazy colorless region that surrounds red blood cells viewed under a microscope.

dif·fu·sate (dĭ-fyŏŏ′zāt′) *n.* See **dialysate.**

dif·fuse (dĭ-fyŏŏs′) *adj.* Not limited to one tissue or location; widespread. —*v.* (dĭ-fyŏŏz′) To spread or to be spread widely, as through a tissue. —**dif·fus′i·ble** (-fyŏŏ′zə-bəl) *adj.*

diffuse abscess *n.* An abscess not enclosed by a well-defined capsule.

diffuse cataract *n.* A congenital cataract that involves only the embryonic nucleus of the lens.

diffuse cutaneous leishmaniasis *n.* A chronic form of leishmaniasis caused by *Leishmania aethiopia* in Ethiopia and Kenya and by various subspecies of *L. mexicana* in Central and South America, and characterized by nonulcerating, non-necrotizing skin lesions that spread over the body. Also called *anergic leishmaniasis, disseminated cutaneous leishmaniasis, leishmaniasis tegumentaria diffusa.*

diffuse idiopathic skeletal hyperostosis *n.* A generalized spinal and extraspinal articular disorder characterized by calcification and ossification of ligaments, particularly of the anterior longitudinal ligament. Also called *ankylosing hyperostosis, Forrestier's disease, hyperostotic spondylosis.*

diffuse mesangial proliferation *n.* See **mesangial proliferative glomerulonephritis.**

diffuse waxy spleen *n.* Amyloid degeneration of the spleen, affecting chiefly the extrasinusoidal tissue spaces of the pulp.

diffusible stimulant *n.* A stimulant that produces a rapid but temporary effect.

dif·fus·ing capacity (dĭ-fyŏŏ′zĭng) *n.* The capacity of the alveolocapillary membrane to transfer gas.

dif·fu·sion (dĭ-fyŏŏ′zhən) *n.* 1. The process of diffusing or the condition of being diffused. 2. The spontaneous intermingling of the particles of two or more substances as a result of random thermal motion. 3. See **dialysis** (sense 1).

diffusion anoxia *n.* See **diffusion hypoxia.**

diffusion hypoxia *n.* An abrupt transient decrease in alveolar oxygen tension when room air is inhaled at the conclusion of a nitrous oxide anesthesia. Also called *diffusion anoxia.*

diffusion respiration *n.* A procedure for maintaining oxygenation of the blood during apnea by intratracheal insufflation of oxygen at high flow rates.

di·flo·ra·sone diacetate (dī-flôr′ə-sōn′) *n.* A corticosteroid used in topical preparations to control or prevent inflammation.

Di·flu·can (dī′flŏŏ′kən) A trademark for the drug fluconazole.

di·flu·ni·sal (dī-flŏŏ′nĭ-săl′, -sôl′) *n.* A salicylic acid derivative with anti-inflammatory, analgesic, and antipyretic actions.

di·gas·tric (dī-găs′trĭk) *adj.* 1. Having two bellies; biventral. Used especially of a muscle with two fleshy parts separated by an intervening tendinous part. 2. Of or relating to the digastric muscle.

digastric fossa *n.* A hollow on the posterior surface of the base of the mandible, on either side of the median plane, giving attachment to the anterior belly of the digastric muscle.

digastric muscle *n.* 1. A muscle with two fleshy bellies separated by a fibrous insertion. 2. A muscle consisting of two bellies united by a central tendon connected to the body of the hyoid bone, with origin from the digastric groove medial to the mastoid process, with insertion into the lower border of the mandible, with nerve supply of the posterior belly from the facial nerve, and of the anterior belly by the mylohyoid nerve, and whose action elevates the hyoid when the mandible is fixed and depresses the mandible when the hyoid is fixed.

digastric triangle *n.* See **submandibular triangle.**

Di·ge·ne·a (dī-jĕ′nē-ə, dī′jə-nē′ə) *n.* A subclass of parasitic flatworms marked by a complex life cycle involving developmental stages in a mollusk intermediate host and an adult stage in a vertebrate and including all of the common flukes of humans and other mammals.

di·gen·e·sis (dī-jĕn′ĭ-sĭs) *n.* Reproduction in distinctive patterns in alternate generations, typically involving alternating sexual and asexual cycles in succeeding host organisms, as seen in malarial parasites and certain trematode flatworms. —**di′ge·net′ic** (-jə-nĕt′ĭk) *adj.*

di·gest (dī-jĕst′, dĭ-) *v.* **1.** To convert food into simpler chemical compounds that can be absorbed and assimilated by the body, as by chemical and muscular action in the alimentary canal. **2.** To soften or disintegrate by means of chemical action, heat, or moisture. —**di·gest′i·bil′i·ty** *n.* —**di·gest′i·ble** *adj.*

di·ges·tant (dī-jĕs′tənt, dĭ-) *adj.* Aiding or stimulating digestion. —*n.* A substance that aids digestion.

di·ges·tion (dī-jĕs′chən, dĭ-) *n.* The process by which food is converted into substances that can be absorbed and assimilated by the body, especially that accomplished in the alimentary canal by the mechanical and enzymatic breakdown of foods into simpler chemical compounds.

di·ges·tive (dī-jĕs′tĭv, dĭ-) *adj.* Of or relating to digestion. —*n.* A digestant.

digestive gland *n.* A gland, such as the liver or pancreas, that secretes into the alimentary canal substances necessary for digestion.

digestive system *n.* The alimentary canal and digestive glands regarded as an integrated system responsible for the ingestion, digestion, and absorption of foodstuffs and the elimination of associated wastes. Also called *alimentary system.*

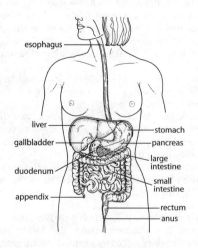

digestive system

digestive tract *n.* See **alimentary canal.**

dig·it (dĭj′ĭt) *n.* A finger or toe; dactyl.

dig·i·tal (dĭj′ĭ-tl) *adj.* **1.** Of or resembling a finger or toe or an impression made by them. **2.** Done or performed with a finger. —**dig′i·tal·ly** *adv.*

digital furrow *n.* Any of the grooves occurring on the palmar surface of a finger joint.

dig·i·tal·in (dĭj′ĭ-tăl′ĭn, -tā′lĭn) *n.* A mixture of glycosides obtained from the leaves and seeds of the common foxglove and used as a cardiotonic.

dig·i·tal·is (dĭj′ĭ-tăl′ĭs) *n.* **1.** A plant of the genus *Digitalis,* which includes the foxgloves, several species of which are a source of cardioactive steroid glycosides used in the treatment of certain heart diseases. **2.** A pharmaceutical that is prepared from the seeds and dried leaves of the purple foxglove, *Digitalis purpurea,* and is prescribed as a cardiac stimulant in the treatment of congestive heart failure and other disorders of the heart.

dig·i·tal·i·za·tion (dĭj′ĭ-tl-ĭ-zā′shən) *n.* The administration of digitalis by a dosage schedule until sufficient amounts are present in the body to produce the desired therapeutic effects.

digital joint *n.* Any of the hinge joints between the phalanges of the fingers or toes. Also called *interphalangeal joint, phalangeal joint.*

digital reflex *n.* See **Hoffmann's sign.**

digital sub·trac·tion angiography (səb-trăk′shən) *n.* A computer-assisted x-ray technique that subtracts images of bone and soft tissue to permit viewing of the cardiovascular system.

dig·i·tate (dĭj′ĭ-tāt′) *or* **dig·i·tat·ed** (-tā′tĭd) *adj.* **1.** Having a digit or digits. **2.** Having fingerlike processes or impressions.

dig·i·ta·tion (dĭj′ĭ-tā′shən) *n.* **1.** Division into fingerlike parts. **2.** A fingerlike part or process.

dig·i·tox·in (dĭj′ĭ-tŏk′sĭn) *n.* A secondary cardioactive glycoside that is derived from and similar in effect to digitalis but that is more completely absorbed from the gastrointestinal tract.

dig·i·tus (dĭj′ĭ-təs) *n.,* pl. **–ti** (-tī′) A digit.

di·glos·si·a (dī-glŏs′ē-ə) *n.* See **bifid tongue.**

dig·ox·in (dĭj-ŏk′sĭn) *n.* A cardioactive steroid glycoside with pharmacological effects similar to digitalis.

di·het·er·o·zy·gote (dī-hĕt′ə-rō-zī′gōt′) *n.* An individual heterozygous for two different gene pairs at two different loci.

di·hy·drate (dī-hī′drāt′) *n.* A chemical compound containing two molecules of water.

di·hy·dric alcohol (dī-hī′drĭk) *n.* An alcohol containing two hydroxyl groups, such as ethylene glycol.

dihydro– *pref.* Relating a molecule with two hydrogen atoms added: *dihydrocodeine.*

di·hy·dro·co·deine bitartrate (dī-hī′drə-kō′dēn′) *n.* A narcotic analgesic derived from codeine, about one-sixth as potent as morphine.

di·hy·dro·fo·lic acid (dī-hī′drə-fō′lĭk, -fŏl′ĭk) *n.* An intermediate formed during the oxidation of tetrahydrofolic acid to folic acid.

di·hy·dro·o·ro·tate (dī-hī′drō-ôr′ə-tāt′) *n.* An intermediate formed during pyrimidine biosynthesis.

di·hy·dro·pte·ro·ic acid (dī-hī′drō-tə-rō′ĭk) *n.* An intermediate formed during the biosynthesis of folic acid; its formation is inhibited by sulfonamides.

di·hy·dro·ta·chys·ter·ol (dī-hī′drō-tə-kĭs′tə-rŏl′, -rōl′) *n. Abbr.* **DHT** A rapidly acting form of vitamin D, prescribed in the treatment of hypocalcemia.

di·hy·dro·tes·tos·ter·one (dī-hī′drō-tĕs-tŏs′tə-rōn′) *n. Abbr.* **DHT** A derivative of testosterone having androgenic activity and anabolic and tumor-suppressing capabilities useful in the treatment of certain breast cancers. Also called *stanolone*.

di·hy·drox·y·ac·e·tone (dī′hī-drŏk′sē-ăs′ĭ-tōn′) *n.* An isomer of glyceraldehyde important in the metabolism of carbohydrates and that is used topically to darken the skin.

di·hy·drox·y·phen·yl·al·a·nine (dī′hī-drŏk′sē-fĕn′əl-ăl′ə-nēn′, -fē′nəl-) *n.* Dopa.

di·i·o·dide (dī-ī′ə-dīd′) *n.* A compound containing two atoms of iodine combined with an element or radical.

di·ke·tone (dī-kē′tōn′) *n.* A compound containing two carbonyl groups.

di·ke·to·pi·per·a·zine (dī-kē′tō-pī-pĕr′ə-zēn′) *n.* **1.** A cyclic dipeptide formed by the dehydration of two molecules of glycine. **2.** Any of various cyclic organic compounds formed by the dehydration of alpha-amino acids other than glycine.

dil. *abbr. Latin* dilue (dilute)

di·lac·er·a·tion (dī-lăs′ə-rā′shən) *n.* **1.** Discission of a cataractous lens. **2.** A displacement of some portion of a developing tooth resulting in a tooth with sharply angulated roots.

Di·la·cor (dĭl′ə-kôr′) A trademark for the drug diltiazem hydrochloride.

Di·lan·tin (dī-lăn′tn) A trademark for the drug phenytoin.

dil·a·ta·tion (dĭl′ə-tā′shən, dī′lə-) *n.* Physiological, pathological, or artificial enlargement of a cavity, canal, blood vessel, or opening.

dilatation and curettage *n.* See dilation and curettage.

dil·a·ta·tor (dĭl′ə-tā′tər, dī′lə-) *n.* See **dilator** (sense 2).

di·late (dī-lāt′, dī′lāt′) *v.* To make or become wider or larger.

di·la·tion (dī-lā′shən, dī-) *n.* **1.** The act of expanding or the condition of being expanded. **2.** Dilatation.

dilation and curettage *n. Abbr.* **D & C** A surgical procedure in which the cervix is expanded using a dilator and the uterine lining scraped with a curette, performed for the diagnosis and treatment of various uterine conditions. Also called *dilatation and curettage*.

dilation and evacuation *n. Abbr.* **D & E** A surgical procedure in which the cervix is dilated and the early products of conception are removed from the uterus.

di·la·tor (dī-lā′tər, dī′lā′-, dī-lā′-) *n.* **1.** An instrument or a substance for enlarging a cavity, canal, blood vessel, or opening. **2.** A muscle that dilates an orifice or a body part, such as a blood vessel or the pupil of the eye. Also called *dilatator*.

Di·lau·did (dĭ-lô′dĭd) A trademark for the drug hydromorphone hydrochloride.

dil·do *or* **dil·doe** (dĭl′dō) *n., pl.* **–dos** *or* **–does** An object that is shaped like and is used as a substitute for an erect penis.

dil·ti·a·zem hydrochloride (dĭl-tī′ə-zĕm′) *n.* A calcium channel blocking agent used to dilate coronary blood vessels.

dil·u·ent (dĭl′yo͞o-ənt) *adj.* Serving to dilute. —*n.* A substance that dilutes the strength of a solution or mixture.

di·lute (dī-lo͞ot′, dī-) *v.* To reduce a solution or mixture in concentration, quality, strength, or purity, as by adding water. —*adj.* Thinned or weakened by diluting.

di·lu·tion (dī-lo͞o′shən, dī-) *n.* **1.** The act of reducing the concentration of a mixture or solution. **2.** A diluted solution.

dim. *abbr. Latin* dimidius (half)

di·me·li·a (dī-mē′lē-ə, -mēl′yə) *n.* Congenital duplication of all or part of a limb.

di·men·hy·dri·nate (dī′mĕn-hī′drə-nāt′) *n.* An antihistamine used to treat motion sickness and allergic disorders.

di·men·sion (dĭ-mĕn′shən, dī-) *n.* **1.** A measure of spatial extent, especially width, height, or length. **2.** Scope or magnitude.

di·mer (dī′mər) *n.* **1.** A molecule consisting of two identical simpler molecules. **2.** A chemical compound consisting of such molecules. —**di·mer′ic** (dī-mĕr′ĭk) *adj.*

di·mer·cap·rol (dī′mər-kăp′rôl, -rōl) *n.* A chelating agent developed as an antidote for lewisite and other arsenical poisons, also used as an antidote for antimony, bismuth, chromium, mercury, gold, and nickel poisoning. Also called *anti-lewisite, British anti-lewisite*.

Di·me·tane (dī′mə-tān′) A trademark for the drug brompheniramine maleate.

di·meth·yl pol·y·si·lox·ane (dī-mĕth′əl pŏl′ē-sĭ-lŏk′-sān′) *n.* A polymer composed of alternating silicon and oxygen atoms and having two methyl groups attached; it can, depending on molecular weight, have properties ranging from oils to plastics.

di·meth·yl·sulf·ox·ide (dī-mĕth′əl-sŭl-fŏk′sīd′) *n.* DMSO.

di·meth·yl·tryp·ta·mine (dī-mĕth′əl-trĭp′tə-mēn′) *n.* DMT.

di·mor·phism (dī-môr′fĭz′əm) *n.* **1.** Existence in two shapes or forms, especially the existence within a species of two distinct forms that differ in one or more characteristics, such as size or shape. **2.** Crystallization of the same substance in two distinct forms. —**di·mor′phic, di·mor′phous** (-fəs) *adj.*

dim·ple (dĭm′pəl) *n.* **1.** A small natural indentation in the chin, cheek, or sacral region, probably due to some developmental fault in the subcutaneous connective tissue or in underlying bone. **2.** A depression of similar appearance resulting from trauma or the contraction of scar tissue. —**dim′ple** *v.*

dim·pling (dĭm′plĭng) *n.* A condition marked by the formation of natural or artificial dimples.

di·ni·tro·phe·nol (dī-nī′trō-fē′nôl′, -nōl′) *n.* Any of six crystalline compounds, especially a highly toxic compound that increases fat metabolism and was formerly used in weight control.

di·ni·tro·phen·yl·hy·dra·zine test (dī-nī′trō-fĕn′əl-hī′drə-zēn′, -zĭn, -fē′nəl-) *n.* A test to determine the presence of ketoacids; used in screening for maple syrup urine disease.

din·ner pad (dĭn′ər) *n.* A pad placed over the pit of the stomach before the application of a plaster jacket, and removed after the plaster has hardened, in order to leave space for varying conditions of abdominal distention.

di·no·flag·el·late (dī′nō-flăj′ə-lĭt, -lāt′, -flə-jĕl′ĭt) *n.* Any of numerous chiefly marine flagellates of the order Dinoflagellata, some species of which produce a potent neurotoxin that may cause severe food poisoning following ingestion of parasitized shellfish.

di·nu·cle·o·tide (dī-nōō′klē-ə-tīd′) *n.* A nucleotide molecule that consists of a combination of two nucleotide units.

di·oe·cious *or* **di·e·cious** (dī-ē′shəs) *adj.* Of or relating to organisms, especially plants, having the male and female reproductive organs borne on separate individuals of the same species; sexually distinct.

–diol *suff.* Relating to a compound having two hydroxyl groups added, especially a glycol: *ethandiol.*

di·op·ter (dī-ŏp′tər) *n. Abbr.* **D.** A unit of measurement of the refractive power of lenses equal to the reciprocal of the focal length measured in meters.

dioptric aberration *n.* See **spherical aberration**.

di·op·trics (dī-ŏp′trĭks) *n.* The branch of optics that deals with the refraction of light. —**di·op′tric** *adj.*

di·ose (dī′ōs, -ōz′) *n.* A monosaccharide containing two carbon atoms.

Di·o·van (dī′ə-văn′) A trademark for the drug valsartan.

di·o·vu·lar (dī-ō′vyə-lər, -ŏv′yə-) *adj.* Of, relating to, or derived from two ova.

di·o·vu·la·to·ry (dī-ō′vyə-lə-tôr′ē, -ŏv′yə-) *adj.* Releasing two ova in one ovarian cycle.

di·ox·ide (dī-ŏk′sīd) *n.* A compound containing two oxygen atoms per molecule.

di·ox·in (dī-ŏk′sĭn) *n.* Any of several carcinogenic or teratogenic heterocyclic hydrocarbons that occur as impurities in petroleum-derived herbicides.

di·ox·y·gen·ase (dī-ŏk′sĭ-jə-nās′, -nāz′) *n.* Any of a group of enzymes that catalyze the insertion of an oxygen molecule into an organic substrate.

DIP *abbr.* distal interphalangeal (as in DIP joint)

di·pep·ti·dase (dī-pĕp′tĭ-dās′, -dāz′) *n.* An enzyme that catalyzes the hydrolysis of dipeptides into their constituent amino acids.

di·pep·tide (dī-pĕp′tīd′) *n.* A peptide that, on hydrolysis, yields two amino acid molecules.

di·pep·ti·dyl carboxypeptidase (dī-pĕp′tĭ-dĭl′) *n.* A proteolytic enzyme that catalyzes the removal of dipeptides from a variety of compounds, as from angiotensin I as it is converted to angiotensin II. Also called *angiotensin-converting enzyme.*

dipeptidyl peptidase *n.* An enzyme that exists in two forms each of which catalyzes the hydrolysis of dipeptides from polypeptides.

Di·pet·a·lo·ne·ma (dī-pĕt′l-ō-nē′mə) *n.* A large genus of filarial worms that are transmitted by a species of gnats to humans and other vertebrates, producing microfilariae in the blood or tissue fluids, and live as adults in deep connective tissue, membranes, or visceral surfaces.

Dipetalonema per·stans (pûr′stănz′) *n.* A filarial worm that produces unsheathed microfilariae in the blood and lives as an adult in the peritoneal, pleural, or pericardial cavities.

Dipetalonema strep·to·cer·ca (strĕp′tə-sûr′kə) *n.* A filarial worm that produces unsheathed microfilariae in the circulating blood and lives as an adult in the dermis and subcutaneous tissues.

di·phal·lus (dī-făl′əs) *n.* A rare congenital anomaly in which the penis or clitoris is partially or completely doubled. —**di·phal′lic** *adj.*

di·pha·sic (dī-fā′zĭk) *adj.* **1.** Having two phases or stages. **2.** Of or being a disorder marked by two distinct phases, such as bipolar disorder.

di·phen·hy·dra·mine (dī′fĕn-hī′drə-mēn′, -mĭn) *n.* An antihistamine usually used to treat respiratory symptoms and allergic conditions, such as hay fever, hives, and allergic rhinitis.

di·phe·nox·y·late hydrochloride (dī′fĭ-nŏk′sĭ-lāt′) *n.* An oral drug that is derived from meperidine hydrochloride and counteracts peristalsis, and that is used primarily in combination with atropine to treat diarrhea.

di·phen·yl (dī-fĕn′əl, -fē′nəl) *n.* See **biphenyl**.

di·phen·yl·a·mine (dī-fĕn′əl-ə-mēn′, -ăm′ĭn, -fē′nəl-) *n.* A colorless crystalline compound used as a stabilizer for plastics and in the manufacture of dyes, explosives, pesticides, and pharmaceuticals.

di·phos·gene (dī-fŏz′jēn′) *n.* A colorless liquid that is used in organic synthesis and whose vapor was used as a poison gas in World War I. Also called *trichlormethyl chloroformate.*

di·phos·phate (dī-fŏs′fāt′) *n.* An ester of phosphoric acid containing two phosphate groups.

diph·the·ri·a (dĭf-thîr′ē-ə, dĭp-) *n.* An acute infectious disease caused by *Corynebacterium diphtheriae,* and characterized by the production of a systemic toxin and the formation of a false membrane on the lining of the mucous membrane of the throat and other respiratory passages, causing difficulty in breathing, high fever, and weakness. The toxin is particularly harmful to the tissues of the heart and central nervous system. —**diph′the·rit′ic** (-thə-rĭt′ĭk), **diph·ther′ic** (-thĕr′ĭk), **diph·the′ri·al** *adj.*

diphtheria antitoxin *n.* The antitoxin specific for the toxin produced by *Corynebacterium diphtheriae.*

diphtheria, tetanus toxoids, and pertussis vaccine *n. Abbr.* **DTP** A vaccine available in three forms: diphtheria and tetanus toxoids plus pertussis vaccine; tetanus-diphtheria toxoids, adult type; and tetanus toxoids; used for active immunization against diphtheria, tetanus, and whooping cough.

diphtheritic membrane *n.* A false membrane formed on mucous surfaces in diphtheria.

diph·the·roid (dĭf′thə-roid′) *n.* **1.** A local infection that resembles diphtheria, especially in the formation of a false membrane, but that is caused by a microorganism other than *Corynebacterium diphtheriae.* Also called *pseudodiphtheria.* **2.** Any of various microorganisms resembling *Corynebacterium diphtheriae.* —**diph′the·roid′** *adj.*

di·phyl·lo·both·ri·a·sis (dī-fĭl′ō-bŏth-rī′ə-sĭs) *n.* Infection with the cestode tapeworm *Diphyllobothrium latum* resulting from ingestion of raw or inadequately cooked fish infected with the larva.

Di·phyl·lo·both·ri·um (dī-fĭl′ō-bŏth′rē-əm) *n.* A large genus of tapeworms, one species of which causes diphyllobothriasis in humans.

di·phy·o·dont (dī-fī′ə-dŏnt′) *adj.* Developing two successive sets of teeth, one deciduous and one permanent, as in humans. —*n.* A diphyodont animal.

di·piv·e·frin hydrochloride (dī-pĭv′ə-frĭn) *n.* An ophthalmic adrenergic that is used in drop form in the initial therapy for controlling intraocular pressure in chronic open-angle glaucoma.

dip·la·cu·sis (dĭp′lə-kōō′sĭs) *n.* A difference in the perception of sound by the ears, either in time or in pitch, so that one sound is heard as two.

di·ple·gia (dī-plē′jə) *n.* Paralysis of corresponding parts on both sides of the body. —**di·ple′gic** *adj. & n.*

diplo– *or* **dipl–** *pref.* **1.** Double: *diplococcus.* **2.** Having double the basic number of chromosomes; diploid: *diplont.*

dip·lo·ba·cil·lus (dĭp′lō-bə-sĭl′əs) *n.* A rod-shaped bacterium occurring in pairs linked end to end.

dip·lo·bac·te·ri·a (dĭp′lō-băk-tîr′ē-ə) *n.* Bacterial cells linked together in pairs.

dip·lo·blas·tic (dĭp′lō-blăs′tĭk) *adj.* Derived from two embryonic germ layers, the ectoderm and the endoderm. Used of invertebrates such as sponges and coelenterates.

dip·lo·car·di·a (dĭp′lō-kär′dē-ə) *n.* A condition in which the lateral halves of the heart are separated by a central fissure.

dip·lo·coc·coid (dĭp′lō-kŏk′oid′) *adj.* Resembling a diplococcus.

dip·lo·coc·cus (dĭp′lō-kŏk′əs) *n., pl.* **-coc·ci** (-kŏk′sī′, -kŏk′ī′) Any of various paired spherical bacteria, including those of the genus *Diplococcus,* some of which are pathogenic. —**dip′lo·coc′cal** (-kŏk′əl), **dip′lo·coc′cic** (-kŏk′sĭk, -kŏk′ĭk) *adj.*

Dip·lo·coc·cus (dĭp′lō-kŏk′əs) *n.* A genus of gram-positive anaerobic encapsulated fermenting bacteria having a somewhat elongated spherical shape.

dip·lo·co·ri·a (dĭp′lō-kôr′ē-ə) *n.* Presence of a double pupil in the eye. Also called *dicoria.*

dip·lo·e (dĭp′lō-ē′) *n.* The central layer of spongy, porous, bony tissue between the hard outer and inner bone layers of the cranium. —**dip′lo·ic** (-lō-ĭk) *adj.*

dip·lo·gen·e·sis (dĭp′lō-jĕn′ĭ-sĭs) *n.* The development of a double fetus or of a fetus with a part or parts doubled.

diploic vein *n.* Any of the veins, designated frontal, anterior temporal, posterior temporal, and occipital, located in the diploe and connected with the cerebral sinuses by emissary veins.

dip·loid (dĭp′loid′) *adj.* Having two sets of chromosomes or double the haploid number of chromosomes in the germ cell, with one member of each chromosome pair derived from the ovum and one from the spermatazoon. The diploid number, 46 in humans, is the normal chromosome complement of an organism's somatic cells. —*n.* A diploid organism or cell.

dip·loi·dy (dĭp′loi′dē) *n.* The state or condition of being diploid.

dip·lo·mate (dĭp′lə-māt′) *n.* One who has received a diploma, especially a physician certified as a specialist by a board of examiners.

dip·lo·my·e·li·a (dĭp′lō-mī-ē′lē-ə) *n.* Complete or incomplete doubling of the spinal cord, sometimes accompanied by a bony septum of the vertebral canal.

dip·lo·ne·ma (dĭp′lə-nē′mə) *n., pl.* **-mas** *or* **-ma·ta** (-mə-tə) The doubled form of the chromosome strand visible at the diplotene stage of meiosis.

di·plop·a·gus (dĭ-plŏp′ə-gəs) *n., pl.* **-gi** (-gī′, -jī′) A pair of equally developed conjoined twins, each with fairly complete bodies, although one or more internal organs may be shared.

di·plo·pi·a (dĭ-plō′pē-ə) *n.* See **double vision.** —**di·plo′pic** (-plō′pĭk, -plŏp′ĭk) *adj.*

dip·lo·sis (dĭ-plō′sĭs) *n.* The formation of the diploid number of chromosomes during fertilization by the fusion of the nuclei of two haploid gametes.

dip·lo·some (dĭp′lə-sōm′) *n.* The pair of centrioles of mammalian cells.

dip·lo·so·mi·a (dĭp′lə-sō′mē-ə) *n.* See **conjoined twins.**

dip·lo·tene (dĭp′lə-tēn′) *n.* A stage of meiotic prophase in which homologous chromosome pairs begin to separate and chiasmata become visible.

di·po·lar ion (dī-pō′lər) *n.* An ion having both a negative and a positive charge, each localized at a different point in the molecule, which thus has both positive and negative poles. Also called *zwitterion.*

di·pole moment (dī′pōl′) *n.* **1.** The product of either charge in an electric dipole with the distance separating them. **2.** The product of the strength of either pole in a magnetic dipole with the distance separating them.

di·pro·pyl·tryp·ta·mine (dī-prō′pĭl-trĭp′tə-mēn′) *n.* DPT.

dip·se·sis (dĭp-sē′sĭs) *n.* Abnormal or excessive thirst. Also called *dipsosis.*

dip·so·gen (dĭp′sə-jən, -jĕn′) *n.* An agent that provokes thirst. —**dip′so·gen′ic** (-jĕn′ĭk) *adj.*

dip·so·ma·ni·a (dĭp′sə-mā′nē-ə, -mān′yə) *n.* An insatiable craving for alcoholic beverages. —**dip′so·ma′ni·ac** (-ăk′) *adj. & n.* —**dip′so·ma·ni′a·cal** (-mə-nī′ə-kəl) *adj.*

dip·so·sis (dĭp-sō′sĭs) *n.* See **dipsesis.**

dip·so·ther·a·py (dĭp′sə-thĕr′ə-pē) *n.* The treatment of disease by controlled abstention from liquids.

Dip·ter·a (dĭp′tər-ə) *n.* An order of insects comprising the true flies, characterized by a single pair of membranous wings and a pair of club-shaped balancing organs, and including many important disease vectors such as the mosquito, tsetse fly, and sandfly.

dip·ter·an (dĭp′tər-ən) *or* **dip·ter·on** (-tə-rŏn′) *n.* A dipterous insect. —**dip′ter·an** *adj.*

dip·ter·ous (dĭp′tər-əs) *adj.* **1.** Of or characteristic of insects of the order Diptera. **2.** Having two wings or winglike appendages.

dip·y·li·di·a·sis (dĭp′ə-lĭ-dī′ə-sĭs) *n.* Infection with *Dipylidium caninum.*

Di·py·lid·i·um ca·ni·num (dī′pī-lĭd′ē-əm kā-nī′nəm, dĭp′ə-) *n.* Tapeworm whose larvae are harbored by dog fleas or by lice.

di·pyr·id·a·mole (dī-pĭr′ĭ-də-mōl′, -pə-rĭd′ə-) *n.* A drug that acts as a coronary vasodilator and is used in the long-term treatment of angina pectoris.

di·rect diplopia (dĭ-rĕkt′, dī-) *n.* See **homonymous diplopia.**

direct flap *n.* A surgical flap that is raised completely and transferred to its recipient site during the same procedure. Also called *immediate flap.*

direct fracture *n.* A bone fracture, especially of the skull, occurring at the point of injury.

direct nuclear division *n.* See **amitosis.**

direct ophthalmoscope *n.* An instrument designed to visualize the interior of the eye, with the instrument relatively close to the subject's eye and the observer viewing an upright magnified image.

di·rec·tor (dĭ-rĕk′tər, dī-) *n.* A smoothly grooved instrument used with a knife to limit the incision of tissues. Also called *staff.*

direct oxidase *n.* See **oxygenase.**

direct percussion *n.* See **immediate percussion.**

direct reacting bilirubin *n.* Serum bilirubin that has been conjugated with glucuronic acid in the liver.

direct transfusion *n.* Transfusion of blood from the donor directly to the recipient. Also called *immediate transfusion.*

direct vision *n.* See **central vision.**

Di·ro·fi·lar·i·a (dī′rō-fə-lâr′ē-ə) *n.* A genus of filarial worms including the heartworm and other species, usually found in mammals other than humans.

dir. prop. *abbr. Latin* directione propria (with proper direction)

dirt-eating *n.* See **geophagy.**

dis– *pref.* **1.** Not: *disjugate.* **2.** Absence of; opposite of: *disorientation.* **3.** Undo; do the opposite of: *dislocate.* **4.** Deprive of; remove: *dismember.*

dis·a·bil·i·ty (dĭs′ə-bĭl′ĭ-tē) *n.* A disadvantage or deficiency, especially a physical or mental impairment that prevents or restricts normal achievement.

dis·a·bled (dĭs-ā′bəld) *adj.* Impaired, as in physical functioning. —*n.* Physically impaired people considered as a group. Often used with *the.*

di·sac·cha·ri·dase (dī-săk′ər-ĭ-dās′, -dāz′) *n.* An enzyme, such as invertase or lactase, that catalyzes the hydrolysis of disaccharides to monosaccharides.

di·sac·cha·ride (dī-săk′ə-rīd′) *n.* Any of a class of carbohydrates, including lactose and sucrose, that yield two monosaccharides upon hydrolysis.

dis·ag·gre·ga·tion (dĭs-ăg′rĭ-gā′shən) *n.* **1.** A breaking up into component parts. **2.** An inability to coordinate various sensations and a failure to observe their mutual relations. —**dis·ag′gre·gate′** *v.*

dis·ar·tic·u·la·tion (dĭs′är-tĭk′yə-lā′shən) *n.* The amputation of a limb through a joint, without the cutting of bone. Also called *exarticulation.* —**dis′ar·tic′u·late′** *v.*

disc (dĭsk) *n.* **1.** Variant of **disk. 2.** A discus.

disc·ec·to·my (dĭs-kĕk′tə-mē) *n.* The partial or complete excision of an intervertebral disk. Also called *discotomy.*

dis·charge (dĭs-chärj′) *v.* **1.** To emit a substance, as by excretion or secretion. **2.** To release a patient from custody or care. **3.** To generate an electrical impulse. Used of a neuron. —*n.* (dĭs′chärj, dĭs-chärj′) **1.** The act of releasing, emitting, or secreting. **2.** A substance that is excreted or secreted. **3.** The generation of an electrical impulse by a neuron.

dis·chro·na·tion (dĭs′krə-nā′shən) *n.* A disturbance in the consciousness of time.

dis·ci·form (dĭs′ə-fôrm′, dĭs′kə-) *adj.* Flat and rounded in shape; discoid.

disciform degeneration *n.* The degeneration of the macula and other areas of the retina, caused by hemorrhage and the proliferation of blood vessels, and resulting in a mass of fibrous tissue and loss of visual acuity.

dis·ci·sion (dĭ-sĭzh′ən) *n.* **1.** The incision of or cutting through a part. **2.** An operation for soft cataracts in which the crystalline capsule is opened and the substance of the crystalline lens is broken up to allow it to be absorbed.

dis·ci·tis (dĭs-kī′tĭs) *n.* Variant of **diskitis.**

dis·cli·na·tion (dĭs′klə-nā′shən) *n.* See **extorsion** (sense 2).

dis·clos·ing agent (dĭ-sklō′zĭng) *n.* A dye used in dentistry as a diagnostic aid, applied to the teeth to reveal the presence of dental plaque.

disclosing solution *n.* A solution that selectively stains all soft debris, pellicle, and bacterial plaque on the teeth.

disco– *or* **disc–***or* **disci–** *pref.* Disk: *discoid.*

dis·co·gen·ic (dĭs′kə-jĕn′ĭk) *adj.* Relating to a disorder originating in or from an intervertebral disk.

dis·co·gram *or* **dis·ko·gram** (dĭs′kə-grăm′) *n.* An x-ray image produced by discography.

dis·cog·ra·phy (dĭ-skŏg′rə-fē) *n.* Examination of the intervertebral disk space using x-rays after injection of contrast media into the disk.

dis·coid (dĭs′koid′)*or* **dis·coi·dal** (dĭ-skoid′l) *adj.* Shaped like or resembling a disk.

discoid lupus er·y·the·ma·to·sus (ĕr′ə-thē′mə-tō′səs, -thĕm′ə-) *n.* Lupus erythematosus in which only cutaneous lesions are present, usually on the face, occurring as atrophic plaques with erythema, hyperkeratosis, follicular plugging, and telangiectasia.

dis·con·tin·u·a·tion test (dĭs′kən-tĭn′yōō-ā′shən) *n.* A test to determine whether a drug is responsible for a reaction; a positive result is obtained if symptoms stop after use of the drug is discontinued.

dis·cop·a·thy (dĭ-skŏp′ə-thē) *n.* Disease of a disk, especially of an intervertebral disk.

dis·co·pla·cen·ta (dĭs′kō-plə-sĕn′tə) *n.* A placenta having discoid shape.

dis·cor·dance (dĭ-skôr′dns) *n.* The presence of a given genetic trait in only one member of a pair of identical twins. —**dis·cor′dant** *adj.*

discordant alternation *n.* An alternation in heart activities that involve either the systemic or pulmonary circuit, but not both.

dis·cot·o·my (dĭ-skŏt′ə-mē) *n.* See **discectomy.**

dis·crete (dĭ-skrēt′) *adj.* Not joined to or incorporated with another; separate; distinct.

dis·cus (dĭs′kəs) *n., pl.* **dis·ci** (dĭs′kī′, dĭs′ī′) A flat circular surface; a disk.

dis·cu·tient (dĭ-skyōō′shənt) *adj.* Causing dispersal or disappearance of a pathological accumulation. —*n.* A discutient agent or drug.

dis·ease (dĭ-zēz′) *n.* A pathological condition of a body part, an organ, or a system resulting from various causes, such as infection, genetic defect, or environmental stress, and characterized by an identifiable group of signs or symptoms.

dis·eased (dĭ-zēzd′) *adj.* **1.** Affected with disease. **2.** Unsound or disordered.

disease determinant *n.* Any of a group of variables, such as specific disease agents and environmental factors, that directly or indirectly influence the frequency or distribution of a disease.

dis·en·gage·ment (dĭs′ĕn-gāj′mənt) *n.* The emergence of the presenting part of the fetus from the vaginal canal during childbirth. —**dis′en·gage′** *v.*

dis·e·qui·lib·ri·um (dĭs-ē′kwə-lĭb′rē-əm, -ĕk′wə-) *n.* The loss or lack of stability or equilibrium.

dis·func·tion (dĭs-fŭngk′shən) *n.* Variant of **dysfunction**.

dis·ger·mi·no·ma (dĭs-jûr′mə-nō′mə) *n.* Variant of **dysgerminoma**.

dish·pan hands (dĭsh′păn′) *pl.n.* A rough, dry, scaly condition of the hands typically caused by sensitivity to or excessive use of household detergents or cleaning agents.

dis·in·fect (dĭs′ĭn-fĕkt′) *v.* To cleanse something so as to destroy or prevent the growth of disease-carrying microorganisms.

dis·in·fec·tant (dĭs′ĭn-fĕk′tənt) *n.* An agent, such as heat, radiation, or a chemical, that disinfects by destroying, neutralizing, or inhibiting the growth of disease-carrying microorganisms. —*adj.* Serving to disinfect.

dis·in·fes·tant (dĭs′ĭn-fĕs′tənt) *n.* An agent that eradicates an infestation, as of vermin.

dis·in·hi·bi·tion (dĭs′ĭn-hə-bĭsh′ən, dĭs-ĭn′-) *n.* **1.** A loss of inhibition, as through the influence of drugs or alcohol. **2.** A temporary loss of an inhibition caused by an unrelated stimulus, such as a loud noise.

dis·in·ser·tion (dĭs′ĭn-sûr′shən) *n.* A tear in the extreme periphery of the retina that ends at the ciliary ring; it may occur as a result of trauma and is common in juvenile retinal detachment.

dis·in·te·gra·tion (dĭs-ĭn′tĭ-grā′shən) *n.* **1.** The breaking up of the component parts of a substance, as in catabolism or decay. **2.** The disorganization or disruption of mental processes in mental illness. **3.** The natural or induced transformation of an atomic nucleus from a more massive to a less massive configuration by the emission of particles or radiation. —**dis·in′te·grate′** *v.*

disintegration constant *n.* See **decay constant**.

dis·joint (dĭs-joint′) *v.* To put out of joint; dislocate.

dis·junc·tion (dĭs-jŭngk′shən) *n.* The separation of homologous chromosomes during meiosis.

disk *or* **disc** (dĭsk) *n.* **1.** A thin, flat, circular object or plate. **2.** See **lamella** (sense 2).

dis·ki·tis *or* **dis·ci·tis** (dĭs-kī′tĭs) *n.* A nonbacterial inflammation of an intervertebral disk or disk space.

dis·ko·gram (dĭs′kə-grăm) *n.* Variant of **discogram**.

disk syndrome *n.* A syndrome that is caused by a compressive radiculopathy from intervertebral disk pressure and combines symptoms of lower back pain, pain in the thigh, and sciatica with wasting and loss of achilles and patellar reflexes.

dis·lo·cate (dĭs′lō-kāt′, dĭs-lō′kāt) *v.* To displace a body part, especially to displace a bone from its normal position.

dis·lo·ca·tion (dĭs′lō-kā′shən) *n.* Displacement of a body part, especially the temporary displacement of a bone from its normal position; luxation.

dislocation fracture *n.* A bone fracture occurring near a joint and causing the bone to dislocate from the joint.

dis·mem·ber (dĭs-mĕm′bər) *v.* To amputate a limb or a part of a limb. —**dis·mem′ber·ment** *n.*

dis·mu·tase (dĭs-myōō′tās, -tāz) *n.* Any of various enzymes that catalyze the reaction of two identical molecules to produce two molecules in different states of oxidation or phosphorylation.

di·so·di·um (dī-sō′dē-əm) *adj.* Containing two atoms of sodium.

dis·or·der (dĭs-ôr′dər) *n.* A disturbance or derangement that affects the function of mind or body. —*v.* To disturb the normal physical or mental health of; disturb or derange.

dis·or·gan·i·za·tion (dĭs-ôr′gə-nĭ-zā′shən) *n.* The destruction of an organ or tissue causing loss of function.

dis·or·gan·ized schizophrenia (dĭs-ôr′gə-nīzd′) *n.* See **hebephrenia**.

dis·o·ri·en·ta·tion (dĭs-ôr′ē-ĕn-tā′shən) *n.* **1.** Loss of one's sense of direction, position, or relationship with one's surroundings. **2.** A temporary or permanent state of confusion regarding place, time, or personal identity.

dis·pen·sa·ble (dĭ-spĕn′sə-bəl) *adj.* Capable of being dispensed, administered, or distributed. Used of a drug.

dis·pen·sa·ry (dĭ-spĕn′sə-rē) *n.* **1.** An office in a hospital or other institution from which medical supplies and medicines are dispensed. **2.** A public institution that dispenses medicines or medical aid. **3.** An outpatient department of a hospital.

dis·pen·sa·to·ry (dĭ-spĕn′sə-tôr′ē) *n.* A book in which the contents, preparation, physiologic action, and therapeutic uses of medicines are described.

dis·pense (dĭ-spĕns′) *v.* To prepare and give out medicines.

dis·perse (dĭ-spûrs′) *v.* **1.** To cause to separate and move in different directions; scatter. **2.** To cause to vanish or disappear.

disperse phase *n.* The particles or droplets in a disperse system.

disperse system *n.* A system, such as a colloid, consisting of a substance dispersed in a medium.

dis·per·sion (dĭ-spûr′zhən) *n.* **1.** The act or process of dispersing. **2.** The state of being dispersed. **3.** Disperse system.

dispersion medium *n.* The continuous medium, such as a gas, liquid, or solid, in which a disperse phase is distributed. Also called *external phase*.

di·spi·reme (dī-spī′rēm′) *n.* The double chromatin coil present during the mitotic telophase.

dis·place·ment (dĭs-plās′mənt) *n.* **1.** Removal from the normal location or position. **2.** A defense mechanism in which there is an unconscious shift of emotions, affect, or desires from the original object to a more acceptable or immediate substitute. **3.** A chemical reaction in which an atom, a radical, or a molecule replaces another in a compound.

dis·sect (dĭ-sĕkt′, dī-, dī′sĕkt′) *v.* **1.** To cut apart or separate tissue, especially for anatomical study. **2.** In surgery, to separate different anatomical structures along natural lines by dividing the connective tissue framework.

dissecting aneurysm *n.* The splitting or dissection of an arterial wall by blood entering through a tear of the inner lining or by interstitial hemorrhage.

dissecting cellulitis *n.* A chronic folliculitis of the scalp.

dis·sec·tion (dĭ-sĕk′shən, dī-) *n.* **1.** The act or an instance of dissecting. **2.** Something that has been dissected, such as a tissue specimen under study.

dissection tubercle *n.* See **postmortem wart.**

dis·sem·i·nat·ed (dĭ-sĕm′ə-nā′tĭd) *adj.* Spread over a large area of a body, a tissue, or an organ.

disseminated cutaneous leishmaniasis *n.* See **diffuse cutaneous leishmaniasis.**

disseminated intravascular coagulation *n. Abbr.* **DIC** A hemorrhagic disorder that occurs following the uncontrolled activation of clotting factors and fibrinolytic enzymes throughout small blood vessels, resulting in tissue necrosis and bleeding. Also called *consumption coagulopathy.*

disseminated lipogranulomatosis *n.* A congenital lipid metabolism disorder developing soon after birth, characterized by swollen joints, diffuse subcutaneous nodules, and the deposition of lipids in cells of affected tissues. Also called *Farber's disease.*

disseminated lupus er·y·the·ma·to·sus (ĕr′ə-thē′mə-tō′səs, -thĕm′ə-) *n.* See **systemic lupus erythematosus.**

disseminated tuberculosis *n.* See **acute tuberculosis.**

dis·sim·u·la·tion (dĭ-sĭm′yə-lā′shən) *n.* Concealment of the truth about a situation, especially about a state of health, as by a malingerer.

dis·so·ci·at·ed anesthesia (dĭ-sō′shē-ā′tĭd, -sē-) *n.* Loss of sensation for pain and temperature without the loss of tactile sense.

dissociated nystagmus *n.* A nystagmus in which the movements of the two eyes are dissimilar in direction, extent, and periodicity.

dis·so·ci·a·tion (dĭ-sō′sē-ā′shən, -shē-) *n.* **1.** The chemical process by which the action of a solvent or a change in physical condition, as in pressure or temperature, causes a molecule to split into simpler groups of atoms, single atoms, or ions. **2.** The separation of an electrolyte into ions of opposite charge. **3.** Separation of a group of related psychological activities into autonomously functioning units, as in the generation of multiple personalities. —**dis·so′ci·ate′** *v.* —**dis·so′ci·a′tive** *adj.*

dissociation sensibility *n.* Loss of the sensibility to pain and temperature with the preservation of the sense of touch.

dissociative anesthesia *n.* A form of general anesthesia characterized by catalepsy, catatonia, and amnesia, but not necessarily involving complete unconsciousness, as that produced by ketamine.

dissociative identity disorder *n.* See **multiple personality disorder.**

dissociative reaction *n.* A psychological reaction characterized by such behavior as amnesia, fugues, sleepwalking, and dream states.

dis·solve (dĭ-zŏlv′) *v.* **1.** To pass or cause to pass into a solution, as salt in water. **2.** To become or cause to

become liquid; melt. **3.** To cause to disintegrate or become disintegrated.

dis·tad (dĭs′tăd′) *adv.* Toward the periphery; in a distal direction.

dis·tal (dĭs′təl) *adj.* **1.** Anatomically located far from a point of reference, such as an origin or a point of attachment. **2.** Situated farthest from the middle and front of the jaw, as a tooth or tooth surface.

distal myopathy *n.* A hereditary myopathy, usually occurring after age 40, that mainly affects the distal portions of the limbs.

dis·tance (dĭs′təns) *n.* The extent of space between two objects or places; an intervening space.

dis·tant flap (dĭs′tənt) *n.* A surgical flap in which the recipient area is distant from, and must be brought into close approximation to, the donor site.

dis·tem·per (dĭs-tĕm′pər) *n.* **1.** An infectious viral disease occurring in dogs, characterized by loss of appetite, a catarrhal discharge from the eyes and nose, vomiting, partial paralysis, and sometimes death. **2.** A similar viral disease of cats characterized by fever, vomiting, diarrhea leading to dehydration, and sometimes death. **3.** Any of various similar mammalian diseases.

dis·tend (dĭ-stĕnd′) *v.* To swell out or expand or cause to swell out or expand from or as if from internal pressure.

dis·ten·tion *or* **dis·ten·sion** (dĭ-stĕn′shən) *n.* The act of distending or the state of being distended.

dis·tich·i·a (dĭ-stĭk′ē-ə) *or* **dis·ti·chi·a·sis** (dĭs′tĭ-kī′ə-sĭs) *n.* A congenital abnormality in which there is an additional row of eyelashes that turn in upon the eye.

dis·till (dĭ-stĭl′) *v.* **1.** To subject a substance to distillation. **2.** To separate a distillate by distillation. **3.** To increase the concentration of, separate, or purify a substance by distillation.

dis·til·late (dĭs′tə-lāt′, -lĭt, dĭ-stĭl′ĭt) *n.* A liquid condensed from vapor in distillation.

dis·til·la·tion (dĭs′tə-lā′shən) *n.* **1.** The evaporation and subsequent collection of a liquid by condensation as a means of purification. **2.** The extraction of the volatile components of a mixture by the condensation and collection of the vapors that are produced as the mixture is heated.

dis·to·buc·cal (dĭs′tō-bŭk′əl) *adj.* Relating to the distal and the buccal surfaces of a tooth.

dis·to·buc·co·oc·clu·sal (dĭs′tō-bŭk′ō-ə-kloo′zəl, -səl) *adj.* Relating to the distal, buccal, and occlusal surfaces of a bicuspid or molar tooth.

dis·to·buc·co·pul·pal (dĭs′tō-bŭk′ō-pŭl′pəl) *adj.* Relating to the angle formed by the junction of a distal, buccal, and pulpal wall of a tooth cavity.

dis·to·cer·vi·cal (dĭs′tō-sûr′vĭ-kəl) *adj.* Relating to the line angle formed by the junction of the distal and gingival walls of a tooth cavity.

dis·to·clu·sal (dĭs′tō-kloo′zəl) *adj.* **1.** Relating to or characterized by distoclusion. **2.** Of or relating to a compound cavity or restoration involving the distal and the occlusal surfaces of a tooth. **3.** Relating to the line angle formed by the distal and the occlusal walls of a tooth cavity.

dis·to·clu·sion (dĭs′tō-kloo′zhən) *n.* A malocclusion in which the lower teeth are distal to the upper teeth.

dis·to·gin·gi·val (dĭs′tō-jĭn′jə-vəl, -jĭn-jī′-) *adj.* Relating to the junction of the distal surface of a tooth and the gingiva.

dis·to·in·ci·sal (dĭs′tō-ĭn-sī′zəl) *adj.* Relating to the angle formed by the junction of the distal and the incisal walls of a cavity in a tooth.

dis·to·la·bi·al (dĭs′tō-lā′bē-əl) *adj.* Relating to the distal and labial surfaces of a tooth.

dis·to·la·bi·o·pul·pal (dĭs′tō-lā′bē-ō-pŭl′pəl) *adj.* Relating to the angle formed by the junction of the distal, labial, and pulpal walls of the incisal part of a tooth cavity.

dis·to·lin·gual (dĭs′tō-lĭng′gwəl) *adj.* Relating to the distal and lingual surfaces of a tooth.

dis·to·lin·guo·oc·clu·sal (dĭs′tō-lĭng′gwō-ə-klōō′zəl, -səl) *adj.* Relating to the distal, lingual, and occlusal surfaces of a bicuspid or molar tooth.

dis·to·mi·a·sis (dĭs′tō-mī′ə-sĭs) *or* **dis·to·ma·to·sis** (-mə-tō′sĭs) *n.* Infection by a trematode or fluke.

dis·to·mo·lar (dĭs′tō-mō′lər) *n.* A supernumerary tooth located behind the third molar.

dis·to·pul·pal (dĭs′tō-pŭl′pəl) *adj.* Relating to the angle formed by the junction of the distal and the pulpal walls of a tooth cavity.

dis·tor·tion (dĭ-stôr′shən) *n.* **1.** A twisting out of normal shape or form. **2.** A psychological defense mechanism that helps to repress or to disguise unacceptable thoughts. **3.** Parataxic distortion. —**dis·tor′tion·al, dis·tor′tion·ar′y** *adj.*

distortion aberration *n.* The faulty formation of an image arising because the magnification of the peripheral part of an object is different from that of the central part when viewed through a lens.

dis·to·ver·sion (dĭs′tō-vûr′zhən) *n.* The tilting of a tooth from its normal position toward the back of the jaw following the curvature of the dental arch.

dis·trac·tion (dĭ-străk′shən) *n.* **1.** A condition or state of mind in which the attention is diverted from an original focus or interest. **2.** Separation of bony fragments or joint surfaces of a limb by extension.

dis·tress (dĭ-strĕs′) *n.* **1.** Mental or physical suffering or anguish. **2.** Severe strain resulting from exhaustion or trauma. —**dis·tress′** *adj.*

dis·tri·bu·tion (dĭs′trə-byōō′shən) *n.* **1.** The extension of the branches of arteries or nerves to the tissues and organs. **2.** The area in which the branches of an artery or a nerve terminate, or the area supplied by such an artery or nerve. **3.** A set of numbers and their frequency of occurrence from measurements within a statistical population. —**dis′tri·bu′tion·al** *adj.*

dis·trix (dĭs′trĭks) *n.* Splitting of the hairs at their ends.

di·sul·fate (dī-sŭl′fāt′) *n.* A compound containing two sulfate ions or radicals.

di·sul·fide (dī-sŭl′fīd′) *n.* A chemical compound containing two sulfur atoms combined with other elements or radicals. Also called *bisulfide.*

disulfide bond *n.* The covalent bond between sulfur atoms that binds two peptide chains or different parts of one peptide chain and is a structural determinant in many protein molecules.

di·sul·fi·ram (dī-sŭl′fə-răm′) *n.* An antioxidant used in the treatment of chronic alcoholism that interferes with the normal metabolic degradation of alcohol in the body, producing an unpleasant reaction when a small quantity of alcohol is consumed.

di·ter·pene (dī-tûr′pēn′) *n.* Any of a class of terpenes with 20 carbon atoms and 4 branched methyl groups.

Di·tro·pan (dī′trə-pən) A trademark for the drug oxybutynin chloride.

Ditt·rich's plug (dĭt′rĭks) *n.* Any of the minute, grayish, ill-smelling masses of bacteria and fatty acid crystals in the sputum in pulmonary gangrene and fetid bronchitis.

di·u·re·sis (dī′ə-rē′sĭs) *n.* Discharge of urine, especially in unusually large amounts.

di·u·ret·ic (dī′ə-rĕt′ĭk) *adj.* Tending to increase the discharge of urine. —*n.* A substance or drug that tends to increase the discharge of urine.

Di·u·ril (dī′ə-rĭl′) A trademark for the drug chlorthiazide.

di·ur·nal (dī-ûr′nəl) *adj.* **1.** Having a 24-hour period or cycle; daily. **2.** Occurring or active during the daytime rather than at night. —**di·ur′nal·ly** *adv.*

di·va·lent (dī-vā′lənt) *adj.* Bivalent. —**di·va′lence, di·va′len·cy** *n.*

di·val·pro·ex sodium (dī-văl′prō-ĕks′) *n.* An anticonvulsant used in the treatment of petit mal and related seizure disorders.

di·var·i·ca·tion (dī-văr′ĭ-kā′shən, dī-) *n.* See **diastasis** (sense 1).

di·ver·gence (dĭ-vûr′jəns, dī-) *n.* **1.** A moving or spreading apart in different directions from a common point. **2.** The degree by which things deviate or spread apart. **3.** A turning of both eyes outward from a common point or of one eye when the other is fixed. **4.** The spreading of branches of the neuron to form synapses with several other neurons. **5.** The evolutionary process by which organisms descended from a common ancestor tend to acquire different forms when living under different conditions. —**di·ver′gent** *adj.*

divergence insufficiency *n.* The condition in which an exophoria or exotropia is more marked for near vision than for far vision.

divergent strabismus *n.* See **exotropia.**

di·ver·tic·u·lec·to·my (dī′vûr-tĭk′yə-lĕk′tə-mē) *n.* Excision of a diverticulum.

di·ver·tic·u·li·tis (dī′vûr-tĭk′yə-lī′tĭs) *n.* Inflammation of a diverticulum, especially of the small pockets in the wall of the colon that fill with stagnant fecal material and become inflamed.

di·ver·tic·u·lo·ma (dī′vûr-tĭk′yə-lō′mə) *n.* A granulomatous mass in the wall of the colon.

di·ver·tic·u·lo·sis (dī′vûr-tĭk′yə-lō′sĭs) *n.* A condition characterized by the presence of numerous diverticula in the colon.

di·ver·tic·u·lum (dī′vûr-tĭk′yə-ləm) *n.,* *pl.* **–la** (-lə) A pouch or sac branching out from a hollow organ or structure. See illustration on page 236. —**di·ver·tic′u·lar** *adj.*

di·vide (dĭ-vīd′) *v.* **1.** To separate or become separated into parts, sections, groups, or branches. **2.** To sector into units of measurement; graduate. **3.** To separate and group according to kind; classify. **4.** To branch out, as a blood vessel. **5.** To undergo cell division.

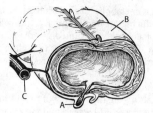

diverticulum
an intestinal diverticulum:
A. diverticulum, B. large intestine, C. blood vessel

div·ing goiter (dī′vĭng) *n.* A freely movable goiter that is sometimes above and sometimes below the sternal notch. Also called *wandering goiter.*

diving reflex *n.* A reflexive response to diving in many aquatic mammals and birds, characterized by physiological changes that decrease oxygen consumption, such as slowed heart rate and decreased blood flow to the abdominal organs and muscles, until breathing resumes. Though less pronounced, the reflex also occurs in humans, upon submersion in water.

div. in par. aeq. *abbr. Latin* divide in partes aequales, dividiatur in partes aequales (divide into equal parts, let there be divided into equal parts)

di·vi·nyl ether (dī-vī′nəl) *n.* A rapidly acting inhalation anesthetic. Also called *vinyl ether.*

di·vi·sion (dĭ-vĭzh′ən) *n.* **1.** The act or process of dividing. **2.** Cell division. **3.** The operation of determining how many times one quantity is contained in another; the inverse of multiplication.

di·vul·sion (dĭ-vŭl′shən) *n.* **1.** The removal of a part by tearing. **2.** The forcible dilation of the walls of a cavity or canal.

di·vul·sor (dĭ-vŭl′sər, -sôr′) *n.* An instrument used for forcible dilation of the urethra or other canal or cavity.

di·zy·got·ic (dī′zī-gŏt′ĭk) *or* **di·zy·gous** (dī-zī′gəs) *adj.* Derived from two separately fertilized eggs. Used especially of fraternal twins.

diz·zi·ness (dĭz′ē-nĭs) *n.* A disorienting sensation such as faintness, light-headedness, or unsteadiness.

DJD *abbr.* degenerative joint disease

Djer·as·si (jə-räs′ē) **Carl** Born 1923. Austrian-born American chemist noted for his work on the development of an oral contraceptive.

DKA *abbr.* diabetic ketoacidosis

dl– *pref.* Containing dextrorotatory and levorotatory forms of a compound. No longer in technical use.

dM *abbr.* decimorgan

DM *abbr.* diabetes mellitus

DMD *abbr.* Doctor of Dental Medicine

DMF (dē′ĕm-ĕf′) *abbr.* decayed, missing, or filled (used for permanent teeth)

DMSO (dē′ĕm-ĕs-ō′) *n.* Dimethyl sulfoxide; a colorless hygroscopic liquid obtained from lignin, used as a penetrant to convey medications into the tissues.

DMT (dē′ĕm-tē′) *n.* Dimethyltryptamine; a synthetic hallucinogenic drug.

DN *abbr.* dibucaine number

DNA (dē′ĕn-ā′) *n.* Deoxyribonucleic acid; a nucleic acid that consists of two long chains of nucleotides twisted together into a double helix and joined by hydrogen bonds between complementary bases adenine and thymine or cytosine and guanine; it carries the cell's genetic information and hereditary characteristics via its nucleotides and their sequence and is capable of self-replication and RNA synthesis.

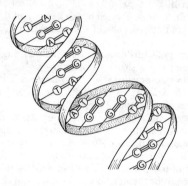

DNA
double helix molecule containing nucleotide bases adenine (A), guanine (G), cytosine (C), and thymine (T)

DNA fingerprint *n.* An individual's unique sequence of DNA base pairs. Also called *genetic fingerprint.*

DNA fingerprinting *n.* A method used to identify multilocus DNA banding patterns that are specific to an individual by exposing a sample of the person's DNA to molecular probes and various analytical techniques such as Southern blot analysis. DNA fingerprinting is often used to provide evidence in criminal law cases. Also called *genetic fingerprinting.*

DNA helix *n.* See **double helix.**

DNA polymorphism *n.* A condition in which one of two different but normal nucleotide sequences can exist at a particular site in a DNA molecule.

DNase (dē-ĕn′ās) *or* **DNAase** (dē′ĕn-ā′ās) *n.* An enzyme that catalyzes the hydrolysis of DNA.

DNA virus *n.* A virus whose nucleic acid core is composed of DNA, such as any of the adenoviruses, papovaviruses, herpesviruses, or poxviruses.

DNP (dē′ĕn-pē′) *n.* Deoxyribonucleoprotein; a complex of DNA and protein that usually yields DNA upon cell disruption and isolation.

DNR *abbr.* do not resuscitate (a physician's order to refrain from initiating a code blue)

DNS *abbr.* Director of Nursing Services; Doctor of Nursing Services

DO *abbr.* Doctor of Osteopathy

DOA *abbr.* dead on admission; dead on arrival

DOB *abbr.* date of birth

do·bu·ta·mine hydrochloride (dō-byōō′tə-mēn′) *n.* A synthetic adrenergic catecholamine used to stimulate myocardial function and increase cardiac output.

Dob·zhan·sky (dəb-zhăn′skē), **Theodosius** 1900–1975. Russian-born American geneticist. His *Genetics and the Origin of the Species* (1937) synthesized Mendel's laws of heredity and Darwinian theory. He is also known for his study of the fruit fly *Drosophilia*, which showed a large degree of genetic variation within a population.

doc (dŏk) *n.* A physician, dentist, or veterinarian.

DOC (dē'ō-sē') *n.* **1.** Deoxycorticosterone; a steroid hormone secreted by the adrenal cortex or produced synthetically and used to treat adrenal insufficiency. **2.** Deoxycholic acid; a bile acid used as a choleretic and digestant and in the synthesis of adrenocortical hormones such as cortisone.

doc·tor (dŏk'tər) *n.* **1.** A person, especially a physician, dentist, or veterinarian, trained in the healing arts and licensed to practice. **2.** A person who has earned the highest academic degree awarded by a university in a specified discipline.

doc·u·sate sodium (dŏk'yə-sāt') *n.* A surface-active agent that, when ingested, decreases the surface tension in the intestinal tract and acts as a stool softener.

DOE *abbr.* dyspnea on exertion

Doerf·ler-Stewart test (dûrf'lər-) *n.* A test that differentiates between functional and organic hearing loss by examining a person's ability to respond to spondee words in the presence of a masking noise.

Döh·le body (dē'lē, dœ'lĕ) *n.* A discrete round or oval body found in neutrophils and associated with infections, burns, trauma, pregnancy, or cancer.

Doi·sy (doi'zē), **Edward Adelbert** 1893–1986. American biochemist. He shared a 1943 Nobel Prize for isolating two forms of vitamin K.

dol (dōl) *n.* A unit for the measurement of the intensity of pain.

dolicho– *pref.* Long: *dolichofacial.*

dol·i·cho·ce·phal·ic (dŏl'ĭ-kō-sə-făl'ĭk) *or* **dol·i·cho·ceph·a·lous** (-sĕf'ə-ləs) *adj.* Having a disproportionately long head.

dol·i·cho·ec·tat·ic artery (dŏl'ĭ-kō-ĕk-tăt'ĭk) *n.* A distorted, dilated, and elongated artery commonly compressing a neural structure.

dol·i·cho·fa·cial (dŏl'ĭ-kō-fā'shəl) *adj.* Having a disproportionately long face.

dol·i·chol (dŏl'ĭ-kôl) *n.* Any of various long-chain unsaturated isoprenoid alcohols found either free or phosphorylated in membranes of the endoplasmic reticulum and Golgi apparatus.

dol·i·cho·pel·lic (dŏl'ĭ-kō-pĕl'ĭk) *or* **dol·i·cho·pel·vic** (-pĕl'vĭk) *adj.* Characterizing or having a disproportionately long pelvis.

dolichopellic pelvis *n.* A pelvis having an anteroposterior diameter longer than its transverse diameter.

dol·i·cho·pro·sop·ic (dŏl'ĭ-kō-prō-sŏp'ĭk) *adj.* Having a disproportionately long face.

doll's eye sign (dŏlz) *n.* Reflex movement of the eyes such that the eyes lower as the head is raised, indicating functional integrity of the nerve pathways involved in eye movement.

Do·lo·bid (dōlə-bĭd') A trademark for the drug diflunisal.

do·lor (dō'lər) *n.* **1.** Pain. **2.** Sorrow; grief. —**do'lo·rif'ic** *adj.*

do·lo·rim·e·try (dō'lə-rĭm'ĭ-trē, dōl'ə-) *n.* The measurement of pain sensitivity or pain intensity.

DOM (dē'ō-ĕm') *n.* 2,5-Dimethoxy-4-methylamphetamine; an hallucinogenic agent that is chemically related to amphetamine. Also called *STP.*

Do·magk (dō'mäk'), **Gerhard** 1895–1964. German biochemist. He won a 1939 Nobel Prize for his work on the antibacterial effect of sulfa drugs but declined the award at the instruction of the German government.

do·main (dō-mān') *n.* One of the homologous regions that make up an immunoglobulin's heavy and light chains and serve specific immunological functions.

dom·i·cil·i·at·ed (dŏm'ĭ-sĭl'ē-ā'tĭd, dō'mĭ-) *adj.* Of or relating to an organism living in close association with humans so that partial domestication results, leading to the organism's dependence on continued association with the human environment.

dom·i·nance (dŏm'ə-nəns) *n.* The condition or state of being dominant.

dominance of genes *n.* A full phenotypic expression of a gene in both heterozygotes and homozygotes.

dom·i·nant (dŏm'ə-nənt) *adj.* **1.** Exercising the most influence or control. **2.** Of, relating to, or being an allele that produces the same phenotypic effect whether inherited with a homozygous or heterozygous allele. —*n.* **1.** A dominant allele or trait. **2.** An organism having a dominant trait.

dominant character *n.* See **dominant trait.**

dominant eye *n.* The eye customarily used for monocular tasks.

dominant gene *n.* A gene that is expressed phenotypically in heterozygous or homozygous individuals.

dominant hemisphere *n.* The cerebral hemisphere that is more involved than the other in governing certain body functions, such as controlling the arm and leg used preferentially in skilled movements.

dominant idea *n.* An idea that governs all the actions and thoughts of the individual.

dominant inheritance *n.* Inheritance in which an allele produces the same phenotypic effect whether inherited with a homozygous or heterozygous allele.

dominant trait *n.* An inherited character determined by a dominant gene. Also called *dominant character.*

Do·nath-Land·stei·ner phenomenon (dō'nāth-lănd'-stī'nər, -nät-) *n.* The hemolysis that occurs in a sample of blood from an individual with paroxysmal hemoglobinuria when the sample is cooled to around 5°C and then warmed.

Don·ders' law (dŏn'dərz) *n.* The principle that the rotation of the eyeball is determined by the distance of the object from the median plane and the line of the horizon.

do·nep·e·zil hydrochloride (dō-nĕp'ə-zĭl') *n.* An acetylcholinesterase inhibitor drug used to treat dementia caused by Alzheimer's disease.

dong quai (dŏong kwā, kwī) *n.* A perennial aromatic herb (*Angelica sinensis*) native to China and Japan, having a root that is used medicinally for gynecological complaints such as premenstrual syndrome, menstrual cramps, and menopausal symptoms.

Don Juan (dŏn wŏn') *n.* A man who is an obsessive seducer of women, especially one who does so out of feelings of impotence or inferiority.

do·nor (dō'nər) *n.* **1.** One from whom blood, tissue, or an organ is taken for use in a transfusion or transplant.

2. A chemical compound that can transfer an atom, a radical, or a particle to an acceptor.

donor card *n.* A card, usually carried on one's person, authorizing the use of one's bodily organs for transplantation in the event of one's death.

Don·o·van body (dŏn′ə-vən, dŭn′-) *n.* See **Leishman-Donovan body.**

don·o·va·no·sis (dŏn′ə-və-nō′sĭs) *n.* A chronic destructive ulceration of the inguinal region and the external genitalia caused by *Calymmatobacterium granulomatis,* which is observed intracellularly as Leishman-Donovan bodies in the infected tissue. Also called *granuloma inguinale.*

do·pa (dō′pə) *n.* Dihydroxyphenylalanine; an amino acid formed in the liver from tyrosine and converted to dopamine in the brain.

do·pa·mine (dō′pə-mēn′) *n.* A monoamine neurotransmitter formed in the brain by the decarboxylation of dopa and essential to the normal functioning of the central nervous system. A reduction in its concentration within the brain is associated with Parkinson's disease. Also called *3-hydroxytyramine.*

do·pa·mi·ner·gic (dō′pə-mə-nûr′jĭk) *adj.* Relating to, involved in, or initiated by the neurotransmitter activity of dopamine or related substances.

dope (dōp) *n.* **1.** A narcotic, especially an addictive narcotic. **2.** An illicit drug, especially marijuana.

dop·ing (dō′pĭng) *n.* The use of a drug or blood product to improve athletic performance.

Dop·pler echocardiography (dŏp′lər) *n.* The use of Doppler ultrasonography to augment echocardiograms that are two-dimensional by allowing velocities to be registered within the echocardiogram.

Doppler effect *n.* An apparent change in the frequency of waves, as of sound or light, occurring when the source and observer are in motion relative to each other, with the frequency increasing when the source and observer approach each other and decreasing when they move apart.

Doppler ultrasonography *n.* Ultrasonography applying the Doppler effect, in which frequency-shifted ultrasound reflections produced by moving targets in the bloodstream, usually red blood cells, are used to determine the direction and velocity of blood flow.

dor·nase al·fa (dôr′nās′ ăl′fə, -nāz′) *n.* A genetically engineered enzyme used to hydrolyze the DNA in bronchial mucus, facilitating its expectoration, in the treatment of cystic fibrosis.

dors– *pref.* Variant of **dorso–.**

dor·sad (dôr′săd′) *adv.* In the direction of the back; dorsally.

dor·sal (dôr′səl) *adj.* **1.** Of, toward, on, in, or near the back or upper surface of an organ, a part, or an organism. **2.** Lying on the back; supine.

dorsal artery of clitoris *n.* Either of two terminal branches of the internal pudendal artery in females.

dorsal artery of foot *n.* An artery that is a continuation of the anterior tibial artery, with branches to the lateral tarsal, arcuate, and dorsal metatarsal arteries, and with anastomoses with the lateral plantar artery to form the plantar arch.

dorsal artery of nose *n.* An artery with origin in the ophthalmic artery, with distribution to the skin of the

side of the nose, and with anastomosis to the angular artery.

dorsal artery of penis *n.* An artery that is the dorsal terminal branch of the internal pudendal artery in males.

dorsal column of spinal cord *n.* See **posterior column of spinal cord.**

dorsal digital artery *n.* Any of the arteries that are the collateral digital branches of the dorsal metatarsal arteries in the foot, and of the dorsal metacarpal arteries in the hand.

dorsal digital nerve *n.* Any of the nerves of the hand supplying skin of the dorsal surface of a finger.

dorsal digital nerve of foot *n.* Any of the nerves of the foot that supply the skin of the proximal and middle phalanges.

dorsal digital vein of toe *n.* Any of the veins that join to form the four common dorsal digital veins, and terminate in the dorsal venous arch.

dorsal flexure *n.* A flexure in the mid-dorsal region in the embryo.

dor·sal·gia (dôr-săl′jə) *n.* Pain in the upper back.

dorsal horn *n.* See **posterior horn** (sense 1, 2).

dorsal interosseous muscle of foot *n.* Any of four muscles with their origins from the sides of the adjacent metatarsal bones, with insertion of the first and the second into the proximal phalanx of the second toe and with insertion of the third and the fourth into the proximal phalanx of the third and the fourth toes, with nerve supply from the lateral plantar nerve, and by whose action the first adducts the second toe, and the second, third, and fourth abduct the second, the third, and the fourth toes.

dorsal interosseous muscle of hand *n.* Any of four muscles with origins from the sides of the adjacent metacarpal bones, with insertion to the proximal phalanges and extensor expansions, with nerve supply from the ulnar nerve, and whose action abducts the index finger, abducts or adducts the middle finger, or abducts the ring finger.

dorsal lateral cutaneous nerve *n.* The continuation of the sural nerve in the foot, supplying the lateral margin and dorsum.

dorsal medial cutaneous nerve *n.* The medial terminal branch of the superficial peroneal nerve, supplying the dorsum of the foot and the dorsal nerves to the toes.

dorsal metacarpal vein *n.* Any of three veins on the back of the hand, draining from the four fingers into the dorsal venous network of the hand.

dorsal metatarsal vein *n.* Any of the veins that arise from the dorsal digital veins forming the dorsal venous arch of the foot.

dorsal nerve of clitoris *n.* The deep terminal branch of the pudendal nerve, supplying especially the glans clitoridis.

dorsal nerve of penis *n.* The deep terminal branch of the pudendal nerve running along the dorsum of the penis, supplying the skin of the penis, the prepuce, and the glans.

dorsal nerve of scapula *n.* A nerve that arises from the fifth to the seventh cervical nerves and supplies the elevator muscle of the scapula and the greater and the lesser rhomboid muscles.

dorsal nucleus *n.* See thoracic nucleus.

dorsal nucleus of vagus *n.* The visceral motor nucleus that is located in the vagal trigone of the floor of the fourth ventricle and gives rise to the parasympathetic fibers of the vagus nerve innervating the heart muscle and the smooth musculature and glands of the respiratory and intestinal tracts.

dorsal root *n.* The sensory root of a spinal nerve. Also called *posterior root.*

dorsal root ganglion *n.* See spinal ganglion.

dorsal scapular artery *n.* An artery with its origin in the subclavian or transverse cervical artery, with distribution to the muscles and skin along the medial border of the scapula, and with anastomoses to the suprascapular and scapular circumflex arteries. Also called *descending scapular artery.*

dorsal scapular vein *n.* A tributary to the subclavian vein or the external jugular vein, accompanying the descending scapular artery.

Dor·set's culture egg medium (dôr′sĭts) *n.* A medium for cultivating *Mycobacterium tuberculosis;* it consists of the whites and yolks of four fresh eggs and a solution of sodium chloride.

dor·si·flex·ion (dôr′sə-flĕk′shən) *n.* The turning of the foot or the toes upward.

dor·si·spi·nal (dôr′sĭ-spī′nəl) *adj.* Relating to or characteristic of the spinal column, especially to its dorsal aspect.

dorso– *or* **dorsi–** *or* **dors–** *pref.* **1.** Back: *dorsad.* **2.** Dorsal: *dorsoventrad.*

dor·so·ceph·a·lad (dôr′sō-sĕf′ə-lăd′) *adv.* Toward the back of the head.

dor·so·lat·er·al (dôr′sō-lăt′ər-əl) *adj.* Of or involving both the back and the side.

dorsolateral fasciculus *n.* A longitudinal bundle of thin, unmyelinated and poorly myelinated fibers capping the apex of the posterior horn of the spinal gray matter, composed of posterior root fibers and short association fibers that connect neighboring segments of the posterior horn. Also called *dorsolateral tract.*

dor·so·lum·bar (dôr′sō-lŭm′bər, -bär′) *adj.* Of or relating to the lower thoracic and upper lumbar vertebral region of the back.

dor·so·sa·cral position (dôr′sō-sā′krəl) *n.* See lithotomy position.

dor·so·ven·trad (dôr′sō-vĕn′trăd) *adv.* Moving from the dorsal to the ventral aspect.

dor·sum (dôr′səm) *n., pl.* **-sa** (-sə) **1.** The back. **2.** The upper, outer surface of an organ, appendage, or part.

dos·age (dō′sĭj) *n.* **1.** Administration of a therapeutic agent in prescribed amounts. **2.** Determination of the amount to be so administered. **3.** The amount so administered.

dose (dōs) *n. Abbr.* **D. 1.** A specified quantity of a therapeutic agent, such as a drug, prescribed to be taken at one time or at stated intervals. **2.** The amount of radiation administered as therapy to a given site. —*v.* **1.** To give or prescribe something, such as medicine, in specified amounts. **2.** To give someone a dose, as of medicine.

do·sim·e·ter (dō-sĭm′ĭ-tər) *n.* An instrument that measures the amount of radiation absorbed in a given period.

do·sim·e·try (dō-sĭm′ĭ-trē) *n.* The accurate measurement of doses, especially of radiation.

dot (dŏt) *n.* A tiny round mark made by or as if by a pointed instrument; a spot.

dot·age (dō′tĭj) *n.* The loss of previously intact mental powers; senility. Also called *anility.*

dou·ble blind experiment (dŭb′əl) *n.* A testing procedure, designed to eliminate biased results, in which the identity of those receiving a test treatment is concealed from both administrators and subjects until after the study is completed.

double bond *n. Symbol* Δ A covalent bond in which two electron pairs are shared between two atoms.

double-channel catheter *n.* A catheter with two lumens, allowing injection and removal of fluid. Also called *two-way catheter.*

double compartment hydrocephalus *n.* A form of hydrocephalus in which accumulations of fluid occur above and below the tentorium cerebelli because of an occlusion of the cerebral aqueduct.

double contrast enema *n.* A procedure consisting of an evacuation with barium enema followed by the injection of air into the rectum.

double-flap amputation *n.* Amputation in which a flap is cut from the soft areas on either side of the limb.

double fracture *n.* A fracture occurring in two sections of the same bone.

double helix *n.* The coiled structure of a double-stranded DNA molecule in which strands linked by hydrogen bonds form a spiral configuration. Also called *DNA helix, Watson-Crick helix.*

double-jointed *adj.* Having unusually flexible joints, especially of the limbs or fingers.

double-masked experiment *n.* A double-blind study in which neither the subject nor the observer knows the identity of the control or variable.

double pneumonia *n.* Pneumonia affecting both lungs.

double product *n.* A measure of the work load of the heart, equal to systolic blood pressure multiplied by heart rate.

double stain *n.* A mixture of two dyes, each of which stains different portions of a tissue or cell.

dou·blet (dŭb′lĭt) *n.* A pairing of two lenses to optically correct a chromatic and spherical aberration.

double vision *n.* A disorder of vision in which a single object appears double. Also called *diplopia.*

dou·bly armed suture (dŭb′lē) *n.* A surgical suture performed with a needle at each end. Also called *cobbler's suture.*

douche (do͞osh) *n.* **1.** A stream of water, often containing medicinal or cleansing agents, that is applied to a body part or cavity for hygienic or therapeutic purposes. **2.** An instrument for applying a douche. —*v.* To cleanse or treat by means of a douche.

Doug·las bag (dŭg′ləs) *n.* A receptacle for collecting expired air to determine oxygen consumption in humans under various work conditions.

Douglas cul-de-sac *n.* See rectouterine pouch.

Douglas pouch *n.* See rectouterine pouch.

Doug·las's fold (dŭg′lə-sĭz) *n.* See rectouterine fold.

dou·la (do͞o′lə) *n.* A woman who assists another woman during labor and provides support to her, the infant, and the family after childbirth.

dow·a·ger's hump (dou′ə-jərz) *n.* An abnormal curvature of the spine that is primarily manifested as a rounded hump in the upper back and that typically affects older women, with the curvature being the result of collapse of the spinal column because of osteoporosis.

down·er (dou′nər) *n.* A depressant or sedative drug, such as a barbiturate or tranquilizer.

Dow·ney cell (dou′nē) *n.* A type of atypical lymphocyte usually occurring in infectious mononucleosis and other viral diseases.

Down syndrome (doun) *or* **Down's syndrome** (dounz) *n.* A congenital disorder, caused by the presence of an extra 21st chromosome, in which the affected person has mild to moderate mental retardation, short stature, and a flattened facial profile. Also called *trisomy 21, trisomy 21 syndrome.*

dox·a·zo·sin mesylate (dŏk-să′zə-sĭn) *n.* An alpha-blocker drug used to treat hypertension and benign prostatic hyperplasia.

dox·e·pin hydrochloride (dŏk′sə-pĭn′) *n.* A tricyclic antidepressant drug.

dox·o·ru·bi·cin (dŏk′sə-rōō′bĭ-sĭn) *n.* An antibiotic obtained from the bacterium *Streptomyces peucetius,* used as an anticancer drug.

dox·y·cy·cline (dŏk′sĭ-sī′klēn′, -klĭn) *n.* An antibacterial derived from tetracycline.

DP *abbr.* Doctor of Podiatry

DPH *abbr.* Diploma in Public Health; Doctor of Public Health; Doctor of Public Hygiene

DPM *abbr.* Doctor of Physical Medicine; Doctor of Podiatric Medicine

DPT[1] *abbr.* diphtheria, pertussis, and tetanus (vaccine)

DPT[2] (dē′pē-tē′) *n.* Dipropyltryptamine; a hallucinogenic drug similar to DMT.

DPT vaccine *n.* See DTP vaccine.

dr *abbr.* dram

DR *abbr.* reaction of degeneration

drachm (drăm) *n.* See dram.

dra·cun·cu·li·a·sis (drə-kŭng′kyə-lī′ə-sĭs) *or* **dra·cun·cu·lo·sis** (-lō′sĭs) *n.* Infestation with *Dracunculus medinensis.* Also called *dracontiasis.*

Dra·cun·cu·lus (drə-kŭng′kyə-ləs) *n.* A genus of nematodes that includes parasitic species such as *Dracunculus medinensis,* which migrates within subcutaneous tissues and forms chronic ulcers in the skin.

draft (drăft) *n.* A measured portion of a liquid or aerosol medication; a dose.

dra·gée (drä-zhā′) *n.* A small, often medicated candy.

drain (drān) *n.* A device, such as a tube, inserted into the opening of a wound or into a body or dental cavity to facilitate discharge of fluid or purulent material. —*v.* To draw off a liquid gradually as it forms.

drain·age (drā′nĭj) *n.* The removal of fluid or purulent material from a wound or body cavity.

drainage tube *n.* A tube inserted into a wound or cavity to facilitate fluid removal.

dram (drăm) *n. Abbr.* **dr 1.** A unit of weight in the US Customary System that is equal to $\frac{1}{16}$ of an ounce or 27.34 grains (1.77 grams). Also called *drachm.* **2.** A unit of apothecary weight that is equal to $\frac{1}{8}$ of an ounce or 60 grains (3.89 grams).

Dram·a·mine (drăm′ə-mēn′) A trademark for the drug dimenhydrinate.

drape (drāp) *v.* To cover, dress, or hang with or as if with cloth in loose folds. —*n.* A cloth arranged over a patient's body during an examination or treatment or during surgery, designed to provide a sterile field around the area.

drawer sign (drôr) *n.* An indication of laxity or a tear in the anterior or posterior cruciate ligaments of the knee in which there is a forward or backward sliding of the tibia. Also called *drawer test.*

dream (drēm) *n.* A series of images, ideas, emotions, and sensations occurring involuntarily in the mind during certain stages of sleep.

dream analysis *n.* A method of diagnosing a patient's mental state by studying his or her dreams. Also called *oneiroscopy.*

dream·y state (drē′mē) *n.* The semiconscious state associated with an epileptic attack.

drep·a·no·cyte (drĕp′ə-na-sīt′, drə-păn′ə-) *n.* See **sickle cell. —drep′a·no·cyt′ic** (-sĭt′ĭk) *adj.*

drepanocytic anemia *n.* See sickle cell anemia.

drep·a·no·cy·to·sis (drĕp′ə-nō-sī-tō′sĭs, drə-păn′ō-) *n.* See sickle cell anemia.

dress (drĕs) *v.* To apply medication, bandages, or other therapeutic materials to an area of the body such as a wound.

dres·sing (drĕs′ĭng) *n.* A therapeutic or protective material applied to a wound.

dressing forceps *n.* A slender forceps for grasping gauze or sutures and removing fragments of necrosed tissue and small foreign bodies in dressing wounds.

Dress·ler beat (drĕs′lər) *n.* A fusion beat interrupting a ventricular tachycardia and, on an electrocardiogram, producing a narrow wave complex.

Drew (drōō), **Charles Richard** 1904–1950. American physician who developed in 1940 a method of efficiently preserving blood plasma for transfusion. He organized and directed blood-plasma programs in the United States and Great Britain, becoming head of the first American Red Cross Blood Bank in 1941.

drift (drĭft) *n.* **1.** A gradual deviation from an original course, model, method, or intention. **2.** Movement of teeth from their normal position in the dental arch because of the loss of contiguous teeth. **3.** See **genetic drift. 4.** A variation or random oscillation about a fixed setting, position, or mode of behavior.

Drin·ker respirator (drĭng′kər) *n.* An airtight metal tank enclosing all the body except the head and forcing the lungs to inhale and exhale by regulating changes in air pressure. Also called *iron lung.*

drip (drĭp) *n.* **1.** The process of forming and falling in drops. **2.** Moisture or liquid such as medication that falls in drops. —*v.* To fall in drops.

drip feed *n.* **1.** Administration of blood, plasma, saline, or sugar solutions, usually intravenously, a drop at a time. **2.** The device or tubes by which such a substance is administered. **3.** The substance administered in this manner.

drive (drīv) *n.* A strong motivating tendency or instinct, especially of sexual or aggressive origin, that prompts activity toward a particular end.

drom·o·graph (drŏm′ə-grăf′, drō′mə-) *n.* An instrument for recording the rate at which blood flows or circulates within the body.

drom·o·ma·ni·a (drŏm′ə-mā′nē-ə, drō′mə-) *n.* An uncontrollable impulse or desire to wander or travel.

drom·o·trop·ic (drŏm′ə-trŏp′ĭk, drō′mə-) *adj.* Relating to or influencing the conductivity of nerve fibers or cardiac muscle fibers.

dro·nab·i·nol (drō-năb′ə-nôl) *n.* The principal psychoactive substance present in *Cannabis sativa* used therapeutically to control nausea and vomiting associated with cancer chemotherapy.

drop (drŏp) *n.* **1.** The smallest quantity of liquid heavy enough to fall in a spherical mass. **2.** A volume of liquid equal to $\frac{1}{76}$ of a teaspoon and regarded as a unit of dosage for medication. **3.** A small globular piece of candy, usually readily dissolved in the mouth. —*v.* To fall, be dispensed, or poured in drops.

drop foot *n.* See **foot-drop.**

drop hand *n.* See **wrist-drop.**

drop·let infection (drŏp′lĭt) *n.* An infection transmitted from one individual to another by droplets of moisture expelled from the upper respiratory tract through sneezing or coughing.

drop·per (drŏp′ər) *n.* A device that produces drops, especially a small tube with a suction bulb at one end for drawing in a liquid and releasing it in drops. Also called *instillator.*

drop·si·cal (drŏp′sĭ-kəl) *adj.* Relating to or suffering from dropsy.

drop·sy (drŏp′sē) *n.* Edema. No longer in technical use.

drows·i·ness (drou′zē-nĭs) *n.* A state of impaired awareness associated with a desire or inclination to sleep. Also called *hypnesthesia.*

DrPH *abbr.* Doctor of Public Health; Doctor of Public Hygiene

drug (drŭg) *n.* **1.** A substance used in the diagnosis, treatment, or prevention of a disease or as a component of a medication. **2.** Such a substance as recognized or defined by the US Food and Drug Administration. **3.** A chemical substance, such as a narcotic or hallucinogen, that affects the central nervous system, causing changes in behavior and often addiction. —*v.* **1.** To administer a drug, especially in an overly large quantity, to an individual. **2.** To stupefy or dull with or as if with a drug; to narcotize.

drug abuse *n.* Habitual use of drugs to alter one's mood, emotion, or state of consciousness.

drug eruption *n.* An eruption caused by ingestion, injection, inhalation, or insertion of a drug, often a result of allergic sensitization. Also called *dermatitis medicamentosa, dermatosis medicamentosa, drug rash.*

drug-fast *adj.* Relating to, characteristic of, or being microorganisms that resist or become tolerant to an antibacterial agent.

drug in·ter·ac·tion (ĭn′tər-ăk′shən) *n.* The pharmacological result, either desirable or undesirable, of drugs interacting with themselves or with other drugs, with endogenous chemical agents, with components of the diet, or with chemicals used in or resulting from diagnostic tests.

drug psychosis *n.* Psychosis caused by ingestion of a drug such as LSD.

drug rash *n.* See **drug eruption.**

drug tetanus *n.* A condition characterized by tonic spasms, caused by strychnine or another tetanic drug. Also called *toxic tetanus.*

drum (drŭm) *n.* See **eardrum.**

drum·head (drŭm′hĕd′) *n.* See **eardrum.**

drum membrane *n.* See **eardrum.**

drum·stick finger (drŭm′stĭk′) *n.* See **clubbed finger.**

drunk·en·ness (drŭng′kə-nĭs) *n.* The condition of being delirious with or as if with alcohol; intoxication.

druse (drōoz) *n.*, *pl.* **dru·sen** (drōo′zən) One of the small hyaline or colloid bodies sometimes occurring behind the retina of the eye.

dry abscess (drī) *n.* The remains of an abscess after the pus is absorbed.

dry cough *n.* A cough not accompanied by expectoration; a nonproductive cough.

dry eye *n.* Keratoconjunctivitis characterized by decreased tear flow and thickening and hardening of the cornea and conjunctiva. Also called *dry-eye syndrome, keratoconjunctivitis sicca.*

dry gangrene *n.* Gangrene that develops as a result of arterial obstruction and is characterized by mummification of the dead tissue and absence of bacterial decomposition. Also called *mummification.*

dry joint *n.* A joint with atrophic desiccating changes.

dry labor *n.* Labor after spontaneous loss of practically all of the amniotic fluid.

dry nurse *n.* A nurse employed to care for but not breast-feed an infant.

dry pleurisy *n.* Pleurisy characterized by a fibrinous exudation, resulting in adhesion between the opposing surfaces of the pleura. Also called *adhesive pleurisy, fibrinous pleurisy, plastic pleurisy.*

dry rale *n.* An auscultative sound produced by a constriction in a bronchial tube or by the presence of a viscid secretion narrowing the lumen of the tube.

dry socket *n.* A painful inflamed condition at the site of extraction of a tooth that occurs when a blood clot fails to form properly or is dislodged.

dry synovitis *n.* Synovitis with little serous or purulent effusion. Also called *synovitis sicca.*

dry vomiting *n.* See **vomiturition.**

Ds The symbol for the element **darmstadtium.**

DSM *abbr.* Diagnostic and Statistical Manual of Mental Disorders

DT *abbr.* delirium tremens; duration tetany

DTaP *abbr.* acellular pertussis vaccine

DTD *abbr.* diastrophic dysplasia

DTIC (dē′tē-ī-sē′) A trademark for the drug dacarbazine.

DTP *abbr.* diphtheria, tetanus, and pertussis (vaccine); distal tingling on percussion (as occurs in Tinel's sign)

DTP vaccine *n.* A vaccine given to infants and children to immunize against diphtheria, tetanus, and pertussis. Also called *DPT vaccine.*

du·al·ism (dōo′ə-lĭz′əm) *n.* **1.** The theory that blood cells have two origins, from the lymphatic system and from the bone marrow. **2.** The view in psychology that the mind and body function separately, without interchange.

DUB *abbr.* dysfunctional uterine bleeding

Du·bin John·son syndrome (dōō′bĭn-jŏn′sən) *n.* An inherited defect in hepatic excretory function marked by an increase of serum bilirubin concentration, an excessive urinary excretion of abnormal proportions of a form of coproporphyrin, a retention of dark pigment by hepatocytes, and the nonvisualization of the gall bladder using a cholecystogram. Also called *chronic idiopathic jaundice.*

dub·ni·um (dōōb′nē-əm) *n. Symbol* **Db** A radioactive synthetic element whose longest-lived isotopes have mass numbers of 258, 261, 262, and 263 with half-lives of 4.2, 1.8, 34, and 30 seconds. Atomic number 105.

Du·bois abscesses (dōō-bwä′) *pl.n.* Small cysts of the thymus, especially associated with congenital syphilis. Also called *thymic abscesses.*

Du·bos (dōō-bôs′, -bō′, dü-), **René Jules** 1901–1982. French-born American bacteriologist noted for his research on natural antibiotics, tuberculosis, and environmental factors in disease.

Du·bo·witz score (dōō′bə-wĭts′) *n.* A method of clinical assessment in the newborn from birth until five days old that includes neurological criteria for the infant's maturity and other physical criteria to determine gestational age.

Du·chenne-Aran disease (dōō-shĕn′-, dü-) *n.* See **progressive muscular atrophy.**

Duchenne-Erb paralysis *n.* See **Erb's palsy.**

Du·chenne's disease (dōō-shĕnz′, dü-) *n.* **1.** See **progressive bulbar paralysis. 2.** See **pseudohypertrophic muscular dystrophy. 3.** See **tabes dorsalis.**

Duchenne's dystrophy *or* **Duchenne's paralysis** *n.* See **pseudohypertrophic muscular dystrophy.**

Du·crey's bacillus (dōō-krāz′) *n.* A gram-negative, rod-shaped bacterium that causes chancroid formation in humans.

duct (dŭkt) *n.* A tubular bodily canal or passage, especially one for carrying a glandular secretion such as bile. —**duct·al** *adj.*

duc·tile (dŭk′təl, -tīl′) *adj.* Easily molded or shaped.

duc·tion (dŭk′shən) *n.* **1.** The act of leading, bringing, or conducting. **2.** The rotation of an eye on the vertical and horizontal axis.

duct·less (dŭkt′lĭs) *adj.* Lacking a duct, as glands that only secrete internally.

ductless gland *n.* See **endocrine gland.**

ducts of Rivinus (dŭkts) *n.* The small ducts of the sublingual salivary glands that open into the mouth on the surface of the sublingual fold.

duc·tule (dŭk′tōōl′) *n.* A small duct. —**duc′tu·lar** (-tə-lər) *adj.*

duc·tus (dŭk′təs) *n., pl.* **ductus** Duct.

ductus ar·te·ri·o·sus (är-tîr′ē-ō′səs) *n.* A fetal vessel that connects the left pulmonary artery with the descending aorta and that normally closes at birth, becoming the arterial ligament. Also called *arterial canal, arterial duct, Botallo's duct.*

ductus ve·no·sus (vē-nō′səs) *n.* A fetal vein that passes through the liver to the inferior vena cava.

due date (dōō) *n.* See **estimated date of confinement.**

Du·gas' test (dōō-gäz′) *n.* A test performed to determine whether an injured shoulder is due to a dislocation or a fracture. If the elbow cannot be made to touch the chest while the hand rests on the opposite shoulder, the injury is a dislocation.

Duh·ring's disease (dōōr′ĭngz, dōō′rĭngz) *n.* See **dermatitis herpetiformis.**

DUI *abbr.* driving under the influence (of alcohol)

Dukes classification (dōōks) *n.* A classification into three stages of the extent of spread of operable carcinoma of the large intestine.

Dukes disease *n.* See **fourth disease.**

Dul·bec·co (dŭl-bĕk′ō), **Renato** Born 1914. Italian-born American virologist. He shared a 1975 Nobel Prize for research on the interaction of tumor viruses and genetic material.

Dul·co·lax (dŭl′kō-lăks′) A trademark for an over-the-counter laxative containing bisacodyl.

dull (dŭl) *adj.* **1.** Lacking responsiveness or alertness; insensitive. **2.** Not intensely or keenly felt, as in pain.

dump·ing syndrome (dŭm′pĭng) *n.* A condition occurring after eating in patients with shunts of the upper alimentary canal and including flushing, sweating, dizziness, weakness, and vasomotor collapse. Also called *postgastrectomy syndrome.*

duodenal ampulla *n.* The dilated portion of the upper part of the duodenum. Also called *duodenal cap.*

duodenal cap *n.* **1.** See **duodenal ampulla. 2.** The first portion of the duodenum, as seen in a roentgenogram or by fluoroscopy. Also called *pyloric cap.*

duodenal fossa *n.* Any of the peritoneal recesses occurring along the duodenum.

duodenal gland *n.* Any of the small, branched, coiled tubular glands situated deeply in the submucosa of the first part of the duodenum and secreting an alkaline mucus that helps neutralize gastric acid in the chyme. Also called *Brunner's gland.*

du·o·de·nec·to·my (dōō′ō-dn-ĕk′tə-mē, dōō-ŏd′n-ĕk′-) *n.* Excision of the duodenum.

du·o·de·ni·tis (dōō′ō-dn-ī′tĭs, dōō-ŏd′n-ī′-) *n.* Inflammation of the duodenum.

duodeno– *pref.* Duodenum: *duodenotomy.*

du·o·de·no·cho·lan·gi·tis (dōō′ə-dē′nō-kō′lăn-jī′tĭs, dōō-ŏd′n-ō-) *n.* Inflammation of the duodenum and the common bile duct.

du·o·de·no·cho·le·cys·tos·to·my (dōō′ə-dē′nō-kō′-lĭ-sĭ-stŏs′tə-mē, dōō-ŏd′n-ō-) *n.* The formation of a fistula between the duodenum and the gallbladder. Also called *duodenocystostomy.*

du·o·de·no·cho·led·o·chot·o·my (dōō′ə-dē′nō-kə-lĕd′ə-kŏt′ə-mē, dōō-ŏd′n-ō-) *n.* Incision into the common bile duct through an adjacent portion of the duodenum.

du·o·de·no·cys·tos·to·my (dōō′ə-dē′nō-sĭ-stŏs′tə-mē, dōō-ŏd′n-ō-) *n.* See **duodenocholecystostomy.**

du·o·de·no·en·ter·os·to·my (dōō′ə-dē′nō-ĕn′tə-rŏs′-tə-mē, dōō-ŏd′n-ō-) *n.* The surgical formation of a passage between the duodenum and another part of the intestinal tract.

du·o·de·no·je·ju·nal flexure (dōō′ə-dē′nō-jə-jōō′nəl, dōō-ŏd′n-ō-) *n.* An abrupt bend in the small intestine at the junction of the duodenum and jejunum.

du·o·de·no·je·ju·nos·to·my (doo'ə-dē'nō-jə-joo'-nŏs'tə-mē, doo-ŏd'n-ō-) *n.* Surgical formation of a passage between the duodenum and the jejunum.

du·o·de·nol·y·sis (doo'ō-dn-ŏl'ĭ-sĭs, doo-ŏd'n-ŏl'-) *n.* The freeing of the duodenum from adhesions by means of surgery.

du·o·de·nor·rha·phy (doo'ə-dn-ôr'ə-fē, doo-ŏd'n-ôr'-) *n.* Suture of a tear or incision in the duodenum.

du·o·de·nos·co·py (doo'ə-dn-ŏs'kə-pē, doo-ŏd'n-ŏs'-) *n.* The examination of the interior of the duodenum through an endoscope.

du·o·de·nos·to·my (doo'ə-dn-ŏs'tə-mē, doo-ŏd'n-ŏs'-) *n.* The surgical establishment of an opening into the duodenum.

du·o·de·not·o·my (doo'ə-dn-ŏt'ə-mē, doo-ŏd'n-ŏt'-) *n.* Incision of the duodenum.

du·o·de·num (doo'ə-dē'nəm, doo-ŏd'n-əm) *n., pl.* **du·o·de·nums** *or* **du·o·de·na** (doo'ə-dē'nə, doo-ŏd'n-ə) The beginning portion of the small intestine, starting at the lower end of the stomach and extending to the jejunum. —**du'o·de'nal** (doo'ə-dē'nəl, doo-ŏd'n-əl) *adj.*

du·plex kidney (doo'plĕks') *n.* A kidney having two pelviocaliceal systems.

duplex uterus *n.* A uterus with a double lumen.

du·pli·ca·tion (doo'plĭ-kā'shən) *n.* The existence or growth into two corresponding parts.

duplication of chromosomes *n.* The occurrence of a repeated section of genes in a chromosome.

Du·puy-Du·temps operation (dü-pwē'dü-täN') *n.* An operation for the correcting of stenosis of the lacrimal duct.

Du·puy·tren's amputation (də-pwē'trənz, -pwē-tränz') *n.* The surgical removal of an arm at the shoulder joint.

Dupuytren's contracture *n.* A disease of the palmar fascia resulting in thickening and contraction of fibrous bands on the palmar surface.

du·ra (door'ə) *n.* See **dura mater**. —**du'ral** *adj.*

dural sheath *n.* An extension of the dura mater that envelops the roots of spinal nerves.

dural sinus *n.* See **sinus of dura mater**.

dura ma·ter (mā'tər, mä-) *n.* The tough fibrous membrane covering the brain and the spinal cord and lining the inner surface of the skull. Also called *dura, pachymeninx.*

du·ra·tion tetany (doo-rā'shən) *n. Abbr.* **DT** A tonic spasm occurring in degenerated muscles upon application of a strong electric current.

Dürck's node (dûrks, dürks) *n.* Any of the small cell infiltrations of the perivascular lymphatic tissue occurring throughout the brain, spinal cord, and meninges in human trypanosomiasis.

dur. dol. *abbr. Latin* durante dolore (while the pain lasts)

Dur·ham rule (dûr'əm) *n.* A 1954 US rule used as a test of criminal responsibility and stating that an individual accused of a crime is not criminally responsible if the unlawful act was the product of mental disease or mental defect.

Dur·i·cef (dyoor'ĭ-sĕf') A trademark for the drug cefadroxil.

Du·ro·ziez symptom (doo-rō'zē-ā', dü-rô-zyā') *n.* A double murmur heard over the femoral artery in cases of aortic insufficiency. Also called *Duroziez murmur.*

dust cell *n.* See **alveolar macrophage**.

Du·ve (doo'və, dü'-), **Christian Marie René Joseph de** Born 1917. British-born Belgian physiologist. He shared a 1974 Nobel Prize for contributions to the understanding of the components of living cells.

du Vi·gneaud (doo vēn'yō), **Vincent** 1901–1978. American biochemist. He won a 1955 Nobel Prize for his work on pituitary hormones.

DVM *abbr.* Doctor of Veterinary Medicine

DVT *abbr.* deep venous thrombosis

dwarf (dwôrf) *n., pl.* **dwarfs** *or* **dwarves** (dwôrvz) An abnormally small person, often having limbs and features not properly proportioned or formed.

dwarf·ism (dwôr'fĭz'əm) *n.* A pathological condition of arrested growth having various causes. Also called *nanism.*

DWI *abbr.* driving while intoxicated

dx *abbr.* diagnosis

Dy The symbol for the element **dysprosium**.

dy·ad (dī'ăd', -əd) *n.* **1.** Two individuals or units regarded as a pair, such as a mother and a daughter. **2.** A divalent atom or radical. **3.** One pair of homologous chromosomes resulting from the division of a tetrad during meiosis.

Dy·a·zide (dī'ə-zīd') A trademark for a drug combination of hydrochlorothiazide and triamterene.

dye (dī) *n.* A substance used to color materials or substances, such as cells, tissues, and microorganisms.

dy·nam·ic equilibrium (dī-năm'ĭk) *n.* See **equilibrium** (sense 2).

dynamic ileus *n.* Obstruction of the bowel caused by spastic contractions of a segment of the bowel. Also called *spastic ileus.*

dynamic psychiatry *n.* See **psychoanalytic psychiatry**.

dynamic psychology *n.* The branch of psychology that concerns itself with the causes and motivations of behavior.

dynamic refraction *n.* Refraction of the eye during accommodation.

dy·nam·ics (dī-năm'ĭks) *n.* **1.** See **kinetics** (sense 1). **2.** Psychodynamics.

dynamic splint *n.* A splint that aids in initiating and performing movements by controlling the plane and range of motion of the injured part. Also called *active splint, functional splint.*

dynamic viscosity *n. Symbol* μ A measure of the molecular frictional resistance of a fluid as calculated using Newton's law.

dynamo– *pref.* Force; energy: *dynamogenesis.*

dy·na·mo·gen·e·sis (dī'nə-mō-jĕn'ĭ-sĭs) *n.* The generation of power, force, or energy, especially muscular or nervous energy.

dy·nam·o·graph (dī-năm'ə-grăf') *n.* An instrument for recording the degree of muscular force.

dy·na·mom·e·ter (dī'nə-mŏm'ĭ-tər) *n.* An instrument for measuring the degree of muscular power. Also called *ergometer.*

Dy·na·pen (dī'nə-pĕn') A trademark for the drug dicloxacillin sodium.

dyne (dīn) *n.* A centimeter-gram-second unit of force, equal to the force required to impart an acceleration of one centimeter per second per second to a mass of one gram.

dy·nein (dī′nēn′, -nē-ĭn) *n.* An ATPase associated with motile structures, especially the microtubules.

dys– *pref.* **1.** Abnormal: *dysplasia.* **2.** Impaired: *dysesthesia.* **3.** Difficult: *dysphonia.* **4.** Bad: *dyspepsia.*

dys·a·cou·si·a *or* **dys·a·cu·si·a** (dĭs′ə-kōō′zē-ə, -zhə, -kyōō′-) *n.* A condition in which ordinary sounds produce discomfort or pain in the ear.

dys·a·cu·sis (dĭs′ə-kōō′sĭs) *n.* **1.** An impairment of hearing that is not primarily a loss of the ability to perceive sound. **2.** Dysacousia.

dys·a·phi·a (dĭs-ā′fē-ə) *n.* An impairment in the sense of touch.

dys·ar·te·ri·ot·o·ny (dĭs′är-tîr′ē-ŏt′ə-nē) *n.* Abnormal blood pressure.

dys·ar·thri·a (dĭs-är′thrē-ə) *n.* Difficulty in articulating words due to emotional stress or to paralysis, incoordination, or spasticity of the muscles used in speaking. —**dys·ar′thric** *adj.*

dys·ar·thro·sis (dĭs′är-thrō′sĭs) *n.* **1.** A deformity, dislocation, or disease of a joint. **2.** A false joint. **3.** A dysarthric condition.

dys·au·to·no·mi·a (dĭs-ô′tə-nō′mē-ə) *n.* **1.** Abnormal functioning of the autonomic nervous system. **2.** Familial dysautonomia.

dys·bar·ism (dĭs′bə-rĭz′əm) *n.* A complex of symptoms resulting from exposure to excessively low or rapidly changing air pressure.

dys·ba·sia (dĭs-bā′zhə) *n.* **1.** Difficulty in walking, especially as the result of a disorder of the nervous system. **2.** Difficulty in or distortion of walking that occurs in persons with mental disorders.

dys·bu·li·a (dĭs-bōō′lē-ə, -byōō′-) *n.* A weakness and uncertainty of willpower. —**dys·bu′lic** *adj.*

dys·cal·cu·li·a (dĭs′kăl-kyōō′lē-ə) *n.* Impairment of the ability to solve mathematical problems, usually resulting from brain dysfunction.

dys·ce·pha·li·a (dĭs′sə-fā′lē-ə, -fāl′yə) *or* **dys·ceph·a·ly** (dĭs-sĕf′ə-lē) *n.* A congenital malformation of the cranium and the bones of the face.

dys·chei·ri·a *or* **dys·chi·ri·a** (dĭs-kī′rē-ə) *n.* The inability to recognize which side of the body has been touched even though there is no apparent loss of sensation. —**dys·chei′ral** *adj.*

dys·che·zi·a (dĭs-kē′zē-ə, -zhə) *n.* The inability to defecate without pain or difficulty.

dys·chon·dro·gen·e·sis (dĭs′kŏn′drō-jĕn′ĭ-sĭs) *n.* Abnormal development of cartilage.

dys·chon·dro·pla·sia (dĭs′kŏn′drō-plā′zhə) *n.* See enchondromatosis.

dys·chon·dros·te·o·sis (dĭs′kŏn-drŏs′tē-ō′sĭs) *n.* A familial bone dysplasia characterized by bowing of the radius, dorsal dislocation of the distal ulna and proximal carpal bones, and mesomelic dwarfism. Also called *Leri-Weill syndrome.*

dys·chro·ma·top·si·a (dĭs-krō′mə-tŏp′sē-ə) *n.* See dichromatism (sense 2).

dys·chro·mi·a (dĭs-krō′mē-ə) *n.* A discoloration, especially of the skin.

dys·co·ri·a (dĭs-kôr′ē-ə) *n.* An abnormality in the shape of the pupil.

dys·cra·sia (dĭs-krā′zhə) *n.* **1.** An abnormal state or disorder of the body, especially of the blood. **2.** Disease. No longer in technical use.

dys·em·bry·o·ma (dĭs-ĕm′brē-ō′mə) *n.* A embryonal tumor having tissues that show more irregular arrangement than typical of such tumors.

dys·en·ce·pha·li·a splanch·no·cys·ti·ca (dĭs-ĕn′sə-fā′lē-ə splăngk′nō-sĭs′tĭ-kə, -fāl′yə) *n.* See **Meckel syndrome.**

dys·en·ter·y (dĭs′ən-tĕr′ē) *n.* An inflammatory disorder of the lower intestinal tract, usually caused by a bacterial, parasitic, or protozoan infection and resulting in pain, fever, and severe diarrhea, often accompanied by the passage of blood and mucus. —**dys′en·ter′ic** *adj.*

dys·er·e·thism (dĭs-ĕr′ə-thĭz′əm) *n.* A condition in which a person responds slowly to stimuli.

dys·er·gia (dĭ-sûr′jə) *n.* The lack of muscular coordination due to a defect in the efferent nerve impulses.

dys·es·the·sia (dĭs′ĭs-thē′zhə) *n.* **1.** Impairment of sensation, especially that of touch. **2.** A condition in which an unpleasant sensation is produced by ordinary stimuli.

dys·fi·brin·o·ge·ne·mi·a (dĭs′fī-brĭn′ə-jə-nē′mē-ə, -fī′brə-nō-) *n.* A familial disorder in which fibrinogens function inadequately resulting in symptoms ranging from bleeding to thrombosis.

dys·func·tion *or* **dis·func·tion** (dĭs-fŭngk′shən) *n.* Abnormal or impaired functioning, especially of a bodily system or organ. —**dys·func′tion·al** *adj.*

dysfunctional uterine bleeding *n. Abbr.* **DUB** Bleeding from the uterus due to an endocrine imbalance.

dys·gam·ma·glob·u·li·ne·mi·a (dĭs-găm′ə-glŏb′yə-lə-nē′mē-ə) *n.* A disorder involving an abnormality in the structure, distribution, or frequency of serum gamma-globulins.

dys·gen·e·sis (dĭs-jĕn′ĭ-sĭs) *n.* Defective or abnormal embryonic development of an organ.

dys·gen·ic (dĭs-jĕn′ĭk) *adj.* Relating to or causing the deterioration of hereditary qualities in offspring.

dys·ger·mi·no·ma *or* **dis·ger·mi·no·ma** (dĭs-jûr′mə-nō′mə) *n.* A rare malignant ovarian neoplasm composed of undifferentiated gonadal germinal cells.

dys·geu·sia (dĭs-gyōō′zhə, -jōō′-) *n.* An impairment or dysfunction of the sense of taste.

dys·gna·thi·a (dĭs-nā′thē-ə) *n.* An abnormality of the mouth that extends beyond the teeth and includes the maxilla, mandible, or both. —**dys·gnath′ic** (-năth′ĭk, -nā′thĭk) *adj.*

dys·gno·si·a (dĭs-nō′zē-ə, -zhə) *n.* A cognitive disorder, especially one resulting from a mental disorder or disease.

dys·graph·i·a (dĭs-grăf′ē-ə) *n.* Impairment of the ability to write, usually caused by brain dysfunction or disease.

dys·har·mon·ic diplacusis (dĭs′här-mŏn′ĭk) *n.* A form of diplacusis in which the same sound is heard with a different pitch in each ear.

dys·he·ma·to·poi·e·sis (dĭs-hē′mə-tō-poi-ē′sĭs, dĭs′hĭ-măt′ə-) *or* **dys·he·mo·poi·e·sis** (dĭs-hē′mə-) *n.* Abnormal formation of blood cells. —**dys·he′ma·to·poi·et′-ic** (dĭs-hē′mə-tō-poi-ĕt′ĭk, -hĭ-măt′ō-) *adj.*

dys·hi·dro·sis (dĭs′hī-drō′sĭs) *n.* **1.** A vesicular eruption that occurs primarily on the hands and feet. Also called *cheiropompholyx, pompholyx.* **2.** Any of various disorders of the sweat glands.

dys·kar·y·o·sis (dĭs-kăr′ē-ō′sĭs) *n.* An abnormality of nuclei seen in exfoliated cells, often cells from the uterine cervix, in which the cytoplasm remains unchanged but the nuclei exhibit hyperchromatism, irregularity or enlargement, or an increase in number. —**dys·kar′y·ot′ic** (-ŏt′ĭk) *adj.*

dys·ker·a·to·ma (dĭs-kĕr′ə-tō′mə) *n.* A skin tumor characterized by dyskeratosis.

dys·ker·a·to·sis (dĭs-kĕr′ə-tō′sĭs) *n.* **1.** Premature keratinization in cells that are not in the keratinizing surface layer of the skin. **2.** Keratinization of the corneal epithelium. —**dys·ker′a·tot′ic** (-tŏt′ĭk) *adj.*

dyskeratosis con·gen·i·ta (kən-jĕn′ĭ-tə) *n.* A genetic disorder marked by nail dystrophy, oral leukoplakia, pigmentation of the cellular connective tissue of the skin, and anemia progressing to pancytopenia.

dys·ki·ne·sia (dĭs′kə-nē′zhə, -kī-) *n.* An impairment in the ability to control movements, characterized by spasmodic or repetitive motions or lack of coordination. —**dys′ki·net′ic** (-nĕt′ĭk) *adj.*

dyskinesia al·ger·a (ăl′jər-ə) *n.* A hysterical condition in which active movement causes pain.

dyskinesia in·ter·mit·tens (ĭn′tər-mĭt′ənz) *n.* Sporadic disability of the limbs due to impaired circulation.

dys·la·li·a (dĭs-lā′lē-ə, -lăl′ē-ə) *n.* An articulation disorder resulting from impaired hearing or structural abnormalities of the articulatory organs.

dys·lec·tic (dĭs-lĕk′tĭk) *adj.* Variant of **dyslexic.**

dys·lex·i·a (dĭs-lĕk′sē-ə) *n.* A learning disorder marked by impairment of the ability to recognize and comprehend written words.

dys·lex·ic (dĭs-lĕk′sĭk) *or* **dys·lec·tic** (-tĭk) *adj.* Of or relating to dyslexia. —*n.* A person who is affected by dyslexia.

dys·lip·i·de·mi·a (dĭs-lĭp′ĭ-dē′mē-ə) *n.* An abnormal concentration of lipids or lipoproteins in the blood.

dys·lo·gi·a (dĭs-lō′jē-ə) *n.* **1.** Difficulty in the expression of ideas or of the ability to speak. **2.** Impairment of the ability to reason or to think logically as a result of a mental disorder.

dys·ma·ture (dĭs′mə-tŏor′, -chŏor′) *adj.* **1.** Of, relating to, or characteristic of faulty embryologic development, often leading to structural and/or functional abnormalities. **2.** Relating to or characteristic of an infant whose birth weight is inappropriately low for its gestational age.

dys·ma·tu·ri·ty (dĭs′mə-tŏor′ĭ-tē, -chŏor′-) *n.* A complex of symptoms occurring in an infant, such as a relative absence of subcutaneous fat, skin wrinkling, prominent fingernails and toenails, and a meconium staining of the skin and the placental membranes, that is associated with postmaturity or placental insufficiency.

dys·me·li·a (dĭs-mē′lē-ə, -mēl′yə) *n.* A congenital abnormality characterized by missing or foreshortened extremities and sometimes spinal abnormalities.

dys·men·or·rhe·a *or* **dys·men·or·rhoe·a** (dĭs-mĕn′ə-rē′ə) *n.* A condition marked by painful menstruation. Also called *menorrhalgia.*

dys·me·tri·a (dĭs-mē′trē-ə, -mĕt′rē-ə) *n.* An inability or impaired ability to accurately control the range of movement in muscular acts.

dys·mim·i·a (dĭs-mĭm′ē-ə) *n.* **1.** An impairment of the ability to use gestures to express oneself. **2.** An inability to imitate.

dys·mne·sia (dĭs-nē′zhə) *n.* A naturally poor or an impaired memory.

dys·mor·phism (dĭs-môr′fĭz′əm) *n.* An anatomical malformation.

dys·mor·pho·gen·e·sis (dĭs-môr′fō-jĕn′ĭ-sĭs) *n.* The process of abnormal tissue formation.

dys·mor·phol·o·gy (dĭs′môr-fŏl′ə-jē) *n.* The branch of clinical genetics concerned with the study of structural defects, especially congenital malformations.

dys·my·o·to·ni·a (dĭs′mī-ə-tō′nē-ə) *n.* Abnormal muscular tonicity.

dys·o·don·ti·a·sis (dĭs′ō-dŏn-tī′ə-sĭs) *n.* A difficulty or irregularity in the eruption of teeth.

dys·on·to·gen·e·sis (dĭs-ŏn′tō-jĕn′ĭ-sĭs) *n.* Defective development as a result of abnormal cell and tissue growth and differentiation. —**dys·on′to·ge·net′ic** (-jə-nĕt′ĭk) *adj.*

dys·o·rex·i·a (dĭs′ə-rĕk′sē-ə) *n.* A diminished, disordered, or unnatural appetite.

dys·os·mi·a (dĭs-ŏz′mē-ə) *n.* An impairment or dysfunction of the sense of smell.

dys·os·to·sis (dĭs′ŏs-tō′sĭs) *n.* The defective formation of bone. Also called *dysosteogenesis.*

dysostosis mul·ti·plex (mŭl′tə-plĕks′) *n.* See **Hurler's syndrome.**

dys·pa·reu·ni·a (dĭs′pə-rōo′nē-ə) *n.* Difficult or painful sexual intercourse.

dys·pep·si·a (dĭs-pĕp′shə, -sē-ə) *n.* Disturbed digestion; indigestion.

dys·pha·gia (dĭs-fā′jə) *or* **dys·pha·gy** (dĭs′fə-jē) *n.* Difficulty in swallowing or inability to swallow. Also called *aglutition, aphagia, odynophagia.* —**dys·phag′ic** (-făj′-ĭk) *adj.*

dys·phag·o·cy·to·sis (dĭs-făg′ə-sī-tō′sĭs) *n.* Disordered phagocytosis, especially failure of cells to ingest and digest bacteria.

dys·pha·sia (dĭs-fā′zhə) *n.* Impairment of speech and verbal comprehension, especially when associated with brain injury. Also called *dysphrasia.*

dys·phe·mi·a (dĭs-fē′mē-ə) *n.* A speech disorder characterized by stammering or stuttering and usually having an emotional or psychological basis.

dys·pho·ni·a (dĭs-fō′nē-ə) *n.* Difficulty in speaking, usually evidenced by hoarseness.

dys·pho·ri·a (dĭs-fôr′ē-ə) *n.* An emotional state marked by anxiety, depression, and restlessness.

dys·phor·ic hypomania (dĭs-fôr′ĭks) *n.* A mood disorder in which an individual who has had a major depressive episode undergoes an episode with some manic symptoms although not so severe or of such duration as to be categorized as manic. Also called *bipolar II.*

dys·phra·sia (dĭs-frā′zhə) *n.* See **dysphasia.**

dys·pig·men·ta·tion (dĭs'pĭg-mən-tā'shən) *n.* An abnormality in the formation or distribution of pigment, especially in the skin.

dys·pla·sia (dĭs-plā'zhə) *n.* Abnormal development or growth of tissues, organs, or cells. —**dys·plas'tic** (-plăs'tĭk) *adj.*

dysplasia ep·i·phys·i·a·lis mul·ti·plex (ĕp'ə-fĭz'ē-ā'-lĭs mŭl'tə-plĕks') *n.* An inherited abnormality affecting bone epiphyses, characterized by difficulty in walking, pain and stiffness of joints, stubby fingers, and often a type of dwarfism.

dysplasia epiphysialis punc·ta·ta (pŭngk-tā'tə) *n.* See **stippled epiphysis.**

dysplastic nevus syndrome *n.* An atypical nevus, usually larger than 5 millimeters in diameter with variable pigmentation and ill-defined borders, marked by melanocytic dysplasia and associated with an increased risk for the development of nonfamilial cutaneous malignant melanoma. Also called *dysplastic nevus.*

dysp·ne·a (dĭsp-nē'ə) *n.* Difficulty in breathing, often associated with lung or heart disease and resulting in shortness of breath. —**dysp·ne'ic** (-nē'ĭk) *adj.*

dys·prax·i·a (dĭs-prăk'sē-ə) *n.* Impairment of the ability to execute purposeful, voluntary movement.

dys·pro·si·um (dĭs-prō'zē-əm, -zhē-əm) *n. Symbol* **Dy** A soft, silvery rare-earth element used in nuclear research. Atomic number 66.

dys·pro·tein·e·mi·a (dĭs-prōt'n-ē'mē-ə, -prō'tē-nē'-) *n.* An abnormality in protein content of the blood, usually in the content of immunoglobulins. —**dys·pro'-tein·e'mic** *adj.*

dys·ra·phism (dĭs'rā-fĭz'əm) *or* **dys·ra·phi·a** (dĭs-rā'fē-ə) *n.* The defective fusion of a raphe, especially of the neural folds.

dys·re·flex·i·a (dĭs'rĭ-flĕk'sē-ə) *n.* Abnormally increased or decreased response to physiologic stimuli. Also called *autonomic dysreflexia.*

dys·rhyth·mi·a (dĭs-rĭth'mē-ə) *n.* An abnormality in an otherwise normal rhythmic pattern.

dys·se·ba·ci·a (dĭs'sə-bā'shē-ə, -shə) *n.* See **seborrheic dermatitis.**

dys·som·ni·a (dĭs-sŏm'nē-ə) *n.* A disturbance in the normal rhythm or pattern of sleep.

dys·sta·sia (dĭs-stā'zhə) *n.* Difficulty in standing. —**dys·stat·ic** (-stăt'ĭk) *adj.*

dys·syn·er·gia (dĭs'sə-nûr'jə) *n.* See **ataxia.**

dyssynergia cer·e·bel·lar·is my·o·clon·i·ca (sĕr'ə-bĕ-lâr'ĭs mī'ō-klŏn'ĭ-kə) *n.* A disease complex characterized by epilepsy, muscle spasms, and gradually increasing tremors.

dyssynergia cerebellaris pro·gres·si·va (prō'grĭ-sī'-və) *n.* See **Hunt's syndrome.**

dys·tax·i·a (dĭs-tăk'sē-ə) *n.* A mild degree of ataxia.

dys·thy·mi·a (dĭs-thī'mē-ə) *n.* A mood disorder characterized by despondency or mild depression. —**dys·thy'mic** *adj.*

dysthymic disorder *n.* A chronic disturbance of mood lasting at least two years in adults or one year in children, characterized by recurrent periods of mild depression and such symptoms as insomnia, tearfulness, and pessimism.

dys·to·ci·a (dĭs-tō'sē-ə, -shē-ə, -shə) *n.* A slow or difficult labor or delivery.

dys·to·ni·a (dĭs-tō'nē-ə) *n.* Abnormal tonicity of tissue. —**dys·ton'ic** (-tŏn'ĭk) *adj.*

dystonia mus·cu·lo·rum de·for·mans (mŭs'kyə-lôr'-əm dē-fôr'mənz) *n.* A disease, especially of children, characterized by muscular contractions that produce distortions of the spine and hips with the muscles being spastic when in action and without tension when at rest.

dystonic reaction *n.* A state of abnormal tension or muscle tone, similar to dystonia, produced as a side effect of certain antipsychotic medications.

dys·to·pi·a (dĭs-tō'pē-ə) *n.* An abnormal position, as of an organ or a body part. Also called *malposition.* —**dys·top'ic** (-tŏp'ĭk) *adj.*

dystrophia un·gui·um (ŭng'gwē-əm) *n.* Dystrophy of the fingernails or toenails.

dystrophic calcification *n.* Calcification of degenerated or necrotic tissue.

dys·tro·phin (dĭs'trə-fĭn) *n.* A structural protein found in small amounts in normal muscle but absent or present in abnormal amounts in individuals with muscular dystrophy.

dys·troph·o·neu·ro·sis (dĭ-strŏf'ō-nŏo-rō'sĭs) *n.* A nervous disorder attributed to poor or improper nutrition.

dys·tro·phy (dĭs'trə-fē) *or* **dys·tro·phi·a** (dĭ-strō'fē-ə) *n.* **1.** A degenerative disorder caused by inadequate or defective nutrition. **2.** Any of several disorders, especially muscular dystrophy, in which the muscles weaken and atrophy. —**dys·troph'ic** (dĭ-strŏf'ĭk, -strō'fĭk) *adj.*

dys·u·ri·a (dĭs-yŏor'ē-ə) *n.* Difficult or painful urination. —**dys·u'ric** (-yŏor'ĭk) *adj.*

dys·ver·sion (dĭs-vûr'zhən) *n.* A turning in any direction, but not a complete turning over.

E

ϵ **1.** The Greek letter *epsilon*. Entries beginning with this character are alphabetized under **epsilon**. **2.** The symbol for **molar absorption coefficient**.

η The Greek letter *eta*. Entries that begin with this character are alphabetized under **eta**.

e *abbr.* electron

ear (îr) *n.* **1.** The organ of hearing, responsible for maintaining equilibrium as well as sensing sound and divided into the external ear, the middle ear, and the inner ear. **2.** The part of this organ that is externally visible. **3.** The sense of hearing.

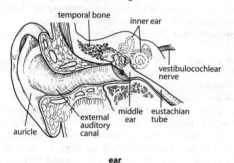

ear

cross section

ear·ache (îr′āk′) *n.* Pain in the ear; otalgia.

ear canal *n.* The narrow, tubelike passage through which sound enters the ear. Also called *external auditory canal*.

ear·drops (îr′drŏps′) *n.* Liquid medicine administered into the ear.

ear·drum (îr′drŭm′) *n.* The thin, semitransparent, oval-shaped membrane that separates the middle ear from the external ear. Also called *drum, drumhead, drum membrane, myringa, myrinx, tympanic membrane, tympanum*.

ear·lobe *or* **ear lobe** (îr′lōb′) *n.* The soft, fleshy, pendulous lower part of the external ear.

ear·ly intervention (ûr′lē) *n. Abbr.* **EI** A process of assessment and therapy provided to children, especially those younger than age 6, to facilitate normal cognitive and emotional development and to prevent developmental disability or delay.

earth (ûrth) *n.* Any of several metallic oxides, such as alumina or zirconia, from which it is difficult to remove oxygen. No longer in technical use.

ear·wax (îr′wăks′) *n.* A waxlike secretion of certain glands lining the canal of the external ear; cerumen.

eat (ēt) *v.* **1.** To take into the body by the mouth for digestion or absorption. **2.** To consume, ravage, or destroy by or as if by ingesting, such as by a disease.

eat·ing disorder (ē′tĭng) *n.* Any of several patterns of severely disturbed eating behavior, especially anorexia nervosa and bulimia, seen mainly in female teenagers and young women.

eating epilepsy *n.* A form of complex precipitated epilepsy in which seizures are provoked by eating.

Ea·ton agent (ēt′n) *n.* Mycoplasma pneumoniae.

Eaton-Lambert syndrome *n.* See **Lambert-Eaton syndrome**.

E·berth (ā′bərt), **Karl Joseph** 1835–1926. German bacteriologist and pathologist who was among the first to identify the bacillus of typhoid fever (1880).

E·bo·la virus (ĭ-bō′lə, ĕb′ə-lə) *n.* An RNA filovirus of African origin that is spread through contact with infected bodily fluids or secretions and causes acute hemorrhagic fever, often leading to death from progressive organ failure.

Eb·stein's anomaly (ĕb′stīnz, ĕp′shtīnz) *n.* Congenital downward displacement of the tricuspid valve into the right ventricle. Also called *Ebstein's disease*.

Ebstein's sign *n.* An indication of pericardial effusion in which percussion shows the cardiohepatic angle to be obtuse to the right cardiac wall.

e·bur·na·tion (ē′bər-nā′shən, ĕb′ər-) *n.* Degeneration of bone into a hard, ivorylike mass, such as occurs at articular surfaces of bones in osteoarthritis.

e·bur·ni·tis (ē′bər-nī′tĭs, ĕb′ər-) *n.* Increased density and hardness of dentin.

EBV *abbr.* Epstein-Barr virus

EB virus (ē′bē′) *n.* See **Epstein-Barr virus**.

ec– *pref.* Out; outside of: *eclabium*.

ec·cen·tric (ĭk-sĕn′trĭk, ĕk-) *adj.* **1.** Departing from a recognized, conventional, or established norm or pattern. **2.** Situated or proceeding away from the center. —*n.* A person of odd or unconventional behavior. —**ec′cen·tric′i·ty** (ĕk′sĕn-trĭs′ĭ-tē) *n.*

eccentric hypertrophy *n.* Hypertrophic growth of the walls of a hollow organ, especially the heart, in which the overall size and volume are enlarged.

eccentric occlusion *n.* The occlusion of the teeth when the lower and upper jaws are not centrical.

ec·cen·tro·chon·dro·pla·sia (ĭk-sĕn′trō-kŏn′drō-plā′-zhə) *n.* Abnormal epiphysial development from eccentric centers of ossification.

ec·chon·dro·ma (ĕk′ən-drō′mə) *n., pl.* **–mas** *or* **–ma·ta** (-mə-tə) A cartilaginous tumor arising as an overgrowth from normally situated cartilage, such as a mass protruding from the articular surface of a bone. Also called *ecchondrosis*.

ec·chy·mo·ma (ĕk′ĭ-mō′mə) *n., pl.* **–mas** *or* **–ma·ta** (-mə-tə) A slight hematoma following a bruise.

ec·chy·mosed (ĕk′ĭ-mōst′, -mōzd′) *adj.* Characterized by or affected with ecchymosis.

ec·chy·mo·sis (ĕk′ĭ-mō′sĭs) *n., pl.* **–ses** (-sēz′) The passage of blood from ruptured blood vessels into subcutaneous tissue, marked by a purple discoloration of the skin. —**ec′chy·mot′ic** (-mŏt′ĭk) *adj.*

ecchymotic mask *n.* A dusky discoloration of the head and neck occurring when the trunk has been subjected to sudden and extreme compression, as in traumatic asphyxia.

Ec·cles (ĕk′əlz), Sir **John Carew** 1903–1997. Australian physiologist. He shared a 1963 Nobel Prize for research on the action of nerve impulses.

ec·crine (ĕk′rĭn, -rīn′, -rēn′) *adj.* **1.** Relating to an eccrine gland or its secretion, as of sweat. **2.** Exocrine.

eccrine gland *or* **eccrine sweat gland** *n.* Any of the numerous small sweat glands distributed over the body's surface that produce a clear aqueous secretion devoid of cytoplasmic constituents and important in regulating body temperature.

eccrine poroma *n.* A poroma of the eccrine glands on the sole of the foot.

ec·cri·sis (ĕk′rĭ-sĭs) *n.* **1.** The excretion of waste products from the body. **2.** A waste product; excrement.

ec·crit·ic (ĭ-krĭt′ĭk) *adj.* Of or promoting the expulsion of waste matter.

ec·cy·e·sis (ĕk′sī-ē′sĭs) *n.* See **ectopic pregnancy.**

ec·dem·ic (ĭk-dĕm′ĭk) *adj.* Of or being a disease that is brought into a region from the outside, neither epidemic nor endemic.

ECF *abbr.* extracellular fluid

ECF-A *abbr.* eosinophil chemotactic factor of anaphylaxis

ECG *abbr.* electrocardiogram; electrocardiograph

ec·go·nine (ĕk′gə-nēn′, -nĭn) *n.* The principal portion of the cocaine molecule, obtainable by hydrolysis.

ech·i·na·ce·a (ĕk′ə-nā′sē-ə, -nā′shə) *n.* Any of several coneflowers of the genus *Echinacea,* whose roots, seeds, and other parts are used in herbal medicine in the belief that they stimulate the immune system.

echino– *or* **echin–** *pref.* Spiny: *echinococcosis.*

e·chi·no·coc·co·sis (ĭ-kī′nə-kə-kō′sĭs) *n., pl.* **–ses** (-sēz) **1.** Infestation with organisms of the genus *Echinococcus.* **2.** Hydatid disease.

e·chi·no·coc·cus (ĭ-kī′nə-kŏk′əs) *n., pl.* **–coc·ci** (-kŏk′sī′, -kŏk′ī′) A tapeworm of the genus *Echinococcus.*

Echinococcus *n.* A genus of parasitic tapeworms, the larvae of which, under certain conditions, infect humans, forming large hydatid cysts in the liver or lungs and causing serious or fatal disease.

echinococcus cyst *n.* See **hydatid cyst.**

ech·o·a·cou·sia (ĕk′ō-ə-kōō′zhə) *n.* A subjective disturbance of hearing in which a sound heard appears to be repeated.

ech·o·a·or·tog·ra·phy (ĕk′ō-ā′ôr-tŏg′rə-fē) *n.* The application of ultrasound techniques to the diagnosis and study of the aorta, particularly the abdominal aorta.

ech·o·car·di·o·gram (ĕk′ō-kär′dē-ə-grăm′) *n.* A visual record produced by echocardiography.

ech·o·car·di·og·ra·phy (ĕk′ō-kär′dē-ŏg′rə-fē) *n.* The use of ultrasound in the diagnosis of cardiovascular lesions and in recording the size, motion, and composition of various cardiac structures. Also called *ultrasound cardiography.* **—ech′o·car′di·o·graph′** (-ə-grăf′) *n.* **—ech′o·car′di·o·graph′ic** *adj.*

ech·o diplacusis (ĕk′ō) *n.* A condition in which sound heard in the affected ear is repeated.

ech·o·en·ceph·a·lo·gram (ĕk′ō-ĕn-sĕf′ə-lə-grăm′, -ə-lō-) *n.* A visual record of the brain that is produced by echoencephalography.

ech·o·en·ceph·a·log·ra·phy (ĕk′ō-ĕn-sĕf′ə-lŏg′rə-fē) *n.* The use of reflected ultrasound in order to create a detailed visual image of the brain. **—ech′o·en·ceph′a·lo·graph′** (-lə-grăf′, -lō-) *n.*

ech·o·gen·ic (ĕk′ō-jĕn′ĭk) *adj.* Containing structures that reflect high-frequency sound waves and thus can be imaged by ultrasound techniques.

ech·o·gram (ĕk′ō-grăm′) *n.* See **sonogram.**

e·chog·ra·phy (ĕ-kŏg′rə-fē) *n.* See **ultrasonography.**

ech·o·la·li·a (ĕk′ō-lā′lē-ə) *n.* **1.** The immediate and involuntary repetition of words or phrases just spoken by others, often a symptom of autism or some types of schizophrenia. Also called *echophrasia.* **2.** An infant's repetition of the sounds made by others, a normal occurrence in childhood development. Also called *echophrasia.* **—ech′o·la′lic** (-lĭk) *adj.*

ech·o·mim·i·a (ĕk′ō-mĭm′ē-ə) *n.* See **echopathy.**

ech·o·mo·tism (ĕk′ō-mō′tĭz′əm) *n.* See **echopraxia.**

e·chop·a·thy (ĕ-kŏp′ə-thē) *n.* A mental disorder in which the words or actions of another are imitated and repeated. Also called *echomimia.*

ech·o·phra·sia (ĕk′ō-frā′zhə) *n.* See **echolalia** (sense 1, 2).

ech·o·prax·i·a (ĕk′ō-prăk′sē-ə) *n.* The involuntary imitation of movements made by another. Also called *echomotism.*

ech·o·vi·rus (ĕk′ō-vī′rəs) *or* **ECHO virus** (ĕk′ō) *n.* Any of a number of retroviruses of the family Picornaviridae, inhabiting the gastrointestinal tract and associated with various diseases, such as viral meningitis, mild respiratory infections, and severe diarrhea in newborns.

Eck fistula (ĕk) *n.* An anastomosis created between the vena cava and the portal vein in order to divert the flow of blood from the intestinal system away from the liver and directly to the heart.

ec·la·bi·um (ĕk-lā′bē-əm) *n.* Eversion of a lip.

e·clamp·si·a (ĭ-klămp′sē-ə) *n.* Coma or convulsions in a patient with preeclampsia, occurring in late pregnancy, during labor, or within 24 hours after parturition. **—e·clamp′tic** (-tĭk) *adj.*

e·clamp·to·gen·ic (ĭ-klămp′tə-jĕn′ĭk) *or* **e·clamp·tog·e·nous** (-tŏj′ə-nəs) *adj.* Causing eclampsia.

e·clipse period (ĭ-klĭps′) *n.* The period of time between infection by a virus and the appearance of the mature virus within the cell.

ec·mne·sia (ĕk-nē′zhə) *n.* Loss of memory for recent events.

eco– *pref.* Ecology; ecological: *ecosystem.*

E. coli (ē kō′lī) *n.* A bacillus *Escherichia coli;* a bacillus normally found in the human gastrointestinal tract and existing as numerous strains, some of which are responsible for diarrheal diseases. Other strains have been used experimentally in molecular biology.

e·col·o·gy (ĭ-kŏl′ə-jē) *n.* **1.** The branch of science that is concerned with the relationships between organisms and their environments. **2.** The relationship between organisms and their environments. **3.** The study of the detrimental effects of modern civilization on the environment, with a view toward their prevention or reversal through conservation. **—e′co·log′i·cal** (ē′kə-lŏj′ĭ-kəl, ĕk′ə-), **e′co·log′ic** (-ĭk) *adj.* **—e·col′o·gist** *n.*

e·con·a·zole (ĭ-kŏn′ə-zōl′) *n.* A broad-spectrum antifungal agent used in the treatment of athlete's foot and related fungal infections.

e·co·sys·tem (ē′kō-sĭs′təm, ĕk′ō-) *n.* An ecological community together with its environment, functioning as a unit.

e·co·tax·is (ē′kə-tăk′sĭs, ĕk′ō-) *n.* The migration of lymphocytes from the thymus and bone marrow into tissues possessing an appropriate microenvironment.

Ec·o·trin (ĕk′ə-trĭn′) A trademark for a preparation of enteric-coated aspirin.

e·co·trop·ic virus (ē′kə-trŏp′ĭk, -trō′pĭk, ĕk′ə-) *n.* An oncornavirus that does not produce disease in its natural host, but does replicate in tissue culture cells derived from the host species.

é·cra·seur (ā-krä-zœr′) *n.* A surgical snare, especially one of great strength for cutting through the base or pedicle of a tumor.

ECS *abbr.* electrocerebral silence

ec·sta·sy (ĕk′stə-sē) *n.* MDMA.

ECT *abbr.* electroconvulsive therapy

ec·tad (ĕk′tăd′) *adv.* Toward the outside; outward.

ec·tal (ĕk′təl) *adj.* Of or situated on the outside; outer; external.

ec·ta·sia (ĕk-tā′zhə) *or* **ec·ta·sis** (ĕk′tə-sĭs) *n.* Dilation or distention of a tubular structure.

–ectasia *or* **–ectasis** *suff.* Dilation: *angiectasia.*

ec·tat·ic (ĕk-tăt′ĭk) *adj.* Of, relating to, or marked by ectasia.

ec·ten·tal (ĕk-tĕn′tl) *adj.* **1.** Relating to both the ectoderm and entoderm. **2.** Of or being the line where the ectoderm and endoderm join.

ect·eth·moid (ĕk-tĕth′moid′) *n.* See **ethmoidal labyrinth.**

ec·thy·ma (ĕk-thī′mə) *n.* A pyogenic infection of the skin due to staphylococci or streptococci and characterized by adherent crusts beneath which ulceration occurs.

ecto– *or* **ect–** *pref.* Outer; external: *ectoparasite.*

ec·to·an·ti·gen (ĕk′tō-ăn′tĭ-jən) *n.* A toxin or other inducer of antibody formation, separate or separable from its source. Also called *exoantigen.*

ec·to·blast (ĕk′tə-blăst′) *n.* See **ectoderm.**

ec·to·car·di·a (ĕk′tō-kär′dē-ə) *n.* Congenital displacement of the heart. Also called *exocardia.*

ec·to·cer·vix (ĕk′tō-sûr′vĭks) *n.* The portion of the uterine cervix extending into the vagina and lined with stratified squamous epithelium.   **—ec′to·cer′vi·cal** (-vĭ-kəl) *adj.*

ec·to·derm (ĕk′tə-dûrm′) *n.* The outermost of the three primary germ layers of an embryo, from which the epidermis, nervous tissue, and sense organs develop. Also called *ectoblast.* **—ec′to·der′mal, ec′to·der′mic** *adj.*

ectodermal dysplasia *n.* Abnormal development or growth of tissues and structures that develop from the ectoderm.

ec·to·der·mo·sis (ĕk′tō-dər-mō′sĭs) *n.,* *pl.* **–ses** (-sēz) A disorder of an organ or tissue developed from the ectoderm.

ec·to·en·zyme (ĕk′tō-ĕn′zīm) *n.* **1.** An enzyme situated on the outer surface of a cell's membrane so that its active site is available to the exterior environment of the cell. **2.** Extracellular enzyme.

ec·tog·e·nous (ĕk-tŏj′ə-nəs) *or* **ec·to·gen·ic** (ĕk′tə-jĕn′ĭk) *adj.* **1.** Having the ability to live and develop

outside a host, as certain pathogenic microorganisms. **2.** Exogenous.

ec·to·mere (ĕk′tə-mîr′) *n.* Any of the blastomeres from which the ectoderm develops.

ec·to·morph (ĕk′tə-môrf′) *n.* An individual having a lean, slightly muscular body build in which tissues derived from the embryonic ectoderm predominate. **—ec′to·mor′phic** *adj.* **—ec′to·mor′phy** *n.*

–ectomy *suff.* Surgical removal: *tonsillectomy.*

ec·top·a·gus (ĕk-tŏp′ə-gəs) *n.* Conjoined twins in which the bodies are joined laterally.

ec·to·par·a·site (ĕk′tə-păr′ə-sīt′) *n.* A parasite that lives on the surface or exterior of the host organism, such as an ectophyte or an ectozoon.   **—ec′to·par′a·sit′ic** (-sĭt′ĭk) *adj.* **—ec′to·par′a·sit·ism** (-sĭ-tĭz′əm, -sī-tĭz′əm) *n.*

ec·to·phyte (ĕk′tə-fīt′) *n.* A plant parasite of the skin, such as ringworm. **—ec·to·phyt′ic** (-fĭt′ĭk) *adj.*

ec·to·pi·a (ĕk-tō′pē-ə) *or* **ec·to·py** (ĕk′tə-pē) *n.* An abnormal location or position of an organ or body part, occurring congenitally or as the result of an injury.

ectopia cor·dis (kôr′dĭs) *n.* A congenital condition in which the heart is exposed on the chest wall because of maldevelopment of the sternum and pericardium.

ectopia len·tis (lĕn′tĭs) *n.* Displacement of the lens of the eye.

ectopia pu·pil·lae con·gen·i·ta (pyōō-pĭl′ē kən-jĕn′ĭ-tə) *n.* Congenital displacement of the pupil of the eye.

ectopia tes·tis (tĕs′tĭs) *n.* See **ectopic testis.**

ec·top·ic (ĕk-tŏp′ĭk) *adj.* **1.** Out of place, as of an organ not in its proper position, or of a pregnancy occurring elsewhere than in the cavity of the uterus. **2.** Of or relating to a heartbeat that has its origin elsewhere than in the sinoatrial node.

ectopic beat *n.* A beat of the heart originating somewhere other than the sinoatrial node.

ectopic pregnancy *n.* Implantation and subsequent development of a fertilized ovum outside the cavity of the uterus. Also called *eccyesis.*

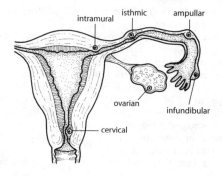

ectopic pregnancy
sites of ectopic pregnancy in the female reproductive system

ectopic schistosomiasis *n.* A clinical form of schistosomiasis that, rather than occurring at the usual site of parasitism, as in the mesenteric vein or hepatic portals, occurs at various unusual sites, such as the skin, brain, or spinal cord.

ectopic tachycardia *n.* Tachycardia originating in a focus other than the sinus node.

ectopic testis *n.* A condition in which the testis has descended but occupies an abnormal position. Also called *ectopia testis, parorchidium.*

ec·to·py (ĕk′tə-pē) *n.* Variant of **ectopia.**

ect·os·te·al (ĕk-tŏs′tē-əl) *adj.* Relating to the external surface of a bone.

ec·tos·to·sis (ĕk′tŏs-tō′sĭs) *n.* **1.** Ossification in cartilage beneath the perichondrium. **2.** The formation of bone beneath the periosteum.

ec·to·therm (ĕk′tə-thûrm′) *n.* An organism that regulates its body temperature largely by exchanging heat with its surroundings; a poikilotherm.

ectothermic (ĕk′tə-thûr′mĭk) *or* **ec·to·ther·mal** (-məl) *or* **ec·to·ther·mous** (-məs) *adj.* Of or relating to an organism that regulates its body temperature largely by exchanging heat with its surrounding environment.

ec·to·thrix (ĕk′tō-thrĭks′) *n.* A fungal parasite, such as certain dermatophytes, forming a sheath of spores on the outside of a hair as well as growing within the hair shaft.

ec·to·zo·on (ĕk′tə-zō′ŏn′) *n.,* *pl.* **-zo·a** (-zō′ə) An animal parasite, such as a flea or louse, living on the exterior of the host organism.

ectro– *pref.* Congenital absence: *ectropody.*

ec·tro·chei·ry *or* **ec·tro·chi·ry** (ĕk′trə-kī′rē) *n.* Congenital absence of all or a part of a hand.

ec·tro·dac·ty·ly (ĕk′trō-dăk′tə-lē) *or* **ec·tro·dac·tyl·i·a** (-dăk-tĭl′ē-ə) *or* **ec·tro·dac·tyl·ism** (-dăk′tə-lĭz′əm) *n.* Congenital absence of one or more fingers or toes.

ec·trog·e·ny (ĕk-trŏj′ə-nē) *n.* Congenital absence of a body part. —**ec′tro·gen′ic** (-trə-jĕn′ĭk) *adj.*

ec·tro·me·li·a (ĕk′trō-mē′lē-ə, mēl′yə) *n.* Congenital absence of one or more limbs. —**ec′tro·mel′ic** (-mĕl′ĭk, -mē′lĭk) *adj.*

ec·tro·pi·on (ĕk-trō′pē-ŏn′, -ən) *n.* A rolling outward of the margin of a body part, especially an eyelid.

ectropion u·ve·ae (yōō′vē-ē′) *n.* Eversion of the pupillary margin. Also called *iridectropium.*

ec·trop·o·dy (ĕk-trŏp′ə-dē) *n.* Congenital absence of all or a part of a foot.

ec·tro·syn·dac·ty·ly (ĕk′trō-sĭn-dăk′tə-lē) *n.* A congenital deformity marked by the absence of one or more digits and by the fusion of others.

ec·ze·ma (ĕk′sə-mə, ĕg′zə-) *n.* An acute or chronic noncontagious inflammation of the skin, characterized chiefly by redness, itching, and the outbreak of lesions that may discharge serous matter and become encrusted and scaly.

eczema her·pet·i·cum (hər-pĕt′ĭ-kəm) *n.* Kaposi's varicelliform eruption.

eczema mar·gi·na·tum (mär′jə-nā′təm) *n.* See **tinea cruris.**

eczema num·mu·lar·e (nŭm′yə-lâr′ē) *n.* Eczema appearing in discrete, coin-shaped patches.

ec·zem·a·toid (ĕg-zĕm′ə-toid′, -zē′mə-) *adj.* Resembling eczema in appearance.

ec·zem·a·tous (ĕg-zĕm′ə-təs, -zē′mə-) *adj.* Of, marked by, or resembling eczema.

eczema vac·ci·na·tum (văk′sə-nā′təm) *n.* A form of generalized vaccinia supervening upon existing atopic dermatitis and accompanied by a high fever, malaise, and enlargement of the lymph nodes.

ED *abbr.* effective dose; erectile dysfunction

EDC *abbr.* estimated date of confinement

E·dec·rin (ə-dĕk′rĭn) A trademark for the drug ethacrynic acid.

Ed·el·man (ĕd′l-mən), **Gerald Maurice** Born 1929. American biochemist. He shared a 1972 Nobel Prize for research on the chemical structure and nature of antibodies.

e·de·ma (ĭ-dē′mə) *n.,* *pl.* **-mas** *or* **-ma·ta** (-mə-tə) An accumulation of an excessive amount of watery fluid in cells, tissues, or serous cavities.

edema ne·o·na·to·rum (nē′ō-nā-tôr′əm) *n.* A diffuse, firm edema occurring in the newborn, beginning usually in the legs and spreading upward.

e·dem·a·tous (ĭ-dĕm′ə-təs) *adj.* Marked by edema.

e·den·tate (ē-dĕn′tāt′) *adj.* Lacking teeth.

e·den·tu·lous (ē-dĕn′chə-ləs) *adj.* Having no teeth; toothless.

e·det·ic acid (ĭ-dĕt′ĭk) *n.* EDTA.

ed·ro·pho·ni·um chloride (ĕd′rə-fō′nē-əm) *n.* A competitive antagonist of skeletal muscle relaxants, such as curare derivatives, used as an antidote for curariform drugs, as a diagnostic agent in myasthenia gravis, and in myasthenic crisis.

EDTA (ē′dē-tē-ā′) *n.* Ethylenediaminetetraacetic acid; a crystalline acid that acts as a strong chelating agent and that forms a sodium salt used as an antidote for metal poisoning and as an anticoagulant.

EEG *abbr.* electroencephalogram

EENT *abbr.* eye, ear, nose, and throat

e·fa·vir·enz (ə-fä′vĭr-ĕnz′) *n.* A non-nucleoside drug used to treat HIV infection.

ef·fect (ĭ-fĕkt′) *n.* **1.** Something brought about by a cause or an agent; a result. **2.** The power to produce an outcome or achieve a result; influence. **3.** A scientific law, hypothesis, or phenomenon. **4.** The condition of being in full force or execution. **5.** Something that produces a specific impression or supports a general design or intention. —*v.* **1.** To bring into existence. **2.** To produce as a result. **3.** To bring about. —**ef·fect′i·ble** *adj.*

ef·fec·tive conjugate (ĭ-fĕk′tĭv) *n.* The conjugate measured from the nearest lumbar vertebra to the pubic symphysis. Also called *false conjugate.*

effective dose *n. Abbr.* **ED** The dose, usually of a drug, that produces a desired effect.

effective half-life *n.* See **half-life** (sense 3).

effective osmotic pressure *n.* The part of the total osmotic pressure of a solution that governs the tendency of its solvent to pass across a boundary, usually a semipermeable membrane.

effective renal blood flow *n. Abbr.* **ERBF** The amount of blood flowing to the parts of the kidney that produce urine.

effective renal plasma flow *n. Abbr.* **ERPF** The amount of plasma flowing to the parts of the kidney that function in the production of urine.

effective temperature *n.* A comfort index or scale that takes into account the temperature of air, its moisture content, and movement.

ef·fec·tor (ĭ-fĕk′tər) *n.* **1.** A muscle, gland, or organ capable of responding to a stimulus, especially a nerve impulse. **2.** A nerve ending that carries impulses to a muscle, gland, or organ and activates muscle contraction or glandular secretion.

ef·fem·i·na·tion (ĭ-fĕm′ə-nā′shən) *n.* The acquisition of feminine characteristics, either physiologically by women, or pathologically by persons of either sex.

ef·fer·ent (ĕf′ər-ənt) *adj.* Directed away from a central organ or section. —*n.* An efferent organ or body part, such as a blood vessel.

efferent duct *n.* Any of the small seminal ducts leading from the testis to the head of the epididymis.

efferent glomerular arteriole *n.* The vessel that carries blood from the glomerular capillary network to the capillary bed of the proximal convoluted tubule.

efferent nerve *n.* A nerve conveying impulses from the central nervous system to the periphery. Also called *centrifugal nerve.*

efferent vessel *n.* **1.** A vein carrying blood from a part. **2.** A lymphatic vessel leaving a lymph node. **3.** An arteriole carrying blood out of a renal glomerulus.

ef·fer·ves·cent salt (ĕf′ər-vĕs′ənt) *n.* Any of the preparations that are made by adding sodium bicarbonate and tartaric and citric acids to a medicinally active salt.

Ef·fex·or (ĕf′ĕk-sôr′) A trademark for the drug venlafaxine hydrochloride.

ef·fi·cien·cy (ĭ-fĭsh′ən-sē) *n.* **1.** The production of the desired effects or results with minimum waste of time, effort, or skill. **2.** A measure of effectiveness; specifically, the useful work output divided by the energy input in any system.

ef·flo·resce (ĕf′lə-rĕs′) *v.* **1.** To blossom; bloom. **2.** To become a powder by losing water of crystallization, as when a hydrated crystal is exposed to air. —**ef′flo·res′-cence** *n.*

ef·flu·vi·um (ĭ-flōō′vē-əm) *n.,*   *pl.* **–vi·ums** *or* **–vi·a** (-vē-ə) **1.** A shedding, especially of hair. **2.** An exhalation, especially one of bad odor or injurious influence. No longer in technical use.

ef·fort syndrome (ĕf′ərt) *n.* See **neurocirculatory asthenia.**

ef·fu·sion (ĭ-fyōō′zhən) *n.* **1.** The escape of fluid from the blood vessels or lymphatics into the tissues or a cavity. **2.** The fluid so escaped.

e·flor·ni·thine hydrochloride (ĭ-flôr′nə-thēn′) *n.* An antineoplastic and antiprotozoal orphan drug used in the treatment of *Pneumocystis carinii* pneumonia in AIDS and of sleeping sickness caused by *Gambian trypanosomia.*

EFM *abbr.* electronic fetal monitoring

EGA *abbr.* estimated gestational age

E·gas Mo·niz (ĕ-gäs′ mô-nēsh′), **Antonio de** 1874–1955. Portuguese neurologist. He shared a Nobel Prize (1949) for advances in brain surgery.

e·gest (ē-jĕst′) *v.* To discharge or excrete from the body.

e·ges·ta (ē-jĕs′tə) *pl.n.* Unabsorbed food residues that are discharged from the digestive tract.

egg (ĕg) *n.* The female sexual cell or gamete; an ovum.

egg albumin *n.* The white of an egg. Also called *ovalbumin.*

egg cluster *n.* One of the clumps of cells that results from the breaking up of the gonadal cords in the ovarian cortex and later develops into a primary ovarian follicle.

egg membrane *n.* Any of the membranes forming the investing envelope of the ovum.

egg white *n.* The albumen of an egg, used especially in cooking.

e·go (ē′gō, ĕg′ō) *n.* In psychoanalytic theory, the division of the psyche that is conscious, most immediately controls thought and behavior, and mediates between the person and external reality.

e·go·bron·choph·o·ny (ē′gō-brŏng-kŏf′ə-nē) *n.* Egophony accompanied by bronchophony.

e·go·cen·tric (ē′gō-sĕn′trĭk, ĕg′ō-) *adj.* Marked by extreme concentration of attention upon oneself; self-centered. —**e′go·cen′tric** *n.*

ego-dystonic *adj.* Repugnant to or at variance with the aims of the ego.

ego ideal *n.* In psychoanalytic theory, the part of one's ego that contains an idealized self based on those people, especially parents and peers, one admires and wishes to emulate.

ego identity *n.* The sense of oneself as a distinct continuous entity.

e·go·ma·ni·a (ē′gō-mā′nē-ə, -mān′yə, ĕg′ō-) *n.* Extreme appreciation or preoccupation with the self.

e·goph·o·ny (ē-gŏf′ə-nē) *n.* A peculiar broken quality of the voice sounds, like the bleating of a goat, heard over lung tissue in cases of pleurisy with effusion. —**e′go·phon′ic** (ē′gə-fŏn′ĭk) *adj.*

ego-syntonic *adj.* Acceptable to the aims of the ego.

e·go·trop·ic (ē′gō-trŏp′ĭk, -trō′pĭk, ĕg′ō-) *n.* Marked by extreme concentration of attention upon oneself.

E·gyp·tian ophthalmia (ĭ-jĭp′shən) *n.* See **trachoma.**

Eh·lers-Dan·los syndrome (ā′lərs-dăn′lŏs, -dän-lōs′) *n.* A hereditary disorder of the connective tissue characterized by overelasticity and friability of the skin, excessive extensibility of the joints, and fragility of the cutaneous blood vessels. Also called *cutis hyperelastica, elastic skin.*

Ehr·lich (âr′lĭкн), **Paul** 1854–1915. German bacteriologist who conducted pioneering research in chemotherapy and developed the chemical Salvarsan as a treatment of syphilis. He is also known for his work in the fields of hematology and immunology, for which he shared a 1908 Nobel Prize.

Ehr·lich·i·a (âr-lĭk′ē-ə) *n.* A genus of bacteria of the order Rickettsiales that occur singly or in inclusions in circulating white blood cells.

ehr·lich·i·o·sis (âr-lĭk′ē-ō′sĭs) *n.* Infection with parasitic leukocytic rickettsiae especially by *Ehrlichia sennetsu,* which produces manifestations in humans similar to those of Rocky Mountain spotted fever.

Ehr·lich's inner body (âr′lĭks) *n.* A round oxyphil body found in red blood cells in hemocytolysis due to a specific blood poison. Also called *Heinz-Ehrlich body.*

EI *abbr.* early intervention

ei·co·sa·noid (ī-kō′sə-noid′) *n.* Any of the physiologically active substances derived from arachidonic acid, including the prostaglandins, leukotrienes, and thromboxanes.

ei·co·sa·pen·ta·e·no·ic acid (ī′kō-sə-pěn′tə-ĭ-nō′ĭk) *n.* *Abbr.* **EPA** An omega-3 fatty acid found in fish oils.

ei·dop·tom·e·try (ī′dŏp-tŏm′ĭ-trē) *n.* The measurement of the acuteness of form vision. No longer in technical use.

eighth cranial nerve *n.* See **vestibulocochlear nerve.**

Eijk·man (īk′män′, āk′-), **Christiaan** 1858–1930. Dutch hygienist and pathologist. He shared a 1929 Nobel Prize for his discovery of the nutrient, later called vitamin B₁ or thiamine, that relieves beriberi.

Ei·ken·el·la cor·ro·dens (ī′kə-něl′ə kə-rō′dənz) *n.* A rod-shaped, gram-negative, facultatively anaerobic bacterium normally in the adult human oral cavity but which may become an opportunistic pathogen, especially in immunocompromised individuals.

ei·ko·nom·e·ter *or* **ei·co·nom·e·ter** (ī′kə-nŏm′ĭ-tər) *n.* **1.** An instrument used for determining the magnifying power of a microscope, or the size of a microscopic object. **2.** An instrument used for detecting aniseikonia.

Ei·me·ri·a (ī-mîr′ē-ə) *n.* A genus of coccidial protozoa that is highly pathogenic, especially in young domesticated mammals and birds.

–ein *suff.* A chemical compound related to a specified compound with a similar name ending in *-in* or *-ine: phthalein.*

Ein·stein (īn′stīn′), **Albert** 1879–1955. German-born American theoretical physicist whose special and general theories of relativity revolutionized modern thought on the nature of space and time and formed a theoretical base for the exploitation of atomic energy. He won a Nobel Prize in 1921 for his explanation of the photoelectric effect.

ein·stein·i·um (īn-stī′nē-əm) *n.* *Symbol* **Es** A radioactive transuranic element synthesized by neutron irradiation of plutonium or other elements. Its longest-lived isotope is Es 254 with a half-life of 275 days. Atomic number 99.

Eint·ho·ven (īnt′hō′vən), **Willem** 1860–1927. Dutch physiologist. He won a 1924 Nobel Prize for his contributions to electrocardiography.

Ein·tho·ven's triangle (īnt′hō′vənz) *n.* An imaginary equilateral triangle having the heart at its center and formed by lines that represent the three standard limb leads of the electrocardiogram.

Ei·sen·meng·er's complex (ī′zən-měng′ərz) *n.* A defect of the interventricular septum with pulmonary hypertension and a consequent right-to-left shunt through the defect.

Eisenmenger syndrome *n.* A condition that is caused by pulmonary hypertension associated with a congenital defect between the two circulations so that a reversed, right-to-left shunt results.

e·jac·u·late (ĭ-jăk′yə-lāt′) *v.* To eject or discharge abruptly, especially to discharge semen in orgasm. —*n.* (ĭ-jăk′yə-lĭt) Semen ejaculated in orgasm.

e·jac·u·la·tion (ĭ-jăk′yə-lā′shən) *n.* The act or process of ejaculating.

e·jac·u·la·ti·o pre·cox (ĭ-jăk′yə-lā′shē-ō prē′kŏks′) *n.* Premature ejaculation.

e·jac·u·la·to·ry (ĭ-jăk′yə-lə-tôr′ē) *adj.* Relating to an ejaculation.

ejaculatory duct *n.* The duct that is formed by the union of the deferent duct and the excretory duct of

the seminal vesicle and opens into the prostatic urethra. Also called *spermiduct.*

e·jec·ta (ĭ-jěk′tə) *n.* Something that has been ejected from the body. Also called *ejection.*

e·jec·tion (ĭ-jěk′shən) *n.* **1.** The act of driving or casting out by physical force from within. **2.** See **ejecta.**

ejection fraction *n.* The blood present in the ventricle at the end of diastole and expelled during the contraction of the heart.

ejection murmur *n.* A systolic murmur ending before the second heart sound and produced by the ejection of blood into the aorta or pulmonary artery.

ejection period *n.* See **sphygmic interval.**

ejection sound *n.* A sharp sound heard on auscultation in early systole over the aortic or pulmonic area when the aorta or pulmonary artery is dilated.

eka– *pref.* One or first, used especially to name undiscovered elements of the periodic table whose characteristics have been postulated: *eka-osmium.*

EKG *abbr.* electrocardiogram; electrocardiograph

EKY *abbr.* electrokymogram

e·lab·o·ra·tion (ĭ-lăb′ə-rā′shən) *n.* **1.** The process of working out in detail by labor and study. **2.** The mental process occurring partly during dreaming and partly during the recalling or telling of a dream, by means of which the latent content of the dream is brought into increasingly more coherent and logical order, resulting in the manifest content of the dream. —**e·lab′o·rate′** *v.*

e·las·tance (ĭ-lăs′təns) *n.* A measure of the tendency of a hollow organ to recoil toward its original dimensions upon removal of a distending or compressing force. It is the reciprocal of compliance.

e·las·tase (ĭ-lăs′tās′, -tāz′) *n.* An enzyme found especially in pancreatic juice that catalyzes the hydrolysis of elastin.

e·las·tic (ĭ-lăs′tĭk) *adj.* Having the property of returning to the original shape after being distorted.

elastic bandage *n.* A stretchable bandage used to create localized pressure.

elastic cartilage *n.* A yellowish flexible cartilage in which the matrix is infiltrated by a network of elastic fibers; it occurs primarily in the external ear, eustachian tube, and some cartilages of the larynx and epiglottis. Also called *yellow cartilage.*

elastic fiber *n.* Any of the fibers 0.2 to 2 micrometers in diameter containing elastin. They branch and anastomose to form networks and fuse to form fenestrated membranes. Also called *yellow fiber.*

e·las·ti·cin (ĭ-lăs′tĭ-sĭn) *n.* See **elastin.**

e·las·tic·i·ty (ĭ-lă-stĭs′ĭ-tē, ē′lă-) *n.* **1.** The condition or property of being elastic; flexibility. **2.** The property of returning to an initial form or state following deformation.

elastic lamella *n.* A thin sheet of elastic fibers, as found in a vein or in the respiratory tract.

elastic lamina of cornea *n.* See **limiting layer of cornea** (sense 2).

elastic layer of cornea *n.* See **limiting layer of cornea** (sense 2).

elastic membrane *n.* A membrane formed of elastic connective tissue fibers, such as that surrounding the arteries.

elastic skin *n.* See **Ehlers-Danlos syndrome.**

elastic tissue *n.* Connective tissue in which elastic fibers predominate.

e·las·tin (ĭ-lăs′tĭn) *n.* An elastic, fibrous mucoprotein, similar to collagen, and the major connective tissue protein of elastic fibers. Also called *elasticin.*

e·las·to·fi·bro·ma (ĭ-lăs′tō-fī-brō′mə) *n.* A nonencapsulated slow-growing mass of poorly cellular, collagenous, fibrous tissue and elastic tissue, occurring usually in subscapular adipose tissue of old persons.

e·las·toid degeneration (ĭ-lăs′toid′) *n.* See **elastosis** (sense 2).

e·las·to·ma (ĭ-lă-stō′mə, ē′lă-) *n.* An inherited disorder of connective tissue characterized by slightly elevated yellowish plaques on the neck, armpits, abdomen, and thighs, associated with angioid streaks of the retina and elastic tissue degeneration in other organs. Also called *pseudoxanthoma elasticum.*

e·las·tor·rhex·is (ĭ-lăs′tə-rĕk′sĭs) *n.* Fragmentation of elastic tissue in which the normal wavy strands appear shredded and clumped.

e·las·to·sis (ĭ-lă-stō′sĭs, ē′lă-) *n.* **1.** A degenerative change in elastic tissue. **2.** The degeneration of connective tissue in the skin, in such a manner that many tissues resemble elastin when stained. Also called *elastoid degeneration.*

elastosis col·loi·da·lis con·glom·er·a·ta (kŏl′oi-dā′lĭs kŏn′glō-bā′tə) *n.* See **colloid acne.**

elastosis per·fo·rans ser·pig·i·no·sa (pûr′fə-rănz′-sər-pĭj′ə-nō′sə) *n.* A disorder of the connective tissue characterized by ring-shaped groups of asymptomatic keratotic papules; the epidermis is thickened around a central plug of keratin, overlying an accumulation of elastic tissue.

el·bow (ĕl′bō′) *n.* **1.** The joint or bend of the arm between the forearm and the upper arm. Also called *cubitus.* **2.** The bony outer projection of this joint. **3.** Something having a bend or an angle that is similar to an elbow.

elbow bone *n.* See **ulna.**

el·bowed bougie (ĕl′bōd′) *n.* A bougie with a sharply angulated bend near its tip.

elbow joint *n.* A compound hinge joint between the humerus and the bones of the forearm. Also called *cubital joint.*

El·de·pryl (ĕl′də-prəl) A trademark for the drug selegiline hydrochloride.

eld·er·care (ĕl′dər-kâr′) *n.* Social and medical programs and facilities intended for the care and maintenance of the aged.

e·lec·tive mutism (ĭ-lĕk′tĭv) *n.* A form of childhood mutism in which the ability to speak is intact, but there is a refusal to speak in almost all social situations.

E·lec·tra complex (ĭ-lĕk′trə) *n.* In psychoanalytic theory, a daughter's unconscious libidinal desire for her father.

e·lec·tri·cal alternation (ĭ-lĕk′trĭ-kəl) *n.* A varied alternation in the activity of the heart indicative of myocardial disease as measured by an electrocardiograph. Also called *electrical alternans.*

electrical axis *n.* The direction of the electromotive force developed in the heart during activation.

electrical failure *n.* Failure in which the cardiac inade-

quacy is secondary to disturbance of the electrical impulse.

electro– *or* **electr–** *pref.* **1.** Electricity; electric; electrically: *electrocautery.* **2.** Electron: *electronegative.*

e·lec·tro·an·al·ge·sia (ĭ-lĕk′trō-ăn′əl-jē′zhə) *n.* Analgesia that is induced by the passage of an electric current.

e·lec·tro·an·es·the·sia (ĭ-lĕk′trō-ăn′ĭs-thē′zhə) *n.* Anesthesia produced by an electric current.

e·lec·tro·car·di·o·gram (ĭ-lĕk′trō-kär′dē-ə-grăm′) *n.* *Abbr.* **ECG, EKG** The curve traced by an electrocardiograph. Also called *cardiogram.*

e·lec·tro·car·di·o·graph (ĭ-lĕk′trō-kär′dē-ə-grăf′) *n.* *Abbr.* **ECG, EKG** An instrument used in the detection and diagnosis of heart abnormalities that measures electrical potentials on the body surface and generates a record of the electrical currents associated with heart muscle activity. Also called *cardiograph.* —**e·lec′-tro·car′di·og′ra·phy** (-kär′dē-ŏg′rə-fē) *n.*

e·lec·tro·cau·ter·i·za·tion (ĭ-lĕk′trō-kô′tər-ĭ-zā′shən) *n.* The cauterization of tissue by an electrocautery.

e·lec·tro·cau·ter·y (ĭ-lĕk′trō-kô′tə-rē) *n.* **1.** An instrument for directing a high-frequency current through a local area of tissue. **2.** A metal cauterizing instrument heated by electricity. **3.** The cauterization of tissue by means of one of these instruments.

e·lec·tro·cer·e·bral silence (ĭ-lĕk′trō-sĕr′ə-brəl, -sə-rē′-) *n.* *Abbr.* **ECS** The absence of electrical activity in the brain measured by an electroencephalogram, indicating cerebral death.

e·lec·tro·chem·i·cal (ĭ-lĕk′trō-kĕm′ĭ-kəl) *adj.* Of or relating to chemical reactions brought about by electricity; galvanochemical.

e·lec·tro·co·ag·u·la·tion (ĭ-lĕk′trō-kō-ăg′yə-lā′shən) *n.* Therapeutic use of a high-frequency electric current to bring about the coagulation and destruction of tissue.

e·lec·tro·coch·le·o·gram (ĭ-lĕk′trō-kŏk′lē-ə-grăm′, -kō′klē-) *n.* The record obtained by electrocochleography of the inner ear.

e·lec·tro·coch·le·og·ra·phy (ĭ-lĕk′trō-kŏk′lē-ŏg′rə-fē) *n.* A measurement of the electrical potentials generated by sound simulation in the inner ear.

e·lec·tro·con·trac·til·i·ty (ĭ-lĕk′trō-kŏn′trăk-tĭl′ĭ-tē) *n.* The power of contraction of muscular tissue in response to an electrical stimulus.

e·lec·tro·con·vul·sive (ĭ-lĕk′trō-kən-vŭl′sĭv) *adj.* Of or relating to a convulsive response to an electrical stimulus.

electroconvulsive therapy *n.* *Abbr.* **ECT** Administration of electric current to the brain through electrodes placed on the head, usually near the temples, in order to induce unconsciousness and brief convulsions. Used in the treatment of certain mental disorders, especially acute depression. Also called *electroshock, electroshock therapy.*

e·lec·tro·cor·ti·co·gram (ĭ-lĕk′trō-kôr′tĭ-kə-grăm′) *n.* The record obtained by electrocorticography.

e·lec·tro·cor·ti·cog·ra·phy (ĭ-lĕk′trō-kôr′tĭ-kŏg′rə-fē) *n.* The technique of measuring the electrical activity of the cerebral cortex.

e·lec·trode (ĭ-lĕk′trōd′) *n.* **1.** A solid electric conductor through which an electric current enters or leaves an electrolytic cell or other medium. **2.** A collector or emitter of electric charge or of electric-charge carriers, as in a semiconducting device.

e·lec·tro·der·mal (ĭ-lĕk′trō-dûr′məl) *adj.* Of or relating to the electrical properties of the skin.

electrodermal audiometry *n.* A form of electrophysiologic audiometry used to determine hearing thresholds by measuring changes in skin resistance as a conditioned response to noise stimuli.

e·lec·tro·der·ma·tome (ĭ-lĕk′trō-dûr′mə-tōm′) *n.* A dermatome powered by electricity.

e·lec·tro·des·ic·ca·tion (ĭ-lĕk′trō-dĕs′ĭ-kā′shən) *n.* Destruction of lesions or sealing off of blood vessels by monopolar high-frequency electric current.

e·lec·tro·di·ag·no·sis (ĭ-lĕk′trō-dī′əg-nō′sĭs) *n.* Determination of the nature of a disease through observation of changes in electrical irritability.

e·lec·tro·di·al·y·sis (ĭ-lĕk′trō-dī-ăl′ĭ-sĭs) *n.* Dialysis at a rate that is increased by the application of an electric potential across the dialysis membrane, used especially to remove electrolytes from a colloidal suspension.

e·lec·tro·en·ceph·a·lo·gram (ĭ-lĕk′trō-ĕn-sĕf′ə-lə-grăm′) *n. Abbr.* **EEG** A graphic record of brain waves as recorded by an electroencephalograph.

e·lec·tro·en·ceph·a·lo·graph (ĭ-lĕk′trō-ĕn-sĕf′ə-lə-grăf′) *n.* An instrument that generates a record of the electrical activity of the brain by measuring electric potentials using electrodes attached to the scalp. —**e·lec′tro·en·ceph′a·lo·graph′ic** *adj.* —**e·lec′tro·en·ceph′a·log′ra·phy** (-lŏg′rə-fē) *n.*

electroencephalographic dysrhythmia *n.* An irregularity in the pattern of a brain-wave tracing.

e·lec·tro·en·dos·mo·sis (ĭ-lĕk′trō-ĕn′dŏz-mō′sĭs) *n.* Endosmosis produced by an electric field.

e·lec·tro·gas·tro·gram (ĭ-lĕk′trō-găs′trə-grăm′) *n.* The record obtained with the electrogastrograph.

e·lec·tro·gas·tro·graph (ĭ-lĕk′trō-găs′trə-grăf′) *n.* A graphic recording of the electrical phenomena associated with gastric secretion and movement. —**e·lec′tro·gas·trog′ra·phy** (-gă-strŏg′rə-fē) *n.*

e·lec·tro·gram (ĭ-lĕk′trə-grăm′) *n.* A graphic record made from the measurement of electrical events in living tissues.

e·lec·tro·he·mo·sta·sis (ĭ-lĕk′trō-hē′mə-stā′sĭs, -hē-mŏs′tə-) *n.* The arrest of hemorrhage by means of a high-frequency current.

e·lec·tro·im·mu·no·dif·fu·sion (ĭ-lĕk′trō-ĭm′yə-nō-dĭ-fyōō′zhən, -ĭ-myōō′-) *n.* An immunochemical method that combines electrophoretic separation with immunodiffusion by incorporating antibody into the support medium.

e·lec·tro·ky·mo·gram (ĭ-lĕk′trō-kī′mə-grăm′) *n. Abbr.* **EKY** The graphic record produced by the electrokymograph. No longer in technical use.

e·lec·tro·ky·mo·graph (ĭ-lĕk′trō-kī′mə-grăf′) *n.* An apparatus for recording the movements of the heart and great vessels by observing changes in the x-ray silhouettes. No longer in technical use.

e·lec·trol·y·sis (ĭ-lĕk-trŏl′ĭ-sĭs, ē′lĕk-) *n.* **1.** Chemical change, especially decomposition, that is produced in an electrolyte by an electric current. **2.** Destruction of

living tissue, especially that of the hair roots, by means of an electric current applied with a needle-shaped electrode.

e·lec·tro·lyte (ĭ-lĕk′trə-līt′) *n.* **1.** A chemical compound that ionizes when dissolved or molten to produce an electrically conductive medium. **2.** Any of various ions, such as sodium or chloride, required by cells to regulate the electric charge and flow of water molecules across the cell membrane.

electrolyte balance *n.* The relative concentrations of ions in the extracellular and intracellular fluids of the body, especially those that are produced from ionized salts.

e·lec·tro·lyt·ic (ĭ-lĕk′trə-lĭt′ĭk) *adj.* **1.** Of or relating to electrolysis. **2.** Produced by electrolysis. **3.** Of or relating to electrolytes. —**e·lec′tro·lyt′i·cal·ly** *adv.*

e·lec·tro·mag·net·ic radiation (ĭ-lĕk′trō-măg-nĕt′ĭk) *n.* Radiation originating in a varying electromagnetic field, such as visible light, radio waves, x-rays, and gamma rays.

e·lec·tro·me·chan·i·cal dissociation (ĭ-lĕk′trō-mə-kăn′ĭ-kəl) *n.* Persistence of electrical activity in the heart without an associated mechanical contraction; it is often a sign of cardiac rupture.

e·lec·tro·mo·tive force (ĭ-lĕk′trō-mō′tĭv) *n. Abbr.* **EMF** The energy per unit charge that is reversibly converted from chemical or other forms of energy into electrical energy in a battery.

e·lec·tro·my·o·gram (ĭ-lĕk′trō-mī′ə-grăm′) *n. Abbr.* **EMG** A graphic record of the electrical activity of a muscle as recorded by an electromyograph.

e·lec·tro·my·o·graph (ĭ-lĕk′trō-mī′ə-grăf′) *n.* An instrument used in diagnosing neuromuscular disorders that produces an audio or visual record of the electrical activity of a skeletal muscle by means of an electrode inserted into the muscle or placed on the skin. —**e·lec′tro·my·og′ra·phy** (-mī-ŏg′rə-fē) *n.*

e·lec·tron (ĭ-lĕk′trŏn′) *n. Abbr.* **e** A stable subatomic particle in the lepton family having a rest mass of 9.1066×10^{-28} gram and a unit negative electric charge of approximately 1.602×10^{-19} coulomb. Also called *negatron.*

e·lec·tro·nar·co·sis (ĭ-lĕk′trō-när-kō′sĭs) *n.* An insensitivity to pain induced for therapeutic purposes by the application of electric current to the body.

e·lec·tro·neg·a·tive (ĭ-lĕk′trō-nĕg′ə-tĭv) *adj.* **1.** Having a negative electric charge. **2.** Tending to attract electrons to form a chemical bond. **3.** Capable of acting as a negative electrode.

e·lec·tro·neu·rog·ra·phy (ĭ-lĕk′trō-nŏŏ-rŏg′rə-fē) *n.* A method of measuring and recording the conduction velocities associated with the electrical stimulation of peripheral nerves.

e·lec·tro·neu·ro·my·og·ra·phy (ĭ-lĕk′trō-nŏŏr′ō-mī-ŏg′rə-fē) *n.* Electromyography in which the peripheral nerves to the muscle under study are stimulated with electric current.

e·lec·tron·ic cell counter (ĭ-lĕk-trŏn′ĭk, ē′lĕk-) *n.* An automatic blood cell counter, sometimes capable of providing multiple simultaneous measurements, as of white blood cells, red blood cells, hemoglobin, and hematocrit.

electronic fetal monitor *n. Abbr.* **EFM** An electronic device used during labor to monitor fetal heartbeat and maternal uterine contractions.

electron microscope *n. Abbr.* **EM** Any of a class of microscopes that use electrons rather than visible light to produce magnified images, especially of objects having dimensions smaller than the wavelengths of visible light, with linear magnification approaching or exceeding one million (10^6).

electron radiography *n.* A radiographic imaging process in which the incident x-rays are converted to a latent charge image and developed by a special printing process to eliminate background fog and image noise.

electron spin resonance *n. Abbr.* **ESR** A spectrometric method, based on measurement of the spins of unpaired electrons in a magnetic field, for detecting and estimating free radicals in organic reactions.

electron transport *n.* The successive passage of electrons from one cytochrome or flavoprotein to another by a series of oxidation-reduction reactions during the aerobic production of ATP, with the electrons originating from an oxidizable substrate and passing to molecular oxygen.

electron volt *n. Abbr.* **eV, ev** A unit of energy equal to the energy acquired by an electron falling through a potential difference of one volt, approximately 1.602×10^{-19} joule.

e·lec·tro·nys·tag·mog·ra·phy (ĭ-lĕk′trō-nĭs′tăg-mŏg′rə-fē) *n. Abbr.* **ENG** A study of the recorded changes in corneoretinal potential caused by movements of the eye, used to assess nystagmus.

e·lec·tro·oc·u·log·ra·phy (ĭ-lĕk′trō-ŏk′yə-lŏg′rə-fē) *n. Abbr.* **EOG** The study and interpretation of electroencephalograms made by moving the eyes a constant distance between two fixed points.

e·lec·tro·pher·o·gram (ĭ-lĕk′trō-fĕr′ə-grăm′) *or* **e·lec·tro·pho·ret·o·gram** (-fə-rĕt′ə-grăm′) *n.* A recording of the separated components of a mixture produced by electrophoresis.

e·lec·tro·phile (ĭ-lĕk′trə-fīl′, -fīl) *or* **e·lec·tro·phil** (-fīl) *n.* A chemical compound or group that is attracted to electrons and that tends to accept electrons. —**e·lec′tro·phil′ic** (-fīl′ĭk) *adj.*

e·lec·tro·pho·re·sis (ĭ-lĕk′trō-fə-rē′sĭs) *n.* **1.** The migration of charged colloidal particles or molecules through a solution under the influence of an applied electric field usually provided by immersed electrodes. Also called *ionophoresis, phoresis.* **2.** A method of separating substances, especially proteins, and analyzing molecular structure based on the rate of movement of each component in a colloidal suspension while under the influence of an electric field. —**e·lec′tro·pho·ret′ic** (-rĕt′ĭk) *adj.*

e·lec·tro·phren·ic respiration (ĭ-lĕk′trō-frĕn′ĭk) *n.* Respiration induced by the application of rhythmic electrical stimulation at the motor points of the phrenic nerve, usually used on individuals whose nervous respiratory center is paralyzed as a result of acute bulbar poliomyelitis.

e·lec·tro·phys·i·ol·o·gy (ĭ-lĕk′trō-fĭz′ē-ŏl′ə-jē) *n.* **1.** The branch of physiology that studies the relationship between electric phenomena and bodily processes. **2.** The electric activity associated with a bodily part or function.

e·lec·tro·ret·i·no·gram (ĭ-lĕk′trō-rĕt′n-ə-grăm′) *n. Abbr.* **ERG** A graphic record of the electrical activity of the retina.

e·lec·tro·ret·i·nog·ra·phy (ĭ-lĕk′trō-rĕt′n-ŏg′rə-fē) *n.* The study and interpretation of electroretinograms.

e·lec·tro·scis·sion (ĭ-lĕk′trō-sĭzh′ən) *n.* The cutting of tissues by an electrocautery knife.

e·lec·tro·shock (ĭ-lĕk′trō-shŏk′) *n.* See **electroconvulsive therapy.** —*v.* To administer electroconvulsive therapy to a person.

electroshock therapy *n. Abbr.* **EST** See **electroconvulsive therapy.**

e·lec·tro·sur·ger·y (ĭ-lĕk′trō-sûr′jə-rē) *n.* The surgical use of high-frequency electric current for cutting or destroying tissue, as in electrocauterization.

e·lec·tro·tax·is (ĭ-lĕk′trō-tăk′sĭs) *n.* Movement of organisms or cells in response to an electric current. Also called *electrotropism.*

e·lec·tro·ther·a·py (ĭ-lĕk′trō-thĕr′ə-pē) *n.* Medical therapy using electric currents. Also called *electrotherapeutics.*

e·lec·trot·o·nus (ĭ-lĕk′trŏt′n-əs, ē′lĕk-) *n.* Alteration in excitability and conductivity of a nerve or muscle during the passage of an electric current through it. —**e·lec′tro·ton′ic** (-trə-tŏn′ĭk) *adj.*

e·lec·trot·ro·pism (ĭ-lĕk′trŏt′rə-pĭz′əm, ē′lĕk-, ĭ-lĕk′trō-trō′-) *n.* See **electrotaxis.**

e·lec·tu·ar·y (ĭ-lĕk′chōō-ĕr′ē) *n.* See **confection.**

el·e·doi·sin (ĕl′ĭ-doi′sĭn) *n.* A protein that is formed in the venom gland of several species of octopuses and is used as a vasodilator and a contraction agent of extravascular smooth muscle.

e·le·i·din (ĭ-lē′ĭ-dn) *n.* A semifluid, acidophilic substance related to keratin and present in the stratum lucidum of the epidermis.

el·e·ment (ĕl′ə-mənt) *n.* **1.** A substance that cannot be reduced to simpler substances by normal chemical means and that is composed of atoms having an identical number of protons in each nucleus. **2.** A fundamental, essential, or irreducible constituent of a composite entity.

el·e·men·ta·ry granules (ĕl′ə-mĕn′tə-rē, -trē) *pl.n.* See **hemoconia.**

elementary particle *n.* **1.** A knoblike body that appears on the luminal surfaces of mitochondrial cristae and is believed to be involved with the electron transport system. **2.** Any of the subatomic particles that compose matter and energy, especially one hypothesized or regarded as an irreducible constituent of matter. Also called *fundamental particle.*

el·e·o·ma (ĕl′ē-ō′mə) *n., pl.* **–mas** *or* **–ma·ta** (-mə-tə) See **lipogranuloma.**

el·e·phan·ti·a·sis (ĕl′ə-fən-tī′ə-sĭs) *n.* Chronic, often extreme enlargement and hardening of cutaneous and subcutaneous tissue, especially of the legs and external genitals, resulting from lymphatic obstruction and usually caused by infestation of the lymph glands and vessels with a filarial worm. —**el′e·phan·ti′ac′** (-tī′ăk′) *adj.*

elephantiasis neu·ro·ma·to·sa (nŏŏ-rō′mə-tō′sə) *n.* Enlargement of a limb due to diffuse neurofibromatosis of the skin and subcutaneous tissue.

elephantiasis nos·tras (nŏs′trəs) *n.* A solid persistent edema of the eyelids and face caused by recurrent erysipelas or injury.

elephantiasis scro·ti (skrō′tī) *n.* See **chyloderma**.

el·e·phan·toid fever (ĕl′ə-făn′toid′, ĕl′ə-fən-toid′) *n.* Lymphangitis and temperature increase that mark the beginning of endemic elephantiasis.

el·e·trip·tan hy·dro·bro·mide (ĕl′ə-trĭp′tăn hī′drō-brō′mīd′) *n.* An oral drug of the triptan class used to treat migraine headaches.

el·e·va·tor (ĕl′ə-vā′tər) *n.* **1.** A surgical instrument used to elevate tissues or to raise a sunken part, such as a depressed fragment of bone. **2.** A dental instrument used to remove teeth or parts of teeth that cannot be gripped with a forceps or to loosen teeth and roots before using forceps.

elevator muscle of angle of mouth *n.* A muscle with origin from the canine fossa of the maxilla, with insertion into the orbicular muscle of the mouth and into the skin at the corner of the mouth, with nerve supply from the facial nerve, and whose action raises the corner of the mouth.

elevator muscle of anus *n.* A muscle formed by the puborectal muscle, the elevator muscle of the prostate, the pubococcygeal muscle, and the iliococcygeal muscle, with origin from the back of the pubis and the spine of the ischium, with insertion into the anococcygeal ligament and the sides of the lower part of the sacrum and coccyx, with nerve supply from the fourth sacral nerve, and whose action draws the anus upward in defecation and supports the pelvic viscera.

elevator muscle of prostate *n.* The most medial muscular fibers of the elevator muscle of the anus in the male.

elevator muscle of scapula *n.* A muscle with origin from the posterior tubercles of the transverse processes of the four upper cervical vertebrae, with insertion into the superior angle of the scapula, with nerve supply from the dorsal nerve of the scapula, and whose action raises the scapula.

elevator muscle of soft palate *n.* A muscle with origin from the temporal bone and the lower part of the auditory tube, with insertion into the soft palate, with nerve supply from the pharyngeal plexus, and whose action raises the soft palate.

elevator muscle of thyroid gland *n.* A band of muscular fibers occasionally passing from the thyrohyoid muscle to the isthmus of the thyroid gland.

elevator muscle of upper eyelid *n.* A muscle with origin from the sphenoid bone, with insertion into the eyelid, tarsal plate, and walls of the eye socket, with nerve supply from the oculomotor nerve, and whose action raises the upper eyelid.

elevator muscle of upper lip *n.* A muscle with origin from the maxilla below the infraorbital foramen, with insertion to the orbicular muscle of the upper lip, with nerve supply from the facial nerve, and whose action elevates the upper lip.

elevator muscle of upper lip and wing of nose *n.* A muscle with origin from the root of the nasal process of the maxilla, with insertion to the ala of the nose and the orbicular muscle of the upper lip, with nerve supply from the facial nerve, and whose action elevates the upper lip and the wing of the nose.

11-cis-ret·i·nal (-sĭs′rĕt′n-ăl′, -ôl′) *n.* The isomer of retinaldehyde that enzymatically combines with opsin to form rhodopsin.

11-ox·y·cor·ti·coid (-ŏk′sē-kôr′tĭ-koid′) *n.* A corticosteroid that contains an alcohol or ketone group.

e·lev·enth cranial nerve (ĭ-lĕv′ənth) *n.* See **accessory nerve**.

e·lim·i·na·tion (ĭ-lĭm′ə-nā′shən) *n.* The process of expelling or removing, especially of waste products from the body.

elimination diet *n.* A diet designed to detect what foodstuffs cause allergic reactions by separate and successive withdrawal of foods from the diet until the food that causes the symptoms is discovered.

El·i·mite (ĕl′ə-mīt′) A trademark for the drug permethrin.

El·i·on (ĕl′ē-ən), **Gertrude Belle** 1918–1999. American drug researcher. She shared a 1988 Nobel Prize for developing drugs to treat leukemia and gout.

ELISA (ĭ-lī′zə) *n.* Enzyme-linked immunosorbent assay; a sensitive immunoassay that uses an enzyme linked to an antibody or antigen as a marker for the detection of a specific protein, especially an antigen or antibody.

e·lix·ir (ĭ-lĭk′sər) *n.* A sweetened aromatic solution of alcohol and water, serving as a vehicle for medicine.

el·lag·ic acid (ĭ-lăj′ĭk) *n.* A yellow crystalline compound that is obtained from tannins and used as a hemostatic.

El·li·ot's operation (ĕl′ē-əts) *n.* A surgical procedure in which the eyeball is trephined at the corneoscleral margin to relieve tension in glaucoma.

el·lip·soi·dal joint (ĭ-lĭp-soid′l, ĕl′ĭp-, ē′lĭp-) *n.* A modified biaxial ball-and-socket joint in which the joint surfaces are elongated or ellipsoidal. Also called *condylar joint*.

el·lip·ti·cal amputation (ĭ-lĭp′tĭ-kəl) *n.* A form of circular amputation in which the sweep of the knife is not exactly vertical to the long axis of the limb.

el·lip·to·cyte (ĭ-lĭp′tə-sīt′) *n.* An elliptical erythrocyte. Also called *ovalocyte*.

el·lip·to·cy·to·sis (ĭ-lĭp′tō-sī-tō′sĭs) *n.* A relatively rare hereditary abnormality of red blood cells in which more than half of the cells are rod forms and elliptocytes. It is often associated with hemolytic anemia. Also called *ovalocytosis*.

El·lis (ĕl′ĭs), **(Henry) Havelock** 1859–1939. British psychologist and writer known for his pioneering works on sexuality, such as *Studies in the Psychology of Sex* (seven volumes, 1897–1928).

el·u·ant *or* **el·u·ent** (ĕl′yŏŏ-ənt) *n.* A substance used as a solvent in the process of elution.

el·u·ate (ĕl′yŏŏ-ĭt, -āt′) *n.* The solution of solvent and dissolved matter resulting from elution.

e·lu·tion (ĭ-lŏŏ′shən) *n.* **1.** The chromatographic process of using a solvent to extract an adsorbed substance from a solid adsorbing medium. **2.** The removal of antibody from the antigen to which it is attached.

EM *abbr.* electron microscope

em– *pref.* Variant of **en–**.

e·ma·ci·a·tion (ĭ-mā′shē-ā′shən) *n.* The process of

losing so much flesh as to become extremely thin; wasting.

em·a·na·tion (ĕm′ə-nā′shən) *n.* **1.** Something that issues from a source; an emission. **2.** Any of several radioactive gases that are isotopes of radon and are products of radioactive decay.

e·mas·cu·la·tion (ĭ-măs′kyə-lā′shən) *n.* The surgical removal of the testes and penis; castration.

em·balm (ĕm-bäm′) *v.* To treat a corpse with preservatives in order to prevent decay.

em·bar·rass (ĕm-băr′əs) *v.* To interfere with or impede (a bodily function or part).

Emb·den-Mey·er·hof pathway (ĕm′dən-mī′ər-hôf′) *n.* The anaerobic metabolic pathway by which glucose, especially the glycogen in human muscle, is converted to lactic acid.

em·be·lin (ĕm′bə-lĭn) *n.* The active principle from the berries of certain species of Asiatic shrubs, formerly used as an anthelmintic.

em·bo·le (ĕm′bə-lē) *n.* Emboly.

em·bo·lec·to·my (ĕm′bə-lĕk′tə-mē) *n.* Surgical removal of an embolus.

em·bol·ic (ĕm-bŏl′ĭk) *adj.* **1.** Relating to, or caused by an embolus or embolism. **2.** Relating to emboly.

em·bo·lism (ĕm′bə-lĭz′əm) *n.* **1.** The obstruction or occlusion of a blood vessel by an embolus. **2.** An embolus.

em·bo·li·za·tion (ĕm′bə-lĭ-zā′shən) *n.* **1.** The process by which a blood vessel or organ is obstructed by an embolus or other mass. **2.** The surgical introduction of various substances into the circulatory system to obstruct specific blood vessels.

em·bo·lo·la·li·a (ĕm′bə-lō-lā′lē-ə) *n.* A speech disorder in which meaningless words or sounds are interjected into sentences. Also called *embolophrasia.*

em·bo·lus (ĕm′bə-ləs) *n., pl.* **–li** (-lī′) A mass, such as an air bubble, detached blood clot, or foreign body, that travels in the bloodstream and lodges in a blood vessel, thus serving to obstruct or occlude such a vessel.

em·bo·ly (ĕm′bə-lē) *n.* The formation of a gastrula from a blastula by invagination.

em·bra·sure (ĕm-brā′zhər) *n.* The sloped valley between two teeth.

em·bro·ca·tion (ĕm′brə-kā′shən) *n.* **1.** The act or process of moistening and rubbing a body part with a liniment or lotion. **2.** A liniment or lotion.

em·bry·ec·to·my (ĕm′brē-ĕk′tə-mē) *n.* Surgical removal of an embryo, especially one implanted outside of the uterus.

em·bry·o (ĕm′brē-ō′) *n., pl.* **–os 1.** An organism in its early stages of development, especially before it has reached a distinctively recognizable form. **2.** An organism at any time before full development, birth, or hatching. **3.** The fertilized egg of a vertebrate animal following cleavage. **4.** In humans, the prefetal product of conception from implantation through the eighth week of development.

embryo– *or* **embry–** *pref.* Embryo: *embryogenesis.*

em·bry·o·blast (ĕm′brē-ə-blăst′) *n.* Any of the germinal disk cells of the inner cell mass in the blastocyst that form the embryo.

em·bry·o·car·di·a (ĕm′brē-ō-kär′dē-ə) *n.* A symptom of heart disease in which the sounds of the heart

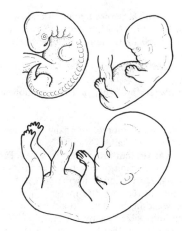

embryo

Clockwise from top left: *human embryo at five, seven, and eight weeks of development*

resemble those of the fetal heart, usually occurring in serious myocardial disease.

em·bry·oc·to·ny (ĕm′brē-ŏk′tə-nē) *n.* See feticide.

em·bry·o·gen·e·sis (ĕm′brē-ō-jĕn′ĭ-sĭs) *or* **em·bry·og·e·ny** (-ŏj′ə-nē) *n.* The development and growth of an embryo, especially the period from the second week through the eighth week following conception. **—em′-bry·o·gen′ic** (-jĕn′ĭk) *adj.*

em·bry·ol·o·gist (ĕm′brē-ŏl′ə-jĭst) *n.* A specialist in embryology.

em·bry·ol·o·gy (ĕm′brē-ŏl′ə-jē) *n.* **1.** The branch of biology that deals with the formation, early growth, and development of living organisms. **2.** The embryonic structure or development of an organism.

em·bry·o·ma (ĕm′brē-ō′mə) *n.* See embryonal tumor.

embryoma of kidney *n.* See Wilms' tumor.

em·bry·on·al carcinoma (ĕm′brē-ə-nəl) *n.* A malignant neoplasm of the testis.

embryonal carcinosarcoma *n.* See blastoma.

embryonal leukemia *n.* See stem cell leukemia.

embryonal rhabdomyosarcoma *n.* A form of rhabdomyosarcoma occurring in infants and children and characterized by the occurrence of malignant tumors of loose, spindle-celled tissue throughout the body.

embryonal tumor *or* **embryonic tumor** *n.* A usually malignant tumor arising during intrauterine or early postnatal development from the rudiments of an organ or from immature tissue and forming immature structures characteristic of the part from which it arises. Also called *embryoma.*

em·bry·on·ic (ĕm′brē-ŏn′ĭk) *or* **em·bry·on·al** (ĕm′brē-ə-nəl) *adj.* Of, relating to, or being an embryo.

embryonic area *n.* The area of the blastoderm on either side of, and immediately cephalic to, the primitive streak where the component cell layers have become thickened.

embryonic disk *n.* **1.** A platelike mass of cells in the blastocyst from which a mammalian embryo develops. Also called *embryonic shield.* **2.** See germinal disk.

embryonic membrane *n.* See fetal membrane.

embryonic shield *n.* See **embryonic disk** (sense 1).

em·bry·on·i·za·tion (ĕm'brē-ŏn'ĭ-zā'shən) *n.* The change of a cell or tissue to an embryonic structure or form.

em·bry·o·noid (ĕm'brē-ə-noid') *adj.* Resembling an embryo.

em·bry·o·ny (ĕm'brē-ə-nē) *n.* The condition of being an embryo.

em·bry·op·a·thy (ĕm'brē-ŏp'ə-thē) *n.* A developmental disorder in an embryo, especially one caused by a disease such as rubella.

em·bry·o·plas·tic (ĕm'brē-ō-plăs'tĭk) *adj.* **1.** Participating in the production of or producing an embryo. **2.** Relating to the formation of an embryo.

em·bry·ot·o·my (ĕm'brē-ŏt'ə-mē) *n.* The cutting of the fetus while in the uterus to aid its removal when delivery is impossible by natural means.

em·bry·o·tox·ic·i·ty (ĕm'brē-ō-tŏk-sĭs'ĭ-tē) *n.* The state of being toxic to an embryo, resulting in abnormal development or death.

em·bry·o·tox·on (ĕm'brē-ō-tŏk'sŏn', -ən) *n.* A congenital opacity of the margin of the cornea.

embryo transfer *n.* After artificial insemination, the process by which the fertilized ovum is transferred at the blastocyst stage to the recipient's uterus.

em·bry·o·troph (ĕm'brē-ə-trŏf', trŏf') *n.* The nutritive material that is supplied to the embryo of a placental mammal during development. —**em·bry·o·troph·ic** (-trŏf'ĭk, -trō'fĭk) *adj.*

em·bry·ot·ro·phy (ĕm'brē-ŏt'rə-fē) *n.* The nutrition of the embryo.

e·med·ul·late (ĭ-mĕd'l-āt', ĭ-mĕd'yə-lāt') *v.* To extract marrow or pith.

e·mei·o·cy·to·sis (ē'mē-ō-sī-tō'sĭs) *n.* Variant of **emiocytosis.**

e·mer·gen·cy medical technician (ĭ-mûr'jən-sē) *n. Abbr.* **EMT** A person trained and certified to appraise and initiate the administration of emergency care for victims of trauma or acute illness before or during transportation of victims to a health care facility.

emergency medicine *n.* The branch of medicine that deals with the evaluation and initial treatment of medical conditions that are caused by trauma or sudden illness.

emergency room *n. Abbr.* **ER** The section of a health care facility intended to provide rapid treatment for victims of sudden illness or trauma.

emergency theory *n.* See **fight-or-flight reaction.**

em·e·sis (ĕm'ĭ-sĭs) *n., pl.* **–ses** (-sēz') The act or process of vomiting.

e·met·ic (ĭ-mĕt'ĭk) *n.* An agent that causes vomiting. —*adj.* Causing vomiting.

em·e·to·ca·thar·tic (ĕm'ĭ-tō-kə-thär'tĭk) *adj.* Causing vomiting and purging.

EMF *abbr.* electromotive force

EMG *abbr.* electromyogram

EMG syndrome *n.* A hereditary disorder that is characterized by exomphalos, macroglossia, and gigantism, often with neonatal hypoglycemia. Also called *Beckwith-Wiedemann syndrome.*

–emia *or* **–hemia** *or* **–aemia** *or* **–haemia** *suff.* Blood: *leukemia.*

e·mic·tion (ĭ-mĭk'shən) *n.* See **urination.**

em·i·gra·tion (ĕm'ĭ-grā'shən) *n.* The passage of white blood cells through the walls of small blood vessels.

em·i·nence (ĕm'ə-nəns) *n.* The projecting prominent part of an organ, especially a bone.

e·mi·o·cy·to·sis *or* **e·mei·o·cy·to·sis** (ē'mē-ō-sī-tō'sĭs) *n.* See **exocytosis** (sense 2).

em·is·sar·y (ĕm'ĭ-sĕr'ē) *n.* Any of various venous channels through the skull that connect the venous sinuses of the dura mater with the veins external to the skull.

emissary vein *n.* Any of the channels of communication between the venous sinuses of the dura mater and the veins of the diploe and the scalp.

e·mis·sion (ĭ-mĭsh'ən) *n.* A discharge of fluid from a living body, usually a seminal discharge.

EMLA (ĕm'lə) A trademark for a drug combination of lidocaine and prilocaine.

em·men·a·gogue (ĭ-mĕn'ə-gôg') *n.* An agent that induces or hastens menstrual flow. Also called *hemagogue.* —**em·men·a·gog·ic** (-gŏj'ĭk) *adj.*

em·men·i·a (ĭ-mĕn'ē-ə, ĭ-mē'nē-ə) *n.* See **menses.** —**em·men·ic** (ĭ-mĕn'ĭk) *adj.*

em·men·i·op·a·thy (ĭ-mĕn'ē-ŏp'ə-thē) *n.* A menstrual disorder.

em·me·tro·pi·a (ĕm'ĭ-trō'pē-ə) *n.* The condition of the normal eye when parallel rays are focused exactly on the retina and vision is perfect. —**em·me·trop·ic** (-trŏp'ĭk, -trō'pĭk) *adj.*

em·o·din (ĕm'ə-dĭn') *n.* A crystalline compound obtained from rhubarb and used as a laxative.

e·mol·lient (ĭ-mŏl'yənt) *adj.* Softening and soothing, especially to the skin. —*n.* An agent that softens or soothes the skin.

e·mo·tion (ĭ-mō'shən) *n.* An intense mental state that arises subjectively rather than through conscious effort and is often accompanied by physiological changes. —**e·mo'tion·al** *adj.*

emotional deprivation *n.* The lack of adequate and appropriate interpersonal and environmental interaction, usually in the early developmental years.

emotional disorder *n.* An emotional illness.

emotional illness *n.* A psychological disorder characterized by irrational and uncontrollable fears, persistent anxiety, or extreme hostility.

emotional intelligence *n.* Intelligence regarding the emotions, especially in the ability to monitor one's own or others' emotions.

e.m.p. *abbr. Latin* ex modo praescripto (in the manner prescribed)

em·pa·thize (ĕm'pə-thīz') *v.* To feel empathy in relation to another person.

em·pa·thy (ĕm'pə-thē) *n.* **1.** Direct identification with, understanding of, and vicarious experience of another person's situation, feelings, and motives. **2.** The projection of one's own feelings or emotional state onto an object or animal. —**em'pa·thet·ic** (-thĕt'ĭk), **em·path'ic** (-păth'ĭk) *adj.*

Em·ped·o·cles (ĕm-pĕd'ə-klēz') Fifth century BC. Greek philosopher who believed all matter is composed of the elemental particles of fire, water, earth, and air and all change is caused by attraction and repulsion.

em·per·i·po·le·sis (ĕm-pĕr'ə-pə-lē'sĭs) *n.* Active penetration by one cell into and through a larger cell.

em·phy·se·ma (ĕm′fĭ-sē′mə, -zē′-) *n.* **1.** A pathological condition of the lungs marked by an abnormal increase in the size of the air spaces, resulting in labored breathing and an increased susceptibility to infection. It can be caused by irreversible expansion of the alveoli or by the destruction of alveolar walls. Also called *pulmonary emphysema.* **2.** An abnormal distention of body tissues caused by retention of air. —**em′phy·sem′a·tous** (-sĕm′ə-təs, -sē′mə-, -zĕm′ə-, -zē′mə-) *adj.* —**em′phy·se′mic** *adj. & n.*

em·pir·ic (ĕm-pîr′ĭk) *n.* **1.** One who is guided by practical experience rather than by precepts or theory. **2.** An unqualified or dishonest practitioner; a charlatan. —*adj.* **1.** Empirical. **2.** Relating to a school of ancient Greek medicine in which a physician relied on experience and precedent in the observation and treatment of disease, and on analogical reasoning in discovering new diseases.

em·pir·i·cal (ĕm-pîr′ĭ-kəl) *adj.* **1.** Relying on or derived from observation or experiment. **2.** Verifiable or provable by means of observation or experiment. **3.** Of or being a philosophy of medicine emphasizing practical experience and observation over scientific theory. —**em·pir′i·cal·ly** *adv.*

empirical formula *n.* A chemical formula that indicates the relative proportions of the elements in a molecule rather than the actual number of atoms of the elements.

em·pir·i·cism (ĕm-pîr′ĭ-sĭz′əm) *n.* **1.** Employment of empirical methods, as in science. **2.** The practice of medicine that disregards scientific theory and relies solely on practical experience. —**em·pir′i·cist** *n.*

empiric risk *n.* Risk that is based only on empirical evidence, not on formal theory or conjecture.

em·pros·thot·o·nos (ĕm′prŏs-thŏt′n-əs) *n.* A tetanic spasm in which the head and feet are drawn forward and the spine arches backward.

em·py·e·ma (ĕm′pī-ē′mə) *n., pl.* **–ma·ta** (-mə-tə) The presence of pus in a body cavity, especially the pleural cavity. —**em′py·e′mic** *adj.*

em·py·e·sis (ĕm′pī-ē′sĭs) *n., pl.* **–ses** (-sēz) A pustular eruption.

EMS *abbr.* electrical muscle stimulation; Emergency Medical Service

EMT *abbr.* emergency medical technician

em·tri·cit·a·bine (ĕm′trĭ-sĭt′ə-bēn′, -sī′tə-) *n.* A nucleoside analog used to treat HIV infection in combination with other antiretroviral drugs.

Em·tri·va (ĕm-trē′və) A trademark for the drug emtricitabine.

e·mul·gent (ĭ-mŭl′jənt) *adj.* Of or being a straining, extracting, or purifying process.

e·mul·si·fi·er (ĭ-mŭl′sə-fī′ər) *n.* An agent used to make an emulsion of a fixed oil.

e·mul·si·fy (ĭ-mŭl′sə-fī′) *v.* To make into an emulsion. —**e·mul′si·fi·ca′tion** (-fĭ-kā′shən) *n.*

e·mul·sion (ĭ-mŭl′shən) *n.* A suspension of small globules of one liquid in a second liquid with which the first will not mix. —**e·mul′sive** *adj.*

e·mul·soid (ĭ-mŭl′soid′) *n.* A colloidal dispersion in which the dispersed particles are more or less liquid, exerting an attraction on and absorbing a certain quantity of the fluid in which they are suspended.

e·munc·to·ry (ĭ-mŭngk′tə-rē) *adj.* Serving to carry waste out of the body; excretory. —*n.* An organ or duct that removes or carries waste from the body.

E-my·cin (ē′mī′sĭn) A trademark for the drug erythromycin.

en– or **em–** *pref.* In; into; within: *enzootic.*

e·nal·a·pril maleate (ĭ-năl′ə-prĭl) *n.* An angiotensin-converting enzyme inhibitor used as an antihypertensive agent.

e·nam·el (ĭ-năm′əl) *n.* The hard, calcareous substance covering the exposed portion of a tooth.

enamel cap *n.* The enamel covering the crown of a tooth.

enamel crypt *n.* The narrow space filled with mesenchyme and located between the dental lamina and an enamel organ.

enamel dysplasia *n.* See **amelogenesis imperfecta.**

enamel germ *n.* The enamel organ of a developing tooth.

enamel layer *n.* See **ameloblastic layer.**

enamel membrane *n.* The internal layer of the enamel organ formed by the enamel cells.

e·nam·e·lo·gen·e·sis (ĭ-năm′ə-lō-jĕn′ĭ-sĭs) *n.* See **amelogenesis.**

e·nam·e·lo·ma (ĭ-năm′ə-lō′mə) *n., pl.* **–mas** *or* **–ma·ta** (-mə-tə) A developmental anomaly in which a small nodule of enamel is below the cementoenamel junction, usually at the bifurcation of molar teeth.

enamel organ *n.* A mass of ectodermal cells budded from the dental lamina. It develops the ameloblast layer of cells which produce the enamel cap of a developing tooth.

enamel rod *n.* Any of several calcified, microscopic rods radiating from the surface of the dentin and forming the substance of tooth enamel.

en·an·them (ĭ-năn′thəm) *or* **en·an·the·ma** (ĕn′ăn-thē′mə) *n.* A mucous membrane eruption, especially one occurring in connection with one of the exanthemas. —**en′an·them′a·tous** (-thĕm′ə-təs, -thē′mə-təs) *adj.*

en·an·the·sis (ĕn′ăn-thē′sĭs) *n.* The skin eruption associated with a general disease, such as scarlatina.

en·an·ti·o·morph (ĭ-năn′tē-ə-môrf′) *n.* Either of a pair of crystals, molecules, or compounds that are mirror images of each other but are not identical. Also called *enantiomer.*

en·ar·thro·di·al (ĕn′är-thrō′dē-əl) *adj.* Of or relating to a ball-and-socket joint.

en·ar·thro·sis (ĕn′är-thrō′sĭs) *n.* See **ball-and-socket joint.**

En·brel (ĕn′brĕl′) A trademark for the drug etanercept.

en·cap·su·late (ĕn-kăp′sə-lāt′) *v.* **1.** To form a capsule or sheath around. **2.** To become encapsulated. —**en·cap′su·la′tion** *n.*

en·ceph·a·lal·gia (ĕn-sĕf′ə-lăl′jə) *n.* Pain in the head; headache.

en·ceph·a·lat·ro·phy (ĕn-sĕf′ə-lăt′rə-fē) *n.* Atrophy of the brain. —**en·ceph′a·la·troph′ic** (-lə-trŏf′ĭk) *adj.*

en·ce·phal·ic (ĕn′sə-făl′ĭk) *adj.* **1.** Of or relating to the brain. **2.** Located within the cranial cavity.

encephalic vesicle *n.* See **cerebral vesicle.**

en·ceph·a·li·tis (ĕn-sĕf′ə-lī′tĭs) *n., pl.* **–lit·i·des** (-lĭt′ĭ-dēz) Inflammation of the brain. Also called *cephalitis.* —**en·ceph′a·lit′ic** (-lĭt′ĭk) *adj.*

en·ceph·a·li·tis le·thar·gi·ca (lə-thär′jĭ-kə) *n.* A viral epidemic encephalitis characterized by apathy, paralysis of an eye muscle, and extreme muscular weakness. Also called *sleeping sickness, von Economo's disease.*

encephalitis per·i·ax·i·a·lis dif·fu·sa (pĕr′ē-ăk′sē-ā′lĭs dĭ-fyōō′sə) *n.* See **Schilder's disease.**

encephalo– *or* **encephal–** *pref.* Brain: *encephalitis.*

en·ceph·a·lo·cele (ĕn-sĕf′ə-lō-sēl′) *n.* A congenital gap in the skull that usually results in a protrusion of brain material. Also called *bifid cranium, cephalocele, craniocele.*

en·ceph·a·lo·cra·ni·o·cu·ta·ne·ous lipomatosis (ĕn-sĕf′ə-lō-krā′nē-ō-kyōō-tā′nē-əs) *n.* A rare syndrome of multiple fibrolipomas or angiofibroma of the face, scalp, and neck present at birth, sometimes with symptomatic intracranial lipomas.

en·ceph·a·lo·fa·cial angiomatosis (ĕn-sĕf′ə-lō-fā′shəl) *n.* See **Sturge-Weber syndrome.**

en·ceph·a·lo·gram (ĕn-sĕf′ə-lə-grăm′, -ə-lō-) *n.* **1.** An x-ray picture of the brain taken by encephalography. **2.** An electroencephalogram.

en·ceph·a·lo·graph (ĕn-sĕf′ə-lə-grăf′, -ə-lō-) *n.* **1.** An encephalogram. **2.** An electroencephalogram.

en·ceph·a·log·ra·phy (ĕn-sĕf′ə-lŏg′rə-fē) *n.* Radiographic examination of the brain in which some of the cerebrospinal fluid is replaced with air or another gas that acts as a contrasting medium. **—en·ceph′a·lo·graph′ic** (-ə-lə-grăf′ĭk, -ə-lō-) *adj.*

en·ceph·a·loid (ĕn-sĕf′ə-loid′) *adj.* **1.** Resembling the brain or its tissue. **2.** Of a relatively soft and nonfibrous consistency. Used of a carcinoma.

en·ceph·a·lo·lith (ĕn-sĕf′ə-lō-lĭth′) *n.* A concretion in the brain or in one of its ventricles. Also called *cerebral calculus.*

en·ceph·a·lo·ma (ĕn-sĕf′ə-lō′mə) *n.,* *pl.* **–mas** *or* **–ma·ta** (-mə-tə) A tumor or swelling of the brain. Also called *cerebroma.*

en·ceph·a·lo·ma·la·cia (ĕn-sĕf′ə-lō-mə-lā′shə) *n.* Softening of brain tissue, usually caused by vascular insufficiency or degenerative changes. Also called *cerebromalacia.*

en·ceph·a·lo·men·in·gi·tis (ĕn-sĕf′ə-lō-mĕn′ĭn-jī′tĭs) *n.* See **meningoencephalitis.**

en·ceph·a·lo·me·nin·go·cele (ĕn-sĕf′ə-lō-mə-nĭng′gə-sēl′) *n.* See **meningoencephalocele.**

en·ceph·a·lo·men·in·gop·a·thy (ĕn-sĕf′ə-lō-mĕn′ĭng-gŏp′ə-thē) *n.* See **meningoencephalopathy.**

en·ceph·a·lo·mere (ĕn-sĕf′ə-lō-mîr′) *n.* See **neuromere.**

en·ceph·a·lom·e·ter (ĕn-sĕf′ə-lŏm′ĭ-tər) *n.* An apparatus for indicating the location of the cortical centers on the skull.

en·ceph·a·lo·my·e·li·tis (ĕn-sĕf′ə-lō-mī′ə-lī′tĭs) *n.* An acute inflammation of the brain and spinal cord.

en·ceph·a·lo·my·e·lo·cele (ĕn-sĕf′ə-lō-mī′ə-lə-sēl′) *n.* A congenital defect in the occipital region with herniation of the meninges, the medulla, and the spinal cord.

en·ceph·a·lo·my·e·lo·neu·rop·a·thy (ĕn-sĕf′ə-lō-mī′ə-lō-nōō-rŏp′ə-thē) *n.* Any of various diseases involving the brain, the spinal cord, and the peripheral nervous system.

en·ceph·a·lo·my·e·lop·a·thy (ĕn-sĕf′ə-lō-mī′ə-lŏp′ə-thē) *n.* Any of various diseases involving both the brain and spinal cord.

en·ceph·a·lo·my·e·lo·ra·dic·u·li·tis (ĕn-sĕf′ə-lō-mī′-ə-lō-rə-dĭk′yə-lī′tĭs) *n.* Inflammation involving the brain, spinal cord, and spinal roots.

en·ceph·a·lo·my·e·lo·ra·dic·u·lop·a·thy (ĕn-sĕf′ə-lō-mī′ə-lō-rə-dĭk′yə-lŏp′ə-thē) *n.* Any of various diseases of the brain, spinal cord, and spinal roots.

en·ceph·a·lo·my·o·car·di·tis (ĕn-sĕf′ə-lō-mī′ō-kär-dī′tĭs) *n.* An acute viral disease characterized by inflammation and degeneration of skeletal and cardiac muscle and lesions of the central nervous system.

encephalomyocarditis virus *n.* A picornavirus that causes a febrile illness with central nervous system involvement in humans.

en·ceph·a·lon (ĕn-sĕf′ə-lŏn′) *n.,* *pl.* **–la** (-lə) See **brain.** **—en·ceph′a·lous** *adj.*

en·ceph·a·lop·a·thy (ĕn-sĕf′ə-lŏp′ə-thē) *n.* Degeneration of brain function, caused by any of various acquired disorders, including metabolic disease, organ failure, inflammation, and chronic infection. Also called *cephalopathy, cerebropathy.* **—en·ceph′a·lo·path′ic** (-lə-păth′ĭk) *adj.*

en·ceph·a·lo·py·o·sis (ĕn-sĕf′ə-lō-pī-ō′sĭs) *n.* Purulent inflammation of the brain.

en·ceph·a·lor·rha·gia (ĕn-sĕf′ə-lō-rā′jə) *n.* See **cerebral hemorrhage.**

en·ceph·a·los·chi·sis (ĕn-sĕf′ə-lŏs′kĭ-sĭs) *n.* Developmental failure of the rostral part of the neural tube to close.

en·ceph·a·lo·scle·ro·sis (ĕn-sĕf′ə-lō-sklə-rō′sĭs) *n.* A hardening of the brain.

en·ceph·a·lo·sis (ĕn-sĕf′ə-lō′sĭs) *n.* Any of various organic diseases of the brain. Also called *cerebrosis.*

en·ceph·a·lot·o·my (ĕn-sĕf′ə-lŏt′ə-mē) *n.* Dissection or incision of the brain.

en·ceph·a·lo·tri·gem·i·nal angiomatosis (ĕn-sĕf′ə-lō-trī-jĕm′ə-nəl) *n.* See **Sturge-Weber syndrome.**

en·chon·dral (ĕn-kŏn′drəl) *adj.* Intracartilaginous.

en·chon·dro·ma (ĕn′kŏn-drō′mə) *n.* A benign cartilaginous growth starting within the medullary cavity of a bone that formed from cartilage. **—en′chon·dro′ma·tous** (-drō′mə-təs, -drŏm′ə-) *adj.*

en·chon·dro·ma·to·sis (ĕn-kŏn′drō-mə-tō′sĭs, ĕn′-kŏn-drō′-) *n.* A congenital but nonfamilial disorder involving tubular bones, especially of the hands and feet, and characterized by a neoplasmlike proliferation of cartilage in the metaphyses that cause distorted growth in length or pathological fractures. Also called *dyschondroplasia, Ollier's disease.*

en·chon·dro·sar·co·ma (ĕn-kŏn′drō-sär-kō′mə) *n.* A malignant neoplasm of cartilage cells derived from an enchondroma or occurring in the same locations.

en·clave (ĕn′klāv′, ŏn′-) *n.* A detached mass of tissue enclosed in tissue of another kind.

en·cod·ing (ĕn-kō′dĭng) *n.* The first of three stages in the memory process, involving processes associated with receiving or registering stimuli through one or more of the senses and modifying that information.

en·cop·re·sis (ĕn′kŏ-prē′sĭs) *n.* The repeated uncontrolled or involuntary passage of feces.

en·coun·ter group (ĕn-koun′tər) *n.* A psychotherapy group in which the participants try to increase their sensitivity and gain insight into their emotions by expressing their own emotions and responding to the emotions of others in the group.

en·cyst (ĕn-sĭst′) *v.* To enclose or become enclosed in a cyst. —**en·cyst′ment, en′cys·ta′tion** *n.*

en·cyst·ed calculus (ĕn-sĭs′tĭd) *n.* A urinary calculus enclosed in a sac developed from the wall of the bladder. Also called *pocketed calculus.*

end– *pref.* Variant of **endo–.**

en·da·me·ba *or* **en·da·moe·ba** (ĕn′də-mē′bə) *n.* Variant of **entameba.**

end·an·gi·i·tis *or* **end·an·ge·i·tis** (ĕn′dăn-jē-ī′tĭs) *or* **en·do·an·gi·i·tis** (ĕn′dō-ăn′jē-) *n.* An inflammation of the tunica intima of a blood vessel. Also called *endovasculitis.*

end·a·or·ti·tis (ĕn′dā-ôr-tī′tĭs) *n.* Inflammation of the intima of the aorta.

end·ar·ter·ec·to·my (ĕn′där-tə-rĕk′tə-mē) *n.* Excision of the inner lining of an artery that is clogged with atherosclerotic buildup.

end·ar·te·ri·tis (ĕn′där-tə-rī′tĭs) *or* **en·do·ar·te·ri·tis** (ĕn′dō-är′tə-) *n.* Inflammation of the intima of an artery.

end artery (ĕnd) *n.* An artery with insufficient anastomoses to maintain viability of the tissue supplied if arterial occlusion occurs. Also called *terminal artery.*

end·au·ral (ĕn-dôr′əl) *adj.* Within the ear.

end·brain (ĕnd′brān′) *n.* See **telencephalon.**

end bud *n.* See **tail bud.**

end bulb *n.* One of the oval or rounded bodies in which a sensory nerve fiber terminates.

end-diastolic volume *n.* The amount of blood present in the ventricle immediately before a cardiac contraction begins; used as a measurement of diastolic function.

en·dem·ic (ĕn-dĕm′ĭk) *adj.* **1.** Prevalent in or restricted to a particular region, community, or group of people. Used of a disease. **2.** Enzootic. —**en·dem′i·cal·ly** *adv.* —**en·dem′ism** *n.*

endemic hematuria *n.* See **schistosomiasis haematobium.**

endemic neuritis *n.* See **beriberi.**

endemic stability *n.* A situation in which all factors influencing disease occurrence are relatively stable, resulting in little fluctuation in disease incidence over time. Also called *enzootic stability.*

endemic typhus *n.* See **murine typhus.**

en·dem·o·ep·i·dem·ic (ĕn-dĕm′ō-ĕp′ĭ-dĕm′ĭk) *adj.* Of or being a temporary large increase in the number of cases of an endemic disease.

end·er·gon·ic (ĕn′dər-gŏn′ĭk) *adj.* Of or relating to a chemical reaction that absorbs energy and therefore cools its surroundings.

en·der·mic (ĕn-dûr′mĭk) *adj.* Acting medicinally by absorption through the skin.

En·ders (ĕn′dərz), **John Franklin** 1897–1985. American bacteriologist. He shared a 1954 Nobel Prize for developing a method of growing the poliomyelitis virus in various tissue cultures.

end-feet (ĕnd′fēt′) *pl.n.* See **axon terminals.**

endo– *or* **end–** *pref.* Inside; within: *endometrium.*

en·do·an·eu·rys·mo·plas·ty (ĕn′dō-ăn′yə-rĭz′mə-plăs′tē) *n.* See **aneurysmoplasty** (sense 1).

en·do·an·eu·rys·mor·rha·phy (ĕn′dō-ăn′yə-rĭz-môr′ə-fē) *n.* See **aneurysmoplasty** (sense 1).

en·do·an·gi·i·tis (ĕn′dō-ăn′jē-ī′tĭs) *n.* Variant of **end-angiitis.**

en·do·ap·pen·di·ci·tis (ĕn′dō-ə-pĕn′dĭ-sī′tĭs) *n.* Simple catarrhal inflammation limited to the mucosal surface of the vermiform appendix.

en·do·ar·te·ri·tis (ĕn′dō-är′tə-rī′tĭs) *n.* Variant of **end-arteritis.**

en·do·bi·ot·ic (ĕn′də-bī-ŏt′ĭk) *adj.* Living as a parasite or symbiont within the tissues of a host.

en·do·blast (ĕn′də-blăst′) *n.* Variant of **entoblast.**

en·do·bron·chi·al tube (ĕn′dō-brŏng′kē-əl) *n.* See **Carlen's catheter.**

endocardial cushion *n.* See **atrioventricular canal cushion.**

endocardial fibroelastosis *n.* A congenital condition characterized by thickening of the inner lining of the left ventricle, thickening and malformation of the cardiac valves, and hypertrophy of the heart.

en·do·car·di·tis (ĕn′dō-kär-dī′tĭs) *n.* Inflammation of the endocardium. —**en′do·car·dit′ic** (-dĭt′ĭk) *adj.*

en·do·car·di·um (ĕn′dō-kär′dē-əm) *n., pl.* **–di·a** (-dē-ə) The thin serous membrane, composed of endothelial and subendothelial tissue, that lines the interior of the heart. —**en′do·car′di·al** *adj.*

en·do·cer·vi·cal (ĕn′dō-sûr′vĭ-kəl) *adj.* **1.** Within a cervix, specifically within the uterine cervix. **2.** Of or relating to the endocervix.

en·do·cer·vi·ci·tis (ĕn′dō-sûr′vĭ-sī′tĭs) *n.* Inflammation of the mucous membrane of the uterine cervix. Also called *endotrachelitis.*

en·do·cer·vix (ĕn′dō-sûr′vĭks) *n.* The mucous membrane of the uterine cervical canal.

en·do·chon·dral bone (ĕn′dō-kŏn′drəl) *n.* See **cartilage bone.**

endochondral ossification *n.* The formation of bone in which a cartilage template is gradually replaced by a bone matrix, as in the formation of long bones or in osteoarthritic ossification of synovial cartilage.

en·do·co·li·tis (ĕn′dō-kə-lī′tĭs) *n.* Simple inflammation of the colon.

en·do·cra·ni·al (ĕn′dō-krā′nē-əl) *adj.* **1.** Within the cranium. **2.** Of or relating to the endocranium.

en·do·cra·ni·um (ĕn′dō-krā′nē-əm) *n., pl.* **–ni·a** (-nē-ə) **1.** The outermost layer of the dura mater. **2.** The inner surface of the skull.

en·do·crine (ĕn′də-krĭn, -krēn′, -krīn′) *adj.* **1.** Secreting internally, most commonly into the systemic circulation. **2.** Of or relating to endocrine glands or the hormones secreted by them. —*n.* **1.** The secretion of an endocrine gland. **2.** An endocrine gland.

endocrine gland *n.* Any of various ductless glands, such as the thyroid, adrenal, or pituitary, having hormonal secretions that pass directly into the bloodstream. Also called *ductless gland.*

endocrine system *n.* The bodily system that consists of the endocrine glands and the hormones they secrete. See illustration on page 262.

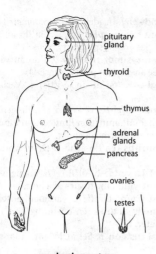

pituitary gland

thyroid

thymus

adrenal glands

pancreas

ovaries

testes

endocrine system

en·do·cri·nol·o·gy (ĕn′də-krə-nŏl′ə-jē) *n.* The study of the glands and hormones of the body and their related disorders. —**en′do·cri′no·log′ic** (-krĭn′ə-lŏj′ĭk), **en′·do·crin′o·log′i·cal** *adj.*

en·do·cri·no·ma (ĕn′də-krə-nō′mə) *n.* A tumor with endocrine tissue that retains the function of the parent organ, usually to an excessive degree.

en·do·cri·nop·a·thy (ĕn′də-krə-nŏp′ə-thē) *n.* A disorder in the function of an endocrine gland and the consequences thereof.

en·do·cys·ti·tis (ĕn′dō-sĭ-stī′tĭs) *n.* Inflammation of the mucous membrane of the bladder.

en·do·cy·to·sis (ĕn′dō-sī-tō′sĭs) *n.* A process of cellular ingestion by which the plasma membrane folds inward to bring substances into the cell. —**en′do·cyt′ic** (-sĭt′ĭk), **en′do·cy·tot′ic** (-sī-tŏt′ĭk) *adj.* —**en′do·cy·tose′** (-tōs′) *v.*

en·do·derm (ĕn′də-dûrm′) *or* **en·to·derm** (ĕn′tə-) *n.* The innermost of the three primary germ layers of an embryo, developing into the gastrointestinal tract, the lungs, and associated structures. Also called *hypoblast.* —**en′do·der′mal** *adj.*

endodermal sinus tumor *n.* A malignant neoplasm occurring in the gonads, in sacrococcygeal teratomas, and in the mediastinum and producing alpha-fetoprotein. Also called *yolk-sac tumor.*

en·do·don·tia (ĕn′dō-dŏn′shə) *n.* Endodontics.

en·do·don·tics (ĕn′dō-dŏn′tĭks) *n.* The branch of dentistry that deals with diseases of the tooth root, dental pulp, and surrounding tissue. —**en′do·don′tic** *adj.* —**en′do·don′tist** *n.*

en·do·en·ter·i·tis (ĕn′dō-ĕn′tə-rī′tĭs) *n.* Inflammation of the intestinal mucous membrane.

en·do·en·zyme (ĕn′dō-ĕn′zīm′) *n.* An enzyme that acts on or is retained within the cell producing it.

en·dog·a·my (ĕn-dŏg′ə-mē) *n.* **1.** Reproduction by the fusion of gametes of similar ancestry. **2.** Marriage within a particular group in accordance with custom or law. —**en·dog′a·mous** *adj.*

en·do·gen·ic toxicosis (ĕn′də-jĕn′ĭk) *n.* See **autointoxication.**

en·dog·e·nous (ĕn-dŏj′ə-nəs) *adj.* **1.** Originating or produced within an organism, tissue, or cell. **2.** Caused by factors within the body. Used of a disease. —**en·dog′e·nous·ly** *adv.* —**en·dog′e·ny** *n.*

endogenous depression *n.* A group of symptoms that resemble depression but are not precipitated by a stressful experience, especially psychomotor agitation or retardation, insomnia and early morning awakening, weight loss, excessive guilt, and lack of reactivity to one's environment.

endogenous hyperglyceridemia *n.* See **type IV familial hyperlipoproteinemia.**

endogenous infection *n.* An infection caused by an infectious agent that is already present in the body, but has previously been inapparent or dormant.

en·do·in·tox·i·ca·tion (ĕn′dō-ĭn-tŏk′sĭ-kā′shən) *n.* Poisoning by an endogenous toxin.

en·do·lymph (ĕn′də-lĭmf′) *n.* The fluid contained in the membranous labyrinth of the inner ear. Also called *Scarpa's fluid.* —**en′do·lym·phat′ic** (-lĭm-făt′ĭk) *adj.*

endolymphatic duct *n.* A small membranous canal connecting with the saccule and utricle of the membranous labyrinth and terminating in the endolymphatic sac.

endolymphatic hydrops *n.* See **Ménière's disease.**

endolymphatic sac *n.* The dilated blind extremity of the endolymphatic duct.

endometrial stromal sarcoma *n.* A rare sarcoma in which the lesions form multiple foci in the myometrium and in vascular spaces in other sites and the tissue and cells resemble endometrial stroma cells.

en·do·me·tri·oid (ĕn′dō-mē′trē-oid′) *adj.* Microscopically resembling endometrial tissue.

endometrioid carcinoma *n.* Adenocarcinoma of the ovary.

endometrioid tumor *n.* A tumor of the ovary containing epithelial or stromal elements resembling endometrial tissue.

en·do·me·tri·o·ma (ĕn′dō-mē′trē-ō′mə) *n.* A circumscribed mass of endometrial tissue occurring outside the uterus in endometriosis.

en·do·me·tri·o·sis (ĕn′dō-mē′trē-ō′sĭs) *n.* A condition, usually resulting in pain and dysmenorrhea, characterized by the abnormal presence of functional endometrial tissue outside the uterus, frequently as cysts containing altered blood.

en·do·me·tri·tis (ĕn′dō-mĭ-trī′tĭs) *n.* Inflammation of the endometrium.

en·do·me·tri·um (ĕn′dō-mē′trē-əm) *n., pl.* **–tri·a** (-trē-ə) The glandular mucous membrane comprising the inner layer of the uterine wall. —**en′do·me′tri·al** *adj.*

en·do·mi·to·sis (ĕn′dō-mī-tō′sĭs) *n.* See **endopolyploidy.** —**en′do·mi·tot′ic** (-tŏt′ĭk) *adj.*

en·do·morph (ĕn′də-môrf′) *n.* An individual having a body build characterized by relative prominence of the abdomen and other soft body parts developed from the embryonic endodermal layer. —**en′do·mor′phic** *adj.* —**en′do·mor′phy** *n.*

En·do·my·ce·ta·les (ĕn′dō-mī′sĭ-tā′lēz) *n.* An order of ascomycetous fungi that includes the yeasts.

en·do·my·o·car·di·al (ĕn′dō-mī′ō-kär′dē-əl) *adj.* Of

or relating to the endocardial and myocardial membrane.

en·do·myo·car·di·al fibrosis *n.* A disorder endemic in parts of Africa, characterized by thickening of the ventricular endocardium by fibrosis.

en·do·my·o·car·di·tis (ĕn′dō-mī′ō-kär-dī′tĭs) *n.* Inflammation of the endocardial and the myocardial membrane.

en·do·my·o·me·tri·tis (ĕn′dō-mī′ō-mĭ-trī′tĭs) *n.* Sepsis involving the tissues of the uterus occurring after a cesarean section.

en·do·mys·i·um (ĕn′dō-mĭs′ē-əm, -mĭz′-) *n.* The fine connective tissue sheath surrounding a muscle fiber.

en·do·neu·ri·tis (ĕn′dō-noŏ-rī′tĭs) *n.* Inflammation of the endoneurium.

en·do·neu·ri·um (ĕn′dō-noŏr′ē-əm) *n., pl.* **–neu·ri·a** (-noŏr′ē-ə) The delicate connective tissue enveloping individual nerve fibers within a peripheral nerve. Also called *Henle's sheath.*

en·do·nu·cle·ase (ĕn′dō-noŏ′klē-ās′, -āz′) *n.* Any of a group of enzymes that catalyze the hydrolysis of phosphodiester bonds between nucleic acids in a DNA molecule or RNA sequence.

en·do·par·a·site (ĕn′dō-păr′ə-sīt′) *n.* A parasite, such as a tapeworm or hookworm, living within the body of its host. **—en′do·par·a·sit′ic** (-sĭt′ĭk) *adj.* **—en′do·par′a·sit·ism** (-sī-tĭz′əm) *n.*

en·do·pep·ti·dase (ĕn′dō-pĕp′tĭ-dās′, -dāz′) *n.* Any of a large group of enzymes that catalyze the hydrolysis of peptide bonds in the interior of a polypeptide chain or protein molecule.

en·do·per·i·car·di·tis (ĕn′dō-pĕr′ĭ-kär-dī′tĭs) *n.* Simultaneous inflammation of the endocardium and the pericardium.

en·do·per·i·my·o·car·di·tis (ĕn′dō-pĕr′ə-mī′ō-kär-dī′tĭs) *n.* Simultaneous inflammation of the heart muscle and of the endocardium and pericardium.

en·do·per·i·to·ni·tis (ĕn′dō-pĕr′ĭ-tn-ī′tĭs) *n.* Superficial inflammation of the peritoneum.

en·do·phle·bi·tis (ĕn′dō-flĭ-bī′tĭs) *n.* Inflammation of the inner lining of a vein.

en·doph·thal·mi·tis (ĕn′dŏf-thəl-mī′tĭs, -thăl-, -dŏp-) *n.* Inflammation of the internal structures of the tissues in the eyeball.

en·do·phyte (ĕn′də-fīt′) *n.* A plant parasite living inside another organism. **—en′do·phyt′ic** (-dō-fĭt′ĭk) *adj.*

en·do·plasm (ĕn′də-plăz′əm) *n.* A central, less viscous portion of the cytoplasm that is distinguishable in certain cells, especially motile cells and protozoa. **—en′do·plas′mic** *adj.*

endoplasmic reticulum *n. Abbr.* **ER** The membrane network in cytoplasm that is composed of tubules or cisternae. Some membranes carry ribosomes on their surfaces while others are smooth.

en·do·pol·y·ploi·dy (ĕn′dō-pŏl′ē-ploi′dē) *n.* A process by which chromosomes replicate without the division of the cell nucleus, resulting in a polyploid nucleus. Also called *endomitosis.* **—en′do·pol′y·ploid′** *adj.*

en·do·rec·tal pull-through procedure (ĕn′dō-rĕk′təl) *n.* Removal of diseased rectal mucosa along with resec-

tion of the lower bowel, followed by anastomosis of the proximal stump to the anus.

en·do·re·du·pli·ca·tion (ĕn′dō-rĭ-doŏ′plĭ-kā′shən) *n.* A form of polyploidy or polysomy characterized by redoubling of chromosomes, giving rise to four-stranded chromosomes at prophase and metaphase.

end organ *n.* The encapsulated termination of a sensory nerve.

en·dor·phin (ĕn-dôr′fĭn) *n.* Any of a group of peptide hormones that bind to opiate receptors and are found mainly in the brain. Endorphins reduce the sensation of pain and affect emotions.

en·dor·phi·ner·gic (ĕn-dôr′fə-nûr′jĭk) *adj.* Of or relating to nerve cells or fibers that employ an endorphin as their neurotransmitter.

en·do·sal·pin·gi·tis (ĕn′dō-săl′pĭn-jī′tĭs) *n.* Inflammation of the mucous membrane lining the eustachian or fallopian tube.

en·do·scope (ĕn′də-skōp′) *n.* An instrument for examining visually the interior of a bodily canal or hollow organ such as the colon, bladder, or stomach. **—en′do·scop′ic** (-skŏp′ĭk) *adj.*

endoscopic biopsy *n.* A biopsy obtained by instruments passed through an endoscope or obtained by a needle introduced under endoscopic guidance.

endoscopic retrograde cholangiopancreatography *n. Abbr.* **ERCP** The use of an endoscope to inspect the pancreatic duct and common bile duct. It may also involve biopsy or the introduction of contrast material for radiographic examination.

en·dos·co·py (ĕn-dŏs′kə-pē) *n.* Examination of the interior of a canal or hollow organ by means of an endoscope. **—en·dos′co·pist** *n.*

en·do·skel·e·ton (ĕn′dō-skĕl′ĭ-tn) *n.* An internal supporting skeleton, derived from the mesoderm, that is characteristic of vertebrates and certain invertebrates. **—en′do·skel′e·tal** (-ĭ-tl) *adj.*

en·dos·mo·sis (ĕn′dŏz-mō′sĭs) *n.* The passage of a fluid inward through a permeable membrane, as of a cell, toward a fluid of higher concentration. **—en′dos·mot′ic** (-mŏt′ĭk) *adj.*

en·do·so·nos·co·py (ĕn′dō-sə-nŏs′kə-pē) *n.* A sonographic study carried out by transducers inserted into the body as miniature probes in the urethra, bladder, or rectum.

en·do·spore (ĕn′də-spôr′) *n.* **1.** A small spore formed within the vegetative cells of some bacteria. **2.** A fungus spore borne within a cell or within the tubular end of a sporophore. **3.** The inner layer of the wall of a spore.

en·do·stat·in (ĕn′dō-stăt′n) *n.* A potent, naturally occurring antiangiogenic protein that inhibits the formation of the blood vessels that feed tumors and is under investigation as a potential cancer therapy.

en·do·ste·i·tis (ĕn′dŏ-stē-ī′tĭs) *or* **en·do·sti·tis** (ĕn′dō-stī′tĭs) *n.* Inflammation of the endosteum or of the medullary cavity of a bone. Also called *central osteitis, perimyelitis.*

en·do·ste·o·ma (ĕn′dŏ-stē-ō′mə) *or* **en·do·sto·ma** (ĕn′dŏ-stō′mə) *n.* A benign tumor of bone tissue in the medullary cavity of a bone.

en·dos·te·um (ĕn-dŏs′tē-əm) *n., pl.* **–te·a** (-tē-ə) The thin layer of cells lining the medullary cavity of a bone. Also called *medullary membrane.* —**en·dos′te·al** *adj.*

en·do·ten·din·e·um (ĕn′dō-tĕn-dĭn′ē-əm) *n.* The fine connective tissue surrounding secondary fascicles of a tendon.

endothelial dystrophy of cornea *n.* The spontaneous loss of corneal endothelium resulting in the accumulation of fluid within the corneal stroma and the epithelium.

endothelial myeloma *n.* See **Ewing's tumor.**

en·do·the·li·oid (ĕn′dō-thē′lē-oid′) *adj.* Resembling endothelium.

en·do·the·li·o·ma (ĕn′dō-thē′lē-ō′mə) *n., pl.* **–mas** *or* **–ma·ta** (-mə-tə) Any of various benign or occasionally malignant neoplasms derived from the endothelial tissue of blood vessels or lymphatic channels.

en·do·the·li·o·sis (ĕn′dō-thē′lē-ō′sĭs) *n.* Proliferation of endothelium.

en·do·the·li·um (ĕn′dō-thē′lē-əm) *n., pl.* **–li·a** (-lē-ə) A thin layer of flat epithelial cells that lines serous cavities, lymph vessels, and blood vessels. —**en′do·the′li·al** *adj.*

en·do·therm (ĕn′də-thûrm′) *n.* An organism that generates heat to maintain its body temperature above the temperature of its surroundings; a homeotherm.

en·do·ther·mic (ĕn′dō-thûr′mĭk) *or* **en·do·ther·mal** (-məl) *adj.* **1.** Of or relating to a chemical reaction during which there is absorption of heat. **2.** Of or relating to an endotherm; warm-blooded. —**en′do·ther′my** *n.*

en·do·tho·rac·ic fascia (ĕn′dō-thə-răs′ĭk) *n.* The extrapleural fascia that lines the wall of the chest, extending over the cupola of the pleura as the suprapleural membrane and forming a thin layer between the diaphragm and the pleura.

en·do·thrix (ĕn′dō-thrĭks′) *n.* A trichophyton, especially *Trichophyton violaceum* or *T. tonsurans,* whose spores and sometimes mycelia characteristically invade the interior of the hair shaft.

en·do·tox·e·mi·a (ĕn′dō-tŏk-sē′mē-ə) *n.* The presence of endotoxins in the blood, which, if derived from gram-negative rod-shaped bacteria, may cause hemorrhages, necrosis of the kidneys, and shock.

en·do·tox·i·co·sis (ĕn′dō-tŏk′sĭ-kō′sĭs) *n.* Poisoning by an endotoxin.

en·do·tox·in (ĕn′dō-tŏk′sən) *n.* A toxin that forms an integral part of the cell wall of certain bacteria and is only released upon destruction of the bacterial cell. Endotoxins are less potent and less specific than most exotoxins and do not form toxoids. Also called *intracellular toxin.* —**en′do·tox′ic** *adj.*

en·do·tra·che·al (ĕn′də-trā′kē-əl) *adj.* Within or passing through the trachea.

endotracheal intubation *n.* The passage of a tube through the nose or mouth into the trachea for maintenance of the airway, as during the administration of anesthesia.

endotracheal tube *n.* A tube inserted into the trachea to provide a passageway for air. Also called *tracheal tube.*

en·do·trach·e·li·tis (ĕn′dō-trăk′ə-lī′tĭs) *n.* See **endocervicitis.**

en·do·vas·cu·lar (ĕn′dō-văs′kyə-lər) *adj.* **1.** Intravascular. **2.** Of or relating to a surgical procedure in which a catheter containing medications or miniature instruments is inserted percutaneously into a blood vessel for the treatment of vascular disease.

en·do·vas·cu·li·tis (ĕn′dō-văs′kyə-lī′tĭs) *n.* See **endangiitis.**

end piece *or* **endpiece.** The terminal part of the tail of a spermatozoon, consisting of the axoneme and the flagellar membrane.

end plate *or* **endplate.** The area of synaptic contact between a motor nerve and a muscle fiber.

end-position nystagmus *n.* A jerky nystagmus occurring in a normal individual when attempts are made to fixate a point at the limits of fixation.

end stage *n.* The final phase of a terminal disease. —**end′-stage′** *adj.*

end-systolic volume *n.* The amount of blood in the ventricle at the end of the cardiac ejection period and immediately preceding ventricular relaxation; used as a measure of systolic function.

end-tidal *adj.* Pertaining to or occurring at the end of a normal exhalation.

–ene *suff.* An unsaturated organic compound, especially one containing a double bond between carbon atoms: *ethylene.*

en·e·ma (ĕn′ə-mə) *n., pl.* **–mas 1.** The injection of liquid into the rectum through the anus for cleansing, for stimulating evacuation of the bowels, or for other therapeutic or diagnostic purposes. **2.** The fluid so injected.

en·er·gy (ĕn′ər-jē) *n.* **1.** The capacity for work or vigorous activity; vigor; power. **2.** The capacity of a physical system to do work.

en·er·vate (ĕn′ər-vāt′) *v.* **1.** To remove a nerve or nerve part. **2.** To cause weakness or a reduction of strength. —**en′er·va′tion** *n.*

en·fu·vir·tide (ĕn-fyōō′vîr-tĭd′) *n.* An antiretroviral drug of the fusion inhibitor class used to treat HIV infection.

ENG *abbr.* electronystagmography

en·gage·ment (ĕn-gāj′mənt) *n.* The entrance of the fetal head or presenting part into the upper opening of the maternal pelvis.

Eng·el·mann's disease (ĕng′əl-mənz, -mänz′) *n.* See **diaphysial dysplasia.**

en·gorge (ĕn-gôrj′) *v.* To fill to excess, as with blood or other fluid. —**en·gorge′ment** *n.*

en·gram (ĕn′grăm′) *n.* A physical alteration thought to occur in living neural tissue in response to stimuli, posited as an explanation for memory. Also called *neurogram.*

en·graph·i·a (ĕn-grăf′ē-ə) *n.* Formation of engrams.

en·keph·a·lin (ĕn-kĕf′ə-lĭn) *n.* Either of two closely related pentapeptides having opiate qualities and occurring especially in the brain and spinal cord.

en·keph·a·li·ner·gic (ĕn-kĕf′ə-lə-nûr′jĭk) *adj.* Of or relating to nerve cells or fibers that employ an enkephalin as their neurotransmitter.

–enoic *suff.* Unsaturated acid, especially one containing at least one double bond: *octadecenoic acid.*

e·nol (ē′nôl′, ē′nōl′) *n.* An organic compound containing a hydroxyl group bonded to a carbon atom that in turn forms a double bond with another carbon atom. —**e·nol′ic** (ē-nōl′ĭk) *adj.*

e·no·lase (ē′nə-lās′, -lāz′) *n.* An enzyme that is present in muscle tissue and that acts in carbohydrate metabolism.

en·oph·thal·mos (ĕn′ŏf-thăl′məs, -mŏs′, -ŏp-) *n.* Recession of the eyeball within the orbit.

en·os·to·sis (ĕn′ŏ-stō′sĭs) *n., pl.* **–ses** (-sēz) A mass of proliferating bone tissue within a bone.

en·si·form (ĕn′sə-fôrm′) *adj.* Sword-shaped; xiphoid.

ensiform cartilage *n.* See **xiphoid process.**

ensiform process *n.* See **xiphoid process.**

en·stro·phe (ĕn′strə-fē) *n.* The turning inward of an eyelid; entropion.

ENT *abbr.* ear, nose, and throat

ent– *pref.* Variant of **ento–.**

en·tad (ĕn′tăd′) *adv.* Toward the interior; inward.

en·tal (ĕn′tl) *adj.* Of or situated on the inside; inner; internal.

en·ta·me·ba *or* **en·ta·moe·ba** (ĕn′tə-mē′bə) *or* **en·da·me·ba** *or* **en·da·moe·ba** (ĕn′də-) *n.* A parasitic ameba of the genus *Entamoeba.*

en·ta·me·bi·a·sis *or* **en·ta·moe·bi·a·sis** (ĕn′tă-mə-bī′ə-sĭs) *n.* Infection with *Entamoeba histolytica.*

Entamoeba *n.* A genus of amebas whose members are parasitic in the cecum and large bowel of humans and many mammals and birds. *E. histolytica,* the only distinct pathogen of the genus, causes amebic dysentery and hepatic amebiasis.

en·ta·sia (ĕn-tā′zhə) *or* **en·ta·sis** (ĕn′tə-sĭs) *n.* See **tonic spasm.**

enter– *pref.* Variant of **entero–.**

en·ter·al (ĕn′tər-əl) *adj.* **1.** Within or by way of the intestine, as distinguished from parenteral. **2.** Enteric. —**en′ter·al·ly** *adv.*

en·ter·al·gia (ĕn′tə-răl′jə) *n.* Severe abdominal pain accompanying spasms of the intestine. —**en′ter·al′gic** (-jĭk) *adj.*

en·ter·ec·ta·sis (ĕn′tə-rĕk′tə-sĭs) *n.* Dilation or distention of the intestine.

en·ter·ec·to·my (ĕn′tə-rĕk′tə-mē) *n.* Surgical removal of a segment of the intestine.

en·ter·el·co·sis (ĕn′tər-əl-kō′sĭs) *n.* Ulceration of the intestine.

en·ter·ic (ĕn-tĕr′ĭk) *adj.* **1.** Of, relating to, or within the intestine. **2.** By way of the intestine; enteral.

enteric-coated *adj.* Relating to an oral preparation of a drug that has been treated so that release is delayed until passage from the stomach into the intestine.

enteric fever *n.* **1.** See **typhoid fever. 2.** See **paratyphoid fever.**

en·ter·i·coid fever (ĕn-tĕr′ĭ-koid′) *n.* A fever resembling the typhoid fever.

enteric orphan virus *n.* Any of various enteroviruses found in humans and other animals whose role in causing disease may not be specifically understood.

enteric tuberculosis *n.* A tuberculous infection of areas of the digestive tract having relative statis or abundant lymphoid tissue resulting from the expectoration and swallowing of tubercle bacilli; it is a complication of open tuberculosis of the lungs.

enteric virus *n.* See **enterovirus.**

en·ter·i·tis (ĕn′tə-rī′tĭs) *n.* Inflammation of the intestinal tract, especially of the small intestine.

enteritis ne·crot·i·cans (nĭ-krŏt′ĭ-kănz′) *n.* Enteritis with necrosis of the intestinal wall caused by *Clostridium welchii.*

entero– *or* **enter–** *pref.* Intestine: *enteritis.*

en·ter·o·a·nas·to·mo·sis (ĕn′tə-rō-ə-năs′tə-mō′sĭs) *n.* See **enteroenterostomy.**

en·ter·o·bac·ter·i·um (ĕn′tə-rō-băk-tîr′ē-əm) *n., pl.* **–i·a** (-ē-ə) Any of various gram-negative rod-shaped bacteria of the family Enterobacteriaceae that includes some pathogens of animals, such as the colon bacillus and salmonella.

en·ter·o·bi·a·sis (ĕn′tə-rō-bī′ə-sĭs) *n.* Infestation of the intestine with the common pinworm *Enterobius vermicularis.*

En·ter·o·bi·us (ĕn′tə-rō′bē-əs) *n.* A genus of nematode worms including the common pinworm.

en·ter·o·cele (ĕn′tə-rō-sēl′) *n.* **1.** A hernial protrusion through a defect in the rectovaginal or vesicovaginal pouch. **2.** An intestinal hernia.

en·ter·o·cen·te·sis (ĕn′tə-rō-sĕn-tē′sĭs) *n.* Surgical puncture of the intestine with a hollow needle to withdraw gas or fluid.

en·ter·o·chro·maf·fin cell (ĕn′tə-rō-krō′mə-fĭn) *n.* See **enteroendocrine cell.**

en·ter·o·clei·sis (ĕn′tə-rō-klī′sĭs) *n.* Occlusion of the lumen of the alimentary canal.

en·ter·oc·ly·sis (ĕn′tə-rŏk′lĭ-sĭs) *n.* See **high enema.**

en·ter·o·coc·cus (ĕn′tə-rō-kŏk′əs) *n., pl.* **–coc·ci** (-kŏk′sī′, -kŏk′ī′) A usually nonpathogenic streptococcus that inhabits the intestine. —**en′ter·o·coc′cal** *adj.*

en·ter·o·coele (ĕn′tə-rō-sēl′) *n.* The coelom formed from a pocketlike outgrowth of the wall of the archenteron, especially in echinoderms and chordates.

en·ter·o·co·li·tis (ĕn′tə-rō-kō-lī′tĭs, -kə-) *n.* Inflammation of the mucous membrane of both the small and large intestine. Also called *coloenteritis.*

en·ter·o·co·los·to·my (ĕn′tə-rō-kə-lŏs′tə-mē) *n.* **1.** The surgical formation of a connection between the small intestine and colon. **2.** The connection itself.

en·ter·o·cyst (ĕn′tə-rō-sĭst′) *n.* A cyst of the wall of the intestine. Also called *enterocystoma.*

en·ter·o·cys·to·cele (ĕn′tə-rō-sĭs′tə-sēl′) *n.* A hernia of the intestine and the bladder wall.

en·ter·o·cys·to·ma (ĕn′tə-rō-sĭ-stō′mə) *n.* See **enterocyst.**

en·ter·o·en·do·crine cell (ĕn′tə-rō-ĕn′də-krĭn, -krēn′, -krīn′) *n.* Any of several types of hormone-secreting cells that are present throughout the epithelium of the digestive tract and that often stain readily with silver or chromium salts. Also called *argentaffin cell, enterochromaffin cell.*

en·ter·o·en·ter·os·to·my (ĕ′tə-rō-ĕn′tə-rŏs′tə-mē) *n.* A surgical connection between two segments of intestine. Also called *enteroanastomosis, intestinal anastomosis.*

en·ter·o·gas·tric reflex (ĕn'tə-rō-găs'trĭk) *n.* Peristaltic contraction of the small intestine induced by the entrance of food into the stomach.

en·ter·o·gas·tri·tis (ĕn'tə-rō-gă-strī'tĭs) *n.* See **gastroenteritis.**

en·ter·o·gas·trone (ĕn'tə-rō-găs'trōn') *n.* A hormone released by the upper intestinal mucosa that inhibits gastric motility and secretion.

en·ter·og·e·nous (ĕn'tə-rŏj'ə-nəs) *adj.* Of intestinal origin.

enterogenous cyanosis *n.* A condition resembling cyanosis, caused by the absorption of nitrites or other toxics from the intestine and by the formation of methemoglobin or sulfhemoglobin in the blood.

enterogenous cyst *n.* A cyst derived from cells sequestered from the primitive foregut, classified histologically as bronchogenic, esophageal, or gastric.

en·ter·o·he·pat·ic circulation (ĕn'tə-rō-hĭ-păt'ĭk) *n.* Circulation of substances such as bile salts, which are absorbed from the intestine and carried to the liver, where they are secreted into the bile and again enter the intestine.

en·ter·o·hep·a·ti·tis (ĕn'tə-rō-hĕp'ə-tī'tĭs) *n.* Inflammation of the intestine and the liver.

en·ter·o·hep·a·to·cele (ĕn'tə-rō-hĕp'ə-tə-sēl', -hĭ-păt'ə-) *n.* A congenital umbilical hernia containing intestine and liver tissue.

en·ter·o·ki·nase (ĕn'tə-rō-kī'nās', -nāz', -kĭn'ās', -āz') *n.* An enzyme secreted by the upper intestinal mucosa that catalyzes the conversion of the inactive trypsinogen to trypsin. Also called *enteropeptidase.*

en·ter·o·ki·ne·sis (ĕn'tə-rō-kə-nē'sĭs, -kī-) *n.* Muscular contraction of the alimentary canal, as in peristalsis. —**en'ter·o·ki·net'ic** (-nĕt'ĭk) *adj.*

en·ter·o·lith (ĕn'tə-rō-lĭth') *n.* An intestinal calculus formed of layers surrounding a nucleus of a hard indigestible substance.

en·ter·o·li·thi·a·sis (ĕn'tə-rō-lĭ-thī'ə-sĭs) *n.* The presence of calculi in the intestine.

en·ter·ol·o·gy (ĕn'tə-rŏl'ə-jē) *n.* The branch of medicine that is concerned with disorders of the intestinal tract.

en·ter·ol·y·sis (ĕn'tə-rŏl'ĭ-sĭs) *n.* The surgical division or removal of intestinal adhesions.

en·ter·o·meg·a·ly (ĕn'tə-rō-mĕg'ə-lē) *n.* See **megaloenteron.**

en·ter·o·mer·o·cele (ĕn'tə-rō-mîr'ə-sēl') *n.* See **femoral hernia.**

en·ter·o·my·co·sis (ĕn'tə-rō-mī-kō'sĭs) *n.* An intestinal disease of fungal origin.

en·ter·on (ĕn'tə-rŏn') *n.* The alimentary canal; the intestines.

en·ter·o·pa·re·sis (ĕn'tə-rō-pə-rē'sĭs, -păr'ĭ-sĭs) *n.* A state of diminished or arrested peristalsis with flaccidity of the intestinal walls.

en·ter·o·path·o·gen (ĕn'tə-rō-păth''ə-jən, -jĕn') *n.* An organism that is capable of producing intestinal disease. —**en'ter·o·path'o·gen'ic** (-jĕn'ĭk) *adj.*

en·ter·op·a·thy (ĕn'tə-rŏp'ə-thē) *n.* A disease of the intestinal tract.

en·ter·o·pep·ti·dase (ĕn'tə-rō-pĕp'tĭ-dās', -dāz') *n.* See **enterokinase.**

en·ter·o·pex·y (ĕn'tə-rō-pĕk'sē) *n.* Surgical fixation of a segment of intestine to the abdominal wall.

en·ter·o·plas·ty (ĕn'tə-rō-plăs'tē) *n.* Reconstructive surgery of the intestine.

en·ter·o·ple·gia (ĕn'tə-rō-plē'jə) *n.* See **paralytic ileus.**

en·ter·op·to·sis (ĕn'tə-rŏp-tō'sĭs) *or* **en·ter·op·to·si·a** (-tō'sē-ə, -zē-ə) *n.* The abnormal descent of the intestines in the abdominal cavity that is usually associated with the downward displacement of other viscera.

en·ter·or·rha·gia (ĕn'tə-rō-rā'jə) *n.* Bleeding within the intestinal tract.

en·ter·or·rha·phy (ĕn'tə-rôr'ə-fē) *n.* Surgical suture of the intestine.

en·ter·or·rhex·is (ĕn'tə-rō-rĕk'sĭs) *n.* Rupture of the intestine.

en·ter·o·sep·sis (ĕn'tə-rō-sĕp'sĭs) *n.* Sepsis occurring or originating in the intestine.

en·ter·o·spasm (ĕn'tə-rō-spăz'əm) *n.* Increased, irregular, and painful peristalsis.

en·ter·o·sta·sis (ĕn'tə-rō-stā'sĭs) *n.* A retardation or arrest of the passage of the intestinal contents, as from obstruction. Also called *intestinal stasis.*

en·ter·o·stat·in (ĕn'tə-rō-stăt'n) *n.* A substance produced in the pancreas that initiates a sensation of fullness, which may lead to decreased food consumption and weight loss.

en·ter·o·stax·is (ĕn'tə-rō-stăk'sĭs) *n.* The oozing of blood from the mucous membrane of the intestine.

en·ter·o·ste·no·sis (ĕn'tə-rō-stə-nō'sĭs) *n.* A narrowing or stricture of the lumen of the intestine.

en·ter·os·to·my (ĕn'tə-rŏs'tə-mē) *n.* **1.** Surgical construction of an opening into the intestine through an incision in the abdominal wall. **2.** The opening itself. —**en'ter·os'to·mal** *adj.*

en·ter·ot·o·my (ĕn'tə-rŏt'ə-mē) *n.* An incision into the intestine.

en·ter·o·tox·i·gen·ic (ĕn'tə-rō-tŏk'sə-jĕn'ĭk) *adj.* Of or being an organism containing or producing an enterotoxin.

en·ter·o·tox·in (ĕn'tə-rō-tŏk'sĭn) *n.* A cytotoxin produced by bacteria that is specific for the mucous membrane of the intestine and causes the vomiting and diarrhea associated with food poisoning.

en·ter·o·trop·ic (ĕn'tə-rō-trŏp'ĭk, -trō'pĭk) *adj.* Attracted to or affecting the intestine.

en·ter·o·vi·rus (ĕn'tə-rō-vī'rəs) *n.* A virus of the genus *Enterovirus.* Also called *enteric virus.*

Enterovirus *n.* A genus of picornaviruses, including polioviruses, coxsackieviruses, and echoviruses, that infect the gastrointestinal tract and often spread to other areas of the body, especially the nervous system. —**en'ter·o·vi'ral** *adj.*

en·ter·o·zo·on (ĕn'tə-rō-zō'ŏn') *n., pl.* **–zo·a** (-zō'ə) An animal, such as a tapeworm or hookworm, that is parasitic in the intestine. —**en'ter·o·zo'ic** *adj.*

en·thal·py (ĕn'thăl'pē, ĕn-thăl'-) *n.* A thermodynamic function of a system, equivalent to the sum of the internal energy of the system plus the product of its volume multiplied by the pressure exerted on it by its surroundings.

en·the·sis (ĕn′thĭ-sĭs) *n.*, *pl.* **–ses** (-sēz) The surgical insertion of synthetic or other inorganic material to replace lost tissue.

en·the·si·tis (ĕn′thĭ-sī′tĭs) *n.* Traumatic disease occurring at the point of attachment of skeletal muscles to bone, where recurring stress causes inflammation and often fibrosis and calcification.

en·the·sop·a·thy (ĕn′thĭ-sŏp′ə-thē) *n.* A disease occurring at the site of attachment of muscle tendons and ligaments to bones or joint capsules. **—en·the′so·path′ic** (ĕn-thē′sə-păth′ĭk) *adj.*

en·thet·ic (ĕn-thĕt′ĭk) *adj.* **1.** Relating to enthesis. **2.** Exogenous.

ento– *or* **ent–** *pref.* Inside; within: *entozoon.*

en·to·blast (ĕn′tə-blăst′) *or* **en·do·blast** (ĕn′də-) *n.* Any of the blastomeres of an embryo from which the endoderm develops.

en·to·cele (ĕn′tə-sēl′) *n.* An internal hernia.

en·to·cho·roi·de·a (ĕn′tō-kə-roi′dē-ə, -kô-) *n.* See **choriocapillary layer.**

en·to·cor·ne·a (ĕn′tō-kôr′nē-ə) *n.* See **limiting layer of cornea** (sense 2).

en·to·derm (ĕn′tə-dûrm′) *n.* Variant of **endoderm.**

en·to·ec·tad (ĕn′tō-ĕk′tăd′) *adv.* From inside or within toward the outside.

en·to·mi·on (ĕn-tō′mē-ŏn′, -ən) *n.*, *pl.* **–mi·a** (-mē-ə) The tip of the mastoid angle of the parietal bone.

en·to·mol·o·gy (ĕn′tə-mŏl′ə-jē) *n.* The study of insects. **—en′to·mo·log′ic** (-mə-lŏj′ĭk), **en′to·mo·log′i·cal** (-ĭ-kəl) *adj.* **—en′to·mol′o·gist** *n.*

en·top·ic (ĕn-tŏp′ĭk) *adj.* Occurring or situated in the normal place.

ent·op·tic (ĕn-tŏp′tĭk) *adj.* Occurring or located within the eyeball.

en·to·ret·i·na (ĕn′tō-rĕt′n-ə) *n.* The internal or nervous portion of the retina, consisting of five layers from the outer plexiform to the nerve fiber layer.

en·to·zo·on (ĕn′tə-zō′ŏn′) *n.*, *pl.* **–zo·a** (-zō′ə) An animal parasite, such as a tapeworm or liver fluke, inhabiting any of the internal organs or tissues. **—en′to·zo′al** *adj.*

en·trails (ĕn′trālz′, -trəlz) *pl.n.* The internal organs, especially the intestines; viscera.

en·trap·ment neuropathy (ĕn-trăp′mənt) *n.* Neuritis in which a neuron is continually irritated by compression created by encroachment or impingement of a nearby anatomical structure.

en·tro·pi·on (ĕn-trō′pē-ŏn′, -ən) *n.* **1.** The inversion or turning inward of a part. **2.** The infolding of the margin of an eyelid.

entropion u·ve·ae (yōō′vē-ē′) *n.* Inversion of the pupillary margin. Also called *iridentropium.*

en·tro·py (ĕn′trə-pē) *n.* **1.** For a closed thermodynamic system, a quantitative measure of the amount of thermal energy not available to do work. **2.** A measure of the disorder or randomness in a closed system. **—en·tro′pic** (ĕn-trō′pĭk, -trŏp′ĭk) *adj.*

en·ty·py (ĕn′tə-pē) *n.* The condition in an early mammalian embryo in which the endoderm covers the embryonic and amniotic ectoderm.

e·nu·cle·ate (ĭ-nōō′klē-āt′) *v.* **1.** To remove something, such as a tumor or an eye, whole and without rupture from an enveloping cover or sac. **2.** To remove a cell's nucleus. **—***adj.* (-ĭt, -āt′) Lacking a nucleus. **—e·nu′cle·a′tion** *n.*

en·u·re·sis (ĕn′yə-rē′sĭs) *n.* The uncontrolled or involuntary discharge of urine.

en·ve·lope (ĕn′və-lōp′, ŏn′-) *n.* An enclosing structure or cover, such as a membrane or the outer coat of a virus.

en·ven·om·a·tion (ĕn-vĕn′ə-mā′shən) *n.* The injection of a poisonous material by sting, spine, bite, or other similar means.

en·vi·ron·ment (ĕn-vī′rən-mənt, -vī′ərn-) *n.* The totality of circumstances surrounding an organism or group of organisms, especially the combination of external physical conditions that affect and influence the growth, development, and survival of organisms. **—en·vi′ron·men′tal** (-mĕn′tl) *adj.*

environmental medicine *n.* The study of the effects of environmental exposure to synthetic chemicals on the immune system.

environmental psychology *n.* The study of how changes in physical space and related physical stimuli can affect the behavior of individuals.

en·zo·ot·ic (ĕn′zō-ŏt′ĭk) *adj.* Prevalent among or restricted to animals of a specific geographic area. Used of a disease. **—***n.* An enzootic disease.

enzootic stability *n.* See **endemic stability.**

en·zy·got·ic (ĕn′zī-gŏt′ĭk) *adj.* Monozygotic.

en·zyme (ĕn′zīm) *n.* Any of numerous proteins or conjugated proteins produced by living organisms and functioning as specialized catalysts for biochemical reactions. **—en′zy·mat′ic** (-zə-măt′ĭk), **en·zy′mic** (-zī′mĭk, -zĭm′ĭk) *adj.*

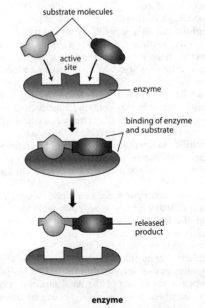

enzyme
Top: *substrate molecules bonding with an enzyme's active site*
Center: *the substrate molecules and enzyme bind to form a single molecule*
Bottom: *the new molecule and unchanged enzyme separate*

enzyme-inhibition theory of narcosis *n.* The theory that narcotics inhibit respiratory enzymes by suppressing the formation of high-energy phosphate bonds within the cell.

enzyme-linked immunosorbent assay *n.* ELISA.

en·zy·mol·o·gy (ĕn′zə-mŏl′ə-jē) *n.* The branch of science that deals with the biochemical nature and activity of enzymes.

en·zy·mol·y·sis (ĕn′zə-mŏl′ĭ-sĭs) *n.* Chemical change or cleavage of a substance by enzymatic action.

en·zy·mop·a·thy (ĕn′zə-mŏp′ə-thē) *n.* Any of various disturbances of enzyme function, such as the genetic deficiency of a specific enzyme.

EOG *abbr.* electro-oculography

e·o·sin (ē′ə-sən) *n.* Any of a class of red acid dyes of the xanthene group used as cytoplasmic stains and as counterstains, especially the sodium and potassium salts of certain of these dyes.

e·o·sin·o·pe·ni·a (ē′ə-sĭn′ə-pē′nē-ə) *n.* A reduction in the normal number of eosinophils present in the blood.

e·o·sin·o·phil (ē′ə-sĭn′ə-fĭl′) *or* **e·o·sin·o·phile** (-fĭl′) *n.* **1.** A type of white blood cell containing cytoplasmic granules that are easily stained by eosin or other acid dyes. Also called *eosinophilic leukocyte, oxyphil, oxyphilic leukocyte.* **2.** A microorganism, cell, or histological element easily stained by eosin or other acid dyes. —**e′o·sin′o·phil′ic** *adj.*

eosinophil adenoma *n.* See **growth hormone-producing adenoma.**

eosinophil chemotactic factor of anaphylaxis *n. Abbr.* **ECF-A** A peptide chemotactic for eosinophils and released from disrupted mast cells.

e·o·sin·o·phil·i·a (ē′ə-sĭn′ə-fĭl′ē-ə) *n.* An increase in the number of eosinophils in the blood. Also called *eosinophilic leukocytosis.*

eosinophilic cellulitis *n.* See **Wells′ syndrome.**

eosinophilic fasciitis *n.* Induration and edema of the connective tissues of the extremities, which usually appears following exertion and is associated with eosinophilia.

eosinophilic granuloma *n.* A lesion having numerous histiocytes that may contain Langerhans granules, eosinophils, and pockets of necrosis. It is usually a solitary bone lesion but may develop in the lung.

eosinophilic leukemia *n.* A form of granulocytic leukemia characterized by abnormal numbers of or a predominance of eosinophilic granulocytes in the tissues and blood.

eosinophilic leukocyte *n.* See **eosinophil** (sense 1).

eosinophilic leukocytosis *n.* See **eosinophilia.**

eosinophilic leukopenia *n.* A condition characterized by a decrease in the number of eosinophilic granulocytes normally present in the blood.

eosinophilic meningitis *n.* See **angiostrongylosis.**

eosinophilic non·al·ler·gic rhinitis (nŏn′ə-lûr′jĭk) *n.* Hyperplastic thickening of the nasal mucosa with abnormal numbers of eosinophils, not attributable to a specific allergen.

eosinophilic pneumonia *n.* A disorder characterized by radiologic evidence of infiltrates accompanied by either peripheral blood eosinophilia or eosinophilic infiltrates in lung tissue.

e·o·sin·o·phil·u·ri·a (ē′ə-sĭn′ə-fĭl-yŏŏr′ē-ə) *n.* The presence of eosinophils in the urine.

ep– *pref.* Variant of **epi–**.

EPA *abbr.* eicosapentaenoic acid

ep·ax·i·al (ĕp-ăk′sē-əl) *adj.* Located above or behind an axis, such as the spinal axis or the axis of a limb.

ep·en·dy·ma (ĭ-pĕn′də-mə) *n., pl.* **–mas** *or* **–ma·ta** (-mə-tə) The epithelial membrane lining the canal of the spinal cord and the ventricles of the brain. —**ep·en′dy·mal** *adj.*

ependymal cell *n.* **1.** A type of neuroglia cell lining the central canal of the spinal cord or the brain. **2.** A cell of the ependymal area of the developing neural tube.

ep·en·dy·mi·tis (ĭ-pĕn′də-mī′tĭs) *n.* Inflammation of the ependyma.

ep·en·dy·mo·blast (ĭ-pĕn′də-mō-blăst′) *n.* An embryonic ependymal cell.

ep·en·dy·mo·cyte (ĭ-pĕn′də-mō-sīt′) *n.* An ependymal cell.

ep·en·dy·mo·ma (ĭ-pĕn′də-mō′mə) *n., pl.* **–mas** *or* **–ma·ta** (-mə-tə) A central nervous system neoplasm made up of relatively undifferentiated ependymal cells. Also called *medulloepithelioma.*

eph·apse (ĕf′ăps′) *n.* A point of contact where two or more nerve cell processes touch but do not form a typical synaptic contact. —**eph·ap′tic** *adj.*

e·phe·bi·at·rics (ĭ-fē′bē-ăt′rĭks) *n.* See **adolescent medicine.**

e·phe·bic (ĭ-fē′bĭk) *adj.* Of or relating to the period of puberty or adolescence.

e·phed·ra (ĭ-fĕd′rə, ĕf′ĭ-drə) *n.* **1.** Any of various mostly shrubby gymnosperms of the genus *Ephedra,* some of which (especially *E. sinica*) are used as a source of ephedrine. **2.** A stimulant derived from a plant of this genus.

e·phed·rine (ĭ-fĕd′rĭn, ĕf′ĭ-drēn′) *n.* An odorless crystalline or powdered alkaloid isolated from shrubs of the genus *Ephedra* or made synthetically and used in the treatment of allergies and asthma.

e·phe·lis (ĭ-fē′lĭs) *n., pl.* **–li·des** (-lĭ-dēz′) Freckle.

epi– *or* **ep–** *pref.* **1.** On; upon: *epineural.* **2.** Over; above: *epibasal.* **3.** Around: *epicystitis.* **4.** Close to; near: *epimer.* **5.** Besides: *epiphenomenon.* **6.** After: *epigenesis.*

ep·i·an·dros·ter·one (ĕp′ē-ăn-drŏs′tə-rōn′) *n.* An inactive isomer of androsterone found normally in urine and in testicular and ovarian tissue.

ep·i·blast (ĕp′ə-blăst′) *n.* The outer layer of a blastula that gives rise to the ectoderm after gastrulation. —**ep′i·blas′tic** *adj.*

ep·i·bleph·a·ron (ĕp′ə-blĕf′ə-rŏn′) *n.* A congenital horizontal fold of skin near the margin of the upper or lower eyelid caused by the abnormal insertion of muscle fibers.

e·pib·o·ly (ĭ-pĭb′ə-lē) *n.* The growth of a rapidly dividing group of cells around a more slowly dividing group of cells, as in the formation of a gastrula.

ep·i·bul·bar (ĕp′ə-bŭl′bər, -bär′) *adj.* Of or being on the eyeball.

ep·i·can·thic fold (ĕp′ĭ-kăn′thĭk) *n.* A fold of skin of the upper eyelid that partially covers the inner corner of the eye. Also called *epicanthus, palpebronasal fold.*

ep·i·car·di·a (ĕp′ĭ-kär′dē-ə) *n.* The lower portion of

the esophagus extending through the diaphragm to the stomach.

ep·i·car·di·um (ĕp′ĭ-kär′dē-əm) *n.*, *pl.* **-di·a** (-dē-ə) The inner layer of the pericardium that is in contact with the surface of the heart. Also called *visceral layer.* —**ep′i·car′di·al** *adj.*

ep·i·con·dy·lal·gia (ĕp′ĭ-kŏn′dl-ăl′jə) *n.* Pain in an epicondyle of the humerus or in the tendons or muscles that originate there.

ep·i·con·dyle (ĕp′ĭ-kŏn′dīl, -dl) *n.* A rounded projection at the end of a bone, located on or above a condyle and usually serving as a place of attachment for ligaments and tendons.

ep·i·con·dy·li·tis (ĕp′ĭ-kŏn′dl-ī′tĭs) *n.* Infection or inflammation of an epicondyle.

ep·i·cra·ni·al muscle (ĕp′ĭ-krā′nē-əl) *n.* The galea aponeurotica together with the occipitofrontal and the temporoparietal muscles inserting into it.

ep·i·cra·ni·um (ĕp′ĭ-krā′nē-əm) *n.*, *pl.* **-ni·ums** or **-ni·a** (-nē-ə) The structures covering the cranium.

ep·i·cri·sis (ĕp′ĭ-krī′sĭs, ĕp′ĭ-krī′sĭs) *n.* A secondary crisis in the course of a disease.

ep·i·crit·ic (ĕp′ĭ-krĭt′ĭk) *adj.* Of, relating to, or mediating the ability to discriminate slight differences in sensory stimuli, especially of touch and temperature.

ep·i·cys·ti·tis (ĕp′ĭ-sĭ-stī′tĭs) *n.* Inflammation of the tissue surrounding the bladder.

ep·i·cys·tot·o·my (ĕp′ĭ-sĭ-stŏt′ə-mē) *n.* See **suprapubic cystotomy.**

ep·i·dem·ic (ĕp′ĭ-dĕm′ĭk) or **ep·i·dem·i·cal** (-ĭ-kəl) *adj.* Spreading rapidly and extensively by infection and affecting many individuals in an area or population at the same time, as of a disease or illness. —*n.* An outbreak or unusually high occurrence of a disease or illness in a population or area.

epidemic gastroenteritis virus *n.* A virus that is the causative agent of epidemic nonbacterial gastroenteritis but whose taxonomic classification remains undetermined. Also called *gastroenteritis virus type A.*

epidemic hemoglobinuria *n.* The presence of hemoglobin or of pigments derived from it in the urine of infants, characterized by cyanosis and jaundice.

epidemic hemorrhagic fever *n.* An acute viral hemorrhagic fever characterized by headache, high fever, sweating, thirst, photophobia, coryza, cough, myalgia, arthralgia, and abdominal pain with nausea and vomiting. This phase lasts from three to six days and is followed by capillary hemorrhages, edema, oliguria, and shock. Also called *Far Eastern hemorrhagic fever, hemorrhagic fever with renal syndrome, Korean hemorrhagic fever, Manchurian hemorrhagic fever.*

ep·i·de·mic·i·ty (ĕp′ĭ-də-mĭs′ĭ-tē) *n.* The ability to spread from one host to others; the state of being epidemic.

epidemic keratoconjunctivitis *n.* A highly infectious follicular conjunctivitis of the eye caused by an adenovirus and characterized by inflammation but little exudate. Also called *virus keratoconjunctivitis.*

epidemic keratoconjunctivitis virus *n.* An adenovirus causing of epidemic keratoconjunctivitis and associated with swimming pool conjunctivitis.

epidemic myalgia *n.* See **epidemic pleurodynia.**

epidemic myositis *n.* See **epidemic pleurodynia.**

epidemic neuromyasthenia *n.* An epidemic disease characterized by stiffness of the neck and back, headache, diarrhea, fever, and localized muscular weakness. Also called *benign myalgic encephalomyelitis, Iceland disease.*

epidemic nonbacterial gastroenteritis *n.* An epidemic, communicable, but rather mild disease of sudden onset caused by epidemic gastroenteritis virus and characterized by fever, abdominal cramps, nausea, vomiting, diarrhea, and headache. Also called *acute infectious nonbacterial gastroenteritis.*

epidemic parotitis *n.* See **mumps.**

epidemic parotitis virus *n.* See **mumps virus.**

epidemic pleurodynia *n.* An epidemic disease that is caused by a coxsackievirus, is characterized by paroxysmal pain in the lower chest, and is accompanied by fever, headache, and malaise. Also called *Bornholm disease, devil's grip, diaphragmatic pleurisy, epidemic myalgia, epidemic myositis.*

epidemic pleurodynia virus *n.* A strain of coxsackievirus that causes epidemic pleurodynia. Also called *Bornholm disease virus.*

epidemic polyarthritis *n.* A mild febrile illness of humans in Australia characterized by polyarthralgia and rash, and caused by the Ross River virus.

epidemic roseola *n.* See **rubella.**

epidemic typhus *n.* A form of typhus characterized by high fever, mental and physical depression, and macular and papular eruptions; it is caused by *Rickettsia prowazekii* and transmitted by body lice.

ep·i·de·mi·ol·o·gy (ĕp′ĭ-dē′mē-ŏl′ə-jē, -dĕm′ē-) *n.* The branch of medicine that deals with the study of the causes, distribution, and control of disease in populations. —**ep′i·de′mi·ol′o·gist** *n.*

epidermal cyst *n.* A cyst formed of a mass of epidermal cells that has been pushed beneath the epidermis as a result of trauma.

ep·i·der·mal·i·za·tion (ĕp′ĭ-dûr′mə-lĭ-zā′shən) *n.* The transformation of glandular or mucosal epithelium into stratified squamous epithelium. Also called *squamous metaplasia.*

epidermal ridge *n.* Any of the ridges of the epidermis of the palms and soles, where the sweat pores open. Also called *skin ridge.*

ep·i·der·mis (ĕp′ĭ-dûr′mĭs) *n.* The nonvascular outer protective layer of the skin, covering the dermis. —**ep′i·der′mal** (-məl), **ep′i·der′mic** *adj.*

ep·i·der·mi·tis (ĕp′ĭ-dər-mī′tĭs) *n.* Inflammation of the epidermis.

ep·i·der·mo·dys·pla·sia (ĕp′ĭ-dûr′mō-dĭs-plā′zhə) *n.* The abnormal growth or development of the epidermis.

epidermodysplasia ver·ru·ci·for·mis (və-roō′sə-fôr′mĭs) *n.* The occurrence of numerous flat warts on the hands, face, neck, and feet.

ep·i·der·moid (ĕp′ĭ-dûr′moid′) *adj.* Composed of or resembling epidermal tissue. —*n.* A cystic tumor made up of abnormal epidermal cells.

epidermoid carcinoma *n.* See **squamous cell carcinoma.**

epidermoid cyst *n.* A cyst of the dermis consisting of keratin and sebum and lined with keratin-forming epithelium.

ep·i·der·mol·y·sis (ĕp′ĭ-dər-mŏl′ĭ-sĭs) *n.* A condition in which the epidermis is loosely attached to the dermis and readily detaches or forms blisters.

epidermolysis bul·lo·sa (bə-lō′sə) *n.* Any of a group of inherited chronic noninflammatory skin diseases in which large blisters and erosions develop after slight trauma.

Ep·i·der·moph·y·ton (ĕp′ĭ-dər-mŏf′ĭ-tŏn′, -tən) *n.* A genus of fungi that is parasitic to human skin and nails and that includes the species believed to be the cause of athlete's foot and tinea cruris.

ep·i·der·mot·ro·pism (ĕp′ĭ-dər-mŏt′rə-pĭz′əm) *n.* Movement toward the epidermis.

ep·i·did·y·mec·to·my (ĕp′ĭ-dĭd′ə-mĕk′tə-mē) *n.* Surgical removal of the epididymis.

ep·i·did·y·mis (ĕp′ĭ-dĭd′ə-mĭs) *n.,* *pl.* **–mi·des** (-mĭ-dēz′) A long, narrow, convoluted tube in the spermatic duct system that lies on the posterior aspect of each testicle and connects with the vas deferens.

ep·i·did·y·mi·tis (ĕp′ĭ-dĭd′ə-mī′tĭs) *n.* Inflammation of the epididymis.

ep·i·did·y·mo-or·chi·tis (ĕp′ĭ-dĭd′ə-mō-ôr-kī′tĭs) *n.* Inflammation of both the epididymis and the testis.

ep·i·did·y·mo·plas·ty (ĕp′ĭ-dĭd′ə-mō-plăs′tē) *n.* Surgical repair of the epididymis.

ep·i·did·y·mot·o·my (ĕp′ĭ-dĭd′ə-mŏt′ə-mē) *n.* Incision into the epididymis.

ep·i·did·y·mo·vas·ec·to·my (ĕp′ĭ-dĭd′ə-mō-və-sĕk′tə-mē, -vā-zĕk′-) *n.* Surgical removal of the epididymis and the vas deferens.

ep·i·did·y·mo·va·sos·to·my (ĕp′ĭ-dĭd′ə-mō-vă-sŏs′tə-mē) *n.* The surgical severing of the vas deferens with anastomosis to the epididymis.

ep·i·du·ral (ĕp′ĭ-doŏr′əl) *adj.* Located on or over the dura mater. —*n.* An injection into the epidural space of the spine.

epidural anesthesia *n.* Regional anesthesia produced by injection of a local anesthetic into the epidural space of the lumbar or sacral region of the spine.

epidural block *n.* **1.** Obstruction of the epidural space by compression, hematoma, or scar tissue. **2.** Epidural anesthesia. Not in technical use.

epidural hematoma *n.* An accumulation of blood between the skull and the dura mater. Also called *extradural hemorrhage.*

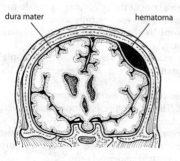

epidural hematoma
frontal section of brain

epidural space *n.* The space between the walls and the dura mater of the vertebral canal.

ep·i·du·rog·ra·phy (ĕp′ĭ-doŏ-rŏg′rə-fē) *n.* Radiographic visualization of the epidural space following the introduction of a radiopaque contrast medium.

ep·i·es·tri·ol (ĕp′ē-ĕs′trī-ôl′, -ōl′, -ĕ-strī′-) *n.* An epimer of estriol found in urine, bile, and the placenta.

ep·i·gas·tral·gia (ĕp′ĭ-gă-străl′jə) *n.* Pain in the epigastric region.

epigastric artery *n.* **1.** An artery with its origin in the external iliac artery and with cremasteric, muscular, and pubic branches; inferior epigastric artery. **2.** An artery with origin in the femoral artery and with distribution to the inguinal glands and integument of the lower abdomen; superficial epigastric artery. **3.** An artery with origin in the medial terminal branch of the internal thoracic artery and with distribution to the abdominal muscles and integument and the falciform ligament; superior epigastric artery.

epigastric fossa *n.* The slight depression in the midline below the sternum. Also called *pit of the stomach.*

epigastric hernia *n.* A hernia through the linea alba above the navel.

ep·i·gas·tri·um (ĕp′ĭ-găs′trē-əm) *n.,* *pl.* **–tri·a** (-trē-ə) The highest of three median regions of the abdomen, lying above the umbilical region and between the hypochondriac regions. —**ep′i·gas′tric** (-trĭk) *adj.*

ep·i·gas·tro·cele (ĕp′ĭ-găs′trə-sēl′) *n.* A hernia located in the epigastric region.

ep·i·gen·e·sis (ĕp′ə-jĕn′ĭ-sĭs) *n.* The theory that an individual is developed by successive differentiation of an unstructured egg rather than by a simple enlarging of a preformed entity. —**ep′i·ge·net′ic** (-jə-nĕt′ĭk) *adj.*

epiglottic cartilage *n.* A thin lamina of elastic cartilage forming the central portion of the epiglottis.

epiglottic fold *n.* Any of the three folds of mucous membrane in the oral cavity that pass between the tongue and the epiglottis.

ep·i·glot·ti·dec·to·my (ĕp′ĭ-glŏt′ĭ-dĕk′tə-mē) *n.* Excision of all or a part of the epiglottis.

ep·i·glot·tis (ĕp′ĭ-glŏt′ĭs) *n.,* *pl.* **–glot·tis·es** *or* **–glot·ti·des** (-glŏt′ĭ-dēz′) The thin elastic cartilaginous structure located at the root of the tongue that folds over the glottis to prevent food and liquid from entering the trachea during the act of swallowing. —**ep′i·glot′tic** *adj.*

ep·i·glot·ti·tis (ĕp′ĭ-glŏ-tī′tĭs) *n.* Inflammation of the epiglottis. —**ep·i·glot·ti·di·tis** (-glŏt′i-dī′tĭs) *n.*

ep·i·ker·a·to·pha·ki·a (ĕp′ĭ-kĕr′ə-tō-fā′kē-ə) *n.* A surgical procedure that modifies optical refractive error through the addition of a donated cornea to the anterior surface of the faulty cornea.

ep·i·late (ĕp′ə-lāt′) *v.* To remove a hair from a part of the body by forcible extraction, electrolysis, or loosening at the root by chemical means.

ep·i·la·tion (ĕp′ə-lā′shən) *n.* The act or result of removing hair, as by mechanical or chemical means. Also called *depilation.*

e·pil·a·to·ry (ĭ-pĭl′ə-tôr′ē) *adj.* Of or relating to the removal of hair. —*n.* See **depilatory.**

ep·i·lem·ma (ĕp′ə-lĕm′ə) *n.* The connective tissue sheath covering a nerve fiber near its termination.

ep·i·lep·sy (ĕp′ə-lĕp′sē) *n.* Any of various neurological disorders characterized by sudden, recurring attacks of motor, sensory, or psychic malfunction with or without loss of consciousness or convulsive seizures. Also called *seizure disorder*.

ep·i·lep·tic (ĕp′ə-lĕp′tĭk) *n.* A person who has epilepsy. —*adj.* **1.** Affected with epilepsy. **2.** Of, relating to, or associated with epilepsy.

ep·i·lep·ti·form (ĕp′ə-lĕp′tə-fôrm′) *adj.* Epileptoid.

ep·i·lep·to·gen·ic (ĕp′ə-lĕp′tə-jĕn′ĭk) *or* **ep·i·lep·tog·e·nous** (ĕp′ə-lĕp-tŏj′ə-nəs) *adj.* Having the capacity to induce epilepsy.

epileptogenic zone *n.* A cortical region of the brain that, when stimulated, produces spontaneous seizure or aura.

ep·i·lep·toid (ĕp′ə-lĕp′toid′) *adj.* Resembling epilepsy or any of its symptoms.

ep·i·man·dib·u·lar (ĕp′ə-măn-dĭb′yə-lər) *adj.* Occurring on the lower jaw.

ep·i·men·or·rha·gia (ĕp′ə-mĕn′ə-rā′jə) *n.* Menstruation that is unusually prolonged and profuse.

ep·i·men·or·rhe·a (ĕp′ə-mĕn′ə-rē′ə) *n.* Unusually frequent menstruation.

ep·i·mer (ĕp′ə-mər) *n.* One of two molecules that differ only in the spatial arrangement around a single carbon atom.

e·pim·er·ase (ĭ-pĭm′ə-rās′, -rāz′) *n.* Any of a class of enzymes that catalyze changes to epimers.

ep·i·mere (ĕp′ə-mîr′) *n.* The dorsal portion of the mesoderm of a chordate embryo that forms skeletal muscles.

ep·i·mor·pho·sis (ĕp′ə-môr-fō′sĭs) *n.* Regeneration of a part of an organism by extensive cell proliferation and differentiation at the cut surface.

ep·i·mys·i·ot·o·my (ĕp′ə-mĭz′ē-ŏt′ə-mē, -mĭzh′ē-) *n.* Incision or sectioning of a muscle within its sheath.

ep·i·mys·i·um (ĕp′ə-mĭz′ē-əm, -mĭzh′ē-) *n., pl.* **–mys·i·a** (-mĭz′ē-ə, -mĭzh′-) The external sheath of connective tissue surrounding a muscle.

ep·i·neph·rine *or* **ep·i·neph·rin** (ĕp′ə-nĕf′rĭn) *n.* **1.** A catecholamine hormone of the adrenal medulla that is the most potent stimulant of the sympathetic nervous system, resulting in increased heart rate and force of contraction, vasoconstriction or vasodilation, relaxation of bronchiolar and intestinal smooth muscle, glycogenolysis, lipolysis, and other metabolic effects. Also called *adrenaline*. **2.** A white to brownish crystalline compound that is isolated from the adrenal glands of certain mammals or synthesized and is used in medicine as a heart stimulant, vasoconstrictor, and bronchial relaxant.

epinephrine reversal *n.* The fall in blood pressure produced by epinephrine following the administration of alpha-blockers.

ep·i·neph·ros (ĕp′ə-nĕf′rŏs′, -rəs) *n.* See **adrenal gland.**

ep·i·neu·ral (ĕp′ə-nŏor′əl) *adj.* Located or positioned on a neural arch of a vertebra.

ep·i·neu·ri·al (ĕp′ə-nŏor′ē-əl) *adj.* Of, relating to, or characteristic of the epineurium.

ep·i·neu·ri·um (ĕp′ə-nŏor′ē-əm) *n., pl.* **–neu·ri·a** (-nŏor′ē-ə) The thick sheath of connective tissue surrounding a nerve trunk.

ep·i·ot·ic center (ĕp′ē-ŏt′ĭk) *n.* The center of ossification that forms the mastoid process.

Ep·i·Pen (ĕp′ĭ-pĕn′) A trademark for a self-injection kit containing epinephrine, used intramuscularly for anaphylactic shock.

ep·i·phar·ynx (ĕp′ə-făr′ĭngks) *n.* See **nasopharynx.**

ep·i·phe·nom·e·non (ĕp′ə-fĭ-nŏm′ə-nŏn′) *n.* An additional condition or symptom occurring in the course of a disease that is not necessarily connected with the disease.

e·piph·o·ra (ĭ-pĭf′ər-ə) *n.* Watering of the eyes due to a blockage of the lacrimal ducts or the excessive secretion of tears.

epiphysial arrest *n.* Premature fusion between epiphysis and diaphysis of a bone.

epiphysial aseptic necrosis *n.* Aseptic necrosis of bony epiphyses that may be due to obstruction of normal blood supply.

epiphysial cartilage *n.* The disk of cartilage between the shaft and the epiphysis of a long bone during its growth. Also called *epiphysial plate*.

epiphysial line *n.* The line of junction of the epiphysis and diaphysis of a long bone where growth in length occurs.

epiphysial plate *n.* See **epiphysial cartilage.**

ep·i·phys·i·ol·y·sis (ĕp′ə-fĭz′ē-ŏl′ĭ-sĭs) *n.* The loosening or separation, either partial or complete, of an epiphysis from the shaft of a bone.

e·piph·y·sis (ĭ-pĭf′ĭ-sĭs) *n., pl.* **-ses** (-sēz′) **1.** The end of a long bone that is originally separated from the main bone by a layer of cartilage but that later becomes united to the main bone through ossification. **2.** See **pineal body.** —**ep′i·phys′i·al** (ĕp′ə-fĭz′ē-əl), **ep′·i·phys′e·al** (ĕp′ə-fĭz′ē-əl, -fə-sē′əl) *adj.*

e·piph·y·si·tis (ĭ-pĭf′ĭ-sī′tĭs) *n.* Inflammation of an epiphysis.

ep·i·pi·al (ĕp′ə-pī′əl, -pē′əl) *adj.* Located or positioned on the pia mater.

epiplo– *pref.* Omentum: *epiploic.*

ep·i·plo·ic (ĕp′ə-plō′ĭk) *adj.* Omental.

epiploic appendix *n.* Any of several small processes or sacs of peritoneum, generally distended with fat and projecting from the serous coat of the large intestine. Also called *epiploic appendage*.

epiploic foramen *n.* The passage below and behind the portal fissure of the liver, connecting the two sacs of the peritoneum.

e·pip·lo·on (ĭ-pĭp′lō-ŏn′) *n., pl.* **–lo·a** (-lō-ə) See **greater omentum.**

ep·i·scle·ra (ĕp′ĭ-sklîr′ə) *n.* The connective tissue layer between sclera and conjunctiva of the eye.

ep·i·scle·ral (ĕp′ĭ-sklîr′əl) *adj.* **1.** Situated on the sclera of the eye. **2.** Of or relating to the episclera.

episcleral artery *n.* Any of numerous small branches of the anterior ciliary arteries that perforate the sclera behind the cornea to supply the iris and ciliary body.

episcleral space *n.* The space between the sheath of eyeball and the sclera. Also called *Tenon's space*.

episcleral vein *n.* Any of a series of small venules in the sclera of the eye close to the corneal margin that empty into the anterior ciliary veins.

ep·i·scle·ri·tis (ĕp′ĭ-sklə-rī′tĭs) *n.* Inflammation of the episcleral tissue.

episio– *pref.* Vulva: *episiotomy.*

e·pis·i·o·per·i·ne·or·rha·phy (ĭ-pĭz′ē-ō-pĕr′ə-nē-ôr′ə-fē, ĭ-pē′zē-) *n.* Suture of the perineum and vulva.

e·pis·i·o·plas·ty (ĭ-pĭz′ē-ō-plăs′tē, ĭ-pē′zē-) *n.* Surgical repair of a defect of the vulva.

e·pis·i·or·rha·phy (ĭ-pĭz′ē-ôr′ə-fē, ĭ-pē′zē-) *n.* Suture of a lacerated vulva.

e·pis·i·o·ste·no·sis (ĭ-pĭz′ē-ō-stə-nō′sĭs, ĭ-pē′zē-) *n.* Contraction or narrowing of the vulvar orifice.

e·pis·i·ot·o·my (ĭ-pĭz′ē-ŏt′ə-mē, ĭ-pē′zē-) *n.* Incision of the perineum during childbirth to ease delivery.

ep·i·some (ĕp′ĭ-sōm′) *n.* A genetic particle within certain cells, especially bacterial cells, that can exist either autonomously in the cytoplasm or as part of a chromosome.

ep·i·spa·di·as (ĕp′ĭ-spā′dē-əs) *or* **ep·i·spa·di·a** (-dē-ə) *n.* A congenital defect in which the urethra opens on the upper penile surface. —**ep′i·spa′di·al** *adj.*

ep·i·sple·ni·tis (ĕp′ĭ-splə-nī′tĭs) *n.* An inflammation of the capsule of the spleen.

e·pis·ta·sis (ĭ-pĭs′tə-sĭs) *n., pl.* **-ses** (-sēz′) **1.** A film that forms over the surface of a urine specimen. **2.** An interaction between nonallelic genes, especially an interaction in which one gene suppresses the expression of another. **3.** The suppression of a bodily discharge or secretion. —**ep′i·stat′ic** (ĕp′ĭ-stăt′ĭk) *adj.*

ep·i·stax·is (ĕp′ĭ-stăk′sĭs) *n., pl.* **-stax·es** (-stăk′sēz′) A nosebleed.

ep·i·ster·nal (ĕp′ĭ-stûr′nəl) *adj.* **1.** Situated over or on the sternum. **2.** Of or relating to the episternum.

ep·i·ster·num (ĕp′ĭ-stûr′nəm) *n.* The broad upper segment of the sternum occasionally fused with the body of the sternum and forming the sternal angle. Also called *manubrium, presternum.*

ep·i·stro·phe·us (ĕp′ĭ-strō′fē-əs) *n.* See **axis** (sense 3).

ep·i·ten·din·e·um (ĕp′ĭ-tĕn-dĭn′ē-əm) *n.* The white fibrous sheath surrounding a tendon.

ep·i·thal·a·mus (ĕp′ə-thăl′ə-məs) *n.* A dorsal segment of the diencephalon containing the habenula and the pineal body.

ep·i·tha·lax·i·a (ĕp′ə-thə-lăk′sē-ə) *n.* The shedding of epithelial cells, especially those that line the intestine.

epithelial dystrophy *n.* Dystrophy of the cornea characterized by opacification of the central cornea and affecting primarily the epithelium and its basement membrane.

ep·i·the·li·al·i·za·tion (ĕp′ə-thē′lē-ə-lĭ-zā′shən) *or* **ep·i·the·li·za·tion** (-thē′lĭ-zā′shən) *n.* The process of covering a denuded surface with epithelium.

ep·i·the·li·al·ize (ĕp′ə-thē′lē-ə-līz′) *or* **ep·i·the·lize** (-thē′līz) *v.* To become covered with epithelial tissue, as of a wound.

epithelial lamina *n.* The layer of modified ependymal cells that forms the inner layer of the choroid tela, facing the ventricle.

epithelial pearl *n.* See **keratin pearl.**

epithelial plug *n.* A mass of epithelial cells temporarily occluding an embryonic opening, most commonly of the nostrils.

ep·i·the·li·oid (ĕp′ə-thē′lē-oid′) *adj.* Of or resembling epithelium.

epithelioid cell *n.* A nonepithelial cell, especially one derived from a macrophage, having characteristics resembling those of an epithelial cell, often found in granulomas associated with tuberculosis.

ep·i·the·li·o·lyt·ic (ĕp′ə-thē′lē-ō-lĭt′ĭk) *adj.* Having a destructive effect on epithelium.

ep·i·the·li·o·ma (ĕp′ə-thē′lē-ō′mə) *n., pl.* **-mas** *or* **-ma·ta** (-mə-tə) A benign or malignant tumor derived from epithelium.

epithelioma ad·e·noi·des cys·ti·cum (ăd′n-oi′dēz sĭs′tĭ-kəm) *n.* See **trichoepithelioma.**

epithelioma cu·nic·u·la·tum (kyōō-nĭk′yə-lā′təm) *n.* A rare form of verrucous carcinoma occurring on the sole of the foot and characterized by a slow-growing, usually nonmetastasizing, warty mass.

ep·i·the·li·o·ma·tous (ĕp′ə-thē′lē-ō′mə-təs) *adj.* Of or relating to an epithelioma.

ep·i·the·li·um (ĕp′ə-thē′lē-əm) *n., pl.* **-li·a** (-lē-ə) *or* **-li·ums** Membranous tissue composed of one or more layers of cells separated by very little intercellular substance and forming the covering of most internal and external surfaces of the body and its organs. —**ep′i·the′li·al** *adj.*

ep·i·the·li·za·tion (ĕp′ə-thē′lĭ-zā′shən) *n.* Variant of epithelialization.

ep·i·tope (ĕp′ĭ-tōp′) *n.* The surface portion of an antigen capable of eliciting an immune response and of combining with the antibody produced to counter that response.

ep·i·trich·i·um (ĕp′ĭ-trĭk′ē-əm) *n.* See **periderm.**

ep·i·tym·pan·ic (ĕp′ĭ-tĭm-păn′ĭk) *adj.* Situated above or located in the upper part of the tympanic cavity or membrane.

ep·i·tym·pa·num (ĕp′ĭ-tĭm′pə-nəm) *n.* See **attic.**

Ep·i·vir (ĕp′ĭ-vîr′) A trademark for the drug lamivudine.

ep·i·zo·ic (ĕp′ĭ-zō′ĭk) *adj.* Living or growing on the external surface of an animal.

ep·i·zo·ol·o·gy (ĕp′ĭ-zō-ŏl′ə-jē) *n.* Epizootiology.

ep·i·zo·on (ĕp′ĭ-zō′ŏn, -ən) *n., pl.* **-zo·a** (-zō′ə) An epizoic organism.

ep·i·zo·ot·ic (ĕp′ĭ-zō-ŏt′ĭk) *adj.* Affecting a large number of animals at the same time within a particular region or geographic area. Used of a disease. —**ep′i·zo·ot′ic** *n.*

ep·i·zo·ot·i·ol·o·gy (ĕp′ĭ-zō-ŏt′ē-ŏl′ə-jē) *n.* **1.** The science dealing with the character, ecology, and causes of diseases in animals, especially epizootic diseases. **2.** The sum of the factors controlling the presence of a disease in an animal population.

e·pler·e·none (əp-lâr′ə-nōn′) *n.* A drug that blocks aldosterone receptors and is used for the treatment of hypertension and congestive heart failure.

e·po·e·tin al·fa (ĭ-pō′ĭ-tĭn ăl′fə) *n.* A recombinant preparation of human erythropoietin used to treat some forms of anemia.

E·po·gen (ē′pə-jən) A trademark for the drug epoetin alfa.

ep·o·nych·i·a (ĕp′ə-nĭk′ē-ə) *n.* An infection affecting the proximal nail fold.

ep·o·nych·i·um (ĕp′ə-nĭk′ē-əm) *n.* **1.** The condensed eleidin-rich areas of the epidermis preceding the formation of nails in the embryo. **2.** The thin skin adhering to the nail at its base.

ep·o·nym (ĕp′ə-nĭm′) *n.* A name of a drug, structure, or disease based on or derived from the name of a person. —**ep′o·nym′ic** *adj.*

ep·o·o·pho·rec·to·my (ĕp′ō-ə-fə-rĕk′tə-mē) *n.* Surgical removal of the epoophoron.

ep·o·oph·o·ron (ĕp′ō-ŏf′ə-rŏn′) *n.* Any of the rudimentary tubules in the mesosalpinx between the ovary and the uterine tube.

ep·ox·y (ĭ-pŏk′sē) *n.* Any of various usually thermosetting resins capable of forming tight cross-linked polymer structures characterized by toughness, strong adhesion, and low shrinkage, used especially in surface coatings and adhesives. —*adj.* Containing an oxygen atom bound to two different atoms linked in some other way, especially a compound containing a ring formed by one oxygen atom and two carbon atoms.

ep·ro·sar·tan mesylate (ĕp′rō-sär′tăn) *n.* An angiotensin II receptor antagonist that is used to treat hypertension.

EPS *abbr.* extrapyramidal symptoms

ep·si·lon (ĕp′sə-lŏn′, -lən) *n.* **1.** *Symbol* ε The fifth letter of the Greek alphabet. **2.** The fifth in a series. —*adj.* **1.** Of or relating to the fifth member of a particular ordered set. **2.** Relating to or characterizing a polypeptide chain that is one of five types of heavy chains present in immunoglobins.

Ep·som salts (ĕp′səm) *pl.n.* Hydrated magnesium sulfate, used as a cathartic and as an agent to reduce inflammation.

Ep·stein-Barr virus (ĕp′stīn-) *n. Abbr.* **EBV** A herpesvirus that is the causative agent of infectious mononucleosis. It is also associated with various types of human cancers. Also called *EB virus.*

Ep·stein's pearls (ĕp′stīnz′) *pl.n.* Multiple small white epithelial inclusion cysts found in the midline of the palate in most newborns.

e·pu·lis (ĭ-pyōō′lĭs) *n.* Inflammatory cellular proliferation or a tumorlike growth of the gum that may be present at birth. —**ep′u·loid′** (ĕp′yə-loid′) *adj.*

e·qua·tion (ĭ-kwā′zhən) *n.* **1.** A statement asserting the equality of two mathematical expressions, usually written as a linear array of symbols that are separated into left and right sides and are joined by an equal sign. **2.** A representation of a chemical reaction, usually written as a linear array in which the symbols and quantities of the reactants are separated from those of the products by an equal sign, arrow, or set of opposing arrows.

equation division *n.* Nuclear division in which each chromosome divides into equal longitudinal halves.

e·qua·to·ri·al plane (ē′kwə-tôr′ē-əl, ĕk′wə-) *n.* The plane that contains all of the centromeres and their spindle attachments during metaphase of mitosis.

equatorial plate *n.* The plane located midway between the poles of a dividing cell during miotic metaphase and touching the centromeres and their spindle attachments.

equatorial staphyloma *n.* A staphyloma occurring in the area of exit of the vortex veins of the eyeball. Also called *scleral staphyloma.*

e·qui·ax·i·al (ē′kwē-ăk′sē-əl) *adj.* Having axes of equal length.

e·quil·i·bra·tion (ĭ-kwĭl′ə-brā′shən) *n.* **1.** The development or maintenance of an equilibrium. **2.** The process of exposing a liquid to a gas that is at a certain partial pressure until the partial pressures of the gas inside and outside the liquid are equal.

e·qui·lib·ri·um (ē′kwə-lĭb′rē-əm, ĕk′wə-) *n.* **1.** A condition in which all influences acting upon it are canceled by others, resulting in a stable, balanced, or unchanging system. **2.** The state of a chemical reaction in which its forward and reverse reactions occur at equal rates so that the concentration of the reactants and products does not change with time. Also called *dynamic equilibrium.* **3.** Mental or emotional balance.

equilibrium dialysis *n.* A method for determining the association constants for hapten-antibody reactions, by placing hapten and antibody in compartments separated by a semipermeable membrane, thereby allowing hapten to diffuse across the membrane until its concentration reaches equilibrium.

e·quine (ē′kwīn′, ĕk′wīn′) *adj.* **1.** Of, relating to, or characteristic of a horse. **2.** Of or belonging to the family Equidae, which includes the horses, asses, and zebras.

eq·ui·no·val·gus (ĕk′wə-nō-văl′gəs, ĭ-kwī′nō-) *n.* Talipes equinovalgus.

eq·ui·no·var·us (ĕk′wə-nō-vâr′əs, ĭ-kwī′nō-) *n.* Talipes equinovarus.

e·qui·tox·ic (ē′kwĭ-tŏk′sĭk, ĕk′wĭ-) *adj.* Having equal toxicity.

e·quiv·a·lent (ĭ-kwĭv′ə-lənt) *adj.* Equal, as in value, force, or meaning.

Er The symbol for the element **erbium.**

ER *abbr.* emergency room; endoplasmic reticulum

Er·a·sis·tra·tus (ĕr′ə-sĭs′trə-təs) fl. c. 250 BC. Greek physician and anatomist. Through observation and dissection he advanced the understanding of the brain, heart, and motor and sensory nerves.

ERBF *abbr.* effective renal blood flow

er·bi·um (ûr′bē-əm) *n. Symbol* **Er** A soft rare-earth element, used in metallurgy and nuclear research. Atomic number 68.

Erb's disease (ûrbz, ĕrps) *n.* See **progressive bulbar paralysis.**

Erb's palsy *n.* Birth palsy in which there is paralysis of the muscles of the upper arm due to a lesion of the brachial plexus or the roots of the fifth and sixth cervical nerves. Also called *Duchenne-Erb paralysis.*

Erb's sign *n.* **1.** An indication of tetany in which the electric excitability of the muscles increases. **2.** See **Erb-Westphal sign.**

Erb-Westphal sign *n.* An indication of tabes and certain other spinal cord diseases and, occasionally, of brain disease in which the patellar tendon reflex is absent. Also called *Erb's sign, Westphal-Erb sign, Westphal's sign.*

ERCP *abbr.* endoscopic retrograde cholangiopancreatography

e·rect (ĭ-rĕkt′) *adj.* **1.** Being in or having a vertical, upright position. **2.** Being in or having a stiff, rigid physiological condition.

e·rec·tile (ĭ-rĕk′təl, -tīl′) *adj.* **1.** Of or relating to tissue capable of filling with blood and becoming rigid. **2.** Capable of being raised to an upright position.

erectile dysfunction *n. Abbr.* **ED** The inability to achieve penile erection or to maintain an erection until ejaculation. Also called *impotence.*

erectile tissue *n.* Tissue with numerous vascular spaces that may become engorged with blood.

e·rec·tion (ĭ-rĕk′shən) *n*. **1.** The firm and enlarged condition of a body organ or part when the erectile tissue surrounding it becomes filled with blood, especially such a condition of the penis or clitoris. **2.** The process of filling with blood.

e·rec·tor (ĭ-rĕk′tər) *n*. A muscle that makes a body part erect. Also called *arrector*.

erector muscle of hair *n*. Any of the bundles of smooth muscle fibers, attached to the deep part of hair follicles, passing outward alongside the sebaceous glands to the papillary layer of the corium, whose action erects hairs.

erector muscle of spine *n*. A muscle with origin from the sacrum, ilium, and spines of the lumbar vertebrae, dividing into three columns that insert into the ribs and vertebrae, with nerve supply from the posterior branches of the spinal nerves, and whose action extends the vertebral column.

e·rep·sin (ĭ-rĕp′sən) *n*. An enzyme complex found in intestinal and pancreatic juices that functions in the breakdown of polypeptides into amino acids.

er·e·thism (ĕr′ə-thĭz′əm) *n*. Abnormal irritability or sensitivity of an organ or body part to stimulation.

erg (ûrg) *n*. The centimeter-gram-second unit of energy or work equal to the work done by a force of one dyne acting over a distance of one centimeter.

ERG *abbr*. electroretinogram

er·ga·sia (ûr-gā′zhə) *n*. The sum of the mental, behavioral, and physiological functions and reactions that make up an individual.

er·gas·to·plasm (ûr-găs′tə-plăz′əm) *n*. See **granular endoplasmic reticulum**.

ergo– *pref*. Work: *ergometer*.

er·go·cal·cif·er·ol (ûr′gō-kăl-sĭf′ə-rôl′, -rōl′) *n*. See **vitamin D₂**.

er·go·graph (ûr′gə-grăf′) *n*. A device for measuring the work capacity of a muscle or group of muscles during contraction. —**er′go·graph′ic** *adj*.

er·gom·e·ter (ûr-gŏm′ĭ-tər) *n*. See **dynamometer**.

er·go·nom·ics (ûr′gə-nŏm′ĭks) *n*. The applied science of equipment design, as for the workplace, intended to maximize productivity by reducing operator fatigue and discomfort.

er·gos·ter·ol (ûr-gŏs′tə-rôl′, -rōl′) *n*. A crystalline sterol synthesized by yeast from sugars or derived from ergot and converted to vitamin D₂ when exposed to ultraviolet radiation.

er·got (ûr′gət, -gŏt′) *n*. **1.** A fungus that infects various cereal plants and forms compact black masses of branching filaments that replace many of the grains of the host plant. **2.** The dried sclerotia of ergot, usually obtained from rye seed and used as a source of several medicinally important alkaloids and as the basic source of lysergic acid.

er·got·a·mine (ûr-gŏt′ə-mēn′, -mĭn) *n*. A crystalline alkaloid derived from ergot that induces vasoconstriction and is used especially in treating migraine.

er·got·ism (ûr′gə-tĭz′əm) *n*. Poisoning caused by consuming ergot-infected grain or grain products, or from excessive use of drugs containing ergot.

Er·lang·er (ûr′lăng′ər), **Joseph** 1874–1965. American physiologist. He shared a 1944 Nobel Prize for developing methods of recording electrical nerve impulses and for his studies on synaptic function.

e·rode (ĭ-rōd′) *v*. **1.** To wear away by or as if by abrasion. **2.** To eat into; ulcerate.

e·rog·e·nous (ĭ-rŏj′ə-nəs) *adj*. **1.** Responsive or sensitive to sexual stimulation, as of particular body parts. **2.** Arousing sexual desire.

erogenous zone *n*. A part of the body that excites sexual feelings when touched or stimulated. Also called *erotogenic zone*.

E·ros or **e·ros** (ĕr′ŏs, îr′-) *n*. **1.** In psychoanalytic theory, the sum of all instincts for self-preservation. **2.** Sexual drive; libido.

E-rosette test *n*. A test to identify T cells by mixing purified human blood lymphocytes with serum and sheep red blood cells; rosettes of red blood cells form around human T cells on incubation.

e·ro·sion (ĭ-rō′zhən) *n*. **1.** Superficial destruction of a surface by friction, pressure, ulceration, or trauma. **2.** The wearing away of a tooth by chemical or abrasive action. Also called *odontolysis*.

e·ro·sive (ĭ-rō′sĭv) *adj*. Causing erosion.

e·rot·ic (ĭ-rŏt′ĭk) *adj*. **1.** Of or concerning sexual love and desire. **2.** Tending to arouse sexual desire. **3.** Dominated by sexual love or desire.

e·rot·i·cism (ĭ-rŏt′ĭ-sĭz′əm) *n*. Sexual excitement.

er·o·tism (ĕr′ə-tĭz′əm) *n*. Eroticism.

e·ro·to·gen·ic (ĭ-rō′tə-jĕn′ĭk, ĭ-rŏt′ə-) *adj*. Causing sexual excitement.

erotogenic zone *n*. See **erogenous zone**.

e·ro·to·ma·ni·a (ĭ-rō′tə-mā′nē-ə, ĭ-rŏt′ə-) *n*. Excessive sexual desire.

er·o·top·a·thy (ĕr′ə-tŏp′ə-thē) *n*. An abnormality of sexual desire. —**e·ro′to·path′ic** (ĭ-rō′tə-păth′ĭk, ĭ-rŏt′ə-) *adj*.

e·ro·to·pho·bi·a (ĭ-rō′tə-fō′bē-ə, ĭ-rŏt′ə-) *n*. An abnormal fear of love, especially sexual feelings and their physical expression.

ERPF *abbr*. effective renal plasma flow

er·rhine (ĕr′īn′) *adj*. Promoting or inducing nasal discharge. —*n*. A medication that promotes or induces such discharge.

er·ror (ĕr′ər) *n*. **1.** A defect or insufficiency in structure or function. **2.** An act, assertion, or decision, especially one made in testing a hypothesis, that unintentionally deviates from what is correct, right, or true.

ERT *abbr*. estrogen replacement therapy

e·ruc·ta·tion (ĭ-rŭk-tā′shən, ē′rŭk-) *n*. The act or an instance of belching.

e·rupt (ĭ-rŭpt′) *v*. **1.** To break through the gums in developing. Used of teeth. **2.** To appear on the skin. Used of a rash or blemish.

e·rup·tion (ĭ-rŭp′shən) *n*. **1.** An appearance of a rash or blemish on the skin. **2.** Such a rash or blemish. **3.** The emergence of a tooth through the gums. —**e·rup′tive** (-tĭv) *adj*.

eruptive xanthoma *n*. A condition affecting individuals with severe hyperlipemia in which groups of waxy yellow or yellowish-brown lesions appear suddenly, especially over extensors of the elbows and knees and on the back and buttocks.

ERV *abbr*. expiratory reserve volume

er·y·sip·e·las (ĕr'ĭ-sĭp'ə-ləs, îr'-) *n.* An acute disease of the skin and subcutaneous tissue caused by a hemolytic bacterium and marked by localized inflammation and fever. Also called *Saint Anthony's fire.* —**er'y·si·pel'a·tous** (-sĭ-pĕl'ə-təs) *adj.*

er·y·sip·e·loid (ĕr'ĭ-sĭp'ə-loid', îr'-) *n.* An infectious disease of the skin that is contracted by handling fish or meat infected with the bacterium *Erysipelothrix rhusiopathiae* and characterized by red lesions on the hands.

Er·y·sip·e·lo·thrix (ĕr'ĭ-sĭp'ə-lō-thrĭks', -sə-pĕl'ə-, îr'-) *n.* A genus of gram-positive rod-shaped bacteria that are parasitic on mammals, birds, and fish; it includes the causative agent of erysipeloid.

er·y·the·ma (ĕr'ə-thē'mə) *n.* Redness of the skin caused by dilatation and congestion of the capillaries, often a sign of inflammation or infection. —**er'y·them'a·tous** (-thĕm'ə-təs, -thē'mə-) *adj.*

erythema ab ig·ne (ăb ĭg'nē) *n.* See **erythema caloricum.**

erythema an·nu·lar·e (ăn'yə-lâr'ē) *n.* Erythema characterized by ringed or rounded lesions.

erythema annulare cen·trif·u·gum (sĕn-trĭf'yə-gəm) *n.* A chronic recurring erythematous eruption consisting of small and large annular lesions that can be distinct from each other or joined together.

erythema ar·thrit·i·cum ep·i·dem·i·cum (är-thrĭt'ĭ-kəm ĕp'ĭ-dĕm'ĭ-kəm) *n.* See **Haverhill fever.**

erythema ca·lo·ri·cum (kə-lôr'ĭ-kəm) *n.* A fine network of pigmented spots or patches that occur primarily on the shins as a result of exposure to radiant heat. Also called *erythema ab igne.*

erythema chron·i·cum mi·grans (krŏn'ĭ-kəm mī'grănz') *n.* A raised erythematous ring on the skin having hard borders and a central clearing, and radiating from the site of an insect bite; it is the characteristic lesion of Lyme disease.

erythema dose *n.* The minimum amount of x-rays or other form of radiation sufficient to produce redness of the skin after application, regarded as the dose that is safe to give at one time.

erythema in·du·ra·tum (ĭn'də-rā'təm) *n.* A chronic disorder characterized by recurrent hard subcutaneous nodules that frequently form necrotic ulcers, usually on the calves and less frequently on the thighs or arms of women. Also called *Bazin's disease, tuberculosis cutis indurativa.*

erythema in·fec·ti·o·sum (ĭn-fĕk'shē-ō'səm) *n.* A mild infectious disease occurring mainly in early childhood, marked by a rosy-red maculopapular rash on the cheeks, often spreading to the trunk and limbs. Fever and arthritis may also be present. Also called *fifth disease.*

erythema i·ris (ī'rĭs) *n.* The erythematous concentric lesion that is characteristic of erythema multiforme. Also called *herpes iris.*

erythema mar·gi·na·tum (mär'jə-nā'təm) *n.* A form of erythema multiforme in which elevated defined bands remain after erythematous patches have cleared; it occurs in rheumatic fever.

erythema mi·grans lin·guae (mī'grănz' lĭng'gwē) *or* **erythema migrans** *n.* See **geographical tongue.**

erythema mul·ti·for·me (mŭl'tə-fôr'mē) *n.* A skin disease associated with allergies, seasonal changes, or drug sensitivities, and characterized by the acute eruption of red macules, papules, or subdermal vesicles on the skin and mucous membranes; the characteristic lesion consists of a papule surrounded by a concentric ring. Also called *herpes iris.*

erythema no·do·sum (nō-dō'səm) *n.* A skin disease associated with joint pain, fever, hypersensitivity, or infection, and characterized by small, painful, pink to blue nodules under the skin and on the shins that tend to recur.

erythema nodosum le·pro·sum (lĕ-prō'səm) *n.* An acute lepromatous reaction with generalized systemic involvement characterized by the formation of painful deep nodules on the face, thighs, and arms, usually seen in undiagnosed, untreated, or neglected cases of leprosy.

erythema per·ni·o (pûr'nē-ō) *n.* See **chilblain.**

er·y·the·ma·to·ve·sic·u·lar (ĕr'ə-thē'mə-tō-vĕ-sĭk'yə-lər, -və-, -thĕm'ə-) *adj.* Relating to or characterized by edema, erythema, and vesiculation, as in allergic contact dermatitis.

erythema tox·i·cum (tŏk'sĭ-kəm) *n.* A skin condition caused by reaction to a toxic and characterized by a widespread erythmatous eruption.

erythema toxicum ne·o·na·to·rum (nē'ō-nā-tôr'əm) *n.* A common temporary eruption of erythema, small papules, and occasionally pustules in newborns, associated with contact dermatitis or hypersensitivity to milk or other allergens.

er·y·thor·bic acid (ĕr'ə-thôr'bĭk) *n.* An optical isomer of ascorbic acid used as an antioxidant.

er·y·thral·gia (ĕr'ə-thrăl'jə) *n.* A mottled reddening of the skin that is usually accompanied by throbbing pain.

er·y·thras·ma (ĕr'ə-thrăz'mə) *n.* A bacterial skin infection characterized by reddish brown, slightly raised patches, especially in the armpits and groin.

e·ryth·re·de·ma (ĭ-rĭth'rĭ-dē'mə) *n.* See **acrodynia** (sense 1).

er·y·thre·mi·a (ĕr'ə-thrē'mē-ə) *n.* A chronic form of polycythemia of unknown cause, characterized by an increase in blood volume and red blood cells, bone marrow hyperplasia, redness or cyanosis of the skin, and enlargement of the spleen. Also called *Osler's disease, Osler-Vaquez disease, polycythemia rubra, polycythemia vera, Vaquez disease.*

er·y·threm·ic myelosis (ĕr'ə-thrĕm'ĭk, -thrē'mĭk) *n.* A neoplastic process involving the erythropoietic tissue, characterized by anemia, irregular fever, splenomegaly, hepatomegaly, hemorrhagic disorders, and the presence of numerous erythroblasts in all stages of maturation in the circulating blood.

er·y·thrism (ĕr'ə-thrĭz'əm) *n.* Redness of the hair with a ruddy freckled complexion. —**er'y·thris'tic** (-thrĭs'tĭk) *adj.*

erythro- *or* **erythr-** *pref.* 1. Red: *erythroid.* 2. Erythrocyte: *erythropoiesis.*

e·ryth·ro·blast (ĭ-rĭth'rə-blăst') *n.* Any of the nucleated cells normally found in bone marrow that develop into red blood cells. —**e·ryth'ro·blast'ic** *adj.*

e·ryth·ro·blas·te·mi·a (ĭ-rĭth′rō-blă-stē′mē-ə) *n.* The presence of an abnormal number of erythroblasts in the blood.

e·ryth·ro·blas·to·pe·ni·a (ĭ-rĭth′rō-blăs′tə-pē′nē-ə) *n.* A decrease in the number of erythroblasts in bone marrow, as seen in aplastic anemia.

e·ryth·ro·blas·to·sis (ĭ-rĭth′rō-blă-stō′sĭs) *n., pl.* **–ses** (-sēz) The abnormal presence of erythroblasts in the blood.

erythroblastosis fe·ta·lis (fē-tā′lĭs) *n.* A severe hemolytic disease of a fetus or newborn caused by production of maternal antibodies for fetal red blood cells, usually involving Rh incompatibility between the mother and fetus. Also called *ABO hemolytic disease of newborn, congenital anemia, hemolytic disease of newborn, neonatal anemia, RH disease.*

e·ryth·ro·blas·tot·ic (ĭ-rĭth′rō-blă-stŏt′ĭk) *adj.* Relating to erythroblastosis, especially erythroblastosis fetalis.

er·y·throc·la·sis (ĕr′ə-thrŏk′lə-sĭs) *n.* The fragmentation or breaking down of red blood cells.

e·ryth·ro·clas·tic (ĭ-rĭth′rō-klăs′tĭk) *adj.* Destructive to red blood cells.

e·ryth·ro·cy·a·no·sis (ĭ-rĭth′rō-sī′ə-nō′sĭs) *n.* A condition caused by exposure to cold and characterized by swelling of the limbs and the appearance of irregular red-blue patches on the skin, occurring especially in girls and women.

e·ryth·ro·cyte (ĭ-rĭth′rə-sīt′) *n.* See **red blood cell.** —**e·ryth′ro·cyt′ic** (-sĭt′ĭk) *adj.*

erythrocyte fragility test *n.* See **fragility test.**

erythrocyte indices *pl.n.* Calculations for determining the average size, hemoglobin content, and concentration of red blood cells, including mean cell volume, mean cell hemoglobin, and mean cell hemoglobin concentration.

erythrocyte sedimentation rate *n. Abbr.* **ESR** See **sedimentation rate.**

e·ryth·ro·cy·the·mi·a (ĭ-rĭth′rō-sī-thē′mē-ə) *n.* See **polycythemia.**

erythrocytic series *n.* The cells in various stages of hemopoiesis in red bone marrow.

e·ryth·ro·cy·tol·y·sin (ĭ-rĭth′rō-sī-tŏl′ĭ-sĭn) *n.* See **hemolysin.**

e·ryth·ro·cy·tol·y·sis (ĭ-rĭth′rō-sī-tŏl′ĭ-sĭs) *n.* See **hemolysis.**

e·ryth·ro·cy·tor·rhex·is (ĭ-rĭth′rō-sī′tə-rĕk′sĭs) *n.* The rupture of red blood cells causing the escape of particles of protoplasm. Also called *erythrorrhexis.*

e·ryth·ro·cy·tos·chi·sis (ĭ-rĭth′rō-sī-tŏs′kĭ-sĭs) *n.* The fragmentation or breaking up of red blood cells into small particles that contain hemoglobin but that morphologically resemble platelets.

e·ryth·ro·cy·to·sis (ĭ-rĭth′rō-sī-tō′sĭs) *n.* An abnormal increase in the number of circulating red blood cells.

e·ryth·ro·de·gen·er·a·tive (ĭ-rĭth′rō-dĭ-jĕn′ər-ə-tĭv) *adj.* Relating to or characterized by degeneration of red blood cells.

e·ryth·ro·der·ma (ĭ-rĭth′rō-dûr′mə) *n.* A skin disease characterized by intense, widespread reddening of the skin, often preceding or associated with exfoliation. Also called *erythrodermatitis.*

erythroderma des·qua·ma·ti·vum (dĕ-skwā′mə-tī′-vəm) *n.* Severe seborrheic dermatitis and erythroderma in newborns or young malnourished children. Also called *Leiner's disease.*

erythroderma pso·ri·at·i·cum (sôr′ē-ăt′ĭ-kəm) *n.* Dermatitis characterized by exfoliation and inflammation similar to that occurring in psoriasis.

e·ryth·ro·der·ma·ti·tis (ĭ-rĭth′rō-dûr′mə-tī′tĭs) *n.* See **erythroderma.**

e·ryth·ro·don·tia (ĭ-rĭth′rō-dŏn′shə) *n.* A reddish or reddish-brown discoloration of the teeth.

e·ryth·ro·dys·es·the·sia syndrome (ĭ-rĭth′rō-dĭs′ĭs-thē′zhə) *n.* A condition caused by continuous infusion therapy and resulting in a tingling sensation of the palms and soles, progressing to severe pain and tenderness with erythema and edema.

e·ryth·ro·gen·e·sis im·per·fec·ta (ĭ-rĭth′rō-jĕn′ĭ-sĭs ĭm′pər-fĕk′tə) *n.* See **congenital hypoplastic anemia.**

e·ryth·ro·gen·ic (ĭ-rĭth′rō-jĕn′ĭk) *adj.* **1.** Inducing a rash or reddening of the skin. **2.** Producing a sensation of the color red. **3.** Relating to the formation of red blood cells.

erythrogenic toxin *n.* See **streptococcus erythrogenic toxin.**

er·y·throid (ĕr′ə-throid′, ĭ-rĭth′roid′) *adj.* **1.** Having a red color, especially of erythrocytes; reddish. **2.** Of or relating to a red blood cell or one of its developmental precursors.

e·ryth·ro·ker·a·to·der·ma (ĭ-rĭth′rō-kĕr′ə-tō-dûr′mə) *n.* A skin condition in which papules and scaly skin form as a result of injury.

erythrokeratoderma var·i·a·bi·lis (văr′ē-ā′bə-lĭs) *n.* A hereditary skin disease characterized by tough, scaly plaques associated with erythroderma that may vary daily in size, shape, and position.

e·ryth·ro·ki·net·ics (ĭ-rĭth′rō-kə-nĕt′ĭks, -kī-) *n.* A study of the kinetics of red blood cells from their generation to destruction.

e·ryth·ro·leu·ke·mi·a (ĭ-rĭth′rō-lōō-kē′mē-ə) *n.* A malignant disorder characterized by the proliferation of erythroblastic and leukoblastic tissues.

e·ryth·ro·leu·ko·sis (ĭ-rĭth′rō-lōō-kō′sĭs) *n.* A condition resembling leukemia that affects both erythroblastic and leukoblastic tissues.

er·y·throl·y·sin (ĕr′ə-thrŏl′ĭ-sĭn) *n.* See **hemolysin.**

er·y·throl·y·sis (ĕr′ə-thrŏl′ĭ-sĭs) *n.* See **hemolysis.**

e·ryth·ro·me·lal·gia (ĭ-rĭth′rō-mə-lăl′jə) *n.* Paroxysmal throbbing and burning pain in the skin, affecting one or both legs and feet, sometimes one or both hands, accompanied by a dusky mottled redness of the parts and associated with polycythemia vera, thrombocytemia, gout, neurological disease, or heavy-metal poisoning. Also called *Mitchell's disease, red neuralgia.*

e·ryth·ro·my·cin (ĭ-rĭth′rə-mī′sĭn) *n.* An antibiotic obtained from a strain of *Streptomyces erythreus,* effective against many gram-positive bacteria and some gram-negative bacteria.

er·y·thron (ĕr′ə-thrŏn′) *n.* The total mass of circulating red blood cells, their precursors, and the tissues that produce them.

e·ryth·ro·ne·o·cy·to·sis (ĭ-rĭth′rō-nē′ō-sī-tō′sĭs) *n.*

The presence of regenerative forms of red blood cells in the blood.

e·ryth·ro·pe·ni·a (ĭ-rĭth′rō-pē′nē-ə) *n.* A deficiency in the number of red blood cells.

e·ryth·ro·pha·gia (ĭ-rĭth′rō-fā′jə) *n.* The destruction of red blood cells by cells such as macrophages.

e·ryth·ro·phag·o·cy·to·sis (ĭ-rĭth′rō-făg′ə-sī-tō′sĭs) *n.* The ingestion of red blood cells by a macrophage or other phagocyte.

e·ryth·ro·phil (ĭ-rĭth′rə-fĭl) *adj.* Erythrophilic. —*n.* A cell or tissue that stains red.

e·ryth·ro·phil·ic (ĭ-rĭth′rə-fĭl′ĭk) *adj.* Having an affinity for a red stain or dye.

e·ryth·ro·pla·ki·a (ĭ-rĭth′rō-plā′kē-ə) *n.* A red, velvety, plaquelike lesion of the mucous membrane, the formation of which often indicates a precancerous condition.

e·ryth·ro·pla·sia (ĭ-rĭth′rō-plā′zhə) *n.* Erythema and dysplasia of the epithelium.

erythroplasia of Quey·rat (kā-rä′) *n.* Carcinoma of the glans penis.

e·ryth·ro·poi·e·sis (ĭ-rĭth′rō-poi-ē′sĭs) *n.* The formation or production of red blood cells. —**e·ryth′ro·poi·et′ic** (-ĕt′ĭk) *adj.*

erythropoietic porphyria *n.* A category of porphyria that includes congenital erythropoietic porphyria and erythropoietic protoporphyria.

erythropoietic protoporphyria *n.* A benign inherited disorder of porphyrin metabolism characterized by enhanced fecal excretion of protoporphyrin and elevated concentration of protoporphyrin in red blood cells, plasma, and feces, with acute solar urticaria or chronic solar eczema appearing quickly upon exposure to sunlight.

e·ryth·ro·poi·e·tin (ĭ-rĭth′rō-poi-ē′tĭn) *n.* **1.** A glycoprotein hormone that stimulates the production of red blood cells by bone marrow. **2.** Epoetin alfa.

e·ryth·ro·pros·o·pal·gia (ĭ-rĭth′rō-prŏs′ə-păl′jə) *n.* See **cluster headache.**

er·y·throp·si·a (ĕr′ə-thrŏp′sē-ə) *n.* A vision abnormality in which all objects appear reddish.

e·ryth·ror·rhex·is (ĭ-rĭth′rə-rĕk′sĭs) *n.* See **erythrocytorrhexis.**

er·y·thru·ri·a (ĕr′ə-throͦor′ē-ə) *n.* The passage of red urine.

Es The symbol for the element **einsteinium.**

es·cape (ĭ-skāp′) *n.* **1.** A gradual effusion from an enclosure; a leakage. **2.** A cardiological situation in which one pacemaker defaults or an atrioventricular conduction fails, and another pacemaker sets the heart's pace for one or more beats.

escape beat *n.* An automatic beat, usually arising from the atrioventricular node or ventricle, but occurring after an expected normal beat has defaulted.

es·caped ventricular contraction (ĭ-skāpt′) *n.* A heartbeat following an abnormally long pause, caused by an impulse in the ventricle.

escape rhythm *n.* Three or more consecutive impulses occurring at a rate that does not exceed the upper limit of the inherent pacemaker of the heart.

es·cap·ism (ĭ-skā′pĭz′əm) *n.* The tendency to escape from daily reality or routine by indulging in daydreaming, fantasy, or entertainment.

es·char (ĕs′kär′) *n.* A dry scab or slough formed on the skin as a result of a burn or by the action of a corrosive or caustic substance.

es·cha·rot·ic (ĕs′kə-rŏt′ĭk) *n.* A caustic or corrosive substance or drug. —*adj.* Producing an eschar.

es·cha·rot·o·my (ĕs′kə-rŏt′ə-mē) *n.* Incision into a burn eschar in order to lessen its pull on the surrounding tissue.

Esch·e·rich·i·a (ĕsh′ə-rĭk′ē-ə) *n.* A genus of aerobic, gram-negative, rod-shaped bacteria widely found in nature; one species, *Escherichia coli*, which normally occurs in human and animal intestines, can cause urogenital tract infections and diarrhea in infants and adults.

es·ci·tal·o·pram oxalate (ĕs′ĭ-tăl′ō-prăm′) *n.* A drug of the SSRI class that is an isomer of citalopram and is used primarily to treat depression.

–esis *suff.* Condition, action, or process: *centesis.*

Es·ka·lith (ĕs′kə-lĭth′) A trademark for a drug containing lithium carbonate.

es·mo·lol hydrochloride (ĕs′mə-lôl′) *n.* A beta-blocker used to treat certain types of tachycardia.

es·o·eth·moi·di·tis (ĕs′ō-ĕth′moi-dī′tĭs) *n.* Inflammation of the lining membrane of the ethmoid sinuses.

es·o·gas·tri·tis (ĕs′ō-gă-strī′tĭs) *n.* Inflammation of the mucous membrane of the stomach.

es·o·mep·ra·zole magnesium (ē′sō-mĕp′rə-zōl′, ĕs′-ō-) *n.* A drug of the proton pump inhibitor class.

e·soph·a·gal·gia (ĭ-sŏf′ə-găl′jə) *n.* Pain in the esophagus. Also called *esophagodynia.*

esophageal achalasia *n.* An esophageal obstruction that develops due to failure of the esophagogastric sphincter to relax, causing the upper esophagus to fill with retained food. Also called *cardiospasm.*

esophageal lead (lēd) *n.* **1.** A lead of an electrocardiograph that has an electrode inserted into the esophagus. **2.** A record that is obtained from such a lead.

esophageal reflux *n.* See **gastroesophageal reflux.**

esophageal speech *n.* A technique for speaking after total laryngectomy involving the swallowing of air and its subsequent expulsion to produce a vibration in the hypopharynx.

esophageal varices *n.* Longitudinal, superficial venous varices at the lower end of the esophagus that are prone to ulceration and massive bleeding.

esophageal vein *n.* Any of several small venous trunks bringing blood from the esophagus and emptying into the brachiocephalic vein or the azygos vein.

e·soph·a·gec·ta·sis (ĭ-sŏf′ə-jĕk′tə-sĭs) *or* **e·soph·a·gec·ta·sia** (-jĭk-tā′zhə) *n.* Dilation of the esophagus.

e·soph·a·gec·to·my (ĭ-sŏf′ə-jĕk′tə-mē) *n.* Excision of all or a part of the esophagus.

e·soph·a·gism (ĭ-sŏf′ə-jĭz′əm) *n.* Esophageal spasm causing dysphagia.

e·soph·a·gi·tis (ĭ-sŏf′ə-jī′tĭs) *n.* Inflammation of the esophagus.

e·soph·a·go·car·di·o·plas·ty (ĭ-sŏf′ə-gō-kär′dē-ō-plăs′tē) *n.* A reconstructive operation on the esophagus and cardiac end of the stomach.

e·soph·a·go·cele (ĭ-sŏf′ə-gō-sēl′) *n.* Protrusion of the mucous membrane of the esophagus through a rupture in the muscular coat.

e·soph·a·go·dyn·i·a (ĭ-sŏf′ə-gō-dĭn′ē-ə) *n.* See **esophagalgia.**

e·soph·a·go·en·ter·os·to·my (ĭ-sŏf′ə-gō-ĕn′tə-rŏs′tə-mē) *n.* The surgical formation of a direct communication between the esophagus and intestine.

e·soph·a·go·gas·trec·to·my (ĭ-sŏf′ə-gō-gă-strĕk′tə-mē) *n.* The removal of a portion of the lower esophagus and proximal stomach for treatment of neoplasms or strictures of those organs, especially lesions at or near the cardioesophageal junction.

e·soph·a·go·gas·tric junction (ĭ-sŏf′ə-gō-găs′trĭk) *n.* The line at the cardiac orifice of the stomach where there is a transition from the stratified squamous epithelium of the esophagus to the simple columnar epithelium of the stomach.

e·soph·a·go·gas·tro·a·nas·to·mo·sis (ĭ-sŏf′ə-gō-găs′trō-ə-năs′tə-mō′sĭs) *n.* See **esophagogastrostomy.**

e·soph·a·go·gas·tro·plas·ty (ĭ-sŏf′ə-gō-găs′trə-plăs′tē) *n.* Surgical repair of the cardiac sphincter of the stomach. Also called *cardioplasty.*

e·soph·a·go·gas·tros·to·my (ĭ-sŏf′ə-gō-gă-strŏs′tə-mē) *n.* Surgical anastomosis of the esophagus to the stomach, usually following esophagogastrectomy. Also called *esophagogastroanastomosis.*

e·soph·a·go·gram (ĭ-sŏf′ə-gə-grăm′) *n.* A radiograph of the esophagus obtained during esophagography.

e·soph·a·gog·ra·phy (ĭ-sŏf′ə-gŏg′rə-fē) *n.* Radiographic visualization of the esophagus using a swallowed radiopaque contrast medium.

e·soph·a·go·ma·la·cia (ĭ-sŏf′ə-gō-mə-lā′shə) *n.* Softening of the walls of the esophagus.

e·soph·a·go·my·ot·o·my (ĭ-sŏf′ə-gō-mī-ŏt′ə-mē) *n.* Treatment of esophageal achalasia by a longitudinal division of the lowest part of the esophageal muscle down to the submucosal layer.

e·soph·a·go·plas·ty (ĭ-sŏf′ə-gə-plăs′tē) *n.* Surgical repair of a defect in the wall of the esophagus.

e·soph·a·go·pli·ca·tion (ĭ-sŏf′ə-gō-plĭ-kā′shən) *n.* Surgery to narrow a dilated esophagus by making longitudinal folds or tucks in its walls.

e·soph·a·gop·to·sis (ĭ-sŏf′ə-gŏp-tō′sĭs, -gō-tō′sĭs) *or* **e·soph·a·gop·to·si·a** (-tō′sē-ə, -zē-ə) *n.* Relaxation and downward displacement of the walls of the esophagus.

e·soph·a·go·scope (ĭ-sŏf′ə-gə-skōp′) *n.* An endoscope for examining the interior of the esophagus.

e·soph·a·gos·co·py (ĭ-sŏf′ə-gŏs′kə-pē) *n.* Examination of the interior of the esophagus by means of an esophagoscope.

e·soph·a·go·spasm (ĭ-sŏf′ə-gə-spăz′əm) *n.* Spasm of the walls of the esophagus.

e·soph·a·go·ste·no·sis (ĭ-sŏf′ə-gō-stə-nō′sĭs) *n.* Stricture or a general narrowing of the esophagus.

e·soph·a·gos·to·my (ĭ-sŏf′ə-gŏs′tə-mē) *n.* The surgical formation of an opening directly into the esophagus from without.

e·soph·a·got·o·my (ĭ-sŏf′ə-gŏt′ə-mē) *n.* An incision through the wall of the esophagus.

e·soph·a·gus *or* **oe·soph·a·gus** (ĭ-sŏf′ə-gəs) *n., pl.* **-gi** (-jī′, -gī′) The portion of the digestive canal between the pharynx and stomach, consisting of a cervical part from the cricoid cartilage to the thoracic inlet, a thoracic part from the thoracic inlet to the diaphragm, and an abdominal part below the diaphragm to the stomach. —**e·soph·a·ge·al** (-jē′əl) *adj.*

es·o·pho·ri·a (ĕs′ə-fôr′ē-ə) *n.* A tendency of the eyes to deviate inward. —**es′o·phor′ic** (-fôr′ĭk) *adj.*

es·o·sphe·noid·i·tis (ĕs′ō-sfē′noi-dī′tĭs) *n.* Osteomyelitis of the sphenoid bone.

es·o·tro·pi·a (ĕs′ə-trō′pē-ə) *n.* The form of strabismus in which the visual axes converge. Also called *convergent strabismus, crossed eyes.* —**es′o·trop′ic** (-trŏp′ĭk, -trō′pĭk) *adj.*

ESP *abbr.* extrasensory perception

es·pun·di·a (ĭ-spŭn′dē-ə) *n.* A type of American leishmaniasis caused by *Leishmania braziliensis* that affects the mucous membranes, particularly of the nose and mouth, resulting in grossly destructive changes. Also called *Breda's disease.*

ESR *abbr.* erythrocyte sedimentation rate; electron spin resonance

es·sen·tial (ĭ-sĕn′shəl) *adj.* **1.** Constituting or being part of the essence of something; inherent. **2.** Basic or indispensable; necessary. **3.** Of, relating to, or being a dysfunctional condition or a disease whose cause is unknown. **4.** Of, relating to, or being a substance that is required for normal functioning but cannot be synthesized by the body and therefore must be included in the diet. —*n.* **1.** Something fundamental. **2.** Something necessary or indispensable. —**es·sen′ti·al′i·ty** (-shē-ăl′ĭ-tē), **es·sen′tial·ness** *n.*

essential amino acid *n.* An alpha-amino acid that is required for protein synthesis but cannot be synthesized by humans and must be obtained in the diet.

essential dysmenorrhea *n.* See **primary dysmenorrhea.**

essential fructosuria *n.* A benign inherited metabolic disorder caused by a deficiency of fructokinase and characterized by the presence of fructose in the blood and urine.

essential hematuria *n.* Hematuria whose cause has not been determined.

essential hypertension *n.* Hypertension without known cause or preexisting renal disease.

essential oil *n.* A volatile oil, usually having the characteristic odor or flavor of the plant from which it is obtained, used to make perfumes and flavorings.

essential pentosuria *n.* A benign inheritable disorder in which there is a regular excretion of pentoses in the urine, especially of xylulose. Also called *primary pentosuria.*

essential pruritus *n.* Itching that occurs independently of skin lesions.

essential tachycardia *n.* Persistent rapid action of the heart that cannot be attributed to any discernible organic lesion.

essential telangiectasia *n.* **1.** Localized capillary dilation of undetermined origin. **2.** See **angioma serpiginosum.**

Es·ser graft (ĕs′ər) *n.* See **inlay graft.**

EST *abbr.* electroshock therapy

es·ta·zo·lam (ĕs-tā′zō-lăm′) *n.* A benzodiazepine drug used to treat insomnia.

es·ter (ĕs′tər) *n.* Any of a class of organic compounds corresponding to the inorganic salts and formed from an organic acid and an alcohol, usually with the elimination of water.

es·ter·ase (ĕs′tə-rās′, -rāz′) *n.* Any of various enzymes that catalyze the hydrolysis of an ester.

es·ter·i·fi·ca·tion (ĕ-stĕr′ə-fĭ-kā′shən) *n.* A chemical reaction resulting in the formation of at least one ester product. —**es·ter′i·fied** (ĕ-stĕr′ə-fīd′) *adj.*

es·the·sia (ĕs-thē′zhə) *n.* Variant of **aesthesia.**

esthesio– *or* **aesthesio–** *pref.* Sensation or perception: *esthesioneurosis.*

es·the·si·od·ic (ĕs-thē′zē-ŏd′ĭk) *adj.* Variant of **aesthesiodic.**

es·the·si·o·gen·e·sis (ĕs-thē′zē-ō-jĕn′ĭ-sĭs) *n.* Variant of **aesthesiogenesis.**

es·the·si·o·gen·ic (ĕs-thē′zē-ō-jĕn′ĭk) *adj.* Variant of **aesthesiogenic.**

es·the·si·om·e·ter (ĕs-thē′zē-ŏm′ĭ-tər) *n.* Variant of **aesthesiometer.**

es·the·si·om·e·try (ĕs-thē′zē-ŏm′ĭ-trē) *n.* Variant of **aesthesiometry.**

es·the·si·o·neu·ro·sis (ĕs-thē′zē-ō-nŏŏ-rō′sĭs) *n.* Variant of **aesthesioneurosis.**

es·the·si·o·phys·i·ol·o·gy (ĕs-thē′zē-ō-fĭz′ē-ŏl′ə-jē) *n.* Variant of **aesthesiophysiology.**

es·thet·ic (ĕs-thĕt′ĭk) *adj.* Variant of **aesthetic.**

es·thet·ics (ĕs-thĕt′ĭks) *n.* Variant of **aesthetics.**

es·ti·mat·ed date of confinement (ĕs′tə-mĭ′tĭd) *n. Abbr.* **EDC** The date at which an infant is expected to be born, calculated from the date of the last menstrual period. Also called *due date.*

estimated gestational age *n. Abbr.* **EGA** The estimated age of a fetus, usually reported in weeks and based on the date of the last menstrual period.

es·ti·val (ĕs′tə-vəl) *adj.* Relating to or occurring in the summer.

es·ti·vo·au·tum·nal (ĕs′tə-vō-ô-tŭm′nəl) *adj.* Relating to or occurring in summer and autumn.

Est·lan·der operation (ĕst′lăn′dər, -län′-) *n.* A procedure to transfer a full-thickness flap of the lip from one side of the lip to the same side of the opposite lip.

Es·trace (ĕs′trās′) A trademark for a drug preparation of conjugated estrogen.

es·tra·di·ol (ĕs′trə-dī′ôl′, -ōl′) *n.* The most potent naturally occurring estrogen.

es·tra·mus·tine phosphate sodium (ĕs′trə-mŭs′tēn′) *n.* An antineoplastic agent that combines the actions of estrogen and nitrogen mustard in the treatment of carcinoma of the prostate.

Es·tra·test (ĕs′trə-tĕst′) A trademark for a drug preparation containing esterified estrogens and methyltestosterone.

es·trin (ĕs′trĭn) *n.* See **estrogen.**

es·tri·ol (ĕs′trī-ôl′, -ōl′, ĕ-strī′-) *n.* A metabolite of estradiol and usually the predominant estrogenic metabolite that is found in the urine of pregnant women. Also called *theelol.*

es·tro·gen *or* **oes·tro·gen** (ĕs′trə-jən) *n.* Any of several natural or synthetic substances formed by the ovary, placenta, testis, and certain plants, that stimulate the female secondary sex characteristics, exert systemic effects such as the growth and maturation of long bones, and are used to treat disorders due to estrogen deficiency and to ameliorate cancers of the breast and prostate. Also called *estrin.*

es·tro·gen·ic (ĕs′trə-jĕn′ĭk) *adj.* **1.** Causing estrus in animals. **2.** Having an action similar to that of an estrogen.

estrogen replacement therapy *n. Abbr.* **ERT** The administration of estrogen, especially in postmenopausal women, to relieve symptoms and conditions associated with estrogen deficiency, such as hot flashes and osteoporosis.

es·trone (ĕs′trōn′) *n.* A metabolite of estradiol, commonly found in urine, having considerably less biological activity than estradiol but similar properties and uses. Also called *theelin.*

es·tro·pi·pate (ĕs′trō-pī′pāt′) *n.* An estrogen compound containing the sulfate of estrone and piperazine, used for estrogen replacement therapy.

es·trous (ĕs′trəs) *adj.* Relating to or being in estrus.

estrous cycle *n.* The recurrent set of physiological and behavioral changes that take place from one period of estrus to another.

es·trus *or* **oes·trus** (ĕs′trəs) *n.* The periodic state of sexual excitement in the female of most mammals, excluding humans, that immediately precedes ovulation and during which the female is most receptive to mating; heat.

e·ta (ā′tə, ē′tə) *n. Symbol* η The seventh letter of the Greek alphabet.

e·tan·er·cept (ĭ-tăn′ər-sĕpt′) *n.* A drug that blocks tumor necrosis factor receptors and is used primarily to treat rheumatoid arthritis.

eth·a·cryn·ic acid (ĕth′ə-krĭn′ĭk) *n.* A diuretic compound used in the treatment of severe edema.

eth·al·de·hyde (ĕ-thăl′də-hīd′) *n.* See **acetaldehyde.**

eth·am·bu·tol (ĕ-thăm′byə-tôl′, -tōl′) *n.* An antibacterial drug used in combination with other drugs in the treatment of pulmonary tuberculosis.

eth·a·no·ic acid (ĕth′ə-nō′ĭk) *n.* See **acetic acid.**

eth·a·nol (ĕth′ə-nôl′, -nōl′) *n.* See **alcohol** (sense 2).

eth·ene (ĕth′ēn) *n.* See **ethylene.**

eth·e·nyl (ĕth′ə-nĭl) *n.* Vinyl.

e·ther (ē′thər) *n.* **1.** Any of a class of organic compounds in which two hydrocarbon groups are linked by an oxygen atom. **2.** An anesthetic ether, especially diethyl ether.

e·the·re·al (ĭ-thîr′ē-əl) *adj.* **1.** Characterized by lightness and insubstantiality; intangible. **2.** Of, relating to, or containing ether. —**e·the′re·al′i·ty** (-ăl′ĭ-tē), **e·the′re·al·ness** *n.* —**e·the′re·al·ly** *adv.*

ethereal oil *n.* See **volatile oil.**

eth·i·cal (ĕth′ĭ-kəl) *adj.* **1.** Of, relating to, or dealing with ethics. **2.** Being in accordance with the accepted principles of right and wrong that govern the conduct of a profession.

eth·ics (ĕth′ĭks) *n.* The rules or standards governing the conduct of a person or the conduct of the members of a profession.

eth·i·nyl estradiol (ĕth′ə-nĭl′) *n.* A synthetic estrogen derivative commonly used in oral contraceptives.

ethmo– *pref.* Ethmoid bone; ethmoid: *ethmoturbinals.*

eth·moid (ĕth′moid′) *or* **eth·moi·dal** (ĕth-moid′l) *adj.* Resembling a sieve. —*n.* The ethmoid bone.

ethmoidal artery *n.* **1.** An artery with origin in the ophthalmic artery, with distribution to the cerebral membranes in the anterior cranial fossa, the anterior ethmoidal cells, frontal sinus, anterior upper part of the nasal mucous membranes, and the skin of the nose; anterior ethmoidal artery. **2.** An artery with origin in the ophthalmic artery and with distribution to the ethmoidal cells and the lateral wall of the nasal cavity; posterior ethmoidal artery.

ethmoidal cell *n.* Any of the cavities in the ethmoid bone that are filled with air and that communicate with the nasal cavity.

ethmoidal crest *n.* **1.** A ridge on the nasal surface of the upper jawbone that attaches to the middle nasal concha. Also called *nasal concha.* **2.** A ridge on the palatine bone to which the middle nasal concha attaches. Also called *nasal concha.*

ethmoidal foramen *n.* Either of two foramina, anterior and posterior, formed by grooves on either edge of the ethmoidal notch of the frontal bone and by similar grooves on the ethmoid bone.

ethmoidal labyrinth *n.* A mass of air cells with thin bony walls forming part of the lateral wall of the nasal cavity. Also called *ectethmoid.*

ethmoidal sinus *n.* Any of the evaginations of the mucous membrane of the middle and superior meatus of the nasal cavity, subdivided into anterior, middle, and posterior sinuses.

ethmoidal vein *n.* Any of the veins that drain the ethmoidal sinuses and pass into the superior ophthalmic vein.

ethmoid bone *n.* A light spongy bone located between the eye sockets, forming part of the walls and septum of the superior nasal cavity, and containing perforations for the passage of olfactory nerve fibers.

eth·moi·dec·to·my (ĕth′moi-dĕk′tə-mē) *n.* Removal of all or a part of the mucosal lining and bony partitions between the ethmoid sinuses.

ethmoid infundibulum *n.* A passage from the middle meatus of the nose communicating with the anterior ethmoidal cells and frontal sinus.

eth·moid·i·tis (ĕth′moi-dī′tĭs) *n.* Inflammation of the ethmoid sinuses.

eth·mo·tur·bi·nal (ĕth′mō-tûr′bə-nəl) *adj.* Relating to the superior and middle nasal conchae.

eth·no·cen·trism (ĕth′nō-sĕn′trĭz′əm) *n.* The tendency to evaluate other groups according to the values and standards of one's own ethnic group, especially with the conviction that one's own ethnic group is superior to the other groups. —**eth′no·cen′tric** (-trĭk) *adj.* —**eth′-no·cen·tric′i·ty** (-sĕn-trĭs′ĭ-tē) *n.*

eth·ox·y (ĕ-thŏk′sē) *n.* The univalent radical C_2H_5O. —*adj.* Relating to or containing the ethoxy radical.

eth·yl (ĕth′əl) *n.* The univalent hydrocarbon radical C_2H_5.

ethyl alcohol *n.* See **alcohol** (sense 2).

eth·yl·ate (ĕth′ə-lāt′) *n.* A compound in which the hydrogen of the hydroxyl group of an alcohol is replaced by a metallic atom, usually sodium or potassium. —*v.* To introduce the ethyl group into a compound. —**eth′-yl·a′tion** *n.*

ethyl chloride *n.* A chemical compound that is a gas at room temperature and a colorless, volatile, flammable or explosive liquid under high pressure. It is used as a local anesthetic, potent inhalation anesthetic, refrigerant, and solvent.

eth·yl·ene (ĕth′ə-lēn′) *n.* **1.** An explosive gas derived from natural gas and petroleum infrequently used as an inhalation anesthetic. Also called *ethene.* **2.** The bivalent hydrocarbon radical C_2H_4 that is isomeric to the ethylidene radical.

eth·yl·ene·di·a·mine·tet·ra·a·ce·tic acid (ĕth′ə-lēn-dī′ə-mēn-tĕt′rə-ə-sē′tĭk) *n.* EDTA.

ethylene glycol *n.* A colorless syrupy alcohol used as an antifreeze in cooling and heating systems.

ethyl ether *n.* See **diethyl ether**.

eth·yl·i·dene (ĕth′ə-lĭ-dēn′, ĕ-thĭl′ĭ-) *n.* The bivalent hydrocarbon radical C_2H_4 that is isomeric to the ethylene radical.

ethyl oxide *n.* See **diethyl ether**.

eth·yl·vi·nyl ether (ĕth′əl-vī′nəl) *n.* A flammable, moderately potent inhalation anesthetic. Also called *vinylethyl ether.*

e·thy·no·di·ol (ĕ-thī′nə-dī′ôl′, -ōl′) *n.* A semisynthetic steroid having similar biophysiological effects as progesterone and administered with an estrogen as an oral contraceptive.

e·thy·nyl (ĕ-thī′nĭl, ĕth′ə-) *n.* The univalent hydrocarbon radical HCC derived from acetylene.

et·i·dro·nate disodium (ĕt′ĭ-drō′nāt′) *n.* A drug that affects bone resorption and is used in the treatment of Paget's disease, heterotopic ossification, and hypercalcemia of malignancy.

e·ti·o·la·tion (ē′tē-ə-lā′shən) *n.* **1.** Paleness or pallor resulting from deprivation of light. **2.** The process of blanching or making pale by withholding light. —**e′ti·o·late′** *v.*

e·ti·ol·o·gy *or* **ae·ti·ol·o·gy** (ē′tē-ŏl′ə-jē) *n.* **1.** The science and study of the causes or origins of disease. **2.** The cause or origin of a disease or disorder as determined by medical diagnosis.

e·to·do·lac (ĭ-tō′də-lăk) *n.* A nonsteroidal anti-inflammatory medication, used especially in the treatment of osteoarthritis.

e·to·po·side (ē′tə-pō′sīd′) *n.* A semisynthetic derivative of podophyllotoxin that is a mitotic inhibitor used in the treatment of refractory testicular tumors and small cell lung cancer.

Eu The symbol for the element **europium**.

eu– *pref.* **1.** Good; well; true: *eupepsia.* **2.** A derivative of a specified substance: *euglobulin.*

Eu·bac·te·ri·um (yōō′băk-tîr′ē-əm) *n.* A genus of anaerobic, nonsporeforming, nonmotile bacteria occurring in the intestinal tract; they attack carbohydrates and may be pathogenic.

eu·ca·lyp·tol (yōō′kə-lĭp′tôl′, -tōl′) *or* **eu·ca·lyp·tole** (-tōl′) *n.* A colorless oily liquid derived from eucalyptus and used in pharmaceuticals.

Eu·car·y·o·tae (yōō-kăr′ē-ō′tē) *n.* Variant of **Eukaryotae**.

eu·car·y·ote (yōō-kăr′ē-ōt, -ē-ət) *n.* Variant of **eukaryote**. —**eu·car′y·ot′ic** (-ŏt′ĭk) *adj.*

eu·chlor·hy·dri·a (yōō′klôr-hī′drē-ə) *n.* The presence of normal amounts of free hydrochloric acid in the gastric juice.

eu·cho·li·a (yōō-kō′lē-ə) *n.* A normal state of the bile in quantity and quality.

eu·chro·ma·tin (yōō-krō′mə-tĭn) *n.* Chromosomal material that consists of uncoiled dispersed threads during interphase, is genetically active, and stains lightly with basic dyes.

eu·cra·sia (yōō-krā′zhə) *n.* **1.** Homeostasis. No longer in technical use. **2.** A condition of reduced susceptibility. No longer in technical use.

eu·di·a·pho·re·sis (yōō-dī′ə-fə-rē′sĭs, -dī-ăf′ə-) *n.* Normal, free sweating.

eu·gen·ic (yōō-jĕn′ĭk) *adj.* **1.** Of or relating to eugenics. **2.** Relating or adapted to the production of good or improved offspring.

eu·gen·ics (yōō-jĕn′ĭks) *n.* The study of hereditary improvement of the human race by controlled selective breeding.

eu·ge·nol (yōō′jə-nôl′, -nōl′) *n.* An aromatic liquid that is made from clove oil and is used as a dental analgesic.

eu·glob·u·lin (yōō-glŏb′yə-lĭn) *n.* A simple protein that is soluble in dilute salt solutions and insoluble in distilled water.

eu·gly·ce·mi·a (yōō′glī-sē′mē-ə) *n.* Normal concentration of glucose in the blood. Also called *normoglycemia.* —**eu′gly·ce′mic** (-mĭk) *adj.*

eu·gna·thi·a (yōō-nā′thē-ə, -năth′ē-ə) *n.* Normal development and function of the system that includes the jaw and the teeth.

eu·gon·ic (yōō-gŏn′ĭk) *adj.* Relating to rapid and relatively luxuriant growth of a bacterial culture, especially that of the tubercle bacillus.

Eu·kar·y·o·tae *or* **Eu·car·y·o·tae** (yōō-kăr′ē-ō′tē) *n.* A superkingdom of organisms characterized by eukaryotic cells; its single-cell members are assigned to the kingdom Protoctista, and its multicellular members are assigned to the kingdoms Fungi, Plantae, and Animalia.

eu·kar·y·ote *or* **eu·car·y·ote** (yōō-kăr′ē-ōt, -ē-ət) *n.* A single-celled or multicellular organism whose cells contain a distinct membrane-bound nucleus. —**eu·kar′y·ot′ic** (-ŏt′ĭk) *adj.*

Eu·len·burg's disease (oi′lən-bûrgz′, -bŏŏrks′) *n.* See **congenital paramyotonia.**

Eu·ler (oi′lər), **Ulf Svante von** 1905–1983. Swedish physiologist. He shared a 1970 Nobel Prize for studies of nerve impulse transmission.

eu·me·tri·a (yōō-mē′trē-ə) *n.* A normal graduation of the strength of nerve impulses to match the intended voluntary movement.

eu·nuch (yōō′nək) *n.* A man or boy whose testes have been removed or have never developed.

eu·nuch·oid (yōō′nə-koid′) *adj.* Partially resembling or having the general characteristics of a eunuch.

eunuchoid gigantism *n.* Gigantism in which testicular secretions are deficient or absent causing deficient sexual development and persistence of prepuberal characteristics.

eu·nuch·oid·ism (yōō′nə-koi-dĭz′əm) *n.* A condition or state in which the testes are present but fail to function normally.

eu·pep·si·a (yōō-pĕp′sē-ə, -shə) *n.* Good digestion.

eu·pep·tic (yōō-pĕp′tĭk) *adj.* **1.** Digesting well; having a good digestion. **2.** Conducive to digestion.

Eu·phor·bi·a pil·u·lif·er·a (yōō-fôr′bē-ə pĭl′yə-lĭf′ər-ə) *n.* A plant that yields substances used in treating asthma, coryza, and angina pectoris.

eu·pho·ret·ic (yōō′fə-rĕt′ĭk) *adj.* Having the capability to produce euphoria.

eu·pho·ri·a (yōō-fôr′ē-ə) *n.* A feeling of great happiness or well-being, commonly exaggerated and not necessarily well founded.

eu·pho·ri·ant (yōō-fôr′ē-ənt) *n.* A drug that tends to produce euphoria. —**eu·pho′ri·ant** *adj.*

eu·plas·tic (yōō-plăs′tĭk) *adj.* Readily transformed into tissue, as in the healing of a wound.

euplastic lymph *n.* Lymph containing relatively few white blood cells but a comparatively high concentration of fibrinogen and tending to become organized with fibrous tissue.

eu·ploid (yōō′ploid′) *adj.* Having a chromosome number that is an exact multiple of the haploid number for the species. —*n.* An organism having a euploid chromosome number. —**eu′ploi′dy** *n.*

eup·ne·a (yōōp-nē′ə) *n.* Easy, free respiration, as is observed normally under resting conditions. —**eup·ne′ic** *adj.*

eu·prax·i·a (yōō-prăk′sē-ə) *n.* Normal ability to perform coordinated movements.

Eu·rax (yōōr′ăks′) A trademark for the drug crotamiton.

eu·rhyth·mi·a (yōō-rĭth′mē-ə) *n.* Harmonious relationships among the separate organs of the body.

eu·ro·pi·um (yōō-rō′pē-əm) *n. Symbol* **Eu** A rare-earth element used as a neutron absorber in nuclear research. Atomic number 63.

eury– *pref.* Wide; broad: *eurycephalic.*

eu·ry·ce·phal·ic (yōōr′ĭ-sə-făl′ĭk) *or* **eu·ry·ceph·a·lous** (-sĕf′ə-ləs) *adj.* Having an unusually broad head.

eu·ryg·nath·ic (yōōr′ĭg-năth′ĭk) *or* **eu·ryg·na·thous** (yōō-rĭg′nə-thəs) *adj.* Having a wide jaw.

eu·ry·on (yōōr′ē-ŏn′) *n.* The extremity on either side of the greatest transverse diameter of the head; it is a point used in craniometry.

eu·ry·o·pi·a (yōōr′ē-ō′pē-ə) *n.* Abnormally wide opening of the eyes.

eu·sta·chian (yōō-stā′shən, -shē-ən, -kē-ən) *adj.* Described by or attributed to Italian anatomist Bartolommeo Eustachio.

eustachian tube *n.* A slender tube that connects the tympanic cavity with the nasal part of the pharynx and that serves to equalize air pressure on either side of the eardrum. Also called *auditory tube, salpinx.*

Eu·sta·chi·o (yōō-stä′kē-ō, ĕ′ōō-stä′kyō), **Bartolomeo** 1520–1574. Italian anatomist. A founder of modern anatomy, he is noted for his descriptions of the human ear and heart.

eu·sys·to·le (yōō-sĭs′tə-lē) *n.* Normal cardiac systole. —**eu′sys·tol′ic** (-sĭ-stŏl′ĭk) *adj.*

eu·tec·tic alloy (yōō-tĕk′tĭk) *n.* An alloy that is generally brittle, easily melted, and subject to tarnish and corrosion, used primarily in dental solders.

eu·tel·e·gen·e·sis (yōō-tĕl′ə-jĕn′ĭ-sĭs) *n.* Artificial insemination by semen from a donor selected because of certain desirable characteristics for the development of superior offspring.

eu·tha·na·sia (yōō′thə-nā′zhə) *n.* **1.** The act or practice of ending the life of an individual suffering from a terminal illness or an incurable condition, as by lethal injection or the suspension of extraordinary medical treatment. **2.** A quiet, painless death.

eu·then·ics (yōo-thĕn′ĭks) *n.* The science concerned with establishing the optimum living conditions for plants, animals, or humans, especially through proper provisioning and environment.

eu·ther·mic (yōo-thûr′mĭk) *adj.* Having, being, or maintaining an optimal temperature.

eu·thy·roid·ism (yōo-thī′roi-dĭz′əm) *n.* **1.** The physiological state characterized by normal serum levels of thyroid hormone. **2.** Normal functioning of the thyroid gland. —**eu·thy′roid′** *adj.*

eu·ton·ic (yōo-tŏn′ĭk) *adj.* Normotonic.

eu·tro·phi·a (yōo-trō′fē-ə) *n.* A state of normal nourishment and growth.

eu·troph·ic (yōo-trŏf′ĭk, -trō′fĭk) *adj.* Relating to, characterized by, or promoting eutrophia.

eV *or* **ev** *abbr.* electron volt

e·vac·u·ant (ĭ-văk′yōo-ənt) *adj.* Causing evacuation, especially of the bowels; purgative. —*n.* A purgative agent.

e·vac·u·ate (ĭ-văk′yōo-āt′) *v.* **1.** To empty or remove the contents of. **2.** To excrete or discharge waste matter, especially of the bowels.

e·vac·u·a·tion (ĭ-văk′yōo-ā′shən) *n.* Discharge of waste materials from the excretory passages of the body, especially from the bowels.

e·vac·u·a·tor (ĭ-văk′yōo-ā′tər) *n.* An instrument for removal of material from a body cavity.

e·vag·i·na·tion (ĭ-văj′ə-nā′shən) *n.* The protrusion of a part or organ from its normal position. —**e·vag′i·nate′** *v.*

ev·a·nes·cent (ĕv′ə-nĕs′ənt) *adj.* Of short duration; passing away quickly.

Ev·ans (ĕv′ənz), **Herbert McLean** 1882–1971. American anatomist who isolated four pituitary hormones and discovered vitamin E (1922).

Evans blue *n.* A diazo dye used to determine blood volume on the basis of the dilution of a standard solution of the dye in the plasma after its intravenous injection; it is also used as a vital stain for following diffusion through blood vessel walls.

e·vap·o·rate (ĭ-văp′ə-rāt′) *v.* **1.** To convert or change into a vapor; volatilize. **2.** To produce vapor. **3.** To draw or pass off in the form of vapor. **4.** To draw moisture away from, as by heating, leaving only the dry solid portion. **5.** To deposit a metal on a substrate by vacuum sublimation. —**e·vap′o·ra′tor** *n.* —**e·vap′o·ra·tiv′i·ty** (-ər-ə-tĭv′ĭ-tē) *n.*

e·vap·o·ra·tion (ĭ-văp′ə-rā′shən) *n.* **1.** A change from liquid to vapor form. **2.** Loss of volume of a liquid by conversion into vapor. Also called *volatilization.*

e·ven·tra·tion (ē′vĕn-trā′shən) *n.* **1.** Protrusion of the omentum or intestine through an opening in the abdominal wall. **2.** Removal of the contents of the abdominal cavity.

eventration of diaphragm *n.* Extreme elevation of part of the diaphragm, which is usually atrophic and abnormally thin.

e·ver·sion (ĭ-vûr′zhən) *n.* A turning outward, as of the eyelid.

e·vert (ĭ-vûrt′) *v.* To turn inside out or outward.

e·vis·cer·a·tion (ĭ-vĭs′ə-rā′shən) *n.* **1.** Removal of the contents of the eyeball, leaving the sclera and sometimes the cornea. **2.** See **exenteration. 3.** Protrusion of the abdominal viscera, as through a defect created by wound dehiscence. —**e·vis′cer·ate′** *v.*

E·vis·ta (ē-vĭs′tə) A trademark for the drug raloxifene.

ev·o·ca·tion (ĕv′ə-kā′shən, ē′və-) *n.* The induction of a particular tissue produced by the action of an evocator during embryogenesis.

ev·o·ca·tor (ĕv′ə-kā′tər, ē′və-) *n.* A factor in the control of morphogenesis in the early embryo. Also called *inductor.*

e·voked response (ĭ-vōkt′) *n.* An alteration in the electrical activity of a particular part of the nervous system as a result of receiving a sensory stimulus.

ev·o·lu·tion (ĕv′ə-lōo′shən, ē′və-) *n.* **1.** A continuing process of change from one state or condition to another or from one form to another. **2.** The theory that groups of organisms change with passage of time, mainly as a result of natural selection, so that descendants differ morphologically and physiologically from their ancestors.

ev·o·lu·tion·ar·y fitness (ĕv′ə-lōo′shə-nĕr′ē) *n.* The probability that the line of descent from an individual with a specific trait will not die out.

evolution of carbon dioxide *n.* An expression of the rate at which carbon dioxide is produced by the body, usually given as the microliters of carbon dioxide produced in 1 hour by 1 milligram dry weight of tissue.

e·vul·sion (ĭ-vŭl′shən) *n.* A forcible pulling out or extraction.

Ew·art's sign (yōo′ərts) *n.* An indication of a large pericardial effusion in which an area of dullness is evident below the angle of the left scapula together with bronchial breathing and bronchophony.

Ew·ing (yōo′ĭng), **James** 1866–1943. American pathologist. An authority on cancer, he established oncology as a clinical specialty.

Ew·ing's tumor (yōo′ĭngz) *n.* A malignant tumor usually occurring before age 20 in males and involving metaphyses of the bones of the extremities. Also called *endothelial myeloma, Ewing's sarcoma.*

ex– *pref.* Outside; out of; away from: *excementosis.*

exa– *pref.* One quintillion (10^{18}): *exagram.*

ex·ac·er·ba·tion (ĭg-zăs′ər-bā′shən) *n.* An increase in the severity of a disease or in any of its signs or symptoms. —**ex·ac′er·bate′** *v.*

ex·am·i·na·tion (ĭg-zăm′ə-nā′shən) *n.* An investigation or inspection for the purpose of diagnosis.

ex·am·ine (ĭg-zăm′ĭn) *v.* **1.** To study or analyze an organic material. **2.** To test or check the condition or health of. **3.** To determine the qualifications, aptitude, or skills of by means of questions or exercises.

ex·an·the·ma (ĕg′zăn-thē′mə) *or* **ex·an·them** (ĭg-zăn′thəm) *n.* **1.** A skin eruption occurring as a symptom of an acute viral or coccal disease. **2.** A disease, such as measles or scarlet fever, accompanied by a skin eruption. —**ex·an′the·mat′ic** (ĭg-zăn′-thə-măt′ĭk), **ex′an·them′a·tous** (ĕg′zăn-thĕm′ə-təs) *adj.*

exanthema su·bi·tum (sōo′bĭ-təm) *n.* A viral disease affecting infants and young children, characterized by a fever that lasts several days and a spotty rash that appears shortly after the fever has subsided. Also called *roseola infantum, sixth disease.*

ex·ar·tic·u·la·tion (ĕk′sär-tĭk′yə-lā′shən) *n.* See **disarticulation.**

ex·ca·la·tion (ĕk′skə-lā′shən) *n.* The absence, suppression, or failure to develop one member of a series, such as a finger or vertebra.

ex·ca·va·tion (ĕk′skə-vā′shən) *n.* 1. A natural cavity, pouch, or recess. 2. A cavity formed artificially or as the result of a pathological process.

excavation of optic disk *n.* The normally occurring depression or pit in the center of the optic disk. Also called *physiologic excavation.*

ex·ca·va·tor (ĕk′skə-vā′tər) *n.* An instrument, such as a sharp spoon or curette, used in scraping out pathological tissue.

Ex·ced·rin (ĕk-sĕd′rĭn) A trademark for an over-the-counter preparation containing acetaminophen alone or combined with caffeine or aspirin or both.

ex·ce·men·to·sis (ĕk′sĭ-mĕn-tō′sĭs) *n.* The outgrowth of cementum on the root surface of a tooth.

ex·cess (ĭk-sĕs′, ĕk′sĕs′) *n.* An amount or quantity beyond what is normal or sufficient; a surplus.

ex·change (ĭks-chānj′) *v.* To substitute one thing for another. —*n.* The act of substituting one thing for another.

exchange transfusion *n.* The removal of most of a patient's blood followed by introduction of an equal amount from donors. Also called *substitution transfusion, total transfusion.*

ex·cip·i·ent (ĭk-sĭp′ē-ənt) *n.* An inert substance used as a diluent or vehicle for a drug.

ex·cise (ĭk-sīz′) *v.* To remove by cutting.

ex·ci·sion (ĭk-sĭzh′ən) *n.* 1. Surgical removal by cutting, as of a tumor or a portion of a structure or organ. Also called *exection.* 2. A recombination event in which a genetic element is removed.

excision biopsy *n.* Excision of an entire lesion for gross and microscopic examination.

ex·cit·a·ble (ĭk-sī′tə-bəl) *adj.* 1. Capable of reacting to a stimulus. Used of a tissue, cell, or cell membrane. 2. Capable of emotional arousal. —**ex·cit′a·bil′i·ty, ex·cit′a·ble·ness** *n.*

excitable area *n.* See **motor cortex.**

ex·ci·ta·tion (ĕk′sī-tā′shən) *n.* 1. The act of increasing the rapidity or the intensity of the physical or mental processes; stimulation. 2. The complete, all-or-none response of a nerve or muscle to an adequate stimulus, ordinarily including propagation of excitation along the membranes of the cell or cells involved.

excitation wave *n.* An electrical wave that propagates along a muscle fiber just before its contraction.

ex·ci·ta·to·ry postsynaptic potential (ĭk-sī′tə-tôr′ē) *n.* A local change in the depolarization produced in the postsynaptic neuronal membrane in response to an excitatory impulse; summation of these depolarizations can lead to discharge of an impulse by the neuron.

ex·cit·ed state (ĭk-sī′tĭd) *n.* The condition of an atom or molecule after absorbing energy from exposure to light, electricity, elevated temperature, or chemical re-

action, and which may be a necessary prelude to a chemical reaction or to the emission of light.

ex·cite·ment (ĭk-sīt′mənt) *n.* An emotional state characterized by its potential for impulsive or poorly controlled activity.

ex·cit·ing eye (ĭk-sī′tĭng) *n.* The injured eye in sympathetic ophthalmia.

ex·ci·to·mo·tor (ĭk-sī′tō-mō′tər) *adj.* Causing or increasing the rapidity of motion.

ex·ci·to·re·flex nerve (ĭk-sī′tō-rē′flĕks′) *n.* A visceral nerve that causes reflex action.

ex·ci·tor nerve (ĭk-sī′tər) *n.* A nerve conducting impulses that stimulate increased function.

ex·clave (ĕk′sklāv′) *n.* An outlying, detached portion of a gland or other part, as of the thyroid or pancreas; an accessory gland.

ex·clu·sion (ĭk-skloō′zhən) *n.* Surgical isolation of a part or segment without removal from the body.

ex·co·ri·ate (ĭk-skôr′ē-āt′) *v.* To scratch or otherwise abrade the skin by physical means. —**ex·co′ri·a′tion** *n.*

ex·cre·ment (ĕk′skrə-mənt) *n.* Waste matter or any excretion cast out of the body, especially feces.

ex·cre·men·ti·tious (ĕk′skrə-mĕn-tĭsh′əs) *adj.* Relating to any cast-out waste material.

ex·cres·cence (ĭk-skrĕs′əns) *n.* An outgrowth from a surface that may be normal, such as a fingernail, or abnormal, such as a wart.

ex·cres·cent (ĭk-skrĕs′ənt) *adj.* Growing out abnormally, excessively, or superfluously.

ex·cre·ta (ĭk-skrē′tə) *pl.n.* Waste matter, such as sweat or feces, discharged from the body. —**ex·cre′tal** *adj.*

ex·crete (ĭk-skrēt′) *v.* To eliminate waste material from the body.

ex·cre·tion (ĭk-skrē′shən) *n.* 1. The act or process of discharging waste matter from the blood, tissues, or organs. 2. The matter, such as urine, feces, or sweat, that is so excreted.

ex·cre·to·ry (ĕk′skrĭ-tôr′ē) *adj.* Of, relating to, or used in excretion.

excretory duct *n.* Any of the various ducts carrying secretion from a gland or fluid from a reservoir.

excretory ductule of lacrimal gland *n.* Any of the ductules that open into the superior fornix of the conjunctival sac.

excretory gland *n.* A gland separating waste material from the blood.

ex·cy·clo·duc·tion (ĭk-sī′klō-dŭk′shən) *n.* The outward rotation of the upper pole of a cornea.

ex·cy·clo·pho·ri·a (ĭk-sī′klō-fôr′ē-ə) *n.* The tendency of the eyes to rotate outward, prevented by the impulse of the eyes to act in coordination. Also called *plus cyclophoria.*

ex·cys·ta·tion (ĕk′sĭ-stā′shən) *n.* Escape from a cyst. Used of encysted parasites.

ex·ec·u·tive function (ĭg-zĕk′yə-tĭv) *n.* The cognitive process that regulates an individual's ability to organize thoughts and activities, prioritize tasks, manage time efficiently, and make decisions. Impairment of executive function is seen in a range of disorders, including some pervasive developmental disorders and nonverbal learning disabilities.

ex·e·mi·a (ĭk-sē′mē-ə) *n.* A condition in which a considerable portion of the blood is temporarily removed from general circulation, as in shock when there is a great accumulation within the abdomen.

ex·en·ceph·a·ly (ĕk′sən-sĕf′ə-lē) *n.* A condition in which the skull is defective, causing exposure or extrusion of the brain. —**ex′en·ce·phal′ic** (-sə-făl′ĭk) *adj.*

ex·en·ter·a·tion (ĕk-sĕn′tə-rā′shən) *n.* The surgical removal of internal organs and tissues, usually the radical removal of the contents of a body cavity. Also called *evisceration.* —**ex·en′ter·ate′** *v.*

ex·en·ter·i·tis (ĕk-sĕn′tə-rī′tĭs) *n.* Inflammation of the peritoneal covering of the intestine.

ex·er·cise (ĕk′sər-sīz′) *n.* Active bodily exertion performed to develop or maintain fitness.

exercise physiology *n.* The study of the body's metabolic response to short-term and long-term physical activity.

ex·er·e·sis (ĕk-sĕr′ĭ-sĭs) *n.* Surgical removal of any part or organ; excision.

ex·er·gon·ic (ĕk′sər-gŏn′ĭk) *adj.* Of or relating to a reaction that releases energy to its surroundings.

ex·fo·li·a·tion (ĕks-fō′lē-ā′shən) *n.* **1.** Detachment and shedding of superficial cells of an epithelium or a tissue surface. **2.** Scaling or desquamation of the horny layer of epidermis. **3.** Loss of deciduous teeth following physiological loss of root structure. **4.** Extrusion of permanent teeth as a result of disease or loss of opposing teeth. —**ex·fo′li·ate′** *v.*

ex·fo·li·a·tive (ĕks-fō′lē-ā′tĭv) *adj.* Marked by exfoliation, desquamation, or profuse scaling.

exfoliative cytology *n.* The microscopic examination of cells that have been shed from a lesion or have been recovered from a tissue for the diagnosis of disease. Also called *cytopathology.*

exfoliative dermatitis *n.* Widespread dermatitis characterized by scaling and shedding of the skin and usually accompanied by redness. Also called *pityriasis rubra.*

exfoliative gastritis *n.* Gastritis with excessive shedding of mucosal epithelial cells.

ex·ha·la·tion (ĕks′hə-lā′shən, ĕk′sə-) *n.* **1.** The act or an instance of breathing out. Also called *expiration.* **2.** The giving forth of gas or vapor. **3.** Something, such as air or vapor, that is exhaled.

ex·hale (ĕks-hāl′, ĕk-sāl′) *v.* **1.** To breathe out. **2.** To emit a gas, vapor, or odor.

ex·haus·tion (ĭg-zôs′chən) *n.* **1.** The inability to respond to stimuli; extreme fatigue. **2.** The act or an instance of using up a supply of something. **3.** The extraction of the active constituents of a drug by treating with water, alcohol, or another solvent.

exhaustion psychosis *n.* A confused emotional state resulting from exhaustion.

ex·hi·bi·tion·ism (ĕk′sə-bĭsh′ə-nĭz′əm) *n.* An abnormal compulsion to expose the genitals with the intent of provoking sexual interest in the viewer. —**ex′hi·bi′tion·ist** *n.*

Ex-Lax (ĕks′lăks′) A trademark for an over-the-counter laxative containing senna.

exo– *pref.* Outside; external: *exoskeleton.*

ex·o·an·ti·gen (ĕk′sō-ăn′tĭ-jən) *n.* See **ectoantigen.**

ex·o·car·di·a (ĕk′sō-kär′dē-ə) *n.* See **ectocardia.**

ex·o·crine (ĕk′sə-krĭn, -krēn, -krīn′) *adj.* **1.** Of or relating to a glandular secretion released externally through a duct to a surface. **2.** Relating to a gland that secretes outwardly through a duct or ducts.

exocrine gland *n.* A gland, such as a sebaceous gland or sweat gland, that releases its secretions to the body's cavities, organs, or surface through a duct.

ex·o·cy·to·sis (ĕk′sō-sī-tō′sĭs) *n., pl.* **-ses** (-sēz′) **1.** The appearance of migrating inflammatory cells in the epidermis. **2.** A process of cellular secretion or excretion in which substances contained in vesicles are discharged from the cell by fusion of the vesicular membrane with the outer cell membrane. Also called *emiocytosis.*

ex·o·de·vi·a·tion (ĕk′sō-dē′vē-ā′shən) *n.* **1.** Exophoria. **2.** Exotropia.

ex·o·don·tia (ĕk′sə-dŏn′shə) *n.* Exodontics.

ex·o·don·tics (ĕk′sə-dŏn′tĭks) *n.* The dental specialty dealing with tooth extraction. —**ex′o·don′tist** *n.*

ex·o·en·zyme (ĕk′sō-ĕn′zīm′) *n.* See **extracellular enzyme.**

ex·o·e·ryth·ro·cyt·ic stage (ĕk′sō-ĭ-rĭth′rə-sĭt′ĭk) *n.* The developmental stage of the malaria parasite in liver parenchyma cells of the vertebrate host before the red blood cells become infected.

ex·og·a·my (ĕk-sŏg′ə-mē) *n.* Sexual reproduction by means of conjugation of two gametes of different ancestry, as in certain protozoan species.

ex·o·gas·tru·la (ĕk′sō-gǎs′trə-lə) *n.* An abnormal embryo in which the primitive gut has been everted.

ex·og·e·nous (ĕk-sŏj′ə-nəs) *adj.* **1.** Originating or produced outside of an organism, tissue, or cell. **2.** Having a cause external to the body. Used of diseases. —**ex·og′e·nous·ly** *adv.*

exogenous fiber *n.* Any of the afferent or efferent nerve fibers by which a given region of the central nervous system is connected with other regions.

exogenous hyperglyceridemia *n.* Persistent hyperglyceridemia due to a retarded rate of removal of dietary chylomicrons from plasma.

ex·om·pha·los (ĕk-sŏm′fə-lŏs′, -ləs) *n.* **1.** Protrusion or rupture of the navel. **2.** See **umbilical hernia. 3.** See **omphalocele.**

ex·on (ĕk′sŏn) *n.* A nucleotide sequence in DNA that carries the code for the final mRNA molecule and thus defines a protein's amino acid sequence. Also called *coding sequence.* —**ex·on′ic** *adj.*

ex·o·nu·cle·ase (ĕk′sō-nōō′klē-ās′, -āz′) *n.* Any of a group of enzymes that catalyze the hydrolysis of single nucleotides from the end of a DNA or RNA chain.

ex·o·pep·ti·dase (ĕk′sō-pĕp′tĭ-dās′, -dāz′) *n.* Any of a group of enzymes that catalyze the hydrolysis of single amino acids from the end of a polypeptide chain.

Ex·o·phi·a·la (ĕk′sō-fī′ə-lə) *n.* A genus of pathogenic fungi including species that cause mycetoma, phaeohyphomycosis, and tinea nigra.

Exophiala jean·sel·me·i (jēn-sĕl′mē-ī′) *n.* A fungus found in cases of mycetoma or phaeohyphomycosis.

Exophiala wer·neck·i·i (wər-nĕk′ē-ī′) *n.* A fungus that causes tinea nigra.

ex·o·pho·ri·a (ĕk′sə-fôr′ē-ə) *n.* A tendency of the eyes to deviate outward. —**ex′o·phor′ic** (-fôr′ĭk) *adj.*

ex·oph·thal·mic (ĕk′səf-thăl′mĭk) *adj.* **1.** Of or relating to exophthalmos. **2.** Marked by prominence of the eyeball.

exophthalmic goiter *n.* Any of various forms of hyperthyroidism, such as Graves' disease, involving enlargement of the thyroid gland and protrusion of the eyeballs.

exophthalmic ophthalmoplegia *n.* Ophthalmoplegia with protrusion of the eyeballs due to orbital edema and contracture of the ocular muscles, incidental to thyroid disorders.

ex·oph·thal·mos (ĕk′səf-thăl′məs) *n.* Abnormal protrusion of the eyeball.

ex·o·phyt·ic (ĕk′sə-fĭt′ĭk) *adj.* Growing outward. Used of a tumor or oral lesion.

ex·o·se·ro·sis (ĕk′sō-sĭ-rō′sĭs) *n.* Serous oozing from the skin surface, as from eczema or abrasion.

ex·o·skel·e·ton (ĕk′sō-skĕl′ĭ-tn) *n.* **1.** All hard parts, such as hair, teeth, and nails, that develop from the ectoderm or mesoderm in vertebrates. **2.** A hard outer structure, such as the shell of an insect, that provides protection or support for an organism.

ex·os·mo·sis (ĕk′sŏz-mō′sĭs, -sŏs-) *n.* The passage of a fluid through a semipermeable membrane toward a solution of lower concentration, especially the passage of water through a cell membrane into the surrounding medium. —**ex′os·mot′ic** (-mŏt′ĭk) *adj.*

ex·os·to·sis (ĕk′sŏ-stō′sĭs) *n.*, *pl.* **-ses** (-sēz) A projection that is capped by cartilage and arises from a bone that develops from cartilage. Also called *hyperostosis, poroma.*

exostosis car·ti·la·gin·e·a (kär′tl-ə-jĭn′ē-ə) *n.* An ossified chondroma arising from the epiphysis or joint surface of a bone.

ex·o·ter·ic (ĕk′sə-tĕr′ĭk) *adj.* Arising outside the organism; of external origin.

ex·o·ther·mic (ĕk′sō-thûr′mĭk) *or* **ex·o·ther·mal** (-məl) *adj.* **1.** Of or relating to a chemical reaction during which heat is released. **2.** Of or relating to the external warmth of the body.

ex·o·tox·ic (ĕk′sō-tŏk′sĭk) *adj.* **1.** Relating to an exotoxin. **2.** Relating to the introduction of an exogenous poison or toxin.

ex·o·tox·in (ĕk′sō-tŏk′sĭn) *n.* A toxin secreted by a microorganism and released into the environment in which it grows. Also called *extracellular toxin.*

ex·o·tro·pi·a (ĕk′sə-trō′pē-ə) *n.* Strabismus in which the visual axis of one eye deviates from that of the other. Also called *divergent strabismus, walleye.*

ex·pan·sion (ĭk-spăn′shən) *n.* **1.** An increase in size. **2.** The spreading out of a structure, such as a tendon.

ex·pec·tant (ĭk-spĕk′tənt) *adj.* Pregnant.

ex·pec·to·rant (ĭk-spĕk′tər-ənt) *adj.* Promoting or facilitating the secretion or expulsion of phlegm, mucus, or other matter from the respiratory tract. —*n.* An expectorant medicine.

ex·pec·to·rate (ĭk-spĕk′tə-rāt′) *v.* **1.** To eject saliva, mucus, or other body fluid from the mouth; spit. **2.** To clear out the chest and lungs by coughing up and spitting out matter. —**ex·pec′to·ra′tion** *n.*

ex·pe·ri·ence (ĭk-spîr′ē-əns) *n.* The feeling of emotions and sensations as opposed to thinking; involvement in what is happening rather than abstract reflection on an event. —**ex·pe′ri·ence** *v.*

ex·per·i·ment (ĭk-spĕr′ə-mənt) *n.* **1.** A test under controlled conditions that is made to demonstrate a known truth, to examine the validity of a hypothesis, or to determine the efficacy of something previously untried. **2.** The process of conducting such a test; experimentation. **3.** An innovative act or procedure. **4.** The result of experimentation. —*v.* (-mĕnt′) **1.** To conduct an experiment. **2.** To try something new, especially in order to gain experience.

ex·per·i·men·tal group (ĭk-spĕr′ə-mĕn′tl) *n.* A group of subjects that are exposed to the variable of a control experiment.

experimental medicine *n.* The scientific investigation of medical problems by experimentation upon animals or by clinical research.

experimental psychology *n.* **1.** The branch of psychology that studies conditioning, learning, perception, motivation, emotion, language, and thinking by conducting experiments under controlled conditions. **2.** Any of the branches of psychology that make extensive use of experimental methods.

experimenter effect *n.* The influence of the experimenter's behavior, personality traits, or expectancies on the results of his or her own research.

ex·pi·ra·tion (ĕk′spə-rā′shən) *n.* See **exhalation** (sense 1).

ex·pi·ra·to·ry (ĭk-spī′rə-tôr′ē) *adj.* Of, relating to, or involving the expiration of air from the lungs.

expiratory reserve volume *n. Abbr.* **ERV** The maximal volume of air, usually about 1000 milliliters, that can be expelled from the lungs after normal expiration. Also called *reserve air, supplemental air.*

expiratory stridor *n.* A singing sound during general anesthesia due to the semi-approximated vocal cords offering resistance to the escape of air.

ex·pire (ĭk-spīr′) *v.* **1.** To breathe one's last breath; die. **2.** To exhale.

ex·pired gas (ĭk-spīrd′) *n.* **1.** A gas that has been expired from the lungs. **2.** See **mixed expired gas.**

ex·plant (ĕk-splănt′) *v.* To transfer living tissue from an organism to an artificial medium for culture. —*n.* (ĕks′plănt′) Tissue so transferred.

ex·plo·ra·tion (ĕk′splə-rā′shən) *n.* An active examination, usually involving endoscopy or a surgical procedure, to determine conditions present as an aid in diagnosis. —**ex·plor′a·to′ry** (ĭk-splôr′ə-tôr′ē) *adj.*

explore (ĭk-splôr′) *v.* To examine for diagnostic purposes.

ex·plor·er (ĭk-splôr′ər) *n.* A sharp, pointed probe used on tooth surfaces to detect caries or other defects.

ex·po·sure keratitis (ĭk-spō′zhər) *n.* See **lagophthalmic keratitis.**

ex·press (ĭk-sprĕs′) *v.* **1.** To press or squeeze out. **2.** To produce a phenotype. Used of a gene.

ex·pressed skull fracture (ĭk-sprĕst′) *n.* A fracture in which part of the bone of the skull is pushed outward.

ex·pres·sion (ĭk-sprĕsh′ən) *n.* **1.** The act of pressing or squeezing out. **2.** The outward manifestation of a mood or disposition by mobility of the facial features;

facies. **3.** The phenotype manifested by a genotype under fixed environmental conditions.

expression vector *n.* A vector, such as a plasmid, yeast, or animal virus genome, used to introduce foreign genetic material into a host cell in order to replicate and amplify the foreign DNA sequences as a recombinant molecule.

ex·pres·sive aphasia (ĭk-sprĕs′ĭv) *n.* See **motor aphasia.**

ex·pul·sive (ĭk-spŭl′sĭv) *adj.* Tending to expel.

expulsive pain *n.* A labor pain associated with contraction of the uterine muscle.

ex·qui·site (ĕk′skwĭ-zĭt, ĭk-skwĭz′ĭt) *n.* Extremely intense, keen, or sharp. Used of pain or tenderness.

ex·san·gui·nate (ĕks-săng′gwə-nāt′) *v.* To deprive of or drain of blood. —**ex·san′gui·na′tion** *n.*

ex·san·guine (ĕks-săng′gwĭn) *adj.* Deprived of blood.

ex·sect (ĕk-sĕkt′) *v.* To excise. No longer in technical use.

ex·sec·tion (ĕk-sĕk′shən) *n.* See **excision.**

ex·sic·cant (ĕk-sĭk′ənt) *n.* Desiccant. —**ex·sic′cant** *adj.*

ex·sic·cate (ĕk′sĭ-kāt′) *v.* To dry up or cause to dry up; desiccate. —**ex′sic·ca′tor** *n.*

ex·sic·ca·tion (ĕk′sĭ-kā′shən) *n.* **1.** The process of being dried up; desiccation. **2.** Removal of water of crystallization.

ex·sorp·tion (ĕk-zôrp′shən) *n.* The movement of substances from the blood into the lumen of the gut.

ex·stro·phy (ĕk′strə-fē) *n.* A congenital turning out or eversion of a hollow organ.

exstrophy of bladder *n.* A congenital gap in the anterior wall of the bladder and the abdominal wall in front of it, with exposure of the posterior wall of the bladder.

exstrophy of cloaca *n.* A developmental anomaly in which an area of intestinal mucosa is interposed between two separate areas of the urinary bladder.

ext. *abbr.* extension; external; extract

ex·tend (ĭk-stĕnd′) *v.* To straighten a limb; unbend.

ex·tended family therapy (ĭk-stĕn′dĭd) *n.* Family therapy that involves family members who are outside the nuclear family but are closely associated with it.

extended radical mastectomy *n.* Surgical removal of the entire breast, the pectoral muscles, and the lymphatic-bearing tissues of the armpit and chest wall.

ex·ten·sion (ĭk-stĕn′shən) *n.* *Abbr.* **ext. 1.** The act of straightening or extending a flexed limb. **2.** A pulling or dragging force exerted on a limb in a distal direction.

ex·ten·sor (ĭk-stĕn′sər) *n.* A muscle that extends or straightens a limb or body part.

extensor dig·i·tor·um brev·is (dĭj′ĭ-tôr′əm brĕv′ĭs) *n.* A muscle with its origin from the dorsal surface of the calcaneus, with insertion by four tendons to those of the long extensor muscle of the toes and by a slip to the base of the proximal phalanx of the big toe, with nerve supply from the deep peroneal nerve, and whose action extends the toes.

extensor hal·lu·cis brevis (hăl′ōō-sĭs, -kĭs) *n.* The medial belly of the short extensor muscle of the toes, whose tendon is inserted into the base of the proximal phalanx of the big toe.

extensor muscle of fingers *n.* A muscle with origin from the lateral epicondyle of the humerus, with insertion into the base of the proximal, middle, and distal phalanges, with nerve supply from the radial nerve, and whose action extends the fingers.

extensor muscle of index finger *n.* A muscle with its origin from the ulna, with insertion to an aponeurosis of the index finger, with nerve supply from the radial nerve, and whose action assists in extending the forefinger.

extensor muscle of little finger *n.* A muscle with its origin from the lateral epicondyle of the humerus, with insertion to the dorsum of the proximal, middle, and distal phalanges of the little finger, with nerve supply from the radial nerve, and whose action extends the little finger.

extensor pol·li·cis brevis (pŏl′ə-sĭs, -kĭs) *n.* A muscle with origin from the trapezium and the flexor retinaculum, with insertion to the proximal phalanx of the thumb, with nerve supply from the median nerve, and whose action abducts the thumb.

extensor retinaculum *n.* A strong fibrous band stretching obliquely across the back of the wrist and binding down the extensor tendons of the fingers and thumb.

ex·te·ri·or·ize (ĭk-stîr′ē-ə-rīz′) *v.* **1.** To turn outward; externalize. **2.** To direct a patient's interest, thoughts, or feelings into a channel leading outside himself or herself. **3.** To expose an internal organ temporarily for observation, or permanently for physiological experiment or surgery.

ex·tern (ĕk′stûrn′) *n.* An advanced student or recent graduate who assists in the medical or surgical care of hospital patients and may reside outside the institution.

ex·ter·nal (ĭk-stûr′nəl) *adj.* *Abbr.* **ext.** Relating to, connected with, or existing on the outside; exterior.

external acoustic pore *n.* The orifice of the ear canal in the tympanic portion of the temporal bone. Also called *external acoustic foramen, external auditory foramen.*

external auditory canal *n.* See **ear canal.**

external auditory foramen *n.* See **external acoustic pore.**

external capsule *n.* A thin lamina of white substance in the brain that separates the claustrum from the putamen.

external carotid nerve *n.* Any of the sympathetic nerve fibers extending upward from the superior cervical ganglion along the external carotid artery, forming the external carotid plexus.

external carotid plexus *n.* An autonomic plexus that is formed by the external carotid nerves, surrounds the external carotid artery, and gives origin to a number of secondary plexuses along the branches of the external carotid artery.

external carotid steal syndrome *n.* Brief ischemic attacks that are marked by dizziness and loss of balance and are caused by insufficient blood supply to the vertebral and basilar arteries.

external conjugate *n.* The distance in a straight line between the depression under the last spinous process of the lumbar vertebrae and the upper edge of the pubic symphysis.

external ear *n.* The outer portion of the ear including the auricle and the passage leading to the eardrum. Also called *outer ear.*

external elastic lamina *n.* A layer of elastic connective tissue lying immediately outside the smooth muscle of the tunica media of an artery. Also called *external elastic layer.*

external fistula *n.* A fistula between a body cavity and the skin.

external fixation *n.* The fixation of a fractured bone by a splint or plastic dressing.

external genitalia *n.* **1.** The vulva of the female. **2.** The penis and scrotum of the male.

external hemorrhoids *pl.n.* Hemorrhoids occurring at the outer side of the external anal sphincter.

external iliac vein *n.* A continuation of the femoral vein above the inguinal ligament, uniting with the internal iliac vein to form the common iliac vein.

external intercostal muscle *n.* Any of the muscles with their origin from the lower border of a rib, with insertion into the upper border of the rib below, with nerve supply from the intercostal nerve, and that contract during inspiration and maintain tension in the intercostal spaces to resist mediolateral movement.

external jugular vein *n.* A vein that is formed by the junction of the posterior auricular and the retromandibular veins, passes down the side of the neck superficial to the sternocleidomastoid muscle, and empties into the subclavian vein.

external nasal vein *n.* Any of several vessels that drain the external nose and empty into the angular vein or the facial vein.

external obturator muscle *n.* A muscle with origin from the margin of the obturator foramen and the adjacent surface of the obturator membrane, with insertion into fossa of the greater trochanter, with nerve supply from the obturator nerve, and whose action rotates the thigh laterally.

external occipital crest *n.* A ridge extending from the external occipital protuberance to the border of the great foramen.

external ophthalmopathy *n.* A disease of the conjunctiva, cornea, or adnexa of the eye.

external ophthalmoplegia *n.* Paralysis affecting one or more of the extrinsic eye muscles.

external phase *n.* See **dispersion medium.**

external pudendal vein *n.* Any of the veins that correspond to the external pudendal arteries, empty into the great saphenous vein or into the femoral vein, and receive the superficial dorsal veins of the penis or clitoris and the anterior scrotal or labial veins.

external respiration *n.* The exchange of respiratory gases in the lungs.

external spermatic artery *n.* See **cremasteric artery.**

external sphincter muscle of anus *n.* A fusiform ring of striated muscular fibers surrounding the anus, attached posteriorly to the coccyx and anteriorly to the central tendon of the perineum.

external traction *n.* A pulling force created by using fixed anchorage outside the oral cavity.

external urethral opening *n.* **1.** The slitlike opening of the urethra in the glans penis. **2.** In the female, the external orifice of the urethra in the vestibule.

external urethrotomy *n.* A urethrotomy via an external opening in the perineum or penile skin.

external version *n.* Version of a fetus performed by external manipulation with both hands.

ex·ter·o·cep·tor (ĕk′stə-rō-sĕp′tər) *n.* One of the peripheral end organs of the afferent nerves in the skin or mucous membranes that respond to stimuli from outside the body. —**ex′ter·o·cep′tive** *adj.*

ex·ter·o·fec·tive (ĕk′stə-rō-fĕk′tĭv) *n.* Relating to the response of the nervous system to external stimuli.

ex·ti·ma (ĕk′stə-mə) *n.* The outermost coat of a blood vessel.

ex·tinc·tion (ĭk-stĭngk′shən) *n.* Progressive reduction in the strength of the conditioned response in successive conditioning trials during which only the conditioned stimulus is presented and the unconditioned stimulus is omitted. See **absorbance.**

ex·tin·guish (ĭk-stĭng′gwĭsh) *n.* To bring about the extinction of a conditioned response.

ex·tir·pa·tion (ĕk′stər-pā′shən) *n.* The surgical removal of an organ, part of an organ, or diseased tissue. —**ex′-tir·pate′** *v.*

ex·tor·sion (ĭk-stôr′shən) *n.* **1.** The outward rotation of a limb or organ. **2.** The outward divergent rotation of the upper poles of the vertical meridian of the cornea of each eye. Also called *disclination, positive declination.*

extra– *or* **extro–** *pref.* Outside; beyond: *extracellular.*

ex·tra·cap·su·lar (ĕk′strə-kăp′sə-lər) *adj.* Outside of a capsule.

extracapsular ankylosis *n.* Stiffness of a joint due to hardening or ossification of the surrounding tissues. Also called *spurious ankylosis.*

extracapsular ligament *n.* Any of the ligaments associated with a synovial joint but separate from and external to its articular capsule.

ex·tra·cel·lu·lar (ĕk′strə-sĕl′yə-lər) *adj.* Located or occurring outside a cell or cells.

extracellular enzyme *n.* An enzyme, such as a digestive enzyme, that functions outside the cell from which it originates. Also called *exoenzyme.*

extracellular fluid *n. Abbr.* **ECF 1.** The interstitial fluid and the plasma, constituting about 20 percent of the weight of the body. **2.** All fluid outside of cells, usually excluding transcellular fluid.

extracellular toxin *n.* See **exotoxin.**

ex·tra·chro·mo·so·mal element (ĕk′strə-krō′mə-sō′-məl) *n.* See **plasmid.**

extrachromosomal inheritance *n.* Inheritance of traits through DNA that is not connected with the chromosomes but rather to DNA from organelles in the cell. Also called *cytoplasmic inheritance.*

ex·tra·cor·po·re·al (ĕk′strə-kôr-pôr′ē-əl) *adj.* Situated or occurring outside the body.

extracorporeal circulation *n.* Circulation of the blood outside the body, as through a heart-lung machine or artificial kidney.

ex·tract (ĭk-străkt′) *v.* **1.** To draw or pull out, using force or effort. **2.** To obtain from a substance by chemical or mechanical action, as by pressure, distillation, or evaporation. **3.** To remove for separate consideration or publication; excerpt. **4.** To determine or calculate the root of a number. —*n.* (ĕk′străkt′) *Abbr.* **ext. 1.** A concentrated preparation of a drug obtained by removing the active constituents of the drug with suitable solvents, evaporating all or nearly all of the solvent, and adjusting the residual mass or powder to the prescribed standard. **2.** A preparation of the essential constituents of a food or a flavoring; a concentrate. —**ex·tract′a·ble, ex·tract′i·ble** *adj.* —**ex·trac′tor** *n.*

extracting forceps *n.* See **dental forceps.**

ex·trac·tion (ĭk-străk′shən) *n.* **1.** The act of extracting or the condition of being extracted. **2.** Something obtained by extracting; an extract. **3.** The removal by withdrawing or pulling out of a tooth from its socket. **4.** Removal of a baby from the genital canal in assisted delivery. **5.** The active portion of a drug.

extraction coefficient *n.* The percentage of a substance removed from the blood or plasma in a single passage through a tissue.

extraction ratio *n.* The fraction of a substance removed from blood flowing through the kidney, calculated using the ratio of the concentrations of the substance in arterial and renal venous plasma.

ex·trac·tive (ĭk-străk′tĭv) *adj.* **1.** Used in or obtained by extraction. **2.** Possible to extract. —*n.* **1.** Something that may be extracted. **2.** A substance present in tissue that can be separated by successive treatment with solvents and recovered by evaporation of the solution; the insoluble portion of an extract.

ex·trac·tor (ĭk-străk′tər) *n.* An instrument that is used for drawing or pulling out any natural part or foreign body.

ex·tra·cys·tic (ĕk′strə-sĭs′tĭk) *adj.* Outside of, or unrelated to, a cyst or bladder.

ex·tra·dur·al hemorrhage (ĕk′strə-dŏor′əl) *n.* See **epidural hematoma.**

ex·tra·em·bry·on·ic (ĕk′strə-ĕm′brē-ŏn′ĭk) *adj.* Located outside of the embryonic body.

ex·tra·oc·u·lar muscle (ĕk′strə-ŏk′yə-lər) *n.* Any of the six small muscles that control movement of the eyeball within the socket.

ex·tra·per·i·to·ne·al fascia (ĕk′strə-pĕr′ĭ-tn-ē′əl) *n.* See **subperitoneal fascia.**

ex·tra·phys·i·o·log·ic (ĕk′strə-fĭz′ē-ə-lŏj′ĭk) *adj.* Outside of the domain of physiology.

ex·tra·py·ram·i·dal (ĕk′strə-pĭ-răm′ĭ-dl) *adj.* Relating to or involving neural pathways situated outside or independent of the pyramidal tracts.

extrapyramidal dyskinesia *n.* Any of various movement disorders caused by disease of the extrapyramidal motor system of the brain and generally characterized by insuppressible, automatic movements that cease only during sleep.

extrapyramidal motor system *n.* Any of the various brain structures affecting bodily movement, excluding the motor neurons, the motor cortex, and the pyramidal tract, and including the corpus striatum, its substantia nigra and subthalamic nucleus, and its connections with the midbrain.

ex·tra·sac·cu·lar hernia (ĕk′strə-săk′yə-lər) *n.* See **sliding hernia.**

ex·tra·sen·so·ry (ĕk′strə-sĕn′sə-rē) *adj.* Being outside the normal range or bounds of the senses.

extrasensory perception *n.* *Abbr.* **ESP** Perception by means other than through the ordinary senses, as in telepathy, clairvoyance, or precognition.

ex·tra·sys·to·le (ĕk′strə-sĭs′tə-lē) *n.* An ectopic, usually premature contraction of one of the chambers of the heart, resulting in momentary cardiac arrhythmia. Also called *premature systole.*

ex·tra·u·ter·ine (ĕk′strə-yōō′tər-ĭn, -tə-rīn′) *adj.* Located or occurring outside the uterus.

ex·trav·a·sate (ĭk-străv′ə-sāt′) *v.* To exude from or pass out of a vessel into the tissues. Used of blood, lymph, or urine. —**ex·trav′a·sate′, ex·trav′a·sa′tion** *n.*

ex·tra·vas·cu·lar (ĕk′strə-văs′kyə-lər) *adj.* **1.** Located or occurring outside a blood or lymph vessel. **2.** Lacking vessels; nonvascular.

extravascular fluid *n.* All fluid outside the blood vessels, comprising both intracellular and transcellular fluids and constituting about 48 percent to 58 percent of the body weight.

ex·trem·i·tas (ĭk-strĕm′ĭ-təs) *n.,* *pl.* **ex·trem·i·ta·tes** (ĭk-strĕm′ĭ-tā′tēz) A limb; extremity.

ex·trem·i·ty (ĭk-strĕm′ĭ-tē) *n.* **1.** An end of an elongated or pointed structure. **2.** A bodily limb or appendage.

ex·trin·sic (ĭk-strĭn′sĭk, -zĭk) *adj.* Of or relating to an organ or structure, especially a muscle, originating outside of the part where it is found or upon which it acts; adventitious. —**ex·trin′si·cal·ly** *adv.*

extrinsic allergic alveolitis *n.* Pneumoconiosis resulting from hypersensitivity to inhaled organic dust.

extrinsic factor *n.* See **vitamin B₁₂.**

extrinsic incubation period *n.* The interval between the acquisition of an infectious agent by a vector and the vector's ability to transmit the agent to other susceptible vertebrate hosts.

extrinsic sphincter *n.* A sphincter formed by circular muscular fibers extraneous to the organ.

extro– *pref.* Variant of **extra–.**

ex·tro·ver·sion *or* **ex·tra·ver·sion** (ĕk′strə-vûr′zhən) *n.* **1.** A turning inside out, as of an organ or part. **2.** Interest in one's environment or in others as opposed to or to the exclusion of oneself.

ex·tro·vert *or* **ex·tra·vert** (ĕk′strə-vûrt′) *n.* An individual interested in others or in the environment as opposed to or to the exclusion of self.

ex·trude (ĭk-strōod′) *v.* **1.** To thrust, force, or press out. **2.** To protrude or project.

ex·tru·sion (ĭk-strōo′zhən) *n.* **1.** A thrusting or forcing out of a normal position. **2.** The eruption or migration of a tooth beyond its normal occlusal position.

ex·tu·ba·tion (ĕk′stōo-bā′shən) *n.* The removal of a tube from an organ, structure, or orifice; specifically, the removal of the tube after intubation of the larynx or trachea.

ex·u·ber·ant (ĭg-zōo′bər-ənt) *adj.* Proliferating or growing excessively.

ex·u·date (ĕks′yōo-dāt′) *n.* A fluid that has exuded out of a tissue or its capillaries due to injury or inflammation.

ex·u·da·tion (ĕks′yōo-dā′shən) *n.* **1.** The act or process of exuding. **2.** An exudate. —**ex′u·da′tive** *adj.*

exudation cyst *n.* A cyst resulting from distention of a closed cavity, such as a bursa, by an excessive secretion of its normal fluid contents.

exudative inflammation *n.* Inflammation in which the distinguishing feature is an exudate, which may be serous, serofibrinous, fibrinous, or mucous.

exudative retinitis *n.* A chronic inflammatory condition of the retina, characterized by the appearance of white or yellowish raised areas encircling the optic disk, due to the accumulation of edematous fluid beneath the retina. Also called *Coats disease.*

ex·ude (ĭg-zōod′, ĭk-sōod′) *v.* To ooze or pass gradually out of a body structure or tissue.

ex·um·bil·i·ca·tion (ĕk′sŭm-bĭl′ĭ-kā′shən) *n.* Protrusion of the navel.

eye (ī) *n.* **1.** An organ of vision or of light sensitivity. **2.** Either of a pair of hollow structures located in bony sockets of the skull, functioning together or independently, each having a lens capable of focusing incident light on an internal photosensitive retina from which nerve impulses are sent to the brain; the organ of vision. **3.** The external, visible portion of this organ together with its associated structures, especially the eyelids, eyelashes, and eyebrows. **4.** The pigmented iris of this organ. **5.** The faculty of seeing; vision.

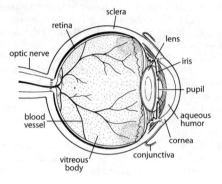

eye
cross section

eye·ball (ī′bôl′) *n.* **1.** The globe-shaped portion of the eye surrounded by the socket and covered externally by the eyelids. Also called *bulb of eye.* **2.** The eye itself.

eye bank *n.* A place where corneas of eyes removed immediately after death are preserved for subsequent keratoplasty.

eye bath *n.* See **eyecup** (sense 1).

eye·brow (ī′brou′) *n.* **1.** The bony ridge that extends over the eye. **2.** The arch of short hairs that covers this ridge.

eye chart *n.* A chart of letters and figures of various sizes, used to test visual acuity.

eye·cup (ī′kŭp′) *n.* **1.** A small cup with a rim contoured to fit the socket of the eye, used for applying a liquid medicine or wash to the eye. Also called *eye bath, eyeglass.* **2.** See **optic cup.**

eyed·ness (īd′nĭs) *n.* A preference for use of one eye rather than the other.

eye·drop·per (ī′drŏp′ər) *n.* A dropper for administering liquid medicines, especially one for dispensing medications into the eye.

eye·glass (ī′glăs′) *n.* **1.** eyeglasses Glasses for the eyes. **2.** A single lens in a pair of glasses; a monocle. **3.** See **eyepiece. 4.** See **eyecup** (sense 1).

eye·ground (ī′ground′) *n.* The fundus of the eye as seen with the ophthalmoscope.

eye·lash (ī′lăsh′) *n.* **1.** Any of the short hairs fringing the edge of the eyelid. Also called *cilium.* **2.** A row of hairs fringing the eyelid.

eyelash sign *n.* An indication of unconsciousness due to functional disease, such as conversion hysteria, rather than cranial trauma or a brain lesion, in which the stroking of the eyelashes will elicit movement of the eyelids.

eye·lid *or* **eye-lid** (ī′lĭd′) *n.* Either of two folds of skin and muscle that can be closed over the exposed portion of the eyeball. Also called *palpebra.*

eye·lift (ī′lĭft′) *n.* Cosmetic plastic surgery of the tissue surrounding the eye to reduce or eliminate folds, wrinkles, and sags.

eye·piece (ī′pēs′) *n.* The compound lens located at the end of a microscope tube nearest the eye. Also called *eyeglass.*

eye·sight (ī′sīt′) *n.* **1.** The faculty of sight; vision. **2.** Range of vision; view.

eye socket *n.* See **orbital cavity.**

eye·strain (ī′strān′) *n.* Pain and fatigue of the eyes, often accompanied by headache, due to prolonged use of the eyes, uncorrected defects of vision, or imbalance of the eye muscles. Also called *asthenopia.*

eye·tooth (ī′tōoth′) *n.* A canine tooth of the upper jaw.

eye·wash (ī′wŏsh′) *n.* A soothing solution for bathing or medicating the eye.

e·zet·i·mibe (ĭ-zĕt′ə-mīb′) *n.* A drug that inhibits the absorption of cholesterol from the intestine and is used to treat primary hypercholesterolemia.

F

F¹ The symbol for the element **fluorine**.

F² *abbr.* Fahrenheit

FAAN *abbr.* Fellow of the American Academy of Nursing

fa·bel·la (fə-bĕl′ə) *n., pl.* **–bel·lae** (-bĕl′ē) A small sesamoid bone in the tendon of the lateral head of the gastrocnemius muscle.

Fab fragment (ĕf′ā-bē′) *n.* The portion of an immunoglobulin molecule that binds the antigen.

Fa·bri·cus ab A·qua·pen·den·te (fă-brĭsh′ē-əs ăb ăk′wə-pĕn-dĕn′tē), **Hieronymus** 1537–1619. Italian anatomist who gave the first detailed descriptions (1603) of the semilunar valves of the veins and established embryology as a medical discipline with his comparative studies of human and animal fetal development.

Fa·bry's disease (fă′brēz) *n.* A sex-linked disorder of glycolipid metabolism characterized by a variety of progressive symptoms including fevers, hypertension, and purple skin lesions, with death resulting from renal, cardiac, or cerebrovascular complications. Also called *angiokeratoma corporis diffusum.*

FACCP *abbr.* Fellow of the American College of Chest Physicians

FACD *abbr.* Fellow of the American College of Dentists

face (fās) *n.* **1.** The front portion of the head, from forehead to chin. **2.** Facies.

face-bow (fās′bō′) *n.* A caliperlike device used in dentistry to record the relationship of the jaws to the temporomandibular joints.

face-lift (fās′lĭft′) *n.* Plastic surgery to remove facial wrinkles, sagging skin, fat deposits, or other visible signs of aging for cosmetic purposes. Also called *rhytidectomy, rhytidoplasty.*

face presentation *n.* Head presentation of the fetus during birth in which the face is the presenting part.

fac·et (făs′ĭt) *n.* **1.** A small smooth area on a bone or other firm structure. **2.** A worn spot on a tooth, produced by chewing or grinding.

fac·e·tec·to·my (făs′ĭ-tĕk′tə-mē) *n.* Excision of a facet, as of a vertebra.

fa·cial (fā′shəl) *adj.* Relating to the face.

facial artery *n.* An artery with origin in the external carotid artery, with branches to the palatine, tonsillar, and glandular branches, the submental, inferior and superior labial, masseteric, buccal, and nasal branches, and the angular artery; external maxillary artery.

facial axis *n.* See **basifacial axis.**

facial bone *n.* Any of the bones surrounding the mouth and nose and contributing to the eye sockets, including the upper jawbones, the zygomatic, nasal, lacrimal, and palatine bones, the inferior nasal concha and the vomer, lower jawbone, and hyoid bone.

facial canal *n.* The bony passage in the temporal bone through which the facial nerve passes to the stylomastoid foramen.

facial hemiplegia *n.* Paralysis of one side of the face.

facial muscle *n.* Any of the numerous muscles supplied by the facial nerve and that attach to and move the skin. Also called *muscle of facial expression.*

facial nerve *n.* Either of a pair of nerves that originate in the pons, traverse the facial canal of the temporal bone, and pass through the parotid gland, reach the facial muscles through various branches, control facial muscles, and relay sensation from the taste buds of the front part of the tongue. Also called *seventh cranial nerve.*

facial palsy *n.* Unilateral paralysis of the facial muscles supplied by the facial nerve. Also called *Bell's palsy, facial paralysis, facioplegia, prosopoplegia.*

facial tic *n.* Involuntary spasmodic movement of the facial muscles. Also called *facial spasm, prosopospasm.*

facial vein *n.* Any of four veins of the face; the anterior, common, deep, and retrimandibular.

–facient *suff.* **1.** Causing; bringing about: *somnifacient.* **2.** Something that causes or brings about: *abortifacient.*

fa·ci·es (fā′shē-ēz′, -shēz) *n., pl.* **facies 1.** Face. **2.** The appearance or expression of the face, especially when typical of a certain disorder or disease. **3.** The general aspect or outward appearance, as of a given growth of flora.

fa·cil·i·ta·tion (fə-sĭl′ĭ-tā′shən) *n.* The enhancement or reinforcement of a reflex or other nerve activity by the arrival of other excitatory impulses at the reflex center.

fac·ing (fā′sĭng) *n.* A tooth-colored material used to hide the buccal or labial surface of a gold crown to give the outward appearance of a natural tooth.

facio– *pref.* Face: *facioplegia.*

fa·ci·o·dig·i·to·gen·i·tal dysplasia (fā′shē-ō-dĭj′ĭ-tō-jĕn′ĭ-tl) *n.* An inherited syndrome characterized by an exaggerated width between the eyes, anteverted nostrils, broad upper lip, saddle-bag scrotum, and lax ligaments resulting in hyperextension of the knee, flat feet, and hyperextensible fingers. Also called *Aarskog-Scott syndrome.*

fa·ci·o·plas·ty (fā′shē-ə-plăs′tē) *n.* Reparative or reconstructive surgery of the face.

fa·ci·o·ple·gia (fā′shē-ō-plē′jə) *n.* See **facial palsy.**

fa·ci·o·scap·u·lo·hu·mer·al muscular dystrophy (fā′shē-ō-skăp′yə-lō-hyoo′mər-əl) *n.* A benign inherited form of dystrophy beginning in childhood and characterized by wasting and weakness primarily of the muscles of the face, shoulder girdle, and arms. Also called *Landouzy-Déjérine dystrophy.*

FACOG *abbr.* Fellow of the American College of Obstetricians and Gynecologists

FACP *abbr.* Fellow of the American College of Physicians; Fellow of the American College of Prosthodontists

FACR *abbr.* Fellow of the American College of Radiologists

FACS *abbr.* Fellow of the American College of Surgeons

FACSM *abbr.* Fellow of the American College of Sports Medicine

fac·ti·tious (făk-tĭsh′əs) *adj.* Produced artificially rather than by a natural process.

fac·tor (făk′tər) *n.* **1.** One that contributes in the cause of an action. **2.** A mathematical component that by multiplication makes up a number or expression. **3.** A gene. **4.** A substance, such as a vitamin, that functions in a specific biochemical reaction or bodily process, such as blood coagulation.

factor I *n.* See **fibrinogen.**

factor II *n.* **1.** See **prothrombin. 2.** See **lipoic acid.**

factor III *n.* See **thromboplastin.**

factor IV *n.* Calcium ions as a factor in the clotting of blood.

factor V *n.* A factor in the clotting of blood, a deficiency of which leads to parahemophilia. Also called *accelerator factor, plasma accelerator globulin, proaccelerin, prothrombin accelerator.*

factor VII *n.* A factor in the clotting of blood that forms a complex with tissue thromboplastin and calcium to activate the prothrombinase, thus acting to accelerate the conversion of prothrombin to thrombin. Also called *convertin, cothromboplastin, proconvertin, serum accelerator, serum accelerator globulin, serum prothrombin conversion accelerator.*

factor VIII *n.* A factor in the clotting of blood, a deficiency of which is associated with hemophilia A. Also called *antihemophilic factor, antihemophilic globulin, antihemophilic globulin A, proserum prothrombin conversion accelerator.*

factor IX *n.* A factor in the clotting of blood necessary for the formation of intrinsic blood thromboplastin; a deficiency of it causes hemophilia B. Also called *antihemophilic globulin B, Christmas factor.*

factor X *n.* See **prothrombinase.**

factor XI *n.* A factor in the clotting of blood, a deficiency of which results in a hemorrhagic tendency. Also called *plasma thromboplastin antecedent.*

factor XII *n.* A factor in the clotting of blood, a deficiency of which results in prolonged clotting time for venous blood. Also called *Hageman factor.*

factor XIII *n.* A factor in the clotting of blood that is converted by thrombin into its active form, which cross-links subunits of the fibrin clot to form insoluble fibrin. Also called *Laki-Lorand factor.*

fac·to·ri·al experiment (făk-tôr′ē-əl) *n.* An experimental design in which two or more series of treatments are tried in all combinations.

facts of life (făkts) *pl.n.* The basic physiological functions involved in sex and reproduction. Often used with *the.*

fac·ul·ta·tive (făk′əl-tā′tĭv) *adj.* **1.** Capable of functioning under varying environmental conditions. Used of certain organisms, such as bacteria that can live with or without oxygen. **2.** Capable of occurring along various pathways or under various conditions.

facultative anaerobe *n.* An organism, such as a bacterium, that can live in the absence as well as in the presence of atmospheric oxygen.

facultative hyperopia *n.* Manifest hyperopia that can be overcome by an effort of accommodation.

facultative parasite *n.* An organism that may either lead an independent existence or live as a parasite.

fac·ul·ty (făk′əl-tē) *n.* A natural or specialized power of a living organism.

FAD *abbr.* flavin adenine dinucleotide

Fa·den suture (fäd′n) *n.* A suture placed between an ocular rectus muscle and the posterior sclera to limit excessive action of the eyeball.

fag·o·py·rism (făg′ō-pī′rĭz′əm, fə-gŏp′ə-) *n.* Photosensitization, mainly in cattle and sheep, caused by ingestion of buckwheat *(Fagopyrum esculentum)* and characterized by irritation of the skin, edema, and a serous exudate.

Fahr·en·heit (făr′ən-hīt′) *adj. Abbr.* **F** Of or relating to a temperature scale that registers the freezing point of water as 32°F and the boiling point as 212°F at one atmosphere of pressure.

fail·ure (fāl′yər) *n.* The inability to function or perform satisfactorily.

failure to thrive *n. Abbr.* **FTT** A significant delay in physical growth of an infant or young child, caused by an organic, psychological, or environmental disturbance.

faint (fānt) *n.* An abrupt, usually brief loss of consciousness; an attack of syncope. *—adj.* Extremely weak; threatened with syncope. *—***faint** *v.*

faith healer (fāth) *n.* One who treats disease with prayer.

fal·cate (făl′kāt′) *adj.* Falciform.

fal·ci·form (făl′sə-fôrm′) *adj.* Curved and tapering to a point; sickle-shaped.

falciform ligament *n.* See **falciform process.**

falciform ligament of liver *n.* A crescent-shaped fold of the peritoneum extending to the surface of the liver from the diaphragm and the anterior abdominal wall.

falciform process *n.* A continuation of the inner border of the sacrotuberous ligament upward and forward on the inner aspect of the ramus of the ischium. Also called *falciform ligament.*

fal·cip·a·rum malaria (făl-sĭp′ər-əm, fôl-) *n.* Malaria caused by *Plasmodium falciparum* and characterized by severe malarial paroxysms that recur about every 48 hours and often by acute cerebral, renal, or gastrointestinal manifestations. Also called *malignant tertian malaria.*

fal·cu·la (făl′kyə-lə) *n.* See **falx cerebelli.**

fal·cu·lar (făl′kyə-lər) *adj.* **1.** Relating to the falx cerebelli. **2.** Falciform.

fall·en arch (fô′lən) *n.* A breaking down of the longitudinal or transverse arch of the foot, resulting in flat foot or spread foot.

fall·ing of womb (fô′lĭng) *n.* See **prolapse of uterus.**

fal·lo·pi·an (fə-lō′pē-ən) *adj.* Described by or attributed to Italian anatomist Gabriello Fallopio.

fallopian tube *or* **Fallopian tube** *n.* Either of a pair of slender tubes from each ovary to the side of the fundus of the uterus, through which the ova pass. Also called *gonaduct, oviduct, salpinx, uterine tube.*

Fal·lo·pi·o (fə-lō′pē-ō), **Gabriele** 1523–1562. Italian anatomist noted for his studies of the human reproductive system. The Fallopian tubes are named for him.

Fal·lot's tetralogy (fă-lōz′) *n.* A congenital malformation of the heart characterized by a defect in the ventricular septum, misplacement of the origin of the aorta, narrowing of the pulmonary artery, and enlargement of the right ventricle. Also called *Fallot's tetrad, tetralogy of Fallot.*

Fallot's triad *n.* Trilogy of Fallot.

false anemia (fôls) *n.* See **pseudoanemia.**

false aneurysm *n.* **1.** A pulsating, encapsulated hematoma communicating with a ruptured vessel. **2.** See **pseudoaneurysm.**

false ankylosis *n.* See **fibrous ankylosis.**

false blepharoptosis *n.* See **pseudoptosis.**

false conjugate *n.* **1.** See **diagonal conjugate. 2.** See **effective conjugate.**

false cyst *n.* See **pseudocyst** (sense 1).

false diverticulum *n.* A diverticulum of the intestine that passes through a defect in the muscular wall of the gut and thus does not include a layer of muscle in its wall.

false hematuria *n.* See **pseudohematuria.**

false hermaphroditism *n.* See **pseudohermaphroditism.**

false image *n.* The image produced in the deviating eye in strabismus.

false joint *n.* A bony junction, usually occurring at the site of a poorly united fracture, that allows abnormal motion. Also called *pseudarthrosis.*

false knot *n.* A knotlike bulge in the umbilical vein causing apparent twisting of the cord.

false membrane *n.* A thick, tough, fibrinous exudate formed on the surface of a mucous membrane or the skin. Also called *croupous membrane, neomembrane, plica, pseudomembrane.*

false negative *n.* A negative test result when the attribute for which the subject is being tested actually exists in that subject. —**false'-neg'a·tive** *adj.*

false-negative reaction *n.* An erroneous or mistakenly negative response.

false neuroma *n.* See **traumatic neuroma.**

false pain *n.* A uterine contraction, preceding and sometimes resembling a true labor pain, but distinguishable from it by the lack of progressive effacement and dilation of the cervix.

false pelvis *n.* See **large pelvis.**

false positive *n.* A positive test result in a subject that does not possess the attribute for which the test is being conducted. —**false'-pos·i·tive** *adj.*

false-positive reaction *n.* An erroneous or mistakenly positive response.

false pregnancy *n.* A usually psychosomatic condition, occurring in both males and females, in which physical symptoms of pregnancy are manifested without conception. Also called *pseudocyesis, pseudopregnancy.*

false rib *n.* Any of the five pairs of lower ribs that do not articulate directly with the sternum.

false suture *n.* A suture whose opposing margins are smooth or contain only a few projections.

false vocal cord *n.* See **vestibular fold.**

false waters *pl.n.* A leakage of fluid before or at the beginning of labor, before amnionic rupture.

fal·si·fi·ca·tion (fôl'sə-fĭ-kā'shən) *n.* The deliberate act of misrepresentation so as to deceive.

falx (fălks, fôlks) *n., pl.* **fal·ces** (făl'sēz', fôl'-) A sickle-shaped anatomical structure.

falx cer·e·bel·li (sĕr'ə-bĕl'ī) *n.* A short process of dura mater projecting from the internal occipital crest below

the tentorium, and bifurcating into two diverging limbs passing to either side of the foramen magnum. Also called *falcula.*

falx cer·e·bri (sĕr'ə-brī) *n.* The scythe-shaped fold of dura mater in the longitudinal fissure between the two cerebral hemispheres.

fam·ci·clo·vir (făm-sī'klō-vîr') *n.* A synthetic nucleoside analog used in the treatment of herpes simplex and herpes zoster infections.

fa·mil·ial (fə-mĭl'yəl) *adj.* Occurring or tending to occur among family members, usually by heredity.

familial aggregation *n.* Occurrence of a trait in more members of a family than can be readily accounted for by chance.

familial Alzheimer's disease *n.* An inherited form of Alzheimer's disease caused by a defect on a particular chromosome.

familial amyloidosis *n.* A hereditary form of amyloidosis associated with familial Mediterranean fever, cold hypersensitivity, various patterns of neuropathy, or amyloid deposits in various organs.

familial benign chronic pemphigus *n.* A recurrent blistering dermatitis, predominantly of the neck, groin, and armpit regions, characterized by vesicles and bullae that become crusted lesions with vesicular borders. Also called *Hailey and Hailey disease.*

familial broad-beta hyperlipoproteinemia *n.* See **type II familial hyperlipoproteinemia.**

familial dysautonomia *n.* A congenital disorder involving the nervous system, especially the functioning of the autonomic nervous system, and including such symptoms as indifference to pain, diminished secretion of tears, poor vasomotor control, motor incoordination, difficulty in swallowing and emotional instability. Also called *Riley-Day syndrome.*

familial fat-induced hyperlipemia *n.* See **type I familial hyperlipoproteinemia.**

familial hemiplegic migraine *n.* A rare inherited migraine disorder characterized by a temporary paralysis of one side of the body followed by severely throbbing headaches and nausea; it occasionally can cause coma.

familial high-density lipoprotein deficiency *n.* See **Tangier disease.**

familial hyperbetalipoproteinemia *n.* See **type II familial hyperlipoproteinemia.**

familial hyperbetalipoproteinemia and hyperprebetalipoproteinemia *n.* See **type III familial hyperlipoproteinemia.**

familial hypercholesterolemia *n.* **1.** See **type II familial hyperlipoproteinemia. 2.** See **hypercholesterolemia** (sense 2).

familial hypercholesterolemia with hyperlipemia *n.* See **type III familial hyperlipoproteinemia.**

familial hyperchylomicronemia *n.* See **type I familial hyperlipoproteinemia.**

familial hyperchylomicronemia with hyperprebetalipoproteinemia *n.* See **type V familial hyperlipoproteinemia.**

familial hyperlipoproteinemia *n.* Any of several inherited disorders of lipoprotein metabolism characterized by changes in serum concentrations of low-density lipoproteins and the lipids associated with them. For some clinical types, see under *type.*

familial hyperprebetalipoproteinemia *n.* See **type IV familial hyperlipoproteinemia.**

familial hypertriglyceridemia *n.* **1.** See **type I familial hyperlipoproteinemia. 2.** See **type IV familial hyperlipoproteinemia.**

familial hypertrophic cardiomyopathy *n.* An inherited, often fatal, heart condition caused by a genetic defect affecting production of myosin.

familial intestinal polyposis *n.* **1.** A hereditary disorder characterized by polyposis of the mucosa of the colon with no associated lesions. Polyps usually form in late childhood and may cover the mucosal surface. **2.** Polyposis of the small or large intestine that is associated with Gardner's, Peutz-Jeghers, Turcot, and Zollinger-Ellison syndromes.

familial Mediterranean fever *n.* See **familial paroxysmal polyserositis.**

familial non·he·mo·lyt·ic jaundice (nŏn′hē-mə-lĭt′ĭk) *n.* Jaundice without evidence of liver damage, biliary obstruction, or hemolysis. Also called *Gilbert's disease.*

familial paroxysmal polyserositis *n.* A hereditary disease that is characterized by transient, recurring attacks of abdominal pain, fever, pleurisy, arthritis, and rash. Also called *familial Mediterranean fever, Mediterranean fever.*

familial periodic paralysis *n.* Any of various inherited forms of periodic paralysis.

familial polyendocrine adenomatosis *n.* An inherited disorder in which functioning tumors occur in more than one endocrine gland, commonly the pancreatic islands and parathyroid glands, often associated with peptic ulcers and gastric hypersecretion.

familial screening *n.* The screening of close relatives of individuals who have diseases that may be latent, as in age-dependent dominant traits, or that may involve risk to offspring, as X-linked traits.

familial spinal muscular atrophy *n.* See **infantile muscular atrophy.**

fam·i·ly (făm′ə-lē, făm′lē) *n.* **1.** A group of blood relatives, especially parents and their children. **2.** A taxonomic category of related organisms ranking below an order and above a genus.

family doctor *n.* See **family physician.**

family medicine *n.* The branch of medicine that deals with the provision of comprehensive health care to individuals regardless of age or sex while placing particular emphasis on the family unit. Also called *family practice.*

family physician *n. Abbr.* **FP** A physician who practices the specialty of family medicine. Also called *family doctor, family practitioner.*

family planning *n.* A program to regulate the number and spacing of children in a family through the practice of contraception or other methods of birth control.

family practice *n. Abbr.* **FP** See **family medicine.**

family practitioner *n. Abbr.* **FP** See **family physician.**

family therapy *n.* A form of psychotherapy in which the interrelationships of family members are examined in group sessions in order to identify and alleviate problems of one or more family members.

fa·mo·ti·dine (fə-mō′tĭ-dēn′) *n.* A histamine H_2 antagonist used in the treatment of duodenal ulcers.

Fam·vir (făm′vîr′) A trademark for the drug famciclovir.

FANA test (ĕf′ā-ĕn-ā′) *n.* See **fluorescent antinuclear antibody test.**

Fan·co·ni's anemia (făn-kō′nēz, făn-) *n.* A type of idiopathic refractory anemia characterized by pancytopenia, hypoplasia of the bone marrow, and congenital anomalies, occurring in members of the same family. Also called *congenital pancytopenia.*

Fanconi's syndrome *n.* A group of renal tubular disorders that includes cystinosis, adult Fanconi's syndrome, and acquired Fanconi's syndrome.

fan·ta·sy (făn′tə-sē, -zē) *n.* Imagery that is more or less coherent, as in dreams and daydreams, yet unrestricted by reality. Also called *phantasia.*

fan·tom (făn′təm) *n.* Variant of **phantom.**

Far·a·beuf's triangle (făr′ə-bœfs′) *n.* A triangle formed by the internal jugular and facial veins and the hypoglossal nerve.

far·ad (făr′əd, -ăd′) *n.* The unit of capacitance in the meter-kilogram-second system equal to the capacitance of a capacitor having a charge of 1 coulomb when a potential difference of 1 volt is applied.

far·a·day (făr′ə-dā′) *n.* The electric charge required to deposit or liberate 1 gram equivalent weight of a substance in electrolysis, approximately 9.6494×10^4 coulombs.

far-and-near suture (făr′ənd-nîr′) *n.* A suture used to approximate fascial edges, in which alternate near and far stiches are used.

Far·ber's disease *or* **Far·ber's syndrome** (fär′bərz) *n.* See **disseminated lipogranulomatosis.**

far·del (fär-dĕl′) *n.* A measurement used in genetic counseling to determine the penalty incurred as a result of the occurrence of a genetic disease in an individual.

Far East·ern hemorrhagic fever (fär ē′stərn) *n.* See **epidemic hemorrhagic fever.**

far·i·na·ceous (făr′ə-nā′shəs) *adj.* Made from, rich in, or consisting of starch.

farm·er's lung (fär′mərz) *n.* An occupational disease characterized by fever and dyspnea, caused by inhalation of organic dust from moldy hay containing spores of actinomycetes and certain fungi.

far point *n.* The farthest point at which an object can be seen distinctly by the eye.

far·sight·ed *or* **far-sight·ed** (fär′sī′tĭd) *adj.* **1.** Able to see distant objects better than objects at close range; hyperopic. **2.** Capable of seeing to a great distance.

far·sight·ed·ness (fär′sī′tĭd-nĭs) *n.* See **hyperopia.**

FAS *abbr.* fetal alcohol syndrome

fas·ci·a (făsh′ē-ə) *n.,* *pl.* **fas·ci·ae** (făsh′ē-ē′, fā′shē-ē) A sheet or band of fibrous connective tissue enveloping, separating, or binding together muscles, organs, and other soft structures of the body. —**fas′ci·al** *adj.*

fascia ad·her·ens (ăd-hîr′ənz, -hĕr′-) *n.* A broad intercellular junction in the intercalated disk of cardiac muscle anchoring actin filaments.

fascia graft *n.* A graft of fibrous tissue, usually the broad fascia.

fas·ci·cle (făs′ĭ-kəl) *n.* See **fasciculus.**

fas·cic·u·lar (fə-sĭk′yə-lər) *or* **fas·cic·u·late** (-lĭt) *or* **fas·cic·u·lat·ed** (-lā′tĭd) *adj.* **1.** Relating to a fasciculus. **2.** Arranged in the form of a bundle or collection of rods.

fascicular degeneration *n.* Muscular degeneration due to atrophy of motor neurons in the spinal cord or brainstem.

fascicular graft *n.* A nerve graft in which each bundle of fibers is approximated and sutured separately.

fas·cic·u·la·tion (fə-sĭk′yə-lā′shən) *n.* **1.** An arrangement of fasciculi. **2.** A coarser form of muscular contraction than fibrillation, consisting of involuntary contractions or twitchings of groups of muscle fibers. —**fas·cic′u·late′** *v.*

fas·cic·u·lus (fə-sĭk′yə-ləs) *n., pl.* **–li** (-lī′) A bundle of anatomical fibers, as of muscle. Also called *fascicle.*

fasciculus grac·i·lis (grăs′ə-lĭs) *n.* The smaller medial subdivision of the posterior funiculus of the spinal cord. Also called *posterior pyramid of medulla.*

fas·ci·ec·to·my (făsh′ē-ĕk′tə-mē, făs′-) *n.* Excision of strips of fascia.

fas·ci·i·tis (făsh′ē-ī′tĭs, făs′-) *n.* **1.** Inflammation in a fascia. **2.** The proliferation of fibroblasts in a fascia.

fascio– *pref.* Fascia: *fasciotomy.*

fas·ci·od·e·sis (făsh′ē-ŏd′ĭ-sĭs, făs′-) *n.* Surgical attachment of fascia to another or to a tendon.

fas·ci·o·la (fə-sē′ə-lə, -sī′-) *n., pl.* **–lae** (-lē′) A small band or group of fibers.

Fasciola *n.* A genus of large digenetic liver flukes that infect mammals.

fas·ci·o·lar (fə-sē′ə-lər, -sī′-) *adj.* Of or relating to a fasciola.

fas·ci·o·li·a·sis (fə-sē′ə-lī′ə-sĭs, -sī′-) *n.* Infection with a liver fluke of the genus *Fasciola.*

fas·ci·o·lop·si·a·sis (făsh′ē-ō-lŏp-sī′ə-sĭs, fə-sī′ō-) *n.* Parasitization or disease caused by any of the flukes of the genus *Fasciolopsis.*

Fas·ci·o·lop·sis (făs′ē-ō-lŏp′sĭs, fə-sī′ō-) *n.* A genus of very large intestinal flukes that includes *Fasciolopsis buski,* a species found in the intestine of humans in eastern and southern Asia.

fas·ci·o·plas·ty (făsh′ē-ə-plăs′tē) *n.* Plastic surgery on a fascia.

fas·ci·or·rha·phy (făsh′ē-ôr′ə-fē) *n.* Suture of a fascia or of an aponeurosis. Also called *aponeurorrhaphy.*

fas·ci·ot·o·my (făsh′ē-ŏt′ə-mē) *n.* Incision through a fascia.

fast[1] (făst) *adj.* **1.** Acting, moving, or being capable of acting or moving quickly. **2.** Accomplished in relatively little time. **3.** Exhibiting resistance to change. Used especially of stained microorganisms that cannot be decolorized. **4.** Firmly fixed or fastened.

fast[2] (făst) *v.* **1.** To abstain from food. **2.** To eat little or abstain from certain foods, especially as a religious discipline. —*n.* **1.** The act or practice of abstaining from or eating very little food. **2.** A period of such abstention or self-denial.

fas·tid·i·ous (fă-stĭd′ē-əs, fə-) *adj.* **1.** Possessing or displaying careful, meticulous attention to detail. **2.** Difficult to please; exacting. **3.** Having complex nutritional requirements. Used of microorganisms.

fas·tig·i·um (fă-stĭj′ē-əm) *n.* **1.** The summit of the roof of the fourth ventricle of the brain. **2.** The acme or period of full development of a disease.

fast rhythm *n.* A brain-wave pattern on an electroencephalogram that occurs at a frequency above 13 hertz.

fast smear *n.* A cytologic smear containing vaginal and cervical scrapings that are mixed, smeared, and fixed immediately.

fast-twitch *adj.* Of or relating to skeletal muscle that is composed of strong, rapidly contracting fibers, adapted for high-intensity, low-endurance activities.

fat (făt) *n.* **1.** Any of various soft, solid, or semisolid organic compounds constituting the esters of glycerol and fatty acids and their associated organic groups. **2.** A mixture of such compounds occurring widely in organic tissue, especially in the adipose tissue of animals and in the seeds, nuts, and fruits of plants. **3.** Adipose tissue. **4.** Obesity; corpulence. —**fat** *adj.*

fa·tal (fāt′l) *adj.* Causing or capable of causing death.

fa·tal·i·ty (fā-tăl′ĭ-tē, fə-) *n.* **1.** A death resulting from an accident or disaster. **2.** One that is killed as a result of such an occurrence.

fa·tal·i·ty rate (fā-tăl′ĭ-tē, fə-) *n.* See **death rate.**

fat cell *n.* Any of various connective tissue cells found in adipose tissue, specialized for the storage of fat, and distended with one or more fat globules, the cytoplasm usually being compressed into a thin envelope, with the nucleus at one point in the periphery. Also called *adipose cell, adipocyte.*

fat embolism *n.* The presence of fat globules that obstruct circulation, usually the result of fractures of a long bone, burns, parturition, or the fatty degeneration of the liver.

fat·i·ga·ble (făt′ĭ-gə-bəl) *adj.* Subject to fatigue. —**fat′i·ga·bil′i·ty** *n.*

fa·tigue (fə-tēg′) *n.* **1.** Physical or mental weariness resulting from exertion. **2.** A sensation of boredom and lassitude due to absence of stimulation, to monotony, or to lack of interest in one's surroundings. **3.** The decreased capacity or complete inability of an organism, organ, or part to function normally because of excessive stimulation or prolonged exertion.

fatigue fracture *n.* A fracture, usually transverse in orientation, that occurs as a result of repeated or unusual endogenous stress.

fat necrosis *n.* Necrosis of adipose tissue, characterized by the formation of small quantities of calcium soaps when fat is hydrolyzed into glycerol and fatty acids. Also called *steatonecrosis.*

fat pad *n.* An accumulation of encapsulated adipose tissue.

fat-soluble *adj.* Soluble in fats or fat solvents.

fat-soluble vitamin *n.* Any of various vitamins soluble in fats or fat solvents.

fat tide *n.* An increase in the fat content of blood and lymph following a meal.

fat·ty (făt′ē) *n.* **1.** Containing or composed of fat. **2.** Characteristic of fat; greasy. **3.** Derived from or chemically related to fat.

fatty acid *n.* Any of a large group of long-chain monobasic organic acids hydrolytically derived from fats.

fatty acid oxidation cycle *n.* The series of reactions by which fatty acids are metabolized by the body to produce energy.

fatty cirrhosis *n.* Early nutritional cirrhosis, especially in alcoholics, in which the liver is enlarged by fatty change with mild fibrosis.

fatty degeneration *n.* The accumulation of fat globules within the cells of an organ, such as the liver or heart, resulting in deterioration of tissue and diminished functioning of the affected organ. Also called *adipose degeneration, steatosis.*

fatty heart *n.* **1.** Fatty degeneration of the myocardium. **2.** Accumulation of fatty tissue on the outer surface of the heart with occasional infiltration of fat between the muscle bundles of the heart wall. Also called *adiposis cardiaca, cor adiposum.*

fatty hernia *n.* See **pannicular hernia.**

fatty infiltration *n.* The abnormal accumulation of fat droplets in the cytoplasm of cells.

fatty kidney *n.* A kidney in which there is a fatty change in the parenchymal cells, especially a fatty degeneration.

fatty liver *n.* Yellow discoloration of the liver due to fatty degeneration of the parenchymal cells.

fatty metamorphosis *n.* The presence of microscopically visible droplets of fat in the cytoplasm of cells.

fatty oil *n.* A nonvolatile oil of animal or plant derivation, chemically a glyceride of a fatty acid, that is not capable of distillation and that is convertible into a soap by substituting the glycerine with an alkaline base.

fau·ces (fô′sēz′) *pl.n.* The passage from the back of the mouth to the pharynx, bounded by the soft palate, the base of the tongue, and the palatine arches.

fau·cial (fô′shəl) *or* **fau·cal** (-kəl) *adj.* Of or relating to the fauces.

faucial tonsil *n.* See **tonsil** (sense 2).

fau·ci·tis (fô-sī′tĭs) *n.* Inflammation of the fauces.

fault·y union (fôl′tē) *n.* Union of a fracture by fibrous tissue without bone formation.

fau·na (fô′nə) *n., pl.* **–nas** *or* **–nae** (-nē′) Animals, especially the animals of a particular region or period, considered as a group.

fa·ve·o·late (fə-vē′ə-lāt′) *adj.* Pitted with cavities; honeycombed.

fa·ve·o·lus (fə-vē′ə-ləs) *n., pl.* -**li** (-lī′) A small pit or depression.

fa·vid (fā′vĭd) *n.* An allergic reaction in the skin observed in favus.

fa·vism (fā′vĭz′əm) *n.* An acute hereditary condition in which the ingestion of certain species of beans, or the inhalation of the pollen of their flowers, causes fever, headache, abdominal pain, severe anemia, prostration, and coma.

fa·vus (fā′vəs) *n.* A severe type of chronic ringworm of the scalp and nails that is caused by various dermatophytes and occurs in humans and certain animals.

FBS *abbr.* fasting blood sugar

FCAP *abbr.* Fellow of the College of American Pathologists

Fc fragment (ĕf-sē′) *n.* The portion of an immunoglobulin molecule that can be crystallized.

FDA *abbr.* Food and Drug Administration

Fe The symbol for the element **iron** (sense 1).

fear (fîr) *n.* A feeling of agitation and dread caused by the presence or imminence of danger.

fe·bric·i·ty (fĭ-brĭs′ĭ-tē) *n.* The condition of having a fever.

feb·ri·fa·cient (fĕb′rə-fā′shənt) *n.* A substance that produces fever. —*adj.* **fe·brif·ic** (fĭ-brĭf′ĭk) Causing or producing fever.

feb·ri·fuge (fĕb′rə-fyōoj′) *n.* An agent that acts to reduce a fever; an antipyretic. —*adj. or* **fe·brif·u·gal** (fĭ-brĭf′yə-gəl, -brĭf′ə-) Acting to reduce fever.

feb·rile (fĕb′rəl, fē′brəl) *adj.* Of, relating to, or characterized by fever; feverish.

febrile convulsion *n.* A convulsion accompanying high fever in infants and young children.

fe·cal (fē′kəl) *adj.* Relating to or composed of feces.

fecal abscess *n.* See **stercoral abscess.**

fecal fistula *n.* See **intestinal fistula.**

fecal impaction *n.* An immovable collection of compressed or hardened feces in the colon or rectum.

fe·ca·lith (fē′kə-lĭth′) *n.* See **coprolith.**

fe·cal·oid (fē′kə-loid′) *adj.* Resembling feces.

fe·ca·lo·ma (fē′kə-lō′mə) *n.* See **coproma.**

fe·cal·u·ri·a (fē′kə-loor′ē-ə) *n.* Commingling of feces with urine passed from the urethra due to a fistula between the intestinal tract and bladder.

fecal vomiting *n.* The vomiting of fecal matter that has been drawn into the stomach from the intestine by spasmodic contractions of the gastric muscles. Also called *copremesis, stercoraceous vomiting.*

fe·ces (fē′sēz) *pl.n.* The matter that is discharged from the bowel during defecation; excrement. Also called *stercus.*

Fech·ner (fĕk′nər, fĕкн′-), **Gustav Theodor** 1801–1887. German psychologist and physicist who studied the relationship between strength of stimulus and intensity of sensation, thereby founding psychophysics.

Fechner-Weber law *n.* See **Weber-Fechner law.**

fec·u·lent (fĕk′yə-lənt) *adj.* Full of foul or impure matter; fecal.

fe·cund (fē′kənd, fĕk′ənd) *adj.* Capable of producing offspring; fertile.

fe·cun·da·tion (fē′kən-dā′shən, fĕk′ən-) *n.* The act of fertilizing; fertilization. —**fe′cun·date′** *v.*

fe·cun·di·ty (fĭ-kŭn′dĭ-tē) *n.* The capacity for producing offspring, especially in abundance.

feed·back (fēd′băk′) *n.* **1.** The return of a portion of the output of a process or system to the input, especially when used to maintain performance or to control a system or process. **2.** The portion of the output so returned. **3.** The return of information about the result of a process or activity.

feedback inhibition *n.* An inhibition of activity due to the production of an end product of the action. Also called *feedback mechanism.*

feeding tube *n.* A flexible tube that is inserted through the pharynx and into the esophagus and stomach and through which liquid food is passed.

fee-for-ser·vice (fē′fər-sûr′vĭs) *adj.* Charging a fee for each service performed.

feel (fēl) *v.* **1.** To perceive through the sense of touch. **2.** To perceive as a physical sensation, as of pain. **3.** To be conscious of a particular physical, mental, or emotional state.

feel·ing (fē′lĭng) *n.* **1.** The sensation involving perception by touch. **2.** A physical sensation, as of pain. **3.** An affective state of consciousness, such as that resulting from emotions, sentiments, or desires.

FEF *abbr.* forced expiratory flow

Feh·ling's solution (fā′lĭngz) *n.* An aqueous solution of copper sulfate, sodium hydroxide, and potassium sodium tartrate used to test for the presence of sugars and aldehydes in a substance, such as urine.

Fel·dene (fĕl′dēn′) A trademark for the drug piroxicam olamine.

fel·la·ti·o (fə-lā′shē-ō′) *n.* Oral stimulation of the penis.

fel·low (fĕl′ō) *n.* **1.** A physician who enters a training program in a medical specialty after completing residency, usually in a hospital or academic setting. **2.** A physician who has attained specified credentials required for admittance to a professional organization.

fel·on (fĕl′ən) *n.* A purulent infection or abscess in the bulbous distal end of a finger. Also called *whitlow.*

felt·work (fĕlt′wûrk′) *n.* **1.** A fibrous network. **2.** A close plexus of nerve fibrils.

Fel·ty's syndrome (fĕl′tēz) *n.* A condition caused by hypersplenism and resulting in rheumatoid arthritis with splenomegaly and leukopenia.

fe·male (fē′māl′) *adj.* Of, relating to, or denoting the sex that produces ova or bears young. —*n.* **1.** A member of the sex that produces ova or bears young. **2.** A woman or girl.

female athlete triad *n.* A group of findings commonly seen in young female athletes, consisting of eating disorders, amenorrhea, and osteoporosis.

female condom *n.* See **condom** (sense 2).

Fe·mar·a (fə-mär′ə) A trademark for the drug letrozole.

fem·i·nin·i·ty complex (fĕm′ə-nĭn′ĭ-tē) *n.* In psychoanalytic theory, the unconscious fear, in boys and men, of castration at the hands of the mother with resultant identification with the imagined aggressor and envious desire for breasts and vagina.

fem·i·ni·za·tion (fĕm′ə-nĭ-zā′shən) *n.* The acquisition of female characteristics by the male. —**fem′i·nize′** (-nīz′) *v.*

fem·o·ral (fĕm′ər-əl) *adj.* Of or relating to the femur or thigh.

femoral artery *n.* **1.** An artery with origin at the continuation of the external iliac artery, with branches to the pudendal, epigastric, circumflex iliac arteries, the deep artery of the thigh, and the descending genicular artery, and terminating in the popliteal artery. **2.** See **deep artery of thigh.**

femoral canal *n.* The medial compartment of the femoral sheath. Also called *crural canal.*

femoral hernia *n.* A hernia through the femoral ring. Also called *crural hernia, enteromerocele, merocele.*

femoral nerve *n.* A nerve that arises from the second, third, and fourth lumbar nerves and supplies the muscles and skin of the anterior region of the thigh.

femoral sheath *n.* The fascia enclosing the femoral vessels of the leg. Also called *crural sheath.*

femoral triangle *n.* A triangular space at the upper part of the thigh, bounded by the sartorius and adductor longus muscles and the inguinal ligament. Also called *Scarpa's triangle.*

femoral vein *n.* A vein that accompanies the femoral artery in the same sheath and becomes the external iliac vein.

fem·o·ro·tib·i·al (fĕm′ə-rō-tĭb′ē-əl) *adj.* Relating to the femur and the tibia.

femto– *pref.* One quadrillionth (10^{-15}): *femtovolt.*

fe·mur (fē′mər) *n., pl.* **fe·murs** *or* **fem·o·ra** (fĕm′ər-ə) **1.** See **thigh. 2.** The long bone of the thigh, and the longest and strongest bone in the human body, situated between the pelvis and the knee and articulating with the hipbone and with the tibia and patella. Also called *thighbone.*

fe·nes·tra (fə-nĕs′trə) *n., pl.* **–trae** (-trē′) **1.** A small anatomical opening, often closed by a membrane. **2.** The opening in a bone made by surgical fenestration. **3.** A specialized opening, as in a surgical instrument. —**fe·nes′tral** *adj.*

fenestra of cochlea *n.* See **round window.**

fenestra of vestibule *n.* See **oval window.**

fen·es·trat·ed (fĕn′ĭ-strā′tĭd) *or* **fen·es·trate** (fĕn′ĭ-strāt′, fĭ-nĕs′trāt′) *adj.* Having fenestrae or windowlike openings.

fenestrated capillary *n.* A blood capillary found in renal glomeruli, intestinal villi, and some glands, in which ultramicroscopic pores of variable size occur.

fenestrated membrane *n.* A sheetlike elastic membrane of the laminae of large arteries made up of fused elastic fibers.

fen·es·tra·tion (fĕn′ĭ-strā′shən) *n.* **1.** An opening in the surface of a structure, as in a membrane. **2.** The surgical creation of such an opening. **3.** The surgical creation of an artificial opening in the bony part of the inner ear to improve or restore hearing.

fen·flu·ra·mine (fĕn-floor′ə-mēn′) *n.* A fluorinated compound that is used in the treatment of refractory obesity.

fen-phen (fĕn′fĕn) *n.* A combination of the drugs fenfluramine and phentermine, formerly prescribed for weight loss, whose use was discontinued because of association with pulmonary hypertension.

fen·ta·nyl (fĕn′tə-nĭl) *n.* A narcotic analgesic used in combination with other drugs before, during, or following surgery.

fentanyl citrate *n.* A narcotic analgesic that acts like morphine, used as a supplementary analgesic agent in general anesthesia.

Fe·o·sol (fē′ə-sôl, -sŏl) A trademark for a preparation of ferrous sulfate.

fer·ment (fûr′mĕnt′) *n.* **1.** An agent, as a yeast, bacterium, mold, or enzyme, that causes fermentation. **2.** Fermentation. —*v.* (fər-mĕnt′) To cause or undergo fermentation.

fer·men·ta·tion (fûr′mən-tā′shən, -mĕn-) *n.* Any of a group of chemical reactions that split complex organic compounds into relatively simple substances, especially the anaerobic conversion of sugar to carbon dioxide and alcohol by yeast.

fer·mi·um (fûr′mē-əm, fĕr′-) *n. Symbol* **Fm** A synthetic radioactive metallic element whose most stable isotope is Fm 257 with a half-life of approx. 100 days. Atomic number 100.

fern·ing (fûr′nĭng) *n.* The formation of a fernlike pattern in a specimen of crystallized cervical mucus secreted at midcycle.

fern test (fûrn) *n.* A test for estrogenic activity in which cervical mucus smears form a fernlike pattern at times when estrogen secretion is elevated, as at the time of ovulation.

fer·re·dox·in (fĕr′ĭ-dŏk′sĭn) *n.* A protein found in green plants, algae, and anaerobic bacteria, containing iron and labile sulfur in equal amounts, and functioning in electron transport reactions in biochemical processes, such as photosynthesis.

Fer·rein's pyramid (fĕr′ĭnz, fĕ-răNz′) *n.* See **medullary ray.**

ferri– *pref.* Iron, especially ferric ion: *ferritin.*

fer·ric (fĕr′ĭk) *adj.* Of, relating to, or containing iron, especially with a valence of 3 or a valence higher than in a corresponding ferrous compound.

ferric chloride test *n.* A test for phenylketonuria in which ferric chloride is added to urine and turns the urine blue-green when phenylketonuria is present.

fer·ri·heme (fĕr′ĭ-hēm′, fĕr′ə-) *n.* See **hematin.**

fer·ri·tin (fĕr′ĭ-tĭn) *n.* An iron-containing protein complex, found principally in the intestinal mucosa, spleen, and liver, that functions as the primary form of iron storage in the body.

ferro– *or* **ferr–** *pref.* **1.** Iron: *ferrokinetics.* **2.** Ferrous iron: *ferroprotein.*

fer·ro·cy·to·chrome (fĕr′ō-sī′tə-krōm′) *n.* A cytochrome containing ferrous iron.

fer·ro·ki·net·ics (fĕr′ō-kə-nĕt′ĭks, -kī-) *n.* The study of iron metabolism using radioactive iron.

fer·ro·pro·tein (fĕr′ō-prō′tēn′) *n.* Any of the proteins, such as heme or cytochrome, that contain iron in a prosthetic group.

fer·rous (fĕr′əs) *adj.* Of, relating to, or containing iron, especially with a valence of 2 or a valence lower than in a corresponding ferric compound.

fer·rous sulfate (fĕr′əs) *adj.* An iron compound used primarily for treating iron-deficiency amemia.

fer·ru·gi·na·tion (fə-rōō′jə-nā′shən) *n.* Deposition of ferric salts in the walls of small blood vessels, usually of the basal ganglia and cerebellum.

fer·ru·gi·nous (fə-rōō′jə-nəs) *adj.* **1.** Associated with or containing iron. **2.** Having the color of iron rust; reddish-brown.

fer·rum (fĕr′əm) *n.* Iron.

fer·tile (fûr′tl) *adj.* **1.** Capable of conceiving and bearing young. **2.** Fertilized. Used of an ovum.

fertile period *n.* The period in the menstrual cycle during which conception is most likely to occur, usually 10 to 18 days after the onset of menstruation.

fer·til·i·ty (fər-tĭl′ĭ-tē) *n.* The state of being fertile, especially the ability to produce young.

fertility factor *n.* See **F plasmid.**

fer·til·i·za·tion (fûr′tl-ĭ-zā′shən) *n.* The union of male and female gametes to form a zygote, a process that begins with the penetration of the secondary oocyte by the spermatozoon and is completed with the fusion of the male and female pronuclei.

fes·ter (fĕs′tər) *v.* **1.** To ulcerate. **2.** To form pus; putrefy. —*n.* An ulcer.

fes·ti·nant (fĕs′tə-nənt) *adj.* Rapid; accelerating.

fes·ti·na·tion (fĕs′tə-nā′shən) *n.* The acceleration of gait noted in Parkinsonism and similar disorders.

fes·toon (fĕ-stōōn′) *n.* A carving in the base material of a denture that simulates the contours of the natural tissue being replaced by the denture.

FET *abbr.* forced expiratory time

fet– *pref.* Variant of **feto–.**

fe·tal (fēt′l) *adj.* Of, relating to, or being a fetus.

fetal age *n.* See **developmental age** (sense 1).

fetal alcohol syndrome *n. Abbr.* **FAS** A complex of birth defects including cardiac, cranial, facial, or neural abnormalities and physical and mental growth retardation, occurring in an infant due to excessive alcohol consumption by the mother during pregnancy.

fetal aspiration syndrome *n.* A syndrome resulting from meconium aspiration by the fetus and often leading to aspiration pneumonia.

fetal distress syndrome *n.* An abnormal condition of a fetus during gestation or at the time of delivery, marked by altered heart rate or rhythm and leading to compromised blood flow or changes in blood chemistry.

fetal dystocia *n.* A difficult delivery due to an abnormality in the shape, size, or position of the fetus.

fetal hemoglobin *n.* The predominant form of hemoglobin in a fetus and a newborn. Normally present in small amounts in an adult, it may be abnormally elevated in certain forms of anemia. Also called *Hemoglobin F.*

fetal hydrops *n.* The abnormal accumulation of serous fluid in fetal tissues, usually fatal to the fetus.

fetal medicine *n.* The branch of medicine that deals with the growth, development, care, and treatment of the fetus and with environmental factors that may harm the fetus.

fetal membrane *n.* A structure or tissue, such as the chorion, amnion, and allantois, developed from the fertilized ovum but not part of the embryo proper. Also called *embryonic membrane.*

fetal placenta *n.* The chorionic portion of the placenta, containing the fetal blood vessels, from which the umbilical cord arises.

fetal souffle *n.* A blowing murmur, synchronous with the fetal heartbeat, sometimes only systolic and sometimes continuous, heard on auscultation over the pregnant uterus. Also called *funic souffle.*

fetal warfarin syndrome *n.* A fetal syndrome caused by administration of warfarin to a pregnant woman and resulting in fetal bleeding, nasal hypoplasia, optic atrophy, and fetal death.

fe·ti·cide (fē′tĭ-sīd′) *n.* Destruction of the embryo or fetus in the uterus. Also called *embryoctony.*

fet·id (fĕt′ĭd, fē′tĭd) *adj.* Having an offensive odor.

fet·ish (fĕt′ĭsh, fē′tĭsh) *n.* **1.** Something, such as an object or nonsexual part of the body, that arouses sexual desire and may become necessary for sexual gratification. **2.** An abnormally obsessive preoccupation or attachment.

fet·ish·ism (fĕt′ĭ-shĭz′əm, fē′tĭ-) *n.* The act of using a fetish for sexual arousal and gratification.

feto– *or* **feti–** *or* **fet–** *pref.* Fetus; fetal: *fetology.*

fe·to·glob·u·lin (fē′tə-glŏb′yə-lĭn) *n.* Any of the plasma globulins of unknown function occurring in small amounts in normal adults and in larger amounts in the fetus, especially in the second trimester of development.

fe·tog·ra·phy (fē-tŏg′rə-fē) *n.* Radiography of the fetus within the uterus.

fe·tol·o·gy (fē-tŏl′ə-jē) *n.* The branch of medicine concerned with the study, diagnosis, and treatment of the fetus, especially within the uterus.

fe·tom·e·try (fē-tŏm′ĭ-trē) *n.* Estimation of the size of the fetus, especially of its head, before delivery.

fe·top·a·thy (fē-tŏp′ə-thē) *n.* Disease in a fetus after the mother's third month of pregnancy.

fe·to·pla·cen·tal (fē′tō-plə-sĕn′tl) *adj.* Relating to the fetus and its placenta.

fe·to·pro·tein (fē′tə-prō′tēn) *n.* Any of several antigens normally present in a fetus and occurring abnormally in adults as a result of certain neoplastic conditions or diseases of the liver.

fe·tor (fē′tər, -tôr′) *n.* A very offensive odor.

fetor ex o·re (ĕks ôr′ē) *n.* See **halitosis.**

fetor he·pat·i·cus (hĭ-păt′ĭ-kəs) *n.* A peculiar odor of the breath in individuals with severe liver disease caused by volatile aromatic substances that accumulate in the blood and urine.

fe·to·scope (fē′tə-skōp′) *n.* **1.** A flexible fiber-optic device that is used to view a fetus in utero. **2.** A type of stethoscope designed for listening to the fetal heartbeat. —**fe·tos′co·py** (fē-tŏs′kə-pē) *n.*

fe·to·tox·ic·i·ty (fē′tō-tŏk-sĭs′ĭ-tē) *n.* Injury to the fetus from a substance that enters the maternal and placental circulation and may cause death or retardation of growth and development.

fet·tle (fĕt′l) *n.* **1.** Proper or sound condition. **2.** Mental or emotional state; spirits.

fe·tus (fē′təs) *n., pl.* –**tus·es** **1.** The unborn young of a viviparous vertebrate having a basic structural resemblance to the adult animal. **2.** In humans, the unborn young from the end of the eighth week after conception to the moment of birth.

fetus pap·y·ra·ce·us (păp′ə-rā′shē-əs, -shəs) *n.* One of twin fetuses that has died and has been pressed against the uterine wall as a result of the growth of the living fetus.

FEV *abbr.* forced expiratory volume

fe·ver (fē′vər) *n.* **1.** Body temperature above the normal of 98.6°F (37°C). Also called *pyrexia.* **2.** Any of various diseases in which there is an elevation of the body temperature above normal.

fever blister *n.* Cold sore.

fe·ver·ish (fē′vər-ĭsh) *adj.* **1.** Having a fever. **2.** Relating to or resembling a fever. **3.** Causing or tending to cause a fever.

fex·o·fen·a·dine hydrochloride (fĕk′sə-fĕn′ə-dēn′) *n.* A nonsedating antihistamine used to treat allergic rhinitis and allergic skin disorders.

F factor *n.* See **F plasmid.**

FFP *abbr.* fresh frozen plasma

FGT *abbr.* female genital tract

fi·ber (fī′bər) *n.* **1.** A slender thread or filament. **2.** Extracellular filamentous structures such as collagenic or elastic connective tissue fibers. **3.** The nerve cell axon with its glial envelope. **4.** An elongated threadlike cell, such as a muscle cell or one of the epithelial cells of the lens of the eye. **5.** Coarse, indigestible plant matter, consisting primarily of polysaccharides such as cellulose, that when eaten stimulates intestinal peristalsis. Also called *roughage.*

fiber optics *n.* An optical system in which light or an image is conveyed by a compact bundle of fine flexible glass or plastic fibers. —**fi′ber-op′tic** *adj.*

fi·ber·scope (fī′bər-skōp′) *n.* A flexible fiber-optic instrument used to view an object or area, such as a body cavity, that would otherwise be inaccessible.

Fi·bi·ger (fē′bē-gər), **Johannes Andreas Grib** 1867–1928. Danish pathologist. The first to produce cancer experimentally, he won a 1926 Nobel Prize.

fibr– *pref.* Variant of **fibro–.**

fi·bre·mi·a (fī-brē′mē-ə) *n.* The presence of formed fibrin in the blood, causing thrombosis or embolism. Also called *inosemia.*

fi·bril (fī′brəl, fĭb′rəl) *or* **fi·bril·la** (fī-brĭl′ə) *n.* A minute fiber.

fi·bril·lar (fī′brə-lər, fĭb′rə-) *or* **fi·bril·lar·y** (-lĕr′ē) *adj.* **1.** Relating to a fibril. **2.** Relating to the fine rapid contractions or twitchings of fibers or of small groups of fibers in skeletal or cardiac muscle.

fibrillary contractions *pl.n.* Abnormal contractions occurring spontaneously in individual muscle fibers, commonly seen a few days after damage to the motor nerves supplying the muscle.

fibrillary tremor *n.* Isolated twitching of the fine strands or fasciculi of a muscle.

fib·ril·late (fĭb′rə-lāt′, fī′brə-) *v.* **1.** To undergo or to cause to undergo fibrillation. **2.** To make or to become fibrillar. —*adj.* Being fibrillated.

fib·ril·lat·ed (fĭb′rə-lā′tĭd, fī′brə-) *adj.* Composed of fibrils.

fib·ril·la·tion (fĭb′rə-lā′shən, fī′brə-) *n.* **1.** Fine, rapid twitching of individual muscle fibers with little or no movement of the muscle as a whole. **2.** The formation of fibrils. **3.** Vermicular twitching, usually slow, of individual muscular fibers, commonly occurring in the atria or ventricles of the heart and in recently denervated skeletal muscle fibers.

fi·bril·lo·gen·e·sis (fī′brə-lō-jĕn′ĭ-sĭs, fīb′rə-, fī-brĭl′-ō-) *n.* The development of fine fibrils normally present in collagen fibers of connective tissue.

fi·brin (fī′brĭn) *n.* An elastic, insoluble, whitish protein derived from fibrinogen by the action of thrombin and forming an interlacing fibrous network in the coagulation of blood. —**fi′brin·ous** *adj.*

fi·brin·ase (fī′brə-nās′, -nāz′) *n.* **1.** Factor XIII. No longer in technical use. **2.** See **plasmin.**

fibrin calculus *n.* A urinary calculus formed primarily from blood fibrinogen.

fibrin/fibrinogen degradation product *n.* Any of several poorly characterized small peptides produced following the action of plasmin on fibrinogen and fibrin.

fibrino– *pref.* Fibrin: *fibrinocellular.*

fi·bri·no·cel·lu·lar (fī′brə-nō-sĕl′yə-lər) *adj.* Composed of fibrin and cells, as in certain exudates resulting from acute inflammation.

fi·brin·o·gen (fī-brĭn′ə-jən) *n.* A protein in the blood plasma that is essential for the coagulation of blood and is converted to fibrin by thrombin and ionized calcium. Also called *factor I.*

fi·brin·o·ge·ne·mi·a (fī-brĭn′ə-jə-nē′mē-ə) *n.* See **hyperfibrinogenemia.**

fi·bri·no·gen·e·sis (fī′brə-nō-jĕn′ĭ-sĭs) *n.* The formation or production of fibrin.

fi·brin·o·gen·ic (fī′brə-nō-jĕn′ĭk) *or* **fi·bri·nog·e·nous**

(fī′brə-nŏj′ə-nəs) *adj.* **1.** Of or relating to fibrinogen. **2.** Producing fibrin.

fi·brin·o·gen·ol·y·sis (fī-brĭn′ə-jə-nŏl′ĭ-sĭs, fī′brə-nō-) *n.* The inactivation or dissolution of fibrinogen in the blood.

fi·brin·o·gen·o·pe·ni·a (fī-brĭn′ə-jĕn′ō-pē′nē-ə) *n.* A decrease in concentration of fibrinogen that is found in the blood.

fi·bri·noid (fī′brə-noid′, fĭb′rə-) *adj.* Of or resembling fibrin. —*n.* A homogenous acellular material that resembles fibrin and is found in the placenta, forms in connective tissue and in the walls of blood vessels in certain diseases, and is sometimes observed in healing wounds and malignant hypertension.

fibrinoid degeneration *or* **fibrinous degeneration** *n.* A form of degeneration in which tissue, such as connective tissue or blood vessels, accumulates deposits of an acidophilic homogeneous material that resembles fibrin when stained.

fi·bri·nol·y·sin (fī′brə-nŏl′ĭ-sĭn) *n.* See **plasmin.**

fi·bri·nol·y·sis (fī′brə-nŏl′ĭ-sĭs) *n., pl.* **-ses** (-sēz′) The breakdown of fibrin, usually by the enzymatic action of plasmin. —**fi′bri·no·lyt′ic** (-nə-lĭt′ĭk) *adj.*

fibrinolytic purpura *n.* Purpura in which the bleeding is associated with rapid fibrinolysis of the clot.

fi·bri·no·pep·tide (fī′brə-nō-pĕp′tīd′) *n.* Either of two peptides released from fibrinogen by thrombin.

fi·bri·no·pu·ru·lent (fī′brə-nō-pyŏor′ə-lənt) *adj.* Relating to pus or suppurative exudate that contains a relatively large amount of fibrin.

fibrinous bronchitis *n.* Inflammation of the bronchial mucous membrane, accompanied by a fibrinous exudation. Also called *pseudomembranous bronchitis.*

fibrinous cataract *n.* See **fibroid cataract.**

fibrinous inflammation *n.* Exudative inflammation in which there is an unusually large amount of fibrin in the exudate.

fibrinous pericarditis *n.* Acute pericarditis accompanied by fibrinous exudate on the serous membrane. Also called *hairy heart.*

fibrinous pleurisy *n.* See **dry pleurisy.**

fibrinous polyp *n.* A mass of fibrin retained within the uterine cavity after childbirth.

fibrinous rhinitis *n.* See **membranous rhinitis.**

fi·bri·nu·ri·a (fī′brə-nŏor′ē-ə) *n.* The passage of urine that contains fibrin.

fibro– *or* **fibr–** *pref.* Fiber, especially fibrous tissue: *fibrocyst.*

fi·bro·ad·e·no·ma (fī′brō-ăd′n-ō′mə) *n.* A benign tumor usually in breast tissue, derived from glandular epithelium and composed of dense epithelial and fibroblastic tissue. Also called *fibroid adenoma.*

fi·bro·ad·i·pose (fī′brō-ăd′ə-pōs′) *adj.* Relating to or containing both fibrous and fatty structures.

fi·bro·a·re·o·lar (fī′brō-ə-rē′ə-lər) *adj.* Of or relating to connective tissue that is both fibrous and areolar.

fi·bro·blast (fī′brə-blăst′) *n.* A stellate or spindle-shaped cell with cytoplasmic processes present in connective tissue, capable of forming collagen fibers. —**fi′bro·blas′tic** *adj.*

fi·bro·car·ci·no·ma (fī′brō-kär′sə-nō′mə) *n.* A hard, slow-growing carcinoma composed primarily of fibrous tissue. Also called *scirrhous carcinoma.*

fi·bro·car·ti·lage (fī′brō-kär′tl-ĭj) *n.* Cartilage that contains numerous thick bundles of collagen fibers.

fi·bro·car·ti·lag·i·nous (fī′brō-kär′tl-ăj′ə-nəs) *adj.* Relating to or composed of fibrocartilage.

fi·bro·cel·lu·lar (fī′brō-sĕl′yə-lər) *adj.* Both fibrous and cellular.

fi·bro·chon·dri·tis (fī′brō-kŏn-drī′tĭs) *n.* Inflammation of a fibrocartilage.

fi·bro·chon·dro·ma (fī′brō-kŏn-drō′mə) *n.* A benign neoplasm of cartilaginous tissue in which there is an abnormally large amount of fibrous stroma.

fi·bro·cyst (fī′brə-sĭst′) *n.* A cystic lesion that is circumscribed by or situated within a conspicuous amount of fibrous connective tissue.

fi·bro·cys·tic (fī′brō-sĭs′tĭk) *adj.* Characterized by increased fibrosis and cystic spaces, especially in glandular tissue.

fibrocystic disease of breast *n.* A benign disease common in women in their thirties, forties, and fifties, marked by small fluid-containing cysts that form in one or both breasts and associated with stromal fibrosis and variable degrees of intraductal epithelial hyperplasia and sclerosing adenosis. Also called *cystic disease of breast.*

fibrocystic disease of pancreas *n.* See **cystic fibrosis.**

fi·bro·cys·to·ma (fī′brō-sĭ-stō′mə) *n.* A benign neoplasm, usually derived from glandular epithelium, characterized by cysts within a conspicuous fibrous stroma.

fi·bro·dys·pla·sia (fī′brō-dĭs-plā′zhə) *n.* Abnormal development of fibrous connective tissue.

fibrodysplasia os·sif·i·cans pro·gres·si·va (ŏ-sĭf′ĭ-kănz′ prō′grĭ-sī′və) *n.* An inherited generalized disorder of connective tissue in which bone replaces tendons, fasciae, and ligaments.

fi·bro·e·las·tic (fī′brō-ĭ-lăs′tĭk) *adj.* Composed of collagen and elastic fibers.

fi·bro·e·las·to·sis (fī′brō-ĭ-lăs′tō′sĭs) *n.* Excessive proliferation of collagenous and elastic fibrous tissue.

fi·bro·en·chon·dro·ma (fī′brō-ĕn′kŏn-drō′mə) *n.* An enchondroma in which the neoplastic cartilage cells are situated within an abundant fibrous stroma.

fi·bro·ep·i·the·li·o·ma (fī′brō-ĕp′ə-thē′lē-ō′mə) *n.* A skin tumor composed of fibrous tissue intersected by thin bands of basal cells of the epidermis.

fi·bro·fol·lic·u·lo·ma (fī′brō-fə-lĭk′yə-lō′mə) *n.* A neoplastic proliferation of the fibrous sheath of the hair follicle, with solid extensions of the epithelium of the follicular infundibulum.

fi·broid (fī′broid′) *adj.* Composed of or resembling fibers or fibrous tissue. —*n.* **1.** A fibroma or myoma occurring especially one that occurs in the uterine wall. **2.** See **fibroleiomyoma.**

fibroid adenoma *n.* See **fibroadenoma.**

fibroid cataract *n.* A sclerotic hardening of the lenticular capsule, following exudative iridocyclitis. Also called *fibrinous cataract.*

fibroid degeneration *or* **fibrous degeneration** *n.* A form of degeneration in which fibrous tissue forms or replaces other tissues.

fi·broid·ec·to·my (fī′broi-dĕk′tə-mē) *n.* Surgical removal of a fibroid tumor.

fibroid induration *n.* See **cirrhosis.**

fi·bro·la·mel·lar liver cell carcinoma (fī′brō-lə-mĕl′-ər) *n.* Carcinoma of the liver in which malignant hepatocytes are intersected by fibrous lamellated bands.

fi·bro·lei·o·my·o·ma (fī′brō-lī′ō-mī-ō′mə) *n.* A leiomyoma containing nonneoplastic collagenous fibrous tissue. Also called *leiomyofibroma, fibroid.*

fi·bro·li·po·ma (fī′brō-lǐ-pō′mə, -lī-) *n.* A lipoma having an abundant amount of fibrous tissue.

fi·bro·ma (fī-brō′mə) *n., pl.* **–mas** *or* **–ma·ta** (-mə-tə) A benign neoplasm that is composed of fibrous connective tissue. —**fi·brom′a·tous** (-brŏm′ə-təs, -brō′mə-) *adj.*

fibroma mol·le grav·i·dar·um (mŏl′ē grăv′ǐ-dâr′əm) *n.* Skin tags or polyps that develop on women during pregnancy and often disappear at term.

fibroma myx·o·ma·to·des (mĭk-sō′mə-tō′dēz) *n.* See **myxofibroma.**

fi·bro·ma·toid (fī-brō′mə-toid′) *adj.* Of or resembling a fibroma.

fi·bro·ma·to·sis (fī-brō′mə-tō′sĭs) *n.* **1.** The occurrence of multiple fibromas, with a relatively large distribution. **2.** Abnormal hyperplasia of a fibrous tissue.

fi·bro·mus·cu·lar (fī′brō-mǔs′kyə-lər) *adj.* Relating to or containing both fibrous and muscular tissues.

fi·bro·my·al·gia (fī′brō-mī-ăl′jə) *n.* A syndrome characterized by chronic pain in the muscles of soft tissues surrounding joints, fatigue, and tenderness at specific sites in the body. Also called *fibromyositis, fibrositis.*

fi·bro·my·ec·to·my (fī′brō-mī-ĕk′tə-mē) *n.* Excision of a fibromyoma.

fi·bro·my·o·ma (fī′brō-mī-ō′mə) *n.* A benign tumor that contains a large amount of fibrous tissue.

fi·bro·my·o·si·tis (fī′brō-mī′ə-sī′tĭs) *n.* Chronic inflammation of a muscle with an overgrowth of the connective tissue.

fi·bro·myx·o·ma (fī′brō-mĭk-sō′mə) *n.* A benign tumor that contains a large amount of mature fibroblasts and connective tissue.

fi·bro·nec·tin (fī′brə-nĕk′tĭn) *n.* A fibrous linking protein that functions as a reticuloendothelial mediated host defense mechanism and is impaired by surgery, burns, infection, neoplasia, and disorders of the immune system.

fi·bro·neu·ro·ma (fī′brō-nŏŏ-rō′mə) *n.* See **neurofibroma.**

fi·bro·pap·il·lo·ma (fī′brō-păp′ə-lō′mə) *n.* A papilloma containing a conspicuous amount of fibrous connective tissue at the base.

fi·bro·pla·sia (fī′brə-plā′zhə) *n.* The formation of fibrous tissue, as normally occurs in the healing of wounds. —**fi′bro·plas′tic** (-plăs′tĭk) *adj.*

fi·bro·re·tic·u·late (fī′brō-rǐ-tĭk′yə-lĭt, -lāt′) *adj.* Relating to or consisting of a network of fibrous tissue.

fi·bro·sar·co·ma (fī′brō-sär-kō′mə) *n.* A malignant tumor derived from fibrous connective tissue and characterized by immature proliferating fibroblasts or undifferentiated anaplastic spindle cells.

fi·bro·se·rous (fī′brō-sîr′əs) *adj.* Composed of fibrous tissue with a serous surface.

fi·bros·ing adenosis (fī′brō-sĭng) *n.* See **sclerosing adenosis.**

fi·bro·sis (fī-brō′sĭs) *n.* The formation of fibrous tissue as a reparative or reactive process. —**fi·brot′ic** (-brŏt′ĭk) *adj.*

fi·bro·sit·ic headache (fī′brə-sĭt′ĭk) *n.* A headache centered in the occipital region due to fibrositis of the occipital muscles.

fi·bro·si·tis (fī′brə-sī′tĭs) *n.* Inflammatory hyperplasia of white fibrous connective tissue, especially surrounding muscles, causing pain and stiffness.

fi·bro·tho·rax (fī′brō-thôr′ăks′) *n.* Fibrosis of the pleural space.

fi·brous (fī′brəs) *adj.* Composed of or characterized by fibroblasts, fibrils, or connective tissue fibers.

fibrous ankylosis *n.* Stiffening of a joint due to the presence of fibrous bands between and about the bones forming the joint. Also called *false ankylosis, pseudankylosis.*

fibrous astrocyte *or* **fibrillary astrocyte** *n.* A stellate cell with long processes found in the white matter of the brain and spinal cord and characterized by bundles of fine filaments in its cytoplasm.

fibrous capsule *n.* A capsule of fibrous cells or tissue, as that surrounding the kidney and thyroid.

fibrous cortical defect *n.* A common small defect of a bone, in which the cortex is filled with fibrous tissue, occurring most frequently in the lower femoral shaft of a child. Also called *nonosteogenic fibroma.*

fibrous dysplasia of bone *n.* A disorder of bone marrow maintenance in which the abnormal proliferation of fibrous tissue causes asymmetric distortion and expansion of bones.

fibrous goiter *n.* A firm hyperplasia of the thyroid and its capsule.

fibrous joint *n.* See **immovable joint.**

fibrous membrane *n.* The outer fibrous part of the capsule of a synovial joint that may be thickened in places to form capsular ligaments.

fibrous tissue *n.* Tissue composed of bundles of collagenous white fibers between which are rows of connective tissue cells.

fibrous tubercle *n.* A tubercle in which fibroblasts proliferate about the periphery, eventually forming a rim or wall of cellular fibrous tissue or collagenous material.

fib·u·la (fĭb′yə-lə) *n., pl.* **–las** *or* **–lae** (-lē′) The outer, narrower, and smaller of the two bones of the human lower leg, extending from the knee to the ankle, and articulating with the tibia above and the tibia and talus below. Also called *calf bone.* —**fib′u·lar** (-lər) *adj.*

fibular artery *n.* See **peroneal artery.**

fibular nerve *n.* Any of the three peroneal nerves: common, deep, and superficial peroneal.

fibular vein *n.* See **peroneal vein.**

fib·u·lar·is brev·is (fĭb′yə-lâr′ĭs brĕv′ĭs) *n.* See **peroneal brevis.**

fibularis lon·gus (lŏn′gəs) *n.* See **peroneal longus.**

fib·u·lo·cal·ca·ne·al (fĭb′yə-lō-kăl-kā′nē-əl) *adj.* Relating to the fibula and the calcaneus.

Fi·coll-Hy·paque technique (fī′kŏl-hī′pāk′) *n.* A centrifugation technique for separating lymphocytes from other formed elements in blood.

fi·co·sis (fī-kō′sĭs) *n.* See **sycosis.**

field block (fēld) *n.* Regional anesthesia produced by

diffusion of a local anesthetic solution into the tissues surrounding a surgical field.

fifth (fĭfth) *adj.* **1.** Coming after fourth, as in order, rank, or time. **2.** Being the outermost digit, as on a hand. —**fifth** *n.*

fifth cranial nerve *n.* See **trigeminal nerve.**

fifth disease *n.* See **erythema infectiosum.**

fight-or-flight reaction *n.* A set of physiological changes, such as increases in heart rate, arterial blood pressure, and blood glucose, initiated by the sympathetic nervous system to mobilize body systems in response to stress. Also called *emergency theory.*

fig·ure (fĭg′yər) *n.* **1.** A form or shape, as of the human body. **2.** A person representing the essential aspects of a particular role.

figure and ground *n.* An aspect of perception in which the perceived is separated into at least two parts, each with different attributes but each influencing the other.

figure eight suture *n.* A suture used to approximate fascial edges, made using crisscross stiches.

figure-of-8 bandage *n.* A bandage applied alternately to two parts, usually two segments of a limb above and below the joint, in such a way that the turns describe the figure 8.

fig wart (fĭg) *n.* See **genital wart.**

fi·la·ceous (fə-lā′shəs) *adj.* Composed of filaments or threadlike structures.

fil·a·ment (fĭl′ə-mənt) *n.* A fibril, fine fiber, or threadlike structure. —**fil′a·men′tous** (-mĕn′təs), **fil′a·men′ta·ry** (-mĕn′tə-rē, -mĕn′trē) *adj.*

fi·lar (fĭl′lər) *adj.* **1.** Relating to a thread or filament. **2.** Composed of filaments or threadlike structures.

fi·lar·i·a (fə-lâr′ē-ə) *n.,* pl. **–i·ae** (-ē-ē′) Any of various threadlike nematode worms of the superfamily Filarioidea parasitic in vertebrates and often transmitted as larvae by biting insects. The adult form lives in the blood and lymphatic tissues, causing inflammation and obstruction that can lead to elephantiasis. —**fi·lar′i·al** (-ē-əl), **fi·lar′i·an** (-ē-ən) *adj.*

Filaria *n.* A genus of nematodes no longer in taxonomic use and whose members are now classified in the family Onchocercidae.

fi·a·ri·a·sis (fĭl′ə-rī′ə-sĭs) *n.* Disease caused by the presence of filariae in the tissues of the body, often resulting in occlusion of the lymphatic channels that can lead to elephantiasis.

fi·lar·i·cide (fə-lâr′ĭ-sīd′) *n.* An agent that kills filariae. —**fi·lar′i·cid′al** (-sīd′l) *adj.*

fi·lar·i·form (fə-lâr′ə-fôrm′) *adj.* **1.** Resembling filariae or other types of small nematode worms. **2.** Thin or hairlike.

Fi·la·tov flap (fə-lä′təf) *or* **Fi·la·tov-Gil·lies flap** (-gĭl′ēz) *n.* See **tubed flap.**

fil·i·al (fĭl′ē-əl) *adj.* **1.** Relating to the relationship of offspring to parents. **2.** In genetics, relating to a generation or the sequence of generations following the parental generation.

filial generation *n.* The generation resulting from a genetically controlled mating that is successive to the parental generation.

fil·i·form (fĭl′ə-fôrm′, fī′lə-) *adj.* Having the form of or resembling a thread or filament.

filiform bougie *n.* A very slender bougie usually used for exploration of strictures or sinus tracts having small diameters.

filiform papilla *n.* Any of numerous elongated conical projections on the back of the tongue.

filled milk (fĭld) *n.* Skim milk with vegetable oils added to substitute for butterfat.

fil·let (fĭl′ĭt) *n.* **1.** A loop of cord or tape used for making traction on a part of the fetus. **2.** A loop-shaped band of fibers, especially the lemniscus.

fill·ing (fĭl′ĭng) *n.* Material, such as amalgam, gold, or a synthetic resin, used to fill a cavity in a tooth.

filling defect *n.* A defect in the contour of part of the gastrointestinal tract, as seen by x-ray after contrast medium has been introduced, indicating the presence of a tumor or foreign body.

film (fĭlm) *n.* **1.** A light-sensitive or x-ray-sensitive substance used in taking photographs or radiographs. **2.** A thin layer or membranous coating.

fi·lo·pres·sure (fĭl′lō-prĕsh′ər) *n.* Temporary pressure on a blood vessel by a ligature.

fi·lo·vi·rus (fē′lō-v′rəs, fĭl′o) *n.* Any of a group of filamentous RNA viruses of the family Filoviridae, including Ebola and Marburg viruses, that are characterized by elongated, branched, curved, or spherical virions and that cause hemorrhagic fevers.

fil·ter (fĭl′tər) *n.* **1.** A porous material through which a liquid or gas is passed in order to separate the fluid from suspended particulate matter. **2.** A device containing such a substance. **3.** Any of various electric, electronic, acoustic, or optical devices used to reject signals, vibrations, or radiations of certain frequencies while passing others. **4.** A translucent screen, used in both diagnostic and therapeutic radiology, that permits the passage of rays having desirable levels of energy. **5.** A device used in spectrophotometric analysis to isolate a segment of the spectrum. —*v.* **1.** To pass a liquid or gas through a filter. **2.** To remove by passing through a filter. **3.** To pass through or as if through a filter.

fil·ter·a·ble (fĭl′tər-ə-bəl, fĭl′trə-) *or* **fil·tra·ble** (-trə-bəl) *adj.* Relating to smaller viruses and some bacteria capable of passing through a fine-pored filter.

fil·ter·ing operation (fĭl′tə-rĭng) *n.* The surgical creation of a fistula between the anterior chamber of the eye and the subconjunctival space, as for glaucoma.

fil·trate (fĭl′trāt′) *v.* To put or go through a filter. —*n.* Material, especially liquid, that has passed through a filter.

fil·tra·tion (fĭl-trā′shən) *n.* The process of passing a liquid through a filter.

filtration angle *n.* The acute angle occurring between the iris and the cornea at the periphery of the anterior chamber of the eye. Also called *angle of the iris, iridocorneal angle.*

filtration coefficient *n.* A measure of a membrane's permeability to water, taking into account both hydraulic and osmotic pressures.

filtration fraction *n.* The portion of blood plasma that enters the kidney and filters through the renal glomerular membranes.

fi·lum (fī′ləm) *n.,* pl. **–la** (-lə) A threadlike anatomical structure; a filament.

filum du·rae ma·tris spi·na·lis (dŏŏr′ē mā′trĭs spī-nā′-lĭs) *n.* The termination of the spinal dura mater, surrounding the terminal filum of the cord and attached to the deep dorsal sacrococcygeal ligament.

fim·bri·a (fĭm′brē-ə) *n., pl.* **–bri·ae** (-brē-ē′) **1.** A fringelike anatomical part or structure. **2.** See **pilus** (sense 2). —**fim′bri·al** *adj.*

fimbria hip·po·cam·pi (hĭp′ə-kăm′pī) *n.* A narrow crest of white matter attached to the medial border of the hippocampus. Also called *corpus fimbriatum.*

fim·bri·ate (fĭm′brē-ĭt, -āt′) *or* **fim·bri·at·ed** (-ā′tĭd) *adj.* Having fimbriae. —**fim′bri·a′tion** *n.*

fim·bri·o·cele (fĭm′brē-ō-sēl′) *n.* A hernia containing fimbriae of the uterine tube.

fi·nal host (fī′nəl) *n.* See **definitive host.**

final motor neuron *n.* See **lower motor neuron.**

fi·nas·ter·ide (fə-năs′tə-rīd′) *n.* A synthetic androgen inhibitor used primarily in men for the treatment of benign prostatic hyperplasia and androgenic alopecia.

fin·ger (fĭng′gər) *n.* One of the five digits of the hand, especially one other than the thumb.

fin·ger·nail (fĭng′gər-nāl′) *n.* The nail on a finger.

finger-nose test *n.* A test of coordination of the arms and hands in which an individual is asked to touch the tip of his or her nose with the index finger.

fin·ger·print (fĭng′gər-prĭnt′) *n.* **1.** An impression on a surface of the curves formed by the ridges on a fingertip, especially such an impression made in ink and used as a means of identification. **2.** A distinctive or identifying mark or characteristic. **3.** An analytical method capable of making fine distinctions between similar compounds. —*v.* **1.** To take fingerprints of. **2.** To identify by a distinctive mark or characteristic.

finger-thumb reflex *n.* See **basal joint reflex.**

fin·ger·tip (fĭng′gər-tĭp′) *n.* The extreme end or tip of a finger.

finger-to-finger test *n.* A test for coordination of the arms and hands in which an individual is asked to bring the index fingers together.

Fin·sen (fĭn′sən), **Niels Ryberg** 1860–1904. Danish physician. He won a 1903 Nobel Prize for developing a method of treating skin diseases with ultraviolet light.

fire (fīr) *v.* To generate an electrical impulse. Used of a neuron.

first (fûrst) *adj.* **1.** Coming before all others in order or location. **2.** Occurring or acting before all others in time; earliest. **3.** Being the innermost digit, especially on a foot. —**first** *n.*

first aid *n.* Emergency treatment administered to an injured or sick person before professional medical care is available. —**first′-aid′** *adj.*

first cranial nerve *n.* See **olfactory nerve.**

first cuneiform bone *n.* See **medial cuneiform bone.**

first-degree burn *n.* A mild burn that produces redness of the skin but no blistering.

first finger *n.* See **index finger.**

first heart sound *n.* The heart sound that occurs with ventricular systole and is produced mainly by closure of the atrioventricular valves.

first molar *n.* The sixth permanent tooth or fourth deciduous tooth in the upper and lower jaw on either side.

Fi·scher (fĭsh′ər), **Hans** 1881–1945. German chemist known for his research on the components of blood. He won a 1930 Nobel Prize for his work on the synthesis of hemin.

Fish·berg concentration test (fĭsh′bərg) *n.* A test of renal water conservation in which urine samples are collected after the individual has abstained from fluids overnight and the specific gravity of the urine is measured.

fish skin (fĭsh) *n.* See **ichthyosis.**

fish·skin disease (fĭsh′skĭn′) *n.* See **ichthyosis.**

fis·sion (fĭsh′ən) *n.* **1.** The act or process of splitting into parts. **2.** The amitotic division of a cell or its nucleus. **3.** An asexual process of reproduction in which a unicellular organism divides into two or more independently maturing daughter cells. **4.** A nuclear reaction in which an atomic nucleus, especially a heavy nucleus such as an isotope of uranium, splits into fragments, usually two of comparable mass, with the evolution of from 100 million to several hundred million electron volts of energy.

fission fungi *pl.n.* See **Schizomycetes.**

fission product *n.* A usually radioactive isotope produced as a result of the fission of a massive atom such as U^{235}.

fis·si·par·i·ty (fĭs′ə-păr′ĭ-tē) *n.* See **schizogenesis.**

fis·sip·a·rous (fĭ-sĭp′ər-əs) *adj.* Reproducing or propagating by fission.

fis·su·ra (fĭ-sŏŏr′ə, -shŏŏr′ə) *n., pl.* **–su·rae** (-sŏŏr′ē, -shŏŏr′ē) **1.** A deep fissure, cleft, or slit. **2.** A particularly deep sulcus of the surface of the brain or spinal cord.

fis·sure (fĭsh′ər) *n.* **1.** A deep furrow, cleft, or slit. **2.** A developmental break or fault in the enamel of a tooth.

fis·sured fracture (fĭsh′ərd) *n.* See **linear fracture.**

fissure of Rolando *or* **Rolando's fissure** *n.* A double S-shaped fissure that extends obliquely upward and backward on the lateral surface of each cerebral hemisphere of the brain and located at the boundary between the frontal and parietal lobes. Also called *central sulcus.*

fissure of round ligament *n.* A cleft on the lower surface of the liver that lodges the round ligament of the liver.

fissure of Syl·vi·us (sĭl′vē-əs) *or* **sylvian fissure** *n.* The deepest and most prominent of the cortical fissures of the brain, extending between frontal and temporal lobes, then back and slightly upward over the lateral aspect of the cerebral hemisphere. Also called *lateral cerebral sulcus.*

fissure of venous ligament *n.* A deep cleft on the posterior surface of the liver between the left and caudate lobes that lodges the venous ligament.

fis·tu·la (fĭs′chə-lə) *n., pl.* **–las** *or* **–lae** (-lē′) An abnormal passage from a hollow organ to the body surface, or from one organ to another.

fis·tu·la·tion (fĭs′chə-lā′shən) *or* **fis·tu·li·za·tion** (-lĭ-zā′shən) *n.* Formation of a fistula in a part of the body.

fis·tu·lec·to·my (fĭs′chə-lĕk′tə-mē) *n.* Surgical removal of a fistula. Also called *syringectomy.*

fis·tu·lot·o·my (fĭs′chə-lŏt′ə-mē) *n.* Incision of a fistula. Also called *syringotomy.*

fis·tu·lous (fĭs′chə-ləs) *or* **fis·tu·lar** (-lər) *adj.* Relating to or containing a fistula.

fit¹ (fĭt) v. To be the proper size and shape. —adj. Physically sound; healthy. —n. The degree of precision with which surfaces are adjusted or adapted to each other in a machine, device, or collection of parts.

fit² (fĭt) n. **1.** A seizure or a convulsion, especially one caused by epilepsy. **2.** The sudden appearance of a symptom such as coughing or sneezing.

fit·ness (fĭt′nĭs) n. **1.** The state or condition of being physically sound and healthy, especially as the result of exercise and proper nutrition. **2.** A state of general mental and physical well-being. **3.** The state of being suitably adapted to an environment.

fitness walking n. The aerobic sport of brisk, rhythmic, vigorous walking, intended to improve cardiovascular efficiency, strengthen the heart, control weight gain, and reduce stress.

5-HT (fīv′ăch′tē′) abbr. 5-hydroxytryptamine

5-hy·drox·y·tryp·ta·mine (-hī-drŏk′sē-trĭp′tə-mēn′) n. Abbr. **5-HT** See **serotonin**.

fix·ate (fĭk′sāt′) v. **1.** To make fixed, stable, or stationary. **2.** To focus one's eyes or attention on something. **3.** To develop a fixation; become excessively attached to a person or thing.

fix·a·tion (fĭk-sā′shən) n. **1.** The condition of being stabilized, firmly attached, or set. **2.** The act or process of stabilizing or attaching something, especially a body part by surgery. **3.** The rapid killing and preservation of tissue elements to retain as nearly as possible the same characteristics they had in the living body. **4.** The conversion of a gas into solid or liquid form by chemical reactions. **5.** In psychoanalytic theory, a strong emotional attachment to a person or thing, especially an attachment formed in childhood or infancy and manifested in disturbed behavior that persists throughout life. **6.** The coordinated positioning and focusing of both eyes on an object.

fixation nystagmus n. A nystagmus manifested during fixation movements of the eyes, arising as opticokinetic nystagmus or resulting from midbrain lesions.

fixation point n. See **point of fixation**.

fix·a·tive (fĭk′sə-tĭv) adj. Serving to fix, bind, or make firm or stable. —n. A substance used for the preservation of tissue or cell specimens.

fix·a·tor (fĭk′sā′tər, fĭk-sā′tər) n. A device that provides rigid immobilization of a fractured bone by means of rods attached to pins that are placed in or through the bone.

fixator muscle n. A muscle that acts as a stabilizer of one part of the body during movement of another part.

fixed drug eruption (fĭxt) n. A drug eruption that recurs at a particular site or sites following the administration of a particular drug.

fixed idea n. An often unreasonable idea or feeling that persists despite evidence to the contrary or efforts to ignore it; an obsession. Also called idée fixe.

fixed macrophage n. See **histiocyte**.

fixed oil n. A nonvolatile oil, especially a fatty oil of vegetable origin.

fixed partial denture n. A denture that is permanently attached to natural teeth or tooth roots for support.

fixed pupil n. A pupil that is unresponsive to stimuli.

fixed-rate pacemaker n. An artificial pacemaker that emits electrical stimuli at a constant frequency regardless of the heart's rhythm.

fixed virus n. Rabies virus that has undergone serial passage through rabbits, thus stabilizing its virulence and incubation period.

flac·cid (flăs′sĭd, flăk′ĭd) adj. Lacking firmness, resilience, or muscle tone. —**flac·cid′i·ty** (-sĭd′ĭ-tē) n.

flagellar antigen n. A heat-labile antigen found in bacterial flagella. Also called H antigen.

flag·el·late (flăj′ə-lĭt, -lāt′, flə-jĕl′ĭt) adj. **1.** Flagellated. **2.** Relating to or caused by a flagellate organism. —n. A member of the class Mastigophora, comprising organisms having a flagellum.

flag·el·lat·ed (flăj′ə-lā′tĭd) adj. Having a flagellum or flagella.

flag·el·la·tion (flăj′ə-lā′shən) n. **1.** Whipping oneself or another as a means of arousing or heightening sexual feeling. **2.** The flagellar arrangement on an organism.

flag·el·lo·sis (flăj′ə-lō′sĭs) n. Infection with flagellated protozoa in the intestinal or genital tract.

fla·gel·lum (flə-jĕl′əm) n., pl. **–gel·la** (-jĕl′ə) A threadlike appendage, especially a whiplike extension of certain cells or organisms that functions as an organ of locomotion. —**fla·gel·lar** (-jĕl′ər) adj.

Flag·yl (flăg′əl) A trademark for the drug metronidazole.

flail (flāl) v. **1.** To move vigorously or erratically; thrash about. **2.** To strike or lash out violently.

flail chest n. The loss of stability of the thoracic cage following multiple fractures of the ribs with or without accompanying fracture of the sternum.

flail joint n. A joint that has an excessive or abnormal degree of mobility.

flange (flănj) n. **1.** A projecting rim or edge. **2.** The part of the denture base that extends from the cervical ends of the teeth to the border of the denture.

flank (flăngk) n. **1.** The side of the body between the pelvis or hip and the last rib; the side. **2.** The section of flesh in that area.

flank position n. A lateral recumbent position in which the lower leg is flexed and the upper leg is extended, with convex extension of the upper side of the body, used for nephrectomy.

flap (flăp) n. Tissue used in surgical grafting that is only partially detached from its donor site so that it continues to be nourished during transfer to the recipient site.

flap amputation n. Amputation in which flaps of muscular and cutaneous tissues are used to cover the end of the bone. Also called flap operation.

flap·less amputation (flăp′lĭs) n. An amputation that does not use tissue to cover the stump.

flap operation n. **1.** See **flap amputation**. **2.** In dental surgery, the detachment of a portion of the mucoperiosteal tissues from an underlying bone or impacted tooth for better access and visibility in examining the area covered by the tissue.

flap·ping tremor (flăp′ing) n. See **asterixis**.

flare (flâr) n. An area of redness on the skin surrounding the primary site of infection or irritation.

flash·back (flăsh′băk′) n. **1.** An unexpected recurrence of the effects of a hallucinogenic drug long after its original use. **2.** A recurring, intensely vivid mental image of a past traumatic experience.

flash blindness (flăsh) *n.* Temporary loss of vision produced when retinal light-sensitive pigments are bleached by light more intense than that to which the retina is physiologically adapted at that moment.

flash method *n.* A method in which milk is sterilized by raising it rapidly to a temperature of 178°F and, after holding it at that temperature for a brief period, rapidly reducing its temperature to 40°F.

flat bone (flăt) *n.* A bone having a thin, flattened shape, as the scapula.

flat chest *n.* A chest in which the anteroposterior diameter is less than the average.

flat condyloma *n.* A secondary syphilitic eruption of flat-topped papules, usually found wherever contiguous folds of skin produce heat and moisture and especially about the anus and genitals. Also called *condyloma latum.*

flat electroencephalogram *n.* An electroencephalogram indicating the absence of electric potentials of cerebral origin, indicative under certain specified conditions of cerebral death. Also called *isoelectric electroencephalogram.*

flat flap *n.* A surgical flap in which the pedicle is left flat or open during transfer rather than tubed. Also called *open flap.*

flat·foot (flăt′fŏŏt′) *n., pl.* **–feet** (-fēt′) A condition in which the arch of the foot is abnormally flattened down so that the entire sole makes contact with the ground. Also called *splayfoot, talipes planus.*

flat pelvis *n.* A pelvis in which the anteroposterior diameter is uniformly contracted, the sacrum being dislocated forward between the iliac bones.

flat plate *n.* A survey radiograph, usually of the abdomen, without use of contrast media and obtained while the patient is recumbent.

flat·u·lence (flăch′ə-ləns) *or* **flat·u·len·cy** (flăch′ə-lən-sē) *n.* The presence of excessive gas in the digestive tract. —**flat′u·lent** *adj.*

fla·tus (flā′təs) *n.* Gas generated in or expelled from the digestive tract, especially from the stomach or intestines.

flat wart *n.* A small, flat, flesh-colored wart that occurs in groups, especially on the faces of young people. Also called *verruca plana.*

flat·worm (flăt′wûrm′) *n.* Any of various worms of the phylum Platyhelminthes, including the parasitic tapeworms and flukes, characteristically having a soft, flat, bilaterally symmetrical body and no body cavity. Also called *platyhelminth.*

fla·vin (flā′vĭn) *or* **fla·vine** (-vēn′) *n.* **1.** Any of various water-soluble yellow pigments, including riboflavin, found in plant and animal tissue as coenzymes of flavoproteins. **2.** A ketone that gives color to various natural yellow pigments.

flavin-adenine dinucleotide *or* **flavine-adenine dinucleotide** *n. Abbr.* **FAD** A derivative of riboflavin that functions in certain oxidation-reduction reactions in the body as a coenzyme of various flavoproteins.

fla·vine (flā′vēn′) *n.* **1.** A brownish-red crystalline powder used as an antiseptic. **2.** Variant of **flavin.**

flavin mononucleotide *or* **flavine mononucleotide** *n. Abbr.* **FMN** A derivative of riboflavin that condenses with adenine nucleotide to form flavin adenine dinucleotide and that acts as a coenzyme of various flavoproteins.

fla·vi·vi·rus (flā′və-vī′rəs) *n.* An arbovirus of the genus *Flavivirus.*

Flavivirus *n.* A genus of arboviruses of the family Togaviridae, the type species of which is the yellow fever virus.

flavo– *or* **flav–** *pref.* **1.** Yellow: *flavin.* **2.** Flavin: *flavoprotein.*

Fla·vo·bac·te·ri·um (flā′vō-băk-tîr′ē-əm) *n.* A genus of gram-negative rod-shaped bacteria occurring in soil and water and characteristically producing yellow, orange, red, or yellow-brown pigments.

fla·vo·en·zyme (flā′vō-ĕn′zīm′) *n.* An enzyme that possesses a flavin nucleotide as coenzyme.

fla·vo·noid (flā′və-noid′) *n.* Any of a large group of phytonutrients that are water-soluble pigments, considered to have antioxidant and anti-inflammatory properties. Also called *bioflavonoid.*

fla·vo·pro·tein (flā′vō-prō′tēn′) *n.* Any of a group of enzymes with flavin bound to protein that acts as dehydrogenases.

flea (flē) *n.* Any of various small, wingless, bloodsucking insects of the order Siphonaptera that have legs adapted for jumping and are parasitic in the hair and feathers of warm-blooded animals.

fle·cai·nide acetate (flĭ-kā′nīd′) *n.* A drug that stabilizes membranes and has local anesthetic activity, used in the treatment of ventricular arrhythmias.

Fle·gel's disease (flā′gəlz) *n.* See **hyperkeratosis lenticularis perstans.**

Flem·ing (flĕm′ĭng), Sir **Alexander** 1881–1955. British bacteriologist who discovered penicillin in 1928. He shared a 1945 Nobel Prize for this achievement.

Flem·ming (flĕm′ĭng), **Walther** 1843–1915. German biologist known for his research on cell division and on the splitting of chromosomes. He coined the term *mitosis.*

flesh (flĕsh) *n.* The soft tissue of the body of a vertebrate, covering the bones and consisting mainly of skeletal muscle and fat. —**flesh′y** *adj.*

flesh fly *n.* Any of various dipterous flies of the family Sarcophagidae whose larvae are parasitic in living animal tissue or feed on carrion.

flesh wound *n.* A wound that penetrates the flesh but does not damage underlying bones or vital organs.

flex (flĕks) *v.* **1.** To bend. **2.** To contract a muscle. **3.** To move a joint so that the parts it connects approach each other.

Flex·e·ril (flĕk′sə-rĭl′) A trademark for the drug cyclobenzaprine hydrochloride.

flex·i·bil·i·tas ce·re·a (flĕk′sə-bĭl′ĭ-təs sîr′ē-ə) *n.* The characteristic rigidity of catalepsy that may be overcome by slight external force but that returns immediately, holding the limb firmly in the new position.

flex·i·ble (flĕk′sə-bəl) *adj.* **1.** Capable of being bent or flexed. **2.** Capable of being bent repeatedly without injury or damage. —**flex′i·bil′i·ty, flex′i·ble·ness** *n.*

flex·ion (flĕk′shən) *n.* **1.** The act of bending a joint or limb in the body by the action of flexors. **2.** The condition of being flexed or bent.

Flex·ner (flĕks′nər), **Simon** 1863–1946. American microbiologist who isolated the bacillus of dysentery (1900), developed a serum for cerebrospinal meningitis (1907), and led the team that identified the cause of poliomyelitis.

Flex·ner's bacillus (flĕks′nərz) *n.* A gram-negative bacterium *Shigella flexneri* that causes severe dysentery in adults and gastroenteritis in infants.

flex·or (flĕk′sər) *n.* A muscle that when contracted acts to bend a joint or limb in the body.

flexor dig·i·ti min·i·mi brev·is man·us (dĭj′ĭ-tī′ mĭn′-ə-mī′ brĕv′ĭs măn′əs, dĭj′ĭ-tē′ mĭn′ə-mē′) *n.* A muscle with origin from the hamate, with insertion to the proximal phalanx of the little finger, with nerve supply from the ulnar nerve, and whose action flexes the proximal phalanx of the little finger.

flexor digiti minimi brevis pedis (pĕd′əs) *n.* A muscle with origin from the base of the metatarsal of the little toe and the sheath of the long peroneal muscle, with insertion to the base of the proximal phalanx of the little toe, with nerve supply from the lateral plantar nerve, and whose action flexes the proximal phalanx of the little toe.

flexor dig·i·tor·um brevis (dĭj′ĭ-tôr′əm) *n.* A muscle with its origin from the calcaneus and the plantar fascia, with insertion to the middle phalanges of the four lateral toes, with nerve supply from the medial plantar nerve, and whose action flexes the four lateral toes.

flexor hal·lu·cis brevis (hăl′ōō-sĭs, -kĭs) *n.* A muscle with origin from the cuboid and the middle and the lateral cuneiform bones, with insertion to the base of the proximal phalanx of the big toe, with nerve supply from the medial and the lateral plantar nerves, and whose action flexes the big toe.

flexor pol·li·cis brevis (pŏl′ə-sĭs, -kĭs) *n.* A muscle with origin from the flexor retinaculum of the wrist and from the ulnar side of the first metacarpal, with insertion to the base of the proximal phalanx of the thumb, with nerve supply from the median and ulnar nerves, and whose action flexes the proximal phalanx of the thumb.

flexor ret·i·nac·u·lum (rĕt′n-ăk′yə-ləm) *n.* A strong fibrous band crossing the front of the carpus and binding down the flexor tendons of the digits and the tendon of the radial flexor muscle of the wrist.

flex·u·ra (flĕk-so͞or′ə, flĕk-shoͦor′ə) *n., pl.* **flex·u·rae** (-soͦor′ē, -shoͦor′ē) A bend; a flexure.

flex·ure (flĕk′shər) *n.* **1.** A bend or curve, as in a tubular organ. **2.** The act or an instance of bending. —**flex′ur·al** *adj.*

Flint's murmur (flĭnts) *n.* A diastolic murmur, similar to that of mitral stenosis, heard at the cardiac apex in some cases of free aortic insufficiency. Also called *Austin Flint murmur.*

float·ers (flō′tər) *pl.n.* Specks or small threads in the visual field, usually perceived to be moving, that are caused by minute aggregations of cells or proteins in the vitreous humor of the eye.

float·ing (flō′tĭng) *adj.* **1.** Completely or partially unattached. **2.** Out of the normal position; unduly movable. Used of certain organs such as the kidney.

floating cartilage *n.* A loose piece of cartilage within a joint cavity that is detached from the articular cartilage or from a meniscus.

floating kidney *n.* A kidney that is displaced and movable. Also called *wandering kidney.*

floating rib *n.* Any of the two lowest pairs of ribs with no anterior attachment to the sternum. Also called *vertebral rib.*

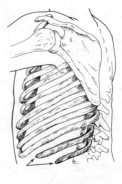

floating rib

floating spleen *n.* A spleen that is palpable because of excessive mobility from a relaxed or lengthened pedicle. Also called *lien mobilis.*

floc·cil·la·tion (flŏk′sə-lā′shən) *n.* An aimless plucking at the bedclothes occurring especially in the delirium of a fever.

floc·cose (flŏk′ōs) *adj.* Growing in short curving filaments or chains, closely but irregularly disposed. Used of certain bacteria.

floc·cu·lar (flŏk′yə-lər) *adj.* Relating to a flocculus, especially to the flocculus of the cerebellum.

floc·cu·la·tion (flŏk′yə-lā′shən) *or* **floc·cu·lence** (flŏk′-yə-ləns) *n.* **1.** The process of becoming flocculent. **2.** Precipitation from solution in the form of fleecy masses. —**floc′cu·late′** *v.*

flocculation reaction *n.* A precipitin test characterized by a flocculent precipitate of antigen and antibody. Also called *flocculation test.*

floc·cu·lent (flŏk′yə-lənt) *adj.* **1.** Having a fluffy or wooly appearance. **2.** Containing numerous shreds or fluffy particles of grayish or white mucus or other material. Used of a fluid such as urine. **3.** Of or being a fluid bacterial culture in which there are numerous colonies either floating in the fluid medium or loosely deposited at the bottom. **4.** Having a soft waxy or wool-like covering, as of certain insects. —**floc′cu·lence** *n.*

floc·cu·lus (flŏk′yə-ləs) *n., pl.* **–li** (-lī′) **1.** A small fluffy mass or tuft. **2.** Either of a pair of small lobes on the posterior border of the cerebellum, forming part of the vestibular part of the cerebellum.

flood·ing (flŭd′ĭng) *n.* A form of desensitization used in behavior therapy in which the patient imagines or is actually exposed to anxiety-producing stimuli.

floor plate (flôr) *n.* The thin ventral portion of the embryonic neural tube that merges with the basal portion of the lateral plates. Also called *ventral plate.*

flo·ra (flôr′ə) *n., pl.* **flo·ras** or **flo·rae** (flôr′ē′) **1.** Plants considered as a group. **2.** The microorganisms that normally inhabit a bodily organ or part.

Flo·rey (flôr′ē), **Howard Walter** 1898–1968. Australian-born British pathologist. He shared a 1945 Nobel Prize for isolating and purifying penicillin.

flor·id (flôr′ĭd) *adj.* Of a bright red or ruddy color. Used of certain skin lesions. —**flo·rid′i·ty** (flə-rĭd′ĭ-tē, flô-) *n.*

florid oral papillomatosis *n.* Diffuse involvement of the lips and oral mucosa with benign squamous papillomas.

Flor·i·nef (flôr′ĭ-něf′) A trademark for the drug fludrocortisone acetate.

flo·ta·tion (flō-tā′shən) *n.* The process of separating different materials, especially minerals, by agitating a pulverized mixture of the materials with water, oil, and chemicals. Differential wetting of the suspended particles causes unwetted particles to be carried by air bubbles to the surface for collection.

flotation method *n.* Any of several procedures for concentrating helminth eggs, when the eggs are difficult to find in direct examination, by use of a liquid of sufficiently high specific gravity.

flow (flō) *v.* **1.** To move or run smoothly with unbroken continuity. **2.** To circulate, as the blood in the body. **3.** To menstruate. —*n.* **1.** The smooth motion characteristic of fluids. **2.** The volume of fluid or gas passing a given point per unit of time. **3.** Menstrual discharge.

flow·ers (flou′ərz) *pl.n.* A fine powder produced by condensation or sublimation of a compound.

flow·me·ter (flō′mē′-tər) *n.* An instrument for monitoring, measuring, or recording the rate of flow, pressure, or discharge of liquids or gases.

Flox·in (flŏk′sĭn) A trademark for the drug ofloxacin.

fl oz or **fl. oz.** *abbr.* fluid ounce

flu (flōō) *n.* Influenza.

flu·con·a·zole (flōō-kŏn′ə-zōl′, -kō′nə-) *n.* A broad-spectrum antifungal agent that is used especially to treat candidiasis and infections caused by *Cryptococcus neoformans.*

fluc·tu·ant (flŭk′chōō-ənt) *n.* Capable of being moved. Used of an abnormal mass such as a tumor or abscess.

flu·dro·cor·ti·sone acetate (flōō′drō-kôr′tĭ-sōn′, -zōn′) *n.* A synthetic mineralocorticoid used to increase blood pressure by lowering the amount of salt the body excretes and to treat adrenocortical insufficiency resulting from Addison's disease.

flu·id (flōō′ĭd) *n.* An amorphous substance whose molecules move freely past one another; a liquid or gas. —*adj.* Of or characteristic of a fluid. —**flu·id′i·ty** (-ĭd′ĭ-tē), **flu′id·ness** *n.*

fluid balance *n.* The difference between the amount of water taken into the body and the amount excreted or lost. Also called *water balance.*

fluid dram *n.* A unit of volume or capacity in the apothecary system, equal to $\frac{1}{8}$ of a fluid ounce or 3.70 milliliters.

flu·id·ex·tract (flōō′ĭd-ĕk′străkt′) *n.* A concentrated alcohol solution of a vegetable drug of such strength that each milliliter contains the equivalent of one gram of the dry form of the drug.

fluid ounce or **fluidounce** *n. Abbr.* **fl oz, fl. oz.** A unit of volume or capacity equal to 8 fluid drams or 29.57 milliliters.

flu·i·drachm (flōō′ĭ-drăm′, flōō′ĭ-drăm′) *n.* A fluid dram.

fluke (flōōk) *n.* See **trematode.**

flu·nis·o·lide (flōō-nĭs′ə-līd′) *n.* An anti-inflammatory corticosteroid administered by inhalation in the treatment of allergies and asthma.

flu·ni·tra·ze·pam (flōō-nĭ-trăz′ə-păm) *n.* A benzodiazepine drug that is illegal in the US but is used elsewhere as a hypnotic and in anesthesia. It is popularly known as the "date rape drug" because its ability to cause semiconciousness and memory blackouts has led to its association with unwanted sexual encounters.

flu·o·cin·o·nide (flōō′ə-sĭn′ə-nīd′) *n.* A corticosteroid used topically as an anti-inflammatory agent.

fluor– *pref.* Variant of **fluoro–.**

fluo·res·ce·in (flōō-rĕs′ē-ĭn, flô-) *n.* An orange-red compound that exhibits intense fluorescence in alkaline solution and is used in ophthalmology to reveal corneal lesions.

fluo·res·cence (flōō-rĕs′əns, flô-) *n.* **1.** The emission of electromagnetic radiation, especially of visible light, stimulated in a substance by the absorption of incident radiation and persisting only as long as the stimulating radiation is continued. **2.** The property of emitting such radiation. —**fluo·res′cent** *adj.*

fluorescent antibody technique *n.* Either of two techniques used to test for antigen with a fluorescent antibody: direct, in which immunoglobulin conjugated with a fluorescent dye is added to tissue and combines with a specific antigen; or indirect, in which unlabeled immunoglobulin is added to tissue and combines with a specific antigen, after which the antigen-antibody complex may be labeled with a fluorescent antibody.

fluorescent antinuclear antibody test *n.* A test for antinuclear antibody components, especially for diagnosis of collagen-vascular diseases. Also called *FANA test.*

fluorescent microscope *n.* A microscope fitted with a source of ultraviolet radiation to aid in the detection and examination of fluorescent specimens.

fluorescent treponemal antibody absorption test *n.* A serologic test for syphilis using a suspension of *Treponema pallidum* as antigen. Also called *FTA-ABS test.*

fluor·i·da·tion (flŏor′ĭ-dā′shən, flôr′-) *n.* The addition of a fluorine compound to drinking water for the purpose of reducing tooth decay. —**fluor′i·date′** *v.*

fluor·ide (flŏor′īd′, flôr′-) *n.* **1.** A compound of fluorine with another element. **2.** The univalent anion of fluorine.

fluoride number *n.* The percent inhibition of pseudocholinesterase produced by fluorides, used to differentiate normal from atypical pseudocholinesterases.

fluor·i·di·za·tion (flŏor′ĭ-dĭ-zā′shən, flôr′-) *n.* The therapeutic use of fluorides to reduce the incidence of dental decay, as by topical application of fluoride agents to the teeth.

fluor·ine (flŏor′ēn′, -ĭn, flôr′-) *n. Symbol* **F** A highly corrosive, toxic, gaseous halogen element. It is a component of many drugs, and its radioisotope is used in functional brain imaging and bone scans. Atomic number 9.

fluoro– or fluor– *pref.* **1.** Fluorine: *fluorosis.* **2.** Fluorescence: *fluoroscope.*

fluor·o·chrome (flŏŏr′ə-krōm′, flôr′-) *n.* Any of a group of fluorescent dyes used to stain tissues and cells for examination by fluorescence microscopy.

fluo·rog·ra·phy (flŏŏ-rŏg′rə-fē, flô-) *n.* See **photofluorography**.

fluo·rom·e·ter (flŏŏ-rŏm′ĭ-tər, flô-) *n.* An instrument for detecting and measuring fluorescence.

fluo·rom·e·try (flŏŏ-rŏm′ĭ-trē, flô-) *n.* An analytic method for detecting and measuring fluorescence in compounds that uses ultraviolet light stimulating the compounds, causing them to emit visible light. —**fluor′o·met′ric** (flŏŏr′ə-mĕt′rĭk, flôr′-) *adj.*

fluor·o·pho·tom·e·try (flŏŏr′ō-fō-tŏm′ĭ-trē, flôr′-) *n.* Measurement of the light emitted by a fluorescent substance, especially that emitted from the interior of the eye after intravenous injection of fluorescein to test the integrity of the retinal vasculature.

fluor·o·quin·o·lone (flŏŏr′ə-kwĭn′ə-lōn′, flôr′-) *n.* Any of a group of broad-spectrum antibiotics that are fluorinated derivatives of quinolone compounds and are especially effective against gram-negative bacteria.

fluor·o·scope (flŏŏr′ə-skōp′, flôr′-) *n.* A device equipped with a fluorescent screen on which the internal structures of an optically opaque object, such as the human body, may be continuously viewed as shadowy images formed by the differential transmission of x-rays through the object. —*v.* To examine the interior of a body with a fluoroscope. —**fluor′o·scop′ic** (-skŏp′ĭk) *adj.*

fluo·ros·co·py (flŏŏ-rŏs′kə-pē, flô-) *n.* Examination by means of a fluoroscope. Also called *radioscopy.*

fluo·ro·sis (flŏŏ-rō′sĭs, flô-) *n.* An abnormal condition caused by excessive intake of fluorine, as from fluoridated drinking water, characterized chiefly by mottling of the teeth. —**fluo·rot′ic** (-rŏt′ĭk) *adj.*

fluor·o·u·ra·cil (flŏŏr′ō-yŏŏr′ə-sĭl, flôr′-) *n.* An antineoplastic agent used especially in the treatment of cancers of the skin, breast, and digestive system.

flu·ox·e·tine hydrochloride (flŏŏ-ŏk′sĭ-tēn′) *n.* An oral antidepressant that is chemically unrelated to other antidepressants.

flu·phen·a·zine (flŏŏ-fĕn′ə-zēn′) *n.* A tranquilizing drug used especially in the form of its hydrochloride in psychotherapy.

flu·ran·dren·o·lide (flŏŏr′ăn-drĕn′ə-līd′, -drē′nə-) *n.* An anti-inflammatory glucocorticoid used in topical preparations.

flu·raz·e·pam hydrochloride (flŏŏ-răz′ə-păm′) *n.* A benzodiazepine drug, usually used to treat insomnia.

flur·bip·ro·fen (flŏŏr-bĭp′rə-fən) *n.* A nonsteroidal anti-inflammatory agent with anti-inflammatory, analgesic, and antipyretic actions.

flush (flŭsh) *v.* **1.** To turn red, as from fever, heat, or strong emotion; blush. **2.** To clean, rinse, or empty with a rapid flow of a liquid, especially water. —*n.* **1.** An act of cleansing or rinsing with a flow of water. **2.** A reddening of the skin, as with fever, emotion, or exertion. **3.** A brief sensation of heat over all or part

of the body. —*adj.* Having surfaces in the same plane; even.

flut·ter (flŭt′ər) *n.* Abnormally rapid pulsation, especially of the atria or ventricles of the heart.

flutter-fibrillation *n.* An electrocardiographic pattern of atrial activity with features of both fibrillation and flutter.

flu·va·stat·in (flŏŏ′və-stăt′n) *n.* A statin drug given to treat hyperlipidemia.

flux (flŭks) *n.* **1.** The discharge of large quantities of fluid material from the body, especially the discharge of watery feces from the intestines. **2.** Material thus discharged from the bowels. **3.** The rate of flow of fluid, particles, or energy through a given surface. **4.** Flux density.

flux density *n.* The rate of flow of fluid, particles, or energy per unit area.

flux·ion·ar·y hyperemia (flŭk′shə-nĕr′ē) *n.* See **active hyperemia**.

fly (flī) *n.* Any of numerous two-winged insects of the order Diptera.

fly blister *n.* A cantharidal blister caused by the vesicating body fluid of certain beetles.

Fm The symbol for the element **fermium.**

FMN *abbr.* flavin mononucleotide

fMRI *abbr.* functional magnetic resonance imaging

foam cell (fōm) *n.* A cell containing lipids in small vacuoles, as seen in leprosy and xanthoma, often a histiocyte.

foam·y virus (fō′mē) *n.* Any of the various retroviruses found in primates and other mammals and characterized by the lacelike changes they cause in monkey kidney cells.

fo·cal (fō′kəl) *adj.* Of or relating to a focus.

focal amyloidosis *n.* See **nodular amyloidosis.**

focal depth *n.* A measure of the power of a lens to produce clear images at different distances from it. Also called *depth of focus.*

focal distance *n.* See **focal length.**

focal epilepsy *n.* An epileptic condition in which disturbance in a localized area of cerebral function causes the twitching of a limb, the occurrence of a somatosensory or special sense phenomenon, or a specific disturbance of complex mental functions. Also called *cortical epilepsy, focal seizure disorder.*

focal glomerulonephritis *n.* Glomerulonephritis affecting only a small proportion of renal glomeruli.

focal infection *n.* A bacterial infection localized in a specific part of the body, such as the tonsils, that may spread to another part of the body.

focal length *n.* The distance from the surface of a lens or mirror to its focal point. Also called *focal distance, focus.*

focal necrosis *n.* The occurrence of numerous, small, fairly well circumscribed foci of necrosis.

focal point *n.* See **focus** (sense 1).

focal reaction *n.* A limited reaction that occurs at the point of entrance of an infecting organism or of an injection. Also called *local reaction.*

focal segmental glomerulosclerosis *n.* Segmental collapse of glomerular capillaries with thickened basement membranes and increased mesangial matrix, seen sometimes in nephrotic syndrome or mesangial proliferative glomerulonephritis.

focal seizure *n.* A seizure that originates from a localized area of the cerebral cortex, involves neurologic symptoms specific to the affected area of the brain, and may progress to a generalized seizure. Also called *partial seizure.*

focal seizure disorder *n.* See **focal epilepsy.**

fo·cus (fō′kəs) *n.,* pl. **–cus·es** or **–ci** (-sī′, -kī′) **1.** A point at which rays of light or other radiation converge or from which they appear to diverge, as after refraction or reflection in an optical system. Also called *focal point.* **2.** See **focal length. 3.** The distinctness or clarity of an image rendered by an optical system. **4.** The state of maximum distinctness or clarity of such an image. **5.** An apparatus used to adjust the focal length of an optical system in order to make an image distinct or clear. **6.** The region of a localized bodily infection or disease. —*v.* **1.** To cause light rays or other radiation to converge on or toward a central point; concentrate. **2.** To render an object or image in clear outline or sharp detail by adjustment of one's vision or an optical device. **3.** To adjust a lens or instrument to produce a clear image. **4.** To converge on or toward a central point of focus; be focused.

Fo·gar·ty catheter (fō′gər-tē) *n.* A catheter with an inflatable balloon near its tip; it is used to remove emboli and thrombi from the cardiovascular system, and to remove stones from the biliary ducts.

fog·ging (fŏg′ĭng) *n.* A method of refracting the eye in which accommodation is relaxed by overcorrection with a convex spherical lens, used in testing vision.

fo·la·cin (fō′lə-sĭn, fŏl′ə-) *n.* See **folic acid.**

fo·late (fō′lāt′) *n.* **1.** A salt or ester of folic acid. **2.** See **folic acid.**

fold (fōld) *n.* **1.** A crease or ridge apparently formed by folding, as of a membrane; a plica. **2.** In the embryo, a transient elevation or reduplication of tissue in the form of a lamina.

fold·ed lung syndrome (fōl′dĭd) *n.* Collapse of part of the lung caught between shrinking fibrous pleura scars, which sometimes results from pleural asbestosis. Also called *round atelectasis.*

Fo·ley catheter (fō′lē) *n.* A catheter held in the bladder by an inflatable balloon.

fo·li·ate papilla (fō′lē-ĭt, -āt′) *n.* Any of the numerous projections that are arranged in several transverse folds on the lateral margins of the tongue just in front of the palatoglossus muscle.

fo·lic acid (fō′lĭk, fŏl′ĭk) *n.* A yellowish-orange compound of the vitamin B complex group, occurring in green plants, fresh fruit, liver, and yeast. Also called *folacin, folate, vitamin B_c.*

folic acid antagonists *pl.n.* Modified pterins, such as aminopterin and amethopterin, that interfere with the action of folic acid and produce the symptoms of a folic acid deficiency.

fo·lie á deux (fô-lē′ ä dœ′, fŏl′ē) *n.* A condition in which symptoms of a mental disorder occur simultaneously in two individuals who share a close relationship or association.

folie du doute (dü dōot′, dōot′) *n.* A mental disorder characterized by extreme indecision, especially concerning everyday matters, and a pathological preoccupation with minute details.

fo·li·nate (fō′lə-nāt′) *n.* A salt or ester of folinic acid.

fo·lin·ic ac·id (fō-lĭn′ĭk) *n.* A compound that acts as a formyl group carrier in transformylation reactions. Also called *citrovorum factor, leucovorin.*

Fo·lin's test (fō′lĭnz) *n.* **1.** A spectrophotometric test used to determine the quantity of uric acid in urine in which a phosphotungstic acid is mixed with a base. **2.** A test used to determine the quantity of urea in urine in which urea is decomposed by boiling with magnesium chloride and the freed ammonia is measured.

fo·li·um (fō′lē-əm) *n.,* pl. **–li·a** (-lē-ə) A broad, thin, leaflike structure, as of the cerebellar cortex.

folk medicine (fōlk) *n.* Traditional medicine as practiced by nonprofessional healers or embodied in local custom or lore, generally involving the use of natural and especially herbal remedies.

fol·lib·er·in (fō-lĭb′ər-ĭn) *n.* See **follicle-stimulating hormone-releasing factor.**

fol·li·cle (fŏl′ĭ-kəl) *n.* **1.** A small bodily cavity or sac. **2.** A crypt or minute cul-de-sac or lacuna, such as the depression in the skin from which the hair emerges. **3.** An ovarian follicle. **4.** A spherical mass of cells usually containing a cavity.

follicle mite *n.* Any of various tiny mites of the genus *Demodex* that infest the hair follicles of mammals.

follicle of the thyroid gland *n.* Any of the small spherical vesicular components of the thyroid gland lined with epithelium and containing a colloid substance that stores thyroid hormones.

follicle-stimulating hormone *n. Abbr.* **FSH** A glycoprotein hormone of the anterior pituitary gland that stimulates the Graafian follicles and assists in follicular maturation and in the secretion of estradiol. It also stimulates the epithelium of the seminiferous tubules and assists in inducing spermatogenesis. Also called *follitropin.*

follicle-stimulating hormone-releasing factor *n. Abbr.* **FRF, FSH-RF** A decapeptide of hypothalamic origin capable of accelerating pituitary secretion of follicle-stimulating hormone. Also called *folliberin, follicle-stimulating hormone-releasing hormone.*

fol·lic·u·lar (fə-lĭk′yə-lər) *adj.* **1.** Relating to, having, or resembling a follicle or follicles. **2.** Affecting or growing out of a follicle or follicles.

follicular atresia *n.* The normal process affecting the ovarian primordial follicles in which death of the ovum results in cystic degeneration followed by cicatricial closure.

follicular cell *n.* An epithelial cell lining a follicle, such as that of the thyroid or ovary.

follicular conjunctivitis *n.* Conjunctivitis characterized by discrete lymphoid follicles in the conjunctival stroma.

follicular cyst *n.* A cyst caused by the retention of secretions in a follicular space due to the blockage of a duct, especially in a Graafian follicle.

follicular cystitis *n.* Chronic cystitis characterized by small mucosal nodules and the formation of lymphoid follicles in the bladder.

follicular dendritic cell *n.* Any of the cells present in aggregates of B cells that trap antigen-antibody complexes on their dendritic processes. Also called *dendritic cell.*

follicular goiter *n.* See **parenchymatous goiter.**

follicular lymphoma *n.* See **nodular lymphoma**.

follicular mucinosis *n.* Mucinosis affecting hair follicles of the face or scalp.

follicular phase *n.* The phase during which the ovarian follicle develops during the menstrual cycle.

follicular stigma *n.* The point where the Graafian follicle will rupture on the surface of the ovary.

fol·lic·u·late (fə-lĭk′yə-lĭt) *or* **fol·lic·u·lat·ed** (-lā′tĭd) *adj.* Having or consisting of a follicle or follicles.

fol·lic·u·li·tis (fə-lĭk′yə-lī′tĭs) *n.* Inflammation of a follicle, especially of a hair follicle.

folliculitis bar·bae (bär′bē) *n.* See **barber's itch**.

folliculitis de·cal·vans (dē-kăl′vănz′) *n.* A papular or pustular inflammation of the hair follicles of the scalp, resulting in scarring and local loss of hair.

folliculitis ke·loi·da·lis (kē′loi-dā′lĭs) *n.* See **acne keloid**.

folliculitis u·ler·y·the·ma·to·sa re·tic·u·la·ta (yōo-lĕr′ə-thē′mə-tō′sə rĭ-tĭk′yə-lā′tə, -thĕm′ə-) *n.* An eruptive folliculitis usually occurring on the cheeks, in which atrophy of the skin creates a network of pitted scars.

fol·lic·u·lo·ma (fə-lĭk′yə-lō′mə) *n., pl.* **–mas** *or* **–ma·ta** (-mə-tə) **1.** Cystic enlargement of a Graafian follicle. **2.** See **granulosa cell tumor**.

fol·lic·u·lo·sis (fə-lĭk′yə-lō′sĭs) *n.* The presence of lymph follicles in abnormally large numbers.

fol·lic·u·lus (fə-lĭk′yə-ləs) *n., pl.* **-li** (-lī′) Follicle.

fol·li·tro·pin (fŏl′ĭ-trō′pĭn) *n.* See **follicle-stimulating hormone**.

fol·low·ing bougie (fŏl′ō-ĭng) *n.* A flexible tapered bougie with a screw tip that is attached to the tailing end of a filiform bougie, allowing the progressive dilation of a passage.

fo·men·ta·tion (fō′mən-tā′shən, -mĕn-) *n.* **1.** A substance or material used as a warm, moist medicinal compress; a poultice. **2.** The therapeutic application of warmth and moisture, as to relieve pain.

fo·mes (fō′mēz) *n., pl.* **fom·i·tes** (fŏm′ĭ-tēz′, fō′mĭ-) Fomite.

fo·mite (fō′mīt′) *n.* An inanimate object or substance, such as clothing, furniture, or soap, that is capable of transmitting infectious organisms from one individual to another.

fon·ta·nel *or* **fon·ta·nelle** (fŏn′tə-nĕl′) *n.* Any of the soft membranous gaps between the incompletely formed cranial bones of a fetus or infant. Also called *soft spot*.

fon·tic·u·lus (fŏn-tĭk′yə-ləs) *n., pl.* **fon·tic·u·li** (-lī′) Fontanel.

food (fōod) *n.* Material, usually of plant or animal origin, that contains essential nutrients, such as carbohydrates, fats, proteins, vitamins, or minerals, and is ingested and assimilated by an organism to produce energy, stimulate growth, and maintain life.

food ball *n.* A gastric concretion formed of vegetable fibers from the seeds and skins of fruits and sometimes containing starch granules and fat globules. Also called *phytobezoar*.

Food Guide Pyramid *n.* A food pyramid devised by the US Department of Agriculture in 1992, in which grains and cereals represent the base beneath layers for fruits and vegetables, meats and dairy products, and fats and sweets at the peak.

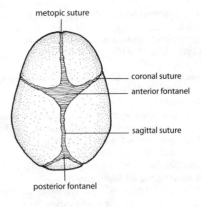

fontanel
anterior and posterior fontanels

food poisoning *n.* **1.** Bacterial food poisoning. **2.** Poisoning caused by ingesting substances, such as certain mushrooms, that contain natural toxins.

food pyramid *n.* A graphic representation of human nutritional needs in the form of a pyramid, in which foods whose recommended daily intake is highest occupy the wider bottom part and foods whose recommended daily intake is lowest occupy the slender top part.

foot (fōot) *n., pl.* **feet** (fēt) **1.** The lower extremity of the vertebrate leg that is in direct contact with the ground in standing or walking. **2.** A unit of length in the US Customary and British Imperial systems equal to 12 inches (30.48 centimeters).

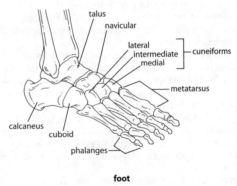

foot
anterior view of bones in the foot

foot-and-mouth disease *n.* An acute, highly contagious degenerative viral disease of cattle and other cloven-hoofed animals, characterized by fever and the eruption of vesicles around the mouth and hoofs. Also called *hoof-and-mouth disease*.

foot-candle *n.* A unit of measure of the intensity of light falling on a surface equal to 1 lumen per square foot. It has been replaced in the International System by the candela (1 lumen per square meter).

foot-drop *n.* Paralysis or weakness of the dorsiflexor muscles of the foot and ankle, resulting in dragging of the foot and toes. Also called *drop foot*.

foot·ling presentation (foõt′lĭng) *n.* Breech presentation of the fetus during birth in which the feet are the presenting part. Also called *foot presentation.*

foot·plate (foõt′plāt′) *n.* **1.** See **base of stapes. 2.** See **pedicel** (sense 2).

foot-pound *n.* A unit of work equal to the energy expended, or work done, in raising a mass of one pound a height of one foot against gravity.

foot-pound-second system *n. Abbr.* **fps system** The British, Canadian, or US system of units based on the foot, the pound, and the second as the fundamental units of length, mass, and time.

foot presentation *n.* See **footling presentation.**

foot process *n.* See **pedicel** (sense 2).

fo·ra·men (fə-rā′mən) *n., pl.* **–ra·mens** *or* **–ram·i·na** (-răm′ə-nə) An aperture or perforation through a bone or a membranous structure. —**fo·ram′i·nal** (-răm′ə-nəl), **fo·ram′i·nous** (-nəs) *adj.*

foramen ce·cum me·dul·lae ob·lon·ga·tae (sē′kəm mĭ-dŭl′ē öb′lŏng-gā′tē) *n.* A small triangular depression at the lower boundary of the pons that marks the upper limit of the median fissure of the medulla oblongata.

foramen mag·num (măg′nəm) *n.* See **great foramen.**

foramen of vena cava *n.* An opening in the right lobe of the central tendon of the diaphragm, transmitting the inferior vena cava and branches of the right phrenic nerve. Also called *quadrate foramen.*

foramen ovale (ō-văl′ē, -vā′lē, -vä′-) *n.* An opening in the septum between the right and left atria of the heart, present in the fetus but usually closed soon after birth.

foramen spi·no·sum (spī-nō′səm) *n.* An opening in the greater wing of the sphenoid bone, in front of the spine, transmitting the middle meningeal artery.

fo·ram·i·na (fə-răm′ə-nə) *n.* A plural of **foramen.**

foraminal node *n.* One of the hepatic nodes next to the epiploic foramen.

Forbes disease (fôrbz) *n.* See **type 3 glycogenosis.**

force (fôrs) *n.* **1.** The capacity to do work or cause physical change; energy, strength, or active power. **2.** A vector quantity that tends to produce an acceleration of a body in the direction of its application.

forced alimentation *n.* See **forced feeding** (sense 1).

forced beat *n.* **1.** A premature beat believed to be precipitated by the preceding normal beat to which it is coupled. **2.** An extrasystole caused by artificial stimulation of the heart.

forced expiratory flow *n. Abbr.* **FEF** The flow of air from the lungs during measurement of forced vital capacity.

forced expiratory time *n. Abbr.* **FET** The time taken to expire a given volume during measurement of forced vital capacity.

forced expiratory volume *n. Abbr.* **FEV** The maximum volume of air that can be expired from the lungs in a specific time interval when starting from maximum inspiration.

forced feeding *n.* **1.** Administration of liquid food through a nasal tube passed into the stomach. Also called *forced alimentation.* **2.** Forcing a person to eat more food than desired. —**force′-feed′** *v.*

forced vital capacity *n. Abbr.* **FVC** Vital capacity measured with subject exhaling as rapidly as possible.

force of mastication *n.* The force created by the dynamic action of the masticatory muscles during the physiological act of chewing. Also called *masticatory force.*

for·ceps (fôr′səps, -sĕps) *n., pl.* **forceps 1.** An instrument resembling a pair of pincers, used for grasping, manipulating, or extracting, especially in surgery. **2.** Either of two bands of white fibers composing the radiation of the corpus callosum to the cerebrum.

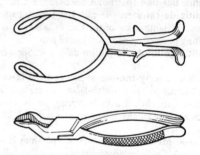

forceps
Top: *obstetrical*
Bottom: *dental*

forceps delivery *n.* The birth of a child assisted by extraction with a forceps designed to grasp the head.

for·ci·pres·sure (fôr′sə-prĕsh′ər) *n.* A method of arresting hemorrhage by compressing a blood vessel with forceps.

Fordyce's spots (fôr′dī′sĭz) *n.* A condition marked by the presence of numerous small yellowish-white granules on the inner surface and border of the lips. Also called *Fordyce's disease.*

fore·arm (fôr′ärm′) *n.* The part of the arm between the wrist and the elbow.

fore·brain (fôr′brān′) *n.* The prosencephalon.

fore·con·scious (fôr′kŏn′shəs) *adj.* Capable of being called into the conscious mind but not currently in the realm of consciousness. —*n.* The part of the psyche that contains thoughts, feelings, and impulses that are not currently part of one's consciousness but that can be readily called into consciousness. Also called *preconscious.*

fore·fin·ger (fôr′fĭng′gər) *n.* See **index finger.**

fore·gut (fôr′gŭt′) *n.* The anterior part of the embryonic alimentary canal of a vertebrate from which the pharynx, lungs, esophagus, stomach, liver, pancreas, and duodenum develop.

fore·head (fôr′hĕd′, -ĭd) *n.* The part of the face between the eyebrows, the normal hairline, and the temples. Also called *brow.*

for·eign body (fôr′ĭn) *n.* An object or entity in the body that has been introduced from outside.

foreign body granuloma *n.* A granuloma caused by the presence of foreign material in tissue.

Fo·rel's decussation (fə-rĕlz′, fô-) *n.* See **tegmental decussation** (sense 2).

fore·milk (fôr′mĭlk′) *n.* See **colostrum.**

fo·ren·sic (fə-rĕn′zĭk) *adj.* Relating to, used in, or appropriate for courts of law or for public discussion or argumentation.

forensic dentistry *n.* **1.** The application of dentistry to legal problems, as in using the teeth for identifying the dead. **2.** The law as it applies to the practice of dentistry. Also called *legal dentistry.*

forensic medicine *n.* The branch of medicine that interprets or establishes the medical facts in civil or criminal law cases. Also called *legal medicine, medical jurisprudence.*

forensic psychiatry *n.* The branch of psychiatry that makes determinations, as regarding fitness to stand trial, the need for commitment, or responsibility for criminal behavior, in a court of law.

forensic psychology *n.* The application of psychology to legal matters in a court of law.

fore·play (fôr′plā′) *n.* The sexual stimulation that precedes intercourse.

fore·skin (fôr′skĭn′) *n.* The loose fold of skin that covers the glans of the penis. Also called *prepuce.*

fore·wa·ters (fôr′wô′tərz) *n.* The amniotic fluid between the presenting part, usually the head, and the intact fetal membranes.

–form *suff.* Having the form of: *plexiform.*

For·mad's kidney (fôr′mădz) *n.* An enlarged and deformed kidney that is sometimes seen in chronic alcoholism.

for·mal·de·hyde (fôr-măl′də-hīd′) *n.* A colorless, gaseous compound that is the simplest aldehyde, used for manufacturing melamine and phenolic resins, fertilizers, dyes, and embalming fluids and in aqueous solution as a preservative and disinfectant.

for·ma·lin (fôr′mə-lĭn) *n.* An aqueous solution of formaldehyde that is 37 percent by weight.

for·ma·lin pigment (fôr′mə-lĭn) *n.* A pigment formed in blood-rich tissues that come in contact with aqueous solutions of formaldehyde that have acidic pH values.

for·mam·i·dase (fôr-măm′ĭ-dās′, -dāz′) *n.* An enzyme that catalyzes the hydrolysis of formylkynurenine to kynurenine and formate, important in the breakdown of tryptophan.

for·mate (fôr′māt′) *n.* A compound, such as a salt or ester of formic acid, that contains the HCOO⁻ radical.

for·ma·ti·o (fôr-mā′shē-ō) *n., pl.* **–ma·ti·o·nes** (-mā′-shē-ō′nēz) A structure of definite shape or cellular arrangement; a formation.

for·ma·tion (fôr-mā′shən) *n.* **1.** The act or process of forming something or of taking form. **2.** Something formed.

forme fruste (fôrm′ frōōst′, früst′) *n., pl.* **formes frustes** (fôrm′ frōōst′, früst′) An incomplete, abortive, or unusual form of a syndrome or disease.

for·mic acid (fôr′mĭk) *n.* A colorless caustic fuming liquid used in dyeing and finishing textiles and paper and in the manufacture of fumigants, insecticides, and refrigerants.

for·mi·ca·tion (fôr′mĭ-kā′shən) *n.* An abnormal sensation as of insects running over or into the skin, associated with cocaine intoxication or disease of the spinal cord and peripheral nerves.

for·mim·i·no·glu·tam·ic ac·id (fôr-mĭm′ə-nō-glōō-tăm′ĭk) *n.* An intermediate that forms during the conversion of histidine to glutamic acid.

for·mu·la (fôr′myə-lə) *n., pl.* **–las** *or* **–lae** (-lē′) **1.** A symbolic representation of the chemical composition or of the chemical composition and structure of a compound. **2.** The chemical compound so represented. **3.** A prescription of ingredients in fixed proportion; a recipe. **4.** A liquid food for infants, containing most of the nutrients in human milk. **5.** A mathematical statement, especially an equation, of a fact, rule, principle, or other logical relation.

for·mu·lar·y (fôr′myə-lĕr′ē) *n.* A book containing a list of pharmaceutical substances along with their formulas, uses, and methods of preparation.

formula weight *n.* See **molecular weight.**

for·myl (fôr′mĭl′) *n.* The univalent radical HCO, characteristic of aldehydes.

for·myl·ase (fôr′mə-lās′, -lāz′) *n.* Formamidase.

for·myl·ky·nu·re·nine (fôr′məl-kī-nŏŏr′ə-nēn′) *n.* An intermediate that is formed during the breakdown of tryptophan.

for·ni·ca·tion (fôr′nĭ-kā′shən) *n.* Sexual intercourse between partners who are not married to each other. **—for′ni·cate′** *v.*

for·nix (fôr′nĭks) *n., pl.* **–ni·ces** (-nĭ-sēz′) **1.** An arch-shaped structure, especially the arch-shaped roof of an anatomical space. **2.** The compact bundle of white fiber by which the hippocampus of each cerebral hemisphere projects to the opposite hippocampus and to the septum, the anterior nucleus of the thalamus, and the mamillary body.

For·res·tier's disease (fôr′ĕ-styāz′) *n.* See **diffuse idiopathic skeletal hyperostosis.**

Forss·mann (fôrs′män′, -mən), **Werner Theodor Otto** 1904–1979. German physician. He shared a 1956 Nobel Prize for developing cardiac catheterization.

For·taz (fôr′tăz′) A trademark for the drug ceftazidime.

Fort Bragg fever (fôrt brăg′) *n.* See **pretibial fever.**

For·to·vase (fôr′tō-vās′) A trademark for the drug saquinavir.

for·ward heart failure (fôr′wərd) *n.* Congestive heart failure resulting from inadequate cardiac output, characterized by weakness, fatigue, and the retention of sodium and water.

Fos·a·max (fŏs′ə-măks′) A trademark for the drug alendronate sodium.

fos·car·net sodium (fŏs-kär′nĭt) *n.* A pyrophosphate analog used to treat herpes simplex infections.

fos·sa (fŏs′ə) *n., pl.* **fos·sae** (fŏs′ē′) A small longitudinal cavity or depression, as in a bone.

fossa of lacrimal gland *n.* A hollow in the orbital plate of the frontal bone, formed by the overhanging margin and zygomatic process and lodging the lacrimal gland.

fossa of vestibule of vagina *n.* The portion of the vestibule of the vagina located between the frenulum of the pudendal lips and the posterior commissure of the vulva. Also called *navicular fossa of vestibule of vagina.*

fos·sette (fŏ-sĕt′) *n.* **1.** A small depression; a dimple. **2.** A small deep ulcer of the cornea.

fos·su·la (fŏs′ə-lə, -yə-lə) *n., pl.* **–lae** (-lē′) A small fossa.

Fos·ter frame (fô′stər) *n.* A reversible bed similar to a Stryker frame.

Foth·er·gill's disease (fŏ*th*′ər-gĭlz′) *n.* **1.** See **anginose scarlatina**. **2.** See **trigeminal neuralgia**.

Fothergill's neuralgia *n.* See **trigeminal neuralgia**.

Fothergill's operation *n.* See **Manchester operation**.

fou·lage (foo-läzh′) *n.* A form of massage in which the muscles are kneaded and pressed.

foun·da·tion (foun-dā′shən) *n.* The basis on which something stands or is supported; a base.

foun·der (foun′dər) *v.* **1.** To stumble, especially to stumble and go lame. Used of horses. **2.** To become ill from overeating. Used of livestock. **3.** To be afflicted with laminitis. Used of horses. —*n.* See **laminitis**.

foun·tain decussation (foun′tən) *n.* See **tegmental decussation** (sense **?**).

fountain syringe *n.* A fluid reservoir with a tube attached to the bottom so that the flow is controlled by gravity, used for vaginal or rectal injections and for irrigating wounds.

4-alpha-D-glu·ca·no·trans·fer·ase (-gloo′kə-nō-trăns′-fə-rās′, -rāz′) *n.* A transferase enzyme that catalyzes the conversion of maltodextrins into amylose and glucose; debranching enzyme.

four·chette (foor-shĕt′) *n.* See **frenulum of pudendal lips**.

4-pyr·i·dox·ic acid (-pĭr′ĭ-dŏk′sĭk) *n.* A crystalline acid found in urine that is the principal metabolic product of pyridoxal.

fourth (fôrth) *adj.* **1.** Coming after third, as in order, place, rank, time, or quality. **2.** Being the digit that is next to and on the outermost side of the third digit, as on a foot. —**fourth** *n.*

fourth cranial nerve *n.* See **trochlear nerve**.

fourth disease *n.* A mild exanthematous disease of childhood resembling scarlatina. Also called *Dukes disease, scarlatinella.*

fourth heart sound *n.* The heart sound occurring in late diastole, corresponding with atrial contraction.

fourth ventricle *n.* An irregular cavity that extends from the obex to a communication with the sylvian aqueduct and is enclosed between the cerebellum dorsally and the tegmentum of rhombencephalon ventrally.

fo·ve·a (fō′vē-ə) *n.,* *pl.* **–ve·ae** (-vē-ē′) **1.** A small pit or cuplike depression in a bone or organ. **2.** The fovea centralis.

fovea cen·tra·lis (sĕn-trā′lĭs) *n.* A depression in the center of the macula of the retina, the area of the most acute vision, where only cones are present and where blood vessels are lacking. Also called *central fovea, central pit.*

fo·ve·ate (fō′vē-āt′, -ĭt) *adj.* Foveolate.

fo·ve·a·tion (fō′vē-ā′shən) *n.* **1.** The state of being pitted or scarred, as occurs in smallpox, chickenpox, or vaccinia. **2.** Any of the pits formed under such conditions.

fo·ve·o·la (fō-vē′ə-lə) *n.,* *pl.* **–las** *or* **–lae** (-lē′) A small fovea. —**fo·ve′o·lar** *adj.*

fo·ve·o·late (fō′vē-ə-lāt′, -lĭt, fō-vē′ə-) *adj.* Having minute pits or small depressions on the surface.

Fow·ler's position (fou′lərz) *n.* An inclined position in which the head of the bed is raised to promote dependent drainage after an abdominal operation.

Fox-Fordyce disease (fŏks′-) *n.* A rare chronic eruption of dry papules and distended ruptured apocrine glands, with intense pruritis and follicular hyperkeratosis of the nipples, armpits, and pubic and chest regions.

fox·glove (fŏks′glŭv′) *n.* Any of several herbs of the genus *Digitalis,* especially *D. purpurea,* having a long cluster of large, tubular, pinkish-purple flowers and leaves that are the source of the drug digitalis.

FP *abbr.* family physician; family practice; family practitioner

F plasmid *n.* The prototype conjugative plasmid associated with conjugation in a strain of *Escherichia coli.* Also called *fertility factor, F factor.*

fps system *abbr.* foot-pound-second system

Fr The symbol for the element **francium**.

Fra·cas·to·ro (frä′kä-stō′rō), **Girolamo** 1483–1553. Italian physician and poet who wrote the poem *Syphilis sive morbus Gallicus* (1530), in which the name *syphilis* was first given to the disease.

frac·tion (frăk′shən) *n.* **1.** An expression that indicates the quotient of two quantities. **2.** A chemical component that is separated by fractionation. **3.** A disconnected piece; a fragment. **4.** An aliquot portion or any portion.

frac·tion·a·tion (frăk′shə-nā′shən) *n.* **1.** The process of dividing or separating into parts; breaking up. **2.** The division of a total therapeutic dose of radiation into small doses to be administered over a period of days or weeks. **3.** The separation of a chemical compound into components, as by distillation.

frac·ture (frăk′chər) *n. Abbr.* **fx 1.** The act or process of breaking. **2.** A break, rupture, or crack, especially in bone or cartilage. —*v.* To cause to break.

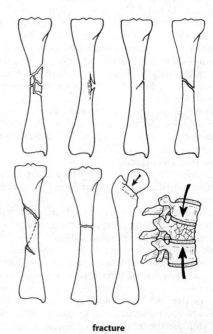

fracture
types of fractures:
Top: *comminuted, greenstick, incomplete, and oblique*
Bottom: *spiral, transverse, impacted, and compression*

fracture by contrecoup *n.* See **contrafissura.**

frag·ile site (frăj′əl) *n.* A nonstaining gap at a specific point on a chromosome that usually involves both chromatids and always appears at exactly the same point on chromosomes of different cells from an individual or kindred.

fragile X-chromosome *n.* An X-chromosome with a fragile site near the end of the long arm, resulting in the appearance of an almost detached fragment.

fragile X syndrome *n.* An X-linked inherited disorder characterized by mental retardation, enlarged testes, and large ears, chin, and forehead in males and mild mental retardation or no effect in females.

fra·gil·i·ty (frə-jĭl′ĭ-tē) *n.* The quality or state of being easily broken or destroyed.

fragility of blood *n.* The increased susceptibility of red blood cells to break down when exposed to varying concentrations of saline.

fragility test *n.* A test to measure the resistance of red blood cells to hemolysis in hypotonic saline solutions. Also called *erythrocyte fragility test.*

frag·ment (frăg′mənt) *n.* **1.** A small part broken off or detached. **2.** An incomplete or isolated portion; a bit. —*v.* (frăg′mĕnt′) To break or separate into fragments.

fram·be·sia (frăm-bē′zhə, -zhē-ə) *n.* See **yaws.**

fram·be·si·o·ma (frăm-bē′zhē-ō′mə, -zē-) *n.* See **mother yaw.**

frame (frām) *n.* Something composed of parts fitted and joined together.

Fran·ces·chet·ti's syndrome (frăn′chĭ-skĕt′ēz, frän′-chĕ-) *n.* See **mandibulofacial dysostosis.**

Fran·ci·sel·la (frăn′sĭ-sĕl′ə) *n.* A genus of coccoid or rod-shaped, gram-negative aerobic bacteria, having some pathogenic species.

Francisella tu·la·ren·sis (tōō′lə-rĕn′sĭs) *n.* A bacterium of the genus *Francisella* that causes tularemia in humans.

fran·ci·um (frăn′sē-əm) *n. Symbol* Fr An extremely unstable radioactive element of the alkali metals, having approx. 19 isotopes, the most stable of which is Fr 223 with a half-life of 21 minutes. Atomic number 87.

frank (frăngk) *adj.* Clearly manifest; clinically evident.

Frank·fort horizontal plane (frăngk′fərt) *n.* See **Frankfort plane.**

Frankfort plane *n.* A standard craniometric reference plane passing through the right and left porion and the left orbitale. Also called *Frankfort horizontal plane.*

Frank·lin (frăngk′lĭn), **Rosalind** 1920–1958. British biophysicist. Her x-ray diffraction studies of DNA led to the description of the full structure of DNA by James Watson and Francis Crick.

Frank-Starling curve *n.* See **Starling's curve.**

fra·ter·nal (frə-tûr′nəl) *adj.* **1.** Of or relating to brothers. **2.** Of, relating to, or being a twin developed from two separately fertilized ova; dizygotic.

fraternal twins *pl.n.* Twins that derive from separately fertilized ova and that have different genetic makeup. They may be of the same or opposite sex.

Fra·zier-Spil·ler operation (frā′zhər-spĭl′ər) *n.* A subtemporal trigeminal rhizotomy.

FRC *abbr.* functional residual capacity

FRCP *abbr.* Fellow of the Royal College of Physicians

FRCS *abbr.* Fellow of the Royal College of Surgeons

freck·le (frĕk′əl) *n.* A small brownish spot on the skin, often turning darker or increasing in number upon exposure to the sun.

Fre·det-Ramstedt operation (frə-dā′-) *n.* See **pyloromyotomy.**

free association (frē) *n.* A psychoanalytic technique in which a patient verbalizes the passing contents of his or her mind without reservation. The verbalized conflicts that emerge provide insights into the unconscious mind that are the basis of the psychoanalyst's interpretations in psychoanalysis.

free energy *n.* A thermodynamic quantity that is the difference between a system's internal energy and the product of its absolute temperature and entropy; the portion of total energy of a natural system that can be used for work.

free flap *n.* An island flap in which the donor vessels are severed and the flap is moved to the recipient site where it is revascularized.

free gingiva *n.* The portion of the gum that surrounds the tooth but is not directly attached to the tooth surface.

free graft *n.* A graft cut free from its attachments and transplanted to another site.

free macrophage *n.* An actively motile macrophage typically found in sites of inflammation.

free nerve endings *pl.n.* Peripheral endings of sensory nerve fibers in which the terminal filaments end freely in the tissue.

free radical *n.* **1.** An uncharged atom or group of atoms having at least one unpaired electron, which makes it highly reactive. **2.** An organic compound having some unpaired valence electrons; a normal byproduct of oxidation reactions in metabolism.

freeze (frēz) *v.* **1.** To pass from the liquid to the solid state by loss of heat. **2.** To make or become congealed, stiffened, or hardened by exposure to cold.

freeze-drying *n.* See **lyophilization.**

Frei·berg's disease (frī′bûrgz′) *n.* Osteochondrosis of the head of the second metatarsal bone.

Frei test (frī) *n.* A skin test for venereal lymphogranuloma that uses antigen prepared from chlamydiae grown in the yolk sac of a chick embryo.

Frej·ka pillow splint (frā′kə) *n.* A pillow splint used for abduction and flexion of the femurs in treating congenital hip dysplasia or dislocation in infants.

frem·i·tus (frĕm′ĭ-təs) *n., pl.* **fremitus** A palpable vibration, as felt by the hand placed on the chest during coughing or speaking.

fre·nal (frē′nəl) *adj.* Relating to or characteristic of a frenum.

French scale *n.* A scale for grading the sizes of sounds, tubules, catheters, and other tubular devices. Also called *Charrière scale.*

fre·nec·to·my (frə-nĕk′tə-mē) *n.* Excision of a frenum.

fre·no·plas·ty (frē′nə-plăs′tē) *n.* Surgical correction of an abnormally attached frenum.

fre·not·o·my (frə-nŏt′ə-mē) *n.* Incision of a frenum, especially of the frenulum of the tongue.

fren·u·lum (frĕn′yə-ləm) *n., pl.* **–la** (-lə) A small frenum or band of fibrous material.

frenulum of clitoris *n.* The line of union of the inner portions of the labia minora on the undersurface of the glans clitoridis.

frenulum of lip *n.* Either of the two folds of mucous membrane extending from the gums to the middle line of the lower or upper lip.

frenulum of prepuce *n.* A fold of mucous membrane passing from the underside of the glans penis to the deep surface of the prepuce.

frenulum of pudendal lips *n.* A small band or fold of mucous membrane forming the posterior margin of the vulva and connecting the posterior ends of the labia majora. Also called *fourchette.*

frenulum of tongue *n.* A fold of mucous membrane extending from the floor of the mouth to the midline of the underside of the tongue.

fre·num (frē'nəm) *n., pl.* **–nums** *or* **–na** (-nə) **1.** A membranous fold of skin or mucous membrane that supports or restricts the movement of a part or organ, such as the small band of tissue connecting the tongue to the floor of the mouth. **2.** An anatomical structure resembling such a fold.

fresh frozen plasma *n. Abbr.* **FFP** Blood plasma frozen within 6 hours of collection.

fret·ting (frĕt'ĭng) *n.* A hole, or worn or polished spot made on metals by abrasion or erosion.

Freud (froid), **Anna** 1895–1982. Austrian-born British psychoanalyst noted for her application of psychoanalysis to child therapy.

Freud, Sigmund 1856–1939. Austrian physician and founder of psychoanalysis who theorized that the symptoms of hysterical patients represent forgotten and unresolved infantile psychosexual conflicts. His psychoanalytic theories profoundly influenced 20th-century thought.

Freud·i·an (froi'dē-ən) *adj.* Relating to or being in accordance with the psychoanalytic theories of Sigmund Freud. —*n.* An individual who accepts the tenets of psychoanalytic theories of Sigmund Freud, especially a psychiatrist who applies Freudian theory and method in conducting psychotherapy.

Freudian slip *n.* A verbal mistake that is thought to reveal an unconscious belief, thought, or emotion.

Freund's adjuvant (froindz) *n.* A substance consisting of killed microorganisms, such as mycobacteria, in an oil and water emulsion that is administered to induce and enhance the formation of antibodies.

Frey's irritation hairs (frīz) *pl.n.* Short hairs of varying degrees of stiffness that are embedded at right angles into the end of a light wooden handle and are used for determining the presence and sensitivity of pressure points of the skin.

FRF *abbr.* follicle-stimulating hormone-releasing factor

fri·a·ble (frī'ə-bəl) *adj.* **1.** Readily crumbled; brittle. **2.** Relating to a dry, brittle growth of bacteria.

fric·tion (frĭk'shən) *n.* **1.** The rubbing of one object or surface against another. **2.** A physical force that resists the relative motion or tendency to such motion of two bodies in contact.

friction sound *n.* The sound heard on auscultation caused by the rubbing together of two opposing serous surfaces that are roughened by an inflammatory exudate. Also called *friction rub.*

Fried·länd·er's bacillus (frēd'lĕn'dərz) *n.* The pathogenic bacterium *Klebsiella pneumoniae* that often causes pneumonia.

Friedländer's pneumonia *n.* A severe form of lobar pneumonia that is caused by infection with Friedländer's bacillus and characterized by swelling of the affected lobe.

Fried·man curve (frēd'mən) *n.* A graphic representation of the hours of labor plotted against cervical dilation in centimeters.

Fried·reich's ataxia (frēd'rīks, -rīкнs) *n.* See **hereditary spinal ataxia.**

Friedreich's disease *n.* See **myoclonus multiplex.**

Friedreich's sign *n.* An indication of adherent pericardium in which previously distended neck veins suddenly collapse with each diastole of the heart.

frig·id (frĭj'ĭd) *adj.* **1.** Extremely cold. **2.** Persistently averse to sexual intercourse.

fri·gid·i·ty (frĭ-jĭd'ĭ-tē) *n.* The state of marked or abnormal sexual indifference.

frôle·ment (frōl-mäн') *n.* **1.** A succession of slow, brushing movements in massage, done with the palm of the hand. **2.** A rustling sound sometimes heard during auscultation in pericardial disease.

frons (frŏnz) *n., pl.* **fron·tes** (frŏn'tēz) Forehead.

front·ad (frŭn'tăd') *adv.* Toward the front or toward the forehead.

fron·tal (frŭn'tl) *adj.* **1.** Of, relating to, directed toward, or situated at the front. **2.** Of or relating to the forehead or frontal bone. **3.** Of or relating to the frontal plane.

frontal area *n.* See **frontal cortex.**

frontal artery *n.* An artery with origin in the ophthalmic artery, with distribution to the anterior portion of the scalp, and with anastomoses to the branches of the supraorbital artery. Also called *supratrochlear artery.*

frontal axis *n.* A line running transversely through the center of the eyeball.

frontal bone *n.* A cranial bone consisting of a vertical portion corresponding to the forehead and a horizontal portion that forms the roofs of the orbital and nasal cavities.

frontal cortex *n.* The cortex of the frontal lobe of the cerebral hemisphere. Also called *frontal area, prefrontal area.*

frontal crest *n.* A ridge arising at the termination of the sagittal sulcus on the cerebral surface of the frontal bone and ending at the foramen cecum.

frontal groove *n.* Any of the three frontal sulci.

frontal gyrus *n.* **1.** A broad convolution on the convexity of the frontal lobe of the cerebrum between the inferior frontal sulcus and the sylvian fissure, divided by branches of the sylvian fissure into three parts; inferior frontal gyrus. **2.** A convolution on the convexity of each frontal lobe of the cerebrum running from front to back between the superior and inferior frontal sulci; middle frontal gyrus. **3.** A broad convolution running from front to back on the medial edges of the convex surface and of each frontal lobe; superior frontal gyrus.

fron·ta·lis (frŭn-tā'lĭs) *adj.* Frontal.

frontal lobe *n.* The largest portion of each cerebral hemisphere, anterior to the central sulcus.

frontal nerve *n.* A branch of the ophthalmic nerve that divides within the eye socket into the supratrochlear and the supraorbital nerves.

frontal plane *n.* See **coronal plane.**

frontal pole *n.* The most anterior promontory of each cerebral hemisphere.

frontal sinus *n.* A hollow formed on either side in the lower part of the squama of the frontal bone, communicating by the ethmoidal infundibulum with the middle meatus of the nasal cavity of the same side.

frontal sulcus *n.* **1.** A sagittal fissure on the outer surface of each frontal lobe of the cerebrum, demarcating the middle from the inferior frontal gyrus; inferior frontal sulcus. **2.** A sagittal fissure dividing the middle frontal gyrus into an upper and lower part; middle frontal sulcus. **3.** A sagittal fissure on the superior surface of each frontal lobe of the cerebrum, forming the lateral boundary of the superior frontal gyrus; superior frontal sulcus.

frontal suture *n.* The suture that lies between the two halves of the frontal bone of a child's skull and is usually obliterated by about the sixth year.

fron·to·an·te·ri·or position (frŭn′tō-ăn-tîr′ē-ər) *n.* A cephalic presentation of the fetus with the forehead directed toward either the right or left front quarter of the mother's pelvis.

fron·to·ma·lar (frŭn′tō-mā′lər, -lär′) *adj.* Of or being frontozygomatic.

fron·to·max·il·lar·y (frŭn′tō-măk′sə-lĕr′ē) *adj.* Relating to or characteristic of both the frontal bone and the maxilla.

fron·to·na·sal (frŭn′tō-nā′zəl) *adj.* Relating to or characteristic of both frontal and nasal bones.

fron·to·oc·cip·i·tal (frŭn′tō-ŏk-sĭp′ĭ-tl) *adj.* **1.** Relating to or characteristic of both the forehead and the occiput. **2.** Relating to or characteristic of both the frontal and occipital bones.

fron·to·pa·ri·e·tal (frŭn′tō-pə-rī′ĭ-təl) *adj.* Relating to or characteristic of both frontal and parietal bones.

fron·to·pos·te·ri·or position (frŭn′tō-pŏ-stîr′ē-ər, -pō-) *n.* A cephalic presentation of the fetus with the forehead directed toward either the right or left rear quarter of the mother's pelvis.

fron·to·tem·po·ral (frŭn′tō-tĕm′pər-əl, -tĕm′prəl) *adj.* Relating to or characteristic of both the frontal and the temporal bones.

fron·to·trans·verse position (frŭn′tō-trănz-vûrs′, -trăns-, -trănz′vûrs′, -trăns′-) *n.* A cephalic presentation of the fetus with the forehead toward either the right or left iliac fossa of the mother's pelvis.

fron·to·zy·go·mat·ic (frŭn′tō-zī′gə-măt′ĭk, -zĭg′ə-) *adj.* Relating to or characteristic of both the frontal and the zygomatic bones.

frost (frôst) *n.* A deposit of minute ice crystals formed when water vapor condenses at a temperature below freezing.

frost·bite (frôst′bīt′) *n.* Injury or destruction of skin and underlying tissue, most often that of the nose, ears, fingers, or toes, resulting from prolonged exposure to freezing or subfreezing temperatures.

frost·ed liver (frŏs′tĭd) *n.* Hyaloserositis of the liver.

Frost-Lang operation (-lăng′) *n.* Insertion of a spherical prosthesis after the enucleation of the eyeball.

Frost suture *n.* An intermarginal suture between the eyelids to protect the cornea.

frot·tage (frô-täzh′) *n.* **1.** Massage; rubbing. **2.** The act of rubbing against the body of another person, as in a crowd, to attain sexual gratification.

fro·zen pelvis (frō′zən) *n.* A condition in which the true pelvis is indurated throughout, especially by carcinoma.

frozen section *n.* A thin slice of tissue that is cut from a frozen specimen and is often used for rapid microscopic diagnosis.

frozen shoulder *n.* Inflammation between the joint capsule and the peripheral articular shoulder cartilage that causes pain whether in motion or at rest. Also called *adhesive capsulitis.*

FRS *abbr.* Fellow of the Royal Society

fructo– *pref.* Denoting a fructose-like configuration, that is, a dextrorotatory compound containing six carbons and including a keto group: *fructoside.*

fruc·to·fu·ra·nose (frŭk′tō-fyŏŏr′ə-nōs′) *n.* A fructose with a furanose ring.

fruc·to·ki·nase (frŭk′tō-kī′nās′, -nāz′, -kĭn′ās′, -āz′) *n.* A liver enzyme that catalyzes the transfer of phosphate groups to fructose.

fruc·tose (frŭk′tōs′, frŏŏk′-) *n.* A very sweet sugar occurring in many fruits and honey and used as a preservative for foodstuffs and as an intravenous nutrient. Also called *fruit sugar, levulose.*

fruc·to·se·mi·a (frŭk′tō-sē′mē-ə, frŏŏk′-) *n.* Presence of fructose in blood. Also called *levulosemia.*

fruc·to·side (frŭk′tə-sīd′, frŏŏk′-) *n.* A glycoside that yields fructose upon hydrolysis.

fruc·to·su·ria (frŭk′tō-sŏŏr′ē-ə, frŏŏk′-) *n.* Presence of fructose in urine.

fruit sugar (frŏŏt) *n.* See **fructose.**

frus·tra·tion (frŭ-strā′shən) *n.* **1.** The condition that results when an impulse or an action is thwarted by an external or an internal force. **2.** The blocking or thwarting of an impulse, purpose, or action.

FSH *abbr.* follicle-stimulating hormone

FSH-RF *abbr.* follicle-stimulating hormone-releasing factor

ft. *or* **ft** *abbr.* foot; *Latin* fiat, fiant (let there be done; let there be made)

FTA-ABS test (ĕf′tē-ā′ā′bē-ĕs′) *n.* See **fluorescent treponemal antibody absorption test.**

FTT *abbr.* failure to thrive

Fuchs epithelial dystrophy (fyŏŏks, fŏŏкнs) *n.* A condition that often develops following endothelial dystrophy, beginning with a thin spreading central accumulation of fluid in the central cornea; it occurs predominantly in elderly women.

fuch·sin (fyŏŏk′sĭn) *or* **fuch·sine** (-sĭn, -sēn′) *n.* Any of various red to purple-red rosanilin dyes used as bacterial and histological stains.

fuch·sin·o·phil (fyŏŏk-sĭn′ə-fĭl′) *adj.* Staining readily with fuchsin. —*n.* A cell or tissue that stains readily with fuchsin. —**fuch·sin′o·phil′ic** *adj.*

fu·cose (fyŏŏ′kōs′) *n.* An aldose present in the polysaccharides associated with some blood groups.

fu·co·si·do·sis (fyŏŏ-kō′sĭ-dō′sĭs) *n.* An inherited metabolic storage disease caused by a deficiency of alpha-fucosidase and the accumulation of glycolipids that contain fructose, and marked by progressive neurologic deterioration, spasticity, tremor, and mild skeletal changes.

fu·gac·i·ty (fyōō-găs′ĭ-tē) *n.* A measure of the tendency of a substance, often a fluid, to move from one phase to another or from one site to another.

–fuge *suff.* One that expels or drives away: *vermifuge.*

fugue (fyōōg) *n.* A pathological amnesiac condition that may persist for several months and usually results from severe mental stress, in which one is apparently conscious of one's actions but has no recollection of them after returning to a normal state.

ful·crum (fŏŏl′krəm, fŭl′-) *n., pl.* **–crums** *or* **–cra** (-krə) **1.** The point or support on which a lever pivots. **2.** An anatomical structure that acts as a hinge or point of support.

ful·gu·rant (fŏŏl′gyər-ənt, -gər-, fŭl′-) *adj.* Characterized by sudden shooting pain.

ful·gu·rat·ing (fŏŏl′gyə-rā′tĭng, -gə-, fŭl′-) *adj.* Lightninglike, especially of sudden shooting pain.

ful·gu·ra·tion (fŏŏl′gyə-rā′shən, -gə-, fŭl′-) *n.* The destruction of tissue, usually malignant tumors, by means of a high-frequency electric current applied with a needlelike electrode.

full denture (fŏŏl) *n.* See **complete denture.**

full·er's earth (fŏŏl′ərz) *n.* A highly absorbent claylike substance consisting of hydrated aluminum silicates, applied moistened with water as a poultice.

full-thickness flap *n.* A surgical flap consisting of the full thickness of the mucosa and submucosa or skin and subcutaneous tissues.

full-thickness graft *n.* A skin graft including the full thickness of the skin and subcutaneous tissue.

ful·mi·nant (fŏŏl′mə-nənt, fŭl′-) *adj.* Occurring suddenly, rapidly, and with great severity or intensity, usually of pain. —**ful′mi·nat′ing** (-nā′tĭng) *adj.*

fu·ma·rase (fyōō′mə-rās′, -rāz′) *n.* An enzyme, occurring in liver and muscle, that catalyzes the conversion of fumaric acid to malic acid.

fu·mar·ic acid (fyōō-măr′ĭk) *n.* An organic acid that is formed from succinic acid and is an intermediate in the Krebs cycle.

fu·mi·gant (fyōō′mĭ-gənt) *n.* A chemical compound used in its gaseous state as a disinfectant.

fu·mi·gate (fyōō′mĭ-gāt′) *v.* To subject to smoke or fumes, usually in order to exterminate pests or disinfect. —**fu′mi·ga′tion** *n.*

fum·ing (fyōō′mĭng) *adj.* Producing or emitting smoke or vapor, as for certain concentrated nitric, sulfuric, and hydrochloric acids.

func·ti·o lae·sa (fŭngk′shē-ō lē′sə) *n.* The loss of the capacity to function.

func·tion (fŭngk′shən) *n.* **1.** The physiological property or the special action of an organ or body part. **2.** Something that is closely related to another thing and is dependent on it for its existence, value, or significance, such as growth resulting from nutrition. **3.** A mathematical variable so related to another that for each value assumed by one there is a value determined for the other. **4.** A rule of correspondence between two sets such that there is a unique element in the second set assigned to each element in the first set. **5.** The general

properties of a substance, depending on its chemical character and relation to other substances, that provide the basis upon which it may be grouped as among acids or bases. **6.** A particular reactive grouping in a molecule.

func·tion·al (fŭngk′shə-nəl) *adj.* **1.** Of or relating to a function. **2.** Affecting the physiological function but not the structure.

functional anatomy *n.* See **physiological anatomy.**

functional blindness *n.* Loss of vision related to conversion hysteria.

functional congestion *n.* Increased flow of blood to an organ while it is functioning. Also called *physiologic congestion.*

functional deafness *n.* See **psychogenic deafness.**

functional disorder *n.* A physical disorder in which the symptoms have no known or detectable organic basis but are believed to be the result of psychological factors such as emotional conflicts or stress. Also called *functional disease.*

functional group *n.* An atom or group of atoms that replaces hydrogen in an organic compound and that defines the structure of a family of compounds and determines the properties of the family.

functional hypertrophy *n.* See **physiologic hypertrophy.**

functional magnetic resonance imaging *n. Abbr.* **fMRI** Magnetic resonance imaging that provides three-dimensional images of the brain based on changes in blood flow and that can be correlated with brain functions.

functional murmur *n.* A cardiac murmur not associated with a heart lesion. Also called *innocent murmur, inorganic murmur.*

functional neurosurgery *n.* The surgical destruction or chronic excitation of a part of the brain as treatment of a physiological or psychological disorder.

functional occlusion *n.* **1.** Tooth contact within functional range of the surfaces of opposing teeth. **2.** Occlusion occurring during biting and chewing.

functional residual capacity *n. Abbr.* **FRC** The volume of gas that remains in the lungs at the end of a normal expiration. Also called *functional residual air.*

functional splint *n.* **1.** A fixed restoration covering all or part of the abutment teeth, used to join two or more teeth into a rigid unit. **2.** See **dynamic splint.**

fun·da·ment (fŭn′də-mənt) *n.* See **anus.**

fun·da·men·tal particle (fŭn′də-měn′tl) *n.* See **elementary particle** (sense 2).

fun·dec·to·my (fŭn-děk′tə-mē) *n.* See **fundusectomy.**

fun·di·form (fŭn′də-fôrm′) *adj.* Having a looped form; sling-shaped.

fun·do·pli·ca·tion (fŭn′dō-plĭ-kā′shən) *n.* The surgical procedure of tucking or folding the fundus of the stomach around the esophagus to prevent reflux, used in the repair of a hiatal hernia.

fun·dus (fŭn′dəs) *n., pl.* **–di** (-dī′) The bottom of or part farthest from the opening of a sac or hollow organ. —**fun′dic** *adj.*

fun·du·sec·to·my (fŭn′də-sěk′tə-mē) *n.* Excision of the fundus of an organ. Also called *fundectomy.*

fundus gland *n.* See **gastric gland.**

fundus of eye *n.* The portion of the interior of the eyeball around the posterior pole, visible through the ophthalmoscope.

fundus of gallbladder *n.* The wide closed end of the gallbladder at the lower border of the liver.

fundus of stomach *n.* The portion of the stomach that lies above the cardiac notch.

fundus of urinary bladder *n.* The base of the bladder, formed by the posterior wall.

fundus of uterus *n.* The upper rounded extremity of the uterus above the openings of the fallopian tubes.

fun·gal (fŭng′gəl) *or* **fun·gous** (-gəs) *adj.* Of, relating to, resembling, or caused by a fungus.

fun·gate (fŭng′gāt′) *v.* To grow rapidly like a fungus. —*adj.* Having the form of or resembling a fungus.

fun·ge·mi·a (fŭn-jē′mē-ə, fŭng-gē′-) *n.* The presence of fungi in the blood.

fun·gi (fŭn′jī, fŭng′gī) *n.* Plural of **fungus.**

Fungi *n.* The kingdom of organisms that is made up of the fungi and includes the yeasts, molds, mildews, and mushrooms.

fun·gi·cide (fŭn′jĭ-sīd′, fŭng′gĭ-) *n.* A chemical substance that destroys or inhibits the growth of fungi. —**fun′gi·cid′al** (-sīd′l) *adj.*

fun·gi·form (fŭn′jə-fôrm′, fŭng′gə-) *adj.* Shaped like a mushroom.

fungiform papilla *n.* Any of many tiny mushroomlike elevations on the back of the tongue, the epithelium of which often have taste buds.

Fungi Im·per·fec·ti (ĭm′pər-fĕk′tī) *n.* A phylum of fungi that are without a sexual stage in their life cycle, reproducing only by asexual spores. Also called *Deuteromycetes.*

fun·gi·stat·ic (fŭn′jĭ-stăt′ĭk, fŭng′gĭ-) *adj.* Having an inhibiting effect upon the growth and reproduction of fungi without destroying them.

fun·gi·tox·ic (fŭn′jĭ-tŏk′sĭk, fŭng′gĭ-) *adj.* Having a toxic effect on fungi.

Fun·gi·zone (fŭn′jə-zōn′) A trademark for the drug amphotericin B.

fun·goid (fŭng′goid′) *adj.* Of, relating to, resembling, or being a fungus.

fun·gos·i·ty (fŭng-gŏs′ĭ-tē) *n.* A fungoid growth.

fun·gous (fŭng′gəs) *adj.* Variant of **fungal.**

fun·gus (fŭng′gəs) *n.,* *pl.* **fun·gi** (fŭn′jī, fŭng′gī) *or* **fun·gus·es** Any of numerous eukaryotic organisms that reproduce by spores. The spores of most fungi grow a network of slender tubes called hyphae that spread into and feed off of dead organic matter or living organisms. The hyphae often produce specialized reproductive bodies, such as mushrooms.

fungus ball *n.* **1.** A compact mass of fungal mycelium and cellular debris produced by bacterial and mycotic infectious agents and residing within a lung cavity. **2.** See **aspergilloma** (sense 2).

fu·nic (fyōō′nĭk) *adj.* Of, relating to, or originating in the umbilical cord.

funic souffle *or* **funicular souffle** *n.* See **fetal souffle.**

funicular graft *n.* A nerve graft in which each funiculus is approximated and sutured separately.

funicular process *n.* The tunica vaginalis surrounding the spermatic cord.

fu·nic·u·li·tis (fyōō-nĭk′yə-lī′tĭs, fə-) *n.* **1.** Inflammation of a funiculus, especially of the spermatic cord. **2.** Inflammation of the portion of a spinal nerve root that lies within the intervertebral canal.

fu·nic·u·lo·pexy (fyōō-nĭk′yə-lō-pĕk′sē, fə-) *n.* The suturing of the spermatic cord to the surrounding tissue to correct an undescended testicle.

fu·nic·u·lus (fyōō-nĭk′yə-ləs, fə-) *or* **fu·ni·cle** (fyōō′nĭ-kəl) *n.,* *pl.* **–li** (-lī′) *or* **–cles** **1.** A slender cordlike strand or band, especially a bundle of nerve fibers in a nerve trunk. **2.** Any of three major divisions of white matter in the spinal cord, consisting of fasciculi. **3.** The umbilical cord. —**fu·nic′u·lar** (-lər) *adj.*

fu·ni·form (fyōō′nə-fôrm′) *adj.* Having a ropelike or cordlike appearance or structure.

fu·nis (fyōō′nĭs) *n.* **1.** See **umbilical cord. 2.** A cordlike structure.

Funk (fŭngk, fōōngk), **Casimir** 1884–1967. Polish-born American biochemist whose research of deficiency diseases led to the discovery of vitamins, which he named in 1912.

fun·nel chest (fŭn′əl) *n.* A hollow at the lower part of the chest caused by a backward displacement of the xiphoid cartilage. Also called *funnel breast, pectus excavatum, pectus recurvatum.*

funnel-shaped pelvis *n.* A pelvis in which the inlet dimensions are normal, but the outlet is contracted in the transverse diameter or in both transverse and anteroposterior diameters.

fun·ny bone (fŭn′ē) *n.* A point on the elbow where the ulnar nerve runs close to the surface and produces a tingling sensation if knocked against bone.

FUO *abbr.* fever of unknown origin

fu·ran (fyōōr′ăn′, fyōō-răn′) *n.* Any of a group of colorless, volatile, heterocyclic organic compounds containing a ring of four carbon atoms and one oxygen atom, used in the synthesis of organics.

fu·ra·nose (fyōōr′ə-nōs′) *n.* A sugar having a cyclic structure resembling that of furan.

fur·cal (fûr′kəl) *adj.* Forked.

fur·ca·tion (fûr-kā′shən) *n.* **1.** A forking, or a forklike part or branch. **2.** The region of a multirooted tooth at which the root divides.

fur·fu·ra·ceous (fûr′fə-rā′shəs, -fyə-) *adj.* Made of or covered with scaly particles, such as dandruff.

fu·ror ep·i·lep·ti·cus (fyōōr′ôr′ ĕp′ə-lĕp′tĭ-kəs) *n.* The sudden unprovoked attacks of intense anger and violence to which individuals with psychomotor epilepsy are occasionally subject.

fu·ro·se·mide (fyōō-rō′sə-mīd′) *n.* A white to yellow crystalline powder used as a diuretic.

fur·row (fûr′ō) *n.* **1.** A rut, groove, or narrow depression. **2.** A deep wrinkle in the skin, as on the forehead.

fur·rowed tongue (fûr′ōd) *n.* A painless condition of the tongue that is marked by numerous longitudinal grooves on the dorsal surface. Also called *scrotal tongue.*

fu·run·cle (fyōōr′ŭng′kəl) *n.* See **boil.** —**fu·run′cu·lar** (fyōō-rŭng′kyə-lər), **fu·run′cu·lous** (-ləs) *adj.*

fu·run·cu·loid (fyŏŏ-rŭng′kyə-loid′) *adj.* Resembling a boil.

fu·run·cu·lo·sis (fyŏŏ-rŭng′kyə-lō′sĭs) *n.* A skin condition characterized by the development of recurring boils or the simultaneous occurrence of a number of furuncles.

fu·run·cu·lus (fyŏŏ-rŭng′kyə-ləs) *n., pl.* **-li** (-lī′) A boil.

fused kidney (fyŏŏzd) *n.* A single anomalous organ produced by congenital fusion of the embryonic kidneys.

fu·si·form (fyŏŏ′zə-fôrm′) *adj.* Tapering at each end; spindle-shaped.

fusiform aneurysm *n.* An elongated, spindle-shaped dilation of an artery.

fusiform gyrus *n.* An extremely long convolution extending lengthwise over the lower surface of the temporal and occipital lobes of the brain.

fu·si·mo·tor (fyŏŏ′zə-mō′tər) *adj.* Of or relating to the motor innervation of intrafusal muscle fibers by efferent neurons of the gray matter of the spinal cord.

fu·sion (fyŏŏ′zhən) *n.* **1.** The act or procedure of liquefying or melting by the application of heat. **2.** The merging of different elements into a union, as of vertebrae. **3.** The mechanism by which both eyes blend slightly different images from each eye into a single image. **4.** The growing together of two or more teeth as a result of the abnormal union of their formative organs. **5.** A nuclear reaction in which nuclei combine to form more massive nuclei with the simultaneous release of energy.

fusion beat *n.* The atrial or ventricular complex in an electrocardiogram when either the atria or the ventricles are activated by two simultaneously invading impulses.

fusion inhibitor *n.* A drug that interferes with the entry of HIV into helper T cells by inhibiting the fusion of the viral and cell membranes.

Fu·so·bac·te·ri·um (fyŏŏ′zō-băk-tîr′ē-əm) *n.* A genus of gram-negative, anaerobic bacteria that produce butyric acid as a major metabolic product and occur in purulent or gangrenous infections.

fu·so·cel·lu·lar (fyŏŏ′zō-sĕl′yə-lər) *adj.* Composed of spindle-shaped cells.

fu·so·spi·ril·lar·y gingivitis (fyŏŏ′zō-spī′rə-lĕr′ē) *n.* See **trench mouth.**

fu·so·spi·ro·chet·al (fyŏŏ′zō-spī′rə-kĕt′l) *adj.* Of, relating to, or caused by the association of fusiform bacteria and spirochetes.

fusospirochetal gingivitis *n.* See **trench mouth.**

Futch·er's line (fŏŏch′ərz) *n.* A line of pigmentation occurring symmetrically and bilaterally along the lateral edge of the biceps muscle.

Fu·ze·on (fyŏŏ′zē-ŏn) A trademark for the drug enfuvirtide.

FVC *abbr.* forced vital capacity

f wave *n.* A pattern of irregular undulations of the base line in an electrocardiogram that is indicative of atrial fibrillation.

F wave *n.* A pattern of regular, rapid atrial waves in an electrocardiogram, indicative of atrial flutter.

fx *abbr.* fracture

G

γ The Greek letter *gamma*. Entries beginning with this character are alphabetized under **gamma**.

g¹ (jē) *n*. A unit of acceleration equal to the acceleration caused by gravity at the earth's surface, about 9.8 meters (32 feet) per second per second.

g² *abbr*. gram

G_{M2} gangliosidosis *n*. See Tay-Sachs disease.

G *abbr*. glucose; gravitational constant; guanine

Ga The symbol for the element **gallium**.

GABA *abbr*. gamma-aminobutyric acid

GABA-alpha (jē'ā-bē'ā-) *n*. A cell receptor that inhibits brain cells from responding to neuronal messages.

gab·a·pen·tin (găb'ə-pĕn'tn) *n*. An oral anticonvulsant chemically related to gamma-aminobutyric acid, used primarily in the treatment of focal seizures and neuralgia, especially after infection with herpes zoster.

gad·o·lin·i·um (găd'l-ĭn'ē-əm) *n*. *Symbol* **Gd** A malleable, ductile metallic rare-earth element, used as a contrast medium for magnetic resonance imaging and as a radioisotope in bone mineral analysis. Atomic number 64.

gag (găg) *v*. **1.** To choke, retch, or undergo a regurgitative spasm. **2.** To prevent from talking. —*n*. An instrument adjusted between the teeth to keep the mouth from closing during operations in the mouth or throat.

gag reflex *n*. Retching or gagging caused by the contact of a foreign body with the mucous membrane of the throat.

gain (gān) *n*. **1.** An increase in amount or degree. **2.** Progress; advancement.

gait (gāt) *n*. A particular way or manner of walking.

Gaj·du·sek (gī'də-shĕk'), **D(aniel) Carleton** Born 1923. American virologist. He shared a 1976 Nobel Prize for research on the origin and spread of infectious diseases.

gal. *abbr*. gallon

ga·lac·ta·cra·sia (gə-lăk'tə-krā'zhə) *n*. Abnormal composition of breast milk.

ga·lac·ta·gogue (gə-lăk'tə-gôg') *n*. An agent that promotes the secretion and flow of milk.

ga·lac·tic (gə-lăk'tĭk) *adj*. **1.** Relating to milk. **2.** Promoting the flow of milk.

galacto– *or* **galact–** *pref*. Milk: *galactotherapy*.

ga·lac·to·bol·ic (gə-lăk'tə-bŏl'ĭk) *adj*. Causing the release or ejection of milk from the breast.

ga·lac·to·cele (gə-lăk'tə-sēl') *n*. A retention cyst that results from occlusion of a lactiferous duct. Also called *lactocele*.

ga·lac·to·ki·nase (gə-lăk'tō-kī'nās', -nāz', -kĭn'ās', -āz') *n*. An enzyme that catalyzes the phosphorylation of galactose in the presence of ATP.

galactokinase deficiency *n*. An inborn error of metabolism due to a congenital deficiency of galactokinase, resulting in increased blood galactose concentration, enlargement of the liver, cataracts, and mental retardation.

ga·lac·to·lip·id (gə-lăk'tō-lĭp'ĭd, -lī'pĭd) *n*. See cerebroside.

ga·lac·to·lip·in (gə-lăk'tō-lĭp'ĭn) *n*. See cerebroside.

ga·lac·to·phore (gə-lăk'tə-fôr') *n*. See lactiferous duct.

ga·lac·to·pho·ri·tis (gə-lăk'tō-fə-rī'tĭs, găl'ək-tŏf'ə-rī'tĭs) *n*. Inflammation of the milk ducts.

gal·ac·toph·o·rous (găl'ək-tŏf'ə-rəs) *adj*. Conveying milk.

galactophorous duct *n*. See lactiferous duct.

ga·lac·to·poi·e·sis (gə-lăk'tə-poi-ē'sĭs) *n*. The production and secretion of milk by the mammary glands. —**ga·lac'to·poi·et'ic** (-ĕt'ĭk) *adj*.

ga·lac·tor·rhe·a (gə-lăk'tə-rē'ə) *n*. **1.** A continued discharge of milk from the breasts between intervals of nursing or after weaning. Also called *lactorrhea*. **2.** Excessive flow of milk during lactation.

gal·ac·tos·am·ine (găl'ək-tō'sə-mēn', gə-lăk-) *n*. An amino-acid derivative of galactose occurring in various mucopolysaccharides.

ga·lac·tos·a·mi·no·gly·can (gə-lăk'tō-sə-mē'nō-glī'-kăn', -săm'ə-nō-) *n*. See mucopolysaccharide.

ga·lac·tose (gə-lăk'tōs') *n*. A monosaccharide commonly occurring in lactose. Also called *brain sugar*.

galactose cataract *n*. A neonatal cataract associated with galactosemia.

ga·lac·to·se·mi·a (gə-lăk'tə-sē'mē-ə) *n*. An inherited metabolic disorder characterized by the deficiency of an enzyme necessary for galactose metabolism and characterized by elevated levels of galactose in the blood and, if untreated, mental retardation and eye and liver abnormalities. —**ga·lac'to·se'mic** *adj*.

galactose tolerance test *n*. A liver function test in which the rate of excretion of galactose following ingestion or an intravenous injection of a known amount is measured.

ga·lac·to·si·dase (gə-lăk'tō-sĭ-dās', -dāz', -lăk-tō'-) *n*. Any of a group of enzymes that catalyze the hydrolysis of a galactoside.

ga·lac·to·side (gə-lăk'tə-sīd') *n*. Any of a group of glycosides that yield galactose on hydrolysis and exist in alpha and beta forms.

ga·lac·to·sis (găl'ək-tō'sĭs) *n*. The formation of milk by the mammary glands.

ga·lac·to·su·ri·a (gə-lăk'tə-sŏŏr'ē-ə, -shŏŏr'-) *n*. Excretion of galactose in urine.

ga·lac·to·syl (gə-lăk'tə-sĭl) *n*. The glycosyl radical of galactose.

ga·lac·to·ther·a·py (gə-lăk'tō-thĕr'ə-pē) *n*. **1.** The treatment of disease by prescription of an exclusive or nearly exclusive milk diet. **2.** The medicinal treatment of a nursing infant by administering to the mother a drug that is excreted in part in her milk. Also called *lactotherapy*.

ga·lac·tu·ro·nan (gə-lăk'tyŏŏ-rə-năn') *n*. A polysaccharide constituent of some pectins that yields galacturonic acid when hydrolyzed.

ga·lan·gal (gə-lăng′gəl) *or* **ga·lan·ga** (-gə) *n.* A plant of eastern Asia, having pungent, aromatic rhizomes used as an aromatic stimulant and carminative.

gal·ba·num (găl′bə-nəm, gôl′-) *n.* A bitter, aromatic gum resin extract that is used therapeutically in incense and medicinally as a counterirritant.

ga·le·a (gā′lē-ə) *n., pl.* **–le·ae** (-lē-ē′) **1.** An anatomical structure shaped like a helmet. **2.** The aponeurosis connecting the occipitofrontal muscle to form the epicranium. **3.** A type of bandage used for covering the head.

Ga·len (gā′lən), AD 130?–200? Greek anatomist, physician, and writer whose theories formed the basis of European medicine until the Renaissance.

ga·len·i·cal (gā-lĕn′ĭ-kəl, gə-) *n.* **1.** A medicinal preparation composed mainly of herbal or vegetable matter. **2.** A remedy prepared according to an official formula. —*adj.* Of, relating to, or being a medicinal preparation made up chiefly of herbal or vegetable matter.

gall¹ (gôl) *n.* See **bile** (sense 1).

gall² (gôl) *n.* A skin sore caused by friction and abrasion. —*v.* To become irritated, chafed, or sore.

gallbladder *or* **gall bladder** *n.* A small, pear-shaped muscular sac, located under the right lobe of the liver, in which bile secreted by the liver is stored until needed by the body for digestion. Also called *cholecyst, cholecystis.*

gallbladder fossa *n.* A depression lodging the gallbladder on the undersurface of the liver anteriorly, between the quadrate and the right lobes.

gall duct *n.* **1.** See **bile duct. 2.** See **common bile duct.**

gal·li·um (găl′ē-əm) *n. Symbol* **Ga** A rare metallic element that is liquid near room temperature and is found as a trace element in coal, bauxite, and other minerals. Atomic number 31.

gallium-67 *n.* A gamma-ray emitting nuclide that has a half-life of 78 hours and is used in its citrate form as a tumor- and inflammation-localizing radiotracer.

gallium-68 *n.* A positron-emitting nuclide having a half-life of 1.13 hours, used as a tracer in brain scanning.

Gal·lo (găl′ō), **Robert Charles** Born 1937. American virologist who was one of the first to identify the virus that causes AIDS and to develop a test for it.

gal·lon (găl′ən) *n. Abbr.* **gal.** A unit of volume in the US Customary System, used in liquid measure, equal to 4 quarts, 231 cubic inches, or 8.3389 pounds of distilled water (3.7853 liters).

gal·lop (găl′əp) *n.* A triple cadence to the heart sounds at rates of 100 beats per minute or more due to an abnormal third or fourth heart sound being heard in addition to the first and second sounds. Also called *gallop rhythm.*

gall·stone (gôl′stōn′) *n.* A concretion in the gallbladder or in a bile duct, composed chiefly of cholesterol, calcium salts, and bile pigments. Also called *biliary calculus, cholelith.*

Gal·va·ni (găl-vä′nē, gäl-), **Luigi** 1737–1798. Italian physiologist and physician who asserted that animal tissues generate electricity. Although proved wrong, his work stimulated research on electricity.

gal·van·ic skin response (găl-văn′ĭk) *n. Abbr.* **GSR** A measure of electrical resistance as a reflection of changes in emotional arousal, taken by attaching electrodes to any part of the skin and recording changes in moment-to-moment perspiration and related activity of the autonomic nervous system.

gal·va·no·chem·i·cal (găl′və-nō-kĕm′ĭ-kəl) *adj.* Of or being electrochemical.

gam– *pref.* Variant of **gamo–.**

Gam·bi·an trypanosomiasis (găm′bē-ən) *n.* An African trypanosomiasis characterized by erythematous patches and local edemas, cramps, tremors, and paresthesia, enlargement of the lymph glands, spleen, and liver, emaciation, and, in later stages, lethargy, coma, and death. Also called *chronic sleeping sickness, chronic trypanosomiasis.*

gam·ete (găm′ēt′, gə-mēt′) *n.* A reproductive cell having the haploid number of chromosomes, especially a sperm or egg capable of fusing with a gamete of the opposite sex to produce a fertilized egg.

gamete intrafallopian transfer *n. Abbr.* **GIFT** A technique of assisted reproduction in which eggs and sperm are inserted directly into a woman's fallopian tubes, where fertilization may occur.

gameto– *or* **gamet–** *pref.* Gamete: *gametogenesis.*

ga·me·to·cide (gə-mē′tə-sīd′) *n.* An agent that is destructive to gametes or gametocytes, especially malarial gametocytes.

ga·me·to·cyte (gə-mē′tə-sīt′) *n.* A cell from which gametes develop by meiotic division, especially a spermatocyte or an oocyte.

ga·me·to·gen·e·sis (gə-mē′tə-jĕn′ĭ-sĭs) *n.* The formation and the development of gametes. —**ga·me′to·gen′ic, gam′e·tog′e·nous** (găm′ĭ-tŏj′ə-nəs) *adj.*

gam·e·toid theory (găm′ĭ-toid′) *n.* The theory that the malignancy of a tumor results from neoplastic cells having developed the characteristics of gametes, so that they multiply and grow autonomously as parasites on the host's tissues.

gam·ma (găm′ə) *n.* **1.** *Symbol* **γ** The third letter of the Greek alphabet. **2.** The third item in a series or system of classification. **3.** The third position from a designated carbon atom in an organic molecule at which an atom or a radical may be substituted. **4.** A unit of magnetic field strength equal to one hundred thousandth (10^5) of an oersted. **5.** A unit of mass equal to one millionth (10^6) of a gram. —*adj.* **1.** Relating to or being the atom or radical group that is in the third position relative to the functional group of atoms in an organic molecule. **2.** Relating to or characterizing a polypeptide chain that is one of five types of heavy chains that may be present in immunoglobins.

gam·ma-a·mi·no·bu·tyr·ic acid (găm′ə-ə-mē′nō-byoo-tîr′ĭk, -ăm′ə-nō-) *n. Abbr.* **GABA** An amino acid that occurs in the central nervous system and that is associated with the transmission of inhibitory nerve impulses.

gamma angle *n.* The angle formed between the line joining the fixation point to the center of the eye and the optic axis.

gamma-benzene hex·a·chlo·ride (hĕk′sə-klôr′īd′) *n.* See **lindane.**

gamma carotene *n.* An isomer of carotene.

gamma fiber *n.* A nerve fiber that has a conduction rate of about 20 meters per second.

gamma globulin *n.* **1.** A protein fraction of blood serum containing many antibodies that protect against bacterial and viral infectious diseases. **2.** A solution of gamma globulin prepared from human blood and administered for passive immunization against measles, German measles, hepatitis A, poliomyelitis, and other infections.

gam·ma-hy·drox·y·bu·ty·rate (găm′ə-hī-drŏk′sē-byōō′tə-rāt′) *n. Abbr.* **GHB** A compound that is a metabolite of gamma-aminobutyric acid, used illegally for its euphoric and sedative effects.

gamma-interferon *n.* A lymphokine produced by macrophages and T cells that is involved in regulation of the immune system and activation of phagocytes.

Gamma Knife A trademark for a radiologic nonsurgical device used in stereotactic radiosurgery.

gamma ray *n.* Electromagnetic radiation emitted from the nucleus of an atom by radioactive decay and having energies in a range from ten thousand (10^4) to ten million (10^7) electron volts.

gam·mop·a·thy (gă-mŏp′ə-thē) *n.* A disturbance in immunoglobulin synthesis.

Gam·na-Gan·dy bodies (găm′nə-găn′dē, -găn-dē′, găm′nä-) *pl.n.* Small firm nodules of fibrous tissue that are impregnated with iron pigment and calcium salts and that occur chiefly in the spleen in such conditions as congestive splenomegaly and sickle cell anemia. Also called *Gamna-Gandy nodules, siderotic nodules.*

Gam·na's disease (găm′nəz, găm′näz) *n.* A form of chronic enlargement of the spleen characterized by conspicuous thickening of the capsule and the presence of Gamna-Gandy bodies.

gamo– *or* **gam–** *pref.* Sexual: *gamogenesis.*

gam·o·gen·e·sis (găm′ə-jĕn′ĭ-sĭs) *n.* The act or process of sexual reproduction.

–gamous *suff.* **1.** Having a specified number of mates: *monogamous.* **2.** Having a specified kind of reproduction or reproductive organs: *heterogamous.*

–gamy *suff.* **1.** Marriage; mate: *monogamy.* **2.** Procreative or propagative union: *heterogamy.*

gan·ci·clo·vir (găn-sī′klō-vîr) *n.* An antiviral agent derived from guanine and used in the prevention and treatment of opportunistic cytomegalovirus infections.

gan·gli·ate (găng′glē-ĭt, -āt′) *or* **gan·gli·at·ed** (-glē-ā′-tĭd) *adj.* Having ganglia.

gangliated nerve *n.* A nerve of the sympathetic nervous system.

gan·gli·ec·to·my (găng′glē-ĕk′tə-mē) *n.* See **ganglionectomy.**

gan·gli·form (găng′glə-fôrm′) *or* **gan·gli·o·form** (-glē-ə-fôrm′) *adj.* Having the form or appearance of a ganglion.

gan·gli·i·tis (găng′glē-ī′tĭs) *n.* See **ganglionitis.**

gan·gli·o·blast (găng′glē-ō-blăst′) *n.* An embryonic cell giving rise to ganglion cells.

gan·gli·o·cyte (găng′glē-ō-sīt′) *n.* See **ganglion cell.**

gan·gli·o·cy·to·ma (găng′glē-ō-sī-tō′mə) *n.* See **ganglioneuroma.**

gan·gli·o·gli·o·ma (găng′glē-ō-glē-ō′mə, -glī-) *n.* See **central ganglioneuroma.**

gan·gli·ol·y·sis (găng′glē-ŏl′ĭ-sĭs) *n.* The dissolution or breaking up of a ganglion.

gan·gli·o·ma (găng′glē-ō′mə) *n.* See **ganglioneuroma.**

gan·gli·on (găng′glē-ən) *n., pl.* **–gli·ons** *or* **–gli·a** (-glē-ə) **1.** A group of nerve cells forming a nerve center, especially one located outside the brain or spinal cord. Also called *neuroganglion.* **2.** A benign tumorlike cyst containing mucopolysaccharide-rich fluid enclosed within fibrous tissue and usually attached to a tendon sheath in the hand, wrist, or foot. Also called *myxoid cyst, synovial cyst.* **—gan′gli·al** *adj.*

gan·gli·on·at·ed (găng′glē-ə-nā′tĭd) *adj.* Having ganglia; gangliate.

ganglion cell *n.* A neuron having its cell body outside the central nervous system. Also called *gangliocyte.*

gan·gli·on·ec·to·my (găng′glē-ə-nĕk′tə-mē) *n.* Excision of a ganglion. Also called *gangliectomy.*

gan·gli·o·neu·ro·ma (găng′glē-ō-nŏŏ-rō′mə) *n.* A benign neoplasm composed of mature ganglionic neurons scattered singly or in clumps within a relatively abundant and dense stroma of neurofibrils and collagenous fibers. Also called *gangliocytoma, ganglioma, neurocytoma.*

gan·gli·on·ic (găng′glē-ŏn′ĭk) *adj.* Relating to a ganglion; ganglial.

ganglionic blockade *n.* Inhibition of nerve impulse transmission at autonomic ganglionic synapses by drugs such as nicotine or hexamethonium.

ganglionic blocking agent *n.* A substance that blocks nerve impulses in autonomic ganglia.

ganglionic layer of cerebellar cortex *n.* See **Purkinje layer.**

ganglionic motor neuron *n.* See **postganglionic motor neuron.**

ganglion im·par (ĭm′pär) *n.* See **coccygeal ganglion.**

gan·gli·on·i·tis (găng′glē-ə-nī′tĭs) *n.* Inflammation of a ganglion. Also called *gangliitis.*

ganglion of autonomic plexuses *n.* Any of the autonomic ganglia located in the plexuses of autonomic fibers.

ganglion of sympathetic trunk *n.* Any of the clusters of postganglionic nerve-cell bodies located at intervals along the sympathetic trunks, including the superior cervical, middle cervical, and cervicothoracic ganglions, the thoracic, lumbar, and sacral ganglions, and the coccygeal ganglion. Also called *paravertebral ganglion.*

gan·gli·on·os·to·my (găng′glē-ə-nŏs′tə-mē) *n.* The surgical formation of an opening into a ganglion.

gan·gli·o·ple·gic (găng′glē-ō-plē′jĭk) *adj.* Paralyzing an autonomic ganglion. **—***n.* An agent that paralyzes an autonomic ganglion.

gan·gli·o·side (găng′glē-ə-sīd′) *n.* Any of a group of glycosphingolipids chemically similar to the cerebrosides, found principally in the surface membrane of nerve cells and in the spleen.

gan·gli·o·si·do·sis (găng′glē-ō-sī-dō′sĭs) *n.* Any of a group of diseases marked by abnormal accumulation of gangliosides within the nervous system.

gan·grene (găng′grēn′, găng-grēn′) *n.* Death and decay of body tissue, often in a limb, caused by insufficient blood supply and usually following injury or disease. **—gan′gre·nous** (găng′grə-nəs) *adj.*

gangrenous stomatitis *n.* Stomatitis characterized by necrosis of the oral tissue.

Gan·ser's syndrome (găn′zərz, gän′-) *n.* A pseudo-psychotic condition typically occurring in individuals feigning insanity and characterized by wrong but related answers to questions.

gap (găp) *n.* **1.** An opening in a structure or surface; a cleft or breach. **2.** An interval or discontinuity in any series or sequence.

gap 1 *n. Abbr.* **G₁** In the somatic cell cycle, the temporary cessation that follows mitosis and indicates a gap in DNA synthesis.

gap 2 *n. Abbr.* **G₂** In the somatic cell cycle, a pause between the completion of DNA synthesis and the onset of the next mitosis.

gap junction *n.* A gap between adjacent cell membranes containing very fine latticelike connections that allow physiologic components to pass directly from cell to cell. Also called *nexus.*

gap phenomenon *n.* A short period in the cycle of atrioventricular or intraventricular conduction during which an impulse is allowed to pass.

Gar·a·my·cin (găr′ə-mī′sĭn) A trademark for the drug gentamicin.

Gard·ner-Dia·mond syndrome (gärd′nər-dī′mənd) *n.* See **autoerythrocyte sensitization syndrome.**

Gard·ner's syndrome (gärd′nərz) *n.* An inherited syndrome characterized by development of multiple tumors, including osteomas of the skull, epidermoid cysts, and fibromas before age 10 and of multiple polyposis predisposing to colon cancer.

gar·gle (gär′gəl) *v.* To force exhaled air through a liquid held in the back of the mouth, with the head tilted back, in order to cleanse or medicate the mouth or throat. —*n.* A medicated fluid used for gargling. Also called *throatwash.*

gar·goyl·ism (gär′goil′ĭz′əm) *n.* A condition characterized by coarsened facial surface and distorted features and associated with Hurler's syndrome and Hunter's syndrome.

Gar·ré's disease (gă-rāz′, gä-) *n.* See **sclerosing osteitis.**

Gärt·ner's bacillus (gĕrt′nərz) *n.* A gram-negative, motile, rod-shaped bacterium of the genus *Salmonella* that causes gastroenteritis in humans.

gas (găs) *n., pl.* **gas·es** *or* **gas·ses 1.** The state of matter distinguished from the solid and liquid states by relatively low density and viscosity, relatively great expansion and contraction with changes in pressure and temperature, the ability to diffuse readily, and the spontaneous tendency to become distributed uniformly throughout any container. **2.** A substance in the gaseous state. **3.** A gaseous fuel, such as natural gas. **4.** Gasoline. **5.** A gaseous asphyxiant, an irritant, or a poison. **6.** A gaseous anesthetic, such as nitrous oxide. **7.** Flatulence. **8.** Flatus. —*v.* **1.** To treat chemically with gas. **2.** To overcome, disable, or kill with poisonous fumes. **3.** To give off gas.

gas abscess *n.* An abscess containing gas caused by *Enterobacter aerogenes, Escherichia coli,* or other gas-forming microorganisms.

gas bacillus *n.* An anaerobic, gram-negative, motile bacterium of the genus *Clostridium* that causes gas gangrene in humans.

gas chromatography *n.* Chromatographic process in which a mixture of gases or vapors are separated by their differential adsorption by a stationary phase.

gas·e·ous (găs′ē-əs, găsh′əs) *adj.* **1.** Of, relating to, or existing as a gas. **2.** Full of or containing gas; gassy.

gas gangrene *n.* A form of gangrene occurring in a wound that is infected with anaerobic bacteria, especially species of *Clostridium,* and characterized by presence of gas in the affected tissue and constitutional septic symptoms.

gas gangrene antitoxin *n.* The antitoxin specific for the toxin of one or more species of *Clostridium* that cause gas gangrene and associated toxemia.

gash (găsh) *v.* To make a long, deep cut in; slash deeply. —*n.* **1.** A long, deep cut. **2.** A deep flesh wound.

gas-liquid chromatography *n. Abbr.* **GLC** A form of gas chromatography in which the stationary phase is a liquid rather than a solid.

gas·om·e·ter (gă-sŏm′ĭ-tər) *n.* An apparatus for measuring gases.

gasometric analysis *n.* The determination of the structure or quantity of a substance by means of measuring its gaseous derivatives.

gas·om·e·try (gă-sŏm′ĭ-trē) *n.* Determination of the relative proportion of gases in a mixture. —**gas′o·met′ric** (găs′ə-mĕt′rĭk) *adj.*

gas peritonitis *n.* Inflammation of the peritoneum accompanied by an intraperitoneal gas.

Gas·ser (găs′ər), **Herbert Spencer** 1888–1963. American physiologist. He shared a 1944 Nobel Prize for research on the functions of nerve fibers.

gas·ser·i·an (gă-sîr′ē-ən) *adj.* Of, relating to, or described by Austrian anatomist Johann Ludwig Gasser (1723–1765).

gasserian ganglion *n.* See **trigeminal ganglion.**

gas·sing (găs′ĭng) *n.* Poisoning by irrespirable or otherwise noxious gases.

gas·ter (găs′tər) *n.* The stomach.

gastr– *pref.* Variant of **gastro–.**

gas·trad·e·ni·tis (gă-străd′n-ī′tĭs) *n.* Inflammation of the glands of the stomach.

gas·tral·gia (gă-străl′jə) *n.* See **gastrodynia.**

gas·trec·ta·sis (gă-strĕk′tə-sĭs) *or* **gas·trec·ta·sia** (găs′trĭk-tā′zhə) *n.* Dilation of the stomach.

gas·trec·to·my (gă-strĕk′tə-mē) *n.* Excision of part or all of the stomach.

gas·tric (găs′trĭk) *adj.* Of, relating to, or associated with the stomach.

gastric analysis *n.* The determination of the pH and acid output of the contents of the stomach.

gastric artery *n.* **1.** Any of four or five small arteries given off from the splenic artery, passing to the greater curvature of the stomach, and anastomosing with other arteries in that region. **2.** An artery with origin in the hepatic artery, with distribution to the pyloric portion of the stomach, and with anastomoses to the left gastric artery; right gastric artery. **3.** An artery with origin in the celiac artery, with distribution to the stomach, the esophagus, and a portion of the left lobe of the liver, and with anastomoses to the esophageal and right gastric arteries; left gastric artery.

gastric bypass *n.* A surgical procedure used for treatment of morbid obesity, consisting of the severance of the upper stomach, anastomosis of the small upper pouch of the stomach to the jejunum, and closure of the distal part of the stomach.

gastric calculus *n.* See **gastrolith.**

gastric digestion *n.* The part of digestion, chiefly of proteins, carried on in the stomach by the enzymes of the gastric juices. Also called *peptic digestion.*

gastric feeding *n.* The administration of food directly into the stomach by a tube inserted either through the nasopharynx and esophagus or directly through the abdominal wall.

gastric fistula *n.* A tract leading from the stomach to the abdominal wall.

gastric fold *n.* Any of the characteristic folds of the mucous membrane lining the stomach.

gastric gland *n.* Any of the branched tubular glands in the mucosa of the fundus and body of the stomach, containing parietal cells that secrete hydrochloric acid and zymogenic cells that produce pepsin. Also called *fundus gland, gastric follicle.*

gastric indigestion *n.* Indigestion in the stomach.

gastric inhibitory polypeptide *n. Abbr.* **GIP** A peptide hormone secreted by the stomach that stimulates insulin release as part of the digestive process.

gastric juice *n.* The colorless, watery, acidic digestive fluid that is secreted by various glands in the mucous membrane of the stomach and consists chiefly of hydrochloric acid, pepsin, rennin, and mucin.

gastric lymphatic follicle *n.* Any of various small lymphoid tissue masses in gastric mucosa.

gastric reflux *n.* See **gastroesophageal reflux.**

gastric secretin *n.* Gastrin.

gastric stapling *n.* Partitioning of the stomach by rows of staples in the treatment of morbid obesity.

gastric tetany *n.* Tetany of muscles of respiration and extremities, associated with gastric disorders.

gastric triangle *n.* See **submandibular triangle.**

gastric ulcer *n.* An ulcer in the mucous membrane of the stomach.

gastric vertigo *n.* Vertigo that is associated with a disease of the stomach. Also called *Trousseau's syndrome.*

gas·trin (găs′trĭn) *n.* Any of the hormones secreted in the pyloric-antral mucosa of the stomach and that stimulate secretion of the parietal cells.

gas·tri·no·ma (găs′trə-nō′mə) *n., pl.* **–mas** or **–ma·ta** (-mə-tə) A gastrin-secreting tumor associated with Zollinger-Ellison syndrome.

gas·tri·tis (gă-strī′tĭs) *n.* Chronic or acute inflammation of the stomach, especially of the mucous membrane of the stomach.

gastritis cys·ti·ca pol·y·po·sa (sĭs′tĭ-kə pŏl′ə-pō′sə, -zə) *n.* Large fixed mucosal polyps arising in the stomach proximal to an old gastroenterostomy.

gastro– or **gastr–** *pref.* Stomach; gastric: *gastritis.*

gas·tro·a·nas·to·mo·sis (găs′trō-ə-năs′tə-mō′sĭs) *n.* Anastomosis of the cardiac and the antral segments of the stomach. Also called *gastrogastrostomy.*

gas·tro·car·di·ac (găs′trō-kär′dē-ăk′) *adj.* Relating to the stomach and the heart.

gas·tro·cele (găs′trə-sēl′) *n.* **1.** The cavity of the gastrula of an embryo. Also called *archenteron.* **2.** Hernia of a portion of the stomach.

gas·troc·ne·mi·us (găs′trŏk-nē′mē-əs, găs′trə-) *n., pl.* **–mi·i** (-mē-ī′) A muscle with its origin from the lateral and medial condyles of the femur, with insertion with the soleus muscle by the Achilles tendon into the lower half of the posterior surface of the calcaneus, with nerve supply from the tibial nerve, and whose action causes plantar flexion of the foot.

gas·tro·col·ic (găs′trō-kŏl′ĭk, -kō′lĭk) *adj.* Relating to the stomach and the colon.

gastrocolic omentum *n.* See **greater omentum.**

gastrocolic reflex *n.* A mass movement of the contents of the colon, often preceded by a similar movement in the small intestine, that sometimes occurs immediately after food enters the stomach.

gas·tro·co·li·tis (găs′trō-kə-lī′tĭs) *n.* Inflammation of the stomach and the colon.

gas·tro·co·los·to·my (găs′trō-kə-lŏs′tə-mē) *n.* The surgical formation of a communication between the stomach and the colon.

gas·tro·du·o·de·nal (găs′trō-dōō′ə-dē′nəl, -dōō-ŏd′-n-əl) *adj.* Relating to the stomach and the duodenum.

gastroduodenal artery *n.* An artery with origin in the hepatic artery and branches to the right gastroepiploic and superior pancreaticoduodenal arteries.

gas·tro·du·o·de·ni·tis (găs′trō-dōō′ō-də-nī′tĭs, -dōō-ŏd′n-ī′-) *n.* Inflammation of the stomach and the duodenum.

gas·tro·du·o·de·nos·co·py (găs′trō-dōō′ə-də-nŏs′kə-pē, -dōō-ŏd′n-ŏs′-) *n.* Visualization of the interior of the stomach and the duodenum by a gastroscope.

gas·tro·du·o·de·nos·to·my (găs′trō-dōō′ə-də-nŏs′tə-mē, -dōō-ŏd′n-ŏs′-) *n.* The surgical formation of a communication between the stomach and the duodenum.

gas·tro·dyn·i·a (găs′trō-dĭn′ē-ə) *n.* Pain in the stomach; a stomach ache. Also called *gastralgia.*

gas·tro·en·ter·ic (găs′trō-ĕn-tĕr′ĭk) *adj.* Relating to the gastrointestinal tract.

gas·tro·en·ter·i·tis (găs′trō-ĕn′tə-rī′tĭs) *n.* Inflammation of the mucous membrane of the stomach and intestines. Also called *enterogastritis.*

gastroenteritis virus type A *n.* See **epidemic gastroenteritis virus.**

gastroenteritis virus type B *n.* See **rotavirus.**

gas·tro·en·ter·o·co·li·tis (găs′trō-ĕn′tə-rō-kō-lī′tĭs, -kə-) *n.* Inflammation of the stomach, small intestines, and colon.

gas·tro·en·ter·ol·o·gy (găs′trō-ĕn′tə-rŏl′ə-jē) *n.* The medical specialty concerned with the function and disorders of the stomach, intestines, and related organs of the gastrointestinal tract. **—gas′tro·en′ter·o·log′ic** (-ə-lŏj′ĭk), **gas′tro·en′ter·o·log′i·cal** *adj.*

gas·tro·en·ter·op·a·thy (găs′trō-ĕn′tə-rŏp′ə-thē) *n.* A disorder of the stomach and intestines.

gas·tro·en·ter·o·plas·ty (găs′trō-ĕn′tə-rō-plăs′tē) *n.* The surgical repair of defects in the stomach and the intestine.

gas·tro·en·ter·op·to·sis (găs′trō-ĕn′tə-rŏp-tō′sĭs) *n.* Downward displacement of the stomach and a portion of the intestine.

gas·tro·en·ter·os·to·my (găs′trō-ĕn′tə-rŏs′tə-mē) *n.* The surgical formation of a new opening between the stomach and the intestine, either anterior or posterior to the mesocolon.

gas·tro·en·ter·ot·o·my (găs′trō-ĕn′tə-rŏt′ə-mē) *n.* Incision into the stomach and the intestine.

gas·tro·ep·i·plo·ic (găs′trō-ĕp′ə-plō′ĭk) *adj.* Relating to the stomach and the greater omentum.

gastroepiploic artery *n.* Gastro-omental artery.

gas·tro·e·soph·a·ge·al (găs′trō-ĭ-sŏf′ə-jē′əl) *adj.* Relating to the stomach and the esophagus.

gastroesophageal hernia *n.* A hiatal hernia into the thorax.

gastroesophageal reflux *n.* A backflow of the contents of the stomach into the esophagus, caused by the relaxation of the lower esophageal sphincter. Also called *esophageal reflux, gastric reflux.*

gastroesophageal reflux disease *n. Abbr.* **GERD** A chronic condition caused by gastroesophageal reflux, characterized by heartburn, acid indigestion, and sometimes reflux esophagitis.

gas·tro·e·soph·a·gi·tis (găs′trō-ĭ-sŏf′ə-jī′tĭs) *n.* Inflammation of the stomach and the esophagus.

gas·tro·e·soph·a·gos·to·my (găs′trō-ĭ-sŏf′ə-gŏs′tə-mē) *n.* The surgical formation of a new opening between the esophagus and the stomach.

gas·tro·gas·tros·to·my (găs′trō-gă-strŏs′tə-mē) *n.* See **gastroanastomosis.**

gas·tro·ga·vage (găs′trō-gə-văzh′) *n.* See **gavage** (sense 1).

gas·tro·gen·ic (găs′trə-jĕn′ĭk) *adj.* Derived from or caused by the stomach.

gas·tro·he·pat·ic (găs′trō-hĭ-păt′ĭk) *adj.* Relating to the stomach and the liver.

gas·tro·il·e·ac reflex (găs′trō-ĭl′ē-ăk′) *n.* Opening of the ileocolic valve when food enters the stomach.

gas·tro·il·e·i·tis (găs′trō-ĭl′ē-ī′tĭs) *n.* Inflammation of the stomach and the ileum.

gas·tro·il·e·os·to·my (găs′trō-ĭl′ē-ŏs′tə-mē) *n.* The surgical formation of a direct communication between the stomach and the ileum.

gas·tro·in·tes·ti·nal (găs′trō-ĭn-tĕs′tə-nəl) *adj. Abbr.* **GI** Relating to the stomach and the intestines.

gastrointestinal tract *n.* The part of the digestive system consisting of the stomach, small intestine, and large intestine.

gas·tro·je·ju·no·col·ic (găs′trō-jə-jōō′nō-kŏl′ĭk, -kō′lĭk) *adj.* Of or relating to the stomach, jejunum, and colon.

gas·tro·je·ju·nos·to·my (găs′trō-jə-jōō′nŏs′tə-mē,-jē′-jōō-) *n.* The surgical formation of a direct communication between the stomach and the jejunum.

gas·tro·li·e·nal (găs′trō-lī′ə-nəl) *adj.* Gastrosplenic.

gas·tro·lith (găs′trə-lĭth′) *n.* A pathological concretion formed in the stomach. Also called *gastric calculus.*

gas·tro·li·thi·a·sis (găs′trō-lĭ-thī′ə-sĭs) *n.* The presence of one or more gastroliths in the stomach.

gas·trol·y·sis (gă-strŏl′ĭ-sĭs) *n.* Surgical division of perigastric adhesions.

gas·tro·ma·la·cia (găs′trō-mə-lā′shə) *n.* Softening of the walls of the stomach.

gas·tro·meg·a·ly (găs′trō-mĕg′ə-lē) *n.* Enlargement of the abdomen or the stomach.

gas·tro·myx·or·rhe·a (găs′trō-mĭk′sə-rē′ə) *n.* Excessive secretion of mucus in the stomach.

gas·tro·o·men·tal artery (găs′trō-ō-mĕn′təl) *n.* **1.** An artery with origin in the gastroduodenal artery, with distribution to the stomach and the greater omentum, and with branches from the left gastroepiploic artery anastomosing with branches of the right and the left gastric arteries; right gastro-omental artery. **2.** An artery with origin in the splenic artery, with distribution to the stomach and the greater omentum, frequently joining the right gastroepiploic artery; left gastro-omental artery.

gas·tro·pa·ral·y·sis (găs′trō-pə-răl′ĭ-sĭs) *n.* Paralysis of the muscular coat of the stomach.

gas·tro·pa·re·sis (găs′trō-pə-rē′sĭs, -păr′ĭ-sĭs) *n.* Mild gastroparalysis.

gas·tro·path·ic (găs′trə-păth′ĭk) *adj.* Of or relating to a disease of the stomach.

gas·trop·a·thy (gă-strŏp′ə-thē) *n.* Any disease of the stomach.

gas·tro·pex·y (găs′trə-pĕk′sē) *n.* The surgical attachment of the stomach to the abdominal wall or to the diaphragm.

gas·tro·phren·ic (găs′trə-frĕn′ĭk) *adj.* Relating to the stomach and the diaphragm.

gas·tro·plas·ty (găs′trə-plăs′tē) *n.* Surgical repair of a defect in the stomach or lower esophagus.

gas·tro·pli·ca·tion (găs′trō-plĭ-kā′shən) *n.* The reduction of stomach size by suturing a fold in the stomach wall. Also called *gastrorrhaphy.*

gas·trop·to·sis (găs′trŏp-tō′sĭs) *n.* Downward displacement of the stomach.

gas·tro·pul·mo·nar·y (găs′trō-pŏŏl′mə-nĕr′ē, -pŭl′-) *adj.* Pneumogastric.

gas·tro·py·lor·ec·to·my (găs′trō-pī′lə-rĕk′tə-mē) *n.* See **pylorectomy.**

gas·tro·py·lor·ic (găs′trō-pī-lôr′ĭk, -pĭ-) *adj.* Relating to the stomach and the pylorus.

gas·tror·rha·gia (găs′trə-rā′jə) *n.* Hemorrhage from the stomach.

gas·tror·rha·phy (gă-strôr′ə-fē) *n.* Suture of a perforation of the stomach. See **gastroplication.**

gas·tror·rhe·a (găs′trə-rē′ə) *n.* Excessive secretion of gastric juice or mucus by the stomach.

gas·tros·chi·sis (gă-strŏs′kĭ-sĭs) *n.* A congenital fissure in the abdominal wall usually accompanied by protrusion of the viscera. Also called *celoschisis.*

gas·tro·scope (găs′trə-skōp′) *n.* An endoscope for examining the inner surface of the stomach. —**gas′tro·scop′ic** (-skŏp′ĭk) *adj.* —**gas·tros′co·pist** (gă-strŏs′kə-pĭst) *n.* —**gas·tros′co·py** (-kə-pē) *n.*

gas·tro·spasm (găs′trə-spăz′əm) *n.* Spasmodic contraction of the walls of the stomach.

gas·tro·splen·ic (găs′trō-splĕn′ĭk) *adj.* Relating to the stomach and the spleen.

gas·tro·stax·is (găs′trō-stăk′sĭs) *n.* The oozing of blood from the mucous membrane of the stomach.

gas·tro·ste·no·sis (găs′trō-stə-nō′sĭs) *n.* Diminution in size of the cavity of the stomach.

gas·tros·to·la·vage (gă-strŏs′tō-lä-văzh′) *n.* Washing out the stomach through a gastric fistula.

gas·tros·to·my (gă-strŏs′tə-mē) *n.* Surgical construction of a permanent opening from the external surface of the abdominal wall into the stomach, usually for inserting a feeding tube.

gas·trot·o·my (gă-strŏt′ə-mē) *n.* An incision into the stomach.

gas·tro·to·nom·e·try (găs′trō-tō-nŏm′ĭ-trē) *n.* The measurement of intragastric pressure.

gas·tro·trop·ic (găs′trō-trŏp′ĭk) *adj.* Affecting the stomach.

gas·tru·la (găs′trə-lə) *n.*, *pl.* **-las** or **-lae** (-lē′) An embryo at the stage following the blastula, consisting of a hollow, two-layered sac of ectoderm and endoderm surrounding an archenteron that communicates with the exterior through the blastopore.

gas·tru·la·tion (găs′trə-lā′shən) *n.* Transformation of the blastula into the gastrula.

gate-control theory *n.* The theory that afferent stimuli, especially pain, entering the substantia gelatinosa, are modulated so that transmission to neurons is blocked by inhibitory agents.

gate·keep·er (gāt′kē′pər) *n.* A primary-care provider, often in the setting of a managed-care organization, who coordinates patient care and provides referrals to specialists, hospitals, laboratories, and other medical services.

Gau·cher's cell (gō-shāz′) *n.* An altered macrophage containing kerasin and derived from the reticuloendothelial system, characteristic of Gaucher's disease.

Gaucher's disease *n.* A rare familial disorder of fat metabolism due to a glucocerebrosidase deficiency and characterized by enlargement of the liver and spleen, lymphadenopathy, and bone destruction. Also called *cerebroside lipidosis, cerebrosidosis.*

gaunt·let bandage (gônt′lĭt, gănt′-) *n.* A figure-of-8 bandage covering the hand and fingers.

gauss (gous) *n.*, *pl.* **gauss** or **gauss·es** The centimeter-gram-second unit of magnetic induction.

gaus·si·an (gou′sē-ən) *adj.* Relating to or described by German mathematician and astronomer Karl Friedrich Gauss (1777-1855).

gauze (gôz) *n.* A bleached, woven cotton cloth, used for dressings, bandages, and absorbent sponges.

ga·vage (gə-väzh′) *n.* 1. The introduction of nutritive material into the stomach by means of a tube. Also called *gastrogavage.* 2. The therapeutic use of a high-potency diet.

Ga·vard's muscle (gə-värz′, gä-) *n.* Oblique fibers in the muscular coat of the stomach.

gay (gā) *adj.* Relating to or having a sexual orientation to persons of the same sex.

gaze nystagmus *n.* A nystagmus occurring in partial gaze paralysis when an attempt is made to look in the direction of the palsy.

G-banding stain *n.* A staining technique in which chromosomes are treated with trypsin, then with Giemsa stain to produce dark heterochromatic regions and light euchromatic regions. Also called *Giemsa chromosome banding stain.*

G cell *n.* An enteroendocrine cell that secretes gastrin, found primarily in the gastric glands of the pyloric cavity mucosa of the stomach.

Gd The symbol for the element **gadolinium**.

Ge The symbol for the element **germanium**.

ge– *pref.* Variant of **geo–**.

Gei·ger counter (gī′gər) *n.* An instrument that measures radiation by detecting radioactive particles as they cross a metal or glass tube filled with gas, causing ionization of the gas molecules and producing an electrical discharge. Also called *Geiger-Müller counter.*

Geiger tube *n.* A metal or glass tube filled with gas and used with a geiger counter.

gel (jĕl) *n.* A colloid in which the disperse phase combines with the dispersion medium to produce a semisolid material. —*v.* 1. To become a gel. 2. To convert a sol into a gel.

gel·a·tin or **gel·a·tine** (jĕl′ə-tn) *n.* A derived protein formed by boiling collagen of animal tissues.

ge·lat·i·nous (jə-lăt′n-əs) *adj.* 1. Of, relating to, or containing gelatin. 2. Resembling gelatin; viscous.

ge·la·tion (jĕ-lā′shən) *n.* 1. Solidification by cooling or freezing. 2. The process of forming a gel. 3. Transformation of a sol into a gel.

gel diffusion precipitin test *n.* Any of various precipitin tests in which the precipitate forms in a gel medium, usually agar, into which one or both reactants have diffused.

ge·lo·sis (jĕ-lō′sĭs) *n.* An extremely firm mass in a tissue, especially in a muscle, with a consistency resembling that of frozen tissue.

gem·el·lip·a·ra (jĕm′ə-lĭp′ər-ə) *n.* A woman who has given birth to twins.

gem·fi·bro·zil (jĕm-fī′brə-zĭl, -fĭb′rə-) *n.* An antihyperlipidemic agent used in the treatment of very high serum triglyceride levels.

gem·i·nate (jĕm′ə-nĭt, -nāt′) *adj.* Occurring in pairs.

gem·i·na·tion (jĕm′ə-nā′shən) *n.* Embryologic partial division of a primordium, as of a single tooth germ forming two teeth.

gem·ma·tion (jĕ-mā′shən) *n.* A form of fission in which the parent cell does not divide, but forms a bud-like cell that separates and begins an independent existence. Also called *budding, bud fission.*

gem·mule (jĕm′yōol) *n.* The small bud that projects from the parent cell during gemmation.

–gen or **–gene** *suff.* 1. Producer: *androgen*. 2. One that is produced: *phosgene*.

ge·na (jē′nə) *n.*, *pl.* **-nae** (-nē) The cheek or lateral side of the face. —**ge′nal** *adj.*

genal gland *n.* See **buccal gland**.

gen·der (jĕn′dər) *n.* 1. The sex of an individual, male or female, based on reproductive anatomy. 2. Sexual identity, especially in relation to society or culture.

gender dysphoria *n.* A persistent unease with having the physical characteristics of one's gender, accompanied by strong identification with the opposite gender and a desire to live as or to become a member of the opposite gender.

gender identity *n.* A person's sense of being male or female, resulting from a combination of genetic and environmental influences.

gender role *n.* The pattern of masculine or feminine behavior of an individual that is defined by a particular culture and that is largely determined by a child's upbringing.

gene (jēn) *n.* A hereditary unit that occupies a specific location on a chromosome, determines a particular characteristic in an organism by directing the formation of a specific protein, and is capable of replicating itself at each cell division.

ge·ne·al·o·gy (jē′nē-ŏl′ə-jē, -ăl′-, jĕn′ē-) *n*. **1.** A record or table of the descent of a person, family, or group from an ancestor or ancestors; a family tree. **2.** The study or investigation of ancestry and family histories.

gene amplification *n*. A cellular process characterized by the production of copies of a gene or genes to amplify the phenotype that the gene confers on the cell.

gene augmentation therapy *n*. A procedure for correcting metabolic deficiencies caused by a missing or defective gene by having a healthy gene produce the necessary product without actually substituting that gene for the flawed or absent gene in the DNA.

gene dosage compensation *n*. The putative mechanism that adjusts the X-linked phenotypes of males and females to compensate for the haploid state in males and the diploid state in females.

gene mapping *n*. The determination of the sequence of genes and their relative distances from one another on a specific chromosome.

gene pool *n*. The collective genetic information contained within a population of sexually reproducing organisms.

gen·er·al (jĕn′ər-əl) *adj*. Of or affecting the entire body. —*n*. General anesthesia.

general-adaptation syndrome *n*. A syndrome in which non-specific reactions of organisms to stress can be grouped into three stages: alarm, resistance, and exhaustion.

general anatomy *n*. The study of the structure and composition of the body as well as of its tissues and fluids.

general anesthesia *n*. Loss of the ability to perceive pain associated with loss of consciousness, produced by anesthetic agents.

general anesthetic *n*. An agent that produces loss of sensation and loss of consciousness.

general duty nurse *n*. A nurse who does not specialize in a particular area of practice but is available for any duty.

general immunity *n*. Immunity that protects the body as a whole.

gen·er·al·ist (jĕn′ər-ə-lĭst) *n*. A physician whose practice is not oriented in a specific medical specialty but instead covers a variety of medical problems.

gen·er·al·i·za·tion (jĕn′ər-ə-lĭ-zā′shən) *n*. **1.** The act or an instance of generalizing. **2.** A principle, a statement, or an idea having general application.

gen·er·al·ize (jĕn′ər-ə-līz′) *v*. **1.** To reduce to a general form, class, or law. **2.** To render indefinite or unspecific. **3.** To infer from many particulars. **4.** To draw inferences or a general conclusion from. **5.** To make generally or universally applicable.

gen·er·al·ized (jĕn′ər-ə-līzd′) *adj*. **1.** Involving an entire organ, as when an epileptic seizure involves all parts of the brain. **2.** Not specifically adapted to a particular environment or function; not specialized. **3.** Generally prevalent.

generalized anaphylaxis *n*. The immediate anaphylactic response of a sensitized individual following his or her inoculation with an antigen. Also called *systemic anaphylaxis*.

generalized anxiety disorder *n*. An anxiety disorder characterized by consistent feelings of anxiety for a period of at least six months and accompanied by symptoms such as fatigue, restlessness, irritability and sleep disturbance.

generalized cortical hyperostosis *n*. See Van Buchem's syndrome.

generalized epilepsy *n*. An epileptic condition characterized by generalized seizures, especially grand mal seizures. Also called *generalized seizure disorder*.

generalized glycogenosis *n*. See type 2 glycogenosis.

generalized seizure *n*. A seizure that originates from multiple brain foci and is characterized by general rather than localized neurologic symptoms, may be tonic-clonic, and may progress from a focal seizure.

generalized seizure disorder *n*. See **generalized epilepsy**.

generalized tonic-clonic epilepsy *n*. See grand mal.

generalized tonic-clonic seizure *n*. See grand mal seizure.

generalized tonic-clonic seizure disorder *n*. See grand mal.

generalized vaccinia *n*. A skin eruption following vaccination for smallpox, seen most commonly in people with previously traumatized skin.

generalized xanthelasma *n*. Xanthoma planum of the neck, trunk, extremities, and eyelids in individuals with normal plasma lipid levels.

general paresis *n*. A brain disease occurring as a late consequence of syphilis, characterized by dementia, progressive muscular weakness, and paralysis. Also called *Bayle's disease, paralytic dementia*.

general practitioner *n*. *Abbr*. **GP** A physician whose practice consists of providing ongoing care covering a variety of medical problems in patients of all ages, often including referral to appropriate specialists.

general stimulant *n*. A stimulant that affects the entire body.

gen·er·a·tion (jĕn′ə-rā′shən) *n*. **1.** A form or stage in the life cycle of an organism. **2.** All of the offspring that are at the same stage of descent from a common ancestor. **3.** The average interval of time between the birth of parents and the birth of their offspring. **4.** A group of individuals born and living about the same time. **5.** A group of generally contemporaneous individuals regarded as having common cultural or social characteristics and attitudes. **6.** The act or process of generating; origination, production, or procreation.

gen·er·a·tive (jĕn′ər-ə-tĭv, -ə-rā′-) *adj*. **1.** Having the ability to originate, produce, or procreate. **2.** Of or relating to the production of offspring.

gen·er·a·tor (jĕn′ə-rā′tər) *n*. One that generates, especially a machine that converts mechanical energy into electrical energy.

ge·ner·ic (jə-nĕr′ĭk) *adj*. **1.** Of or relating to a genus. **2.** Relating to or descriptive of an entire group or class; general. **3.** Of or relating to a drug sold under or identified by its official nonproprietary or chemical name. —*n*. A drug sold under its generic name.

generic name *n*. **1.** The official nonproprietary name of a drug, under which it is licensed and identified by the manufacturer. **2.** The first name of the two-part

Latin taxonomic name of an organism, which specifies the biological genus. **3.** A designation formerly used to indicate the class or type of a compound.

gen·e·sis (jĕn′ĭ-sĭs) *n., pl.* **–ses** (-sēz′) The coming into being of something; the origin.

–genesis *suff.* Origin; production: *biogenesis.*

gene-splicing *n.* The process in which fragments of DNA from one or more different organisms are combined to form recombinant DNA and are made to function within the cells of a host organism.

gene therapy *n.* A technique for the treatment of genetic disease in which a gene that is absent or defective is replaced by a healthy gene.

ge·net·ic (jə-nĕt′ĭk) *or* **ge·net·i·cal** (-ĭ-kəl) *adj.* **1.** Of or relating to genetics or genes. **2.** Affecting or affected by genes, as a disorder or deficiency. **3.** Of, relating to, or influenced by the origin or development of something; ontogenic.

ge·net·i·cal·ly modified organism (jə-nĕt′ĭ-kə-lē) *n. Abbr.* **GMO** An organism whose genetic characteristics have been altered by the insertion of a modified gene or a gene from another organism using the techniques of genetic engineering.

genetic amplification *n.* A process for increasing specific DNA sequences, especially to increase the proportion of plasmid DNA to bacterial DNA.

genetic association *n.* The occurrence together in a population, more often than can be readily explained by chance, of two or more traits of which at least one is known to be genetic.

genetic code *n.* The sequence of nucleotides that is the basis of heredity in the DNA molecule of a chromosome and that specifies the amino acid sequence in the synthesis of proteins.

genetic counseling *n.* The counseling of prospective parents on the probabilities and dangers of inherited diseases occurring in their offspring and on the diagnosis and treatment of such diseases.

genetic disease *n.* A disease caused by the absence of a gene or by products of a defective gene.

genetic dominant *adj.* Of, relating to, or characteristic of a pattern of inheritance of an autosomal trait that is expressed by a gene that always manifests itself phenotypically.

genetic drift *n.* Random fluctuations in the frequency of the appearance of a gene in a small isolated population, presumably owing to chance rather than natural selection. Also called *drift.*

genetic engineering *n.* Scientific alteration of the structure of genetic material in a living organism using recombinant DNA, employed for such purposes as creating bacteria that synthesize insulin.

genetic female *n.* **1.** An individual with a normal female karyotype, including two X-chromosomes. **2.** An individual whose cell nuclei contain Barr bodies.

genetic fingerprint *n.* See **DNA fingerprint.**

genetic fingerprinting *n.* See **DNA fingerprinting.**

genetic fitness *n.* The reproductive success of a genotype, usually measured as the number of offspring produced by an individual that survive to reproductive age relative to the average for the population.

genetic immunity *n.* See **innate immunity.**

ge·net·i·cist (jə-nĕt′ĭ-sĭst) *n.* A specialist in genetics.

genetic lethal *n.* A disorder that prevents effective reproduction by those affected, such as Klinefelter syndrome.

genetic load *n.* The aggregate of deleterious genes that are carried, mostly hidden, in the genome of a population and that may be transmitted to descendants.

genetic male *n.* **1.** An individual with one X-chromosome and one Y-chromosome, the normal male karyotype. **2.** An individual whose cell nuclei do not contain Barr bodies.

genetic map *n.* A graphic representation of the genes or mutable sites on a chromosome.

genetic marker *n.* A gene phenotypically associated with a particular, easily identified trait and used to identify an individual or cell carrying that gene.

genetic psychology *n.* The study of the influence of genetic factors on personality development.

ge·net·ics (jə-nĕt′ĭks) *n.* The branch of biology that deals with heredity, especially the mechanisms of hereditary transmission and the variation of inherited traits among similar or related organisms.

genetic screening *n.* The analysis of DNA samples to detect the presence of a gene or genes associated with an inherited disorder.

ge·net·o·troph·ic (jə-nĕt′ō-trŏf′ĭk, -trō′fĭk) *adj.* **1.** Of or relating to genetics and nutrition. **2.** Of or relating to inherited individual differences in nutritional requirements.

ge·ni·al (jĭ-nī′əl) *or* **ge·ni·an** (-ən) *adj.* Of or relating to the chin.

genial tubercle *n.* See **mental spine.**

gen·ic (jē′nĭk, jĕn′ĭk) *adj.* Of, relating to, produced by, or being genes or a gene.

–genic *suff.* **1.** Producing; generating: *carcinogenic.* **2.** Produced or generated by: *cryptogenic.* **3.** Suitable for production or reproduction by a specified medium: *photogenic.*

ge·nic·u·lar (jə-nĭk′yə-lər) *adj.* Of or relating to the knee joint.

genicular vein *n.* Any of the veins that accompany the genicular arteries, drain blood from structures around the knee, and end in the popliteal vein.

ge·nic·u·late (jə-nĭk′yə-lĭt) *or* **ge·nic·u·lat·ed** (-lā′tĭd) *adj.* **1.** Bent abruptly, as a knee. **2.** Of, relating to, or being the geniculate body or geniculate ganglion. **3.** Having kneelike joints; able to bend at an abrupt angle.

geniculate body *n.* **1.** Lateral geniculate body. **2.** Medial geniculate body.

geniculate ganglion *n.* A ganglion of the intermediate nerve located within the facial canal and containing sensory neurons that innervate taste buds on the front two-thirds of the tongue.

geniculate neuralgia *n.* A severe stabbing pain deep in the ear. Also called *Hunt's neuralgia, neuralgia facialis vera.*

ge·nic·u·lum (jə-nĭk′yə-ləm) *n., pl.* **-la** (-lə) **1.** A small kneelike anatomical structure. **2.** A sharp bend in an organ.

–genin *suff.* Relating to a steroid, often one that is toxic: *sapogenin.*

ge·ni·o·glos·sus (jē′nē-ō-glŏs′əs) *n*. Either of a pair of lingual muscles with origin in the mandible, with insertion to the lingual fascia below the mucous membrane and epiglottis, with nerve supply from the hypoglossal nerve, and whose action depresses and protrudes the tongue.

ge·ni·o·hy·oid (jē′nē-ō-hī′oid′) *n*. A muscle with origin in the mandible, with insertion to the hyoid bone, with nerve supply from the first and second cervical nerve, whose action draws the hyoid forward or depresses the jaw when the hyoid is fixed.

ge·ni·on (jə-nī′ŏn′, -ən) *n*. The point at the tip of the mental spine of the mandible.

ge·ni·o·plas·ty (jē′nē-ō-plăs′tē, jə-nī′ə-) *n*. See **mentoplasty**.

ge·nis·te·in (jə-nĭs′tē-ĭn, -nĭs′tēn′) *n*. A phytoestrogen found in soy, having antioxidant and anticancer properties.

gen·i·tal (jĕn′ĭ-tl) *adj*. **1**. Of or relating to biological reproduction. **2**. Of or relating to the genitalia. **3**. Of or relating to the stage of psychosexual development in psychoanalytic theory beginning in puberty and during which the genitals become the focus of sexual gratification. —*n*. A reproductive organ, especially one of the external sex organs.

genital cord *n*. One of a pair of mesenchymal ridges bulging into the caudal part of the celom of an embryo and containing the wolffian and müllerian ducts as well as the primordium of the broad ligaments and uterine walls in the female.

genital corpuscle *n*. Any of the encapsulated nerve endings in skin of the genitalia and nipples.

genital herpes *n*. A highly contagious, sexually transmitted viral infection caused by herpesvirus type two and characterized by painful lesions in the genital and anal regions.

gen·i·ta·li·a (jĕn′ĭ-tā′lē-ə, -tāl′yə) *pl.n*. The reproductive organs, especially the external sex organs.

gen·i·tal·i·ty (jĕn′ĭ-tăl′ĭ-tē) *n*. **1**. In psychoanalytic theory, the genital components of sexuality. **2**. The capacity for erotic sensation in genitalia.

genital organ *n*. Any of the organs of reproduction or generation, including, in the female, the vulva, clitoris, ovaries, uterine tubes, uterus, and vagina, and in the male, the penis, scrotum, testes, epididymides, deferent ducts, seminal vesicles, prostate, and bulbourethral glands.

genital phase *n*. In psychoanalytic theory, the final stage of psychosexual development, reached in puberty, when erotic interest and activity are focused on a sexual partner.

genital ridge *n*. See **gonadal ridge**.

gen·i·tals (jĕn′ĭ-tlz) *pl.n*. Genitalia.

genital tract *n*. The genital passages of the urogenital system.

genital wart *n*. A pointed papilloma usually on the skin or mucous membranes of the anus and external genitalia, and caused by a virus transmitted through sexual contact. Also called *condyloma acuminatum, fig wart, moist wart, pointed wart, venereal wart, verruca acuminata*.

gen·i·to·cru·ral (jĕn′ĭ-tō-krōōr′əl) *adj*. Genitofemoral.

gen·i·to·fem·o·ral (jĕn′ĭ-tō-fĕm′ər-əl) *adj*. Relating to or involving the genitalia and the thigh; genitocrural.

genitofemoral nerve *n*. A nerve that arises from the first and second lumbar nerves, passes distad along the anterior surface of the psoas major muscle, and divides into genital and femoral branches.

gen·i·to·u·ri·nar·y (jĕn′ĭ-tō-yōōr′ə-nĕr′ē) *adj*. *Abbr*. **GU** Of or relating to the genital and urinary organs or their functions.

genitourinary system *n*. See **urogenital system**.

gen·o·cop·y (jĕn′ə-kŏp′ē) *n*. A trait that is a phenotypic copy of a genetic trait but is caused by a mechanism other than genotype expression.

gen·o·der·ma·to·sis (jĕn′ō-dûr′mə-tō′sĭs, jē′nō-) *n*. A skin condition of genetic origin.

ge·nome (jē′nōm′) *or* **ge·nom** (-nŏm) *n*. A complete haploid set of chromosomes with its associated genes. —**ge·nom′ic** (-nŏm′ĭk) *adj*.

ge·no·mics (jē-nō′mĭks) *n*. The study of all of the nucleotide sequences, including structural genes, regulatory sequences, and noncoding DNA segments, in the chromosomes of an organism.

ge·no·spe·cies (jē′nə-spē′shēz, -sēz, jĕn′ə-) *pl.n*. A group of organisms that can interbreed.

ge·no·tox·ic (jē′nō-tŏk′sĭk) *adj*. Damaging to DNA and thereby capable of causing mutations or cancer.

gen·o·type (jĕn′ə-tīp′, jē′nə-) *n*. **1**. The genetic constitution of an organism or a group of organisms. **2**. A group or class of organisms having the same genetic constitution. —**gen′o·typ′i·cal** (-tĭp′ĭ-kəl) *adj*.

–genous *suff*. **1**. Producing; generating: *hematogenous*. **2**. Produced by or produced in a specified manner: *exogenous*.

gen·ta·mi·cin sulfate *or* **gen·ta·my·cin sulfate** (jĕn′tə-mī′sĭn) *n*. A broad-spectrum antibiotic derived from an actinomycete used in the treatment of various infections.

gen·tian·o·phil (jĕn′shə-nō-fĭl′) *or* **gen·tian·o·phile** (-fīl′, -fĭl′) *adj*. Staining readily with gentian violet. —**gen′tian·o·phil′ic** *adj*.

gen·tian·o·pho·bic (jĕn′shə-nō-fō′bĭk) *adj*. Not staining or staining poorly with gentian violet.

gen·tian violet (jĕn′shən) *n*. Any of several basic dyes that are derivatives of pararosaniline, especially a dark green or greenish mixture that is used as a biological stain and as a bactericide, a fungicide, and an anthelmintic.

ge·nu (jē′nōō, jĕn′yōō) *n*., *pl*. **gen·u·a** (jĕn′yōō-ə) **1**. Knee. **2**. An anatomical structure resembling the angular shape of a flexed knee.

gen·u·al (jĕn′yōō-əl) *adj*. Genicular.

gen·u·cu·bi·tal position (jĕn′yōō-kyōō′bĭ-tl) *n*. See **knee-elbow position**.

gen·u·pec·to·ral position (jĕn′yōō-pĕk′tər-əl) *n*. See **knee-chest position**.

genu re·cur·va·tum (rē′kûr-vā′təm) *n*. The backward curvature of the knee; hyperextension of the knee.

ge·nus (jē′nəs) *n*., *pl*. **gen·er·a** (jĕn′ər-ə) A taxonomic category ranking below a family and above a species and generally consisting of a group of species exhibiting similar characteristics.

genu val·gum (văl′gəm) *n*. Knock-knee.

genu var·um (vâr′əm) *n.* Bowleg.

–geny *suff.* Production; generation; origin: *ontogeny.*

geo– *or* **ge–** *pref.* Earth: *geophagia.*

Ge·o·cil·lin (jē′-ə-sĭl′ĭn) A trademark for the drug carbenicillin.

ge·ode (jē′ōd′) *n.* A cystlike space with or without an epithelial lining, usually observed in subarticular bone in arthritic disorders.

ge·o·graph·i·cal tongue (jē′ə-grăf′ĭ-kəl) *n.* A chronic inflammation of the tongue characterized by distinct somewhat circular groupings of lesions bounded by a white band. Also called *benign migratory glossitis, erythema migrans linguae, pityriasis linguae.*

ge·o·met·ric isomerism (jē′ə-mĕt′rĭk) *n.* A form of isomerism displayed by unsaturated compounds or by ring compounds, where rotation about a carbon bond is restricted, as in *cis* and *trans* configurations.

geometric mean *n.* The *n*th root, usually the positive *n*th root, of a product of *n* factors.

ge·oph·a·gy (jē-ŏf′ə-jē) *or* **ge·oph·a·gism** (-jĭz′əm) *or* **ge·o·pha·gia** (jē′ə-fā′jə) *n.* The eating of earthy substances, such as clay or chalk, that is practiced as a custom or for dietary or subsistence reasons. Also called *dirt-eating.* —**ge·oph′a·gist** *n.*

ge·ot·ri·cho·sis (jē-ŏt′rĭ-kō′sĭs, jē′ō-trĭ-) *n.* An infection of the lungs or of the mouth and intestines caused by the fungus *Geotrichum candidum.*

ger– *pref.* Variant of **gero–.**

GERD *abbr.* gastroesophageal reflux disease

ger·i·at·ric (jěr′ē-ăt′rĭk) *adj.* **1.** Of or relating to geriatrics. **2.** Of or relating to old age or to the aging process. —*n.* An old person.

ger·i·at·rics (jěr′ē-ăt′rĭks) *n.* The branch of medicine that deals with the diagnosis and treatment of diseases and problems specific to old age. —**ger′i·a·tric′ian** (jěr′ē-ə-trĭsh′ən) *n.*

germ (jûrm) *n.* **1.** A small mass of protoplasm or cells from which a new organism or one of its parts may develop. **2.** A microorganism, especially a pathogen.

ger·ma·ni·um (jər-mā′nē-əm) *n. Symbol* **Ge** A brittle crystalline gray-white metalloid element, used in certain optical glasses and dental alloys and as an intestinal astringent in veterinary medicine. Atomic number 32.

Ger·man measles (jûr′mən) *n.* See **rubella.**

German measles virus *n.* See **rubella virus.**

germ cell *n.* An ovum or a sperm cell or one of their developmental precursors. Also called *sex cell.*

ger·mi·cide (jûr′mĭ-sīd′) *n.* An agent that kills germs, especially pathogenic microorganisms; a disinfectant. —**ger′mi·cid′al** (-sīd′l) *adj.*

ger·mi·nal (jûr′mə-nəl) *adj.* **1.** Of, relating to, or having the nature of a germ cell. **2.** Of, relating to, or occurring in the earliest stage of development of an embryo or organism.

germinal area *n.* The place in the blastoderm where embryonic development is initiated.

germinal cell *n.* A cell from which other cells are derived, especially a dividing cell in the embryonic neural tube.

germinal center of Flem·ming (flěm′ĭng) *n.* A spherical mass in the center of a lymph node that contains actively proliferating B cells.

germinal disk *n.* A flattened, disklike region of cells from which the embryo develops in the fertilized ovum of many vertebrate species. Also called *embryonic disk.*

germinal epithelium *n.* See **surface epithelium.**

germinal localization *n.* The determination in very young embryos of the presumptive areas for specific organs or structures.

germinal membrane *n.* See **blastoderm.**

germinal pole *n.* See **animal pole.**

ger·mi·na·tive layer (jûr′mə-nā′tĭv) *n.* See **Malpighian layer.**

ger·mi·no·ma (jûr′mə-nō′mə) *n.* A neoplasm derived from germinal tissue.

germ layer *n.* Any of the three primary cellular layers, the ectoderm, endoderm, or mesoderm, into which most animal embryos differentiate and from which the organs and tissues of the body develop.

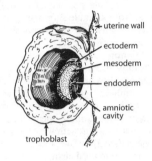

germ layer
endoderm and adjacent germ layers

germ line *n.* Cells from which gametes are derived.

germ membrane *n.* See **blastoderm.**

germ plasm *n.* **1.** The cytoplasm of a germ cell, especially that part containing the chromosomes. **2.** Germ cells as distinguished from other body cells. **3.** Hereditary material; genes.

germ theory *n.* The doctrine holding that infectious diseases are caused by the activity of microorganisms within the body.

gero– *or* **ger–** *pref.* Old age: *geroderma.*

ger·o·der·ma (jěr′ō-dûr′mə) *n.* Thinning of the skin accompanied by the loss of elasticity and subcutaneous fat, as in the aging process.

ger·o·don·tics (jěr′ə-dŏn′tĭks) *n.* The branch of dentistry that deals with the diagnosis, prevention, and treatment of dental diseases and problems specific to old people.

ger·o·mor·phism (jěr′ō-môr′fĭz′əm) *n.* A condition of appearing prematurely old or aged.

ge·ron·tal (jě-rŏn′tl) *adj.* Relating to or characteristic of old age.

geronto– *or* **geront–** *pref.* Old age: *gerontology.*

ger·on·tol·o·gy (jěr′ən-tŏl′ə-jē) *n.* The scientific study of the biological, psychological, and sociological phenomena that are associated with old age and aging. —**ger′on·tol′o·gist** *n.*

ger·on·tox·on (jěr′ŏn-tŏk′sŏn′, -sən) *n.* See **arcus cornealis.**

Ge·ro·ta's capsule (gə-rō′təz, gā-) *n.* See **renal fascia.**

Ge·sell (gĭ-zĕl′), **Arnold Lucius** 1880–1961. American psychologist and pediatrician noted for his research on child development.

ges·ta·gen (jĕs′tə-jən, -jĕn′) *n.* A substance, such as a steroid hormone, that affects the uterus in a manner similar to progesterone.

ge·stalt *or* **Ge·stalt** (gə-shtält′, -shtôlt′, -stält′, -stôlt′) *n., pl.* **–stalts** *or* **–stalt·en** (-shtält′n, -shtôlt′n, -stält′n, -stôlt′n) A physical, biological, psychological, or symbolic configuration or pattern of elements so unified as a whole that its properties cannot be derived from a simple summation of its parts. Also called *gestalt phenomenon.*

ge·stalt·ism (gə-shtäl′tĭz′əm, -shtôl′-, -stäl′-, -stôl′-) *n.* The school or theory of psychology that emphasizes the wholeness and organized structure of every psychological, physiological, and behavioral experience, maintaining that experiences are not reducible and thus cannot be derived from a simple summation of perceptual elements such as sensation and response. Also called *Gestalt psychology.*

gestalt phenomenon *n.* See **gestalt.**

Gestalt psychology *n.* See **gestaltism.**

gestalt therapy *n.* Psychotherapy with individuals or groups that emphasizes treatment of the person as a whole, including a person's biological components and their organic functioning, perceptual configuration, and interrelationships with the external world.

ges·ta·tion (jĕ-stā′shən) *n.* The period of fetal development from conception until birth; pregnancy.

ges·ta·tion·al age (jĕ-stā′shə-nəl) *n.* See **estimated gestational age.**

gestational edema *n.* The occurrence of a generalized and excessive accumulation of fluid in the tissues due to pregnancy.

gestational proteinuria *n.* Proteinuria during or under the influence of pregnancy and in the absence of hypertension, edema, renal infection, or known intrinsic renovascular disease.

gestational psychosis *n.* A psychotic reaction associated with pregnancy.

ges·to·sis (jĕ-stō′sĭs) *n., pl.* **ges·to·ses** (jĕ-stō′sēz) A toxemic disorder of pregnancy.

GFR *abbr.* glomerular filtration rate

GH *abbr.* growth hormone

GHB *abbr.* gamma-hydroxybutyrate

Ghon's tubercle (gŏnz, gônz, gōnz) *n.* The pulmonary lesion of primary tuberculosis. Also called *Ghon's focus, Ghon's primary lesion.*

ghost cell *n.* **1.** A dead cell in which the outline remains visible, but whose nucleus and cytoplasmic structures are not stainable. **2.** A red blood cell after loss of its hemoglobin.

ghost corpuscle (gōst) *n.* See **achromocyte.**

GHRF *or* **GH-RF** *abbr.* growth hormone-releasing factor

GI *abbr.* gastrointestinal; Gingival Index

Gia·not·ti-Cros·ti syndrome (jə-nŏt′ē-krŏs′tē) *n.* A disease of young children caused by infection with hepatitis B virus, characterized by eruptions of reddish or discolored papules on the face, buttocks, and limbs and by malaise and low-grade fever. Also called *papular acrodermatitis of childhood.*

gi·ant axonal neuropathy (jī′ənt) *n.* A generalized disorder of neurofilaments marked by progressive peripheral neural degeneration in childhood.

giant cell *n.* An unusually large cell, especially a large multinucleated phagocytic cell.

giant cell arteritis *n.* See **temporal arteritis.**

giant cell carcinoma *n.* A malignant epithelial neoplasm characterized by large undifferentiated cells.

giant cell fibroma *n.* A form of irritation fibroma, occurring most frequently on the gums of young adults, composed of fibroblasts with large stellate or multiple nuclei.

giant cell granuloma *n.* A non-neoplastic lesion of the gums or jaw bones, characterized by a proliferation of granulation tissue containing many multinucleated giant cells.

giant cell myeloma *n.* See **giant cell tumor of bone.**

giant cell pneumonia *n.* A rare complication of measles, in which multinucleated giant cells line the alveoli. Also called *Hecht's pneumonia, interstitial giant cell pneumonia.*

giant cell sarcoma *n.* A malignant giant cell tumor of bone.

giant cell tumor of bone *n.* A sometimes malignant osteolytic tumor composed of multinucleated giant cells and ovoid or spindle-shaped cells. It occurs most frequently in an end of a long tubular bone. Also called *giant cell myeloma, osteoclastoma.*

giant cell tumor of tendon sheath *n.* A nodule, possibly inflammatory, that usually develops from the flexor sheath of the fingers and thumb and is composed of fibrous tissue, multinucleated giant cells, and lipid- and hemosiderin-containing macrophages. Also called *localized nodular tenosynovitis.*

giant condyloma *n.* A large, often recurrent genital wart in the preputial sac of the penis of uncircumcised men. Also called *Buschke-Löwenstein tumor.*

gi·ant·ism (jī′ən-tĭz′əm) *n.* **1.** The quality or condition of being great in size. **2.** See **gigantism** (sense 2).

giant urticaria *n.* See **angioneurotic edema.**

Gi·ar·di·a (jē-är′dē-ə) *n.* A genus of flagellated, usually nonpathogenic protozoa that are parasitic in the intestines of vertebrates including humans and most domestic animals.

gi·ar·di·a·sis (jē′är-dī′ə-sĭs) *n.* A condition in which the intestines are infected with the protozoan *Giardia lamblia.* Also called *lambliasis.*

gib·bos·i·ty (gĭ-bŏs′ĭ-tē) *n.* **1.** The condition of being gibbous. **2.** A rounded hump or protuberance.

gib·bous (gĭb′əs) *adj.* **1.** Characterized by convexity; protuberant. **2.** Having a hump; humpbacked.

gib·bus (gĭb′əs) *n.* The hump of a deformed spine.

Gib·son murmur (gĭb′sən) *n.* The typical continuous rumbling murmur associated with patent ductus arteriosus. Also called *machinery murmur.*

Giem·sa chromosome banding stain (gēm′zə) *n.* See **G-banding stain.**

Giemsa stain *n.* A mixture of glycerin, methanol, methylene azure, and eosin used to stain chromosomes, blood cell producing tissues, and certain species of spirochetes and protozoans.

Gier·ke's disease (gîr′kəz) *n.* See **type 1 glycogenosis.**

Gif·ford's operation (gĭf′ərdz) *n.* See **delimiting keratotomy.**

GIFT *abbr.* gamete intrafallopian transfer

giga– *pref.* One billion (10^9): *gigahertz.*

gi·gan·tism (jī-găn′tĭz′əm) *n.* **1.** The quality or state of being gigantic; abnormally large size. **2.** Excessive growth of the body or any of its parts, especially as a result of oversecretion of the growth hormone by the pituitary gland. Also called *giantism.*

giganto– *or* **gigant–** *pref.* Huge: *gigantomastia.*

gi·gan·to·mas·ti·a (jī-găn′tō-măs′tē-ə) *n.* Extreme hypertrophy of the breast.

Gil·bert (gĭl′bərt), **Walter** Born 1932. American biologist. He shared a 1980 Nobel Prize for developing methods of mapping the structure and function of DNA.

Gil·bert's disease *or* **Gil·bert's syndrome** (zhĕl-bĕrz′) *n.* See **familial nonhemolytic jaundice.**

gill arch (gĭl) *n.* See **branchial arch.**

Gilles de la Tour·ette's disease *or* **Gilles de la Tourette's syndrome** (zhĕl də lä tŏŏ-rĕts′) *n.* See **Tourette's syndrome.**

gill slit *n.* One of several rudimentary invaginations in the embryonic surface, present during development of air-breathing vertebrates and corresponding to the functional gill slits of aquatic species.

gin·gi·va (jĭn′jə-və, jĭn-jī′-) *n., pl.* **–vae** (-vē′) See **gum**[2]. —**gin′gi·val** (jĭn′jə-vəl, jĭn-jī′-) *adj.*

Gingival Index *n. Abbr.* **GI** An index of periodontal disease that relates to the severity and location of the lesion.

gingival crevice *n.* See **gingival sulcus.**

gingival margin *n.* The top edge or crest of the gingiva surrounding a tooth.

gingival massage *n.* Stimulation of the gingiva by rubbing or rhythmic pressure.

Gingival-Periodontal Index *n. Abbr.* **GPI** An index of gingivitis, gingival irritation, and advanced periodontal disease.

gingival sulcus *n.* The narrow space or groove between the surface of the tooth and the free gingiva. Also called *gingival crevice, subgingival space.*

gin·gi·vec·to·my (jĭn′jə-vĕk′tə-mē) *n.* Surgical removal of gum tissue. Also called *gum resection.*

gin·gi·vi·tis (jĭn′jə-vī′tĭs) *n.* Inflammation of the gums, characterized by redness and swelling.

gingivo– *or* **gingiv–** *pref.* Gingiva: *gingivoplasty.*

gin·gi·vo·glos·si·tis (jĭn′jə-vō-glô-sī′tĭs) *n.* Inflammation of the tongue and the gums.

gin·gi·vo·lin·guo·ax·i·al (jĭn′jə-vō-lĭng′gwō-ăk′sē-əl) *adj.* Of or relating to the angle formed by the gingival, lingual, and axial walls of a cavity.

gin·gi·vo·os·se·ous (jĭn′jə-vō-ŏs′ē-əs) *adj.* Of or relating to the gum tissue and its underlying bone.

gin·gi·vo·plas·ty (jĭn′jə-vō-plăs′tē) *n.* The surgical reshaping and recontouring of the gum tissue for cosmetic, physiological, or functional purposes.

gin·gi·vo·sis (jĭn′jə-vō′sĭs) *n.* See **chronic desquamative gingivitis.**

gin·gi·vo·sto·ma·ti·tis (jĭn′jə-vō-stō′mə-tī′tĭs) *n.* Inflammation of the gums and the mucous membrane of the oral cavity.

gin·gly·form (jĭng′glə-fôrm, gĭng′-) *adj.* Ginglymoid.

gin·gly·mo·ar·thro·di·al (jĭng′glə-mō-är-thrō′dē-əl, gĭng′-) *adj.* Relating to or resembling a hinge joint and a sliding joint.

gin·gly·moid (jĭng′glə-moid′, gĭng′-) *adj.* Of, relating to, or resembling a hinge joint, such as the elbow.

ginglymoid joint *n.* See **hinge joint.**

gin·gly·mus (jĭng′glə-məs, gĭng′-) *n.* A hinge joint.

gink·go (gĭng′kō) *n.* A deciduous tree (*Ginkgo biloba*) native to China, from whose leaves an extract is prepared that is thought by some to have curative properties.

GIP *abbr.* gastric inhibitory polypeptide

gir·dle (gûr′dl) *n.* **1.** Something that encircles like a belt. **2.** An elasticized, flexible undergarment worn over the waist and hips. **3.** The pelvic or pectoral girdle.

girdle anesthesia *n.* Anesthesia distributed as a band encircling the abdomen.

girdle sensation *n.* See **zonesthesia.**

git·a·lin (jĭt′l-ĭn, jĭ-tā′lĭn, -tăl′ĭn) *n.* **1.** A crystalline glycoside obtained from digitalis. **2.** An amorphous mixture of the glycosides obtained from digitalis.

gla·bel·la (glə-bĕl′ə) *n., pl.* **–bel·lae** (-bĕl′ē) **1.** The smooth area between the eyebrows just above the nose. **2.** The most forward projecting point of the forehead in the midline of the supraorbital ridges. Also called *mesophryon.*

gla·brate (glā′brāt′, -brĭt) *adj.* Glabrous.

gla·brous (glā′brəs) *adj.* Having no hairs or projections, especially on body parts that normally have hair; smooth.

glad·i·o·lus (glăd′ē-ō′ləs) *n., pl.* **–lus·es** *or* **–li** (-lī) The large middle section of the sternum.

gland (glănd) *n.* **1.** A cell, a group of cells, or an organ that produces a secretion for use in or for elimination from the body. **2.** Any of various organs, such as lymph nodes, that resemble true glands but perform a nonsecretory function.

glan·di·lem·ma (glăn′də-lĕm′ə) *n.* The capsule of a gland.

gland of auditory tube *n.* Any of the mucus-secreting glands situated near the pharyngeal end of the eustachian tube.

gland of Moll *n.* See **ciliary gland.**

glan·du·la (glăn′jə-lə) *n., pl.* **–lae** (-lē′) A small gland.

glandula glom·i·for·mis (glŏm′ə-fôr′mēz) *n.* Any of the tubular glands of the skin that have a blind extremity coiled into the form of a ball or glomerulus.

glan·du·lar (glăn′jə-lər) *adj.* **1.** Of, relating to, affecting, or resembling a gland or its secretion. **2.** Functioning as a gland. **3.** Having glands. **4.** Resulting from the abnormal function of a gland or glands.

glandular epithelium *n.* Epithelium made up of cells that produce secretions.

glan·dule (glăn′jōōl) *n.* A small gland.

glan·du·lous (glăn′jə-ləs) *adj.* Glandular.

glans (glănz) *n., pl.* **glan·des** (glăn′dēz) **1.** A conical vascular body forming the distal end of the penis. **2.** A conical vascular body forming the distal end of the clitoris.

glans cli·tor·i·dis (klĭ-tôr′ĭ-dĭs, klī-) *n.* The small mass of erectile tissue at the tip of the clitoris.

glans penis *n.* The conical expansion of the corpus spongiosum that forms the head of the penis.

Glanz·mann's thrombasthenia (glănz′mənz, glänts′-mänz) *n.* An inherited hemorrhagic disorder characterized by normal or prolonged bleeding time, normal coagulation time but defective clot retraction, and normal platelet count but morphologic or functional abnormality of platelets. Also called *Glanzmann's disease.*

gla·se·ri·an fissure (glă-zîr′ē-ən) *n.* See **petrotympanic fissure.**

Glas·gow Coma Scale (glăs′gō) *n.* A scale for measuring level of consciousness, especially after a head injury, in which scoring is determined by three factors: amount of eye opening, verbal responsiveness, and motor responsiveness.

glass (glăs) *n.* **1.** Any of a large class of materials with highly variable mechanical and optical properties that solidify from the molten state without crystallization, are typically made by silicates fusing with boric oxide, aluminum oxide, or phosphorus pentoxide, are generally hard, brittle, and transparent or translucent, and are considered to be supercooled liquids rather than true solids. **2.** Something usually made of glass, such as a window, mirror, or drinking vessel. **3. glasses** A pair of lenses mounted in a light frame, used to correct faulty vision or protect the eyes. Also called *spectacles.* **4.** A device, such as a monocle or spyglass, containing a lens or lenses and used as an aid to vision.

glass eye *n.* **1.** An artificial eye fashioned of glass. **2.** An eye whose iris is whitish, pale, or colorless.

glass·y degeneration (glăs′ē) *n.* See **hyaline degeneration.**

glassy membrane *n.* **1.** A clear, highly refractive basement membrane between the granular layer and the internal capsule of a maturing ovarian follicle. **2.** See **hyaline membrane.**

Glau·ber's salt (glou′bərz) *n.* A colorless hydrated sodium sulfate used as a cathartic and diuretic.

glau·co·ma (glou-kō′mə, glô-) *n.* Any of a group of eye diseases characterized by abnormally high intraocular fluid pressure, damaged optic disk, hardening of the eyeball, and partial to complete loss of vision. —**glau·co′ma·tous** (-kō′mə-təs) *adj.*

glaucomatous cataract *n.* A nuclear opacity usually seen in absolute glaucoma.

glaucomatous cup *n.* A deep depression of the optic disk caused by glaucoma. Also called *glaucomatous excavation.*

glaucomatous halo *n.* **1.** A yellowish ring surrounding the optic disk, indicating atrophy of the choroid in glaucoma. **2.** A circle of illumination seen around lights, caused by corneal edema in glaucoma.

GLC *abbr.* gas-liquid chromatography

gleet (glēt) *n.* **1.** Inflammation of the urethra resulting from chronic gonorrhea and characterized by a mucopurulent discharge. **2.** The discharge that is characteristic of this inflammation. Also called *medorrhea.* —**gleet′y** *adj.*

Glenn's operation (glĕnz) *n.* Surgical anastomosis between the superior vena cava and the right main pulmonary artery to increase pulmonary blood flow as a correction for tricuspid atresia.

gle·no·hu·mer·al ligament (glē′nō-hyōō′mər-əl, glĕn′-ō-) *n.* Any of three fibrous bands that reinforce the articular capsule of the shoulder joint and are attached to the margin of the glenoid cavity of the scapula and to the neck of the humerus.

gle·noid (glē′noid′, glĕn′oid′) *adj.* Relating to the articular depression of the scapula entering into the formation of the shoulder joint.

glenoid cavity *n.* The hollow in the head of the scapula into which the head of the humerus sits to make the shoulder joint. Also called *glenoid fossa.*

gli·a (glē′ə, glī′ə) *n.* See **neuroglia.**

glia cell *n.* Any of the cells of the neuroglia; a glial cell.

gli·a·din (glī′ə-dĭn) *n.* Any of a class of simple proteins separable from wheat and rye glutens.

gli·al cell (glē′əl, glī′əl) *n.* Any of the cells making up the neuroglia, especially the astrocytes, oligodendroglia, and microglia.

glid·ing joint (glī′dĭng) *n.* See **plane joint.**

glio– *or* **gli–** *pref.* Neuroglia: *glioma.*

gli·o·blast (glē′ə-blăst′, glī′-) *n.* An early neural cell developing from the early ependymal cell of the neural tube.

gli·o·blas·to·ma (glē′ō-blă-stō′mə, glī′-) *n.* A glioma consisting chiefly of undifferentiated anaplastic cells frequently arranged radially about an irregular focus of necrosis, usually occurring in the cerebrum of adults. Also called *grade IV astrocytoma.*

glioblastoma mul·ti·for·me (mŭl′tə-fôr′mē) *n.* A virulent brain cancer that is usually fatal.

gli·o·ma (glē-ō′mə, glī-) *n.*, *pl.* **-mas** *or* **-ma·ta** (-mə-tə) A tumor that originates in the neuroglia of the brain or the spinal cord. —**gli·om′a·tous** (-ŏm′ə-təs, -ō′mə-) *adj.*

gli·o·ma·to·sis (glē-ō′mə-tō′sĭs, glī-) *n.* Neoplastic growth of neuroglial cells in the brain or spinal cord, especially one of relatively large size or having multiple foci. Also called *neurogliomatosis.*

gli·o·neu·ro·ma (glē′ō-nōō-rō′mə, glī′-) *n.* A ganglioneuroma derived from neurons, containing numerous glial cells and fibers in the matrix.

gli·o·sar·co·ma (glē′ō-sär-kō′mə, glī′-) *n.* A glioma consisting of immature, undifferentiated, pleomorphic, spindle-shaped cells with hyperchromatic nuclei and poorly formed fibrillary processes.

gli·o·sis (glē-ō′sĭs, glī-) *n.* Excessive proliferation of the neuroglia.

glip·i·zide (glĭp′ĭ-zīd′) *n.* An oral sulfonylurea having hypoglycemic activity and used therapeutically as an antidiabetic.

glis·so·ni·tis (glĭs′ə-nī′tĭs) *n.* Inflammation of Glisson's capsule.

Glis·son's capsule (glĭs′ənz) *n.* See **perivascular fibrous capsule.**

glob·al (glō′bəl) *adj.* **1.** Having the shape of a globe; spherical. **2.** Of or involving the entire earth; worldwide. **3.** Comprehensive; total. **4.** Of or relating to the eyeball. —**glob′al·ly** *adv.*

global aphasia *n.* The loss of the ability to express and understand speech and other forms of communication. Also called *total aphasia.*

glo·bin (glō′bĭn) *n.* The protein that is a constituent of hemoglobin. Also called *hematohiston.*

glo·boid cell leukodystrophy (glō′boid′) *n.* An inherited metabolic encephalopathy of infancy with rapidly progressive cerebral degeneration, massive loss of myelin, severe astrocytic gliosis, and infiltration of the white matter with characteristic multinucleate globoid cells. Also called *Krabbe's disease.*

glo·bo·side (glō′bə-sīd′) *n.* A glycosphingolipid, especially a ceramide tetrasaccharide, that is found in the kidneys, red blood cells, blood serum, liver, and spleen, and, in one form of gangliosidosis, accumulates in tissues.

glob·ule (glŏb′yōōl) *n.* A small spherical body, especially a drop of liquid. —**glob′u·lar** (-yə-lər) *adj.*

glob·u·lin (glŏb′yə-lĭn) *n.* Any of a family of proteins that are precipitated from plasma by ammonium sulfate and may be further fractionated into many subgroups that differ with respect to associated lipids or carbohydrates.

glob·u·li·nu·ri·a (glŏb′yə-lə-nŏŏr′ē-ə) *n.* Excretion of globulin in the urine.

glo·bus (glō′bəs) *n., pl.* **–bi** (-bī′) **1.** A round or spherical body. **2.** Any of the brown bodies sometimes found in the granulomatous lesions of leprosy.

globus hys·ter·i·cus (hĭ-stĕr′ĭ-kəs) *n.* A sensation as of having a lump or ball in the throat, symptomatic of hysteria.

globus pal·li·dus (păl′ĭ-dəs) *n.* The inner and lighter gray portion of the lentiform nucleus of the brain. Also called *pallidum.*

glo·mal (glō′məl) *adj.* Of or involving a glomus.

glo·man·gi·o·ma (glō-măn′jē-ō′mə, glō′măn-) *n.* See **glomus tumor.**

glo·man·gi·o·sis (glō-măn′jē-ō′sĭs, glō′măn-) *n.* The occurrence of multiple complexes of small vascular channels, each resembling a glomus.

glo·mec·to·my (glō-mĕk′tə-mē) *n.* Excision of a glomus tumor.

glo·mer·u·lar (glō-mĕr′yə-lər) *adj.* Relating to or affecting a glomerulus or the glomeruli.

glomerular filtration rate *n. Abbr.* **GFR** The volume of water filtered out of the plasma through glomerular capillary walls into Bowman's capsules per unit of time.

glomerular nephritis *n.* See **glomerulonephritis.**

glom·er·ule (glŏm′ə-rōōl′, glŏm′yə-) *n.* A glomerulus. —**glo·mer′u·late** (glō-mĕr′yə-lĭt) *adj.*

glo·mer·u·li·tis (glō-mĕr′yə-lī′tĭs) *n.* Inflammation of a glomerulus, especially of the renal glomeruli, as in glomerulonephritis.

glo·mer·u·lo·ne·phri·tis (glō-mĕr′yə-lō-nə-frī′tĭs) *n.* Renal disease that is marked by bilateral inflammatory changes in glomeruli that are not the result of kidney infection. Also called *glomerular nephritis.*

glo·mer·u·lop·a·thy (glō-mĕr′yə-lŏp′ə-thē) *n.* Disease of the renal glomeruli.

glo·mer·u·lo·sa cell (glō-mĕr′yə-lō′sə, -zə) *n.* A cell of the zona glomerulosa of the adrenal cortex that is the source of aldosterone.

glo·mer·u·lo·scle·ro·sis (glō-mĕr′yə-lō-sklə-rō′sĭs) *n.* Hyaline deposits or scarring within the renal glomeruli, a degenerative process occurring in association with renal arteriosclerosis or diabetes.

glo·mer·u·lus (glō-mĕr′yə-ləs) *n., pl.* **–li** (-lī′) **1.** A small cluster or intertwined mass. **2.** A tuft of capillaries situated within a Bowman's capsule at the end of a renal tubule in the vertebrate kidney that filters waste products from the blood and thus initiates urine formation. **3.** The twisted secretory portion of a sweat gland. **4.** A nerve ending consisting of a cluster of dendritic ramifications and axon terminals surrounded by a glial sheath.

glo·mus (glō′məs) *n., pl.* **glom·er·a** (glŏm′ər-ə) **1.** A small globular body. **2.** A small body surrounded by many nerve fibers, consisting of an anastomosis between fine arterioles and veins and functioning as a regulation mechanism in the flow of blood, control of temperature, and conservation of heat in a particular organ or part.

glomus cho·roi·de·um (kô-roi′dē-əm, kə-) *n.* The marked enlargement of the choroid plexus of the lateral ventricle of the brain at the junction of the central part with the inferior horn.

glomus jug·u·lar·e (jŭg′yə-lâr′ē) *n.* A microscopic collection of chemoreceptor tissue in the adventitia of the bulb of the jugular vein.

glomus jugulare tumor *n.* See **chemodectoma.**

glomus tumor *n.* A painful tumor composed of specialized pericytes that are usually arranged in single encapsulated nodular masses that occur almost exclusively in the skin. Also called *angiomyoneuroma, angioneuromyoma, glomangioma.*

glos·sa (glô′sə) *n., pl.* **glos·sas** *or* **glos·sae** (glô′sē) The tongue.

glos·sal (glô′səl) *adj.* Of or relating to the tongue.

glos·sal·gia (glô-săl′jə) *n.* See **glossodynia.**

glos·sec·to·my (glô-sĕk′tə-mē) *n.* Excision or amputation of the tongue. Also called *lingulectomy.*

Glos·si·na (glô-sī′nə) *n.* A genus of bloodsucking dipterous flies comprising the tsetse flies of tropical and subtropical Africa; they serve as vectors of the pathogenic trypanosomes that cause various forms of African trypanosomiasis.

glos·si·tis (glô-sī′tĭs) *n.* Inflammation of the tongue. —**glos·sit′ic** (-sĭt′ĭk) *adj.*

glossitis ar·e·a·ta ex·fo·li·a·ti·va (âr′ē-ā′tə ĕks-fō′lē-ə-tī′və) *n.* Geographical tongue.

glosso– *or* **gloss–** *pref.* Tongue: *glossospasm.*

glos·so·cele (glôs′ə-sēl′) *n.* Protrusion of the tongue from the mouth due to its excessive size.

glos·so·dyn·i·a (glôs′ō-dĭn′ē-ə) *n.* A burning or painful sensation in the tongue. Also called *glossalgia.*

glos·so·ep·i·glot·tic (glô′sō-ĕp′ĭ-glŏt′ĭk) *or* **glos·so·ep·i·glot·tid·e·an** (-glō-tĭd′ē-ən) *adj.* Relating to the tongue and the epiglottis.

glos·so·hy·al (glô′sō-hī′əl) *adj.* Hyoglossal.

glos·so·la·li·a (glô′sə-lā′lē-ə) *n.* Fabricated, nonmeaningful speech, especially associated with trances or certain schizophrenic syndromes.

glos·sop·a·thy (glô-sŏp′ə-thē) *n.* A disease of the tongue.

glos·so·pha·ryn·geal (glôs′ō-fə-rĭn′jəl, -făr′ən-jē′əl) *adj.* Relating to the tongue and pharynx.

glossopharyngeal breathing *n.* Respiration unaided by the primary muscles of respiration, the air being forced into the lungs by use of the tongue and muscles of the pharynx.

glossopharyngeal nerve *n.* Either of a pair of nerves that emerge from the medulla, supply sensation to the pharynx and the back third of the tongue, and carry motor fibers to the stylopharyngeal muscle and parasympathetic fibers to the otic ganglion. Also called *ninth cranial nerve.*

glos·so·plas·ty (glô′sə-plăs′tē) *n.* Reparative or plastic surgery of the tongue.

glos·sor·rha·phy (glô-sôr′ə-fē) *n.* Suture of a wound of the tongue.

glos·so·spasm (glô′sə-spăz′əm) *n.* Spasmodic contraction of the tongue.

glos·sot·o·my (glô-sŏt′ə-mē) *n.* Incision of the tongue.

glos·so·trich·i·a (glô′sō-trĭk′ē-ə) *n.* See **hairy tongue.**

glot·tal (glŏt′l) *adj.* Of or relating to the glottis.

glot·tic (glŏt′ĭk) *adj.* **1.** Of or relating to the tongue. **2.** Of or relating to the glottis.

glot·tis (glŏt′ĭs) *n.,* pl. **glot·tis·es** or **glot·ti·des** (glŏt′-ĭ-dēz′) The vocal apparatus of the larynx, consisting of the true vocal cords and the rima glottidis.

glot·ti·tis (glŏ-tī′tĭs) *n.* Inflammation of the glottic portion of the larynx.

glove anesthesia (glŭv) *n.* Loss of sensation in an area that would be covered by a glove.

glove box *n.* An enclosed workspace equipped with gloved openings that allow manipulation in the interior, designed to prevent contamination of the product, the environment, or the worker.

glov·er's suture (glŭv′ərz) *n.* A continuous suture in which each stitch is passed through the loop of the preceding one.

Glu *abbr.* glutamic acid; glutamine

glu·ca·gon (gloo′kə-gŏn′) *n.* A polypeptide hormone secreted by alpha cells that initiates a rise in blood sugar levels by stimulating the breakdown of glycogen by the liver.

glu·ca·go·no·ma (gloo′kə-gŏ-nō′mə) *n.* A glucagon-secreting tumor, usually derived from pancreatic islet cells.

glu·can (gloo′kăn′, -kən) *n.* A polysaccharide, such as cellulose, that is a polymer of glucose.

gluco– or **gluc–** *pref.* Glucose: *glucagon.*

glu·co·cer·e·bro·side (gloo′kō-sĕr′ə-brə-sīd′, -sə-rē′-) *n.* See **glucosylceramide.**

glu·co·cor·ti·coid (gloo′kō-kôr′tĭ-koid′) *n.* Any of a group of anti-inflammatory steroidlike compounds, such as hydrocortisone, that are produced by the adrenal cortex, are involved in carbohydrate, protein, and fat metabolism, and are used as anti-inflammatory agents. —**glu′co·cor′ti·coid′** *adj.*

glu·co·fu·ra·nose (gloo′kō-fyoŏr′ə-nōs′) *n.* A cyclic glucose in which an oxygen atom links carbons located at particular positions in the ring.

glu·co·gen·e·sis (gloo′kō-jĕn′ĭ-sĭs) *n.* The formation of glucose through the breakdown of glycogen. —**glu′-co·gen′ic** *adj.*

glu·co·ki·nase (gloo′kō-kī′nās′, -nāz′, -kĭn′ās′, -āz′) *n.* A liver enzyme that uses ATP to catalyze the phosphorylation of glucose to glucose-6-phosphate during glycogenesis.

glu·co·ki·net·ic (gloo′kō-kə-nĕt′ĭk, -kī-) *adj.* Having the ability to activate glucose, especially by breaking down stored glycogen so as to increase glucose concentrations in the blood.

glu·co·lip·id (gloo′kō-lĭp′ĭd, -lī′pĭd) *n.* Any of various glycolipids that contain glucose.

Glucometer (gloo-kŏm′ĭ-tər) A trademark for a portable monitor used to measure blood glucose levels.

glu·co·ne·o·gen·e·sis (gloo′kə-nē′ə-jĕn′ĭ-sĭs) *n.* The formation of glucose, especially by the liver, from non-carbohydrate sources, such as amino acids. Also called *glyconeogenesis.*

glu·con·ic acid (gloo-kŏn′ĭk) *n.* An acid formed from the oxidation of glucose and other sugars.

Glu·co·phage (gloo′kō-fāj′) A trademark for the drug metformin.

glu·co·pro·tein (gloo′kō-prō′tēn′) *n.* A glycoprotein in which glucose is the carbohydrate.

glu·co·py·ra·nose (gloo′kō-pī′rə-nōs′) *n.* A cyclic form of glucose containing a pyranose ring.

glu·co·sa·mine (gloo-kō′sə-mēn′, gloo′kō-sə-mēn′) *n.* An amino derivative of glucose that is found especially in polysaccharides such as chitin and in cell membranes.

glu·co·san (gloo′kə-săn′) *n.* **1.** A polysaccharide yielding glucose upon hydrolysis. **2.** Any of several anhydrides of glucose.

glu·cose (gloo′kōs′) *n.* A monosaccharide sugar in the blood that serves as the major energy source of the body; it occurs in most plant and animal tissue. Also called *blood sugar.*

glucose-6-phosphatase *n.* A liver enzyme that catalyzes the hydrolysis of glucose-6-phosphate to glucose and inorganic phosphate, thus allowing glucose in the liver to enter the blood.

glucose-6-phosphate *n.* An essential intermediate formed from glucose and ATP during the metabolism of glucose.

glucose-6-phosphate dehydrogenase *n.* An enzyme that catalyzes the oxidation of glucose-6-phosphate during glucose metabolism.

glucose oxidase method *n.* A highly specific method for measuring glucose in serum or plasma by reacting the test fluid with glucose oxidase in which gluconic acid and hydrogen peroxide are formed.

glu·cose·phos·phate isomerase deficiency (gloo′kōs-fŏs′fāt′) *n.* An inherited enzyme deficiency characterized by chronic homolytic anemia. Also called *phosphohexose isomerase deficiency.*

glucose tolerance test *n.* A test for evaluating the body's capability to metabolize glucose and based upon the ability of the liver to absorb and store excess glucose as glycogen.

glucose transport maximum *n.* The maximal rate of reabsorption of glucose from the glomerular filtrate.

glu·co·si·dase (gloo-kō′sĭ-dās′, -dāz′) *n.* Any of various enzymes that catalyze glucoside hydrolysis.

glu·co·side (gloo′kə-sīd′) *n.* A glycoside, the sugar component of which is glucose. —**glu′co·sid′ic** (-sĭd′-ĭk) *adj.*

glu·co·su·ri·a (gloo′kə-soŏr′ē-ə, -shoŏr′-) *n.* Excretion of glucose in the urine, especially in elevated quantities. Also called *glycosuria.*

glu·co·syl·cer·a·mide (gloo′kə-sĭl-sə-răm′īd′, -sûr′ə-mīd′) *n.* A glycolipid containing a fatty acid, glucose, and sphingosine. Also called *glucocerebroside.*

glu·co·syl·trans·fer·ase (glo͞o′kə-sĭl-trăns′fə-rās′, -rāz′) *n.* Any of various enzymes that catalyze the transfer of glucosyl groups from one compound to another compound.

Glu·co·trol (glo͞o′kə-trōl′) A trademark for the drug glipizide.

glu·cu·ro·nate (glo͞o-kyo͝or′ə-nāt′) *n.* A salt or ester of glucuronic acid.

glu·cu·ron·ic acid (glo͞o′kyə-rŏn′ĭk) *n.* The uronic acid of glucose that conjugates various substances in the liver so as to detoxify or inactivate them.

glu·cu·ron·i·dase (glo͞o′kyə-rŏn′ĭ-dās′, -dāz′) *n.* An enzyme that catalyzes the hydrolysis of various glucuronides, especially one that catalyzes the hydrolysis of the beta form of a glucuronide.

glu·cu·ro·nide (glo͞o-kyo͝or′ə-nīd′) *n.* Any of various derivatives of glucuronic acid that often combine with toxic organic compounds and are excreted.

glue-sniffing *n.* The inhalation of fumes from plastic cements, the solvents of which, such as toluene, xylene, and benzene, induce central nervous system stimulation followed by depression.

glu·ta·mate (glo͞o′tə-māt′) *n.* **1.** A salt of glutamic acid. **2.** An ester of glutamic acid.

glu·tam·ic acid (glo͞o-tăm′ĭk) *n.* *Abbr.* **Glu** A nonessential amino acid occurring widely in plant and animal tissue and having a salt, monosodium glutamate, that is used as a flavor-intensifying seasoning.

glutamic-oxaloacetic transaminase *n.* *Abbr.* **GOT** See SGOT.

glutamic-pyruvic transaminase *n.* *Abbr.* **GPT** See SGPT.

glu·tam·i·nase (glo͞o-tăm′ə-nās′) *n.* An enzyme found in kidneys and in other tissues that catalyzes the breakdown of glutamine to ammonia and glutamic acid.

glu·ta·mine (glo͞o′tə-mēn′) *n.* *Abbr.* **Glu** A nonessential amino acid that occurs widely in proteins and blood and other tissue and is metabolized to yield urinary ammonia. Also called *glutaminic acid.*

glu·tam·i·nyl (glo͞o-tăm′ə-nĭl) *n.* The univalent radical $C_5H_9N_2O_2$ of glutamine.

glu·tam·o·yl (glo͞o-tăm′ō-ĭl) *n.* The divalent radical $C_5H_7NO_2$ of glutamic acid.

glu·tam·yl (glo͞o-tăm′əl, glo͞o′tə-mĭl′) *n.* The radical $OCCH_2CH_2CH(NH_2)CO$ of glutamic acid.

glu·tar·ic acid (glo͞o-tăr′ĭk) *n.* An acid formed during the catabolism of tryptophan.

glu·ta·thi·one (glo͞o′tə-thī′ōn′) *n.* A tripeptide of the amino acids glycine, cystine, and glutamic acid occurring widely in plant and animal tissues and forming reduced and oxidized forms important in biological oxidation-reduction reactions.

glu·te·al (glo͞o′tē-əl, glo͞o-tē′-) *adj.* Of or relating to the buttocks.

gluteal artery *n.* **1.** An artery with origin in the internal iliac artery, with distribution to the hip joint and gluteal region; inferior gluteal artery. **2.** An artery with origin in the internal iliac artery, with distribution to the gluteal region; superior gluteal artery.

gluteal fold *n.* A prominent fold on the back of the upper thigh that marks the upper limit of the thigh from the lower limit of the buttock.

gluteal furrow *n.* The groove between the buttock and thigh.

glu·ten (glo͞ot′n) *n.* A mixture of insoluble plant proteins occurring in cereal grains, chiefly corn and wheat, used as an adhesive and as a flour substitute.

gluten enteropathy *n.* See celiac disease.

gluten-sensitive enteropathy *n.* See celiac disease.

glu·te·o·fem·o·ral (glo͞o′tē-ō-fĕm′ər-əl) *adj.* Relating to the buttocks and the thighs.

gluteofemoral bursa *n.* See intermuscular gluteal bursa.

glu·te·o·in·gui·nal (glo͞o′tē-ō-ĭng′gwə-nəl) *adj.* Relating to the buttocks and the groin.

glu·teth·i·mide (glo͞o-tĕth′ə-mīd′) *n.* A nonbarbiturate sedative and hypnotic drug.

glu·te·us (glo͞o′tē-əs, glo͞o-tē′-) *n.*, *pl.* **glu·te·i** (glo͞o′-tē-ī′, glo͞o-tē′ī′) Any of the three large muscles of each buttock, especially the gluteus maximus, that extend, abduct, and rotate the thigh.

gluteus max·i·mus (măk′sə-məs) *n.* A muscle with origin from the ilium, the sacrum and the coccyx, and the sacrotuberous ligament, with insertion to the iliotibial band of the broad fascia and the gluteal ridge of the femur, with nerve supply from the inferior gluteal nerve, and whose action extends the thigh.

gluteus me·di·us (mē′dē-əs) *n.* A muscle with origin in the ilium, with insertion to the surface of the greater trochanter, with nerve supply from the superior gluteal nerve, and whose action abducts and rotates the thigh.

gluteus min·i·mus (mĭn′ə-məs) *n.* A muscle with origin from the ilium, with insertion to the greater trochanter, with nerve supply from the superior gluteal nerve, and whose action abducts the thigh.

glu·ti·nous (glo͞ot′n-əs) *adj.* Adhesive; sticky. —**glu′ti·nous·ness, glu′ti·nos′i·ty** (-ŏs′ĭ-tē) *n.*

glu·ti·tis (glo͞o-tī′tĭs) *n.* Inflammation of the muscles of the buttock.

Gly *abbr.* glycine

gly·bu·ride (glī′byo͝or-īd′) *n.* A sulfonylurea drug used to treat non-insulin-dependent diabetes mellitus.

gly·can (glī′kăn′, -kən) *n.* See polysaccharide.

gly·ce·mi·a (glī-sē′mē-ə) *n.* The presence of glucose in the blood.

gly·ce·mic index (glī-sē′mĭk) *n.* An index that measures the ability of a given food to elevate blood sugar.

glyc·er·al·de·hyde (glĭs′ə-răl′də-hīd′) *n.* A sweet colorless crystalline solid that is an intermediate compound in carbohydrate metabolism.

gly·cer·ic acid (glĭ-sĕr′ĭk) *n.* A colorless syrupy acid obtained from oxidation of glycerol.

glyceric aciduria *n.* A metabolic disorder caused by an enzyme deficiency, resulting in the excretion of glyceric and oxalic acids in the urine and ultimately leading to oxalosis.

glyc·er·i·dase (glĭs′ər-ĭ-dās′, -dāz′) *n.* Any of various enzymes that catalyze the hydrolysis of glycerides.

glyc·er·ide (glĭs′ə-rīd′) *n.* A natural or synthetic ester of glycerol and fatty acids.

glyc·er·in *or* **glyc·er·ine** (glĭs′ər-ĭn) *n.* Glycerol or a preparation of glycerol.

glyc·er·ol (glĭs′ə-rôl′, -rōl′) *n.* A sweet syrupy fluid obtained by the saponification of fats and fixed oils, used as a solvent, a skin emollient, and as a vehicle and sweetening agent; it is also used by injection or in suppository form for constipation and orally to reduce ocular tension.

glyc·er·yl (glĭs′ər-əl) *n.* A trivalent radical obtained from glycerol by the removal of hydroxyl groups.

gly·cine (glī′sēn′, -sĭn) *n. Abbr.* **Gly** A nonessential amino acid derived from the alkaline hydrolysis of gelatin and used as a nutrient and dietary supplement, also used in biochemical research and in the treatment of certain myopathies.

glycine am·i·di·no·trans·fer·ase (ăm′ĭ-dē′nō-trăns′-fə-rās′, -rāz′, ăm′ĭ-dĭn′ō-) *n.* An enzyme that catalyzes the transfer of an amidine group from arginine to glycine during creatine synthesis.

gly·ci·nu·ri·a (glī′sə-nŏŏr′ē-ə) *n.* The presence of large amounts of glycine in the urine, associated with certain kidney disorders.

glyco– *pref.* **1.** Sugar: *glycoprotein.* **2.** Glycogen: *glycogenesis.*

gly·co·ca·lyx (glī′kō-kā′lĭks, -kăl′ĭks) *n.* An outer filamentous coating of carbohydrate-rich molecules on the surface of certain cells.

gly·co·cho·late (glī′kō-kō′lāt′, -kōl′āt′) *n.* A salt or ester of glycocholic acid.

gly·co·cho·lic acid (glī′kō-kō′lĭk) *n.* A crystalline acid occurring in bile and formed through the conjugation of cholic acid and glycine.

gly·co·gen (glī′kə-jən) *n.* A polysaccharide that is the main form of carbohydrate storage in animals and occurs mainly in liver and muscle tissue; it is readily converted to glucose. Also called *animal starch.* —**gly′co·gen′ic** (-jĕn′ĭk) *adj.*

glycogen acanthosis *n.* Elevated gray-white plaques in the distal mucosa of the esophagus, with epithelium thickened by the proliferation of large glycogen-filled squamous cells.

gly·co·gen·e·sis (glī′kə-jĕn′ĭ-sĭs) *n.* The formation of glycogen. —**gly′co·ge·net′ic** (-jə-nĕt′ĭk) *adj.*

glycogen granule *n.* A granule of glycogen occurring in a cell as an alpha granule or a beta granule.

gly·co·gen·ol·y·sis (glī′kə-jə-nŏl′ĭ-sĭs) *n.* The hydrolysis of glycogen to glucose. —**gly′co·gen′o·lyt′ic** (-jĕn′-ə-lĭt′ĭk) *adj.*

gly·co·ge·no·sis (glī′kə-jə-nō′sĭs) *n.* Any of various inheritable diseases caused by enzyme deficiencies and characterized by the abnormal accumulation of glycogen in tissue. Also called *dextrinosis, glycogen storage disease.*

gly·cog·e·nous (glī-kŏj′ə-nəs) *adj.* Relating to glycogenesis; glycogenetic.

glycogen storage disease *n.* See **glycogenosis.**

glycogen synthase *n.* An enzyme that catalyzes the transfer of glucose from UDP-glucose to glycogen.

gly·col (glī′kôl′, -kōl′) *n.* **1.** Any of various alcohols containing two hydroxyl groups. **2.** Ethylene glycol.

gly·col·al·de·hyde (glī′kôl-ăl′də-hīd′, -kōl-) *n.* A diose believed to be an intermediate in the metabolism of carbohydrates and proteins.

gly·col·ic acid (glī-kŏl′ĭk) *n.* A colorless crystalline compound found in sugar beets, cane sugar, and unripe grapes that is used in pharmaceuticals and pesticides.

glycolic aciduria *n.* Excessive excretion of glycolic acid in the urine.

gly·co·lip·id (glī′kə-lĭp′ĭd) *n.* A lipid, such as a cerebroside, that contains carbohydrate groups.

gly·co·lyl (glī′kə-lĭl′) *n.* The univalent radical, $HOCH_2CO$, of glycolic acid.

gly·col·y·sis (glī-kŏl′ə-sĭs) *n.* The ATP-generating metabolic process of most cells in which carbohydrates are converted to pyruvic acid. —**gly′co·lyt′ic** (glī′kə-lĭt′ĭk) *adj.*

gly·co·ne·o·gen·e·sis (glī′kə-nē′ə-jĕn′ĭ-sĭs) *n.* See **gluconeogenesis.**

gly·co·pe·ni·a (glī′kə-pē′nē-ə) *n.* A deficiency of any or all sugars in an organ or a tissue.

gly·co·pep·tide (glī′kō-pĕp′tīd′) *n.* Glycoprotein.

gly·co·phil·i·a (glī′kə-fĭl′ē-ə) *n.* A condition in which there is a distinct tendency to develop hyperglycemia after ingestion of glucose.

gly·co·pro·tein (glī′kō-prō′tēn′) *n.* Any of a group of conjugated proteins that contain a carbohydrate as the nonprotein component.

gly·co·pty·a·lism (glī′kō-tī′ə-lĭz′əm) *n.* See **glycosialia.**

gly·co·pyr·ro·late (glī′kō-pîr′ə-lāt′) *n.* A parasympatholytic compound used as premedication to general anesthesia, as an antagonist to the bradycardic effects of neostigmine during curare reversal, and as an adjunct in the treatment of peptic ulcer.

gly·cor·rha·chi·a (glī′kə-rā′kē-ə, -răk′ē-ə) *n.* The presence of sugar in the cerebrospinal fluid.

gly·cor·rhe·a (glī′kə-rē′ə) *n.* Discharge of sugar from the body, as in glucosuria, especially in unusually large quantities.

gly·cos·a·mi·no·gly·can (glī′kōs-ə-mē′nō-glī′kăn′) *n.* See **mucopolysaccharide.**

gly·co·se·cre·to·ry (glī′kō-sĭ-krē′tə-rē) *adj.* Causing or involved in the secretion of glycogen.

gly·co·si·a·li·a (glī′kō-sī-ā′lē-ə, -ăl′ē-ə) *n.* Sugar in the saliva. Also called *glycoptyalism.*

gly·co·si·a·lor·rhe·a (glī′kō-sī′ə-lō-rē′ə) *n.* An excessive secretion of saliva that contains sugar.

gly·co·side (glī′kə-sīd′) *n.* Any of a group of organic compounds, occurring abundantly in plants, that yield a sugar and one or more nonsugar substances on hydrolysis. —**gly′co·sid′ic** (-sĭd′ĭk) *adj.*

gly·co·sphin·go·lip·id (glī′kō-sfĭng′gō-lĭp′ĭd) *n.* A lipid derived from a ceramide that contains a carbohydrate such as glucose or galactose.

gly·co·stat·ic (glī′kə-stăt′ĭk) *adj.* Promoting or maintaining a steady supply of glycogen in muscle, liver, and other tissues.

gly·co·su·ri·a (glī′kə-sŏŏr′ē-ə, -shŏŏr′-) *n.* **1.** See **glucosuria.** **2.** Excretion of carbohydrates in the urine. —**gly′co·su′ric** *adj.*

gly·co·syl (glī′kə-sĭl′) *n.* A univalent radical resulting from detachment of a hydroxyl group from the hemiacetal of a cyclic glucose.

gly·co·sy·lat·ed hemoglobin (glī-kō′sə-lā′tĭd) *n.* Any of four hemoglobin fractions that together account for less than 4 percent of the total hemoglobin in the blood.

gly·co·sy·la·tion (glī′kə-sə-lā′shən) *n.* The addition of glycosyl groups to a protein to form a glycoprotein.

gly·co·syl·trans·fer·ase (glī′kə-sĭl-trăns′fə-rās′, -rāz′) *n.* An enzyme that catalyzes the transfer of glycosyl groups from one compound to another.

gly·co·troph·ic (glī′kə-trŏf′ĭk, -trō′fĭk) *or* **gly·co·trop·ic** (-trŏp′ĭk, -trō′pĭk) *adj.* Tending to antagonize the action of insulin and cause hyperglycemia.

glycotropic factor *n.* A principle in extracts of the anterior lobe of the pituitary gland that raises blood sugar levels and antagonizes the action of insulin. Also called *insulin-antagonizing factor.*

glyc·u·re·sis (glĭk′yə-rē′sĭs, glī′kyə-) *n.* Glycosuria.

gly·cu·ro·nate (glī-kyoōr′ə-nāt′) *n.* A salt or ester of a uronic acid, especially glucuronic acid.

gly·cyl (glī′səl) *n.* A univalent acyl radical of glycine.

gm. *abbr.* gram

GMO *abbr.* genetically modified organism

GMP (jē′ĕm-pē′) *n.* A nucleotide composed of guanine, ribose, and one phosphate group that is formed during protein synthesis. Also called *guanine ribonucleotide, guanylic acid.*

gnat (năt) *n.* Any of various small, biting, two-winged flies, such as a biting midge or black fly.

gnath·ic (năth′ĭk) *adj.* Relating to the jaw or alveolar process.

gnath·i·on (năth′ē-ŏn′, nā′thē-) *n.* The most inferior point of the mandible in the midline.

gnatho– *or* **gnath–** *pref.* Jaw: *gnathoplasty.*

gnath·o·dy·nam·ics (năth′ō-dī-năm′ĭks) *n.* The study of the relationship of the magnitude and direction of the forces involved in mastication.

gnath·o·dy·na·mom·e·ter (năth′ō-dī′nə-mŏm′ĭ-tər) *n.* A device for measuring biting pressure. Also called *bite gauge.*

gnath·o·log·ic·al (năth′ō-lŏj′ĭ-kəl) *adj.* Of or relating to gnathodynamics.

gnath·o·plas·ty (năth′ə-plăs′tē) *n.* Reparative surgery of the jaw.

Gna·thos·to·ma (nă-thŏs′tə-mə) *n.* A genus of nematode worms with multiple-host aquatic life cycles.

gna·thos·to·mi·a·sis (nă-thŏs′tə-mī′ə-sĭs, năth′ō-stō-) *n.* A migrating edema or creeping eruption caused by subcutaneous infection with larvae of *Gnathostoma spinigerum,* usually contracted by eating undercooked fish.

–gnathous *suff.* Characterized by a specified kind of jaw: *anisognathous.*

gno·si·a (nō′sē-ə, -zē-ə) *n.* The perceptive faculty enabling one to recognize the form and the nature of persons and things.

gno·to·bi·ol·o·gy (nō′tō-bī-ŏl′ə-jē) *n.* The study of organisms or conditions that are either free of germs or associated only with known or specified germs.

gno·to·bi·o·ta (nō′tō-bī-ō′tə) *n.* The aggregate of specified microorganisms with which a germ-free laboratory animal or plant has been infected.

gno·to·bi·ote (nō′tō-bī′ōt′) *n.* A germ-free animal infected with one or more microorganisms in order to study the microorganism in a controlled situation.

gno·to·bi·ot·ic (nō′tō-bī-ŏt′ĭk) *adj.* **1.** Of or relating to gnotobiology. **2.** Free of germs or associated only with known and specified germs.

gno·to·bi·ot·ics (nō′tō-bī-ŏt′ĭks) *n.* Gnotobiology.

GnRH *abbr.* gonadotropin-releasing hormone

gob·let cell (gŏb′lĭt) *n.* A mucus-secreting epithelial cell that distends with mucin before secretion and collapses to a goblet shape after secretion. Also called *beaker cell.*

goi·ter (goi′tər) *n.* A noncancerous enlargement of the thyroid gland, visible as a swelling at the front of the neck, that is often associated with iodine deficiency. —**goi′trous** (-trəs) *adj.*

goi·tro·gen·ic (goi′trə-jĕn′ĭk) *adj.* Causing goiter.

gold (gōld) *n. Symbol* **Au** A soft yellow element that resists corrosion and is the most malleable and ductile metal, used to treat rheumatoid arthritis and intravenously in liver imaging. Atomic number 79.

gold sodium thi·o·mal·ate (thī′ō-măl′āt′, -mā′lāt′) *n.* An intravenous drug containing two salts of the element gold, used to treat rheumatoid arthritis.

Gold·blatt kidney (gōld′blăt′) *n.* A kidney whose arterial blood supply has been reduced, associated with arterial hypertension.

Goldblatt phenomenon *n.* Hypertension occurring as a result of the partial occlusion of a renal artery.

Gold·flam disease (gōld′flăm, gôlt′flăm) *n.* See **myasthenia gravis.**

Gold·stein (gōld′stēn), **Joseph Leonard** Born 1940. American biochemist. He shared a 1985 Nobel Prize for discoveries related to cholesterol metabolism.

Gold·stein's toe sign (gōld′stīnz) *n.* Increased space between the big toe and its neighbor, seen in Down syndrome and, occasionally, cretinism.

Gol·gi (gôl′jē), **Camillo** 1844?–1926. Italian histologist. He shared a 1906 Nobel Prize for research on the structure of the nervous system.

Golgi apparatus *n.* See **Golgi complex.**

Golgi cell *n.* A neuron with short dendrites and with either a long axon or an axon that breaks into processes a short distance from the cell body.

Golgi complex *n.* A complex of parallel, flattened saccules, vesicles, and vacuoles that lies adjacent to the nucleus of a cell and is concerned with the formation of secretions within the cell. Also called *Golgi apparatus.*

Golgi-Maz·zo·ni corpuscle (-măt-sō′nē) *n.* An encapsulated sensory nerve ending similar to a lamellated corpuscle but simpler in structure and found in the subcutaneous tissue of the fingertips.

Gol·gi's stain (gôl′jēz) *n.* Any of several methods for staining nerve cells, nerve fibers, and neuroglia in which fixed tissue is impregnated with silver nitrate and potassium dichromate resulting in the complete staining of some nerve cells while other cells are not stained at all.

Golgi tendon organ *n.* A proprioceptive sensory nerve ending embedded among the fibers of a tendon, often near the musculotendinous junction. Also called *neurotendinous spindle.*

Golgi type I neuron *n.* A nerve cell having a long axon that leaves the gray matter of the central nervous system, of which it forms a part.

Golgi type II neuron *n.* A nerve cell having a short axon that ramifies in the gray matter of the central nervous system.

go·mit·o·li (gō-mĭt′ə-lē) *pl.n.* Intricately coiled capillary vessels present largely in the upper infundibular stem of the stalk of the pituitary gland and comprising a portion of the pituitary portal circulation.

gom·pho·sis (gŏm-fō′sĭs) *n.*, *pl.* **-ses** (-sēz) A type of immovable articulation, as of a tooth inserted into its bony socket. Also called *peg-and-socket joint.*

gon– *pref.* Variant of **gono–**.

go·nad (gō′năd) *n.* An organ that produces gametes, especially a testis or an ovary. —**go·nad′al** (gō-năd′l), **go·nad′ic** *adj.*

gonadal cord *n.* Any of the columns of germinal and follicle cells entering the embryonic ovarian cortex.

gonadal dysgenesis *n.* Defective embryonic development of the gonads.

gonadal ridge *n.* An elevation of thickened mesothelium and underlying mesenchyme on the ventromedial border of the embryonic mesonephros in which the primordial germ cells become embedded and establish it as the primordium of the testis or the ovary. Also called *genital ridge.*

go·nad·ec·to·my (gō′nə-dĕk′tə-mē) *n.* Excision of an ovary or a testis.

go·nad·o·crin (gō-năd′ə-krĭn′) *n.* Any of the peptides that stimulate release of follicle-stimulating hormone and luteinizing hormone from the pituitary.

go·nad·o·lib·er·in (gō-năd′ō-lĭb′ər-ĭn, gŏn′ə-dō-) *n.* **1.** See **gonadotropin-releasing factor. 2.** See **luteinizing hormone/follicle-stimulating hormone-releasing factor.**

gon·a·dop·a·thy (gŏn′ə-dŏp′ə-thē) *n.* A disease affecting the gonads.

go·nad·o·rel·in hydrochloride (gō-năd′ə-rĕl′ĭn) *n.* A synthetic gonadotropin-releasing hormone used to evaluate the functional capacity of the gonadotrophs of the anterior pituitary gland.

go·nad·o·troph (gō-năd′ə-trŏf′, -trōf′, gŏn′ə-dō-) *n.* A cell of the anterior lobe of the pituitary gland that affects certain cells of the ovary or the testis.

go·nad·o·trop·ic (gō-năd′ə-trŏp′ĭk, -trō′pĭk) *or* **go·nad·o·troph·ic** (-trŏf′ĭk, -trō′fĭk) *adj.* **1.** Of or relating to the actions of a gonadotropin. **2.** Promoting the growth or function of the gonads.

go·nad·o·tro·pin (gō-năd′ə-trō′pĭn, -trŏp′ĭn) *or* **go·nad·o·tro·phin** (-trō′fĭn, -trō′pĭn) *n.* A hormone that stimulates the growth and activity of the gonads, especially any of several pituitary hormones that stimulate the function of the ovaries and testes. Also called *gonadotropic hormone.*

gonadotropin-releasing factor *n.* A substance that is produced by the hypothalamus and stimulates the release of gonadotropin by the anterior lobe of the pituitary gland. Also called *gonadoliberin.*

gonadotropin-releasing hormone *n. Abbr.* **GnRH** A hormone produced by the hypothalamus that stimulates the anterior pituitary gland to begin secreting luteinizing hormone and follicle-stimulating hormone. Also called *luliberin, luteinizing hormone-releasing hormone.*

gon·a·duct (gŏn′ə-dŭkt′) *n.* **1.** See **seminal duct. 2.** See **fallopian tube.**

go·nal·gia (gō-năl′jə) *n.* Pain in the knee.

gon·an·gi·ec·to·my (gŏn′ăn-jē-ĕk′tə-mē) *n.* See **vasectomy.**

gon·ar·thri·tis (gŏn′är-thrī′tĭs) *n.* Inflammation of the knee joint.

gon·ar·throt·o·my (gŏn′är-thrŏt′ə-mē) *n.* Incision into the knee joint.

gon·e·cyst (gŏn′ĭ-sĭst′) *or* **gon·e·cys·tis** (gŏn′ĭ-sĭs′tĭs) *n.* See **seminal vesicle.**

gon·e·cys·to·lith (gŏn′ĭ-sĭs′tə-lĭth′) *n.* A concretion or calculus in a seminal vesicle.

Go·nin operation (gō-năN′, gô-) *n.* Treatment of retinal detachment by closure of the break in the retina through cauterization.

gonio– *pref.* Angle: *goniometer.*

go·ni·om·e·ter (gō′nē-ŏm′ĭ-tər) *n.* **1.** An optical instrument for measuring crystal angles, as between crystal faces. **2.** See **arthrometer.**

go·ni·on (gō′nē-ŏn′) *n.*, *pl.* **-ni·a** (-nē-ə) The outer point on either side of the lower jaw at which the jawbone angles upward.

go·ni·o·punc·ture (gō′nē-ə-pŭngk′chər) *n.* An operation for congenital glaucoma in which a puncture is made in the filtration angle.

go·ni·o·scope (gō′nē-ə-skōp′) *n.* An ophthalmoscope used to examine the angle of the anterior chamber of the eye.

go·ni·os·co·py (gō′nē-ŏs′kə-pē) *n.* Examination of the angle of the anterior chamber of the eye with a gonioscope or with a contact prism lens.

go·ni·o·syn·ech·i·a (gō′nē-ō-sə-nĕk′ē-ə) *n.* Adhesion of the iris to the posterior surface of the cornea in the angle of the anterior chamber of the eye.

go·ni·ot·o·my (gō′nē-ŏt′ə-mē) *n.* Surgical opening of Schlemm's canal by way of the angle of the anterior chamber of the eye to treat congenital glaucoma.

go·ni·tis (gō-nī′tĭs) *n.* Inflammation of the knee.

gono– *or* **gon–** *pref.* Sexual; reproductive: *gonophore.*

gon·o·cele (gŏn′ə-sēl′) *n.* A cystic lesion of the epididymis or rete testis, resulting from obstruction and containing secretions from the testis.

gon·o·cide (gŏn′ə-sīd′) *n.* An agent that destroys gonococci. Also called *gonococcicide.*

gonococcal conjunctivitis *n.* Severe conjunctivitis that is caused by gonococci and marked by intense swelling of the conjunctiva and eyelids and by a profuse purulent discharge.

gon·o·coc·ce·mi·a (gŏn′ə-kŏk-sē′mē-ə) *n.* The presence of gonococci in the blood.

gon·o·coc·cic (gŏn′ə-kŏk′ĭk, -kŏk′sĭk) *adj.* Relating to the gonococcus.

gon·o·coc·ci·cide (gŏn′ə-kŏk′sĭ-sīd′) *n.* See **gonocide.**

gon·o·coc·cus (gŏn′ə-kŏk′əs) *n.*, *pl.* **-coc·ci** (-kŏk′sī′, -kŏk′ī′) The bacterium *Neisseria gonorrhoeae,* which is the causative agent of gonorrhea. —**gon′o·coc′cal** *adj.*

gon·o·phore (gŏn′ə-fôr′) *n.* A structure, such as an oviduct, that stores or conducts sex cells.

gon·or·rhe·a (gŏn′ə-rē′ə) *n.* A sexually transmitted disease caused by gonococci and affecting mucous membrane chiefly of the genital and urinary tracts, marked by an acute purulent discharge and painful or difficult urination, though women often have no symptoms. —**gon′or·rhe′al, gon′or·rhe′ic** *adj.*

gonorrheal ophthalmia *n.* Acute purulent conjunctivitis due to gonococcal infection.

Gon·y·au·lax cat·a·nel·la (gŏn′ē-ô′lăks′ kăt′ə-nĕl′ə) *n.* A marine dinoflagellate protozoan that produces a powerful toxin that accumulates in the tissues of mussels and other filter-feeding shellfish; it may cause fatal poisoning in humans who have eaten contaminated shellfish.

Good·ell's sign (gŏŏd′əlz) *n.* An indication of pregnancy in which the cervix and vagina soften.

Good·pas·ture (gŏŏd′păs′chər), **Ernest William** 1886–1960. American pathologist who developed the technique for cultivating viruses and rickettsia in fertile chicken eggs, thus enabling the development of a number of vaccines.

Good·pas·ture's syndrome (gŏŏd′păs′chərz) *n.* Glomerulonephritis associated with circulating antibodies against basement-membrane antigens; it may be preceded by hemoptysis.

goof·ball *or* **goof ball** (gŏŏf′bôl′) *n.* A barbiturate or tranquilizer in the form of a pill, especially when taken for nonmedical purposes.

goose bumps (gŏŏs) *pl.n.* Momentary roughness of the skin caused by erection of the papillae in response to cold or fear. Also called *cutis anserina, goose flesh, goose pimples.*

gor·get (gôr′jĭt) *n.* A surgical director or guide with a wide groove for use in lithotomy.

Gor·lin-Chau·dhry-Moss syndrome (gôr′lĭn-chô′drē-môs′) *n.* A rare congenital condition associated with craniofacial dysostosis, patent ductus arteriosus, hypertrichosis, hypoplasia of the labia majora, and dental and ocular abnormalities.

Gor·lin's syndrome (gôr′lĭnz) *n.* See **basal-cell nevus syndrome.**

Gor·man's syndrome (gôr′mənz) *n.* A disorder characterized by hemangiomatosis of the skeletal system with or without involvement of the overlying skin and resulting in osteolysis and fibrous replacement of bone.

go·se·rel·in acetate (gō′sə-rĕl′ĭn) *n.* A synthetic peptide analog of gonadotropin-releasing hormone used primarily to treat cancer of the breast and prostate, endometriosis, and infertility.

gos·sy·pol (gŏs′ə-pôl′, -pōl′) *n.* A toxic pigment obtained from cottonseed oil and detoxified by heating, shown to inhibit sperm production.

GOT *abbr.* glutamic-oxaloacetic transaminase

gouge (gouj) *n.* A strong curved chisel used in bone surgery.

Gou·ley's catheter (gŏŏ′lēz) *n.* A curved steel instrument grooved on its inferior surface so that it can be passed over a guide inserted through a urethral stricture.

goun·dou (gŏŏn′dŏŏ) *n.* A disease characterized by exostoses of the nasal processes of the maxillary bones, thus causing swelling on each side of the nose; it is endemic in West Africa and considered to be a consequence of yaws.

gout (gout) *n.* An inherited disorder of uric-acid metabolism occurring mostly in men, marked by painful inflammation of the joints, especially of the feet and hands, and arthritic attacks resulting from elevated levels of uric acid in the blood and the deposition of urate crystals around the joints. The condition can become chronic and result in deformity. —**gout′y** *adj.*

gown (goun) *n.* A robe or smock worn in operating rooms and other parts of hospitals as a guard against contamination.

GP *abbr.* general practitioner

GPI *abbr.* Gingival-Periodontal Index

GPT *abbr.* glutamic-pyruvic transaminase

gr *or* **gr.** *abbr.* grain; gram

Graaf·i·an follicle *or* **graaf·i·an follicle** (grä′fē-ən, grăf′-ē-) *n.* A mature ovarian follicle in which the oocyte attains its full size and the surrounding follicular cells are permeated by one or more fluid-filled cavities. Also called *secondary follicle, vesicular ovarian follicle.*

grac·i·lis muscle (grăs′ə-lĭs) *n.* A muscle with origin in the ramus of the pubis, with insertion to the shaft of the tibia, with nerve supply from the obturator nerve, and whose action adducts the thigh, flexes the knee, and rotates the leg medially.

grad. *abbr. Latin* gradatim (gradually)

grade I astrocytoma *n.* See **astrocytoma.**

grade II astrocytoma *n.* See **astroblastoma.**

grade III astrocytoma *n.* See **astroblastoma.**

grade IV astrocytoma *n.* See **glioblastoma.**

gra·di·ent (grā′dē-ənt) *n.* **1.** The rate at which a physical quantity, such as temperature or pressure, changes relative to change in a given variable, especially distance. **2.** A series of progressively increasing or decreasing differences in the growth rate, metabolism, or physiological activity of a cell, an organ, or an organism.

grad·u·at·ed (grăj′ŏŏ-ā′tĭd) *adj.* Marked with or divided into intervals, as of volume or temperature, for use in measurement.

graduated tenotomy *n.* Partial incisions of the tendon of an eye muscle performed to correct a slight degree of strabismus.

Grae·fe's operation (grā′fəz) *n.* **1.** The removal of a cataract by a limbal incision coupled with a capsulotomy and an iridectomy. **2.** An iridectomy for the treatment of glaucoma.

Graefe's sign *or* **von Graefe's sign** (vŏn) *n.* An indication of Graves' disease in which the upper eyelid does not evenly follow the downward movement of the eyeball, but instead lags or moves jerkily.

graft (grăft) *v.* To transplant or implant tissue surgically into a body part to replace a damaged part or compensate for a defect. —*n.* **1.** Material, especially living tissue or an organ, surgically attached to or inserted into a body part to replace a damaged part or compensate for a defect. **2.** The procedure of implanting or transplanting such material. **3.** The configuration or condition resulting from such a procedure.

graft-versus-host disease *n.* A type of incompatibility reaction of transplanted cells against host tissues that possess an antigen not possessed by the donor. Also called *graft-versus-host reaction.*

Gra·ham Steell's murmur (grā′əm stēlz′) *n.* An early diastolic murmur caused by pulmonary insufficiency secondary to pulmonary hypertension.

grain (grān) *n.* **1.** A small, dry, one-seeded fruit of a cereal grass, having the fruit and the seed walls united. **2.** The fruits of cereal grasses especially after having been harvested, considered as a group. **3.** A relatively small discrete particulate or crystalline mass. **4.** *Abbr.*

gr. A unit of weight in the US Customary System, an avoirdupois unit that is equal to 0.002286 ounce (0.065 gram).

gram (grăm) *n. Abbr.* **g, gm., gr.** A metric unit of mass equal to 15.432 grains, one thousandth (10^{-3}) of a kilogram, or 0.035 ounce.

Gram (grăm, gräm), **Hans Christian Joachim** 1853–1938. Danish physician who developed (1884) Gram's stain as a method of distinguishing types of bacteria.

–gram *suff.* Something written or drawn; a record: *cardiogram.*

gram calorie *n.* See **calorie** (sense 3).

gram-centimeter *n.* A unit of measurement equal to the energy exerted, or work done, when a mass of 1 gram is raised a height of 1 centimeter.

gram equivalent *n.* **1.** The weight of a substance, usually in grams, that combines or reacts with a standard weight of a reference element or compound. **2.** The atomic or molecular weight in grams of an atom or group of atoms involved in a reaction divided by the valence.

gram·i·ci·din (grăm′ĭ-sīd′n) *n.* An antibiotic produced by a *Bacillis* bacterium and used to treat certain gram-positive bacteria infections.

gram-ion *n.* The weight in grams of an ion that is equal to the sum of the atomic weights of the atoms making up the ion.

gram-meter *n.* A unit of energy equal to 100 gram-centimeters.

gram-molecular weight *n.* See **mole**[3] (sense 2).

gram molecule *n.* See **mole**[3] (sense 1).

gram-negative *or* **Gram-negative** *adj.* Of, relating to, or being a bacterium that does not retain the violet stain used in Gram's method.

gram-positive *or* **Gram-positive** *adj.* Of, relating to, or being a bacterium that retains the violet stain that is used in Gram's method.

Gram's stain (grămz) *n.* A staining technique used to classify bacteria in which a bacterial specimen is first stained with crystal violet, then treated with an iodine solution, decolorized with alcohol, and counterstained with safranine. Gram-positive bacteria retain the violet stain; gram-negative bacteria do not. Also called *Gram's method.*

grand·daugh·ter cyst (grăn′dô′tər) *n.* A cyst that sometimes develops within a daughter cyst.

grand mal (grănd′ mäl′, măl′) *n.* A severe epilepsy characterized by seizures involving tonic-clonic spasms and by the loss of consciousness. Also called *generalized tonic-clonic epilepsy, generalized tonic-clonic seizure disorder, grand mal epilepsy, major epilepsy.*

grand mal seizure *n.* A sudden attack or convulsion characterized by generalized muscle spasms and loss of consciousness; it is recurrent in grand mal. Also called *generalized tonic-clonic seizure.*

Gra·nit (grä-nēt′), **Ragnar Arthur** 1900–1991. Finnish-born Swedish physiologist. He shared a 1967 Nobel Prize for research on the human eye.

granul– *pref.* Variant of **granulo–**.

gran·u·lar (grăn′yə-lər) *adj.* **1.** Composed or appearing to be composed of granules or grains. **2.** Relating to or containing particles having a strong affinity for nuclear stains, as in certain bacteria.

granular cell tumor *n.* A slow-growing benign tumor that often involves the peripheral nerves in skin, mucosa, or connective tissue. Also called *granular cell myoblastoma.*

granular conjunctivitis *n.* See **trachoma**.

granular endoplasmic reticulum *n.* Endoplasmic reticulum in which the cisternae are studded with ribosomes, associated with the synthesis of proteins. Also called *ergastoplasm.*

granular layer *n.* **1.** The deeper of the two layers of the cortex of the cerebellum, containing many granule cells whose dendrites synapse with incoming highly branched nerve fibers but whose axons form synapses with dendrites of Purkinje cells, basket cells, and stellate cells; granular layer of the cerebellar cortex. **2.** A layer of somewhat flattened cells containing granules of keratohyalin and eleidin, lying just above the prickle cell layer of the epidermis; granular layer of the epidermis. **3.** The layer of small cells that forms the wall of an ovarian follicle; granular layer of a vesicular ovarian follicle.

granular leukoblast *n.* See **promyelocyte**.

granular leukocyte *n.* A mature white blood cell having granules in its cytoplasm.

granular ophthalmia *n.* See **trachoma**.

gran·u·la·ti·o (grăn′yə-lā′shē-ō) *n., pl.* **–la·ti·o·nes** (-lā′shē-ō′nēz) Granulation.

gran·u·la·tion (grăn′yə-lā′shən) *n.* **1.** The process of forming grains or granules. **2.** The state or appearance of having grains or granules. **3.** Small, fleshy, beadlike protuberances, consisting of outgrowths of new capillaries, on the surface of a wound that is healing. Also called *granulation tissue.* **4.** The formation of these protuberances.

gran·ule (grăn′yōōl) *n.* **1.** A small grain or pellet; a particle. **2.** A cellular or cytoplasmic particle, especially one that stains readily. **3.** A very small pill, usually coated with gelatin or sugar.

granule cell *n.* One of the small neurons of the cortex of the cerebellum and cerebrum.

granulo– *or* **granul–** *pref.* Granule; granular: *granulocyte.*

gran·u·lo·cyte (grăn′yə-lō-sīt′) *n.* Any of a group of white blood cells having granules in the cytoplasm. **—gran′u·lo·cyt′ic** (-sĭt′ĭk) *adj.*

granulocyte-macrophage colony-stimulating factor *n.* A naturally occurring protein that stimulates the production of granulocytes and macrophages by stem cells and is used as a drug by some immunosuppressed individuals.

granulocytic leukemia *n.* See **myelogenous leukemia**.

granulocytic sarcoma *n.* A malignant tumor of immature myeloid cells, associated with granulocytic leukemia. Also called *myeloid sarcoma.*

granulocytic series *n.* The cells in various stages of granulopoietic development in the bone marrow.

gran·u·lo·cy·to·pe·ni·a (grăn′yə-lō-sī′tə-pē′nē-ə) *n.* A condition characterized by an abnormally low number of granular white blood cells in the blood. Also called *granulopenia.*

gran·u·lo·cy·to·poi·e·sis (grăn′yə-lō-sī′tə-poi-ē′sĭs) *n.* See **granulopoiesis.** —**gran′u·lo·cy′to·poi·et′ic** (-ĕt′ĭk) *adj.*

gran·u·lo·cy·to·sis (grăn′yə-lō-sī-tō′sĭs) *n.* A condition characterized by an abnormally large number of granulocytes in blood or tissues.

gran·u·lo·ma (grăn′yə-lō′mə) *n., pl.* **-mas** *or* **-ma·ta** (-mə-tə) A mass of inflamed granulation tissue, usually associated with ulcerated infections. —**gran′u·lo′ma·tous** (-mə-təs) *adj.*

granuloma in·gui·na·le (ĭng′gwə-nā′lē) *n.* See **donovanosis.**

granuloma mul·ti·for·me (mŭl′tə-fôr′mē) *n.* A chronic granulomatous annular eruption of the skin on the upper body in older adults in central Africa.

gran·u·lo·ma·to·sis (grăn′yə-lō′mə-tō′sĭs) *n.* Any of various conditions marked by multiple granulomas.

granulomatosis dis·ci·for·mis chron·i·ca et pro·gres·si·va (dĭs′ə-fôr′mĭs krŏn′ĭ-kə ĕt prō′grĭ-sī′və) *n.* See **Miescher's granulomatosis.**

granulomatosis sid·e·rot·i·ca (sĭd′ə-rŏt′ĭ-kə) *n.* Granulomatosis in which firm brown nodules that contain iron are present in an enlarged spleen.

granulomatous colitis *n.* Colitis that is characterized by granulomas.

granulomatous encephalomyelitis *n.* A disease causing necrosis and granulomas in brain tissue.

granulomatous enteritis *n.* See **Crohn's disease.**

granulomatous inflammation *n.* A form of proliferative inflammation characterized by the formation of granulomas.

granuloma trop·i·cum (trŏp′ĭ-kəm) *n.* See **yaws.**

gran·u·lo·mere (grăn′yə-lō-mîr′) *n.* The central part of a blood platelet. Also called *chromomere.*

gran·u·lo·pe·ni·a (grăn′yə-lō-pē′nē-ə) *n.* See **granulocytopenia.**

gran·u·lo·plas·tic (grăn′yə-lō-plăs′tĭk) *adj.* Forming granules.

gran·u·lo·poi·e·sis (grăn′yə-lō-poi-ē′sĭs) *n.* The formation of granulocytes. Also called *granulocytopoiesis.* —**gran′u·lo·poi·et′ic** (-ĕt′ĭk) *adj.*

gran·u·lo·sa cell (grăn′yə-lō′sə) *n.* A cell lining the vesicular ovarian follicle that becomes a luteal cell after ovulation.

granulosa cell tumor *n.* A benign or malignant tumor of the ovary developing from the granular layer of the Graafian follicle and frequently secreting estrogen. Also called *folliculoma.*

gran·u·lose (grăn′yə-lōs′) *adj.* Having a surface covered with granules.

gran·u·lo·sis (grăn′yə-lō′sĭs) *n.* The formation of a mass of granules.

granulosis ru·bra na·si (rōō′brə nā′zī) *n.* A condition marked by redness, papules, and occasional vesicles of the skin of the nose and face, resulting from blockage and inflammation of the sweat ducts.

–graph *suff.* An instrument for writing, drawing, or recording: *cardiograph.*

graph·an·es·the·sia (grăf′ăn-ĭs-thē′zhə) *n.* Loss of the ability to recognize figures traced on the skin, as with a pencil-shaped piece of wood.

graph·or·rhe·a (grăf′ə-rē′ə) *n.* The writing of long lists of meaningless words, as occurs in some manic disorders.

–graphy *suff.* 1. A writing or representation produced in a specified manner or by a specified process: *tomography.* 2. A writing about or a representation of a specified thing: *ophthalmography.*

grasp reflex *or* **grasp·ing reflex** (grăs′pĭng) *n.* An involuntary bending of the fingers in response to tactile and tendon stimulation on the palm, producing an uncontrollable grasp, and associated with frontal lobe brain lesions.

grat·tage (gră-täzh′, grə-) *n.* Scraping or brushing an ulcer or surface that has granulations to stimulate the healing process.

grave (grāv) *adj.* Serious or dangerous, as a symptom or disease.

grav·el (grăv′əl) *n.* Sandlike concretions of uric acid, calcium oxalate, and mineral salts formed in the passages of the biliary and urinary tracts.

Graves' disease (grāvz) *n.* A condition usually caused by excessive thyroid hormone and characterized by an enlarged thyroid gland, protrusion of eyeballs, a rapid heartbeat, and nervous excitability. Also called *Basedow's disease, Parry's disease.*

grav·id (grăv′ĭd) *adj.* Carrying eggs or developing young. —**gra·vid′i·ty** (grə-vĭd′ĭ-tē), **grav′id·ness** *n.*

grav·i·da (grăv′ĭ-də) *n., pl.* **–das** *or* **–dae** (-dē′) A pregnant woman.

gra·vid·ic (grə-vĭd′ĭk) *adj.* Taking place during pregnancy.

gravid uterus *n.* The uterus in pregnancy.

gra·vim·e·ter (gră-vĭm′ĭ-tər, grăv′ə-mē′-) *n.* 1. See **hydrometer.** 2. An instrument used to measure variations in a gravitational field. —**gra·vim′e·try** (gră-vĭm′ĭ-trē, grə-) *n.*

grav·i·met·ric (grăv′ə-mĕt′rĭk) *adj.* 1. Relating to or determined by weight. 2. Relating to measurement of variations in a gravitational field.

gravimetric analysis *n.* The determination of the quantities of the constituents of a compound.

grav·i·re·cep·tor (grăv′ə-rĭ-sĕp′tər) *n.* Any of various specialized receptor organs and nerve endings in the inner ear, joints, tendons, and muscles, that give the brain information about body position, equilibrium, and the direction of gravitational forces.

grav·i·ta·tion (grăv′ĭ-tā′shən) *n.* 1. The natural phenomenon of attraction between massive bodies. 2. The act or process of moving under the influence of this attraction. 3. A movement toward a source of attraction.

grav·i·ta·tion·al constant (grăv′ĭ-tā′shə-nəl) *n. Abbr.* **G** The constant in Newton's law of gravitation that yields the attractive force between two bodies when multiplied by the product of the masses of the two bodies and divided by the square of the distance between them. Also called *newtonian constant of gravitation.*

gravitational ulcer *n.* A leg ulcer that is slow to heal because of the position of the extremity and the incompetence of the valves of the varicosed veins.

gray (grā) *n. Abbr.* **Gy** A unit for a specific absorbed dose of radiation equal to 100 rads.

Gray, Henry 1825?–1861. British anatomist whose work *Anatomy, Descriptive and Surgical* (1858), known as *Gray's Anatomy,* remains a standard text.

gray cataract *n.* A cataract of gray color usually occurring in senile, mature, or cortical cataracts.

gray column *n.* Any of the three masses of gray matter that extend longitudinally through the center of each lateral half of the spinal cord and appear as gray horns in transverse sections.

gray degeneration *n.* The degeneration of the white substance of the spinal cord, the fibers of which lose their myelin sheaths and become darker in color.

gray fiber *n.* See **unmyelinated fiber.**

gray hepatization *n.* The second stage of hepatization of the lung tissue in pneumonia, when the yellowish-gray exudate is beginning to degenerate before breaking down.

gray induration *n.* A lung condition occurring during and after pneumonia, marked by an increase in fibrous connective tissue in the alveoli.

gray matter *n.* Brownish-gray nerve tissue, especially of the brain and spinal cord, composed of nerve cell bodies and their dendrites and some supportive tissue. Also called *gray substance, substantia grisea.*

gray scale *n.* Gray-scale ultrasonography.

gray-scale ultrasonography *n.* Ultrasonography that displays small differences in an acoustical impedance as if they were different shades of gray.

gray substance *n.* See **gray matter.**

gray syndrome *n.* A potentially fatal syndrome of infants caused by transplacental effects of chloramphenicol administered to the mother and resulting in the infant's gray appearance at birth and during the neonatal period. Also called *gray-baby syndrome.*

great auricular nerve (grāt) *n.* A nerve arising from the second and third cervical nerves and supplying the skin of part of the ear, the adjacent portion of the scalp, cheek, and angle of the jaw.

great cardiac vein *n.* A tributary of the coronary sinus that begins at the apex of the heart and runs in the anterior interventricular sulcus.

great cerebral vein *n.* A vein formed by the junction of the two internal cerebral veins and passes between the corpus callosum and the pineal gland to continue into the straight sinus.

great·er curvature of stomach (grā′tər) *n.* The convex lateral border of the stomach to which the greater omentum is attached.

greater occipital nerve *n.* The medial branch of the dorsal ramus of the second cervical nerve that is mainly cutaneous and supplies the back part of the scalp.

greater omentum *n.* A peritoneal fold passing from the stomach to the transverse colon, hanging like an apron in front of the intestines. Also called *caul, epiploon, gastrocolic omentum, velum.*

greater palatine foramen *n.* An opening in the rear corner of the hard palate opposite the last molar tooth. Also called *posterior palatine foramen.*

greater palatine nerve *n.* A branch of the pterygopalatine ganglion supplying the mucosa and glands of the hard palate and the front part of the soft palate.

greater petrosal nerve *n.* The parasympathetic root of the pterygopalatine ganglion, a branch of the facial nerve running on the temporal bone to the pterygopalatine ganglion.

greater posterior rectus muscle of head *n.* A muscle with origin from the spinous process of the axis, with insertion into the occipital bone, with nerve supply from the first cervical nerve, and whose action rotates the head and draws it backward.

greater psoas muscle *n.* A muscle with origin from the bodies of the vertebrae and the intervertebral disks from the twelfth thoracic to the fifth lumbar vertebrae and from the transverse processes of the lumbar vertebrae, with insertion into the femur, with nerve supply from the lumbar plexus, and whose action flexes the thigh. Also called *psoas major.*

greater rhomboid muscle *n.* A muscle with origin from the spinous processes and supraspinous ligaments of the first four thoracic vertebrae, with insertion into the scapula below the spine, with nerve supply from the dorsal nerve of the scapula, and whose action draws the scapula toward the vertebral column.

greater splanchnic nerve *n.* A nerve that arises from the fifth or sixth to the ninth or tenth thoracic sympathetic ganglia and passes along the thoracic vertebrae to join the celiac plexus.

greater trochanter *n.* A strong process overhanging the root of the neck of the femur, giving attachment to the gluteus medius and minimus muscles, the piriform muscle, the internal and external obturator muscles, and the gemelli muscles.

greater vestibular gland *n.* See **Bartholin's gland.**

greater zygomatic muscle *n.* A muscle with origin from the zygomatic bone anterior to the temporozygomatic suture, with insertion into the muscles at the angle of the mouth, with nerve supply from the facial nerve, and whose action draws the upper lip up and to the side.

great foramen *n.* The large orifice in the base of the skull through which the spinal cord passes to the cranial cavity and becomes continuous with the medulla oblongata. Also called *foramen magnum.*

great muscle *n.* Any of the three vastus muscles: intermediate vastus, lateral vastus, and medial vastus.

great saphenous vein *n.* A vein formed by the union of the dorsal vein of the big toe and the dorsal venous arch of the foot and empties into the femoral vein in the upper part of the femoral triangle.

Green·field's disease (grēn′fēldz′) *n.* The late-infantile form of metachromatic leukodystrophy.

green·ie (grē′nē) *n.* An amphetamine pill that is green in color.

green soap (grēn) *n.* A translucent, yellowish-green soft or liquid soap made chiefly from vegetable oils and used in the treatment of skin disorders.

green·stick fracture (grēn′stĭk′) *n.* A fracture in which one side of the bone is broken and the other side is bent.

greg·a·rine (grĕg′ə-rīn′) *n.* Any of various sporozoan protozoans of the order Gregarinida that are parasitic within the digestive tracts of various invertebrates.

—*adj.* Of or belonging to the order Gregarinida. —**greg·a·rin·i·an** (-rĭn′ē-ən) *adj.*

Greig's syndrome (grĕg) *n.* See **ocular hypertelorism.**

grenz rays (grĕnts) *pl.n.* Very soft x-rays, closely allied to ultraviolet rays in their wavelength and in their biological action upon tissues.

grief (grēf) *n.* Deep mental anguish, as that arising from bereavement.

grind·ing (grīn′dĭng) *n.* The pathological wearing away of tooth substance by mechanical means.

grinding-in *n.* The correction of occlusal problems or tooth imperfections by grinding.

gripe (grīp) *v.* To have sharp pains in the bowels. —*n.* **1. gripes** Sharp, spasmodic pains in the bowels. **2.** A firm hold; a grasp.

grippe *or* **grip** (grĭp) *n.* See **influenza.**

gris·e·o·ful·vin (grĭz′ē-ə-fŭl′vĭn) *n.* An antibiotic administered orally for the treatment of ringworm and other fungal infections of the skin, hair, and nails.

Grit·ti-Stokes amputation (grē′tē-stōks′) *n.* Amputation of the leg through the knee in which the patella is preserved and applied to the end of the femur. Also called *Stokes' amputation.*

groin (groin) *n.* The crease or hollow at the junction of the inner part of each thigh with the trunk, together with the adjacent region and often including the external genitals.

groove (grōōv) *n.* A rut, groove, or narrow depression or channel in a surface.

groove of nail matrix *n.* The cutaneous furrow in which the lateral border of a nail is situated.

Gross (grōs), **Samuel David** 1805–1884. American surgeon and educator who wrote widely influential medical treatises, including *A System of Surgery* (1859).

gross anatomy *n.* The study of the structures of the body that can be seen with the naked eye. Also called *macroscopic anatomy.*

ground bundle (ground) *n.* See **proper fasciculus.**

ground lamella *n.* See **interstitial lamella.**

ground state *n.* The state of least possible energy in a physical system, as of atoms or molecules.

ground substance *n.* **1.** The amorphous intercellular material in which the cells and fibers of connective tissue are embedded, composed of proteoglycans, plasma constituents, metabolites, water, and ions present between cells and fibers. Also called *matrix.* **2.** See **hyaloplasm.**

group (grōōp) *n.* **1.** An assemblage of persons or objects gathered or located together; an aggregation. **2.** A class or collection of related objects or entities. **3.** Two or more atoms that behave so that are regarded as behaving as a single chemical unit. —*v.* **1.** To place or arrange in a group. **2.** To belong to or form a group.

group agglutination *n.* The clumping of antibodies specific for a group of antigens common to several bacteria, each of which possesses its own specific antigen.

group agglutinin *n.* An agglutinin specific for a group antigen. Also called *cross-reacting agglutinin, minor agglutinin, partial agglutinin.*

group antigen *n.* Any of several antigens that are shared by related genera of microorganisms.

group A streptococcus *n.* A common but virulent streptococcus that kills the tissue it infects and produces toxins that trigger a form of shock that affects the vital organs.

group home *n.* A small supervised residential facility, as for mentally ill people, in which residents typically participate in daily tasks and are often free to come and go voluntarily.

group practice *n.* The practice of medicine by a group of physicians, each of whom is usually confined to some special field but all of whom share a common facility.

group therapy *n.* A form of psychotherapy that involves sessions guided by a therapist and attended by several clients who confront their personal problems together. The interaction among clients is considered to be an integral part of the therapy.

grow (grō) *v.* **1.** To increase in size by a natural process. **2.** To develop and reach maturity. **3.** To be capable of growth; thrive.

grow·ing pains (grō′ĭng) *pl.n.* Pains in the limbs and joints of children or adolescents, frequently occurring at night and often attributed to rapid growth but arising from various unrelated causes.

growth (grōth) *n.* **1.** The process of growing. **2.** Full development; maturity. **3.** An increase, as in size, number, value, or strength. **4.** Something that grows or has grown. **5.** An abnormal mass of tissue, such as a tumor, growing in or on an organism.

growth factor *n.* A substance that affects the growth of an organism.

growth hormone *n. Abbr.* **GH** A polypeptide hormone secreted by the anterior lobe of the pituitary gland that promotes growth of the body, especially by stimulating release of somatomedin, and that influences the metabolism of proteins, carbohydrates, and lipids. Also called *human growth hormone, pituitary growth hormone, somatotropin.*

growth hormone-producing adenoma *n.* A tumor that may secrete both growth hormone and prolactin, causing gigantism or acromegaly. Also called *acidophil adenoma, eosinophil adenoma.*

growth hormone-releasing factor *or* **growth hormone-releasing hormone** *n. Abbr.* **GHRF, GH-RF** See **somatoliberin.**

growth line *n.* Any of various dense transverse lines observed in radiographs of long bones, representing bone regrowth after temporary cessation of longitudinal growth. Also called *Harris' line.*

growth-onset diabetes *n.* Insulin-dependent diabetes.

growth rate *n.* Absolute or relative growth increase, expressed in units of time.

Gru·ber (grü′bər), **Max von** 1853–1927. Austrian bacteriologist noted for his work in serum diagnosis, including the discovery (1896) of the specific agglutination of bacteria by the blood serum of immunized animals.

gru·mous (grōō′məs) *adj.* Thick and lumpy, as clotting blood.

gry·po·sis (grə-pō′sĭs, grī-) *n.* An abnormal curvature, as of the nails.

GSR *abbr.* galvanic skin response

GSW *abbr.* gunshot wound

gt. *abbr.* gutta

GTP (jē′tē-pē′) *n.* Guanosine triphosphate; a nucleotide similar to ATP, composed of guanine, ribose, and three phosphate groups, and necessary for the synthesis of proteins.

gtt. *abbr. Latin* guttae (drops)

GU *abbr.* genitourinary

guai·a·col (gwī′ə-kôl′, -kŏl′) *n.* A yellowish, oily, aromatic substance derived from guaiacum or wood creosote and used chiefly as an expectorant, a local anesthetic, and an antiseptic.

guai·fen·e·sin (gwī-fĕn′ə-sĭn) *n.* An expectorant drug used to thin mucus and sputum.

gua·nase (gwä′nās′, gwä′nāz′) *n.* See **guanine deaminase.**

gua·na·zo·lo (gwä′nə-zō′lō) *n.* See **azaguanine.**

gua·neth·i·dine (gwä-nĕth′ĭ-dēn′) *n.* A drug used as its sulfate salt in the treatment of hypertension.

gua·nine (gwä′nēn′) *n. Abbr.* **G** A purine base that is an essential constituent of both RNA and DNA.

guanine deaminase *n.* A liver enzyme that catalyzes the conversion of guanine to xanthine. Also called *guanase.*

guanine deoxyribonucleotide *n.* See **deoxyguanylic acid.**

guanine ribonucleotide *n.* See **GMP.**

gua·no·sine (gwä′nə-sēn′, -sĭn) *n.* A nucleoside consisting of guanine and ribose.

guanosine 3′,5′-monophosphate *n.* Cyclic GMP.

guanosine monophosphate *n.* Cyclic GMP.

guanosine triphosphate *n.* GTP.

gua·nyl·ic acid (gwä-nĭl′ĭk) *n.* See **GMP.**

guarded *adj.* Watched over; supervised, as of the condition of a patient.

guarding *n.* A spasm of muscles that minimizes the motion or agitation of sites that are affected by injury or disease.

guar gum (gwär) *n.* A water-soluble paste made from the seeds of the guar plant and used as a thickener and stabilizer in foods and pharmaceuticals.

gu·ber·nac·u·lum (goo′bər-năk′yə-ləm) *n., pl.* **–la** (-lə) A fibrous cord connecting two structures.

gubernaculum den·tis (dĕn′tĭs) *n.* A band of connective tissue uniting the tooth sac with the gum.

gubernaculum tes·tis (tĕs′tĭs) *n.* A mesenchymal column of tissue that connects the fetal testis to the developing scrotum and that is involved in testicular descent.

Gué·rin (gā-răn′, -răN′), **Camille** 1872–1961. French bacteriologist. With Albert Calmette he developed (c. 1921) the Bacillus Calmette-Guérin vaccine for immunization against tuberculosis.

guide (gīd) *n.* A device or instrument by which something is led into its proper course, such as a grooved director or a catheter guide.

Guil·lain-Bar·ré syndrome (gē-yăn′bə-rā′, gē-yăN′-) *n.* See **acute idiopathic polyneuritis.**

guil·lo·tine (gĭl′ə-tēn′, gē′ə-) *n.* A ring-shaped instrument with a sliding knifeblade running through it, used in cutting off an enlarged tonsil.

guin·ea pig (gĭn′ē) *n.* Any of various small, short-eared domesticated rodents of the genus *Cavia*, having variously colored hair and no visible tail. They are widely kept as pets and often used as experimental animals.

guinea worm *n.* A long, threadlike nematode of tropical Asia and Africa that is a subcutaneous parasite of humans and other mammals and causes ulcerative lesions on the legs and feet.

Gulf War syndrome (gŭlf) *n.* A medical condition affecting some veterans of the Gulf War, characterized by fatigue, headache, joint pain, skin rashes, nausea, and respiratory disorders, and attributed to reactions to drugs and vaccines, infectious diseases, or exposure to chemicals, radiation, and smoke from oil fires.

gul·let (gŭl′ĭt) *n.* **1.** The esophagus. **2.** The throat.

Gull·strand (gŭl′stränd′), **Allvar** 1862–1930. Swedish ophthalmologist. He won a 1911 Nobel Prize for his study of the dioptrics of the human eye.

gum[1] (gŭm) *n.* **1.** Any of various viscous substances that are exuded by certain plants and trees and dry into water-soluble, noncrystalline, brittle solids. **2.** A similar plant exudate, such as a resin. **3.** Any of various adhesives made from such exudates or other sticky substance.

gum[2] (gŭm) *n.* The firm connective tissue covered by mucous membrane that envelops the alveolar arches of the jaw and surrounds the bases of the teeth. Also called *gingiva.* —*v.* To chew food with toothless gums.

gum·boil (gŭm′boil′) *n.* A small boil or abscess on the gum, often resulting from tooth decay.

gum line *n.* The position of the margin of the gum in relation to teeth in the dental arch.

gum·ma (gŭm′ə) *n., pl.* **gum·mas** *or* **gum·ma·ta** (gŭm′ə-tə) A small, rubbery granuloma having a necrotic center and an inflamed, fibrous capsule. It is characteristic of an advanced stage of syphilis. Also called *syphiloma.* —**gum′ma·tous** *adj.*

gummatous abscess *n.* An abscess due to the softening and breaking down of a gumma, especially in bone. Also called *syphilitic abscess.*

gum resection *n.* See **gingivectomy.**

Gunn's dot (gŭnz) *n.* Any of the minute glistening white or yellowish nonpathogenic spots usually occurring on the posterior part of a fundus.

Gunn's sign *n.* An indication of arteriolar sclerosis observed ophthalmoscopically, in which the underlying vein at arteriovenous crossings is compressed. Also called *Marcus Gunn's sign.*

gun·stock deformity (gŭn′stŏk′) *n.* A deformity of the elbow, resulting from condylar fracture at the elbow in which the forearm deviates toward the midline of the body when extended.

Gün·ther's disease (goon′tərz, gün′-) *n.* See **congenital erythropoietic porphyria.**

Günz·berg's test (günts′bərgz, -bĕrks′) *n.* A test for detecting hydrochloric acid utilizing phloroglucinol and vanillin, which produce a bright red color in the presence of the acid.

gur·gling rale (gûr′glĭng) *n.* A coarse sound heard in auscultation over large cavities or the trachea when nearly filled with secretions.

gur·ney (gûr′nē) *n., pl.* **–neys** A metal stretcher with wheeled legs, used for transporting patients.

gus·ta·tion (gŭ-stā′shən) *n.* **1.** The act of tasting. **2.** The sense of tasting.

gus·ta·to·ry (gŭs′tə-tôr′ē) *or* **gus·ta·tive** (-tə-tĭv) *adj.* Of or relating to the sense of taste.

gustatory cell *n.* See **taste cell**.

gustatory hyperesthesia *n.* See **hypergeusia**.

gustatory hyperhidrosis *n.* Sweating of the lips, nose, and forehead that occurs after eating certain foods.

gustatory rhinorrhea *n.* Watery nasal discharge associated with stimulation of the sense of taste.

gut (gŭt) *n.* **1.** The alimentary canal or a portion thereof, especially the intestine or stomach. **2.** The embryonic digestive tube, consisting of the foregut, the midgut, and the hindgut. **3. guts** The bowels; entrails; viscera. **4.** A thin, tough cord made from the intestines of animals, usually sheep, and used as a suture material in surgery.

Guth·rie test (gŭth′rē) *n.* A bacterial inhibition assay for measuring serum phenylalanine, used to detect phenylketonuria in the newborn.

gut·ta (gŭt′ə) *n., pl.* **gut·tae** (gŭt′ē′) *Abbr.* **gt** A drop, as of liquid medicine.

gut·ta-per·cha (gŭt′ə-pûr′chə) *n.* A rubbery substance from the latex of any of several tropical trees, used as a temporary filling material in dentistry and in the manufacture of orthopedic splints.

gutta-percha point *n.* A cone of a gutta percha compound used for filling root canals in conjunction with a cement, paste, or plastic.

guttat. *abbr. Latin* guttatim (drop by drop)

gut·tate (gŭt′āt′) *or* **gut·tat·ed** (-ā′tĭd) *adj.* **1.** Having the shape of or resembling drops, as certain cutaneous lesions. **2.** Spotted as if by drops.

gut·ter fracture (gŭt′ər) *n.* A long, narrow, depressed fracture of the skull.

gutter wound *n.* A tangential wound that makes a surface furrow without breaking the skin.

gut·tur·al (gŭt′ər-əl) *adj.* Of or relating to the throat.

Gy *abbr.* gray

GYN *abbr.* gynecology

gyn– *pref.* Variant of **gyno–**.

gy·nan·drism (gī-năn′drĭz′əm, jĭ-) *n.* A developmental abnormality characterized by hypertrophy of the clitoris and union of the labia majora, simulating in appearance the penis and scrotum.

gy·nan·dro·blas·to·ma (gī-năn′drō-blă-stō′mə, jĭ-) *n.* **1.** Arrhenoblastoma. **2.** An ovarian tumor with characteristics of an arrhenoblastoma and a granulosa cell tumor and producing simultaneous androgenic and estrogenic effects.

gy·nan·droid (gī-năn′droid′, jĭ-) *n.* A woman affected with gynandrism.

gy·nan·dro·mor·phism (gī-năn′drə-môr′fĭz′əm, jĭ-) *n.* The occurrence of both male and female characteristics in an organism.

gy·nan·dro·mor·phous (gī-năn′drə-môr′fəs, jĭ-) *adj.* Having both male and female characteristics.

Gy·na·zole (gī′nə-zōl′) A trademark for the drug butoconazole nitrate.

–gyne *suff.* Female reproductive organ: *androgyne*.

gy·ne·cic (jī-nē′sĭk, -nĕs′ĭk, jĭ-) *adj.* Relating to or associated with women.

gyneco– *or* **gynec–** *pref.* Woman: *gynecology*.

gy·ne·cog·ra·phy (jĭn′ĭ-kŏg′rə-fē, gī′nĭ-) *n.* See **hysterosalpingography**.

gyn·e·coid (gī′nĭ-koid′, jĭn′ĭ-) *adj.* Characteristic of a woman.

gynecoid pelvis *n.* The normal female pelvis.

gy·ne·col·o·gist (gī′nĭ-kŏl′ə-jĭst, jĭn′ĭ-) *n.* A physician specializing in gynecology.

gy·ne·col·o·gy (gī′nĭ-kŏl′ə-jē, jĭn′ĭ-) *n. Abbr.* **GYN** The branch of medicine dealing with the administration of health care to women, especially the diagnosis and treatment of disorders affecting the female reproductive organs. —**gy′ne·co·log′i·cal** (-kə-lŏj′ĭ-kəl), **gy′ne·co·log′ic** *adj.*

gyn·e·co·mas·ti·a (gī′nĭ-kō-măs′tē-ə, jĭn′ĭ-) *n.* Abnormal enlargement of the male mammary glands, sometimes to the point of secreting milk.

gyn·e·cop·a·thy (gī′nĭ-kŏp′ə-thē, jĭn′ĭ-) *n.* Any of various diseases specific to women.

gyn·e·pho·bi·a (gī′nĭ-fō′bē-ə, jĭn′ĭ-) *n.* An abnormal or irrational fear of women.

gyno– *or* **gyn–** *pref.* **1.** Woman; female: *gynandromorphism*. **2.** Female reproductive organ or system: *gynoplastics*.

gyn·o·gen·e·sis (gī′nə-jĕn′ĭ-sĭs, jĭn′ə-) *n.* The development of an embryo that contains only maternal chromosomes because the egg has been activated by sperm without fusion of the egg and sperm nuclei.

gy·no·plas·tics (gī′nə-plăs′tĭks, jĭn′ə-) *or* **gyn·o·plas·ty** (jĭn′ə-plăs′tē, gī′nə-, jĭ′-) *n.* The reparative or reconstructive surgery of the female reproductive organs.

gy·rate (jī′rāt′) *v.* **1.** To revolve around a fixed point or axis. **2.** To revolve in or as if in a circle or spiral. —*adj.* In rings; coiled or convoluted. —**gy·ra′tion** *n.*

gyrate atrophy of choroid and retina *n.* Progressive atrophy of the choriocapillary layer of the eye, the pigmentary epithelium, and the retina with associated ornithinuria.

gy·rec·to·my (jī-rĕk′tə-mē) *n.* Excision of a cerebral gyrus.

gyri in·su·lae (ĭn′sə-lē′, -syə-) *pl.n.* The long gyrus of the insula and the short gyrus of the insula considered together.

gy·rose (jī′rōs) *adj.* Marked by irregular curved lines like the surface of a cerebral hemisphere.

gy·ro·spasm (jī′rə-spăz′əm) *n.* A condition characterized by spasmodic rotary movements of the head.

gy·rus (jī′rəs) *n., pl.* **-ri** (-rī′) A rounded ridge, as on the surfaces of the cerebral hemispheres.

gyrus for·ni·ca·tus (fôr′nĭ-kā′təs) *n.* The horseshoe-shaped cortical convolution bordering the hilus of the cerebral hemisphere.

H

h The symbol for **Planck's constant.**

H The symbol for the element **hydrogen.**

HA1 virus (āch′ā-wŭn′) *n.* Variant of **hemadsorption virus type 1.**

HA2 virus (āch′ā-tōō′) *n.* Variant of **hemadsorption virus type 2.**

haar·schei·be tumor (här′shī′bə) *n.* Hamartoma of the hair disk. Also called *trichodiscoma.*

ha·be·na (hă-bē′nə) *n., pl.* **–nae** (-nē) **1.** A frenum or a restricting fibrous band. **2.** See **habenula** (sense 3). —**ha·be′nal, ha·be′nar** (-nər) *adj.*

ha·ben·u·la (hă-běn′yə-lə) *n., pl.* **–lae** (-lē′) **1.** A frenulum. **2.** The stalk of the pineal gland. No longer in technical use. **3.** A circumscript cell mass embedded in the posterior end of the medullary stria of the thalamus, from which it receives most of its afferent fibers. Also called *habena, pedunculus of pineal body.* —**ha·ben′u·lar** *adj.*

hab·it (hăb′ĭt) *n.* **1.** A recurrent, often unconscious, pattern of behavior that is acquired through frequent repetition. **2.** Physical constitution. **3.** An addiction, especially to a narcotic drug.

habit-forming *adj.* Capable of leading to physiological or psychological dependence.

habit spasm *n.* See **tic.**

ha·bit·u·al abortion (hə-bĭch′ōō-əl) *n.* Three or more consecutive spontaneous abortions that occur at about the same stage of pregnancy.

ha·bit·u·ate (hə-bĭch′ōō-āt′) *v.* **1.** To accustom by frequent repetition or prolonged exposure. **2.** To cause physiological or psychological habituation, as to a drug. **3.** To experience psychological habituation.

ha·bit·u·a·tion (hə-bĭch′ōō-ā′shən) *n.* **1.** The process of habituating or the state of being habituated. **2.** Physiological tolerance to a drug resulting from repeated use. **3.** Psychological dependence on a drug. **4.** The decline of a conditioned response following repeated exposure to the conditioned stimulus.

hab·i·tus (hăb′ĭ-təs) *n., pl.* **habitus** The physical and constitutional characteristics of an individual, especially the tendency to develop a certain disease.

Haeck·el (hĕk′əl), **Ernst** 1834–1919. German philosopher and naturalist who supported Darwin's theory and mapped a genealogical tree relating all animal life.

Haeck·el's law (hĕk′əlz) *n.* See **biogenetic law.**

haem– *pref.* Variant of **hemo–.**

haema– *pref.* Variant of **hemo–.**

Hae·ma·phy·sa·lis (hē′mə-fī′sə-lĭs, hĕm′ə-) *n.* A genus of small eyeless widely distributed ticks that are important vectors of certain disease-causing bacteria, protozoa, and viruses.

haemat– *pref.* Variant of **hemato–.**

haemato– *pref.* Variant of **hemato–.**

–haemia *suff.* Variant of **–emia.**

haemo– *pref.* Variant of **hemo–.**

Hae·moph·i·lus *or* **He·moph·i·lus** (hē-mŏf′ə-ləs) *n.* A genus of aerobic to facultatively anaerobic parasitic bacteria of the family Brucellaceae that contain minute, gram-negative, rod-shaped cells.

Haemophilus ae·gyp·ti·us (ĭ-jĭp′shē-əs) *n.* Koch-Weeks bacillus.

Haemophilus du·crey·i (dōō-krā′ī′) *n.* Ducrey's bacillus.

Haemophilus in·flu·en·zae (ĭn′flōō-ĕn′zē) *n.* A gram-negative, rod-shaped bacterium of the genus *Haemophilus,* especially Haemophilus influenzae type b, that occurs in the human respiratory tract and causes acute respiratory infections, acute conjunctivitis, and purulent meningitis. Also called *Pfeiffer's bacillus.*

Haemophilus influenzae type b *n. Abbr.* **Hib** A gram-negative, rod-shaped bacterium of the genus *Haemophilus* that is found in the human respiratory tract and causes acute respiratory infections, such as pneumonia, and other diseases, especially meningitis in young children. Haemophilus influenzae type b is the most common pathogenic form.

Haemophilus influenzae type b conjugate vaccine *n.* See **Hib vaccine.**

Haff·kine (hăf′kĭn), **Waldemar Mordecai Wolfe** 1860–1930. Russian bacteriologist known for his work in India on inoculations against cholera and plague.

haf·ni·um (hăf′nē-əm) *n. Symbol* **Hf** A metallic element found with zirconium and used in nuclear reactor control rods and in tungsten alloys used in filaments. Atomic number 72.

Hage·man factor (hä′gə-mən) *n.* See **factor XII.**

H agglutinin *n.* An agglutinin formed as the result of stimulation by, and reaction with a thermolabile antigen that is present in the flagella of motile microorganisms.

Hah·ne·mann (hä′nə-mən, -män′), **(Christian Friedrich) Samuel** 1755–1843. German physician and founder of homeopathy. He postulated that medicine produces symptoms in healthy people that are similar to those that it relieves in sick people.

Hai·ley and Hai·ley disease (hā′lē) *n.* See **familial benign chronic pemphigus.**

hair (hâr) *n.* **1.** Any of the cylindrical, keratinized, often pigmented filaments characteristically growing from the epidermis of a mammal. **2.** A growth of such filaments, as that forming the coat of an animal or covering the scalp of a human. **3.** One of the fine hairlike processes of a sensory cell.

hair·ball (hâr′bôl′) *n.* A small mass of hair located in the stomach or intestine of an animal, such as a cat, resulting from an accumulation of small amounts of hair that are swallowed each time the animal licks its coat. Also called *pilobezoar, trichobezoar.*

hair bulb *n.* The lower expanded extremity of a hair that fits like a cap over the hair papilla at the bottom of the hair follicle.

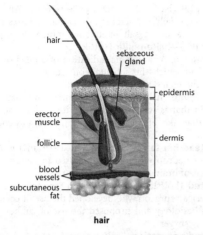

hair

hair cast *n.* A small, nodular accretion of epithelial cells and keratinous debris, appearing along the shaft of a hair and resulting from failure of the internal root sheath to disintegrate.

hair cell *n.* A cell with hairlike processes, especially one of the sensory epithelial cells present in the organ of Corti.

hair disk *n.* A highly innervated area of skin around a hair follicle consisting of a thickened layer of epithelial cells in which unmyelinated terminals of a single axon ramify.

hair follicle *n.* A deep narrow pit that is formed by the tubular invagination of the epidermis and corium and encloses the root of the hair.

hair·line (hâr′līn′) *n.* The outline of the growth of hair on the head, especially across the front.

hairline fracture *n.* A fracture in which the fragments do not separate because the line of break is so fine. Also called *capillary fracture.*

hair papilla *n.* A knoblike vascular indentation of the bottom of a hair follicle, on which the hair bulb fits.

hair root *n.* The part of a hair that is embedded in a hair follicle.

hair·y (hâr′ē) *adj.* **1.** Covered with hair or hairlike projections. **2.** Consisting of or resembling hair.

hairy cell *n.* White blood cells having multiple processes and characteristically present in hairy cell leukemia where they replace bone marrow.

hairy cell leukemia *n.* A lymphocytic leukemia, usually originating with B cells, and characterized by splenomegaly and cells with a ciliated appearance in the spleen, bone marrow, liver, and blood. Also called *leukemic reticuloendotheliosis.*

hairy heart *n.* See **fibrinous pericarditis.**

hairy leukoplakia *n.* A white raised lesion having keratin projections on its surface and appearing on the tongue and occasionally on the buccal mucosa of patients with AIDS.

hairy mole *n.* A nevus covered with a growth of hair.

hairy tongue *n.* A benign condition of the tongue that is marked by elongation and often staining of the filiform papillae. Also called *glossotrichia, trichoglossia.*

hal– *pref.* Variant of **halo–.**

ha·la·tion (hā-lā′shən) *n.* **1.** Blurring of the visual image due to glare from strong illumination. **2.** A blurring or spreading of light around bright areas on a photographic image.

hal·cin·o·nide (hăl-sĭn′ə-nīd′) *n.* A corticosteroid used in topical preparations as an anti-inflammatory agent.

Hal·ci·on (hăl′sē-ən) A trademark for the drug triazolam.

Hal·dane (hôl′dān′, -dən) Family of Scottish intellectuals and scientists, including **John Scott Haldane** (1860–1936), a physiologist noted for his studies of the exchange of gases during respiration; and his son **John Burdon Sanderson Haldane** (1892–1964), a geneticist.

Hal·dane effect (hôl′dān′) *n.* The promotion of carbon dioxide dissociation that results from the oxygenation of hemoglobin.

Hal·dol (hăl′dôl′, -dŏl′, -dōl′) A trademark for the drug haloperidol.

half and half nail (hăf) *n.* Division of the nail by a transverse line into a proximal dull white part and a distal pink or brown part. It is seen in uremia.

half-life *n.* **1.** The time required for half the nuclei of a specific radionuclide or radioactive substance to undergo radioactive decay. Also called *physical half-life.* **2.** The time required for half the quantity of a drug or other substance deposited in a living organism to be metabolized or eliminated by normal biological processes. Also called *biological half-life.* **3.** The time required for the radioactivity of material taken in by or administered to an organism to be reduced to half its initial value by a combination of biological elimination processes and radioactive decay. Also called *effective half-life.*

half·way house (hăf′wā′) *n.* A rehabilitation facility for individuals, such as mental patients or substance abusers, who no longer require the complete facilities of a hospital or other institution but who are not yet prepared to return to their communities.

hal·ide (hăl′īd′, hā′līd′) *n.* A chemical compound of a halogen with a more electropositive element or group.

hal·i·ste·re·sis (hăl′ĭ-stə-rē′sĭs, hə-lĭs′tə-) *n.* A deficiency of lime salts in the bones.

hal·i·to·sis (hăl′ĭ-tō′sĭs) *n.* The condition of having foul-smelling breath. Also called *fetor ex ore.*

hal·i·tus (hăl′ĭ-təs) *n.* An exhalation, as of a breath or vapor.

Hall (hôl), **Granville Stanley** 1844–1924. American psychologist who established an experimental psychology laboratory at Johns Hopkins University (1882), founded child psychology, and profoundly influenced educational psychology.

Hal·ler (hä′lər), **Albrecht von** 1708–1777. Swiss physiologist whose investigations into the structure of nerves and the relationship of nerves to muscles form the basis of modern neurology. Haller also discovered the role of bile in digesting fats and developed a botanical taxonomic system.

Hal·ler's circle (hăl′ərz, hä′lərz) *n.* A network of branches of the short ciliary arteries on the sclera around the point of entrance of the optic nerve.

Hal·ler·vor·den-Spatz syndrome (hăl′lər-vôr′dn-shpätz′, hä′lər-) *or* **Hallervorden syndrome** *n.* An inherited syndrome in which the nerve fibers connecting the striatum and globus pallidus are completely demyelinated.

Hal·lion's test (äl-yôɴz′) *n.* A test of collateral circulation in cases of aneurysm, in which the main artery and vein of a limb are compressed; the veins of the hand or foot swell up if the collateral circulation is impeded.

Hal·lo·peau's disease (ä-lə-pōz′, -lô-) *n.* **1.** See **acrodermatitis continua. 2.** See **pemphigus vegetans** (sense 2). **3.** See **lichen sclerosus et atrophicus.**

hal·lu·cal (hăl′ə-kəl, -yə-) *adj.* Relating to the first digit of the foot.

hal·lu·ci·na·tion (hə-loō′sə-nā′shən) *n.* **1.** False or distorted perception of objects or events with a compelling sense of their reality, usually resulting from a mental disorder or drug. **2.** The objects or events so perceived. —**hal·lu′ci·nate′** *v.*

hal·lu·ci·na·to·ry (hə-loō′sə-nə-tôr′ē) *adj.* **1.** Of or characterized by hallucination. **2.** Inducing or causing hallucination.

hal·lu·ci·no·gen (hə-loō′sə-nə-jən) *n.* A substance that induces hallucination. —**hal·lu′cin·o·gen′ic** (-jĕn′ĭk) *adj.*

hal·lu·ci·no·sis (hə-loō′sə-nō′sĭs) *n.* An abnormal condition or a mental state that is characterized by hallucination.

hal·lux (hăl′əks) *n., pl.* **hal·lu·ces** (hăl′yə-sēz′, hăl′ə-) **1.** The big toe. **2.** A homologous or similar digit on the hind foot of certain mammals.

hallux do·lo·ro·sus (dō′lə-rō′səs) *n.* A condition, associated with flatfoot, in which walking causes severe pain in the metatarsophalangeal joint of the big toe.

hallux flex·us (flĕk′səs) *n.* Hammer toe of the big toe.

hallux rig·i·dus (rĭj′ĭ-dəs) *n.* A condition in which there is stiffness in the metatarsophalangeal joint of the big toe.

hallux val·gus (văl′gəs) *n.* Deviation of the tip or main axis of the big toe toward the outer side of the foot.

hallux var·us (vâr′əs) *n.* Deviation of the main axis of the big toe to the inner side of the foot.

ha·lo (hā′lō) *n., pl.* **–los** *or* **–loes 1.** A reddish yellow ring surrounding the optic disk, caused by an expansion of the scleral ring that makes the deeper structures visible. **2.** Glaucomatous halo. **3.** A ring of light surrounding a luminous body.

halo– *or* **hal–** *pref.* **1.** Salt: *halophilic.* **2.** Halogen: *halide.*

Hal·og (hăl′ŏg′) A trademark for the drug halcinonide.

hal·o·gen (hăl′ə-jən) *n.* Any of a group of five chemically related nonmetallic elements including fluorine, chlorine, bromine, iodine, and astatine.

ha·lom·e·ter (hă-lŏm′ĭ-tər, hā-) *n.* **1.** An instrument used to measure the diffraction halo of a red blood cell. **2.** An instrument for measuring ocular halos.

halo nevus *n.* A usually benign, sometimes multiple, melanotic nevus that involutes, producing a pigmented center that is surrounded by a uniformly depigmented zone. Also called *leukoderma acquisitum centrifugum, Sutton's disease.*

hal·o·per·i·dol (hăl′ō-pĕr′ĭ-dôl′, -dōl′) *n.* A tranquilizer used especially in the treatment of psychotic disorders, including schizophrenia.

hal·o·phil (hăl′ə-fĭl) *or* **hal·o·phile** (-fīl′) *n.* An organism, especially a microorganism, that requires a high concentration of salt in its environment for optimal growth. —**hal′o·phil′ic** (-fĭl′ĭk) *adj.*

halo sign *n.* A radiologic indication of a dead or dying fetus in which the subcutaneous fat layer is elevated over the fetal skull.

hal·o·thane (hăl′ə-thān′) *n.* A colorless, nonflammable liquid that is widely used as an inhalation anesthetic and that takes effect rapidly and can be rapidly counteracted.

Hal·stead-Rei·tan battery (hôl′stĕd′-rī′tăn′) *n.* An array of neuropsychological tests used to determine the effects of brain damage on behavior.

Hal·sted (hôl′stəd, -stĕd′), **William Stewart** 1852–1922. American surgeon who developed the use of cocaine in anesthesiology and proposed the use of rubber gloves during surgery.

Hal·sted's operation (hôl′stədz, -stĕdz′) *n.* **1.** An operation for the radical correction of inguinal hernia. **2.** See **radical mastectomy.**

Halsted's suture *n.* A suture placed through the subcuticular fascia, used for exact skin approximation.

ha·mar·ti·a (hä′mär-tē′ə, hə-mär′shē-ə) *n.* A developmental defect characterized by the abnormal arrangement or combination of tissues normally present in a specific area.

ha·mar·to·blas·to·ma (hə-mär′tō-blă-stō′mə) *n.* A malignant tumor of undifferentiated anaplastic cells derived from a hamartoma.

ham·ar·to·ma (hăm′är-tō′mə) *n., pl* **–mas** *or* **–ma·ta** (-mə-tə) A benign tumorlike malformation resulting from faulty development in an organ and composed of an abnormal mixture of tissue elements that develop and grow at the same rate as normal elements but are not likely to compress adjacent tissue. —**ham′ar·tom′a·tous** (-tŏm′ə-təs, -tō′mə-) *adj.*

ha·mate (hā′māt′) *n.* A bone on the medial side of the carpus, articulating with the fourth and fifth metacarpal, triquetrum, lunate, and capitate bones. Also called *unciform bone.*

Ham·bur·ger's law (hăm′bûr′gərz) *n.* The principle that, under acidic conditions, albumins and phosphates in the blood pass from red blood cells to serum and chlorides pass from serum to red blood cells while, under basic conditions, the reverse occurs.

Ham·il·ton (hăm′əl-tən), **Alice** 1869–1970. American toxicologist and physician known for her research on occupational poisons and her book *Industrial Poisons in the United States* (1925).

Ham·man-Rich syndrome (hăm′ən-rĭch′) *n.* A syndrome involving acute or chronic interstitial fibrosis of the lung and giving rise to serious right-sided heart failure and cor pulmonale.

Ham·man's syndrome (hăm′ənz) *n.* Spontaneous mediastinal emphysema resulting from rupture of alveoli. Also called *Hamman's disease.*

ham·mer (hăm′ər) *n.* See **malleus.**

hammer finger *n.* See **baseball finger.**

ham·mer·toe *or* **hammer toe** (hăm′ər-tō′) *n.* A toe, usually the second, that is permanently flexed downward, resulting in a clawlike shape.

Ham's test (hămz) *n.* See **acidified serum test**.

ham·string (hăm′strĭng′) *n.* **1.** Any of the tendons at the rear hollow of the human knee. **2. hamstrings** The hamstring muscle. **3.** The large tendon in the back of the hind tarsal joint of the quadruped.

hamstring muscle *n.* Any of the three muscles constituting the back of the upper leg that serve to flex the knee joint, adduct the leg, and extend the thigh.

ham·u·lar (hăm′yə-lər) *adj.* Hook-shaped; unciform.

ham·u·lus (hăm′yə-ləs) *n., pl.* **–li** (-lī′) A small hooklike projection or process, as at the end of a bone.

hand (hănd) *n.* **1.** The terminal part of the human arm located below the forearm, used for grasping and holding and consisting of the wrist, palm, four fingers, and an opposable thumb. **2.** A homologous or similar part in other animals.

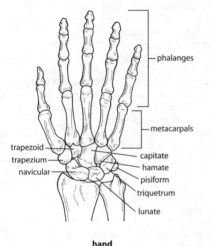

hand
dorsal view of bones in the hand

hand·ed (hăn′dĭd) *adj.* Of, relating to, or characterizing the dexterity, preference, or size with respect to a hand or hands.

hand·ed·ness (hăn′dĭd-nĭs) *n.* **1.** A preference for using one hand as opposed to the other. **2.** The chirality of a molecule.

hand-foot-and-mouth disease *n.* An exanthematous eruption of the fingers, toes, palms, and soles, accompanied by often painful blistering and ulceration of the buccal mucous membrane, tongue, and soft palate, caused by a coxsackievirus.

hand·i·cap (hăn′dē-kăp′) *n.* A physical, emotional, or mental condition that interferes with one's normal functioning.

H & P *abbr.* history and physical (examination)

Hand-Schüller-Christian disease (hănd′-) *n.* A progressive disease beginning in childhood that is marked by protruding eyeballs, diabetes insipidus, and a softening and destruction of bone, especially the skull, and is caused by abnormal cholesterol metabolism. Also called *Christian's disease, Schüller's disease*.

hang·man's fracture (hăng′mənz) *n.* A fracture or dislocation fracture of the cervical vertebrae near the base of the skull.

hang·nail (hăng′nāl′) *n.* A small piece of dead skin at the side or the base of a fingernail that is partly detached from the rest of the skin.

Han·sen (hăn′sən, hän′-), **Gerhard Henrik Armauer** 1746–1845. Norwegian physician and bacteriologist who discovered (1869) the leprosy bacillus.

Han·sen's bacillus (hăn′sənz) *n.* An aerobic, nonmotile, gram-positive bacterium *Mycobacterium leprae* that causes leprosy in humans.

Hansen's disease *n.* See **leprosy**.

han·ta·vi·rus (hăn′tə-vī′rəs) *n.* A type of virus carried by rodents causing severe respiratory infections in humans and, in some cases, hemorrhaging, kidney disease, and death.

H antigen *n.* See **flagellar antigen**.

haph·al·ge·sia (hăf′əl-jē′zhə) *n.* Pain caused by slight touch.

haplo– *pref.* **1.** Simple: *haploprotein*. **2.** Single: *haplotype*.

hap·loid (hăp′loid′) *adj.* Having the same number of sets of chromosomes as a germ cell, or half the diploid number of a somatic cell. The haploid number (23 in humans) is the normal chromosome complement of germ cells. —*n.* A haploid organism or cell. —**hap′-loi′dy** (-loi′dē) *n.*

hap·lo·scope (hăp′lə-skōp′) *n.* An instrument for presenting separate views to each eye so that they may be seen as one integrated view. —**hap′lo·scop′ic** (-skŏp′-ĭk) *adj.*

hap·lo·sis (hăp-lō′sĭs) *n.* Reduction of the diploid number of chromosomes by one half during meiosis, resulting in the haploid number.

hap·lo·type (hăp′lə-tīp′) *n.* **1.** The set of alleles that determine different antigens but are closely linked on one chromosome and inherited as a unit, providing a distinctive genetic pattern used in histocompatibility testing. **2.** The antigenic phenotype determined by closely linked genes that are inherited as a unit from one parent.

hap·py-pup·pet syndrome (hăp′ē-pŭp′ĭt) *n.* A congenital syndrome of unknown cause that is characterized by mental retardation, ataxic movements, hypotonia, epileptic seizures, prolonged and easily provoked spasms of laughter, prognathism, and an open-mouthed facial expression.

Haps·burg jaw (hăps′bûrg′, häps′bŏŏrk′) *n.* A prognathous jaw, often accompanied by an overdeveloped lower lip.

Hapsburg lip *n.* A projecting overdeveloped lower lip, often accompanied by a prognathous jaw.

hap·ten (hăp′tən) *n.* A substance that is capable of reacting with a specific antibody but cannot induce the formation of antibodies unless bound to a carrier protein or other molecule. Also called *incomplete antigen, partial antigen*.

hap·tic (hăp′tĭk) *adj.* Of or relating to the sense of touch; tactile.

hap·tics (hăp′tĭks) *n.* The science that deals with the sense of touch.

hap·to·glo·bin (hăp′tə-glō′bĭn) *n.* A plasma protein that is a normal constituent of blood serum and functions in the binding of free hemoglobin in the bloodstream.

Ha·ra·da's syndrome (hə-rä′dəz) *n.* A syndrome of unknown cause, usually occurring in young adults, that is characterized by bilateral fundal edema, retinal detachment, and inflammation of the choroid, ciliary body, and iris of the eye as well as by temporary or permanent loss of hearing and visual acuity, and by graying and loss of hair.

hard chancre (härd) *n.* See **chancre.**

hard corn *pl.n.* A corn located over a toe joint. Also called *heloma durum.*

hard·en·ing of arteries (här′dn-ĭng) *n.* The condition of arteriosclerosis.

hard palate *n.* The anterior part of the palate, consisting of the bony palate covered above by the mucous membrane of the nose, and below by the mucoperiosteum of the roof of the mouth.

hard pulse *n.* A pulse that strikes forcibly against the tip of the finger and is difficult to compress, indicating hypertension.

hard rays *pl.n.* Radiation of short wavelength and great penetrability.

hard tubercle *n.* A nonnecrotic tubercle.

hard ulcer *n.* See **chancre.**

Har·dy-Rand-Ritter test (här′dē-rănd′-) *n.* A test for color-vision deficiency similar to the Ishihara test.

Hardy-Wein·berg law (-wīn′bərg) *n.* A fundamental principle in population genetics stating that the genotype frequencies and gene frequencies of a large, randomly mating population remain constant provided immigration, mutation, and selection do not take place.

hare·lip (hâr′lĭp′) *n.* See **cleft lip.**

har·le·quin fetus (här′lĭ-kwĭn, -kĭn) *n.* A newborn, usually premature collodian baby whose symptoms are severe.

har·mon·ic mean (här-mŏn′ĭk) *n.* The reciprocal of the arithmetic mean of the reciprocals of a specified set of numbers.

harmonic suture *n.* See **plane suture.**

Har·ris' line (här′ĭ-sĭz) *n.* See **growth line.**

Har·ri·son's groove (hăr′ĭ-sənz) *n.* A groove in the chest manifesting a deformity of the ribs caused by the pull of the diaphragm on ribs weakened by rickets or by other softening of the bone.

Hart·line (härt′līn′), **Haldan Keffer** 1903–1983. American biophysicist. He shared a 1967 Nobel Prize for research on the physiological and electrical activities of the optic nerve and the eye.

Hart·man·nel·la (härt′mə-nĕl′ə) *n.* A free-living ameba commonly found in soil, sewage, and water and known to invade invertebrates such as snails and oysters; it is considered to be a causative agent of primary amebic meningoencephalitis.

Hart·mann's operation (härt′mənz) *n.* Resection of the rectosigmoid colon with closure of the rectal stump and colostomy.

Hart·nup disease (härt′nəp) *n.* A congenital metabolic disorder characterized by aminoaciduria, a pellagralike, light-sensitive skin rash, and a temporary cerebellar ataxia. Also called *Hartnup syndrome, H disease.*

har·vest bug (här′vĭst) *n.* See **chigger** (sense 1).

harvest mite *n.* See **chigger** (sense 1).

Har·vey (här′vē), **William** 1578–1657. English physician, anatomist, and physiologist who discovered the circulation of blood in the human body (1628).

hash (hăsh) *n.* Hashish.

Ha·shi·mo·to's disease (hăsh′ĭ-mō′tōz, hä′shē-) *n.* An autoimmune disease of the thyroid gland, resulting in diffuse goiter, infiltration of the thyroid gland with lymphocytes, and hypothyroidism. Also called *Hashimoto's thyroiditis, lymphadenoid goiter, struma lymphomatosa.*

hash·ish (hăsh′ēsh′, -ĭsh, hă-shēsh′, hä-) *n.* A purified resin prepared from the flowering tops of the female cannabis plant and smoked or chewed as a narcotic or an intoxicant.

Has·sall's concentric corpuscle (hăs′ôlz, -əlz) *n.* See **thymic corpuscle.**

has·si·um (hä′sē-əm) *n. Symbol* **Hs** A radioactive synthetic element whose longest-lived isotopes have mass numbers of 264 and 265 with half-lives of 0.08 millisecond and 2 milliseconds. Atomic number 108.

haus·tra·tion (hô-strā′shən) *n.* **1.** The formation of a haustrum. **2.** A haustrum.

haus·trum (hô′strəm) *n., pl.* **haus·tra** (hô′strə) Any of a series of saccules or pouches, especially of the colon. —**haus′tral** *adj.*

HAV *abbr.* hepatitis A virus

Hav·er·hill fever (hāv′rəl, hā′vər-əl) *n.* An infection by *Streptobacillus moniliformis* marked by initial chills and high fever gradually subsiding and followed by arthritis usually in the larger joints and spine, and by a rash occurring chiefly over the joints and on the extensor surfaces of the extremities. Also called *erythema arthriticum epidemicum.*

Ha·vers (hā′vərz, hăv′ərz), **Clopton** 1655?–1702. English physician and anatomist known for his studies of the minute structure of bone.

ha·ver·sian canal (hə-vûr′zhən) *n.* Any of various canals in compact bone through which blood vessels, nerve fibers, and lymphatics pass.

haversian lamella *n.* See **concentric lamella.**

haversian space *n.* A space in compact bone formed by the enlargement of a haversian canal.

haversian system *n.* See **osteon.**

Haw·orth (hou′ərth, härth), Sir **Walter Norman** 1883–1950. British biochemist. He shared a 1937 Nobel Prize for his research on carbohydrates and vitamin C.

Ha·yem-Wi·dal syndrome (ä-yĕm′vē-däl′, ä-yän′-) *n.* Acquired hemolytic anemia characterized by jaundice, anemia, moderate enlargement of the spleen, increased fragility of red blood cells, and increased concentrations of urobilin in the urine.

hay fever (hā) *n.* An allergic condition affecting the mucous membranes of the upper respiratory tract and the eyes, usually characterized by nasal discharge, sneezing, and itchy, watery eyes and usually caused by an abnormal sensitivity to airborne pollen.

Hay·garth's nodes (hā′gärths′) *pl.n.* Bony growths in the area of the finger joints occurring in rheumatoid arthritis, leading to ankylosis and associated with lateral deflection of the fingers toward the ulnar side.

Hb *abbr.* hemoglobin

HB *abbr.* hepatitis B vaccine

Hb A *abbr.* hemoglobin A

HB$_c$Ag *abbr.* hepatitis B core antigen

HB$_s$Ag *abbr.* hepatitis B surface antigen

H band *n.* The pale area in the center of the A band of a striated muscle fiber.

Hb AS *abbr.* hemoglobin A and hemoglobin S (heterozygous state) (the sickle cell trait)

Hb Bart's *abbr.* Bart's hemoglobin

Hb C *abbr.* hemoglobin C

HBe *or* **HB$_e$Ag** *abbr.* hepatitis B e antigen

Hb F *n.* A form of hemoglobulin present in high concentrations in the fetal stage of development but normally diminishing to a low concentration in children and adults except in certain anemias, leukemia, and hemoglobin disorders.

Hb H *abbr.* hemoglobin H

Hb M *abbr.* hemoglobin M

HBP *abbr.* high blood pressure

Hb S *abbr.* hemoglobin S

HBV *abbr.* hepatitis B virus

HCFA *abbr.* Health Care Financing Administration

HCG *abbr.* human chorionic gonadotropin

HCS *abbr.* human chorionic somatomammotropic hormone

Hct *abbr.* hematocrit

HCTZ *abbr.* hydrochlorothiazide

HCV *abbr.* hepatitis C virus

h.d. *abbr. Latin* hora decubitus (before sleep, at bedtime)

H disease *n.* See **Hartnup disease.**

HDL *abbr.* high-density lipoprotein

HDL cholesterol *n.* See **high-density lipoprotein.**

HDRV *abbr.* human diploid cell rabies vaccine

HDV *abbr.* hepatitis D virus

He The symbol for the element **helium.**

head (hĕd) *n.* **1.** The uppermost or forwardmost part of the human body, containing the brain and the eyes, ears, nose, mouth, and jaws. **2.** The analogous part of various vertebrate and invertebrate animals. **3.** The pus-containing tip of an abscess, boil, or pimple. **4.** The rounded proximal end of a long bone. **5.** The end of a muscle that is attached to the less movable part of the skeleton.

head·ache (hĕd′āk′) *n.* A pain in the head. Also called *cephalalgia.*

head cap *n.* See **acrosomal cap.**

head cold *n.* A common cold mainly affecting the mucous membranes of the nasal passages, characterized by congestion, headache, and sneezing.

head-dropping test *n.* A test used in the diagnosis of disease of the extrapyramidal system in which the head of a person in supine position is lifted by the examiner with one hand and allowed to fall into the other; in healthy individuals, the head falls suddenly, like a dead weight, whereas in extrapyramidal disease, it falls slowly.

head fold *n.* A ventral folding of the cephalic extremity in the embryonic disk, so that the brain lies in a rostral direction to the mouth and pericardium.

heal (hēl) *v.* **1.** To restore to health or soundness; cure. **2.** To become well; return to sound health.

heal·ing by first intention (hē′lĭng) *n.* Healing by fibrous adhesion, without suppuration or formation of granulation tissue. Also called *primary adhesion, primary union.*

healing by second intention *n.* Union of two granulating surfaces that is accompanied by suppuration and delayed closure. Also called *secondary adhesion, secondary union.*

healing by third intention *n.* The slow filling of a wound, cavity, or ulcer by granulations, with subsequent formation of scar tissue.

health (hĕlth) *n.* **1.** The overall condition of an organism at a given time. **2.** Soundness, especially of body or mind; freedom from disease or abnormality.

health care *or* **healthcare** *n.* The prevention, treatment, and management of illness and the preservation of mental and physical well-being through the services offered by the medical and allied health professions. —*adj.* **health-care** Of or relating to health care.

health food *n.* A food believed to be highly beneficial to health, especially a food grown organically and free of chemical additives.

health·ful (hĕlth′fəl) *adj.* **1.** Conducive to good health; salutary. **2.** Healthy. —**health′ful·ness** *n.*

health insurance *n.* Insurance against expenses incurred through illness of the insured.

health maintenance organization *n.* An HMO.

health·y (hĕl′thē) *adj.* **1.** Being in good health. **2.** Conducive to good health; healthful. **3.** Indicative of sound, rational thinking or frame of mind. —**health′i·ly** *adv.* —**health′i·ness** *n.*

hear (hîr) *v.* To perceive (sound) by the ear.

hear·ing (hîr′ĭng) *n.* The sense by which sound is perceived; the capacity to hear.

hearing aid *n.* A small electronic apparatus that amplifies sound and is worn in or behind the ear to compensate for impaired hearing.

hearing dog *n.* A dog trained to assist a deaf or hearing-impaired person by signaling the occurrence of certain sounds, such as a ringing telephone.

hearing-impaired *adj.* **1.** Having a diminished or defective sense of hearing, but not deaf; hard of hearing. **2.** Completely incapable of hearing; deaf. —*n.* Persons who are deficient in hearing or are deaf.

hearing impairment *n.* A reduction or defect in the ability to perceive sound.

heart (härt) *n.* **1.** The chambered, muscular organ in vertebrates that pumps blood received from the veins into the arteries, thereby maintaining the flow of blood through the entire circulatory system. See illustration on page 352. **2.** A similarly functioning structure in invertebrates.

heart attack *n.* Acute myocardial infarction typically resulting from an occlusion or obstruction of a coronary artery and characterized by sudden, severe pain in the chest that often radiates to the shoulder, arm, or jaw.

heart·beat (härt′bēt′) *n.* A single complete pulsation of the heart.

heart block *n.* A condition in which faulty transmission of the impulses that control the heartbeat results in a lack of coordination in the contraction of the atria and ventricles of the heart.

heart·burn (härt′bûrn′) *n.* A burning sensation, usually centered in the middle of the chest near the sternum,

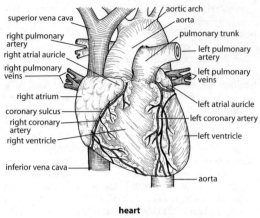

superior vena cava
right pulmonary artery
right atrial auricle
right pulmonary veins
right atrium
coronary sulcus
right coronary artery
right ventricle
inferior vena cava

aortic arch
aorta
pulmonary trunk
left pulmonary artery
left pulmonary veins
left atrial auricle
left coronary artery
left ventricle
aorta

heart
anterior view

caused by the reflux of acidic stomach fluids that enter the lower end of the esophagus. Also called *acid reflux, cardialgia, pyrosis.*

heart disease *n.* A structural or functional abnormality of the heart, or of the blood vessels supplying the heart, that impairs its normal functioning.

heart failure *n.* **1.** A condition marked by weakness, edema, and shortness of breath that is caused by the inability of the heart to maintain adequate blood circulation in the peripheral tissues and the lungs. Also called *cardiac insufficiency, congestive heart failure, myocardial insufficiency.* **2.** The resulting clinical syndrome, consisting of shortness of breath, pitting edema, enlarged tender liver, engorged neck veins, and pulmonary rales.

heart-lung machine *n.* An apparatus through which the blood is temporarily diverted, especially during heart surgery, to oxygenate it and pump it throughout the body.

heart massage *n.* See **cardiac massage.**

heart rate *n. Abbr.* **HR** The number of heartbeats per unit of time, usually expressed as beats per minute.

heart sac *n.* See **pericardium.**

heart sound *n.* Any of the sounds heard on auscultation over the heart, usually referred to as first, second, third, or fourth heart sound. Also called *cardiac sound.*

heat (hēt) *n.* **1.** A form of energy associated with the motion of atoms or molecules and capable of being transmitted through solid and fluid media by conduction, through fluid media by convection, and through empty space by radiation. **2.** The sensation or perception of such energy as warmth or hotness. **3.** An abnormally high bodily temperature, as from a fever. **4.** Estrus.

heat capacity *n.* The amount of heat required to raise the temperature of one mole or one gram of a substance by one degree Celsius without change of phase. Also called *thermal capacity.*

heat cramps *pl.n.* Painful muscle spasms following hard work in intense heat, caused by loss of salt and water from profuse sweating.

heat exhaustion *n.* A condition caused by exposure to heat, marked by prostration, weakness, and collapse, resulting from unrecognized or unavoidable dehydration. Also called *heat prostration.*

heat-labile *adj.* Destroyed or altered by heat.

heat lamp *n.* A lamp that emits infrared light and produces heat, used to apply topical heat to the skin for therapeutic purposes.

heat prostration *n.* See **heat exhaustion.**

heat rash *n.* An inflammatory skin condition caused by obstruction of the ducts of the sweat glands, resulting from exposure to high heat and humidity and marked by the eruption of small, red papules accompanied by an itching or prickling sensation. Also called *miliaria, miliaria rubra, prickly heat, strophulus, tropical lichen.*

heat shock protein *n.* Any of a group of cellular proteins that are produced under conditions of heat stress and help to stabilize other cellular proteins exposed to high temperatures.

heat stroke *n.* A severe condition caused by impairment of the body's temperature-regulating abilities, resulting from prolonged exposure to excessive heat and characterized by cessation of sweating, severe headache, high fever, hot dry skin, and, in serious cases, collapse and coma.

heat urticaria *n.* See **cholinergic urticaria.**

heav·y chain (hĕv′ē) *n.* The larger of the two types of polypeptide chains in immunoglobulins, consisting of an antigen-binding portion having a variable amino acid sequence, and a constant region that defines the antibody class.

heavy chain disease *n.* Any of several disorders of lymphocytes that are characterized by the presence of high-molecular-weight polypeptides, especially gamma-globulins, in serum and urine and by symptoms similar to those of malignant lymphoma.

heavy eye *n.* The eye that is affected in severe uniocular myopia.

heavy hydrogen *n.* See **deuterium.**

heavy-ion treatment *n.* A cancer treatment method in which cancer cells are bombarded with the positively-charged nuclei of ions of carbon, neon, and other elements in order to kill the cells.

he·be·phre·ni·a (hē′bə-frē′nē-ə, -frĕn′ē-ə) *n.* A schizophrenia, usually starting at puberty, characterized by foolish mannerisms, senseless laughter, delusions, hallucinations, and regressive behavior. Also called *disorganized schizophrenia, hebephrenic schizophrenia.* —**he′be·phren′ic** (-frĕn′ĭk, -frē′nĭk) *adj.*

Heb·er·den (hĕb′ər-dn), **William** 1710–1801. British physician who gave the first clinical description (1768) of angina pectoris.

Heb·er·den's nodes (hĕb′ər-dənz) *pl.n.* Small bony growths found on the terminal phalanges of the fingers in osteoarthritis.

he·bet·ic (hĭ-bĕt′ĭk) *adj.* Of or relating to youth.

heb·e·tude (hĕb′ĭ-tōōd′) *n.* Dullness of mind; mental lethargy. —**heb′e·tu′di·nous** (-tōōd′n-əs) *adj.*

he·bi·at·rics (hē′bē-ăt′rĭks) *n.* See **adolescent medicine.**

hec·a·ter·o·mer·ic (hĕk′ə-tĕr′ō-mĕr′ĭk) *or* **hec·a·to·mer·ic** (-tō-mĕr′ĭk) *or* **hec·a·tom·er·al** (-tŏm′ər-əl) *adj.* Having an axon that divides and gives off processes to both sides of the spinal cord. Used of a spinal neuron.

Hecht's pneumonia (hĕkts) *n.* See **giant cell pneumonia.**

hecto– *or* **hect–** *pref.* One hundred (10^2): *hectogram.*

he·don·ics (hĭ-dŏn′ĭks) *n.* The branch of psychology

that studies pleasant and unpleasant sensations and states of mind.

hed·ro·cele (hĕd′rə-sēl′) *n.* Prolapse of the intestine through the anus.

heel (hēl) *n.* **1.** The rounded posterior portion of the foot under and behind the ankle. **2.** A similar anatomical part, such as the rounded base of the palm.

heel bone *n.* See **calcaneus.**

heel tendon *n.* See **Achilles tendon.**

Heer·fordt's disease (hâr′fôrts′) *n.* See **uveoparotid fever.**

Heg·glin's anomaly (hĕg′lĭnz) *n.* A hereditary disorder characterized by basophilic structures in most granulocytes, faulty maturation of platelets, and thrombocytopenia. Also called *May-Hegglin anomaly.*

height (hīt) *n. Abbr.* **ht 1.** The distance from the base of something to the top. **2.** Stature, especially of the human body.

height of contour *n.* The line encircling a tooth or other structure at its greatest bulge or diameter with respect to a selected path of insertion.

Heim·lich (hīm′lĭk′), **Henry J(ay)** Born 1920. American surgeon who in 1974 developed the Heimlich maneuver, a technique of ejecting an obstruction from the trachea of a choking victim.

Heimlich maneuver *n.* An emergency technique used to eject an object, such as food, from the trachea of a choking person. The technique employs a firm upward thrust just below the rib cage to force air from the lungs up through the trachea, thus dislodging the obstruction.

Hei·ne-Me·din disease (hī′nə-mād′n) *n.* See **acute anterior poliomyelitis.**

Heinz-Ehr·lich body (hīnz′âr′lĭk) *n.* See **Ehrlich's inner body.**

He·La cell (hē′lə) *n.* Any of the cells of the first continuously cultured human carcinoma strain, originally obtained from cancerous cervical tissue and maintained for use in studying cellular processes.

hel·i·cal (hĕl′ĭ-kəl, hē′lĭ-) *adj.* **1.** Of or having the shape of a helix; spiral. **2.** Having a shape approximating that of a helix.

hel·i·cine (hĕl′ĭ-sēn′, hē′lĭ-) *adj.* Of or relating to a helix; helical.

helicine artery *n.* Any of the coiled arteries in the erectile tissue of the penis.

hel·i·coid (hĕl′ĭ-koid′, hē′lĭ-) *adj.* Arranged in or having the general shape of a flattened coil or spiral.

hel·i·co·pod gait (hĕl′ĭ-kō-pŏd′) *n.* A gait seen in some hysterical disorders, in which the feet describe half circles. Also called *helicopodia.*

hel·i·co·tre·ma (hĕl′ĭ-kō-trē′mə) *n.* An opening at the apex of the cochlea that connects the vestibular canal and the scala tympani.

he·li·en·ceph·a·li·tis (hē′lē-ĕn-sĕf′ə-lī′tĭs) *n.* Inflammation of the brain following sunstroke.

he·li·um (hē′lē-əm) *n. Symbol* **He** An inert gaseous element used in liquid form as a cryogen and as a substitute for nitrogen in artificial breathing mixtures for deep-sea diving and workers in high-pressure conditions. Atomic number 2.

he·lix (hē′lĭks) *n., pl.* **-lix·es** *or* **hel·i·ces** (hĕl′ĭ-sēz′, hē′lĭ-) **1.** A spiral form or structure. **2.** The folded rim of

skin and cartilage around most of the outer ear. **3.** A three-dimensional curve that lies on a cylinder or cone, so that its angle to a plane perpendicular to the axis is constant.

Hel·lin's law (hĕl′ĭnz) *n.* The principle that twins occur once in 89 births, triplets once in 89² births, and quadruplets once in 89³ births.

hel·minth (hĕl′mĭnth′) *n.* A worm, especially a parasitic roundworm or tapeworm.

hel·min·tha·gogue (hĕl-mĭn′thə-gŏg′) *n.* See **anthelmintic.**

hel·min·them·e·sis (hĕl′mĭn-thĕm′ĭ-sĭs) *n.* The vomiting or oral expulsion of intestinal worms.

hel·min·thi·a·sis (hĕl′mĭn-thī′ə-sĭs) *n., pl.* **-ses** (-sēz′) A disease that is caused by infestation with parasitic worms.

hel·min·thic (hĕl-mĭn′thĭk) *adj.* **1.** Of or relating to worms, especially parasitic worms. **2.** Tending to expel worms. —*n.* See **anthelmintic.**

hel·min·tho·ma (hĕl′mĭn-thō′mə) *n., pl.* **-mas** *or* **-ma·ta** (-mə-tə) A tumor of granulomatous tissue caused by a parasitic worm.

Hel·min·tho·spo·ri·um (hĕl-mĭn′thō-spôr′ē-əm) *n.* A genus of rapidly growing, saprobic fungi that are common laboratory contaminants.

he·lo·ma (hē-lō′mə) *n., pl.* **-mas** *or* **-ma·ta** (-mə-tə) See **corn.**

heloma du·rum (do͝or′əm) *n.* See **hard corn.**

heloma mol·le (mŏl′ē) *n.* See **soft corn.**

he·lot·o·my (hē-lŏt′ə-mē) *n.* Treatment of a corn or corns by surgery.

help·er cell (hĕl′pər) *n.* A T cell that promotes the activation and functions of B cells and other T cells. Also called *helper T cell.*

helper virus *n.* A virus whose replication aids the development of a defective virus into a fully infectious agent.

hem– *pref.* Variant of **hemo–.**

hema– *pref.* Variant of **hemo–.**

he·ma·cy·tom·e·ter (hē′mə-sī-tŏm′ĭ-tər) *n.* See **hemocytometer.**

he·mad·sorp·tion (hē′măd-zôrp′shən, -sôrp′-) *n.* The adherence of an agent or substance to the surface of a red blood cell.

hemadsorption virus type 1 *or* **HA1 virus** (āch′ā-wŭn′) *n.* See **parainfluenza 3 virus.**

hemadsorption virus type 2 *or* **HA2 virus** (āch′ā-to͞o′) *n.* See **parainfluenza 1 virus.**

he·mag·glu·ti·na·tion (hē′mə-glo͞ot′n-ā′shən) *n.* The agglutination of red blood cells caused by an antibody either for red blood cell antigens or for antigens that coat red blood cells or by the presence of viruses or other microbes. —**he′mag·glu′ti·nate′** *v.*

hemagglutination inhibition test *n.* A test to determine the amount of a specific antigen in a blood serum sample. Also called *HI test.*

he·mag·glu·ti·nin (hē′mə-glo͞ot′n-ĭn) *n.* A substance that causes agglutination of red blood cells.

he·ma·gogue (hē′mə-gŏg′) *n.* **1.** An agent that promotes the flow of blood. **2.** See **emmenagogue.** —**he′ma·gog′ic** (-gŏj′ĭk) *adj.*

he·mal (hē′məl) *adj.* **1.** Of or relating to the blood or blood vessels. **2.** Relating to or located on the side of the body that contains the heart and principal blood vessels.

hemal arch *n.* Any of three or four V-shaped bones located ventral to the bodies of the third to sixth coccygeal vertebrae and usually enclosing the ventral caudal artery and vein.

he·mal·um (hē-măl′əm) *n.* A solution of hematoxylin and alum used as a nuclear stain in histology, especially with eosin as a counterstain.

he·mam·e·bi·a·sis (hē′măm-ə-bī′ə-sĭs) *n.* An infection of red blood cells with ameboid forms of parasites, as in malaria.

he·ma·nal·y·sis (hē′ə-năl′ĭ-sĭs) *n.* Analysis of the blood, especially by chemical methods.

he·man·gi·ec·ta·sis (hē′măn-jē-ĕk′tə-sĭs) *n.* Dilation of the blood vessels.

hemangio– or **hemangi–** *pref.* Blood vessel: *hemangioma.*

he·man·gi·o·blast (hĭ-măn′jē-ō-blăst′) *n.* A primitive embryonic cell of mesodermal origin that produces cells giving rise to vascular endothelium, reticuloendothelial elements, and blood-forming cells.

he·man·gi·o·blas·to·ma (hĭ-măn′jē-ō-blă-stō′mə) *n.* A benign, slowly growing, cerebellar neoplasm composed of capillary-forming endothelial cells. Also called *angioblastoma.*

he·man·gi·o·en·do·the·li·o·blas·to·ma (hĭ-măn′jē-ō-ĕn′dō-thē′lē-ō-blă-stō′mə) *n.* A hemangioendothelioma in which the endothelial cells occur in an immature form.

he·man·gi·o·en·do·the·li·o·ma (hĭ-măn′jē-ō-ĕn′dō-thē′lē-ō′mə) *n.* A neoplasm derived from blood vessels, marked by prominent endothelial cells that occur singly or in aggregates and line vascular tubes.

he·man·gi·o·fi·bro·ma (hĭ-măn′jē-ō-fī-brō′mə) *n.* A hemangioma having a fibrous tissue framework.

he·man·gi·o·ma (hĭ-măn′jē-ō′mə) *n.,* *pl.* **–mas** or **–ma·ta** (-mə-tə) A congenital benign skin lesion consisting of dense, usually elevated masses of dilated blood vessels.

he·man·gi·o·ma·to·sis (hĭ-măn′jē-ō-mə-tō′sĭs) *n.* The presence of multiple hemangiomas.

he·man·gi·o·per·i·cy·to·ma (hĭ-măn′gē-ō-pĕr′ĭ-sī-tō′mə) *n.* A rare vascular, usually benign neoplasm composed of round and spindle cells presumably derived from pericytes.

he·man·gi·o·sar·co·ma (hĭ-măn′jē-ō-sär-kō′mə) *n.* A rare malignant neoplasm characterized by rapidly proliferating anaplastic cells derived from blood vessels and lining blood-filled spaces.

he·ma·pher·e·sis (hē′mə-fĕr′ə-sĭs, hĕm′ə-) *n.* See apheresis.

he·mar·thro·sis (hē′mär-thrō′sĭs, hĕm′är-) *n.* Accumulation of blood in a joint or joint cavity.

he·ma·te·in (hē′mə-tē′ĭn, hē′mə-tēn′) *n.* A reddish-brown crystalline compound used as an indicator and a biological stain.

he·ma·tem·e·sis (hē′mə-tĕm′ĭ-sĭs, hĕm′ə-, hē′mə-tə-mē′sĭs) *n.* The vomiting of blood.

he·mat·en·ceph·a·lon (hē′mə-tĕn-sĕf′ə-lŏn′) *n.* See cerebral hemorrhage.

he·mat·ic (hĭ-măt′ĭk) *adj.* Of, relating to, resembling,

containing, or acting on blood. —*n.* See **hematinic.**

he·ma·ti·dro·sis (hē′mə-tĭ-drō′sĭs, hĕm′ə-) *n.* The excretion of blood or blood pigment in the sweat. Also called *hemidrosis.*

he·ma·tin (hē′mə-tĭn) *n.* A blue to blackish-brown compound formed in the oxidation of hemoglobin and containing ferric iron. Also called *ferriheme, oxyheme, oxyhemochromogen.*

hematin chloride *n.* See **hemin.**

he·ma·ti·ne·mi·a (hē′mə-tə-nē′mē-ə) *n.* The presence of heme in the blood.

he·ma·tin·ic (hē′mə-tĭn′ĭk) *adj.* **1.** Acting to improve the quality of blood, as by increasing hemoglobin concentration or stimulating red blood cell formation. **2.** Of or relating to hematin. —*n.* A drug that improves the quality of blood, as by increasing hemoglobin concentration. Also called *hematic.*

hemato– or **hemat–** or **haemat–** or **haemato–** *pref.* Blood: *hematology.*

he·ma·to·blast (hē′mə-tə-blăst′, hĭ-măt′ə-) *n.* An immature undifferentiated blood cell.

he·ma·to·cele (hē′mə-tə-sēl′, hĭ-măt′ə-) *n.* **1.** An effusion of blood into a canal or a cavity of the body. **2.** See **hemorrhagic cyst.**

he·ma·to·ceph·a·ly (hē′mə-tō-sĕf′ə-lē, hĭ-măt′ə-) *n.* An effusion of blood within the brain.

he·ma·to·che·zi·a (hē′mə-tō-kē′zē-ə, hĭ-măt′ə-) *n.* The passage of bloody stools.

he·ma·to·chy·lu·ri·a (hē′mə-tō-kī-lo̅o̅r′ē-ə, hĭ-măt′ō-) *n.* The presence of blood and chyle in the urine.

he·ma·to·col·po·me·tra (hē′mə-tō-kŏl′pō-mē′trə, hĭ-măt′ō-) *n.* The accumulation of blood in the uterus and vagina.

he·ma·to·col·pos (hē′mə-tō-kŏl′pəs, hĭ-măt′ō-) *n.* The accumulation of menstrual blood in the vagina. Also called *retained menstruation.*

he·mat·o·crit (hĭ-măt′ə-krĭt′) *n. Abbr.* **Hct 1.** The percentage by volume of packed red blood cells in a given sample of blood after centrifugation. **2.** A centrifuge used to determine the volume of blood cells and plasma in a given sample of blood.

he·ma·to·cyst (hē′mə-tō-sĭst′, hĭ-măt′ə-) *n.* See **hemorrhagic cyst.**

he·ma·to·cys·tis (hē′mə-tō-sĭs′tĭs, hĭ-măt′ə-) *n.* An effusion of blood into the bladder.

he·ma·to·cy·tu·ri·a (hē′mə-tō-sī-to̅o̅r′ē-ə, hĭ-măt′ō-) *n.* The presence of red blood cells in the urine.

he·ma·to·gen·e·sis (hē′mə-tə-jĕn′ĭ-sĭs, hĭ-măt′ə-) or **he·mo·gen·e·sis** (hē′mə-) *n.* See **hematopoiesis.** —**he′ma·to·gen′ic, he′ma·to·ge·net′ic** *adj.*

hematogenetic calculus *n.* A greenish or dark brown calculus formed around the teeth.

he·ma·tog·e·nous (hē′mə-tŏj′ə-nəs) *adj.* **1.** Producing blood. **2.** Originating in or spread by the blood.

hematogenous jaundice *n.* See **hemolytic jaundice.**

he·ma·to·his·ton (hē′mə-tō-hĭs′tŏn′, hĭ-măt′ə-) *n.* See **globin.**

he·ma·toid (hē′mə-toid′, hĕm′ə-) *adj.* Resembling blood.

he·ma·toi·din (hē′mə-toid′n) *n.* A ironless pigment derived from hemoglobin and formed within tissues, chemically similar to bilirubin.

he·ma·tol·o·gist (hē′mə-tŏl′ə-jĭst) *n.* A physician specializing in hematology.

he·ma·tol·o·gy (hē′mə-tŏl′ə-jē) *n.* The science of the blood and blood-producing organs. —**he′ma·to·log′ic** (-tə-lŏj′ĭk), **he′ma·to·log′i·cal** *adj.*

he·ma·to·lym·phan·gi·o·ma (hē′mə-tō-lĭm-făn′jē-ō′mə) *n.* A congenital tumor consisting of lymphatic vessels and blood vessels.

he·ma·tol·y·sis (hē′mə-tŏl′ĭ-sĭs) *n.* Variant of **hemolysis**.

he·ma·to·ma (hē′mə-tō′mə) *n., pl.* –**mas** *or* –**ma·ta** (-mə-tə) A localized swelling filled with blood resulting from a break in a blood vessel.

he·ma·to·me·tra (hē′mə-tō-mē′trə, hĭ-măt′ə-) *n.* A collection or retention of blood in the uterine cavity. Also called *hemometra*.

he·ma·tom·e·try (hē′mə-tŏm′ĭ-trē) *n.* Examination of the blood to determine the total number and relative proportions of various blood cells and the percentage of hemoglobin.

he·ma·tom·phal·o·cele (hē′mə-tŏm-făl′ə-sēl′, -tŏm′fə-lō-sēl′) *n.* An umbilical hernia in which there is an effusion of blood.

he·ma·to·my·e·li·a (hē′mə-tō-mī-ē′lē-ə, hĭ-măt′ə-) *n.* Hemorrhage into the substance of the spinal cord, usually caused by trauma. Also called *hematorrhachis interna, myelapoplexy, myelorrhagia.*

he·ma·to·my·e·lo·pore (hē′mə-tō-mī′ə-lə-pôr′, hĭ-măt′ə-) *n.* The formation of porosities in the spinal cord as a result of hemorrhages.

he·ma·to·pa·thol·o·gy (hē′mə-tō-pă-thŏl′ə-jē, hĭ-măt′ō-) *n.* The branch of pathology dealing with diseases of the blood and the blood-producing organs. Also called *hemopathology.*

he·ma·to·plas·tic (hē′mə-tō-plăs′tĭk, hĭ-măt′ə-) *adj.* Hemoplastic.

he·ma·to·poi·e·sis (hē′mə-tō-poi-ē′sĭs, hĭ-măt′ə-) *or* **he·mo·poi·e·sis** (hē′mə-) *n.* The formation of blood or blood cells in the living body. Also called *hematogenesis, sanguification.* —**he′ma·to·poi·et′ic** (-ĕt′ĭk) *adj.*

hematopoietic gland *n.* An organ involved in the formation of blood or blood cells, such as the spleen.

hematopoietic system *n.* The blood-making organs, principally the bone marrow and lymph nodes.

he·ma·to·por·phy·rin (hē′mə-tō-pôr′fə-rĭn, hĭ-măt′ə-) *n.* A porphyrin that does not contain iron and is formed when heme or hemoglobin is decomposed by an acid. Also called *hemoporphyrin.*

he·ma·top·si·a (hē′mə-tŏp′sē-ə, hĕm′ə-) *n.* Hemorrhage into the eye.

he·ma·tor·rha·chis (hē′mə-tôr′ə-kĭs) *n.* A spinal hemorrhage. Also called *hemorrhachis.*

hematorrhachis ex·ter·na (ĭk-stûr′nə) *n.* Hemorrhage into the spinal canal external to the spinal cord, either within or outside the dura.

hematorrhachis in·ter·na (ĭn-tûr′nə) *n.* See **hematomyelia**.

he·ma·to·sal·pinx (hē′mə-tō-săl′pĭngks, hĭ-măt′ə-) *n.* A collection of blood in a tube, as in a fallopian tube, associated with tubal pregnancy. Also called *hemosalpinx.*

he·ma·to·sper·ma·to·cele (hē′mə-tō-spûr′mə-tə-sēl′, -spər-măt′ə-, hĭ-măt′ə-) *n.* A spermatocele that contains blood.

he·ma·to·sper·mi·a (hē′mə-tō-spûr′mē-ə, hĭ-măt′ə-) *n.* See **hemospermia**.

he·ma·to·stat·ic (hē′mə-tō-stăt′ĭk, hĭ-măt′ə-) *adj.* Characterized or caused by stagnation or arrest of blood in the vessels.

he·ma·to·stax·is (hē′mə-tō-stăk′sĭs, hĭ-măt′ə-) *n.* Spontaneous bleeding caused by a disease of the blood.

he·ma·tos·te·on (hē′mə-tŏs′tē-ŏn′, -ən) *n.* Bleeding in the medullary cavity of a bone.

he·ma·to·tox·ic (hē′mə-tō-tŏk′sĭk, hĭ-măt′ə-) *adj.* Variant of **hemotoxic**.

he·ma·to·tox·in (hē′mə-tō-tŏk′sĭn, hĭ-măt′ə-) *n.* See **hemotoxin**.

he·ma·to·tra·che·los (hē′mə-tō-trə-kē′lŏs′, -kē′ləs, hĭ-măt′ə-) *n.* Distention of the uterine cervix with accumulated blood.

he·ma·to·trop·ic (hē′mə-tō-trŏp′ĭk, -trō′pĭk, hĭ-măt′ə-) *adj.* Hemotropic.

he·ma·to·tym·pa·num (hē′mə-tō-tĭm′pə-nəm, hĭ-măt′ə-) *n.* See **hemotympanum**.

he·ma·tox·y·lin (hē′mə-tŏk′sə-lĭn) *n.* A yellow or red crystalline compound used in histological dyes and as an indicator.

hematoxylin-eosin stain *n.* A widely used, two-stage stain for cells in which hematoxylin is followed by a counterstain of red eosin so that the nuclei stain a deep blue-black and the cytoplasm stains pink.

he·ma·to·zo·on (hē′mə-tō-zō′ŏn′, hĭ-măt′ə-) *n., pl.* –**zo·a** (-zō′ə) A parasitic protozoan or similar organism that lives in the blood. —**he′ma·to·zo′al, he′ma·to·zo′ic** *adj.*

he·ma·tu·ri·a (hē′mə-tŏor′ē-ə) *n.* The presence of blood in the urine. Also called *hematuresis.* —**he′ma·tu′ric** *adj.*

heme (hēm) *n.* The deep red, oxygen-carrying, nonprotein, ferrous component of hemoglobin. Also called *reduced hematin.*

hem·er·a·lo·pi·a (hĕm′ər-ə-lō′pē-ə) *n.* A visual defect marked by the inability to see as clearly in bright light as in dim light. Also called *day blindness.*

hemi– *pref.* Half: *hemicardia.*

–hemia *suff.* Variant of **–emia**.

hem·i·ac·e·tal (hĕm′ē-ăs′ĭ-tăl′) *n.* Any of a class of compounds containing an alkyl group, especially when formed as intermediates during the preparation of acetals from aldehydes or ketones.

hem·i·a·geu·sia (hĕm′ē-ə-gyōo′zhə, -jōo′-) *n.* Loss of taste on one side of the tongue. Also called *hemigeusia.*

hem·i·al·gia (hĕm′ē-ăl′jə) *n.* Pain affecting one half of the body.

hem·i·a·my·os·the·ni·a (hĕm′ē-ā-mī′əs-thē′nē-ə, -ə-mī′-) *n.* See **hemiparesis**.

hem·i·an·al·ge·sia (hĕm′ē-ăn′əl-jē′zhə) *n.* Loss of sensibility to pain on one side of the body.

hem·i·an·en·ceph·a·ly (hĕm′ē-ăn′ən-sĕf′ə-lē) *n.* Congenital defect of one side of the brain.

hem·i·an·es·the·sia (hĕm′ē-ăn′ĭs-thē′zhə) *n.* Loss of tactile sensibility on one side of the body. Also called *unilateral anesthesia.*

hem·i·a·nop·si·a (hĕm′ē-ə-nŏp′sē-ə) *or* **hem·i·a·no·pi·a** (-nō′pē-ə) *n.* Loss of vision in one half of the visual field of one or both eyes. —**hem′i·a·nop′tic** (-nŏp′-tĭk) *adj.*

hem·i·an·os·mi·a (hĕm′ē-ăn-ŏz′mē-ə) *n.* Loss of the sense of smell in one of the nostrils.

hem·i·a·prax·i·a (hĕm′ē-ə-prăk′sē-ə) *n.* Apraxia affecting one side of the body.

hem·i·ar·thro·plas·ty (hĕm′ē-är′thrə-plăs′tē) *n.* Arthroplasty in which one joint surface is replaced with an artificial material, usually metal.

hem·i·a·tax·i·a (hĕm′ē-ə-tăk′sē-ə) *n.* Ataxia affecting one side of the body.

hem·i·ath·e·to·sis (hĕm′ē-ăth′ĭ-tō′sĭs) *n.* Athetosis affecting one hand only or one hand and one foot only.

hem·i·at·ro·phy (hĕm′ē-ăt′rə-fē) *n.* Atrophy of one side of a body part or organ.

hem·i·az·y·gos vein (hĕm′ē-ăz′ĭ-gŏs′, -ā-zī′gŏs′) *n.* A continuation of the left ascending lumbar vein, ascending along the left side of the lower thoracic vertebrae to the eighth vertebra, where it crosses the midline behind the aorta, thoracic duct, and esophagus, and empties into the azygos vein.

hem·i·bal·lis·mus (hĕm′ē-bə-lĭz′məs) *or* **hem·i·bal·lism** (-băl′ĭz′əm) *n.* Violent writhing and muscle spasms involving one side of the body, usually caused by a lesion of the subthalamic nucleus of the opposite side of the brain.

hem·i·block (hĕm′ē-blŏk′) *n.* Arrest of the cardiac impulse in one of the two main divisions of the left branch of the atrioventricular trunk.

he·mic (hē′mĭk) *adj.* Of or relating to the blood.

hem·i·car·di·a (hĕm′ĭ-kär′dē-ə) *n.* **1.** Either lateral half of the heart, including the atrium and ventricle. **2.** A congenital malformation of the heart in which only two of the usual four chambers are formed.

hem·i·cel·lu·lose (hĕm′ĭ-sĕl′yə-lōs′, -lōz′) *n.* Any of several polysaccharides that are more complex than a sugar and less complex than cellulose and found in plant cell walls.

hem·i·cen·trum (hĕm′ĭ-sĕn′trəm) *n.* One of the two lateral halves of a vertebra.

hem·i·ceph·a·lal·gia (hĕm′ē-sĕf′ə-lăl′jə) *n.* Headache affecting one side of the head, characteristic of migraine. Also called *hemicrania.*

hem·i·ce·pha·li·a (hĕm′ē-sə-fā′lē-ə, -făl′yə) *n.* Congenital failure of the cerebrum to develop normally, usually with the cerebellum and basal ganglia in rudimentary form.

hem·i·cho·re·a (hĕm′ē-kô-rē′ə, -kə-) *n.* Chorea affecting the muscles on one side of the body.

he·mic murmur (hē′mĭk) *n.* A cardiac or vascular murmur heard in anemic persons who have no valvular lesion.

hem·i·co·lec·to·my (hĕm′ē-kə-lĕk′tə-mē) *n.* Surgical removal of the right or left side of the colon.

hem·i·cra·ni·a (hĕm′ĭ-krā′nē-ə) *n.* **1.** See **migraine. 2.** See **hemicephalalgia.**

hem·i·cra·ni·o·sis (hĕm′ĭ-krā′nē-ō′sĭs) *n.* Enlargement of one side of the cranium.

hem·i·des·mo·some (hĕm′ĭ-dĕz′mə-sōm′, -dĕs′-) *n.* Any of the specialized structures representing half

desmosomes that occur on the basal surface of certain stratified squamous epithelial cells.

hem·i·di·a·pho·re·sis (hĕm′ē-dī′ə-fə-rē′sĭs, -dī-ăf′ə-) *n.* Sweating on one side of the body. Also called *hemidrosis, hemihidrosis.*

hem·i·dro·sis[1] (hĕm′ĭ-drō′sĭs, hē′mĭ-) *n.* See **hematidrosis.**

hem·i·dro·sis[2] (hĕm′ĭ-drō′sĭs) *n.* See **hemidiaphoresis.**

hem·i·dys·es·the·sia (hĕm′ē-dĭs′ĭs-thē′zhə) *n.* Dysesthesia affecting one side of the body.

hem·i·dys·tro·phy (hĕm′ĭ-dĭs′trə-fē) *n.* Underdevelopment of one side of the body.

hem·i·ec·tro·me·li·a (hĕm′ē-ĕk′trō-mē′lē-ə) *n.* Defective development of limbs on a side of the body.

hem·i·ep·i·lep·sy (hĕm′ē-ĕp′ə-lĕp′sē) *n.* Epilepsy in which the convulsive movements are confined to one side of the body.

hem·i·fa·cial (hĕm′ĭ-fā′shəl) *adj.* Relating to one side of the face.

hem·i·gas·trec·to·my (hĕm′ĭ-gă-strĕk′tə-mē) *n.* Excision of the distal half of the stomach.

hem·i·geu·sia (hĕm′ĭ-gyōō′zhə, -jōō′-) *n.* See **hemiageusia.**

hem·i·glos·sec·to·my (hĕm′ĭ-glô-sĕk′tə-mē) *n.* Surgical removal of one half of the tongue.

hem·i·glos·si·tis (hĕm′ĭ-glô-sī′tĭs) *n.* A vesicular eruption on one side of the tongue and the corresponding inner surface of the cheek.

hem·i·gna·thi·a (hĕm′ĭ-nā′thē-ə, -năth′ē-ə) *n.* Defective development of one side of the mandible.

hem·i·hi·dro·sis (hĕm′ē-hī-drō′sĭs) *n.* See **hemidiaphoresis.**

hem·i·hyp·al·ge·sia (hĕm′ĭ-hī′păl-jē′zhə) *n.* Partial loss of sensibility to pain affecting one side of the body.

hem·i·hy·per·es·the·sia (hĕm′ĭ-hī′pər-ĭs-thē′zhə) *n.* Increased sensibility to tactile stimulation and pain on one side of the body.

hem·i·hy·per·i·dro·sis (hĕm′ĭ-hī′pər-ĭ-drō′sĭs) *n.* Excessive sweating on one side of the body.

hem·i·hy·per·to·ni·a (hĕm′ĭ-hī′pər-tō′nē-ə) *n.* Increased muscular tone on one side of the body.

hem·i·hy·per·tro·phy (hĕm′ĭ-hī-pûr′trə-fē) *n.* Hypertrophy of one side of the face or body.

hem·i·hyp·es·the·sia (hĕm′ĭ-hī′pĭs-thē′zhə) *n.* Diminished sensibility on one side of the body.

hem·i·hy·po·to·ni·a (hĕm′ĭ-hī′pō-tō′nē-ə) *n.* Partial loss of muscular tone on one side of the body.

hem·i·lam·i·nec·to·my (hĕm′ĭ-lăm′ə-nĕk′tə-mē) *n.* Surgical removal of a portion of a vertebral lamina.

hem·i·lar·yn·gec·to·my (hĕm′ĭ-lăr′ən-jĕk′tə-mē) *n.* Excision of one side of the larynx.

hem·i·lat·er·al (hĕm′ĭ-lăt′ər-əl) *adj.* Relating to one lateral half, as of an organ.

he·min (hē′mĭn) *n.* The reddish-brown crystalline chloride of heme produced when hemoglobin reacts with certain reagents in a test for the presence of blood. Also called *hematin chloride.*

hem·i·op·ic pupillary reaction (hĕm′ē-ŏp′ĭk, -ō′pĭk) *n.* See **Wernicke's reaction.**

hem·i·par·an·es·the·sia (hĕm′ĭ-păr′ăn-ĭs-thē′zhə) *n.*

Anesthesia of one lower extremity or of the lower part of one side of the body.

hem·i·par·a·ple·gia (hĕm′ĭ-păr′ə-plē′jə) *n.* Paralysis of one leg.

hem·i·pa·re·sis (hĕm′ē-pə-rē′sĭs, -păr′ĭ-sĭs) *n.* Slight paralysis or weakness affecting one side of the body. Also called *hemiamyosthenia.*

hem·i·pel·vec·to·my (hĕm′ĭ-pĕl-vĕk′tə-mē) *n.* Amputation of an entire leg together with one lateral half of the pelvis on the same side. Also called *interpelviabdominal amputation.*

hem·i·ple·gia (hĕm′ĭ-plē′jə) *n.* Paralysis affecting only one side of the body. —**hem′i·ple′gic** (-jĭk) *adj.*

hemiplegic gait *n.* The walk of hemiplegics, characterized by swinging the affected leg in a half circle.

hem·i·sen·so·ry (hĕm′ĭ-sĕn′sə-rē) *n.* Loss of sensation on one side of the body.

hem·i·spasm (hĕm′ĭ-spăz′əm) *n.* A spasm affecting one or more muscles of one side of the face or body.

hem·i·sphere (hĕm′ĭ-sfîr′) *n.* **1.** A half of a symmetrical spherical structure as divided by a plane of symmetry. **2.** Either of the lateral halves of the cerebrum; a cerebral hemisphere. —**hem′i·spher′ic** (-sfîr′ĭk, -sfĕr′-), **hem′i·spher′i·cal** *adj.*

hem·i·sys·to·le (hĕm′ĭ-sĭs′tə-lē) *n.* Contraction of the left ventricle following every second atrial contraction, producing one pulse to every two heartbeats.

hem·i·tho·rax (hĕm′ĭ-thôr′ăks′) *n.* One side of the chest.

hem·i·ver·te·bra (hĕm′ĭ-vûr′tə-brə) *n.* A congenital defect of the spine in which one side of a vertebra fails to develop completely.

hem·i·zy·gos·i·ty (hĕm′ĭ-zī-gŏs′ĭ-tē) *n.* The state of having unpaired genes in an otherwise diploid cell; men are normally hemizygous for the genes on the X-chromosome.

hem·i·zy·gote (hĕm′ĭ-zī′gōt′) *n.* An individual hemizygous with respect to one or more specified genes.

hem·i·zy·got·ic (hĕm′ĭ-zī-gŏt′ĭk) *adj.* Hemizygous.

hem·i·zy·gous (hĕm′ĭ-zī′gəs) *adj.* Having unpaired genes in an otherwise diploid cell.

hemo– *or* **hema–** *or* **hem–** *or* **haemo–** *or* **haema–** *or* **haem–** *pref.* Blood: *hemocyte.*

he·mo·blast (hē′mə-blăst′) *n.* See **hemocytoblast.**

he·mo·blas·to·sis (hē′mə-blă-stō′sĭs) *n.* Proliferation of the blood-forming tissues.

he·mo·ca·ther·e·sis (hē′mō-kă-thĕr′ĭ-sĭs, -thîr′-, -kăth′-ə-rē′-) *n.* Destruction of blood cells, especially of red blood cells. —**he′mo·cath′e·ret′ic** (-kăth′ə-rĕt′ĭk) *adj.*

he·moc·cult (hē′mə-kŭlt′) *n.* A qualitative test for hidden blood in the stool, based upon detecting the peroxidase activity of hemoglobin.

he·mo·cho·le·cyst (hē′mə-kō′lĭ-sĭst′) *n.* **1.** A cyst containing blood and bile. **2.** A nontraumatic hemorrhage or an accumulation of old blood in the gallbladder. No longer in technical use.

he·mo·cho·le·cys·ti·tis (hē′mə-kō′lĭ-sĭ-stī′tĭs) *n.* Inflammation and hemorrhage of the gallbladder.

he·mo·cho·ri·al placenta (hē′mə-kôr′ē-əl) *n.* A placenta, as in humans, in which maternal blood is in direct contact with the chorion.

he·mo·chro·ma·to·sis (hē′mə-krō′mə-tō′sĭs) *n.* A hereditary disorder of iron metabolism characterized by excessive accumulation of iron in tissues, diabetes mellitus, liver dysfunction, and a bronze skin pigmentation. Also called *bronzed disease.*

he·moc·la·sis (hē-mŏk′lə-sĭs) *n.* The rupture, hemolysis, or destruction of red blood cells. —**he′mo·clas′tic** (hē′mə-klăs′tĭk) *adj.*

he·mo·con·cen·tra·tion (hē′mō-kŏn′sən-trā′shən) *n.* A decrease in plasma volume resulting in an increase in the concentration of red blood cells in blood.

he·mo·co·nia (hē′mə-kō′nē-ə) *n.* Small refractive particles in the blood, thought to be lipid material associated with fragmented stroma from red blood cells. Also called *elementary granules.*

he·mo·co·ni·o·sis (hē′mō-kō′nē-ō′sĭs) *n.* An abnormal amount of hemoconia in blood.

he·mo·cyte (hē′mə-sīt′) *n.* A cellular component or formed element of the blood.

he·mo·cy·to·blast (hē′mə-sī′tə-blăst′) *n.* A stem cell derived from the embryonic mesenchyme and considered to be capable of developing into any type of blood cell. Also called *hemoblast, lymphoidocyte.*

he·mo·cy·to·cath·er·e·sis (hē′mə-sī′tō-kă-thĕr′ĭ-sĭs, -thîr′-, -kăth′ə-rē′-) *n.* The destruction of red blood cells, as by hemolysis.

he·mo·cy·tol·y·sis (hē′mō-sī-tŏl′ĭ-sĭs) *n.* The dissolution of blood cells.

he·mo·cy·tom·e·ter (hē′mō-sī-tŏm′ĭ-tər) *n.* An instrument for counting the blood cells in a measured volume of blood. Also called *hemacytometer.*

he·mo·cy·tom·e·try (hē′mō-sī-tŏm′ĭ-trē) *n.* The counting of blood cells.

he·mo·cy·to·trip·sis (hē′mō-sī′tə-trĭp′sĭs) *n.* The fragmentation or disintegration of blood cells by means of mechanical trauma.

he·mo·di·ag·no·sis (hē′mō-dī′əg-nō′sĭs) *n.* Diagnosis by examination of the blood.

he·mo·di·al·y·sis (hē′mō-dī-ăl′ĭ-sĭs) *n.* A procedure for removing metabolic waste products or toxic substances from the bloodstream by dialysis.

he·mo·di·a·lyz·er (hē′mō-dī′ə-lī′zər) *n.* A machine for performing hemodialysis in acute or chronic renal failure. Also called *artificial kidney.*

he·mo·di·lu·tion (hē′mō-dī-lōō′shən, -dĭ-) *n.* An increase in the volume of plasma, resulting in a reduced concentration of red blood cells in blood.

he·mo·dy·nam·ics (hē′mə-dī-năm′ĭks) *n.* The study of the forces involved in the circulation of blood. —**he′mo·dy·nam′·ic** *adj.*

he·mo·en·do·the·li·al placenta (hē′mō-ĕn′dō-thē′lē-əl) *n.* A placenta in which the trophoblast becomes so attenuated that maternal blood is separated from fetal blood only by the endothelium of the chorionic capillaries.

he·mo·fil·tra·tion (hē′mō-fĭl-trā′shən) *n.* A process similar to hemodialysis, by which blood is dialyzed using ultrafiltration and simultaneous reinfusion of physiologic saline solution.

he·mo·flag·el·late (hē′mō-flăj′ə-lāt′, -lĭt, -flə-jĕl′ĭt) *n.* A flagellate protozoan, such as a trypanosome, that is parasitic in the blood.

he·mo·fus·cin (hē′mō-fŭs′ĭn) *n.* A brown pigment derived from hemoglobin and occasionally occurring in urine along with hemosiderin.

he·mo·gen·e·sis (hē′mə-jĕn′ĭ-sĭs) *n.* Variant of **hematogenesis.**

he·mo·gen·ic (hē′mə-jĕn′ĭk) *adj.* Hemoplastic.

he·mo·glo·bin (hē′mə-glō′bĭn) *n. Abbr.* **Hb, Hgb** The red respiratory protein of red blood cells that transports oxygen as oxyhemoglobin from the lungs to the tissues, where the oxygen is readily released and the oxyhemoglobin becomes hemoglobin. —**he′mo·glo′·bi·nous** *adj.*

hemoglobin A *n. Abbr.* **Hb A** The hemoglobin present in normal adults.

hemoglobin C *n. Abbr.* **Hb C** An abnormal hemoglobin in which lysine has replaced glutamic acid causing reduced plasticity of the red blood cells.

hemoglobin C disease *n.* An inherited anemia characterized by an excessive destruction of red blood cells, an enlarged spleen, and target cells and hemoglobin C in the blood.

hemoglobin disease *n.* Any of several inherited diseases characterized by the presence of various abnormal hemoglobin molecules in the blood.

he·mo·glo·bi·ne·mi·a (hē′mə-glō′bə-nē′mē-ə) *n.* The presence of free hemoglobin in the blood plasma.

Hemoglobin F *n.* See **fetal hemoglobin.**

hemoglobin H *n. Abbr.* **Hb H** An abnormal hemoglobin that cannot effectively transport oxygen; it is usually associated with a thalassemialike syndrome.

hemoglobin H disease *n.* An inherited disease characterized by moderate anemia and red blood cell abnormalities, with red blood cells containing Bart's hemoglobin being replaced by cells containing hemoglobin H.

hemoglobin M *n. Abbr.* **Hb M** A group of abnormal hemoglobins in which a single amino acid substitution favors the formation of methemoglobin and is thus associated with methemoglobinemia.

he·mo·glo·bi·nol·y·sis (hē′mə-glō′bə-nŏl′ĭ-sĭs) *n.* The destruction or chemical lysis of hemoglobin.

he·mo·glo·bi·nop·a·thy (hē′mə-glō′bə-nŏp′ə-thē) *n.* A disorder caused by or associated with the presence of abnormal hemoglobins in the blood.

he·mo·glo·bi·no·phil·ic (hē′mə-glō′bə-nə-fĭl′ĭk) *adj.* Of or relating to microorganisms that cannot be cultured except in the presence of hemoglobin.

hemoglobin S *n. Abbr.* **Hb S** An abnormal hemoglobin in which valine has replaced glutamic acid causing the hemoglobin to become less soluble under decreasing oxygen concentrations and to polymerize into crystals that distort the red blood cells into a sickle shape. Also called *sickle cell hemoglobin.*

he·mo·glo·bi·nu·ri·a (hē′mə-glō′bə-nŏŏr′ē-ə) *n.* The presence of free hemoglobin in the urine. —**he′mo·glo′bi·nu′ric** *adj.*

hemoglobinuric nephrosis *n.* Acute oliguric renal failure associated with hemoglobinuria, following an incompatible blood transfusion.

he·mo·gram (hē′mə-grăm′) *n.* A record of the findings from an examination of the blood, especially with

reference to the numbers, proportions, and morphological features of the formed elements.

he·mo·his·ti·o·blast (hē′mō-hĭs′tē-ə-blăst′) *n.* A primitive mesenchymal cell believed to be capable of developing into a histiocyte or into any of the various types of blood cells, including monocytes.

he·mo·lith (hē′mə-lĭth′) *n.* A concretion in the wall of a blood vessel.

he·mo·lymph (hē′mə-lĭmf′) *n.* The blood and lymph considered as a circulating tissue.

he·mol·y·sate (hĭ-mŏl′ĭ-sāt′) *n.* The product resulting from the lysis of red blood cells.

he·mol·y·sin (hĭ-mŏl′ĭ-sĭn, hē′mə-lī′-) *n.* An agent or a substance, such as an antibody or a bacterial toxin, that causes the destruction of red blood cells, thereby liberating hemoglobin. Also called *erythrocytolysin, erythrolysin.*

he·mo·ly·sin·o·gen (hē′mə-lī-sĭn′ə-jən, hĭ-mŏl′ĭ-sĭn′-ə-jən) *n.* The antigenic material in red blood cells that stimulates the formation of hemolysin.

hemolysin unit *n.* The smallest quantity of inactivated immune serum that will sensitize a suspension of red blood cells so that complement will cause complete hemolysis.

he·mol·y·sis (hĭ-mŏl′ĭ-sĭs, hē′mə-lī′sĭs) *or* **he·ma·tol·y·sis** (hē′mə-tŏl′ĭ-sĭs) *n.* The destruction or dissolution of red blood cells, with release of hemoglobin. Also called *erythrocytolysis, erythrolysis.*

he·mo·lyt·ic (hē′mə-lĭt′ĭk) *adj.* Destructive to red blood cells; hematolytic.

hemolytic anemia *n.* Anemia resulting from the abnormal destruction of red blood cells, as in response to certain toxic or infectious agents and in certain inherited blood disorders.

hemolytic disease of newborn *n.* See **erythroblastosis fetalis.**

hemolytic jaundice *n.* Jaundice resulting from the lysis of red blood cells and the consequent increased production of bilirubin, as in response to toxic or infectious agents or in immune disorders. Also called *hematogenous jaundice.*

hemolytic splenomegaly *n.* Splenomegaly associated with congenital hemolytic jaundice.

hemolytic uremic syndrome *n.* A syndrome in which hemolytic anemia and thrombocytopenia occur with acute renal failure, marked in children by sudden gastrointestinal bleeding, urine that contains red blood cells and is scanty in volume, and microangiopathic hemolytic anemia; in adults it is associated with complications of pregnancy following normal delivery, with oral contraceptive use, or with infection.

he·mo·lyze (hē′mə-līz′) *v.* To undergo or cause to undergo hemolysis.

he·mo·me·di·as·ti·num (hē′mō-mē′dē-ə-stī′nəm) *n.* Blood in the mediastinum.

he·mo·me·tra (hē′mō-mē′trə) *n.* See **hematometra.**

he·mo·ne·phro·sis (hē′mō-nə-frō′sĭs) *n.* Blood in the pelvis of the kidney.

he·mo·pa·thol·o·gy (hē′mō-pă-thŏl′ə-jē) *n.* See **hematopathology.**

he·mop·a·thy (hē-mŏp′ə-thē) *n.* Any of various abnormal conditions or diseases of the blood or the blood-forming tissues.

he·mo·per·fu·sion (hē'mō-pər-fyŏŏ'zhən) *n.* The passage of blood through columns of adsorptive material, such as activated charcoal, to remove toxic substances from the blood.

he·mo·per·i·car·di·um (hē'mō-pĕr'ĭ-kär'dē-əm) *n.* Blood in the pericardial sac.

he·mo·per·i·to·ne·um (hē'mō-pĕr'ĭ-tn-ē'əm) *n.* Blood in the peritoneal cavity.

he·mo·pex·in (hē'mō-pĕk'sĭn) *n.* A serum protein that is part of the beta-globulin fraction and functions in binding heme and porphyrins.

he·mo·phil (hē'mə-fĭl') *or* **he·mo·phile** (-fĭl') *n.* A microorganism that grows well in media containing blood.

he·mo·phil·i·a (hē'mə-fĭl'ē-ə, -fēl'yə) *n.* Any of several hereditary blood-coagulation disorders, manifested almost exclusively in males, in which the blood fails to clot normally because of a deficiency or an abnormality of one of the clotting factors.

hemophilia A *n.* Hemophilia due to deficiency of factor VIII, characterized by prolonged clotting time, decreased formation of thromboplastin, and diminished conversion of prothrombin.

hemophilia B *n.* A clotting disorder of blood resembling hemophilia A, caused by hereditary deficiency of factor IX. Also called *Christmas disease.*

he·mo·phil·i·ac (hē'mə-fĭl'ē-ăk', -fē'lē-) *n.* A person who is affected with hemophilia.

he·mo·phil·ic (hē'mə-fĭl'ĭk) *adj.* **1.** Of or affected by hemophilia. **2.** Growing well in blood or in a culture medium containing blood. Used of certain bacteria.

He·moph·i·lus (hĭ-mŏf'ə-ləs) *n.* Variant of **Haemophilus.**

he·mo·pho·bi·a (hē'mə-fō'bē-ə) *n.* An abnormal fear of blood.

he·mo·pho·re·sis (hē'mō-fə-rē'sĭs) *n.* Blood convection or irrigation of the tissues.

he·moph·thal·mi·a (hē'mŏf-thăl'mē-ə) *or* **he·moph·thal·mus** (-məs) *n.* An effusion of blood into the eyeball.

he·mo·plas·tic (hē'mə-plăs'tĭk) *adj.* Of or relating to the formation of blood cells.

he·mo·pleu·ro·pneu·mo·nia syndrome (hē'mə-plŏŏr'ō-nŏŏ-mōn'yə) *n.* A respiratory syndrome characterized by fever, spitting of blood, shortness of breath, and moderate tachycardia.

he·mo·pneu·mo·per·i·car·di·um (hē'mə-nŏŏ'mō-pĕr'ĭ-kär'dē-əm) *n.* Blood and air in the pericardial space. Also called *pneumohemopericardium.*

he·mo·pneu·mo·tho·rax (hē'mə-nŏŏ'mō-thôr'ăks') *n.* The accumulation of air and blood in the pleural cavity. Also called *pneumohemothorax.*

he·mo·poi·e·sis (hē'mə-poi-ē'sĭs) *n.* Variant of **hematopoiesis.**

he·mo·por·phy·rin (hē'mō-pôr'fə-rĭn) *n.* See **hematoporphyrin.**

he·mo·pre·cip·i·tin (hē'mō-prĭ-sĭp'ĭ-tĭn) *n.* An antibody that combines with and precipitates soluble antigenic material from red blood cells.

he·mo·pro·tein (hē'mə-prō'tēn') *n.* A conjugated protein containing a metal-porphyrin compound as the prosthetic group.

he·mop·ty·sis (hĭ-mŏp'tĭ-sĭs) *n.* The spitting of blood derived from the lungs or from the bronchial tubes.

he·mor·rha·chis (hĭ-môr'ə-kĭs) *n.* See **hematorrhachis.**

hem·or·rhage (hĕm'ər-ĭj) *n.* An escape of blood from the blood vessels, especially when excessive. Also called *hemorrhea.* —**hem'or·rhage** *v.* —**hem'or·rhag'-ic** (hĕm'ə-răj'ĭk) *adj.*

hem·or·rha·gen·ic (hĕm'ər-ə-jĕn'ĭk) *adj.* Causing or producing hemorrhage.

hemorrhagic ascites *n.* The presence of blood-stained serous fluid in the peritoneal cavity.

hemorrhagic colitis *n.* Abdominal cramps and bloody diarrhea, without fever, attributed to a self-limited infection by a strain of *Escherichia coli.*

hemorrhagic cyst *n.* A cyst containing blood or resulting from the encapsulation of a hematoma. Also called *blood cyst, hematocele, hematocyst.*

hemorrhagic disease of newborn *n.* A syndrome marked by spontaneous internal or external bleeding with hypoprothrombinemia and by markedly elevated bleeding and clotting times, usually occurring between the third and sixth day after birth.

hemorrhagic endovasculitis *n.* Endothelial and medial hyperplasia of placental blood vessels with thrombosis, fragmentation, and diapedesis of red blood cells resulting in stillbirth or fetal developmental disorders.

hemorrhagic fever *n.* A syndrome that occurs in perhaps 20 percent to 40 percent of infections by certain arboviruses and is marked by high fever, scattered petechiae, bleeding from the gastrointestinal tract and other organs, hypotension, and shock.

hemorrhagic fever with renal syndrome *n.* See **epidemic hemorrhagic fever.**

hemorrhagic infarct *n.* An infarct that is red because of the infiltration of blood from collateral vessels into the necrotic area. Also called *red infarct.*

hemorrhagic measles *n.* See **black measles.**

hemorrhagic plague *n.* The hemorrhagic form of bubonic plague.

hemorrhagic rickets *n.* Bone changes occurring in infantile scurvy, characterized by subperiosteal hemorrhage and deficient osteoid tissue formation.

hemorrhagic shock *n.* Hypovolemic shock resulting from acute hemorrhage marked by hypotension, tachycardia, oliguria, and pale, cold skin.

hem·or·rhag·in (hĕm'ə-răj'ĭn, -rā'jĭn) *n.* Any of a group of toxins found in certain venoms and plant poisons that cause degeneration and lysis of endothelial cells in capillaries and small vessels, thereby producing small hemorrhages in tissues.

hem·or·rhe·a (hĕm'ə-rē'ə) *n.* See **hemorrhage.**

hem·or·rhoid (hĕm'ə-roid') *n.* **1.** An itching or painful mass of dilated veins in swollen anal tissue. **2. hemorrhoids** The pathological condition in which such painful masses occur. Also called *piles.*

hem·or·rhoi·dal (hĕm'ə-roid'l) *adj.* **1.** Of or relating to hemorrhoids. **2.** Relating to certain arteries and veins supplying the region of the rectum and anus.

hemorrhoidal vein *n.* Any of the three rectal veins.

hem·or·rhoid·ec·to·my (hĕm′ə-roi-dĕk′tə-mē) *n.* Surgical removal of hemorrhoids.

he·mo·sal·pinx (hē′mō-săl′pĭngks) *n.* See **hematosalpinx.**

he·mo·sid·er·in (hē′mō-sĭd′ər-ĭn) *n.* An insoluble protein that contains iron and that is produced by phagocytic digestion of hematin and found as granules in most tissues, especially in the liver.

he·mo·sid·er·o·sis (hē′mō-sĭd′ə-rō′sĭs) *n.* Abnormal accumulation of hemosiderin in tissue.

he·mo·sper·mi·a (hē′mə-spûr′mē-ə) *n.* The presence of blood in the seminal fluid. Also called *hematospermia.*

he·mo·sta·sis (hē′mə-stā′sĭs, hē-mŏs′stə-) *n.* **1.** The stoppage of bleeding or hemorrhage. **2.** The stoppage of blood flow through a blood vessel or body part. **3.** The stagnation of blood.

he·mo·stat (hē′mə-stăt′) *n.* **1.** An agent, such as a chemical, that stops bleeding. **2.** An instrument for arresting hemorrhage by compression of the bleeding vessel.

he·mo·stat·ic (hē′mə-stăt′ĭk) *adj.* **1.** Arresting the flow of blood within the vessels. **2.** Arresting hemorrhage. —*n.* A hemostatic device or agent.

hemostatic forceps *n.* A forceps with a catch for locking the blades, used for seizing the end of a blood vessel to control hemorrhage.

he·mo·ther·a·py (hē′mə-thĕr′ə-pē) *or* **he·mo·ther·a·peu·tics** (-thĕr′ə-pyōō′tĭks) *n.* The treatment of disease by the use of blood or blood derivatives, as in transfusion.

he·mo·tho·rax (hē′mə-thôr′ăks′) *n.* Blood in the pleural cavity.

he·mo·tox·ic (hē′mə-tŏk′sĭk) *or* **he·ma·to·tox·ic** (hē′-mə-tō-, hĭ-măt′ə-) *adj.* **1.** Causing blood poisoning. **2.** Hemolytic.

he·mo·tox·in (hē′mə-tŏk′sĭn) *n.* A substance, especially one produced by a bacterium, that destroys red blood cells. Also called *hematotoxin.*

he·mo·troph (hē′mə-trŏf′, -trōf′) *n.* The nutritive materials supplied to the embryo through the placenta from the maternal bloodstream.

he·mo·trop·ic (hē′mə-trŏp′ĭk, -trō′pĭk) *adj.* Of or relating to the mechanism by which blood cells, especially red blood cells, attract phagocytic cells.

he·mo·tym·pa·num (hē′mə-tĭm′pə-nəm) *n.* The presence of blood in the tympanic cavity of the middle ear. Also called *hematotympanum.*

Hench (hĕnch), **Philip Showalter** 1896–1965. American physician. He shared a 1950 Nobel Prize for discoveries concerning adrenocortical hormones.

Hen·der·son-Has·sel·balch equation (hĕn′dər-sən-hăs′əl-bălk′, -hä′səl-bälкн′) *n.* An equation expressing the pH of a buffer solution as a function of the concentration of the weak acid or base and the salt components of the buffer.

Hen·der·so·nu·la to·ru·loi·de·a (hĕn′dər-sə-nyōō′lə tôr′yə-loi′dē-ə) *n.* A species of black yeast capable of producing infections of the toenails as well as of the skin of the feet.

Hen·dra virus (hĕn′drə) *n.* A paramyxovirus that causes encephalitis in humans and is transmitted from animals.

Hen·le (hĕn′lə), **Friedrich Gustav Jacob** 1809–1885. German anatomist whose works, including *Handbuch der Rationellen Pathologie* (1846–1852), integrated the study of pathology and physiology. He is also known for advancing histology with his microscopic anatomical examinations.

Hen·le's ampulla (hĕn′lēz) *n.* The enlarged end of the vas deferens. Also called *ampulla of vas deferens.*

Henle's fissures *n.* Minute spaces filled with connective tissue between the muscular fibers of the heart.

Henle's loop *n.* See **nephronic loop.**

Henle's sheath *n.* See **endoneurium.**

Henle's tubule *n.* The straight descending and ascending portions of renal tubules forming Henle's loop.

He·noch-Schön·lein purpura (hä′nôk-, -nôкн-) *n.* A form of nonthrombocytopenic purpura occurring most commonly in boys and associated with pain or swelling of the joints, colic, vomiting of blood, passage of bloody stools, and sometimes inflammation of the kidneys. Also called *allergic purpura, anaphylactoid purpura, Schönlein-Henoch purpura, Schönlein's disease.*

hen·ry (hĕn′rē) *n., pl.* **–rys** *or* **–ries** (-rēz) *Abbr.* **H** The unit of inductance in which an induced electromotive force of one volt is produced when the current is varied at the rate of one ampere per second.

Hen·ry's law (hĕn′rēz) *n.* The principle that at equilibrium the amount of gas dissolved in a given volume of liquid is directly proportional to the partial pressure of that gas in the gas phase.

Hen·sen (hĕn′zən), **(Christian Andreas) Viktor** 1835–1924. German physiologist noted for his research in embryology and his studies of the sense organs.

Hen·sen's cell (hĕn′sənz, -zənz) *n.* One of the supporting cells in the spiral organ.

Hensen's node *n.* See **primitive node.**

he·par (hē′pär) *n., pl.* **he·pat·a** (hĭ-păt′ə) The liver.

hep·a·rin (hĕp′ər-ĭn) *n.* A complex organic acid that is found especially in lung and liver tissue, has a mucopolysaccharide as its active constituent, prevents platelet agglutination and blood clotting, and is used in the form of its sodium salt in the treatment of thrombosis. —**hep′a·rin′i·za′tion** (-ə-rĭn′ĭ-zā′shən) *n.* —**hep′a·rin·ize′** (-ər-ə-nīz′) *v.*

hep·a·ri·tin sulfate (hĕp′ər-ĭ-tn) *n.* A polysaccharide containing the same repeating disaccharide groups as heparin, it accumulates in persons with certain mucopolysaccharidoses.

hepat– *pref.* Variant of **hepato–.**

hep·a·tal·gia (hĕp′ə-tăl′jə) *n.* Pain in the liver. Also called *hepatodynia.*

hep·a·ta·tro·phi·a (hĕp′ə-tə-trō′fē-ə) *or* **hep·a·tat·ro·phy** (-tăt′rə-fē) *n.* Atrophy of the liver.

hep·a·tec·to·my (hĕp′ə-tĕk′tə-mē) *n.* Excision of liver tissue.

he·pat·ic (hĭ-păt′ĭk) *adj.* **1.** Of, relating to, or resembling the liver. **2.** Acting on or occurring in the liver. —*n.* A drug that acts on the liver.

hepatic artery *n.* **1.** An artery with origin in the celiac artery, with branches to the right gastric, gastroduodenal, and proper hepatic arteries; common hepatic artery. **2.** An artery with origin in the common hepatic artery, and with branches to the right and left hepatic arteries; proper hepatic artery.

hepatic coma *n.* A coma occurring in advanced cirrhosis, hepatitis, poisoning, or other liver disease.

hepatic duct *n.* **1.** Left hepatic duct. **2.** Right hepatic duct.

hepatic encephalopathy *n.* See **portal-systemic encephalopathy.**

hepatic flexure *n.* See **right colic flexure.**

hepatic lobule *n.* A polygonal histologic unit of the liver, consisting of masses of liver cells arranged around a central vein that is a terminal branch of one of the hepatic veins, and at whose periphery branches of the portal vein, hepatic artery, and bile duct are located.

hepatico– *pref.* Liver, hepatic: *hepaticotomy.*

he·pat·i·co·do·chot·o·my (hĭ-păt′ĭ-kō-dō-kŏt′ə-mē) *n.* Incision into the common bile duct and the hepatic duct.

he·pat·i·co·du·o·de·nos·to·my (hĭ-păt′ĭ-kō-dōō′ə-dn-ŏs′tə-mē, -dōō-ŏd′n-ŏs′-) *n.* The surgical formation of a communication between a hepatic duct and the duodenum.

he·pat·i·co·en·ter·os·to·my (hĭ-păt′ĭ-kō-ĕn′tə-rŏs′tə-mē) *n.* The surgical formation of a communication between a hepatic duct and the intestine.

he·pat·i·co·gas·tros·to·my (hĭ-păt′ĭ-kō-gă-strŏs′tə-mē) *n.* The surgical formation of a communication between a hepatic duct and the stomach.

he·pat·i·co·li·thot·o·my (hĭ-păt′ĭ-kō-lĭ-thŏt′ə-mē) *n.* Surgical removal of one or more calculi from a hepatic duct.

he·pat·i·co·lith·o·trip·sy (hĭ-păt′ĭ-kō-lĭth′ə-trĭp′sē) *n.* The crushing of a biliary calculus in a hepatic duct.

he·pat·i·cos·to·my (hĭ-păt′ĭ-kŏs′tə-mē) *n.* The surgical formation of an opening into a hepatic duct.

he·pat·i·cot·o·my (hĭ-păt′ĭ-kŏt′ə-mē) *n.* Incision into a hepatic duct.

hepatic porphyria *n.* A category of porphyria that includes porphyria cutanea tarda, variegate porphyria, and coproporphyria.

hepatic portal vein *n.* See **portal vein.**

hepatic vein *n.* Any of the veins that carry from the liver the blood collected from the hepatic artery and portal vein and that terminate in three large veins, designated right, middle, and left, that open into the inferior vena cava below the diaphragm.

hep·a·tit·ic (hĕp′ə-tĭt′ĭk) *adj.* Of, relating to, or characterized by hepatitis.

hep·a·ti·tis (hĕp′ə-tī′tĭs) *n., pl.* **–tit·i·des** (-tĭt′ĭ-dēz′) Inflammation of the liver, caused by infectious or toxic agents and characterized by jaundice, fever, liver enlargement, and abdominal pain.

hepatitis A *n.* A form of viral hepatitis caused by an enterovirus that does not persist in the blood serum, is transmitted by ingestion of infected food and water, and has a shorter incubation and milder symptoms than hepatitis B. Also called *infectious hepatitis.*

hepatitis B *n.* A form of viral hepatitis caused by a DNA virus that often persists in the blood serum and can cause chronic liver damage. Hepatitis B is usually transmitted by infected blood products (as through

transfusion), by contaminated needles, or by exposure to infected bodily fluids through sexual intercourse. Also called *serum hepatitis.*

hepatitis B core antigen *n. Abbr.* **HB$_c$Ag** A core protein antigen of the hepatitis B virus found on the Dane particle and also in hepatocyte nuclei in hepatitis B infections.

hepatitis B e antigen *n. Abbr.* **HBe, HB$_e$Ag** A core protein antigen of the hepatitis B virus distinct from hepatitis B core antigen, associated with infectivity.

hepatitis B surface antigen *n. Abbr.* **HB$_s$Ag** An antigen derived from the surface of the hepatitis B virus that is present in the blood in active hepatitis B infection. Also called *Australia antigen.*

hepatitis B vaccine *n. Abbr.* **HB** A vaccine prepared from the inactivated surface antigen of the hepatitis B virus and used to immunize against hepatitis B.

hepatitis C *n.* A form of viral hepatitis that is caused by an RNA virus that is transmitted primarily by blood and blood products, as in blood transfusions or intravenous drug use, and sometimes through sexual contact. Most cases of non-A, non-B hepatitis are of this type.

hepatitis D *n.* A form of viral hepatitis caused by an RNA virus that can only invade cells in the presence of hepatitis B virus. It is usually more severe than other forms of hepatitis, is transmitted sexually or by exposure to infected blood or blood products, and is most prevalent in tropical and subtropical areas of the Mediterranean basin. Also called *delta hepatitis.*

hepatitis delta virus *n.* Causative agent of acute or chronic viral hepatitis type D. Also called *delta agent, delta antigen.*

hepatitis E *n.* A self-limited, acute hepatitis caused by a calicivirus, having symptoms similar to those of hepatitis A and spread via contaminated drinking water and food. It is endemic in developing countries and has occurred in epidemics in regions of Asia, Africa, and Central America.

hepatitis G *n.* A form of viral hepatitis caused by an RNA virus and often found in conjunction with hepatitis C infection.

hep·a·ti·za·tion (hĕp′ə-tĭ-zā′shən) *n.* The conversion of a loose tissue into a firm mass like the substance of the liver, especially such a conversion of lung tissue in pneumonia.

hepato– *or* **hepat–** *pref.* Liver: *hepatitis.*

hep·a·to·blas·to·ma (hĕp′ə-tō-blă-stō′mə) *n.* A malignant neoplasm occurring in young children, primarily in the liver, composed of tissue resembling embryonic hepatic epithelium.

hep·a·to·car·ci·no·ma (hĕp′ə-tō-kär′sə-nō′mə) *n.* See **hepatocellular carcinoma.**

he·pat·o·cele (hĭ-păt′ə-sēl′, hĕp′ə-tō-) *n.* Hernial protrusion of part of the liver through the abdominal wall or through the diaphragm.

hep·a·to·cel·lu·lar carcinoma (hĕp′ə-tō-sĕl′yə-lər, hĭ-păt′ō-) *n.* A carcinoma derived from parenchymal cells of the liver. Also called *hepatocarcinoma, malignant hepatoma.*

hepatocellular jaundice *n.* Jaundice caused by injury, inflammation, or liver cell failure.

hep·a·to·cho·lan·gi·o·je·ju·nos·to·my (hĕp′ə-tō-kō-lăn′jē-ō-jə-jŏo′nŏs′tə-mē, -jē′jŏo-) *n.* Surgical union of the hepatic duct to the jejunum.

hep·a·to·cho·lan·gi·os·to·my (hĕp′ə-tō-kō-lăn′jē-ŏs′tə-mē) *n.* The surgical formation of an opening into the common bile duct to establish drainage.

hep·a·to·cho·lan·gi·tis (hĕp′ə-tō-kō′lăn-jī′tĭs) *n.* Inflammation of the liver and bile ducts.

hep·a·to·cys·tic (hĕp′ə-tō-sĭs′tĭk) *adj.* Relating to the liver and gallbladder.

hep·a·to·cyte (hĕp′ə-tə-sīt′, hĭ-păt′ə-) *n.* A parenchymal liver cell.

hep·a·to·dyn·i·a (hĕp′ə-tō-dĭn′ē-ə) *n.* See **hepatalgia**.

hep·a·to·en·ter·ic (hĕp′ə-tō-ĕn-tĕr′ĭk) *adj.* Relating to the liver and the intestine.

hep·a·tof·u·gal (hĕp′ə-tŏf′yə-gəl, -tō-fyŏo′-) *adj.* Flowing away from the liver.

hep·a·to·gas·tric (hĕp′ə-tō-găs′trĭk) *adj.* Relating to the liver and the stomach.

hep·a·to·gen·ic (hĕp′ə-tə-jĕn′ĭk) *or* **hep·a·tog·e·nous** (-tŏj′ə-nəs) *adj.* Formed or originating in the liver.

hepatogenous jaundice *n.* Jaundice resulting from liver disease, not from changes in the blood.

hep·a·tog·ra·phy (hĕp′ə-tŏg′rə-fē) *n.* Radiographic examination of the liver.

hep·a·toid (hĕp′ə-toid′) *adj.* Resembling the liver.

hep·a·to·jug·u·lar reflux (hĕp′ə-tō-jŭg′yə-lər, hĭ-păt′ə-) *n.* An elevation of venous pressure, visible in the jugular veins and measurable in the veins of the arm, that is produced in active or impending congestive heart failure by firm pressure with the flat hand over the abdomen.

hep·a·to·len·tic·u·lar degeneration (hĕp′ə-tō-lĕn-tĭk′yə-lər, hĭ-păt′ō-) *n.* See **Wilson's disease**.

hep·a·to·lith (hĕp′ə-tə-lĭth′) *n.* A concretion in the liver.

hep·a·to·li·thec·to·my (hĕp′ə-tō-lĭ-thĕk′tə-mē) *n.* Surgical removal of a calculus from the liver.

hep·a·to·li·thi·a·sis (hĕp′ə-tō-lĭ-thī′ə-sĭs) *n.* The presence of calculi in the liver.

hep·a·tol·o·gy (hĕp′ə-tŏl′ə-jē) *n.* The branch of medical science concerned with the liver and its diseases.

hep·a·tol·y·sin (hĕp′ə-tŏl′ĭ-sĭn) *n.* A cytolysin that destroys parenchymal liver cells.

hep·a·to·ma (hĕp′ə-tō′mə) *n., pl.* **-mas** *or* **-ma·ta** (-mə-tə) A usually malignant tumor occurring in the liver.

hep·a·to·ma·la·cia (hĕp′ə-tō-mə-lā′shə) *n.* Softening of the liver.

hep·a·to·meg·a·ly (hĕp′ə-tō-mĕg′ə-lē, hĭ-păt′ə-) *n.* The abnormal enlargement of the liver. Also called *megalohepatia*.

hep·a·to·mel·a·no·sis (hĕp′ə-tō-mĕl′ə-nō′sĭs) *n.* Deep pigmentation of the liver.

hep·a·tom·phal·o·cele (hĕp′ə-tŏm-făl′ō-sēl′, -tŏm′fə-lō-) *n.* Umbilical hernia with liver involvement.

hep·a·to·neph·ric (hĕp′ə-tō-nĕf′rĭk) *adj.* Relating to the liver and the kidney.

hepatonephric syndrome *n.* See **hepatorenal syndrome**.

hep·a·top·a·thy (hĕp′ə-tŏp′ə-thē) *n.* A disease or disorder of the liver. —**hep′a·to·path′ic** (hĕp′ə-tō-păth′ĭk, hĭ-păt′ō-) *adj.*

hep·a·to·pet·al (hĕp′ə-tō-pĕt′l) *adj.* Flowing toward the liver.

hep·a·to·pex·y (hĕp′ə-tə-pĕk′sē) *n.* Surgical anchoring of the liver to the abdominal wall.

hep·a·to·pneu·mon·ic (hĕp′ə-tō-nŏo-mŏn′ĭk) *adj.* Relating to the liver and the lungs.

hep·a·to·por·tal (hĕp′ə-tō-pôr′tl) *adj.* Relating to the portal system of the liver.

hep·a·to·pul·mo·nar·y (hĕp′ə-tō-pŏol′mə-nĕr′ē, -pŭl′-) *adj.* Hepatopneumonic.

hep·a·to·re·nal (hĕp′ə-tō-rē′nəl) *adj.* Relating to the liver and the kidney.

hepatorenal syndrome *n.* A condition in which acute renal failure occurs with disease of the liver or biliary tract, the cause of which is believed to be either a decrease in renal blood flow or damage to both the liver and the kidneys as from carbon tetrachloride poisoning or leptospirosis. Also called *hepatonephric syndrome*.

hep·a·tor·rha·phy (hĕp′ə-tôr′ə-fē) *n.* Suture of a wound of the liver.

hep·a·tor·rhex·is (hĕp′ə-tō-rĕk′sĭs) *n.* Rupture of the liver.

hep·a·tos·co·py (hĕp′ə-tŏs′kə-pē) *n.* Examination of the liver.

hep·a·to·sple·ni·tis (hĕp′ə-tō-splĭ-nī′tĭs) *n.* Inflammation of the liver and the spleen.

hep·a·to·sple·nog·ra·phy (hĕp′ə-tō-splĭ-nŏg′rə-fē) *n.* Radiographic visualization of the liver and the spleen following the injection of a contrast medium.

hep·a·to·sple·no·meg·a·ly (hĕp′ə-tō-splē′nō-mĕg′ə-lē, -splĕn′ō-) *n.* The enlargement of the liver and of the spleen.

hep·a·to·sple·nop·a·thy (hĕp′ə-tō-splĭ-nŏp′ə-thē) *n.* A disease of the liver and spleen.

hep·a·tot·o·my (hĕp′ə-tŏt′ə-mē) *n.* Incision into the liver.

hep·a·to·tox·e·mi·a (hĕp′ə-tō-tŏk-sē′mē-ə) *n.* Autointoxication originating in the liver.

hep·a·to·tox·ic (hĕp′ə-tō-tŏk′sĭk) *adj.* Damaging or destructive to the liver.

hep·a·to·tox·in (hĕp′ə-tō-tŏk′sĭn, hĭ-păt′ō-) *n.* A toxin that is destructive to liver parenchyma.

hepta– *or* **hept–** *pref.* **1.** Seven: *heptameter.* **2.** Containing seven atoms, molecules, or groups: *heptane.*

hep·tane·di·o·ic acid (hĕp′tān-dī-ō′ĭk) *n.* See **pimelic acid**.

hep·tose (hĕp′tōs′, -tōz′) *n.* A monosaccharide containing seven carbon atoms in a molecule.

herb·al·ist (ûr′bə-lĭst, hûr′-) *n.* **1.** One who grows, collects, or specializes in the use of herbs, especially medicinal herbs. **2.** See **herb doctor**.

herb·al medicine (ûr′bəl, hûr′-) *n.* **1.** The study or use of medicinal herbs to prevent and treat diseases and ailments or to promote health and healing. **2.** A drug or preparation made from a plant or plants and used for any such purposes.

herb doctor (ûrb, hûrb) *n.* One who practices healing with herbs. Also called *herbalist*.

Her·bert's operation (hûr′bərts) *n.* An operation for creating a filtering cicatrix in glaucoma by cutting and displacing a wedge-shaped scleral flap.

Her·cep·tin (hûr-sĕp′tn) A trademark for the drug trastuzumab.

herd immunity (hûrd) *n.* **1.** Resistance to the spread of infectious disease in a group because susceptible members are few, making transmission from an infected member unlikely. **2.** The immunologic status of a population, determined by the ratio of resistant to susceptible members and their distribution.

he·red·i·tar·y (hə-rĕd′ĭ-tĕr′ē) *adj.* Transmitted or capable of being transmitted genetically from parent to offspring.

hereditary angioneurotic edema *n.* A hereditary condition manifested by recurring episodes of edema of the skin, mucous membranes, or viscera and associated with either a deficiency of an esterase inhibitor of one of the components of complement or a functionally inactive form of the inhibitor.

hereditary cerebellar ataxia *n.* A disease of later childhood and early adult life marked by ataxic gait, hesitating and explosive speech, nystagmus, and sometimes optic neuritis.

hereditary cerebral leukodystrophy *n.* See **Merzbacher-Pelizaeus disease.**

hereditary chorea *n.* A chronic disorder characterized by choreic movements in the face and extremities, accompanied by a gradual loss of the mental faculties ending in dementia. Also called *Huntington's chorea, Huntington's disease.*

hereditary hemorrhagic telangiectasia *n.* An inherited disease, usually beginning after puberty, characterized by multiple telangiectases and by fragile capillaries that break easily and bleed into the skin and mucous membranes. Also called *Rendu-Osler-Weber disease, Rendu-Osler-Weber syndrome.*

hereditary hypertrophic neuropathy *n.* An inherited chronic sensorimotor multiple neuropathy characterized by the progressive swelling and mucoid degeneration of peripheral nerves. Also called *Déjérine's disease.*

hereditary lymphedema *n.* Permanent pitting edema, usually confined to the lower extremities. Also called *trophedema.*

hereditary multiple exostoses *pl.n.* An inherited disturbance of enchondral bone growth in which multiple osteochondromas of long bones appear during childhood, with shortening of the radius and fibula. Also called *diaphysial aclasis, osteochondromatosis.*

hereditary opalescent dentin *n.* See **dentinogenesis imperfecta.**

hereditary progressive arthro-ophthalmopathy *n.* A hereditary disease marked by progressive myopia and abnormal epiphysial development in vertebrae and long bones. Also called *Stickler syndrome.*

hereditary spherocytosis *n.* A congenital defect in the cell membrane of red blood cells resulting in thickened, fragile red blood cells that are susceptible to spontaneous hemolysis and marked by chronic anemia, reticulocytosis, mild jaundice, and fever and abdominal pain. Also called *chronic acholuric jaundice, chronic familial jaundice, congenital hemolytic anemia, congenital hemolytic jaundice, spherocytic anemia.*

hereditary spinal ataxia *n.* Sclerosis of the posterior and lateral columns of the spinal cord, occurring in children and characterized by ataxia in the lower extremities that spreads to the upper extremities and is followed by paralysis and contractures. Also called *Friedreich's ataxia.*

he·red·i·ty (hə-rĕd′ĭ-tē) *n.* **1.** The genetic transmission of characteristics from parent to offspring. **2.** One's genetic constitution.

heredo– *pref.* Heredity; hereditary: *heredofamilial.*

her·e·do·fa·mil·ial (hĕr′ĭ-dō-fə-mĭl′yəl) *adj.* Relating to an inherited condition present in more than one member of a family. No longer in technical use.

her·e·do·mac·u·lar degeneration (hĕr′ĭ-dō-măk′yə-lər) *n.* Inherited macular degeneration.

her·i·ta·bil·i·ty (hĕr′ĭ-tə-bĭl′ĭ-tē) *n.* **1.** The quality of being heritable. **2.** The proportion of phenotypic variance attributable to variance in genotypes.

her·i·ta·ble (hĕr′ĭ-tə-bəl) *adj.* **1.** Capable of being passed from one generation to the next; hereditary. **2.** Capable of inheriting or taking by inheritance.

her·maph·ro·dite (hər-măf′rə-dīt′) *n.* An individual having the reproductive organs and many of the secondary sex characteristics of both sexes. —**her·maph′-ro·dit′ic** (-dĭt′ĭk) *adj.*

her·maph·ro·dit·ism (hər-măf′rə-dī-tĭz′əm) *n.* The presence of both ovarian and testicular tissue in an individual.

her·met·ic (hər-mĕt′ĭk) *or* **her·met·i·cal** (-ĭ-kəl) *adj.* Completely sealed, especially against the escape or entry of air. —**her·met′i·cal·ly** *adv.*

her·ni·a (hûr′nē-ə) *n.,* *pl.* –**ni·as** The protrusion of an organ or other bodily structure through the wall that normally contains it. —**her′ni·al** *adj.*

hernial sac *n.* The peritoneal envelope of a hernia.

her·ni·ate (hûr′nē-āt′) *v.* To protrude through an abnormal bodily opening. —**her′ni·a′tion** *n.*

her·ni·at·ed (hûr′nē-ā′tĭd) *adj.* Of or relating to a bodily structure that has protruded through an abnormal opening in the wall that contains it.

herniated disk *n.* The protrusion of a degenerated or fragmented intervertebral disk into the intervertebral foramen, compressing the nerve root. Also called *protruded disk, ruptured disk.*

hernio– *pref.* Hernia: *herniology.*

her·ni·oid (hûr′nē-oid′) *adj.* Resembling a hernia.

her·ni·o·plas·ty (hûr′nē-ə-plăs′tē) *n.* Surgical correction of a hernia.

her·ni·or·rha·phy (hûr′nē-ôr′ə-fē) *n.* Surgical correction of a hernia by suturing.

her·ni·ot·o·my (hûr′nē-ŏt′ə-mē) *n.* The surgical correction of a hernia by cutting through a band of tissue that constricts it. Also called *celotomy.*

he·ro·ic (hĭ-rō′ĭk) *adj.* Relating to a risky medical procedure that may endanger the patient but also has a possibility of being successful, whereas lesser action would result in failure.

her·o·in (hĕr′ō-ĭn) *n.* A white, odorless, bitter, crystalline compound that is derived from morphine and is a highly addictive narcotic. Also called *diacetylmorphine.*

her·o·in·ism (hĕr′ō-ĭ-nĭz′əm) *n.* Addiction to heroin.

He·roph·i·lus (hə-rŏf′ə-ləs) fl. c. 300 BC. Greek anatomist and surgeon. A pioneer of dissection, he compared the human anatomy to that of other animals and gave detailed descriptions of the brain, liver, spleen, and sexual organs.

her·pan·gi·na (hûr′păn-jī′nə, hûr-păn′jə-) *n.* A mild disease of children caused by a coxsackievirus and marked by fever, dysphagia, and vesicopapular lesions of the mucous membranes of the throat.

her·pes (hûr′pēz) *n.* Any of several viral diseases causing the eruption of small blisterlike vesicles on the skin or mucous membranes, especially herpes simplex or herpes zoster. —**her·pet′ic** (hər-pĕt′ĭk) *adj.*

herpes encephalitis *n.* Encephalitis caused by the herpes simplex virus.

herpes ges·ta·ti·o·nis (jĕ-stā′shē-ō′nĭs) *n.* A rare polymorphous skin eruption of unknown origin occurring in late pregnancy that is more common on the extremities than on the trunk. It may recur during each subsequent pregnancy.

herpes iris *n.* **1.** See **erythema iris. 2.** See **erythema multiforme.**

herpes sim·plex (sĭm′plĕks′) *n.* **1.** A recurrent viral disease that is caused by herpesvirus type one and is marked by fluid-containing vesicles on the mouth, lips, or face; cold sore. **2.** A recurrent viral disease that is caused by herpesvirus type two and is marked by fluid-containing vesicles on the genitals.

her·pes·vi·rus (hûr′pēz-vī′rəs) *n.* Either of two types of DNA-containing animal viruses of the genus *Herpesvirus*, herpesvirus type one or herpesvirus type two, which form inclusion bodies within the nuclei of host cells. Also called *herpes simplex virus.*

Herpesvirus *n.* A genus of viruses of the family Herpetoviridae including the causative agents of genital herpes and shingles.

herpes zoster *n.* See **shingles.**

herpes zoster virus *n.* See **varicella-zoster virus.**

herpetic keratitis *n.* Inflammation of the cornea or of the cornea and conjunctiva caused by herpesvirus type one. Also called *herpetic keratoconjunctivitis.*

herpetic whitlow *n.* A painful infection of the finger, caused by herpesvirus and often accompanied by lymphangitis and regional adenopathy.

her·pet·i·form (hûr-pĕt′ə-fôrm′) *adj.* Of or resembling herpes.

herpetiform aphthae *n.* Aphthae characterized by numerous ulcers clustered in groups of vesicles.

Her·pe·to·vir·i·dae (hûr′pĭ-tō-vîr′ĭ-dē′) *n.* A family of morphologically similar viruses, all of which contain double-stranded DNA, whose infections produce characteristic inclusion bodies.

her·pe·to·vi·rus (hûr′pĭ-tō-vī′rəs) *n.* A virus belonging to the family Herpetoviridae.

Her·plex (hûr′plĕks′) A trademark for the drug idoxuridine.

her·sage (ĕr-säzh′) *n.* Surgical separation of the individual fibers of a nerve trunk.

Hers disease (ârz, ĕrs) *n.* See **type 6 glycogenosis.**

Her·shey (hûr′shē), **Alfred Day** 1908–1997. American biologist. He shared a 1969 Nobel Prize for investigating the mechanism of viral infection in living cells.

hertz (hûrts) *n., pl.* **hertz** *Abbr.* **Hz** A unit of frequency equal to 1 cycle per second.

Herx·hei·mer's reaction (hûrks′hī′mərz, hĕrks′-) *n.* An inflammatory reaction in tissues infected by spirochetes, as in syphilis or Lyme disease, induced in certain cases by treatment with salvarsan, mercury, or antibiotics. Also called *Jarisch-Herxheimer reaction.*

Heschl's gyrus (hĕsh′əlz) *n.* See **transverse temporal gyrus.**

hes·i·tan·cy (hĕz′ĭ-tən-sē) *n.* An involuntary delay or inability in starting the urinary stream.

Hess (hĕs), **Walter Rudolf** 1881–1973. Swiss physiologist. He shared a 1949 Nobel Prize for his research on the brain's control of the body.

Hes·sel·bach's hernia (hĕs′əl-bäks′, -bäкнs′) *n.* A hernia with diverticula through the cribriform fascia, presenting a lobular outline.

Hesselbach's triangle *n.* See **inguinal triangle.**

het·er·ax·i·al (hĕt′ə-răk′sē-əl) *adj.* Having mutually perpendicular axes of unequal length.

het·er·es·the·sia (hĕt′ər-ĭs-thē′zhə) *n.* A variation in the degree of the sensory response to a cutaneous stimulus as the stimulus crosses different areas on the surface of the skin.

hetero– *or* **heter–** *pref.* Other; different: *heterocellular.*

het·er·o·ag·glu·ti·nin (hĕt′ə-rō-ə-glōot′n-ĭn) *n.* A hemagglutinin that agglutinates red blood cells in one or more species other than the species from which it was derived.

het·er·o·an·ti·bod·y (hĕt′ə-rō-ăn′tĭ-bŏd′ē) *n.* An antibody that is specific for antigens originating in species other than that of the antibody producer.

het·er·o·an·ti·se·rum (hĕt′ə-rō-ăn′tĭ-sîr′əm) *n.* An antiserum developed in one animal species against antigens or cells of another species.

het·er·o·blas·tic (hĕt′ə-rō-blăs′tĭk) *adj.* Developing from more than a single type of tissue.

het·er·o·cel·lu·lar (hĕt′ə-rō-sĕl′yə-lər) *adj.* Formed of cells of different kinds.

het·er·o·chro·mat·ic (hĕt′ə-rō-krō-măt′ĭk) *adj.* **1.** Of or relating to heterochromatin. **2.** Of or characterized by different colors; varicolored. **3.** Consisting of different wavelengths or frequencies.

het·er·o·chro·ma·tin (hĕt′ə-rō-krō′mə-tĭn) *n.* The part of the chromonema that remains tightly coiled and condensed during interphase and thus stains readily.

het·er·o·chro·mi·a (hĕt′ə-rō-krō′mē-ə) *n.* A difference in coloration in two structures or two parts of the same structure that are normally alike in color.

het·er·o·chro·mic uveitis (hĕt′ə-rō-krō′mĭk) *n.* Pigmentary changes in the iris with inflammation of the anterior uvea.

het·er·o·chro·mo·some (hĕt′ə-rō-krō′mə-sōm′) *n.* **1.** A chromosome composed primarily of heterochromatin. **2.** See **allosome.**

het·er·o·chro·mous (hĕt′ə-rō-krō′məs) *adj.* Having an abnormal difference in coloration.

het·er·o·chro·ni·a (hĕt′ə-rō-krō′nē-ə) *n.* The origin or development of tissues or organs at an unusual time or out of the regular sequence. —**het′er·o·chron′ic** (-krŏn′ĭk), **het′er·och·ro·nous** (hĕt′ə-rŏk′rə-nəs) *adj.*

het·er·o·clad·ic anastomosis (hĕt′ə-rō-klăd′ĭk) *n.* A surgical connection between branches of different arteries.

het·er·o·crine (hĕt′ə-rə-krĭn, -krēn′) *adj.* Secreting two or more kinds of material.

het·er·o·cy·clic (hĕt′ə-rō-sī′klĭk, -sĭk′lĭk) *adj.* Containing more than one kind of atom joined in a ring.

het·er·o·cy·to·trop·ic (hĕt′ə-rō-sī′tə-trŏp′ĭk, -trō′pĭk) *adj.* Having an affinity for cells of a different species. Used of an antibody.

heterocytotropic antibody *n.* A cytotropic antibody similar in activity to a homocytotropic antibody but having affinity for cells of a different species.

het·er·od·ro·mous (hĕt′ə-rŏd′rə-məs) *adj.* Moving in the opposite direction.

het·er·oe·cious (hĕt′ə-rē′shəs) *adj.* Spending different stages of a life cycle on different, usually unrelated hosts. Used of parasites such as rust fungi and tapeworms. —**het′er·oe′cism** (-sĭz′əm) *n.*

het·er·o·er·o·tism (hĕt′ə-rō-ĕr′ə-tĭz′əm) *n.* See **alloerotism.** —**het′er·o·e·rot′ic** (-ĭ-rŏt′ĭk) *adj.*

het·er·o·gam·ete (hĕt′ə-rō-găm′ēt′, -gə-mēt′) *n.* Either of two conjugating gametes that differ in structure or behavior, such as the small motile male spermatozoon and the larger nonmotile female ovum.

het·er·o·ga·met·ic (hĕt′ə-rō-gə-mĕt′ĭk) *adj.* Producing dissimilar gametes, such as those of human males, who produce two types of spermatozoa, one bearing the X-chromosome and the other bearing the Y-chromosome.

het·er·og·a·mous (hĕt′ə-rŏg′ə-məs) *adj.* Relating to heterogamy.

het·er·og·a·my (hĕt′ə-rŏg′ə-mē) *n.* The state or condition in which conjugating gametes are dissimilar in structure and size as well as in function.

het·er·o·ge·ne·i·ty (hĕt′ə-rō′jə-nē′ĭ-tē) *n.* The quality or state of being heterogeneous.

het·er·o·ge·ne·ous (hĕt′ər-ə-jē′nē-əs, -jēn′yəs) *adj.* Composed of parts having dissimilar characteristics or properties.

heterogeneous nuclear RNA *n.* See **hnRNA.**

heterogeneous radiation *n.* Radiation consisting of different frequencies, various energies, or a variety of particles.

heterogeneous system *n.* A chemical system that contains various distinct and mechanically separable parts or phases, such as a suspension.

het·er·o·gen·e·sis (hĕt′ə-rō-jĕn′ĭ-sĭs) *n.* The production of offspring unlike the parents.

het·er·o·ge·net·ic (hĕt′ə-rō-jə-nĕt′ĭk) *adj.* Relating to heterogenesis.

heterogenetic antigen *n.* An antigen occurring in several different phylogenetically unrelated species. Also called *heterophil antigen.*

heterogenetic parasite *n.* A parasite whose life cycle involves an alternation of generations.

het·er·o·gen·ic (hĕt′ə-rō-jĕn′ĭk) *or* **het·er·o·ge·ne·ic** (-jə-nē′ĭk) *adj.* Relating to different gene constitutions, especially with respect to different species.

heterogenic en·ter·o·bac·te·ri·al antigen (ĕn′tə-rō-băk-tîr′ē-əl) *n.* See **common antigen.**

het·er·o·ge·note (hĕt′ə-rō-jē′nōt′) *n.* A microorganism containing an exogenous piece of genetic material that differs from the corresponding region of its original genome, but in a limited way resembles a heterozygote.

het·er·og·e·nous (hĕt′ə-rŏj′ə-nəs) *adj.* Not arising within the body; derived from another individual or species.

heterogenous vaccine *n.* Vaccine prepared from microorganisms obtained from a source other than the person who is to be vaccinated.

het·er·o·graft (hĕt′ə-rō-grăft′) *n.* A type of tissue graft in which the donor and recipient are of different species. Also called *heterologous graft, heteroplastic graft, heterotransplant, xenograft.*

het·er·o·kar·y·on (hĕt′ər-ə-kăr′ē-ŏn′, -ən) *n.* A cell having two or more genetically different nuclei.

het·er·o·ki·ne·sis (hĕt′ə-rō-kə-nē′sĭs, -kī-) *n.* Differential distribution of X-chromosomes and Y-chromosomes during meiotic cell division.

het·er·o·la·li·a (hĕt′ə-rō-lā′lē-ə) *n.* A form of aphasia characterized by habitual substitution of meaningless or inappropriate words for those intended. Also called *heterophasia, heterophemia.*

het·er·o·lat·er·al (hĕt′ə-rō-lăt′ər-əl) *adj.* Originating in a corresponding part of an opposite side.

het·er·ol·o·gous (hĕt′ə-rŏl′ə-gəs) *adj.* **1.** Of or relating to cytologic or histological elements not normally occurring in a designated part of the body. **2.** Derived from a different species, as a graft or transplant. **3.** Immunologically related but not identical. Used of certain cells and antiserums.

heterologous graft *n.* See **heterograft.**

heterologous stimulus *n.* A stimulus that acts upon any part of the sensory apparatus or a nerve tract.

heterologous tumor *n.* A tumor composed of a tissue unlike that from which it develops.

het·er·ol·o·gy (hĕt′ə-rŏl′ə-jē) *n.* Lack of correspondence between bodily parts, as in structure or development, arising from differences in origin.

het·er·ol·y·sis (hĕt′ə-rŏl′ĭ-sĭs, -ə-rō-lī′sĭs) *n., pl.* **–ses** (-sēz′) Dissolution or digestion of cells or proteins from one species by a lytic agent from a different species. —**het′er·o·lyt′ic** (-ə-rō-lĭt′ĭk) *adj.*

het·er·o·mer·ic (hĕt′ə-rō-mĕr′ĭk) *adj.* **1.** Having a different chemical composition. **2.** Of or relating to spinal neurons that have processes passing over to the opposite side of the cord.

heteromeric cell *n.* See **commissural cell.**

het·er·o·met·a·pla·sia (hĕt′ə-rō-mĕt′ə-plā′zhə) *n.* Tissue transformation resulting in the production of a tissue that is foreign to the part where it is produced.

het·er·o·met·ric autoregulation (hĕt′ə-rō-mĕt′rĭk) *n.* Autoregulation of the strength of ventricular contraction that occurs in direct relation to the end diastolic fiber length, as in law of the heart.

het·er·o·me·tro·pi·a (hĕt′ə-rō-mĭ-trō′pē-ə) *n.* A condition in which the degree of refraction in each eye is dissimilar.

het·er·o·mor·pho·sis (hĕt′ə-rō-môr′fə-sĭs, -môr-fō′-sĭs) *n.* **1.** The development of one tissue from a tissue of another kind or type. **2.** The embryonic development of a tissue or an organ inappropriate to its site.

het·er·o·mor·phous (hĕt′ə-rō-môr′fəs) *adj.* Differing from the normal type.

het·er·on·o·mous (hĕt′ə-rŏn′ə-məs) *adj.* Differing in development or manner of specialization. —**het′er·on′o·my** *n.*

het·er·on·y·mous diplopia (hĕt′ə-rŏn′ə-məs) *n.* A form of double vision in which the false image is on the same side as the healthy eye. Also called *crossed diplopia*.

heteronymous hemianopsia *n.* See **crossed hemianopsia**.

het·er·op·a·thy (hĕt′ə-rŏp′ə-thē) *n.* Abnormal sensitivity to stimuli.

het·er·oph·a·gy (hĕt′ə-rŏf′ə-jē) *n.* Digestion within a cell of a substance taken in by phagocytosis from the cell's environment.

het·er·o·pha·sia (hĕt′ə-rō-fā′zhə) *n.* See **heterolalia**.

het·er·o·phe·mi·a (hĕt′ə-rō-fē′mē-ə) *n.* See **heterolalia**.

het·er·o·phil (hĕt′ə-rō-fĭl′) *or* **het·er·o·phile** (-fīl′) *n.* A granulocyte; in humans, a neutrophil. —*adj.* Relating to heterogenetic antigens or to antibodies directed against such antigens.

heterophil antigen *n.* See **heterogenetic antigen**.

het·er·o·pho·ni·a (hĕt′ə-rō-fō′nē-ə) *n.* **1.** The change of voice at puberty. **2.** An abnormality in the voice sounds.

het·er·o·pho·ri·a (hĕt′ə-rō-fôr′ē-ə) *n.* A tendency of the eyes to deviate from the parallel.

het·er·oph·thal·mus (hĕt′ə-rŏf-thăl′məs, -ŏp-) *n.* A difference in the appearance of the two eyes.

Het·er·oph·y·es (hĕt′ə-rŏf′ē-ēz′) *n.* A genus of trematode worms parasitic in fish-eating birds and mammals, including humans.

het·er·o·phy·i·a·sis (hĕt′ə-rō-fī-ī′ə-sĭs) *n.* Infection with trematodes of the genus *Heterophyes*.

het·er·o·pla·sia (hĕt′ə-rō-plā′zhə) *n.* **1.** The development of cytologic and histologic elements that are not normal for the organ or part in which they occur. **2.** Malposition of tissue or a part that is otherwise normal.

het·er·o·plas·tic (hĕt′ə-rō-plăs′tĭk) *adj.* **1.** Relating to or manifesting heteroplasia. **2.** Relating to tissue transplantation from one species to another.

heteroplastic graft *n.* See **heterograft**.

het·er·o·plas·ty (hĕt′ər-ə-plăs′tē) *n.* The surgical grafting of tissue obtained from one individual or species to another.

het·er·o·ploid (hĕt′ər-ə-ploid′) *adj.* Having a chromosome number that is not a whole-number multiple of the haploid chromosome number for that species. —**het′er·o·ploid′** *n.*

het·er·o·ploi·dy (hĕt′ər-ə-ploi′dē) *n.* The state of an individual or cell possessing a chromosome number other than the normal diploid number.

het·er·o·pyk·no·sis (hĕt′ə-rō-pĭk-nō′sĭs) *n.* A state of variable density between chromosomes of different cells or between individual chromosomes.

het·er·o·sex·u·al (hĕt′ə-rō-sĕk′shoō-əl) *adj.* Sexually oriented to persons of the opposite sex. —*n.* A heterosexual person.

het·er·o·sex·u·al·i·ty (hĕt′ə-rō-sĕk′shoō-ăl′ĭ-tē) *n.* Erotic attraction, predisposition, or sexual behavior between persons of the opposite sex.

het·er·o·sug·ges·tion (hĕt′ə-rō-səg-jĕs′chən, -sə-jĕs′-) *n.* Suggestion received from another person.

het·er·o·tax·i·a (hĕt′ə-rō-tăk′sē-ə) *n.* Abnormal arrangement of organs or parts of the body in relation to one another.

het·er·o·tax·ic (hĕt′ə-rō-tăk′sĭk) *adj.* Abnormally placed or arranged.

het·er·o·to·ni·a (hĕt′ə-rō-tō′nē-ə) *n.* A state of abnormality or variation in tension or tone.

het·er·o·to·pi·a (hĕt′ər-ə-tō′pē-ə) *or* **het·er·ot·o·py** (hĕt′ə-rŏt′ə-pē) *n.* **1.** Displacement of an organ or other body part to an abnormal location. **2.** Displacement of gray matter, usually into the deep cerebral white matter. —**het′er·o·top′ic** (-tŏp′ĭk) *adj.*

het·er·o·trans·plant (hĕt′ə-rō-trăns′plănt′) *n.* See **heterograft**.

het·er·o·trans·plan·ta·tion (hĕt′ə-rō-trăns′plăn-tā′shən) *n.* The transplantation of a heterograft.

het·er·o·tri·cho·sis (hĕt′ə-rō-trĭ-kō′sĭs) *n.* Hair growth of variegated color.

het·er·o·troph (hĕt′ər-ə-trŏf′, -trōf′) *n.* An organism that cannot synthesize its own food and is dependent upon complex organic substances for nutrition. —**het′er·o·troph′ic** (-trŏf′ĭk, -trō′fĭk) *adj.* —**het′er·ot′ro·phy** (-ə-rŏt′rə-fē) *n.*

het·er·o·tro·pi·a (hĕt′ə-rō-trō′pē-ə) *n.* See **strabismus**.

het·er·o·typ·ic (hĕt′ə-rō-tĭp′ĭk) *or* **het·er·o·typ·i·cal** (-ĭ-kəl) *adj.* Of a different or unusual type or form.

heterotypical chromosome *n.* See **allosome**.

heterotypic cortex *n.* See **allocortex**.

het·er·o·xan·thine (hĕt′ə-rō-zăn′thēn′, -thĭn) *n.* A product of purine metabolism occurring in urine.

het·er·ox·e·nous (hĕt′ə-rŏk′sə-nəs) *adj.* Relating to digenesis; digenetic.

heteroxenous parasite *n.* A parasite that has more than one obligatory host in its life cycle.

het·er·o·zy·gos·i·ty (hĕt′ə-rō-zī-gŏs′ĭ-tē) *n.* The state of being heterozygous.

het·er·o·zy·gote (hĕt′ə-rō-zī′gōt′) *n.* An organism that has different alleles at a particular gene locus on homologous chromosomes.

het·er·o·zy·gous (hĕt′ər-ə-zī′gəs) *adj.* **1.** Having different alleles at one or more corresponding chromosomal loci. **2.** Of or relating to a heterozygote.

HEV *abbr.* hepatitis E virus

hexa– *or* **hex–** *pref.* **1.** Six: *hexagram.* **2.** Containing six atoms, molecules, or groups: *hexose.*

hex·a·chlo·ro·phene (hĕk′sə-klôr′ə-fēn′) *or* **hex·a·chlo·ro·phane** (-fān′) *n.* An almost odorless white powder that is used as a disinfectant and as an antibacterial agent in soaps.

hex·ad (hĕk′săd′) *n.* **1.** A group or series of six. **2.** An element or radical having a valence of six.

hex·a·dac·ty·ly (hĕk′sə-dăk′tə-lē) *or* **hex·a·dac·tyl·ism** (-lĭz′əm) *n.* The presence of six digits on one or both hands or feet.

hex·a·dec·a·no·ic acid (hĕk′sə-dĕk′ə-nō′ĭk) *n.* See **palmitic acid**.

hex·a·mer (hĕk′sə-mər) *n.* **1.** A polymer molecule composed of six monomers. **2.** A capsomer with six structural subunits.

hex·ane (hĕk′sān′) *n.* A colorless, flammable liquid, derived from the distillation of petroleum and used as a solvent.

hex·i·tol (hĕk′sĭ-tôl′, -tōl′) *n.* The sugar alcohol obtained on the reduction of a hexose.

hex·o·ki·nase (hĕk′sə-kī′nās′, -nāz′, -kĭn′ās′, -āz′) *n.* A transferase enzyme present in yeast, muscle, and other tissues, that acts during carbohydrate metabolism to catalyze the transfer of phosphate from ATP to glucose and other hexoses.

hexokinase method *n.* A highly specific method for determining the concentration of glucose in serum or plasma by spectrophotometrically measuring the NADP formed from hexokinase-catalyzed transformations of glucose and various intermediates.

hex·one base (hĕk′sōn′) *n.* See histone base.

hex·os·a·mine (hĕk-sō′sə-mēn′, hĕk′sō-săm′ēn′) *n.* The amine derivative of a hexose formed by replacing a hydroxyl group with an amino group.

hex·os·a·min·i·dase (hĕk′sō-sə-mĭn′ĭ-dās′, -dāz′) *n.* Any of at least four enzymes, each of which is the catalyst for the removal of hexose residues from specific oligosaccharides; deficiencies of these enzymes can cause certain metabolic disorders.

hex·o·san (hĕk′sə-săn′) *n.* Any of several polysaccharides that yield a hexose when hydrolyzed.

hex·ose (hĕk′sōs′) *n.* Any of various simple sugars, such as glucose and fructose, that have six carbon atoms per molecule.

hexose phosphatase *n.* An enzyme that catalyzes the hydrolysis of a hexose phosphate to a hexose.

hex·u·lose (hĕks′yə-lōs′) *n.* See ketohexose.

hex·yl (hĕk′səl) *n.* The univalent hydrocarbon radical, C_6H_{13}.

hex·yl·caine hydrochloride (hĕk′səl-kān′) *n.* A local anesthetic agent used for surface application, infiltration, or nerve block.

hex·yl·re·sor·ci·nol (hĕk′səl-rĭ-zôr′sə-nôl′, -nōl′) *n.* A yellowish-white crystalline phenol used as an antiseptic and anthelmintic.

Hey·er-Pu·denz valve (hā′ər-pyōō′dĕnz′) *n.* A valve used in the shunting procedure to relieve hydrocephaly, in which a ventricular catheter leads the cerebrospinal fluid into a pump through which the fluid passes down a distal catheter into the right atrium of the heart.

Hey·mans (hī′mənz, ā-mäns′), **Corneille Jean François** 1892–1968. Belgian physiologist. He won a 1938 Nobel Prize for determining the role of the aortic sinus in the regulation of respiration.

Hey·rov·sky (hā′rŏf-skē), **Jaroslav** 1890–1967. Czech chemist. He won a 1959 Nobel Prize for the development of polarography.

Hf The symbol for the element **hafnium**.

Hg The symbol for the element **mercury**.

Hgb *abbr.* hemoglobin

HGH *abbr.* human growth hormone

H-graft anastomosis *n.* The side-to-side surgical grafting of adjacent blood vessels using a straight connecting conduit.

hiatal hernia *n.* A hernia in which part of the stomach protrudes through the esophageal opening of the diaphragm. Also called *hiatus hernia*.

hi·a·tus (hī-ā′təs) *n.*, *pl.* **hiatus** *or* **–tus·es 1.** An aperture or fissure in an organ or a body part. **2.** A foramen. —**hi·a′tal** *adj.*

hiatus e·so·pha·ge·us (ē′sə-fā′jē-əs) *n.* The opening in the diaphragm between the central tendon and the aortic foramen through which the esophagus and the two vagus nerves pass.

hiatus hernia *n.* See **hiatal hernia**.

hiatus sa·phe·nus (sə-fē′nəs) *n.* The opening in the broad fascia through which the saphenous vein passes to enter the femoral vein. Also called *oval fossa*.

hiatus sem·i·lu·nar·is (sĕm′ē-lōō-nâr′ĭs) *n.* A groove in the lateral wall of the middle meatus of the nasal cavity, into which the maxillary sinus, the frontonasal duct, and the middle ethmoid cells open.

Hib *abbr.* Haemophilus influenzae type b

hi·ber·no·ma (hī′bər-nō′mə) *n.,* *pl.* **–mas** *or* **–ma·ta** (-mə-tə) A rare type of benign tumor in humans, consisting of brown fat that resembles the fat in certain hibernating animals.

Hib vaccine (hĭb) *n.* A conjugate vaccine that provides immunization against infections that are caused by *Haemophilus influenzae* type b, especially bacterial meningitis and pneumonia in children. Also called *Haemophilus influenzae type b conjugate vaccine.*

hic·cup *or* **hic·cough** (hĭk′əp) *n.* A spasm of the diaphragm causing sudden inhalation interrupted by spasmodic closure of the glottis, producing a characteristic noise. —**hic′cup, hic′cough** *v.*

hidr– *pref.* Variant of **hidro–**.

hi·drad·e·ni·tis (hī-drăd′n-ī′tĭs, hī-) *n.* Inflammation of the sweat glands.

hidradenitis sup·pu·ra·ti·va (sŭp′yə-rə-tī′və) *n.* Inflammation of the apocrine sweat glands of the perianal, axillary, and genital areas, producing chronic abscesses or sinuses.

hi·drad·e·no·ma (hī-drăd′n-ō′mə, hī-) *n.* A benign tumor derived from epithelial cells of sweat glands.

hidro– *or* **hidr–** *pref.* **1.** Sweat: *hidropoiesis.* **2.** Sweat glands: *hidrocystoma.*

hi·dro·cys·to·ma (hī′drō-sĭ-stō′mə) *n.* A cystic form of hidradenoma. Also called *syringocystoma.*

hi·dro·poi·e·sis (hī′drō-poi-ē′sĭs) *n.* The formation of sweat. —**hi′dro·poi·et′ic** (-ĕt′ĭk) *adj.*

hi·dros·che·sis (hī-drŏs′kĭ-sĭs, hī-) *n.* The suppression of sweating.

hi·dro·sis (hī-drō′sĭs, hī-) *n.,* *pl.* **–ses** (-sēz) **1.** The formation and excretion of sweat. **2.** Sweat, especially in excessive or abnormal amounts. —**hi·drot′ic** (-drŏt′ĭk) *adj.*

hidrotic ectodermal dysplasia *n.* A congenital dystrophy of nails and hair characterized by thickened nails, sparse or absent scalp hair, and often associated with a thickening of skin on palms and soles.

high blood pressure (hī) *n. Abbr.* **HBP** Hypertension.

high calorie diet *n.* A diet containing more than 4,000 calories per day.

high-density lipoprotein *n. Abbr.* **HDL** A lipoprotein that contains relatively small amounts of cholesterol and triglycerides and is associated with a decreased risk of atherosclerosis and coronary artery disease. Also called *alpha-lipoprotein, HDL cholesterol.*

high endothelial postcapillary venule *n.* Any of a group of venules located in the lymph nodes, tonsils, and aggregated lymphatic follicles, having a high-walled endothelium through which blood lymphocytes migrate into the lymphatic parenchyma.

high enema *n.* An enema instilled high up into the colon. Also called *enteroclysis.*

high-energy *adj.* **1.** Of or relating to elementary particles with energies exceeding hundreds of thousands of electron volts. **2.** Yielding a large amount of energy upon undergoing chemical reaction. **3.** Vigorous; dynamic.

high-energy phosphate bond *n.* A phosphate linkage that is present in certain intermediates of carbohydrate metabolism and containing the energy used in metabolic processes or transferred or stored. Also called *high-energy phosphate.*

high·est intercostal vein (hī′ĭst) *n.* A vein that drains the first intercostal space into either the vertebral vein or the brachiocephalic vein.

High·more's body (hī′môrz′) *n.* A mass of fibrous tissue continuous with the tunica albuginea, projecting into the testis from its posterior border.

high-pressure oxygen *n.* See **hyperbaric oxygen.**

high steppage gait *n.* A gait in which the foot is raised high to avoid catching a drooping foot and is then brought down suddenly in a flapping manner, often due to paralysis of the peroneal and anterior tibial muscles.

Hi·gou·me·na·ki·a sign (hē′gōō-mä′nə-kē-ə) *n.* An indication of late-stage congenital syphilis in which there is sternoclavicular swelling.

hi·lar (hī′lər) *adj.* Of or relating to a hilum.

hi·li·tis (hī-lī′tĭs) *n.* Inflammation of the lining membrane of a hilum.

Hill (hĭl), **Archibald Vivian** 1886–1977. British physiologist. He shared a 1922 Nobel Prize for his investigation of heat production in muscles and nerves.

hill·ock (hĭl′ək) *n.* A small protuberance or elevation, as from an organ, a tissue, or other structure.

Hill operation *n.* A surgical procedure used to prevent esophageal reflux.

Hill's equation (hĭlz) *n.* An expression of the percentage of oxygen in the blood based on the pressure of oxygen gas being administered and the rate at which hemoglobin releases oxygen.

Hill's sign *n.* An indication of aortic insufficiency in which systolic blood pressure is higher in the legs than in the arms.

Hil·ton's law (hĭl′tənz) *n.* The principle that the nerve supplying a joint also supplies both the muscles that move the joint and the skin covering the articular insertion of those muscles.

Hilton's white line *n.* See **white line of anal canal.**

hi·lum (hī′ləm) *n., pl.* **-la** (-lə) A depression or slit-like opening through which nerves, ducts, or blood vessels enter and leave in an organ or a gland. Also called *porta.* —**hi′lar** (-lər) *adj.*

hi·lus cell (hī′ləs) *n.* A cell in the hilum of the ovary that produces androgens and thus is functionally analogous to an interstitial cell.

hind·brain (hīnd′brān′) *n.* See **rhombencephalon.**

hind·gut (hīnd′gŭt′) *n.* **1.** The large intestine, rectum, and anal canal. **2.** The caudal or terminal part of the embryonic gut.

hind·wa·ter (hīnd′wô′tər) *n.* **1.** See **hydrorrhea gravidarum. 2.** The amniotic fluid behind the fetus as it emerges from the birth canal.

hinge (hĭnj) *n.* A jointed or flexible device that allows the turning or pivoting of a part, such as a door or lid, on a stationary frame.

hinged flap *n.* A turnover flap transferred by lifting it over onto its pedicle as though the pedicle was a hinge.

hinge joint *n.* A uniaxial joint in which a broad, transversely cylindrical convexity on one bone fits into a corresponding concavity on the other, allowing motion in one plane only, as in the elbow. Also called *ginglymoid joint.*

hinge region *n.* **1.** The portion of a crystalline form of tRNA that deforms to an L shape under electron microscopy. **2.** A short sequence of amino acids that lies at the base of each of the heavy chain regions of an immunoglobin and facilitates flexible movement of the molecule.

Hin·kle (hĭng′kəl), **Beatrice Moses** 1874–1953. American psychiatrist who cofounded the first psychotherapy clinic in the United States (1908).

hip (hĭp) *n.* **1.** The lateral prominence of the pelvis from the waist to the thigh. **2.** The hip joint.

hip·bone (hĭp′bōn′) *n.* Either of two large flat bones formed by the fusion of ilium, ischium, and pubis, constituting the lateral half of the pelvis and articulating with its fellow, with the sacrum, and with the femur. Also called *coxa, innominate bone.*

hip joint *n.* The ball-and-socket joint formed by the head of the femur and the cup-shaped cavity of the hipbone. Also called *coxa.*

Hip·pel's disease (hĭp′əlz) *n.* See **Lindau's disease.**

hip·po·cam·pal fissure (hĭp′ə-kăm′pəl) *n.* See **hippocampal sulcus.**

hippocampal gyrus *n.* See **parahippocampal gyrus.**

hippocampal sulcus *n.* A shallow groove between the dentate gyrus and the parahippocampal gyrus. Also called *hippocampal fissure.*

hip·po·cam·pus (hĭp′ə-kăm′pəs) *n., pl.* **-pi** (-pī′) The complex, internally convoluted structure that forms the medial margin of the cortical mantle of the cerebral hemisphere, borders the choroid fissure of the lateral ventricle, is composed of two gyri with their white matter, and forms part of the limbic system. —**hip′po·cam′pal** (-pəl) *adj.*

Hip·poc·ra·tes (hĭ-pŏk′rə-tēz′) Called "the Father of Medicine." 460?–377? BC. Greek physician who laid the foundations of scientific medicine by freeing medical study from the constraints of philosophical speculation and superstition. He is traditionally but inaccurately considered the author of the Hippocratic oath.

hip·po·crat·ic facies (hĭp′ə-krăt′ĭk) *n.* A pinched expression of the face, with sunken eyes, hollow cheeks and temples, and relaxed lips, observed in one dying after an exhausting illness. Also called *hippocratic face.*

hippocratic finger *n.* See **clubbed finger.**

hippocratic nail *n.* The coarse curved nail of a clubbed finger.

Hippocratic Oath *n.* An oath of ethical professional behavior sworn by new physicians and attributed to Hippocrates.

hippocratic suc·cus·sion sound (sə-kŭsh′ən) *n.* A splashing sound heard on auscultation in a patient with hydropneumothorax or pyopneumothorax.

hip·pus (hĭp′əs) *n.* Spasmodic, rhythmical dilation and constriction of the pupil, independent of illumination, convergence, or psychic stimuli.

hir·cus (hûr′kəs) *n.*, *pl.* **–ci** (-sī′) **1.** The odor of the armpits. **2.** See **tragus** (sense 1, 2).

Hirsch·feld's canal (hûrsh′fĕldz′) *n.* Any of various canals that extend vertically through alveolar bone between roots of mandibular and maxillary incisor and maxillary bicuspid teeth. Also called *interdental canal.*

Hirsch·o·witz syndrome (hûr′shə-wĭts′) *n.* A dermatological syndrome in which acanthosis nigricans occurs in association with hypovitaminosis; it responds well to topical applications of retinoic acid.

Hirsch·sprung's disease (hîrsh′sprŭngz′) *n.* See **congenital megacolon.**

hir·sute (hûr′sōōt′, hîr′-, hər-sōōt′) *adj.* Covered with hair; hairy.

hir·sut·ism (hûr′sōō-tĭz′əm, hîr′-, hər-sōō′-) *n.* The presence of excessive body and facial hair, especially in women.

hi·ru·di·cide (hĭ-rōō′dĭ-sīd′) *n.* An agent that kills leeches.

hir·u·din (hĭ-rōōd′n, hîr′ə-dən, -yə-) *n.* A substance extracted from the salivary glands of leeches and used as an anticoagulant.

Hir·u·din·e·a (hîr′ə-dĭn′ē-ə, -yə-) *n.* A class of worms, comprising the leeches that feed on blood and tissue exudates of vertebrates.

Hi·ru·do (hĭ-rōō′dō) *n.* A genus of leeches that includes the species most commonly used in medicine.

His *abbr.* histidine

His (hĭs), **Wilhelm** 1863–1934. German anatomist who is known for his investigations of the heart. He described (1893) the atrioventricular trunk, also called the His bundle.

His bundle *n.* See **bundle of His.**

His bundle electrogram *n.* An electrogram that is recorded from the atrioventricular trunk during cardiac catheterization.

His's line (hĭs′ĭz) *n.* An imaginary line extending from the tip of the anterior nasal spine to the hindmost point on the posterior margin of the foramen magnum, dividing the face into an upper and a lower part.

hist– *pref.* Variant of **histo–.**

His·ta·log test (hĭs′tə-lôg′) *n.* A test for measuring maximal production of gastric acidity or anacidity using betazole hydrochloride.

his·tam·i·nase (hĭ-stăm′ə-nās′, -nāz′, hĭs′tə-mə-) *n.* An enzyme that inactivates histamine and is found in the digestive system.

his·ta·mine (hĭs′tə-mēn′, -mĭn) *n.* A physiologically active depressor amine found in plant and animal tissue, derived from histidine by decarboxylation and released from cells in the immune system as part of an allergic reaction. It is a powerful stimulant of gastric secretion, constrictor of bronchial smooth muscle, and vasodilator. —**his′ta·min′ic** (-mĭn′ĭk) *adj.*

his·ta·mine-fast (hĭs′tə-mēn-făst′, -mĭn-) *adj.* Of or relating to the absence of the normal response to histamine, especially regarding gastric anacidity.

his·ta·mi·ne·mi·a (hĭs′tə-mə-nē′mē-ə, hĭ-stăm′ə-) *n.* The presence of histamine in the blood.

histamine test *n.* A test for measuring maximal production of gastric acidity or anacidity, in which, after the administration of an antihistamine, histamine acid phosphate is injected subcutaneously and the gastric contents are then analyzed.

histaminic headache *n.* See **cluster headache.**

his·ta·mi·nu·ri·a (hĭs′tə-mə-nōōr′ē-ə) *n.* The excretion of histamine in the urine.

his·ti·dase (hĭs′tĭ-dās′, -dāz′) *n.* See **histidine ammonia-lyase.**

his·ti·di·nase (hĭs′tĭ-də-nās′, -nāz′) *n.* See **histidine ammonia-lyase.**

his·ti·dine (hĭs′tĭ-dēn′, -dĭn) *n. Abbr.* **His** An amino acid that is essential for tissue growth and repair.

histidine ammonia-lyase *n.* An enzyme that catalyzes the deamination of histidine to urocanate. Also called *histidase, histidinase.*

histidine decarboxylase *n.* An enzyme that catalyzes the decarboxylation of histidine to histamine.

his·ti·di·ne·mi·a (hĭs′tĭ-də-nē′mē-ə) *n.* A hereditary disorder characterized by an elevation of histidine levels in the blood, excretion of histidine in the urine due to deficient histidase activity, and often manifested clinically by mild mental retardation.

his·ti·di·nu·ri·a (hĭs′tĭ-də-nōōr′ē-ə) *n.* The excretion of excessive histidine in the urine.

his·ti·dyl (hĭs′tĭ-dĭl′) *n.* The univalent radical, $C_6H_8N_3O_2$, of histidine.

histio– *pref.* Body tissue: *histioblast.*

his·ti·o·blast (hĭs′tē-ə-blăst′) *n.* A tissue-forming cell. Also called *histoblast.*

his·ti·o·cyte (hĭs′tē-ə-sīt′) *n.* A relatively inactive, immobile macrophage found in normal connective tissue. Also called *fixed macrophage, histocyte.* —**his′ti·o·cyt′ic** (-sĭt′ĭk) *adj.*

histiocytic medullary reticulosis *n.* A rapidly fatal lymphoma, characterized by fever, jaundice, pancytopenia, and enlargement of the liver, spleen, and lymph nodes. The affected organs show focal necrosis and hemorrhage, with proliferation of histiocytes and with phagocytosis of the red blood cells.

his·ti·o·cy·to·ma (hĭs′tē-ō-sī-tō′mə) *n.*, *pl.* **–mas** or **–ma·ta** (-mə-tə) A tumor composed of histiocytes.

his·ti·o·cy·to·sis (hĭs′tē-ō′sī-tō′sĭs) *n.*, *pl.* **–ses** (-sēz) Abnormal multiplication of histiocytes. Also called *histocytosis.*

histiocytosis X *n.* Any of a group of disorders of unknown cause characterized by histiocytic proliferation, including Hand-Schüller-Christian disease.

his·ti·o·gen·ic (hĭs′tē-ō-jĕn′ĭk) *adj.* Histogenous.

his·ti·oid (hĭs′tē-oid′) *adj.* Variant of **histoid.**

histo– *or* **hist–** *pref.* Body tissue: *histogenesis.*

his·to·blast (hĭs′tə-blăst′) *n.* See **histioblast.**

his·to·chem·is·try (hĭs′tō-kĕm′ĭ-strē) *n.* The branch of science that deals with the chemical composition of the cells and tissues of the body.

his·to·com·pat·i·bil·i·ty (hĭs′tō-kəm-păt′ə-bĭl′ĭ-tē) *n.* A state or condition in which the absence of immunologic interference permits the grafting of tissue or the transfusion of blood without rejection.

histocompatibility antigen *n.* Any of various antigens on the surface of cell membranes that serve to identify a cell as self or nonself and are used to determine whether a tissue graft or transfusion will be accepted by a recipient.

histocompatibility gene *n.* A gene that is part of the major histocompatibility complex and is responsible for the production of a histocompatibility antigen.

his·to·cyte (hĭs′tə-sīt′) *n.* See **histiocyte.**

his·to·cy·to·sis (hĭs′tō-sī-tō′sĭs) *n.* See **histiocytosis.**

his·to·dif·fer·en·ti·a·tion (hĭs′tō-dĭf′ə-rĕn′shē-ā′shən) *n.* The morphologic appearance of tissue characteristics that occur during embryonic development of the embryo.

his·to·gen·e·sis (hĭs′tō-jĕn′ĭ-sĭs) *n.* The formation and development of the tissues of the body. —**his′to·ge·net′ic** (-jə-nĕt′ĭk), **his′to·gen′ic** (-jĕn′ĭk) *adj.*

his·tog·e·nous (hĭ-stŏj′ə-nəs) *adj.* Formed by tissues; histogenetic.

his·toid (hĭs′toid′) *or* **his·ti·oid** (hĭs′tē-oid′) *adj.* Resembling the structure of one of the tissues of the body. Used of the histologic structure of a tumor.

histoid leprosy *n.* A lepromatous leprosy characterized by lesions that resemble dermatofibromas or other spindle-cell tumors.

histoid tumor *n.* A type of connective tumor that is composed of a single type of differentiated tissue.

his·to·in·com·pat·i·bil·i·ty (hĭs′tō-ĭn′kəm-păt′ə-bĭl′ĭ-tē) *n.* A state of immunologic dissimilarity sufficient to cause rejection of homograft transplants.

histologic accommodation *n.* Change in the shape of cells to meet altered physical conditions.

his·tol·o·gy (hĭ-stŏl′ə-jē) *n.* The science concerned with the minute structure of tissues and organs in relation to their function. Also called *microanatomy.* —**his′to·log′i·cal** (hĭs′tə-lŏj′ĭ-kəl), **his′to·log′ic** *adj.* —**his·tol′o·gist** *n.*

his·tol·y·sis (hĭ-stŏl′ĭ-sĭs) *n.* The breakdown and disintegration of tissue. —**his′to·lyt′ic** (hĭs′tə-lĭt′ĭk) *adj.*

his·to·ma (hĭ-stō′mə) *n., pl.* **-mas** *or* **–ma·ta** (-mə-tə) A benign tumor having cytologic and histologic elements closely similar to those of normal tissue from which the tumor cells derive.

his·to·met·a·plas·tic (hĭs′tō-mĕt′ə-plăs′tĭk) *adj.* Stimulating the transformation of tissue from one type to another.

his·tone (hĭs′tōn′) *n.* Any of several small simple proteins that are most commonly found in association with the DNA in chromatin and contain a high proportion of basic amino acids.

histone base *n.* The alpha-amino acids arginine, histidine, and lysine that are basic because of their respective side chains of guanidine, imidazole, and an amine group. Also called *hexone base.*

his·to·nu·ri·a (hĭs′tō-nŏŏr′ē-ə) *n.* The excretion of histone in the urine.

his·to·path·o·gen·e·sis (hĭs′tō-păth′ə-jĕn′ĭ-sĭs) *n.* The development of tissue in relation to disease.

his·to·pa·thol·o·gy (hĭs′tō-pə-thŏl′ə-jē, -pă-) *n.* The science concerned with the cytologic and histologic structure of abnormal or diseased tissue.

his·to·phys·i·ol·o·gy (hĭs′tō-fĭz′ē-ŏl′ə-jē) *n.* The microscopic study of tissues in relation to their physiological functions.

His·to·plas·ma cap·su·la·tum (hĭs′tə-plăz′mə kăp′sə-lā′təm) *n.* A parasitic fungus causing histoplasmosis in humans and other mammals.

his·to·plas·min (hĭs′tə-plăz′mĭn) *n.* An antigenic extract of *Histoplasma capsulatum* used in immunological tests for histoplasmosis.

his·to·plas·mo·ma (hĭs′tō-plăz-mō′mə) *n., pl.* **–mas** *or* **–ma·ta** (-mə-tə) An infectious granuloma of the lung caused by *Histoplasma capsulatum.*

his·to·plas·mo·sis (hĭs′tō-plăz-mō′sĭs) *n., pl.* **–ses** (-sēz) An infectious disease caused by the inhalation of spores of *Histoplasma capsulatum,* most often asymptomatic but occasionally producing acute pneumonia or an influenzalike illness and spreading to other organs and systems in the body. Also called *Darling's disease.*

his·tor·rhex·is (hĭs′tə-rĕk′sĭs) *n.* Breakdown of tissue by a process other than infection.

his·to·tome (hĭs′tə-tōm′) *n.* See **microtome.**

his·tot·o·my (hĭ-stŏt′ə-mē) *n.* See **microtomy.**

his·to·tox·ic (hĭs′tō-tŏk′sĭk) *adj.* Poisonous to tissues.

histotoxic anoxia *n.* Anoxia due to the inability of tissue cells to utilize oxygen.

his·to·troph·ic (hĭs′tō-trŏf′ĭk, -trō′fĭk) *adj.* Nourishing or favoring the formation of tissue.

his·to·trop·ic (hĭs′tō-trŏp′ĭk, -trō′pĭk) *adj.* Attracted to tissues. Used of certain parasites, stains, and chemical compounds.

Hitch·ings (hĭch′ĭngz), **George Herbert** 1905–1998. American biochemist. He shared a 1988 Nobel Prize for developing drugs to treat leukemia and gout.

HI test (āch′ī′) *n.* See **hemagglutination inhibition test.**

Hit·zig (hĭt′sĭk′, -sĭкн′), **(Julius) Eduard** 1838–1907. German physiologist. By using electrodes in different locations of the cortex to stimulate different muscle contractions (1870), he was able to prove the localization of cerebral function.

HIV (āch′ī-vē′) *n.* Human immunodeficiency virus; a retrovirus that causes AIDS by infecting helper T cells of the immune system. The most common serotype, HIV-1, is distributed worldwide, while HIV-2 is primarily confined to West Africa. Also called *AIDS virus, human T-cell leukemia virus type III, human T-cell lymphotrophic virus type III, lymphadenopathy-associated virus.*

hives (hīvz) *pl.n.* See **urticaria.**

Hiv·id (hĭv′ĭd) A trademark for the drug zalcitabine.

HI *abbr.* latent hyperopia

HLA *abbr.* human leukocyte antigen

HLA complex *n.* See **major histocompatibility complex.**

HLA typing (āch′ĕl-ā′) *n.* A method for determining compatibility for bone marrow transplantation using the tissue of unrelated donors and recipients.

Hm *abbr.* manifest hyperopia

HMD *abbr.* hyaline membrane disease

HMG *abbr.* human menopausal gonadotropin

HMO (āch′ĕm-ō′) *n.* A corporation that is financed by insurance premiums and has member physicians and professional staff who provide curative and preventive medicine within certain financial, geographic, and professional limits to enrolled volunteer members and their families.

hnRNA (āch′ĕn-är′ĕn-ā′) *n.* An extrachromosomal RNA molecule found in the nucleus, especially RNA transcribed from DNA rather than other RNA and the proteins produced from such RNA.

Ho The symbol for the element **holmium**.

hoarse (hôrs) *adj.* **1.** Rough or grating in sound, as of a voice. **2.** Having or characterized by a husky, grating voice.

hob·nail cell (hŏb′nāl′) *n.* A cell in a mesonephroma having a round expansion of clear cytoplasm projecting into the lumen of neoplastic tubules and a narrow, basal part containing the nucleus.

hobnail liver *n.* A nodular appearance of the liver surface due to cirrhosis.

Hodg·kin (hŏj′kĭn), Sir **Alan Lloyd** 1914–1998. British physiologist. He shared a 1963 Nobel Prize for research on the action of nerve impulses.

Hodgkin, Dorothy Mary Crowfoot 1910–1994. Egyptian-born British chemist. She won a 1964 Nobel Prize for determining the structure of compounds needed to combat pernicious anemia.

Hodgkin, Thomas 1798–1866. British physician who developed criteria for classifying the malignancy of a cancer. He was the first to describe (1832) Hodgkin's disease.

Hodg·kin's disease (hŏj′kĭnz) *n.* A malignant, progressive, sometimes fatal disease of unknown etiology that is marked by enlargement of the lymph nodes, spleen, and liver and is often accompanied by anemia and fever.

Hodg·son's disease (hŏj′sənz) *n.* Dilation of the aortic arch associated with aortic valve insufficiency.

Hof·fa's operation (hôf′əz) *n.* An operation for treating congenital dislocation of the hip, consisting of hollowing out the acetabulum and reducing the head of the femur after severing the muscles inserted into the upper portion of the bone.

Hoff·mann's sign (hôf′mənz) *n.* **1.** Severe pain in the trigeminal nerve in response to mild mechanical stimulation, characteristic of latent tetany. **2.** Flexion of the terminal phalanx of the thumb and of the second and third phalanges of the other fingers when one of the middle fingertips is flicked. Also called *digital reflex, Hoffmann's reflex.*

Hof·meis·ter's operation (hôf′mī′stərz) *n.* Partial gastrectomy with anastomosis to the jejunum.

hol– *pref.* Variant of **holo–**.

ho·lan·dric (hō-lăn′drĭk, hŏ-) *adj.* Relating to a trait encoded by a gene or genes located on the Y-chromosome and therefore occurring only in males.

holandric gene *n.* See **Y-linked gene**.

hole of retina *n.* A break in the continuity of the neural and pigmented layers of the retina that allows them to separate.

ho·lism (hō′lĭz′əm) *n.* **1.** The theory that living matter or reality is made up of organic or unified wholes that are greater than the simple sum of their parts. **2.** A holistic investigation or system of treatment. —**ho·lis′tic** (hō-lĭs′tĭk) *adj.*

holistic medicine *n.* An approach to medical care that emphasizes the study of all aspects of a person's health, including psychological, social, and economic influences on health status.

Hol·len·horst plaques (hŏl′ən-hôrst′) *pl.n.* Glittering orange-yellow atheromatous emboli in the retinal arterioles containing cholesterin crystals, indicative of cardiovascular disease.

Hol·ley (hŏl′ē), **Robert William** 1922–1993. American biochemist. He shared a 1968 Nobel Prize for the study of genetic codes.

hol·low back (hŏl′ō) *n.* See **lordosis**.

hollow bone *n.* See **pneumatic bone**.

Holmes-Adie syndrome (hōmz′-, hōlmz′-) *n.* A syndrome of unknown etiology that is characterized by tonic pupillary reactions in which tendon reflexes are absent or diminished. Also called *Adie's pupil, Adie syndrome, Holmes-Adie pupil, pupillotonic pseudostrabismus.*

hol·mi·um (hōl′mē-əm) *n. Symbol* **Ho** A soft malleable rare-earth element. Atomic number 67.

holo– *or* **hol–** *pref.* Whole; entirely: *holoblastic.*

hol·o·blas·tic (hŏl′ə-blăs′tĭk, hō′lə-) *adj.* Exhibiting cleavage in which the entire egg separates into individual blastomeres.

hol·o·cord (hŏl′ə-kôrd′, hō′lə-) *adj.* Of, relating to, or characteristic of the spinal cord throughout its length.

hol·o·crine (hŏl′ə-krĭn, -krīn′, -krēn′, hō′lə-) *adj.* Of or relating to a gland whose output consists of disintegrated secretory cells along with the secretory product itself.

holocrine gland *n.* A gland whose secretion consists of its own disintegrated secretory cells along with its secretory product.

hol·o·di·a·stol·ic (hŏl′ō-dī′ə-stŏl′ĭk, hō′lō-) *adj.* Relating to or lasting throughout the diastole portion of a heartbeat.

hol·o·en·dem·ic (hŏl′ō-ĕn-dĕm′ĭk, hō′lō-) *adj.* Endemic in the entire population of a given area.

hol·o·en·zyme (hŏl′ō-ĕn′zīm′, hō′lō-) *n.* An active, complex enzyme consisting of an apoenzyme and a coenzyme.

hol·o·gram (hŏl′ə-grăm′, hō′lə-) *n.* A three-dimensional diffraction pattern of the image of an object made using holography.

ho·log·ra·phy (hō-lŏg′rə-fē) *n.* A method of producing a three-dimensional image of an object by recording on a photographic plate or film the pattern of interference formed by a split laser beam and then illuminating the pattern either with a laser or with ordinary light.

hol·o·gyn·ic (hŏl′ō-jĭn′ĭk, -gī′nĭk, hō′lə-) *adj.* Relating to or being a trait passed only to successive generations of females.

hol·o·phyt·ic (hŏl′ō-fĭt′ĭk, hō′lō-) *adj.* Not requiring the ingestion of exogenous organic substances for nutrition; obtaining nourishment in the manner of a green plant. Used of certain protozoans capable of photosynthesis.

hol·o·pros·en·ceph·a·ly (hŏl′ō-prŏs′ĕn-sĕf′ə-lē, hō′lō-) *n.* Failure of the forebrain to divide into hemispheres or lobes causing insufficient development of facial characteristics such as the nose, lips, and palate; in severe cases, cyclopia can occur.

hol·o·ra·chis·chi·sis (hŏl'ō-rə-kĭs'kĭ-sĭs, hō'lō-) *n.* Spina bifida in which the entire spinal column is open.

hol·o·sys·tol·ic (hŏl'ō-sĭ-stŏl'ĭk, hō'lō-) *adj.* Relating to or lasting throughout the systole of a heartbeat.

hol·o·type (hŏl'ə-tīp', hō'lə-) *n.* The specimen used as the basis of the original published description of a taxonomic group and later designated as the type specimen.

hol·o·zo·ic (hŏl'ə-zō'ĭk, hō'lə-) *adj.* Obtaining nourishment by the ingestion of organic material, as animals do. Used of certain protozoans.

Hol·ter monitor (hōl'tər) *n.* A portable device used to measure the electrical activity of the heart over an extended period of time, allowing detection of intermittent arrhythmias and other electrical disturbances.

Holt·house's hernia (hōlt'hou'zĭz) *n.* An inguinal hernia with extension of the loop of the intestine along the inguinal ligament.

hom– *pref.* Variant of **homo–**.

Ho·mans' sign (hō'mănz') *n.* An indication of incipient or established thrombosis in the leg veins in which slight pain occurs at the back of the knee or calf when, with the knee bent, the ankle is slowly and gently dorsiflexed.

ho·mat·ro·pine (hō-măt'rō-pēn') *n.* An anticholinergic drug that is used in its bromide form to dilate the pupil of the eye and in combination with hydrocodone to prevent overdosage of that drug. Also called *mandelytropine*.

hom·ax·i·al (hō-măk'sē-əl) *adj.* Having all axes of equal length.

home·bound (hōm'bound') *adj.* Restricted or confined to home, as of an invalid.

homeo– *pref.* Like; similar: *homeostasis*.

ho·me·o·box gene (hō'mē-ə-bŏks') *n.* A DNA sequence in a homeotic gene that encodes for a specific sequence of amino acids in a protein.

ho·me·o·met·ric autoregulation (hō'mē-ə-mĕt'rĭk) *n.* Autoregulation of the strength of ventricular contraction by mechanisms or agents that do not depend upon change in the end diastolic fiber length.

ho·me·o·mor·phous (hō'mē-ə-môr'fəs) *adj.* Having a similar shape, but not necessarily of the same composition, as of the crystal form of unlike chemical compounds.

ho·me·op·a·thy (hō'mē-ŏp'ə-thē) *n.* A system for treating disease based on the administration of minute doses of a drug that in massive amounts produces symptoms in healthy persons similar to those of the disease. —**ho'me·o·path'ic** (-ə-păth'ĭk) *adj.* —**ho'me·o·path', ho'me·op'a·thist** *n.*

ho·me·o·pla·sia (hō'mē-ə-plā'zhə) *n.* **1.** The growth of new tissue having the same form and properties as normal tissue. **2.** The tissue formed in this manner. —**ho'me·o·plas'tic** (-plăs'tĭk) *adj.*

ho·me·o·sta·sis (hō'mē-ō-stā'sĭs) *n.* **1.** The ability or tendency of an organism or a cell to maintain internal equilibrium by adjusting its physiological processes. **2.** The processes used to maintain such bodily equilibrium. —**ho'me·o·stat'ic** (-stăt'ĭk) *adj.*

ho·me·o·ther·a·py (hō'mē-ō-thĕr'ə-pē) *or* **ho·me·o·ther·a·peu·tics** (-thĕr'ə-pyoo'tĭks) *n.* The treatment or prevention of disease using homeopathic principles. —**ho'me·o·ther'a·peu'tic** *adj.*

ho·me·o·ther·mic (hō'mē-ə-thûr'mĭk) *or* **ho·moi·o·ther·mic** (hō-moi'ə-) *adj.* Maintaining a relatively constant body temperature that is independent of the temperature of the surrounding environment.

ho·me·ot·ic gene (hō'mē-ŏt'ĭk) *n.* Any of a family of genes that results in a significant change in the embryonic development of a body part that is homologous to one usually found elsewhere.

homo– *or* **hom–** *pref.* Same; like: *homotype*.

ho·mo·bi·o·tin (hō'mə-bī'ə-tĭn) *n.* A homologue of biotin that acts as an active antagonist of biotin for some bacteria and as a replacement for biotin in certain functions for other organisms.

ho·mo·blas·tic (hō'mə-blăs'tĭk) *adj.* Relating to or developing from a single type of tissue.

ho·mo·car·no·sine (hō'mə-kär'nə-sēn') *n.* A dipeptide occurring in the human brain and formed from gamma-aminobutyric acid and histidine.

ho·mo·clad·ic anastomosis (hō'mə-klăd'ĭk) *n.* A surgical connection between branches of an artery.

ho·mo·cys·te·ine (hō'mə-sĭs'tə-ēn', -ĭn, -tē-) *n.* An amino acid that is a homologue of cysteine, is produced by the demethylation of methionine, and forms a complex with serine that metabolizes to produce cysteine and homoserine.

ho·mo·cys·tine (hō'mə-sĭs'tēn') *n.* An amino acid resulting from the oxidation of homocysteine and excreted in the urine in homocystinuria.

ho·mo·cys·ti·ne·mi·a (hō'mə-sĭs'tə-nē'mē-ə) *n.* The presence of an excess of homocystine in plasma.

ho·mo·cys·ti·nu·ri·a (hō'mə-sĭs'tə-noor'ē-ə) *n.* An inherited metabolic disorder caused by a deficiency of an enzyme important in the metabolism of homocystine and characterized by the excretion of homocystine in the urine, mental retardation, dislocation of the crystalline lens of the eye, sparse blond hair, and cardiovascular and skeletal deformities.

ho·mo·cy·to·trop·ic (hō'mō-sī'tə-trŏp'ĭk, -trō'pĭk) *adj.* Relating to or having an affinity for cells of the species in which it originated, as of an antibody.

homocytotropic antibody *n.* An antibody that has an affinity for mast cells of the same or of a closely related species and that, upon combining with a specific antigen, triggers the release of pharmacological mediators of anaphylaxis from the cells to which it attaches. Also called *reaginic antibody*.

ho·mo·ga·met·ic (hō'mō-gə-mĕt'ĭk) *adj.* Producing gametes containing only one type of sex chromosome.

ho·mog·a·my (hō-mŏg'ə-mē) *n.* Reproduction within a group that perpetuates qualities or traits that distinguish the group from a larger group of which it is part. Also called *inbreeding*.

ho·mo·ge·ne·ous (hō'mə-jē'nē-əs, -jĕn'yəs) *adj.* **1.** Of the same or similar nature or kind. **2.** Uniform in structure or composition throughout, as of a chemical mixture.

homogeneous radiation *n.* Radiation consisting of a narrow band of frequencies of the same energy or of a single type of particle.

homogeneous system *n.* A chemical system the parts of which cannot be mechanically separated and which has uniform physical properties throughout its mass or volume.

ho·mo·gen·e·sis (hō′mə-jĕn′ĭ-sĭs) *n.* Reproduction in which the offspring are similar to the parents.

ho·mo·ge·note (hō′mə-jē′nōt′) *n.* A partially diploid bacterial zygote in which the diploid region contains a specific locus where the corresponding alleles are identical.

ho·mog·e·nous (hə-mŏj′ə-nəs, hō-) *adj.* Of or exhibiting homogeny.

ho·mo·gen·tis·ic acid (hō′mō-jĕn-tĭz′ĭk) *n.* An intermediate of the metabolic breakdown of tyrosine and phenylalanine; it occurs in the urine in cases of alkaptonuria. Also called *alkapton.*

ho·mo·gen·ti·su·ri·a (hō′mō-jĕn′tĭ-sŏŏr′ē-ə) *n.* See alkaptonuria.

ho·mog·e·ny (hə-mŏj′ə-nē, hō-) *n.* Similarity of structure between organs or parts, possibly of dissimilar function, that are related by common descent.

ho·mo·graft (hō′mə-grăft′, hŏm′ə-) *n.* See allograft.

ho·moi·o·ther·mic (hō-moi′ə-thûr′mĭk) *adj.* Variant of homeothermic.

ho·mo·lat·er·al (hō′mə-lăt′ər-əl) *adj.* Ipsilateral.

ho·mol·o·gous (hə-mŏl′ə-gəs, hō-) *adj.* **1.** Corresponding or similar in position, value, structure, or function. **2.** Similar in structure and evolutionary origin, though not necessarily in function. **3.** Relating to the correspondence between an antigen and the antibody produced in response to it. **4.** Having the same morphology and linear sequence of gene loci as another chromosome. **5.** Belonging to or being a series of organic compounds each successive member of which differs from the preceding member by a constant increment, especially by an added CH_2 group.

homologous chromosome *n.* Either member of a single pair of chromosomes.

homologous graft *n.* See allograft.

homologous stimulus *n.* A stimulus acting only upon nerve terminations in a special sense organ.

homologous tumor *n.* A tumor composed of tissue of the same sort as that from which it develops.

ho·mo·logue *or* **hom·o·log** (hŏm′ə-lôg′, hō′mə-) *n.* Something homologous, as an organ or part.

ho·mol·y·sin (hō-mŏl′ĭ-sĭn) *n.* A sensitizing, hemolytic antibody formed as the result of stimulation by an antigen derived from an animal of the same species.

ho·mol·y·sis (hō-mŏl′ĭ-sĭs) *n.* **1.** Lysis of a cell by extracts of the same type of tissue. **2.** Lysis of red blood cells by homolysin and complement. **3.** Decomposition of a chemical compound into two uncharged atoms or radicals.

ho·mo·mor·phic (hō′mə-môr′fĭk, hŏm′ə-) *adj.* **1.** Of, relating to, or characterized by a similarity of form but different structure. **2.** Relating to two or more structures of similar size and form, usually of synaptic chromosomes.

ho·mon·o·mous (hō-mŏn′ə-məs, hə-) *adj.* Relating to parts having similar form and structure, and arranged in a series, such as fingers and toes.

ho·mon·y·mous (hō-mŏn′ə-məs, hə-) *adj.* **1.** Having the same name. **2.** Relating to the same sides of a field of vision.

homonymous diplopia *n.* A form of double vision in which the false image is on the same side as the affected eye, due to convergent squint or muscle paralysis. Also called *direct diplopia.*

homonymous hemianopsia *n.* Hemianopsia of the right or left halves of the visual field of both eyes. Also called *lateral hemianopsia.*

ho·mo·phil (hō′mə-fĭl′) *adj.* Relating to or characteristic of an antibody that reacts only with the antigen that caused it to be formed.

ho·mo·plas·tic (hō′mə-plăs′tĭk, hŏm′ə-) *adj.* Of, relating to, or derived from another individual of the same species, as of a tissue graft.

homoplastic graft *n.* See allograft.

ho·mo·plas·ty (hō′mə-plăs′-tē) *n.* Surgical repair using grafts from an individual of the same species.

ho·mo·pol·y·mer (hō′mə-pŏl′ə-mər) *n.* A polymer composed of identical monomeric units.

hom·or·gan·ic (hŏm′ôr-găn′ĭk, hō′môr-) *adj.* **1.** Produced by the same organ. **2.** Produced by homologous organs.

ho·mo·ser·ine (hō′mə-sĕr′ēn′) *n.* An amino acid formed in the conversion of methionine to cysteine.

ho·mo·sex·u·al (hō′mə-sĕk′shōō-əl, -mō-) *adj.* Of, relating to, or having a sexual orientation to persons of the same sex. —*n.* A homosexual person; a gay man or a lesbian.

ho·mo·sex·u·al·i·ty (hō′mə-sĕk′shōō-ăl′ĭ-tē, -mō-) *n.* **1.** Sexual orientation to persons of the same sex. **2.** Sexual activity with another of the same sex.

ho·mo·ton·ic (hō′mə-tŏn′ĭk) *adj.* Having uniform tension, as of muscular contraction.

ho·mo·top·ic (hō′mə-tŏp′ĭk) *adj.* Relating to or occurring in the same or corresponding place or part of the body.

ho·mo·type (hō′mə-tīp′, hŏm′ə-) *n.* A part or organ that has the same structure or function as another, especially to a corresponding one on the opposite side of the body. —**ho′mo·typ′ic** (-tĭp′ĭk), **ho′mo·typ′i·cal** *adj.*

homotypic cortex *n.* See isocortex.

ho·mo·va·nil·lic acid (hō′mō-və-nĭl′ĭk, hŏm′ō-) *n.* A dopamine metabolite occurring in human urine.

ho·mo·zy·gos·i·ty (hō′mō-zī-gŏs′ĭ-tē, hŏm′ō-) *n.* The condition of having identical genes at one or more loci in homologous chromosome segments.

ho·mo·zy·gote (hō′mō-zī′gōt′, -mə-, hŏm′ə-) *n.* An organism that has the same alleles at a particular gene locus on homologous chromosomes.

ho·mo·zy·gous (hō′mō-zī′gəs, -mə-, hŏm′ə-) *adj.* Having the same alleles at one or more gene loci on homologous chromosome segments.

homozygous by descent *adj.* Possessing two genes at a given locus that are descended from a single source, such as may occur in inbreeding.

ho·mun·cu·lus (hō-mŭng′kyə-ləs, hə-) *n., pl.* **-li** (-lī′) **1.** A diminutive human. **2.** A miniature, fully formed individual which adherents of the early biological theory of preformation believed to be present in the sperm cell.

hon·ey·comb lung (hŭn′ē-kōm′) *n.* The radiological and gross appearance of the lungs resulting from diffuse fibrosis and cystic dilation of bronchioles.

Hong Kong influenza (hŏng′ kŏng′) *n.* Influenza that is caused by a serotype of influenza virus type A; it was first identified in Hong Kong during the 1968 epidemic. Also called *Hong Kong flu.*

hoof-and-mouth disease *n.* See **foot-and-mouth disease.**

Hooke's law (hŏŏks) *n.* The principle that the stress applied to stretch or compress a body is proportional to the strain or to the change in length thus produced, so long as the limit of elasticity of the body is not exceeded.

hook·worm (hŏŏk′wûrm′) *n.* Any of numerous small parasitic nematodes of the family Ancylostomatidae having hooked mouthparts with which they fasten themselves to the intestinal walls of various hosts, including humans.

hookworm disease *n.* A disease resulting from infestation with hookworms and usually marked by abdominal discomfort, diarrhea, and anemia.

Hoo·ver's sign (hŏŏ′vərz) *n.* **1.** An indication of compensatory movement in legs in which a supine individual, when asked to raise one leg, involuntarily exerts counterpressure with the heel of the opposite leg even if that leg is paralyzed, or if the individual attempts to lift a paralyzed leg, counterpressure is made with the heel of the other leg. **2.** An indication of a change in the contour of the diaphragm as a result of intrathoracic conditions in which movement of the costal margins of the diaphragm changes during respiration.

Hop·kins (hŏp′kĭnz), Sir **Frederick Gowland** 1861–1947. British biochemist. He shared a 1929 Nobel Prize for discovery of growth-promoting vitamins.

hor. decub. *abbr. Latin* hora decubitus (before sleep, at bedtime)

hor·de·o·lum (hôr-dē′ə-ləm) *n., pl.* **-la** (-lə) See **sty.**

hore·hound (hôr′hound′) *n.* **1.** An aromatic Eurasian plant whose leaves yield a bitter extract that is used as a cough remedy. **2.** A candy or preparation flavored with this extract.

hor·i·zon·tal fissure of cerebellum (hôr′ĭ-zŏn′tl) *n.* A deep cleft encircling the cerebellum.

horizontal maxillary fracture *n.* A horizontal fracture occurring at the base of the upper jawbone above the apices of the teeth. Also called *LeFort I fracture.*

horizontal overlap *n.* The projection of either the upper anterior or the upper posterior teeth or both beyond their antagonists in a horizontal direction. Also called *overjet.*

horizontal plane *n.* A plane crossing the body at right angles to the coronal and sagittal planes. Also called *transverse plane.*

horizontal transmission *n.* Transmission of infection by contact.

hor·mone (hôr′mōn′) *n.* **1.** A substance, usually a peptide or steroid, produced by one tissue and conveyed by the bloodstream to another to effect physiological activity, such as growth or metabolism. **2.** A synthetic compound that acts like a hormone in the body. —**hor·mon′al** (-mō′nəl) *adj.*

hormone replacement therapy *n. Abbr.* **HRT** The therapeutic administration of estrogen and progesterone, especially to postmenopausal women, to reduce symptoms and signs of estrogen deficiency such as hot flashes and osteoporosis.

hor·mo·no·gen·e·sis (hôr-mō′nə-jĕn′ĭ-sĭs) *n.* The formation of hormones. —**hor·mo′no·gen′ic** *adj.*

hor·mo·no·poi·e·sis (hôr-mō′nə-poi-ē′sĭs) *n.* The production of hormones. —**hor·mo′no·poi·et′ic** (-ĕt′ĭk) *adj.*

horn (hôrn) *n.* **1.** One of the hard, usually permanent structures projecting from the head of certain mammals, such as cattle, consisting of a bony core covered with a sheath of keratinous material. **2.** A hard protuberance that is similar to or suggestive of a horn. **3.** The hard, smooth keratinous material forming the outer covering of animal horns. **4.** Any of the major subdivisions of the lateral ventricle in the cerebral hemisphere of the brain: the frontal horn, occipital horn, and temporal horn. Also called *cornu.*

Hor·ner's pupil (hôr′nərz) *n.* A pupil that is constricted due to impairment of the sympathetic nerve of the dilator muscle of the pupil.

Horner's syndrome *n.* A syndrome caused by a lesion in the sympathetic nervous system, especially the cervical chain or central pathways, and characterized by drooping upper eyelid, pupillary contraction, absence of sweating, and receding eyeball.

Horner's teeth *n.* Incisor teeth having a hypoplastic groove running horizontally across them.

Horner-Trantas dot *n.* Any of the small, white, calcareouslike cellular infiltrates occurring on the edge of the conjunctiva in vernal conjunctivitis.

horn·y (hôr′nē) *adj.* **1.** Made of horn or a similar substance. **2.** Tough and calloused, as of skin.

horny layer *n.* See **stratum corneum.**

ho·rop·ter (hô-rŏp′tər) *n.* The sum of all points in space whose images form at corresponding points on the plane of the retina.

hor·rip·i·la·tion (hô-rĭp′ə-lā′shən, hŏ-) *n.* The bristling of body hair, as from cold; goose bumps.

horse·rad·ish peroxidase (hôrs′răd′ĭsh) *n.* An enzyme used in immunohistochemistry to label the antigen-antibody complex.

horse·shoe fistula (hôrs′shŏŏ′, hôrsh′-) *n.* An anal fistula partially encircling the anus and opening at both ends on the cutaneous surface.

horseshoe kidney *n.* The union of the lower, or occasionally the upper, extremities of the kidneys by a tissue band extending across the vertebral column.

hor. som. *abbr. Latin* hora somni (before sleep, at bedtime)

Hor·te·ga cell (ôr-tā′gə) *n.* See **microglia.**

hos·pice (hŏs′pĭs) *n.* A program or facility that provides palliative care and attends to the emotional, spiritual, social, and financial needs of terminally ill patients at a facility or at a patient's home.

hos·pi·tal (hŏs′pĭ-tl) *n.* An institution that provides medical, surgical, or psychiatric care and treatment for the sick or the injured.

hospital formulary *n.* A compilation of pharmaceuticals and other information that reflects the current clinical judgment of a hospital's medical staff.

hos·pi·tal·ist (hŏs′pĭt-l-ĭst) *n.* A physician, usually an internist, who specializes in the care of hospitalized patients.

hos·pi·tal·i·za·tion (hŏs′pĭ-tl-ĭ-zā′shən) *n.* **1.** The act of placing a person in a hospital as a patient. **2.** The condition of being hospitalized. **3.** Insurance that fully or partially covers one's hospital expenses.

hospital record *n.* The medical record for a patient generated during a period of hospitalization, usually including written accounts of consultants' opinions as well as nurses' observations and treatments.

host (hōst) *n.* **1.** The animal or plant on which or in which a parasitic organism lives. **2.** The recipient of a transplanted tissue or organ.

hot flash (hŏt) *n.* A sudden, brief sensation of heat, often over the entire body, caused by a transient dilation of the blood vessels of the skin and experienced by some menopausal women. Also called *hot flush.*

hot spot *n.* A region in a gene in which there is a high rate of mutation. Its existence depends on the size of the region concerned, the readiness with which the mutation can be detected, and the possibility that selection against mutants at that point is less than that against mutants elsewhere.

Houns·field (hounz′fēld′), **Godfrey Newbold** 1919–2004. British engineer and inventor. He shared a 1979 Nobel Prize for development of the CAT scan x-ray technique.

hour·glass contraction (our′glăs′) *n.* Constriction of the middle portion of a hollow organ, such as the stomach or the uterus.

hourglass murmur *n.* A murmur in which there are two areas of maximum loudness, one preceding and the other following a softer midpoint. Its graph resembles an hourglass.

hourglass stomach *n.* A condition in which there is an abnormal constriction of the stomach wall dividing it into two cavities, cardiac and pyloric.

house·bound (hous′bound′) *adj.* Confined to one's home, as by illness.

house call (hous) *n.* A professional visit made to a home, especially by a physician.

house·maid's knee (hous′mādz′) *n.* Swelling and inflammation of the bursa in front of the patella just beneath the skin that is caused by trauma, such as that caused by excessive kneeling. Also called *prepatellar bursitis.*

house officer *n.* An intern or resident who is employed by a hospital to provide service to patients during the period the intern or resident is receiving training in a medical specialty.

house physician *n.* **1.** A physician, especially an intern or a resident who cares for hospitalized patients under the supervision of the surgical and medical staff of a hospital. **2.** A physician employed by a hotel or another establishment.

house staff *n.* The physicians and surgeons in specialty training at a hospital who care for patients under the direction and responsibility of attending staff.

Hous·say (ōō-sī′), **Bernardo Alberto** 1887–1971. Argentine physiologist. He shared a 1947 Nobel Prize for research on pituitary hormones.

How·ell-Jol·ly body (hou′əl-zhô-lē′) *n.* A spherical

granule often observed in the stroma of a red blood cell, especially after a splenectomy.

How·ship's lacuna (hou′shĭps) *n.* Any of the tiny depressions, pits, or irregular grooves in bone that is being resorbed by osteoclasts. Also called *resorption lacuna.*

HPI *abbr.* history of present illness

HPL *abbr.* human placental lactogen

HPV *abbr.* human papilloma virus

HR *abbr.* heart rate

HRT *abbr.* hormone replacement therapy

h.s. *abbr. Latin* hora somni (before sleep, at bedtime)

Hs The symbol for the element **hassium.**

ht *abbr.* height

Ht *abbr.* total hyperopia

HTLV (āch′tē-ĕl-vē′) *n.* Human T-cell lymphotropic virus; any of a group of lymphotropic retroviruses that have a selective affinity for certain T cells and are associated with adult T cell leukemia and lymphoma. One type, HTLV-III, causes AIDS. Also called *human T-cell leukemia virus.*

HTLV-I *n.* Human T-cell lymphotropic virus type I; a retrovirus that causes diseases similar to multiple sclerosis.

HTLV-III *n.* Human T-cell lymphotropic virus type III; HIV.

Hu·bel (hyōō′bəl), **David Hunter** Born 1926. American neurobiologist. He shared a 1981 Nobel Prize for studies on the organization and functioning of the brain, particularly with respect to vision.

Hug·gins (hŭg′ĭnz), **Charles Brenton** 1901–1997. Canadian-born American surgeon. He shared a 1966 Nobel Prize for research in hormone treatment for cancer of the prostate.

hum (hŭm) *n.* A low, continuous murmur blended of many sounds.

hu·man antihemophilic factor (hyōō′mən) *n.* A lyophilized concentrate of factor VIII that is obtained from fresh normal human plasma and used as a hemostatic agent in hemophilia. Also called *antihemophilic globulin.*

human chorionic gonadotropin *n. Abbr.* **HCG** See **chorionic gonadotropin.**

human chorionic so·ma·to·mam·mo·trop·ic hormone (sō′mə-tə-măm′ə-trŏp′ĭk, -trō′pĭk, sə-măt′ə-)*or* **human chorionic so·ma·to·mam·mo·tro·pin** (-măm′ə-trō′pĭn, -mə-mŏt′rə-pĭn) *n. Abbr.* **HCS** See **human placental lactogen.**

human diploid cell rabies vaccine *n. Abbr.* **HDRV** Rabies vaccine composed of inactive virus prepared from fixed rabies virus cultured on human diploid cells.

human gamma globulin *n.* A preparation of human plasma proteins containing antibodies of normal adults.

human genetics *n.* The study of the genetic aspects of humans as a species.

Human Genome Project *n.* An international research effort to map and identify the role of all genes in the human genome.

human growth hormone *n. Abbr.* **HGH** See **growth hormone.**

human immunodeficiency virus *n.* HIV.

human insulin *n.* A protein that has the normal structure of insulin produced by the human pancreas but that is prepared by recombinant DNA techniques and by semisynthetic processes.

human leukocyte antigen *n. Abbr.* **HLA** A gene product of the major histocompatibility complex; these antigens have been shown to have a strong influence on human allotransplantation, transfusions in refractory patients, and certain disease associations.

human menopausal gonadotropin *n. Abbr.* **HMG** An injectable preparation that is obtained from the urine of menopausal women, has biological activity similar to that of follicle-stimulating hormone, and is used with chorionic gonadotropin to induce ovulation.

human papilloma virus *n. Abbr.* **HPV** A DNA virus of the genus *Papillomavirus,* certain types of which cause cutaneous and genital warts in humans, including condyloma acuminatum. Other types are associated with severe cervical intraepithelial neoplasia and with anogenital and laryngeal carcinomas. Also called *infectious papilloma virus, infectious warts virus, verruca vulgaris virus.*

human placental lactogen *n. Abbr.* **HPL** A hormone that is isolated from human placentas, that has a biological activity that weakly mimics the activity of somatropin and prolactin, and that is secreted into maternal circulation. Also called *chorionic growth hormone-prolactin, human chorionic somatomammotropic hormone, placental growth hormone.*

human plasma protein fraction *n.* A sterile solution of selected proteins removed by fractionation from the blood plasma of adult human donors and used to augment blood volume.

human T-cell leukemia virus *n.* See **HTLV.**

human T-cell leukemia virus type III *n.* See **HIV.**

human T-cell lymphotrophic virus type III *n.* See **HIV.**

Hu·ma·trope (hōō′mə-trōp′) A trademark for the drug somatropin.

hu·mer·al (hyōō′mər-əl) *adj.* **1.** Of, relating to, or located in the region of the humerus or the shoulder. **2.** Relating to or being a body part analogous to the humerus.

hu·mer·o·ra·di·al (hyōō′mə-rō-rā′dē-əl) *adj.* Relating to or characterizing the humerus and the radius, especially the ratio of the length of one to the length of the other.

hu·mer·o·scap·u·lar (hyōō′mə-rō-skăp′yə-lər) *adj.* Relating to the humerus and the scapula.

hu·mer·o·ul·nar (hyōō′mə-rō-ŭl′nər) *adj.* Relating to the humerus and the ulna, especially the ratio of the length of one to the length of the other.

hu·mer·us (hyōō′mər-əs) *n., pl.* **–mer·i** (-mə-rī′) The long bone of the arm or forelimb, extending from the shoulder to the elbow.

hu·mid·i·ty (hyōō-mĭd′ĭ-tē) *n.* Dampness, especially of the air.

hu·mor (hyōō′mər) *n.* **1.** A body fluid, such as blood, lymph, or bile. **2.** Aqueous humor. **3.** Vitreous humor. **4.** One of the four fluids of the body, blood, phlegm, choler, and black bile, whose relative proportions were thought in ancient and medieval physiology to determine a person's disposition and general health. **5.** A person's characteristic disposition or temperament. **6.** An often temporary state of mind; a mood.

hu·mor·al (hyōō′mər-əl) *adj.* **1.** Relating to body fluids, especially serum. **2.** Relating to or arising from any of the bodily humors.

humoral immunity *n.* The component of the immune response involving the transformation of B cells into plasma cells that produce and secrete antibodies to a specific antigen.

hump·back (hŭmp′băk′) *or* **hunch·back** (hŭnch′-) *n.* See **kyphosis.**

Hu·mu·lin (hyōō′myə-lĭn) A trademark for a drug preparation of insulin.

hun·ger (hŭng′gər) *n.* **1.** A strong desire or need for food. **2.** The discomfort, weakness, or pain caused by a prolonged lack of food. **3.** A strong desire or craving, as for affection.

hunger contractions *pl.n.* Strong contractions of the stomach associated with hunger pains.

hunger pain *n.* Pain or discomfort in the epigastrium associated with hunger.

Hun·ner's ulcer (hŭn′ərz) *n.* A focal lesion involving all layers of the bladder wall in chronic interstitial cystitis.

Hun·ter (hŭn′tər), **John** 1728–1793. British surgeon who founded pathological anatomy in England.

Hun·ter's canal (hŭn′tərz) *n.* See **adductor canal.**

Hunter's syndrome *n.* A metabolic deficiency syndrome caused by a lack of certain sulfatase and by an inability to break down mucopolysaccharides and characterized by the presence of mucopolysaccharides in connective tissue. Also called *type II mucopolysaccharidosis.*

Hun·ting·ton's chorea (hŭn′tĭng-tənz) *n.* See **hereditary chorea.**

Huntington's disease *n.* See **hereditary chorea.**

Hunt's neuralgia (hŭnts) *n.* See **geniculate neuralgia.**

Hunt's syndrome *n.* **1.** A tremor beginning in one extremity and gradually increasing in intensity until it involves other parts of the body. Also called *dyssynergia cerebellaris progressiva.* **2.** Facial paralysis, otalgia, and herpes zoster resulting from viral infection of the seventh cranial nerve and geniculate ganglion. **3.** A form of juvenile paralysis associated with primary atrophy of the pallidal system.

Hur·ler's syndrome (hûr′lərz) *n.* A hereditary defect in mucopolysaccharide metabolism characterized by the excretion of dermatan sulfate and heparitin sulfate in the urine, abnormal development of skeletal cartilage and bone, corneal clouding, enlarged liver and spleen, mental retardation and sometimes deafness, and a coarsened facial surface with flattened nose and enlarged lips. Also called *dysostosis multiplex, Hurler's disease, lipochondrodystrophy, type I mucopolysaccharidosis.*

hur·loid facies (hûr′loid′) *n.* The coarse gargoylelike facial appearance characteristic of the mucopolysaccharidoses and mucolipidoses.

Hürth·le cell (hûr′tl, hürt′lə) *n.* A thyroid follicular cell that is enlarged and has acidophilic cytoplasm, especially present in adenomas.

Hürthle cell carcinoma *n.* A malignant neoplasm of the thyroid gland.

Hürthle cell tumor *n.* A benign or malignant tumor of the thyroid gland.

Hutch·in·son-Gil·ford syndrome *or* **Hutch·in·son-Gil·ford disease** (hŭch′ĭn-sən-gĭl′fərd) *n.* See **progeria.**

Hutch·in·son's crescentic notch (hŭch′ĭn-sənz) *n.* The semilunar notch on the incisal edge of the upper middle incisors in Hutchinson's teeth.

Hutchinson's facies *n.* The facial expression produced by the drooping eyelids and motionless eyes in ophthalmoplegia.

Hutchinson's freckle *n.* See **malignant lentigo.**

Hutchinson's mask *n.* A sensation often associated with tabes dorsalis in which the face feels as if it is covered with a mask or cobwebs.

Hutchinson's pupil *n.* Dilation of one pupil when the other is contracted, resulting from compression of the third nerve due to meningeal hemorrhage at the base of the brain.

Hutchinson's teeth *n.* A condition of the teeth characteristic of congenital syphilis, in which the incisal edge is notched and narrower than the neck area at the gums.

Hutchinson's triad *n.* A triad seen in congenital syphilis, consisting of parenchymatous keratitis, labyrinthine disease, and Hutchinson's teeth.

Hux·ley (hŭks′lē), **Andrew Fielding** Born 1917. British physiologist. He shared a 1963 Nobel Prize for research on nerve cells.

Huxley, Thomas Henry 1825–1895. British biologist who championed Darwin's theory of evolution. His works include *Evidence as to Man's Place in Nature* (1863) and *Science and Culture* (1881).

hx *abbr.* (medical) history

hyal– *pref.* Variant of **hyalo–.**

hy·a·lin (hī′ə-lĭn) *or* **hy·a·line** (-lĭn, -līn′) *n.* **1.** The uniform matrix of hyaline cartilage. **2.** A translucent product of some forms of tissue degeneration.

hy·a·line (hī′ə-lĭn, -līn′) *adj.* Resembling glass, as in translucence or transparency; glassy. —*n.* **1.** Something that is translucent or transparent. **2.** Variant of **hyalin.**

hyaline body *n.* A homogeneous eosinophilic inclusion body in the cytoplasm of an epithelial cell.

hyaline cartilage *n.* Semitransparent opalescent cartilage that forms most of the fetal skeleton and that consists of cells that synthesize a surrounding matrix of hyaluronic acid, collagen, and protein; in the adult, it is found in the trachea, larynx, and joint surfaces.

hyaline degeneration *n.* Any of several degenerative processes that affect various cells and tissues, resulting in the formation of rounded masses or broad bands of homogeneous acidophilic substances that have a glassy appearance. Also called *glassy degeneration, hyalinosis.*

hyaline membrane *n.* The thin, clear basement membrane between the inner fibrous layer of a hair follicle and its outer root sheath. Also called *glassy membrane.*

hyaline membrane disease *n. Abbr.* **HMD** See **respiratory distress syndrome.**

hyaline tubercle *n.* A fibrous tubercle in which the cellular fibrous tissue and collagenous material alter and merge into a fairly homogeneous, firm, acellular mass.

hy·a·lin·i·za·tion (hī′ə-lĭn′ĭ-zā′shən) *n.* The formation of hyalin. —**hy′a·lin·ized** (hī′ə-lə-nīzd′) *adj.*

hy·a·li·no·sis (hī′ə-lə-nō′sĭs) *n.* See **hyaline degeneration.**

hy·a·li·nu·ri·a (hī′ə-lə-nŏŏr′ē-ə) *n.* The excretion of hyalin or hyaline casts in the urine.

hy·a·li·tis (hī′ə-lī′tĭs) *n.* Inflammation of the vitreous humor of the eye in which the inflammatory changes extend into the avascular vitreous from adjacent structures. Also called *vitreitis.*

hyalo– *or* **hyal–** *pref.* **1.** Glass: *hyalophagia.* **2.** Glassy; hyaline: *hyaloplasm.* **3.** Hyalin: *hyalosis.*

hy·al·o·gen (hī-ăl′ə-jən) *n.* Any of various insoluble substances related to mucoids occurring in structures such as cartilage, vitreous humor, and hydatid cysts and yielding sugars on hydrolysis.

hy·a·lo·hy·pho·my·co·sis (hī′ə-lō-hī′fō-mī-kō′sĭs) *n.* An infection caused by a fungus having colorless mycelium that usually occurs as a result of indwelling catheters, steroid therapy, immunosuppressive drugs or cytotoxins, or the body's decreased resistance to postsurgical infection.

hy·a·loid (hī′ə-loid′) *adj.* Glassy or transparent in appearance; hyaline.

hyaloid artery *n.* The terminal branch of the primitive ophthalmic artery, which forms in the embryo an extensive ramification in the primary vitreous and vascular tunic around the lens and which is usually atrophied by the time of birth.

hyaloid body *n.* See **vitreous body.**

hyaloid fossa *n.* A depression on the front surface of the vitreous body in which the lens lies.

hyaloid membrane *n.* See **vitreous membrane.**

hy·a·lo·mere (hī′ə-lō-mîr′) *n.* The peripheral area of a blood platelet that remains clear after staining.

Hy·a·lom·ma (hī′ə-lŏm′ə) *n.* A genus of large ixodid ticks that parasitize domestic animals and a wide variety of wild animals and serve as vectors for a variety of pathogens in humans and animals.

hy·a·lo·pha·gia (hī′ə-lō-fā′jə) *n.* The eating or chewing of glass.

hy·a·lo·plasm (hī′ə-lō-plăz′əm) *n.* The clear, fluid portion of cytoplasm as distinguished from the granular and netlike components. Also called *ground substance.*

hy·a·lo·se·ro·si·tis (hī′ə-lō-sîr′ō-sī′tĭs) *n.* Inflammation of a serous membrane producing a fibrinous exudate that eventually becomes hyalinized, resulting in a relatively thick, glistening, white or gray-white coating.

hy·a·lo·sis (hī′ə-lō′sĭs) *n.* A degenerative change in the vitreous humor of the eye.

hy·al·o·some (hī-ăl′ə-sōm′) *n.* An oval or round structure within a cell nucleus that stains faintly but otherwise resembles a nucleolus.

hy·a·lu·ro·nate (hī′ə-lŏŏr′ə-nāt′) *n.* A salt or ester of hyaluronic acid.

hy·a·lu·ron·ic acid (hī′ə-lŏŏ-rŏn′ĭk) *n.* A mucopolysaccharide that is found in spaces around tissue, the synovial fluid of joints, and the vitreous humor of the eyes and that acts as a binding, lubricating, and protective agent.

hy·a·lu·ron·i·dase (hī′ə-lŏŏ-rŏn′ĭ-dās′, -dāz′) *n.* Any of three enzymes that catalyze the hydrolysis of hyaluronic acid, thus increasing the tissue permeability to fluids. One or more of these enzymes occur in the testes and in spermatozoa.

H-Y antigen *n.* An antigen factor, dependent on the Y-chromosome, responsible for differentiating the human embryo into the male phenotype by inducing the embryonic gonad to develop into a testis.

hy·brid·o·ma (hī′brĭ-dō′mə) *n.* A cell hybrid produced in vitro by the fusion of a lymphocyte that produces antibodies and a myeloma tumor cell. It proliferates into clones that produce a continuous supply of a specific antibody.

Hy·co·dan (hī′kə-dăn′) A trademark for the drug hydrocodone bitartrate, combined with a bromide form of homatropine to prevent overdosage.

hy·dan·to·in (hī-dăn′tō-ĭn) *n.* A crystalline substance derived from urea or allantoin.

hy·da·tid (hī′də-tĭd) *n.* **1.** A hydatid cyst. **2.** The encysted larva of *Echinococcus granulosus.* **3.** An abnormal vascular structure that is usually filled with fluid.

hydatid cyst *n.* A cyst formed as a result of infestation by larvae of the tapeworm *Echinococcus granulosus.* Also called *echinococcus cyst.*

hydatid disease *n.* An infection, usually of the liver or the lungs, with the larvae of an *Echinococcus* tapeworm, and characterized by the formation of hydatid cysts.

hydatid fremitus *n.* See **hydatid thrill.**

hy·da·tid·i·form (hī′də-tĭd′ə-fôrm′) *adj.* Having the form or appearance of a hydatid.

hydatidiform mole *n.* A vesicular or polycystic placental mass resulting from the proliferation of the trophoblast and the hydropic degeneration and avascularity of the chorionic villi, usually indicative of an abnormal pregnancy. Also called *mole.*

hy·da·tid·o·cele (hī′də-tĭd′ə-sēl′) *n.* A cystic mass formed in the scrotum and composed of one or more hydatids.

hy·da·ti·do·ma (hī′də-tĭ-dō′mə) *n., pl.* **–mas** *or* **–ma·ta** (-mə-tə) A benign neoplasm in which there is prominent formation of hydatids.

hy·da·ti·do·sis (hī′də-tĭ-dō′sĭs) *n.* The diseased state caused by the presence of hydatid cysts.

hy·da·ti·dos·to·my (hī′də-tĭ-dŏs′tə-mē) *n.* Surgical evacuation of a hydatid cyst.

hydatid thrill *n.* The trembling or vibratory sensation felt by the hand when examining a hydatid cyst. Also called *hydatid fremitus.*

hydr– *pref.* Variant of **hydro–.**

hy·dra·gogue (hī′drə-gôg′) *n.* Any of a class of cathartics that aid in the removal of edematous fluids and thus promote the discharge of watery fluid from the bowels.

hy·dral·a·zine (hī-drăl′ə-zēn′) *n.* A crystalline compound whose hydrochloride form is used in the treatment of hypertension.

hy·dram·ni·os (hī-drăm′nē-ŏs′) *n.* The presence of an excessive amount of amniotic fluid. Also called *polyhydramnios.*

hy·dran·en·ceph·a·ly (hī′drăn-ən-sĕf′ə-lē) *n.* The congenital absence of the cerebral hemispheres in which the space in the cranium that they normally occupy is filled with fluid.

hy·drar·gyr·i·a (hī′drär-jĭr′ē-ə, -jī′rē-ə) *or* **hy·drar·gy·rism** (hī-drär′jə-rĭz′əm) *n.* See **mercury poisoning.**

hy·drar·gy·rum (hī-drär′jə-rəm) *n.* See **mercury.**

hy·drar·thro·sis (hī′drär-thrō′sĭs) *n.* An effusion of serous fluid into a joint cavity. **—hy′drar·thro′di·al** (-thrō′dē-əl) *adj.*

hy·drase (hī′drās′, -drāz′) *n.* See **hydratase.**

hy·dras·tine (hī-drăs′tēn′, -tĭn) *n.* A poisonous white alkaloid obtained from the yellow root of a woodland plant and formerly used locally to treat inflammation of mucous membranes.

hy·dra·tase (hī′drə-tāz′, -tāz′) *n.* Any of various lyases that catalyze the addition or removal of water from a substrate. Also called *hydrase.*

hy·drate (hī′drāt′) *n.* A solid compound containing water molecules combined in a definite ratio as an integral part of a crystal. **—v. 1.** To rehydrate. **2.** To supply water to a person or thing in order to restore or maintain fluid balance.

hy·dra·tion (hī-drā′shən) *n.* **1.** The addition of water to a chemical molecule without hydrolysis. **2.** The process of providing an adequate amount of liquid to bodily tissues.

hy·dre·mi·a (hī-drē′mē-ə) *n.* An increase in blood volume occurring because of excessive plasma or water with or without a reduction in the concentration of blood proteins.

hy·dren·ceph·a·lo·cele (hī′drĕn-sĕf′ə-lō-sēl′) *or* **hy·dro·en·ceph·a·lo·cele** (hī′drō-ĕn-) *or* **hy·dro·ceph·a·lo·cele** (hī′drō-sĕf′-) *n.* A protrusion of a sac containing brain substance and a watery fluid through a cleft in the skull.

hy·dren·ceph·a·lo·me·nin·go·cele (hī′drĕn-sĕf′ə-lō-mə-nĭng′gə-sēl′) *n.* A protrusion of a sac containing meninges, brain substance, and spinal fluid through a cleft in the skull.

hy·dric (hī′drĭk) *adj.* Of or relating to hydrogen in a chemical grouping, as in a molecule.

hy·dride (hī′drīd′) *n.* A compound of hydrogen with another, more electropositive element or group.

hydro– *or* **hydr–** *pref.* **1.** Water; liquid: *hydrocephalus.* **2.** Hydrogen: *hydrochloride.*

hy·dro·a (hī-drō′ə) *n.* A vesicular eruption, especially of the skin.

hydroa vac·cin·i·for·me (văk-sĭn′ə-fôr′mē) *n.* A hereditary recurrent eruption of bullae as a result of exposure to the sun that primarily affects male children or young men.

hy·dro·bleph·a·ron (hī′drō-blĕf′ə-rŏn′) *n.* A fluid-filled swelling of the eyelid.

hy·dro·cal·y·co·sis (hī′drō-kăl′ĭ-kō′sĭs) *n.* A rare symptomless anomaly of the renal calix in which it is dilated as a result of an obstruction of the infundibulum; it may result in infection.

hy·dro·car·bon (hī′drə-kär′bən) *n.* An organic compound, such as benzene and methane, that contains only carbon and hydrogen.

hy·dro·cele (hī′drə-sēl′) *n.* A pathological accumulation of serous fluid in a bodily cavity, especially in the scrotal pouch.

hy·dro·ce·lec·to·my (hī′drə-sĭ-lĕk′tə-mē) *n.* Excision of a hydrocele.

hydrocele spinalis *n.* See **spina bifida.**

hy·dro·ceph·a·lo·cele (hī′drō-sĕf′ə-lō-sēl′) *n.* Variant of **hydrencephalocele.**

hy·dro·ceph·a·lus (hī′drō-sĕf′ə-ləs) *or* **hy·dro·ceph·a·ly** (-lē) *n.* A usually congenital condition in which an abnormal accumulation of fluid in the cerebral ventricles causes enlargement of the skull and compression of the brain, destroying much of the neural tissue. —**hy′-dro·ce·phal′ic** (-sə-făl′ĭk), **hy′dro·ceph′a·loid′** *adj.*

hydrocephalus ex vac·u·o (ĕks văk′yoō-ō) *n.* A hydrocephalic condition resulting from the loss or atrophy of brain tissue.

hy·dro·chlo·ric acid (hī′drə-klôr′ĭk) *n.* A clear, colorless, fuming, poisonous, highly acidic aqueous solution of hydrogen chloride, normally present in a dilute form in gastric juice, and used in a variety of laboratory processes.

hy·dro·chlo·ride (hī′drə-klôr′īd′) *n.* A compound resulting from the reaction of hydrochloric acid with an organic base.

hy·dro·chlo·ro·thi·a·zide (hī′drə-klôr′ə-thī′ə-zīd′, -zĭd) *n. Abbr.* **HCTZ** A diuretic that is used alone or in combination with other drugs primarily to treat hypertension.

hy·dro·cho·le·cys·tis (hī′drō-kō′lĭ-sĭs′tĭs) *n.* The effusion of serous fluid into the gallbladder.

hy·dro·cho·le·re·sis (hī′drō-kō′lə-rē′sĭs) *n.* The increased output of watery bile having a low specific gravity, viscosity, and solids content. —**hy′dro·cho′-le·ret′ic** (-rĕt′ĭk) *adj.*

hy·dro·cir·so·cele (hī′drō-sûr′sə-sēl′) *n.* A condition in which a hydrocele of the scrotal pouch and a variocele occur together.

hy·dro·co·done bitartrate (hī′drə-kō′dōn) *n.* A narcotic drug related to codeine, used as an analgesic and antitussive.

hy·dro·col·loid (hī′drə-kŏl′oid′) *n.* **1.** A substance that forms a gel with water. **2.** Such a substance used to take dental impressions, especially one derived from marine kelp.

hy·dro·col·po·cele (hī′drō-kŏl′pə-sēl′) *n.* The accumulation of watery fluid or mucous fluid in the vagina. Also called *hydrocolpos.*

hy·dro·cor·ti·sone (hī′drə-kôr′tĭ-sōn′, -zōn′) *n.* **1.** A steroid hormone produced by the adrenal cortex that regulates carbohydrate metabolism and maintains blood pressure. Also called *cortisol.* **2.** A preparation of this hormone obtained from natural sources or produced synthetically and used to treat inflammatory conditions and adrenal failure.

Hy·dro·cor·tone (hī′drə-kôr′tōn′) A trademark for the drug hydrocortisone.

hy·dro·cy·an·ic acid (hī′drō-sī-ăn′ĭk) *n.* An aqueous solution of hydrogen cyanide that is a poisonous weak acid. Also called *prussic acid.*

hy·dro·cyst (hī′drə-sĭst′) *n.* A cyst having clear watery contents.

hy·dro·en·ceph·a·lo·cele (hī′drō-ĕn-sĕf′ə-lō-sēl′) *n.* Variant of **hydrencephalocele.**

hy·dro·gel (hī′drə-jĕl′) *n.* A colloidal gel in which the particles are dispersed in water.

hy·dro·gen (hī′drə-jən) *n. Symbol* **H** A colorless, highly flammable gaseous element, the most abundant in the universe, used in ammonia and methanol synthesis, in the hydrogenation of organic materials, and as a reducing atmosphere. Atomic number 1.

hydrogen-1 *n.* The most abundant isotope of hydrogen, having atomic mass 1. Also called *protium.*

hydrogen-2 *n.* See **deuterium.**

hydrogen-3 *n.* See **tritium.**

hy·drog·e·nase (hī-drŏj′ə-nās′, -nāz′) *n.* An enzyme in certain microorganisms that catalyzes the formation of hydrogen.

hy·dro·gen·a·tion (hī′drə-jə-nā′shən, hī-drŏj′ə-) *n.* The addition of hydrogen to a compound, especially to solidify an unsaturated fat or fatty acid.

hydrogen bond *n.* A chemical bond in which a hydrogen atom of one molecule is attracted to an electronegative atom, especially a nitrogen, oxygen, or fluorine atom, usually of another molecule.

hydrogen bromide *n.* An irritating colorless gas used in the manufacture of barbiturates and synthetic hormones.

hydrogen chloride *n.* A colorless, fuming, corrosive, very soluble, suffocating gas that forms hydrochloric acid in solution.

hydrogen cyanide *n.* A colorless, volatile, extremely poisonous flammable liquid miscible in water and used in the manufacture of dyes and fumigants.

hydrogen donor *n.* A substance or compound that gives up or transfers a hydrogen atom to another substance.

hydrogen peroxide *n.* A colorless, heavy, strongly oxidizing liquid that is capable of reacting explosively with combustibles and is used principally in aqueous solution as a mild antiseptic, a bleaching agent, an oxidizing agent, and a laboratory reagent. Also called *hydroperoxide.*

hydrogen sulfide *n.* A colorless, flammable poisonous gas that has a characteristic rotten-egg odor, is formed in the decomposition of organic matter containing sulfur, and is used as an antiseptic, a bleach, and a reagent.

hydrogen transport *n.* The enzymatic transfer of hydrogen from a hydrogen donor to an acceptor through an oxidation-reduction reaction.

hy·dro·ki·net·ic (hī′drō-kə-nĕt′ĭk, -kī-) *or* **hy·dro·ki·net·i·cal** (-ĭ-kəl) *adj.* Of or relating to the kinetic energy and motion of fluids.

hy·dro·lase (hī′drə-lās′, -lāz′) *n.* An enzyme that catalyzes the hydrolysis of a substrate through the addition of water.

hy·dro·ly·ase (hī′drō-lī′ās′, -āz′) *n.* Any of a class of lyase enzymes that catalyze the removal of water from a molecule leading to formation of new double bonds within the affected molecule.

hy·drol·y·sate (hī-drŏl′ĭ-sāt′, hī′drə-lī′-) *or* **hy·drol·y·zate** (-zāt′) *n.* A product of hydrolysis.

hy·drol·y·sis (hī-drŏl′ĭ-sĭs) *n.* Decomposition of a chemical compound by reaction with water, such as the dissociation of a dissolved salt or the catalytic conversion of starch to glucose. —**hy′dro·lyt′ic** (-drə-lĭt′ĭk) *adj.* —**hy′dro·lyze′** (-drə-līz′) *v.*

hy·dro·ma (hī-drō′mə) *n.* See **hygroma.**

hy·dro·me·nin·go·cele (hī′drō-mə-nĭng′gə-sēl′) *n.* A fluid-filled protrusion of the meninges of the brain or spinal cord through a defect in the skull or vertebral column.

hy·drom·e·ter (hī-drŏm′ĭ-tər) *n.* An instrument used to determine specific gravity, especially a sealed graduated tube, weighted at one end, that sinks in a fluid to a depth indicating the fluid's specific gravity. Also called *gravimeter.* —**hy′dro·met′ric** (hī′drə-mĕt′-rĭk) *adj.* —**hy·drom′e·try** *n.*

hy·dro·me·tra (hī′drō-mē′trə) *n.* The accumulation of thin mucus or other watery fluid in the uterus.

hy·dro·me·tro·col·pos (hī′drō-mē′trō-kŏl′pəs) *n.* The accumulation and distention of the uterus and vagina by a fluid other than blood or pus.

hy·dro·mi·cro·ceph·a·ly (hī′drō-mī′krō-sĕf′ə-lē) *n.* Microcephaly associated with an increase in cerebrospinal fluid.

hy·dro·mor·phone hydrochloride (hī′drō-môr′fōn′) *n.* A synthetic derivative of morphine used as a respiratory sedative and analgesic that is more potent than morphine.

hy·drom·pha·lus (hī-drŏm′fə-ləs) *n.* A cystic tumor at the navel, usually a vitellointestinal cyst.

hy·dro·my·e·li·a (hī′drō-mī-ē′lē-ə) *n.* A dilation of the central canal of the spinal cord caused by an increase of fluid.

hy·dro·my·e·lo·cele (hī′drō-mī′ə-lō-sēl′) *n.* The protrusion of a saclike portion of spinal cord containing cerebrospinal fluid through a spina bifida.

hy·dro·my·o·ma (hī′drō-mī-ō′mə) *n.* A leiomyoma that contains cystlike areas of proteinaceous fluid.

hy·dro·ne·phro·sis (hī′drō-nə-frō′sĭs) *n.* The dilation of the pelvis and calices of one or both kidneys because of the accumulation of urine resulting from obstruction to urine outflow. Also called *uronephrosis.* —**hy′dro·ne·phrot′ic** (-frŏt′ĭk) *adj.*

hy·dro·per·i·car·di·tis (hī′drō-pĕr′ĭ-kär-dī′tĭs) *n.* Pericarditis accompanied by an effusion of serous fluid into the pericardial cavity.

hy·dro·per·i·car·di·um (hī′drō-pĕr′ĭ-kär′dē-əm) *n.* The noninflammatory accumulation of watery fluid in the pericardial cavity.

hy·dro·per·i·to·ne·um (hī′drō-pĕr′ĭ-tn-ē′əm) *n.* See ascites.

hy·dro·per·ox·ide (hī′drō-pə-rŏk′sīd′) *n.* See hydrogen peroxide.

hy·dro·phil·i·a (hī′drə-fĭl′ē-ə) *n.* **1.** A tendency of the blood and tissues to absorb fluid. **2.** The ability to combine with or attract water.

hy·dro·phil·ic (hī′drə-fĭl′ĭk) *adj.* Having an affinity for water; readily absorbing or dissolving in water.

hy·dro·pho·bi·a (hī′drə-fō′bē-ə) *n.* **1.** An abnormal fear of water. **2.** Rabies.

hy·dro·pho·bic (hī′drə-fō′bĭk, -fŏb′ĭk) *adj.* **1.** Repelling, tending not to combine with, or unable to dissolve in water. **2.** Of or exhibiting hydrophobia.

hy·drop·ic degeneration (hī-drŏp′ĭk) *n.* See cloudy swelling.

hy·dro·pneu·ma·to·sis (hī′drō-nōō′mə-tō′sĭs) *n.* Presence of gas and liquid in tissues.

hy·dro·pneu·mo·go·ny (hī′drō-nōō-mō′gə-nē) *n.* The injection of air into a joint to determine the amount of effusion.

hy·dro·pneu·mo·per·i·car·di·um (hī′drō-nōō′mō-pĕr′ĭ-kär′dē-əm) *n.* The accumulation of serous fluid and gas in the pericardial sac. Also called *pneumohydropericardium.*

hy·dro·pneu·mo·per·i·to·ne·um (hī′drō-nōō′mō-pĕr′ĭ-tn-ē′əm) *n.* The accumulation of serous fluid and gas in the peritoneal cavity. Also called *pneumohydroperitoneum.*

hy·dro·pneu·mo·tho·rax (hī′drō-nōō′mō-thôr′ăks′) *n.* The accumulation of fluid and gas in the pleural cavity. Also called *pneumohydrothorax.*

hy·drops (hī′drŏps′) *n.* The excessive accumulation of serous fluid in tissues or cavities of the body.

hy·dro·py·o·ne·phro·sis (hī′drō-pī′ō-nə-frō′sĭs) *n.* The accumulation of purulent urine in the pelvis and calices of the kidneys, usually the result of bacterial infection following obstruction of the ureter.

hy·dro·qui·none (hī′drō-kwĭ-nōn′, -kwĭn′ōn′) *n.* A white crystalline compound used as an antioxidant, a stabilizer, and a reagent. Also called *hydroquinol.*

hy·dror·rhe·a (hī′drə-rē′ə) *n.* A profuse watery discharge from any part of the body, such as the nose.

hydrorrhea grav·i·dar·um (grăv′ĭ-dâr′əm) *n.* The discharge of a watery fluid from the vagina during pregnancy. Also called *hindwater.*

hy·dro·sal·pinx (hī′drō-săl′pĭngks) *n.* The accumulation of serous fluid in the fallopian tube.

hy·dro·sar·co·cele (hī′drō-sär′kə-sēl′) *n.* A chronic swelling of the testis accompanied by a hydrocele.

hy·dro·sol (hī′drə-sôl′, -sŏl′) *n.* A colloid with water as the dispersing medium.

hy·dro·stat·ic (hī′drə-stăt′ĭk) *or* **hy·dro·stat·i·cal** (-ĭ-kəl) *adj.* Of or relating to fluids at rest or under pressure.

hy·dro·sy·rin·go·my·e·li·a (hī′drō-sə-rĭng′gō-mī-ē′lē-ə) *n.* See syringomyelia.

hy·dro·tax·is (hī′drə-tăk′sĭs) *n.* Movement of a cell or an organism in response to moisture.

hy·dro·ther·a·py (hī′drə-thĕr′ə-pē) *n.* External use of water in the medical treatment of certain diseases.

hy·dro·thi·o·ne·mi·a (hī′drō-thī′ə-nē′mē-ə) *n.* The presence of hydrogen sulfide in the blood.

hy·dro·thi·o·nu·ri·a (hī′drō-thī′ə-nōōr′ē-ə) *n.* The presence of hydrogen sulfide in the urine.

hy·dro·tho·rax (hī′drə-thôr′ăks′) *n.* The accumulation of serous fluid in one or both pleural cavities.

hy·drot·ro·pism (hī-drŏt′rə-pĭz′əm) *n.* Growth or movement in a sessile organism toward or away from water.

hy·dro·tu·ba·tion (hī′drō-tōō-bā′shən) *n.* The injection of liquid medication or saline solution through the cervix into the uterine cavity and fallopian tubes for therapeutic purposes.

hy·dro·u·re·ter (hī′drō-yōō-rē′tər, -yōōr′ĭ-) *n.* The distention of the ureter with urine due to blockage. Also called *uroureter.*

hy·dro·var·i·um (hī′drō-vâr′ē-əm) *n.* The accumulation of fluid in the ovary.

hy·drox·ide (hī-drŏk′sīd′) *n.* A chemical compound containing the hydroxyl group, especially one that releases a hydroxyl group when dissolved.

hydroxy– *pref.* Having, adding, or substituting a hydroxyl radical in a compound: *hydroxyapatite.*

hy·drox·y·ap·a·tite (hī-drŏk′sē-ăp′ə-tīt′) *n.* The principal bone salt that provides the compressional strength of vertebrate bone.

hy·drox·y·ky·nu·re·ni·nu·ri·a (hī-drŏk′sē-kī-nōōr′ə-nĭ-nōōr′ē-ə) *n.* An inherited abnormality in tryptophan metabolism believed to be due to a defect in kynureninase and characterized by mild mental retardation, migrainelike headaches, and urinary excretion of excessive amounts of kynurenine and xanthurenic acid.

hy·drox·yl (hī-drŏk′sĭl) *n.* The univalent radical or group OH, a characteristic component of bases, certain acids, phenols, alcohols, carboxylic and sulfonic acids, and amphoteric compounds.

hy·drox·yl·ase (hī-drŏk′sə-lās′, -lāz′) *n.* Any of various enzymes that catalyze the formation of hydroxyl groups by oxidation of the substrate.

hy·drox·y·meth·yl (hī-drŏk′sē-mĕth′əl) *n.* See **methylol.**

hy·drox·y·phen·yl·u·ri·a (hī-drŏk′sē-fĕn′ə-lŏŏr′ē-ə, -fē′nə-) *n.* The presence of tyrosine and phenylalanine in the urine as a result of a deficiency of ascorbic acid.

hy·drox·y·pro·line (hī-drŏk′sē-prō′lēn′) *n.* An amino acid produced during the hydrolysis of collagen.

hy·drox·y·pro·li·ne·mi·a (hī-drŏk′sē-prō′lĭ-nē′mē-ə) *n.* An inherited metabolic disorder characterized by high hydroxyproline concentrations in plasma and urine and severe mental retardation.

hy·drox·y·u·re·a (hī-drŏk′sē-yŏŏ-rē′ə) *n.* An antineoplastic drug that suppresses the production of blood cell precursors in the bone marrow and is used in the treatment of certain leukemias, carcinomas, and sickle cell anemia.

hy·drox·y·zine (hī-drŏk′sĭ-zēn′) *n.* A drug given in its salt forms both orally and intramuscularly, used as a sedative and antihistamine.

hy·dru·ri·a (hī-drŏŏr′ē-ə) *n.* See **polyuria.** —**hy·dru′ric** (-drŏŏr′ĭk) *adj.*

hy·giene (hī′jēn′) *n.* **1.** The science that deals with the promotion and preservation of health. Also called *hygienics.* **2.** The conditions and practices that serve to promote or preserve health, as those followed for personal hygiene. —**hy·gien′ist** (hī-jē′nĭst, hī-jĕn′ĭst) *n.*

hy·gien·ic (hī-jĕn′ĭk, -jē′nĭk) *adj.* **1.** Of or relating to hygiene. **2.** Tending to promote or preserve health. **3.** Sanitary.

hy·gien·ics (hī-jĕn′ĭks, -jē′nĭks) *n.* See **hygiene.**

hygro– *or* **hygr–** *pref.* Moisture; liquid; humidity: *hygroscopic.*

hy·gro·ma (hī-grō′mə) *n.*, *pl.* **–mas** *or* **–ma·ta** (-mə-tə) A cystic swelling containing a serous fluid. Also called *hydroma.*

hy·grom·e·try (hī-grŏm′ĭ-trē) *n.* See **psychrometry.**

hy·gro·scop·ic (hī′grə-skŏp′ĭk) *adj.* Readily absorbing moisture, as from the atmosphere.

hy·men (hī′mən) *n.* A membranous fold of tissue that partly or completely occludes the external vaginal orifice. —**hy′men·al** *adj.*

hymenal caruncle *n.* Any of the various tabs or projections surrounding the vaginal orifice after rupture of the hymen.

hy·men·ec·to·my (hī′mə-nĕk′tə-mē) *n.* Excision of the hymen.

hy·men·i·tis (hī′mə-nī′tĭs) *n.* An inflammation of the hymen.

hy·men·ol·o·gy (hī′mə-nŏl′ə-jē) *n.* The branch of anatomy and physiology that deals with the structure, function, and diseases of the membranes of the body.

hy·men·ot·o·my (hī′mə-nŏt′ə-mē) *n.* The surgical division of a hymen.

hy·o·ep·i·glot·tic (hī′ō-ĕp′ĭ-glŏt′ĭk) *or* **hy·o·ep·i·glot·tid·e·an** (-glŏ-tĭd′ē-ən) *adj.* Of or relating to the hyoid bone and the epiglottis.

hy·o·glos·sal membrane (hī′ō-glô′səl) *n.* A delicate fibrous membrane extending between the hyoid bone and the tongue.

hy·o·glos·sus (hī′ō-glŏs′əs) *n.* A muscle with origin from the hyoid bone, with insertion to the side of the tongue, with nerve supply from the hypoglossal nerve, and whose action retracts and pulls down the side of the tongue.

hy·oid (hī′oid′) *adj.* **1.** Shaped like the letter U. **2.** Of or relating to the hyoid bone. —*n.* The hyoid bone.

hyoid arch *n.* The second postoral arch in the branchial arch series.

hyoid bone *n.* A U-shaped bone at the base of the tongue that supports the muscles of the tongue.

hy·o·scine (hī′ə-sēn′) *n.* See **scopolamine.**

hy·o·scy·a·mine (hī′ə-sī′ə-mēn′) *n.* A poisonous white crystalline alkaloid isometric with atropine and having similar uses but more potent effects.

hyp– *pref.* Variant of **hypo–.**

hyp·a·cu·sis (hĭp′ə-kŏŏ′sĭs, -kyŏŏ′-, hī′pə-) *or* **hy·po·a·cu·sis** (hī′pō-ə-) *n.* A hearing impairment associated with a deficiency in the peripheral neurosensory or conductive organs of hearing.

hyp·al·bu·mi·ne·mi·a (hĭp′ăl-byŏŏ′mə-nē′mē-ə, hī′-păl-) *n.* Variant of **hypoalbuminemia.**

hyp·al·ge·sia (hĭp′ăl-jē′zhə, hī′păl-) *or* **hy·po·al·ge·sia** (hī′pō-ăl-) *n.* Diminished sensitivity to pain. —**hyp′al·ge′sic** (-zĭk) *adj.*

hyp·am·ni·os (hĭ-păm′nē-ŏs′, hī-) *n.* The presence of an abnormally small amount of amniotic fluid.

hyp·an·a·ki·ne·sis (hĭ-păn′ə-kə-nē′sĭs, -kī-, hī-) *n.* A diminution of the normal movements of the gastric or intestinal tracts.

hyper– *pref.* **1.** Over; above; beyond: *hyperflexion.* **2.** Excessive; excessively: *hyperhydration.*

hy·per·a·cid·i·ty (hī′pər-ə-sĭd′ĭ-tē) *n.* Abnormally high acidity, as of the stomach.

hy·per·ac·tive (hī′pər-ăk′tĭv) *adj.* **1.** Highly or excessively active, as a gland. **2.** Having behavior characterized by constant overactivity. **3.** Afflicted with attention deficit disorder.

hy·per·ac·tiv·i·ty (hī′pər-ăk-tĭv′ĭ-tē) *n.* A general restlessness or excess of movement, as that in children with minimal brain dysfunction or hyperkinesis.

hy·per·a·cu·sis (hī′pər-ə-kŏŏ′sĭs, -kyŏŏ′-) *n.* Abnormally acute hearing due to heightened irritability of the sensory neural mechanism.

hy·per·ad·e·no·sis (hī′pər-ăd′n-ō′sĭs) *n.* Enlargement of glands, especially of the lymph glands.

hy·per·ad·i·po·sis (hī′pər-ăd′ə-pō′sĭs) *n.* Excessive accumulation of body fat; extreme adiposis.

hy·per·a·dre·no·cor·ti·cal·ism (hī′pər-ə-drē′nō-kôr′-tĭ-kə-lĭz′əm) *n.* Excessive secretion of adrenocortical hormones, especially cortisol. Also called *hypercortisolism.*

hy·per·aes·the·sia (hī′pər-ĭs-thē′zhə) *n.* Variant of **hyperesthesia.**

hy·per·al·dos·ter·on·ism (hī′pər-ăl-dŏs′tə-rō-nĭz′əm, -ăl′dō-stēr′ə-) *n.* See **aldosteronism**.

hy·per·al·ge·sia (hī′pər-ăl-jē′zhə) *n.* Extreme sensitivity to pain. —**hy′per·al·ge′sic** (-zĭk) *adj.*

hy·per·al·i·men·ta·tion (hī′pər-ăl′ə-měn-tā′shən) *n.* The administration of nutrients by intravenous feeding, especially to individuals unable to take in food through the alimentary tract.

hy·per·am·y·la·se·mi·a (hī′pər-ăm′ə-lā-sē′mē-ə) *n.* The presence of an excess of amylase in the blood serum, as in acute pancreatitis.

hy·per·an·a·ki·ne·sia (hī′pər-ăn′ə-kə-nē′zhə, -kī-) *or* **hy·per·an·a·ki·ne·sis** (-sĭs) *n.* **1.** Excessive activity of a body part; hyperactivity. **2.** Excessive gastric or intestinal movements.

hy·per·a·phi·a (hī′pər-ā′fē-ə, -ăf′ē-ə) *n.* Extreme sensitivity to touch. —**hy′per·aph′ic** (-ăf′ĭk) *adj.*

hy·per·bar·ic (hī′pər-băr′ĭk) *adj.* Of, relating to, producing, operating, or occurring at pressures higher than normal atmospheric pressure. —**hy′per·bar′i·cal·ly** *adv.*

hyperbaric chamber *n.* A compartment capable of high-pressure oxygenation, used to treat decompression sickness and anaerobic infections.

hyperbaric oxygen *n.* Oxygen at a pressure that is above one atmosphere. Also called *high-pressure oxygen.*

hy·per·bar·ism (hī′pər-băr′ĭz′əm) *n.* Disturbances to the body resulting from the pressure of ambient gases at greater than normal atmospheric pressure.

hy·per·be·ta·lip·o·pro·tein·e·mi·a (hī′pər-bā′tə-lĭp′-ō-prō′tē-nē′mē-ə, -lī′pō-) *n.* An abnormally high concentration of beta-lipoproteins in the blood.

hy·per·bil·i·ru·bi·ne·mi·a (hī′pər-bĭl′ĭ-rōō′bə-nē′mē-ə) *n.* An abnormally high concentration of bilirubin in the blood.

hy·per·cal·ce·mi·a (hī′pər-kăl-sē′mē-ə) *n.* An abnormally high concentration of calcium in the blood.

hy·per·cal·ci·u·ri·a (hī′pər-kăl′sē-yōōr′ē-ə) *n.* The excretion of abnormally high concentrations of calcium in the urine.

hy·per·cap·ni·a (hī′pər-kăp′nē-ə) *n.* An increased concentration of carbon dioxide in the blood. Also called *hypercarbia.*

hy·per·ce·men·to·sis (hī′pər-sē′měn-tō′sĭs, -sĭ-měn′) *n.* An overgrowth of cementum on the root of a tooth possibly caused by localized trauma or inflammation, metabolic dysfunction, or developmental defects.

hy·per·chlo·re·mi·a (hī′pər-klôr-ē′mē-ə) *n.* An abnormally large amount of chloride ions in the blood. Also called *chloremia.*

hy·per·chlor·hy·dri·a (hī′pər-klôr-hī′drē-ə) *n.* The presence of an abnormal amount of hydrochloric acid in the stomach. Also called *chlorhydria.*

hy·per·cho·les·ter·ol·e·mi·a (hī′pər-kə-lěs′tər-ə-lē′mē-ə) *or* **hy·per·cho·les·ter·e·mi·a** (-tə-rē′mē-ə) *n.* **1.** An abnormally high concentration of cholesterol in the blood. **2.** A familial disorder that is characterized by an abnormally high concentration of cholesterol in the blood. Also called *familial hypercholesterolemia.*

hy·per·cho·li·a (hī′pər-kō′lē-ə) *n.* A condition in which an abnormally large amount of bile is formed in the liver.

hy·per·chro·ma·tism (hī′pər-krō′mə-tĭz′əm) *n.* **1.** Ex-

cessive formation of skin pigment. Also called *hyperchromia.* **2.** A condition in which cells or parts of cells, especially cell nuclei, stain more intensely than normal. Also called *hyperchromasia.* —**hy′′per·chro·mat′ic** (-krə-măt′ĭk) *adj.*

hy·per·chro·mic (hī′pər-krō′mĭk) *adj.* Of, relating to, or characterized by an increase in light absorption, especially of ultraviolet light. —**hy′per·chro·mic′i·ty** (-mĭs′ĭ-tē) *n.*

hyperchromic anemia *n.* Anemia characterized by an increase in the ratio of the weight of hemoglobin to the volume of the red blood cell.

hy·per·chy·li·a (hī′pər-kī′lē-ə) *n.* An excessive secretion of gastric juice.

hy·per·chy·lo·mi·cro·ne·mi·a (hī′pər-kī′lō-mī′krə-nē′mē-ə) *n.* An increase in the serum concentration of chylomicrons.

hy·per·cor·ti·sol·ism (hī′pər-kôr′tĭ-zôl-ĭz′əm) *n.* See **hyperadrenocorticalism**.

hy·per·cry·es·the·sia (hī′pər-krī′ĭs-thē′zhə) *n.* Excessive sensitivity to cold. Also called *hypercryalgesia.*

hy·per·cu·pre·mi·a (hī′pər-kōō-prē′mē-ə, -kyōō-) *n.* An abnormally high concentration of copper in the blood.

hy·per·cy·a·not·ic (hī′pər-sī′ə-nŏt′ĭk) *adj.* Characterized by extreme cyanosis.

hy·per·cy·the·mi·a (hī′pər-sī-thē′mē-ə) *n.* See **polycythemia**.

hy·per·cy·to·sis (hī′pər-sī-tō′sĭs) *n.* An abnormal increase in the number of cells in the blood or the tissues, especially of white blood cells.

hy·per·dac·ty·ly (hī′pər-dăk′tə-lē) *n.* See **polydactyly**.

hy·per·di·crot·ic (hī′pər-dī-krŏt′ĭk) *adj.* Characterized by excess dicrotism.

hy·per·e·che·ma (hī′pər-ĭ-kē′mə) *n.* The auditory magnification or exaggeration of a sound.

hy·per·em·e·sis (hī′pər-ěm′ĭ-sĭs) *n.* Excessive vomiting. —**hy′per·e·met′ic** (-ĭ-mět′ĭk) *adj.*

hyperemesis grav·i·dar·um (grăv′ĭ-dâr′əm) *n.* Severe, intractable vomiting during pregnancy, usually in the first trimester.

hy·per·e·mi·a (hī′pə-rē′mē-ə) *n.* An increase in the quantity of blood flow to a body part; engorgement. —**hy′per·e′mic** (-mĭk) *adj.*

hy·per·en·ceph·a·ly (hī′pər-ən-sěf′ə-lē) *n.* The absence or deficient development of the fetal cranial vault causing the incompletely formed brain to be exposed.

hy·per·e·o·sin·o·phil·i·a (hī′pər-ē′ə-sĭn′ə-fĭl′ē-ə) *n.* An abnormally high increase in the number of eosinophilic granulocytes in the blood or tissues.

hy·per·e·o·sin·o·phil·ic syndrome (hī′pər-ē′ə-sĭn′ə-fĭl′ĭk) *n.* A syndrome in which the concentration of eosinophils increases in peripheral blood with later infiltration into bone marrow, heart, and other organ systems, accompanied by nocturnal sweating, coughing, anorexia, weight loss, itching, skin lesions, and symptoms of Löffler's endocarditis.

hy·per·er·ga·sia (hī′pər-ûr-gā′zhə) *n.* Increased or excessive functional activity.

hy·per·er·gia (hī′pər-ûr′jə) *or* **hy·per·er·gy** (hī′pə-rûr′jē) *or* **hyp·er·gia** (hī-pûr′jə) *n.* An altered state of reactivity in which allergic response is heightened. —**hy′per·er′gic** (-jĭk) *adj.*

hy·per·e·ryth·ro·cy·the·mi·a (hī′pər-ĭ-rĭth′rō-sī-thē′-mē-ə) *n.* See **polycythemia.**

hy·per·es·o·pho·ri·a (hī′pər-ĕs′ə-fôr′ē-ə) *n.* The tendency of one eye to deviate upward and inward.

hy·per·es·the·sia *or* **hy·per·aes·the·sia** (hī′pər-ĭs-thē′-zhə) *n.* An abnormal or pathological increase in sensitivity to sensory stimuli, as of the skin to touch or the ear to sound. Also called *oxyesthesia.* —**hy′per·es·thet′-ic** (-thĕt′ĭk) *adj.*

hy·per·ex·o·pho·ri·a (hī′pər-ĕk′sə-fôr′ē-ə) *n.* The tendency of one eye to deviate upward and outward.

hy·per·ex·ten·sion (hī′pər-ĭk-stĕn′shən) *n.* Extension of a joint beyond its normal range of motion. —**hy′-per·ex·tend′** (-ĭk-stĕnd′) *v.*

hyperextension-hyperflexion injury *n.* Violence to the body causing the unsupported head to rapidly hyperextend and hyperflex the neck, as in whiplash injury.

hy·per·fer·re·mi·a (hī′pər-fə-rē′mē-ə) *n.* An abnormally high concentration of iron in the blood.

hy·per·fi·brin·o·ge·ne·mi·a (hī′pər-fī-brĭn′ə-jə-nē′-mē-ə) *n.* An increased level of fibrinogen in the blood. Also called *fibrinogenemia.*

hy·per·fi·bri·nol·y·sis (hī′pər-fī′brə-nŏl′ĭ-sĭs) *n.* Markedly increased fibrinolysis.

hy·per·flex·ion (hī′pər-flĕk′shən) *n.* Flexion of a limb or part beyond its normal range. —**hy′per·flex′** *v.*

hy·per·func·tion·al occlusion (hī′pər-fŭngk′shə-nəl) *n.* Occlusal stress of a tooth or the teeth exceeding normal physiological demands.

hy·per·gal·ac·to·sis (hī′pər-găl′ək-tō′sĭs) *n.* The excessive secretion of milk.

hy·per·gam·ma·glob·u·li·ne·mi·a (hī′pər-găm′ə-glŏb′yə-lə-nē′mē-ə) *n.* An increased concentration of gamma globulins in the plasma, such as is frequently observed in chronic infectious diseases.

hy·per·gen·e·sis (hī′pər-jĕn′ĭ-sĭs) *n.* An excessive development or redundancy of the parts or organs of the body. —**hy′per·ge·net′ic** (-jə-nĕt′ĭk) *adj.*

hy·per·gen·i·tal·ism (hī′pər-jĕn′ĭ-tl-ĭz′əm) *n.* Abnormally overdeveloped genitalia.

hy·per·geu·sia (hī′pər-gyoo′zhə, -joo′-) *n.* Abnormal acuteness of the sense of taste. Also called *gustatory hyperesthesia, oxygeusia.*

hy·per·gia (hī-pûr′jə) *n.* Variant of **hyperergia.** —**hy·per′gic** *adj.*

hy·per·glan·du·lar (hī′pər-glăn′jə-lər) *adj.* Characterized by overactivity or increased size of a gland or glands.

hy·per·glob·u·li·a (hī′pər-glŏ-byoo′lē-ə) *n.* See **polycythemia.**

hy·per·glob·u·li·ne·mi·a (hī′pər-glŏb′yə-lə-nē′mē-ə) *n.* A condition characterized by abnormally large amounts of globulins in the blood.

hy·per·gly·ce·mi·a (hī′pər-glī-sē′mē-ə) *n.* The presence of an abnormally high concentration of glucose in the blood. —**hy′per·gly·ce′mic** (-mĭk) *adj.*

hy·per·glyc·er·i·de·mi·a (hī′pər-glĭs′ə-rĭ-dē′mē-ə) *n.* A condition characterized by an elevated concentration of glycerides in the blood.

hy·per·gly·ci·ne·mi·a (hī′pər-glī′sə-nē′mē-ə) *n.* A hereditary disorder that is marked by an elevated concentration of glycine in the blood and is usually present within chylomicrons.

hyperglycinemia with hyperglycinuria *n.* A hereditary, usually fatal metabolic disorder generally appearing shortly after birth and characterized by vomiting, metabolic acidosis, ketonuria, osteoporosis, periodic thrombocytopenia, neutropenia, mental retardation, and neuropsychiatric dysfunction. Also called *glycinemia.*

hy·per·gly·ci·nu·ri·a (hī′pər-glī′sə-nŏŏr′ē-ə) *n.* An abnormally high level of glycine in the urine.

hy·per·gly·co·gen·ol·y·sis (hī′pər-glī′kə-jə-nŏl′ĭ-sĭs) *n.* Excessive glycogenolysis.

hy·per·gly·cor·rha·chi·a (hī′pər-glī′kə-rā′kē-ə, -răk′-ē-ə) *n.* The presence of excessive amounts of sugar in the cerebrospinal fluid.

hy·per·gly·co·su·ri·a (hī′pər-glī′kə-sŏŏr′ē-ə, -shŏŏr′-) *n.* The persistent excretion of abnormally large amounts of glucose in the urine.

hy·per·go·nad·ism (hī′pər-gō′năd-ĭz′əm, -gŏn′ə-dĭz′-əm) *n.* A condition marked by the enhanced secretion of gonadal hormones.

hy·per·go·nad·o·tro·pic (hī′pər-gō-năd′ə-trŏp′ĭk, -trō′pĭk) *adj.* Of or involving increased production or excretion of gonadotropic hormones.

hypergonadotropic eunuchoidism *n.* Eunuchoidism of gonadal origin, commonly accompanied by enhanced levels of pituitary gonadotropins in the blood and urine, as in Klinefelter's syndrome.

hy·per·he·mo·glo·bi·ne·mi·a (hī′pər-hē′mə-glō′bə-nē′mē-ə) *n.* A condition marked by an unusually large amount of hemoglobin in the blood.

hy·per·hi·dro·sis (hī′pər-hī-drō′sĭs, -hĭ-) *or* **hy·per·i·dro·sis** (hī′pər-ĭ-) *n.* Excessive or profuse perspiration. Also called *polyhidrosis.* —**hy′per·hi·drot′ic** (-drŏt′ĭk) *adj.*

hy·per·hy·dra·tion (hī′pər-hī-drā′shən) *n.* Excess water content of the body.

hy·per·i·cin (hī-pĕr′ĭ-sĭn) *n.* A drug, produced synthetically or as an extract of Saint John's wort, used as an antidepressant and antiviral agent.

hy·per·im·mu·no·glob·u·lin E syndrome (hī′pər-ĭm′yə-nō-glŏb′yə-lĭn, -ĭ-myoo′-) *n.* An immunodeficiency disorder characterized by high plasma levels of a particular immunoglobin, a white blood cell chemotactic defect, and recurrent staphylococcal infections at various sites including the skin and upper respiratory tract. Also called *Job's syndrome.*

hy·per·in·fec·tion (hī′pər-ĭn-fĕk′shən) *n.* Infection by very large numbers of organisms as a result of immunologic deficiency.

hy·per·in·su·lin·ism (hī′pər-ĭn′sə-lə-nĭz′əm) *n.* A condition marked by excessive secretion of insulin by the islets of Langerhans, resulting in hypoglycemia; the symptoms are similar to those of insulin shock, though more chronic in character.

hy·per·in·vo·lu·tion (hī′pər-ĭn′və-loo′shən) *n.* See **superinvolution.**

hy·per·i·so·ton·ic (hī′pər-ī′sə-tŏn′ĭk) *adj.* Having the higher osmotic pressure of two solutions.

hy·per·ka·le·mi·a (hī′pər-kā-lē′mē-ə) *n.* An abnormally high concentration of potassium ions in the blood. Also called *hyperpotassemia.*

hy·per·ka·le·mic periodic paralysis (hī′pər-kā-lē′-mĭk) *n.* An inherited form of periodic paralysis in which the serum potassium concentration is elevated during attacks. Onset occurs in infancy and condition is marked by frequent but mild attacks with myotonia often present.

hy·per·ker·a·to·sis (hī′pər-kĕr′ə-tō′sĭs) *n., pl.* **–ses** (-sēz) Hypertrophy of the cornea or the horny layer of the skin. Also called *hyperkeratinization.* —**hy′per·ker′-a·tot′ic** (-tŏt′ĭk) *adj.*

hyperkeratosis len·tic·u·lar·is per·stans (lĕn-tĭk′yə-lâr′ĭs pûr′stănz′) *n.* An inherited skin disorder with onset in midlife, marked by small keratotic papules of the tops of the feet and on the legs, with pinpoint keratotic papules of the palms and soles. Also called *Flegel's disease.*

hy·per·ke·to·ne·mi·a (hī′pər-kē′tə-nē′mē-ə) *n.* The presence of elevated concentrations of ketone bodies in the blood.

hy·per·ke·to·nu·ri·a (hī′pər-kē′tə-nŏŏr′ē-ə) *n.* An increase in the urinary excretion of ketonic compounds.

hy·per·ki·ne·mi·a (hī′pər-kə-nē′mē-ə) *n.* A condition marked by an abnormally large cardiac output.

hy·per·ki·ne·sia (hī′pər-kə-nē′zhə, -kī-) *or* **hy·per·ki·ne·sis** (-sĭs) *n.* **1.** Pathologically increased muscular movement. **2.** Hyperactivity, especially in children. —**hy′per·ki·net′ic** (-nĕt′ĭk) *adj.*

hyperkinetic syndrome *n.* A childhood or adolescent disorder characterized by excessive activity, emotional instability, significantly reduced attention span, and an absence of shyness and fear, and that occasionally develops in individuals with brain injury, mental defect, or epilepsy.

hy·per·lac·ta·tion (hī′pər-lăk-tā′shən) *n.* Continuance of lactation beyond the normal period.

hy·per·leu·ko·cy·to·sis (hī′pər-lōō′kə-sī-tō′sĭs) *n.* An unusually large increase in number and proportion of white blood cells in blood or tissues.

hy·per·li·pe·mi·a (hī′pər-lĭ-pē′mē-ə, -lī-) *n.* See **hyperlipidemia.**

hy·per·lip·i·de·mi·a (hī′pər-lĭp′ĭ-dē′mē-ə) *or* **hy·per·lip·oi·de·mi·a** (-lĭp′oi-dē′mē-ə) *n.* An excess of lipids in the blood. Also called *hyperlipemia, lipemia, lipidemia.*

hy·per·lip·o·pro·tein·e·mi·a (hī′pər-lĭp′ō-prō′tē-nē′-mē-ə, -lī′pō-) *n.* A condition marked by an abnormally high level of lipoproteins in the blood.

hy·per·li·po·sis (hī′pər-lĭ-pō′sĭs) *n.* **1.** An extreme accumulation of fat in the body. **2.** An extreme degree of fatty degeneration.

hy·per·li·thu·ri·a (hī′pər-lĭ-thŏŏr′ē-ə) *n.* An excessive excretion of uric acid in the urine.

hy·per·lu·cent lung (hī′pər-lōō′sənt) *n.* The radiographic finding that one lung is less dense than the other normal lung, as from infection or a bronchial foreign body.

hy·per·ly·si·ne·mi·a (hī′pər-lī′sə-nē′mē-ə) *n.* A hereditary disorder characterized by an abnormal increase of lysine in the blood and associated with mental retardation, convulsions, and anemia.

hy·per·ly·si·nu·ri·a (hī′pər-lī′sə-nŏŏr′ē-ə) *n.* A form of aminoaciduria characterized by abnormally high concentrations of lysine in the urine.

hy·per·mag·ne·se·mi·a (hī′pər-măg′nĭ-sē′mē-ə) *n.* An abnormally large concentration of magnesium in the blood serum.

hy·per·mas·ti·a (hī′pər-măs′tē-ə) *n.* **1.** Excessive enlargement of mammary glands. **2.** See **polymastia.**

hy·per·ma·ture cataract (hī′pər-mə-chŏŏr′, -tŏŏr′) *n.* A cataract in which the lens becomes either dehydrated and flattened or liquid and soft, with the nucleus at the bottom of the capsule.

hy·per·men·or·rhe·a (hī′pər-mĕn′ə-rē′ə) *n.* Excessively prolonged or profuse menstrual flow. Also called *menorrhagia, menostaxis.*

hy·per·me·tab·o·lism (hī′pər-mĭ-tăb′ə-lĭz′əm) *n.* An abnormal increase in metabolic rate.

hy·per·me·tri·a (hī′pər-mē′trē-ə) *n.* An ataxic muscle disorder characterized by overreaching the intended object or goal.

hy·per·me·tro·pi·a (hī′pər-mĭ-trō′pē-ə) *n.* See **hyperopia.**

hy·perm·ne·sia (hī′pərm-nē′zhə) *n.* Exceptionally exact or vivid memory, especially as associated with certain mental illnesses.

hy·per·my·o·to·ni·a (hī′pər-mī′ə-tō′nē-ə) *n.* Extreme or excessive muscular tonicity.

hy·per·my·ot·ro·phy (hī′pər-mī-ŏt′rə-fē) *n.* Hypertrophy of muscular tissue.

hy·per·na·tre·mi·a (hī′pər-nə-trē′mē-ə) *n.* An abnormally high plasma concentration of sodium ions.

hy·per·ne·o·cy·to·sis (hī′pər-nē′ō-sī-tō′sĭs) *n.* A form of hyperleukocytosis characterized by an increase in immature white blood cells in the blood.

hy·per·o·nych·i·a (hī′pə-rō-nĭk′ē-ə) *n.* Hypertrophy of the nails.

hy·per·o·pi·a (hī′pə-rō′pē-ə) *n. Abbr.* **H** An abnormal condition of the eye in which vision is better for distant objects than for near objects. It results from the eyeball being too short for light rays to properly focus on the retina, thus forming a blurred image. Also called *farsightedness, hypermetropia.* —**hy′per·ope′** (hī′pə-rōp′) *n.* —**hy′per·o′pic** (-ō′pĭk, -ŏp′ĭk) *adj.*

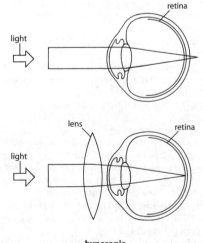

hyperopia
Top: *hyperopic vision*
Bottom: *corrected vision*

hyperopic astigmatism *n.* Astigmatism in which one meridian is hyperopic while the one at a right angle to it is without refractive error.

hy·per·o·rex·i·a (hī′pə-rō-rĕk′sē-ə) *n.* See **bulimia**.

hy·per·or·tho·cy·to·sis (hī′pər-ôr′thō-sī-tō′sĭs) *n.* Hyperleukocytosis in which percentages of the various types of white blood cells are within the normal range and immature forms are not observed.

hy·per·os·mi·a (hī′pər-ŏz′mē-ə) *n.* An exaggerated or abnormally acute sense of smell.

hy·per·os·mo·lal·i·ty (hī′pər-ŏz′mə-lăl′ĭ-tē) *n.* The abnormal increase in the osmolality of a solution, especially a body fluid.

hy·per·os·mo·lar·i·ty (hī′pər-ŏz′mə-lăr′ĭ-tē) *n.* The abnormal increase in the osmolarity of a solution, especially a body fluid, as occurs in dehydration.

hy·per·os·mot·ic (hī′pər-ŏz-mŏt′ĭk) *adj.* Of, relating to, or characterized by increased osmosis.

hy·per·os·te·oi·do·sis (hī′pər-ŏs′tē-oi-dō′sĭs) *n.* Excessive formation of osteoid.

hy·per·os·to·sis (hī′pər-ŏ-stō′sĭs) *n.*, *pl.* **-ses** (-sēz) **1.** Excessive or abnormal thickening or growth of bone tissue. **2.** See **exostosis**. —**hy′per·os·tot′ic** (hī′pər-ŏ-stŏt′ĭk) *adj.*

hyperostosis cor·ti·ca·lis de·for·mans (kôr′tĭ-kā′lĭs dē-fôr′mănz′) *n.* A hereditary disorder marked by irregular thickening of skull and bone cortex with thickening and widening of the shafts of long bones and elevated levels of serum alkaline phosphatase.

hyperostosis fron·ta·lis in·ter·na (frŭn-tā′lĭs ĭn-tûr′nə) *n.* The abnormal deposition of bone on the frontal bone of the skull; it most commonly affects women and is seen in Morgagni's syndrome.

hyperostotic spondylosis *n.* See **diffuse idiopathic skeletal hyperostosis**.

hy·per·o·var·i·an·ism (hī′pər-ō-vâr′ē-ə-nĭz′əm) *n.* A condition of sexual precocity in girls due to premature development of the ovaries accompanied by the secretion of ovarian hormones.

hy·per·ox·al·u·ri·a (hī′pər-ŏk′sə-lŏŏr′ē-ə) *n.* The presence of an unusually large amount of oxalic acid or oxalates in the urine.

hy·per·ox·i·a (hī′pər-ŏk′sē-ə) *n.* **1.** An excess of oxygen in tissues and organs. **2.** A higher than normal oxygen tension, such as that produced by breathing air or oxygen at greater than atmospheric pressures.

hy·per·par·a·sit·ism (hī′pər-păr′ə-sī-tĭz′əm, -sī-) *n.* A condition in which a secondary parasite develops within a previously existing parasite.

hy·per·par·a·thy·roid·ism (hī′pər-păr′ə-thī′roi-dĭz′-əm) *n.* An increase in the secretory activity of the parathyroid glands, causing generalized osteitis fibrosa cystica, elevated serum calcium, decreased serum phosphorus, and increased excretion of both calcium and phosphorus.

hy·per·pep·sin·i·a (hī′pər-pĕp-sĭn′ē-ə) *n.* The presence of excess pepsin in gastric juice.

hy·per·per·i·stal·sis (hī′pər-pĕr′ĭ-stôl′sĭs, -stăl′-) *n.* A condition marked by excessive rapidity of the passage of food through the stomach and intestine.

hy·per·pha·gia (hī′pər-fā′jə) *n.* Abnormally increased appetite for and consumption of food, thought to be associated with a lesion or injury in the hypothalamus.

hy·per·pha·lan·gism (hī′pər-fə-lăn′jĭz′əm, -fā-) *n.* The presence of a supernumerary phalanx or phalanges in a digit. Also called *polyphalangism*.

hy·per·phen·yl·al·a·ni·ne·mi·a (hī′pər-fĕn′əl-ăl′ə-nə-nē′mē-ə, -fē′nəl-) *n.* Abnormally high blood levels of phenylalanine, possibly associated with elevated tyrosine levels, seen especially in newborns.

hy·per·pho·ne·sis (hī′pər-fō-nē′sĭs) *n.* A noticeable increase in the perceived sound in auscultation or percussion.

hy·per·pho·ri·a (hī′pər-fôr′ē-ə) *n.* A tendency of the visual axis of one eye to deviate upward.

hy·per·phos·pha·ta·se·mi·a (hī′pər-fŏs′fə-tə-sē′mē-ə) *n.* An abnormally high concentration of alkaline phosphatase in the blood.

hy·per·phos·pha·te·mi·a (hī′pər-fŏs′fə-tē′mē-ə) *n.* An abnormally high concentration of phosphates in the blood.

hy·per·phos·pha·tu·ri·a (hī′pər-fŏs′fə-tŏŏr′ē-ə) *n.* An increased excretion of phosphates in the urine.

hy·per·pig·men·ta·tion (hī′pər-pĭg′mən-tā′shən) *n.* Excessive pigmentation, especially of the skin.

hy·per·pi·tu·i·ta·rism (hī′pər-pĭ-tŏŏ′ĭ-tə-rĭz′əm) *n.* **1.** Pathologically excessive production of anterior pituitary hormones, especially somatotropin. **2.** The condition resulting from an excess of pituitary hormones, such as gigantism in children and acromegaly in adults. —**hy′per·pi·tu′i·tar′y** (-tĕr′ē) *adj.*

hy·per·pla·sia (hī′pər-plā′zhə) *n.* An abnormal increase in cells in a tissue or organ, excluding tumor formation, whereby the bulk of the tissue or organ is increased. —**hy′per·plas′tic** (-plăs′tĭk) *adj.*

hyperplastic gingivitis *n.* Gingivitis that persists for a long period and is characterized by the proliferation of fibrous connective tissue causing enlarged firm gums. Also called *proliferative gingivitis*.

hyperplastic polyp *n.* A benign small sessile polyp of the large bowel with lengthening and cystic dilation of mucosal glands. Also called *metaplastic polyp*.

hy·per·ploid (hī′pər-ploid′) *adj.* Having a chromosome number that is greater than but is not an exact multiple of the normal euploid number. —*n.* An organism having a hyperploid chromosome number. —**hy′per·ploi′dy** *n.*

hy·perp·ne·a (hī′pərp-nē′ə, hī′pər-nē′ə) *n.* Abnormally deep and rapid breathing. —**hy′perp·ne′ic** (-ĭk) *adj.*

hy·per·po·lar·ize (hī′pər-pō′lə-rīz′) *v.* To cause an increase in polarity, as across a cell membrane. —**hy′per·po′lar·i·za′tion** (-pō′lər-ĭ-zā′shən) *n.*

hy·per·po·ne·sis (hī′pər-pō-nē′sĭs) *n.* Exaggerated activity in the motor portion of the nervous system.

hy·per·po·tas·se·mi·a (hī′pər-pə-tă-sē′mē-ə) *n.* See **hyperkalemia**.

hy·per·prax·i·a (hī′pər-prăk′sē-ə) *n.* Excessive activity; restlessness.

hy·per·pre·be·ta·lip·o·pro·tein·e·mi·a (hī′pər-prē′-bā′tə-lĭp′ō-prō′tē-nē′mē-ə) *n.* Increased concentrations of very low-density lipoproteins in the blood.

hy·per·pro·in·su·li·ne·mi·a (hī′pər-prō-ĭn′sə-lə-nē′-mē-ə) *n.* Elevated levels of proinsulin or proinsulinlike material in the blood.

hy·per·pro·lac·ti·ne·mi·a (hī′pər-prō-lăk′tə-nē′mē-ə) *n.* An elevated level of prolactin in the blood.

hy·per·pro·li·ne·mi·a (hī′pər-prō′lə-nē′mē-ə) *n.* A hereditary metabolic disorder characterized by elevated proline concentrations in the blood and by urinary excretion of proline, hydroxyproline, and glycine.

hy·per·pro·tein·e·mi·a (hī′pər-prō′tē-nē′mē-ə, -tē-ə-nē′-) *n.* An abnormally high concentration of protein in the blood.

hy·per·pro·te·o·sis (hī′pər-prō′tē-ō′sĭs) *n.* A condition due to excessive protein in the diet.

hy·per·py·rex·i·a (hī′pər-pī-rěk′sē-ə) *n.* Abnormally high fever. —**hy′per·py·rex′i·al, hy′per·py·ret′ic** (-rět′ĭk) *adj.*

hy·per·re·ac·tive malarious splenomegaly (hī′pər-rē-ăk′tĭv) *n.* A syndrome marked by persistent splenomegaly, exceptionally high levels of malaria antibody, and hepatic sinusoidal lymphocytosis, possibly caused by a disturbance in T cell control of the humoral response to recurrent malaria. Also called *tropical splenomegaly syndrome.*

hy·per·re·flex·i·a (hī′pər-rĭ-flěk′sē-ə) *n.* An exaggerated response of the deep tendon reflexes, usually resulting from injury to the central nervous system or metabolic disease. Also called *autonomic dysreflexia.*

hy·per·res·o·nance (hī′pər-rěz′ə-nəns) *n.* Greater than normal resonance, often of a lower pitch, on percussion of the body.

hy·per·sal·i·va·tion (hī′pər-săl′ə-vā′shən) *n.* See **ptyalism.**

hy·per·sar·co·si·ne·mi·a (hī′pər-sär′kə-sə-nē′mē-ə) *n.* See **sarcosinemia.**

hy·per·se·cre·to·ry (hī′pər-sĭ-krē′tə-rē) *adj.* Of or relating to excessive production of a bodily secretion. —**hy′per·se·crete′** *v.* —**hy′per·se·cre′tion** *n.*

hy·per·sen·si·tive (hī′pər-sěn′sĭ-tĭv) *adj.* Responding excessively to the stimulus of a foreign agent, such as an allergen; abnormally sensitive. —**hy′per·sen′si·tive·ness, hy′per·sen′si·tiv′i·ty** (-tĭv′ĭ-tē) *n.*

hy·per·sen·si·ti·za·tion (hī′pər-sěn′sĭ-tĭ-zā′shən) *n.* The act of inducing hypersensitiveness.

hy·per·som·ni·a (hī′pər-sŏm′nē-ə) *n.* A condition in which one sleeps for an excessively long time but is normal in the waking intervals.

hy·per·splen·ism (hī′pər-splěn′ĭz′əm, -splē′nĭz′əm) *n.* A condition in which the hemolytic action of the spleen is greatly increased.

hy·per·sthe·ni·a (hī′pər-sthē′nē-ə) *n.* An excess of muscular tension or muscular strength. —**hy′per·sthen′ic** (-sthěn′ĭk) *adj.*

hy·per·sthe·nu·ri·a (hī′pər-sthē-no͝or′ē-ə) *n.* Excretion of urine of unusually high specific gravity and concentration of solutes, resulting usually from loss or deprivation of water.

hy·per·tel·o·rism (hī′pər-těl′ə-rĭz′əm) *n.* Abnormal distance between two paired organs.

hy·per·ten·sion (hī′pər-těn′shən) *n.* **1.** Persistent high blood pressure. **2.** Arterial disease in which chronic high blood pressure is the primary symptom.

hy·per·ten·sive (hī′pər-těn′sĭv) *adj.* **1.** Of or characterized by abnormally increased blood pressure. **2.** Causing an increase in blood pressure. —*n.* A person having or susceptible to high blood pressure.

hypertensive arteriopathy *n.* Arterial degeneration resulting from hypertension.

hypertensive arteriosclerosis *n.* A progressive increase in the muscle and elastic tissue of the arterial walls resulting from hypertension.

hypertensive retinopathy *n.* A retinal condition that occurs in accelerated hypertension and that is characterized by arteriolar constriction, flame-shaped hemorrhages, cotton-wool patches, progressive severity of star-shaped edematous spot at the macula, and papilledema.

hy·per·ten·sor (hī′pər-těn′sər, -sôr′) *n.* An agent or drug that raises blood pressure.

hy·per·the·co·sis (hī′pər-thē-kō′sĭs) *n.* Diffuse hyperplasia of the epithelioid cells of the corpus luteum.

hy·per·the·li·a (hī′pər-thē′lē-ə, -thēl′yə) *n.* See **polythelia.**

hy·per·ther·mal·ge·sia (hī′pər-thûr′məl-jē′zhə) *n.* Extreme sensitivity to heat.

hy·per·ther·mi·a (hī′pər-thûr′mē-ə) *n.* Abnormally high body temperature, usually resulting from infection, medication, or head injury, and sometimes brought about intentionally to treat diseases, especially certain cancers. —**hy′per·ther′mal** *adj.*

hy·per·throm·bi·ne·mi·a (hī′pər-thrŏm′bə-nē′mē-ə) *n.* An abnormal increase of thrombin in the blood, frequently leading to intravascular coagulation.

hy·per·thy·mism (hī′pər-thī′mĭz′əm) *n.* Excessive activity of the thymus gland. —**hy′per·thy′mic** *adj.*

hy·per·thy·roid·ism (hī′pər-thī′roi-dĭz′əm) *n.* **1.** Pathologically excessive production of thyroid hormones. **2.** The condition resulting from excessive activity of the thyroid gland, characterized by increased basal metabolism. —**hy′per·thy′roid** *adj.*

hy·per·thy·rox·i·ne·mi·a (hī′pər-thī-rŏk′sə-nē′mē-ə) *n.* An elevated concentration of thyroxine in the blood.

hy·per·to·ni·a (hī′pər-tō′nē-ə) *n.* Extreme tension of the muscles or arteries.

hy·per·ton·ic (hī′pər-tŏn′ĭk) *adj.* **1.** Having extreme muscular or arterial tension; spastic. **2.** Having the higher osmotic pressure of two solutions. —**hy′per·to·nic′i·ty** (-tə-nĭs′ĭ-tē, -tō-) *n.*

hy·per·tri·cho·sis (hī′pər-trĭ-kō′sĭs) *n.* Growth of hair in excess of the normal.

hy·per·tri·glyc·er·i·de·mi·a (hī′pər-trī-glĭs′ər-ĭ-dē′-mē-ə) *n.* An elevated triglyceride concentration in the blood.

hypertrophic arthritis *n.* See **osteoarthritis.**

hypertrophic gastritis *n.* See **Ménétrièr's disease.**

hypertrophic hypersecretory gastropathy *n.* Nodular thickenings of the gastric mucosa with acid hypersecretion and frequently with peptic ulceration that is not associated with a gastrin-secreting tumor.

hypertrophic pulmonary osteoarthropathy *n.* Expansion of the distal ends or entire shafts of the long bones, which is sometimes associated with erosion of the articular cartilages, thickening and villous proliferation of the synovial membranes, and often with finger clubbing. Also called *Bamberger-Marie disease, Marie's disease.*

hypertrophic pyloric stenosis *n.* Muscular hypertrophy of the pyloric sphincter associated with projectile vomiting appearing two to three weeks after birth. Also called *congenital pyloric stenosis.*

hypertrophic rhinitis *n.* Chronic rhinitis with permanent thickening of the mucous membrane.

hy·per·tro·phy (hī-pûr′trə-fē) *n.* A nontumorous enlargement of an organ or a tissue as a result of an increase in the size rather than the number of constituent cells. —*v.* To grow or cause to grow abnormally large. —**hy′per·tro′phic** (-trō′fĭk, -trŏf′ĭk) *adj.*

hy·per·tro·pi·a (hī′pər-trō′pē-ə) *n.* Upward deviation of the visual axis of one eye.

hy·per·u·ri·ce·mi·a (hī′pər-yŏŏr′ĭ-sē′mē-ə) *n.* An unusually high concentration of uric acid in the blood. —**hy′per·u′ri·ce′mic** *adj.*

hy·per·val·i·ne·mi·a (hī′pər-văl′ə-nē′mē-ə, -vā′lə-) *n.* An abnormally high concentration of valine in the blood, as in maple syrup urine disease.

hy·per·vas·cu·lar (hī′pər-văs′kyə-lər) *adj.* Containing an excessive number of blood vessels.

hy·per·ven·ti·la·tion (hī′pər-věn′tl-ā′shən) *n.* Abnormally fast or deep respiration resulting in the loss of carbon dioxide from the blood, thereby causing a decrease in blood pressure and sometimes fainting. —**hy′per·ven′ti·late′** *v.*

hyperventilation tetany *n.* Tetany caused by forced breathing due to a reduction in the carbon dioxide in the blood.

hy·per·vi·ta·min·o·sis (hī′pər-vī′tə-mə-nō′sĭs) *n.* Any of various abnormal conditions in which the physiological effect of a vitamin is produced to a pathological degree by excessive intake of the vitamin.

hy·per·vo·le·mi·a (hī′pər-vŏ-lē′mē-ə) *n.* An abnormally increased volume of blood. —**hy′per·vo·le′mic** *adj.*

hy·pes·the·sia (hī′pĭs-thē′zhə) *n.* Variant of **hypoesthesia**.

hy·pha (hī′fə) *n., pl.* **–phae** (-fē) A long, slender, usually branched filament of fungal mycelium.

hyp·he·do·ni·a (hĭp′hĭ-dō′nē-ə, hĭp′-) *n.* An abnormal lessening of the capacity to experience pleasure.

hy·phe·ma (hī-fē′mə) *n.* Hemorrhage into the anterior chamber of the eye.

hy·phe·mi·a (hī-fē′mē-ə) *n.* **1.** Hyphema. **2.** See **oligemia**.

hyp·hi·dro·sis (hĭp′hī-drō′sĭs, hĭp′-) *n.* Variant of **hypohidrosis**.

hyp·na·gog·ic *or* **hyp·no·gog·ic** (hĭp′nə-gŏj′ĭk, -gō′jĭk) *adj.* **1.** Inducing sleep; soporific. **2.** Of or relating to the state of drowsiness preceding sleep. **3.** Relating to the images or hallucinations sometimes perceived during this state.

hyp·na·gogue (hĭp′nə-gôg′) *n.* A drug or an agent that induces sleep.

hyp·nap·a·gog·ic (hĭp-năp′ə-gŏj′ĭk, -gō′jĭk) *adj.* **1.** Causing wakefulness; preventing sleep. **2.** Of or relating to a state similar to the hypnagogic through which the mind passes while coming out of sleep.

3. Relating to the images or hallucinations sometimes perceived during this state.

hyp·nes·the·sia (hĭp′nĭs-thē′zhə) *n.* See **drowsiness**.

hypno– *or* **hypn–** *pref.* **1.** Sleep: *hypnolepsy.* **2.** Hypnosis: *hypnoanalysis.*

hyp·no·a·nal·y·sis (hĭp′nō-ə-năl′ĭ-sĭs) *n.* The use of hypnosis and psychoanalytic techniques.

hyp·no·gen·e·sis (hĭp′nō-jĕn′ĭ-sĭs) *n.* The process of inducing or entering sleep or a hypnotic state. —**hyp′no·gen′ic** *adj.*

hypnogenic spot *n.* A pressure-sensitive point on the body of certain susceptible persons that when pressed causes the induction of sleep.

hyp·noid (hĭp′noid′) *or* **hyp·noi·dal** (hĭp-noid′l) *adj.* Of or resembling hypnosis or sleep.

hyp·no·lep·sy (hĭp′nə-lĕp′sē) *n.* See **narcolepsy**.

hyp·no·pho·bi·a (hĭp′nə-fō′bē-ə) *n.* An abnormal fear of falling asleep. —**hyp′no·pho′bic** *adj.*

hyp·no·pom·pic (hĭp′nə-pŏm′pĭk) *adj.* Of or relating to the partially conscious state that precedes complete awakening from sleep.

hyp·no·sis (hĭp-nō′sĭs) *n., pl.* **–ses** (-sēz) **1.** A trancelike state resembling somnambulism, usually induced by another person, in which the subject may experience forgotten or suppressed memories, hallucinations, and heightened suggestibility. **2.** A sleeplike state or condition. **3.** Hypnotism.

hyp·no·ther·a·py (hĭp′nō-thĕr′ə-pē) *n.* **1.** Therapy using hypnosis, especially for chronic pain. **2.** Treatment of disease by inducing prolonged sleep.

hyp·not·ic (hĭp-nŏt′ĭk) *adj.* **1.** Of or relating to hypnotism or hypnosis. **2.** Inducing or tending to induce sleep; soporific. —*n.* An agent that causes sleep.

hyp·no·tism (hĭp′nə-tĭz′əm) *n.* **1.** The theory or practice of inducing hypnosis. **2.** The act of inducing hypnosis. —**hyp′no·tist** *n.*

hyp·no·tize (hĭp′nə-tīz′) *v.* To put a person into a state of hypnosis. —**hyp′no·tiz′a·ble** *adj.* —**hyp′no·ti·za′tion** (-tĭ-zā′shən) *n.*

hy·po (hī′pō) *n.* **1.** A hypodermic syringe. **2.** A hypodermic injection.

hypo– *or* **hyp–** *pref.* **1.** Below; beneath; under: *hypochondriac.* **2.** Less than normal; deficient: *hypofunction.* **3.** In the lowest state of oxidation: *hypoxanthine.*

hy·po·a·cid·i·ty (hī′pō-ə-sĭd′ĭ-tē) *n.* A lower than normal degree of acidity.

hy·po·a·cu·sis (hī′pō-ə-kōō′sĭs, -kyōō′-) *n.* Variant of **hypacusis**.

hy·po·ad·re·nal·ism (hī′pō-ə-drē′nə-lĭz′əm, -drĕn′ə-) *n.* Reduced adrenocortical function.

hy·po·al·bu·mi·ne·mi·a (hī′pō-ăl-byōō′mə-nē′mē-ə) *or* **hyp·al·bu·mi·ne·mi·a** (hĭp′ăl-, hī′păl-) *n.* An abnormally low level of albumin in the blood.

hy·po·al·dos·ter·o·nu·ri·a (hī′pō-ăl-dŏs′tər-ə-nŏŏr′-ē-ə) *n.* Abnormally low levels of aldosterone in the urine.

hy·po·al·ge·sia (hī′pō-ăl-jē′zhə) *n.* Variant of **hypalgesia**.

hy·po·al·i·men·ta·tion (hī′pō-ăl′ə-mĕn-tā′shən) *n.* A condition of insufficient nourishment.

hy·po·al·ler·gen·ic (hī′pō-ăl′ər-jĕn′ĭk) *adj.* Having a decreased tendency to provoke an allergic reaction.

hy·po·az·o·tu·ri·a (hī′pō-ăz′ə-tŏor′ē-ə) *n.* The excretion of abnormally small quantities of nonprotein nitrogenous material, especially urea, in the urine.

hy·po·bar·ic (hī′pə-băr′ĭk) *adj.* **1.** Relating to ambient gas pressures below one atmosphere. **2.** Less dense than diluent or medium. Used of solutions.

hy·po·bar·ism (hī′pə-băr′ĭz′əm) *n.* Dysbarism resulting from greater gas pressure within the body than in the surrounding medium, so that gas in body cavities tends to expand and gases dissolved in body fluids tend to come out of solution as bubbles.

hy·po·ba·rop·a·thy (hī′pō-bə-rŏp′ə-thē) *n.* Sickness produced by reduced barometric pressure.

hy·po·be·ta·lip·o·pro·tein·e·mi·a (hī′pō-bā′tə-lĭp′ō-prō′tē-nē′mē-ə, -lī′pō-) *n.* Abnormally low levels of beta-lipoproteins in the plasma.

hy·po·blast (hī′pə-blăst′) *n.* See **endoderm.** —**hy′po·blas′tic** *adj.*

hy·po·cal·ce·mi·a (hī′pō-kăl-sē′mē-ə) *n.* Abnormally low levels of calcium in blood. —**hy′po·cal·ce′mic** *adj.*

hy·po·cal·ci·fi·ca·tion (hī′pō-kăl′sə-fĭ-kā′shən) *n.* Deficient calcification of bone or teeth.

hy·po·cap·ni·a (hī′pō-kăp′nē-ə) *n.* The presence of abnormally low levels of carbon dioxide in blood. Also called *hypocarbia.*

hy·po·chlo·re·mi·a (hī′pō-klôr-ē′mē-ə) *n.* An abnormally low concentration of chloride ions in the blood. —**hy′po·chlo·re′mic** *adj.*

hy·po·chlor·hy·dri·a (hī′pō-klôr-hī′drē-ə) *n.* An abnormally low level of hydrochloric acid in the stomach.

hy·po·chlo·rite (hī′pə-klôr′īt′) *n.* A salt or ester of hypochlorous acid.

hy·po·chlo·rous acid (hī′pə-klôr′əs) *n.* A weak but strongly oxidizing acid produced by the reaction of chlorine and water and used as a bleaching agent, disinfectant, and chlorinating agent.

hy·po·chlor·u·ri·a (hī′pō-klôr-yŏor′ē-ə) *n.* The excretion of abnormally small quantities of chloride ions in the urine.

hy·po·cho·les·ter·ol·e·mi·a (hī′pō-kə-lĕs′tər-ə-lē′mē-ə) *n.* Abnormally low levels of cholesterol in the blood.

hy·po·chon·dri·a (hī′pə-kŏn′drē-ə) *n.* The conviction that one is or is likely to become ill, often accompanied by physical symptoms, when illness is neither present nor likely. Also called *hypochondriasis.*

hy·po·chon·dri·ac (hī′pə-kŏn′drē-ăk′) *n.* A person afflicted with hypochondria. —*adj.* **1.** Relating to or afflicted with hypochondria. **2.** Relating to or located in the left or right hypochondrium. —**hy′po·chon·dri′a·cal** (-kŏn-drī′ə-kəl) *adj.*

hypochondriacal melancholia *n.* Melancholia accompanied by many physical complaints, most of which have little or no basis in fact.

hy·po·chon·dri·a·sis (hī′pə-kən-drī′ə-sĭs) *n., pl.* **–ses** (-sēz′) See **hypochondria.**

hy·po·chon·dri·um (hī′pə-kŏn′drē-əm) *n., pl.* **–dri·a** (-drē-ə) The upper lateral region of the abdomen on either side of the epigastrium and below the lower ribs.

hy·po·chon·dro·pla·sia (hī′pō-kŏn′drō-plā′zhə) *n.* Congenital dwarfism that is similar to but is milder than achondroplasia, is not familial, and is not evident until midchildhood, in which the skull and facial features remain normal.

hy·po·chro·ma·sia (hī′pō-krō-mā′zhə) *n.* See **hypochromia.**

hy·po·chro·mat·ic (hī′pō-krō-măt′ĭk) *adj.* Containing a small or abnormally low amount of pigment.

hy·po·chro·ma·tism (hī′pō-krō′mə-tĭz′əm) *n.* **1.** The condition or state of being hypochromatic. **2.** See **hypochromia.**

hy·po·chro·mi·a (hī′pō-krō′mē-ə) *n.* An anemic condition in which the percentage of hemoglobin in red blood cells is abnormally low. Also called *hypochromasia, hypochromatism.* —**hy′po·chro′mic** *adj.*

hypochromic anemia *n.* Anemia characterized by a decrease in the ratio of the weight of hemoglobin to the volume of the red blood cell.

hy·po·chy·li·a (hī′pō-kī′lē-ə) *n.* Deficiency of gastric juice.

hy·po·com·ple·men·te·mi·a (hī′pō-kŏm′plə-mən-tē′mē-ə) *n.* A hereditary or acquired condition in which a component of blood complement is lacking or is reduced.

hy·po·cor·ti·coid·ism (hī′pō-kôr′tĭ-koi-dĭz′əm) *n.* See **adrenocortical insufficiency.**

hy·po·cu·pre·mi·a (hī′pō-kŏo-prē′mē-ə, -kyŏo-) *n.* Abnormally low levels of copper in the blood.

hy·po·cy·the·mi·a (hī′pō-sī-thē′mē-ə) *n.* Abnormally low numbers of red blood cells, white blood cells, and other formed elements of the blood.

hy·po·dac·ty·ly (hī′pō-dăk′tə-lē) *n.* The condition of having fewer than five digits on a hand or foot.

Hy·po·der·ma (hī′pə-dûr′mə) *n.* A genus of botflies whose larvae cause a creeping eruption in humans.

hy·po·der·ma·to·sis (hī′pə-dûr′mə-tō′sĭs) *n.* Infection of cattle, sheep, and humans with larvae of flies of the genus *Hypoderma.*

hy·po·der·mic (hī′pə-dûr′mĭk) *adj.* **1.** Of or relating to the layer just beneath the epidermis. **2.** Relating to the hypodermis. **3.** Injected beneath the skin. —*n.* **1.** A hypodermic injection. **2.** A hypodermic needle. **3.** A hypodermic syringe. —**hy′po·der′mi·cal·ly** *adv.*

hypodermic injection *n.* A subcutaneous, intracutaneous, intramuscular, or intravenous injection by means of a hypodermic syringe and needle.

hypodermic needle *n.* **1.** A hollow needle used with a hypodermic syringe. **2.** A hypodermic syringe including the needle.

hypodermic syringe *n.* A syringe with a calibrated barrel, plunger, and tip, used with a hypodermic needle for hypodermic injections and for aspiration.

hypodermic tablet *n.* A tablet that dissolves completely in water to form an injectable solution.

hy·po·der·mis (hī′pə-dûr′mĭs) *or* **hy·po·derm** (hī′pə-dûrm′) *n.* **1.** An epidermal layer of cells that secretes an overlying chitinous cuticle, as in arthropods. **2.** See **tela subcutanea.**

hy·po·der·moc·ly·sis (hī′pə-dûr-mŏk′lĭ-sĭs) *n.* Subcutaneous injection of a saline or other solution.

hy·po·don·tia (hī′pō-dŏn′shə) *n.* A usually congenital condition of having fewer than the normal number of teeth. Also called *oligodontia.*

hy·po·dy·nam·ic (hī′pō-dī-năm′ĭk) *adj.* Possessing or exhibiting subnormal power or force.

hy·po·ec·cri·sis (hī′pō-ĕk′rĭ-sĭs) *n.* Abnormally reduced excretion of waste matter. —**hy′po·ec·crit′ic** (-ĭ-krĭt′ĭk) *adj.*

hy·po·er·gia (hī′pō-ûr′jə) *or* **hy·po·er·gy** (hī′pō-ûr′jē) *n.* See **hyposensitivity.**

hy·po·es·o·pho·ri·a (hī′pō-ĕs′ə-fôr′ē-ə) *n.* The downward and inward deviation of the eyeball.

hy·po·es·the·sia (hī′pō-ĭs-thē′zhə) *or* **hy·pes·the·sia** (hī′pĭs-) *n.* Partial loss of sensitivity to sensory stimuli; diminished sensation. —**hy′pes·the′sic** (-thē′zĭk), **hy′pes·thet′ic** (-thĕt′ĭk) *adj.*

hy·po·ex·o·pho·ri·a (hī′pō-ĕk′sə-fôr′ē-ə) *n.* The outward and downward deviation of the eyeball.

hy·po·fer·re·mi·a (hī′pō-fə-rē′mē-ə) *n.* Deficiency of iron in the blood.

hy·po·fi·brin·o·ge·ne·mi·a (hī′pō-fī-brĭn′ə-jə-nē′mē-ə) *n.* Abnormally low levels of serum fibrinogen.

hy·po·func·tion (hī′pō-fŭngk′shən) *n.* Diminished, abnormally low, or inadequate functioning.

hy·po·ga·lac·ti·a (hī′pō-gə-lăk′tē-ə, -shē-ə) *n.* Abnormally low milk secretion.

hy·po·ga·lac·tous (hī′pō-gə-lăk′təs) *adj.* Producing or secreting a less than normal amount of milk.

hy·po·gam·ma·glob·u·li·ne·mi·a (hī′pō-găm′ə-glŏb′-yə-lə-nē′mē-ə) *n.* **1.** Decreased quantity of the gamma fraction of serum globulin. **2.** A decreased quantity of immunoglobulins in the blood.

hy·po·gan·gli·on·o·sis (hī′pō-găng′glē-ə-nō′sĭs) *n.* A reduction in the number of ganglionic nerve cells, especially of the ganglia of the myenteric plexus.

hypogastric artery *n.* The internal iliac artery.

hypogastric nerve *n.* Either of the two nerve trunks designated right and left that lead from the superior hypogastric plexus into the pelvis to join the inferior hypogastric plexuses.

hypogastric vein *n.* A vein that runs from the sciatic region to the pelvis where it joins the external iliac vein to form the common iliac vein and drains most of the territory supplied by the internal iliac artery. Also called *internal iliac vein.*

hy·po·gas·tri·um (hī′pə-găs′trē-əm) *n., pl.* **–tri·a** (-trē-ə) See **pubic region.** —**hy′po·gas′tric** *adj.*

hy·po·gas·tros·chi·sis (hī′pō-gă-strŏs′kĭ-sĭs) *n.* An abdominal fissure limited to the hypogastric region.

hy·po·gen·e·sis (hī′pə-jĕn′ĭ-sĭs) *n.* Underdevelopment of parts or organs of the body. —**hy′po·ge·net′ic** (-jə-nĕt′ĭk) *adj.*

hy·po·gen·i·tal·ism (hī′pə-jĕn′ĭ-tl-ĭz′əm) *n.* Partial or complete failure of the genitalia to develop, often as a consequence of hypogonadism.

hy·po·geu·sia (hī′pə-gyōō′zhə, -jōō′-) *n.* Impairment of the sense of taste.

hy·po·glos·sal (hī′pə-glô′səl) *adj.* **1.** Of or relating to the area under the tongue. **2.** Of or relating to the hypoglossal nerve.

hypoglossal canal *n.* The canal through which the hypoglossal nerve emerges from the skull. Also called *anterior condyloid foramen.*

hypoglossal nerve *n.* Either of a pair of nerves that arise from the medulla, pass through the hypoglossal canal, and supply muscles of the tongue and the styloglossus, hyoglossus, and genioglossus muscles. Also called *twelfth cranial nerve.*

hypoglossal nucleus *n.* The motor nucleus innervating the musculature of the tongue, located in the medulla oblongata near the midline.

hy·po·glot·tis (hī′pə-glŏt′ĭs) *n.* The undersurface of the tongue.

hy·po·gly·ce·mi·a (hī′pō-glī-sē′mē-ə) *n.* An abnormally low concentration of glucose in the blood.

hy·po·gly·ce·mic (hī′pō-glī-sē′mĭk) *adj.* **1.** Of or relating to hypoglycemia. **2.** Lowering the concentration of glucose in the blood. Used of a drug.

hy·po·gly·co·gen·ol·y·sis (hī′pō-glī′kə-jə-nŏl′ĭ-sĭs) *n.* Diminished or deficient glycogenolysis.

hy·po·gly·cor·rha·chi·a (hī′pō-glī′kə-rā′kē-ə, -răk′ē-ə) *n.* An abnormally low concentration of glucose in the cerebrospinal fluid.

hy·pog·na·thous (hī-pŏg′nə-thəs, hī′pō-năth′əs) *adj.* Having a congenitally underdeveloped lower jaw.

hy·po·go·nad·ism (hī′pō-gō′năd-ĭz′əm, -gŏn′ə-dĭz′-əm) *n.* Inadequate functioning of the testes or ovaries as manifested by deficiencies in gametogenesis or the secretion of gonadal hormones.

hy·po·go·nad·o·tro·pic (hī′pō-gō-năd′ə-trŏp′ĭk, -trō′-pĭk) *adj.* Of or associated with inadequate secretion of gonadotropins.

hypogonadotropic hypogonadism *n.* Defective gonadal development or function due to inadequate secretion of pituitary gonadotropins. Also called *hypogonadotropic eunuchoidism.*

hy·po·hi·dro·sis (hī′pō-hī-drō′sĭs, -hĭ-) *or* **hyp·hi·dro·sis** (hīp′hī-drō′sĭs, -hĭ-, hĭp′-) *n.* Diminished perspiration. —**hy′po·hi·drot′ic** (-drŏt′ĭk) *adj.*

hy·po·ka·le·mi·a (hī′pō-kā-lē′mē-ə) *n.* An abnormally low concentration of potassium ions in the blood. Also called *hypopotassemia.*

hy·po·ka·le·mic periodic paralysis (hī′pō-kə-lē′mĭk) *n.* An inherited form of periodic paralysis characterized by attacks in which the serum potassium level is low and respiratory paralysis may occur. Onset usually occurs between the ages of 7 and 21 years.

hy·po·ki·ne·sis (hī′pō-kə-nē′sĭs, -kī-) *or* **hy·po·ki·ne·sia** (-nē′zhə) *n.* Diminished or abnormally slow movement. Also called *hypomotility.* —**hy′po·ki·net′ic** (-nĕt′ĭk) *adj.*

hy·po·ley·dig·ism (hī′pō-lī′dĭg-ĭz′əm) *n.* Subnormal secretion of androgens by the interstitial cells.

hy·po·mag·ne·se·mi·a (hī′pō-măg′nə-sē′mē-ə) *n.* An abnormally low level of magnesium in the blood.

hy·po·ma·ni·a (hī′pə-mā′nē-ə, -mān′yə) *n.* A mild, nonpsychotic form of mania that is characterized by increased levels of energy, physical activity, and talkativeness.

hy·po·mas·ti·a (hī′pō-măs′tē-ə) *n.* Atrophy or abnormal smallness of the mammary glands.

hy·po·mel·a·no·sis of Ito (hī′pō-mĕl′ə-nō′sĭs) *n.* See **incontinentia pigmenti achromiens.**

hy·po·men·or·rhe·a (hī′pō-mĕn′ə-rē′ə) *n.* A diminution of the flow or a shortening of the duration of menstruation.

hy·po·mere (hī′pə-mîr′) *n.* **1.** The portion of the myotome that forms muscle of the body wall and that is innervated by a branch of a spinal nerve. **2.** The somatic and splanchnic layers of the lateral mesoderm that give rise to the lining of the celom.

hy·po·me·tab·o·lism (hī′pō-mĭ-tăb′ə-lĭz′əm) *n.* An abnormal decrease in metabolic rate.

hy·po·me·tri·a (hī′pō-mē′trē-ə) *n.* An ataxic muscle disorder marked by underreaching an intended object or goal.

hy·pom·ne·sia (hī′pŏm-nē′zhə) *n.* Impaired memory.

hy·po·morph (hī′pə-môrf′) *n.* A person whose standing height is short in proportion to the sitting height, owing to shortness of limb.

hy·po·mo·til·i·ty (hī′pō-mō-tĭl′ĭ-tē) *n.* See **hypokinesis.**

hy·po·my·e·li·na·tion (hī′pō-mī′ə-lə-nā′shən) *n.* Defective formation of myelin in the spinal cord and brain. Also called *hypomyelinogenesis.*

hy·po·my·o·to·ni·a (hī′pō-mī′ə-tō′nē-ə) *n.* Diminished muscular tonicity.

hy·po·myx·i·a (hī′pō-mĭk′sē-ə) *n.* Diminished secretion of mucus.

hy·po·na·tre·mi·a (hī′pō-nə-trē′mē-ə) *n.* Abnormally low concentration of sodium ions in blood.

hy·po·ne·o·cy·to·sis (hī′pō-nē′ō-sī-tō′sĭs) *n.* Leukopenia associated with the presence of immature and young white blood cells.

hy·po·nych·i·um (hī′pō-nĭk′ē-əm) *n.* The epithelium of the nail bed, especially its posterior part in the region of the lunula. **—hy′po·nych′i·al** *adj.*

hy·pon·y·chon (hī-pŏn′ĭ-kŏn′) *n.* Ecchymosis beneath a fingernail or toenail.

hy·po·or·tho·cy·to·sis (hī′pō-ôr′thō-sī-tō′sĭs) *n.* Leukopenia in which the numbers of the various types of white blood cells are within normal range and no immature cells are found in the blood.

hy·po·pan·cre·a·tism (hī′pō-păng′krē-ə-tĭz′əm) *n.* A condition of diminished secretory activity of the pancreas.

hy·po·par·a·thy·roid·ism (hī′pō-păr′ə-thī′roi-dĭz′-əm) *n.* A condition due to diminution or absence of the secretion of the parathyroid hormones.

hy·po·pha·lan·gism (hī′pō-fə-lăn′jĭz′əm) *n.* Congenital absence of one or more phalanges of a digit.

hy·po·pha·ryn·ge·al diverticulum (hī′pō-fə-rĭn′jē-əl, -jəl, -făr′ĭn-jē′əl) *n.* A pulsion diverticulum of the laryngopharynx. Also called *Zenker's diverticulum.*

hy·po·phar·ynx (hī′pō-făr′ĭngks) *n.* See **laryngopharynx.**

hy·po·pho·ne·sis (hī′pō-fō-nē′sĭs) *n.* A noticeable diminution of the perceived sound in auscultation or percussion.

hy·po·pho·ri·a (hī′pə-fôr′ē-ə) *n.* A tendency of the visual axis of one eye to sink below that of the other.

hy·po·phos·pha·ta·sia (hī′pō-fŏs′fə-tā′zhə) *n.* An abnormally low concentration of alkaline phosphatase in the blood.

hy·po·phos·pha·te·mi·a (hī′pō-fŏs′fə-tē′mē-ə) *n.* Abnormally low concentrations of phosphates in the blood.

hy·po·phos·pha·tu·ri·a (hī′pō-fŏs′fə-toŏr′ē-ə) *n.* Abnormally low urinary excretion of phosphates.

hy·poph·y·sec·to·my (hī-pŏf′ĭ-sĕk′tə-mē) *n.* Excision or destruction of the pituitary gland.

hy·poph·y·si·al *or* **hy·poph·y·se·al** (hī-pŏf′ĭ-sē′əl, -zē′, hī′pə-fĭz′ē-əl) *adj.* Of or relating to a pituitary gland.

hypophysial cachexia *n.* See **Simmonds disease.**

hypophysial fossa *n.* See **pituitary fossa.**

hy·po·phys·i·o·priv·ic *or* **hy·po·phys·e·o·priv·ic** (hī′-pō-fĭz′ē-ō-prĭv′ĭk) *adj.* Of or being the condition in which the pituitary gland is functionally inactive or in which it is absent, as after hypophysectomy.

hy·po·phys·i·o·trop·ic *or* **hy·po·phys·e·o·trop·ic** (hī′-pō-fĭz′ē-ō-trŏp′ĭk, -trō′pĭk) *adj.* Of or relating to a hormone that acts on the pituitary gland.

hy·poph·y·sis (hī-pŏf′ĭ-sĭs) *n., pl.* **-ses** (-sēz′) See **pituitary gland.**

hy·poph·y·si·tis (hī-pŏf′ĭ-sī′tĭs) *n.* Inflammation of the pituitary gland.

hy·po·pi·e·sis (hī′pō-pī-ē′sĭs) *n.* See **hypotension** (sense 1).

hy·po·pig·men·ta·tion (hī′pō-pĭg′mən-tā′shən) *n.* Diminished pigmentation, especially of the skin.

hy·po·pi·tu·i·ta·rism (hī′pō-pĭ-toō′ĭ-tə-rĭz′əm) *n.* **1.** Deficient or diminished production of pituitary hormones. **2.** The condition resulting from a deficiency in pituitary hormone, especially growth hormone, characterized by dwarfism in children. **—hy′po·pi·tu′i·tar′y** (-tĕr′ē) *adj.*

hy·po·pla·sia (hī′pō-plā′zhə) *n.* **1.** Incomplete or arrested development of an organ or part. **2.** Atrophy due to destruction of some of the elements of a tissue or organ. **—hy′po·plas′tic** (-plăs′tĭk) *adj.*

hypoplastic anemia *n.* Progressive nonregenerative anemia resulting from greatly depressed, inadequately functioning bone marrow that may lead to aplastic anemia.

hy·po·ploid (hī′pō-ploid′) *adj.* Having a chromosome number that is one or more lower than the normal haploid number of chromosomes characteristic for the species. **—hy′po·ploi′dy** *n.*

hy·pop·ne·a (hī-pŏp′nē-ə, hī′pō-nē′ə) *n.* Abnormally slow or shallow breathing. **—hy′pop·ne′ic** *adj.*

hy·po·po·si·a (hī′pə-pō′zē-ə) *n.* A condition characterized by an abnormally low fluid consumption.

hy·po·po·tas·se·mi·a (hī′pō-pə-tă-sē′mē-ə) *n.* See **hypokalemia.**

hy·po·prax·i·a (hī′pō-prăk′sē-ə) *n.* Deficient activity.

hy·po·pro·tein·e·mi·a (hī′pō-prō′tē-nē′mē-ə, -tē-ə-nē′-) *n.* Abnormally low levels of total protein in the blood.

hy·po·pro·throm·bi·ne·mi·a (hī′pō-prō-thrŏm′bə-nē′mē-ə) *n.* Abnormally low levels of prothrombin in the blood.

hy·po·pty·a·lism (hī′pō-tī′ə-lĭz′əm) *n.* See **hyposalivation.**

hy·po·py·on (hī-pō′pē-ŏn′) *n.* The presence of pus or a puslike fluid in the anterior chamber of the eye.

hy·po·re·flex·i·a (hī′pō-rĭ-flĕk′sē-ə) *n.* Decreased response of the deep tendon reflexes, usually resulting from injury to the central nervous system or metabolic disease.

hy·po·re·ni·ne·mi·a (hī′pō-rē′nə-nē′mē-ə) *n.* Abnormally low levels of renin in the blood.

hy·po·ri·bo·fla·vin·o·sis (hī′pō-rī′bō-flā′və-nō′sĭs) *n.* See **ariboflavinosis.**

hy·po·sal·i·va·tion (hī′pō-săl′ə-vā′shən) *n.* Abnormally reduced salivation. Also called *hypoptyalism.*

hy·po·scle·ral (hī′pō-sklîr′əl) *adj.* Situated beneath the sclerotic coat of the eyeball.

hy·po·sen·si·tiv·i·ty (hī′pō-sĕn′sĭ-tĭv′ĭ-tē) *n.* Less than normal sensitivity to a foreign agent, such as an allergen, in which the response is unusually delayed or lessened in degree. Also called *hypoergia.* —**hy′po·sen′si·tive** *adj.*

hy·po·sen·si·tize (hī′pō-sĕn′sĭ-tīz′) *v.* To make less sensitive, as to an allergen.

hy·pos·mi·a (hī-pŏz′mē-ə) *n.* A diminished or deficient sense of smell.

hy·po·so·mat·o·tro·pism (hī′pō-sə-măt′ə-trō′pĭz′əm, -sō′mə-tə-) *n.* Deficient secretion of somatotropin.

hy·po·spa·di·as (hī′pō-spā′dē-əs) *or* **hy·po·spa·di·a** (-dē-ə) *n.* **1.** A developmental anomaly of the urethra in which a part of the urethral canal is open on the undersurface of the penis or on the perineum. **2.** A similar anomaly in which the urethra opens into the vagina. —**hy′po·spa′di·ac′** (-ăk′) *adj.*

hy·pos·ta·sis (hī-pŏs′tə-sĭs) *n., pl.* **-ses** (-sēz′) **1.** A settling of solid particles in a fluid. **2.** Sediment. **3.** See **hypostatic congestion. 4.** A condition in which the action of one gene conceals or suppresses the action of another gene that is not its allele but that affects the same part or biochemical process in an organism. —**hy′po·stat′ic** (hī′pə-stăt′ĭk) *adj.*

hypostatic congestion *n.* Congestion caused by poor circulation and resulting in the settling of venous blood in the lower part of an organ or the body. Also called *hypostasis.*

hypostatic ectasia *n.* Dilation of a blood vessel, usually a vein, in a dependent portion of the body, as in varicose veins of the leg.

hypostatic pneumonia *n.* Pulmonary congestion due to the stagnation of blood in the dependent portions of the lungs in old persons or in those who are ill and lie in the same position for long periods.

hy·po·sthe·ni·a (hī′pəs-thē′nē-ə) *n.* Abnormal lack of strength. —**hy′po·sthen′ic** (-pəs-thĕn′ĭk) *adj.*

hy·pos·the·nu·ri·a (hī-pŏs′thə-no͞or′ē-ə) *n.* Excretion of urine of low specific gravity due to an inability of the tubules of the kidneys to produce concentrated urine.

hy·po·sto·mi·a (hī′pə-stō′mē-ə) *n.* Microstomia in which the oral opening is a small vertical slit.

hy·po·tel·or·ism (hī′pō-tĕl′ə-rĭz′əm) *n.* Abnormal closeness of the eyes.

hy·po·ten·sion (hī′pə-tĕn′shən) *n.* **1.** Abnormally low arterial blood pressure. Also called *hypopiesis.* **2.** Reduced pressure or tension of any kind, as of the intraocular or cerebrospinal fluids.

hy·po·ten·sive (hī′pə-tĕn′sĭv) *adj.* **1.** Of or characterized by low blood pressure. **2.** Causing a reduction in blood pressure.

hy·po·ten·sor (hī′pə-tĕn′sər, -sôr′) *n.* See **depressor** (sense 4).

hypothalamic infundibulum *n.* The apical portion of the tuber cinereum extending into the stalk of the pituitary gland.

hy·po·thal·a·mo·hy·po·phys·i·al portal system (hī′-pō-thăl′ə-mō-hī′pə-fĭz′ē-əl, -zē′-, -hī-pŏf′ĭ-sē′əl) *n.* A system of veins that originate in the hypothalamus and

pass through the pituitary gland and into its anterior lobe, where they branch into a capillary bed and convey releasing factors to the anterior lobe.

hy·po·thal·a·mus (hī′pō-thăl′ə-məs) *n.* The part of the brain that lies below the thalamus, forming the major portion of the ventral region of the diencephalon, and that regulates bodily temperature, certain metabolic processes, and other autonomic activities. —**hy′po·tha·lam′ic** (-thə-lăm′ĭk) *adj.*

hy·po·the·nar (hī′pō-thē′när′, -nər, hī-pŏth′ə-) *n.* The fleshy mass at the medial side of the palm. Also called *antithenar.* —**hy′po·the′nar** *adj.*

hy·po·ther·mi·a (hī′pə-thûr′mē-ə) *n.* Abnormally low body temperature. —**hy′po·ther′mic** (-mĭk) *adj.*

hy·poth·e·sis (hī-pŏth′ĭ-sĭs) *n., pl.* **-ses** (-sēz′) A tentative explanation that accounts for a set of facts and can be tested by further investigation. —**hy′po·thet′i·cal** (hī′pə-thĕt′ĭ-kəl) *adj.*

hy·po·throm·bi·ne·mi·a (hī′pō-thrŏm′bə-nē′mē-ə) *n.* Abnormally low levels of thrombin in the blood, leading to bleeding without clotting.

hy·po·thy·mi·a (hī′pō-thī′mē-ə) *n.* A state of diminished emotional response, as in depression.

hy·po·thy·mic (hī′pō-thī′mĭk) *adj.* Relating to hypothymia or hypothymism.

hy·po·thy·mism (hī′pō-thī′mĭz′əm) *n.* Reduced or inadequate functioning of the thymus.

hy·po·thy·roid·ism (hī′pō-thī′roi-dĭz′əm) *n.* **1.** Insufficient production of thyroid hormones. **2.** A pathological condition resulting from thyroid insufficiency, which may lead to cretinism or myxedema. —**hy′po·thy′roid** *adj.*

hy·po·to·ni·a (hī′pō-tō′nē-ə) *n.* **1.** Reduced tension or pressure, as of the intraocular fluid in the eyeball. **2.** Relaxation of the arteries. **3.** A condition in which there is diminution or loss of muscular tonicity, resulting in stretching of the muscles beyond their normal limits.

hy·po·ton·ic (hī′pō-tŏn′ĭk) *adj.* **1.** Having less than normal tone or tension, as of muscles or arteries. **2.** Having a lower osmotic pressure than a reference solution. —**hy′po·to·nic′i·ty** (-tə-nĭs′ĭ-tē) *n.*

hy·po·tox·ic·i·ty (hī′pō-tŏk-sĭs′ĭ-tē) *n.* The quality of being only slightly toxic.

hy·po·tri·cho·sis (hī′pō-trĭ-kō′sĭs) *n.* A less than normal amount of hair on the head or body.

hy·pot·ro·phy (hī-pŏt′rə-fē) *n.* Progressive degeneration of an organ or tissue caused by loss of cells.

hy·po·tro·pi·a (hī′pə-trō′pē-ə) *n.* Downward deviation of the visual axis of one eye.

hy·po·tym·pa·num (hī′pō-tĭm′pə-nəm) *n.* The lower part of the cavity of the middle ear.

hy·po·u·ri·ce·mi·a (hī′pō-yo͝or′ĭ-sē′mē-ə) *n.* Abnormally reduced blood concentration of uric acid.

hy·po·u·ri·cu·ri·a (hī′pō-yo͝or′ĭ-kyo͝or′ē-ə) *n.* Abnormally low levels of uric acid in the urine.

hy·po·ven·ti·la·tion (hī′pə-vĕn′tl-ā′shən) *n.* Reduced or deficient ventilation of the lungs, resulting in reduced aeration of blood in the lungs and an increased level of carbon dioxide in the blood.

hy·po·vi·ta·min·o·sis (hī′pō-vī′tə-mə-nō′sĭs) *n.* Insufficiency of one or more essential vitamins.

hy·po·vo·le·mi·a (hī''pō-vŏ-lē′mē-ə) *n.* See **oligemia.** —**hy′po·vo·le′mic** *adj.*

hypovolemic shock *n.* Shock caused by a reduction in the volume of blood, as from hemorrhage.

hy·po·vo·li·a (hī′pō-vō′lē-ə) *n.* Diminished water content or volume, as of extracellular fluid.

hy·po·xan·thine (hī′pō-zăn′thēn′) *n.* A purine present in muscle and other tissues, formed during uric acid synthesis.

hy·pox·e·mi·a (hī′pŏk-sē′mē-ə) *n.* Insufficient oxygenation of arterial blood. —**hy′pox·e′mic** *adj.*

hy·pox·i·a (hī-pŏk′sē-ə, hĭ-) *n.* Insufficient levels of oxygen in blood or tissue. —**hy·pox′ic** *adj.*

hypoxic hypoxia *n.* Hypoxia resulting from a defective mechanism of oxygenation in the lungs, as is caused by a low tension of oxygen, by abnormal pulmonary function, or by a right-to-left shunt in the heart. Also called *anoxic anoxia.*

hypoxic nephrosis *n.* Acute oliguric renal failure following hemorrhage, burns, shock, or other causes of hypovolemia and reduced renal blood flow.

hyp·sar·rhyth·mi·a *or* **hyp·sa·rhyth·mi·a** (hĭp′sə-rĭth′-mē-ə) *n.* The abnormal and characteristically random electroencephalogram often found in babies with infantile spasms, associated with mental retardation. —**hyp′sar·rhyth′moid′** (-moid′) *adj.*

hys·ter·al·gia (hĭs′tə-răl′jə) *n.* The occurence of pain in the uterus. Also called *hysterodynia, metralgia, metrodynia.*

hys·ter·a·tre·sia (hĭs′tər-ə-trē′zhə) *n.* Atresia of the uterine cavity, usually resulting from inflammatory endocervical adhesions.

hys·ter·ec·to·my (hĭs′tə-rĕk′tə-mē) *n.* Surgical removal of part or all of the uterus.

hys·ter·e·sis (hĭs′tə-rē′sĭs) *n., pl.* **-ses** (-sēz) The lagging of an effect behind its cause, as when the change in magnetism of a body lags behind changes in the magnetic field. —**hys′ter·et′ic** (-rĕt′ĭk) *adj.*

hys·ter·eu·ry·sis (hĭs′tər-yōōr′ĭ-sĭs) *n.* Dilation of the lower segment and cervical canal of the uterus.

hys·ter·i·a (hĭ-stĕr′ē-ə, -stĭr′-) *n.* **1.** A psychiatric disorder characterized by the presentation of a physical ailment without an organic cause. **2.** Excessive or uncontrollable emotion, such as fear. —**hys·ter′ic** (hĭ-stĕr′ĭk), **hys·ter′i·cal** (hĭ-stĕr′ĭ-kəl) *adj.*

hys·ter·ic (hĭ-stĕr′ĭk) *n.* **1.** A person suffering from hysteria. **2. hysterics** A fit of uncontrollable laughing or crying.

hysterical personality *n.* A personality disorder marked by immaturity, dependence, self-centeredness, and vanity, with a craving for attention, activity, or excitement, and behavior that is markedly unstable or manipulative.

hysterical psychosis *n.* An acute psychosis accompanied by the symptoms of hysteria.

hystero– *or* **hyster–** *pref.* **1.** Uterus: *hysterectomy.* **2.** Hysteria: *hysteroid.*

hys·ter·o·cat·a·lep·sy (hĭs′tə-rō-kăt′l-ĕp′sē) *n.* Hysteria with cataleptic manifestations.

hys·ter·o·cele (hĭs′tə-rō-sēl′) *n.* **1.** An abdominal or perineal hernia containing part or all of the uterus. **2.** Protrusion of the uterine contents into a weakened, bulging area of the uterine wall.

hys·ter·o·clei·sis (hĭs′tə-rō-klī′sĭs) *n., pl.* **-ses** (-sēz′) Surgical occlusion of the uterus.

hys·ter·o·dyn·i·a (hĭs′tə-rō-dĭn′ē-ə) *n.* See **hysteralgia.**

hys·ter·o·ep·i·lep·sy (hĭs′tə-rō-ĕp′ə-lĕp′sē) *n.* Hysteria that is accompanied by convulsions resembling epileptic seizures.

hys·ter·o·gen·ic (hĭs′tə-rō-jĕn′ĭk) *adj.* Causing hysterical symptoms or reactions.

hys·ter·o·gram (hĭs′tə-rō-grăm′) *n.* **1.** An x-ray of the uterus, usually using contrast media. **2.** A graphic record of the strength of uterine contractions during labor.

hys·ter·o·graph (hĭs′tə-rō-grăf′) *n.* An apparatus for recording hysterograms.

hys·ter·og·ra·phy (hĭs′tə-rŏg′rə-fē) *n.* **1.** Radiography of a uterine cavity filled with contrast medium. **2.** The procedure of recording uterine contractions during labor.

hys·ter·oid (hĭs′tə-roid′) *adj.* Resembling or simulating hysteria.

hys·ter·o·lith (hĭs′tə-rō-lĭth′) *n.* See **uterolith.**

hys·ter·ol·y·sis (hĭs′tə-rŏl′ĭ-sĭs) *n., pl.* **-ses** (-sēz′) The severing or separation of adhesions of the uterus.

hys·ter·om·e·ter (hĭs′tə-rŏm′ĭ-tər) *n.* A graduated sounding instrument for measuring the depth of the uterine cavity. Also called *uterometer.*

hys·ter·o·my·o·ma (hĭs′tə-rō-mī-ō′mə) *n.* A myoma of the uterus.

hys·ter·o·my·o·mec·to·my (hĭs′tə-rō-mī′ə-mĕk′tə-mē) *n.* Surgical removal of a uterine myoma.

hys·ter·o·my·ot·o·my (hĭs′tə-rō-mī-ŏt′ə-mē) *n.* Incision into the uterine muscles.

hys·ter·o·o·o·pho·rec·to·my (hĭs′tə-rō-ō′ə-fə-rĕk′tə-mē) *n.* Surgical removal of the uterus and ovaries.

hys·ter·op·a·thy (hĭs′tə-rŏp′ə-thē) *n.* A disease or disorder of the uterus. —**hys′ter·o·path′ic** (-rō-păth′ĭk) *adj.*

hys·ter·o·pex·y (hĭs′tə-rō-pĕk′sē) *n.* Surgical fixation of a misplaced or abnormally movable uterus. Also called *uterofixation, uteropexy.*

hys·ter·o·plas·ty (hĭs′tə-rō-plăs′tē) *n.* See **uteroplasty.**

hys·ter·or·rha·phy (hĭs′tə-rôr′ə-fē) *n.* Repair of a torn or lacerated uterus by suturing.

hys·ter·or·rhex·is (hĭs′tə-rō-rĕk′sĭs) *n.* Rupture of the uterus.

hys·ter·o·sal·pin·gec·to·my (hĭs′tə-rō-săl′pĭn-jĕk′tə-mē) *n.* Surgical removal of the uterus and one or both oviducts.

hys·ter·o·sal·pin·gog·ra·phy (hĭs′tə-rō-săl′pĭng-gŏg′rə-fē, -pĭn-) *n.* The radiography of the uterus and oviducts that follows an injection of a radiopaque material. Also called *gynecography, hysterotubography, metrosalpingography, uterosalpingography, uterotubography.*

hys·ter·o·sal·pin·go·o·o·pho·rec·to·my (hĭs′tə-rō-săl-pĭng′gō-ō′ə-fə-rĕk′tə-mē) *n.* Excision of the uterus, oviducts, and ovaries.

hys·ter·o·sal·pin·gos·to·my (hĭs′tə-rō-săl′pĭng-gŏs′tə-mē, -pĭn-) *n.* Surgical restoration of a connection between the uterus and an occluded fallopian tube.

hys·ter·o·scope (hĭs′tə-rō-skōp′) *n.* An endoscope used in direct visual examination of the uterine cavity. Also called *metroscope, uteroscope.*

hys·ter·os·co·py (hĭs′tə-rŏs′kə-pē) *n.* Visual inspection of the uterine cavity with an endoscope. Also called *uteroscopy.*

hys·ter·o·spasm (hĭs′tə-rō-spăz′əm) *n.* Spasm of the uterus.

hys·ter·ot·o·my (hĭs′tə-rŏt′ə-mē) *n.* Incision of the uterus. Also called *uterotomy.*

hys·ter·o·tra·che·lec·to·my (hĭs′tə-rō-trā′kə-lĕk′tə-mē, -trăk′ə-) *n.* The surgical removal of the uterine cervix.

hys·ter·o·tra·che·lo·plas·ty (hĭs′tə-rō-trā′kə-lō-plăs′-tē, hĭs′tə-rō-trăk′ə-) *n.* Surgical repair of the uterine cervix.

hys·ter·o·tra·che·lor·rha·phy (hĭs′tə-rō-trā′kə-lôr′ə-fē, -trăk′ə-) *n.* Repair of a lacerated uterine cervix by suturing.

hys·ter·o·tra·che·lot·o·my (hĭs′tə-rō-trā′kə-lŏt′ə-mē, -trăk′ə-) *n.* Incision of the uterine cervix.

hys·ter·o·tu·bog·ra·phy (hĭs′tə-rō-tōō-bŏg′rə-fē) *n.* See **hysterosalpingography.**

Hy·tone (hī′tōn′) A trademark for a topical preparation of the drug hydrocortisone.

Hy·trin (hī′trĭn′) A trademark for the drug terazosin hydrochloride.

Hy·zaar (hī′zär′) A trademark for a drug containing a combination of losartan potassium and hydrochlorothiazide.

Hz *abbr.* hertz

I

ι The Greek letter *iota.* Entries beginning with this character are alphabetized under **iota.**

I 1. The symbol for the element **iodine** (sense 1). **2. i** The symbol for **current** (sense 2).

I 131 uptake test *n.* A test of thyroid function in which iodine-131 is given orally and 24 hours later the amount present in the thyroid gland is measured and compared with normal levels.

–ia *suff.* Disease; pathological or abnormal condition: *anoxia.*

IAP *abbr.* intermittent acute porphyria

–iasis *suff.* A pathological condition characterized or produced by: *teniasis.*

i·at·ric (ī-ăt′rĭk) *adj.* Of or relating to medicine or a physician.

–iatric *suff.* Of or relating to a specified kind of medical practice, treatment, or healing: *geriatric.*

–iatrics *suff.* Medical treatment: *pediatrics.*

i·at·ro·gen·ic (ī-ăt′rə-jĕn′ĭk) *adj.* Induced in a patient by a physician's activity, manner, or therapy.

–iatry *suff.* Medical treatment: *psychiatry.*

I band *n.* A pale band of actin on each side of the Z line of a striated muscle fiber.

i·ban·dro·nate sodium (ī-băn′drə-nāt′) *n.* A synthetic drug analog of pyrophosphate that inhibits bone resorption, taken monthly to treat osteoporosis in postmenopausal women.

IBD *abbr.* inflammatory bowel disease

ibn Zuhr (ĭb′ən zŏŏr′) See **Avenzoar.**

i·bo·ga·ine (ĭ-bō′gə-ēn′, -ĭn) *n.* A white powdery substance that can act as a hallucinogen, a memory stimulant, or a dopamine blocker. It stems the craving for heroin and cocaine without causing dependency.

i·bu·pro·fen (ī′byōō-prō′fən) *n.* A nonsteroidal anti-inflammatory medication used especially in the treatment of arthritis and commonly taken for its analgesic and antipyretic properties.

–ic *suff.* **1.** Of or characterized by: *carbonic.* **2.** Having a valence higher than that of a specified element in compounds or ions named with adjectives ending in *–ous: ferric.* **3.** Of or relating to an acid: *sulfuric acid.*

ICD *abbr.* International Classification of Diseases of the World Health Organization

ICDA *abbr.* International Classification of Diseases, Adapted for Use in the United States

Ice·land disease (īs′lənd) *n.* See **epidemic neuromyasthenia.**

I cell *n.* See **inclusion cell.**

ice pack (īs) *n.* A folded sac filled with crushed ice and applied to sore or swollen parts of the body to reduce pain and inflammation.

ICF *abbr.* intracellular fluid

i·chor (ī′kôr′, ī′kər) *n.* A watery, acrid discharge from a wound or ulcer. —**i′chor·ous** (ī′kər-əs) *adj.*

i·chor·oid (ī′kə-roid′) *adj.* Relating to a thin, purulent discharge.

i·chor·rhe·a (ī′kə-rē′ə) *n.* A discharge that is profuse and ichorous.

ich·thy·ism (ĭk′thē-ĭz′əm) *n.* See **ichthyotoxism.**

ichthyo– or **ichthy–** *pref.* Fish: *ichthyoid.*

ich·thy·oid (ĭk′thē-oid′) *n.* A fish or fishlike vertebrate. —*adj.* or **ich·thy·oi·dal** (ĭk′thē-oid′l) Characteristic of or resembling a fish.

ich·thy·o·si·form erythroderma (ĭk′thē-ō′sə-fôrm′) *n.* Variant of **congenital ichthyosiform erythroderma.**

ich·thy·o·sis (ĭk′thē-ō′sĭs) *n.* A congenital, often hereditary skin disease characterized by dry, thickened, scaly skin. Also called *alligator skin, fish skin, fishskin disease, ichthyosis sauroderma.*

ichthyosis lin·e·ar·is cir·cum·scrip·ta (lĭn′ē-âr′ĭs sûr′kəm-skrĭp′tə) *n.* An inherited skin disorder present at birth or appearing in infancy, that is characterized by redness and scaling that moves from place to place about the body and that shows a peripheral double-edged scale.

ichthyosis sau·ro·der·ma (sôr′ə-dûr′mə) *n.* See **ichthyosis.**

ichthyosis sim·plex (sĭm′plĕks′) *n.* See **ichthyosis vulgaris.**

ichthyosis u·ter·i (yōō′tə-rī′) *n.* The transformation of the columnar epithelium of the endometrium into stratified squamous epithelium.

ichthyosis vul·gar·is (vŭl-gâr′ĭs) *n.* An inherited condition appearing in childhood and characterized by fine scales on the trunk and extremities. Also called *ichthyosis simplex.*

ich·thy·ot·ic (ĭk′thē-ŏt′ĭk) *adj.* Of, relating to, or characterized by ichthyosis.

ich·thy·o·tox·ism (ĭk′thē-ō-tŏk′sĭz′əm) *n.* Poisoning by a toxic substance derived from fish. Also called *ichthyism.*

ICP *abbr.* intracranial pressure

–ics *suff.* **1.** Science; art; study; knowledge; skill: *pharmaceutics.* **2.** Actions, activities, or practices of: *macrobiotics.*

ICSH *abbr.* interstitial cell-stimulating hormone

ic·tal (ĭk′təl) *adj.* Relating to or caused by a stroke or seizure.

ic·ter·ic (ĭk-tĕr′ĭk) *adj.* **1.** Relating to or affected with jaundice. **2.** Used to treat jaundice. —*n.* A remedy for jaundice.

ictero– *pref.* Icterus: *icterogenic.*

ic·ter·o·gen·ic (ĭk′tə-rō-jĕn′ĭk) *adj.* Causing jaundice.

ic·ter·o·hep·a·ti·tis (ĭk′tə-rō-hĕp′ə-tī′tĭs) *n.* Inflammation of the liver with jaundice as a prominent symptom.

ic·ter·oid (ĭk′tə-roid′) *adj.* Having the appearance of being jaundiced.

ic·ter·us (ĭk′tər-əs) *n.* See **jaundice.**

icterus grav·is (grăv′ĭs) *n.* See **malignant jaundice.**

icterus index *n.* A calculation indicating the level of bilirubin in serum or plasma, in which the intensity of the color of a specimen is compared with that of a standard solution using a colorimeter.

icterus ne·o·na·to·rum (nē′ō-nā-tôr′əm) *n.* See **jaundice of newborn.**

ic·tus (ĭk′təs) *n., pl.* **ictus** *or* **–tus·es** A sudden attack, stroke, or seizure.

ICU *abbr.* intensive care unit

ICU psychosis (ī′sē-yōō′) *n.* Psychosis only occurring after admission to an intensive care unit.

id (ĭd) *n.* In psychoanalytic theory, the division of the psyche that is totally unconscious and serves as the source of instinctual impulses and demands for immediate satisfaction of primitive needs.

ID *abbr.* infecting dose

–id *suff.* Body; particle: *chromatid.*

IDDM *abbr.* insulin-dependent diabetes mellitus

–ide *suff.* **1.** Group of related chemical compounds: *monosaccharide.* **2.** Binary compound: *sodium chloride.* **3.** Chemical element with properties similar to another: *lanthanide.*

i·de·a (ī-dē′ə) *n.* Something, such as a thought or conception, that potentially or actually exists in the mind as a product of mental activity.

i·de·al (ī-dē′əl, ī-dēl′) *n.* **1.** A conception of something in its absolute perfection. **2.** One that is regarded as a standard or model of perfection or excellence.

ideal gas *n.* A gas that, when kept at a constant temperature, would obey gas laws exactly. No known gas is an ideal gas.

idea of reference *n.* The belief that other people's statements or acts have special reference to oneself when in fact they do not.

i·de·a·tion (ī′dē-ā′shən) *n.* The formation of ideas or mental images. —**i′de·ate′** *v.* —**i′de·a′tion·al** *adj.*

ideational apraxia *or* **i·de·a·to·ry apraxia** (ī′dē-ə-tôr′ē) *n.* A form of apraxia characterized by the inability to use an object properly due to impairment in the perception of its function or purpose.

i·dée fixe (ē-dā fēks′) *n., pl.* **i·dées fixes** (ē-dā fēks′) A fixed idea; an obsession.

i·den·ti·cal (ī-děn′tĭ-kəl) *adj.* **1.** Exactly equal and alike. **2.** Of or relating to a twin or twins developed from the same fertilized ovum and having the same genetic makeup and closely similar appearance; monozygotic.

identical twins *pl.n.* Twins derived from the same fertilized ovum that at an early stage of development becomes separated into independent̂ly growing cell aggregations, giving rise to two individuals of the same sex, identical genetic makeup, and closely similar appearance.

i·den·ti·fi·ca·tion (ī-děn′tə-fĭ-kā′shən) *n.* **1.** A person's association with the qualities, characteristics, or views of another person or group. **2.** An unconscious process by which a person transfers the response appropriate to a particular person or group to a different person or group.

i·den·ti·ty (ī-děn′tĭ-tē) *n.* **1.** The set of behavioral or personal characteristics by which an individual is recognizable as a member of a group. **2.** The distinct personality of an individual regarded as a persisting entity; individuality.

identity crisis *n.* A psychosocial state or condition of disorientation and role confusion occurring especially in adolescents as a result of conflicting pressures and expectations and often producing acute anxiety.

identity disorder *n.* A disorder occurring in late adolescence and characterized by feelings of uncertainty and distress due to issues such as long-term goals, sexual orientation and behavior, morality, and religious identification.

ideo– *pref.* Idea: *ideology.*

i·de·o·ki·net·ic apraxia (ī′dē-ō-kə-nět′ĭk, -kī-, ĭd′ē-) *n.* Apraxia in which simple acts cannot be performed because the connections between the cortical centers that control volition and the motor cortex are interrupted. Also called *ideomotor apraxia, transcortical apraxia.*

i·de·ol·o·gy (ī′dē-ŏl′ə-jē, ĭd′ē-) *n.* The body of ideas reflecting the social needs and aspirations of an individual, a group, a class, or a culture.

i·de·o·mo·tor (ī′dē-ə-mō′tər, ĭd′ē-) *adj.* Of or relating to an unconscious or involuntary bodily movement made in response to a thought or an idea rather than to a sensory stimulus.

ideomotor apraxia *n.* See **ideokinetic apraxia.**

idio– *pref.* **1.** One's own; private; personal: *idiosyncrasy.* **2.** Distinct; separate: *idioventricular.*

id·i·o·ag·glu·ti·nin (ĭd′ē-ō-ə-glōōt′n-ĭn) *n.* An agglutinin that occurs in the blood of a person or animal without the injection of a stimulating antigen or without the passive transfer of antibodies.

id·i·o·cy (ĭd′ē-ə-sē) *n.* The state or condition of being an idiot; profound mental retardation.

id·i·o·gram (ĭd′ē-ə-grăm′) *n.* A diagrammatic representation of chromosome morphology characteristic of a species or a population.

id·i·o·het·er·o·ag·glu·ti·nin (ĭd′ē-ō-hět′ə-rō-ə-glōōt′-n-ĭn) *n.* An idioagglutinin that occurs in the blood of one animal, but that is capable of combining with the antigenic material from an animal of another species.

id·i·o·het·er·ol·y·sin (ĭd′ē-ō-hět′ə-rŏl′ĭ-sĭn, -rō-lī′sĭn) *n.* An idiolysin occurring in the blood of one species, but capable of combining with the red blood cells of another species, thereby causing hemolysis when complement is present.

id·i·o·i·so·ag·glu·ti·nin (ĭd′ē-ō-ī′sō-ə-glōōt′n-ĭn) *n.* An idioagglutinin occurring in the blood of an animal and capable of agglutinating cells from an animal of the same species.

id·i·o·i·sol·y·sin (ĭd′ē-ō-ī-sŏl′ĭ-sĭn, -ī′sə-lī′sĭn) *n.* An idiolysin occurring in the blood of an animal and capable of combining with red blood cells from an animal of the same species, thereby causing hemolysis when complement is present.

id·i·ol·y·sin (ĭd′ē-ŏl′ĭ-sĭn, ĭd′ē-ə-lī′sĭn) *n.* A lysin that occurs in the blood of a person or an animal without the injection of a stimulating antigen or the passive transfer of antibodies.

id·i·o·mus·cu·lar contraction (ĭd′ē-ō-mŭs′kyə-lər) *n.* See **myoedema.**

id·i·o·path·ic (ĭd′ē-ə-păth′ĭk) *adj.* **1.** Of or relating to a disease having no known cause; agnogenic. **2.** Of or relating to a disease that is not the result of any other disease.

idiopathic aldosteronism *n.* See **primary aldosteronism.**

idiopathic epilepsy *n.* Epilepsy without evident cause.

idiopathic hypercalcemia of infants *n.* Persistent hypercalcemia of unknown cause occurring in very young children and associated with osteosclerosis, renal insufficiency, and sometimes hypertension.

idiopathic hypertrophic osteoarthropathy *n.* Osteoarthropathy that is not a consequence of pulmonary or other progressive lesions.

idiopathic hypertrophic subaortic stenosis *n.* Obstruction of the flow of blood out of the left ventricle due to hypertrophy of the ventricular septum.

idiopathic megacolon *n.* Megacolon resulting in constipation, associated with faulty bowel habits and thin musculature of the colon.

idiopathic neuralgia *n.* Nerve pain that has no apparent cause.

idiopathic pulmonary hemosiderosis *n.* Repeated attacks of difficulty in breathing and hemoptysis leading to the deposition of abnormal amounts of hemosiderin in the lungs. Also called *Ceelen-Gellerstadt syndrome.*

idiopathic retroperitoneal fibrosis *n.* A benign disorder of unknown cause characterized by the proliferation of retroperitoneal connective tissue, usually causing obstruction of the ureters. Also called *Ormond's disease.*

idiopathic thrombocytopenic purpura *n. Abbr.* **ITP** A systemic illness of unknown cause, characterized by extensive ecchymoses and hemorrhages from mucous membranes, deficiencies in the numbers of platelets, anemia, and extreme weakness. Also called *immune thrombocytopenic purpura, purpura hemorrhagica, thrombocytopenic purpura, Werlhof's disease.*

id·i·op·a·thy (ĭd′ē-ŏp′ə-thē) *n.* **1.** A disease of unknown origin or cause. **2.** A primary disease arising spontaneously with no apparent external cause.

id·i·o·syn·cra·sy (ĭd′ē-ō-sĭng′krə-sē) *n.* **1.** A structural or behavioral trait peculiar to an individual or a group. **2.** A physiological or temperamental peculiarity. **3.** An unusual individual reaction to food or a drug. —**id′i·o·syn·crat′ic** (-sĭn-krăt′ĭk) *adj.*

id·i·ot (ĭd′ē-ət) *n.* A person of profound mental retardation having a mental age below three years and generally being unable to learn connected speech or guard against common dangers. The term belongs to a classification system no longer in use and is now considered offensive. —**id′i·ot′ic** (-ŏt′ĭk) *adj.*

idiot savant (să-vänt′) *n., pl.* **idiot savants** A mentally retarded person who exhibits genius in a highly specialized area, such as mathematics.

id·i·o·type (ĭd′ē-ə-tīp′) *n.* A determinant that confers on an immunoglobulin molecule an antigenic individuality that is analogous to the individuality of the molecule's antibody activity.

id·i·o·ven·tric·u·lar (ĭd′ē-ō-věn-trĭk′yə-lər) *adj.* Relating to or associated with the cardiac ventricles.

idioventricular rhythm *n.* A slow independent cardiac rhythm under control of an ectopic ventricular center. Also called *ventricular rhythm.*

i·dox·u·ri·dine (ī′dŏks-yoͦor′ĭ-dēn′) *n. Abbr.* **IDU** A pyrimidine analog that produces both antiviral and anticancer effects by interfering with DNA synthesis and is used locally for the treatment of keratitis from herpes simplex or vaccinia.

IDU *abbr.* idoxuridine

IF *abbr.* initiation factor

IFN *abbr.* interferon

Ig *abbr.* immunoglobulin

IgA *abbr.* immunoglobulin A

IgD *abbr.* immunoglobulin D

IgE *abbr.* immunoglobulin E

IGF *abbr.* insulinlike growth factor

IgG *abbr.* immunoglobulin G

IgM *abbr.* immunoglobulin M

ig·ni·punc·ture (ĭg′nə-pŭngk′chər) *n.* Surgical closing of a break in the retina due to retinal separation by cauterizing the site of the break with a hot needle.

IH *abbr.* infectious hepatitis

IL *abbr.* interleukin

il–¹ *pref.* Variant of **in–¹**.

il–² *pref.* Variant of **in–²**.

IL-1 *abbr.* interleukin-1

IL-2 *abbr.* interleukin-2

IL-3 *abbr.* interleukin-3

ILA *abbr.* insulinlike activity

Ile *abbr.* isoleucine

il·e·ac¹ (ĭl′ē-ăk′) *adj.* Of, relating to, or having the nature of ileus.

il·e·ac² (ĭl′ē-ăk′) *adj.* Of, relating to, or involving the ileum.

il·e·al (ĭl′ē-əl) *adj.* Of or relating to the ileum.

ileal artery *n.* Any of the arteries with their origin in the superior mesenteric artery, with distribution to the ileum, and with anastomoses to the other branches of the superior mesenteric artery.

ileal veins *pl.n.* See **jejunal and ileal veins.**

il·e·ec·to·my (ĭl′ē-ĕk′tə-mē) *n.* Surgical removal of the ileum.

il·e·i·tis (ĭl′ē-ī′tĭs) *n.* Inflammation of the ileum.

ileo– *pref.* Ileum: *ileotomy.*

il·e·o·ce·cal (ĭl′ē-ō-sē′kəl) *adj.* Relating to the ileum and the cecum.

ileocecal opening *n.* The opening of the terminal ileum into the large intestine at the transition between the cecum and the ascending colon.

ileocecal valve *n.* The bilabial prominence of the terminal ileum into the large intestine at the cecocolic junction in cadavers; it appears as a truncated cone with a star-shaped orifice in the living. Also called *ileocolic valve.*

il·e·o·ce·cos·to·my (ĭl′ē-ō-sē-kŏs′tə-mē) *n.* Surgical construction of an opening between the ileum and the cecum. Also called *cecoileostomy.*

il·e·o·co·lic (ĭl′ē-ō-kō′lĭk, -kŏl′ĭk) *adj.* Relating to the ileum and the colon.

ileocolic artery *n.* An artery with origin in the superior mesenteric artery, with distribution to the terminal part of the ileum, cecum, vermiform appendix, and ascending colon, and with anastomoses to the right colic and ileal arteries.

ileocolic valve *n.* See **ileocecal valve.**

ileocolic vein *n.* A tributary of the superior mesenteric vein that drains the terminal ileum, appendix, cecum, and the lower part of the ascending colon.

il·e·o·co·li·tis (ĭl′ē-ō-kə-lī′tĭs) *n.* Inflammation of the mucous membrane of the ileum and the colon.

ileocolitis ul·cer·o·sa chron·i·ca (ŭl′sə-rō′sə krŏn′ĭ-kə) *n.* A chronic form of ileocolitis characterized by mild intermittent fever, anorexia, anemia, slight diarrhea, dull pain in the iliac region, and rapid pulse.

il·e·o·co·los·to·my (ĭl′ē-ō-kə-lŏs′tə-mē) *n.* Surgical construction of an opening between the ileum and the colon.

il·e·o·cys·to·plas·ty (ĭl′ē-ō-sĭs′tə-plăs′tē) *n.* Surgical reconstruction of the bladder using an isolated intestinal segment to augment bladder capacity.

il·e·o·il·e·os·to·my (ĭl′ē-ō-ĭl′ē-ŏs′tə-mē) *n.* Surgical construction of an opening between two segments of the ileum.

il·e·o·je·ju·ni·tis (ĭl′ē-ō-jə-jōō′nī′tĭs, -jē′jōō-, -jĕj′ōō-) *n.* A chronic inflammatory condition involving the jejunum and parts or most of the ileum.

il·e·o·pex·y (ĭl′ē-ō-pĕk′sē) *n.* Surgical fixation of the ileum.

il·e·o·proc·tos·to·my (ĭl′ē-ō-prŏk-tŏs′tə-mē) *n.* Surgical construction of an opening between the ileum and the rectum.

il·e·or·rha·phy (ĭl′ē-ôr′ə-fē) *n.* Suturing of the ileum.

il·e·o·sig·moid·os·to·my (ĭl′ē-ō-sĭg′moi-dŏs′tə-mē) *n.* Surgical construction of an opening between the ileum and the sigmoid colon.

il·e·os·to·my (ĭl′ē-ŏs′tə-mē) *n.* **1.** Surgical construction of an artificial excretory opening through the abdominal wall into the ileum. **2.** The opening created by such a surgical procedure.

il·e·ot·o·my (ĭl′ē-ŏt′ə-mē) *n.* Incision into the ileum.

il·e·um (ĭl′ē-əm) *n., pl.* **–e·a** (-ē-ə) The third and terminal portion of the small intestine, extending from the jejunum to the cecum.

il·e·us (ĭl′ē-əs) *n.* Intestinal obstruction causing severe colicky pain, vomiting, constipation, and often fever and dehydration.

ileus sub·par·ta (sŭb-pär′tə) *n.* The obstruction of the large intestine by pressure of the pregnant uterus.

il·i·ac (ĭl′ē-ăk′) *adj.* Of, relating to, or situated near the ilium.

iliac artery *n.* **1.** One of two terminal branches of the abdominal aorta, becoming the internal iliac artery and giving off the external iliac artery; common iliac artery. **2.** An artery with its origin in the common iliac artery, with branches to the inferior epigastric and deep circumflex iliac arteries, becoming the femoral artery at the inguinal ligament; external iliac artery. **3.** An artery with its origin in the common iliac artery, with branches to the iliolumbar, lateral sacral, obturator, superior gluteal, inferior gluteal, umbilical, superior vesical, inferior vesical, and middle rectal arteries, usually dividing into anterior and posterior arteries; hypogastric artery, internal iliac artery.

iliac bone *n.* See **ilium.**

iliac bursa *n.* A subtendinous bursa at the insertion of the iliopsoas muscle into the lesser trochanter.

iliac colon *n.* The portion of the descending colon that lies in the left iliac fossa, between the crest of the left ilium and the pelvic brim.

iliac crest *n.* The long, curved upper border of the wing of the ilium.

iliac muscle *n.* A muscle with its origin from the iliac fossa, with insertion to the tendon of the psoas muscle, the anterior surface of the lesser trochanter, and the capsule of the hip joint, with nerve supply from the lumbar plexus, and whose action flexes the thigh and rotates it medially.

iliac region *n.* See **inguinal region.**

ilio– *pref.* Ilium: *iliofemoral.*

il·i·o·coc·cyg·e·al (ĭl′ē-ō-kŏk-sĭj′ē-əl) *adj.* Relating to the ilium and the coccyx.

iliococcygeal muscle *n.* The posterior part of the elevator muscle of the anus.

il·i·o·cos·tal muscle (ĭl′ē-ō-kŏs′təl) *n.* The lateral division of the erector muscle of the spine, having three subdivisions: the lumbar iliocostal muscle, the thoracic iliocostal muscle, and the cervical iliocostal muscle.

il·i·o·fem·o·ral (ĭl′ē-ō-fĕm′ər-əl) *adj.* Relating to the ilium and the femur.

iliofemoral ligament *n.* A triangular ligament attached by its apex to the lower front spine of the ilium and rim of the acetabulum, and by its base to the front intertrochanteric line of the femur. The strong medial band is attached to the lower part of the intertrochanteric line. Also called *Y ligament, Y-shaped ligament.*

iliofemoral triangle *n.* See **Bryant's triangle.**

il·i·o·hy·po·gas·tric nerve (ĭl′ē-ō-hī′pə-găs′trĭk) *n.* A nerve that arises from the first lumbar nerve and supplies the abdominal muscles and the skin of the lower part of the anterior abdominal wall.

il·i·o·in·gui·nal (ĭl′ē-ō-ĭng′gwə-nəl) *adj.* Relating to the inguinal region and the groin.

ilioinguinal nerve *n.* A nerve that arises from the first lumbar nerve, passes through the superficial inguinal ring, and supplies the skin of the upper medial thigh and of the scrotum or of the labia majora.

il·i·o·lum·bar (ĭl′ē-ō-lŭm′bər, -bär′) *adj.* Relating to the iliac and the lumbar regions.

iliolumbar artery *n.* An artery with its origin in the inner branch of the abdominal aorta, with distribution to the pelvic muscles and bones, and with anastomoses to the deep circumflex iliac, obturator, and lumbar arteries.

iliolumbar vein *n.* A vein that accompanies the iliolumbar artery and anastomoses with the lumbar and deep circumflex iliac veins.

il·i·o·pec·tin·e·al (ĭl′ē-ō-pĕk-tĭn′ē-əl) *adj.* Relating to the ilium and the pubic bone.

iliopectineal line *n.* See **terminal line.**

il·i·o·pso·as muscle (ĭl′ē-ō-sō′əs) *n.* A compound muscle consisting of the iliac muscle and the greater psoas muscle.

il·i·o·tib·i·al band (ĭl′ē-ō-tĭb′ē-əl) *n.* A fibrous reinforcement of the broad fascia on the lateral surface of the thigh, extending from the crest of the ilium to the lateral condyle of the tibia.

il·i·o·tro·chan·ter·ic (ĭl′ē-ō-trō′kən-tĕr′ĭk) *adj.* Relating to the ilium and the great trochanter of the femur.

iliotrochanteric ligament *n.* The strong lateral band of the iliofemoral ligament, attached to the tubercle at the upper part of the intertrochanteric line.

il·i·um (ĭl′ē-əm) *n.,* *pl.* **–i·a** (-ē-ə) The uppermost and widest of the three bones constituting either of the lateral halves of the pelvis. Also called *iliac bone.*

ill (ĭl) *adj.* **1.** Not healthy; sick. **2.** Not normal, as a condition; unsound. —*n.* A disease or illness, especially of animals.

ill·ness (ĭl′nĭs) *n.* Disease of body or mind; poor health; sickness.

il·lu·sion (ĭ-loo′zhən) *n.* **1.** An erroneous perception of reality. **2.** An erroneous concept or belief. **3.** The condition of being deceived by a false perception or belief. **4.** Something, such as a fantastic plan or desire, that causes an erroneous belief or perception. —**il·lu′sion·al,** **il·lu′sion·ar′y** (-zhə-nĕr′ē) *adj.*

IM *abbr.* internal medicine; intramuscular

im–[1] *pref.* Variant of **in–**[1].

im–[2] *pref.* Variant of **in–**[2].

im·age (ĭm′ĭj) *n.* **1.** An optically formed duplicate or other representative reproduction of an object, especially an optical reproduction of an object formed by a lens or mirror. **2.** A mental picture of something not real or present. **3.** An exact copy of data in a computer file transferred to another medium. —*v.* **1.** To make or produce a likeness of. **2.** To picture something mentally; imagine. **3.** To translate photographs or other pictures by computer into numbers that can be transmitted to a remote location and then reconverted into pictures by another computer. **4.** To visualize something, as by magnetic resonance imaging.

im·age·ry (ĭm′ĭj-rē) *n.* **1.** A set of mental pictures or images. **2.** A technique in behavior therapy in which the patient is conditioned to use pleasant fantasies to counteract the unpleasant feelings associated with anxiety.

im·ag·ing (ĭm′ĭ-jĭng) *n.* **1.** Visualization of internal body organs, tissues, or cavities using specialized instruments and techniques for diagnostic purposes. **2.** The use of mental images to influence bodily processes, especially to control pain.

i·ma·go (ĭ-mā′gō, ĭ-mä′-) *n.,* *pl.* **–goes** *or* **–gi·nes** (-gə-nēz′) **1.** An insect in its sexually mature adult stage after metamorphosis. **2.** An often idealized image of a person, usually a parent, that is formed in childhood and persists unconsciously into adulthood. **3.** See **archetype** (sense 2).

im·bal·ance (ĭm-băl′əns) *n.* **1.** A lack of balance, as in distribution or functioning. **2.** Lack of equality in some aspect of binocular vision, as in strabismus.

im·be·cile (ĭm′bə-sĭl, -səl) *n.* A person of moderate to severe mental retardation having a mental age of from three to seven years and generally being capable of some degree of communication and performance of simple tasks under supervision. The term belongs to a classification system no longer in use and is now considered offensive. —**im′be·cil′i·ty** (-sĭl′ĭ-tē) *n.*

im·bi·bi·tion (ĭm′bə-bĭsh′ən) *n.* Absorption of fluid by a solid or colloid that results in swelling.

im·bri·cate (ĭm′brĭ-kāt′) *or* **im·bri·cat·ed** (-kā′tĭd) *adj.* Having the edges overlapping in a regular arrangement like roof tiles or the scales of a fish. —**im′bri·ca′tion** *n.*

imid– *or* **imido–** *pref.* Imide: *imidazole.*

im·id·az·ole (ĭm′ĭ-dăz′ōl′) *n.* An organic crystalline base that is an inhibitor of histamine.

im·ide (ĭm′īd′) *n.* A compound derived from ammonia and containing the bivalent NH group combined with a bivalent acid group or two monovalent acid groups.

im·i·do (ĭm′ĭ-dō′) *adj.* Of or relating to imides or an imide.

im·i·dole (ĭm′ĭ-dōl′) *n.* See **pyrrole.**

im·ine (ĭm′ēn, -ĭn, ĭ-mēn′) *n.* A compound derived from ammonia and containing the bivalent NH group combined with a bivalent nonacid group.

im·i·no (ĭm′ə-nō′) *adj.* Of or relating to imines or an imine.

imino– *pref.* Imine: *iminoglycinuria.*

imino acid *n.* Any of various organic acids occasionally occurring as intermediates in the metabolism of amino acids and containing both an acid group and a bivalent imino group.

im·i·no·gly·ci·nu·ri·a (ĭm′ə-nō-glī′sə-nŏor′ē-ə) *n.* A benign inborn error of amino acid transport, causing glycine, proline, and hydroxyproline to be excreted in the urine.

i·mip·ra·mine hydrochloride (ĭ-mĭp′rə-mēn′) *n.* A tricyclic antidepressant drug also used to treat enuresis.

imipramine pam·o·ate (păm′ō-āt′) *n.* A tricyclic antidepressant drug also used to treat enuresis.

Im·i·trex (ĭm′ĭ-trĕks′) A trademark for the drug sumatriptan and its succinate form.

im·ma·ture (ĭm′ə-choor′, -toor′) *adj.* Not fully grown or developed.

immature cataract *n.* Partial opacity of the lens.

im·me·di·ate allergy (ĭ-mē′dē-ĭt) *n.* Hypersensitivity that becomes evident within seconds or minutes after contact with an antigen, reaches its peak within an hour or so, then recedes.

immediate auscultation *n.* The direct application of an examiner's ear to the surface of a patient's body in order to listen to the internal sounds of the body.

immediate denture *n.* A complete or partial denture constructed for insertion immediately following the removal of natural teeth.

immediate flap *n.* See **direct flap.**

immediate percussion *n.* Percussion performed directly with the finger or a plexor, without the intervention of another finger or pleximeter. Also called *direct percussion.*

immediate reaction *n.* An allergic or immune response that begins within a period lasting from a few minutes to about an hour after exposure to an antigen to which the individual has been sensitized.

immediate transfusion *n.* See **direct transfusion.**

im·med·i·ca·ble (ĭ-mĕd′ĭ-kə-bəl) *adj.* Incurable.

im·mer·sion (ĭ-mûr′zhən, -shən) *n.* **1.** The placing of a body under water or other liquid. **2.** The use of a fluid on a microscope slide in order to exclude air from between the glass slide and the bottom lens. —**im·merse′** (ĭ-mûrs′) *v.*

immersion foot *n.* See **trench foot.**

immersion objective *n.* A high-powered objective used with a liquid between the lens and the specimen on the slide.

im·mis·ci·ble (ĭ-mĭs′ə-bəl) *adj.* Incapable of being mixed or blended, as oil and water. —**im·mis′ci·bil′i·ty** *n.*

im·mo·bile (ĭ-mō′bəl, -bēl′, -bīl′) *adj.* **1.** Immovable; fixed. **2.** Not moving; motionless. —**im′mo·bil′i·ty** (-bĭl′-ĭ-tē) *n.*

im·mo·bi·lize (ĭ-mō′bə-līz′) *v.* **1.** To render immobile. **2.** To fix the position of a joint or fractured limb, as with a splint or a cast. —**im·mo′bi·li·za′tion** (-lĭ-zā′shən) *n.*

im·mo·tile (ĭ-mōt′l, ĭ-mō′tīl′) *adj.* Not moving or lacking the ability to move.

immotile cilia syndrome *n.* An inherited syndrome caused by the absence of dynein structures and the subsequent inability of cilia to beat effectively and marked by recurrent sinopulmonary infections, reduced fertility in women, and sterility in men.

im·mov·a·ble joint (ĭ-mo͞o′və-bəl) *n.* A union of two bones by fibrous tissue, such as a syndesmosis or gomphosis, in which there is no joint cavity and little motion is possible. Also called *fibrous joint, synarthrodia, synarthrodial joint, synarthrosis.*

im·mune (ĭ-myo͞on′) *adj.* **1.** Of, relating to, or having resistance to infection by a specific pathogen. **2.** Relating to the mechanism of sensitization in which the reactivity is so altered by previous contact with an antigen that the responsive tissues respond quickly upon subsequent contact.

immune adsorption *n.* **1.** The removal of antibody from antiserum by specific antigen, with aggregation of the antigen-antibody complex followed by separation of that complex by means of centrifugation or filtration. **2.** The similar removal of antigen by a specific antiserum.

immune body *n.* Antibody. No longer in technical use.

immune complex *n.* Any of various complexes of an antigen and an antibody in the blood, to which complement may also be fixed, and which may form a precipitate.

immune complex disease *n.* A disease caused by the deposition of antigen-antibody or antigen-antibody-complement complexes on the surface of cells, resulting in the development of chronic or acute inflammation, which may be manifested by vasculitis, endocarditis, neuritis, or glomerulonephritis.

immune deficiency *n.* See **immunodeficiency.**

immune electron microscopy *n.* The use of an electron microscope to examine viral specimens bound to specific antibody.

immune fetal hydrops *n.* A combination of edema and ascites in a fetus, due to erythroblastosis fetalis.

immune reaction *n.* The reaction resulting from the recognition and binding of an antigen by its specific antibody or by a previously sensitized lymphocyte. Also called *immunoreaction.*

immune response *n.* An integrated bodily response to an antigen, especially one mediated by lymphocytes and involving recognition of antigens by specific antibodies or previously sensitized lymphocytes.

immune response gene *n.* A gene in the major histocompatibility complex that controls a cell's immune response to specific antigens.

immune serum *n.* See **antiserum.**

immune serum globulin *n.* A sterile solution of globulins derived from pooled human blood that contains antibodies that are normally present in the blood of adults, used as a passive immunizing agent against rubella, measles, and hepatitis A and as treatment for hypogammaglobulinemia.

immune surveillance *n.* See **immunological surveillance.**

immune system *n.* The integrated body system of organs, tissues, cells, and cell products that differentiates self from nonself and neutralizes potentially pathogenic organisms or substances.

immune thrombocytopenic purpura *n.* See **idiopathic thrombocytopenic purpura.**

im·mu·ni·fa·cient (ĭ-myo͞o′nə-fā′shənt) *adj.* Producing immunity.

im·mu·ni·ty (ĭ-myo͞o′nĭ-tē) *n.* **1.** The quality or condition of being immune. **2.** Inherited, acquired, or induced resistance to infection by a specific pathogen.

im·mu·nize (ĭm′yə-nīz′) *v.* **1.** To render immune. **2.** To produce immunity in, as by inoculation. —**im′mu·ni·za′tion** (-nĭ-zā′shən) *n.*

immuno– *pref.* Immune; immunity: *immunohistochemistry.*

im·mu·no·ad·ju·vant (ĭm′yə-nō-ăj′ə-vənt, ĭ-myo͞o′-) *n.* See **adjuvant** (sense **?**).

im·mu·no·as·say (ĭm′yə-nō-ăs′ā, ĭ-myo͞o′-) *n.* A laboratory or clinical technique that uses the specific binding between an antigen and its homologous antibody to identify and quantify a substance in a sample. Also called *immunochemical assay.*

im·mu·no·blast (ĭm′yə-nō-blăst′, ĭ-myo͞o′-) *n.* An antigenically stimulated white blood cell.

im·mu·no·blas·tic lymphadenopathy (ĭm′yə-nō-blăs′tĭc, ĭ-myo͞o′-) *n.* See **angioimmunoblastic lymphadenopathy.**

im·mu·no·blot (ĭm′yə-nō-blŏt′, ĭ-myo͞o′-) *n.* A laboratory procedure, such as Western blot analysis, in which proteins that have been separated by electrophoresis are transferred onto nitrocellulose sheets and are identified by their reaction with labeled antibodies.

im·mu·no·chem·i·cal assay (ĭm′yə-nō-kĕm′ĭ-kəl, ĭ-myo͞o′-) *n.* See **immunoassay.**

im·mu·no·chem·is·try (ĭm′yə-nō-kĕm′ĭ-strē, ĭ-myo͞o′-) *n.* The chemistry of immunologic phenomena, as of antigen-antibody reactions.

im·mu·no·com·pe·tent (ĭm′yə-nō-kŏm′pĭ-tənt, ĭ-myo͞o′-) *adj.* Having the normal bodily capacity to develop an immune response following exposure to an antigen. —**im′mu·no·com′pe·tence** *n.*

im·mu·no·com·pro·mised (ĭm′yə-nō-kŏm′prə-mīzd, ĭ-myo͞o′-) *adj.* Incapable of developing a normal immune response, usually as a result of disease, malnutrition, or immunosuppressive therapy.

im·mu·no·con·glu·ti·nin (ĭm′yə-nō-kŏn-glo͞ot′n-ĭn, ĭ-myo͞o′-) *n.* An autoantibodylike immunoglobulin formed in animals or in humans against their own complement after injection of complexes that contain complement or of sensitized bacteria.

im·mu·no·cyte (ĭm′yə-nō-sīt′, ĭ-myo͞o′-) *n.* A white blood cell capable of producing antibodies.

im·mu·no·cy·to·chem·is·try (ĭm′yə-nō-sī′tō-kĕm′ĭ-strē, ĭ-myoō′-) *n.* The study of cell constituents by immunologic methods, such as the use of fluorescent antibodies.

im·mu·no·de·fi·cien·cy (ĭm′yə-nō-dĭ-fĭsh′ən-sē, ĭ-myoō′-) *n.* A disorder or deficiency of the normal immune response. Also called *immune deficiency.* —**im′·mu·no·de·fi′cient** *adj.*

immunodeficiency syndrome *n.* A syndrome associated with an immunological deficiency or disorder and characterized primarily by an increased susceptibility to infection.

im·mu·no·de·pres·sion (ĭm′yə-nō-dĭ-prĕsh′ən, ĭ-myoō′-) *n.* See **immunosuppression.**

im·mu·no·dif·fu·sion (ĭm′yə-nō-dĭ-fyoō′zhən, ĭ-myoō′-) *n.* A technique for studying reactions between antigens and antibodies by observing precipitates formed by the combination of specific antigens and antibodies that have diffused in a gel in which they have been separately placed.

im·mu·no·e·lec·tro·pho·re·sis (ĭm′yə-nō-ĭ-lĕk′trə-fə-rē′sĭs, ĭ-myoō′-) *n.* The separation and identification of proteins based on differences in their electrophoretic mobility through agar or a similar medium and in their reactivity with antibodies.

im·mu·no·en·hance·ment (ĭm′yə-nō-ĕn-hăns′mənt, ĭ-myoō′-) *n.* The potentiating effect of immunoenhancers such as specific antibodies in establishing or in delaying rejection of an allograft.

im·mu·no·en·hanc·er (ĭm′yə-nō-ĕn-hăn′sər, ĭ-myoō′-) *n.* A substance that increases an immune response.

im·mu·no·fluo·res·cence (ĭm′yə-nō-floō-rĕs′əns, -flô-, ĭ-myoō′-) *n.* Any of various methods that use antibodies chemically linked to a fluorescent dye to identify or quantify antigens in a tissue sample.

im·mu·no·fluo·res·cent stain (ĭm′yə-nō-floō-rĕs′ənt, -flô-, ĭ-myoō′-) *n.* A staining method in which an antibody or antigen combines selectively with a fluorescent substance, thus labeling the immunogenic substance and indicating its presence.

im·mu·no·gen (ĭm′yə-nə-jən, -jĕn′, ĭ-myoō′-) *n.* See **antigen.**

im·mu·no·ge·net·ics (ĭm′yə-nō-jə-nĕt′ĭks) *n.* The branch of immunology that is concerned with the molecular and genetic basis of the immune response. —**im′mu·no·ge·net′i·cist** (-ĭ-sĭst) *n.*

im·mu·no·gen·ic (ĭm′yə-nō-jĕn′ĭk, ĭ-myoō′-) *adj.* Producing an immune response.

im·mu·no·ge·nic·i·ty (ĭm′yə-nō-jə-nĭs′ĭ-tē, ĭ-myoō′-) *n.* See **antigenicity.**

im·mu·no·glob·u·lin (ĭm′yə-nō-glŏb′yə-lĭn, ĭ-myoō′-) *n. Abbr.* **Ig** Any of a group of large glycoproteins secreted by plasma cells in vertebrates that function as antibodies in the immune response by binding the specific antigens.

immunoglobulin A *n. Abbr.* **IgA** The class of antibodies produced predominantly against ingested antigens, found in body secretions such as saliva, sweat, and tears, and functioning to prevent attachment of viruses and bacteria to epithelial surfaces.

immunoglobulin D *n. Abbr.* **IgD** The class of antibodies found only on the surface of B cells and possibly func-

tioning as antigen receptors to initiate differentiation of B cells into plasma cells.

immunoglobulin E *n. Abbr.* **IgE** The class of antibodies produced in the lungs, skin, and mucous membranes and responsible for allergic reactions.

immunoglobulin G *n. Abbr.* **IgG** The most abundant class of antibodies found in blood serum and lymph and active against bacteria, fungi, viruses, and foreign particles. Immunoglobulin G antibodies trigger action of the complement system.

immunoglobulin M *n. Abbr.* **IgM** The class of antibodies found in circulating body fluids and the first antibodies to appear in response to an initial exposure to an antigen.

im·mu·no·his·to·chem·is·try (ĭm′yə-nō-hĭs′tō-kĕm′-ĭ-strē, ĭ-myoō′-) *n.* Microscopic localization of specific antigens in tissues by staining with antibodies labeled with fluorescent or pigmented material.

immunological mechanism *n.* The collection of cells, chiefly lymphocytes and cells of the reticuloendothelial system, that function in establishing active acquired immunity. Also called *defense mechanism.*

immunological paralysis *n.* Lack of specific antibody production after exposure to large doses of the antigen.

immunological surveillance *n.* A theory that the immune system continually recognizes and removes malignant cells that arise during one's life. Also called *immune surveillance.*

immunological tolerance *n.* Acquired specific failure of the immunological mechanism to respond to a given antigen, induced by exposure to the antigen.

immunologic pregnancy test *n.* Any of various pregnancy tests to detect increased human chorionic gonadotropin in plasma or urine by immunologic methods such as latex particle agglutination, radioimmunoassay, and radioreceptor assays.

im·mu·nol·o·gist (ĭm′yə-nŏl′ə-jĭst) *n.* A specialist in immunology.

im·mu·nol·o·gy (ĭm′yə-nŏl′ə-jē) *n.* The branch of biomedicine that is concerned with the structure and function of the immune system, innate and acquired immunity, and laboratory techniques involving the interaction of antigens with antibodies. —**im′mu·no·log′ic** (-nə-lŏj′ĭk), **im′mu·no·log′i·cal** *adj.*

im·mu·no·per·ox·i·dase technique (ĭm′yə-nō-pə-rŏk′sĭ-dās′, -dāz′, ĭ-myoō′-) *n.* An enzymatic antigen detection technique that uses horseradish peroxidase to label antigen-antibody complexes in tissues and is commonly used in pathology to demonstrate hormones, unique tissue-specific antigens, structural proteins, tissue enzymes, oncofetal antigens, and microorganisms and viruses.

im·mu·no·po·ten·ti·a·tion (ĭm′yə-nō-pə-tĕn′shē-ā′-shən, ĭ-myoō′-) *n.* Enhancement of the immune response by increasing the speed and extent of its development and by prolonging its duration.

im·mu·no·po·ten·ti·a·tor (ĭm′yə-nō-pə-tĕn′shē-ā′tər, ĭ-myoō′-) *n.* An agent that on inoculation enhances the immune response.

im·mu·no·pre·cip·i·ta·tion (ĭm′yə-nō-prĭ-sĭp′ĭ-tā′-shən, ĭ-myoō′-) *n.* The precipitation of sensitized antigen as the result of the interaction of antigen with a specific antibody in solution.

im·mu·no·pro·lif·er·a·tive disorder (ĭm′yə-nō-prə-lĭf′ə-rā′tĭv, ĭ-myōō′-) *n.* A disorder characterized by the production of an abnormally high number of antibody-producing cells, especially those associated with autoallergic disturbances and gamma-globulin abnormalities.

im·mu·no·re·ac·tion (ĭm′yə-nō-rē-ăk′shən, ĭ-myōō′-) *n.* See **immune reaction.** —**im′mu·no·re·ac′tive** (-tĭv) *adj.* —**im′mu·no·re′ac·tiv/i·ty** *n.*

im·mu·no·sor·bent (ĭm′yə-nō-zôr′bənt, ĭ-myōō′-) *n.* An antibody used to remove specific antigen, or an antigen used to remove specific antibody, from solution or suspension.

im·mu·no·stim·u·lant (ĭm′yə-nō-stĭm′yə-lənt, ĭ-myōō′-) *n.* An agent that stimulates the immune system.

im·mu·no·sup·pres·sant (ĭm′yə-nō-sə-prĕs′ənt, ĭ-myōō′-) *n.* An agent that suppresses the body's immune response.

im·mu·no·sup·pres·sion (ĭm′yə-nō-sə-prĕsh′ən, ĭ-myōō′-) *n.* Suppression of the immune response, as by drugs or radiation, in order to prevent the rejection of grafts or transplants or to control autoimmune diseases. Also called *immunodepression.* —**im′mu·no·sup·pres/sive** *adj.*

im·mu·no·ther·a·py (ĭm′yə-nō-thĕr′ə-pē, ĭ-myōō′-) *n.* Treatment of disease by inducing, enhancing, or suppressing an immune response. —**im′mu·no·ther′a·peu/tic** (-pyōō′tĭk) *adj.* —**im′mu·no·ther′a·pist** *n.*

im·mu·no·tox·in (ĭm′yə-nō-tŏk′sĭn, ĭ-myōō′-) *n.* A hybrid molecule formed by binding a toxin to a monoclonal antibody, used to destroy tumor cells.

im·mu·no·trans·fu·sion (ĭm′yə-nō-trăns-fyōō′zhən, ĭ-myōō′-) *n.* A transfusion of blood from a donor who has been immunized by injections of an antigen prepared from microorganisms isolated from the recipient; the recipient then gains passive immunity from the antibodies formed in the donor.

I·mo·di·um (ĭ-mō′dē-əm) A trademark for the drug loperamide.

im·pact·ed (ĭm-păk′tĭd) *adj.* **1.** Wedged together at the broken ends. Used of a fractured bone. **2.** Placed in the alveolus in a manner prohibiting eruption into a normal position. Used of a tooth. **3.** Packed in or wedged in such a manner so as to fill or block an organ or a passage.

impacted fetus *n.* A fetus that because of its large size or narrowing of the pelvic canal has become wedged and incapable of spontaneous advance or recession.

impacted fracture *n.* A bone fracture in which one of the fragments is driven into another fragment.

im·pac·tion (ĭm-păk′shən) *n.* The process or condition of being impacted.

im·paired (ĭm-pârd′) *adj.* Having a physical or mental disability.

im·pair·ment (ĭm-pâr′mənt) *n.* Weakening, damage, or deterioration, especially as a result of injury or disease. —**im·pair/** *v.*

im·par (ĭm′pär) *adj.* Of, relating to, or being an unpaired anatomical part.

im·pat·ent (ĭm-păt′nt, -pāt′nt) *adj.* Not open; closed.

im·ped·i·ment (ĭm-pĕd′ə-mənt) *n.* **1.** Something that impedes; a hindrance or an obstruction. **2.** An organic defect preventing clear articulation of speech.

im·per·fect fungus (ĭm-pûr′fĭkt) *n.* Any of various fungi of the phylum Fungi Imperfecti, including *Aspergillus, Candida, Cryptococcus,* and other human pathogens.

imperfect stage *n.* The asexual phase in the life cycle of a fungus.

im·per·fo·rate (ĭm-pûr′fər-ĭt) *adj.* Lacking a normal opening.

imperforate anus *n.* See **anal atresia.**

im·per·fo·ra·tion (ĭm-pûr′fə-rā′shən) *n.* The condition of being abnormally occluded or closed.

im·per·me·a·ble (ĭm-pûr′mē-ə-bəl) *adj.* Impossible to permeate; not permitting passage. —**im·per′me·a·bil/i·ty, im·per′me·a·ble·ness** *n.*

im·pe·tig·i·nous (ĭm′pĭ-tĭj′ə-nəs) *adj.* Of or relating to impetigo.

im·pe·ti·go (ĭm′pĭ-tī′gō) *n., pl.* **-gos** A contagious skin infection caused by staphylococcal or streptococcal bacteria and characterized by the eruption of superficial pustules that rupture and form thick yellow crusts, usually on the face; it is most commonly seen in children. Also called *impetigo contagiosa, impetigo vulgaris.*

impetigo her·pet·i·for·mis (hər-pĕt′ə-fôr′mĭs) *n.* A rare pyoderma occurring most commonly in pregnant women as an eruption of small, closely aggregated pustules accompanied by fever and fatigue.

impetigo ne·o·na·to·rum (nē′ō-nā-tôr′əm) *n.* A skin disorder in infants characterized by widely disseminated bullous lesions appearing soon after birth and caused by staphylococcal infection, occasionally complicated by streptococcal infection. Also called *dermatitis exfoliativa infantum, pemphigus gangrenosus.*

impetigo vul·gar·is (vŭl-gâr′ĭs) *n.* See **impetigo.**

im·pinge·ment syndrome (ĭm-pĭnj′mənt) *n.* A group of symptoms in the shoulder including progressive pain and impaired function, resulting from injury to the rotator cuff caused by encroachment of surrounding bony structures and ligaments.

im·plant (ĭm-plănt′) *v.* **1.** To insert or embed an object or a device surgically. **2.** To graft or insert a tissue within the body. **3.** To become attached to and embedded in the uterine lining. Used of a fertilized egg. —*n.* (ĭm′plănt′) Something implanted, especially a surgically implanted tissue or device.

im·plan·ta·tion (ĭm′plăn-tā′shən) *n.* **1.** The act or an instance of implanting. **2.** The condition of being implanted. **3.** The process by which a fertilized egg implants in the uterine lining.

implant denture *n.* A denture that receives its stability from a substructure which is partially or wholly implanted in the bone under the soft tissues.

im·plant·ed suture (ĭm-plăn′tĭd) *n.* A suture created by passing a pin through each lip of a wound, parallel to the line of incision, and then looping the pins together with stitches.

im·plo·sion (ĭm-plō′zhən) *n.* **1.** A type of behavior therapy in which the patient is repeatedly subjected to anxiety-arousing stimuli while the therapist attempts to extinguish the patient's anxiety and anxious behavior and replace them with more appropriate responses. **2.** A bursting inward rather than outward.

im·po·tence (ĭm′pə-təns) *or* **im·po·ten·cy** (-tən-sē) *n.* **1.** The quality or condition of being impotent. **2.** See **erectile dysfunction.**

im·po·tent (ĭm′pə-tənt) *adj.* **1.** Incapable of sexual intercourse, often because of an inability to achieve or sustain an erection. **2.** Sterile. Used of males.

im·preg·nate (ĭm-prĕg′nāt) *v.* **1.** To make pregnant; to cause to conceive; inseminate. **2.** To fertilize an ovum. **3.** To fill throughout; saturate. —**im′preg·na′tion** *n.* —**im·preg′na′tor** *n.*

im·pres·sion (ĭm-prĕsh′ən) *n.* **1.** An effect, a feeling, or an image retained as a consequence of experience. **2.** A mark or indentation made by the pressure of one organ on the surface of another. **3.** An imprint of the teeth and surrounding tissues, formed with a plastic material that hardens into a mold for use in making dentures, inlays, or plastic models.

im·pres·sive aphasia (ĭm-prĕs′ĭv) *n.* See **sensory aphasia.**

im·print·ing (ĭm′prĭn′tĭng) *n.* A learning process occurring early in the life of a social animal in which a specific behavior pattern is established through association with a parent or other role model.

im·pulse (ĭm′pŭls′) *n.* **1.** A sudden pushing or driving force. **2.** A sudden wish or urge that prompts an unpremeditated act or feeling; an abrupt inclination. **3.** The electrochemical transmission of a signal along a nerve fiber that produces an excitatory or inhibitory response at a target tissue.

impulse control disorder *n.* Any of various types of mental disorders, such as substance abuse and pathological gambling, characterized by a tendency to gratify an immediate desire or impulse regardless of the consequences to one's self or to others.

im·pul·sion (ĭm-pŭl′shən) *n.* An urge to perform certain actions without regard for internal or social constraints.

im·pul·sive (ĭm-pŭl′sĭv) *adj.* **1.** Inclined or tending to act on impulse rather than thought. **2.** Motivated by or resulting from impulse. —**im·pul′sive·ness, im′pul·siv′i·ty** *n.*

im·pure flutter (ĭm-pyŏor′) *n.* A mixture of atrial flutter and fibrillation waves in the electrocardiogram.

Im·u·ran (ĭm′yə-răn′) A trademark for the drug azathioprine.

IMV *abbr.* intermittent mandatory ventilation

In The symbol for the element **indium.**

in–[1] *or* **il–** *or* **im–** *or* **ir–** *pref.* Not: *invertebrate.* Before *l,* **in–** is usually assimilated to *il-,* before *r* to *ir-,* and before *b, m,* and *p* to *im-.*

in–[2] *or* **il–** *or* **im–** *or* **ir–** *pref.* In; into; within: *intubation.* Before *l,* **in–** is usually assimilated to *il-,* before *r* to *ir-,* and before *b, m,* and *p* to *im-.*

–in *suff.* **1.** Neutral chemical compound: *inulin.* **2.** Pharmaceutical: *rifampin.* **3.** Antibiotic: *penicillin.* **4.** Antigen: *tuberculin.* **5.** Variant of –ine (sense 1).

in·ac·ti·vate (ĭn-ăk′tə-vāt′) *v.* **1.** To render nonfunctional. **2.** To make quiescent. —**in·ac′ti·va′tion** *n.*

in·ac·ti·vat·ed poliovirus vaccine (ĭn-ăk′tə-vā′tĭd) *n. Abbr.* **IPV** See **poliovirus vaccine** (sense 1).

in·ac·tive repressor (ĭn-ăk′tĭv) *n.* See **aporepressor.**

in·ad·e·quate personality (ĭn-ăd′ĭ-kwĭt) *n.* A personality disturbance characterized by an inability to cope with the social, emotional, occupational, and intellectual demands of life.

inadequate stimulus *n.* A stimulus too weak to evoke a response. Also called *subthreshold stimulus.*

in·an·i·mate (ĭn-ăn′ə-mĭt) *adj.* Not having the qualities associated with active, living organisms; not animate. —**in·an′i·mate·ness** *n.*

in·a·ni·tion (ĭn′ə-nĭsh′ən) *n.* Exhaustion, as from lack of nourishment or vitality.

in·ap·pe·tence (ĭn-ăp′ĭ-təns) *n.* Lack of desire or appetite. —**in·ap′pe·tent** *adj.*

in·ar·tic·u·late (ĭn′är-tĭk′yə-lĭt) *adj.* **1.** Uttered without the use of normal words or syllables; incomprehensible as speech or language. **2.** Unable to speak; speechless. **3.** Unable to speak with clarity or eloquence. **4.** Not having joints or segments. —**in′ar·tic′u·late·ness, in′ar·tic′u·la·cy** (-lə-sē) *n.*

in·as·sim·i·la·ble (ĭn′ə-sĭm′ə-lə-bəl) *adj.* Not capable of being utilized for the nutrition of the body.

in·born (ĭn′bôrn′) *adj.* **1.** Possessed by an organism at birth. **2.** Inherited or hereditary.

inborn error of metabolism *n.* Any of a group of congenital disorders caused by an inherited defect in a single specific enzyme that results in a disruption or abnormality in a specific metabolic pathway.

in·bred (ĭn′brĕd′) *adj.* **1.** Produced by inbreeding. **2.** Fixed in the character or disposition as if inherited; deep-seated.

in·breed·ing (ĭn′brē′dĭng) *n.* **1.** See **homogamy. 2.** The continued breeding of closely related individuals so as to preserve desirable traits in a stock.

in·car·cer·at·ed (ĭn-kär′sə-rā′tĭd) *adj.* Trapped or confined, as a hernia.

incarcerated hernia *n.* See **irreducible hernia.**

in·cest (ĭn′sĕst′) *n.* **1.** Sexual relations between persons who are so closely related that their marriage is illegal or forbidden by custom. **2.** The statutory crime of sexual relations with such a near relative.

in·ces·tu·ous (ĭn-sĕs′chōo-əs) *adj.* **1.** Of, involving, or suggestive of incest. **2.** Having committed incest.

in·ci·dence (ĭn′sĭ-dəns) *n.* **1.** The extent or rate of occurrence, especially the number of new cases of a disease in a population over a period of time. **2.** The arrival of radiation or a projectile at a surface. —**in′ci·dent** *adj.*

in·ci·den·tal parasite (ĭn′sĭ-dĕn′tl) *n.* A parasite living on a host other than its normal host.

incident point *n.* The point at which a light ray enters an optical system.

in·ci·sal (ĭn-sī′zəl) *adj.* Relating to the cutting edges of the incisor and cuspid teeth.

incisal guide angle *n.* The angle formed with the horizontal plane by drawing a line in the sagittal plane between incisal edges of the maxillary and the mandibular central incisors when the teeth are in centric occlusion.

in·cise (ĭn-sīz′) v. To cut into with a sharp instrument.

in·cised wound (ĭn-sīzd′) n. A wound characterized by a clean cut, as by a sharp instrument.

in·ci·sion (ĭn-sĭzh′ən) n. **1.** A cut into a body tissue or organ, especially one made during surgery. **2.** The scar resulting from such a cut.

in·ci·sion·al hernia (ĭn-sĭzh′ə-nəl) n. A hernia occurring through an incision or scar.

incision biopsy n. Removal of only a part of a lesion for gross and microscopic examination.

in·ci·sive (ĭn-sī′sĭv) adj. **1.** Having the power to cut. **2.** Relating to the incisor teeth.

incisive bone n. The anterior and inner portion of the upper jawbone. Also called *intermaxillary bone, premaxillary bone.*

incisive canal n. Any of several bony canals that lead from the floor of the nasal cavity into the incisive fossa on the palatal surface of the maxilla and convey the nasopalatine nerves and branches of the greater palatine arteries. Also called *incisor canal.*

incisive foramen n. Any of usually four openings of the incisive canals into the incisive fossa of the hard palate.

incisive fossa n. The depression in the midline of the bony palate behind the central incisors into which the incisive canals open.

incisive papilla n. A slight elevation of the mucosa at the front extremity of the raphe of the palate.

in·ci·sor (ĭn-sī′zər) n. Any of the four teeth adapted for cutting or gnawing, having a chisel-shaped crown and a single conical root and located in the front part of both jaws in both deciduous and permanent dentitions.

incisor canal n. See **incisive canal.**

in·ci·sure (ĭn-sī′zhər) n. An indentation at the edge of a structure; a notch. —**in·ci′su·ral** adj.

in·cli·na·tion (ĭn′klə-nā′shən) n. **1.** A deviation or the degree of deviation from the horizontal or vertical; a slant. **2.** The deviation of the long axis of a tooth from perpendicular. **3.** A tendency toward a certain condition or character. **4.** A characteristic disposition to do, prefer, or favor one thing rather than another; a propensity.

in·clu·sion (ĭn-kloō′zhən) n. **1.** A nonliving mass, such as a droplet of fat, in the cytoplasm of a cell. **2.** The process by which a foreign or heterogenous structure is misplaced in another tissue.

inclusion body n. An abnormal structure in a cell nucleus or cytoplasm having characteristic staining properties and associated especially with certain viral infections, such as rabies and smallpox.

inclusion body disease n. See **cytomegalic inclusion disease.**

inclusion body encephalitis n. A usually fatal disease that appears to result from persistent measles virus infection, causing inflammation in both the white and gray matter and characterized by the presence of nuclear inclusion bodies.

inclusion cell n. A cultured skin fibroblast containing membrane-bound inclusions. Also called *I cell.*

inclusion cell disease n. See **mucolipidosis II.**

inclusion conjunctivitis n. A conjunctivitis caused by *Chlamydia trachomatis* and often affecting newborns but also contracted by adults in swimming pools or from sexual contact, characterized by enlarged papilla on the inner eyelids and purulent discharge. Also called *swimming pool conjunctivitis.*

in·com·pat·i·ble (ĭn′kəm-păt′ə-bəl) adj. **1.** Incapable of associating or blending or of being associated or blended because of disharmony, incongruity, or antagonism. **2.** Producing an undesirable effect when used in combination with a particular substance, as a medicine in combination with alcohol. **3.** Not suitable for combination or administration because of immunological differences, as blood types. —**in′com·pat·i·bil′i·ty** (ĭn′kəm-păt′ə-bĭl′ĭ-tē) n.

in·com·pe·tence (ĭn-kŏm′pĭ-təns) or **in·com·pe·ten·cy** (-tən-sē) n. **1.** The quality of being incompetent or incapable of performing a function, as the failure of the cardiac valves to close properly. **2.** The condition of being not legally qualified, as to stand trial. **3.** The inability to distinguish right from wrong or to manage one's affairs.

in·com·pe·tent (ĭn-kŏm′pĭ-tənt) adj. **1.** Inadequate for or unsuited to a particular purpose or application. **2.** Incapable of proper functioning. **3.** Not qualified in legal terms.

incompetent cervical os n. A defect in the muscular ring at the isthmus of the uterus, allowing premature dilation of the cervix during pregnancy.

in·com·plete abortion (ĭn′kəm-plēt′) n. Abortion in which all of the products of conception are not expelled from the uterus.

incomplete antibody n. See **serum agglutinin.**

incomplete antigen n. See **hapten.**

incomplete dominance n. A heterozygous condition in which both alleles at a gene locus are partially expressed and which often produces an intermediate phenotype.

incomplete fistula n. See **blind fistula.**

incomplete foot presentation n. Breech presentation of the fetus during birth in which a single foot is the presenting part.

incomplete fracture n. A fracture in which the line of fracture does not include the entire bone.

in·con·stant (ĭn-kŏn′stənt) adj. **1.** Changing or varying, especially often and without discernible pattern or reason. **2.** Relating to a structure that normally may or may not be present.

in·con·ti·nence (ĭn-kŏn′tə-nəns) n. **1.** The inability to control excretory functions. **2.** Lack of restraint in sexual relations; immoderation.

in·con·ti·nent (ĭn-kŏn′tə-nənt) adj. **1.** Lacking normal voluntary control of excretory functions. **2.** Lacking sexual restraint; unchaste.

in·con·ti·nen·tia pig·men·ti (ĭn-kŏn′tə-nĕn′shə pĭg-mĕn′tī) n. An inherited developmental defect of the skin marked by pigmented lesions in linear, zebra-stripe, and other configurations and often involving other structures such as the central nervous system. Also called *Bloch-Sulzberger syndrome.*

incontinentia pigmenti a·chro·mi·ens (ə-krō′mē-əns) n. An inherited skin disorder characterized by the appearance of macules with less than normal pigmentation in a swirling or marble pattern, and associated with other abnormalities of the nerves, eyes, muscles, and bones. Also called *hypomelanosis of Ito.*

in·co·or·di·na·tion (ĭn′kō-ôr′dn-ā′shən) *n.* See **ataxia.**

in·cre·ment (ĭn′krə-mənt, ĭng′-) *n.* **1.** The process of increasing in number, size, quantity, or extent. **2.** Something added or gained. **3.** A small positive or negative change in the value of a variable. —**in′cre·men′tal** (-mĕn′tl) *adj.*

in·cre·tion (ĭn-krē′shən) *n.* **1.** The process of internal secretion characteristic of endocrine glands. **2.** The product of this process; a hormone.

in·crust·a·tion (ĭn′krŭ-stā′shən) *n.* **1.** The formation of a crust or a scab. **2.** A coating of hardened exudate or other material on a body or body part.

in·cu·bate (ĭn′kyə-bāt′, ĭng′-) *v.* **1.** To maintain eggs, organisms, or living tissue at optimal environmental conditions for growth and development. **2.** To maintain a chemical or biochemical system under specific conditions in order to promote a particular reaction.

in·cu·ba·tion (ĭn′kyə-bā′shən, ĭng′-) *n.* **1.** The act of incubating or the state of being incubated. **2.** The maintenance of controlled environmental conditions for the purpose of favoring the growth or development of microbial or tissue cultures. **3.** The maintenance of an infant, especially a premature infant, in an environment of controlled temperature, humidity, and oxygen concentration in order to provide optimal conditions for growth and development. **4.** The development of an infection from the time the pathogen enters the body until signs or symptoms first appear.

incubation period *n.* **1.** See **latent period** (sense 2). **2.** See **incubative stage.**

in·cu·ba·tive stage (ĭn′kyə-bā′tĭv, ĭng′-) *n.* The primary stage of certain infectious diseases during which prodromal symptoms appear. Also called *incubation period, latent stage, prodromal stage.*

in·cu·ba·tor (ĭn′kyə-bā′tər, ĭng′-) *n.* **1.** An apparatus in which environmental conditions, such as temperature and humidity, can be controlled, often used for growing bacterial cultures, hatching eggs artificially, or providing suitable conditions for a chemical or biological reaction. **2.** An apparatus for maintaining an infant, especially a premature infant, in an environment of controlled temperature, humidity, and oxygen concentration.

in·cu·bus (ĭn′kyə-bəs, ĭng′-) *n., pl.* **–bus·es** *or* **–bi** (-bī′) **1.** An evil spirit believed to have sexual intercourse with women as they sleep. **2.** A nightmare. **3.** An oppressive or nightmarish burden.

in·cu·dal (ĭng′kyə-dl, ĭng-kyōōd′l) *adj.* Relating to the incus.

in·cu·dec·to·my (ĭng′kyə-dĕk′tə-mē) *n.* Surgical removal of the incus.

in·cu·do·mal·le·al (ĭng′kyə-dō-măl′ē-əl, ĭng-kyōō′-) *adj.* Relating to the incus and the malleus.

in·cu·do·sta·pe·di·al (ĭng′kyə-dō-stā-pē′dē-əl, ĭng-kyōō′-) *adj.* Relating to the incus and the stapes.

in·cur·a·ble (ĭn-kyōōr′ə-bəl) *adj.* Being such that a cure is impossible; not curable.

in·cur·va·tion (ĭn′kûr-vā′shən) *n.* A curvature that turns inward.

in·cus (ĭng′kəs) *n., pl.* **in·cu·des** (ĭng-kyōō′dēz) The middle of the three ossicles in the middle ear, located between the malleus and the stapes and composed of a body and two limbs. Also called *anvil.*

in·cy·clo·pho·ri·a (ĭn-sī′klə-fôr′ē-ə) *n.* The tendency of the eyes to rotate inward, prevented by the impulse of the eyes to act in coordination. Also called *minus cyclophoria.*

in d. *abbr. Latin* in dies (daily)

in·dane·di·one (ĭn′dān-dī′ōn′) *n.* Any of a class of rapidly acting, orally administered anticoagulants.

in·dap·a·mide (ĭn-dăp′ə-mīd′) *n.* A loop diuretic used to treat edema associated with congestive heart failure, hepatic cirrhosis, and renal disease.

in·den·ta·tion (ĭn′dĕn-tā′shən) *n.* A notch, a pit, or a depression.

in·de·pen·dent practice association (ĭn′dĭ-pĕn′dənt) *n.* An IPA.

In·der·al (ĭn′də-rôl′) A trademark for the drug propranolol.

in·dex (ĭn′dĕks′) *n., pl.* **–dex·es** *or* **–di·ces** (-dĭ-sēz′) **1.** A guide, standard, indicator, symbol, or number indicating the relation of one part or thing to another in respect to size, capacity, or function. **2.** A core or mold used to record or maintain the relative position of a tooth or teeth to one another or to a cast. **3.** A guide, usually made of plaster, used to reposition teeth, casts, or parts. **4.** The index finger. —**in′dex′** *v.*

index case *n.* See **proband.**

index extensor muscle *n.* A muscle with origin from the dorsal surface of the ulna, with insertion to the dorsal extensor aponeurosis of the index finger, with nerve supply from the radial nerve, and whose action assists in extending the forefinger.

index finger *n.* The finger next to the thumb. Also called *first finger, forefinger.*

in·di·can (ĭn′dĭ-kăn′) *n.* A potassium salt found in sweat and urine and formed by the conversion of tryptophan to indole by intestinal bacteria.

in·di·can·i·dro·sis (ĭn′dĭ-kăn′ĭ-drō′sĭs) *n.* The excretion of indican in the sweat.

in·di·can·u·ri·a (ĭn′dĭ-kə-nŏŏr′ē-ə) *n.* The presence of excessive amounts of indican in the urine.

in·di·ca·tion (ĭn′dĭ-kā′shən) *n.* **1.** Something that points to or suggests the proper treatment of a disease, as that demanded by its cause or symptoms. **2.** Something indicated as necessary or expedient, as in the administration of a drug. **3.** The degree indicated by a measuring instrument.

in·di·ca·tor (ĭn′dĭ-kā′tər) *n.* **1.** One that indicates, especially a pointer or an index. **2.** An instrument used to monitor the operation or condition of an engine, an electrical network, or another physical system; a meter or gauge. **3.** The needle, dial, or other registering device on such an instrument. **4.** Any of various substances, such as litmus or phenolphthalein, that indicate the presence, absence, or concentration of another substance or the degree of reaction between substances by means of a characteristic change, especially in color.

in·dif·fer·ent (ĭn-dĭf′ər-ənt, -dĭf′rənt) *adj.* **1.** Characterized by a lack of partiality; unbiased. **2.** Not active or involved; neutral. **3.** Undifferentiated, as cells or tissue.

indifferent gonad *n.* The primordial organ in an embryo before its differentiation into testis or ovary.

indifferent tissue *n.* Undifferentiated, nonspecialized embryonic tissue.

in·di·gest·ed (ĭn′dĭ-jĕs′tĭd, -dī-) *adj.* Not digested; being undigested.

in·di·ges·tion (ĭn′dĭ-jĕs′chən, -dī-) *n.* **1.** The inability to digest or a difficulty in properly digesting food in the alimentary tract. **2.** Abdominal discomfort or illness resulting from this inability or difficulty.

in·di·go carmine (ĭn′dĭ-gō′) *n.* Sodium indigotindisulfonate; a blue dye used for measurement of kidney function and as a stain for Negri bodies.

in·din·a·vir (ĭn-dĭn′ə-vîr) *n.* A protease-inhibiting drug usually used in combination with other drugs to suppress the replication of HIV.

in·dir·ect fracture (ĭn′dĭ-rĕkt′, -dī-) *n.* A fracture, especially of the skull, that occurs at a point other than the point of impact or injury.

indirect hemagglutination test *n.* See **passive hemagglutination**.

indirect nuclear division *n.* See **mitosis** (sense 1).

indirect ophthalmoscope *n.* An instrument designed to visualize the interior of the eye, with the instrument at arm's length from the subject's eye and the observer viewing an inverted image through a convex lens located between the instrument and the subject's eye.

indirect reacting bilirubin *n.* Serum bilirubin that has not been conjugated with glucuronic acid in the liver.

indirect transfusion *n.* Transfusion of blood previously obtained from a donor.

indirect vision *n.* See **peripheral vision**.

in·dis·pose (ĭn′dĭ-spōz′) *v.* To cause to be or feel ill; sicken.

in·di·um (ĭn′dē-əm) *n. Symbol* **In** A soft malleable metallic element found primarily in ores of zinc, used in making dental alloys and in its radioisotope forms in diagnostic radiology. Atomic number 49.

in·di·vid·u·al psychology (ĭn′də-vĭj′ōō-əl) *n.* A theory of human behavior emphasizing the drive to overcome feelings of inferiority by compensation and the need to achieve personal goals that have value for society.

in·di·vid·u·a·tion (ĭn′də-vĭj′ōō-ā′shən) *n.* **1.** The act or process of becoming distinct or individual, especially the process by which social individuals become differentiated one from the other. **2.** In Jungian psychology, gradual integration and unification of the self through the resolution of successive layers of psychological conflict. **3.** The formation of distinct organs or structures through the interaction of adjacent tissues in an embryo.

individuation field *n.* The region within which an organizer influences the rearrangement of primordial tissues so that a complete embryo is formed.

In·do·cin (ĭn′də-sĭn′) A trademark for the drug indomethacin.

in·do·cy·a·nine green (ĭn′dō-sī′ə-nēn′) *n.* A green dye that binds serum albumin and is used in determining blood volume and liver function.

in·dol·ac·e·tu·ri·a (ĭn′dō-lăs′ĭ-tōōr′ē-ə) *n.* Excessive amount of indoleacetic acid in the urine.

in·dole (ĭn′dōl′) *n.* **1.** A white crystalline compound obtained from coal tar or various plants and found in the intestines and feces as a product of the bacterial decomposition of tryptophan. Also called *ketole.* **2.** Any of various derivatives of this compound.

in·dole·a·ce·tic acid (ĭn′dō-lə-sē′tĭk) *n.* A plant hormone that stimulates growth.

in·dole·am·ine *or* **in·dol·am·ine** (ĭn′dō-lăm′ēn, ĭn′dō-lə-mēn′) *n.* Any of various indole derivatives, such as serotonin, containing a primary, secondary, or tertiary amine group.

in·do·lent (ĭn′də-lənt) *adj.* **1.** Disinclined to exert oneself; habitually lazy. **2.** Causing little or no pain, as a tumor. **3.** Slow to heal, grow, or develop, as an ulcer; inactive.

indolent bubo *n.* An indurated enlargement of an inguinal node.

in·do·meth·a·cin (ĭn′dō-mĕth′ə-sĭn) *n.* A nonsteroidal anti-inflammatory, antipyretic, and analgesic drug used especially in the treatment of some forms of arthritis.

in·dox·yl (ĭn-dŏk′səl) *n.* A product of intestinal bacterial degradation of indoleacetic acid, excreted in the urine.

in·dox·yl·u·ri·a (ĭn-dŏk′səl-yōōr′ē-ə) *n.* The presence of indoxyl, especially indoxyl sulfate, in the urine.

in·duce (ĭn-dōōs′) *v.* **1.** To bring about or stimulate the occurrence of something, such as labor. **2.** To initiate or increase the production of an enzyme or other protein at the level of genetic transcription. **3.** To produce an electric current or a magnetic charge by induction.

in·duced abortion (ĭn-dōōst′) *n.* Abortion caused intentionally by the administration of drugs or by mechanical means.

induced enzyme *n.* An enzyme produced by a cell in response to the accumulation or addition of a particular substance.

induced hypotension *n.* The deliberate acute reduction of arterial blood pressure to reduce blood loss during surgery, either by pharmacological means or by presurgical withdrawal of blood which is returned to the circulation postsurgically. Also called *controlled hypotension.*

induced radioactivity *n.* See **artificial radioactivity**.

in·duc·er (ĭn-dōō′sər) *n.* **1.** One that induces, especially a molecule that is usually a substrate of a specific enzyme pathway, combining with an active repressor produced by a regulator gene to deactivate the repressor. **2.** A part or structure in an embryo that influences the differentiation of another part.

in·duc·i·ble enzyme (ĭn-dōō′sə-bəl) *n.* An enzyme that is normally present in minute quantities within a cell, but whose concentration increases dramatically when a substrate compound is added.

in·duct (ĭn-dŭkt′) *v.* To produce an electric current or a magnetic charge by induction.

in·duc·tion (ĭn-dŭk′shən) *n.* **1.** The process of initiating or increasing the production of an enzyme or other protein at the level of genetic transcription. **2.** The period from the first administration of anesthesia to the establishment of a depth of anesthesia adequate for surgery. **3.** The change in form or shape caused by the action of one tissue of an embryo on adjacent tissues or parts, as by the diffusion of hormones. **4.** A modification imposed upon the offspring by the action of environment on the germ cells of one or both parents. **5.** The generation of electromotive force in a closed circuit by a varying magnetic flux through the circuit.

induction period *n.* The interval between an initial injection of an antigen and the appearance of demonstrable antibodies in the blood.

in·duc·tor (ĭn-dŭk'tər) *n.* **1.** Something that inducts, especially a device that functions by or introduces inductance into a circuit. **2.** See **evocator. 3.** See **organizer.**

in·du·rat·ed (ĭn'də-rā'tĭd, -dyə-) *adj.* Hardened, as a soft tissue that becomes extremely firm.

in·du·ra·tion (ĭn'də-rā'shən, -dyə-) *n.* **1.** The hardening of a normally soft tissue or organ, especially the skin, because of inflammation, infiltration of a neoplasm, or an accumulation of blood. **2.** A focus or region of abnormally hardened tissue.

in·du·ra·tive (ĭn'də-rā'tĭv, -dyə-) *adj.* Relating to, causing, or characterized by induration.

in·du·si·um gris·e·um (ĭn-doō'zē-əm grĭs'ē-əm) *n.* The supracallosal gyrus.

in·dus·tri·al disease (ĭn-dŭs'trē-əl) *n.* **1.** A pathological condition resulting from exposure to a toxin discharged by a business or industry into the environment. **2.** An occupational disease.

in·dwell·ing (ĭn'dwĕl'ĭng) *adj.* Placed or implanted within the body, as a catheter or electrode.

–ine *suff.* **1.** *or* **–in** A chemical substance: *bromine, amine, quinine.* **2.** Amino acid: *glycine.*

in·e·bri·ant (ĭn-ē'brē-ənt) *adj.* Serving to intoxicate. *—n.* An intoxicant.

in·e·bri·a·tion (ĭn-ē'brē-ā'shən) *n.* The condition of being intoxicated, as with alcohol.

in·ert (ĭn-ûrt') *adj.* **1.** Sluggish in action or motion; lethargic. **2.** Not readily reactive with other chemical elements; forming few or no chemical compounds. **3.** Having no pharmacologic or therapeutic action.

inert gas *n.* See **noble gas.**

in·er·tia (ĭ-nûr'shə) *n.* **1.** The tendency of a body to resist acceleration; the tendency of a body at rest to remain at rest or of a body in motion to stay in motion in a straight line unless acted on by an outside force. **2.** Resistance or disinclination to motion, action, or change.

inertia time *n.* The interval elapsing between the reception of the stimulus from a nerve and the contraction of the muscle.

in ex·tre·mis (ĭn ĕk-strē'mĭs) *adv.* At the point of death.

in·fan·cy (ĭn'fən-sē) *n.* **1.** The earliest period of childhood, especially before the ability to walk has been acquired. **2.** The state of being an infant.

in·fant (ĭn'fənt) *n.* A child in the earliest period of life, especially before he or she can walk.

in·fan·ti·cide (ĭn-făn'tĭ-sīd') *n.* **1.** The act of killing an infant. **2.** The practice of killing newborns.

in·fan·tile (ĭn'fən-tīl', -tĭl) *adj.* **1.** Of or relating to infants or infancy. **2.** Displaying or suggesting a lack of maturity; extremely childish.

infantile acropustulosis *n.* A cyclical papulopustular crusting eruption that appears in the 10 months after birth and subsides at about 2 years of age.

infantile autism *n.* See **autism.**

infantile cortical hyperostosis *n.* A painful thickening of membrane surrounding soft bone tissue, especially in the mandible, the clavicles, and the shafts of long bones, following fever and usually appearing before six months of age and disappearing during childhood. Also called *Caffey's disease, Caffey's syndrome.*

infantile digital fibromatosis *n.* See **recurring digital fibroma of childhood.**

infantile eczema *n.* Eczema in infants.

infantile fibrosarcoma *n.* A rapidly growing but infrequently metastasizing fibrosarcoma that usually appears on the extremities in the first year of life.

infantile muscular atrophy *n.* Progressive muscular wasting due to degeneration of motor neurons in the anterior horns of the spinal cord, with onset usually in the first year of life. Also called *familial spinal muscular atrophy, infantile progressive spinal muscular atrophy.*

infantile neuroaxonal dystrophy *n.* A disorder in infants or young children characterized by slow progressive mental and neurological deterioration

infantile osteomalacia *n.* See **rickets.**

infantile paralysis *n.* See **poliomyelitis.**

infantile progressive spinal muscular atrophy *n.* See **infantile muscular atrophy.**

infantile purulent conjunctivitis *n.* See **ophthalmia neonatorum.**

infantile scurvy *n.* An acute form of scurvy in infants resulting from malnutrition, marked by pallor, fetid breath, coated tongue, diarrhea, and subperiosteal hemorrhages. Also called *Barlow's disease.*

infantile sexuality *n.* In psychoanalytic theory, the overlapping oral, anal, and phallic phases of psychosexual development that occur during the first 5 years of life.

infantile spasm *n.* Brief muscular spasms in infants, usually lasting from one to three seconds and often appearing as nodding spasms.

in·fan·til·ism (ĭn'fən-tl-ĭz'əm, ĭn-făn'tl-) *n.* **1.** A state of arrested development in an adult, characterized by retention of infantile mentality, accompanied by stunted growth and sexual immaturity, and often by dwarfism. **2.** Extreme immaturity, as in behavior or character.

infant mortality rate *n.* The ratio of the number of deaths in the first year of life to the number of live births occurring in the same population during the same period of time.

in·farct (ĭn'färkt', ĭn-färkt') *n.* An area of tissue that undergoes necrosis as a result of obstruction of local blood supply, as by a thrombus or an embolus. **—in·farct'ed** *adj.*

in·farc·tion (ĭn-färk'shən) *n.* **1.** The formation or development of an infarct. **2.** An infarct.

in·fect (ĭn-fĕkt') *v.* **1.** To contaminate with a pathogenic microorganism or agent. **2.** To communicate a pathogen or disease to another organism. **3.** To invade and produce infection in an organ or body part.

in·fect·ed abortion (ĭn-fĕk′tĭd) *n*. Abortion complicated by infection of the genital tract.

in·fec·tion (ĭn-fĕk′shən) *n*. **1.** Invasion by and multiplication of pathogenic microorganisms in a bodily part or tissue, which may produce subsequent tissue injury and progress to overt disease through a variety of cellular or toxic mechanisms. **2.** An instance of being infected. **3.** An agent or a contaminated substance responsible for one's becoming infected. **4.** The pathological state resulting from having been infected. **5.** An infectious disease.

infection-exhaustion psychosis *n*. A psychosis that occurs following an acute infection, shock, or chronic intoxication.

infection immunity *n*. Relative immunity to severe infection by a particular pathogen as a result of a chronic low-grade infection induced earlier by the same pathogen. Also called *premunition*.

in·fec·tious (ĭn-fĕk′shəs) *adj*. **1.** Capable of causing infection. **2.** Caused by or capable of being transmitted by infection. **3.** Caused by a pathogenic microorganism or agent. —**in·fec′tious·ness** *n*.

infectious disease *n*. A disease resulting from the presence and activity of a pathogenic microbial agent.

infectious eczematoid dermatitis *n*. A form of dermatitis caused by the spreading of purulent material that exudes from the site of an infection.

infectious endocarditis *n*. Endocarditis due to infection by microorganisms, such as bacteria or fungi. Also called *infective endocarditis*.

infectious hepatitis *n*. *Abbr.* **IH** See **hepatitis A.**

infectious mononucleosis *n*. A common, acute, infectious disease, usually affecting young people, caused by Epstein-Barr virus and characterized by fever, swollen lymph nodes, sore throat, and lymphocyte abnormalities.

infectious papilloma virus *n*. See **human papilloma virus.**

infectious polyneuritis *n*. See **acute idiopathic polyneuritis.**

infectious warts virus *n*. See **human papilloma virus.**

in·fec·tive (ĭn-fĕk′tĭv) *adj*. Capable of producing infection; infectious. —**in·fec′tive·ness, in′fec·tiv′i·ty** *n*.

infective embolism *n*. See **pyemic embolism.**

infective endocarditis *n*. See **infectious endocarditis.**

in·fe·ri·or (ĭn-fîr′ē-ər) *adj*. **1.** Low or lower in order, degree, or rank. **2.** Low or lower in quality, value, or estimation. **3.** Second-rate; poor. **4.** Situated below or directed downward. **5.** In human anatomy, situated nearer the soles in relation to a reference point. —**in·fe′ri·or′i·ty** (-ôr′ĭ-tē) *n*.

inferior alveolar nerve *n*. A terminal branch of the mandibular nerve that is distributed to the lower teeth, periosteum, and gums of the mandible.

inferior anastomotic vein *n*. An inconstant vein passing from the superficial middle cerebral vein into the transverse sinus.

inferior artery of knee *n*. **1.** An artery with origin in the popliteal artery, with distribution to the knee joint, and with anastomosis to the lateral superior genicular artery; lateral inferior artery of knee. **2.** An artery with its origin in the popliteal artery, with distribution to the knee joint, and with anastomosis to the medial superior genicular arteries; medial inferior artery of knee.

inferior basal vein *n*. A tributary to the common basal vein, draining the medial and posterior part of the inferior lobe in each lung.

inferior cerebellar peduncle *n*. A large bundle of nerve fibers extending up under the lateral recess of the rhomboid fossa, then curving steeply backward into the cerebellum. Also called *restiform body*.

inferior cerebral vein *n*. Any of the veins that drain the undersurface of the cerebral hemispheres and empty into the cavernous and transverse sinuses.

inferior cervical cardiac nerve *n*. A nerve passing from the cervicothoracic ganglion of the sympathetic trunk to the cardiac plexus.

inferior choroid vein *n*. A vein that drains the lower part of the choroid plexus of the lateral ventricle into the basal vein.

inferior cluneal nerve *n*. Any of the branches of the posterior femoral cutaneous nerve supplying the skin of the lower half of the gluteal region.

inferior constrictor muscle of pharynx *n*. A muscle with origin in the outer surfaces of the thyroid and cricoid cartilages, with insertion to the pharyngeal raphe in the wall of the pharynx, with nerve supply from the pharyngeal plexus, and whose action narrows the lower part of the pharynx in swallowing.

inferior dental plexus *n*. A plexus that is formed by branches of the inferior alveolar nerve interlacing before they supply the teeth and gives off dental and gingival branches.

inferior epigastric vein *n*. A vein that corresponds to the inferior epigastric artery and empties into the external iliac vein.

inferior ganglion of glossopharyngeal nerve *n*. See **petrous ganglion.**

inferior ganglion of vagus *n*. A large sensory ganglion of the vagus nerve, in front of the internal jugular vein.

inferior ge·mel·lus muscle (jə-mĕl′əs) *n*. A muscle with its origin from the tuberosity of the ischium, with insertion to the tendon of the internal obturator muscle, with nerve supply from the sacral plexus, and whose action rotates the thigh laterally.

inferior gluteal nerve *n*. A nerve that arises from the fifth lumbar nerve and the first and second sacral nerves and supplies the gluteus maximus muscle.

inferior gluteal vein *n*. Any of the accompanying veins of the inferior gluteal artery uniting into a common trunk that empties into the internal iliac vein.

inferiority complex *n*. A persistent sense of inadequacy or the tendency to diminish oneself, sometimes resulting in excessively aggressive behavior through overcompensation.

inferior labial vein *n*. A tributary of the facial vein that drains the lower lip.

inferior laryngeal nerve *n*. The terminal branch of the recurrent laryngeal nerve, supplying all the laryngeal muscles except the cricothyroid and the mucosa below the vocal cords.

inferior laryngeal vein *n*. A vein that passes from the lower larynx to the plexus thyroideus impar.

inferior lateral cutaneous nerve of arm *n.* A branch of the radial nerve supplying the skin of the lower lateral aspect of the arm.

inferior limb *n.* See **lower extremity**.

inferior lingual muscle *n.* An intrinsic muscle of the tongue, cylindrical in shape, occupying the underpart on either side of the tongue.

inferior longitudinal fasciculus *n.* A bundle of long association fibers running the length of the occipital and temporal lobes of the cerebrum, parallel in part with the inferior horn of the lateral ventricle.

inferior medullary velum *n.* A thin sheet of white matter attached along the peduncle of the flocculus and to the nodulus of the vermis.

inferior mesenteric lymph node *n.* Any of the nodes along the inferior mesenteric artery and its branches that drain the upper part of the rectum, the sigmoid colon, and the descending colon.

inferior mesenteric plexus *n.* An autonomic plexus that is derived from the aortic plexus, surrounds the inferior mesenteric artery, and branches to the descending colon, sigmoid, and rectum.

inferior mesenteric vein *n.* A vein that is the continuation of the superior rectal vein at the brim of the pelvis, ascends to the left of the aorta behind the peritoneum, and empties into the splenic vein or into the superior mesenteric vein.

inferior oblique muscle *n.* A muscle with origin from the orbital plate of the maxilla, with insertion into the sclera between the superior and lateral rectus muscles, with nerve supply from the oculomotor nerve, and whose action directs the pupil of the eye upward and outward.

inferior oblique muscle of head *n.* A muscle with origin in the spinous process of the axis, with insertion into the transverse process of the atlas, with nerve supply from the suboccipital nerve, and whose action rotates the head.

inferior ophthalmic vein *n.* Any of the veins that originate in the lower eyelid and empty into the angular vein.

inferior petrosal sinus *n.* A paired sinus of the dura mater that connects the cavernous sinus with the superior bulb of the internal jugular vein.

inferior phrenic vein *n.* A vein that drains the diaphragm and empties on the right side into the vena cava and on the left side into the left suprarenal vein.

inferior pulmonary vein *n.* **1.** The vein returning blood from the inferior lobe of the left lung to the left atrium; left inferior pulmonary vein. **2.** The vein returning blood from the inferior lobe of the right lung to the left atrium; right inferior pulmonary vein.

inferior rectal nerve *n.* Any of several branches of the pudendal nerve that pass to the external sphincter muscle of the anus and that supply the skin of the anal region.

inferior rectal vein *n.* Any of the veins that pass to the internal pudendal vein from the venous plexus around the anal canal.

inferior rectus muscle *n.* A muscle with origin from the inferior part of the tendinous ring, with insertion into the sclera of the eye, with nerve supply from the oculomotor nerve, and whose action directs the pupil downward and medialward.

inferior retinaculum of extensor muscles *n.* A V-shaped ligament restraining the extensor tendons of the foot, distal to the ankle joint.

inferior sagittal sinus *n.* An unpaired dural sinus in the lower margin of the falx cerebri.

inferior salivary nucleus *n.* A group of preganglionic parasympathetic motor neurons located in the medulla oblongata dorsal to the ambiguous nucleus; its axons govern secretion from the parotid gland by way of the otic ganglion.

inferior tarsal muscle *n.* A poorly developed smooth muscle in the lower eyelid that acts to widen the palpebral fissure.

inferior temporal line *n.* The lower of two curved lines on the parietal bone, marking the limit of attachment of the temporal muscle.

inferior temporal sulcus *n.* The sulcus on the basal aspect of the temporal lobe, separating the fusiform gyrus from the inferior temporal gyrus on its lateral side.

inferior thalamic peduncle *n.* A large fiber bundle emerging from the anterior part of the thalamus in the ventral direction.

inferior thal·a·mo·stri·ate vein (thăl′ə-mō-strī′āt′) *n.* Any of the tributaries to the basal vein that drain the thalamus and striate body and exit through the anterior perforated substance.

inferior thyroid vein *n.* A vein that is formed by veins from the isthmus and lateral lobe of the thyroid gland and the plexus thyroideus impar, terminating in the left brachiocephalic vein.

inferior vein of cerebellar hemisphere *n.* Any of several veins draining the lower cerebellar hemispheres and terminating in the petrosal vein.

inferior vein of eyelid *n.* Any of the tributaries of the superior ophthalmic vein draining the upper eyelid.

inferior vein of vermis *n.* A vein that runs along the lower surface of the vermis, ends in the straight sinus, and drains part of the cerebellum.

inferior vena cava *n. Abbr.* **IVC** A large vein formed by the union of the two common iliac veins that receives blood from the lower limbs and the pelvic and abdominal viscera and empties into the right atrium of the heart. Also called *postcava.*

in·fer·tile (ĭn-fûr′tl) *adj.* Not capable of initiating, sustaining, or supporting reproduction.

in·fer·til·i·ty (ĭn′fər-tĭl′ĭ-tē) *n.* **1.** Absent or diminished fertility. **2.** The persistent inability to achieve conception and produce an offspring.

in·fest (ĭn-fĕst′) *v.* **1.** To live as a parasite in or on tissues or organs or on the skin and its appendages. **2.** To inhabit or overrun in numbers large enough to be harmful, threatening, or obnoxious. —**in′fes·ta′tion** *n.*

in·fib·u·late (ĭn-fĭb′yə-lāt′) *v.* To close off or obstruct the genitals of an individual, especially by sewing together the labia majora in females or fastening the prepuce in males, so as to prevent sexual intercourse.

in·fil·trate (ĭn-fĭl′trāt′, ĭn′fĭl-) *v.* **1.** To cause a liquid to permeate a substance by passing through its interstices or pores. **2.** To permeate a porous substance with a liquid or gas. —*n.* An abnormal substance that accumulates gradually in cells or body tissues.

in·fil·tra·tion (ĭn′fĭl-trā′shən) *n.* **1.** The act or process of infiltrating. **2.** The state of being infiltrated. **3.** The gas, fluid, or dissolved matter that has entered a substance, cell, or tissue. —**in·fil′tra·tive** (-trə-tĭv) *adj.*

infiltration anesthesia *n.* See **local anesthesia.**

in·fi·nite distance (ĭn′fə-nĭt) *n.* A distance of 20 feet or more, at which light rays entering the eyes are practically parallel.

in·firm (ĭn-fûrm′) *adj.* Weak in body, especially from old age or disease; feeble.

in·fir·ma·ry (ĭn-fûr′mə-rē) *n.* A place for the care of the infirm, sick, or injured, especially a small hospital or clinic in an institution or school.

in·fir·mi·ty (ĭn-fûr′mĭ-tē) *n.* **1.** A bodily ailment or weakness, especially one brought on by old age. **2.** A condition or disease producing weakness. **3.** A failing or defect in a person's character.

in·flam·ma·tion (ĭn′flə-mā′shən) *n.* A localized protective reaction of tissue to irritation, injury, or infection, characterized by pain, redness, swelling, and sometimes loss of function. —**in·flame′** *v.*

in·flam·ma·to·ry (ĭn-flăm′ə-tôr′ē) *adj.* Characterized or caused by inflammation.

inflammatory bowel disease *n. Abbr.* **IBD** Any of several incurable and debilitating diseases of the gastrointestinal tract characterized by inflammation and obstruction of parts of the intestine.

inflammatory carcinoma *n.* Carcinoma of the breast that causes edema, hyperemia, tenderness, and rapid enlargement of the breast.

inflammatory lymph *n.* Euplastic lymph that collects on the surface of an acutely inflamed membrane or cutaneous wound. Also called *plastic lymph.*

inflammatory papillary hyperplasia *n.* Closely arranged papules of the palatal mucosa underlying an ill-fitting denture. Also called *palatal papillomatosis.*

inflammatory pseudotumor *n.* A tumorlike mass that is composed of fibrous or granulation tissue infiltrated by inflammatory cells.

inflammatory rheumatism *n.* Acute inflammation of several joints simultaneously, as with rheumatic fever.

in·fla·tion (ĭn-flā′shən) *n.* **1.** Distention with a fluid or gas. **2.** The act of distending an organ or body part with a fluid or gas.

in·flec·tion (ĭn-flĕk′shən) *n.* An inward bending.

in·flu·en·za (ĭn′flo͞o-ĕn′zə) *n.* An acute contagious viral infection, commonly occurring in epidemics or pandemics, and characterized by inflammation of the respiratory tract and by the sudden onset, fever, chills, muscular pain, headache, and severe prostration. Also called *grippe.* —**in′flu·en′zal** *adj.*

influenza A *n.* Influenza caused by infection with a strain of influenza virus type A.

influenza B *n.* Influenza caused by infection with influenza virus type B.

influenza C *n.* Influenza caused by infection with a strain of influenza virus type C.

influenzal pneumonia *n.* **1.** Pneumonia that occurs in conjunction with influenza. **2.** Pneumonia caused by *Haemophilus influenzae.*

influenza virus *n.* Any of three viruses of the genus *Influenzavirus* designated type A, type B, and type C, that cause influenza and influenzalike infections.

In·flu·en·za·vi·rus (ĭn′flo͞o-ĕn′zə-vī′rəs) *n.* A genus of the Orthomyxoviridae family, including viruses that cause influenza A and B; each type has a stable nucleoprotein group antigen that is common to all strains of the type, but distinct from that of the other type.

influenza virus type A *n.* A myxovirus of the genus *Influenzavirus,* antigenically varying from influenza virus type B and influenza virus type C, that causes acute respiratory illness in humans and infections in birds and certain other animals.

influenza virus type B *n.* A myxovirus of the genus *Influenzavirus,* antigenically varying from influenza virus type A and influenza virus type C, that causes various respiratory illnesses in humans.

influenza virus type C *n.* A myxovirus of the genus *Influenzavirus,* antigenically varying from influenza virus type A and influenza virus type B, that causes respiratory illness in humans.

influenza virus vaccine *n.* A vaccine containing influenza virus, usually several strains of the virus, prepared in chick embryos and used to immunize against influenza.

in·formed consent (ĭn-fôrmd′) *n.* Consent by a patient to a surgical or medical procedure or participation in a clinical study after achieving an understanding of the relevant medical facts and the risks involved.

in·for·mo·some (ĭn-fôr′mə-sōm′) *n.* Any of the bodies composed of mRNA and protein that are found in the cytoplasm of animal cells.

infra– *pref.* Inferior to, below, or beneath: *infrasonic.*

in·fra·bulge (ĭn′frə-bŭlj′) *n.* **1.** The portion of the crown of a tooth gingival to the height of contour. **2.** The area of a tooth where the retentive portion of a clasp of a removable partial denture is placed.

in·fra·cla·vic·u·lar fossa (ĭn′frə-klə-vĭk′yə-lər) *n.* A triangular depression bounded by the clavicle and the adjacent borders of the deltoid and greater pectoral muscles. Also called *infraclavicular triangle.*

in·fra·clu·sion (ĭn′frə-klo͞o′zhən) *n.* A condition in which a tooth has failed to erupt to the plane of occlusion. Also called *infraocclusion, infraversion.*

in·frac·tion (ĭn-frăk′shən) *n.* A bone fracture, especially one without displacement.

in·fra·den·ta·le (ĭn′frə-dĕn-tā′lē) *n.* In craniometrics, the apex of the septum between the mandibular central incisors.

in·fra·di·an (ĭn-frā′dē-ən, ĭn′frə-dē′ən) *adj.* Relating to biological variations or rhythms occurring in cycles less frequent than every 24 hours.

in·fra·mam·il·lar·y (ĭn′frə-măm′ə-lĕr′ē) *adj.* Situated below a nipple.

in·fra·mar·gin·al (ĭn′frə-mär′jə-nəl) *adj.* Situated below a margin or edge.

in·fra·max·il·lar·y (ĭn′frə-măk′sə-lĕr′ē) *adj.* Of or relating to the lower jaw; mandibular.

in·fra·na·sal depression (ĭn′frə-nā′zəl) *n.* See **philtrum.**

in·fra·nod·al extrasystole (ĭn′frə-nōd′l) *n.* See **ventricular extrasystole.**

in·fra·oc·clu·sion (ĭn′frə-ə-klōō′zhən) *n.* See **infraclusion.**

in·fra·or·bit·al artery (ĭn′frə-ôr′bĭ-tl) *n.* An artery with origin in the maxillary artery, with distribution to the upper canine and incisor teeth, the inferior rectus and inferior oblique muscles, the lower eyelid, lacrimal sac, and upper lip, and with anastomoses to the branches of the ophthalmic, facial, superior labial, transverse facial, and buccal arteries.

infraorbital canal *n.* A canal that runs beneath the orbital margin of the maxilla from the infraorbital groove to the infraorbital foramen and transmits the infraorbital artery and nerve.

infraorbital foramen *n.* The external opening of the infraorbital canal on the front surface of the body of the maxilla.

infraorbital nerve *n.* The continuation of the maxillary nerve into the eye socket, traversing the infraorbital canal to supply the upper incisors, canines, premolars, upper gums, lower eyelid and conjunctiva, and part of the nose and upper lip.

in·fra·psy·chic (ĭn′frə-sī′kĭk) *adj.* Originating below the level of consciousness, as an idea or action.

in·fra·red (ĭn′frə-rĕd′) *adj.* **1.** Of or relating to the range of invisible radiation wavelengths from about 750 nanometers, just longer than red in the visible spectrum, to 1 millimeter, on the border of the microwave region. **2.** Generating, using, or sensitive to infrared radiation. —*n.* Infrared light or the infrared part of the spectrum.

infrared microscope *n.* A microscope equipped with infrared transmitting optics and capable of measuring the infrared absorption of minute samples with the aid of photoelectric cells.

in·fra·son·ic (ĭn′frə-sŏn′ĭk) *adj.* Generating or using waves or vibrations with frequencies below that of audible sound.

in·fra·spi·na·tus (ĭn′frə-spī-nā′təs) *n.* A muscle with origin from the infraspinous fossa of the scapula, with insertion to the great tubercle of the humerus, with nerve supply from the suprascapular nerve, and whose action extends the arm and rotates it laterally.

infraspinatus bursa *n.* The bursa between the tendon of the infraspinatus muscle and the capsule of the shoulder joint.

in·fra·spi·nous fossa (ĭn′frə-spī′nəs) *n.* The hollow on the dorsal aspect of the scapula inferior to the spine, giving attachment chiefly to the infraspinatus muscle.

in·fra·tem·po·ral crest (ĭn′frə-tĕm′pər-əl, -tĕm′prəl) *n.* A rough ridge marking the angle of union of the temporal and infratemporal surfaces of the greater wing of the sphenoid bone.

infratemporal fossa *n.* The cavity on the side of the skull bounded laterally by the zygomatic arch and by the ramus of the mandible. Also called *zygomatic fossa.*

in·fra·troch·le·ar nerve (ĭn′frə-trŏk′lē-ər) *n.* A branch of the nasociliary nerve, supplying the skin of the eyelids and the root of the nose.

in·fra·ver·sion (ĭn′frə-vûr′zhən) *n.* **1.** The downward turning of one eye. **2.** The rotation of both eyes downward. **3.** See **infraclusion.**

infundibular stem *n.* The neural component of the pituitary stalk, containing nerve tracts passing from the hypothalamus to the nervous lobe. Also called *infundibular stalk.*

in·fun·dib·u·lec·to·my (ĭn′fən-dĭb′yə-lĕk′tə-mē) *n.* Excision of the conus arteriosus, especially of hypertrophied myocardium encroaching on the ventricular outflow tract.

in·fun·dib·u·li·form (ĭn′fən-dĭb′yə-lə-fôrm′) *adj.* Resembling or shaped like a funnel.

in·fun·dib·u·lo·fol·lic·u·li·tis (ĭn′fən-dĭb′yə-lō-fə-lĭk′yə-lī′tĭs) *n.* Inflammation of the superficial part of the hair follicle that is located above the opening of the sebaceous gland.

in·fun·dib·u·lo·ma (ĭn′fən-dĭb′yə-lō′mə) *n., pl.* **–mas** or **–ma·ta** (-mə-tə) A piloid astrocytoma in tissues adjacent to the third ventricle of the cerebrum.

in·fun·dib·u·lum (ĭn′fən-dĭb′yə-ləm) *n., pl.* **–la** (-lə) **1.** A funnel or funnel-shaped structure or passage. **2.** The infundibulum of the fallopian tube. **3.** The expanding portion of a calix as it opens into the pelvis of the kidney. **4.** See **conus arteriosus. 5.** A termination of a bronchiole in the alveolus. **6.** Termination of the cochlear canal beneath the cupola. **7.** The funnel-shaped, unpaired prominence of the base of the hypothalamus behind the optic chiasm, continuous below with the stalk of the pituitary gland. —**in′fun·dib′u·lar** (-lər), **in′fun·dib′u·late′** (-lāt′, -lĭt) *adj.*

infundibulum of uterine tube *n.* The funnellike expansion of the abdominal extremity of a fallopian tube.

in·fuse (ĭn-fyōōz′) *v.* **1.** To steep or soak without boiling in order to extract soluble elements or active principles. **2.** To introduce a solution into the body through a vein for therapeutic purposes.

in·fu·sion (ĭn-fyōō′zhən) *n.* **1.** The process of steeping a substance in water to extract its soluble principles. **2.** A medicinal preparation from such a process. **3.** Introduction of a solution into the body through a vein for therapeutic purposes. **4.** The solution introduced in such a manner.

infusion-aspiration drainage *n.* The continuous infusion of antibiotics into a cavity while fluid is being drained from the cavity.

in·ges·ta (ĭn-jĕs′tə) *pl.n.* Ingested matter, especially food taken into the body through the mouth.

in·ges·tion (ĭn-jĕs′chən) *n.* **1.** The act of taking food and drink into the body by the mouth. **2.** The taking in of particles by a phagocytic cell. —**in·gest′** (-jĕst′) *v.* —**in·ges′tive** (-jĕs′tĭv) *adj.*

in·gra·ves·cent (ĭn′grə-vĕs′ənt) *adj.* Becoming increasingly severe.

in·grow·ing (ĭn′grō′ĭng) *adj.* Growing inward or into a part of the body, especially into the flesh.

in·grown (ĭn′grōn′) *adj.* Grown abnormally into the flesh.

ingrown hair *n.* A hair that grows at an abnormal angle and turns back into the skin, causing the formation of a pustule or papule.

ingrown nail *n.* A toenail, one edge of which has grown abnormally into the nail fold. Also called *ingrown toenail.*

in·growth (ĭn′grōth′) *n.* Something that grows inward or into a part of the body.

in·guen (ĭng′gwĕn′) *n., pl.* **in·gui·na** (ĭng′gwə-nə) See **inguinal region.**

in·gui·nal (ĭng′gwə-nəl) *adj.* **1.** Of or located in the groin. **2.** Relating to the left or right inguinal region of the abdomen.

inguinal canal *n.* The oblique passage through the layers of the lower abdominal wall that transmits the spermatic cord in the male and the round ligament in the female.

inguinal hernia *n.* A hernia into the inguinal canal.

inguinal ligament *n.* A fibrous band formed by the lower border of the aponeurosis of the external oblique muscle that extends from the upper front spine of the ilium to the pubic tubercle. Also called *Poupart's ligament.*

inguinal region *n.* The lower lateral region of the abdomen on either side of the pubic region. Also called *iliac region, inguen.*

inguinal triangle *n.* The triangular area in the lower abdominal wall bounded by the inguinal ligament below, by the rectus muscle of the abdomen medially, and by the inferior epigastric vessels laterally. Also called *Hesselbach's triangle, inguinal trigone.*

in·gui·no·cru·ral (ĭng′gwə-nō-krŏŏr′əl) *adj.* Relating to the groin and the thigh.

in·gui·no·dyn·i·a (ĭng′gwə-nō-dĭn′ē-ə) *n.* Pain in the groin.

in·gui·no·la·bi·al (ĭng′gwə-nō-lā′bē-əl) *adj.* Relating to the groin and the labium.

in·gui·no·per·i·to·ne·al (ĭng′gwə-nō-pĕr′ĭ-tn-ē′əl) *adj.* Relating to the groin and the peritoneum.

in·gui·no·scro·tal (ĭng′gwə-nō-skrōt′l) *adj.* Relating to the groin and the scrotum.

INH (ī′ĕn′āch′) *abbr.* isoniazid

in·ha·lant (ĭn-hā′lənt) *adj.* Used in or for inhaling. —*n.* Something that is inhaled, especially a drug that is delivered to the respiratory passages by a nebulizer or an aerosol container.

in·ha·la·tion (ĭn′hə-lā′shən) *n.* **1.** The act or an instance of inhaling. **2.** A solution of a drug or a combination of drugs administered to the respiratory passages as a nebulized mist.

inhalation analgesia *n.* Loss of the sense of pain due to the inhalation of a vapor or gas that depresses the central nervous system, as nitrous oxide.

inhalation anesthesia *n.* General anesthesia resulting from breathing of anesthetic gases or vapors.

inhalation anesthetic *n.* A gas or a vaporous liquid that produces general anesthesia when breathed.

inhalation therapy *n.* The therapeutic use of gases or of aerosols by inhalation.

in·ha·la·tor (ĭn′hə-lā′tər) *n.* **1.** See **respirator** (sense 1). **2.** See **inhaler.**

in·hale (ĭn-hāl′) *v.* **1.** To breathe in; inspire. **2.** To draw something such as smoke or a medicinal mist into the lungs by breathing; inspire.

in·hal·er (ĭn-hā′lər) *n.* A device that produces a vapor to ease breathing or is used to medicate by inhalation, especially a small nasal applicator containing a volatile medicament. Also called *inhalator.*

in·her·ent (ĭn-hîr′ənt, -hĕr′-) *adj.* Occurring as a natural part or consequence.

inherent immunity *n.* See **innate immunity.**

in·her·it (ĭn-hĕr′ĭt) *v.* To receive a trait from one's parents by genetic transmission.

in·her·it·a·ble (ĭn-hĕr′ĭ-tə-bəl) *adj.* Capable of being inherited. —**in·her′it·a·bil′i·ty** *n.*

in·her·i·tance (ĭn-hĕr′ĭ-təns) *n.* **1.** The process of genetic transmission of traits from parents to offspring. **2.** A characteristic so inherited. **3.** The sum of characteristics genetically transmitted from parents to offspring.

in·her·i·ted character (ĭn-hĕr′ĭ-tĭd) *n.* A single attribute of an animal or plant transmitted at one locus from generation to generation in accordance with genetic principles.

in·hib·in (ĭn-hĭb′ĭn) *n.* A peptide hormone secreted by the follicular cells of the ovary and the Sertoli cells of the testis that inhibits secretion of follicle stimulating hormone from the anterior pituitary.

in·hib·it (ĭn-hĭb′ĭt) *v.* **1.** To hold back; restrain. **2.** To suppress or restrain a behavioral process, an impulse, or a desire consciously or unconsciously. **3.** To prevent or decrease the rate of a chemical reaction. **4.** To decrease, limit, or block the action or function of something in the body, as an enzyme or organ. —**in·hib′i·to′ry** (-tôr′ē) *adj.*

in·hi·bi·tion (ĭn′hə-bĭsh′ən, ĭn′ə-) *n.* **1.** The act of inhibiting or the state of being inhibited. **2.** Something that restrains, blocks, or suppresses. **3.** The conscious or unconscious restraint of a behavioral process, a desire, or an impulse. **4.** Any of a variety of processes that are associated with the gradual attenuation, masking, and extinction of a previously conditioned response. **5.** The condition in which or the process by which a reaction is inhibited. **6.** The condition in which or the process by which an enzyme is inhibited.

in·hib·i·tor *or* **in·hib·it·er** (ĭn-hĭb′ĭ-tər) *n.* **1.** A substance that restrains or retards physiological, chemical, or enzymatic action. **2.** A nerve whose stimulation represses activity.

inhibitory fiber *n.* Any of the nerve fibers that inhibit either the activity of the nerve cells with which they have synaptic connections or the activity of the effector tissue in which they terminate.

inhibitory nerve *n.* A nerve conveying impulses that diminish functional activity in a part.

inhibitory obsession *n.* An obsession involving an impediment to action, usually representing a phobia.

inhibitory postsynaptic potential *n.* A local change in the degree of hyperpolarization of the postsynaptic membrane of a neuron in response to the arrival of an inhibitory impulse.

in·i·on (ĭn′ē-ən) *n.* The most prominent projecting point of the occipital bone at the base of the skull.

in·i·ti·at·ing agent (ĭ-nĭsh′ē-ā′tĭng) *n.* See **promoting agent.**

in·i·ti·a·tion (ĭ-nĭsh′ē-ā′shən) *n.* **1.** The act or an instance of initiating. **2.** The condition of being initiated. **3.** The first stage of tumor induction by a carcinogen in which cells are altered so that they are likely to form a tumor upon subsequent exposure to a promoting agent.

initiation factor *n.* *Abbr.* **IF** Any of several soluble proteins involved in the initiation of protein synthesis and released from the ribosome as it progresses into chain elongation.

i·ni·tis (ĭ-nī′tĭs) *n.* **1.** Inflammation of fibrous tissue. **2.** See **myositis.**

in·ject (ĭn-jĕkt′) *v.* **1.** To introduce a substance, such as a drug or vaccine, into a body part. **2.** To treat by means of injection.

in·ject·a·ble (ĭn-jĕk′tə-bəl) *adj.* Capable of being injected. Used of a drug. —*n.* A drug or medicine that can be injected.

in·jec·tant (ĭn-jĕk′tənt) *n.* A substance injected, as into the skin.

in·ject·ed (ĭn-jĕk′tĭd) *adj.* **1.** Of or relating to a substance introduced into the body. **2.** Of or relating to a blood vessel that is visibly distended with blood.

in·jec·tion (ĭn-jĕk′shən) *n.* **1.** The act of injecting a substance into a tissue, vessel, canal, or organ. **2.** Something that is injected, especially a dose of liquid medicine injected into the body. **3.** Congestion or hyperemia.

in·ju·ry (ĭn′jə-rē) *n.* **1.** Damage, harm, or loss, as from trauma. **2.** A particular form of hurt, damage, or loss.

in·lay (ĭn′lā′, ĭn-lā′) *n.* **1.** A solid filling, as of gold or porcelain, fitted to a cavity in a tooth and cemented into place. **2.** A graft of bone, skin, or other tissue. **3.** An orthomechanical device inserted into a shoe.

inlay graft *n.* A skin graft wrapped around a stent of dental compound and inserted into a prepared surgical pocket. Also called *Esser graft.*

in·let (ĭn′lĕt′, -lĭt) *n.* A passage leading into a cavity.

in·nate (ĭ-nāt′, ĭn′āt′) *adj.* Possessed at birth; inborn. —**in·nate′ness** *n.*

innate immunity *n.* Immunity that occurs naturally as a result of a person's genetic constitution or physiology and does not arise from a previous infection or vaccination. Also called *genetic immunity, inherent immunity, native immunity, natural immunity, nonspecific immunity.*

in·ner cell mass (ĭn′ər) *n.* The mass at the embryonic pole of the blastocyst concerned with the formation of the body of the embryo.

inner ear *n.* The portion of the ear within the temporal bone that is involved in hearing and balance and includes the semicircular canals, vestibule, and cochlea. Also called *internal ear, labyrinth.*

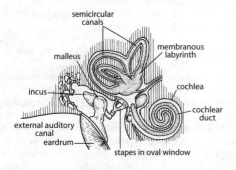

semicircular canals
membranous labyrinth
malleus
incus
cochlea
external auditory canal
eardrum
cochlear duct
stapes in oval window

inner ear
inner ear cross section

in·ner·most intercostal muscle (ĭn′ər-mōst) *n.* A layer of muscle parallel to the internal intercostal muscle but separated from it by the intercostal vessels and nerves.

in·ner·vate (ĭ-nûr′vāt′, ĭn′ər-) *v.* **1.** To supply an organ or a body part with nerves. **2.** To stimulate a nerve, muscle, or body part to action.

in·ner·va·tion (ĭn′ər-vā′shən) *n.* **1.** The arrangement or distribution of nerves to an organ or body part. **2.** The amount or degree of stimulation of a muscle or organ by nerves. —**in′ner·va′tion·al** (-shə-nəl) *adj.*

in·nid·i·a·tion (ĭ-nĭd′ē-ā′shən) *n.* The growth and multiplication of abnormal cells in a new location to which they have been transported by means of lymph or the bloodstream.

in·no·cent (ĭn′ə-sənt) *adj.* Not apparently harmful; benign.

innocent murmur *n.* See **functional murmur.**

in·noc·u·ous (ĭ-nŏk′yōō-əs) *adj.* Having no adverse effect; harmless.

in·nom·i·nate (ĭ-nŏm′ə-nĭt) *adj.* **1.** Having no name. **2.** Anonymous.

innominate artery *n.* An artery with origin in the arch of the aorta and with branches to the right subclavian and the right common carotid arteries. Also called *brachiocephalic trunk.*

innominate bone *n.* See **hipbone.**

innominate cartilage *n.* See **cricoid cartilage.**

innominate vein *n.* See **brachiocephalic vein.**

in·oc·u·la·ble (ĭ-nŏk′yə-lə-bəl) *adj.* **1.** Transmissible by inoculation. **2.** Susceptible to a disease transmitted by inoculation. **3.** That can be used in an inoculation. —**in·oc′u·la·bil′i·ty** *n.*

in·oc·u·lant (ĭ-nŏk′yə-lənt) *n.* See **inoculum.**

in·oc·u·late (ĭ-nŏk′yə-lāt′) *v.* **1.** To introduce a serum, a vaccine, or an antigenic substance into the body of a person or an animal, especially as a means to produce or boost immunity to a specific disease. **2.** To implant microorganisms or infectious material into or on a culture medium. **3.** To communicate a disease to a living organism by transferring its causative agent into the organism. —**in·oc′u·la′tive** *adj.*

in·oc·u·la·tion (ĭ-nŏk′yə-lā′shən) *n.* The act or an instance of inoculating, especially the introduction of an antigenic substance or vaccine into the body to produce immunity to a specific disease.

in·oc·u·lum (ĭ-nŏk′yə-ləm) *n.,* *pl.* **–lums** *or* **–la** (-lə) The microorganisms or other material used in an inoculation. Also called *inoculant.*

in·op·er·a·ble (ĭn-ŏp′ər-ə-bəl, -ŏp′rə-) *adj.* Unsuitable for a surgical procedure. —**in·op′er·a·bil′i·ty** *n.*

in·or·gan·ic (ĭn′ôr-găn′ĭk) *n.* **1.** Not formed by or involving organic life or the products of organic life. **2.** Not composed of organic matter. **3.** Of or relating to compounds not containing carbon to hydrogen bonds. —**in′or·gan′i·cal·ly** *adv.*

inorganic acid *n.* Any of various acids that do not contain carbon atoms.

inorganic chemistry *n.* The chemistry of compounds not containing carbon.

inorganic compound *n.* A compound that does not contain hydrocarbon groups.

inorganic murmur *n.* See **functional murmur.**

in·os·a·mine (ĭ-nō′sə-mēn′) *n.* An inositol in which a hydroxyl group is replaced by an amino group.

in·os·co·py (ĭ-nŏs′kə-pē) *n.* The microscopic examination of biological materials after dissecting or chemically digesting the fibrillary elements and strands of fibrin.

in·os·cu·late (ĭn-ŏs′kyə-lāt′) v. **1.** To unite parts such as blood vessels, nerve fibers, or ducts by small openings. **2.** To unite so as to be continuous; blend.

in·o·se·mi·a (ĭn′ō-sē′mē-ə) n. **1.** The presence of inositol in the blood. **2.** See **fibremia.**

in·o·sine (ĭn′ə-sēn′, -sĭn, ī′nə-) n. A nucleoside formed by the deamination of adenosine or the hydrolysis of inosinic acid.

inosine pran·o·bex (prăn′ə-bĕks′) n. An antiviral agent formed from a complex containing inosine.

in·o·sin·ic acid (ĭn′ə-sĭn′ĭk, ī′nə-) n. Inosine phosphate; a nucleotide that is found in muscle and other tissues.

in·o·si·tol (ĭ-nō′sĭ-tôl′, -tōl′, ī-nō′-) n. Any of nine isomeric alcohols especially one found in plant and animal tissue and classified as a member of the vitamin B complex.

in·o·si·tu·ri·a (ĭn′ō-sĭ-tŏor′ē-ə) n. The presence of inositol in the urine.

in·o·trop·ic (ĭn′ə-trŏp′ĭk, -trō′pĭk, ī′nə-, ē′nə-) adj. Affecting the contraction of muscle, especially heart muscle.

in·pa·tient (ĭn′pā′shənt) n. A patient who is admitted to a hospital or clinic for treatment that requires at least one overnight stay.

in·quest (ĭn′kwĕst′) n. **1.** A legal inquiry into the cause of violent or mysterious death. **2.** The finding based on such an inquiry.

in·sane (ĭn-sān′) adj. Of, exhibiting, or afflicted with insanity.

in·san·i·ty (ĭn-săn′ĭ-tē) n. **1.** Persistent mental disorder or derangement. Not in scientific use. **2.** Unsoundness of mind sufficient in the judgment of a civil court to render a person unfit to maintain a contractual or other legal relationship or to warrant commitment to a mental health facility. **3.** In most criminal jurisdictions, a degree of mental malfunctioning considered to be sufficient to relieve the accused of legal responsibility for the act committed.

in·scrip·tion (ĭn-skrĭp′shən) n. The main part of a prescription, indicating the drug or drugs and the quantity of each to be used in the mixture.

in·sect (ĭn′sĕkt′) n. **1.** Any of numerous usually small arthropod animals of the class Insecta, having an adult stage characterized by three pairs of legs and a body segmented into head, thorax, and abdomen and usually having two pairs of wings. **2.** Any of various similar arthropod animals, such as spiders, centipedes, or ticks.

in·sec·ti·cide (ĭn-sĕk′tĭ-sīd′) n. A chemical substance that kills insects. —**in·sec′ti·cid′al** (-sīd′l) adj.

in·se·cure (ĭn′sĭ-kyŏor′) adj. **1.** Lacking emotional stability; not well-adjusted. **2.** Lacking self-confidence; plagued by anxiety. —**in′se·cu′ri·ty** (-kyŏor′ĭ-tē) n.

in·sem·i·nate (ĭn-sĕm′ə-nāt′) v. To introduce or inject semen into the reproductive tract of a female. —**in·sem′i·na′tion** n.

in·se·nes·cence (ĭn′sĭ-nĕs′əns) n. The process of becoming old; senescence.

in·sen·si·ble (ĭn-sĕn′sə-bəl) adj. **1.** Having lost consciousness, especially temporarily; unconscious. **2.** Lacking physical sensation or the power to react, as to pain or cold; numb.

insensible perspiration n. Perspiration that evaporates before it is perceived as moisture on the skin.

in·ser·tion (ĭn-sûr′shən) n. **1.** The point or mode of attachment of a skeletal muscle to the bone or other body part that it moves. **2.** The placing of a dental prosthesis in the mouth.

in·ser·tion·al mutagenesis (ĭn-sûr′shə-nəl) n. Mutation caused by the insertion of new genetic material into a normal gene.

insertion sequence n. Any of several discrete DNA sequences that repeat at various sites on a bacterial chromosome, on certain plasmids, and on bacteriophages and that can move from one site to another on the chromosome, to another plasmid in the same bacterium, or to a bacteriophage.

in·sid·i·ous (ĭn-sĭd′ē-əs) adj. Being a disease that progresses with few or no symptoms to indicate its gravity. —**in·sid′i·ous·ly** adv.

in·sight (ĭn′sīt′) n. Understanding, especially an understanding of the motives and reasons behind one's actions. —**in′sight·ful** (ĭn′sīt′fəl, ĭn-sīt′-) adj.

in si·tu (ĭn sī′tŏo) adj. **1.** In the original position. **2.** Confined to the site of origin. —**in situ** adv.

in·sol·u·ble (ĭn-sŏl′yə-bəl) adj. Not soluble.

in·som·ni·a (ĭn-sŏm′nē-ə) n. Chronic inability to fall asleep or remain asleep for an adequate length of time.

in·som·ni·ac (ĭn-sŏm′nē-ăk′) n. One who suffers from insomnia. —adj. Having or causing insomnia.

in·sorp·tion (ĭn-sôrp′shən) n. Movement of substances from the intestinal tract into the blood.

in·sper·sion (ĭn-spûr′zhən) n. The act of sprinkling with a fluid or a powder.

in·spi·ra·tion (ĭn′spə-rā′shən) n. The inhalation of air into the lungs.

in·spi·ra·to·ry (ĭn-spīr′ə-tôr′ē) adj. Of, relating to, or used for the drawing in of air.

inspiratory capacity n. The volume of air that can be inhaled after normal inspiration. Also called *complementary air.*

inspiratory reserve volume n. Abbr. **IRV** The maximal volume of air that can be inhaled after a normal inspiration. Also called *complemental air.*

inspiratory stridor n. A crowing sound during the inspiratory phase of respiration during general anesthesia due to relaxation of the laryngeal muscles.

in·spire (ĭn-spīr′) v. To draw in breath; to inhale.

in·spired gas (ĭn-spīrd′) n. A gas that has been inhaled; specifically, an inhaled gas after it has been humidified at body temperature.

in·spis·sate (ĭn-spĭs′āt′, ĭn′spĭ-sāt′) v. To undergo thickening or cause to thicken, as by evaporation or the absorption of fluid. —**in′spis·sa′tion** n.

In·spra (ĭn′sprə) A trademark for the drug eplerenone.

in·star (ĭn′stär′) n. Any of the successive nymphal stages in the metamorphosis of insects or the stages of larval change by successive molts.

in·step (ĭn′stĕp′) n. The arched middle part of the foot between toes and ankle.

in·still (ĭn-stĭl′) v. To pour in drop by drop. —**in′stil·la′tion** (ĭn′stə-lā′shən) n.

in·stil·la·tor (ĭn′stə-lā′tər) n. See **dropper.**

in·stinct (ĭn′stĭngkt′) *n.* **1.** An inborn pattern of behavior that is characteristic of a species and is often a response to specific environmental stimuli. **2.** A powerful motivation or impulse. —**in·stinc′tive, in·stinc′tu·al** (ĭn-stĭngk′chōō-əl) *adj.*

in·sti·tu·tion·a·lize (ĭn′stĭ-tōō′shə-nə-līz′) *v.* To place a person in the care of an institution, especially one providing care for the disabled or mentally ill. —**in′sti·tu′tion·al·i·za′tion** (-shə-nə-lĭ-zā′shən) *n.*

in·stru·ment (ĭn′strə-mənt) *n.* A tool or implement, as for surgery.

in·stru·men·tar·i·um (ĭn′strə-mən-târ′ē-əm) *n., pl.* **-i·a** (-ē-ə) A collection of instruments and other equipment that are used for a surgical operation or for a medical procedure.

in·su·date (ĭn′sōō-dāt′) *n.* Fluid swelling within an arterial wall.

in·suf·fi·cien·cy (ĭn′sə-fĭsh′ən-sē) *n.* **1.** An inability of a bodily part or an organ to function normally. **2.** A moral or mental incompetence. **3.** An inadequate supply.

insufficiency disease *n.* See **deficiency disease.**

insufficiency of eyelids *n.* A condition in which the eyelids are closed only by conscious effort and are not fully closed during sleep.

in·suf·fi·cient (ĭn′sə-fĭsh′ənt) *adj.* **1.** Not sufficient. **2.** Incapable of proper functioning.

in·suf·flate (ĭn′sə-flāt′, ĭn-sŭf′lāt′) *v.* **1.** To blow into, especially to fill the lungs of an asphyxiated person with air, or to blow a medicated vapor, powder, or anesthetic into the lungs, or into any cavity or orifice of the body. **2.** To treat by blowing a medicated powder, gas, or vapor into a bodily cavity. —**in′suf·fla′tor** *n.*

in·suf·fla·tion (ĭn′sə-flā′shən) *n.* **1.** The act or an instance of insufflating. **2.** A finely powdered or liquid inhalant drug.

insufflation anesthesia *n.* The maintenance of inhalation anesthesia by delivery of anesthetic gases or vapors directly to the airway of an individual.

in·su·la (ĭn′sə-lə, ĭns′yə-) *n., pl.* **-lae** (-lē′) **1.** Island. **2.** A circumscribed body or patch on the skin. **3.** See **island of Reil.**

in·su·lar (ĭn′sə-lər, ĭns′yə-) *adj.* Of or being an isolated tissue or island of tissue.

in·su·lin (ĭn′sə-lĭn) *n.* **1.** A polypeptide hormone that is secreted by the islets of Langerhans, helps regulate the metabolism of carbohydrates and fats, especially the conversion of glucose to glycogen, and promotes protein synthesis and the formation and storage of neutral lipids. **2.** Any of various pharmaceutical preparations containing this hormone that are derived from the pancreas of certain animals or produced through genetic engineering and are used parenterally in the medical treatment and management of insulin-dependent diabetes mellitus.

insulin-antagonizing factor *n.* See **glycotropic factor.**

insulin-dependent diabetes mellitus *n. Abbr.* **IDDM** See **diabetes mellitus** (sense 1).

in·su·li·ne·mi·a (ĭn′sə-lə-nē′mē-ə) *n.* An abnormally large concentration of insulin in the blood.

in·su·lin·like activity (ĭn′sə-lĭn-līk′) *n. Abbr.* **ILA** A measure of the substances, usually in plasma, that exert

biological effects similar to those of insulin in various bioassays.

insulinlike growth factor *n. Abbr.* **IGF** See **somatomedin.**

in·su·lin·o·gen·e·sis (ĭn′sə-lĭn′ə-jĕn′ĭ-sĭs) *n.* Production of insulin by the islets of Langerhans. —**in′su·lin′o·gen′ic, in′su·lo·gen′ic** (ĭn′sə-lō-gĕn′ĭk) *adj.*

in·su·li·no·ma (ĭn′sə-lə-nō′mə) *n., pl.* **-mas** or **-ma·ta** (-mə-tə) An islet cell adenoma that secretes insulin. Also called *insuloma.*

insulin pump *n.* A portable device for people with diabetes that injects insulin at programmed intervals in order to regulate blood sugar levels.

insulin resistance *n.* A state of diminished effectiveness of insulin in lowering the levels of blood sugar, usually resulting from insulin binding by antibodies, and associated with such conditions as obesity, ketoacidosis, and infection.

insulin shock *n.* Acute hypoglycemia usually resulting from an overdose of insulin and characterized by sweating, trembling, dizziness, and, if left untreated, convulsions and coma.

in·su·li·tis (ĭn′sə-lī′tĭs) *n.* A histologic change in the islets of Langerhans characterized by edema and the infiltration of small numbers of white blood cells.

in·su·lo·ma (ĭn′sə-lō′mə) *n., pl.* **-mas** or **-ma·ta** (-mə-tə) See **insulinoma.**

in·sult (ĭn′sŭlt′) *n.* A bodily injury, irritation, or trauma.

in·sus·cep·ti·bil·i·ty (ĭn′sə-sĕp′tə-bĭl′ĭ-tē) *n.* The state or condition of not being susceptible to a disease or infection; immunity. —**in′sus·cep′ti·ble** *adj.*

In·tal (ĭn′tāl′) A trademark for the drug cromolyn sodium.

int. cib. *abbr. Latin* inter cibos (between meals)

in·te·gra·tion (ĭn′tĭ-grā′shən) *n.* **1.** The state of combination or the process of combining into completeness and harmony. **2.** The organization of the psychological or social traits and tendencies of a personality into a harmonious whole. **3.** A physiological increase or building up, as by accretion or anabolism. **4.** A recombination event in which a genetic element is inserted.

in·te·gra·tive (ĭn′tĭ-grā′tĭv) *adj.* **1.** Tending or serving to integrate. **2.** Relating to a multidisciplinary, holistic approach to medicine that combines conventional treatments with alternative therapies such as homeopathy or naturopathy.

in·teg·ri·ty (ĭn-tĕg′rĭ-tē) *n.* The state of being unimpaired; soundness or wholeness.

in·teg·u·ment (ĭn-tĕg′yōō-mənt) *n.* **1.** The enveloping membrane of the body, including the dermis, epidermis, hair, nails, and sebaceous, sweat, and mammary glands. **2.** The membrane, capsule, skin, or other covering of a body or a part. —**in·teg′u·men·ta·ry** (-mĕn′tə-rē, -mĕn′trē) *adj.*

integumentary system *n.* The bodily system consisting of the skin and its associated structures, such as the hair, nails, sweat glands, and sebaceous glands.

in·tel·lec·tu·al·i·za·tion (ĭn′tl-ĕk′chōō-ə-lĭ-zā′shən) *n.* **1.** The act or process of intellectualizing. **2.** An unconscious means of protecting oneself from the emotional stress and anxiety that is associated with confronting painful personal fears or problems by excessive reasoning.

in·tel·lec·tu·al·ize (ĭn'tl-ĕk'chōō-ə-līz') *v.* **1.** To furnish a rational structure or meaning for. **2.** To engage in intellectualization.

in·tel·li·gence (ĭn-tĕl'ə-jəns) *n.* **1.** The capacity to acquire and apply knowledge, especially toward a purposeful goal. **2.** An individual's relative standing on two quantitative indices, namely measured intelligence, as expressed by an intelligence quotient, and effectiveness of adaptive behavior.

intelligence quotient *n. Abbr.* **IQ** An index of measured intelligence expressed as the ratio of tested mental age to chronological age, multiplied by 100.

in·ten·sive care (ĭn-tĕn'sĭv) *n.* Continuous and closely monitored health care that is provided to critically ill patients.

intensive care unit *n. Abbr.* **ICU** A specialized section of a hospital containing the equipment, medical and nursing staff, and monitoring devices necessary to provide intensive care. Also called *critical care unit.*

in·ten·tion (ĭn-tĕn'shən) *n.* **1.** An aim that guides action. **2.** The process by which or the manner in which a wound heals. —**in·ten'tion·al** *adj.*

intention spasm *n.* A spasmodic contraction of the muscles occurring when a voluntary movement is attempted.

intention tremor *n.* A tremor that occurs when a voluntary movement is made. Also called *volitional tremor.*

inter– *pref.* **1.** Between; among: *interdental.* **2.** In the midst of; within: *interoceptor.*

in·ter·al·ve·o·lar septum (ĭn'tər-ăl-vē'ə-lər) *n.* The close-meshed capillary network covered by thin alveolar epithelial cells that intervenes between adjacent pulmonary alveoli.

in·ter·arch distance (ĭn'tər-ärch') *n.* The vertical distance between the maxillary and mandibular arches under specific conditions of vertical dimensions.

in·ter·ar·tic·u·lar (ĭn'tər-är-tĭk'yə-lər) *adj.* Situated between two joint surfaces.

interarticular cartilage *n.* See **articular disk.**

interarticular fibrocartilage *n.* See **articular disk.**

in·ter·a·tri·al septum (ĭn'tər-ā'trē-əl) *n.* The wall between the atria of the heart.

in·ter·bod·y (ĭn'tər-bŏd'ē) *adj.* Located or performed between the bodies of two adjacent vertebrae.

in·ter·brain (ĭn'tər-brān') *n.* See **diencephalon.**

in·ter·ca·dence (ĭn'tər-kād'ns) *n.* The occurrence of an extra beat between the two regular pulse beats. —**in'ter·ca'dent** *adj.*

in·ter·ca·lar·y (ĭn-tûr'kə-lĕr'ē, ĭn'tər-kăl'ə-rē) *adj.* Occurring between two others, as an upstroke between two normal pulse beats in a pulse tracing.

intercalary neuron *n.* A neuron running between and connecting two other neurons. Also called *internuncial neuron.*

in·ter·ca·lat·ed (ĭn-tûr'kə-lā'tĭd) *adj.* Inserted between two others; interposed. —**in·ter'ca·late'** *v.*

intercalated disk *n.* An undulating double membrane separating adjacent cells in cardiac muscle fibers.

intercalated duct *n.* One of the minute ducts leading from the acini in glands such as the salivary gland.

in·ter·cap·il·lar·y glomerulosclerosis (ĭn'tər-kăp'ə-lĕr'ē) *n.* See **diabetic glomerulosclerosis.**

in·ter·ca·pit·u·lar vein (ĭn'tər-kə-pĭch'ə-lər) *n.* Any of the veins connecting the dorsal and palmar veins in the hand or the dorsal and plantar veins in the foot.

in·ter·ca·rot·id body (ĭn'tər-kə-rŏt'ĭd) *n.* See **carotid body.**

in·ter·car·pal joint (ĭn'tər-kär'pəl) *n.* See **carpal joint.**

intercarpal ligaments *n.* Any of three sets of short fibrous bands that bind together the two rows of carpal bones.

in·ter·cav·er·nous sinus (ĭn'tər-kăv'ər-nəs) *n.* Either of the anterior or posterior anastomoses between the cavernous sinuses.

in·ter·cel·lu·lar (ĭn'tər-sĕl'yə-lər) *adj.* Located among or between cells.

intercellular bridge *n.* One of the slender cytoplasmic strands connecting adjacent cells. Also called *cell bridge, cytoplasmic bridge.*

intercellular canaliculus *n.* Any of various fine channels between adjoining secretory cells.

in·ter·cil·i·um (ĭn'tər-sĭl'ē-əm) *n.* Glabella.

in·ter·cla·vic·u·lar (ĭn'tər-klə-vĭk'yə-lər) *adj.* Between or connecting the clavicles.

in·ter·cos·tal (ĭn'tər-kŏs'təl) *adj.* Located or occurring between the ribs. —*n.* A space, muscle, or part situated between the ribs.

intercostal artery *n.* **1.** An artery with origin in the costocervical trunk, with distribution to the structures of the first and second intercostal spaces, and with anastomoses to the intercostal branches of the internal thoracic artery; anterior intercostal artery. **2.** Any of nine pairs of arteries arising from the thoracic aorta and distributed to the nine lower intercostal spaces, spinal column, spinal cord, and muscles and integument of the back, with anastomoses to the branches of the musculophrenic, internal thoracic, superior epigastric, subcostal, and lumbar arteries; posterior intercostal artery.

intercostal membrane *n.* Any of the membranous layers between the ribs.

intercostal nerve *n.* Any of the ventral branches of the thoracic nerves.

intercostal space *n.* The interval between each rib.

in·ter·cos·to·bra·chi·al nerve (ĭn'tər-kŏs'tō-brā'kē-əl, -brăk'ē-) *n.* Any of the branches of the second and third intercostal nerves that pass to the skin of the medial side of the arm.

in·ter·course (ĭn'tər-kôrs') *n.* **1.** Dealings or communications that occur between persons or groups. **2.** Sexual intercourse.

in·ter·cri·co·thy·rot·o·my (ĭn'tər-krī'kō-thī-rŏt'ə-mē) *n.* See **cricothyrotomy.**

in·ter·cur·rent (ĭn'tər-kûr'ənt) *adj.* Occurring in addition to and usually altering the course of another disease.

in·ter·cus·pa·tion (ĭn'tər-kŭ-spā'shən) *n.* **1.** The cusp-to-fossa relationship of the upper and lower posterior teeth to one another. **2.** The interlocking or fitting together of the cusps of opposing teeth. Also called *interdigitation.*

in·ter·den·tal (ĭn'tər-dĕn'tl) *adj.* **1.** Located or made for use between the teeth. **2.** Of or relating to the relationship between the proximal surfaces of the teeth of the same arch.

interdental canal *n.* See **Hirschfeld's canal.**

interdental papilla *n.* The gums filling the interproximal space between adjacent teeth.

interdental septum *n.* The bony separation between adjacent teeth in a dental arch.

interdental splint *n.* A splint for a fractured jaw consisting of two metal or acrylic resin bands wired to the teeth of the upper and lower jaws and then fastened together to prevent motion.

in·ter·den·ti·um (ĭn′tər-dĕn′shē-əm) *n.* The interval between any two contiguous teeth.

in·ter·dig·it (ĭn′tər-dĭj′ĭt) *n.* The area of the hand or foot lying between adjacent digits.

in·ter·dig·i·tat·ing cell (ĭn′tər-dĭj′ĭ-tā′tĭng) *n.* A cell with dendritic processes occurring primarily in thymus-dependent areas of the lymph nodes and spleen.

in·ter·dig·i·ta·tion (ĭn′tər-dĭj′ĭ-tā′shən) *n.* **1.** The interlocking of toothed or tonguelike processes. **2.** The processes thus interlocked. **3.** Infoldings of adjacent cell or plasma membranes. **4.** See **intercuspation** (sense 2).

in·ter·face (ĭn′tər-fās′) *n.* A surface forming a common boundary between adjacent regions or bodies.

in·ter·fa·cial canal (ĭn′tər-fā′shəl) *n.* Any of the various intercellular spaces between desmosomes.

in·ter·fer·ence (ĭn′tər-fîr′əns) *n.* **1.** The variation of wave amplitude that occurs when waves of the same or nearly the same frequency come together. **2.** The condition in which infection of a cell by one virus prevents superinfection by another virus. **3.** The condition in which superinfection by a second virus prevents effects that would result from infection by either virus alone, even though both viruses persist.

in·ter·fer·on (ĭn′tər-fîr′ŏn′) *n.* *Abbr.* **IFN** Any of a group of glycoproteins that are produced by different cell types in response to various stimuli, such as exposure to viruses, and that block viral replication in newly infected cells and, in some cases, modulate specific cellular functions.

in·ter·ic·tal (ĭn′tər-ĭk′təl) *adj.* Of or relating to an interval between convulsions or seizures.

in·ter·im denture (ĭn′tər-ĭm) *n.* A dental prosthesis that is used for a short period of time for esthetics or occlusal support or to condition the patient to accept an artificial substitute for missing natural teeth. Also called *temporary denture.*

in·ter·ki·ne·sis (ĭn′tər-kə-nē′sĭs, -kī-) *n.* See **interphase.**

in·ter·lam·i·nar jelly (ĭn′tər-lăm′ə-nər) *n.* The gelatinous material between ectoderm and endoderm that serves as the substrate on which mesenchymal cells migrate.

in·ter·leu·kin (ĭn′tər-lōō′kĭn) *n.* Any of a class of lymphokines that act to stimulate, regulate, or modulate lymphocytes such as T cells.

interleukin-1 *n.* *Abbr.* **IL-1** Any of a group of cytokines, released by macrophages and other cells, that induce the production of interleukin-2 by helper T cells and stimulate the inflammatory response.

interleukin-2 *n.* *Abbr.* **IL-2** A lymphokine that is released by helper T cells in response to an antigen and interleukin-1 and stimulates the proliferation of helper T cells.

interleukin-3 *n.* *Abbr.* **IL-3** A lymphokine, released by helper T cells in response to an antigen or mitogen, that stimulates the growth of blood stem cells and lymphoid cells such as macrophages and mast cells.

in·ter·lo·bar artery (ĭn′tər-lō′bər, -bär′) *n.* Any of the branches of segmental arteries of the kidney that run between the renal lobes and give rise to the arcuate arteries.

interlobar duct *n.* One of the ducts draining the secretion of the lobe of a gland and formed by the junction of several interlobular ducts.

interlobar vein of kidney *n.* Any of the veins that parallel the interlobar arteries, receive blood from the arcuate veins, and terminate in the renal vein.

in·ter·lo·bi·tis (ĭn′tər-lō-bī′tĭs) *n.* Inflammation of the pleura separating two pulmonary lobes.

in·ter·lob·u·lar artery (ĭn′tər-lŏb′yə-lər) *n.* **1.** Any of the arteries that pass between lobules of an organ. **2.** Any of the terminal branches of the hepatic artery passing between the hepatic lobules. **3.** Any of the branches of the interlobar arteries of the kidney passing outward through the cortex and supplying the glomeruli.

interlobular duct *n.* One of the ducts leading from a lobule of a gland and formed by the junction of several intercalated ducts.

interlobular emphysema *n.* Interstitial emphysema in the connective tissue septa between the pulmonary lobules.

interlobular pleurisy *n.* Pleurisy that is limited to the sulci between the pulmonary lobes.

interlobular vein of kidney *n.* Any of the veins that parallel the interlobular arteries, drain the peritubular capillary plexus, and empty into the arcuate veins of the kidney.

interlobular vein of liver *n.* Any of the terminal branches of the portal vein that course between the lobules and empty into the liver sinusoids.

in·ter·max·il·lar·y bone (ĭn′tər-măk′sə-lĕr′ē) *n.* See **incisive bone.**

intermaxillary suture *n.* The line of union of the two upper jawbones.

in·ter·me·di·ar·y nerve (ĭn′tər-mē′dē-ĕr′ē) *n.* A root of the facial nerve containing sensory fibers from the anterior portion of the tongue. Also called *intermediate nerve.*

in·ter·me·di·ate (ĭn′tər-mē′dē-ĭt) *adj.* Lying or occurring in a middle position or state. —*n.* A substance formed in the course of a chemical reaction or the synthesis of a desired end product that then participates in the process until it is either deactivated or consumed.

intermediate an·te·bra·chi·al vein (ăn′tē-brā′kē-əl) *n.* A vein that begins at the base of the dorsum of the thumb, curves around the radial side, ascends the middle of the forearm, and just below the bend of the elbow divides into the intermediate basilic and the intermediate cephalic veins.

intermediate basilic vein *n.* The medial branch of the

intermediate antebrachial vein that joins the basilic vein.

intermediate care *n.* **1.** A level of medical care in a hospital that is intermediate between intensive and basic care. **2.** A level of care for nonacutely ill, disabled, or elderly individuals.

intermediate cephalic vein *n.* The lateral branch of the intermediate antebrachial vein that joins the cephalic vein near the elbow.

intermediate cubital vein *n.* A vein that passes across the bend of the elbow from the cephalic vein to the basilic vein.

intermediate cuneiform bone *n.* A tarsal bone articulating with the medial and lateral cuneiform, navicular, and second metatarsal bones. Also called *middle cuneiform bone, second cuneiform bone.*

intermediate dorsal cutaneous nerve *n.* The lateral terminal branch of the superficial peroneal nerve, supplying the dorsum of the foot and the dorsal nerves to the toes.

intermediate great muscle *n.* See **intermediate vastus muscle.**

intermediate host *n.* A host in which a parasite goes through its larval or developmental stages.

intermediate lamella *n.* See **interstitial lamella.**

intermediate nerve *n.* See **intermediary nerve.**

intermediate supraclavicular nerve *n.* One of several nerves arising from the cervical plexus that pass down across the clavicle to supply the skin in the infraclavicular region. Also called *middle supraclavicular nerve.*

intermediate vas·tus muscle (văs′təs) *n.* A muscle with origin from the shaft of the femur, with insertion into the tibial tuberosity, with nerve supply from the femoral nerve, and whose action extends the leg. Also called *intermediate great muscle.*

in·ter·me·din (ĭn′tər-mēd′n) *n.* See **melanocyte-stimulating hormone.**

in·ter·me·di·o·lat·er·al nucleus (ĭn′tər-mē′dē-ō-lăt′-ər-əl) *n.* The cell column that forms the lateral horn of the gray matter of the spinal cord, extending from the first thoracic through the second lumbar segment, and containing the autonomic motor neurons that give rise to the preganglionic fibers of the sympathetic system.

in·ter·me·di·o·me·di·al nucleus (ĭn′tər-mē′dē-ō-mē′-dē-əl) *n.* A small group of visceral motor neurons immediately ventral to the thoracic nucleus in the thoracic and the upper two lumbar segments of the spinal cord, giving rise to the preganglionic fibers of the sympathetic nervous system.

in·ter·me·di·us (ĭn′tər-mē′dē-əs) *n.* An anatomical element or organ between right and left or lateral and medial structures.

in·ter·men·stru·al pain (ĭn′tər-měn′strōō-əl) *n.* **1.** Pelvic discomfort occurring at the midpoint of the menstrual cycle. **2.** See **mittelschmerz.**

in·ter·met·a·car·pal joint (ĭn′tər-mět′ə-kär′pəl) *n.* Any of the joints between the bases of the second, third, fourth, and fifth metacarpal bones.

in·ter·met·a·tar·sal joint (ĭn′tər-mět′ə-tär′səl) *n.* Any of the joints between the bases of the five metatarsal bones.

in·ter·mit·tent (ĭn′tər-mĭt′nt) *adj.* **1.** Stopping and starting at intervals. **2.** Marked by intervals of complete quietude occurring between two periods of activity. —**in′ter·mit′tence** *n.*

intermittent acute porphyria *n. Abbr.* **IAP** Porphyria caused by overproduction of delta-aminolevulinic acid, with greatly increased urinary excretion of it and of porphobilinogen, due to a deficiency of porphobilinogen deaminase. It is characterized by intermittent acute attacks of hypertension, abdominal colic, psychosis, and neuropathy. Also called *acute intermittent porphyria.*

intermittent claudication *n.* A condition caused by ischemia of the leg muscles due to sclerosis and narrowing of the arteries, characterized by attacks of lameness and pain and brought on by walking. Also called *Charcot's syndrome.*

intermittent cramp *n.* See **tetany.**

intermittent explosive disorder *n.* A disorder of impulse control characterized by several episodes in which aggressive impulses are released and expressed in serious assault or destruction of property although no such impulsiveness or aggressiveness is shown between episodes.

intermittent mandatory ventilation *n. Abbr.* **IMV** Mechanical application of positive pressure at a determined frequency to the airway so as to increase tidal volume.

intermittent positive pressure breathing *n. Abbr.* **IPPB** See **controlled mechanical ventilation.**

intermittent positive pressure ventilation *n.* See **controlled mechanical ventilation.**

intermittent tetanus *n.* See **tetany.**

in·ter·mus·cu·lar gluteal bursa (ĭn′tər-mŭs′kyə-lər) *n.* Any of several small bursae located between the tendon of the gluteus maximus and the rough line of the shaft of the femur. Also called *gluteofemoral bursa.*

intermuscular septum *n.* Any of the aponeurotic sheets separating various muscles of the extremities, including the anterior and posterior crural septa, the lateral and medial femoral septa, and the lateral and medial humeral septa.

in·tern *or* **in·terne** (ĭn′tûrn′) *n.* An advanced student or recent graduate who assists in the medical or surgical care of hospital patients and who resides within that institution. —*v.* To train or to serve as an intern. —**in′tern·ship′** *n.*

in·ter·nal (ĭn-tûr′nəl) *adj.* **1.** Located, acting, or effective within the body. **2.** Of, relating to, or located within the limits or surface; inner.

internal acoustic pore *n.* The inner opening of the internal acoustic meatus on the posterior surface of the temporal bone. Also called *internal acoustic foramen, internal auditory foramen.*

internal adhesive pericarditis *n.* See **concretio cordis.**

internal auditory artery *n.* See **artery of labyrinth.**

internal auditory foramen *n.* See **internal acoustic pore.**

internal auditory vein *n.* See **labyrinthine vein.**

internal capsule *n.* A layer of white matter separating the caudate nucleus and thalamus from the lentiform nucleus and serving as the major route by which the cerebral cortex is connected with the brainstem and the spinal cord.

internal carotid nerve *n.* A sympathetic nerve extending upward from the superior cervical ganglion along the internal carotid artery, forming the internal carotid plexus.

internal carotid plexus *n.* An autonomic plexus that surrounds the internal carotid artery in the carotid canal and in the cavernous sinus and sends branches to the tympanic plexus, sphenopalatine ganglion, abducens and oculomotor nerves, the cerebral vessels, and the ciliary ganglion.

internal cerebral vein *n.* Either of two paired veins that pass caudally near the midline in the choroid tela of the third ventricle and unite to form the great cerebral vein.

internal conjugate *n.* See **conjugate.**

internal ear *n.* See **inner ear.**

internal elastic lamina *n.* A fenestrated layer of elastic tissue that is the outermost part of the intima of an artery. Also called *internal elastic layer.*

internal fistula *n.* A fistula that is located between two internal organs.

internal fixation *n.* The stabilization of fractured bony parts by direct fixation to one another with surgical wires, screws, pins, or plates.

internal hemorrhage *n.* Bleeding into organs or cavities of the body. Also called *concealed hemorrhage.*

internal hemorrhoids *pl.n.* Hemorrhoids beneath the mucous membrane of the anal sphincter.

internal iliac artery *n.* See **iliac artery** (sense 3).

internal iliac vein *n.* See **hypogastric vein.**

internal intercostal muscle *n.* Any of the muscles with their origin from the lower border of a rib, with insertion into the upper border of the rib below, with nerve supply from the intercostal nerve, and that contract during expiration and serve to maintain a tension in the intercostal spaces that resists mediolateral movement.

in·ter·nal·ize (ĭn-tûr′nə-līz′) *v.* **1.** To make internal, personal, or subjective. **2.** To take in and adopt as an integral part of one's attitudes or beliefs. —**in·ter′nal· i·za′tion** (-nə-lĭ-zā′shən) *n.*

internal jugular vein *n.* A vein that is a continuation of the sigmoid sinus of the dura mater and unites behind the cartilage of the first rib with the subclavian vein to form the brachiocephalic vein.

internal medicine *n. Abbr.* **IM** The branch of medicine that deals with the diagnosis and nonsurgical treatment of diseases in adults.

internal obturator muscle *n.* A muscle with origin from the pelvic surface of the obturator membrane and the margin of the obturator foramen, with insertion into the medial surface of the greater trochanter, with nerve supply from the sacral plexus, and whose action rotates the thigh laterally.

internal occipital crest *n.* A ridge running from the internal occipital protuberance to the posterior margin of the great foramen, giving attachment to the falx cerebelli.

internal ophthalmopathy *n.* A disease of the retina, lens, or other internal structure of the eye.

internal ophthalmoplegia *n.* Paralysis affecting only the ciliary muscle and the iris of the eye.

internal phase *n.* The particles contained in a colloid solution.

internal pudendal artery *n.* An artery with origin in the internal iliac artery and with branches to the inferior rectal, perineal, posterior scrotal or labial, and urethral arteries, the artery of the bulb of the penis or vestibule, the deep artery of the penis or clitoris, and the dorsal artery of the penis or clitoris.

internal pudendal vein *n.* A tributary of the internal iliac vein that accompanies the internal pudendal artery and drains the perineum.

internal respiration *n.* See **tissue respiration.**

internal secretion *n.* A secretion that is produced by an endocrine gland and discharged directly into the bloodstream; a hormone.

internal spermatic artery *n.* See **testicular artery.**

internal sphincter muscle of anus *n.* A smooth muscle ring formed by an increase of the circular fibers of the rectum, situated at the upper end of the anal canal.

internal thoracic vein *n.* Either of usually two veins that accompany each internal thoracic artery, fusing together at the upper part of the chest and emptying into the brachiocephalic vein.

internal traction *n.* A pulling force created by using one of the cranial bones, above the point of fracture, for anchorage.

internal urethral opening *n.* The internal opening of the urethra, at the anterior and inferior angle of the trigone.

internal version *n.* Version of a fetus performed with one hand inside the uterus.

in·ter·na·sal suture (ĭn′tər-nā′zəl) *n.* The line of union between the two nasal bones.

in·ter·na·tion·al insulin unit (ĭn′tər-năsh′ə-nəl) *n.* The activity contained in $\frac{1}{22}$ milligram of the international standard of zinc-insulin crystals.

International System of Units *n. Abbr.* **SI** A complete, coherent system of units used for scientific work, in which the fundamental quantities are length, time, electric current, temperature, mass, luminous intensity, and amount of substance.

international unit *n. Abbr.* **IU** **1.** The quantity of a biologically active substance, such as a hormone or vitamin, that is required to produce a specific response. **2.** A unit of potency for similarly active substances that is based on this quantity and is accepted as an international standard.

in·terne (ĭn′tûrn′) *n.* Variant of **intern.**

in·ter·neu·ron (ĭn′tər-no͝or′ŏn′) *n.* A nerve cell found entirely within the central nervous system that acts as a link between sensory neurons and motor neurons. —**in′ter·neu′ro·nal** (-no͝or′ə-nəl, -no͝o-rō′-) *adj.*

in·ter·nist (ĭn-tûr′nĭst) *n.* A physician specializing in internal medicine.

internodal segment *n.* The portion of a myelinated nerve fiber between two successive nodes.

in·ter·node (ĭn′tər-nōd′) *n.* **1.** A section or part between two nodes. **2.** An internodal segment. —**in′- ter·nod′al** (-nōd′l) *adj.*

in·ter·nu·cle·ar (ĭn′tər-nōō′klē-ər) *adj.* **1.** Located or occurring between nuclei. **2.** Located between nerve cell groups in the brain or retina.

in·ter·nun·cial (ĭn′tər-nŭn′shəl) *adj.* Linking two neurons in a neuronal pathway.

internuncial neuron *n.* See **intercalary neuron.**

in·ter·oc·clu·sal distance (ĭn′tər-ə-klōō′zəl) *n.* The vertical distance between the occluding surfaces of the upper and lower teeth when the mandible is in the resting position.

in·ter·o·cep·tor (ĭn′tər-ō-sĕp′tər) *n.* A specialized sensory nerve receptor that receives and responds to stimuli originating from within the body. —**in′ter·o·cep′-tive** *adj.*

in·ter·os·se·ous (ĭn′tər-ŏs′ē-əs) *or* **in·ter·os·se·al** (-əl) *adj.* Connecting or lying between bones.

interosseous artery *n.* **1.** An artery with origin in the ulnar artery and with branches to the anterior and posterior interosseous arteries; common interosseous artery. **2.** An artery with origin in the common interosseous artery and with distribution to the deep posterior compartment of the forearm; posterior interosseous artery. **3.** An artery with origin in the common interosseous artery, with distribution to the deep anterior forearm, and with anastomoses to the posterior interosseous artery; anterior interosseous artery. **4.** An artery with origin in the posterior interosseous artery, with distribution to the elbow joint, and with anastomoses to the branches of the deep brachial artery and the inferior ulnar collateral artery; recurrent interosseous artery.

interosseous cartilage *n.* See **connecting cartilage.**

interosseous nerve of leg *n.* A nerve branching off from one of the muscular branches of the tibial nerve and passing down over the posterior surface of the interosseous membrane, supplying it and the two bones of the leg.

in·ter·pa·ri·e·tal suture (ĭn′tər-pə-rī′ĭ-təl) *n.* See **sagittal suture.**

in·ter·par·ox·ys·mal (ĭn′tər-păr′ək-sĭz′məl) *adj.* Relating to or occurring between successive paroxysms of a disease.

in·ter·pe·dun·cu·lar fossa (ĭn′tər-pĭ-dŭng′kyə-lər) *n.* A deep depression that is found on the inferior surface of the mesencephalon between the two cerebral peduncles.

interpeduncular nucleus *n.* A median ovoid cell group located at the base of the midbrain tegmentum between the left and right cerebral peduncles, receiving the retroflex fasciculus from the habenula and projecting to the raphe nuclei and the central gray substance of the midbrain.

in·ter·pel·vi·ab·dom·i·nal amputation (ĭn′tər-pĕl′vē-ăb-dŏm′ə-nəl) *n.* See **hemipelvectomy.**

in·ter·pha·lan·ge·al joint (ĭn′tər-fə-lăn′jē-əl, -fā-) *n.* See **digital joint.**

in·ter·phase (ĭn′tər-fāz′) *n.* The stage of a cell between two successive mitotic or meiotic divisions. Also called *interkinesis.*

in·ter·phy·let·ic (ĭn′tər-fī-lĕt′ĭk) *adj.* Transitional in form between two kinds of cells during the course of metaplasia.

in·ter·pleu·ral space (ĭn′tər-plŏŏr′əl) *n.* See **mediastinum** (sense 2).

in·ter·po·lat·ed extrasystole (ĭn-tûr′pə-lā′tĭd) *n.* A ventricular contraction that occurs between two normal heartbeats.

in·ter·pre·ta·tion (ĭn-tûr′prĭ-tā′shən) *n.* **1.** The act or process of explaining the meaning of something. **2.** A psychotherapist's explanation of the meaning of a patient's remarks, dreams, memories, experiences, and behavior. —**in·ter′pret** *v.*

in·ter·prox·i·mal (ĭn′tər-prŏk′sə-məl) *adj.* Situated between adjoining surfaces.

interproximal space *n.* The space between adjacent teeth in a dental arch.

in·ter·pu·pil·lar·y (ĭn′tər-pyōō′pə-lĕr′ē) *adj.* Occurring between the pupils of the eyes, referring especially to the distance between the pupils.

in·ter·ra·dic·u·lar alveoloplasty (ĭn′tər-rə-dĭk′yə-lər) *n.* Surgical removal of bone and collapse of the cortical plates to modify the alveolar contour.

interradicular space *n.* The space between the roots of multirooted teeth.

in·ter·rupt·ed suture (ĭn′tə-rŭp′tĭd) *n.* A suture in which each stitch is made from a separate piece of material and fixed by tying the ends together.

in·ter·sex·u·al (ĭn′tər-sĕk′shōō-əl) *adj.* Having both male and female characteristics, including in varying degrees reproductive organs and secondary sexual characteristics, as a result of an abnormality of the sex chromosomes or a hormonal imbalance during embryogenesis.

in·ter·space (ĭn′tər-spās′) *n.* A space between two things; an interval. —**in′ter·space′** *v.* —**in′ter·spa′tial** (-spā′shəl) *adj.*

in·ter·spi·nal muscle (ĭn′tər-spī′nəl) *n.* Any of the paired muscles between the spinous processes of adjacent vertebrae, subdivided into cervical, thoracic, and lumbar muscles.

interspinal plane *n.* A horizontal plane passing through the anterior superior iliac spines, marking the boundary between the lateral and umbilical regions and between the inguinal and pubic regions.

in·ter·stice (ĭn-tûr′stĭs) *n., pl.* **–stic·es** (-stĭ-sēz′, -sĭz) A small area, space, or hole in the substance of an organ or tissue.

in·ter·sti·tial (ĭn′tər-stĭsh′əl) *adj.* Relating to or situated in the small, narrow spaces between tissues or parts of an organ.

interstitial cell *n.* A cell that occurs between the germ cells of the gonads and that may furnish the male sex hormone. Also called *Leydig cell.*

interstitial cell-stimulating hormone *n. Abbr.* **ICHS** See luteinizing hormone.

interstitial cystitis *n.* A chronic inflammatory condition of unknown cause involving the mucosa and muscular tissue of the bladder and resulting in reduced bladder capacity.

interstitial disease *n.* A disease that chiefly affects the connective tissue framework of an organ.

interstitial emphysema *n.* **1.** The presence of air in the pulmonary tissues due to rupture of the air cells. **2.** The presence of air or gas in the connective tissue.

interstitial fluid *n.* The fluid in spaces between the tissue cells.

interstitial gastritis *n.* Inflammation of the stomach involving the submucous and muscle coats.

interstitial giant cell pneumonia *n.* See **giant cell pneumonia**.

interstitial growth *n.* Growth originating in different centers within a structure or an area, characteristic of tissues formed of nonrigid materials.

interstitial hernia *n.* A hernia in which the protrusion is between any two of the layers of the abdominal wall.

interstitial keratitis *n.* See **parenchymatous keratitis**.

interstitial lamella *n.* One of the lamellae of partially resorbed osteons occurring between newer, complete osteons. Also called *ground lamella, intermediate lamella*.

interstitial nephritis *n.* Nephritis in which the interstitial connective tissue is chiefly affected.

interstitial neuritis *n.* Inflammation of the connective tissue framework of a nerve.

interstitial plasma cell pneumonia *n.* See **pneumocystosis**.

interstitial pregnancy *n.* See **intramural pregnancy**.

interstitial tissue *n.* See **connective tissue**.

in·ter·sti·ti·um (ĭn′tər-stĭsh′ē-əm) *n.* An interstice.

in·ter·tar·sal joint (ĭn′tər-tär′səl) *n.* See **tarsal joint**.

in·ter·trans·verse muscle (ĭn′tər-trănz-vûrs′, -trănz′vûrs′) *n.* Any of the paired muscles between the transverse processes of adjacent vertebrae, designated anterior and posterior muscles in the cervical region, lateral and medial in the lumbar region, and single in the thoracic region.

in·ter·tri·go (ĭn′tər-trī′gō′) *n.* Dermatitis occurring between folds or juxtaposed surfaces of the skin and caused by sweat retention, moisture, warmth, and the overgrowth of resident microorganisms.

in·ter·tro·chan·ter·ic crest (ĭn′tər-trō′kən-tĕr′ĭk, -kăn) *n.* The rounded ridge that connects the greater and the lesser trochanter of the femur and that marks the junction of the neck and shaft of the bone.

intertrochanteric line *n.* A rough line that separates the neck and shaft of the femur anteriorly. Also called *spiral line*.

in·ter·tu·ber·cu·lar plane (ĭn′tər-tŏŏ-bûr′kyə-lər) *n.* An Addison's clinical plane passing horizontally through the iliac tubercles and usually cutting the fifth lumbar vertebra. Also called *intertubercular line*.

in·ter·u·re·ter·ic fold (ĭn′tər-yŏŏr′ĭ-tĕr′ĭk) *n.* A fold of mucous membrane extending from the orifice of the ureter of one side to that of the other side. Also called *Mercier's bar*.

in·ter·val (ĭn′tər-vəl) *n.* **1.** A space between two objects, points, or units. **2.** The amount of time between two specified instants, events, or states.

interval phase *n.* Ovulation.

in·ter·ve·nous tubercle (ĭn′tər-vē′nəs) *n.* A projection on the wall of the right atrium of the heart between the orifices of the venae cavae.

in·ter·ven·tion (ĭn′tər-vĕn′shən) *n.* Interference so as to modify a process or situation. —**in′ter·vene′** (ĭn′tər-vēn′) *v.*

in·ter·ven·tric·u·lar foramen (ĭn′tər-vĕn-trĭk′yə-lər) *n.* The short, often slitlike passage that on both the left and the right sides connects the third ventricle in the

diencephalon with the lateral ventricle in the cerebral hemisphere. Also called *Monro's foramen, porta*.

interventricular septum *n.* The wall between the ventricles of the heart.

in·ter·ver·te·bral (ĭn′tər-vûr′tə-brəl, -vûr-tē′-) *adj.* Located between vertebrae.

intervertebral disk *n.* Any of the disks between the bodies of adjacent vertebrae. Also called *intervertebral cartilage*.

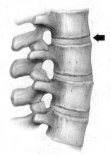

intervertebral disk
profile of lumbar intervertebral disks

intervertebral foramen *n.* Any of the openings into the vertebral canal bounded by the pedicles of adjacent vertebrae above and below, the vertebral bodies in front, and the articular processes behind.

intervertebral vein *n.* Any of numerous veins accompanying the spinal nerves, emptying in the neck into the vertebral vein, in the thorax into the intercostal vein, and in the lumbar and sacral regions into the lumbar and sacral veins.

in·ter·vil·lous lacuna (ĭn′tər-vĭl′əs) *n.* One of the spaces in the placenta that contain maternal blood and into which the chorionic villi project.

intervillous space *n.* Any of the spaces between placental villi containing maternal blood.

in·tes·ti·nal (ĭn-tĕs′tə-nəl) *adj.* Of, relating to, or constituting the intestine.

intestinal anastomosis *n.* See **enteroenterostomy**.

intestinal angina *n.* See **abdominal angina**.

intestinal artery *n.* See **jejunal artery**.

intestinal atresia *n.* Congenital absence or closure of the lumen of the small intestine involving the ileum, jejunum, or duodenum.

intestinal digestion *n.* The part of digestion carried on in the intestine, affecting all foodstuffs, including starches, fats, and proteins.

intestinal emphysema *n.* A condition marked by gas cysts in the intestinal mucous membrane, sometimes causing intestinal obstruction. Also called *pneumatosis cystoides intestinalis*.

intestinal fistula *n.* A tract leading from the lumen of the bowel to the exterior. Also called *fecal fistula, stercoral fistula*.

intestinal gland *n.* Any of the tubular glands in the mucous membrane of the small and large intestines. Also called *intestinal follicle, Lieberkühn's crypt, Lieberkühn's follicle*.

intestinal lipodystrophy *n.* See **Whipple's disease**.

intestinal stasis *n.* See **enterostasis**.

intestinal villus *n.* Any of the many projections of the mucous membrane of the intestine that serve as sites of absorption and that are leaf-shaped in the duodenum and become shorter, more finger-shaped, and sparser in the ileum.

in·tes·tine (ĭn-tĕs′tĭn) *n.* The portion of the alimentary canal extending from the stomach to the anus and, in humans and other mammals, consisting of two segments, the small intestine and the large intestine. Often used in the plural.

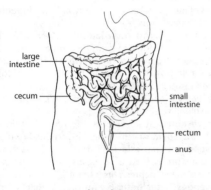

intestine

in·ti·ma (ĭn′tə-mə) *n.,* *pl.* **–mas** *or* **–mae** (-mē′) The innermost coat of an organ. —**in′ti·mal** *adj.*

in·ti·mi·tis (ĭn′tə-mī′tĭs) *n.* Inflammation of an intima, as in endangiitis.

in·toe (ĭn′tō) *n.* See **metatarsus varus**.

in·tol·er·ance (ĭn-tŏl′ər-əns) *n.* Extreme sensitivity or allergy to a drug, food, or other substance. —**in·tol′er·ant** *adj.*

in·tor·sion (ĭn-tôr′shən) *n.* **1.** The inward rotation of a limb or an organ. **2.** The inward convergent rotation of the upper pole of the vertical meridian of each eye. Also called *conclination, negative declination.*

in·tor·tor (ĭn-tôr′tər) *n.* A muscle that serves to turn a part medially.

in·tox·i·cant (ĭn-tŏk′sĭ-kənt) *n.* An agent that intoxicates, especially an alcoholic beverage. —**in·tox′i·cant** *adj.*

in·tox·i·cate (ĭn-tŏk′sĭ-kāt′) *v.* To stupefy or excite, as by the action of a chemical substance such as alcohol.

in·tox·i·ca·tion (ĭn-tŏk′sĭ-kā′shən) *n.* **1.** The pathological state produced by a drug, serum, alcohol, or any toxic substance; poisoning. **2.** Acute alcoholism. **3.** A state of mental excitement or emotional frenzy.

intra– *pref.* Within: *intramedullary.*

in·tra-a·or·tic balloon device (ĭn′trə-ā-ôr′tĭk) *n.* An inflatable balloon placed into the descending aorta to assist the heart in pumping blood.

intra-aortic balloon pump *n.* A pump connected to a balloon device that is inserted into the descending aorta to provide temporary assistance to the heart in the management of left ventricular failure.

in·tra-ar·te·ri·al (ĭn′trə-är-tîr′ē-əl) *adj.* Within arteries or an artery.

in·tra-a·tri·al block (ĭn′trə-ā′trē-əl) *n.* Impaired conduction of a nerve impulse through the atria, manifested by widened and often notched P waves.

intra-atrial conduction *n.* The conduction of the cardiac impulse through the atrial muscle tissue, represented by the P wave. Also called *atrial conduction.*

in·tra·cap·su·lar ankylosis (ĭn′trə-kăp′sə-lər) *n.* Stiffness of a joint due to the presence of bony or fibrous adhesions between the articular surfaces of the joint.

intracapsular ligament *n.* Any of the ligaments located within and separate from the articular capsule of a synovial joint.

in·tra·car·di·ac (ĭn′trə-kär′dē-ăk′) *adj.* Within the heart.

intracardiac catheter *n.* See **cardiac catheter**.

in·tra·car·ti·lag·i·nous (ĭn′trə-kär′tl-ăj′ə-nəs) *adj.* Occurring within a cartilage or cartilaginous tissue.

in·tra·cath·e·ter (ĭn′trə-kăth′ĭ-tər) *n.* A plastic tube, usually attached to a puncturing needle, inserted into a blood vessel for infusion, injection, or pressure monitoring.

in·tra·cav·i·tar·y (ĭn′trə-căv′ĭ-tĕr′ē) *adj.* Within an organ or body cavity.

in·tra·cel·lu·lar (ĭn′trə-sĕl′yə-lər) *adj.* Occurring or situated within a cell or cells.

intracellular canaliculus *n.* A fine canal formed by invagination of a cell membrane into the cytoplasm of a cell.

intracellular fluid *n.* *Abbr.* **ICF** The fluid within the tissue cells.

intracellular toxin *n.* See **endotoxin**.

in·tra·cer·e·bral (ĭn′trə-sĕr′ə-brəl, -sə-rē′-) *adj.* Existing within the cerebrum.

in·tra·cer·vi·cal (ĭn′trə-sûr′vĭ-kəl) *adj.* Existing within a cervix; endocervical.

I·sor·dil (ī′sôr-dĭl′) A trademark for the drug isosorbide dinitrate.

in·tra·cor·po·re·al (ĭn′trə-kôr-pôr′ē-əl) *adj.* **1.** Existing within the body. **2.** Existing within a corpus.

in·tra·cra·ni·al (ĭn′trə-krā′nē-əl) *adj.* Within the cranium.

intracranial cavity *n.* See **cranial cavity**.

intracranial hemorrhage *n.* The escape of blood within the cranium due to the loss of integrity of vascular channels and frequently leading to formation of a hematoma.

intracranial pressure *n.* *Abbr.* **ICP** Pressure within the cranial cavity.

in·trac·ta·ble (ĭn-trăk′tə-bəl) *adj.* **1.** Difficult to manage or govern; stubborn. **2.** Difficult to alleviate, remedy, or cure. —**in·trac′ta·bil′i·ty** *n.*

in·tra·cu·ta·ne·ous (ĭn′trə-kyōō-tā′nē-əs) *adj.* Within the skin; intradermal.

intracutaneous reaction *n.* A skin reaction following the intracutaneous injection of an antigen to which the individual has been sensitized, as in the tuberculin test. Also called *intradermal reaction.*

in·trad (ĭn′trăd′) *adv.* Toward the inner part; inward.

in·tra·der·mal (ĭn′trə-dûr′məl) *adj.* Within or between the layers of the skin.

intradermal nevus *n.* A nevus having nests of melanocytes occurring in the dermis but not at the epidermal-dermal junction.

intradermal reaction *n.* See **intracutaneous reaction**.

intradermal test *n.* A test for hypersensitivity or allergy in which a small amount of the suspected allergen is injected into the skin.

in·tra·em·bry·on·ic (ĭn′trə-ĕm′brē-ŏn′ĭk) *adj.* Within the embryo.

in·tra·fal·lo·pi·an (ĭn′trə-fə-lō′pē-ən) *adj.* Located or occurring within the fallopian tubes.

in·tra·fi·lar (ĭn′trə-fī′lər) *adj.* Situated within the meshes of a network.

in·tra·fu·sal (ĭn′trə-fyōo′zəl) *adj.* Relating to the structures within a muscle spindle.

intrafusal fiber *n.* Any of the muscle fibers present within a neuromuscular spindle.

in·tra·lig·a·men·tar·y pregnancy (ĭn′trə-lĭg′ə-měn′-tə-rē, -měn′trē) *n.* An ectopic pregnancy developing within the broad ligament.

in·tra·lob·u·lar duct (ĭn′trə-lŏb′yə-lər) *n.* One of the ducts contained within a lobule of a gland.

in·tra·med·ul·lar·y (ĭn′trə-měd′l-ĕr′ē, -mə-dŭl′ə-rē) *adj.* **1.** Within the bone marrow. **2.** Within the spinal cord. **3.** Within the medulla oblongata.

in·tra·mu·ral (ĭn′trə-myoor′əl) *adj.* Occurring or situated within the walls of a cavity or organ.

intramural hematoma *n.* A hematoma in the wall of a structure, such as the bowel or bladder, usually resulting from trauma.

intramural pregnancy *n.* An ectopic pregnancy developing in the uterine portion of the fallopian tube. Also called *interstitial pregnancy.*

in·tra·mus·cu·lar (ĭn′trə-mŭs′kyə-lər) *adj.* *Abbr.* **IM** Within a muscle.

in·tra·na·sal (ĭn′trə-nā′zəl) *adj.* Within the nose.

intranasal anesthesia *n.* **1.** Insufflation anesthesia in which an anesthetic is added to inhaled air as it passes through the nose or nasopharynx. **2.** Anesthesia of nasal passages by topical application of an anesthetic solution to nasal mucosa.

in·tra·oc·u·lar (ĭn′trə-ŏk′yə-lər) *adj.* Within the eyeball.

intraocular pressure *n.* The pressure of the intraocular fluid within the eye.

intraocular tension *n.* *Abbr.* **Tn** The pressure within the eyeball, measured by the resistance of the tunics of the eye to indentation.

in·tra·o·ral (ĭn′trə-ôr′əl) *adj.* Within the mouth.

intraoral anesthesia *n.* **1.** Insufflation anesthesia in which an anesthetic is added to inhaled air passing through the mouth. **2.** Anesthesia of the mouth and associated structures by topical application of anesthetic solutions to oral mucosa.

in·tra·pa·ri·e·tal sulcus (ĭn′trə-pə-rī′ĭ-təl) *n.* A horizontal sulcus extending from the postcentral sulcus and dividing into two branches to form with the postcentral sulcus a figure H that divides the parietal lobe into a superior and an inferior lobule.

in·tra·pa·rot·id plexus (ĭn′trə-pə-rŏt′ĭd) *n.* Any of the branches of the facial nerve passing through the substance of the parotid gland, connected by looped anastomoses. Also called *pes anserinus.*

in·tra·par·tum (ĭn′trə-pär′təm) *adj.* Occurring during labor and delivery.

intrapartum hemorrhage *n.* Hemorrhage occurring in the course of normal labor and delivery.

in·tra·psy·chic (ĭn′trə-sī′kĭk) *adj.* Existing or taking place within the mind or psyche.

in·tra·u·ter·ine (ĭn′trə-yōo′tər-ĭn, -tə-rīn′) *adj.* Within the uterus.

intrauterine amputation *n.* See **congenital amputation.**

intrauterine contraceptive *n.* An intrauterine device.

intrauterine device *n.* *Abbr.* **IUD** A birth control device, such as a plastic or metallic loop, ring, or spiral, that is inserted into the uterus to prevent implantation of a fertilized egg in the uterine lining.

intrauterine fracture *n.* A fracture of one or more fetal bones that occurs before birth.

intrauterine growth restriction *n.* See **intrauterine growth retardation.**

intrauterine growth retardation *n.* *Abbr.* **IUGR** Birth weight that is below the tenth percentile for gestational age. Also called *intrauterine growth restriction.*

in·trav·a·sa·tion (ĭn-trăv′ə-sā′shən) *n.* Entry of foreign matter into a blood vessel.

in·tra·vas·cu·lar (ĭn′trə-văs′kyə-lər) *adj.* Within one or more blood vessels.

in·tra·ve·nous (ĭn′trə-vē′nəs) *adj.* *Abbr.* **IV** Within or administered into a vein. —**in′tra·ve′nous·ly** *adv.*

intravenous anesthesia *n.* General anesthesia in which venipuncture is used as a means of injecting central nervous system depressants into the bloodstream.

intravenous anesthetic *n.* An agent that produces anesthesia when injected into the bloodstream via venipuncture.

intravenous bolus *n.* A large volume of fluid or dose of a drug given intravenously and rapidly at one time.

intravenous drip *n.* The continuous introduction of a solution intravenously, a drop at a time.

intravenous pyelogram *n.* *Abbr.* **IVP** A radiologic study in which intravenous injection of a radiopaque contrast medium that is excreted by the kidneys allows visualization of the renal pelvices and urinary tract.

intravenous urography *n.* X-ray examination of kidneys, ureters, and bladder following the injection of a contrast agent into a vein.

in·tra·ven·tric·u·lar block (ĭn′trə-věn-trĭk′yə-lər) *n.* Delayed conduction of an impulse within the ventricular conducting system or myocardium.

intraventricular conduction *n.* The conduction of the cardiac impulse through the ventricular muscle tissue. Also called *ventricular conduction.*

in·tra·vi·tal (ĭn′trə-vīt′l) *adj.* Occurring in or performed on a living organism.

intravital stain *n.* A stain absorbed by living cells after injection into the body.

in·tra vi·tam (ĭn′trə vī′tăm) *adv.* During life.

in·trin·sic (ĭn-trĭn′zĭk) *adj.* **1.** Of or relating to the essential nature of a thing. **2.** Situated within or belonging solely to the organ or body part on which it acts. Used of certain nerves and muscles.

intrinsic factor *n.* A relatively small mucoprotein secreted by the parietal cells of gastric glands and required for adequate absorption of vitamin B_{12} for production of red blood cells. Also called *Castle's intrinsic factor.*

intrinsic reflex *n.* A reflex muscular contraction elicited by the application of a stimulus, usually stretching, to the muscle.

intrinsic sphincter *n.* A thickening of the circular fibers of the tunica muscularis of an organ.

intro– *pref.* **1.** In; into: *intromission*. **2.** Inward: *introspection*.

in·tro·duce (ĭn′trə-do͞os′) *v.* **1.** To put inside or into; insert or inject. **2.** To bring in and establish in a new place or environment.

in·tro·duc·er (ĭn′trə-do͞o′sər) *n.* An instrument or stylet used to insert a catheter, an endotracheal tube, or similar flexible device into the body.

in·tro·flec·tion *or* **in·tro·flex·ion** (ĭn′trə-flĕk′shən) *n.* A bending inward.

in·tro·i·tus (ĭn-trō′ĭ-təs) *n., pl.* **introitus** The entrance into a canal or hollow organ, such as the vagina.

in·tro·jec·tion (ĭn′trə-jĕk′shən) *n.* The process of incorporating the characteristics of a person or object unconsciously into one's psyche, often as a defense mechanism. —**in′tro·ject′** *v.*

in·tro·mis·sion (ĭn′trə-mĭsh′ən) *n.* The act or process of intromitting. —**in′tro·mis′sive** (-mĭs′ĭv) *v.*

in·tro·mit (ĭn′trə-mĭt′) *v.* To cause or permit to enter; introduce or admit.

in·tro·mit·tent (ĭn′trə-mĭt′ənt) *adj.* Conveying or sending into a body or cavity.

in·tron (ĭn′trŏn) *n.* A segment of a gene situated between exons that does not function in coding for protein synthesis.

In·tro·pin (ĭn′trə-pĭn′) A trademark for a medicinal preparation of dopamine.

in·tro·spec·tion (ĭn′trə-spĕk′shən) *n.* Contemplation of one's own thoughts, feelings, and sensations; self-examination. —**in′tro·spect′** *v.* —**in′tro·spec′tive** (-tĭv) *adj.*

in·tro·sus·cep·tion (ĭn′trō-sə-sĕp′shən) *n.* See **intussusception**.

in·tro·ver·sion (ĭn′trə-vûr′zhən, -shən) *n.* **1.** The act or process of introverting or the condition of being introverted. **2.** The direction of or tendency to direct one's thoughts and feelings toward oneself. —**in′tro·ver′sive** (-vûr′sĭv) *adj.*

in·tro·vert (ĭn′trə-vûrt′, ĭn′trə-vûrt′) *v.* **1.** To turn or direct inward. **2.** To concentrate one's interests upon oneself. **3.** To turn a tubular organ or part inward upon itself. —*n.* (ĭn′trə-vûrt′) **1.** One whose thoughts and feelings are directed toward oneself. **2.** An anatomical structure that is capable of being introverted.

in·tro·vert·ed (ĭn′trə-vûr′tĭd) *adj.* Marked by interest in or preoccupation with oneself or one's own thoughts as opposed to others or the environment.

in·tu·bate (ĭn′to͞o-bāt′) *v.* To insert a tube into a hollow organ or body passage. —**in′tu·ba′tion** *n.*

in·tu·i·tive stage (ĭn-to͞o′ĭ-tĭv) *n.* A stage of development, usually occurring between 4 and 7 years of age, in which a child's thought processes are determined by the most prominent aspects of the stimuli to which he or she is exposed, rather than by some form of logical thought.

in·tu·mesce (ĭn′to͞o-mĕs′) *v.* **1.** To swell or expand; enlarge. **2.** To bubble up, especially from the effect of heating.

in·tu·mes·cence (ĭn′to͞o-mĕs′əns) *n.* **1.** The act or process of swelling or the condition of being swollen. **2.** A swollen organ or body part. —**in′tu·mes′cent** *adj.*

in·tus·sus·cept (ĭn′tə-sə-sĕpt′) *v.* To take within, as in telescoping one part of the intestine into another; invaginate.

in·tus·sus·cep·tion (ĭn′tə-sə-sĕp′shən) *n.* **1.** Invagination, especially an infolding of one part of the intestine into another. **2.** Assimilation of new substances into the existing components of living tissue. Also called *introsusception*. —**in′tus·sus·cep′tive** (-tĭv) *adj.*

in·tus·sus·cep·tum (ĭn′tə-sə-sĕp′təm) *n.* The part of the bowel that is invaginated within another part in an intussusception.

in·tus·sus·cip·i·ens (ĭn′tə-sə-sĭp′ē-ənz) *n.* The part of the bowel into which another part is invaginated in an intussusception.

in·u·lase (ĭn′yə-lās′) *n.* An enzyme that catalyzes the conversion of inulin to fructose.

in·u·lin (ĭn′yə-lĭn) *n.* A fructose polysaccharide derived from the rhizomes of *Inula helenium* or *I. elecampane*, and other plants.

inulin clearance *n.* A method for determining the rate of filtration in the renal glomeruli, since inulin is completely filterable through them and is neither excreted nor reabsorbed by the renal tubules.

in·unc·tion (ĭn-ŭngk′shən) *n.* The process of applying and rubbing in an ointment.

in u·ter·o (ĭn yo͞o′tə-rō) *adj.* In the uterus. —**in utero** *adv.*

in·vag·i·nate (ĭn-văj′ə-nāt′) *v.* To infold or become infolded so as to form a hollow space within a previously solid structure, as in the formation of a gastrula from a blastula.

in·vag·i·na·tion (ĭn-văj′ə-nā′shən) *n.* **1.** The act or process of invaginating or the condition of being invaginated. **2.** An invaginated organ or part. **3.** The infolding of a portion of the outer layer of a blastula in the formation of a gastrula.

in·va·lid (ĭn′və-lĭd) *n.* One who is incapacitated by a chronic illness or disability. —*adj.* Incapacitated by illness or injury.

in·va·sive (ĭn-vā′sĭv) *adj.* **1.** Marked by the tendency to spread, especially into healthy tissue, as a tumor. **2.** Of or relating to a medical procedure in which a part of the body is entered, as by puncture or incision. —**in·va′sive·ness** *n.*

in·ver·sion (ĭn-vûr′zhən) *n.* **1.** The act of inverting or the state of being inverted. **2.** Conversion of a substance in which the direction of optical rotation is reversed. **3.** The taking on of the gender role of the opposite sex. **4.** A chromosomal defect in which a segment of the chromosome breaks off and reattaches in the reverse direction.

inversion of uterus *n.* A turning of the uterus inside out, usually following childbirth.

in·vert (ĭn-vûrt′) *v.* **1.** To turn inside out or upside down. **2.** To reverse the position, order, or condition of. **3.** To subject to inversion. —*n.* (ĭn′vûrt′) Something inverted.

in·ver·tase (ĭn-vûr′tās′, ĭn′vər-tās′, -tāz′) *n.* An enzyme that catalyzes the hydrolysis of sucrose into glucose and fructose. Also called *beta-fructofuranosidase, invertin, saccharase, sucrase*.

in·ver·te·brate (ĭn-vûr′tə-brĭt, -brāt′) *adj.* **1.** Lacking a backbone or spinal column; not vertebrate. **2.** Of or relating to invertebrates. —*n.* An animal, such as an insect or a mollusk, that lacks a backbone or spinal column.

in·vert·ed testis (ĭn-vûr′tĭd) *n.* A testis that is rotated in the scrotum, with the epididymis directed anteriorly.

in·ver·tin (ĭn-vûr′tn) *n.* See **invertase.**

in·ver·tor (ĭn-vûr′tər) *n.* A muscle that turns a body part such as the foot inward.

invert sugar *n.* A mixture of equal parts of glucose and fructose resulting from the hydrolysis of sucrose, found naturally in fruits and honey, and produced artificially for use in the food industry.

in·vest·ing cartilage (ĭn-vĕs′tĭng) *n.* See **articular cartilage.**

in·vet·er·ate (ĭn-vĕt′ər-ĭt) *adj.* **1.** Firmly and long established; deep-rooted. **2.** Persisting in an ingrained habit; habitual. —**in·vet′er·a·cy** (-ər-ə-sē) *n.*

in·vi·a·ble (ĭn-vī′ə-bəl) *adj.* Unable to survive or develop normally.

in·vis·ca·tion (ĭn′vĭ-skā′shən) *n.* **1.** Smearing with mucilaginous matter. **2.** The mixing of food with buccal secretions during chewing.

in vi·tro (ĭn vē′trō) *adj.* In an artificial environment outside a living organism. —**in vi′tro** *adv.*

in vitro fertilization *n. Abbr.* **IVF** Fertilization of an egg outside the body of a female by the addition of sperm, as a means of producing a zygote.

in vi·vo (vē′vō) *adj.* Within a living organism. —**in vivo** *adv.*

in vivo fertilization *n.* Fertilization of a ripe egg within the uterus of a fertile donor female, rather than in an artificial medium, for subsequent nonsurgical transfer to an infertile recipient.

in·vo·lu·crum (ĭn′və-lōō′krəm) *n., pl.* **–cra** (-krə) An enveloping sheath or membrane, such as the sheath of new bone that forms around a sequestrum.

in·vol·un·tar·y (ĭn-vŏl′ən-tĕr′ē) *adj.* **1.** Not subject to control of the volition. **2.** Acting or done without or against one's will.

involuntary muscle *n.* Any of the smooth muscles, except for the cardiac muscle, not under control of the will.

in·vo·lu·tion (ĭn′və-lōō′shən) *n.* **1.** A decrease in size of an organ, as of the uterus following childbirth. **2.** The ingrowth and curling inward of a group of cells, as in the formation of a gastrula from a blastula. **3.** A progressive decline or degeneration of normal physiological functioning occurring as a result of the aging process. Also called *catagenesis.* —**in′vo·lu′tion·al** *adj.*

involutional melancholia *n.* A form of depression that occurs in late middle age, sometimes accompanied by paranoia.

involutional psychosis *n.* A mental disturbance occurring during menopause or later life, characterized chiefly by depression.

i·o·ce·tam·ic acid (ī′ō-sĭ-tăm′ĭk) *n.* A radiopaque contrast medium used as a diagnostic aid when administered internally.

iod– *pref.* Variant of **iodo–.**

i·o·da·mide (ī-ō′də-mīd′) *n.* A radiopaque contrast medium used as a diagnostic aid.

i·o·dide (ī′ə-dīd′) *n.* A compound of iodine with a more electropositive element or group.

i·o·dim·e·try (ī′ō-dĭm′ĭ-trē) *n.* The determination of the amount of iodine in a compound or of the amount consumed in a reaction by titrating with a standard solution.

i·o·di·nate (ī′ə-də-nāt′) *v.* To treat or combine with iodine or a compound of iodine.

i·o·dine (ī′ə-dīn′, -dĭn, -dēn) *n.* **1.** *Symbol* **I** A poisonous halogen element having compounds used as germicides, antiseptics, and food supplements, with numerous radioactive isotopes, which are used in diagnosis and treatment of thyroid diseases and neuroendocrine tumors. Atomic number 53. **2.** A liquid containing iodine dissolved in ethyl alcohol, used as an antiseptic for wounds.

iodine-123 *n.* A radioisotope of iodine with a pure gamma emission and a physical half-life of 13.1 hours, used for studies of thyroid metabolism.

iodine-125 *n.* A radioisotope of iodine with a half-life of 60 days that is used as a tracer in thyroid studies and as therapy in hyperthyroidism.

iodine-131 *n.* A radioisotope of iodine that emits beta and gamma rays, has a half-life of 8.05 days, and is used as a tracer in thyroid studies and as therapy in hyperthyroidism and thyroid cancer.

iodine-fast *adj.* Of or relating to hyperthyroidism unresponsive to iodine therapy.

iodine-induced hyperthyroidism *n.* See **Jod-Basedow phenomenon.**

iodine stain *n.* A stain used to detect a variety of polysaccharides, such as cellulose, chitin, and glycogen, in which potassium iodide reacts with starch to produce a blue color.

i·o·din·o·phil (ī′ə-dĭn′ə-fĭl) *or* **i·o·din·o·phile** (-fīl′) *n.* A histologic element that stains readily with iodine. —*adj.* Iodinophilous.

i·o·din·oph·i·lous (ī′ə-də-nŏf′ə-ləs) *adj.* Staining readily with iodine.

i·o·dip·a·mide (ī′ə-dĭp′ə-mīd′) *n.* A radiopaque contrast medium used for diagnostic tests for the biliary system.

i·o·dism (ī′ə-dĭz′əm) *n.* Poisoning by iodine, characterized by severe coryza, an acneform eruption, weakness, salivation, and foul breath.

i·o·dize (ī′ə-dīz′) *v.* To treat or combine with iodine or an iodide. —**i′o·di·za′tion** (-dĭ-zā′shən) *n.*

i·o·dized oil (ī′ə-dīzd′) *n.* An iodine addition product of vegetable oils that is used as a radiopaque contrast medium in hysterosalpingography.

iodo– *or* **iod–** *pref.* Iodine: *iodotherapy.*

i·o·do·chlor·hy·drox·y·quin (ī-ō′də-klôr′hī-drŏk′sĭ-kwĭn′) *or* **i·o·do·chlor·o·hy·drox·y·quin·o·line** (-klôr′-ō-hī-drŏk′sĭ-kwĭn′ə-lēn′, -lĭn) *n.* A compound used topically as a local antibacterial agent and in the treatment of a wide range of dermatoses, intravaginally in the treatment of *Trichomonas vaginalis* vaginitis, and internally in the treatment of mild or asymptomatic intestinal amebiasis.

i·o·do·der·ma (ī-ō′də-dûr′mə) *n.* An eruption of follicular papules and pustules or a granulomatous lesion caused by iodine toxicity or sensitivity.

i·o·do·hip·pu·rate sodium (ī-ō′də-hĭp′yə-rāt′) *n.* A radiopaque compound administered intravenously and orally for diagnostic applications such as retrograde urography and renography.

i·o·do·meth·a·mate sodium (ī-ō′də-mĕth′ə-māt′) *n.* An organic iodine radiopaque compound that is used in intravenous urography and retrograde pyelography.

i·o·dom·e·try (ī′ō-dŏm′ĭ-trē) *n.* An analytical technique involving titrations in which the sudden appearance or disappearance of iodine marks the end point. —**i′o′do·met′ric** (ī-ō′də-mĕt′rĭk) *adj.*

i·o·do·phil·i·a (ī-ō′də-fĭl′ē-ə) *n.* An affinity for iodine, as manifested by some white blood cells in certain conditions.

i·o·dop·sin (ī′ə-dŏp′sĭn) *n.* A violet, light-sensitive visual pigment found in the cones of the retina. Also called *visual violet.*

i·o·do·py·ra·cet (ī-ō′də-pī′rə-sĕt′) *n.* A radiopaque contrast medium used intravenously in urography and also used to determine renal plasma flow and renal tubular excretory mass.

i·o·do·ther·a·py (ī-ō′də-thĕr′ə-pē) *n.* Medical treatment with iodine.

i·o·do·thy·ro·nine (ī-ō′də-thī′rə-nēn′, -nĭn) *n.* Any of the iodinated derivatives of thyronine.

i·o·dox·a·mate meglumine (ī′ə-dŏk′sə-māt′) *n.* A radiopaque contrast medium that is used primarily for cholecystography.

i·o·du·ri·a (ī′ə-dŏŏr′ē-ə) *n.* The excretion of iodine in the urine.

i·on (ī′ən, ī′ŏn′) *n.* An atom or a group of atoms that has acquired a net electric charge by gaining or losing one or more electrons.

ion channel *n.* See **channel** (sense 2).

ion exchange *n.* A reversible chemical reaction occurring between an insoluble solid and a solution during which ions may be interchanged, used in the separation of radioactive isotopes.

ion exchanger *n.* A polymer containing charged groups to which other charged mobile ions become attached or replaced, used in chromatography.

ion-exchange resin *n.* An insoluble polymer containing charged groups or ions that can be exchanged for charged groups or ions present in a surrounding solution.

i·on·ic (ī-ŏn′ĭk) *adj.* Of, containing, or involving an ion or ions.

i·on·i·za·tion (ī′ə-nĭ-zā′shən) *n.* **1.** The formation of or separation into ions by heat, electrical discharge, radiation, or chemical reaction; electrolytic dissociation. **2.** See **iontophoresis.**

ionization chamber *n.* A chamber for detecting ionization of the enclosed gas, used for determining the intensity of ionizing radiation.

i·on·ize (ī′ə-nīz′) *v.* To dissociate atoms or molecules into electrically charged atoms or radicals. —**i′on·iz′er** *n.*

i·on·i·zing radiation (ī′ə-nī′zĭng) *n.* High-energy radiation capable of producing ionization in substances through which it passes.

i·on·o·phore (ī-ŏn′ə-fôr) *n.* Any of a group of organic compounds that form a complex with an ion and transport it across a membrane.

i·on·o·pho·re·sis (ī-ŏn′ə-fə-rē′sĭs) *n.* See **electrophoresis** (sense 1). —**i·on′o·pho·ret′ic** (ī-ŏn′ə-fə-rĕt′ĭk) *adj.*

i·on·to·pho·re·sis (ī-ŏn′tə-fə-rē′sĭs) *n.* The use of an electric current to introduce the ions of a medicament into bodily tissues. Also called *ionization.* —**i·on′to·pho·ret′ic** (-rĕt′ĭk) *adj.*

i·o·pam·i·dol (ī′ə-păm′ĭ-dôl′) *n.* A diagnostic radiopaque contrast medium used in myelography, urography, and ventriculography.

i·o·pa·no·ic acid (ī′ə-pə-nō′ĭk) *n.* A radiopaque iodine compound used as a contrast medium in cholecystography.

i·o·phen·dyl·ate (ī′ə-fĕn′dl-āt′) *n.* An absorbable iodized fatty acid of low viscosity that is used for roentgenography of the spinal cord, biliary tree, sinuses, and body cavities.

i·o·ta (ī-ō′tə) *n. Symbol* ι The ninth letter of the Greek alphabet.

i·o·thal·a·mate sodium (ī′ə-thăl′ə-māt′) *n.* The sodium salt of iothalamic acid, used as a radiopaque contrast medium.

i·o·tha·lam·ic acid (ī′ō-thə-lăm′ĭk) *n.* A white powder that is slightly soluble in water and is used as a radiopaque contrast medium.

i·ox·ag·late (ī′ŏks-ăg′lāt′) *n.* A diagnostic radiopaque contrast medium used in angiography, aortography, and urography.

IPA (ī′pē′ā′) *n.* An independent group of physicians and other health-care providers that are under contract to provide services to members of different HMOs, as well as other insurance plans, usually at a fixed fee per patient.

ip·e·cac (ĭp′ĭ-kăk′) *n.* A preparation that is made from the dried roots and rhizomes of the shrub *Cephaelis ipecacuanha* that is used to induce vomiting.

i·po·date sodium (ī′pə-dāt′) *n.* A radiopaque contrast medium used in cholecystography and cholangiography.

IPPB *abbr.* intermittent positive pressure breathing

ip·ra·tro·pi·um bromide (ĭp′rə-trō′pē-əm) *n.* An inhalant drug, chemically related to atropine, used to treat bronchospasm.

i·pro·ni·a·zid (ī′prə-nī′ə-zĭd) *n.* A compound used as an antidepressant and formerly used in the treatment of tuberculosis.

ip·si·lat·er·al (ĭp′sə-lăt′ər-əl) *adj.* Located on or affecting the same side of the body.

IPV *abbr.* inactivated poliovirus vaccine

IQ *abbr.* intelligence quotient

Ir The symbol for the element **iridium.**

ir–¹ *pref.* Variant of **in–**[1].

ir–² *pref.* Variant of **in–**[2].

ir·be·sar·tan (ĭr′bə-sär′tn) *n.* An oral drug that is an angiotensin II receptor antagonist used to treat hypertension.

ir·i·dec·to·my (ĭr′ĭ-dĕk′tə-mē, ī′rĭ-) *n.* Surgical removal of part of the iris of the eye.

ir·i·dec·tro·pi·um (ĭr′ĭ-dĕk-trō′pē-əm, ī′rĭ-) *n.* See **ectropion uveae.**

ir·i·den·clei·sis (ĭr'ĭ-děn-klī'sĭs, ī'rĭ-) *n.* Confinement of a portion of the iris in a wound of the cornea as a surgical measure in treating glaucoma to permit drainage of the aqueous humor, thereby reducing intraocular pressure.

ir·i·den·tro·pi·um (ĭr'ĭ-děn-trō'pē-əm, ī'rĭ-) *n.* See **entropion uveae.**

ir·i·de·re·mi·a (ĭr'ĭ-də-rē'mē-ə, ī'rĭ-) *n.* An iris so rudimentary that it appears to be absent.

i·rid·e·sis (ĭ-rĭd'ĭ-sĭs, ī'rĭ-dē'sĭs) *n.* Ligature of a portion of the iris brought out through an incision in the cornea. Also called *iridodesis.*

i·rid·ic (ĭ-rĭd'ĭk, ī-rĭd'-) *adj.* Of or relating to the iris.

i·rid·i·um (ĭ-rĭd'ē-əm) *n. Symbol* **Ir** A hard, brittle, corrosion-resistant metallic element, whose radioisotope is used in the treatment of tumors. Atomic number 77.

irido– or **irid–** *pref.* Iris of the eye: *iridectomy.*

ir·i·do·a·vul·sion (ĭr'ĭ-dō-ə-vŭl'shən, ī'rĭ-) *n.* A tearing away of the iris.

ir·i·do·cele (ĭr'ĭ-dō-sēl', ĭ-rĭd'ə-, ĭ-rĭd'ə-) *n.* Protrusion of a portion of the iris through a corneal defect.

ir·i·do·cho·roid·i·tis (ĭr'ĭ-dō-kôr'oi-dī'tĭs, ī'rĭ-) *n.* Inflammation of both the iris and choroid.

ir·i·do·col·o·bo·ma (ĭr'ĭ-dō-kŏl'ə-bō'mə, ī'rĭ-) *n.* A coloboma or congenital defect of the iris.

ir·i·do·cor·ne·al angle (ĭr'ĭ-dō-kôr'nē-əl, ī'rĭ-) *n.* See **filtration angle.**

iridocorneal endothelial syndrome *n.* A syndrome characterized by glaucoma, iris atrophy, decreased corneal endothelium, anterior peripheral adhesion of the iris to the lens capsule, and multiple iris nodules. Also called *Cogan-Reese syndrome, iris-nevus syndrome.*

ir·i·do·cy·clec·to·my (ĭr'ĭ-dō-sī-klěk'tə-mē, -sī-klěk'-, ī'rĭ-) *n.* Removal of the iris and the ciliary body.

ir·i·do·cy·cli·tis (ĭr'ĭ-dō-sī-klī'tĭs, -sī-, ī'rĭ-) *n.* Inflammation of the iris and the ciliary body.

ir·i·do·cy·clo·cho·roid·i·tis (ĭr'ĭ-dō-sī'klō-kôr'oi-dī'tĭs, ī'rĭ-) *n.* Inflammation of the iris, the ciliary body, and the choroid.

ir·i·do·cys·tec·to·my (ĭr'ĭ-dō-sī-stěk'tə-mē, ī'rĭ-) *n.* The surgical creation of an artificial pupil in which the border of the iris and a portion of the lens capsule are drawn out through an incision in the cornea and cut off.

ir·i·dod·e·sis (ĭr'ĭ-dŏd'ĭ-sĭs, ī'rĭ-) *n.* See **iridesis.**

ir·i·do·di·al·y·sis (ĭr'ĭ-dō-dī-ăl'ĭ-sĭs, ī'rĭ-) *n.* Separation of the iris from its ciliary attachment.

ir·i·do·di·as·ta·sis (ĭr'ĭ-dō-dī-ăs'tə-sĭs, ī'rĭ-) *n.* A defect of the peripheral border of the iris with an intact pupil.

ir·i·do·di·la·tor (ĭr'ĭ-dō-dī-lā'tər, -dī'lā'-, -dī-lā'-, ī'rĭ-) *n.* **1.** The dilator muscle of the pupil. **2.** An agent that causes dilation of the pupil.

ir·i·do·do·ne·sis (ĭr'ĭ-dō-dō-nē'sĭs) *n.* Agitated motion of the iris.

ir·i·do·ki·ne·sis (ĭr'ĭ-dō-kə-nē'sĭs, -kī-, ī'rĭ-) *or* **ir·i·do·ki·ne·sia** (-zhə) *n.* The movement of the iris in contracting and dilating the pupil. —**ir'i·do·ki·net'ic** (-nět'ĭk) *adj.*

ir·i·dol·o·gy (ĭr'ĭ-dŏl'ə-jē, ī'rĭ-) *n.* The study of the iris of the eye, especially as associated with disease.

ir·i·do·ma·la·cia (ĭr'ĭ-dō-mə-lā'shə, ī'rĭ-) *n.* Degenerative softening of the iris.

ir·i·do·mes·o·di·al·y·sis (ĭr'ĭ-dō-měz'ō-dī-ăl'ĭ-sĭs, ī'rĭ-) *n.* Surgical separation of adhesions around the inner margin of the iris.

ir·i·do·mo·tor (ĭr'ĭ-dō-mō'tər, ī'rĭ-) *adj.* Of or relating to the movements of the iris.

ir·i·don·co·sis (ĭr'ĭ-dŏng-kō'sĭs, ī'rĭ-) *n.* Thickening of the iris.

ir·i·don·cus (ĭr'ĭ-dŏng'kəs, ī'rĭ-) *n.* A tumefaction of the iris.

ir·i·do·pa·ral·y·sis (ĭr'ĭ-dō-pə-răl'ĭ-sĭs, ī'rĭ-) *n.* See **iridoplegia.**

ir·i·dop·a·thy (ĭr'ĭ-dŏp'ə-thē, ī'rĭ-) *n.* Pathological lesions in the iris.

ir·i·do·ple·gia (ĭr'ĭ-dō-plē'jə, ī'rĭ-) *n.* Paralysis of the sphincter of iris. Also called *iridoparalysis.*

ir·i·dop·to·sis (ĭr'ĭ-dŏp-tō'sĭs, ī'rĭ-) *n.* Prolapse of the iris.

ir·i·dor·rhex·is (ĭr'ĭ-dō-rěk'sĭs, ī'rĭ-) *n.* The tearing away of the iris from its peripheral attachment.

ir·i·dos·chi·sis (ĭr'ĭ-dŏs'kĭ-sĭs, ī'rĭ-) *n.* The separation of the anterior layer of the iris from the posterior layer, with ruptured anterior fibers floating in the aqueous humor.

ir·i·do·scle·rot·o·my (ĭr'ĭ-dō-sklə-rŏt'ə-mē, ī'rĭ-) *n.* Incision of the sclera and the iris.

ir·i·do·ste·re·sis (ĭr'ĭ-dō-stə-rē'sĭs, ī'rĭ-) *n.* The loss or absence of all or part of the iris.

ir·i·dot·a·sis (ĭr'ĭ-dŏt'ə-sĭs, ī'rĭ-) *n.* Surgical stretching of the iris in the treatment of glaucoma.

ir·i·dot·o·my (ĭr'ĭ-dŏt'ə-mē, ī'rĭ-) *n.* Incision of the iris to form an artificial pupil. Also called *corotomy, iritomy, irotomy.*

i·ris (ī'rĭs) *n., pl.* **i·ris·es** *or* **i·ri·des** (ī'rĭ-dēz', ĭr'ĭ-) The round pigmented contractile membrane of the eye that is perforated in the center by the pupil, forms the front part of the vascular tunic, and is attached on the margin to the ciliary body. —**i'ri·dal** (ī'rĭ-dl, ĭr'ĭ-), **i·rid'i·al** (ĭ-rĭd'ē-əl, ĭ-rĭd'-), **i·rid'i·an** *adj.*

iris-nevus syndrome *n.* See **iridocorneal endothelial syndrome.**

iris pit *n.* A coloboma affecting the stroma of the iris with the pigment epithelium intact.

i·rit·ic (ī-rĭt'ĭk, ĭ-rĭt'-) *adj.* Of or relating to the iris.

i·ri·tis (ī-rī'tĭs) *n.* Inflammation of the iris.

i·rit·o·my (ī-rĭt'ə-mē) *n.* See **iridotomy.**

i·ron (ī'ərn) *n.* **1.** *Symbol* **Fe** A lustrous, malleable, ductile, magnetic or magnetizable metallic element. Atomic number 26. **2.** A dietary supplement or medication containing an iron salt, such as ferrous sulfate. —*adj.* Made of or containing iron.

iron-59 *n.* An iron isotope that is a beta emitter with a half-life of 45.1 days and is used as a tracer in the study of iron metabolism.

iron deficiency anemia *n.* A form of hypochromic microcytic anemia due to the dietary lack of iron or to a loss of iron from chronic bleeding.

iron lung *n.* See **Drinker respirator.**

iron-storage disease *n.* Any of various diseases characterized by the storage of excess iron in the parenchyma of many organs, as in idiopathic hemochromatosis or transfusion hemosiderosis.

i·rot·o·my (ī-rŏt′ə-mē) *n.* See **iridotomy**.

ir·ra·di·ate (ĭ-rā′dē-āt′) *v.* **1.** To expose to radiation, as for diagnostic or therapeutic purposes. **2.** To treat with radiation.

ir·ra·di·a·tion (ĭ-rā′dē-ā′shən) *n.* **1.** Exposure or subjection to the action of radiation for diagnostic or therapeutic purposes. **2.** Medical treatment by exposure to radiation. **3.** The spread of a nervous impulse beyond the usual path of conduction.

ir·ra·tion·al (ĭ-răsh′ə-nəl) *adj.* Not rational; marked by a lack of accord with reason or sound judgment.

ir·re·duc·i·ble (ĭr′ĭ-dōō′sə-bəl) *adj.* **1.** Impossible to reduce to a desired, simpler, or smaller form or amount. **2.** Incapable of being made chemically simpler, or of being replaced, hydrogenated, or reduced in positive charge. —**ir′re·duc′i·bil′i·ty** *n.*

irreducible hernia *n.* A hernia that cannot be reduced without surgery. Also called *incarcerated hernia*.

ir·reg·u·lar (ĭ-rĕg′yə-lər) *adj.* **1.** Not straight, uniform, or symmetrical, as facial features. **2.** Of uneven rate, occurrence, or duration, as a heartbeat. **3.** Deviating from a type; atypical.

irregular astigmatism *n.* Astigmatism in which different parts of the same meridian have different degrees of curvature.

irregular bone *n.* Any of a group of bones having peculiar or complex forms, such as the vertebrae.

irregular dentin *n.* See **tertiary dentin**.

ir·re·spon·sive (ĭr′ĭ-spŏn′sĭv) *adj.* **1.** Not responsive, as to treatment or stimuli. **2.** Not responding or answering readily.

ir·re·sus·ci·ta·ble (ĭr′ĭ-sŭs′ĭ-tə-bəl) *adj.* Incapable of being resuscitated or revived.

ir·re·vers·i·ble pulpitis (ĭr′ĭ-vûr′sə-bəl) *n.* Chronic inflammation of the dental pulp.

ir·ri·gate (ĭr′ĭ-gāt′) *v.* To wash out a cavity or wound with a fluid.

ir·ri·ta·bil·i·ty (ĭr′ĭ-tə-bĭl′ĭ-tē) *n.* **1.** The capacity to respond to stimuli. **2.** Abnormal or excessive sensitivity to stimuli of an organism, organ, or body part.

ir·ri·ta·ble (ĭr′ĭ-tə-bəl) *adj.* **1.** Capable of reacting to a stimulus. **2.** Abnormally sensitive to a stimulus.

irritable bowel syndrome *n.* A chronic disorder characterized by motor abnormalities of the small and large intestines, causing variable symptoms including cramping, abdominal pain, constipation, and diarrhea. Also called *irritable colon, spastic colon*.

irritable heart *n.* See **neurocirculatory asthenia**.

ir·ri·tant (ĭr′ĭ-tənt) *adj.* Causing irritation, especially physical irritation. —*n.* A source of irritation.

ir·ri·ta·tion (ĭr′ĭ-tā′shən) *n.* **1.** Extreme incipient inflammatory reaction of the body tissues to an injury. **2.** The normal response of a nerve or muscle to a stimulus. **3.** The evocation of a reaction in the body tissues by the application of a stimulus. —**ir′ri·ta′tive** (-tā′tĭv) *adj.*

irritation fibroma *n.* Slow-growing fibrous nodules on the oral mucosa, resulting from irritation caused by cheek biting or objects such as dentures and fillings.

ir·rup·tion (ĭ-rŭp′shən) *n.* The act or process of breaking through to a surface.

IRV *abbr.* inspiratory reserve volume

Ir·vine-Gass syndrome (ûr′vīn′găs′) *n.* A syndrome of the eye characterized by macular edema and loss of vision following cataract surgery.

is– *pref.* Variant of **iso–**.

is·aux·e·sis (ĭ′sôg-zē′sĭs, -sôk-sē′-) *n.* Growth of parts at the same rate as growth of the whole.

is·che·mi·a (ĭ-skē′mē-ə) *n.* Decreased blood supply to a bodily organ, tissue, or part caused by constriction or obstruction of the blood vessels. —**i·sche′mic** *adj.*

ischemic contracture of left ventricle *n.* The irreversible contraction of the left ventricle of the heart as a complication of a cardiopulmonary bypass operation. Also called *stone heart*.

ischemic hypoxia *n.* Tissue hypoxia resulting from slower circulation through the tissues so that oxygen tension in capillaries is less than normal, even though saturation, content, and tension in arteries are normal. Also called *stagnant anoxia*.

ischemic necrosis *n.* Necrosis caused by hypoxia resulting from local deprivation of blood supply.

is·chi·ad·ic spine (ĭs′kē-ăd′ĭk) *n.* See **sciatic spine**.

ischial bone *n.* See **ischium**.

ischial bursa *n.* The bursa between the gluteus maximus and the tuberosity of the ischium.

is·chi·al·gia (ĭs′kē-ăl′jə) *n.* Pain in the ischium. Also called *ischiodynia*.

ischiatic hernia *n.* A hernia through the sacrosciatic foramen.

is·chi·dro·sis (ĭs′kĭ-drō′sĭs) *n.* See **anhidrosis**.

ischio– *pref.* Ischium: *ischiovertebral*.

is·chi·o·cap·su·lar (ĭs′kē-ō-kăp′sə-lər) *adj.* Relating to the ischium and the capsular ligament of the hip joint.

is·chi·o·cav·er·no·sus (ĭs′kē-ō-kăv′ər-nō′səs) *n.* A muscle with origin from the ramus of the ischium, with insertion into the corpus cavernosum of the penis or of the clitoris, with nerve supply from the perineal nerve, and whose action compresses the crus of the penis or of the clitoris and forces blood in its sinuses into the distal part of the corpus cavernosum.

is·chi·o·cele (ĭs′kē-ō-sēl′) *n.* See **sciatic hernia**.

is·chi·o·coc·cyg·e·al (ĭs′kē-ō-kŏk-sĭj′ē-əl) *adj.* Relating to the ischium and the coccyx.

is·chi·o·dyn·i·a (ĭs′kē-ō-dĭn′ē-ə) *n.* See **ischialgia**.

is·chi·o·fem·o·ral (ĭs′kē-ō-fĕm′ər-əl) *adj.* Relating to the ischium and the femur.

is·chi·o·fib·u·lar (ĭs′kē-ō-fĭb′yə-lər) *adj.* **1.** Relating to the ischium and the fibula. **2.** Connecting the ischium and the fibula.

is·chi·o·ni·tis (ĭs′kē-ə-nī′tĭs) *n.* An inflammation of the ischium.

is·chi·o·pub·ic (ĭs′kē-ō-pyōō′bĭk) *adj.* Of or relating to the ischium and the pubic bone.

is·chi·o·tib·i·al (ĭs′kē-ō-tĭb′ē-əl) *adj.* **1.** Relating to the ischium and the tibia. **2.** Connecting the ischium and the tibia.

is·chi·o·ver·te·bral (ĭs′kē-ō-vûr′tə-brəl, ĭs′kē-ō-vər-tē′-brəl) *adj.* Of or relating to the ischium and the vertebral column.

is·chi·um (ĭs′kē-əm) *n.,* *pl.* **–chi·a** (-kē-ə) The lowest of the three major bones that constitute each half of the pelvis, distinct at birth but later becoming fused with the ilium and pubis. Also called *ischial bone.* **—is′-chi·ad′ic** (-ăd′ĭk) *adj.* **—is′chi·al** (-əl) *adj.* **—is′chi·at′ic** (-ăt′ĭk) *adj.*

is·chu·ret·ic (ĭs′kyoo-rĕt′ĭk) *adj.* Relating to or relieving ischuria.

is·chu·ri·a (ĭs-kyoor′ē-ə) *n.* Retention or suppression of urine.

Ish·i·ha·ra test (ĭsh′ĭ-hä′rə) *n.* A test for color-vision deficiency employing a series of plates on which numbers or letters are printed in dots of primary colors surrounded by dots of other colors; the figures are discernible by individuals with normal color vision.

is·land (ī′lənd) *n.* An isolated tissue or group of cells that is separated from the surrounding tissues by a groove or is marked by a difference in structure or function.

island flap *n.* A surgical flap in which the pedicle consists solely of the supplying blood vessels.

island of Reil (rīl) *n.* An oval region of the cerebral cortex, lateral to the lentiform nucleus, and buried in the fissure of sylvius. Also called *insula.*

islands of Langerhans *n.* See **islets of Langerhans.**

is·let (ī′lĭt) *n.* A small island.

islet cell *n.* One of the endocrine cells making up the islets of Langerhans.

islets of Langerhans *pl.n.* Irregular clusters of endocrine cells scattered throughout the tissue of the pancreas that secrete insulin and glucagon. Also called *islands of Langerhans.*

–ism *suff.* **1.** Action, process; practice: *vegetarianism.* **2.** Characteristic behavior or quality: *puerilism.* **3.** State; condition; quality: *senilism.* **4.** State or condition resulting from an excess of something specified: *strychninism.* **5.** Doctrine; theory; system of principles: *Darwinism.*

–ismus *suff.* Spasm; contraction: *strabismus.*

iso– *or* **is–** *pref.* **1.** Equal; uniform: *isobar.* **2.** Isomeric: *isopropyl.* **3.** Characterized by sameness with respect to species: *isoantigen.* **4.** Characterized by sameness with respect to genotype: *isograft.*

i·so·ag·glu·ti·na·tion (ī′sō-ə-gloot′n-ā′shən) *n.* The agglutination of the red blood cells of an individual by antibodies in the serum of another individual of the same species. Also called *isohemagglutination.*

i·so·ag·glu·ti·nin (ī′sō-ə-gloot′n-ĭn) *n.* An isoantibody normally present in the serum of an individual that causes the agglutination of the red blood cells of another individual of the same species. Also called *isohemagglutinin.*

i·so·ag·glu·tin·o·gen (ī′sō-ăg′loo-tĭn′ə-jən) *n.* An isoantigen that on exposure to its corresponding isoantibody causes agglutination of the red blood cells to which it is attached.

i·so·am·y·lase (ī′sō-ăm′ə-lās′, -lāz′) *n.* An enzyme that catalyzes the cleavage of branching sections in glycogen, amylopectin, and certain dextrins.

i·so·an·ti·bod·y (ī′sō-ăn′tĭ-bŏd′ē) *n.* An antibody produced by or derived from a member of the same species as that in which the antigen was raised. Also called *alloantibody.*

i·so·an·ti·gen (ī′sō-ăn′tĭ-jən) *n.* An antigenic substance present in some members of a species and capable of stimulating antibody production in those members that lack it. Also called *alloantigen.*

i·so·bar (ī′sə-bär′) *n.* **1.** Any of two or more kinds of atoms having the same atomic mass but different atomic numbers. **2.** A line on a weather map connecting points of equal atmospheric pressure.

i·so·bar·ic (ī′sə-bär′ĭk, -bär′-) *adj.* **1.** Having equal weights or pressures. **2.** Of or relating to solutions having the same density as the diluent or medium.

i·so·cap·ni·a (ī′sə-kăp′nē-ə) *n.* A state in which the arterial carbon dioxide pressure remains constant or unchanged.

i·so·cel·lu·lar (ī′sə-sĕl′yə-lər) *adj.* Composed of cells of equal size or of similar character.

i·so·chro·mat·ic (ī′sə-krō-măt′ĭk) *adj.* Of uniform color.

i·so·chro·mat·o·phil (ī′sə-krō-măt′ə-fīl′) *adj.* Having an equal affinity for the same stain. Used of cells and tissues.

i·so·chro·mo·some (ī′sə-krō′mə-sōm′) *n.* A chromosomal aberration in which two daughter chromosomes are formed, each lacking one chromosome arm but with the other arm doubled.

i·so·chro·ni·a (ī′sə-krō′nē-ə) *n.* **1.** The state of having the same chronaxie. **2.** Agreement, with respect to time, rate, or frequency, among processes.

i·soch·ro·nous (ī-sŏk′rə-nəs) *adj.* Occurring during the same time.

i·so·cit·rate dehydrogenase (ī′sə-sĭt′rāt′) *n.* Either of two enzymes that catalyze the oxidative decarboxylation of isocitrate during the Krebs cycle.

i·so·cit·ric acid (ī′sə-sĭt′rĭk) *n.* An isomer of citric acid that is an intermediate in the Krebs cycle.

i·so·co·ri·a (ī′sō-kôr′ē-ə) *n.* Equality in the size of the two pupils.

i·so·cor·tex (ī′sō-kôr′tĕks′) *n.* The larger part of the cerebral cortex, that is distinguished from the allocortex by having a larger number of nerve cells arranged in six layers. Also called *homotypic cortex, neocortex, neopallium.*

i·so·cy·a·nate (ī′sō-sī′ə-nāt′, -nət) *n.* Any of a family of nitrogenous chemicals that are used in industry and can cause respiratory disorders, especially asthma, if inhaled.

i·so·cy·tol·y·sin (ī′sō-sī-tŏl′ĭ-sĭn) *n.* A cytolysin that reacts with the cells of certain other animals of the same species, but not with the cells of the individual that formed it.

i·so·dac·tyl·ism (ī′sō-dăk′tə-lĭz′əm) *n.* A condition in which each of the fingers or toes is approximately equal in length.

i·so·dense (ī′sə-dĕns′) *adj.* Having a radiodensity similar to that of another or adjacent tissue.

i·so·dy·nam·ic (ī′sō-dī-năm′ĭk) *adj.* **1.** Having equal force or strength. **2.** Of or relating to foods or other materials that liberate the same amount of energy on combustion. **3.** Connecting points of equal magnetic intensity.

i·so·e·lec·tric electroencephalogram (ī′sō-ĭ-lĕk′trĭk) *n.* See **flat electroencephalogram.**

isoelectric line *n.* Base line on an electrocardiogram.

isoelectric period *n.* The period in the electrocardiogram between the end of the S wave and the beginning of the T wave, during which electrical forces neutralize each other so that there is no difference in potential under the two electrodes.

isoelectric point *n.* The pH at which the electrolyte concentration of an amphoteric substance such as protein is electrically zero because the concentration of its cation form equals the concentration of its anion form.

i·so·en·er·get·ic (ī′sō-ĕn′ər-jĕt′ĭk) *adj.* Exerting equal force; equally active.

i·so·en·zyme (ī′sō-ĕn′zīm′) *n.* See **isozyme.** —**i′so·en·zy′mic** (-zī′mĭk, -zĭm′ĭk) *adj.*

i·so·er·y·throl·y·sis (ī′sō-ĕr′ə-thrŏl′ĭ-sĭs) *n.* A condition in which red blood cells are destroyed by isoantibodies.

i·so·flu·rane (ī′sō-floõr′ān′) *n.* A halogenated ether with potent anesthetic action.

i·so·fla·vone (ī′sō-flā′vōn′) *n.* A flavonoid that is found in soy.

iso·gam·ete (ī′sō-găm′ēt′, -gə-mēt′) *n.* A gamete that has the same size and structure as the one with which it unites.

i·sog·a·my (ī-sŏg′ə-mē) *n.* Conjugation between gametes of equal size and structure, or between individual cells alike in all respects. —**i·sog′a·mous** *adj.*

i·so·ge·ne·ic (ī′sō-jə-nē′ĭk) *or* **i·so·gen·ic** (-jĕn′ĭk) *adj.* Relating to a group of individuals or to a strain of animals genetically alike with respect to specified gene pairs.

isogeneic graft *n.* See **syngraft.**

isogeneic homograft *n.* See **syngraft.**

i·so·gen·e·sis (ī′sō-jĕn′ĭ-sĭs) *n.* Similarity in development or origin.

i·sog·e·nous (ī-sŏj′ə-nəs) *adj.* Having the same or similar origin, as organs or parts derived from the same embryonic tissue.

i·so·graft (ī′sə-grăft′) *n.* See **syngraft.**

i·so·he·mag·glu·ti·na·tion (ī′sō-hē′mə-gloõt′n-ā′shən) *n.* See **isoagglutination.**

iso·he·mag·glu·ti·nin (ī′sō-hē′mə-gloõt′n-ĭn) *n.* See **isoagglutinin.**

i·so·he·mo·ly·sin (ī′sō-hĭ-mŏl′ĭ-sĭn, -hē′mə-lī′-) *n.* An isolysin that reacts with red blood cells.

i·so·he·mol·y·sis (ī′sō-hĭ-mŏl′ĭ-sĭs, -hē′mə-lī′sĭs) *n.* Isolysis in which there is dissolution of red blood cells as a result of the reaction between an isolysin and a specific antigen in or on the cells.

i·so·i·co·ni·a (ī′sō-ī-kō′nē-ə) *n.* A condition in which the two retinal images are of equal size. —**i′so·i·con′ic** (-kŏn′ĭk) *adj.*

i·so·im·mu·ni·za·tion (ī′sō-ĭm′yə-nĭ-zā′shən) *n.* The development of specific antibodies as a result of antigenic stimulation using material derived from the red blood cells of another individual of the same species.

i·so·ki·net·ic exercise (ī′sō-kə-nĕt′ĭk, -kī-) *n.* Exercise performed using a specialized apparatus that provides variable resistance to a movement, so that no matter how much effort is exerted, the movement takes place at a constant speed.

i·so·la·ble (ī′sə-lə-bəl) *adj.* Possible to isolate.

i·so·late (ī′sə-lāt′) *v.* **1.** To set apart or cut off from others. **2.** To place in quarantine. **3.** To separate a pure strain from a mixed bacterial or fungal culture. **4.** To separate or remove a chemical substance out of a combined mixture. **5.** To separate experiences or memories from the emotions relating to them. —*n.* (-lĭt, -lāt′) A bacterial or fungal strain that has been isolated. —**i′so·la′tor** *n.*

isolated explosive disorder *n.* A disorder of impulse control characterized by a single episode in which an individual commits a violent catastrophic act that is disproportionate to any stress and that has a serious affect on others.

isolated proteinuria *n.* Proteinuria in an individual who is asymptomatic, has normal renal function and urinary sediment, and has no manifestation of systemic disease upon initial examination.

i·so·la·tion (ī′sə-lā′shən) *n.* The act of isolating or the state of being isolated.

i·so·lec·i·thal (ī′sə-lĕs′ə-thəl) *adj.* Having the yolk evenly distributed throughout the egg.

i·so·leu·cine (ī′sə-loõ′sēn′) *n. Abbr.* **Ile** An essential amino acid that is isomeric with leucine.

i·sol·o·gous (ī-sŏl′ə-gəs) *adj.* Syngeneic.

isologous graft *n.* See **syngraft.**

i·sol·y·sin (ī-sŏl′ĭ-sĭn, ī′sə-lī′sĭn) *n.* An antibody that combines with, sensitizes, and causes complement-fixation and the dissolution of the cells that contain the specific isoantigen.

i·sol·y·sis (ī-sŏl′ĭ-sĭs) *n.* Lysis or dissolution of cells as a result of the reaction between an isolysin and a specific antigen in or on the cells. —**i′so·lyt′ic** (ī′sə-lĭt′ĭk) *adj.*

i·so·mal·tose (ī′sō-môl′tōs′, -tōz′) *n.* A disaccharide that is an isomer of maltose.

i·so·mer (ī′sə-mər) *n.* **1.** Any of two or more substances that are composed of the same elements in the same proportions but differ in properties because of differences in the arrangement of atoms. **2.** Any of two or more nuclei with the same mass number and atomic number that have different radioactive properties and can exist in any of several energy states for a measurable period of time. —**i′so·mer′ic** (-mĕr′ĭk) *adj.*

i·som·er·ase (ī-sŏm′ə-rās′) *n.* One of a group of enzymes that catalyzes the conversion of one isomer into another.

i·som·er·ism (ī-sŏm′ə-rĭz′əm) *n.* **1.** The phenomenon of the existence of isomers. **2.** The complex of chemical and physical phenomena characteristic of or attributable to isomers. **3.** The state or condition of being an isomer.

i·som·er·i·za·tion (ī-sŏm′ər-ĭ-zā′shən) *n.* A process in which one isomer is formed from another. —**i·som′er·ize′** (-ə-rīz′) *v.*

i·so·met·ric (ī′sə-mĕt′rĭk) *adj.* **1.** Of or exhibiting equality in dimensions or measurements. **2.** Of, relating to, or being a crystal system of three equal axes lying at right angles to each other. **3.** Of or involving muscular contraction against resistance in which the length of the muscle remains the same.

isometric exercise *n.* Exercise performed by the exertion of effort against a resistance that strengthens and tones the muscle without changing the length of the muscle fibers.

isometric period of cardiac cycle *n.* The period in the cardiac cycle, extending from the closing of the atrioventricular valves to the opening of the semilunar valves, in which the muscle fibers do not shorten.

isometrics *n.* Isometric exercise.

isometric scale *n.* A radiopaque strip of metal calibrated in centimeters, placed between the buttocks of an individual to be x-rayed, used to measure anteroposterior diameters of the pelvis.

i·so·me·tro·pi·a (ī′sō-mĭ-trō′pē-ə) *n.* Equality of refraction in both eyes.

i·so·morph (ī′sə-môrf′) *n.* An object, an organism, or a substance exhibiting isomorphism.

i·so·mor·phic (ī′sə-môr′fĭk) *adj.* **1.** Having a similar structure or appearance but being of different ancestry. **2.** Related by an isomorphism.

isomorphic response *n.* See **Köbner's phenomenon.**

i·so·mor·phism (ī′sə-môr′fĭz′əm) *n.* **1.** A similarity in form, as in organisms of different ancestry. **2.** A close similarity in the crystalline structure of two or more substances of similar chemical composition. —**i′so·mor′phous** *adj.*

i·so·ni·a·zid (ī′sə-nī′ə-zĭd) *n. Abbr.* **INH** An antibacterial compound that is used in the treatment of tuberculosis.

i·sop·a·thy (ī-sŏp′ə-thē) *n.* **1.** The treatment of disease by means of the causal agent or a product of the same disease. **2.** The treatment of a diseased organ by the use of an extract from a similar organ of a healthy animal.

i·so·per·i·stal·tic anastomosis (ī′sō-pĕr′ĭ-stôl′tĭk) *n.* A surgical connection between segments of intestine that allows the contents to flow in a normal direction.

i·soph·a·gy (ī-sŏf′ə-jē) *n.* Autolysis.

i·so·pho·ri·a (ī′sə-fôr′ē-ə) *n.* A state of equality in the tension of the vertical muscles of each eye.

i·so·plas·tic (ī′sə-plăs′tĭk) *adj.* Syngeneic.

isoplastic graft *n.* See **syngraft.**

i·so·pre·cip·i·tin (ī′sō-prī-sĭp′ĭ-tĭn) *n.* An antibody that combines with and precipitates soluble antigenic material in the plasma or serum of another member, but not all members, of the same species.

i·so·prene (ī′sə-prēn′) *n.* A colorless volatile hydrocarbon that is the naturally occurring basis of isoprenoids and that is used in the production of synthetic rubber.

i·so·pre·noid (ī′sə-prē′noid′) *n.* A polymer whose carbon skeleton consists wholly or partly of isoprene units joined end to end.

i·so·pro·pyl alcohol (ī′sə-prō′pəl) *n.* A clear, colorless, flammable, mobile liquid used in antifreeze compounds, in lotions and cosmetics, and as a solvent for gums, shellac, and essential oils.

i·sop·ter (ī-sŏp′tər) *n.* A curve of equal retinal sensitivity in the visual field designated by a fraction, the numerator being the diameter of the test object, and the denominator being the testing distance.

I·sop·tin (ī-sŏp′tn) A trademark for the drug verapamil.

i·sor·rhe·a (ī′sə-rē′ə) *n.* A state of physiological equilibrium between the intake and output of water and solutes.

i·sos·bes·tic point (ī′səs-bĕs′tĭk) *n.* A spectroscopic wavelength at which the absorbance of two substances, one of which can be converted into the other, is the same.

i·so·sex·u·al (ī′sə-sĕk′shoō-əl) *adj.* **1.** Relating to the existence of characteristics or feelings of both sexes in one person. **2.** Relating to or being characteristics or feelings consistent with the sex of an individual.

i·sos·mot·ic (ī′sŏz-mŏt′ĭk, -sŏs-) *adj.* Of or exhibiting equal osmotic pressure.

i·so·sor·bide di·nit·rate (ī′sō-sôr′bīd′ dī-nī′trāt′) *n.* A nitrate vasodilator drug administered orally and sublingually for the treatment and prevention of angina pectoris.

I·sos·po·ra (ī-sŏs′pər-ə) *n.* A genus of coccidia whose species are parasitic chiefly in mammals and include a species capable of causing a mucous diarrhea, anorexia, nausea, and abdominal pain in humans.

i·sos·po·ri·a·sis (ī-sŏs′pə-rī′ə-sĭs) *n.* Infection with coccidium of the genus *Isospora.*

i·sos·the·nu·ri·a (ī-sŏs′thə-noōr′ē-ə, ī′sō-sthē-) *n.* A condition in chronic renal disease in which the kidneys cannot form urine with a higher or a lower specific gravity than that of protein-free plasma.

i·so·sul·fan blue (ī′sō-sŭl′fən) *n.* A dye used to mark lymphatic vessels during lymphography.

i·so·ther·mal (ī′sə-thûr′məl) *adj.* Of, relating to, or indicating equal or constant temperatures.

i·so·tone (ī′sə-tōn′) *n.* One of two or more atoms whose nuclei have the same number of neutrons but different numbers of protons.

i·so·to·ni·a (ī′sə-tō′nē-ə) *n.* A condition of tonic equality, in which the tension or osmotic pressure in two substances or solutions is the same.

i·so·ton·ic (ī′sə-tŏn′ĭk) *adj.* **1.** Of equal tension. **2.** Isosmotic. **3.** Having the same concentration of solutes as the blood. **4.** Of or involving muscular contraction in which the muscle remains under relatively constant tension while its length changes. —**i′so·to·nic′i·ty** (-tə-nĭs′ĭ-tē) *n.*

isotonic exercise *n.* Exercise in which isotonic muscular contraction is used to strengthen muscles and improve joint mobility.

i·so·tope (ī′sə-tōp′) *n.* One of two or more atoms having the same atomic number but different mass numbers. —**i′so·top′ic** (-tŏp′ĭk) *adj.*

i·so·tret·i·no·in (ī′sō-trĕt′n-oin) *n.* A chemical compound that inhibits the secretion of sebum and is used in the treatment of severe forms of acne.

i·so·trop·ic (ī′sə-trŏp′ĭk, -trō′pĭk) *adj.* Identical in all directions. —**i·sot′ro·py** (ī-sŏt′rə-pē), **i·sot′ro·pism** (-rə-pĭz′əm) *n.*

i·so·type (ī′sə-tīp′) *n.* An antigenic marker that occurs in all members of a subclass of an immunoglobulin class. —**i′so·typ′ic** (-tĭp′ĭk) *adj.*

i·so·va·le·ric·ac·i·de·mi·a (ī′sō-və-lîr′ĭ-kăs′ĭ-dē′mē-ə, -lĕr′-) *n.* An inherited disorder of leucine metabolism marked by excessive production of isovaleric acid upon protein ingestion or during infectious episodes and resulting in severe metabolic acidosis.

i·so·vo·lu·mic (ī′sō-və-loo′mĭk) *or* **i·so·vol·u·met·ric** (-vŏl′yoo-mĕt′rĭk) *adj.* Occurring without an associated alteration in volume, especially relating to an early stage in ventricular systole.

i·so·zyme (ī′sə-zīm′) *n.* Any of a group of enzymes that are similar in catalytic properties but are differentiated by variations in physical properties, such as isoelectric point. Also called *isoenzyme.*

is·sue (ĭsh′oo) *n.* **1.** A discharge, as of blood or pus. **2.** A lesion, a wound, or an ulcer that produces a discharge of this sort.

isth·mec·to·my (ĭs-mĕk′tə-mē, ĭsth-) *n.* Excision of the midportion of the thyroid.

isth·mic (ĭs′mĭk) *or* **isth·mi·an** (ĭs′mē-ən) *adj.* Relating to an anatomical isthmus.

isth·mo·pa·ral·y·sis (ĭs′mō-pə-răl′ĭ-sĭs) *n.* Paralysis of the soft palate and of muscles forming the isthmus of the fauces. Also called *isthmoplegia.*

isth·mus (ĭs′məs) *n.,* *pl.* **–mus·es** *or* **–mi** (-mī′) A constriction or narrow passage connecting two larger parts of an organ or other anatomical structure.

isthmus of auditory tube *n.* The narrowest portion of the auditory tube at the junction of the cartilaginous and bony portions. Also called *isthmus of eustachian tube.*

isthmus of fauces *n.* The constricted space that connects the cavity of the mouth and the pharynx.

isthmus of thyroid *n.* The central part of the thyroid gland that joins the two lateral lobes.

isthmus of uterine tube *n.* The narrow portion of the uterine tube adjoining the uterus.

isthmus of uterus *n.* An elongated narrow part of the uterus at the junction of the body of the uterus and the cervix.

I·su·prel (ī′sə-prəl) A trademark for the drug isoproterenol hydrochloride.

itch (ĭch) *n.* **1.** An irritating skin sensation causing a desire to scratch. **2.** Any of various skin disorders, such as scabies, marked by intense irritation and itching. —*v.* To feel, have, or produce an itch.

itch mite *n.* A parasitic mite that burrows into the skin and causes scabies.

itch·y (ĭch′ē) *adj.* Having or causing an itching sensation.

–ite[1] *suff.* **1.** A part of an organ, body, or bodily part: *somite.* **2.** Product: *metabolite.*

–ite[2] *suff.* A salt or ester of an acid named with an adjective ending in *-ous: sulfite.*

i·ter (ī′tər) *n.* A passage leading from one anatomical part to another. —**i′ter·al** (-tər-əl) *adj.*

–itis *suff.* Inflammation or disease of: *laryngitis.*

I·to's nevus (ē′tōz′) *n.* Pigmentation of the skin that is innervated by lateral branches of the supraclavicular nerve and by the lateral cutaneous nerve of the arm, caused by the presence of scattered melanocytes in the dermis.

ITP *abbr.* idiopathic thrombocytopenic purpura

it·ra·con·a·zole (ĭt′rə-kŏn′ĭ-zōl) *n.* A broad-spectrum antifungal agent administered orally to treat systemic fungal infections and onychomycosis.

IU *abbr.* international unit

IUCD *abbr.* intrauterine contraceptive device

IUD *abbr.* intrauterine device

IUGR *abbr.* intrauterine growth retardation

–ium *suff.* Chemical element or group: *californium.*

IV *abbr.* intravenous; intravenously; intraventricular

IVC *abbr.* inferior vena cava

IVF *abbr.* in vitro fertilization

i·vo·ry exostosis (ī′və-rē, īv′rē) *n.* A small, rounded, extremely dense tumor arising from a bone, usually one of the cranial bones.

IVP *abbr.* intravenous pyelogram

Ix·o·des (ĭk-sō′dēz′) *n.* A genus of hard-bodied ticks, many species of which are parasitic on humans and animals.

Ixodes dam·mi·ni (dăm′ə-nī′) *n.* A species of *Ixodes* that is a vector of Lyme disease and human babesiosis in the United States.

ix·o·di·a·sis (ĭk′sō-dī′ə-sĭs) *n.* **1.** Skin lesions caused by the bites of certain ticks. **2.** A disease, such as Rocky Mountain fever, that is transmitted by ticks.

ix·od·ic (ĭk-sŏd′ĭk) *adj.* Relating to or caused by ticks.

ix·od·id (ĭk-sŏd′ĭd, -sō′dĭd) *n.* A member of the family Ixodidae.

Ix·od·i·dae (ĭk-sŏd′ĭ-dē′) *n.* A family of hard-bodied ticks, species of which transmit many important human and animal paralytical diseases.

J

J *abbr.* joule

Ja·bou·lay's method (zhä-boo-lāz′) *n.* A surgical method of linking arteries by splitting the cut ends a short distance and then suturing the flaps together with the inner coats touching each other.

jack·et (jăk′ĭt) *n.* **1.** A fixed bandage that is applied around the body to immobilize the spine. **2.** An artificial crown of a tooth that is composed of fired porcelain or acrylic resin.

Jack·son (jăk′sən), **John Hughlings** 1835–1911. British neurologist whose connection of certain epileptic symptoms to specific locations in the brain advanced the understanding of epilepsy.

jack·so·ni·an epilepsy (jăk-sō′nē-ən) *n.* A form of focal epilepsy in which a seizure progresses from the distal to the proximal muscles of a limb.

Jack·son's membrane (jăk′sənz) *n.* A thin vascular membrane that covers the anterior surface of the ascending colon from the cecum to the right flexure and that may cause the bowel to kink and become obstructed.

Ja·cob (zhä-kôb′), **François** Born 1920. French geneticist. He shared a 1965 Nobel Prize for the study of regulatory activity in body cells.

Ja·co·bi (jə-kō′bē), **Abraham** 1830–1919. German-born American physician who established a children's clinic in New York (1860) and is considered the founder of American pediatrics. His wife, **Mary Corinna Putnam Jacobi** (1842–1906), also a physician, helped expand opportunities for women in medical education.

jac·ti·ta·tion (jăk′tĭ-tā′shən) *n.* Extreme restlessness or tossing in bed, as with some forms of acute disease.

Ja·das·sohn-Le·wan·dow·sky syndrome (yä′däs-zōn-lĕv′ən-dŏv′skē, -lā′vän-dôf′skē) *n.* See **pachyonychia congenita.**

Jadassohn-Tièche nevus (-tyĕsh′) *n.* See **blue nevus.**

Jae·ger's test types (yā′gərz, yĕg′ərz) *pl.n.* Printed letters of different sizes used for testing the acuity of near vision.

Ja·kob-Creutzfeldt disease (yä′kôp-) *n.* See **Creutzfeldt-Jakob disease.**

jam (jăm) *v.* **1.** To block, congest, or clog. **2.** To crush or bruise.

JAMA *abbr. Journal of the American Medical Association*

Jane·way lesion (jān′wā′) *n.* A small erythematous or hemorrhagic lesion seen in some cases of bacterial endocarditis, usually on the palm or the sole.

jan·i·ceps (jăn′ĭ-sĕps′) *n.* A set of conjoined twins whose heads are fused together, with the faces looking in opposite directions.

Jan·sky-Bielschowsky disease (jăn′skē, yän′-) *n.* The early juvenile type of cerebral sphingolipidosis. Also called *Bielschowsky's disease.*

Jan·sky's classification (jăn′skēz, yän′-) *n.* The classification of the blood groups of humans into I, II, III, and IV, now designated, respectively, as O, A, B, and AB.

Ja·nus green B (jā′nəs) *n.* A basic dye used as a histological stain.

Jap·a·nese B encephalitis (jăp′ə-nēz′) *n.* An epidemic encephalitis or encephalomyelitis of Japan, Siberia, and other parts of Asia, caused by a virus of the genus *Flavivirus.*

Japanese B encephalitis virus *n.* A mosquito-borne virus of the genus *Flavivirus* capable of causing febrile response and sometimes encephalitis.

Japanese river fever *n.* See **scrub typhus.**

jar·gon aphasia (jär′gən) *n.* A form of aphasia in which nonsense syllables are uttered or in which several words are run together as one.

Ja·risch-Herxheimer reaction (yä′rĭsh-) *n.* See **Herxheimer's reaction.**

jaun·dice (jôn′dĭs, jän′-) *n.* Yellowish discoloration of the whites of the eyes, skin, and mucous membranes caused by deposition of bile salts in these tissues, occurring as a symptom of various diseases, such as hepatitis, that affect the processing of bile. Also called *icterus.*

jaundice of newborn *n.* **1.** A mild temporary jaundice in newborn infants that is caused mainly by functional immaturity of the liver. **2.** A severe, sometimes fatal form of jaundice in newborn infants that is caused by pathological conditions such as congenital blockage of the common bile duct, erythroblastosis fetalis, and septic pylephlebitis. Also called *icterus neonatorum, Ritter's disease.*

Ja·velle water *or* **Ja·vel water** (zhə-vĕl′) *n.* An aqueous solution of potassium or sodium hypochlorite, used as a disinfectant and bleaching agent.

jaw (jô) *n.* **1.** Either of two bony structures that form the framework of the mouth and hold the teeth. **2.** The mandible or maxilla or the part of the face covering these bones. —**jaw′less** *adj.*

jaw·bone (jô′bōn′) *n.* The maxilla or, especially, the mandible.

jaw reflex *n.* A spasmodic contraction of the temporal muscles following a downward tap on the loosely hanging mandible and seen in lesions of the corticospinal tract.

jaw-winking syndrome *n.* An increase in the width of the eyelids that occurs during chewing, sometimes accompanied by a rhythmic raising of the upper lid when the mouth is open and its subsequent drooping when the mouth is closed. Also called *Marcus Gunn phenomenon.*

Jean·selme's nodules (zhän-sĕlmz′) *pl.n.* Tertiary yaws characterized by the occurrence of nodules on the arms and legs, usually near the joints.

Je·ghers-Peutz syndrome (jā′gərz-) *n.* See **Peutz-Jeghers syndrome.**

je·ju·nal (jə-jōō′nəl) *adj.* Relating to the jejunum.

jejunal and ileal veins *pl.n.* The veins that drain the jejunum and ileum and terminate in the superior mesenteric vein. Also called *ileal veins.*

jejunal artery *n.* Any of various arteries with their origin in the superior mesenteric artery, with distribution to the jejunum, and with anastomoses with one another and with the ileal arteries. Also called *intestinal artery.*

je·ju·nec·to·my (jə-jōō′nĕk′tə-mē, jĕj′ōō-) *n.* Excision of all or a part of the jejunum.

je·ju·ni·tis (jə-jōō′nī′tĭs, jĕj′ōō-) *n.* Inflammation of the jejunum.

jejuno– *or* **jejun–** *pref.* Jejunum: *jejunotomy.*

je·ju·no·co·los·to·my (jə-jōō′nō-kə-lŏs′tə-mē, jĕj′ōō-) *n.* The surgical creation of an opening or passage between the jejunum and the colon.

je·ju·no·il·e·al (jə-jōō′nō-ĭl′ē-əl, jĕj′ōō-) *adj.* Relating to the jejunum and the ileum.

jejunoileal bypass *n.* Anastomosis of the upper jejunum to the terminal ileum for treating morbid obesity. Also called *bowel bypass, jejunoileal shunt.*

je·ju·no·il·e·i·tis (jə-jōō′nō-ĭl′ē-ī′tĭs, jĕj′ōō-) *n.* Inflammation of the jejunum and the ileum.

je·ju·no·il·e·os·to·my (jə-jōō′nō-ĭl′ē-ŏs′tə-mē, jĕj′ōō-) *n.* The surgical creation of an opening or passage between the jejunum and the ileum.

je·ju·no·je·ju·nos·to·my (jə-jōō′nō-jə-jōō′nŏs′tə-mē, jĕj′ōō-nō-jĕj′ōō-) *n.* Surgical creation of an opening or passage between two portions of jejunum.

je·ju·no·plas·ty (jə-jōō′nə-plăs′tē) *n.* A corrective surgical procedure on the jejunum.

je·ju·nos·to·my (jə-jōō′nŏs′tə-mē, jĕj′ōō-) *n.* The surgical creation of an opening from the abdominal wall into the jejunum, usually with a stoma on the abdominal wall.

je·ju·not·o·my (jə-jōō′nŏt′ə-mē, jĕj′ōō-) *n.* Incision into the jejunum.

je·ju·num (jə-jōō′nəm) *n.,* pl. **–na** (-nə) The section of the small intestine between the duodenum and the ileum.

jel·ly (jĕl′ē) *n.* A semisolid resilient substance usually containing some form of gelatin in solution.

jel·ly·fish (jĕl′ē-fĭsh′) *n.,* pl. **jellyfish** *or* **–fish·es 1.** Any of numerous marine coelenterates of the class Scyphozoa, some poisonous species of which, notably the Portuguese man-of-war, produce a toxin that can be injected into the skin by nematocysts on the tentacles, causing linear wheals. **2.** Any of various similar or related coelenterates.

Jen·ner (jĕn′ər), **Edward** 1749–1823. British physician and vaccination pioneer who found that smallpox could be prevented by inoculation with the substance from cowpox lesions.

Jen·sen's disease (yĕn′sənz) *n.* See **retinochoroiditis juxtapapillaris.**

jerk (jûrk) *v.* To make spasmodic motions. —*n.* **1.** A sudden reflexive or spasmodic muscular movement. See **deep reflex. 2. jerks** Involuntary convulsive twitching often resulting from excitement. Often used with *the.*

jerk·y nystagmus (jûr′kē) *n.* A nystagmus in which there is a slow drift of the eyes in one direction, followed by a rapid recovery movement.

Jer·ne (yĕr′nə), **Niels Kai** 1911–1994. Danish immunologist. He shared a 1984 Nobel Prize for pioneering immunology research.

jet injection (jĕt) *n.* The injection of a liquid drug by means of a device that uses high pressure to force the liquid to penetrate the skin or mucous membrane without the use of a needle.

jet lag *or* **jetlag** *n.* A temporary disruption of normal circadian rhythm caused by high-speed travel across several time zones typically in a jet aircraft, resulting in fatigue and varied constitutional symptoms. —**jet′-lagged′** *adj.*

Jex-Blake (jĕks′blāk′), **Sophia** 1840–1912. British physician. After successfully lobbying for legislation permitting women to practice medicine (1876), she became the first licensed woman physician in Great Britain (1877).

jig·ger (jĭg′ər) *n.* **1.** See **chigger** (sense 1). **2.** See **chigoe.**

jim-jams (jĭm′jămz′) *pl.n.* **1.** The jitters. **2.** Delirium tremens.

Job's syndrome (jōbz) *n.* See **hyperimmunoglobulin E syndrome.**

Jo·cas·ta complex (jō-kăs′tə) *n.* In psychoanalytic theory, a mother's libidinous fixation on a son.

jock itch *n.* See **tinea cruris.**

Jod-Basedow phenomenon (yŏd′-) *n.* Induction of thyrotoxicosis in a previously normal individual as a result of exposure to large quantities of iodine. Also called *iodine-induced hyperthyroidism.*

Jof·froy's sign (zhô-frwäz′) *n.* **1.** An indication of exophthalmic goiter in which the facial muscles remain immobile when the eyeballs are rolled upward. **2.** An indication of the early stages of brain disease in which an individual is unable to mentally compute simple mathematical calculations.

jog·ger's amenorrhea (jŏg′ərz) *n.* Temporary cessation of menstruation because of strenuous daily exercise such as jogging.

Jo·hann·sen (yō-hän′sən), **Wilhelm Ludwig** 1857–1927. Danish botanist and geneticist who was a pioneer in the field of experimental genetics.

john·ny (jŏn′ē) *n.* A loose short-sleeved gown opening in the back, worn by patients undergoing medical treatment or examination.

joint (joint) *n.* A point of articulation between two or more bones, especially such a connection that allows motion. See illustration on page 434.

joint capsule *n.* See **articular capsule.**

joint of foot *n.* Any of the joints of the foot, including the ankle joint and the tarsal, tarsometatarsal, intermetatarsal, metatarsophalangeal, and interphalangeal joints.

joint of hand *n.* Any of the joints of the hand, including the wrist joint and the carpal, carpometacarpal, intermetacarpal, metacarpophalangeal, and interphalangeal joints.

Jo·liot-Cu·rie (zhô-lyō′kyōōr′ē, -kyōō-rē′, -kü-), **Irène** 1897–1956. French physicist. She shared a 1935 Nobel Prize with her husband, **Frédéric Joliot-Curie** (1900–1958), for synthesizing new radioactive elements.

Jou·bert's syndrome (zhōō-bĕrz′) *n.* A syndrome of neurological disorders caused by agenesis of the vermis of the brain and characterized by attacks of tachypnea or prolonged apnea, abnormal eye movements, ataxia, and mental retardation.

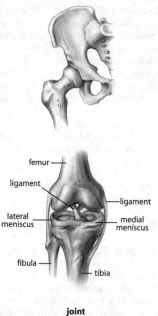

joint
Top: *hip ball-and-socket joint*
Bottom: *anterior view of knee joint*

femur
ligament
ligament
lateral meniscus
medial meniscus
fibula
tibia

joule (jōōl) *n. Abbr.* **J 1.** The International System unit of electrical, mechanical, and thermal energy. **2.** A unit of electrical energy equal to the work done when a current of 1 ampere is passed through a resistance of 1 ohm for 1 second. **3.** A unit of energy equal to the work done when a force of 1 newton acts through a distance of 1 meter.

jowl¹ (joul) *n.* **1.** The jaw, especially the lower jaw. **2.** The cheek.

jowl² (joul) *n.* The flesh under the lower jaw, especially when plump or flaccid.

J point *n.* The point marking the end of the QRS complex and the beginning of the following part that merges into the T wave in an electrocardiogram.

JRA *abbr.* juvenile rheumatoid arthritis

ju·gal (jōō′gəl) *adj.* **1.** Connected like a yoke. **2.** Relating to the zygomatic bone.

jugal bone *n.* See **zygomatic bone.**

ju·ga·le (jōō-gā′lē) *n.* The point at which the temporal and frontal processes of the zygomatic bone meet. Also called *jugal point.*

jug·u·lar (jŭg′yə-lər) *adj.* Of, relating to, or located in the region of the neck or throat. —*n.* A jugular vein.

jugular foramen *n.* A passage between the temporal bone and the occipital bone, containing the internal jugular vein, the inferior petrosal sinus, the glossopharyngeal, vagus, and accessory nerves, and the meningeal branches of the ascending pharyngeal and occipital arteries.

jugular fossa *n.* An oval depression near the rear border of the petrous portion of the temporal bone in which the beginning of the internal jugular vein lies.

jugular ganglion *n.* **1.** The upper, smaller of the two ganglia on the glossopharyngeal nerve as it traverses the jugular foramen. Also called *superior ganglion of glossopharyngeal nerve.* **2.** A small sensory ganglion on the vagus nerve as it traverses the jugular foramen. Also called *superior ganglion of vagus.*

jugular gland *n.* See **signal node.**

jugular nerve *n.* A communicating branch between the superior cervical ganglion of the sympathetic trunk and the superior ganglion of the vagus nerve and the inferior ganglion of the glossopharyngeal nerve.

jugular pulse *n.* The pulse in the right internal jugular vein at the root of the neck.

jugular vein *n.* Any of the three jugular veins: anterior, external, and internal.

jug·u·lo·di·gas·tric node (jŭg′yə-lō-dī-găs′trĭk) *n.* A prominent lymph node in the deep lateral cervical group lying below the digastric muscle and anterior to the internal jugular vein and receiving lymphatic drainage from the pharynx, palatine tonsil, and tongue. Also called *subdigastric node.*

jug·u·lo·o·mo·hy·oid node (jŭg′yə-lō-ō′mō-hī′oid′) *n.* A lymph node of the deep lateral cervical group that lies above the omohyoid muscle and anterior to the internal jugular vein, receives lymphatic drainage from the submental, submandibular, and deep anterior cervical nodes, and whose efferent vessels go to other deep lateral cervical nodes.

ju·gum (jōō′gəm) *n., pl.* **–gums** *or* **-ga** (-gə) **1.** A ridge or furrow connecting two structures. Also called *yoke.* **2.** A type of forceps.

juice (jōōs) *n.* **1.** A fluid naturally contained in plant or animal tissue. **2.** A bodily secretion, especially that secreted by the glands of the stomach and intestines.

jump flap (jŭmp) *n.* A distant flap transferred in stages via an intermediate carrier, as an abdominal flap that is first attached to the wrist and later brought to the face.

junc·tion (jŭngk′shən) *n.* **1.** The act or process of joining or the condition of being joined. **2.** A place where two things join or meet, especially a place where two things come together and one terminates. **3.** A transition layer or boundary between two different materials or between physically different regions in a single material. —**junc′tion·al** *adj.*

junctional epithelium *n.* A circular arrangement of epithelial cells occurring at the base of the gingival sulcus and attached to both the tooth and the subepithelial connective tissue.

junction nevus *n.* A nevus consisting of nests of melanocytes at the junction of the epidermis and dermis that appear as a small, slightly raised, flat, nonhairy, dark-brown or black tumor.

junc·tu·ra (jŭngk-chōōr′ə, -tōōr′-) *n., pl.* **junc·tu·rae** (-chōōr′ē, -tōōr′-) A juncture.

junc·ture (jŭngk′chər) *n.* The point, line, or surface of union of two parts.

Jung (yŏŏng), **Carl Gustav** 1875–1961. Swiss psychiatrist who founded analytical psychology and came up with the concepts of extraversion and introversion and the notion of the collective unconscious.

Jung·i·an (yŏŏng′ē-ən) *adj.* **1.** Relating to or described by Carl Gustav Jung. **2.** Maintaining Jung's psychological theories.

jun·gle fever (jŭng′gəl) *n.* See **malaria.**

junk DNA (jŭngk) *n.* DNA that does not code for proteins or their regulation but is thought to be involved in the evolution of new genes and in gene repair, and constitutes approximately 95 percent of the human genome.

junk food *n.* Any of various prepackaged snack foods high in calories but low in nutritional value.

ju·ve·nile cataract (jōō′və-nīl′, -nəl) *n.* A soft cataract occurring in a child or young adult, usually congenital or resulting from trauma.

juvenile cell *n.* See **metamyelocyte.**

juvenile diabetes *n.* Insulin-dependent diabetes.

juvenile muscular atrophy *n.* Slowly progressive proximal muscular weakness accompanied by fasciculation, wasting, and lower motor neuron disease, with onset usually between 2 and 17 years.

juvenile myoclonic epilepsy *n.* A form of epilepsy that occurs in adolescents, usually upon awakening, and is characterized by jerks of the shoulder muscles and by seizures that have a clonic phase, followed by a tonic phase, then by a return to clonus.

juvenile-onset diabetes *n.* Insulin-dependent diabetes.

juvenile osteomalacia *n.* See **rickets.**

juvenile palmo-plantar fibromatosis *n.* Fibromatosis that occurs in children as a single poorly demarcated nodule on the palm or the sole.

juvenile papillomatosis *n.* A form of fibrocystic disease of the breast in young women, with florid and sclerosing adenosis that microscopically may suggest carcinoma.

juvenile pelvis *n.* A pelvis justo minor in which the bones are slender.

juvenile polyp *n.* A smoothly rounded mucosal hamartoma of the large intestine, which may be multiple and cause rectal bleeding, especially in the first decade of life.

juvenile retinoschisis *n.* A hereditary retinoschisis occurring in children under the age of 10 and characterized by cyst development within the nerve fiber layer of the retina, often with macular involvement.

juvenile rheumatoid arthritis *n. Abbr.* JRA Chronic inflammatory arthritis that begins in childhood, characterized by swelling, tenderness, and pain in one or more joints and by lymph node and splenic enlargement. Also called *Still's disease.*

juvenile xanthogranuloma *n.* A skin condition characterized by single or multiple reddish to yellow papules caused by infiltration of the skin by histiocytes and Touton giant cells, usually found in young children. Also called *nevoxanthoendothelioma.*

jux·ta·ep·i·phys·i·al (jŭk′stə-ĕp′ə-fĭz′ē-əl) *adj.* Close to or adjoining an epiphysis.

jux·ta·glo·mer·u·lar (jŭk′stə-glō-mĕr′yə-lər) *adj.* Close to or adjoining a renal glomerulus.

juxtaglomerular cell *n.* A cell occurring in the kidney and producing renin.

juxtaglomerular granule *n.* Any of the stainable osmophilic secretory granules present in the juxtaglomerular cells, closely resembling zymogen granules.

jux·ta·po·si·tion (jŭk′stə-pə-zĭsh′ən) *n.* The state of being placed or situated side by side.

K

κ The Greek letter *kappa*. Entries beginning with this character are alphabetized under **kappa**.

K¹ The symbol for the element **potassium**.

K² *abbr.* kelvin

ka·la-a·zar (kä′lə-ə-zär′) *n.* See **visceral leishmaniasis**.

ka·le·mi·a (kā-lē′mē-ə) *n.* The presence of potassium in the blood.

kalio– *or* **kal–** *or* **kali–** *pref.* Potassium: *kaliopenia.*

ka·li·o·pe·ni·a (kā′lē-ō-pē′nē-ə, kăl′ē-) *n.* A low potassium concentration in the blood.

ka·li·um (kā′lē-əm) *n.* See **potassium**.

kal·lak (kăl′ăk) *n.* A pustular dermatitis, occurring especially among the Eskimos.

kal·li·din I (kăl′ĭ-dn) *n.* See **bradykinin**.

kallidin II *n.* See **bradykininogen**.

kal·li·kre·in (kăl′ĭ-krē′ĭn) *n.* An enzyme present in blood plasma, lymph, urine, saliva, pancreatic juices, and other body fluids that catalyzes the proteolysis of bradykininogen to bradykinin. Also called *kininogenase.*

kal·u·re·sis (kăl′yŏŏ-rē′sĭs, kāl′-) *or* **ka·li·u·re·sis** (kā′-lē-yŏŏ-rē′sĭs, kăl′ē-) *n.* The excretion of increased amounts of potassium in the urine. —**kal′u·ret′ic** (-rĕt′ĭk) *adj.*

kan·a·my·cin (kăn′ə-mī′sĭn) *n.* A water-soluble broad-spectrum antibiotic obtained from the soil bacterium *Streptomyces kanamyceticus.*

Kan·ner's syndrome (kăn′ərz) *n.* See **autism**.

Kan·trex (kăn′trĕks′) A trademark for the drug kanamycin.

ka·o·lin (kā′ə-lĭn) *n.* A fine white clay that, when powdered, is used as a demulcent and adsorbent and, in dentistry, as an agent that confers opacity and toughness to porcelain teeth.

ka·o·lin·o·sis (kā′ə-lə-nō′sĭs) *n.* Pneumoconiosis that is caused by the inhalation of clay dust.

Ka·o·pec·tate (kā′ə-pĕk′tāt′) A trademark for the compound kaolin.

Ka·po·si's sarcoma (kə-pō′sēz, kăp′ə-) *n. Abbr.* **KS** A cancer characterized by bluish-red nodules on the skin, usually on the lower extremities, that often occurs in people with AIDS.

Kaposi's varicelliform eruption *n.* A rare condition, occurring most commonly in children, that is characterized by high fever and the widespread eruption of vesicles that become pitlike and pus-filled ; it is a complication of vaccinia together with atopic dermatitis.

kap·pa (kăp′ə) *n. Symbol* **κ** The tenth letter of the Greek alphabet. —*adj.* Relating to or characterizing a polypeptide chain that is one of two types of light chains present in immunoglobins.

kappa angle *n.* The angle between the axis of the pupil and the visual axis.

Kar·nof·sky scale (kär-nŏf′skē) *n.* A performance scale that rates a person's normal activities and that can be used to evaluate a patient's progress after a therapeutic procedure.

Kar·ta·ge·ner's syndrome (kär′tə-gā′nərz, kär-tä′gə-nərz) *n.* A syndrome of disorders in which complete transposition of the viscera is associated with bronchiectasis and chronic sinusitis. Also called *Kartagener's triad.*

karyo– *or* **caryo–** *pref.* Cell nucleus: *karyogamy.*

kar·y·o·cyte (kăr′ē-ə-sīt′) *n.* An immature normoblast.

kar·y·og·a·my (kăr′ē-ŏg′ə-mē) *n.* The coming together and fusing of cell nuclei, as in fertilization. —**kar′y·o·gam′ic** (-ə-găm′ĭk) *adj.*

kar·y·o·gen·e·sis (kăr′ē-ə-jĕn′ĭ-sĭs) *n.* Formation of the nucleus of a cell. —**kar′y·o·gen′ic** (-jĕn′ĭk) *adj.*

kar·y·o·ki·ne·sis (kăr′ē-ō-kə-nē′sĭs) *n.* See **mitosis** (sense 1). —**kar′y·o·ki·net′ic** (-nĕt′ĭk) *adj.*

kar·y·o·lymph (kăr′ē-ə-lĭmf′) *n.* The colorless gel or liquid component of the cell nucleus in which stainable elements are suspended, now known to be euchromatin. Also called *nuclear hyaloplasm.*

kar·y·ol·y·sis (kăr′ē-ŏl′ĭ-sĭs) *n.* The dissolution of the nucleus of a cell by swelling or necrosis with the loss of its affinity for staining with basic dyes. —**kar′y·o·lyt′ic** (-ə-lĭt′ĭk) *adj.*

kar·y·o·mi·cro·some (kăr′ē-ō-mī′krə-sōm′) *n.* Any of the minute particles or granules that make up the substance of the cell nucleus.

kar·y·o·mor·phism (kăr′ē-ō-môr′fĭz′əm) *n.* The development of a cell nucleus. —*adj.* Of, relating to, or resembling the nuclear shapes of cells, especially white blood cells.

kar·y·on (kăr′ē-ŏn′) *n.* See **nucleus** (sense 1).

kar·y·o·phage (kăr′ē-ə-fāj′) *n.* An intracellular parasite that phagocytizes the cell nucleus it infects.

kar·y·o·plasm (kăr′ē-ə-plăz′əm) *n.* See **nucleoplasm**.

kar·y·o·plast (kăr′ē-ə-plăst′) *n.* A cell nucleus surrounded by a narrow band of cytoplasm and a plasma membrane.

kar·y·o·pyk·no·sis (kăr′ē-ō-pĭk-nō′sĭs) *n.* A cytologic condition caused by shrinkage of the nucleus of a cell with the condensation of the chromatin into structureless masses, as in superficial or cornified cells of stratified squamous epithelium.

kar·y·or·rhex·is (kăr′ē-ō-rĕk′sĭs) *n.* A stage of cellular necrosis in which the fragments of the nucleus fragments and its chromatin are distributed irregularly throughout the cytoplasm.

kar·y·o·some (kăr′ē-ə-sōm′) *n.* An aggregation of chromatin in the nucleus of a cell not undergoing mitosis.

kar·y·o·type (kăr′ē-ə-tīp′) *n.* **1.** The characterization of the chromosomal complement of an individual or a species, including number, form, and size of the chromosomes. **2.** A photomicrograph of chromosomes arranged according to a standard classification. —*v.* To classify and array the chromosome complement of an organism or a species according to the arrangement, number, size, shape, or other characteristics of the chromosomes.

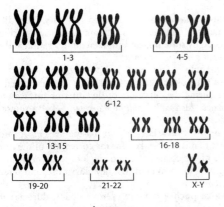

karyotype
of a normal human cell

Ka·sai operation (kä-sī′) *n.* See **portoenterostomy.**

Ka·shin-Bek disease (kä′shĭn-bĕk′) *n.* A form of generalized osteoarthrosis endemic in certain areas of Asia and possibly caused by eating wheat infected with the fungus *Fusarium sporotrichiella.*

kat *abbr.* katal

kat·al (kăt′l) *n.* *Abbr.* **kat** A unit of measurement that expresses the activity of a catalyst in moles per second, such as the amount of an enzyme needed to transform one mole of substrate per second.

Kat·a·ya·ma disease (kăt′ə-yä′mə, kä′tə-) *n.* See **schistosomiasis japonicum.**

Katayama syndrome *n.* See **schistosomiasis japonicum.**

Katz (kăts), **Bernard** 1911–2003. German-born British physiologist. He shared a 1970 Nobel Prize for the study of nerve impulse transmission.

ka·va (kä′və) *n.* A dietary supplement derived from the roots of the shrub *Piper methysticum,* used as a sedative.

Ka·wa·sa·ki disease (kä′wə-sä′kē) *n.* See **mucocutaneous lymph node syndrome.**

Kay·ser-Flei·scher ring (kī′zər-flī′shər) *n.* A greenish-yellow pigmented ring encircling the cornea.

kcal *abbr.* kilocalorie

K-Dur (kā′dûr′) A trademark for an oral preparation of sustained-release potassium chloride.

Kearns-Sayre syndrome (kûrnz′sâr′) *n.* A syndrome usually occurring before the age of 20 and characterized by pigmentary retinal dystrophy, cardiomyopathy, and varied cranial nerve impairment.

Kef·lex (kĕf′lĕks′) A trademark for the drug cephalexin.

Ke·gel exercise (kā′gəl) *n.* Any of various exercises involving controlled contraction and release of the muscles at the base of the pelvis, used especially as a treatment for urinary incontinence.

Kel·ly's operation (kĕl′ēz) *n.* **1.** The surgical correction of retroversion of the uterus by plication of the uterosacral ligaments. **2.** The surgical correction of

stress-related urinary incontinence by placing sutures beneath the bladder neck.

ke·loid *or* **che·loid** (kē′loid′) *n.* A red, raised formation of fibrous scar tissue caused by excessive tissue repair in response to trauma or incision.

ke·loi·do·sis (kē′loi-dō′sĭs) *n.* The presence of multiple keloids.

ke·lo·plas·ty (kē′lə-plăs′tē) *n.* The surgical removal of a scar or keloid.

kel·vin (kĕl′vĭn) *n.* *Abbr.* **K** A unit of temperature in the Kelvin scale equal to $\frac{1}{273.16}$ of the absolute temperature of the triple point of pure water.

Kelvin scale *n.* An absolute scale of temperature in which each degree equals one kelvin. Water freezes at 273.15 K and boils at 373.15 K. Also called *absolute scale.*

Ken·a·log (kĕn′ə-lôg′) A trademark for the drug triamcinolone.

Ken·dall (kĕn′dl), **Edward Calvin** 1886–1972. American biochemist. He shared a 1950 Nobel Prize for discoveries concerning the hormones of the adrenal cortex.

Ken·drew (kĕn′drōō′), **John Cowdery** 1917–1997. British biologist. He shared the 1962 Nobel Prize for chemistry for determining the molecular structure of blood components.

Ken·ny's treatment (kĕn′ēz) *n.* Sister Kenny's treatment for poliomyelitis.

keph·a·lin (kĕf′ə-lĭn) *n.* Variant of **cephalin.**

ker·a·sin (kĕr′ə-sĭn) *n.* A cerebroside found in brain tissue and containing fatty acid, sphingosine, and galactose.

kerat– *pref.* Variant of **kerato–.**

ker·a·tan sulfate (kĕr′ə-tăn′) *n.* Any of several mucopolysaccharides in cartilage, bone, connective tissue, and the cornea. Also called *keratosulfate.*

ker·a·tec·ta·sia (kĕr′ə-tĕk-tā′zhə) *n.* A thinning and herniation of the cornea.

ker·a·tec·to·my (kĕr′ə-tĕk′tə-mē) *n.* Excision of a portion of the cornea.

ke·rat·ic (kĕ-răt′ĭk, kə-) *adj.* Horny.

ker·a·tin (kĕr′ə-tĭn) *n.* Any of a group of scleroproteins or albuminoids that contain large amounts of sulfur and are the chief structural constituents of hair, nails, and other horny tissues.

ker·a·tin·ase (kĕr′ə-tn-ās′, -āz′) *n.* Any of various enzymes that catalyze the hydrolysis of keratin.

ker·a·tin·i·za·tion (kĕr′ə-tn-ĭ-zā′shən) *n.* The conversion of squamous epithelial cells into a horny material, such as nails. Also called *cornification.*

ke·rat·i·no·cyte (kə-răt′n-ə-sīt′, kĕr′ə-tĭn′ə-) *n.* An epidermal cell that produces keratin.

ke·rat·i·no·some (kə-răt′n-ə-sōm′, kĕr′ə-tĭn′ə-) *n.* A membrane-bound granule in the upper layers of the prickle cell layer of certain stratified squamous epithelia. Also called *membrane-coating granule.*

ke·rat·i·nous (kə-răt′n-əs) *adj.* **1.** Relating to or resembling keratin. **2.** Horny.

keratinous cyst *n.* A keratin-containing epithelial cyst.

keratin pearl *n.* A focus of central keratinization found within concentric layers of abnormal squamous cells, occurring in squamous cell carcinoma. Also called *epithelial pearl.*

ker·a·ti·tis (kĕr′ə-tī′tĭs) *n., pl.* **–tit·i·des** (-tĭt′ĭ-dēz′) Inflammation of the cornea.

keratitis sic·ca (sĭk′ə) *n.* Inflammation of the conjunctiva and cornea of the eye with decreased tears.

kerato– *or* **kerat–** *or* **cerato–** *or* **cerat–** *pref.* 1. Horn; horny: *keratosis.* 2. Cornea: *keratectomy.*

ker·a·to·ac·an·tho·ma (kĕr′ə-tō-ăk′ən-thō′mə) *n.* A rapidly growing skin tumor having a central keratin mass and usually occurring on exposed areas, invading the dermis but remaining localized and usually healing spontaneously.

ker·a·to·cele (kĕr′ə-tō-sēl′) *n.* A herniation of Descemet's membrane through a defect in the outer layer of the cornea.

ker·a·to·con·junc·ti·vi·tis (kĕr′ə-tō-kən-jŭngk′tə-vī′tĭs) *n.* Inflammation of the cornea and conjunctiva resulting from hypersensitivity of corneal and conjunctival epithelium to an endogenous toxin.

keratoconjunctivitis sic·ca (sĭk′ə) *n.* See **dry eye.**

ker·a·to·co·nus (kĕr′ə-tō-kō′nəs) *n.* A conical protrusion of the center of the cornea caused by noninflammatory thinning of the stroma and usually affecting both eyes. Also called *conical cornea.*

ker·a·to·cyte (kĕr′ə-tō-sīt′) *n.* A fibroblastic stromal cell of the cornea.

ker·a·to·der·ma (kĕr′ə-tō-dûr′mə) *n.* 1. A horny covering or growth, especially of the skin. 2. A generalized thickening of the stratum corneum.

keratoderma blen·nor·rhag·i·cum (blĕn′ə-răj′ĭ-kəm) *n.* See **keratosis blennorrhagica.**

keratoderma plan·tar·e sul·ca·tum (plăn-târ′ē sŭl-kā′təm) *n.* Thickening of the skin's horny layer and the formation of fissures on the soles. Also called *cracked heel.*

ker·a·to·ep·i·the·li·o·plas·ty (kĕr′ə-tō-ĕp′ə-thē′lē-ō-plăs′tē) *n.* Keratoplasty in which corneal epithelium is transplanted with minimal supporting tissue.

ker·a·tog·e·nous (kĕr′ə-tŏj′ə-nəs) *adj.* Relating to or causing the growth of cells that form horny tissue.

keratogenous membrane *n.* See **nail bed.**

ker·a·to·glo·bus (kĕr′ə-tō-glō′bəs) *n.* See **anterior megalophthalmus.**

ker·a·to·hy·a·lin (kĕr′ə-tō-hī′ə-lĭn) *n.* A colorless translucent protein present in the granules of the granular layer of the epidermis.

keratohyalin granule *n.* Any of the irregularly shaped granules present in the cells of the granular layer of the epidermis.

ker·a·toid (kĕr′ə-toid′) *adj.* 1. Horny. 2. Resembling corneal tissue.

keratoid exanthema *n.* A symptom occurring in the secondary stage of yaws and consisting of patches of fine, light-colored, furfuraceous desquamation scattered irregularly over the limbs and trunk.

ker·a·to·lep·tyn·sis (kĕr′ə-tō-lĕp-tĭn′sĭs) *n.* The surgical removal of the surface of the cornea and covering of the area with conjunctiva from the anterior surface of the eyeball for cosmetic reasons.

ker·a·to·leu·ko·ma (kĕr′ə-tō-lōō-kō′mə) *n.* A white corneal opacity.

ker·a·tol·y·sis (kĕr′ə-tŏl′ĭ-sĭs) *n.* 1. The separation or loosening of the horny layer of the epidermis. 2. A

skin disease characterized by a periodic shedding of the epidermis. —**ker′a·to·lyt′ic** (-tō-lĭt′ĭk) *adj.*

ker·a·to·ma (kĕr′ə-tō′mə) *n.* 1. See **callosity.** 2. A horny tumor.

ker·a·to·ma·la·cia (kĕr′ə-tō-mə-lā′shə) *n.* A condition, usually in children with vitamin A deficiency, characterized by softening and subsequent ulceration and perforation of the cornea.

ker·a·tome (kĕr′ə-tōm′) *n.* Variant of **keratotome.**

ker·a·tom·e·ter (kĕr′ə-tŏm′ĭ-tər) *n.* An instrument for measuring the curvature of the anterior surface of the cornea. Also called *ophthalmometer.* —**ker′a·tom′e·try** *adj.*

ker·a·to·mi·leu·sis (kĕr′ə-tō-mə-lōō′sĭs) *n.* A procedure that is undertaken for the correction of the refraction of the cornea by removing a deep corneal lamella, freezing it, forming it to a new curvature, and then replacing it.

ker·a·to·pach·y·der·ma (kĕr′ə-tō-păk′ĭ-dûr′mə) *n.* A syndrome of congenital deafness characterized by the formation of bandlike constrictions of the fingers and hyperkeratosis of the skin of the palms, soles, elbows, and knees appearing in childhood.

ker·a·top·a·thy (kĕr′ə-tŏp′ə-thē) *n.* A noninflammatory disease of the cornea.

ker·a·to·pha·ki·a (kĕr′ə-tō-fā′kē-ə) *n.* Keratoplasty in which corneal tissue from a donor is frozen, reshaped, and transplanted into the corneal stroma of the recipient to modify refractive error.

ker·a·to·plas·ty (kĕr′ə-tō-plăs′tē) *n.* Surgical replacement of an opaque portion of the cornea with a piece of cornea having the same size and shape. Also called *corneal graft.*

ker·a·to·pros·the·sis (kĕr′ə-tō-prŏs-thē′sĭs) *n.* An acrylic plastic replacement for the central area of an opacified cornea.

ker·a·to·rhex·is *or* **ker·a·tor·rhex·is** (kĕr′ə-tō-rĕk′sĭs) *n.* Rupture of the cornea due to trauma or a perforating ulcer.

ker·a·to·scle·ri·tis (kĕr′ə-tō-sklə-rī′tĭs) *n.* Inflammation of the cornea and the sclera.

ker·a·to·scope (kĕr′ə-tō-skōp′) *n.* An instrument that is marked with lines or circles for use in examining the curvature of the cornea. Also called *Placido's disk.*

ker·a·tos·co·py (kĕr′ə-tŏs′kə-pē) *n.* Examination of the anterior surface of the cornea to determine the character and amount of corneal astigmatism.

ker·a·tose (kĕr′ə-tōs′) *adj.* Relating to or characterized by keratosis.

ker·a·to·sis (kĕr′ə-tō′sĭs) *n., pl.* **–ses** (-sēz) The excessive growth of horny tissue of the skin. —**ker′a·tot′ic** (-tŏt′ĭk) *adj.*

keratosis blen·nor·rhag·i·ca (blĕn′ə-răj′ĭ-kə) *n.* The formation of pustules and crusts on the skin, usually affecting the palms, soles, toes, and glans penis, associated with Reiter's syndrome. Also called *keratoderma blennorrhagicum.*

keratosis fol·lic·u·lar·is (fə-lĭk′yə-lâr′ĭs) *n.* A hereditary eruptive skin disorder, beginning usually in childhood, in which keratotic papules originating from the hair follicles coalesce to form crusty and warty patches. Also called *Darier's disease.*

keratosis pi·lo·ris a·troph·i·cans fa·ci·e·i (pī-lôr′ĭs ə-trŏf′ĭ-kănz′ fā′sē-ē′ī′) *n.* A disorder occurring in early infancy and characterized by erythema and the formation of horny plugs on the outer portions of the eyebrows with destruction of hair follicles.

ker·a·to·sul·fate (kĕr′ə-tō-sŭl′fāt′) *n.* See **keratan sulfate.**

ker·a·to·tome (kĕr′ə-tō-tōm′) *or* **ker·a·tome** (kĕr′ə-tōm′) *n.* A knife used for incisions of the cornea.

ker·a·tot·o·my (kĕr′ə-tŏt′ə-mē) *n.* Incision of the cornea.

ke·ri·on (kîr′ē-ŏn′) *n.* Fungal infection of the hair follicles accompanied by secondary bacterial infection and marked by raised, usually pus-filled and spongy lesions.

Ker·ley B line (kûr′lē) *n.* Any of several fine horizontal lines a few centimeters above the angle in the chest x-ray that is made by the recess between the ribs and the lateral-most portion of the diaphragm.

ker·nic·ter·us (kûr-nĭk′tər-əs) *n.* A grave form of jaundice of the newborn characterized by very high levels of unconjugated bilirubin in the blood and by yellow staining and degenerative lesions in the cerebral gray matter. Also called *nuclear jaundice.*

Ker·nig's sign (kûr′nĭgz) *n.* An indication of meningitis in which complete extension of the leg at the knee is impossible when the individual lies on the back and flexes the thigh at a right angle to the axis of the trunk.

ker·oid (kĕr′oid′) *adj.* Horny.

ke·ta·mine (kē′tə-mēn′) *n.* A general anesthetic given intravenously or intramuscularly in the form of its hydrochloride that produces catatonia and profound analgesia with little relaxation of the skeletal muscles.

keto– *or* **ket–** *pref.* Ketone; ketone group: *ketosis.*

ke·to acid (kē′tō) *n.* A compound containing a ketone and a carboxyl group.

ke·to·ac·i·do·sis (kē′tō-ăs′ĭ-dō′sĭs) *n.* Acidosis caused by the increased production of ketone bodies, as in diabetic acidosis.

ke·to·ac·i·du·ri·a (kē′tō-ăs′ĭ-dōŏr′ē-ə) *n.* Excessive amounts of keto acids in the urine.

ke·to·co·na·zole (kē′tō-kō′nə-zōl′) *n.* An antifungal agent effective on a variety of fungi and used to treat systemic and topical fungal infections.

ke·to·gen·e·sis (kē′tō-jĕn′ĭ-sĭs) *n.* The formation of ketone bodies, as in diabetes mellitus. —**ke′to·gen′ic** *adj.*

ketogenic diet *n.* A high-fat, low-carbohydrate diet that includes normal amounts of protein.

ke·to·hep·tose (kē′tō-hĕp′tōs′) *n.* A seven-carbon sugar containing a ketone group.

ke·to·hex·ose (kē′tō-hĕk′sōs′) *n.* A six-carbon sugar containing a ketone group, such as fructose. Also called *hexulose.*

ke·tol (kē′tôl′, -tōl′) *n.* A compound having an alcohol and ketone group.

ke·tole (kē′tōl′) *n.* See **indole** (sense 1).

ke·to·lyt·ic (kē′tō-lĭt′ĭk) *adj.* Relating to or causing the decomposition of ketones. Used especially of the oxidation products of glucose and similar substances.

ke·tone (kē′tōn′) *n.* Any of a class of organic compounds having a carbonyl group linked to a carbon atom in each of two hydrocarbon radicals.

ketone body *n.* A ketone-containing substance, such as acetoacetic acid, that is an intermediate product of fatty acid metabolism, tends to accumulate in the blood, and is excreted in the urine of individuals affected by starvation or uncontrolled diabetes mellitus. Also called *acetone body.*

ke·to·ne·mi·a (kē′tə-nē′mē-ə) *n.* The presence of detectable levels of ketone bodies in the plasma.

ke·to·nu·ri·a (kē′tə-nōŏr′ē-ə) *n.* An excessive concentration of ketone bodies in the urine.

ke·tose (kē′tōs′) *n.* Any of various carbohydrates containing a ketone group.

ke·to·sis (kē-tō′sĭs) *n., pl.* **-ses** (-sēz) A pathological increase in the production of ketone bodies, as in uncontrolled diabetes mellitus.

Kew garden fever (kyōō) *n.* See **rickettsialpox.**

key-in-lock maneuver *n.* A method by which obstetrical forceps are used to rotate the fetal head.

kg *abbr.* kilogram

khi (kī) *n.* Variant of **chi**[1].

Kho·ra·na (kō-rä′nə), **Har Gobind** Born 1922. Indian-born American biochemist. He shared a 1968 Nobel Prize for the study of genetic codes.

kibe (kīb) *n.* A chapped or inflamed area on the skin, especially on the heel, due to exposure to cold.

kid·ney (kĭd′nē) *n., pl.* **-neys** Either of a pair of organs in the dorsal region of the vertebrate abdominal cavity, functioning to maintain proper water and electrolyte balance, regulate acid-base concentration, and filter the blood of metabolic wastes, which are then excreted as urine.

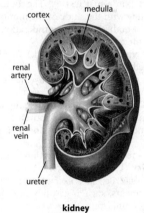

kidney
cutaway view of kidney

kidney stone *n.* A small hard mass in the kidney that forms from deposits chiefly of phosphates and urates. Also called *nephrolith.*

Kien·böck's disease (kēn′bĕks′, -bœks′) *n.* Osteolysis of the lunate bone following trauma to the wrist.

Kier·nan's space (kîr′nənz) *n.* Interlobular space in the liver.

Kies·sel·bach's area (kē′səl-bäks′) *n.* An area on the anterior portion of the nasal septum rich in capillaries and often the site of nosebleeds.

killed (kĭld) *adj.* Of, relating to, or containing microorganisms or viruses that have been killed or inactivated so as to be incapable of causing infection.

kill·er cell (kĭl′ər) *n.* A large differentiated T cell that attacks and lyses target cells bearing specific antigens. Also called *cytotoxic T cell, killer T cell, null cell.*

kilo– *pref.* One thousand (10^3): *kilogram.*

kil·o·cal·o·rie (kĭl′ə-kăl′ə-rē) *n. Abbr.* **kcal** See **calorie** (sense 2).

kil·o·gram (kĭl′ə-grăm′) *n. Abbr.* **kg** The base unit of mass in the International System of Units, equal to 1,000 grams (2.2046 pounds).

kilogram calorie *n.* See **calorie** (sense 2).

kilogram-meter *n.* A unit of energy and work in the meter-kilogram-second system, equal to the work performed by a one-kilogram force acting through a distance of one meter.

Kim·mel·stiel-Wilson disease (kĭm′əl-stēl′-) *n.* Nephrotic syndrome and hypertension in diabetics associated with diabetic glomerulosclerosis. Also called *Kimmelstiel-Wilson syndrome.*

kin– *pref.* Variant of **kino–**.

kin·an·es·the·sia (kĭn′ăn-ĭs-thē′zhə) *n.* A disturbance of deep nerve sensitivity characterized by an inability to perceive direction or extent of movement.

ki·nase (kī′nās′, -nāz′, kĭn′ās′, -āz′) *n.* **1.** An enzyme that catalyzes the conversion of a proenzyme to an active enzyme. **2.** A various enzyme that catalyzes the transfer of a phosphate group from a donor, such as ADP or ATP, to an acceptor.

kin·dred (kĭn′drĭd) *n.* A group of related persons, such as a clan or tribe.

kin·e·mat·ics (kĭn′ə-măt′ĭks) *n.* The branch of mechanics dealing with the study of the motion of a body or a system of bodies without consideration given to its mass or the forces acting on it.

kin·e·mat·ic viscosity (kĭn′ə-măt′ĭk) *n. Symbol* ***ν*** A measure used in fluid flow studies, usually expressed as the dynamic viscosity divided by the density of the fluid.

kin·e·sal·gia (kĭn′ĭ-săl′jə) *or* **ki·ne·si·al·gia** (kĭ-nē′sē-ăl′jə) *n.* Pain caused by muscular movement.

kinesi– *or* **kine–** *or* **kines–** *or* **kinesio–** *pref.* Movement: *kinesimeter.*

ki·ne·sia (kə-nē′zhə, kī-) *n.* See **motion sickness**.

ki·ne·si·at·rics (kə-nē′zē-ăt′rĭks) *n.* See **kinesitherapy**.

ki·ne·sics (kə-nē′zĭks, kī-) *n.* The study of nonverbal bodily movements, such as gestures and facial expressions, as communication.

ki·ne·si·ol·o·gy (kə-nē′zē-ŏl′ə-jē, kī-) *n.* The study of muscular movement, especially the mechanics of human motion. —**kin′e·sim′e·ter** (kĭn′ĭ-sĭm′ĭ-tər, kī′nĭ-) *n.*

ki·ne·si·o·neu·ro·sis (kə-nē′zē-ō-nŏŏ-rō′sĭs, kī-) *n.* A functional nervous disease that is characterized by tics, spasms, or other motor disorders.

ki·ne·sis (kə-nē′sĭs, kī-) *n., pl.* **-ses** (-sēz′) Motion or physical movement, especially movement that is induced by stimulation.

ki·ne·si·ther·a·py (kə-nē′sə-thĕr′ə-pē, kī-) *n.* The treatment of disease by means of passive and active movements, such as massage and exercise. Also called *kinesiatrics.*

kin·es·the·sia (kĭn′ĭs-thē′zhə, kī′nĭs-) *n.* **1.** The sense that detects bodily position, weight, or movement of the muscles, tendons, and joints. **2.** The sensation of moving in space. —**kin′es·thet′ic** (-thĕt′ĭk) *adj.*

kin·es·the·si·om·e·ter (kĭn′ĭs-thē′zē-ŏm′ĭ-tər, kī′nĭs-) *n.* An instrument for determining the degree of muscular sensation in response to movement, weight, and position.

kinesthetic sense *n.* See **myesthesia**.

ki·net·ic (kə-nĕt′ĭk, kī-) *adj.* Of, relating to, or produced by motion.

kinetic energy *n.* The energy possessed by a body because of its motion, equal to one half the mass of the body times the square of its speed.

ki·net·ics (kə-nĕt′ĭks, kī-) *n.* **1.** The branch of mechanics concerned with the effects of forces on the motion of a body or system of bodies, especially of forces that do not originate within the system itself. Also called *dynamics.* **2.** The branch of chemistry concerned with the rates of change in the concentration of reactants in a chemical reaction.

kineto– *pref.* Movement: *kinetoplast.*

ki·net·o·car·di·o·gram (kə-nĕt′ō-kär′dē-ə-grăm′, -nē′tō-, kī-) *n.* A graphic recording of the vibrations of the chest wall produced by cardiac activity. —**ki·net′o·car′di·o·graph′** (-grăf′) *adj.*

ki·net·o·chore (kə-nĕt′ə-kôr′, -nē′tə-, kī-) *n.* See **centromere**.

ki·net·o·gen·ic (kə-nĕt′ə-jĕn′ĭk, -nē′tə-, kī-) *adj.* Causing or producing motion.

ki·net·o·plast (kə-nĕt′ə-plăst′, -nē′tə-, kī-) *n.* An independently replicating rod-shaped structure lying near the base of the flagellum in certain parasitic protozoans.

ki·nin (kī′nĭn) *n.* Any of various polypeptides, such as bradykinin, that act locally to induce vasodilation and contraction of smooth muscle.

ki·nin·o·gen (kī-nĭn′ə-jən, -jĕn′) *n.* The inactive globulin precursor of a plasma kinin.

ki·nin·o·gen·ase (kī-nĭn′ə-jə-nās′, -nāz′) *n.* See **kallikrein**.

kink (kĭngk) *n.* **1.** A tight curl, twist, or bend in a length of thin material. **2.** A painful muscle spasm, as in the neck; a crick. **3.** A mental peculiarity; a quirk. **4.** Peculiarity or deviation in sexual behavior or taste. —*v.* To form or cause to form a kink or kinks.

kink·y-hair disease (kĭng′kē-hâr′) *n.* A congenital metabolic defect manifested by short, sparse, poorly pigmented kinky hair and associated with failure to thrive, physical and mental retardation, and progressive deterioration of the brain. Also called *Menkes syndrome.*

kino– *or* **kin–** *pref.* Movement: *kinocilium.*

ki·no·cil·i·um (kī′nō-sĭl′ē-əm) *n.* A cilium, usually motile, having nine peripheral double microtubules and two single central ones.

Kin·sey (kĭn′zē), **Alfred Charles** 1894–1956. American sexologist and zoologist noted for his 1948 study, *Sex-*

ual Behavior in the Human Male, popularly known as "The Kinsey Report." Kinsey's survey, which was based upon thousands of interviews, revealed a greater variety of sexual behavior than had previously been suspected, and generated much controversy among both the scientific community and the general public.

kin·ship (kĭn′shĭp′) *n.* Connection by blood, marriage, or adoption; family relationship.

kiss·ing disease (kĭs′ĭng) *n.* Infectious mononucleosis.

kiss of life (kĭs) *n.* Mouth-to-mouth resuscitation.

Ki·ta·sa·to (kē′tä-zä′tō), **Shibasaburo** 1852–1931. Japanese bacteriologist. Among his achievements are the isolation (1889) of the causative bacillus of tetanus, the development of vaccines to protect against tetanus and anthrax, and the isolation (1894) of the bacillus of bubonic plague.

Klebs (klāps), **Edwin** 1894–1913. German pathologist who described (1883) the causative bacillus of diphtheria, later isolated by Friedrich Löffler.

Kleb·si·el·la (klĕb′zē-ĕl′ə) *n.* A genus of bacteria of the family Enterobacteriaceae containing nonmotile, gram-negative, frequently encapsulated rods that are arranged singly, in pairs, or in short chains. It includes some human pathogens.

Klebsiella pneu·mo·ni·ae (noo-mō′nē-ē′) *n.* Friedlander's bacillus.

Klebs-Löff·ler bacillus (klĕbz′lĕf′lər, klāps′lœf′lər) *n.* A gram-positive, nonmotile, rod-shaped bacterium *Corynebacterium diphtheriae* that causes diphtheria in humans and produces an exotoxin that causes tissue degeneration.

Klein (klīn), **Melanie** 1882–1960. Austrian-born British psychoanalyst who first introduced play therapy and was the first to use psychoanalysis to treat young children.

klep·to·ma·ni·a (klĕp′tə-mā′nē-ə, -mān′yə) *n.* An obsessive impulse to steal regardless of economic need, usually arising from an unconscious symbolic value associated with the stolen item. —**klep′to·ma′ni·ac′** (-nē-ăk′) *adj.*

Kline·fel·ter's syndrome (klīn′fĕl′tərz) *n.* A chromosomal anomaly in males characterized by the presence of two X-chromosomes and one Y-chromosome, causing reduced testicular size, seminiferous tubule dysgenesis, and infertility. Also called *XXY syndrome.*

Klip·pel-Feil syndrome (klĭ-pĕl′fīl′, -fēl′) *n.* A congenital syndrome of anatomical defects that is characterized by a short neck, extensive fusion of the cervical vertebrae, and abnormalities of the brainstem and the cerebellum.

Klip·pel's disease (klĭ-pĕlz′) *n.* See **arthritic general pseudoparalysis.**

Klon·o·pin (klŏn′ə-pĭn′) A trademark for the drug clonazepam.

K-Lor (kā′lôr′) A trademark for an oral preparation of potassium chloride.

Klug (klŭg, kloog), **Aaron** Born 1926. Lithuanian-born British biochemist. He won a 1982 Nobel Prize for research on the structure of viruses and particles of proteins and nucleic acids.

Klump·ke's paralysis (klŭmp′kēz) *n.* Brachial plexus injury often caused by trauma at birth and resulting in atrophic paralysis of the forearm and small muscles of the hand. Also called *Klumpke-Déjérine syndrome.*

knee (nē) *n.* **1.** The joint between the thigh and the lower leg, formed by the articulation of the femur and the tibia and covered anteriorly by the patella. **2.** The region of the leg that encloses and supports this joint.

knee·cap (nē′kăp′) *n.* See **patella** (sense 1).

knee-chest position *n.* A prone position in which the individual rests on the knees and upper part of the chest, assumed for gynecologic or rectal examination. Also called *genupectoral position.*

knee-elbow position *n.* A prone position in which the patient rests on the knees and elbows, assumed for a rectal or gynecologic examination or an operation. Also called *genucubital position.*

knee jerk *n.* See **patellar reflex.**

knee-jerk reflex *n.* See **patellar reflex.**

knee joint *n.* A compound condylar joint consisting of the joint between the condyles of the femur and the condyles of the tibia, and the articulation between the femur and the patella.

knee presentation *n.* Breech presentation of the fetus during birth in which a knee is the presenting part.

knee reflex *n.* See **patellar reflex.**

Kniest syndrome (knēst) *n.* An inherited syndrome characterized by short limbs, round face with central depression, enlargement and stiffness of joints, and contracture of fingers, and often including cleft palate, scoliosis, retinal detachment and myopia, and deafness; it is a form of metatropic dwarfism.

knit·ting (nĭt′ĭng) *n.* The physiological process by which the fragments of a broken bone are united or the edges of a wound are closed.

knock-knee (nŏk′nē′) *n.* A deformity of the legs in which the knees are abnormally close together and the ankles are spread widely apart.

knock·out mouse (knŏk′out′) *n.* A transgenic mouse that has been genetically engineered to exhibit mutations in specific genes.

knot (nŏt) *n.* **1.** A compact intersection of interlaced material, as of cord, ribbon, or rope. **2.** A protuberant growth or swelling in a tissue, such as a gland.

knuck·le (nŭk′əl) *n.* **1.** The prominence of the dorsal aspect of a joint of a finger, especially of one of the joints that connect the fingers to the hand. **2.** A rounded protuberance formed by the bones in a joint. **3.** A kink or loop of intestine, as in a hernia.

knuck·le·bone (nŭk′əl-bōn′) *n.* A knobbed bone, as of a knuckle or joint.

knuckle pads *n.* An atavistic congenital condition in which thick pads of skin appear over the proximal phalangeal joints.

Köb·ner's phenomenon (kœb′nərz) *n.* An isomorphic cutaneous reaction occurring in response to trauma and affecting previously uninvolved sites in patients with psoriasis, lichen planus, and flat warts. Also called *isomorphic response.*

Koch (kôk, kôкн), **Robert** 1843–1910. German bacteriologist who discovered the cholera bacillus and the bacterial cause of anthrax. He won a 1905 Nobel Prize for developing tuberculin.

Ko·cher (kôʹkər, -кнər), **Emil Theodor** 1841–1917. Swiss surgeon. He won a 1909 Nobel Prize for work on the thyroid gland.

Koch's bacillus (kôks, kôкнs) *n.* **1.** See **tubercle bacillus.** **2.** A gram-negative bacterium *Vibrio cholerae* that produces a soluble exotoxin that may be the causative agent of Asiatic cholera in humans. Also called *comma bacillus.*

Koch's postulates *pl.n.* The series of conditions that must be met in order to establish a microorganism as the causative agent of a disease, namely: it must be present in all cases of the disease; inoculations of its pure cultures must produce the disease in susceptible animals; and from these it must again be isolated and propagated in pure cultures.

Koch-Weeks bacillus (-wēksʹ) *n.* A gram-negative, rod-shaped, parasitic bacterium *Haemophilus aegyptius* that causes acute conjunctivitis.

Kock pouch (kôk) *n.* An ileostomy with a reservoir and valved opening surgically created from doubled loops of ileum.

Köh·ler (kœʹlər), **Georges J.F.** 1946–1995. German immunologist. He shared a 1984 Nobel Prize for the development of a technique for producing monoclonal antibodies.

Köh·ler's disease (kōʹlərz, kœʹ-) *n.* Osteochondrosis of the tarsal navicular bone or of the patella.

Kohl·rausch's muscle (kōlʹrou'shĭz) *n.* Any of the longitudinal muscles of the rectal wall.

koi·lo·cyte (koiʹlə-sīt') *n.* A squamous cell, often binucleate and having a perinuclear hole, characteristic of genital warts.

koi·lo·cy·to·sis (koi'lō-sī-tōʹsĭs) *n.* A condition of certain cells characterized by perinuclear vacuolation.

koi·lo·nych·i·a (koi'lō-nĭkʹē-ə) *n.* A nail deformity characterized by concavity of the outer surface of the nail. Also called *celonychia, spoon nail.*

ko·lyt·ic (kō-lĭtʹĭk) *adj.* Relating to or characterized by an inhibitory action.

Kon·do·le·on operation (kŏn'dō-lēʹŏn) *n.* Excision of strips of subcutaneous connective tissue for the relief of elephantiasis.

Kop·lik's spots (kŏpʹlĭks) *pl.n.* Small red spots on the mucous membrane of the cheek, with a minute bluish-white speck in the center, regarded as symptomatic of measles.

Ko·re·an hemorrhagic fever (kə-rēʹən, kô-) *n.* See **epidemic hemorrhagic fever.**

Korn·berg (kôrnʹbûrg'), **Arthur** Born 1918. American biochemist. He shared a 1959 Nobel Prize for work on the biological synthesis of nucleic acids.

Ko·rot·koff sounds (kə-rŏtʹkôf, kô-) *pl.n.* The sounds heard over an artery when blood pressure is determined by the auscultatory method.

Ko·rot·koff's test (kə-rŏtʹkôfs, kô-) *n.* A test of collateral circulation in cases of aneurysm, in which the artery is compressed above the aneurysm; if blood pressure in the distal circulation is fairly high, the collateral circulation is good.

Kor·sa·koff's syndrome (kôrʹsə-kôfs') *n.* A syndrome that is marked by confusion and severe impairment of memory for which the patient compensates by

confabulation; it is often viewed as the psychological component of Wernicke-Korsakoff syndrome. Also called *Korsakoff's psychosis, polyneuritic psychosis.*

Kr The symbol for the element **krypton.**

Krab·be's disease (krăbʹēz) *n.* See **globoid cell leukodystrophy.**

Krae·pe·lin (krĕpʹə-lēn'), **Emil** 1856–1926. German psychiatrist whose classification system of mental disorders formed the foundation for the standard diagnostic text in the field of psychiatry, the *Diagnostic and Statistical Manual* (DSM).

Kras·ke's operation (krăsʹkēz, krä'skəz) *n.* Removal of the coccyx and excision of the left wing of the sacrum to afford approach for resection of the rectum in cases of cancer or stenosis.

krau·ro·sis vul·vae (krô-rōʹsĭs vŭlʹvē) *n.* Atrophy and shrinkage of the skin of the vagina and vulva often accompanied by a chronic inflammatory reaction in the deeper tissues. Also called *leukokraurosis.*

Krebs (krĕbz, krĕps), **Sir Hans Adolf** 1900–1981. German-born British biochemist who discovered (1936) the Krebs cycle. He shared a 1953 Nobel Prize for investigations into metabolic processes.

Krebs cycle (krĕbz) *n.* A series of enzymatic reactions in aerobic organisms involving oxidative metabolism of acetyl units and producing high-energy phosphate compounds, which serve as the main source of cellular energy. Also called *citric acid cycle, tricarboxylic acid cycle.*

Krebs-Hen·se·leit cycle (-hĕnʹzə-līt') *n.* See **urea cycle.**

Krebs ornithine cycle *n.* See **urea cycle.**

Krebs urea cycle *n.* See **urea cycle.**

Krogh (krôg, krôкн), **(Schack) August Steenberg** 1874–1949. Danish physiologist. He won a 1920 Nobel Prize for the discovery of the regulation of the capillaries' motor mechanism.

Kru·ken·berg's amputation (krooʹkĭn-bûrgz') *n.* A cineplastic amputation at the carpus with the distal end of the forearm used to create a forklike stump.

Krukenberg's spindle *n.* A vertical fusiform area of melanin pigmentation on the posterior surface of the cornea in the pupillary area.

Krukenberg's tumor *n.* A malignant tumor of the ovary that usually occurs bilaterally and in association with mucous carcinoma of the stomach.

kryp·ton (krĭpʹtŏn') *n. Symbol* **Kr** A largely inert gaseous element used in gas fluorescent lamps, whose artificial radioisotope is used in diagnostic imaging. Atomic number 36.

KS *abbr.* Kaposi's sarcoma

KUB (kā'yōoʹbē') *n.* An x-ray of the kidneys, ureter, and bladder.

Kufs disease (kŭfs, koofs) *n.* The adult type of cerebral sphingolipidosis.

Kuhn (koon), **Richard** 1900–1967. Austrian chemist. He won a 1938 Nobel Prize for research on carotenoids and vitamins but declined the award by order of the Nazi government.

Küm·mell's spondylitis (kĭmʹəlz, küʹməlz) *n.* Late post-traumatic collapse of a vertebral body.

Kupf·fer cell (koopʹfər) *n.* Macrophages lining the walls of the hepatic sinusoids.

ku·ru (kŏŏr′ŏŏ) *n.* A progressive, fatal spongiform encephalopathy, probably caused by a slow-acting virus, that is endemic to certain peoples of New Guinea and may be transmitted through cannibalism.

Kuss·maul breathing (kŏŏs′moul) *n.* A abnormal respiratory pattern characeized by rapid, deep breathing, often seen in patients with metabolic acidosis.

Kussmaul respiration *n.* Deep, rapid respiration characteristic of diabetic acidosis or other conditions causing acidosis. Also called *Kussmaul-Kien respiration.*

Kuss·maul's coma (kŏŏs′moulz) *n.* See **diabetic coma.**

Kussmaul's disease *n.* See **polyarteritis nodosa.**

Kussmaul's sign *n.* An indication of cardiac tamponade in which an increase in venous distention and pressure occurs during inspiration.

Kveim antigen (kvām) *n.* A saline suspension of human sarcoid tissue prepared from the spleen of an individual with active sarcoidosis and used in the Kveim test.

Kveim test *n.* An intradermal test for the detection of sarcoidosis, performed by injecting Kveim antigen and examining skin biopsies after three and six weeks; a positive test is indicated by typical nodules showing evidence of sarcoid tissue.

kwa·shi·or·kor (kwä′shē-ôr′kôr′) *n.* A severe malnutrition of infants and young children, primarily in tropical and subtropical regions, caused by deficiency in the quality and quantity of protein in the diet and characterized by anemia, edema, potbelly, depigmentation of the skin, loss or change in hair color, hypoalbuminemia, and bulky stools containing undigested food.

Kwell (kwĕl) A trademark for the drug lindane.

ky·ma·tism (kī′mə-tĭz′əm) *n.* See **myokymia.**

ky·mo·graph (kī′mə-grăf′) *n.* An instrument that is used for recording variations in pressure, as of the blood, or in tension, as of a muscle, by means of a pen or stylus that marks a rotating drum. —**ky′mo·graph′ic** *adj.* —**ky′mo·gram′** (-grăm′) *n.* —**ky·mog′ra·phy** (-mŏg′rə-fē) *n.*

kyn·u·re·nic acid (kĭn′yŏŏ-rē′nĭk, -rĕn′ĭk, kīn′-) *n.* A crystalline acid occurring in the urine as a product of the metabolism of tryptophan.

kyn·u·re·nin·ase (kī′nyŏŏ-rē′nə-nās′, -nāz′, -rĕn′ə-, kĭn′yŏŏ-) *n.* A liver enzyme that catalyzes the formation of alanine and anthranilic acid during tryptophan metabolism.

kyn·u·re·nine (kĭn-yŏŏr′ə-nēn′, kĭn-, kī′nyŏŏ-rē′nĭn, -rĕn′ĭn, kĭn′yŏŏ-) *n.* An amino acid that is a precursor of kynurenic acid and that is excreted in small amounts in the urine as a product of the metabolism of tryptophan.

ky·phos (kī′fŏs′) *n.* The convex part of the back produced by kyphosis; the hump.

ky·pho·sco·li·o·sis (kī′fō-skō′lē-ō′sĭs, -skŏl′ē-) *n.* A condition in which the spinal disorders of kyphosis and scoliosis occur together.

ky·pho·sis (kī-fō′sĭs) *n.* Abnormal rearward curvature of the spine, resulting in a protuberant upper back. Also called *humpback.* —**ky·phot′ic** (-fŏt′ĭk) *adj.*

kyphotic pelvis *n.* Backward curvature of the lumbar spine causing contraction of pelvic measurements.

L

λ **1.** The Greek letter *lambda*. Entries beginning with this character are alphabetized under **lambda.** **2.** The symbol for **decay constant.** **3.** The symbol for Ostwald's solubility coefficient. **4.** The symbol for **wavelength.**

L– *pref.* Of or relating to the configuration of L-glyceraldehyde, a compound that is chosen as the basis for stereochemical nomenclature because it is the simplest carbohydrate that can form optical isomers: L-*lactic acid.*

L *abbr.* left; limes (used with a lower case letter or a plus sign, or used with a subscript letter or plus sign as a symbol for various doses of toxin); *or* **l** liter

l– *pref.* **l–** To the left; levo: *l*-lactic acid.

La The symbol for the element **lanthanum.**

la belle in·dif·fer·ence (lä bĕl′ ăɴ-dē-fä-räɴs′) *n.* A naive, inappropriate lack of emotion or concern for the perceptions by others of one's disability, usually seen in persons with conversion disorder. Also called *belle indifference.*

la·bet·a·lol hydrochloride (lə-bĕt′ə-lôl′, -lōl′) *n.* An alpha- and beta-blocker that is used in the treatment of hypertension.

la·bi·al (lā′bē-əl) *adj.* Relating to the lips or labia.

labial artery *n.* **1.** An artery with origin in the facial artery, with distribution to the lower lip, and with anastomoses to the chin and lower lip arteries; inferior labial artery. **2.** An artery with origin in the facial artery, with distribution to the upper lip and to the nasal septum, and with anastomoses to the sphenopalatine artery; superior labial artery.

labial hernia *n.* See **cremnocele.**

labial splint *n.* An appliance made to conform to the outer aspect of the dental arch and used in the management of jaw and facial injuries.

labial vein *n.* **1.** Any of the veins that pass from the labia majora to the pudendal veins, such as the anterior labial and posterior labial veins. **2.** Either of the two veins that drain the lips: inferior labial vein and superior labial.

labia ma·jo·ra (mə-jôr′ə) *pl.n.* The two outer rounded folds of adipose tissue that lie on either side of the vaginal opening and that form the external lateral boundaries of the vulva.

labia mi·no·ra (mə-nôr′ə) *pl.n.* The two thin inner folds of skin within the vestibule of the vagina enclosed within the cleft of the labia majora.

labia o·ris (ôr′ĭs) *pl.n.* The lips of the mouth.

la·bile (lā′bīl′, -bəl) *adj.* **1.** Receptive to change; adaptable. **2.** Constantly undergoing or likely to undergo change, as a chemical compound; unstable. —**la·bil′i·ty** (-bĭl′ĭ-tē) *n.*

labio– *pref.* Labial: *labiodental.*

la·bi·o·cer·vi·cal (lā′bē-ō-sûr′vĭ-kəl) *adj.* Relating to the labial or the buccal surface of the neck of a tooth.

la·bi·o·cho·re·a (lā′bē-ō-kô-rē′ə, -kə-) *n.* A chronic spasm of the lips that interferes with speech.

la·bi·o·cli·na·tion (lā′bē-ō-klə-nā′shən) *n.* Inclination of a tooth more toward the lips than is normal.

la·bi·o·den·tal (lā′bē-ō-dĕn′tl) *adj.* **1.** Relating to the lips and teeth. **2.** Articulated with the lower lip and upper teeth, as the sounds (f) and (v).

la·bi·o·gin·gi·val (lā′bē-ō-jĭn′jə-vəl, -jĭn-jī′-) *adj.* Relating to the point of junction of the labial border and the gingival line on the distal or mesial surface of an incisor tooth.

la·bi·o·glos·so·la·ryn·geal (lā′bē-ō-glô′sō-lə-rĭn′jəl, -lăr′ən-jē′əl) *adj.* Of or relating to the lips, tongue, and larynx.

la·bi·o·glos·so·pha·ryn·geal (lā′bē-ō-glô′sō-fə-rĭn′jəl, -făr′ən-jē′əl) *adj.* Relating to the lips, tongue, and pharynx.

la·bi·o·graph (lā′bē-ə-grăf′) *n.* An instrument used for recording the movements of the lips during speech.

la·bi·o·men·tal (lā′bē-ō-mĕn′tl) *adj.* Relating to the lower lip and the chin.

la·bi·o·na·sal (lā′bē-ō-nā′zəl) *adj.* Relating to the upper lip and the nose or to both lips and the nose.

la·bi·o·pal·a·tine (lā′bē-ō-păl′ə-tīn′) *adj.* Relating to the lips and the palate.

la·bi·o·place·ment (lā′bē-ō-plās′mənt) *n.* The positioning of a tooth more toward the lips than normal.

la·bi·o·plas·ty (lā′bē-ə-plăs′tē) *n.* Plastic surgery on a lip.

la·bi·o·ver·sion (lā′bē-ō-vûr′zhən) *n.* Displacement of an anterior tooth from the normal line of occlusion toward the lips.

la·bi·um (lā′bē-əm) *n., pl* **–bi·a** (-bē-ə) **1.** A lip or lip-shaped anatomical structure. **2.** Any of four folds of tissue of the female external genitalia.

la·bor (lā′bər) *n.* The physical efforts of expulsion of the fetus and the placenta from the uterus during parturition. —*v.* To undergo the efforts of childbirth.

lab·o·ra·to·ry (lăb′rə-tôr′ē) *n.* **1.** A room or building equipped for scientific research. **2.** A place where drugs and chemicals are manufactured. **3.** A place for practice, observation, or testing.

laboratory diagnosis *n.* Diagnosis based on the results of laboratory analyses, including microscopic, bacteriologic, or biopsy studies.

labor pains *pl.n.* Rhythmical uterine contractions that, under normal conditions, increase in intensity, frequency, and duration, and culminate in vaginal delivery of the infant.

lab·ro·cyte (lăb′rə-sīt′) *n.* See **mast cell.**

la·brum (lā′brəm) *n., pl.* **–bra** (-brə) A lip-shaped anatomical edge, rim, or structure.

lab·y·rinth (lăb′ə-rĭnth′) *n.* **1.** A group of complex interconnecting anatomical cavities. **2.** See **inner ear.**

lab·y·rin·thec·to·my (lăb′ə-rĭn-thĕk′tə-mē) *n.* Excision of the labyrinth of the ear.

lab·y·rin·thine (lăb′ə-rĭn′thĭn, -thēn′) *adj.* Of, relating to, resembling, or constituting a labyrinth.

labyrinthine angiospasm *n.* See **Lermoyez syndrome.**

labyrinthine fluid *n.* The fluid separating the osseous and the membranous labyrinths of the inner ear.

labyrinthine nystagmus *n.* See **vestibular nystagmus.**

labyrinthine vein *n.* Either of two veins that accompany each labyrinthine artery, drain the inner ear, and empty into the transverse sinus or the inferior petrosal sinus. Also called *internal auditory vein.*

labyrinthine vertigo *n.* See **Ménière's disease.**

lab·y·rin·thi·tis (lăb′ə-rĭn-thī′tĭs) *n.* Inflammation of the inner ear, sometimes accompanied by vertigo. Also called *otitis interna.*

lab·y·rin·thot·o·my (lăb′ə-rĭn-thŏt′ə-mē) *n.* Incision into the labyrinth of the ear.

lac (lăk) *n.* **1.** Milk. **2.** A whitish, milky looking liquid.

lac·er·ate (lăs′ə-rāt′) *v.* To rip, cut, or tear. —*adj.* (-rĭt, -rāt′) **1.** Torn; mangled. **2.** Wounded.

lac·er·at·ed (lăs′ə-rā′tĭd) *adj.* Cut or wounded in a jagged manner.

lacerated wound *n.* A wound caused by laceration.

lac·er·a·tion (lăs′ə-rā′shən) *n.* **1.** A jagged wound or cut. **2.** The process or act of tearing tissue.

la·cer·tus (lə-sûr′təs) *n., pl.* **-ti** (-tī′) **1.** The muscular part of the upper arm from the shoulder to the elbow. **2.** A fibrous band related to a muscle.

lach·ry·ma·tion (lăk′rə-mā′shən) *n.* Variant of **lacrimation.**

lach·ry·ma·tor *or* **lac·ri·ma·tor** (lăk′rə-mā′tər) *n.* Tear gas.

lach·ry·ma·to·ry (lăk′rə-mə-tôr′ē) *adj.* Variant of **lacrimatory.**

lac·ri·mal *or* **lach·ry·mal** (lăk′rə-məl) *adj.* **1.** Of or relating to tears. **2.** Of, relating to, or constituting the glands that produce tears.

lacrimal apparatus *n.* The system that secretes and drains tears into the nasal cavity, consisting of the lacrimal gland, the lacrimal lake, the lacrimal duct, the lacrimal sac, and the nasolacrimal duct.

lacrimal artery *n.* An artery with its origin in the ophthalmic artery, with distribution to the lacrimal gland, the lateral and superior rectus muscles, the upper eyelid, forehead, and temporal fossa.

lacrimal bone *n.* A thin irregularly rectangular plate forming part of the medial wall of the eye socket behind the frontal process of the maxilla.

lacrimal canal *n.* See **lacrimal duct.**

lacrimal caruncle *n.* A small reddish body at the medial angle of the eye, containing modified sebaceous and sweat glands.

lacrimal duct *n.* A curved canal beginning at the margin of each eyelid near the medial commissure, and emptying with the duct from the other eye into the lacrimal sac. Also called *lacrimal canal.*

lacrimal fold *n.* A fold of mucous membrane guarding the lower opening of the nasolacrimal duct.

lacrimal gland *n.* An almond-shaped gland that secretes tears into ducts that empty onto the surface of the conjunctiva of the eye.

lacrimal lake *n.* The small cistern-like area of the conjunctiva at the medial angle of the eye, in which the tears collect after bathing the front surface of the eyeball and the conjunctival sac.

lacrimal nerve *n.* A branch of the ophthalmic nerve, supplying the upper eyelid, conjunctiva, and lacrimal gland.

lacrimal papilla *n.* A slight projection from the margin of each eyelid near the medial commissure, in the center of which is the opening of the lacrimal duct.

lacrimal punctum *n.* The minute circular opening of the lacrimal duct on the margin of each eyelid near the medial commissure.

lacrimal sac *n.* The upper portion of the nasolacrimal duct into which the two lacrimal ducts empty. Also called *dacryocyst, tear sac.*

lacrimal vein *n.* A vein that drains the lacrimal gland, and empties into the superior ophthalmic vein.

lac·ri·ma·tion *or* **lach·ry·ma·tion** (lăk′rə-mā′shən) *n.* The secretion of tears, especially in excess.

lac·ri·ma·tor (lăk′rə-mā′tər) *n.* Variant of **lachrymator.**

lac·ri·ma·to·ry *or* **lach·ry·ma·to·ry** (lăk′rə-mə-tôr′ē) *adj.* Causing the secretion of tears.

lac·ri·mot·o·my (lăk′rə-mŏt′ə-mē) *n.* Incision of the lacrimal duct or sac.

La Crosse encephalitis (lə krôs′) *n.* An often fatal infection of the brain caused by a virus occasionally present in the bloodstream of birds and transmitted to humans by the mosquito *Aedes triseriatus.*

lact– *pref.* Variant of **lacto–.**

lac·tac·i·de·mi·a (lăk-tăs′ĭ-dē′mē-ə) *n.* See **lacticacidemia.**

lac·tac·i·do·sis (lăk-tăs′ĭ-dō′sĭs) *n.* Acidosis caused by increased lactic acid.

lac·tal·bu·min (lăk′tăl-byōō′mĭn) *n.* The albumin contained in milk and obtained from whey.

lac·tam (lăk′tăm′) *n.* An amide formed from amino carboxylic acids containing a keto group in a ring configuration, as seen in purines, pyrimidines, and antibiotics. It is tautomeric to lactim.

lac·tase (lăk′tās′) *n.* A galactosidase occurring in the intestine that catalyzes the hydrolysis of lactose into glucose and galactose.

lac·tate[1] (lăk′tāt′) *v.* To secrete or produce milk.

lac·tate[2] (lăk′tāt′) *n.* A salt or ester of lactic acid.

lactate dehydrogenase *n. Abbr.* **LDH** Any of a class of enzymes found in the liver, kidneys, striated muscle, and heart muscle that catalyze the reversible conversion of pyruvate and lactate.

lac·tat·ed Ringer's injection (lăk′tā′tĭd) *n.* A sterile solution of calcium chloride, potassium chloride, sodium chloride, and sodium lactate in water, given intravenously as a systemic alkalizer and as a fluid and electrolyte replenisher.

lactated Ringer's solution *n.* A solution containing sodium chloride, potassium chloride, calcium chloride, and sodium lactate in distilled water, used for the same purposes as Ringer's solution.

lac·ta·tion (lăk-tā′shən) *n.* **1.** The secretion or formation of milk by the mammary glands. **2.** The period during which the mammary glands secrete milk. —**lac·ta′tion·al** *adj.*

lactation amenorrhea *n.* Physiological suppression of menstruation while nursing.

lac·te·al (lăk′tē-əl) *adj.* **1.** Of, relating to, or resembling milk. **2.** Of or relating to a lacteal. —*n.* Any of numerous minute intestinal lymph-carrying vessels that convey chyle from the intestine to lymphatic circulation and thereby to the thoracic duct. Also called *chyle vessel.*

lac·tes·cent (lăk-tĕs′ənt) *adj.* **1.** Becoming milky. **2.** Milky. **3.** Secreting or yielding a milky juice, as certain plants and insects.

lacti– *n.* Variant of **lacto–.**

lac·tic (lăk′tĭk) *adj.* Of, relating to, or derived from milk.

lactic acid *n.* A syrupy, water-soluble liquid existing in three isomeric forms: one in muscle tissue and blood as a result of anaerobic glucose metabolism, a second in sour milk and wines, and a third used in foods, beverages, and pharmaceuticals.

lac·tic·ac·i·de·mi·a (lăk′tĭk-ăs′ĭ-dē′mē-ə) *n.* The presence of dextrorotatory lactic acid in the blood. Also called *lactacidemia.*

lac·tif·er·ous (lăk-tĭf′ər-əs) *adj.* Producing, secreting, or conveying milk.

lactiferous duct *n.* Any of the ducts that drain the lobes of the mammary gland at the nipple. Also called *galactophore, galactophorous duct, mammary duct, mamillary duct, milk duct.*

lactiferous sinus *n.* A circumscribed spindle-shaped dilation of the lactiferous duct just before it enters the nipple of the breast.

lac·ti·fuge (lăk′tə-fyo͞oj′) *adj.* Causing the arrest of the secretion of milk.

lac·tig·e·nous (lăk-tĭj′ə-nəs) *adj.* Producing milk.

lac·tig·er·ous (lăk-tĭj′ər-əs) *adj.* Lactiferous.

lac·tim (lăk′tĭm) *n.* A hydroxy imide compound characterized by an enolic group in a ring configuration. It is tautameric with lactam.

lacto– *or* **lact–** *or* **lacti–** *pref.* **1.** Milk: *lactoglobulin.* **2.** Lactose: *lactase.* **3.** Lactic acid: *lactate.*

lac·to·ba·cil·lus (lăk′tō-bə-sĭl′əs) *n.* Any of various rod-shaped, nonmotile, aerobic bacteria of the genus *Lactobacillus* that ferment lactic acid from sugars and are the causative agents in the souring of milk.

lac·to·cele (lăk′tə-sēl′) *n.* See **galactocele.**

lac·to·fla·vin (lăk′tə-flā′vĭn, lăk′tə-flā′-) *n.* See **riboflavin.**

lac·to·gen (lăk′tə-jən, -jĕn′) *n.* An agent that stimulates lactation.

lac·to·gen·e·sis (lăk′tə-jĕn′ĭ-sĭs) *n.* The production of milk by the mammary glands.

lac·to·gen·ic (lăk′tə-jĕn′ĭk) *adj.* Inducing lactation.

lactogenic hormone *n.* See **prolactin.**

lac·to·glob·u·lin (lăk′tō-glŏb′yə-lĭn) *n.* The globulin present in milk, comprising from 50 to 60 percent of bovine whey protein.

lac·tone (lăk′tōn′) *n.* An anhydride formed by the removal of a water molecule from the hydroxyl and carboxyl radicals of hydroxy acids. —**lac·ton′ic** (-tŏn′ĭk) *adj.*

lac·to·pro·tein (lăk′tō-prō′tēn′) *n.* A protein normally present in milk.

lac·tor·rhe·a (lăk′tə-rē′ə) *n.* See **galactorrhea** (sense 1).

lac·tose (lăk′tōs′) *n.* **1.** A disaccharide in milk that hydrolyzes to yield glucose and galactose. Also called *milk*

sugar. **2.** A white crystalline substance obtained from whey and used in infant foods and in pharmaceuticals as a diluent and excipient. Also called *milk sugar.*

lactose intolerance *n.* The inability to digest lactose, resulting from deficiency of the enzyme lactase and sometimes causing diarrhea or other gastrointestinal symptoms.

lac·to·su·ri·a (lăk′tə-so͝or′ē-ə, -sho͝or′-) *n.* The presence of lactose in the urine.

lac·to·ther·a·py (lăk′tō-thĕr′ə-pē) *n.* See **galactotherapy** (sense 2).

lac·to·tro·pin (lăk′tō-trō′pĭn) *n.* See **prolactin.**

la·cu·na (lə-kyo͞o′nə) *n., pl.* **–nas** *or* **–nae** (-nē) **1.** An anatomical cavity, space, or depression, especially in a bone. **2.** An empty space or a missing part; a gap; a defect. **3.** An abnormal space between the strata or between the cellular elements of the epidermis. **4.** See **corneal space. —la·cu′nal** *adj.*

lacuna mag·na (măg′nə) *n.* A recess on the roof of the navicular fossa of the urethra, formed by a fold of mucous membrane.

la·cu·nar (lə-kyo͞o′nər) *adj.* **1.** Of or relating to a lacuna; lacunal. **2.** Of or relating to a temporary absence of manifestation of a symptom.

lacunar amnesia *n.* A condition in which memory is partially lost or the memory of isolated events is lost.

lacunar ligament *n.* A curved fibrous band that forms the medial boundary of the femoral canal.

la·cu·nule (lə-kyo͞o′no͞ol′) *n.* A very small lacuna.

la·cus (lā′kəs) *n., pl.* **lacus** A lake.

lad·der splint (lăd′ər) *n.* A flexible splint consisting of two stout parallel wires with finer cross wires.

Ladd-Frank·lin (lăd′-frăngk′lĭn), **Christine** 1847–1930. American psychologist and logician noted for her work on the theory of color vision.

Laën·nec (lā-nĕk′), **René Théophile Hyacinthe** 1781–1826. French physician who invented the stethoscope (ca. 1819).

Laën·nec's cirrhosis (lā-nĕks′) *n.* Cirrhosis in which normal liver lobules are replaced by small regeneration nodules, sometimes containing fat, separated by fibrous tissue strands. Also called *portal cirrhosis.*

la·e·trile (lā′ĭ-trĭl′, -trəl) *n.* A drug derived from amygdalin from apricot pits and purported to have antineoplastic properties.

La·fo·ra body (lə-fôr′ə) *n.* An intraneuronal inclusion body composed of acid mucopolysaccharides, seen in familial myoclonic epilepsy.

Lafora body disease *n.* See **myoclonus epilepsy.**

La·fo·ra's disease (lə-fôr′əz) *n.* See **myoclonus epilepsy.**

la·ge·na (lə-jē′nə) *n., pl.* **la·ge·nae** (-nē) One of the three parts of the membranous labyrinth of the inner ear of nonmammalian vertebrates.

lag·ging (lăg′ĭng) *n.* Retarded or diminished movement of the affected side of the chest in pulmonary tuberculosis.

lag·oph·thal·mi·a (lăg′ŏf-thăl′mē-ə) *or* **lag·oph·thal·mos** (-mŏs′) *n.* A condition in which it is difficult or impossible to close the eyelids completely. —**lag′oph·thal′mic** (lăg′ŏf-thăl′mĭk) *adj.*

lagophthalmic keratitis *n.* Inflammation and irritation of the cornea caused by an inability to close the eyelids. Also called *exposure keratitis.*

La·grange's operation (lə-grän′jĭz) *n.* A combined iridectomy and sclerectomy that is performed in glaucoma for the purpose of forming a filtering cicatrix.

LAK cell (lăk) *n.* A white blood cell produced by cultivation of lymphocytes with interleukin-2 and used experimentally to shrink malignant tumors.

lake¹ (lāk) *n.* A small collection of fluid.

lake² (lāk) *n.* A pigment consisting of organic coloring matter with an inorganic, usually metallic base or carrier, used in dyes, inks, and paints. —*v.* To cause blood plasma to become red as a result of the release of hemoglobin from the red blood cells.

La·ki-Lo·rand factor (lăk′ĭ-lə-rănd′) *n.* See **factor XIII.**

lak·y (lā′kē) *adj.* Having a transparent, bright-red appearance. Used of serum or plasma containing hemoglobin from hemolyzed red blood cells.

lal·ling (lăl′ĭng) *n.* A form of stammering in which the speech is almost unintelligible.

lal·o·che·zi·a (lăl′ō-kē′zē-ə) *n.* Emotional relief gained by using indecent or vulgar language.

lal·o·ple·gia (lăl′ō-plē′jə) *n.* Paralysis of the muscles involved in speech.

La·marck (lə-märk′, lä-), Chevalier de **Jean Baptiste Pierre Antoine de Monet** 1744–1829. French naturalist noted for his theories on evolution by adaptative modification and for classifying animals into vertebrates and invertebrates.

La·maze (lə-mäz′), **Ferdinand** 1891–1957. French obstetrician who in the 1950s developed a method of childbirth preparation using behavioral training to reduce pain and anxiety in labor.

Lamaze method *n.* A method of childbirth in which the expectant mother is prepared psychologically and physically to give birth without the use of pain-relieving drugs. —**La·maze** *adj.*

lamb·da (lăm′də) *n.* **1.** *Symbol* **λ** The 11th letter of the Greek alphabet. **2.** The craniometric point at the junction of the sagittal and lambdoid sutures. —*adj.* Of, relating to, or characterizing a polypeptide chain that is one of two types of light chains present in immunoglobins.

lamb·doid (lăm′doid′) *adj.* **1.** Having the shape of the Greek letter lambda. **2.** Relating to the deeply serrated suture.

lambdoid suture *n.* The line of union between the occipital and the parietal bones of the skull.

Lam·bert-Eaton syndrome (lăm′bərt-) *n.* Progressive proximal muscle weakness in individuals with carcinoma, in the absence of dermatomyositis or polymyositis. Also called *carcinomatous myopathy, Eaton-Lambert syndrome.*

Lam·bli·a (lăm′blē-ə) *n.* Giardia.

lam·bli·a·sis (lăm-blī′ə-sĭs) *n.* See **giardiasis.**

Lam·bri·nu·di operation (lăm′brə-noo′dē) *n.* A triple arthrodesis done to prevent foot drop.

LAMB syndrome (lăm) *n.* A syndrome of dermatological disorders characterized by the appearance of lentigines, atrial and mucocutaneous myxomas, and blue nevi. Also called *NAME syndrome.*

lame (lām) *adj.* **1.** Disabled so that movement, especially walking, is difficult or impossible. **2.** Marked by pain or rigidity. —*v.* To cause to become lame; cripple.

la·mel·la (lə-mĕl′ə) *n.*, *pl.* **–mel·las** *or* **–mel·lae** (-mĕl′-ē′) **1.** A thin scale, plate, or layer of bone or tissue, as around the minute vascular canals in bone. **2.** A medicated gelatin disk, used instead of a solution for application to the conjunctiva. Also called *disk.* —**la·mel′lar** *adj.*

lamellar bone *n.* A bone in which the tubular lamellae are formed, which are characterized by parallel spirally arranged collagen fibers.

lamellar cataract *n.* A congenital cataract in which opacity is limited to layers of the lens external to the nucleus. Also called *zonular cataract.*

lamellar ichthyosis *n.* An inherited form of ichthyosis that is present at birth and is characterized by large, coarse scales over most of the body and thickened palms and soles; it is associated with ectropion.

la·mel·late (lə-mĕl′āt′, lăm′ə-lāt′) *adj.* **1.** Having, composed of, or arranged in lamellae. **2.** Resembling a lamella. —**lam′el·la·ted** *adj.* —**lam′el·la′tion** *n.*

lamellated corpuscle *n.* Any of numerous small oval bodies that are sensitive to pressure, are found in the skin of the fingers and elsewhere, are formed of concentric layers of connective tissue. Also called *pacinian corpuscle.*

la·mel·li·po·di·um (lə-mĕl′ə-pō′dē-əm) *n.*, *pl.* **-di·a** (-dē-ə) A sheetlike cytoplasmic extension produced by migrating polymorphonuclear white blood cells that permits movement along a substrate.

lam·i·na (lăm′ə-nə) *n.*, *pl.* **–nas** *or* **–nae** (-nē′) **1.** A thin plate, sheet, or layer. **2.** A thin layer of bone, membrane, or other tissue. —**lam′i·nar, lam′i·nal** *adj.*

lamina fus·ca scle·rae (fŭs′kə sklîr′ē) *n.* A thin layer of pigmented connective tissue on the inner surface of the sclera of the eye, connecting it with the choroid.

lam·i·na·gram (lăm′ə-nə-grăm′) *n.* A film taken by a laminagraph.

lam·i·na·graph (lăm′ə-nə-grăf′) *n.* An x-ray machine that uses a technique in which tissues above and below the level of a suspected lesion are blurred out to emphasize a specific area.

lam·i·nag·ra·phy (lăm′ə-năg′rə-fē) *n.* See **tomography.**

lamina of lens *n.* One of a series of concentric layers composed of the lens fibers that make up the substance of the lens of the eye.

lamina of vertebral arch *n.* The flattened posterior portion of the vertebral arch from which the spinous process extends. Also called *neurapophysis.*

lamina pro·pri·a mu·co·sae (prō′prē-ə myoo-kō′sē) *n.* The layer of connective tissue underlying the epithelium of a mucous membrane.

lam·i·nar·i·a (lăm′ə-nâr′ē-ə) *n.* Any of a genus of kelp applied to the cervical os to stimulate dilation.

lamina tec·ti mes·en·ceph·a·li (tĕk′tī mĕs′ĕn-sĕf′ə-lī′) *n.* The roofplate of the mesencephalon formed by the quadrigeminal bodies. Also called *tectum mesencephali.*

lam·i·nat·ed clot (lăm′ə-nā′tĭd) *n.* A clot formed in a succession of layers, as occurs in the natural course of an aneurysm.

laminated epithelium *n.* See **stratified epithelium.**

lam·i·nec·to·my (lăm′ə-nĕk′tə-mē) *n.* Excision of a vertebral lamina. Also called *rachiotomy.*

lam·i·ni·tis (lăm′ə-nī′tĭs) *n.* Inflammation of a lamina. Also called *founder.*

lam·i·not·o·my (lăm′ə-nŏt′ə-mē) *n.* Surgical division of one or more vertebral laminae.

la·miv·u·dine (lə-mĭv′yōō-dēn′) *n.* An antiretroviral drug that is a nucleoside analog and inhibits replication of HIV.

lamp (lămp) *n.* A device that generates light, heat, or therapeutic radiation.

la·nat·o·side (lə-nătʹə-sīd′) *n.* Any of three cardioactive glycosides, designated A, B, and C, that are obtained from the leaves of *Digitalis lanata.*

lance (lăns) *n.* See **lancet.** —*v.* To make an incision in, as with a lancet.

Lance·field classification (lăns′fēld′) *n.* A serologic classification of hemolytic streptococci, dividing them into groups A to O.

lan·cet (lăn′sĭt) *n.* A surgical knife with a short, wide, pointed double-edged blade, used especially for making punctures and small incisions. Also called *lance.*

lan·ci·nat·ing (lăn′sə-nā′tĭng) *adj.* Characterized by a sensation of cutting, piercing, or stabbing.

Lan·dau-Kleff·ner syndrome (lăn′dou-klĕf′nər) *n.* A syndrome occurring in children and characterized by generalized and psychomotor seizures, associated with acquired aphasia. Also called *acquired epileptic aphasia.*

Lan·dou·zy-Déjérine dystrophy (lăn-dōō′zē-, lăn-dōō-zē′-) *n.* See **facioscapulohumeral muscular dystrophy.**

Lan·dry-Guillain-Barré syndrome *n.* See **acute idiopathic polyneuritis.**

Lan·dry's paralysis (lăn′drēz, lăn-drēz′) *n.* See **acute ascending paralysis.**

Landry syndrome *n.* See **acute idiopathic polyneuritis.**

Land·ström's muscle (lănd′strœmz′) *n.* Microscopic muscle fibers that are attached to the eyelids and to the anterior orbital fascia, and that draw the eyeball forward and the lids backward.

Lang·en·beck's triangle (lăng′ən-bĕks′, läng′-) *n.* A triangle formed by lines drawn from the superior iliac spine to the surface of the great trochanter and to the neck of the femur.

Lang·er·hans (läng′ər-häns′), **Paul** 1847–1888. German pathologist known especially for his histological studies of the skin and pancreas. The islets of Langerhans are named for him.

Langerhans cell *n.* **1.** Any of the dendritic cells of the interstitial spaces of the mammalian epidermis that appear rod- or racket-shaped and are similar to melanocytes but cannot oxidize phenols. **2.** See **centroacinar cell.**

Langerhans granule *n.* A membrane-bound granule that exhibits a characteristic platelike arrangement of particles.

lan·o·lin (lăn′ə-lĭn) *n.* A fatty substance obtained from wool and used in soaps, cosmetics, and ointments.

La·nox·in (lə-nŏk′sĭn) A trademark for the drug digoxin.

lan·so·pra·zole (lăn-sō′prə-zōl′) *n.* A drug of the proton pump inhibitor class.

Lan·ter·man's incisure (län′tər-mänz′) *n.* See **Schmidt-Lanterman incisure.**

lan·tern jaw (lăn′tərn) *n.* **1.** A lower jaw that protrudes beyond the upper jaw. **2.** A long, thin jaw that gives the face a gaunt appearance.

lan·tha·nide (lăn′thə-nīd′) *n.* Any of the chemically related elements with atomic numbers 57 through 71. Also called *rare earth, rare-earth element.*

lan·tha·num (lăn′thə-nəm) *n. Symbol* **La** A soft malleable metallic rare-earth element used in glass manufacture. Atomic number 57.

la·nu·gi·nous (lə-nōō′jə-nəs) *or* **la·nu·gi·nose** (-nōs′) *adj.* Being covered with soft, short hair; downy.

la·nu·go (lə-nōō′gō,) *n., pl.* **–gos** The fine, soft hair that grows on a fetus and is present on a newborn. Also called *lanugo hair.*

laparo– *pref.* **1.** Loin: *laparotomy.* **2.** Abdomen: *laparocele.*

lap·a·ro·cele (lăp′ə-rə-sēl′) *n.* See **abdominal hernia.**

lap·a·ror·rha·phy (lăp′ə-rôr′ə-fē) *n.* See **celiorrhaphy.**

lap·a·ro·scope (lăp′ər-ə-skōp′) *n.* A slender, tubular endoscope that is inserted through an incision in the abdominal wall to examine or perform minor surgery within the abdominal or pelvic cavities. Also called *peritoneoscope.*

lap·a·ros·co·py (lăp′ə-rŏs′kə-pē) *n.* **1.** Examination of the interior of the abdomen by a laparoscope. **2.** A surgical procedure using laparoscopy.

lap·a·rot·o·my (lăp′ə-rŏt′ə-mē) *n.* **1.** Surgical incision into the abdominal cavity through the loin or flank. **2.** See **celiotomy.**

laparotomy pad *n.* A pad made from several layers of gauze folded into a rectangular shape and used especially as a sponge for packing off the viscera in abdominal operations. Also called *abdominal pad.*

lap·i·ni·za·tion (lăp′ə-nĭ-zā′shən) *n.* The weakening of a vaccine by passage through a series of rabbits. —**lap′i·nize′** (-nīz′) *v.*

large bowel (lärj) *n.* See **large intestine.**

large calorie *n. Abbr.* **C, Cal** See **calorie** (sense 2).

large cell carcinoma *n.* A bronchogenic carcinoma composed of large undifferentiated cells.

large cell lymphoma *n.* Lymphoma composed of large mononuclear cells of undetermined type.

large intestine *n.* The portion of the intestine that extends from the ileum to the anus, forming an arch around the convolutions of the small intestine and including the cecum, colon, rectum, and anal canal. Also called *large bowel.*

large muscle of helix *n.* A narrow band of muscular fibers on the anterior border of the helix arising from the spine and inserted at the point where the helix becomes transverse.

large pelvis *n.* An expanded portion of pelvis above the brim. Also called *false pelvis, pelvis major.*

large pudendal lips *pl.n.* The labia majora.

Lar·i·am (lâr′ē-əm) A trademark for the drug mefloquine.

La·ron type dwarfism (lä-rŏn′) *n.* Dwarfism in which somatomedin is absent and somatotropin plasma levels are high.

Lar·rey's amputation (lə-rāz′) *n.* Amputation of the arm at the shoulder joint.

lar·va (lär′və) *n., pl.* **-vas** *or* **-vae** (-vē) **1.** The newly hatched, wingless, often wormlike form of many insects before metamorphosis. **2.** The newly hatched, earliest stage of any of various animals that undergo metamorphosis, differing markedly in form and appearance from the adult. —**lar′val** *adj.*

larva cur·rens (kûr′ənz) *n.* Creeping eruption caused by rapidly moving larvae of *Strongyloides stercoralis*, typically extending from the anal area down the upper thighs.

larva mi·grans (mī′grănz′) *n., pl.* **larvae mi·gran·tes** (mī-grăn′tēz′) A larval worm, typically a nematode, that wanders in the host tissues but does not develop to the adult stage.

lar·vate (lär′vāt′) *adj.* Being masked or concealed, as a of a disease that has undeveloped, absent, or atypical symptoms.

lar·vi·cide (lär′vĭ-sīd′) *n.* An agent that kills insect larvae. —**lar′vi·cid′al** (-sīd′l) *adj.*

laryng– *pref.* Variant of **laryngo–**.

la·ryn·geal (lə-rĭn′jəl, lăr′ən-jē′əl) *or* **la·ryn·gal** (lə-rĭng′gəl) *adj.* Of, relating to, affecting, or near the larynx.

laryngeal artery *n.* **1.** An artery with origin in the inferior thyroid artery, with distribution to the muscles and mucous membrane of the larynx, and with anastomosis to the superior laryngeal artery; inferior laryngeal artery. **2.** An artery with origin in the superior thyroid artery, with distribution to the muscles and mucous membrane of the larynx, and with anastomoses to a branch of the superior thyroid artery and the terminal branches of the inferior laryngeal artery; superior laryngeal artery.

laryngeal papillomatosis *n.* A condition characterized by multiple squamous cell papillomas of the larynx, seen most commonly in young children, usually due to infection by the human papilloma virus transmitted at birth from the maternal genital warts.

laryngeal prominence *n.* See **Adam's apple**.

laryngeal stenosis *n.* A narrowing or a stricture of the larynx.

laryngeal syncope *n.* A psychiatric condition characterized by unusual sensations in the throat and by attacks of coughing that are followed by a brief period of unconsciousness.

lar·yn·gec·to·my (lăr′ən-jĕk′tə-mē) *n.* Surgical removal of part or all of the larynx.

lar·yn·gem·phrax·is (lăr′ĭn-jĕm-frăk′sĭs) *n.* Obstruction or closure of the larynx.

lar·yn·gis·mus (lăr′ĭn-jĭz′məs) *n.* Spasmodic narrowing or closure of the rima glottidis.

laryngismus stri·du·lus (strī′jə-ləs, strĭj′ə-) *n.* A spasmodic closure of the glottis that lasts a few seconds and is followed by noisy inspiration. Also called *pseudocroup*.

lar·yn·gi·tis (lăr′ĭn-jī′tĭs) *n.* Inflammation of the larynx. —**lar′yn·git′ic** (-jĭt′ĭk) *adj.*

laryngitis stri·du·lo·sa (strī′jə-lō′sə, strĭj′ə-) *n.* A catarrhal inflammation of the larynx in children, marked by night attacks of laryngismus stridulus.

laryngo– *or* **laryng–** *pref.* Larynx: *laryngoscope.*

la·ryn·go·cele (lə-rĭng′gə-sēl′) *n.* An air sac connected to the larynx through the ventricle, often bulging outward into the tissue of the neck, especially during coughing.

la·ryn·go·fis·sure (lə-rĭng′gō-fĭsh′ər) *n.* Surgical opening of the larynx that is usually made through the midline of the thyroid cartilage. Also called *laryngotomy, thyrotomy.*

lar·yn·gol·o·gy (lăr′ĭn-gŏl′ə-jē) *n.* The branch of medicine dealing with the study and treatment of disorders of the larynx, pharynx, and fauces. —**lar′yn·gol′o·gist** *n.*

la·ryn·go·pa·ral·y·sis (lə-rĭng′gō-pə-răl′ĭ-sĭs) *n.* Paralysis of the laryngeal muscles. Also called *laryngoplegia.*

lar·yn·gop·a·thy (lăr′ĭn-gŏp′ə-thē) *n.* A disease of the larynx.

la·ryn·go·pha·ryn·geal (lə-rĭng′gō-fə-rĭn′jəl, -făr′ĭn-jē′əl) *adj.* **1.** Relating to the larynx and the pharynx. **2.** Relating to the laryngopharynx.

la·ryn·go·phar·yn·gec·to·my (lə-rĭng′gō-făr′ĭn-jĕk′tə-mē) *n.* Surgical resection or excision of the larynx and the pharynx.

la·ryn·go·phar·yn·gi·tis (lə-rĭng′gō-făr′ĭn-jī′tĭs) *n.* Inflammation of the larynx and the pharynx.

la·ryn·go·phar·ynx (lə-rĭng′gō-făr′ĭngks) *n.* The part of the pharynx that lies below the aperture of the larynx and behind the larynx and that extends to the esophagus. Also called *hypopharynx.*

lar·yn·goph·o·ny (lăr′ĭn-gŏf′ə-nē) *n.* The voice sounds heard in auscultation of the larynx.

la·ryn·go·plas·ty (lə-rĭng′gə-plăs′tē) *n.* Reparative or plastic surgery of the larynx.

la·ryn·go·ple·gia (lə-rĭng′gō-plē′jə) *n.* See **laryngoparalysis**.

la·ryn·go·pto·sis (lə-rĭng′gō-tō′sĭs) *n.* An abnormally low position of the larynx.

la·ryn·go·rhi·nol·o·gy (lə-rĭng′gō-rī-nŏl′ə-jē) *n.* The branch of medical science that deals with the larynx and the nose.

la·ryn·go·scope (lə-rĭng′gə-skōp′, -rĭn′jə-) *n.* A tubular endoscope that is inserted through the mouth and into the larynx and that is used for examining the interior of the larynx. —**la·ryn′go·scop′ic** (-skŏp′ĭk), **la·ryn′go·scop′i·cal** *adj.*

lar·yn·gos·co·py (lăr′ĭn-gŏs′kə-pē) *n.* Examination of the larynx by means of a laryngoscope.

la·ryn·go·spasm (lə-rĭng′gə-spăz′əm) *n.* Spasmodic closure of the larynx.

la·ryn·go·ste·no·sis (lə-rĭng′gō-stə-nō′sĭs) *n.* Stricture or narrowing of the larynx.

lar·yn·gos·to·my (lăr′ĭn-gŏs′tə-mē) *n.* Surgical creation of a permanent opening into the larynx.

lar·yn·got·o·my (lăr′ĭn-gŏt′ə-mē) *n.* See **laryngofissure**.

la·ryn·go·tra·che·al (lə-rĭng′gō-trā′kē-əl) *adj.* Relating to the larynx and the trachea.

la·ryn·go·tra·che·i·tis (lə-rĭng′gō-trā′kē-ī′tĭs) *n.* Inflammation of the larynx and the trachea.

la·ryn·go·tra·che·o·bron·chi·tis (lə-rĭng′gō-trā′kē-ō-brŏn-kī′tĭs, -brŏng-) *n.* An acute respiratory infection involving the larynx, trachea, and bronchi. Also called *croup.*

la·ryn·go·tra·che·ot·o·my (lə-rĭng′gō-trā′kē-ŏt′ə-mē) *n.* Incision of the larynx and trachea.

la·ryn·go·xe·ro·sis (lə-rĭng′gō-zĭ-rō′sĭs) *n.* Abnormal dryness of the laryngeal mucous membrane.

lar·ynx (lăr′ĭngks) *n.,* *pl.* **lar·ynx·es** *or* **la·ryn·ges** (lə-rĭn′jēz) The part of the respiratory tract between the pharynx and the trachea, having walls of cartilage and muscle and containing the vocal cords enveloped in folds of mucous membrane.

La·sègue's sign (lə-sĕgz′, lä-) *n.* An indication of lumbar root or sciatic nerve irritation in which dorsiflexion of the ankle of an individual lying supine with the hip flexed causes pain or muscle spasm in the posterior thigh.

lase (lāz) *v.* To cut, divide, or dissolve a substance with a laser.

la·ser (lā′zər) *n.* Any of several devices that convert incident electromagnetic radiation of mixed frequencies to discrete frequencies of highly amplified and coherent ultraviolet, visible, or infrared radiation; used in surgery to cut and dissolve tissue.

laser-assisted in situ keratomileusis *n.* LASIK.

Lash·ley (lăsh′lē), **Karl Spencer** 1890–1958. American neuropsychologist known for his contributions to the study of localization of brain functions.

LA·SIK (lā′zĭk) *n.* Eye surgery in which the surface of the cornea is reshaped using a laser, performed to correct certain refractive disorders such as myopia.

La·six (lā′sĭks) A trademark for the drug furosemide.

Las·sa fever (lä′sə) *n.* A highly fatal form of epidemic hemorrhagic fever caused by Lassa virus and marked by high fever, sore throat, severe muscle aches, skin rash with hemorrhages, headache, abdominal pain, vomiting, and diarrhea. Also called *Lassa hemorrhagic fever.*

Lassa virus *n.* A virus of the genus *Arenavirus* that causes Lassa fever.

las·si·tude (lăs′ĭ-tōōd′) *n.* A state or feeling of weariness, diminished energy, or listlessness.

la·tah (lä′tə) *n.* A nervous disorder characterized by an exaggerated physical response to being startled or to unexpected suggestion.

la·ten·cy (lāt′n-sē) *n.* 1. The state of being latent. 2. In conditioning, the period of apparent inactivity between the time the stimulus is presented and the moment a response occurs. 3. See **latency period.**

latency period *n.* In psychoanalytic theory, the fourth stage of psychosexual development, extending from about age 5 to puberty, when a child apparently represses sexual urges and prefers to associate with members of the same sex. It is preceded by the phallic stage and followed by the genital stage. Also called *latency, latency period.*

la·tent (lāt′nt) *adj.* 1. Present or potential but not evident or active. 2. In a dormant or hidden stage, as an infection. 3. Undeveloped but capable of normal growth under the proper conditions. 4. Present in the unconscious mind but not consciously expressed.

latent allergy *n.* Hypersensitivity that causes no signs or symptoms but can be detected through immunological testing.

latent content *n.* The hidden meaning of a dream, fantasy, or thought that can be revealed through interpretation of its images or through free association in psychoanalysis.

latent diabetes *n.* A mild form of diabetes mellitus in which the individual displays no overt symptoms, but has abnormal responses to various diagnostic tests. Also called *chemical diabetes.*

latent gout *n.* The presence of abnormally large amounts of uric acid in the blood without the symptoms of gout. Also called *masked gout.*

latent homosexuality *n.* A sexual tendency toward members of the same sex that is not consciously recognized or not expressed overtly.

latent hyperopia *n.* *Abbr.* **Hl** Hyperopia that can be overcome by accommodation and can only be revealed by administration of a mydriatic drug.

latent learning *n.* Learning that is not the result of determined effort and is not evident at the time it occurs, but remains latent until a need for it arises.

latent nystagmus *n.* A jerky nystagmus that is brought out by covering one eye.

latent period *n.* 1. The period elapsing between the application of a stimulus and the obvious response, such as the contraction of a muscle. 2. The interval between exposure to an infectious organism or a carcinogen and the clinical appearance of disease. Also called *incubation period.*

latent reflex *n.* A reflex considered as normal but which usually appears only under a pathological condition that makes its manifestation more likely.

latent schizophrenia *n.* A condition characterized by symptoms of schizophrenia but lacking a psychotic schizophrenic episode.

latent stage *n.* See **incubative stage.**

latent tetany *n.* Tetany manifested only when certain diagnostic procedures are used.

late-onset diabetes *n.* See **diabetes mellitus** (sense 2).

lat·er·ad (lăt′ə-răd′) *adv.* Toward the side.

lat·er·al (lăt′ər-əl) *adj.* 1. Relating to or situated at or on the side. 2. Situated or extending away from the median plane of the body. 3. Relating to the left or right lateral region of the abdomen. —*n.* A lateral part, position, or appendage. —**lat′er·al·ly** *adv.*

lateral aberration *n.* The distance between the paraxial focus of central rays on the optic axis in spherical aberration.

lateral ampullar nerve *n.* A branch of the utriculoampullar nerve that supplies the ampullary crest of the lateral semicircular duct of the ear.

lateral cartilage of nose *n.* The cartilage located in the lateral wall of the nose above the alar cartilage.

lateral cerebral sulcus *n.* See **fissure of Sylvius.**

lateral column of spinal cord *n.* A slight protrusion of the gray matter of the spinal cord into the lateral funiculus of either side, especially in the thoracic region where it encloses preganglionic motor neurons of the sympathetic division of the autonomic nervous system.

lateral cord of brachial plexus *n.* A fasciculus formed by the anterior divisions of the superior and middle trunks, giving rise to the lateral pectoral nerve and terminating by dividing into the musculocutaneous nerve and the lateral root of the median nerve.

lateral cuneiform bone *n.* A tarsal bone, articulating with the intermediate cuneiform, cuboid, and navicular bones and the second, third, and fourth metatarsal bones. Also called *third cuneiform bone.*

lateral cutaneous nerve of calf *n.* A nerve that arises from the common peroneal nerve and is distributed to the skin of the calf.

lateral cutaneous nerve of forearm *n.* A terminal cutaneous branch of the musculocutaneous nerve that supplies the skin of the radial side of the forearm.

lateral cutaneous nerve of thigh *n.* A nerve that arises from the second and third lumbar nerves and supplies the skin of the anterolateral and lateral surfaces of the thigh.

lateral fold *n.* Any of the ventral foldings of the lateral margins of the embryonic disk that establish the definitive embryonic body form.

lateral funiculus *n.* The lateral white column of the spinal cord between the points of exit and entry of the anterior and posterior nerve roots.

lateral geniculate body *n.* The lateral mass of a pair of small oval masses that protrude slightly from the posteroinferior aspects of the thalamus, serving as a processing station in the major pathway from the retina to the cerebral cortex.

lateral hemianopsia *n.* See **homonymous hemianopsia.**

lateral hermaphroditism *n.* Hermaphroditism in which a testis is present on one side of the body and an ovary on the other.

lateral humeral epicondylitis *n.* See **tennis elbow.**

lat·er·al·i·ty (lăt′ə-răl′ĭ-tē) *n.* Preferential use of limbs of one side of the body.

lat·er·al·i·za·tion (lăt′ər-ə-lĭ-zā′shən) *n.* Localization of function attributed to either the right or left side of the brain.

lateral longitudinal stria *n.* A thin longitudinal band of nerve fibers accompanied by gray matter located near each outer edge of the upper surface of the corpus callosum under the cingulate gyrus.

lateral nystagmus *n.* A nystagmus in which the eyes oscillate from side to side.

lateral plane *n.* An Addison's clinical plane passing vertically on either side through a point on the interspinal halfway between the anterior portion of the iliac crest and the median plane.

lateral plantar nerve *n.* One of the two terminal branches of the tibial nerve, dividing into superficial and deep branches, supplying the skin of the lateral aspect of the sole and certain toes, and innervating certain muscles of the plantar part of the foot.

lateral plate *n.* One of two nonsegmented masses of mesoderm on either side of the embryonic disk.

lateral pterygoid muscle *n.* A muscle whose inferior head has origin from the pterygoid process, and whose superior head has origin from the sphenoid bone, with insertion into the mandible and the articular disk, with nerve supply from the lateral pterygoid branch of the trigeminal nerve, and whose action brings the jaw forward and opens it.

lateral rectus muscle *n.* A muscle with origin from the lateral part of the tendinous ring bridging the superior orbital fissure, with insertion into the sclera of the eye, with nerve supply from the abducens nerve, and whose action directs the pupil laterally. See **rectus lateralis.**

lateral rectus muscle of head *n.* A muscle with origin from the transverse process of the atlas, with insertion into the occipital bone, with nerve supply from the first cervical nerve, and whose action inclines the head to one side.

lateral recumbent position *n.* See **Sims' position.**

lateral region *n.* The region of the abdomen lying on either side of the umbilical region and between the hypochondriac and inguinal regions.

lateral sacral vein *n.* Any of the veins that accompany the lateral sacral artery and empty into the internal iliac vein on either side.

lateral spinal sclerosis *n.* An amyotrophic lateral sclerosis in which degeneration of the lateral tracts of the spinal cord causes spastic paraplegia.

lateral supraclavicular nerve *n.* Any of the several branches of the cervical plexus that descend to the skin over the acromion and deltoid region. Also called *posterior supraclavicular nerve.*

lateral thalamic peduncle *n.* The massive group of fibers that emerges from the laterodorsal side of the thalamus to join the radiate crown.

lateral thoracic vein *n.* A tributary of the axillary vein, draining the lateral thoracic wall and communicating with the thoracoepigastric and intercostal veins.

lateral ventricle *n.* A horseshoe-shaped cavity conforming to the general shape of each cerebral hemisphere and communicating with the third ventricle.

late rickets (lāt) *n.* See **osteomalacia.**

latero– *pref.* Side; lateral: *lateroversion.*

lat·er·o·de·vi·a·tion (lăt′ə-rō-dē′vē-ā′shən) *n.* A bending or a displacement to one side.

lat·er·o·duc·tion (lăt′ə-rō-dŭk′shən) *n.* Movement to one side, as of an eye.

lat·er·o·flex·ion (lăt′ə-rō-flĕk′shən) *n.* A bending or curvature to one side.

lat·er·o·tor·sion (lăt′ə-rō-tôr′shən) *n.* A twisting to one side, especially the turning of the eyeball to the left or right on its anteroposterior axis.

lat·er·o·tru·sion (lăt′ə-rō-trōō′zhən) *n.* The outward thrust given by the muscles of chewing to the condyle during movement of the mandible.

lat·er·o·ver·sion (lăt′ə-rō-vûr′zhən) *n.* A turning to one side, as of the uterus.

late systole *n.* See **prediastole.**

late-term *adj.* Occurring or performed after the twentieth week of gestation in humans.

la·tex (lā′tĕks′) *n.* **1.** The colorless or milky sap of certain plants, such as the poinsettia, that coagulates on exposure to air. **2.** An emulsion of rubber or plastic globules in water, used in adhesives and synthetic rubber products. —**la′tex′** *adj.*

latex agglutination test *n.* A passive agglutination test in which antigen is adsorbed onto latex particles.

lath·y·rism (lăth′ə-rĭz′əm) *n.* A disease of humans and animals caused by eating legumes of the genus *Lathyrus* and characterized by spastic paralysis, hyperesthesia, and paresthesia.

la·tis·si·mus dor·si (lă-tĭs′ə-məs dôr′sī) *n.* A muscle with origin from the spinous processes of the lower thoracic and lumbar vertebrae, the median ridge of the sacrum, and the outer lip of the iliac crest, with insertion into the humerus, with nerve supply from the thoracodorsal nerve, and whose action adducts the arm, rotates it medially, and extends it.

Lat·ro·dec·tus (lăt′rə-děk′təs) *n.* A genus of small spiders, including the black widow, capable of inflicting highly poisonous, neurotoxic bites.

LATS *abbr.* long-acting thyroid stimulator

la·tus (lā′təs, lăt′əs) *n., pl.* **lat·er·a** (lăt′ər-ə) Flank.

laud·a·ble (lô′də-bəl) *adj.* Healthy; favorable.

lau·da·num (lôd′n-əm) *n.* A tincture of opium, formerly used as a drug.

laugh·ing gas (lăf′ĭng) *n.* Nitrous oxide, especially as used as an anesthetic.

Lau·rence-Moon-Bardet-Biedl syndrome (lôr′əns-mōōn′-) *n.* A combination of the Laurence-Moon syndrome and the Bardet-Biedl syndrome.

Laurence-Moon syndrome *n.* An inherited syndrome attributed to recessive mutations of two genes on the same chromosome and characterized by mental retardation, pigmentary retinopathy, hypogenitalism, and spastic paraplegia.

lau·ric acid (lôr′ĭk) *n.* A fatty acid occurring in laurel, coconut, and palm oils.

lau·ryl alcohol (lôr′əl) *n.* A colorless solid alcohol used in synthetic detergents and pharmaceuticals.

lav·age (lăv′ĭj, lä-väzh′) *n.* A washing, especially of a hollow organ such as the stomach or lower bowel, with repeated injections of water.

La·ve·ran (lăv′ə-răɴ′, läv-räɴ′), **Charles Louis Alphonse** 1845–1922. French pathologist. He won a 1907 Nobel Prize for investigating the role of protozoa in the generation of disease.

law (lô) *n.* **1.** A rule of conduct or procedure established by custom, agreement, or authority. **2.** A set of rules or principles for a specific area of a legal system. **3.** A piece of enacted legislation. **4.** A formulation describing a relationship observed to be invariable between or among phenomena for all cases in which the specified conditions are met. **5.** A generalization based on consistent experience or results.

law of contiguity *n.* The principle that when two ideas or psychologically perceived events have once occurred in close association, they are likely to occur in close association again, the subsequent occurrence of one tending to elicit the other.

law of excitation *n.* The principle that a motor nerve responds to the alteration of value of an electric current from moment to moment.

law of independent assortment *n.* See Mendel's law (sense 2).

law of inverse square *n.* The principle that the intensity of radiation is inversely proportional to the square of the distance from the source of radiation to the irradiated surface.

law of large numbers *n.* The rule or theorem that a large number of items chosen at random from a population will, on the average, have the characteristics of the population. Also called *Bernoulli's law.*

law of partial pressures *n.* See Dalton's law.

law of recapitulation *n.* See biogenetic law.

law of referred pain *n.* The principle that pain arises only from irritation of nerves that are sensitive to painful stimuli applied to the surface of the body.

law of segregation *n.* See Mendel's law (sense 1).

law of similars *n.* A principle of homeopathic medicine stating that a drug capable of producing morbid symptoms in a healthy person will cure similar symptoms occurring as a manifestation of disease.

law of heart *n.* The principle that the energy released by the heart when it contracts is a function of the length of its muscle fibers at the end of diastole. Also called *Starling's law.*

law·ren·ci·um (lô-rĕn′sē-əm, lō-) *n. Symbol* **Lr** A radioactive synthetic element produced from californium and having isotopes with mass numbers 253 through 260 and half-lives of 650 milliseconds to 3 minutes; atomic number 103.

lax·a·tive (lăk′sə-tĭv) *n.* A food or drug that stimulates evacuation of the bowels. —*adj.* Stimulating evacuation of the bowels.

lay·er (lā′ər) *n.* A single thickness of a material covering a surface or forming an overlying part or segment. —*v.* To divide or form into layers.

layer of rods and cones *n.* The retinal layer containing visual receptors. Also called *bacillary layer.*

la·zy eye (lā′zē) *n.* See amblyopia.

LBBB *abbr.* left bundle branch block

LBT *abbr.* lupus band test

LCAT *abbr.* lecithin cholesterol acyltransferase

LCAT deficiency *n.* A rare inherited condition due to very low lecithin cholesterol acyltransferase activity, characterized by corneal opacities, anemia, proteinuria, and the accumulation of unesterfied cholesterol in plasma and tissues.

LD *abbr.* lethal dose; learning disability

LDH *abbr.* lactate dehydrogenase

LDL *abbr.* low-density lipoprotein

LDL cholesterol *n.* See low-density lipoprotein.

L-do·pa (ĕl′dō′pə) *n.* The levorotatory form of dopa, used to treat Parkinson's disease. Also called *levodopa.*

L dose *n.* Any of a group of terms indicating the relative activity, potency, or combining effect of the diphtheria toxin with an antitoxin.

LE *abbr.* lower extremity; lupus erythematosus

leach·ing (lē′chĭng) *n.* See lixiviation. —**leach** *v.*

lead¹ (lēd) *n.* **1.** Any of the conductors designed to detect changes in electrical potential when situated in or on the body and connected to an instrument that registers and records these changes, such as an electrocardiograph. **2.** A record made from the current supplied by one of these conductors.

lead² (lĕd) *n. Symbol* **Pb** A soft ductile dense metallic element. Atomic number 82.

lead encephalopathy (lĕd) *n.* A rapidly developing encephalopathy caused by the ingestion of lead compounds and seen particularly in early childhood, marked by convulsion, delirium, hallucination, and other cerebral symptoms related to chronic lead poisoning. Also called *lead encephalitis.*

lead line (lĕd) *n.* An irregular dark deposit in the gums occurring in lead poisoning.

lead poisoning (lĕd) *n.* Acute or chronic poisoning by lead or any of its salts, with the acute form marked by gastroenteritis and encephalopathy and the chronic form characterized by anemia and damage to the gastrointestinal tract and nervous system. Also called *saturnism*.

Lear complex (lîr) *n*. In psychoanalytic theory, a father's libidinous fixation on a daughter.

learned drive (lûrnd) *n*. See **motive**.

learned helplessness *n*. A laboratory model of depression in which exposure to a series of unforeseen adverse situations gives rise to a sense of helplessness or an inability to cope with or devise ways to escape such situations, even when escape is possible.

learn·ing (lûr′nĭng) *n*. **1.** The act, process, or experience of gaining knowledge or skill. **2.** Knowledge or skill gained through schooling or study. **3.** Behavioral modification, especially through experience or conditioning.

learning disability *n*. *Abbr.* **LD** A disorder in the basic cognitive and psychological processes involved in using language or performing mathematical calculations, affecting persons of normal intelligence, and not the result of emotional disturbance or impairment of sight or hearing. Also called *learning disorder*. —**learn′ing-dis·a′bled** *adj*.

leath·er-bot·tle stomach (lĕth′ər-bŏt′l) *n*. Marked thickening and rigidity of the stomach wall, with reduced capacity of the lumen.

Le·ber's hereditary optic atrophy (lā′bərz) *n*. The degeneration of the optic nerve and papillomacular bundle with resulting rapid loss of central vision, occurring most often in males.

Le·boy·er (lə-bwä-yā′), **Frederick** Born 1918. French obstetrician who developed a radical method of childbirth called "painless birth," based on his idea that newborns have the ability to experience a full range of emotions.

LE cell *abbr.* lupus erythematosus cell

LE cell test (ĕl′ē′) *n*. See **lupus erythematosus cell test**.

lec·i·thal (lĕs′ə-thəl) *adj*. Relating to or having a yolk.

lec·i·thin (lĕs′ə-thĭn) *n*. Any of a group of phospholipids that on hydrolysis yield two fatty acid molecules and a molecule each of glycerophosphoric acid and choline. They are found in nervous tissue, especially myelin sheaths and egg yolk, and in the plasma membrane of plant and animal cells.

lec·i·thin·ase (lĕs′ə-thə-nās′, -nāz′) *n*. See **phospholipase**.

lecithin-sphingomyelin ratio *n*. The ratio of lecithin to sphingomyelin present in amniotic fluid, used to determine fetal pulmonary maturity.

lec·i·tho·blast (lĕs′ə-thō-blăst′) *n*. One of the cells proliferating to form the yolk-sac entoderm.

lec·tin (lĕk′tĭn) *n*. Any of several plant glycoproteins that bind to specific carbohydrate groups on the cell membranes, used in the laboratory to stimulate proliferation of lymphocytes and to agglutinate red blood cells.

Led·er·berg (lĕd′ər-bûrg′, lā′dər-), **Joshua** Born 1925. American geneticist. He shared a 1958 Nobel Prize for work with genetic mechanisms.

leech (lēch) *n*. Any of various chiefly aquatic bloodsucking or carnivorous annelid worms of the class Hirudinea, one species of which (*Hirudo medicinalis*) was formerly used by physicians to bleed patients. —*v*. To bleed with leeches.

Leeu·wen·hoek or **Leu·wen·hoek** (lā′vən-hook′, lā′ü-wən-hook′) **Anton van** 1632–1723. Dutch naturalist and microscopy pioneer. His careful observations resulted in accurate descriptions of bacteria, spermatozoa, and red blood cells.

LE factor *n*. Any of the antinuclear immunoglobulins that are in the plasma of persons with disseminated lupus erythematosus.

Le·Fort I fracture (lə-fôr′) *n*. See **horizontal maxillary fracture**.

LeFort II fracture *n*. See **pyramidal fracture**.

LeFort III fracture *n*. See **craniofacial disjunction fracture**.

left atrioventricular valve (lĕft) *n*. See **mitral valve**.

left brachiocephalic vein *n*. A vein that receives the left vertebral, internal thoracic, superior intercostal, inferior thyroid, and other veins.

left brain *n*. The cerebral hemisphere to the left of the corpus callosum, controlling the right side of the body.

left-brained *adj*. **1.** Having the left brain dominant. **2.** Of or relating to the thought processes, such as logic and calculation, generally associated with the left brain. **3.** Of or relating to a person whose behavior is dominated by logic, analytical thinking, and verbal communication rather than emotion and creativity.

left colic flexure *n*. The bend at the junction of the transverse and the descending colon. Also called *splenic flexure*.

left colic vein *n*. A tributary of the inferior mesenteric vein, accompanying the left colic artery and draining the left flexure and the descending colon.

left-eyed *adj*. Tending to use the left eye instead of the right when doing work or using an instrument that permits the use of one eye only.

left-footed *adj*. Tending to use the left leg instead of the right.

left gastric vein *n*. A vein that arises from a union of veins from both surfaces of the gastric cardia and empties into the portal vein.

left gastro-omental vein *n*. A vein that runs along the greater curvature of the stomach and empties into the splenic vein. Also called *left gastroepiploic vein*.

left-handed *adj*. Using the left hand more skillfully or easily than the right.

left heart *n*. The left atrium and left ventricle.

left hepatic duct *n*. The duct that drains bile from the left half of the liver.

left lobe of liver *n*. The lobe of the liver separated from the right lobe above and in front by the falciform ligament, and separated from the quadrate and caudate lobes by the fissure for the round ligament and by the fissure for the venous ligament.

left lymphatic duct *n*. See **thoracic duct**.

left ovarian vein *n*. A vein that begins at the pampiniform plexus at the hilum of the ovary and empties into the left renal vein.

left suprarenal vein *n*. A vein that passes downward from the hilum of the left adrenal gland to open into the left renal vein.

left testicular vein *n*. A vein that originates from the pampiniform plexus and joins the left renal vein.

left-to-right shunt *n*. **1.** A diversion of blood from the left side of the heart to the right, as through a septal defect. **2.** A diversion of blood from the systemic circulation to the pulmonary circulation, as through a patent ductus arteriosus.

left umbilical vein *n.* A vein that returns blood from the placenta to the fetus, traversing the umbilical cord to pass into the liver, where it is joined by the portal vein.

left ventricle *n.* The chamber on the left side of the heart that receives the arterial blood from the left atrium and contracts to force it into the aorta.

left ventricular ejection time *n. Abbr.* **LVET** The time measured from onset to notch of the carotid pulse.

left ventricular failure *n.* Congestive heart failure marked by pulmonary congestion and edema.

left ventricular opening *n.* An opening that leads from the left atrium into the left ventricle of the heart. Also called *mitral orifice.*

leg (lĕg) *n.* **1.** One of the two lower limbs of the human body, especially the part between the knee and the foot. **2.** A supporting part resembling a leg in shape or function.

le·gal blindness (lē′gəl) *n.* Visual acuity of less than 6/60 or 20/200 using Snellen test types, or visual field restriction to 20 degrees or less.

legal dentistry *n.* See **forensic dentistry.**

legal medicine *n.* See **forensic medicine.**

Legg-Calvé-Perthes disease (lĕg′-) *n.* See **osteochondritis deformans juvenilis.**

Legg's disease *n.* See **osteochondritis deformans juvenilis.**

Legg-Perthes disease *n.* See **osteochondritis deformans juvenilis.**

Le·gion·el·la (lē′jə-nĕl′ə) *n.* A genus of gram-negative bacilli that includes the species that causes Legionnaires' disease.

Legionella boze·man·i·i (bōz-mǎn′ē-ī′) *n.* A bacillus of the genus *Legionella* that causes pneumonia in humans.

Legionella mic·da·de·i (mǐk-dā′dē-ī′) *n.* A gram-negative bacillus of the genus *Legionella* that causes Pittsburgh pneumonia.

Legionella pneu·mo·phil·i·a (nōō′mə-fǐl′ē-ə) *n.* A bacillus of the genus *Legionella* and the causative agent of Legionnaires' disease.

Le·gion·naires′ disease (lē′jə-nârz′) *n.* An acute, sometimes fatal respiratory disease caused by *Legionella pneumophila* and characterized by severe pneumonia, headache, and a dry cough. Also called *legionellosis.*

Lei·ner's disease (lī′nərz) *n.* See **erythroderma desquamativum.**

leio– *pref.* Smooth: *leiodermia.*

lei·o·der·mi·a (lī′ō-dûr′mē-ə) *n.* Smooth, glossy skin.

lei·o·my·o·fi·bro·ma (lī′ō-mī′ō-fī-brō′mə) *n.* See **fibroleiomyoma.**

lei·o·my·o·ma (lī′ō-mī-ō′mə) *n.* A benign tumor derived from smooth muscle, occurring most often in the uterus.

lei·o·my·o·sar·co·ma (lī′ō-mī′ō-sär-kō′mə) *n.* A malignant neoplasm derived from smooth muscle.

Leish·man-Donovan body (lēsh′mən-) *n.* An intracytoplasmic, nonflagellated, leishmanial form of certain intracellular flagellates. Also called *amastigote, Donovan body.*

Leish·man·i·a (lēsh-mǎn′ē-ə, -mā′nē-ə) *n.* A genus of flagellate protozoa, several species of which cause leishmanisis; all species are indistinguishable morphologically but may be separated by their serological reactions, by their geographic distribution, by their developmental patterns in their sandfly hosts, and by their clinical manifestations of leishmaniasis.

Leishmania ae·thi·o·pi·ca (ē′thē-ō′pǐ-kə) *n.* The protozoan that causes cutaneous leishmaniasis in Ethiopia and Kenya.

Leishmania bra·zil·i·en·sis (brə-zǐl′ē-ĕn′sǐs) *n.* The protozoan that includes subspecies that cause mucocutaneous leishmaniasis.

Leishmania don·o·van·i (dǒn′ə-vǎn′ī, -vā′nī) *n.* The protozoan that includes subspecies that cause visceral leishmaniasis.

Leishmania mex·i·ca·na (mĕk′sǐ-kā′nə) *n.* The protozoan that includes subspecies that cause cutaneous leishmaniasis and diffuse cutaneous leishmaniasis.

leish·man·i·a·sis (lēsh′mə-nī′ə-sǐs) *n.* **1.** An infection caused by the flagellated protozoa of the genus *Leishmania* transmitted to humans by bloodsucking sand flies. **2.** A disease, such as kala-azar caused by flagellated protozoa of the genus *Leishmania.*

leishmaniasis re·cid·i·vans (rǐ-sǐd′ə-vənz) *n.* A cutaneous leishmaniasis caused by *Leishmania tropica* and characterized by a partially healing lesion, intense granuloma production, and development of lesions that produce granulomatous tissue that does not heal sometimes for many years. Also called *lupoid leishmaniasis.*

leishmaniasis teg·u·men·tar·i·a dif·fu·sa (tĕg′yə-mən-târ′ē-ə dǐ-fyōō′sə) *n.* See **diffuse cutaneous leishmaniasis.**

Leishmania trop·i·ca (trǒp′ǐ-kə) *n.* The protozoan that includes subspecies that cause anthroponotic cutaneous leishmaniasis.

Le·jeune syndrome (lə-zhœn′) *n.* See **cri-du-chat syndrome.**

Le·loir (lə-lwär′, lĕ-), **Luis Federico** 1906–1987. French-born Argentine biochemist. He won a 1970 Nobel Prize for the discovery of sugar nucleotides and their role in the biosynthesis of carbohydrates.

Lem·bert suture (län-bĕr′) *n.* A continuous or interrupted suture for intestinal surgery that includes the collagenous submucosal layer but does not enter the lumen of the intestine.

lem·mo·blast (lĕm′ō-blăst′) *n.* A cell developing from the neural crest in an embryo, capable of forming a cell of the neurolemma sheath.

lem·mo·cyte (lĕm′ō-sīt′) *n.* Any of the cells that form the neurilemma.

lem·nis·cus (lĕm-nǐs′kəs) *n., pl.* **–nis·ci** (-nǐs′ī′, -nǐs′-kī′, -nǐs′kē) A bundle of nerve fibers ascending from sensory nuclei in the spinal cord and the rhombencephalon to the thalamus.

Le·nè·gre's syndrome (lə-nĕg′rəz) *n.* A condition in which damage of the cardiac conduction system occurs due to a sclerodegenerative lesion.

length (lĕngkth, lĕngth, lĕnth) *n.* The linear distance between two points.

len·i·tive (lĕn′ĭ-tĭv) *adj.* Capable of easing pain or discomfort. —*n.* A lenitive medicine.

Len·nox-Gas·taut syndrome (lĕn′əks-gă-stō′, -gä-) *n.* A generalized myoclonic astatic epilepsy that occurs in children as a result of various cerebral afflictions such as perinatal hypoxia, cerebral hemorrhage, encephalitis, and maldevelopment or metabolic disorders of the brain; it is characterized by mental retardation and generalized tonic seizures or akinetic attacks. Also called *Lennox syndrome.*

lens (lĕnz) *n., pl.* **lens·es 1.** A ground or molded piece of glass, plastic, or other transparent material with opposite surfaces either or both of which are curved, by means of which light rays are refracted so that they converge or diverge to form an image. **2.** A transparent, biconvex body of the eye between the iris and the vitreous humor that focuses light rays entering through the pupil to form an image on the retina. —**lensed** *adj.*

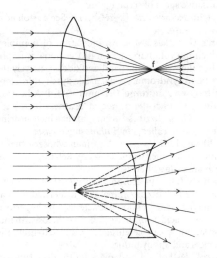

lens

Light passing through a double-convex lens (top) *and a double-concave lens. In each drawing,* f *indicates focus.*

lens·ec·to·my (lĕn-zĕk′tə-mē) *n.* Surgical removal of the lens, usually done by puncture incision through the ciliary disk during vitrectomy.

lens pit *n.* Either of a pair of depressions in the superficial ectoderm of the embryonic head where the lens develops.

lens stars *pl.n.* Congenital cataracts with opacities along the suture lines of the lens of the eye.

lens vesicle *n.* The ectodermal invagination in the embryo that forms opposite the optic cup and is the lens primordium. Also called *lenticular vesicle.*

len·ti·co·nus (lĕn′tĭ-kō′nəs) *n.* A conical projection of the anterior or posterior surface of the lens, occurring as a developmental anomaly.

len·tic·u·lar (lĕn-tĭk′yə-lər) *adj.* **1.** Of or relating to a lens. **2.** Shaped like a biconvex lens.

lenticular ansa *n.* The tortuous efferent pathway of the pallidum in the brain.

lenticular astigmatism *n.* Astigmatism due to a defect in the curvature, position, or index of refraction of the lens.

lenticular capsule *n.* The capsule enclosing the lens of the eye.

lenticular cataract *n.* A cataract in which the opacity is confined to the lens.

lenticular nucleus *n.* See **lentiform nucleus.**

lenticular process of incus *n.* A knob at the tip of the long limb of the incus of the ear, articulating with the stapes. Also called *orbiculare.*

lenticular vesicle *n.* See **lens vesicle.**

len·tic·u·lo·pap·u·lar (lĕn-tĭk′yə-lō-păp′yə-lər) *adj.* Of or relating to an eruption with dome-shaped or lens-shaped papules.

len·tic·u·lus (lĕn-tĭk′yə-ləs) *n., pl.* **–li** (-lī′) An intraocular lens of inert plastic placed in the anterior chamber of the eye, behind the iris, or clipped to the iris after cataract extraction.

len·ti·form (lĕn′tə-fôrm′) *adj.* Shaped like a biconvex lens; lenticular.

lentiform nucleus *n.* The large, cone-shaped mass of gray matter that forms the central core of the cerebral hemisphere, whose convex base is formed by the putamen and whose apical part consists of the globus pallidus. Also called *lenticular nucleus.*

len·tig·i·no·sis (lĕn-tĭj′ə-nō′sĭs) *n.* Multiple lentigines.

len·ti·glo·bus (lĕn′tĭ-glō′bəs) *n.* A rare congenital anomaly in which the posterior surface of the lens has a prominent spheroid elevation.

len·ti·go (lĕn-tī′gō) *n., pl.* **–tig·i·nes** (-tĭj′ə-nēz′) A small, flat, pigmented spot on the skin.

len·ti·vi·rus (lĕn′tə-vī′rəs) *n.* A virus of the genus *Lentivirus* and the family Retroviridae that causes diseases with a long latent period and a slow, progressive course, as HIV.

le·o·nine (lē′ə-nīn) *adj.* Relating to a lion.

le·on·ti·a·sis (lē′ən-tī′ə-sĭs) *n.* The ridges and furrows on the forehead and cheeks of patients who have advanced lepromatous leprosy, giving a leonine appearance. Also called *leonine facies.*

leop·ard retina (lĕp′ərd) *n.* See **tessellated fundus.**

lep·er (lĕp′ər) *n.* One who has leprosy.

le·pid·ic (lə-pĭd′ĭk) *adj.* Relating to scales or a scaly covering layer.

lep·o·thrix (lĕp′ə-thrĭks′) *n.* See **trichomycosis axillaris.**

lep·re·chaun·ism (lĕp′rĭ-kŏn′ĭz′əm) *n.* A rare genetic disorder characterized by mental and physical retardation, emaciation, endocrine disorders, hirsutism, and facial features dominated by large wide-set eyes and large low-set ears.

lep·rid (lĕp′rĭd) *n.* A skin lesion that is characteristic of leprosy.

lep·ro·ma (lĕ-prō′mə) *n., pl.* **–mas** or **–ma·ta** (-mə-tə) A circumscribed, discrete nodular skin lesion characteristic of leprosy. —**lep·ro′ma·tous** (-mə-təs) *adj.*

lepromatous leprosy *n.* Leprosy that is contagious until treated and is characterized by lepromas, macular lesions having ill-defined borders, and, in advanced cases, nerve involvement and destructive lesions of the face, mouth, throat, and larynx.

lep·ro·min (lĕp′rə-mĭn) *n.* An extract of human tissue infected with *Mycobacterium leprae* and used in skin tests to classify the stage and type of leprosy.

lepromin test *n.* A test to evaluate leprosy using an intradermal injection of a lepromin; the test classifies the stage of leprosy based on reaction and differentiates tuberculoid leprosy, in which there is a positive delayed reaction at the injection site, from lepromatous leprosy, in which there is no reaction despite the active infection.

lep·ro·sar·i·um (lĕp′rə-sâr′ē-əm) *n., pl.* **–i·ums** *or* **–i·a** (-ē-ə) A hospital for the treatment of leprosy.

lep·ro·stat·ic (lĕp′rə-stăt′ĭk) *adj.* Having the capability to inhibit the growth of *Mycobacterium leprae*.

lep·ro·sy (lĕp′rə-sē) *n.* A chronic, mildly contagious granulomatous disease of tropical and subtropical regions, caused by the bacillus *Mycobacterium leprae*, characterized by ulcers of the skin, bone, and viscera and leading to loss of sensation, paralysis, gangrene, and deformation. It occurs in two principal types: lepromatous and tuberculoid. Also called *Hansen's disease*. —**lep′rous** (lĕp′rəs), **lep·rot′ic** (lĕ-prŏt′ĭk) *adj.*

–lepsy *or* **-lepsis** *suff.* Seizure: *narcolepsy*.

lepto– *or* **lept–** *pref.* Slender; thin; fine: *leptocyte*.

lep·to·ceph·a·lous (lĕp′tə-sĕf′ə-ləs) *adj.* Having an abnormally small head.

lep·to·ceph·a·ly (lĕp′tə-sĕf′ə-lē) *n.* A malformation characterized by an abnormally small cranium.

lep·to·cyte (lĕp′tə-sīt′) *n.* An abnormally thin or flattened red blood cell having a central rounded pigmented area, a middle pigmentless zone, and a pigmented edge.

lep·to·cy·to·sis (lĕp′tō-sī-tō′sĭs) *n.* The presence of leptocytes in the blood.

lep·to·dac·ty·lous (lĕp′tō-dăk′tə-ləs) *adj.* Having abnormally slender fingers and toes.

lep·to·me·nin·ges (lĕp′tō-mə-nĭn′jēz) *n.* The pia mater and arachnoid considered as one unit enveloping the brain and spinal cord. Also called *pia-arachnoid*. —**lep′to·me·nin′ge·al** (-jē-əl) *adj.*

lep·to·men·in·gi·tis (lĕp′tō-mĕn′ĭn-jī′tĭs) *n.* A condition in which the leptomeninges are inflamed. Also called *pia-arachnitis*.

lep·to·mo·nad (lĕp′tō-mō′năd′, lĕp-tŏm′ə-năd′) *n.* A parasitic flagellate of the genus *Leptomonas*.

Lep·tom·o·nas (lĕp-tŏm′ə-nəs, lĕp′tō-mō′nəs) *n.* A genus of parasitic flagellates commonly found in the digestive tract of insects.

lep·ton (lĕp′tŏn′) *n.* Any of a family of elementary particles that participate in the weak interaction, including the electron and its associated neutrino.

lep·to·so·mat·ic (lĕp′tə-sō-măt′ĭk) *or* **lep·to·som·ic** (-sō′mĭk) *adj.* Having a slender, light, or thin body.

Lep·to·spi·ra (lĕp′tō-spī′rə) *n.* A genus of aerobic spirochetes of the order Spirochaetales, consisting of thin, tightly coiled cells, many species of which cause leptospirosis.

lep·to·spi·ral jaundice (lĕp′tə-spī′rəl) *n.* Jaundice associated with infection by spirochetes of the genus *Leptospira*.

lep·to·spi·ro·sis (lĕp′tō-spī-rō′sĭs) *n.* Any of a group of infectious diseases that are caused by spirochetes of the genus *Leptospira*, are characterized by jaundice and fever, and are transmitted to humans by contact with the urine of infected animals.

lep·to·spi·ru·ri·a (lĕp′tə-spī-ro͞or′ē-ə) *n.* The presence of spirochetes of the genus *Leptospira* in the urine.

lep·to·tene (lĕp′tə-tēn′) *n.* The early stage of prophase in meiosis in which the replicated chromosomes contract and become visible as long filaments well separated from one another.

Lep·to·trich·i·a (lĕp′tō-trĭk′ē-ə) *n.* A genus of anaerobic, gram-negative, filamentous bacteria that naturally occur in the oral cavity but can occur in the genitourinary tract.

Lep·to·trom·bid·i·um (lĕp′tō-trŏm-bĭd′ē-əm) *n.* A genus of trombiculid mites that serve as vectors of tsutsugamushi disease in China, Southeast Asia, Australia, and various islands in the Pacific Ocean.

Leptotrombidium ak·a·mu·shi (ăk′ə-mo͞o′shē, ä′kə-) *n.* A species of mite thought to be a reservoir for the causative agent of scrub typhus.

Le·riche's syndrome (lə-rēsh′shĭz) *n.* See **aortoiliac occlusive disease**.

Le·ri's sign (lā-rēz′) *n.* An indication of hemiplegia in which the voluntary flexion of the elbow is impossible when the wrist on the paralyzed side is passively flexed.

Leri-Weill syndrome (-vĕl′) *n.* See **dyschondrosteosis**.

Ler·moy·ez syndrome (lĕr-mwä-yā′) *n.* A hearing disorder in which the degree of deafness increases until an attack of dizziness occurs, after which hearing improves. Also called *labyrinthine angiospasm*.

les·bi·an (lĕz′bē-ə-n) *n.* A woman whose sexual orientation is to other women. —*adj.* Relating to or being a lesbian. —**les′bi·an·ism** *n.*

Lesch-Ny·han syndrome (lĕsh′nī′ən) *n.* A metabolic disorder that occurs in males, is associated with an enzyme deficiency, and is characterized by hyperuricemia and uric acid urolithiasis, choreoathetosis, mental retardation, spastic cerebral palsy, and self-mutilation of fingers and lips by biting.

Les·col (lĕs′kōl′) A trademark for the drug fluvastatin.

le·sion (lē′zhən) *n.* **1.** A wound or an injury. **2.** A localized pathological change in a bodily organ or tissue. **3.** An infected or diseased patch of skin.

less·er curvature of stomach (lĕs′ər) *n.* The border of the stomach to which the lesser omentum is attached.

lesser occipital nerve *n.* A nerve that arises from the second and third cervical nerves and supplies skin of the auricle of the ear and adjacent portion of scalp.

lesser omentum *n.* A peritoneal fold passing from the margins of the portal fissure to the lesser curvature of the stomach and to the upper border of the duodenum. Also called *omentulum*.

lesser palatine foramen *n.* Any of the openings on the hard palate of the palatine canals passing through the palatine bone and transmitting the smaller palatine nerves and vessels. Also called *anterior palatine foramen*.

lesser palatine nerve *n.* Either of two or any of three branches of the pterygopalatine ganglion that contain sensory fibers of the maxillary and facial nerves and that supply the mucosa and the glands of the soft palate and uvula.

lesser peritoneal cavity *n.* See **omental bursa**.

lesser petrosal nerve *n.* The parasympathetic root of the otic ganglion, derived from the tympanic plexus.

lesser rhomboid muscle *n.* A muscle with origin from the spinous processes of particular cervical vertebrae, with insertion into the scapula above the spine, with nerve supply from the dorsal scapular nerve, and whose action draws the scapula toward the vertebral column and slightly upward.

lesser splanchnic nerve *n.* A nerve that arises from the last two thoracic sympathetic ganglia and passes to the aorticorenal ganglion.

Les·ser's triangle (lĕs′ərz) *n.* The space between the bellies of the digastric muscle and the hypoglossal nerve.

lesser trochanter *n.* A pyramidal process that projects from the shaft of the femur and receives insertion of the iliopsoas muscle.

lesser vestibular gland *n.* Any of the small branched tubular mucous glands opening on the surface of the vestibule between the orifices of the vagina and the urethra.

lesser zygomatic muscle *n.* A muscle with origin from the zygomatic bone, with insertion into the orbicular muscle of the mouth, with nerve supply from the facial nerve, and whose action draws the upper lip upward and outward.

let-down (lĕt′doun′) *n.* A physiologic reflex in lactating females, activated usually in response to sucking or crying by an infant, in which milk previously secreted into the alveoli of the breasts is released into the ducts that lead to the nipple.

le·thal (lē′thəl) *adj.* **1.** Capable of causing death. **2.** Of, relating to, or causing death.

lethal dose *n. Abbr.* **LD** The dose of a chemical or biological preparation that is likely to cause death.

lethal factor *n.* A gene mutation or chromosomal structural change that when expressed causes death before sexual maturity.

lethal gene *n.* A gene whose expression results in the death of the organism.

lethal midline granuloma *n.* A destructive granulomatous lesion usually arising in the nose or paranasal sinuses and ending in death. Also called *malignant granuloma*.

lethal mutation *n.* A mutant trait that leads to a phenotype incapable of effective reproduction.

leth·ar·gy (lĕth′ər-jē) *n.* **1.** A state of sluggishness, inactivity, and apathy. **2.** A state of unconsciousness resembling deep sleep.

let·ro·zole (lĕt′rə-zōl′) *n.* A nonsteroidal aromatase inhibitor drug used to treat breast cancer in postmenopausal women.

Let·ter·er-Si·we disease (lĕt′ər-ər-sī′wē, -sē′və) *n.* See **nonlipid histiocytosis**.

Leu *abbr.* leucine

leuc– *pref.* Variant of **leuko–**.

leu·cine (lōō′sēn′) *n. Abbr.* **Leu** An essential amino acid derived from the hydrolysis of protein by pancreatic enzymes during digestion and necessary for optimal growth in infants and children and for the maintenance of nitrogen balance in adults.

leu·ci·nu·ri·a (lōō′sə-nŏor′ē-ə) *n.* The presence of leucine in the urine.

leuco– *pref.* Variant of **leuko–**.

leu·co·cyte (lōō′kə-sīt′) *n.* Variant of **leukocyte**.

leu·co·cy·to·sis (lōō′kə-sī-tō′sĭs) *n.* Variant of **leukocytosis**.

leu·co·der·ma (lōō′kə-dûr′mə) *n.* Variant of **leukoderma**.

leu·co·pe·ni·a (lōō′kə-pē′nē-ə) *n.* Variant of **leukopenia**.

leu·cor·rhe·a (lōō′kə-rē′ə) *n.* Variant of **leukorrhea**.

leu·cot·o·my (lōō-kŏt′ə-mē) *n.* Variant of **leukotomy**.

leu·co·vo·rin (lōō′kə-vôr′ĭn, lōō-kŏv′ər-ĭn) *n.* See **folinic acid**.

leuk– *pref.* Variant of **leuko–**.

leu·ka·phe·re·sis (lōō′kə-fə-rē′sĭs) *n.* The removal of a quantity of white blood cells from the blood of a donor with the remaining portions of the blood retransfused into the donor.

leu·ke·mi·a (lōō-kē′mē-ə) *n.* Any of various acute or chronic neoplastic diseases of the bone marrow in which unrestrained proliferation of white blood cells occurs and which is usually accompanied by anemia, impaired blood clotting, and enlargement of the lymph nodes, liver, and spleen. —**leu·ke′mic** *adj.*

leukemia cu·tis (kyōō′tĭs) *n.* Leukemia characterized by sometimes nodular yellow-brown, red, blue-red, or purple skin lesions, associated with infiltrations or accumulations of leukemic cells in the skin.

leukemic reticuloendotheliosis *n.* See **hairy cell leukemia**.

leukemic retinopathy *n.* A condition of the retina occurring in all types of leukemia and characterized by the presence of a yellow-orange fundus, engorgement and tortuosity of retinal veins, scattered hemorrhages, and edema of the retina and optic disk.

leu·ke·mid (lōō-kē′mĭd) *n.* Any of various nonspecific cutaneous lesions that are associated with leukemia but that are not accumulations of leukemic cells.

leu·ke·mo·gen (lōō-kē′mə-jən, -jĕn′) *n.* A factor that is known or attributed to be a cause of leukemia.

leu·ke·mo·gen·e·sis (lōō-kē′mə-jĕn′ĭ-sĭs) *n.* Induction, development, and progression of a leukemic disease.

leu·ke·mo·gen·ic (lōō-kē′mə-jĕn′ĭk) *adj.* **1.** Of or relating to leukemogenesis. **2.** Of, relating to, or characterized by a leukemogen.

leu·ke·moid (lōō-kē′moid′) *adj.* Having the various signs and symptoms of leukemia.

leukemoid reaction *n.* A moderate, advanced, or sometimes extreme degree of leukocytosis that is similar or possibly identical to that occurring in leukemia but is due to some other cause.

Leu·ke·ran (lōō′kə-răn′) A trademark for the drug chlorambucil.

leuko– *or* **leuk–** *or* **leuco–** *or* **leuc–** *pref.* **1.** White; colorless: *leukoderma*. **2.** Leukocyte: *leukopenia*.

leu·ko·ag·glu·ti·nin (lōō′kō-ə-glōot′n-ĭn) *n.* An antibody that agglutinates leukocytes.

leu·ko·blast (lōō′kə-blăst′) *n.* An immature white blood cell that is formed during the transition from lymphoidocyte to promyelocyte. Also called *proleukocyte*. —**leu′ko·blas′tic** *adj.*

leu·ko·blas·to·sis (lōō′kō-blă-stō′sĭs) *n.* The abnormal proliferation of immature white blood cells, especially in granulocytic and lymphocytic leukemia.

leu·ko·ci·din (lōō′kə-sīd′n, lōō-kō′sĭ-dn) *n*. A substance, produced by certain species of *Staphylococcus* and *Streptococcus* bacteria, that can destroy or lyse white blood cells.

leu·ko·cyte *or* **leu·co·cyte** (lōō′kə-sīt′) *n*. See **white blood cell.** —**leu′ko·cyt′ic** (-sĭt′ĭk) *adj*.

leu·ko·cy·to·blast (lōō′kə-sī′tə-blăst′) *n*. A white blood cell precursor.

leu·ko·cy·to·clas·tic vasculitis (lōō′kə-sī′tə-klăs′tĭk) *n*. Acute cutaneous vasculitis that is characterized by purpura, especially of the legs, and by exudation of neutrophils and sometimes fibrin around dermal venules, with extravasation of red blood cells.

leu·ko·cy·to·gen·e·sis (lōō′kə-sī′tə-jĕn′ĭ-sĭs) *n*. Formation and development of white blood cells.

leu·ko·cy·tol·y·sin (lōō′kə-sī-tŏl′ĭ-sĭn) *n*. A substance that destroys or lyses white blood cells. Also called *leukolysin.*

leu·ko·cy·tol·y·sis (lōō′kə-sī-tŏl′ĭ-sĭs) *n*. The destruction or lysis of white blood cells. —**leu′ko·cy′to·lyt′ic** (-sī′tə-lĭt′ĭk) *adj*.

leu·ko·cy·to·ma (lōō′kə-sī-tō′mə) *n*. A fairly well circumscribed, nodular, dense accumulation of white blood cells.

leu·ko·cy·to·pe·ni·a (lōō′kə-sī′tə-pē′nē-ə) *n*. See **leukopenia.**

leu·ko·cy·to·pla·ni·a (lōō′kə-sī′tə-plā′nē-ə) *n*. The movement of white blood cells from blood vessels, through serous membranes, or in tissues.

leu·ko·cy·to·poi·e·sis (lōō′kə-sī′tə-poi-ē′sĭs) *n*. See **leukopoiesis.**

leu·ko·cy·to·sis *or* **leu·co·cy·to·sis** (lōō′kə-sī-tō′sĭs) *n*., *pl*. **-ses** (-sēz) An abnormally large increase in the number of white blood cells in the blood, often occurring during an acute infection or inflammation. —**leu′ko·cy·tot′ic** (-tŏt′ĭk) *adj*.

leu·ko·cy·to·tax·i·a (lōō′kə-sī′tə-tăk′sē-ə) *n*. **1.** The active ameboid movement of white blood cells, especially of neutrophilic granulocytes, toward or away from microorganisms or substances formed in inflamed tissue. Also called *leukotaxia, leukotaxis.* **2.** The property of attracting or of repelling white blood cells. —**leu′ko·cy′to·tac′tic** (-tăk′tĭk) *adj*.

leu·ko·cy·to·tox·in (lōō′kə-sī′tə-tŏk′sĭn) *n*. A substance that causes degeneration and necrosis of white blood cells. Also called *leukotoxin.*

leu·ko·cy·tu·ri·a (lōō′kə-sī-tŏŏr′ē-ə) *n*. The presence of white blood cells in urine.

leu·ko·der·ma *or* **leu·co·der·ma** (lōō′kə-dûr′mə) *n*. Partial or total loss of skin pigmentation, often occurring in patches. Also called *leukopathia, piebald skin, vitiligo.*

leukoderma ac·qui·si·tum cen·trif·u·gum (ăk′wĭ-sī′təm sĕn-trĭf′yə-gəm) *n*. See **halo nevus.**

leu·ko·dys·tro·phy (lōō′kō-dĭs′trə-fē) *n*. Degeneration of the white matter of the brain characterized by demyelination and glial reaction, probably related to defects of lipid metabolism. Also called *leukoencephalopathy.*

leu·ko·e·de·ma (lōō′kō-ĭ-dē′mə) *n*. A benign abnormality of the buccal mucosa characterized by a filmy, opalescent-to-whitish gray, wrinkled epithelium similar to that seen in leukoplakia.

leu·ko·en·ceph·a·li·tis (lōō′kō-ĕn-sĕf′ə-lī′tĭs) *n*. Inflammation of the white matter of the brain.

leu·ko·en·ceph·a·lop·a·thy (lōō′kō-ĕn-sĕf′ə-lŏp′ə-thē) *n*. See **leukodystrophy.**

leu·ko·e·ryth·ro·blas·to·sis (lōō′kō-ĭ-rĭth′rō-blă-stō′sĭs) *n*. An anemic condition resulting from space-occupying lesions in the bone marrow and characterized by the presence of immature granular leukocytes and nucleated erythrocytes in the circulating blood. Also called *myelophthisic anemia.*

leu·ko·ko·ri·a (lōō′kō-kôr′ē-ə) *n*. A condition characterized by a reflective white mass within the eye that gives the appearance of white pupil.

leu·ko·krau·ro·sis (lōō′kō-krô-rō′sĭs) *n*. See **kraurosis vulvae.**

leu·ko·lym·pho·sar·co·ma (lōō′kō-lĭm′fō-sär-kō′mə) *n*. See **leukosarcoma.**

leu·kol·y·sin (lōō-kŏl′ĭ-sĭn) *n*. See **leukocytolysin.**

leu·ko·ma (lōō-kō′mə) *n., pl.* **-mas** *or* **-ma·ta** (-mə-tə) A dense white opacity of the cornea. —**leu·kom′a·tous** (lōō-kŏm′ə-təs) *adj*.

leu·ko·my·e·lop·a·thy (lōō′kō-mī′ə-lŏp′ə-thē) *n*. Any of various diseases involving the white matter of the spinal cord.

leu·kon (lōō′kŏn′) *n*. The total mass of circulating white blood cells, their precursors, and the leukopoietic cells from which they arise.

leu·ko·ne·cro·sis (lōō′kō-nə-krō′sĭs) *n*. See **white gangrene.**

leu·ko·nych·i·a (lōō′kō-nĭk′ē-ə) *n*. The occurrence of white spots or patches under the nails due to the presence of air bubbles between the nail and its bed.

leu·ko·path·i·a (lōō′kō-păth′ē-ə) *n*. See **leukoderma.**

leu·ko·pe·de·sis (lōō′kō-pĭ-dē′sĭs) *n*. The movement of white blood cells through the walls of capillaries and into the tissues.

leu·ko·pe·ni·a *or* **leu·co·pe·ni·a** (lōō′kə-pē′nē-ə) *n*. An abnormally low number of white blood cells in the circulating blood. Also called *leukocytopenia.* —**leu′ko·pe′nic** *adj*.

leukopenic index *n*. A number indicating a significant decrease in the white blood cell count after ingestion of food to which a person is hypersensitive.

leukopenic leukemia *n*. A form of lymphocytic leukemia, granulocytic leukemia, or monocytic leukemia in which the number of white blood cells in the blood is normal or only slightly low.

leu·ko·pla·ki·a (lōō′kə-plā′kē-ə) *n*. A condition characterized by white spots or patches on mucous membranes, especially of the mouth and vulva. Also called *leukoplasia, smoker's patch, smoker's tongue.*

leukoplakia vul·vae (vŭl′vē) *n*. A patchy, white, atrophic thickening and keratinization of the vulvar epithelium, associated with papillary hypertrophy.

leu·ko·pla·sia (lōō′kə-plā′zhə) *n*. See **leukoplakia.**

leu·ko·poi·e·sis (lōō′kō-poi-ē′sĭs) *n*. The formation and development of the various types of white blood cells. Also called *leukocytopoiesis.* —**leu′ko·poi·et′ic** (-ĕt′ĭk) *adj*.

leu·kor·rhe·a *or* **leu·cor·rhe·a** (lōō'kə-rē'ə) *n.* A thick, whitish discharge from the vagina or cervical canal. Also called *leukorrhagia.*

leu·ko·sar·co·ma (lōō'kō-sär-kō'mə) *n.* A type of lymphoma characterized by large numbers of abnormal lymphocyte precursors in the blood. Also called *leukolymphosarcoma.*

leu·ko·sar·co·ma·to·sis (lōō'kō-sär-kō'mə-tō'sĭs) *n.* A condition characterized by numerous widespread sarcomas composed of leukemic cells and by the presence of leukemic cells in the blood.

leu·ko·sis (lōō-kō'sĭs) *n.* The abnormal proliferation of one or more of the leukopoietic tissues.

leu·ko·tax·i·a (lōō'kə-tăk'sē-ə) *n.* See **leukocytotaxia** (sense 1). —**leu'ko·tac'tic** (-tăk'tĭk) *adj.*

leu·ko·tax·ine (lōō'kə-tăk'sēn', -sĭn) *n.* A crystalline nitrogenous material produced in injured, acutely degenerating tissue and found in inflammatory exudates that increases the permeability of capillaries and the migration of white blood cells.

leu·ko·tax·is (lōō'kə-tăk'sĭs) *n.* See **leukocytotaxia** (sense 1).

leu·kot·ic (lōō-kŏt'ĭk) *adj.* Relating to, characterized by, or manifesting leukosis.

leu·kot·o·my *or* **leu·cot·o·my** (lōō-kŏt'ə-mē) *n.* Incision into the white matter of the frontal lobe of the brain.

leu·ko·tox·in (lōō'kō-tŏk'sĭn) *n.* See **leukocytotoxin.**

leu·ko·trich·i·a (lōō'kə-trĭk'ē-ə) *n.* Whiteness of the hair.

leu·ko·tri·ene (lōō'kə-trī'ēn') *n.* Any of a group of physiologically active substances that possibly function as mediators of inflammation and as participants in allergic responses.

leu·pro·lide acetate (lōō'prō-līd') *n.* A synthetic polypeptide analog of naturally occurring gonadotropin-releasing hormone used in the treatment of advanced prostate cancer.

Lev·a·quin (lĕv'ə-kwĭn') A trademark for the drug levofloxacin.

lev·ar·te·re·nol (lĕv'är-tîr'ə-nôl', -nōl', -tĕr'-) *n.* See **norepinephrine.**

le·va·tor (lə-vā'tər) *n., pl.* **lev·a·to·res** (lĕv'ə-tôr'ēz) **1.** A surgical instrument for lifting the depressed fragments of a fractured skull. **2.** A muscle that raises a body part.

lev·el (lĕv'əl) *n.* **1.** Relative position or rank on a graded scale, such as mental or emotional development. **2.** A relative degree, as of intensity or concentration.

Le·vi-Mon·tal·ci·ni (lē'vē-mŏn'tl-chē'nē, lĕ'vē-môn'-täl-), **Rita** Born 1909. Italian-American developmental biologist. She shared a 1986 Nobel Prize for the discovery of the nerve growth factor.

Le·vin tube (lə-vĭn') *n.* A tube that is inserted through the nose into the upper alimentary canal and is used to facilitate intestinal decompression.

Le·vi·tra (lə-vē'trə) A trademark for the drug vardenefil hydrochloride.

levo– *or* **lev–** *pref.* **1.** To the left: *levorotation.* **2.** Levorotatory: *levulose.*

le·vo·bu·no·lol hydrochloride (lē'vō-byōō'nə-lôl') *n.*

A beta-blocker administered as eyedrops for the treatment of chronic open-angle glaucoma and ocular hypertension.

le·vo·car·di·a (lē'və-kär'dē-ə) *n.* Situs inversus of the viscera but with normal positioning of the heart on the left, usually associated with congenital cardiac lesions.

le·vo·cli·na·tion (lē'və-klə-nā'shən) *n.* See **levotorsion** (sense 2).

le·vo·do·pa (lē'və-dō'pə) *n.* See **L-dopa.**

le·vo·duc·tion (lē'və-dŭk'shən) *n.* The rotation of one or both eyes to the left.

le·vo·flox·a·cin (lē'vō-flôks'ə-sĭn) *n.* A synthetic broad-spectrum antibiotic of the fluoroquinolone class.

le·vo·nor·ges·trel (lē'və-nôr-jĕs'trəl) *n.* The levorotatory form of norgestrel, used primarily in oral contraceptives and morning-after pills.

Lev·o·phed (lĕv'ə-fĕd') A trademark for a drug preparation of norepinephrine.

le·vo·ro·ta·tion (lē'və-rō-tā'shən) *n.* A counterclockwise rotation, especially of the plane of polarized light.

le·vo·ro·ta·to·ry (lē'və-rō'tə-tôr'ē) *or* **le·vo·ro·ta·ry** (-rō'tə-rē) *adj.* **1.** Turning or rotating the plane of polarization of light to the left (counterclockwise). **2.** Of or relating to a chemical solution that rotates such a plane to the left.

lev·or·pha·nol tartrate (lĕ-vôr'fə-nôl') *n.* An addictive drug used primarily as an analgesic with action similar to morphine.

le·vo·thy·rox·ine sodium (lē'və-thī-rŏk'sēn', -sĭn) *n.* An isomer of thyroxine in a salt form, used to treat thyroxine deficiency.

le·vo·tor·sion (lē'və-tôr'shən) *n.* **1.** See **sinistrotorsion.** **2.** Rotation of the upper pole of the cornea to the left. Also called *levoclination.*

le·vo·ver·sion (lē'və-vûr'zhən) *n.* **1.** A turning toward the left. **2.** Rotation of both eyes to the left.

Le·vox·yl (lə-vŏk'sĭl) A trademark for a drug preparation of thyroxine.

Lev's syndrome (lĕvz) *n.* A condition in which bundle-branch block occurs but the myocardium and coronary arteries are normal and in which there is fibrosis or calcification of the cardiac conducting system, involving the membranous septum, the apex of the muscular septum, and the mitral and aortic rings of the heart.

lev·u·lose (lĕv'yə-lōs', -lōz') *n.* See **fructose.**

lev·u·lo·se·mi·a (lĕv'yə-lō-sē'mē-ə, -lōz') *n.* See **fructosemia.**

Lex·a·pro (lĕk'sə-prō') A trademark for the drug escitalopram oxalate.

Ley·dig (lā'dĭкн'), **Franz** 1821–1908. German anatomist who described (1850) the interstitial cell in a study of the testes and published important works in the field of histology.

Leydig cell *n.* See **interstitial cell.**

LGA *abbr.* large for gestational age

LH *abbr.* luteinizing hormone

Lher·mitte-Du·clos disease (lâr'mĭt-dōō-klō', lĕr-mĕt'-dü-klō') *n.* A disease occurring chiefly in adults characterized by abnormal development and enlargement of the cerebellum and an increase in intracranial pressure.

Lher·mitte's sign (lâr′mĭts, lĕr-mēts′) *n.* An indication of multiple sclerosis and of disorders of the cervical cord, especially compression, in which sudden electric-like shocks extend down the spine when the head is flexed.

LH/FSH-RF *abbr.* luteinizing hormone/follicle-stimulating hormone-releasing factor

LHRH *abbr.* luteinizing hormone-releasing hormone

Li The symbol for the element **lithium**.

Li (lē), **Choh Hao** 1913–1987. Chinese-born American chemist known for isolating and analyzing a number of hormones secreted by the pituitary gland.

li·bid·i·nous (lĭ-bĭd′n-əs) *adj.* Having or exhibiting lustful desires; lascivious.

li·bi·do (lĭ-bē′dō, -bī′-) *n., pl.* **-dos 1.** The psychic and emotional energy associated with instinctual biological drives. **2.** Sexual desire. **3.** Manifestation of the sexual drive.

Lib·man-Sacks endocarditis (lĭb′mən-săks′) *n.* A form of vegetative endocarditis found in association with systemic lupus erythematosus. Also called *atypical verrucous endocarditis, Libman-Sacks syndrome, nonbacterial verrucous endocarditis.*

Lib·ri·um (lĭb′rē-əm) A trademark for the drug chlordiazepoxide hydrochloride.

lice (līs) *n.* Plural of **louse**.

li·censed practical nurse (lī′sənst) *n. Abbr.* **LPN** A nurse who has completed a practical nursing program and is licensed by a state to provide routine patient care under the direction of a registered nurse or a physician.

licensed vocational nurse *n. Abbr.* **LVN** A licensed practical nurse who is permitted by license to practice in California or Texas.

li·chen (lī′kən) *n.* Any of various skin diseases characterized by patchy eruptions of small, firm papules.

li·chen·i·fi·ca·tion (lī-kĕn′ə-fĭ-kā′shən, lī′kə-nə-) *n.* Thickening of the skin with hyperkeratosis caused by chronic inflammation resulting from prolonged scratching or irritation.

lichen myx·e·de·ma·to·sus (mĭk′sĭ-dē′mə-tō′səs) *n.* A skin condition characterized by the widespread eruption of papules or plaques of mucinous edema caused by the deposition of acid mucopolysaccharides in the skin. Also called *papular mucinosis.*

lichen nit·i·dus (nĭt′ĭ-dəs) *n.* A skin condition characterized by minute, asymptomatic, whitish or pinkish, flat-topped skin papules that may occur in conjunction with lichen planus.

li·chen·oid (lī′kə-noid′) *adj.* Resembling lichen.

lichenoid dermatosis *n.* A chronic skin eruption characterized by hardening and thickening of the skin with the accentuation of normal skin markings.

lichenoid keratosis *n.* A solitary benign skin papule or plaque having microscopic features resembling lichen planus.

lichen pla·nus (plā′nəs) *n.* A skin condition characterized by the eruption of flat-topped, shiny, violaceous papules on flexor surfaces, male genitalia, and the mucosa of the oral cavity. Also called *lichen ruber planus.*

lichen scle·ro·sus et a·troph·i·cus (sklə-rō′səs ĕt ə-trŏf′ĭ-kəs) *n.* A skin eruption consisting of white atrophic papules that may contain a central depression or a black keratotic plug. Also called *Hallopeau's disease.*

lichen scrof·u·lo·so·rum (skrŏf′yə-lə-sôr′əm) *n.* See **papular tuberculid.**

lichen sim·plex (sĭm′plĕks′) *n.* A skin condition characterized by small, intensely pruritic papules.

lichen stri·a·tus (strī-ā′təs) *n.* A skin condition seen primarily in children and marked by a self-limited papular eruption having lesions arranged in linear groups, usually on one extremity.

lichen ur·ti·ca·tus (ûr′tĭ-kā′təs) *n.* A form of urticaria occurring in children and characterized by the eruption of papular lesions or small papules and vesicles. Also called *papular urticaria.*

Li·dex (lī′dĕks′) A trademark for the drug fluocinonide.

li·do·caine (lī′də-kān′) *n.* A synthetic amide used as a local anesthetic.

lie (lī) *n.* The manner or position in which something is situated, especially the relation that the long axis of a fetus bears to that of its mother.

Lie·ber·kühn (lē′bər-kyōōn′, -kün′), **Johann Nathanael** 1711–1756. German anatomist known for discovering the intestinal glands.

Lie·ber·kühn's crypt (lē′bər-kyōōnz′, -künz′) *n.* See **intestinal gland.**

Lieberkühn's follicle *n.* See **intestinal gland.**

lie detector *n.* A polygraph used to detect possible deception during an interrogation.

li·en (lī′ən, -ĕn′) *n.* The spleen.

li·e·nal (lī′ə-nəl) *adj.* Splenic.

lienal artery *n.* An artery with its origin in the celiac trunk, with branches to the pancreatic, left gastroepiploic, short gastric, and splenic arteries. Also called *splenic artery.*

lien mo·bi·lis (mō′bə-lĭs) *n.* See **floating spleen.**

lienteric diarrhea *n.* Diarrhea in which undigested food appears in the stools.

li·en·ter·y (lī′ən-tĕr′ē) *n.* The passage of undigested or partially digested food in the stool. —**li′en·ter′ic** (lī′-ən-tĕr′ĭk) *adj.*

life (līf) *n., pl.* **lives** (līvz) **1.** The property or quality that distinguishes living organisms from dead organisms and inanimate matter, manifested in functions such as metabolism, growth, reproduction, and response to stimuli or adaptation to the environment originating from within the organism. **2.** The characteristic state or condition of a living organism. **3.** Living organisms considered as a group. **4.** A living being, especially a person.

life care *or* **life·care** (līf′kâr′) *n.* The provision of services for elderly people, including housing, health care, and social activities.

life cycle *n.* **1.** The characteristic course of developmental changes through which an organism passes from its inception as a fertilized zygote to its mature state, during which another zygote may be produced. **2.** A progression through a series of differing stages of development.

life expectancy *n.* The number of years that one is expected to live as determined by statistics.

life instinct *n.* In psychoanalytic theory, the instinct of self-preservation and sexual procreation.

life science *n.* Any of several branches of science, such as biology, medicine, anthropology, or ecology, that deals with living organisms and their organization, life processes, and relationships to each other and their environment. Also called *bioscience.*

life span *n.* **1.** A lifetime. **2.** The average or maximum length of time an organism, a material, or an object can be expected to survive or last.

life stress *n.* Events or experiences that produce severe strain, such as failure on the job, marital separation, and loss of a loved person.

life·style *or* **life-style** (līf′stīl′) *n.* A way of life or style of living that reflects the attitudes and values of a person or group.

life support *n.* A life-support system.

life-support system *n.* **1.** Equipment that creates a viable environment under conditions otherwise incompatible with life. **2.** Medical equipment that augments or substitutes for an essential bodily function, such as respiration or excretion, enabling a patient who otherwise might not survive to live.

life table *n.* A representation of the survivorship of a defined population.

life·time (līf′tīm′) *n.* **1.** The period of time during which an individual is alive. **2.** The period of time during which property, an object, a process, or a phenomenon exists or functions.

Li-Frau·meni cancer syndrome (lē′frou-mā′nē) *n.* A familial breast cancer syndrome that occurs in young women and that is associated with the occurrence of soft-tissue sarcomas in children and other cancers in close relatives.

lig·a·ment (lĭg′ə-mənt) *n.* **1.** A band or sheet of tough fibrous tissue connecting two or more bones, cartilages, or other structures, or serving as support for fasciae or muscles. **2.** A fold of peritoneum supporting any of the abdominal viscera. **3.** The cordlike remains of a fetal vessel or other structure that has lost its original lumen. —**lig′a·men′tal** (-mĕn′tl), **lig′a·men′tous** *adj.*

ligament of head of femur *n.* A flattened ligament that passes from the fovea in the head of the femur to the borders of the acetabular notch. Also called *round ligament of femur.*

lig·a·men·to·pex·is (lĭg′ə-mĕn′tə-pĕk′sĭs) *or* **lig·a·men·to·pex·y** (-mĕn′tə-pĕk′sē) *n.* A shortening of a ligament of the uterus.

lig·a·men·tum (lĭg′ə-mĕn′təm) *n., pl.* **-ta** (-tə) The cordlike remains of a structure that has lost its original lumen.

li·gand (lī′gənd, lĭg′ənd) *n.* An ion, a molecule, or a molecular group that binds to another chemical entity to form a larger complex.

li·gase (lī′gās′, -gāz′) *n.* Any of a class of enzymes, including the carboxylases, that catalyze the linkage of two molecules, generally utilizing ATP as the energy donor. Also called *synthetase.*

li·gate (lī′gāt′) *v.* To tie or bind with a ligature.

li·ga·tion (lī-gā′shən) *n.* **1.** The act of binding or of applying a ligature. **2.** The state of being bound. **3.** Something that binds; a ligature.

lig·a·ture (lĭg′ə-choor′, -chər) *n.* **1.** The act of tying or binding. **2.** A cord, wire, or bandage used in surgery to close vessels or tie off ducts. **3.** A thread, wire, or cord used in surgery to close vessels or tie off ducts.

light (līt) *n.* **1.** Electromagnetic radiation that has a wavelength in the range from about 4,000 (violet) to about 7,700 (red) angstroms and may be perceived by the normal unaided human eye. **2.** Electromagnetic radiation of any wavelength.

light adaptation *n.* The adjustment of the eye under increased illumination, in which the sensitivity to light is reduced. Also called *photopic adaptation.*

light-adapted eye *n.* An eye that has been exposed to light of relatively high intensity and has undergone adjustments of photochemical change and constriction of the pupil. Also called *photopic eye.*

light chain *n.* The smaller of the two types of polypeptide chains in immunoglobulins, consisting of an antigen-binding portion with a variable amino acid sequence, and a constant region with an amino acid sequence that is relatively unchanging.

light·en·ing (līt′n-ĭng) *n.* The sensation of decreased abdominal distention during the latter weeks of pregnancy following the descent of the fetal head into the pelvic inlet.

light reflex *n.* **1.** Contraction of the pupil of the eye in response to an increase in light. **2.** A circular red light reflected from the retina of the eye. Also called *red reflex.* **3.** See **cone of light.**

light treatment *n.* See **phototherapy.**

limb (lĭm) *n.* **1.** One of the paired jointed extremities of the body; an arm or a leg. **2.** A segment of such a jointed structure.

limb bud *n.* A mesenchymal outgrowth covered with ectoderm on the flank of an embryo that gives rise to either the forelimb or the hindlimb.

limb-girdle muscular dystrophy *n.* A progressive inherited disorder that usually begins in preadolescents and is characterized by symptoms similar to those present in facioscapulohumeral muscular dystrophy with the pelvic girdle often being the most severely affected part.

lim·bic (lĭm′bĭk) *adj.* **1.** Of, relating to, or characterized by a limbus. **2.** Of or relating to the limbic system.

limbic system *n.* A group of deep brain structures, common to all mammals and including the hippocampus, amygdala, gyrus fornicatus, and connecting structures, associated with olfaction, emotion, motivation, behavior, and various autonomic functions.

limb lead (lēd) *n.* **1.** Any of the three standard leads used in electrocardiography, having one electrode attached to the chest and another to a limb. **2.** A unipolar lead in which one electrode is placed on a limb. **3.** A record obtained from such leads.

lim·bus (lĭm′bəs) *n., pl.* **-bi** (-bī′) An edge, border, or fringe of an anatomical part.

lime¹ (līm) *n.* **1.** A spiny evergreen shrub or tree (*Citrus aurantifolia*) native to Asia and having leathery leaves, fragrant white flowers, and edible fruit. **2.** The egg-shaped fruit of this plant, having a green rind and acid juice used as flavoring.

lime² *n.* (līm) **1.** Any of various mineral and industrial forms of calcium oxide differing chiefly in water content and percentage of constituents such as silica, alumina, and iron. **2.** See **calcium oxide**.

li·men (lī′mən) *n.*, *pl.* **li·mens** *or* **lim·i·na** (lĭm′ə-nə) **1.** The threshold of a physiological or psychological response. **2.** The external opening of a canal; an entrance. —**lim′i·nal** (lĭm′ə-nəl) *adj.*

limen in·su·lae (ĭn′sə-lē′) *n.* The transitional band located between the anterior portion of the gray matter of the island of Reil and the posterior perforated substance, formed by a narrow strip of olfactory cortex.

limen na·si (nā′zī) *n.* A ridge marking the boundary between the nasal cavity proper and the vestibule of the nose.

li·mes (lī′mēz) *n.*, *pl.* **lim·i·tes** (lĭm′ĭ-tēz′) *Abbr.* **L** A boundary, limit, or threshold.

lim·i·nal (lĭm′ə-nəl) *adj.* Relating to a threshold.

lim·it (lĭm′ĭt) *n.* **1.** The point, edge, or line beyond which something cannot or may not proceed. **2.** A confining or restricting object, agent, or influence. **3.** The greatest or least amount, number, or extent allowed or possible. —*v.* **1.** To confine or restrict within a boundary or bounds. **2.** To fix definitely; to specify. —**lim′it·a·ble** *adj.*

limit dextrin *n.* Any of various branched polysaccharide fragments that remain following the hydrolysis of starch.

limit dextrinase *n.* An enzyme that catalyzes the hydrolysis of polysaccharides, especially completing the digestion of starch or the conversion of glycogen to glucose.

lim·it·ing layer of cornea (lĭm′ĭ-tĭng) *n.* **1.** A basement membrane that lies between the outer layer of stratified epithelium and the proper substance of the cornea; anterior limiting layer of the cornea. Also called *Bowman's membrane*. **2.** A basement membrane that lies between the proper substance and the endothelial layer of the cornea; posterior limiting layer of the cornea. Also called *Descemet's membrane, elastic lamina of cornea, elastic layer of cornea, entocornea, vitreous membrane*.

limp (lĭmp) *n.* An irregular, jerky, or awkward gait; a claudication. —*v.* To walk lamely, especially with irregularity, as if favoring one leg.

lim·u·lus·ly·sate test (lĭm′yə-ləs-lī′sāt′) *n.* A test for the rapid detection of meningitis that is caused by gram-negative bacteria.

Lin·co·cin (lĭng′kə-sĭn) A trademark for the drug lincomycin hydrochloride.

lin·co·my·cin hydrochloride (lĭng′kə-mī′sĭn) *n.* An antibiotic derived from cultures of the bacterium *Streptomyces lincolnensis* and used in the treatment of certain penicillin-resistant infections.

linc·ture (lĭngk′chər)*or* **linc·tus** (-təs) *n.* A confection.

lin·dane (lĭn′dān) *n.* A white crystalline powder used chiefly as an agricultural pesticide but also used topically in the treatment of scabies and pediculosis. Also called *gamma-benzene hexachloride*.

Lin·dau's disease (lĭn′douz′) *n.* A hereditary disease characterized by hemangiomas of the retina, the cere-

bellum and occasionally the spinal cord, and also sometimes associated with cysts or hamartomas of the kidney, adrenal glands, or other organs. Also called *angiophacomatosis, Hippel's disease, retinocerebral angiomatosis, von Hippel-Lindau disease, von Hippel-Lindau syndrome*.

line (līn) *n.* **1.** The path traced by a moving point. **2.** A thin continuous mark, as that made by a pen, pencil, or brush applied to a surface. **3.** A crease in the skin, especially on the face; a wrinkle. **4.** In anatomy, a long narrow mark, strip, or streak distinguished from adjacent tissue by color, texture, or elevation. **5.** A real or imaginary mark positioned in relation to fixed points of reference. **6.** A border, boundary, or demarcation. **7.** A contour or an outline. **8.** A mark used to define a shape or represent a contour. **9.** Any of the marks that make up the formal design of a picture. **10.** A cable, rope, string, cord, or wire. **11.** A general method, manner, or course of procedure. **12.** A manner or course of procedure determined by a specified factor. **13.** An official or prescribed policy. **14.** Ancestry or lineage. **15.** A series of persons, especially from one family, who succeed each other.

lin·e·a (lĭn′ē-ə) *n.*, *pl.* **-e·ae** (-ē-ē′) A line.

linea al·ba (ăl′bə) *n.* A fibrous band that runs vertically along the center of the anterior abdominal wall and receives the attachments of the oblique and transverse abdominal muscles. Also called *white line*.

linea as·pe·ra (ăs′pə-rə) *n.* A longitudinal ridge running down the posterior surface of the shaft of the femur, affording attachment to various muscles including the vastus medialis, adductor longus, adductor magnus, adductor brevis, vastus lateralis, and short head of the biceps.

line angle *n.* **1.** The junction of two surfaces of the crown of a tooth. **2.** The junction of two surfaces of a tooth cavity.

linea ni·gra (nī′grə, nĭg′rə) *n.* The linea alba in pregnancy, which then becomes pigmented.

lin·e·ar (lĭn′ē-ər) *adj.* Of, relating to, or resembling a line; straight.

linear accelerator *n.* **1.** An electron, a proton, or a heavy-ion accelerator in which the paths of the particles accelerated are essentially straight lines rather than circles or spirals. **2.** A device that produces high energy photons (x-rays) on charged particles for use in radiation therapy.

linear atrophy *n.* Stretch marks.

linear fracture *n.* A fracture that runs parallel to the long axis of a bone. Also called *fissured fracture*.

line of demarcation *n.* A zone of inflammatory reaction separating gangrenous from healthy tissue.

line of fixation *n.* An imaginary line joining the optical point of fixation with the fovea and passing through the nodal point.

lin·gua (lĭng′gwə) *n.*, *pl.* **-guae** (-gwē′) **1.** The tongue. **2.** A tonguelike anatomical structure.

lingua ge·o·graph·i·ca (jē′ə-grăf′ĭ-kə) *n.* Geographical tongue.

lin·gual (lĭng′gwəl) *adj.* **1.** Of or relating to the tongue or any tonguelike part; glossal. **2.** Next to or toward the tongue.

lingual artery *n.* An artery with origin in the carotid artery, with distribution to the undersurface of the tongue, terminating as the deep artery of the tongue, and with branches to the suprahyoid and dorsal lingual branches and the sublingual artery.

lingual follicle *n.* Any of the collections of lymphoid tissue in the mucosa of the pharyngeal part of the tongue that form the lingual tonsil.

lingual goiter *n.* A tumor of thyroid tissue involving the embryonic rudiment at the base of the tongue.

lingual gyrus *n.* A short horizontal convolution on the inferomedial aspect of the occipital and temporal lobes of the brain, demarcated from the fusiform gyrus by the collateral sulcus and from the cuneus by the calcarine sulcus. Also called *medial occipitotemporal gyrus.*

lingual nerve *n.* A branch of the mandibular nerve that is distributed to the front two thirds of the tongue and supplies the mucous membrane of the floor of the mouth.

lingual papilla *n.* Any of the papillae on the tongue: conical, filiform, fungiform, and vallate.

lingual tonsil *n.* A collection of lymphoid follicles on the posterior portion of the dorsum of the tongue.

lingual vein *n.* A vein that receives blood from the tongue, from the sublingual and the submandibular glands, and from the muscles of the floor of the mouth and that empties into the internal jugular vein or the facial vein.

lingua ni·gra (nī′grə, nĭg′rə) *n.* Black tongue.

lingua pli·ca·ta (plĭ-kā′tə) *n.* Furrowed tongue.

Lin·guat·u·la (lĭng-gwăch′yə-lə) *n.* A genus of endoparasitic bloodsucking arthropods commonly known as tongue worms and found in lungs or air passages of various vertebrates, including humans.

lin·guat·u·li·a·sis (lĭng-gwăch′yə-lī′ə-sĭs) *n.* Infection with a tongue worm of the genus *Linguatula.*

lin·gui·form (lĭng′gwə-fôrm′) *adj.* Tongue-shaped.

lin·gu·la (lĭng′gyə-lə) *n., pl.* **-lae** (-lē′) Any of several tongue-shaped processes.

lin·gu·lar (lĭng′gyə-lər) *adj.* Of or relating to a lingula.

lin·gu·lec·to·my (lĭng′gyə-lĕk′tə-mē) *n.* **1.** Excision of the lingular portion of the left upper lobe of the lung. **2.** See **glossectomy**.

linguo– *pref.* Tongue: *linguoversion.*

lin·guo·clu·sion (lĭng′gwə-kloo′zhən) *n.* Displacement of a tooth toward the interior of the dental arch, or toward the tongue.

lin·guo·pap·il·li·tis (lĭng′gwō-păp′ə-lī′tĭs) *n.* Small painful ulcers involving the papillae on the tongue margins.

lin·guo·ver·sion (lĭng′gwə-vûr′zhən) *n.* Malposition of a tooth, lingual to the normal position.

lin·i·ment (lĭn′ə-mənt) *n.* A liquid preparation rubbed into the skin or gums as a counterirritant, rubefacient, anodyne, or cleansing agent.

li·ni·tis (lĭ-nī′tĭs, lī-) *n.* Inflammation of cellular tissue, especially of the perivascular tissue of the stomach.

linitis plas·ti·ca (plăs′tĭ-kə) *n.* Thickening and fibrous proliferation in the wall of the stomach caused by the infiltration of scirrhous carcinoma.

link·age (lĭng′kĭj) *n.* An association between two or more genes such that the traits they control tend to be inherited together.

linkage disequilibrium *n.* The nonrandom association between two or more alleles such that certain combinations of alleles are more likely to occur together on a chromosome than other combinations of alleles.

linkage group *n.* A pair or set of genes on a chromosome that tend to be inherited together.

linkage marker *n.* A locus at which there is a high probability of heterozygotes.

linked (lĭngkt) *adj.* Exhibiting linkage.

link·er (lĭng′kər) *n.* A fragment of synthetic DNA containing a restriction site that may be used for splicing of genes.

Lin·nae·us (lĭ-nē′əs, -nā′-), **Carolus** Known as "Karl Linné." 1707–1778. Swedish botanist and founder of the modern binomial classification system for plants and animals.

lin·o·le·ic acid (lĭn′ə-lē′ĭk) *n.* An unsaturated fatty acid considered essential to the human diet.

lip (lĭp) *n.* **1.** Either of two fleshy folds that surround the opening of the mouth. **2.** A liplike structure bounding or encircling a bodily cavity or groove.

lip– *pref.* Variant of **lipo–**.

lip·ase (lĭp′ās′, lī′pās′) *n.* Any of a group of lipolytic enzymes that cleave a fatty acid residue from the glycerol residue in a neutral fat or a phospholipid.

lip·ec·to·my (lĭ-pĕk′tə-mē, lī-) *n.* Excision of subcutaneous fatty tissue.

lip·e·de·ma (lĭp′ĭ-dē′mə) *n.* Chronic swelling, usually of the lower extremities, caused by the widespread, even distribution of subcutaneous fat and fluid.

lip·e·dem·a·tous alopecia (lĭp′ĭ-dĕm′ə-təs) *n.* Hair loss characterized by itching, soreness, or tenderness of the scalp, thickening of the scalp, and thinning and shortening of the hair.

li·pe·mi·a (lĭ-pē′mē-ə) *n.* See **hyperlipidemia**.

lipemia ret·i·na·lis (rĕt′n-ā′lĭs) *n.* A creamy appearance of the retinal blood vessels that occurs when the concentration of lipids in the blood surpasses five percent.

li·pe·mic (lĭ-pē′mĭk) *adj.* Relating to lipemia.

lip·id (lĭp′ĭd, lī′pĭd) *or* **lip·ide** (lĭp′īd′, lī′pīd′) *n.* Any of a group of organic compounds, including the fats, oils, waxes, sterols, and triglycerides, that are insoluble in water but soluble in common organic solvents, are oily to the touch, and together with carbohydrates and proteins constitute the principal structural material of living cells. —**lip·id′ic** *adj.*

lip·i·de·mi·a (lĭp′ĭ-dē′mē-ə) *or* **lip·oi·de·mi·a** (lĭp′oi-) *n.* See **hyperlipidemia**.

lipid granulomatosis *n.* See **xanthomatosis**.

lipid histiocytosis *n.* Histiocytosis with cytoplasmic accumulation of lipid.

lip·i·do·sis (lĭp′ĭ-dō′sĭs) *n., pl.* **–ses** (-sēz) An inborn or acquired disorder of the lipid metabolism.

lipid pneumonia *or* **lipoid pneumonia** *n.* Inflammatory and fibrotic changes in the lungs due to the inhalation of various fatty substances, or due to accumulation in the lungs of endogenous lipid material following the fracture of a bone.

lipid proteinosis *n.* An inherited lipid metabolism disorder characterized by deposits of a protein-lipid complex on the labial mucosa and sublingual and faucial areas, and by papillomatous eyelid lesions.

Lip·i·tor (lĭp′ə-tôr′) A trademark for the drug atorvastatin calcium.

Lip·mann (lĭp′mən), **Fritz Albert** 1899–1986. German-born American biochemist. He shared a 1953 Nobel Prize for studies of metabolic processes.

lipo– *or* **lip–** *pref.* Fat; fatty; fatty tissue: *lipolysis.*

lip·o·ar·thri·tis (lĭp′ō-är-thrī′tĭs) *n.* Inflammation of the periarticular fatty tissues of the knee.

lip·o·ate (lĭp′ō-āt′) *n.* A salt or ester of lipoic acid.

lip·o·at·ro·phy (lĭp′ō-ăt′rə-fē) *n.* The loss of subcutaneous fat.

lip·o·blast (lĭp′ə-blăst′) *n.* An embryonic fat cell.

lip·o·blas·to·ma (lĭp′ō-blă-stō′mə) *n.* **1.** See **liposarcoma. 2.** A tumor, usually occurring in infants, composed of embryonal fat cells separated into distinct lobules.

lip·o·blas·to·ma·to·sis (lĭp′ō-blă-stō′mə-tō′sĭs) *n.* A diffuse form of lipoblastoma that infiltrates locally but does not metastasize.

lip·o·cele (lĭp′ə-sēl′) *n.* Presence of fatty tissue, without intestine, in a hernia sac. Also called *adipocele.*

lip·o·cere (lĭp′ə-sîr′) *n.* See **adipocere.**

lip·o·chon·dro·dys·tro·phy (lĭp′ō-kŏn′drə-dĭs′trə-fē) *n.* See **Hurler's syndrome.**

lip·o·chrome (lĭp′ə-krōm′) *n.* **1.** A pigmented lipid, such as lutein. **2.** Any of several yellow pigments resembling carotene and xanthophyll that are frequently found in the serum, skin, adrenal cortex, corpus luteum, and arteriosclerotic plaques, and in the liver, spleen, and adipose tissue.

lip·o·crit (lĭp′ə-krĭt′) *n.* A procedure for separating and volumetrically analyzing the amount of lipid in the blood or other body fluid.

lip·o·cyte (lĭp′ə-sīt′) *n.* A fat-storing stellate cell of the liver.

lip·o·der·moid (lĭp′ō-dûr′moid′) *n.* A congenital, yellowish-white, fatty, benign tumor located beneath the conjunctiva of the eye.

lip·o·dys·tro·phy (lĭp′ō-dĭs′trə-fē) *n.* Defective metabolism of fat.

lip·o·e·de·ma (lĭp′ō-ĭ-dē′mə) *n.* Edema of subcutaneous fat, which causes painful swellings, especially of the legs in women.

lip·o·fi·bro·ma (lĭp′ō-fī-brō′mə) *n.* A benign neoplasm of fibrous connective tissue, with conspicuous numbers of adipose cells.

lip·o·fus·cin (lĭp′ō-fŭs′ĭn, -fyoo′sĭn) *n.* Brown pigment granules representing lipid-containing residues of lysosomal digestion.

lip·o·fus·ci·no·sis (lĭp′ə-fŭs′ə-nō′sĭs, -fyoo′sə-) *n.* Abnormal storage of any one of a group of fatty pigments.

lip·o·gen·e·sis (lĭp′ə-jĕn′ĭ-sĭs) *n.* **1.** Production of fat, either fatty degeneration or fatty infiltration. Also called *adipogenesis.* **2.** The normal deposition of fat or the conversion of carbohydrate or protein to fat. —**lip′o·gen′ic** (-jĕn′ĭk), **li·pog′e·nous** (lĭ-pŏj′ə-nəs) *adj.*

lip·o·gran·u·lo·ma (lĭp′ō-grăn′yə-lō′mə) *n.* A nodule of granulomatous inflammation, associated with lipid deposits in tissues. Also called *eleoma.*

lip·o·gran·u·lo·ma·to·sis (lĭp′ō-grăn′yə-lō′mə-tō′sĭs) *n.* **1.** A condition marked by the presence of lipogranulomas. **2.** A local inflammatory reaction to the necrosis of adipose tissue.

li·po·ic acid (lĭ-pō′ĭk) *n.* An organic acid produced by cells of certain microorganisms and essential to oxidative decarboxylation of pyruvate to acetyl-CoA during metabolism. Also called *factor II.*

lip·oid (lĭp′oid′, lī′poid′) *adj.* Resembling fat; adipoid. —*n.* Lipid. No longer in technical use.

lip·oi·de·mi·a (lĭp′oi-dē′mē-ə) *n.* Variant of **lipidemia.**

lipoid granuloma *n.* A granuloma characterized by large mononuclear phagocytes that contain lipid.

lipoid nephrosis *n.* See **membranous glomerulonephritis.**

lip·oi·do·sis (lĭp′oi-dō′sĭs) *n.* Lipidosis.

li·pol·y·sis (lĭ-pŏl′ĭ-sĭs, lī-) *n., pl.* **–ses** (-sēz′) The hydrolysis of lipids. —**lip′o·lyt′ic** (lĭp′ə-lĭt′ĭk, lī′pə-) *adj.*

li·po·ma (lĭ-pō′mə, lī-) *n., pl.* **–mas** *or* **–ma·ta** (-mə-tə) A benign tumor composed chiefly of fat cells.

lipoma sar·co·ma·to·des (sär-kō′mə-tō′dēz) *n.* Liposarcoma.

li·po·ma·toid (lĭ-pō′mə-toid′) *adj.* Resembling a lipoma. Used of accumulations of adipose tissue not thought to be neoplastic.

li·po·ma·to·sis (lĭ-pō′mə-tō′sĭs) *n.* See **adiposis.**

li·po·ma·tous (lĭ-pō′mə-təs) *adj.* Relating to, manifesting the features of, or characterized by the presence of a lipoma.

lipomatous infiltration *n.* Nonencapsulated adipose tissue forming a lipomalike mass, usually in the interatrial septum of the heart, where it may cause arrythmia and sudden death.

lip·o·me·nin·go·cele (lĭp′ō-mə-nĭng′gə-sēl′) *n.* An intraspinal lipoma associated with a spina bifida.

lip·o·mu·co·pol·y·sac·cha·ri·do·sis (lĭp′ō-myoo′kō-pŏl′ē-săk′ə-rĭ-dō′sĭs) *n.* See **mucolipidosis I.**

lip·o·pe·ni·a (lĭp′ə-pē′nē-ə) *n.* An abnormally small amount or a deficiency of lipids in the body.

lip·o·phage (lĭp′ə-fāj′) *n.* A cell that ingests fat.

lip·o·pha·gic (lĭp′ə-fā′jĭk, -făj′ĭk) *adj.* Of or relating to lipophagy.

lipophagic granuloma *n.* A lesion formed as a result of the inflammatory reaction provoked by pockets of necrosis in subcutaneous fat, as in certain types of traumatic injury.

li·poph·a·gy (lĭ-pŏf′ə-jē, lĭp′ə-fā′jē) *n.* The ingestion of fat by a lipophage.

lip·o·phil (lĭp′ə-fĭl′) *n.* A substance having an affinity for, tending to combine with, or capable of dissolving in lipids. —**lip′o·phil′ic** *adj. & n.*

lip·o·pol·y·sac·cha·ride (lĭp′ō-pŏl′ē-săk′ə-rīd′, lī′pō-) *n.* Any of a group of polysaccharides in which a lipid constitutes a portion of the molecule.

lip·o·pro·tein (lĭp′ō-prō′tēn′, lī′pō-) *n.* Any of a group of conjugated proteins that have at least one lipid component and are the principal means by which lipids are transported in the blood.

lipoprotein lipase *n.* An enzyme that cleaves one fatty acid from a triacylglycerol.

lip·o·sar·co·ma (lĭp′ō-sär-kō′mə) *n.* A malignant tumor consisting chiefly of immature, anaplastic lipoblasts of varying sizes, usually occurring in association with a rich network of capillaries. Also called *lipoblastoma.*

lip·o·sculp·ture (lĭp′ō-skŭlp′chər, lī′pō-) *n.* Liposuction that uses ultrasound to break fat into small sections before removal.

li·po·sis (lĭ-pō′sĭs) *n.* **1.** See **adiposis. 2.** Fatty infiltration of tissue, with neutral fats being present in the cells.

lip·o·sol·u·ble (lĭp′ō-sŏl′yə-bəl) *adj.* Soluble in fats or fat solvents.

lip·o·some (lĭp′ə-sōm′, lī′pə-) *n.* An artificial microscopic vesicle consisting of an aqueous core enclosed in one or more phospholipid layers, used to convey vaccines, drugs, enzymes, or other substances to target cells or organs.

lip·o·suc·tion (lĭp′ō-sŭk′shən, lī′pō-) *n.* A usually cosmetic surgical procedure in which excess subcutaneous fat is removed from a specific area of the body, such as the thighs or abdomen, by means of suction.

lip·o·troph·ic (lĭp′ō-trŏf′ĭk, -trō′fĭk) *adj.* Of or relating to lipotrophy.

li·pot·ro·phy (lĭ-pŏt′rə-fē) *n.* An increase of fat in the body.

lip·o·tro·pin (lĭp′ə-trō′pĭn, lī′pə-) *n.* A hormone produced by the anterior pituitary gland that promotes the utilization of fat by the body and is a precursor to the endorphins.

lip·o·vac·cine (lĭp′ō-văk-sēn′ -văk′sēn′) *n.* A vaccine having a vegetable oil as a vehicle.

li·pox·y·gen·ase (lĭ-pŏk′sĭ-jə-nās′, -nāz′) *n.* An enzyme that catalyzes oxidation of unsaturated fatty acids with oxygen to yield peroxides. Also called *lipoxidase.*

lip·ping (lĭp′ĭng) *n.* Formation of a liplike structure, as at the articular end of a bone in osteoarthritis.

lip reflex *n.* A pouting movement of the lips in young infants occurring in response to tapping near the angle of the mouth.

li·pu·ri·a (lĭ-pŏor′ē-ə) *n.* Excretion of fat in the urine. Also called *adiposuria.* —**li·pu′ric** *adj.*

liq·ue·fa·cient (lĭk′wə-fā′shənt) *n.* An agent capable of causing a solid to become liquid.

liq·ue·fac·tion (lĭk′wə-făk′shən) *n.* **1.** The process of liquefying. **2.** The state of being liquefied.

liq·ue·fac·tive necrosis (lĭk′wə-făk′tĭv) *n.* Necrosis marked by a circumscribed lesion consisting of the fluid remains of necrotic tissue that was digested by enzymes. Also called *colliquative necrosis.*

li·ques·cent (lĭ-kwĕs′ənt) *adj.* Becoming or tending to become liquid; melting.

liq·uid (lĭk′wĭd) *n.* **1.** The state of matter in which a substance exhibits a characteristic readiness to flow, little or no tendency to disperse, and relatively high incompressibility. **2.** Matter or a specific body of matter in this state. —*adj.* **1.** Of or being a liquid. **2.** Having been liquefied, especially melted by heating or condensed by cooling. **3.** Flowing readily; fluid. —**liq′uid·ly** *adv.*

liquid-liquid chromatography *n.* Chromatography in which both the moving phase and the stationary (or reverse-moving) phase are liquids.

liq·uor (lĭk′ər) *n.* **1.** An aqueous solution, especially of a medicinal substance. **2.** An alcoholic beverage made by distillation rather than by fermentation. **3.** (lī′kwôr, lĭk′wôr) In anatomical nomenclature, a term for any of several body fluids.

Lis·franc's joint (lĭs-frănks′, lēs-fräɴ′) *n.* See **tarsometatarsal joint.**

Li Shih-Chen (lē′ shər′chŭn′) 1518–1593. Chinese biologist and pharmacist whose *Great Pharmacopoeia* (1596) became the standard text of Chinese herbal medicine.

li·sin·o·pril (lī-sĭn′ə-prĭl′) *n.* An ACE inhibitor drug used in the treatment of hypertension and congestive heart failure.

lisp (lĭsp) *n.* A speech defect or mannerism characterized by mispronunciation of the sounds (s) and (z) as (th) and (*th*). —*v.* To speak with a lisp.

lis·sen·ce·pha·li·a (lĭs′ĕn-sə-fā′lē-ə, -fāl′yə) *or* **lis·sen·ceph·a·ly** (-sĕf′ə-lē) *n.* See **agyria.** —**lis′sen·ce·phal′ic** (-sə-făl′ĭk) *adj.*

lis·sive (lĭs′ĭv) *adj.* Having the property of relieving muscle spasm without causing flaccidity.

lis·so·tric·ic (lĭs′ə-trĭk′ĭk) *or* **lis·so·trich·ous** (-trĭk′əs) *adj.* Having straight hair.

Lis·ter (lĭs′tər), **Joseph** First Baron Lister. 1827–1912. British surgeon who demonstrated in 1865 that carbolic acid was an effective antiseptic agent and introduced it to the surgical process.

Lis·te·ri·a (lĭ-stîr′ē-ə) *n.* A genus of aerobic parasitic bacteria containing small, coccoid, gram-positive rods that tend to form chains of three to five members. They are found in the feces of humans and other animals, on vegetation, and in silage.

lis·te·ri·o·sis (lĭ-stîr′ē-ō′sĭs) *n.* A bacterial disease caused by *Listeria monocytogenes,* affecting wild and domestic animals and occasionally humans and characterized by fever, meningitis, and encephalitis.

Lis·ter's method (lĭs′tərz) *n.* Antiseptic surgery, as first advocated by English surgeon Joseph Lister. Also called *listerism.*

Lis·ting's law (lĭs′tĭngz) *n.* The principle that when the eye turns from looking at one object and fixes upon another, it revolves about an axis perpendicular to a plane cutting both the former and the present lines of vision.

li·ter (lē′tər) *n. Abbr.* **L, l** A unit of volume equal to 1000 cubic centimeters or to 1 cubic decimeter (1.0567 quarts).

–lith *suff.* Mineral concretion; calculus: *cystolith.*

lith·a·gogue (lĭth′ə-gôg′) *n.* An agent that causes the dislodgment or expulsion of calculi, especially urinary calculi. —**lith′a·gogue′** *adj.*

li·thec·to·my (lĭ-thĕk′tə-mē) *n.* See **lithotomy.**

li·thi·a·sis (lĭ-thī′ə-sĭs) *n., pl.* **–ses** (-sēz′) The formation of calculi of any kind, especially biliary or urinary calculi.

lith·i·um (lĭth′ē-əm) *n. Symbol* **Li** A soft, highly reactive metallic element whose carbonate form is used in psychopharmacology. Atomic number 3.

lithium carbonate *n.* A lithium salt used in the treatment of depression and mania associated with bipolar disorder.

litho– *or* **lith–** *pref.* Mineral concretion; calculus: *lithotomy.*

lith·o·clast (lĭth′ə-klăst′) *n.* See **lithotrite.**

lith·o·di·al·y·sis (lĭth′ō-dī-ăl′ĭ-sĭs) *n.* The fragmentation or dissolution of a calculus.

lith·o·gen·e·sis (lĭth′ə-jĕn′ĭ-sĭs) *n.* The formation of calculi.

lith·o·gen·ic (lĭth′ə-jĕn′ĭk) *adj.* Promoting the formation of calculi.

li·thog·e·nous (lĭ-thŏj′ə-nəs) *adj.* Forming or promoting the development of calculi.

li·thol·a·pax·y (lĭ-thŏl′ə-păk′sē, lĭth′ə-lə-) *n.* The procedure of crushing of a stone in the bladder and washing out the fragments through a catheter.

li·thol·y·sis (lĭ-thŏl′ĭ-sĭs) *n.* The dissolution of urinary calculi.

lith·o·lyt·ic (lĭth′ə-lĭt′ĭk) *n.* An agent that dissolves calculi. —**lith′o·lyt′ic** *adj.*

lith·o·ne·phri·tis (lĭth′ō-nə-frī′tĭs) *n.* Inflammation of the kidney due to irritation by calculi.

lith·o·pe·di·on (lĭth′ə-pē′dē-ŏn′) *n.* A dead fetus, usually extrauterine, that has become calcified.

lith·o·scope (lĭth′ə-skōp′) *n.* See **cystoscope.**

Lith·o·stat (lĭth′ə-stăt′) A trademark for the drug acetohydroxamic acid.

li·thot·o·my (lĭ-thŏt′ə-mē) *n.* Surgical removal of a calculus, especially from the urinary tract. Also called *lithectomy.*

lithotomy position *n.* A supine position in which the hips and knees are fully flexed with the legs spread apart and raised and the feet resting in straps. Also called *dorsosacral position.*

lith·o·trip·sy (lĭth′ə-trĭp′sē) *n.* The procedure of crushing a stone in the urinary bladder or urethra. Also called *lithotrity.*

lith·o·trip·ter (lĭth′ə-trĭp′tər) *n.* A device that pulverizes kidney stones by passing shock waves through a water-filled tub in which the patient sits. The procedure creates stone fragments small enough to be expelled in the urine.

lith·o·trip·tic (lĭth′ə-trĭp′tĭk) *n.* An agent that effects the dissolution of a calculus. —**lith′o·trip′tic** *adj.*

lith·o·trip·tos·co·py (lĭth′ə-trĭp-tŏs′kə-pē) *n.* The crushing of a stone in the bladder while viewing directly through a cystoscope.

lith·o·trite (lĭth′ə-trīt′) *n.* An instrument used to crush a stone present in the bladder or urethra. Also called *lithoclast.*

li·thot·ri·ty (lĭ-thŏt′rĭ-tē) *n.* See **lithotripsy.**

lith·u·re·sis (lĭth′yoō-rē′sĭs) *n.* The passage of small calculi in the urine.

lit·mus (lĭt′məs) *n.* A water-soluble blue powder derived from lichens that changes to red with increasing acidity and to blue with increasing basicity.

litmus paper *n.* An unsized white paper impregnated with litmus and used as a pH or acid-base indicator.

litmus test *n.* A test for chemical acidity or basicity using litmus paper.

Lit·ten's phenomenon (lĭt′nz) *n.* See **diaphragm phenomenon.**

lit·ter (lĭt′ər) *n.* **1.** A flat supporting framework, such as a piece of canvas stretched between parallel shafts, for carrying a disabled or dead person; a stretcher. **2.** The offspring produced at one birth by a multiparous mammal. Also called *brood.*

Little Leaguer's elbow *n.* Epicondylitis of the elbow at the origin of the flexor muscles of the forearm due to throwing; usually seen in children or adolescents.

Lit·tre's hernia (lē′trəz, lē-trāz′) *n.* See **parietal hernia.**

Litz·mann obliquity (lĭts′mən, -män′) *n.* Inclination of the fetal head so that the biparietal diameter is oblique in relation to the plane of the pelvic brim, the posterior parietal bone presenting to the birth canal. Also called *posterior asynclitism.*

live (līv) *adj.* **1.** Having life; alive. **2.** Capable of replicating in a host's cells. **3.** Containing living microorganisms or viruses capable of replicating in a host's cells.

li·ve·do (lĭ-vē′dō) *n.* A bluish discoloration of the skin. Also called *suggillation.*

liv·e·doid (lĭv′ĭ-doid′) *adj.* Relating to or resembling livedo.

livedoid dermatitis *n.* A reddish-blue mottled condition of skin caused by inflammation of the cutaneous blood vessels.

livedo re·tic·u·lar·is (rĭ-tĭk′yə-lâr′ĭs) *n.* A purplish network-patterned discoloration of the skin caused by dilation of capillaries and venules.

liv·er (lĭv′ər) *n.* The largest gland of the body, lying beneath the diaphragm in the upper right portion of the abdominal cavity, which secretes bile and is active in the formation of certain blood proteins and in the metabolism of carbohydrates, fats, and proteins.

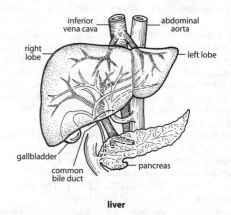

inferior vena cava — abdominal aorta — right lobe — left lobe — gallbladder — common bile duct — pancreas

liver

liver acinus *n.* The smallest functional unit of the liver, comprising all the liver parenchyma, composed of segments of several hepatic lobules, and having as its central axis a terminal branch of the portal vein, hepatic artery, and bile duct.

liver spot *n.* See **age spot.**

live vaccine *n.* A vaccine prepared from living attenuated organisms or from viruses that have been attenuated but can still replicate the cells of the host organism.

liv·id (lĭv′ĭd) *adj.* Having a black-and-blue or a leaden or ashy-gray color, as in discoloration from a contusion, congestion, or cyanosis.

liv·ing will (lĭv′ĭng) *n.* A will in which the signer requests not to be kept alive by medical life-support systems in the event of a terminal illness.

li·vor (lī′vôr, -vər) *n.* The livid discoloration of the skin on the dependent parts of a body after death.

lix·iv·i·a·tion (lĭk-sĭv′ē-ā′shən) *n.* The removal of the soluble constituents of a substance by the action of a percolating liquid. Also called *leaching.* —**lix·iv′i·ate′** (lĭk-sĭv′ē-āt′) *v.*

LLL *abbr.* left lower lobe (of the lung)

LLQ *abbr.* left lower quadrant (of the abdomen)

LM *abbr.* Licentiate in Midwifery

LMP *abbr.* last menstrual period

LNPF *abbr.* lymph node permeability factor

load (lōd) *n.* A departure from normal body content, as of water, salt, or heat. A positive load is a quantity in excess of the normal; a negative load is a deficit.

load·ing (lō′dĭng) *n.* The administration of a substance for the purpose of testing metabolic function.

Lo·a lo·a (lō′ə lō′ə) *n.* A threadlike worm, a species of the family Onchocercidae indigenous to the western part of equatorial Africa. It is the causative agent of loiasis.

lo·bar (lō′bər, -bär′) *adj.* Of or relating to a lobe or lobes.

lobar pneumonia *n.* Pneumonia affecting one or more lobes of the lung, commonly due to infection by *Streptococcus pneumoniae.*

lo·bate (lō′bāt′) *adj.* **1.** Divided into lobes. **2.** Lobe-shaped. —**lo′bate′ly** *adv.*

lobe (lōb) *n.* **1.** A rounded projection, especially a rounded, projecting anatomical part, such as the lobe of the ear. **2.** A subdivision of a body organ or part bounded by fissures, connective tissue, or other structural boundaries. **3.** One of the larger divisions of the crown of a tooth, formed from a distinct point of calcification.

lo·bec·to·my (lō-bĕk′tə-mē) *n.* Excision of a lobe of an organ or a gland.

lo·bi·tis (lō-bī′tĭs) *n.* Inflammation of a lobe.

lo·bo·po·di·um (lō′bə-pō′dē-əm) *n.*, *pl.* **–di·a** (-dē-ə) A thick, cylindrical pseudopodium.

lo·bot·o·my (lə-bŏt′ə-mē, lō-) *n.* **1.** Incision into a lobe. **2.** The division of one or more nerve tracts in a lobe of the cerebrum.

lob·ster-claw deformity (lŏb′stər-clô′) *n.* A deformity of a hand or foot in which the middle digits are missing or fused.

lobular glomerulonephritis *n.* See **membranoproliferative glomerulonephritis.**

lob·u·late (lŏb′yə-lāt′) *or* **lob·u·lat·ed** (-lā′tĭd) *adj.* Divided into lobules.

lob·ule (lŏb′yōōl) *n.* **1.** A small lobe. **2.** A section or subdivision of a lobe. —**lob′u·lar** (-yə-lər), **lob′u·lose′** (-yə-lōs′) *adj.*

lobule of epididymis *n.* Any of the coiled portions of the efferent ducts constituting the head of the epididymis and joining the duct of the epididymis.

lob·u·lus (lŏb′yə-ləs) *n.*, *pl.* **lob·u·li** (-lī′) A lobule.

lo·bus (lō′bəs) *n.*, *pl.* **–bi** (-bī) Lobe.

lobus az·y·gos (ăz′ĭ-gŏs′, ā-zī′-) *n.* A small accessory lobe sometimes found on the upper part of the right lung, separated from the rest of the upper lobe by a deep groove lodging the azygos vein.

LOC *abbr.* loss of consciousness

lo·cal (lō′kəl) *adj.* Affecting or confined to a specific part of the body; not general or systemic. —*n.* Local anesthesia.

local anaphylaxis *n.* The immediate, temporary, localized anaphylactic response of a sensitized individual following injection of an antigen into the skin.

local anesthesia *n.* Regional anesthesia produced by direct infiltration of local anesthetic solution into the surgical site. Also called *infiltration anesthesia.*

local anesthetic *n.* An agent that, when applied directly to mucous membranes or when injected about the nerves, produces loss of sensation by inhibiting nerve excitation or conduction.

local asphyxia *n.* Stagnation of the circulation, sometimes resulting in localized gangrene, especially of the fingers.

local death *n.* Death of a part of the body or of a tissue by necrosis.

local flap *n.* A surgical flap that is transferred to an adjacent area.

local immunity *n.* Natural or acquired immunity to an infectious agent that is limited to a particular organ or tissue.

lo·cal·i·za·tion (lō′kə-lĭ-zā′shən) *n.* **1.** Limitation to a specific area. **2.** The reference of a sensation to its point of origin. **3.** The determination of the location of a pathological process.

lo·cal·ized (lō′kə-līzd′) *adj.* Restricted or limited to a specific part.

localized nodular tenosynovitis *n.* See **giant cell tumor of tendon sheath.**

localized scleroderma *n.* See **morphea.**

lo·cal·iz·ing symptom (lō′kə-lī′zĭng) *n.* A symptom indicating clearly the location of the diseased area.

local reaction *n.* See **focal reaction.**

local stimulant *n.* A stimulant whose action is confined to the part to which it is applied.

lo·ca·tor (lō′kā′tər) *n.* An instrument or apparatus for finding the position of a foreign object in tissue.

lo·chi·a (lō′kē-ə, lŏk′ē-ə) *pl.n.* The normal uterine discharge of blood, tissue, and mucus from the vagina after childbirth. —**lo′chi·al** *adj.*

lo·chi·o·me·tra (lō′kē-ə-mē′trə) *n.* Distention of the uterus with retained lochia.

lo·chi·o·me·tri·tis (lō′kē-ə-mĭ-trī′tĭs) *n.* See **puerperal metritis.**

lo·chi·or·rhe·a (lō′kē-ə-rē′ə) *n.* A profuse flow of the lochia. Also called *lochiorrhagia.*

locked knee *n.* A disorder of the knee joint that prevents the leg from being fully extended, usually resulting from damage to the semilunar cartilage.

lock·jaw (lŏk′jô′) *n.* **1.** See **tetanus** (sense 1). **2.** See **trismus.**

lo·co·mo·tor (lō′kə-mō′tər) *or* **lo·co·mo·tive** (-mō′tĭv) *adj.* Of or relating to movement from one place to another.

locomotor ataxia *n.* See **tabes dorsalis.**

loc·u·lar (lŏk′yə-lər) *adj.* Divided into or having loculi.

loc·u·late (lŏk′yə-lāt′) *adj.* Having or containing numerous loculi.

loc·u·la·tion (lŏk′yə-lā′shən) *n.* The process that results in the formation of a loculus or of loculi.

loc·ule (lŏk′yōōl) *or* **loc·u·lus** (-yə-ləs) *n.* A small cavity or compartment within an organ or a part of an animal.

lo·cus (lō′kəs) *n., pl.* **-ci** (-sī′, -kē, -kī′) **1.** A place; site. **2.** The position that a given gene occupies on a chromosome.

locus of control *n.* A theoretical construct designed to assess a person's perceived control over his or her own behavior. The classification *internal locus* indicates that the person feels in control of events; *external locus* indicates that others are perceived to have that control.

Lo·dine (lō′dēn′) A trademark for the drug etodolac.

Loeb's deciduoma (lōbz) *n.* A mass of decidual tissue that is produced in the uterus in the absence of a fertilized ovum by adminstration of mechanical or hormonal stimulation.

Loe·wi (lō′ē, lœ′vē), **Otto** 1873–1961. German-born American pharmacologist. He shared a 1936 Nobel Prize for work on the chemical transmission of nerve impulses.

Löff·ler (lĕf′lər, lœf′-), **Friedrich August Johannes** 1852–1915. German bacteriologist who isolated (1884) the bacillus that is the causative agent of diphtheria, previously described by Edwin Klebs.

Löff·ler's endocarditis (lĕf′lərz, lœf′-) *n.* Endocarditis of obscure cause characterized by progressive congestive heart failure, multiple systemic emboli, and eosinophilia.

log·ag·no·sia (lŏg′ăg-nō′zhə) *n.* See **aphasia**.

log·am·ne·sia (lŏg′ăm-nē′zhə) *n.* See **aphasia**.

log·a·pha·sia (lŏg′ə-fā′zhə) *n.* Aphasia of articulation.

log·as·the·ni·a (lŏg′ăs-thē′nē-ə) *n.* See **aphasia**.

logo– *or* **log–** *pref.* Word; speech: *logoplegia.*

log·o·ple·gia (lŏg′ə-plē′jə) *n.* Paralysis of the organs of speech.

log·or·rhe·a (lŏg′ə-rē′ə) *n.* Excessive use of words.

–logy *suff.* Science; theory; study: *dermatology.*

lo·i·a·sis (lō-ī′ə-sĭs) *n.* A chronic disease caused by infestation of the subcutaneous connective tissue of the body with the worm *Loa loa* and characterized by hyperemia, exudation of fluid, and a creeping sensation in the tissues with intense itching.

loin (loin) *n.* The part of the body on either side of the spinal column between the ribs and the pelvis.

Lo·mo·til (lō′mə-tĭl′) A trademark for a drug combination of diphenoxylate hydrochloride and atropine.

Long (lông), **Crawford Williamson** 1815–1878. American surgeon and pioneer anesthetist who was among the first (1842) to use ether as an anesthetic.

long abductor muscle of thumb *n.* A muscle with origin from the posterior surfaces of the radius and the ulna, with insertion to the base of the first metacarpal bone, with nerve supply from the radial nerve, and whose action abducts the thumb and assists in extending it.

long-acting thyroid stimulator *n. Abbr.* **LATS** A substance that is present in the blood of hyperthyroid patients and that exerts a prolonged stimulatory effect on the thyroid gland.

long axis *n.* A line parallel to an object lengthwise, as in the body the imaginary line that runs vertically through the head down to the space between the feet.

long bone *n.* One of the elongated bones of the extremities, consisting of a tubular shaft, which is composed of compact bone surrounding a central marrow-filled cavity, and two expanded portions that usually serve as articulation points.

long ciliary nerve *n.* One of two or three branches of the nasociliary nerve, supplying the ciliary muscles, the iris, and the cornea.

long elevator muscle of rib *n.* Any of the muscles with insertion into the second rib below their origin, with nerve supply from the intercostal nerve, and whose actions raise the ribs.

lon·gev·i·ty (lŏn-jĕv′ĭ-tē) *n.* Duration of an individual life beyond the norm for the species.

long extensor muscle of big toe *n.* A muscle with its origin from the tibia, with insertion to the base of the big toe, with nerve supply from the anterior tibial nerve, and whose action extends the big toe.

long extensor muscle of thumb *n.* A muscle with origin from the ulna, with insertion into the base of the thumb, with nerve supply from the radial nerve, and whose action extends the distal phalanx of the thumb.

long extensor muscle of toes *n.* A muscle with its origin from the tibia and the upper margin of the fibula, with insertion by four tendons to the bases of the phalanges of the second to fifth toes, with nerve supply from the deep branch of the peroneal nerve, and whose action extends the four toes.

long flexor muscle of big toe *n.* A muscle with its origin from the fibula, with insertion to the base of the big toe, with nerve supply from the medial plantar nerve, and whose action flexes the big toe.

long flexor muscle of thumb *n.* A muscle with its origin from the radius, with insertion to a phalanx of the thumb, with nerve supply from the median palmar interosseous nerve, and whose action flexes the distal phalanx of the thumb.

long flexor muscle of toes *n.* A muscle with its origin in the middle third of the tibia, with insertion to the bases of the four lateral toes, with nerve supply from the tibial nerve, and whose action flexes the second to the fifth toes.

long gyrus of insula *n.* The most posterior and longest of the slender and relatively straight gyri that compose the insula of the brain.

lon·gis·si·mus cap·i·tis muscle (lŏn-jĭs′ə-məs căp′ĭ-tĭs) *n.* A muscle with origin from the upper thoracic vertebrae and the lower and middle cervical vertebrae, with insertion into the mastoid process, with nerve supply from the dorsal branches of the cervical nerves, and whose action keeps the head erect and draws it backward or to one side.

lon·gi·tu·di·nal (lŏn′jĭ-tōōd′n-əl) *adj.* Running in the direction of the long axis of the body or any of its parts.

longitudinal aberration *n.* The distance separating the focus of paraxial and peripheral rays on the optic axis in spherical aberration.

longitudinal fissure of cerebrum *n.* A deep cleft separating the two hemispheres of the cerebrum, but bridged by the corpus callosum and the hippocampal commissure.

longitudinal fracture *n.* A fracture that follows the long axis of the bone.

longitudinal lie *n.* An anatomical relationship in which the long axis of the fetus is longitudinal and roughly parallel to the long axis of the mother.

longitudinal ligament *n.* Either of two extensive fibrous bands, anterior and posterior, that connect the bodies of the vertebrae by attachment to the intervertebral disks.

longitudinal muscle *n.* Either of the lingual muscles: inferior lingual and superficial lingual.

longitudinal pontine bundle *n.* Any of the massive bundles of corticifugal fibers passing longitudinally through the ventral part of the pons.

longitudinal raphe of tongue *n.* See **median groove of tongue**.

long muscle of head *n.* A muscle with origin from the third to sixth cervical vertebrae, with insertion into the basilar process of the occipital bone, with nerve supply from the cervical plexus, and whose action twists or bends the neck forward.

long muscle of neck *n.* A muscle whose medial portion arises from the third thoracic to the fifth cervical vertebrae and is inserted into the second to fourth cervical vertebrae, whose superolateral portion arises from the third to the fifth cervical vertebrae and is inserted into the anterior tubercle of the atlas, and whose inferolateral portion arises from the first to the third thoracic vertebrae and is inserted into the fifth and sixth cervical vertebrae; whose nerve supply for all three portions is from the ventral branches of the cervical nerve, and whose action for all three portions twists and bends the neck forward.

long palmar muscle *n.* A muscle with origin from the humerus, with insertion into the flexor retinaculum and the palmar fascia, with nerve supply from the median nerve, and whose action tenses the palmar fascia and flexes the hand and forearm.

long Q-T syndrome *n.* An inherited cardiac disorder in which a defect in potassium ion channels interferes with the transmission of electrical signals to the heart muscle, producing a prolonged Q-T interval on an electrocardiogram and sometimes causing cardiac arrhythmias.

long radial extensor muscle of wrist *n.* A muscle with origin from the humerus, with insertion to the base of the second metacarpal bone, with nerve supply from the radial nerve, and whose action extends and deviates the wrist toward the radius.

long-term care facility *n.* See **skilled nursing facility**.

long-term memory *n.* *Abbr.* **LTM** The phase of the memory process considered the permanent storehouse of retained information.

long thoracic nerve *n.* A nerve that arises from the fifth, sixth, and seventh cervical nerves, descends the neck behind the brachial plexus, and is distributed to the anterior serratus muscle.

Lon·i·ten (lŏn′ĭ-tn) A trademark for the drug minoxidil.

loop (lo͞op) *n.* **1.** A curve or bend in a cord or other cylindrical body, forming an oval or circular ring. **2.** A type of loop-shaped intrauterine device.

loop diuretic *n.* A class of diuretic agents that act by inhibiting reabsorption of sodium and chloride.

loop of Henle *n.* See **nephronic loop**.

loop of spinal nerves *n.* Any of the various connecting branches between the ventral branches of the spinal nerves.

loose (lo͞os) *adj.* **1.** No longer fixed or fully attached, as a tooth. **2.** Not compact or dense in arrangement or structure. **3.** Not taut or rigid. **4.** Of or relating to a cough that is accompanied by the production of mucus. **5.** Characterized by the unrestrained movement of bodily fluids, especially in the gastrointestinal tract.

loose-jointed *adj.* **1.** Having freely articulated, highly mobile joints. **2.** Limber or agile in movement.

loos·en·ing of association (lo͞o′sə-nĭng) *n.* A manifestation of a severe thought disorder characterized by the lack of an obvious connection between one thought or phrase and the next.

lo·per·a·mide hydrochloride (lō-pĕr′ə-mīd′) *n.* An over-the-counter drug that inhibits intestinal motility and is used to treat diarrhea.

Lo·pid (lō′pĭd) A trademark for the drug gemfibrozil.

Lo·pres·sor (lə-prĕs′ər) A trademark for the drug metoprolol tartrate.

Lo·prox (lō′prŏks′) A trademark for the drug ciclopirox olamine.

Lo·rain-Lé·vi syndrome (lə-rān′lā-vē′, lô-răn′-) *n.* See **pituitary dwarfism**.

lor·at·a·dine (lôr-ăt′ə-dēn′) *n.* A nonsedating antihistamine used to treat allergic rhinitis and other allergic disorders.

lor·az·e·pam (lôr-ăz′ə-păm′) *n.* A whitish powder that acts as a sedative and antianxiety agent and is used therapeutically to control seizures.

lor·do·sco·li·o·sis (lôr′dō-skō′lē-ō′sĭs, -skŏl′ē-) *n.* A combined backward and lateral curvature of the spine.

lor·do·sis (lôr-dō′sĭs) *n.* An abnormal forward curvature of the spine in the lumbar region. Also called *hollow back, saddle back.* —**lor·dot′ic** (-dŏt′ĭk) *adj.*

lo·sar·tan potassium (lō-sär′tăn) *n.* An oral drug that was the first in the angiotensin II receptor antagonist class, used to treat hypertension.

Lo·ten·sin (lō-tĕn′sĭn) A trademark for the drug benazepril hydrochloride.

lo·tion (lō′shən) *n.* **1.** A medicated preparation consisting of a liquid suspension or dispersion intended for external application. **2.** Any of various externally applied cosmetic liquids.

Lo·tri·min (lō′trə-mĭn′) A trademark for the drug clotrimazole.

Lou Geh·rig's disease (lo͞o′ gĕr′ĭgz) *n.* See **amyotrophic lateral sclerosis**.

loupe (lo͞op) *n.* A small magnifying lens.

louse (lous) *n., pl.* **lice** (līs) Any of numerous small, flat-bodied, wingless biting or sucking insects of the orders Mallophaga or Anoplura, many of which are external parasites on humans.

lo·va·stat·in (lō′və-stăt′n) *n.* A statin drug that is isolated from a strain of *Aspergillus terreus*, used to treat hyperlipidemia.

love handle (lŭv) *n.* A deposit of fat at the waistline. Often used in the plural.

low blood pressure (lō) *n.* Hypotension.

low calorie diet *n.* A diet of 1,200 calories or less per day.

low-compliance bladder *n.* A urinary bladder that has high pressure at low volumes in the absence of activity of the detrusor muscle.

low-density lipoprotein *n. Abbr.* **LDL** A lipoprotein that contains relatively high amounts of cholesterol and is associated with an increased risk of atherosclerosis and coronary artery disease. Also called *LDL cholesterol, beta-lipoprotein.*

low·er airway (lō′ər) *n.* The portion of the respiratory tract that extends from the subglottis through the terminal bronchioles.

lower esophageal sphincter *n.* A ring of smooth muscle fibers at the junction of the esophagus and stomach. Also called *cardiac sphincter.*

lower extremity *n.* The hip, thigh, leg, ankle, or foot. Also called *inferior limb, pelvic limb.*

lower motor neuron *n.* A motor neuron whose cell body is located in the brainstem or the spinal cord and whose axon innervates skeletal muscle fibers. Also called *final motor neuron.*

lower uterine segment *n.* The isthmus of the uterus, the lower extremity of which joins with the cervical canal and during pregnancy expands to become the lower part of the uterine cavity.

Lowe's syndrome (lōz) *n.* See **oculocerebrorenal syndrome.**

low·est splanchnic nerve (lō′ĭst) *n.* A nerve containing the sympathetic fibers for the renal plexus, usually contained in the lesser splanchnic nerve, but occasionally existing as an independent nerve.

Lowe-Ter·rey-Mac·Lach·lan syndrome (lō′tĕr′ē-mə-kläk′lən) *n.* See **oculocerebrorenal syndrome.**

lox·os·ce·lism (lŏk-sŏs′ə-lĭz′əm) *n.* A condition produced by the bite of the brown recluse spider of North America and characterized by a gangrenous slough at the site of bite, nausea, malaise, fever, hemolysis, and thrombocytopenia.

loz·enge (lŏz′ĭnj) *n.* A small, medicated candy intended to be dissolved slowly in the mouth to lubricate and soothe irritated tissues of the throat.

Lo·zi·er (lō′zē-ər), **Clemence Sophia Harned** 1813–1888. An American physician who, in 1863, founded the New York Medical College and Hospital for Women.

Lo·zol (lō′zôl′) A trademark for the drug indapamide.

LP *abbr.* lumbar puncture

LPN *abbr.* licensed practical nurse

Lr The symbol for the element **lawrencium.**

LRH *abbr.* luteinizing hormone-releasing hormone

LSA *abbr.* Licentiate of the Society of Apothecaries

LSD (ĕl′ĕs-dē′) *n.* Lysergic acid diethylamide; a crystalline compound derived from lysergic acid and used as a powerful hallucinogenic drug. Also called *acid, lysergide.*

LTH *abbr.* luteotropic hormone

LTM *abbr.* long-term memory

L-tryp·to·phan (ĕl′trĭp′tə-făn′) *n.* An isomer of the amino acid tryptophan that is a precursor in the for-mation of serotonin and is used as a dietary supplement outside the US.

Lu The symbol for the element **lutetium.**

lu·cid·i·ty (lōō-sĭd′ĭ-tē) *n.* Clarity, especially mental clarity.

lu·cif·u·gal (lōō-sĭf′yə-gəl) *adj.* Avoiding or repelled by light.

lu·cip·e·tal (lōō-sĭp′ĭ-tl) *adj.* Seeking or attracted to light.

lude (lōōd) *n.* A pill or tablet that contains the drug methaqualone.

Lud·wig's angina (lōōd′vĭgz) *n.* Cellulitis of the submandibular spaces of the mouth, usually spreading to the sublingual and submental spaces.

Ludwig's ganglion *n.* A small group of parasympathetic neurons in the interatrial septum of the heart.

Lu·er syringe (lōō′ər) *n.* A glass syringe with a metal tip and locking device to secure the needle, used for hypodermic and intravenous purposes.

lu·es (lōō′ēz) *n., pl.* **lues** Syphilis. —**lu·et′ic** (-ĕt′ĭk) *adj.*

luetic mask *n.* A brownish-yellow pigmentation, occurring in blotches on the forehead, temples, and sometimes cheeks of patients with tertiary syphilis.

LUL *abbr.* left upper lobe (of the lung)

lu·lib·er·in (lōō-lĭb′ər-ĭn) *n.* See **gonadotropin-releasing hormone.**

lum·ba·go (lŭm-bā′gō) *n.* A painful condition of the lower back, as one resulting from muscle strain or a slipped disk.

lum·bar (lŭm′bər, -bär′) *adj.* Of, near, or situated in the part of the back and sides between the lowest ribs and the pelvis.

lumbar artery *n.* **1.** Any of four or five pairs of arteries with origin in the abdominal aorta, with distribution to the lumbar vertebrae, muscles of the back, and the abdominal wall, and with anastomoses to the intercostal, subcostal, superior and inferior epigastric, deep circumflex iliac, and iliolumbar arteries. **2.** An artery with origin in the median sacral artery, with distribution to the sacrum and iliac muscle, and with anastomosis to the iliac artery; lowest lumbar artery.

lumbar flexure *n.* The normal ventral curve of the vertebral column in the lumbar region.

lumbar ganglion *n.* Any of four or more ganglions on either side of the greater psoas muscle, forming the abdominopelvic portion of the sympathetic trunk with the sacral and coccygeal ganglions.

lumbar hernia *n.* A protrusion between the last rib and the iliac crest where the transverse muscle is covered by the latissimus dorsi.

lumbar iliocostal muscle *n.* A muscle with its origin from the erector muscle of the spine, with insertion to the lower six ribs, with nerve supply from the branches of the thoracic and lumbar nerves, and whose action extends, abducts, and rotates the lumbar vertebrae.

lum·bar·i·za·tion (lŭm′bər-ĭ-zā′shən) *n.* Sacral development of the fifth lumbar vertebra.

lumbar nerve *n.* Any of five nerves on either side that emerge from the lumbar portion of the spinal cord.

lumbar plexus *n.* **1.** A nerve plexus formed by the ventral branches of the first four lumbar nerves and lying in the substance of the psoas muscle. **2.** A lymphatic plexus formed of about twenty lymph nodes and connecting vessels situated along the aorta and the common iliac vessels.

lumbar puncture n. Abbr. **LP** Puncture into the subarachnoid space of the lumbar region for diagnostic or therapeutic purposes. Also called rachicentesis, rachiocentesis, spinal puncture, spinal tap.

lumbar quadrate muscle n. A muscle with origin from the iliac crest, the iliolumbar ligament, and the lower lumbar vertebrae, with insertion into the twelfth rib and the upper lumbar vertebrae, with nerve supply from the upper lumbar nerve, and whose action abducts the trunk. Also called quadrate muscle of loins.

lumbar rib n. A rib articulating with the transverse process of the first lumbar vertebra; occurring only occasionally.

lumbar splanchnic nerve n. Any of the branches from the lumbar sympathetic trunks that pass anteriorly to join the celiac, intermesenteric, aortic, and superior hypogastric plexuses.

lumbar triangle n. An area in the posterior abdominal wall, the site of occasional herniation, bounded by the edges of the latissimus dorsi and external oblique muscles and the iliac crest. Also called Petit's lumbar triangle.

lumbar vein n. Any of five veins that accompany the lumbar arteries, drain the posterior body wall and lumbar vertebral venous plexuses, and terminate in the ascending lumbar vein, the inferior vena cava, or in the iliolumbar vein.

lum·bo·co·los·to·my (lŭm′bō-kə-lŏs′tə-mē) n. The formation of a permanent opening into the colon through an incision in the lumbar region.

lum·bo·cos·tal (lŭm′bō-kŏs′təl) adj. Relating to the lumbar and hypochondriac regions.

lumbocostal ligament n. A strong band that unites the twelfth rib with the tips of the transverse processes of the first and second lumbar vertebrae.

lum·bo·cos·to·ab·dom·i·nal triangle (lŭm′bō-kŏs′-tō-ăb-dŏm′ə-nəl) n. An irregular area bounded by the inferior posterior serratus muscle, the abdominal internal and external oblique muscles, and the erector muscle of the spine.

lum·bo·in·gui·nal (lŭm′bō-ĭng′gwə-nəl) adj. Relating to the lumbar and inguinal regions.

lum·bo·sa·cral (lŭm′bō-sā′krəl) adj. Relating to the lumbar vertebrae and the sacrum.

lum·bri·cal muscle of foot (lŭm′brĭ-kəl) n. Any of four muscles of whose origin the first is from the tendon to the second toe of the long flexor muscle of the toes, and the second, third, and fourth are from adjacent sides of all four tendons of this muscle; with insertion into the extensor tendon of each of the four lateral toes; with nerve supply from two plantar nerves, and whose actions serve to flex the proximal phalanges and to extend the middle and distal phalanges.

lumbrical muscle of hand n. Any of four muscles whose origins are from the finger and hand tendons, with insertion into the extensor tendon on the dorsum of each of the four fingers; with nerve supply from the median

and ulnar nerves; and whose actions flex the proximal phalanges and extend the middle and distal phalanges.

lum·bri·cid·al (lŭm′brĭ-sīd′l) adj. Destructive to intestinal worms.

lum·bri·cide (lŭm′brĭ-sīd′) n. An agent that kills intestinal worms.

lum·bri·coid (lŭm′brĭ-koid′) adj. Of or resembling a roundworm.

lum·bri·co·sis (lŭm′brĭ-kō′sĭs) n. Infestation with intestinal worms.

lum·bri·cus (lŭm′brĭ-kəs) n. The roundworm, Ascaris lumbricoides.

lum·bus (lŭm′bəs) n., pl. **–bi** (-bī) The loin.

lu·men (loo′mən) n., pl. **lumens** or **–mi·na** (-mə-nə) **1.** The inner open space or cavity of a tubular organ, as of a blood vessel. **2.** The unit of luminous flux in the International System of Units, equal to the amount of light given out through a solid angle by a source of one candela intensity radiating equally in all directions. —**lu′men·al, lu′min·al** adj.

lu·mi·nes·cence (loo′mə-nĕs′əns) n. **1.** The emission of light that does not derive energy from the temperature of the emitting body, as in fluorescence and bioluminescence. **2.** The light so emitted.

lu·mi·nif·er·ous (loo′mə-nĭf′ər-əs) adj. Generating, yielding, or transmitting light.

lu·mi·no·phore (loo′mə-nə-fôr′) n. An atom or atomic grouping that when present in an organic compound increases the ability of the compound to luminesce.

lu·mi·nous (loo′mə-nəs) adj. Emitting light, especially emitting self-generated light.

lu·mi·rho·dop·sin (loo′mə-rō-dŏp′sĭn) n. An intermediate formed during the bleaching of rhodopsin by light.

lump·ec·to·my (lŭm-pĕk′tə-mē) n. See **tylectomy.**

lu·nar (loo′nər) adj. **1.** Relating to the moon or to a month. **2.** Lunate. **3.** Containing silver.

lu·nate (loo′nāt′) adj. Shaped like a crescent.

lunate bone n. The second of three bones forming the proximal row of bones in the wrist between the scaphoid and triquetrum bones and articulating with the radius, scaphoid, triquetrum, hamate, and capitate bones. Also called semilunar bone.

lung (lŭng) n. Either of the two saclike organs of respiration that occupy the pulmonary cavity of the thorax and in which aeration of the blood takes place. It is common for the right lung, which is divided into three lobes, to be slightly larger than the left, which has two lobes. See illustration on page 472.

lung·worm (lŭng′wûrm′) n. Any of various nematode worms, especially of the family Metastrongylidae, that are parasitic in the lungs of mammals.

lu·nu·la (loon′yə-lə) n., pl. **–lae** (-lē′) A small crescent-shaped structure or marking, especially the proximal region at the base of a fingernail that resembles a half-moon.

lu·pi·form (loo′pə-fôrm′) adj. Lupoid.

lu·poid (loo′poid′) adj. Resembling lupus.

lupoid hepatitis n. An active chronic hepatitis that is characterized by jaundice with liver cell damage and by positive lupus erythematosus cell tests, but that does

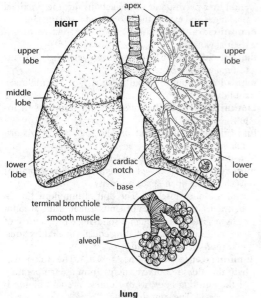

lung
Top: *right and left lungs*
Bottom: *detail showing terminal respiratory units of bronchial tree*

not present the physical manifestations of systemic lupus erythematosus.

lupoid leishmaniasis *n.* See **leishmaniasis recidivans.**

lupoid sycosis *n.* A papular or pustular inflammation of the hair follicles that causes scarring and hair loss, especially in the area of the beard. Also called *ulerythema sycosiforme.*

Lu·pron (lōō′prŏn′) A trademark for the drug leuprolide acetate.

lu·pus (lōō′pəs) *n.* **1.** Systemic lupus erythematosus. **2.** Any of various chronic skin conditions characterized by ulcerative lesions that spread over the body. No longer in scientific use.

lupus band test *n. Abbr.* **LBT** A direct immunofluorescent technique for demonstrating a band of immunoglobulins at the dermal-epidermal junction of the skin of patients with lupus erythematosus.

lupus er·y·the·ma·to·sus (ĕr′ə-thē′mə-tō′səs, -thĕm′-ə-) *n.* **1.** *Abbr.* **LE** A chronic disease of unknown origin characterized by red, scaly lesions or patches on the face and upper portion of the trunk. **2.** Systemic lupus erythematosus.

lupus erythematosus cell *n. Abbr.* **LE cell** A polymorphonuclear white blood cell that has ingested another cell's nuclear material after that cell has been denatured by a substance present in the blood of individuals who have systemic lupus erythematosus.

lupus erythematosus cell test *n.* A test for systemic lupus erythematosus in which characteristic lupus erythematosus cells are formed by incubation of blood or bone marrow of an affected individual or by the action of an affected individual's serum on normal white blood cells. Also called *LE cell test.*

lupus erythematosus pro·fun·dus (prō-fŭn′dəs) *n.* A chronic cutaneous form of lupus erythematosus giving rise to deep-seated, firm, rubbery nodules that sometimes become ulcerated, usually on the face.

lupus hy·per·troph·i·cus (hī′pər-trŏf′ĭ-kəs) *n.* A form of lupus vulgaris in which the tubercles are grouped into prominent hypertrophic nodules with deep-seated scarring, usually on the chin. Also called *lupus tumidus.*

lupus mil·i·ar·is dis·sem·i·na·tus fa·ci·e·i (mĭl′ē-âr′-ĭs dĭ-sĕm′ə-nā′təs fā′shē-ē′ī) *n.* A milletlike papular eruption of the central part of the face.

lupus nephritis *n.* Glomerulonephritis that occurs with systemic lupus erythematosus and is characterized by hematuria progressing to renal failure.

lupus per·ni·o (pûr′nē-ō) *n.* Sarcoid lesions that resemble those of frostbite and that involve the ears and hands.

lupus tu·mi·dus (tōō′mĭ-dəs) *n.* See **lupus hypertrophicus.**

lupus vul·gar·is (vŭl-gâr′ĭs) *n.* Cutaneous tuberculosis with characteristic reddish-brown ulcerating nodular lesions on the face, particularly the nose and ears.

LUQ *abbr.* left upper quadrant (of the abdomen)

Lu·ri·a (lōŏr′ē-ə), **Salvador Edward** 1912–1991. Italian-born American biologist. He shared a 1969 Nobel Prize for investigating the mechanism of viral infection in living cells.

Lusch·ka's bursa (lōŏsh′kəz) *n.* See **pharyngeal bursa.**

Luschka's duct *n.* One of the glandlike tubular structures occurring in the wall of the gallbladder, especially in the area covered with peritoneum.

lu·sus na·tu·rae (lōō′səs nə-tōŏr′ē) *n.* A conspicuous congenital abnormality.

lu·te·al (lōō′tē-əl) *adj.* Of, relating to, or involving the corpus luteum.

luteal cell *n.* See **lutein cell.**

luteal phase *n.* The portion of the menstrual cycle that begins with the formation of the corpus luteum and ends with the start of the menstrual flow, usually 14 days in length.

lu·te·in (lōō′tē-ĭn, -tēn′) *n.* **1.** A yellow carotenoid pigment found widely in nature; xanthophyll. **2.** A dried preparation of corpus luteum.

lutein cell *n.* A cell of the corpus luteum of the ovary. Also called *luteal cell.*

lu·te·in·i·za·tion (lōō′tē-ə-nĭ-zā′shən) *n.* The transformation of the mature ovarian follicle into a corpus luteum. —**lu′te·in·ize′** (lōō′tē-ə-nīz′) *v.*

lu·te·in·iz·ing hormone (lōō′tē-ə-nī′zĭng) *n. Abbr.* **LH** A hormone produced by the anterior lobe of the pituitary gland that stimulates ovulation and the development of the corpus luteum in the female and the production of testosterone by the interstitial cells of the testis in the male. Also called *interstitial cell-stimulating hormone, lutropin.*

luteinizing hormone/follicle-stimulating hormone-releasing factor *n. Abbr.* **LH/FSH-RF** The decapeptide isolated from pig hypothalami that is used to stimulate the release of luteinizing hormone and follicle-stimulating hormone in constant proportions. Also called *gonadoliberin.*

luteinizing hormone-releasing hormone *n. Abbr.* **LHRH, LRH** See **gonadotropin-releasing hormone.**

Lu·tem·bach·er's syndrome (loo′təm-băk′ərz, -bä′-kərz) *n.* A congenital cardiac abnormality consisting of mitral stenosis, an enlarged right atrium, and a defect of the interatrial septum of the heart.

lu·te·o·hor·mone (loo′tē-ō-hôr′mōn′) *n.* See **progesterone** (sense 1).

lu·te·ol·y·sis (loo′tē-ŏl′ĭ-sĭs) *n.* Degeneration or destruction of ovarian luteinized tissue.

lu·te·o·ma (loo′tē-ō′mə) *n., pl.* **–mas** or **–ma·ta** (-mə-tə) An ovarian tumor of granulosa- or theca-cell origin in which luteinization has occurred.

lu·te·o·pla·cen·tal shift (loo′tē-ō-plə-sĕn′təl) *n.* The shift from the corpus luteum to the placenta as the site of production of estrogen and progesterone in amounts that are sufficient to maintain pregnancy in humans.

lu·te·o·trop·ic (loo′tē-ə-trŏp′ĭk, -trō′pĭk) or **lu·te·o·troph·ic** (-trŏf′ĭk, -trō′fĭk) *adj.* Having an affect on the development and function of the corpus luteum.

luteotropic hormone *n. Abbr.* **LTH** See **prolactin.**

lu·te·o·tro·pin (loo′tē-ə-trō′pĭn) *n.* See **prolactin.**

lu·te·ti·um or **lu·te·ci·um** (loo-tē′shē-əm) *n. Symbol* **Lu** A rare-earth element, used in nuclear research. Atomic number 71.

lu·tro·pin (loo′trə-pĭn′) *n.* See **luteinizing hormone.**

Lutz·o·my·ia (loot′zō-mī′yə) *n.* A genus of sand flies or midges of the family Psychodidae that serve as vectors of leishmaniasis and Oroya fever.

Lutz-Splen·do·re-Almeida disease (lŭts′splĕn-dôr′ē-, loots′-) *n.* See **paracoccidioidomycosis.**

lux (lŭks) *n., pl.* **lux·es** or **lu·ces** (loo′sēz) *Abbr.* **lx** The International System unit of illumination, equal to one lumen per square meter. Also called *candle-meter, meter-candle.*

lux·ate (lŭk′sāt′) *v.* To put out of joint; dislocate. **—lux·a′tion** *n.*

Lux·ol fast blue (lŭk′sôl′) *n.* Any of a group of closely related copper phthalocyanine dyes used as stains for myelin in nerve fibers.

LVET *abbr.* left ventricular ejection time

LVH *abbr.* left ventricular hypertrophy

LVN *abbr.* licensed vocational nurse

Lwoff (lwôf), **André Michel** 1902–1994. French microbiologist. He shared a 1965 Nobel Prize for the study of regulatory activity in body cells.

ly·ase (lī′ās′) *n.* Any of a group of enzymes that catalyze the formation of double bonds by removing chemical groups from a substrate without hydrolysis or catalyze the addition of chemical groups to double bonds.

ly·can·thro·py (lī-kăn′thrə-pē) *n.* The delusion that one is a wolf.

ly·co·pene (lī′kə-pēn′) *n.* A red pigment found in blood, the reproductive organs, tomatoes, and palm oils and considered chemically to be the parent substance from which all natural carotenoid pigments are derived.

ly·co·pe·ne·mi·a (lī′kə-pē-nē′mē-ə) *n.* A condition in which there is a high concentration of lycopene in the blood, producing yellowish-orange pigmentation of the skin, due to excessive consumption of lycopene-containing fruits and berries.

ly·co·per·do·no·sis (lī′kə-pûr′də-nō′sĭs) *n.* A respiratory disease caused by inhaling the spores of the puffballs *Lycoperdon pyriforme* and *L. bovista.*

Ly·ell's disease (lī′əlz) *n.* See **staphylococcal scalded skin syndrome.**

ly·ing-in (lī′ĭng-ĭn′) *n., pl.* **ly·ings-in** (lī′ĭngz-) or **ly·ing-ins** A state attending childbirth. **—adj.** Of or intended for use during childbirth.

Lyme arthritis (līm) *n.* Arthritis associated with Lyme disease.

Lyme disease *n.* An inflammatory disease caused by the spirochete *Borrelia burgdorferi* transmitted by ticks and characterized initially by a rash followed by flulike symptoms including fever, joint pain, and headache; if untreated, it can result in chronic arthritis and nerve and heart dysfunction.

lymph (lĭmf) *n.* A clear, watery, sometimes faintly yellowish fluid derived from body tissues that contains white blood cells and circulates throughout the lymphatic system, returning to the venous bloodstream through the thoracic duct. Lymph acts to remove bacteria and certain proteins from the tissues, transport fat from the small intestine, and supply mature lymphocytes to the blood.

lymph– *pref.* Variant of **lympho–.**

lym·phad·e·nec·to·my (lĭm-făd′n-ĕk′tə-mē) *n.* Excision of one or more lymph nodes.

lym·phad·e·ni·tis (lĭm-făd′n-ī′tĭs, lĭm′fə-də-nī′-) *n.* Inflammation of one or more lymph nodes.

lymphadeno– or **lymphaden–** *pref.* Lymph node: *lymphadenectomy.*

lym·phad·e·nog·ra·phy (lĭm-făd′n-ŏg′rə-fē) *n.* Radiography of an enlarged lymph node following the injection of a radiopaque substance into the node.

lym·phad·e·noid (lĭm-făd′n-oid′) *adj.* Of, resembling, or derived from a lymph node.

lymphadenoid goiter *n.* See **Hashimoto's disease.**

lym·phad·e·no·ma (lĭm-făd′n-ō′mə) *n.* A tumorlike enlargement of a lymph node. No longer in technical use.

lym·phad·e·nop·a·thy (lĭm-făd′n-ŏp′ə-thē, lĭm′fə-dn-) *n.* A chronic, abnormal enlargement of the lymph nodes, usually associated with disease.

lymphadenopathy-associated virus *n. Abbr.* **LAV** See **HIV.**

lym·phad·e·no·sis (lĭm-făd′n-ō′sĭs) *n.* The basic underlying proliferative process that results in enlargement of lymph nodes.

lym·pha·gogue (lĭm′fə-gôg′) *n.* An agent that increases the formation and flow of lymph.

lym·phan·gi·al (lĭm-făn′jē-əl) *adj.* Of or relating to a lymphatic vessel.

lym·phan·gi·ec·ta·sis (lĭm-făn′jē-ĕk′tə-sĭs) or **lym·phan·gi·ec·ta·sia** (lĭm-făn′jē-ĭk-tā′zhə) *n.* Dilation of the lymphatic vessels. Also called *lymphectasia.* **—lym·phan′gi·ec·tat′ic** (-ĭk-tăt′ĭk) *adj.*

lym·phan·gi·ec·to·my (lĭm-făn′jē-ĕk′tə-mē) *n.* Excision of a lymphatic vessel.

lymphangio– or **lymphangi–** pref. Lymphatic vessel: *lymphangiography.*

lym·phan·gi·o·en·do·the·li·o·ma (lĭm-făn′jē-ō-ĕn′-dō-thē′lē-ō′mə) *n.* A tumor consisting of irregular groups of endothelial cells with aggregates of tubate structures possibly derived from lymphatic vessels.

lym·phan·gi·og·ra·phy (lĭm-făn′jē-ŏg′rə-fē) *n.* Radiography of the lymph nodes and lymphatic vessels following the injection of a radiopaque substance. Also called *lymphography.* —**lym·phan′gi·o·gram′** (-ə-grăm′) *n.*

lym·phan·gi·ol·o·gy (lĭm-făn′jē-ŏl′ə-jē) *n.* The branch of medical science concerned with the lymphatic system. Also called *lymphology.*

lym·phan·gi·o·ma (lĭm-făn′jē-ō′mə) *n.* A benign tumorlike mass of lymphatic vessels or channels that vary in size, are frequently greatly dilated, and are lined with normal endothelial cells.

lym·phan·gi·o·phle·bi·tis (lĭm-făn′jē-ō-flĭ-bī′tĭs) *n.* Inflammation of the lymphatic vessels and the veins.

lym·phan·gi·o·plas·ty (lĭm-făn′jē-ə-plăs′tē) *n.* Surgical alteration of lymphatic vessels.

lym·phan·gi·o·sar·co·ma (lĭm-făn′jē-ō-sär-kō′mə) *n.* An angiosarcoma in which the tumor cells originate from the endothelial cells of lymphatic vessels.

lym·phan·gi·ot·o·my (lĭm-făn′jē-ŏt′ə-mē) *n.* Incision of lymphatic vessels.

lym·phan·gi·tis (lĭm′făn-jī′tĭs) *or* **lym·phan·gi·i·tis** (lĭm-făn′jē-ī′tĭs) *n.* Inflammation of the lymphatic vessels.

lym·pha·phe·re·sis (lĭm′fə-fə-rē′sĭs) *n.* See **lymphocytapheresis.**

lym·phat·ic (lĭm-făt′ĭk) *adj.* Of or relating to lymph, a lymph node, or a lymphatic vessel. —*n.* A lymphatic vessel.

lymphatic corpuscle *n.* Variant of **lymph corpuscle.**

lymphatic duct *n.* Either of the two terminal lymph vessels that convey lymph to the bloodstream: right and left.

lymphatic leukemia *n.* See **lymphocytic leukemia.**

lym·phat·i·cos·to·my (lĭm-făt′ĭ-kŏs′tə-mē) *n.* Surgical construction of an opening into a lymphatic duct.

lymphatic plexus *n.* A network of lymphatic capillaries that usually lack valves and join to form one or more larger lymphatic vessels that drain to lymph nodes.

lymphatic sinus *n.* Any of the channels in a lymph node crossed by a reticulum of cells and fibers and bounded by littoral cells.

lymphatic system *n.* The interconnected system of spaces and vessels between body tissues and organs by which lymph circulates throughout the body.

lymphatic tissue *n.* Tissue consisting of a network of reticular fibers and cells, the meshes of which are occupied by lymphocytes. Also called *adenoid tissue, lymphoid tissue.*

lymphatic vessel *n.* Any of the vascular channels that transport lymph throughout the lymphatic system and freely anastomose with one another. Also called *absorbent vessel.*

lym·pha·ti·tis (lĭm′fə-tī′tĭs) *n.* Inflammation of the lymphatic vessels or lymph nodes.

lym·pha·tol·y·sis (lĭm′fə-tŏl′ĭ-sĭs) *n.* The destruction or dissolution of the lymphatic vessels or the lymphoid tissue. —**lym′pha·to·lyt′ic** (-tə-lĭt′ĭk) *adj.*

lymph capillary *n.* One of the minute vessels of the lymphatic system.

lymph corpuscle *or* **lymphatic corpuscle** *or* **lymphoid corpuscle** *n.* A mononuclear type of white blood cell formed in lymph nodes, other lymphoid tissue, and blood.

lym·phec·ta·sia (lĭm′fĭk-tā′zhə) *n.* See **lymphangiectasis.**

lym·phe·de·ma (lĭm′fĭ-dē′mə) *n.* Swelling, especially in subcutaneous tissues, as a result of obstruction of lymphatic vessels or lymph nodes, with accumulation of lymph in the affected region.

lym·phe·mi·a (lĭm-fē′mē-ə) *n.* The presence of unusually large numbers of lymphocytes or their precursors in the blood.

lymph follicle *or* **lymphatic follicle** *n.* Any of the spherical masses of lymphoid cells frequently having a more lightly staining center. Also called *lymph nodule.*

lymph gland *n.* See **lymph node.**

lymph node *n.* Any of the small, oval or round bodies, located along the lymphatic vessels, that supply lymphocytes to the bloodstream and remove bacteria and foreign particles from the lymph. Also called *lymph gland, lymphoglandula, lymphonodus.*

lymph node permeability factor *n. Abbr.* **LNPF** A substance released by stimulated or damaged lymphocytes that increases capillary permeability and the accumulation of mononuclear cells.

lymph nodule *n.* See **lymph follicle.**

lympho– *or* **lymph–** *pref.* Lymphatic system; lymph: *lymphocyte.*

lym·pho·blast (lĭm′fə-blăst′) *n.* An immature cell that gives rise to a lymphocyte. Also called *lymphocytoblast.* —**lym′pho·blas′tic** *adj.*

lymphoblastic leukemia *n.* A type of lymphocytic leukemia characterized by abnormal, often immature, lymphocytic cells or by the presence of unusually large numbers of immature lymphocytes occurring together with adult lymphocytes.

lymphoblastic lymphoma *n.* A diffuse malignant lymphoma in children, composed of T-cells that have convoluted nuclei.

lym·pho·blas·to·ma (lĭm′fō-blă-stō′mə) *n.* A form of malignant lymphoma composed chiefly of lymphoblasts.

lym·pho·blas·to·sis (lĭm′fō-blă-stō′sĭs) *n.* The presence of lymphoblasts in the peripheral blood.

lym·pho·cy·ta·phe·re·sis (lĭm′fō-sī′tə-fə-rē′sĭs) *n.* Removal of lymphocytes from donated blood, with the remainder of the blood retransfused into the donor. Also called *lymphapheresis.*

lym·pho·cyte (lĭm′fə-sīt′) *n.* Any of the nearly colorless cells formed in lymphoid tissue, as in the lymph nodes, spleen, thymus, and tonsils, constituting between 22 and 28 percent of all white blood cells in the blood of a normal adult human. They function in the development of immunity and include two specific types, B cells and T cells. —**lym′pho·cyt′ic** (-sĭt′-ĭk) *adj.*

lym·pho·cy·the·mi·a (lĭm′fə-sī-thē′mē-ə) *n.* See **lymphocytosis.**

lymphocytic choriomeningitis virus *n.* A virus of the genus *Arenavirus* that is the causative agent of lymphocytic choriomeningitis.

lymphocytic leukemia *n.* Leukemia characterized by the proliferation and enlargement of lymphoid tissue in various sites and by increased numbers of lymphocytic cells in the blood and in various tissues and organs. Also called *lymphatic leukemia, lymphoid leukemia.*

lymphocytic leukocytosis *n.* See **lymphocytosis.**

lymphocytic leukopenia *n.* See **lymphopenia.**

lymphocytic series *n.* The cells at various states of lymphopoietic development in lymphoid tissue. Also called *lymphoid series.*

lym·pho·cy·to·blast (lĭm′fō-sī′tə-blăst′) *n.* See **lymphoblast.**

lym·pho·cy·to·ma (lĭm′fō-sī-tō′mə) *n., pl.* **–mas** *or* **–ma·ta** (-mə-tə) **1.** A circumscribed nodule or mass of mature lymphocytes, having the appearance of a neoplasm. **2.** A malignant lymphoma whose cells closely resemble mature lymphocytes.

lymphocytoma cu·tis (kyōō′tĭs) *n.* A benign skin nodule caused by dense infiltration of the dermis by lymphocytes and histiocytes, often forming lymphoid follicles.

lym·pho·cy·to·pe·ni·a (lĭm′fō-sī′tə-pē′nē-ə) *n.* See **lymphopenia.**

lym·pho·cy·to·poi·e·sis (lĭm′fō-sī′tə-poi-ē′sĭs) *n.* Formation of lymphocytes.

lym·pho·cy·to·sis (lĭm′fō-sī-tō′sĭs) *n.* A condition marked by an abnormal increase in the number of lymphocytes in the bloodstream, usually resulting from infection or inflammation. Also called *lymphocythemia, lymphocytic leukocytosis.* **—lym′pho·cy·tot′ic** (-tŏt′ĭk) *adj.*

lym·pho·duct (lĭm′fə-dŭkt′) *n.* A lymphatic vessel.

lym·pho·ep·i·the·li·o·ma (lĭm′fō-ĕp′ə-thē′lē-ō′mə) *n.* A poorly differentiated squamous cell carcinoma involving lymphoid tissue in the region of the tonsils and the nasopharynx.

lym·pho·gen·e·sis (lĭm′fə-jĕn′ĭ-sĭs) *n.* The production of lymph.

lym·phog·e·nous (lĭm-fŏj′ə-nəs) *or* **lym·pho·gen·ic** (lĭm′fə-jĕn′ĭk) *adj.* **1.** Originating from or spread through lymph or the lymphatic system. **2.** Producing lymph or lymphocytes.

lym·pho·glan·du·la (lĭm′fō-glăn′jə-lə) *n.* See **lymph node.**

lym·pho·gran·u·lo·ma (lĭm′fō-grăn′yə-lō′mə) *n.* **1.** Any of several unrelated diseases in which the pathological processes result in the formation of granulomas or granulomalike lesions, especially in various groups of lymph nodes which then become conspicuously enlarged. **2.** Hodgkin's disease. No longer in technical use.

lym·pho·gran·u·lo·ma·to·sis (lĭm′fō-grăn′yə-lō′mə-tō′sĭs) *n.* Any of various conditions characterized by the occurrence of multiple and widely distributed lymphogranulomas.

lym·phog·ra·phy (lĭm-fŏg′rə-fē) *n.* See **lymphangiography.**

lym·phoid (lĭm′foid′) *adj.* Of or relating to lymph or the lymphatic tissue where lymphocytes are formed.

lymphoid corpuscle *n.* Variant of **lymph corpuscle.**

lym·phoid·ec·to·my (lĭm′foi-dĕk′tə-mē) *n.* Excision of lymphoid tissue.

lymphoid hypophysitis *n.* An acute anterior pituitary lymphocytic reaction that is characterized clinically by signs and symptoms of anterior pituitary insufficiency.

lymphoid leukemia *n.* See **lymphocytic leukemia.**

lym·phoi·do·cyte (lĭm-foi′də-sīt′) *n.* See **hemocytoblast.**

lymphoid series *n.* See **lymphocytic series.**

lymphoid tissue *n.* See **lymphatic tissue.**

lym·pho·kine (lĭm′fə-kīn′) *n.* Any of various soluble substances, released by sensitized lymphocytes on contact with specific antigens, that act by stimulating activity of monocytes and macrophages.

lym·pho·ki·ne·sis (lĭm′fō-kə-nē′sĭs) *n.* **1.** The circulation of lymph in the lymphatic vessels and through lymph nodes. **2.** The movement of lymph in the semicircular canals.

lym·phol·o·gy (lĭm-fŏl′ə-jē) *n.* See **lymphangiology.**

lym·pho·ma (lĭm-fō′mə) *n., pl.* **–mas** *or* **–ma·ta** (-mə-tə) Any of various usually malignant neoplasms of lymphatic and reticuloendothelial tissues that occur as circumscribed solid tumors and that are composed of cells that resemble lymphocytes, plasma cells, or histiocytes. Also called *malignant lymphoma.* **—lym·pho′ma·toid′, lym·pho′ma·tous** (-təs) *adj.*

lymphomatoid granulomatosis *n.* A disease characterized by granulomatous proliferations of atypical white blood cells, plasma cells, and histiocytes that invade and destroy the small arteries of the lung, skin, kidneys, and nervous system; it usually affects adult men and may develop into lymphoma. Also called *polymorphic reticulosis.*

lym·pho·ma·to·sis (lĭm-fō′mə-tō′sĭs) *n., pl.* **–ses** (-sēz) Any of various conditions characterized by the occurrence of multiple, widely distributed lymphomas in the body.

lym·pho·myx·o·ma (lĭm′fō-mĭk-sō′mə) *n.* A soft nonmalignant tumor containing lymphoid tissue in a matrix of loose areolar connective tissue.

lym·pho·no·dus (lĭm′fō-nō′dəs) *n.* See **lymph node.**

lym·phop·a·thy (lĭm-fŏp′ə-thē) *n.* A disease of the lymphatic vessels and lymph nodes.

lym·pho·pe·ni·a (lĭm′fə-pē′nē-ə) *n.* A reduction in the number of lymphocytes in the blood. Also called *lymphocytic leukopenia, lymphocytopenia.*

lym·pho·plas·ma·phe·re·sis (lĭm′fō-plăz′mə-fə-rē′sĭs) *n.* Removal of lymphocytes and plasma from donated blood, with the remainder of the blood retransfused into the donor.

lym·pho·poi·e·sis (lĭm′fō-poi-ē′sĭs) *n.* The formation of lymphocytes. **—lym′pho·poi·et′ic** (-ĕt′ĭk) *adj.*

lym·pho·re·tic·u·lo·sis (lĭm′fō-rĭ-tĭk′yə-lō′sĭs) *n.* Proliferation of the reticuloendothelial cells of the lymph nodes.

lym·phor·rhe·a (lĭm′fə-rē′ə) *n.* An escape of lymph from ruptured, torn, or cut lymphatic vessels. Also called *lymphorrhagia.*

lym·phor·rhoid (lĭm′fə-roid′) *n.* A dilation of a lymph channel, resembling a hemorrhoid.

lym·pho·sar·co·ma (lĭm′fō-sär-kō′mə) *n.* A diffuse malignant lymphoma.

lym·pho·sar·co·ma·to·sis (lĭm′fō-sär-kō′mə-tō′sĭs) *n.* A condition characterized by the presence of multiple, widely distributed lymphosarcomas in the body.

lym·phos·ta·sis (lĭm-fŏs′tə-sĭs) *n.* Obstruction of the normal flow of lymph.

lym·pho·tax·is (lĭm′fə-tăk′sĭs) *n.* The property of attracting or repelling lymphocytes.

lym·pho·tox·ic·i·ty (lĭm′fō-tŏk-sĭs′ĭ-tē) *n.* The potential of an antibody in the serum of an allograft recipient to react directly with the lymphocytes or other cells of an allograft donor to produce a hyperacute type of graft rejection.

lym·pho·tox·in (lĭm′fə-tŏk′sĭn) *n.* A lymphokine that is toxic to certain susceptible target cells.

lymph varix *n.* Formation of varices or cysts in the lymph nodes resulting from obstruction in the efferent lymphatic vessels.

lymph vessel *n.* A lymphatic vessel.

Ly·nen (lē′nən, lü′-), **Feodor** 1911–1979. German biochemist. He shared a 1964 Nobel Prize for research on cholesterol and fatty acid metabolism.

lyo– *pref.* Dispersion; dissolution: *lyophilic.*

Ly·on (lī′ən), **Mary Frances** Born 1925. British geneticist whose research on mice led to her formulation of the Lyon hypothesis.

Lyon hypothesis *n.* The hypothesis that one X-chromosome is inactive during interphase in normal females and is represented in interphase cell nuclei as the sex chromatin body.

Ly·on·i·za·tion (lī′ə-nĭ-zā′shən) *n.* The phenomenon in which heterozygous females do not phenotypically express their X-linked recessive genotype or do so only randomly. Also called *X-inactivation.*

ly·o·phil (lī′ə-fĭl′) *or* **ly·o·phile** (-fīl′) *adj.* Lyophilic. —*n.* A lyophilic substance.

ly·o·phil·ic (lī′ə-fĭl′ĭk) *adj.* Characterized by strong attraction between the colloid medium and the dispersion medium of a colloidal system.

ly·oph·i·li·za·tion (lī-ŏf′ə-lĭ-zā′shən) *n.* The process of isolating a solid substance from solution by freezing the solution and vaporizing the ice away under vacuum conditions. Also called *freeze-drying.* —**ly·oph′i·lize′** (-līz′) *v.*

ly·o·phobe (lī′ə-fōb′) *adj.* Lyophobic. —*n.* A lyophobic substance.

ly·o·pho·bic (lī′ə-fō′bĭk) *adj.* Characterized by a lack of attraction between the colloid medium and the dispersion medium of a colloidal system.

ly·o·trop·ic (lī′ə-trŏp′ĭk, -trō′pĭk) *adj.* Lyophilic.

ly·pres·sin (lī-prĕs′ĭn) *n.* An antidiuretic and vasopressor substance obtained from the pituitary glands of swine.

Lys *abbr.* lysine

lys– *pref.* Variant of **lyso–.**

ly·sate (lī′sāt′) *n.* The cellular debris and fluid produced by lysis.

lyse (līs, līz) *or* **lyze** (līz) *v.* To undergo or cause to undergo lysis.

ly·se·mi·a (lī-sē′mē-ə) *n.* Disintegration or dissolution of red blood cells and the occurrence of hemoglobin in the plasma and in the urine.

Ly·sen·ko (lĭ-sĕng′kō, -syĕn′kə), **Trofim** 1898–1976. Soviet biologist and agronomist known for his mistaken belief in the genetic theory that acquired characteristics can be inherited.

ly·ser·gic acid (lĭ-sûr′jĭk, lī-) *n.* A crystalline alkaloid derived from ergot and used in medical research as a psychotomimetic agent.

lysergic acid di·eth·yl·am·ide (dī′ĕth-əl-ăm′īd′) *n.* LSD.

ly·ser·gide (lĭ-sûr′jīd′, lī-) *n.* See **LSD.**

ly·sin (lī′sĭn) *n.* **1.** An antibody that is capable of causing the destruction or dissolution of red blood cells, bacteria, or other cellular elements. **2.** A substance that causes lysis.

ly·sine (lī′sēn′, -sĭn) *n. Abbr.* **Lys** An essential amino acid derived from the hydrolysis of proteins and required by the body for optimum growth.

ly·si·ne·mi·a (lī′sə-nē′mē-ə) *n.* Increased concentration of lysine in the blood, associated with mental and physical retardation.

ly·sin·o·gen (lī-sĭn′ə-jən, -jĕn′) *n.* An antigen that stimulates the formation of a specific lysin.

ly·si·no·gen·ic (lī′sə-nō-jĕn′ĭk) *adj.* Of or having the property of a lysinogen.

ly·si·nu·ri·a (lī′sə-noŏr′ē-ə) *n.* The presence of lysine in the urine.

ly·sis (lī′sĭs) *n., pl.* **–ses** (-sēz) **1.** The gradual subsiding of the symptoms of an acute disease; a form of the recovery process. **2.** The dissolution or destruction of cells, such as blood cells or bacteria, as by the action of a specific lysin.

–lysis *suff.* Decomposition; dissolving; disintegration: *hydrolysis.*

lyso– *or* **lys–** *pref.* Lysis: *lysin.*

ly·so·gen (lī′sə-jən) *n.* **1.** An agent capable of inducing lysis. **2.** A bacterium in a state of lysogeny.

ly·so·gen·e·sis (lī′sə-jĕn′ĭ-sĭs) *n.* Lysin production.

ly·so·gen·ic (lī′sə-jĕn′ĭk) *adj.* **1.** Causing or having the power to cause lysis. **2.** Of or relating to a bacterium in a state of lysogeny.

lysogenic bacterium *n.* A bacterium whose genome includes the genome of a temperate bacteriophage.

ly·so·ge·nic·i·ty (lī′sə-jə-nĭs′ĭ-tē) *n.* The property of being lysogenic.

ly·sog·e·nize (lī-sŏj′ĭ-nīz′) *v.* To make lysogenic. —**ly·sog′e·ni·za′tion** (-nĭ-zā′shən) *n.*

ly·sog·e·ny (lī-sŏj′ə-nē) *n.* The fusion of the nucleic acid of a bacteriophage with that of a host bacterium so that the potential exists for the newly integrated genetic material to be transmitted to daughter cells at each subsequent cell division.

ly·so·ki·nase (lī′sə-kī′nās′, -nāz′) *n.* An activator agent, such as streptokinase, urokinase, or staphylokinase, that produces plasmin by indirect or multiple-stage action on plasminogen.

lysosomal disease *n.* A disease caused by the inadequate functioning of a lysosomal enzyme and usually characterized by an excess or an absence of storage of a vital cellular component.

ly·so·some (lī′sə-sōm′) *n.* A membrane-bound organelle in the cytoplasm of most cells containing various hydrolytic enzymes that function in intracellular digestion. —**ly′so·so′mal** *adj.*

ly·so·zyme (lī′sə-zīm′) *n.* An enzyme occurring naturally in egg white, human tears, saliva, and other body fluids, capable of destroying the cell walls of certain bacteria and thereby acting as a mild antiseptic. Also called *muramidase.*

lys·sa (lĭs′ə) *n.* Rabies. No longer in technical use. —**lys′sic** *adj.*

Lys·sa·vi·rus (lĭs′ə-vī′rəs) *n.* A genus of viruses that includes the rabies virus group.

–lyte *suff.* A substance that can be decomposed by a specified process: *electrolyte.*

lyt·ic (lĭt′ĭk) *adj.* **1.** Of, relating to, or causing lysis. **2.** Of or relating to a lysin.

–lytic *suff.* Of, relating to, or causing a specified kind of decomposition: *lymphatolytic.*

lytic cocktail *n.* A mixture of drugs injected intravenously to produce sedation, analgesia, amnesia, hypotension, hypothermia, and blockade of the functions of the sympathetic and parasympathetic nervous systems during surgical anesthesia.

lyze (līz) *v.* Variant of **lyse.**

–lyze *suff.* To cause or undergo lysis: *hydrolyze.*

M

μ **1.** The Greek letter **mu.** Entries beginning with this character are alphabetized under *mu.* **2.** The symbol for **micro-. 3.** The symbol for **dynamic viscosity.**

μμ The symbol for **micromicro-.**

μCi *abbr.* microcurie

μg *abbr.* microgram

μm *abbr.* micrometer; micron

m *abbr.* mass; meter

M *abbr.* molar; molarity; morgan; myopia

mμ *abbr.* millimicron

m– *abbr. meta–*

mA *abbr.* milliampere

MA *abbr.* medical assistant; mental age

MAA *abbr.* macroaggregated albumin

Maa·lox (mā′lŏks′) A trademark for a preparation containing simethicone, aluminum hydroxide, and magnesium hydroxide that is used as an antacid and antiflatulent.

Mace *or* **MACE** (mās) An alternate trademark for Chemical Mace, an aerosol used to immobilize an attacker temporarily.

mac·er·ate (măs′ə-rāt′) *v.* **1.** To make soft by soaking or steeping in a liquid. **2.** To separate into constituents by soaking. —*n.* A substance prepared or produced by macerating.

mac·er·a·tion (măs′ə-rā′shən) *n.* **1.** Softening by soaking in a liquid. **2.** Softening of the tissues after death by autolysis, especially of a stillborn fetus.

Mac·ew·en's sign (mə-kyōō′ənz) *n.* An indication of hydrocephalus in which percussion of the skull generates a cracked-pot sound.

Macewen's triangle *n.* See **suprameatal triangle.**

Ma·che unit (măk′ə, mä′kə) *n. Abbr.* **Mu** A unit of measure of radium emanation. One thousand Mache units equal the amount of emanation in equilibrium with $\frac{1}{2000}$ milligram of radium.

ma·chin·er·y murmur (mə-shē′nə-rē, -shēn′rē) *n.* See **Gibson murmur.**

Mac·leod (mə-kloud′), **John James Rickard** 1876–1935. British physiologist. He shared a 1923 Nobel Prize for the discovery and successful clinical application of insulin.

mac·ren·ceph·a·ly (măk′rĕn-sĕf′ə-lē) *n.* Hypertrophy of the brain.

macro– *or* **macr–** *pref.* **1.** Large: *macronucleus.* **2.** Long: *macrobiotic.* **3.** Inclusive: *macroamylase.*

mac·ro·ad·e·no·ma (măk′rō-ăd′n-ō′mə) *n.* A pituitary adenoma that is larger than ten millimeters in diameter.

mac·ro·ag·gre·gat·ed albumin (măk′rō-ăg′rĭ-gā′tĭd) *n. Abbr.* **MAA** Conglomerate human serum albumin in a suspension, often radiolabeled and used to scan the lungs.

mac·ro·am·y·lase (măk′rō-ăm′ə-lās′, -lāz′) *n.* A serum amylase in which the enzyme is present as a complex joined to a globulin, resulting in a complex that has a high molecular weight that inhibits its renal excretion.

mac·ro·am·y·la·se·mi·a (măk′rō-ăm′ə-lā-sē′mē-ə) *n.* Hyperamylasemia in which a portion of serum amylase exists as macroamylase.

mac·ro·bi·ot·ics (măk′rō-bī-ŏt′ĭks) *n.* The theory or practice of promoting well-being and longevity, principally by means of a diet consisting chiefly of whole grains and beans and restricted amounts of liquids and noncereal foods. —**mac′ro·bi·ot′ic** *adj.*

mac·ro·blast (măk′rə-blăst′) *n.* An abnormally large erythroblast.

mac·ro·ble·phar·i·a (măk′rō-blĕ-fâr′ē-ə) *n.* Abnormal largeness of the eyelids.

mac·ro·car·di·a (măk′rō-kär′dē-ə) *n.* See **cardiomegaly.**

mac·ro·ceph·a·ly (măk′rō-sĕf′ə-lē) *or* **mac·ro·ce·pha·li·a** (-sə-fā′lē-ə, -fāl′yə) *n.* Abnormal largeness of the head. Also called *megacephaly, megalocephaly.* —**mac′ro·ce·phal′ic** (-sə-fāl′ĭk)**, mac′ro·ceph′a·lous** *adj.*

mac·ro·chei·li·a *or* **mac·ro·chi·li·a** (măk′rō-kī′lē-ə) *n.* **1.** Abnormal largeness of the lips. **2.** A condition of permanent swelling of the lip that results from greatly distended lymphatic spaces.

mac·ro·chei·ri·a *or* **mac·ro·chi·ri·a** (măk′rō-kī′rē-ə) *n.* Abnormal largeness of the hands. Also called *cheiromegaly, megalocheiria.*

mac·ro·co·lon (măk′rō-kō′lən) *n.* A sigmoid colon of unusual length.

mac·ro·cor·ne·a (măk′rō-kôr′nē-ə) *n.* An unusually large cornea. Also called *megalocornea.*

mac·ro·cra·ni·um (măk′rō-krā′nē-əm) *n.* An enlarged skull, especially from enlargement of the bones containing the brain, as seen in hydrocephalus.

mac·ro·cry·o·glob·u·li·ne·mi·a (măk′rō-krī′ō-glŏb′-yə-lə-nē′mē-ə) *n.* The presence in the peripheral blood of a type of hemagglutinin that agglutinates red blood cells at cold temperatures.

mac·ro·cyte (măk′rə-sīt′) *n.* An abnormally large red blood cell, especially one associated with pernicious anemia. —**mac′ro·cyt′ic** (-sĭt′ĭk) *n.*

mac·ro·cy·the·mi·a (măk′rō-sī-thē′mē-ə) *n.* See **macrocytosis.**

macrocytic anemia *n.* Anemia in which the average size of the red blood cells in circulation is greater than normal.

mac·ro·cy·to·sis (măk′rō-sī-tō′sĭs) *n., pl.* **–ses** (-sēz) The presence of unusually large numbers of macrocytes in the blood. Also called *macrocythemia.*

mac·ro·dac·ty·ly (măk′rō-dăk′tə-lē) *n.* Abnormal enlargement of one or more fingers or toes.

Mac·ro·dan·tin (măk′rō-dăn′tn) A trademark for the drug nitrofurantoin.

mac·ro·don·tia (măk′rə-dŏn′shə) *n.* A condition in which the teeth are abnormally large. Also called *megadontism, megalodontia.*

mac·ro·ga·mete (măk'rō-găm'ēt, -gə-mēt') *n.* The larger of a pair of conjugating gametes, usually the female, in an organism that reproduces by heterogamy. Also called *megagamete*.

mac·ro·ga·me·to·cyte (măk'rō-gə-mē'tə-sīt') *n.* The female gametocyte or mother cell that produces a macrogamete.

mac·ro·gen·i·to·so·mi·a (măk'rō-jĕn'ĭ-tə-sō'mē-ə) *n.* Excessive bodily and genital development.

macrogenitosomia pre·cox (prē'kŏks') *n.* A disorder in which gonadal maturation and the growth spurt in height typical of adolescence occur in the first decade of life.

ma·crog·li·a (mă-krŏg'lē-ə) *n.* See **astrocyte**.

mac·ro·glob·u·lin (măk'rō-glŏb'yə-lĭn) *n.* A plasma globulin of high molecular weight.

mac·ro·glob·u·li·ne·mi·a (măk'rō-glŏb'yə-lə-nē'mē-ə) *n.* An abnormally large number of macroglobulins in the blood serum.

mac·ro·glos·si·a (măk'rō-glŏ'sē-ə) *n.* Enlargement of the tongue. Also called *megaloglossia, pachyglossia*.

mac·ro·gna·thi·a (măk'rō-nā'thē-ə, măk'rŏg-) *n.* Enlargement or elongation of the jaw.

mac·ro·lide (măk'rə-līd') *n.* A class of antibiotics that are produced by a species of *Streptomyces,* are characterized by a large lactone ring that is linked to one or more sugars, and act by inhibiting protein synthesis.

mac·ro·mas·ti·a (măk'rō-măs'tē-ə) *n.* Abnormal largeness of the breasts.

mac·ro·me·li·a (măk'rō-mē'lē-ə) *n.* A condition in which one or more of the extremities is enlarged. Also called *megalomelia*.

mac·ro·mere (măk'rə-mî') *n.* A large blastomere.

mac·ro·mol·e·cule (măk'rō-mŏl'ĭ-kyōōl') *n.* A very large molecule, such as a protein, consisting of many smaller structural units linked together.

mac·ro·mon·o·cyte (măk'rō-mŏn'ə-sīt') *n.* An unusually large monocyte.

mac·ro·my·e·lo·blast (măk'rō-mī'ə-lə-blăst') *n.* An abnormally large myeloblast.

mac·ro·nor·mo·blast (măk'rō-nôr'mə-blăst') *n.* A large normoblast.

mac·ro·nu·cle·us (măk'rō-nōō'klē-əs) *n.* The larger of two nuclei present in ciliate protozoans, which controls the nonreproductive functions of the cell. —**mac'ro·nu'cle·ar** *adj.*

mac·ro·nu·tri·ent (măk'rō-nōō'trē-ənt) *n.* A nutrient required in large amounts for the normal growth and development of an organism.

mac·ro·nych·i·a (măk'rō-nĭk'ē-ə) *n.* Abnormal largeness of the fingernails or toenails.

mac·ro·pe·nis (măk'rō-pē'nĭs) *n.* An abnormally large penis. Also called *megalopenis*.

mac·ro·phage (măk'rə-fāj') *n.* Any of the large phagocytic cells found in the reticuloendothelial system. —**mac'ro·phag'ic** (-fāj'ĭk) *adj.*

mac·roph·thal·mi·a (măk'rŏf-thăl'mē-ə) *n.* See **megalophthalmus**.

mac·ro·po·di·a (măk'rə-pō'dē-ə) *n.* Abnormal largeness of the feet. Also called *megalopodia*.

mac·ro·pol·y·cyte (măk'rō-pŏl'ĭ-sīt') *n.* An unusually

large neutrophilic leukocyte that contains a multisegmented nucleus.

mac·ro·pro·so·pi·a (măk'rō-prə-sō'pē-ə) *n.* A face overly large in proportion to the cranial vault.

mac·ro·rhin·i·a (măk'rō-rĭn'ē-ə) *n.* Excessive size of the nose.

mac·ro·scop·ic (măk'rə-skŏp'ĭk) *or* **mac·ro·scop·i·cal** (-ĭ-kəl) *adj.* **1.** Large enough to be perceived or examined by the unaided eye. **2.** Relating to observations made by the unaided eye.

macroscopic anatomy *n.* See **gross anatomy**.

ma·cros·co·py (mă-krŏs'kə-pē) *n.* Examination with the naked eye.

mac·ro·sig·moid (măk'rō-sĭg'moid') *n.* Enlargement or dilation of the sigmoid colon.

mac·ro·so·mi·a (măk'rə-sō'mē-ə) *n.* Abnormally large size of the body.

mac·ro·sto·mi·a (măk'rə-stō'mē-ə) *n.* Abnormal largeness of the mouth.

mac·ro·ti·a (mă-krō'shē-ə, -shə) *n.* Excessive enlargement of the auricle of the ear.

mac·u·la (măk'yə-lə) *n., pl.* **–las** *or* **–lae** (-lē') **1.** *also* **mac·ule** (-yōōl') A discolored spot or area on the skin that is not elevated above the surface and is characteristic of certain conditions, such as smallpox, purpura, or roseola. **2.** An opaque spot on the cornea. **3.** The macula lutea. —**mac'u·lar** *adj.*

macula ad·her·ens (ăd-hîr'ənz, -hĕr'-) *n.* See **desmosome**.

macula a·troph·i·ca (ə-trŏf'ĭ-kə) *n.* An atrophic glistening white spot in the skin.

macula ce·ru·le·a (sə-rōō'lē-ə) *n.* A bluish stain on the skin caused by the bites of fleas or lice. Also called *blue spot*.

macula cor·ne·ae (kôr'nē-ē') *n.* A corneal opacity.

macula cri·bro·sa (krĭ-brō'sə) *n.* One of three areas, inferior, middle, and superior, on the wall of the vestibule of the labyrinth of the ear, through which nerve filaments pass to portions of the membranous labyrinth.

macula den·sa (dĕn'sə) *n.* A densely packed group of modified epithelial cells in the distal tubule of a nephron, adjacent to the juxtaglomerular cells.

macula fla·va (flā'və) *n.* A yellowish spot at the anterior end of the rima glottidis where the two vocal folds join.

macula lu·te·a (lōō'tē-ə) *n., pl.* **maculae lu·te·ae** (lōō'-tē-ē') A minute yellowish area containing the fovea centralis located near the center of the retina of the eye, at which visual perception is most acute. Also called *macula retinae, Soemmering's spot, yellow spot*.

macular amyloidosis *n.* Cutaneous amyloidosis characterized by itchy symmetrical brown reticular maculas and the deposition of amyloid as small subepidermal globules.

macular area *n.* The portion of the retina used for central vision.

macular degeneration *n.* Degeneration of the macula lutea characterized by spots of pigmentation and causing a reduction or loss of central vision.

macula ret·i·nae (rĕt'n-ē') *n.* See **macula lutea**.

macular leprosy *n.* Tuberculoid leprosy characterized by lesions that are small, hairless, and dry and that appear erythematous in light skin and hypopigmented or copper-colored in dark skin.

macula sac·cu·li (săk′yə-lī′) *n.* The oval sensory area in the anterior wall of the saccule of the ear where the saccular nerve filaments are attached.

mac·u·late (măk′yə-lāt′) *v.* To spot or blemish. —*adj.* (-lĭt) Spotted or blotched.

macula u·tric·u·li (yōō-trĭk′yə-lī′) *n.* The area in the lower wall of the utricle of the ear where the utricular nerve filments are attached.

mac·ule (măk′yōol′) *n.* Variant of **macula** (sense 1).

mac·u·lo·cer·e·bral (măk′yə-lō-sĕr′ə-brəl, -sə-rē′brəl) *adj.* Of or relating to a nervous disease that is characterized by degenerative lesions in both the retina and the brain.

mac·u·lo·er·y·them·a·tous (măk′yə-lō-ĕr′ə-thĕm′ə-təs, -thē′mə-) *adj.* Relating to lesions that are erythematous and macular.

maculopapular erythroderma *n.* A skin condition characterized by the appearance of reddish maculas and papules.

mac·u·lo·pap·ule (măk′yə-lō-păp′yōol) *n.* A lesion with a sessile base that slopes from a papule in the center. —**mac·u·lo·pap′u·lar** (-yə-lər) *adj.*

mac·u·lop·a·thy (măk′yə-lŏp′ə-thē) *n.* Any of various pathological conditions of the macula lutea.

mad (măd) *adj.* **1.** Angry; resentful. **2.** Suffering from a disorder of the mind; insane. **3.** Affected by rabies; rabid.

mad·a·ro·sis (măd′ə-rō′sĭs) *n.* See **milphosis**.

mad cow disease *n.* See **bovine spongiform encephalopathy**.

Ma·de·lung's deformity (măd′ə-lŭngz′, mä′də-) *n.* A deformity of the wrist due to a curvature of the lower extremity of the radius.

Madelung's disease *n.* The symmetrical deposition of fatty tissue on the upper part of the back, shoulders, and neck.

Mad Hatter syndrome *n.* A complex of disorders resulting from chronic mercury poisoning that includes stomatitis, diarrhea, ataxia, tremor, hyperreflexia, sensorineural impairment, and emotional instability.

mad·ness (măd′nĭs) *n.* The quality or condition of being insane.

Mad·u·ra boil (măj′ər-ə) *n.* See **mycetoma** (sense 1).

Mad·u·rel·la (măd′ə-rĕl′ə, măd′yə-) *n.* A genus of the Fungi Imperfecti that includes a number of species that cause maduromycosis and two species, *M. grisea* and *M. mycetomi*, that cause mycetoma.

mad·u·ro·my·co·sis (măd′ə-rō-mī-kō′sĭs, măd′yə-) *n.* Mycetoma that is caused by a varied group of fungi and is characterized by the formation of swellings and sinuses that discharge oily pus.

mag·got (măg′ət) *n.* The legless, soft-bodied, wormlike larva of any of various flies of the order Diptera, often found in decaying matter.

mag·ic bullet (măj′ĭk) *n.* A drug, therapy, or preventive therapy that cures or prevents a disease.

mag·is·tral (măj′ĭ-strəl) *adj.* Prepared as specified by a physician's prescription. Used of medicine.

mag·ma (măg′mə) *n.* **1.** A mixture of finely divided solids with enough liquid to produce a pasty mass. **2.** A

suspension of particles in a liquid, such as milk of magnesia.

mag·ne·sia (măg-nē′zhə) *n.* Magnesium oxide.

mag·ne·si·um (măg-nē′zē-əm, -zhəm) *n. Symbol* **Mg** A light metallic element that burns with a brilliant white flame, used in various analgesic, antiseptic, anticonvulsant, and antacid pharmaceuticals. Atomic number 12.

magnesium hydroxide *n.* A white powder used as an antacid and a laxative.

magnesium oxide *n.* A white powdery compound having a high melting point (2,800°C), used in food packaging, cosmetics, and pharmaceuticals.

magnesium salicylate *n.* A sodium-free salicylate derivative with anti-inflammatory, analgesic, and antipyretic actions, used for relief of mild to moderate pain.

magnesium sulfate *n.* A colorless crystalline compound used as a cathartic and applied locally as an anti-inflammatory agent.

mag·net·ic resonance (măg-nĕt′ĭk) *n.* The absorption of specific frequencies of radio and microwave radiation by atoms placed in a magnetic fielding.

magnetic resonance imaging *n. Abbr.* **MRI** The use of a nuclear magnetic resonance spectrometer to produce electronic images of specific atoms and molecular structures in solids, especially human cells, tissues, and organs.

mag·ne·to·en·ceph·a·log·ra·phy (măg-nē′tō-ĕn-sĕf′ə-lŏg′rə-fē) *n.* An imaging technique that is used to detect electromagnetic and metabolic shifts occurring in the brain during trauma.

mag·net therapy (măg′nĭt) *n.* An alternative medical therapy in which the placement of magnets or magnetic devices on the skin is thought to prevent or treat symptoms of disease, especially pain.

mag·ni·fi·ca·tion (măg′nə-fĭ-kā′shən) *n.* **1.** The act of magnifying or the state of being magnified. **2.** Something that has been magnified; an enlarged representation, image, or model. **3.** The ratio of the size of an image to the size of an object.

mag·ni·fy (măg′nə-fī′) *v.* To increase the apparent size of, especially with a lens.

mag·no·cel·lu·lar (măg′nō-sĕl′yə-lər) *adj.* Composed of large cells.

maid·en·head (mād′n-hĕd′) *n.* **1.** The condition or quality of being a maiden; virginity. **2.** The hymen.

main·stream·ing (mān′strē′mĭng) *n.* The process of integrating physically or intellectually disadvantaged students into regular school classes. —**main′stream′** *v.*

main·tain·er (mān-tā′nər) *n.* A device used to hold or keep teeth in a given position.

main·te·nance (mān′tə-nəns) *n.* The extent to which a patient continues good health practices without professional supervision, as distinguished from adherence or compliance.

maintenance drug therapy *n.* In chemotherapy, the systematic reduction of the dosage of a drug to a level that maintains protection against exacerbation of the condition.

Ma·joc·chi's disease (mə-yŏk′ēz, mä-yō′kēz) *n.* See **purpura annularis telangiectodes**.

ma·jor agglutinin (mā′jər) *n.* The specific agglutinin present in greatest quantity in an antiserum and developed as a result of immunization. Also called *chief agglutinin.*

major duodenal papilla *n.* A slight elevation marking the opening of the commmon bile duct and pancreatic duct into the duodenum.

major epilepsy *n.* See grand mal.

major histocompatibility complex *n. Abbr.* **MHC** A chromosomal segment that codes for cell-surface histocompatibility antigens and is the principal determinant of tissue type and transplant compatibility. Also called *HLA complex.*

major hysteria *n.* A syndrome characterized by a first stage of aura, a second stage of epileptoid convulsions, a third stage of tonic and clonic spasms, a fourth stage of dramatic behavior, and a fifth stage of delirium.

major salivary gland *n.* Any of three salivary glands, the parotid gland, the submandibular gland, and the sublingual gland, which are the largest of the oral cavity and secrete the most saliva.

major sublingual duct *n.* See Bartholin's duct.

mal (măl, mäl) *n.* A disease or disorder.

mal– *pref.* **1.** Bad; badly: *malpractice.* **2.** Abnormal; abnormally: *malformation.*

ma·la (mā′lə) *n., pl.* **–lae** (-lē) The cheek.

mal·ab·sorp·tion (măl′ăb-zôrp′shən) *n.* Defective or inadequate absorption of nutrients from the intestinal tract.

malabsorption syndrome *n.* A nutritional syndrome caused by any of various disorders in which there is ineffective absorption of nutrients from the gastrointestinal tract, characterized by diverse conditions such as diarrhea, weakness, edema, lassitude, weight loss, poor appetite, protuberant abdomen, pallor, bleeding tendencies, and muscle cramps.

ma·la·cia (mə-lā′shə) *n.* A softening or loss of consistency in any of the organs or tissues. Also called *malacosis, mollities.*

mal·a·co·pla·ki·a (măl′ə-kō-plā′kē-ə) *n.* A rare lesion in the mucosa of the urinary bladder, characterized by mottled yellow and gray soft plaques and nodules that consist of numerous macrophages and calcospherites.

mal·a·co·sis (măl′ə-kō′sĭs) *n.* See malacia.

mal·a·cot·ic (măl′ə-kŏt′ĭk) *adj.* Relating to or characterized by malacia.

mal·ad·just·ed (măl′ə-jus′tĭd) *adj.* Inadequately adjusted to the demands or stresses of daily living.

mal·ad·just·ment (măl′ə-jŭst′mənt) *n.* **1.** Faulty or inadequate adjustment. **2.** Inability to adjust to the demands of interpersonal relationships and the stresses of daily living.

mal·a·dy (măl′ə-dē) *n.* A disease, disorder, or ailment.

mal·aise (mă-lāz′, -lĕz′) *n.* A vague feeling of bodily discomfort, as at the beginning of an illness.

mal·a·lign·ment (măl′ə-līn′mənt) *n.* Displacement of a tooth or teeth from a normal position in the dental arch.

ma·lar (mā′lər, -lär′) *adj.* Of or relating to the cheekbone or the cheek. —*n.* The cheekbone.

malar bone *n.* See zygomatic bone.

ma·lar·i·a (mə-lâr′ē-ə) *n.* An infectious disease characterized by cycles of chills, fever, and sweating, caused by the parasitic infection of red blood cells by a protozoan of the genus *Plasmodium,* which is transmitted by the bite of an infected female anopheles mosquito. Also called *jungle fever, paludism, swamp fever.* —**ma·lar′i·al, ma·lar′i·an, ma·lar′i·ous** *adj.*

ma·lar·i·ae malaria (mə-lâr′ē-ē′) *n.* Malaria with paroxysms that recur every fourth day after the previous paroxysm, counting inclusively, caused by the schizogony and invasion of new red blood cells by *Plasmodium malariae.* Also called *quartan malaria.*

malarial crescent *n.* A gametocyte of the protozoan *Plasmodium falciparum,* whose presence in human red blood cells is evidence of malaria.

malar process *n.* See zygomatic process of maxilla.

Ma·las·se·zi·a (măl′ə-sē′zē-ə, -sā′-) *n.* Pityrosporum.

mal·as·sim·i·la·tion (măl′ə-sĭm′ə-lā′shən) *n.* Incomplete or imperfect assimilation of nutrients by the body.

mal·ate (măl′āt′, mā′lāt′) *n.* A salt or ester of malic acid.

malate dehydrogenase *n.* An enzyme that catalyzes, by means of NAD or NADP, the dehydrogenation of malate to oxaloacetate or the decarboxylation of maleate to pyruvate.

mal·ax·a·tion (măl′ăk-sā′shən) *n.* **1.** The formation of ingredients into a mass for pills and plasters. **2.** A kneading technique in massage.

mal de mer (măl′ də mâr′) *n.* See seasickness.

male (māl) *adj.* Of, relating to, or designating the sex that has organs to produce spermatozoa for fertilizing ova. —*n.* **1.** A member of the sex that begets young by fertilizing ova. **2.** A man or boy.

ma·le·ate (mā′lē-āt′, mə-lē′ət) *n.* **1.** A salt of maleic acid. **2.** An ester of maleic acid.

ma·le·ic acid (mə-lē′ĭk) *n.* A colorless crystalline dibasic acid that is an isomer of fumaric acid and is used as an oil and fat preservative.

male pattern baldness *n.* A progressive, diffuse loss of scalp hair in men that begins in the twenties or early thirties, depends on the presence of the androgenic hormone testosterone, and is caused by a combination of genetic and hormonal factors. Also called *alopecia hereditaria, androgenetic alopecia, male pattern alopecia, patterned alopecia.*

mal·e·rup·tion (măl′ĭ-rŭp′shən) *n.* Faulty eruption of a tooth or teeth.

male Turner's syndrome *n.* See Noonan's syndrome.

mal·for·ma·tion (măl′fôr-mā′shən) *n.* Abnormal or anomalous formation or structure; deformity.

mal·formed (măl-fôrmd′) *adj.* Abnormally or faultily formed.

mal·func·tion (măl-fŭngk′shən) *v.* **1.** To fail to function. **2.** To function improperly. —*n.* **1.** Failure to function. **2.** Faulty or abnormal functioning.

Mal·gaigne's luxation (măl-gĕn′yəz, măl-) *n.* Partial dislocation of the head of the radius of the arm beneath the annular ligament of the radius. Also called *nursemaid's elbow.*

Mal·herbe's calcifying epithelioma (mä-lĕrbz′) *n.* See pilomatrixoma.

mal·ic acid (măl′ĭk, mā′lĭk) *n.* A colorless crystalline intermediate in the Krebs cycle that occurs naturally in a variety of unripe fruit and is used as a flavoring and in the aging of wine.

ma·lig·nan·cy (mə-lĭg′nən-sē) *n.* **1.** The state or quality of being malignant. **2.** A malignant tumor.

ma·lig·nant (mə-lĭg′nənt) *adj.* **1.** Threatening to life, as a disease; virulent. **2.** Tending to metastasize; cancerous. Used of a tumor.

malignant anemia *n.* See **pernicious anemia**.

malignant bubo *n.* The bubo associated with bubonic plague.

malignant ciliary epithelioma *n.* A malignant proliferation of ciliary epithelium that frequently includes the infiltration of the pigmented layer. Also called *adult medulloepithelioma*.

malignant dyskeratosis *n.* Dyskeratosis that is likely to occur in precancerous or malignant lesions.

malignant fibrous histiocytoma *n.* A deeply situated tumor, especially on the extremities of adults, frequently recurring after surgery and metastasizing to the lungs.

malignant granuloma *n.* See **lethal midline granuloma**.

malignant hepatoma *n.* See **hepatocellular carcinoma**.

malignant histiocytosis *n.* A rapidly fatal form of lymphoma characterized by fever, jaundice, pancytopenia, and enlargement of the liver, spleen, and lymph nodes.

malignant hypertension *n.* Severe hypertension that runs a rapid course, causing necrosis of arteriolar walls and hemorrhagic lesions.

malignant hyperthermia *n.* Rapid onset of extremely high fever with muscle rigidity occurring during the administration of general anesthesia, precipitated in genetically susceptible persons especially by halothane or succinylcholine.

malignant jaundice *n.* Jaundice accompanied by high fever and delirium, seen in severe hepatitis and other extensive diseases of the liver. Also called *icterus gravis*.

malignant lentigo *n.* A precancerous brown or black lesion of the skin, often present in older persons, that appears on areas exposed to the sun, is irregular in shape, and is slow growing. Also called *Hutchinson's freckle*.

malignant lymphoma *n.* See **lymphoma**.

malignant melanoma *n.* See **melanoma**.

malignant melanoma in si·tu (ĭn sī′tōō, sē′-) *n.* A melanoma limited to the epidermis and composed of atypical melanocytes that may be round with abundant cytoplasm.

malignant nephrosclerosis *n.* Nephrosclerosis occurring in malignant hypertension.

malignant tertian malaria *n.* See **falciparum malaria**.

malignant tumor *n.* A tumor that invades surrounding tissues, is usually capable of producing metastases, may recur after attempted removal, and is likely to cause death unless adequately treated.

ma·lin·ger (mə-lĭng′gər) *v.* To feign illness or other incapacity in order to avoid duty or work.

mal·in·ter·dig·i·ta·tion (măl′ĭn-tər-dĭj′ĭ-tā′shən) *n.* Faulty intercuspation of teeth.

mal·le·a·ble (măl′ē-ə-bəl) *adj.* **1.** Capable of being shaped or formed, as by hammering or pressure. **2.** Easily controlled or influenced; tractable.

mal·le·o·in·cu·dal (măl′ē-ō-ĭng′kyə-dl, ĭng-kyōod′l) *adj.* Relating to the malleus and the incus in the middle ear.

mal·le·o·lus (mə-lē′ə-ləs) *n., pl.* **mal·le·o·li** (-lī′) A rounded bony prominence, such as those on either side of the ankle joint. —**mal·le′o·lar** (-lər) *adj.*

mal·le·ot·o·my (măl′ē-ŏt′ə-mē) *n.* **1.** The surgical division of the malleus. **2.** The surgical division of the ligaments holding the malleoli of the ankle in apposition.

mal·let finger (măl′ĭt) *n.* See **baseball finger**.

mal·le·us (măl′ē-əs) *n., pl.* **mal·le·i** (măl′ē-ī′) The hammer-shaped bone that is the outermost of the three auditory ossicles, articulating with the body of the incus. Also called *hammer*.

Mal·lo·ry body (măl′ə-rē) *n.* A poorly defined accumulation of eosinophilic material in the cytoplasm of damaged liver cells in certain forms of cirrhosis.

Mal·lo·ry's triple stain (măl′ə-rēz) *n.* A stain, made up of three acid dyes, used to differentially color components of tissue, especially connective tissue.

Mallory-Weiss lesion (-wīs′) *n.* Laceration of the gastric cardia, as seen in Mallory-Weiss syndrome. Also called *Mallory-Weiss tear*.

Mallory-Weiss syndrome *n.* A disorder of the lower end of the esophagus caused by severe retching and vomiting and characterized by laceration associated with bleeding, or by penetration into the mediastinum, with subsequent inflammation.

Mallory-Weiss tear *n.* See **Mallory-Weiss lesion**.

mal·nour·ished (măl-nûr′ĭsht) *adj.* Affected by improper nutrition or an insufficient diet.

mal·nour·ish·ment (măl-nûr′ĭsh-mənt) *n.* Malnutrition.

mal·nu·tri·tion (măl′nōō-trĭsh′ən) *n.* Poor nutrition because of an insufficient or poorly balanced diet or faulty digestion or utilization of foods.

mal·oc·clu·sion (măl′ə-klōō′zhən) *n.* Faulty contact between the upper and lower teeth when the jaw is closed.

ma·lo·nic acid (mə-lō′nĭk, -lŏn′ik) *n.* A white crystalline dicarboxylic acid derived from malic acid and used in the manufacture of barbiturates.

mal·o·nyl-CoA (măl′ə-nĭl′-) *n.* The condensation product of malonic acid and coenzyme A and an intermediate in fatty acid synthesis.

Mal·pi·ghi (măl-pē′gē, mäl-), **Marcello** 1628–1694. Italian anatomist who pioneered the use of a microscope in the study of anatomy and discovered the capillary system.

mal·pigh·i·an (măl-pĭg′ē-ən) *adj.* Of, relating to, or described by the Italian anatomist Marcello Malpighi.

malpighian body *n.* See **malpighian corpuscle** (sense 2).

malpighian capsule *n.* **1.** See **Bowman's capsule**. **2.** A thin fibrous membrane enveloping the spleen and continuing over the vessels entering at the hilus.

malpighian corpuscle *n.* **1.** See **renal corpuscle**. **2.** Any of numerous small nodular masses of lymphoid tissue attached to the sides of the smaller arterial branches in the spleen. Also called *malpighian body, splenic lymph follicle*.

Malpighian layer *n.* The basal layer of the epidermis and the prickle cell layer considered as one unit. Also called *germinative layer.*

malpighian pyramid *n.* See **renal pyramid.**

malpighian stigma *n.* Any of the points where the smaller veins of the spleen enter the larger veins.

mal·po·si·tion (măl′pə-zĭsh′ən) *n.* See **dystopia.**

mal·prac·tice (măl-prăk′tĭs) *n.* Improper or negligent treatment of a patient, as by a physician, resulting in injury, damage, or loss.

mal·pres·en·ta·tion (măl′prĕz-ən-tā′shən) *n.* Presentation of a part of a fetus other than the back of the head during parturition.

mal·ro·ta·tion (măl′rō-tā′shən) *n.* Failure of normal rotation of all or part of an organ or system, such as the intestinal tract or spinal cord, during embryonic development.

MALT (môlt) *n.* Mucosal-associated with lymphoid tissue; rare type of lymphoma of the stomach that may be associated with infection by the bacteria *Helicobacter pylori.* Also called *MALT lymphoma.*

Mal·ta fever (môl′tə) *n.* See **brucellosis.**

mal·tase (môl′tās′, -tāz′) *n.* An enzyme that catalyzes the hydrolysis of maltose to glucose.

mal·tose (môl′tōs′, -tōz′) *n.* A white crystalline sugar formed during the digestion of starch.

mal·un·ion (măl-yōōn′yən) *n.* Incomplete union or union in a faulty position after a fracture or wound.

ma·mil·la (mă-mĭl′ə) *n., pl.* **–mil·lae** (-mĭl′ē) 1. A small rounded elevation resembling the female breast. **2.** See **nipple.**

mam·il·lar·y (măm′ə-lĕr′ē) *adj.* Relating to or shaped like a nipple.

mamillary body *n.* A small round paired cell group that protrudes into the interpeduncular fossa from the inferior aspect of the hypothalamus, receives a major bundle of hippocampal fibers from the fornix, and projects fibers to the anterior thalamic nuclei and into the tegmentum of the brainstem.

mamillary duct *n.* See **lactiferous duct.**

mamillary line *n.* An imaginary vertical line passing through the center of the nipple. Also called *nipple line.*

mam·il·late (măm′ə-lāt′) *or* **mam·mil·lat·ed** (-lā′tĭd) *adj.* Having nipplelike projections.

mam·il·la·tion (măm′ə-lā′shən) *n.* 1. A nipplelike projection. **2.** The condition of having such projections.

ma·mil·li·form (mă-mĭl′ə-fôrm′) *adj.* Nipple-shaped.

ma·mil·lo·tha·lam·ic fascicle (mə-mĭl′ō-thə-lăm′ĭk, măm′ə-lō-) *n.* A thick compact bundle of nerve fibers that passes from the mamillary body on either side to the anterior nucleus of the thalamus. Also called *Vicq d'Azyr's bundle.*

mam·ma (măm′ə) *n., pl.* **mam·mae** (măm′ē) A mammary gland.

mam·mal·gia (mă-măl′jə) *n.* See **mastodynia.**

mam·ma·plas·ty *or* **mam·mo·plas·ty** (măm′ə-plăs′tē) *n.* Reconstructive or cosmetic plastic surgery to alter the size or shape of the breast.

mam·ma·ry (măm′ə-rē) *adj.* Of or relating to a breast or mamma.

mammary artery *n.* The internal thoracic artery or the lateral thoracic artery.

mammary duct *n.* See **lactiferous duct.**

mammary fold *n.* See **mammary ridge.**

mammary gland *n.* Any of the milk-producing apocrine glands typically occurring in pairs in female mammals and consisting of lobes containing clusters of alveoli with a system of ducts to convey the milk to an external nipple or teat.

mammary line *n.* A transverse line drawn between the two nipples.

mammary ridge *n.* A bandlike thickening of ectoderm in the embryo extending from just below the axilla to the inguinal region and giving rise to the mammary glands. Also called *mammary fold, milk line.*

mam·mec·to·my (mă-mĕk′tə-mē) *n.* See **mastectomy.**

mam·mi·form (măm′ə-fôrm′) *adj.* Resembling a breast; breast-shaped.

mam·mil·la (mă-mĭl′ə) *n., pl.* **-mil·lae** (-mĭl′ē) 1. A nipple or teat. **2.** A nipple-shaped protuberance.

mam·mil·la·plas·ty (mă-mĭl′ə-plăs′tē) *n.* Plastic surgery of the nipple and areola of the breast. Also called *theleplasty.*

mam·mil·late (măm′ə-lāt) *or* **mam·mil·lat·ed** (-lā′tĭd) *adj.* 1. Having nipples or mammillae. **2.** Shaped like a nipple or mammilla.

mam·mil·li·tis (măm′ə-lī′tĭs) *n.* Inflammation of the nipple.

mam·mi·tis (mă-mī′tĭs) *n.* See **mastitis.**

mammo– *pref.* Breast; mammary gland: *mammogram.*

mam·mo·gram (măm′ə-grăm′) *n.* An x-ray image of the breast produced by mammography.

mam·mog·ra·phy (mă-mŏg′rə-fē) *n.* Radiographic examination of the breasts for diagnostic purposes.

mam·mo·plas·ty (măm′ə-plăs′tē) *n.* Variant of **mammaplasty.**

mam·mose (măm′ōs′) *adj.* Having large breasts.

mam·mot·o·my (mă-mŏt′ə-mē) *n.* See **mastotomy.**

mam·mo·trop·ic (măm′ə-trŏp′ĭk, -trō′pĭk) *or* **mam·mo·troph·ic** (-trŏf′ĭk, -trō′fĭk) *adj.* Having a stimulating effect upon the development, growth, or function of the mammary glands.

man·aged care (măn′ĭjd) *n.* Any arrangement for health care in which an organization, such as an HMO, another type of doctor-hospital network, or an insurance company, acts as intermediate between the person seeking care and the physician.

Man·ches·ter operation (măn′chĕs′tər, -chĭ-stər) *n.* A vaginal operation for prolapsed uterus consisting of cervical amputation and parametrial fixation of the cervical ligament of the uterus. Also called *Fothergill's operation.*

Man·chu·ri·an hemorrhagic fever (măn-chŏŏr′ē-ən) *n.* See **epidemic hemorrhagic fever.**

man·del·ic acid (măn-dĕl′ĭk) *n.* An acid that has both antibacterial and bacteriostatic properties, used in treating urinary tract infections.

man·de·lyt·ro·pine (măn′də-lĭt′rō-pēn′) *n.* See **homatropine.**

man·di·ble (măn′də-bəl) *n.* A U-shaped bone forming the lower jaw, articulating with the temporal bone on either side. Also called *submaxilla.* —**man·dib′u·lar** (-dĭb′yə-lər) *adj.*

mandibular arch *n.* The first postoral arch in the series of branchial arches. Also called *mandibular process.*

mandibular cartilage *n.* A cartilaginous bar in the embryonic mandibular arch whose proximal end becomes ossified to form the malleus. Also called *Meckel's cartilage.*

mandibular dentition *n.* See **dental arch** (sense 2).

mandibular fossa *n.* A deep hollow in the squamous portion of the temporal bone at the base of the zygomatic process in which the condyle of the mandible rests. Also called *glenoid fossa.*

mandibular joint *n.* The joint between the head of the mandible and the mandibular fossa and articular tubercle of the temporal bone. Also called *temporomandibular joint.*

mandibular nerve *n.* The third division of the trigeminal nerve, formed by the union of the sensory fibers from the trigeminal ganglion and the motor root in the oval foramen through which the nerve emerges, and having meningeal, masseteric, deep temporal, lateral and medial pterygoid, buccal, auriculotemporal, lingual, and inferior alveolar branches.

mandibular node *n.* Any of the facial lymph nodes located by the facial artery near the point where it crosses the mandible.

mandibular process *n.* See **mandibular arch.**

man·dib·u·lo·ac·ral dysplasia (măn-dĭb′yə-lō-ăk′rəl) *n.* A hereditary disorder characterized by dental crowding, ulceration and wasting of the skin on the hands and feet, softening and destruction of the bones, and stiff joints.

man·dib·u·lo·fa·cial (măn-dĭb′yə-lō-fā′shəl) *adj.* Relating to the mandible and the face.

mandibulofacial dysostosis *n.* A syndrome that includes various malformations of specialized structures in the head and neck, including notched eyelid fissures, hypoplasia of the mandible, enlarged mouth with high or cleft palate and incorrectly positioned teeth, and atypical hair growth. Also called *Franceschetti's syndrome.*

man·dib·u·lo·oc·u·lo·fa·cial (măn-dĭb′yə-lō-ŏk′yə-lō-fā′shəl) *adj.* Relating to the mandible and the orbital part of the face.

man·drel *or* **man·dril** (măn′drəl) *n.* **1.** A shaft on which a working tool is mounted, as in a dental drill. **2.** See **mandrin.**

man·drin (măn′drĭn) *n.* A stiff wire or stylet inserted into a soft catheter to give it shape and firmness while passing through a hollow tubular structure. Also called *mandrel.*

ma·neu·ver (mə-nōō′vər) *n.* A movement or procedure that involves skill and dexterity. —*v.* To manipulate into a desired position or toward a predetermined goal.

man·ga·nese (măng′gə-nēz′, -nēs′) *n. Symbol* **Mn** A brittle metallic element, having several allotropes. It is alloyed with steel to increase strength. Atomic number 25.

mange (mānj) *n.* Any of several chronic skin diseases of mammals caused by parasitic mites and characterized by skin lesions, itching, and loss of hair. —**mang′y** (mān′jē) *adj.*

ma·ni·a (mā′nē-ə, mān′yə) *n.* A manifestation of bipolar disorder characterized by profuse and rapidly changing ideas, exaggerated gaiety, and excessive physical activity.

–mania *suff.* An abnormal compulsion or an extreme love for: *pyromania.*

ma·ni·ac (mā′nē-ăk′) *n.* An insane person.

ma·ni·a·cal (mə-nī′ə-kəl) *or* **ma·ni·ac** (mā′nē-ăk′) *adj.* Suggestive of or afflicted with insanity.

man·ic (măn′ĭk) *adj.* Relating to, affected by, or resembling mania.

manic-depressive *adj.* Of, relating to, or affected by bipolar disorder. —*n.* A person who is afflicted with bipolar disorder.

manic-depressive illness *n.* See **bipolar disorder.**

man·i·fes·ta·tion (măn′ə-fĕ-stā′shən) *n.* An indication of the existence, reality, or presence of something, especially an illness.

man·i·fest content (măn′ə-fĕst′) *n.* The content of a dream, fantasy, or thought as it is remembered and reported in psychoanalysis.

manifest hyperopia *n. Abbr.* **Hm** Hyperopia that can be measured by convex lenses without paralyzing accommodation with a mydriatic drug.

man·i·fest·ing heterozygote (măn′ə-fĕs′tĭng) *n.* An organism heterozygous for what is ordinarily a recessive condition and, as a result of special mechanisms, such as Lyonization, with phenotypic manifestations. Also called *manifesting carrier.*

ma·nip·u·late (mə-nĭp′yə-lāt′) *v.* To handle and move in an examination or for therapeutic purposes.

ma·nip·u·la·tion (mə-nĭp′yə-lā′shən) *n.* **1.** The act or the practice of manipulating. **2.** The state of being manipulated.

man·ner·ism (măn′ə-rĭz′əm) *n.* A distinctive behavioral trait; an idiosyncrasy.

man·ni·tol (măn′ĭ-tôl′, -tōl′) *n.* A white, crystalline, water-soluble, slightly sweet alcohol, used as a dietary supplement and dietetic sweetener and in medical tests of renal function.

man·nose (măn′ōs′) *n.* A monosaccharide obtained from various plants by the oxidation of mannitol.

man·no·si·do·sis (măn′ə-sĭ-dō′sĭs) *n.* An inherited disorder caused by the deficiency of an enzyme necessary for the metabolism of mannose and characterized by mental retardation, kyphosis, and an enlarged tongue, with the accumulation of mannose in the body tissues.

ma·nom·e·ter (mə-nŏm′ĭ-tər) *n.* **1.** An instrument that is used for measuring the pressure of liquids and gases. **2.** A sphygmomanometer. —**man′o·met′ric** (măn′ə-mĕt′rĭk), **man′o·met′ri·cal** *adj.* —**ma·nom′e·try** *n.*

man. pr. *abbr. Latin* mane primo (early morning, first thing in the morning)

Man·son (măn′sən), Sir **Patrick** 1844–1922. Scottish parasitologist. One of the founders (1899) of the London School of Tropical Medicine, he introduced (1877) the hypothesis that the mosquito is host to the malaria parasite.

Man·son·el·la (măn′sə-nĕl′ə) *n.* A genus of filarial worms that are found chiefly in Central and South America and cause mansonelliasis.

Mansonella per·stans (pûr′stănz′) *n.* A species of *Mansonella* found in tropical Africa and in northern South America that infests human peritoneal and other body cavities but is only mildly pathogenic; it is transmitted by a biting midge.

Mansonella strep·to·cer·ca (strĕp′tə-sûr′kə) *n.* A species of *Mansonella* found in central and western Africa that causes a lichenoid condition or edema of the skin and that is transmitted by a species of biting midge.

man·so·nel·li·a·sis (măn′sə-nĕl-ī′ə-sĭs) *n.* Infection with a species of filarial worms of the genus *Mansonella,* transmitted by biting midges of the genus *Culicoides;* the adult worms live in the serous cavities, especially the peritoneal cavity, in mesenteric and perivisceral adipose tissue, and in the skin.

Man·so·ni·a (măn-sō′nē-ə) *n.* A genus of mosquitoes that includes species that transmit the filarial worms associated with filariasis and elephantiasis in southeast Asia and Indonesia.

Man·son's disease (măn′sənz) *n.* See **schistosomiasis mansoni.**

man·tle (măn′tl) *n.* **1.** A covering layer of tissue. **2.** See **pallium.**

mantle radiotherapy *n.* The use of radiotherapy with protection of uninvolved radiosensitive structures or organs.

Man·toux test (măn-tōō′, män-) *n.* A tuberculin test in which a small amount of tuberculin is injected under the skin.

man·u·al ventilation (măn′yōō-əl) *n.* A method of assisted or controlled ventilation in which the hands are used to generate airway pressures.

ma·nu·bri·um (mə-nōō′brē-əm, -nyōō′-) *n., pl.* **–bri·a** (-brē-ə) **1.** The upper segment of the sternum with which the clavicle and the first two pairs of ribs articulate. **2.** See **episternum. 3.** The portion of the malleus that is embedded in the tympanic membrane and extends downward, inward, and backward from the neck of the malleus.

ma·nus (mā′nəs, măn′əs) *n., pl.* **manus 1.** The distal part of the arm, including the carpus, metacarpus, and digits. **2.** The hand.

man·y-tailed bandage (mĕn′ē-tāld′) *n.* A large oblong cloth, applied to the thorax or abdomen, with ends cut into narrow strips that are tied or overlapped and pinned. Also called *Scultetus bandage.*

MAO *abbr.* monoamine oxidase

MAOI *abbr.* monoamine oxidase inhibitor

map (măp) *n.* **1.** The human face. **2.** A genetic map. —*v.* **1.** To make a map of. **2.** To locate a gene or DNA sequence in a specific region of a chromosome in relation to known genes or DNA sequences.

ma·ple syr·up urine disease (mā′pəl sĭr′əp, sûr′-) *n.* A hereditary metabolic disorder that is due to a deficiency of decarboxylase enzyme that leads to elevated concentrations of leucine, isoleucine, and valine in the blood and urine, and is characterized by the urine having an odor that is similar to that of maple syrup, severe mental retardation, and seizures. Also called *branched chain ketoaciduria.*

map·ping function (măp′ĭng) *n.* A mathematical formula that relates distances on a gene map to recombination frequencies; its graphic rendering shows that the recombination value of two genes is never greater than

50 percent regardless of how far apart the genes are on a chromosome.

ma·pro·ti·line hydrochloride (mə-prōt′l-ēn′) *n.* An antidepressant that is chemically similar to tricyclic antidepressants and that inhibits neuronal reuptake of norepinephrine.

map unit *n.* A measure of distance between two linked genes corresponding to a recombination frequency of one percent.

Ma·ra·ñon's sign (mär′ən-yōnz′) *n.* An indication of Graves' disease in which a vasomotor reaction occurs following stimulation of the skin over the throat.

ma·ran·tic (mə-răn′tĭk) *adj.* Marasmic.

ma·ras·mus (mə-răz′məs) *n.* Chronic wasting of body tissues, especially in young children, commonly due to prolonged dietary deficiency of protein and calories. Also called *athrepsia.* —**ma·ras′mic** *adj.*

mar·ble bone disease (mär′bəl) *n.* See **osteopetrosis.**

marble bones *n.* See **osteopetrosis.**

Mar·burg virus (mär′bûrg′) *n.* A virus that is considered to contain RNA and that is known to cause Marburg virus disease but whose taxonomic classification remains undetermined.

Marburg virus disease *n.* An often fatal infection of humans by the Marburg virus that is characterized by severe fever, diarrhea, a maculopapular rash, and hemorrhaging.

Mar·cac·ci's muscle (mär-kät′chēz) *n.* A sheet of smooth muscle fibers underlying the areola and nipple of the mammary gland.

march fracture (märch) *n.* A fatigue fracture occurring in a metatarsal bone of the foot.

march hemoglobinuria *n.* Hemoglobinuria occurring after prolonged or heavy physical exercise.

Mar·chia·fa·va-Bi·gna·mi disease (mär′kyə-fä′və-bĭnyä′mē, -bē-) *n.* Degeneration of the corpus callosum, characterized by mental deterioration, dementia, and convulsions, and occurring predominately in chronic alcoholics.

Marchiafava-Mi·che·li syndrome (-mē-kě′lē) *n.* See **paroxysmal nocturnal hemoglobinuria.**

Mar·cus Gunn phenomenon *or* **Mar·cus Gunn syndrome** (mär′kəs gŭn′) *n.* See **jaw-winking syndrome.**

Marcus Gunn's sign *n.* See **Gunn's sign.**

mar·fan·oid (mär′fə-noid′) *adj.* Characteristic of or resembling the symptoms of Marfan's syndrome.

Mar·fan's syndrome (mär′fănz) *n.* A hereditary disorder principally affecting the connective tissues of the body, manifested in varying degrees by excessive bone elongation and joint flexibility and by abnormalities of the eye and cardiovascular system.

mar·gin (mär′jĭn) *n.* **1.** A border or edge, as of an organ. **2.** A limit in a condition or process, beyond or below which something is no longer possible or acceptable. **3.** An amount that is allowed but that is beyond what is needed. **4.** A measure, quantity, or degree of difference.

mar·gin·al (mär′jə-nəl) *adj.* **1.** Of, relating to, located at, or constituting a margin, a border, or an edge. **2.** Marginally within a lower standard or limit of quality. **3.** Relating to or located at the fringe of consciousness. —**mar′gin·al′i·ty** (-jə-năl′ĭ-tē) *n.*

marginal gyrus *n.* The superior frontal gyrus.

marginal sinus of placenta *n.* Any of the discontinuous venous lakes at the margin of the placenta.

mar·gin·a·tion (mär′jə-nā′shən) *n.* The adhesion of white blood cells to the endothelial cells of blood vessels that occurs at the site of an injury during the early phases of inflammation.

margin of safety *n.* The amount between a therapeutic dose and a lethal dose of a drug.

mar·gi·no·plas·ty (mär′jə-nō-plăs′tē) *n.* Plastic or reparative surgery of the tarsal border of an eyelid.

Ma·rie's disease (mə-rēz′, mä-) *n.* **1.** See **acromegaly. 2.** See **hypertrophic pulmonary osteoarthropathy.**

Marie-Strümpell disease *n.* See **ankylosing spondylitis.**

mar·i·jua·na *or* **mar·i·hua·na** (măr′ə-wä′nə) *n.* **1.** The cannabis plant. **2.** A preparation made from the dried flower clusters and leaves of the cannabis plant, usually smoked or eaten to induce euphoria.

Mar·i·nol (măr′ĭ-nôl′) A trademark for the drug dronabinol.

mark (märk) *n.* **1.** A spot or line on a surface, visible through difference in color or elevation from that of the surrounding area. **2.** A distinctive trait or property. —*v.* **1.** To make a visible trace or impression on, as occurs with a spot or dent. **2.** To form, make, or depict by making a mark. **3.** To distinguish or characterize.

mark·er (mär′kər) *n.* **1.** One that marks or serves as a mark. **2.** A physiological substance, such as human chorionic gonadotropin or alpha-fetoprotein, that may indicate disease when present in abnormal amounts in the serum, as that caused by a malignancy. Also called *biomarker.* **3.** A genetic marker.

marker trait *n.* A trait that may be of little importance in itself but which facilitates the detection or understanding of a particular disease.

mar·mo·rat·ed (mär′mə-rā′tĭd) *adj.* Having a marbled or streaked appearance.

Ma·ro·teaux-La·my syndrome (măr′ə-tō′lä-mē′, mä-rô-) *n.* An inherited defect in mucopolysaccharide metabolism characterized by excretion of dermatan sulfate in the urine, retarded growth, lumbar kyphosis, sternal protrusion, knock-knee, and usually enlargement of the liver and spleen. Also called *type VI mucopolysaccharidosis.*

mar·row (măr′ō) *n.* **1.** Bone marrow. **2.** The spinal cord.

marsh gas *n.* See **methane.**

mar·su·pi·al·i·za·tion (mär-soo′pē-ə-lĭ-zā′shən) *n.* Surgical alteration of a cyst or similar enclosed cavity by making an incision and suturing the flaps to the adjacent tissue, creating a pouch.

Mar·tin (mär′tn), **Lillien Jane** 1851–1943. American psychologist who is noted for her pioneering work in gerontology.

mas·cu·line (măs′kyə-lĭn) *n.* **1.** Of or relating to men or boys; male. **2.** Suggestive or characteristic of a man.

masculine pelvis *n.* **1.** A pelvis justo minor in which the bones are large and heavy. **2.** In a female, a slight degree of funnel-shaped pelvis in which the shape approximates that of the male pelvis.

masculine uterus *n.* See **prostatic utricle.**

mas·cu·lin·i·ty (măs′kyə-lĭn′ĭ-tē) *n.* **1.** The quality or condition of being masculine. **2.** Something traditionally considered to be characteristic of a male.

mas·cu·lin·ize (măs′kyə-lə-nīz′) *v.* **1.** To give a masculine appearance or character to. **2.** To cause a female to assume masculine characteristics, as through hormonal imbalance. —**mas′cu·lin·i·za′tion** (-lə-nĭ-zā′shən) *n.*

mas·cu·lin·o·vo·blas·to·ma (măs′kyə-lĭn-ō′vō-blăs-tō′mə) *n.* An ovarian neoplasm that causes varying degrees of masculinization.

MASH *abbr.* Mobile Army Surgical Hospital

mask (măsk) *n.* **1.** A covering for the nose and mouth that is used for inhaling oxygen or an anesthetic. **2.** A covering that is worn over the nose and mouth, as by a surgeon or dentist, to prevent infection. **3.** A facial bandage. **4.** Something, often a trait, that disguises or conceals. **5.** Any of a variety of conditions producing alteration or discoloration of the skin of the face. **6.** An expressionless appearance of the face seen in certain diseases, such as Parkinsonism. —*v.* **1.** To cover with a protective mask. **2.** To cover in order to conceal, protect, or disguise.

masked (măskt) *adj.* **1.** Latent or hidden, as a symptom or disease. **2.** Having masklike markings on the head or face. **3.** Having the anatomy of the next developmental form outlined beneath the integument, as in certain insect pupae.

masked gout *n.* See **latent gout.**

masked virus *n.* A virus ordinarily occurring in the host in a noninfective state but which may be activated by special procedures.

mask·ing (măs′kĭng) *n.* **1.** The concealment or the screening of one sensory process or sensation by another. **2.** An opaque covering used to camouflage the metal parts of a prosthesis.

mask·like face (măsk′līk′) *n.* See **Parkinson's facies.**

mask of pregnancy *n.* See **chloasma.**

Mas·low (măz′lō), **Abraham** 1908–1970. American psychologist and a founder of humanistic psychology who developed a model of human motivation in which a higher need is expressed only after lower needs are fulfilled.

mas·och·ism (măs′ə-kĭz′əm) *n.* **1.** The act or an instance of deriving sexual gratification from being physically or emotionally abused. **2.** A psychological disorder in which sexual gratification is derived from being physically or emotionally abused. **3.** The act or an instance of deriving pleasure from being offended, dominated, or mistreated. **4.** The tendency to seek such mistreatment. —**mas′och·ist** *n.* —**mas′och·is′tic** *adj.*

masochistic personality *n.* A personality disorder characterized by the exploitation or infliction of pain on others or oneself so as to gain personal satisfaction or pleasure.

masque bi·liaire (măsk′ bēl-yâr′) *n.* Hyperpigmentation occurring in the skin around the eyes of middle-aged women, unrelated to systemic disease.

mass (măs) *n.* **1.** A unified body of matter with no specific shape. **2.** A grouping of individual parts or elements that compose a unified body of unspecified size or quantity. **3.** The physical volume or bulk of a solid body. **4.** *Abbr.* **m** The measure of the quantity of matter that a body or an object contains. The mass of the body is not dependent on gravity and therefore is different from but proportional to its weight. **5.** A thick, pasty pharmacological mixture containing drugs from which pills are formed. **6.** One of the seven fundamental SI units, the kilogram. **7.** See **massa**.

mas·sa (măs′ə) *n., pl.* **-sae** (măs′ē) A lump or aggregation of coherent material. Also called *mass*.

mas·sage (mə-säzh′ -säj′) *n.* **1.** The rubbing or kneading of parts of the body especially to aid circulation, relax the muscles, or provide sensual stimulation. **2.** An act or instance of such rubbing or kneading. *—v.* **1.** To give a massage to. **2.** To treat by means of a massage.

massage parlor *n.* An establishment that offers therapeutic massage.

massage therapy *n.* The systematic application of massage to treat muscle pain or dysfunction.

masseteric artery *n.* An artery with its origin in the maxillary artery, with distribution to the deep surface of the masseter muscle.

masseteric nerve *n.* A muscular branch of the mandibular nerve passing to the medial surface of the masseter muscle, which it supplies.

mas·se·ter (mə-sē′tər) *n.* A muscle with origin from the inferior border and medial surface of the zygomatic arch, with insertion into the lateral surface of the ramus of the mandible, with nerve supply from the masseteric nerve, and whose action closes the jaw during chewing. *—*mas·se·ter·ic (măs′ĭ-tĕr′ĭk) *adj.*

mass hysteria *n.* **1.** Spontaneous, en masse development of identical physical or emotional symptoms among a group of individuals, as in a classroom of schoolchildren. **2.** A socially contagious frenzy of irrational behavior in a group of people that occurs as a reaction to an event.

mas·sive (măs′ĭv) *adj.* **1.** Large in comparison with the usual amount. **2.** Affecting a large area of bodily tissue; widespread and severe.

mas·so·ther·a·py (măs′ō-thĕr′ə-pē) *n.* The therapeutic use of massage.

mass peristalsis *n.* Brief forcible peristaltic movements that move the contents through long segments of the large intestine.

mast- *pref.* Variant of **masto-**.

mas·tad·e·ni·tis (măs′tă-dn-ī′tĭs) *n.* See **mastitis**.

mas·tad·e·no·ma (măs′tă-dn-ō′mə) *n.* A benign tumor of the breast.

Mas·tad·e·no·vi·rus (mă-stăd′n-ō-vī′rəs) *n.* A genus of adenoviruses including many species that infect humans, some of which cause respiratory infections and acute follicular conjunctivitis.

mas·tal·gia (mă-stăl′jə) *n.* See **mastodynia**.

mas·tat·ro·phy (mă-stăt′rə-fē) *n.* Atrophy or wasting of the breasts.

mast cell *n.* A cell found in connective tissue that contains numerous basophilic granules and releases substances such as heparin and histamine in response to injury or inflammation of bodily tissues. Also called *labrocyte, mastocyte*.

mast cell leukemia *n.* See **basophilic leukemia**.

mas·tec·to·my (mă-stĕk′tə-mē) *n.* Surgical removal of all or part of a breast, sometimes including excision of the underlying pectoral muscles and regional lymph nodes, usually performed as a treatment for cancer. Also called *mammectomy*.

mas·ter gland (măs′tər) *n.* See **pituitary gland**.

Mas·ter's test (măs′tərz) *n.* See **two-step exercise test**.

Master's two-step exercise test *n.* See **two-step exercise test**.

mas·ti·cate (măs′tĭ-kāt′) *v.* To chew food. *—*mas′ti·ca′tion *n.*

mas·ti·ca·to·ry (măs′tĭ-kə-tôr′ē) *adj.* **1.** Of, relating to, or used in mastication. **2.** Adapted for chewing. *—n.* A medicinal substance that is chewed to increase salivation.

masticatory force *n.* See **force of mastication**.

masticatory system *n.* The organs and structures primarily functioning in mastication, including jaws and jaw muscles, teeth, temporomandibular joints, tongue, lips, cheeks, and mucous membranes.

mas·ti·gote (măs′tĭ-gōt′) *n.* A flagellated protozoan of the class Mastigophora.

mas·ti·tis (mă-stī′tĭs) *n.* Inflammation of the breast. Also called *mammitis, mastadenitis*.

mast leukocyte *n.* See **basophilic leukocyte**.

masto- *or* **mast-** *pref.* Breast; mammary gland; nipple: *mastectomy*.

mas·to·cyte (măs′tə-sīt′) *n.* See **mast cell**.

mas·to·cy·to·ma (măs′tō-sī-tō′mə) *n., pl.* **-mas** *or* **-ma·ta** (-mə-tə) An accumulation or nodule of mast cells that resembles a tumor.

mas·to·cy·to·sis (măs′tō-sī-tō′sĭs) *n., pl.* **-ses** (-sēz) A condition characterized by the abnormal proliferation of mast cells in the tissues.

mas·to·dyn·i·a (măs′tə-dĭn′ē-ə) *n.* Pain in the breast. Also called *mammalgia, mastalgia*.

mas·toid (măs′toid′) *n.* The mastoid process. *—adj.* **1.** Of or relating to the mastoid process, antrum, or sinuses. **2.** Shaped like a breast or nipple.

mastoid antrum *n.* A cavity in the petrous portion of the temporal bone that communicates with the mastoid sinuses and epitympanic recess of the middle ear. Also called *tympanic antrum*.

mastoid bone *n.* See **mastoid process** (sense 1).

mastoid canaliculus *n.* The canal that extends from the jugular fossa through the mastoid process and transmits the auricular branch of the vagus nerve.

mastoid cell *n.* See **mastoid sinus**.

mas·toid·ec·to·my (măs′toi-dĕk′tə-mē) *n.* Surgical removal of mastoid sinuses or part or all of the mastoid process.

mastoid emissary vein *n.* A vein that connects the sigmoid sinus with the occipital vein or with one of the tributaries of the outer jugular vein by way of the mastoid foramen.

mas·toi·de·o·cen·te·sis (măs-toi′dē-ō-sĕn-tē′sĭs) *n.* Surgical puncture of the mastoid sinuses and the mastoid antrum.

mastoid foramen *n.* An opening at the rear of the mastoid process, transmitting a small artery to the dura mater and an emissary vein to the sigmoid sinus.

mas·toid·i·tis (măs′toi-dī′tĭs) *n.* Inflammation of the mastoid process and mastoid sinuses.

mas·toid·ot·o·my (măs′toi-dŏt′ə-mē) *n.* Incision into the subperiosteum or the mastoid process of the temporal bone.

mastoid part *n.* The portion of the petrous part of the temporal bone bearing the mastoid process.

mastoid part *n.* The portion of the petrous part of the temporal bone bearing the mastoid process.

mastoid process *n.* **1.** A conical protuberance of the posterior portion of the temporal bone that is situated behind the ear and serves as a site of muscle attachment. Also called *mastoid bone.* **2.** The part of the first pharyngeal arch in the embryo, developing into the upper jaw in the embryo.

mastoid sinus *n.* Any of numerous air-filled spaces of various sizes in the mastoid process. Also called *mastoid cell.*

mas·to·oc·cip·i·tal (măs′tō-ŏk-sĭp′ĭ-tl) *adj.* Relating to the mastoid portion of the temporal bone and to the occipital bone.

mas·to·pa·ri·e·tal (măs′tō-pə-rī′ĭ-təl) *adj.* Relating to the mastoid portion of the temporal bone and to the parietal bone.

mas·top·a·thy (mă-stŏp′ə-thē) *n.* Any of various diseases of the breasts.

mas·to·pex·y (măs′tə-pĕk′sē) *n.* Plastic surgery to correct sagging breasts. Also called *mazopexy.*

mas·to·pla·sia (măs′tə-plā′zhə) *n.* Enlargement of the breast. Also called *mazoplasia.*

mas·to·plas·ty (măs′tə-plăs′tē) *n.* Plastic surgery of the breast.

mas·top·to·sis (măs′tŏp-tō′sĭs, -tō-tō′sĭs) *n.* Sagging of the breasts.

mas·tor·rha·gia (măs′tə-rā′jə) *n.* Hemorrhage from a breast.

mas·to·scir·rhus (măs′tō-skĭr′əs, -sĭr′əs) *n.* A scirrhous carcinoma of the breast.

mas·to·squa·mous (măs′tō-skwā′məs, -skwä′-) *adj.* Relating to the mastoid and the squamous portions of the temporal bone.

mas·tot·o·my (mă-stŏt′ə-mē) *n.* Incision of the breast. Also called *mammotomy.*

mas·tur·bate (măs′tər-bāt′) *v.* To perform an act of masturbation.

mas·tur·ba·tion (măs′tər-bā′shən) *n.* Excitation of one's own or another's genital organs, usually to orgasm, by manual contact or means other than sexual intercourse.

Mat·as operation (măt′əs) *n.* See **aneurysmoplasty** (sense 1).

match·ing (măch′ĭng) *n.* The process of comparing a study group and a comparison group in an epidemiological study with respect to extraneous or confounding factors such as age, sex, or breed.

mate (māt) *n.* **1.** A spouse. **2.** Either of a pair of animals or birds that associate in order to propagate. **3.** Either of a pair of animals brought together for breeding. —*v.* **1.** To become joined in marriage. **2.** To be paired for reproducing; breed. **3.** To copulate.

ma·te·ri·a al·ba (mə-tîr′ē-ə ăl′bə) *n.* A white cheeselike accumulation of food debris, microorganisms, desquamated epithelial cells, and blood cells deposited around the teeth at the gumline.

materia med·i·ca (mĕd′ĭ-kə) *n.* The branch of medical science that deals with the origin, preparation, dosage, and administration of drugs.

ma·ter·nal (mə-tûr′nəl) *adj.* **1.** Relating to or characteristic of a mother. **2.** Inherited from one's mother.

maternal dystocia *n.* A difficult delivery caused by an abnormality in the mother.

maternal placenta *n.* The part of the placenta derived from uterine tissue. Also called *uterine placenta.*

ma·ter·ni·ty (mə-tûr′nĭ-tē) *n.* **1.** The state of being a mother; motherhood. **2.** The feelings or characteristics associated with being a mother; motherliness. **3.** A maternity ward. —*adj.* Relating to pregnancy, childbirth, or the first months of motherhood.

maternity ward *n.* The department of a hospital that provides care for women during pregnancy and childbirth as well as for newborn infants.

mat·ing (mā′tĭng) *n.* The pairing of a male and a female for the purpose of reproduction.

mat·ri·cal (măt′rĭ-kəl) *adj.* Of or relating to a matrix.

mat·ri·cide (măt′rĭ-sīd′) *n.* The act of killing one's mother. —**mat′ri·cid′al** (-sīd′l) *adj.*

mat·ri·cli·nous (măt′rĭ-klī′nəs) *adj.* Having predominantly maternal hereditary traits.

mat·ri·lin·e·al (măt′rə-lĭn′ē-əl) *adj.* Relating to, based on, or tracing ancestral descent through the maternal line.

ma·trix (mā′trĭks) *n., pl.* **ma·trix·es** *or* **ma·tri·ces** (mā′-trĭ-sēz′, măt′rĭ-) **1.** A surrounding substance within which something else originates, develops, or is contained. **2.** The womb. **3.** The formative cells or tissue of a fingernail, toenail, or tooth. **4.** See **ground substance**. **5.** A specially shaped instrument, plastic material, or metal strip for holding and shaping the material used in filling a tooth cavity.

matrix band *n.* A metal or plastic band secured around the crown of a tooth to confine the restorative material filling a cavity.

matrix calculus *n.* A urinary calculus containing calcium salts and consisting primarily of an organic matrix composed of a mucoprotein and a sulfated mucopolysaccharide; it is usually associated with chronic infection.

matrix un·guis (ŭng′gwĭs) *n.* See **nail bed**.

mat·ter (măt′ər) *n.* **1.** Something that occupies space and can be perceived by one or more senses. **2.** A specific type of substance. **3.** Discharge or waste, such as pus or feces, from a living organism.

mat·tress suture (măt′rĭs) *n.* A suture made with a double stitch that forms a loop about the tissue on both sides of a wound and produces eversion of the edges.

Mat·u·lane (măch′ə-lān′) A trademark for procarbazine hydrochloride.

mat·u·rate (măch′ə-rāt′) *v.* **1.** To mature, ripen, or develop. **2.** To suppurate.

mat·u·ra·tion (măch′ə-rā′shən) *n.* **1.** The process of becoming mature. **2.** Production or discharge of pus. **3.** The processes by which gametes are formed, including the reduction of chromosomes in a germ cell from the diploid number to the haploid number by meiosis. **4.** The final differentiation processes in biological systems, such as the attainment of total functional capability by a cell, a tissue, or an organ. —**mat′u·ra′tion·al** *adj.*

maturation arrest *n.* The cessation of complete differentiation of cells at an immature stage.

maturation division *n.* Either of the two successive cell divisions of meiosis, with only one duplication of the chromosomes, that results in the formation of haploid gametes.

ma·ture (mə-cho͞or′, -too̅r′) *adj.* **1.** Having reached full natural growth or development. **2.** Of, relating to, or characteristic of full mental or physical development. —*v.* To evolve toward or reach full development.

mature bacteriophage *n.* The complete infective form of a bacteriophage.

mature cataract *n.* A cataract in which the entire lens is opaque and swollen.

mature-onset diabetes *n.* Non-insulin-dependent diabetes mellitus.

ma·tu·ri·ty (mə-cho͞or′ĭ-tē, -too̅r′-) *n.* **1.** The state or quality of being fully grown or developed. **2.** The state or quality of being mature.

maturity-onset diabetes *n.* Non-insulin-dependent diabetes mellitus.

Mau·rer's dot (mou′rərz) *n.* Any of the fine granular precipitates or irregular cytoplasmic particles usually present in red blood cells infected with the trophozoites of *Plasmodium falciparum.*

Mau·riac's syndrome (môr′ē-äks′, môr-yäks′) *n.* Dwarfism that is accompanied by obesity and enlargement of the liver and spleen in children with poorly controlled diabetes mellitus.

Mau·ri·ceau's maneuver (mô-rē-sōz′) *n.* A method of delivering the head in an assisted breech delivery in which the infant's body is supported by the right forearm while traction is made upon the shoulders by the left hand.

Mauth·ner's sheath (mout′nərz) *n.* See **axolemma.**

Max·air (măk′sâr′) A trademark for the drug pirbuterol acetate.

max·il·la (măk-sĭl′ə) *n., pl.* **max·il·las** *or* **max·il·lae** (măk-sĭl′ē) Either of a pair of irregularly shaped bones of the skull, fusing in the midline, supporting the upper teeth, and forming part of the eye sockets, hard palate, and nasal cavity; upper jaw.

max·il·lar·y (măk′sə-lĕr′ē) *adj.* Of or relating to a jaw or jawbone, especially the upper one. —*n.* A jawbone.

maxillary antrum *n.* See **maxillary sinus.**

maxillary artery *n.* An artery with its origin in the external carotid artery and branches to the deep auricular, anterior tympanic, middle meningeal, inferior alveolar, masseteric, deep temporal, buccal, superior posterior alveolar, infraorbital, descending palatine arteries, the artery of the pterygoid canal, and the sphenopalatine artery; internal maxillary artery.

maxillary dentition *n.* See **dental arch** (sense 2).

maxillary gland *n.* See **submandibular gland.**

maxillary nerve *n.* The second division of the trigeminal nerve, passing from the trigeminal ganglion into the pterygopalatine fossa, where it continues forward to give off the zygomatic nerve and enter the eye socket.

maxillary process *n.* A thin plate projecting from the upper border of the lower nasal concha, articulating with the maxilla and partly closing the orifice of the maxillary sinus.

maxillary sinus *n.* An air cavity in the body of the maxilla, communicating with the middle meatus of the nose. Also called *antrum of Highmore, maxillary antrum.*

maxillary vein *n.* A posterior continuation of the pterygoid plexus, joining the superficial temporal vein to form the retromandibular vein.

max·il·lo·den·tal (măk-sĭl′ō-dĕn′tl) *adj.* Relating to the upper jaw and its teeth.

max·il·lo·fa·cial (măk-sĭl′ō-fā′shəl) *adj.* Relating to or involving the maxilla and the face.

max·il·lo·man·dib·u·lar (măk-sĭl′ō-măn-dĭb′yə-lər) *adj.* Relating to or involving the maxilla and the mandible.

max·il·lot·o·my (măk′sə-lŏt′ə-mē) *n.* Surgical sectioning of the maxilla to allow movement of all or a part of the maxilla into the desired position.

max·i·mal (măk′sə-məl) *adj.* **1.** Of, relating to, or consisting of a maximum. **2.** Being the greatest possible.

maximal dose *n.* The largest quantity of a drug that an adult can safely take within a given period.

maximal permissible dose *n. Abbr.* **MPD** The largest dose of radiation to which members of a population may be exposed without harmful effects.

max·i·mum (măk′sə-məm) *n., pl.* **–mums** *or* **–ma** (-mə) **1.** The greatest possible quantity or degree. **2.** The greatest quantity or degree reached or recorded; the upper limit of variation. **3.** The time or period during which the highest point or degree is attained. —*adj.* **1.** Having or being the greatest quantity or the highest degree attained or attainable. **2.** Of, relating to, or making up a maximum.

maximum breathing capacity *n. Abbr.* **MBC** The volume of gas that can be breathed in 15 seconds when a person breathes as deeply and quickly as possible. Also called *maximum voluntary ventilation.*

maximum velocity *n.* **1.** The maximum rate of an enzymatic reaction that can be achieved by progressively increasing the substrate concentration. **2.** The maximum initial rate of shortening of a myocardial fiber that can be obtained under zero load. Used to evaluate the contractility of the fiber.

maximum voluntary ventilation *n.* See **maximum breathing capacity.**

Max·i·pime (măk′sə-pēm′) A trademark for the drug cefepime hydrochloride.

Max·zide (măks′zīd′) A trademark for a drug containing hydrochlorothiazide and triamterene, used for hypertension.

May·er-Rokitansky-Küs·ter-Hau·ser syndrome (mī′ər-; -küs′tər-hou′zər) *n.* Congenital absence of the vagina or presence of a short vaginal pouch and absence of the uterus but with normal ovaries. Also called *Rokitansky-Küster-Hauser syndrome.*

May·er's reflex (mī′ərz) *n.* See **basal joint reflex.**

May-Hegglin anomaly (mā′-) *n.* See **Hegglin's anomaly.**

Ma·yo (mā′ō), **William James** 1861–1939. American surgeon who with his brother, **Charles Horace Mayo** (1865–1939), founded the Mayo Clinic, a renowned medical center in Rochester, Minnesota.

Mayo-Rob·son's position (-rŏb′sənz) *n.* A supine position with a thick pad under the loins to elevate the lumbocostal region, used in gallbladder surgery.

Ma·yo's operation (mā′ōz) *n.* An operation for the radical correction of umbilical hernia.

May-White syndrome *n.* Progressive myoclonus epilepsy accompanied by lipomas, deafness, and ataxia.

mazo– *pref.* Breast: *mazoplasia.*

ma·zo·pex·y (mā′zə-pĕk′sē) *n.* See **mastopexy.**

ma·zo·pla·sia (mā′zə-plā′zhə) *n.* See **mastoplasia.**

Mb *abbr.* myoglobin

M band *n.* See **M line.**

MBC *abbr.* maximum breathing capacity

MC *or* **MCh** *abbr. Latin* Magister Chirurgiae (Master of Surgery); Medical Corps

Mc·Ar·dle-Schmid-Pear·son disease (mə-kär′dl-shmĭt′pîr′sən) *n.* See **type 5 glycogenosis.**

Mc·Ar·dle's disease (mə-kär′dlz) *n.* See **type 5 glycogenosis.**

MCAT *abbr.* Medical College Admissions Test

Mc·Bur·ney's point (mək-bûr′nēz) *n.* A point above the anterior superior spine of the ilium, located on a straight line joining that process and the umbilicus, where pressure of the finger elicits tenderness in acute appendicitis.

Mc·Clin·tock (mə-klĭn′tək, -tŏk′), **Barbara** 1902–1992. American genetic botanist. She won a 1983 Nobel Prize for discovering that genes are mobile within the chromosomes of a plant cell.

Mc·Col·lum (mə-kŏl′əm), **Elmer** 1879–1967. American biochemist and nutritionist who first classified vitamins, distinguishing between fat-soluble (A) vitamins and water-soluble (B) vitamins.

Mc·Dou·gall (mək-dōō′gəl), **William** 1871–1938. British-born American psychologist who theorized that human behavior is determined by both instinctive and intentional strivings.

Mc·Dow·ell (mək-dou′əl), **Ephraim** 1771–1830. American surgeon who performed (1809) the first recorded ovariotomy.

mcg *abbr.* microgram

MCH *abbr.* mean cell hemoglobin

MCHC *abbr.* mean cell hemoglobin concentration

mCi *abbr.* millicurie

Mc·Mur·ray test (mək-mûr′ē) *n.* A test for injury to meniscal structures of the knee in which the lower leg is rotated while the leg is extended; pain and a cracking in the knee indicates meniscal injury.

MCP *abbr.* metacarpophalangeal

MCS *abbr.* multiple chemical sensitivity

MCV *abbr.* mean corpuscular volume

Mc·Vay's operation (mək-vāz′) *n.* Surgical repair of femoral hernias by suture of the transverse muscle of the abdomen and its associated fasciae to the pectineal ligament.

Md The symbol for the element **mendelevium.**

MD *abbr. Latin* Medicinae Doctor (Doctor of Medicine); muscular dystrophy

MDF *abbr.* myocardial depressant factor

MDI *abbr.* metered dose inhaler

MDMA (ĕm′dē-ĕm-ā′) *n.* 3,4-Methylenedioxymethamphetamine; a mescaline analog.

ME *abbr.* medical examiner

mead·ow dermatitis (mĕd′ō) *n.* A phototoxic dermatitis in which a streaky eruption develops where the skin comes in contact with a plant and then is exposed to sunlight. Also called *phytophlyctodermatitis, phytophotodermatitis.*

Mead·ows's syndrome (mĕd′ōz) *n.* A disease of the myocardium that develops during pregnancy or the puerperium.

meal[1] (mēl) *n.* **1.** The edible whole or coarsely ground grains of a cereal grass. **2.** A granular substance produced by grinding.

meal[2] (mēl) *n.* **1.** The food served and eaten in one sitting. **2.** A customary time or occasion of eating food.

mean (mēn) *n.* **1.** Something having a position, quality, or condition midway between extremes; a medium. **2.** A number that typifies a set of numbers, such as a geometric mean or an arithmetic mean. **3.** The average value of a set of numbers. —*adj.* **1.** Occupying a middle or intermediate position between two extremes. **2.** Intermediate in size, extent, quality, time, or degree; medium.

mean calorie *n. Abbr.* **cal** See **calorie** (sense 4).

mean cell hemoglobin *n. Abbr.* **MCH** The hemoglobin content of the average red blood cell, calculated from the hemoglobin therein and the red cell count in erythrocyte indices.

mean cell hemoglobin concentration *n. Abbr.* **MCHC** The average hemoglobin concentration in a given volume of packed red blood cells.

mean corpuscular volume *n. Abbr.* **MCV** The average volume of red blood cells in erythrocyte indices, calculated from the hematocrit and the red blood cell count.

mea·sles (mē′zəlz) *n.* **1.** An acute contagious viral disease usually occurring in childhood and characterized by eruption of red spots on the skin, fever, and catarrhal symptoms. Also called *rubeola.* **2.** Black measles. **3.** Any of several other diseases, especially German measles, that cause similar but milder symptoms. **4.** A disease of cattle and swine caused by tapeworm larvae.

measles immune globulin *n.* A sterile solution of globulins prepared from human immune serum globulin that contains the concentration and type of antibodies needed to protect a person from measles without causing the disease.

measles, mumps, rubella vaccine *n. Abbr.* **MMR** A vaccine containing a combination of live attenuated measles, mumps, and rubella viruses in an aqueous suspension.

measles virus *n.* An RNA virus of the genus *Morbillivirus* that causes measles in humans. Also called *rubeola virus.*

measles virus vaccine *n.* A vaccine containing live attenuated strains of measles virus prepared in chick embryo cell cultures and used to immunize against measles.

meas·ure (mĕzh′ər) *n.* **1.** Dimensions, quantity, or capacity as ascertained by comparison with a standard. **2.** A reference standard or sample used for the quantitative comparison of properties. **3.** A unit specified by a scale, such as a degree, or by variable conditions, such as room temperature. **4.** A system of measurement, such as the metric system. **5.** A device used for measuring. **6.** The act of measuring. **7.** An evaluation or a basis of comparison. **8.** Extent or degree. **9.** A definite quantity that has been measured out. —*v.* **1.** To ascertain the dimensions, quantity, or capacity of. **2.** To mark, lay out, or establish dimensions for by measuring. **3.** To bring into comparison. **4.** To mark off or apportion, usually with reference to a given unit of measurement. **5.** To serve as a measure of.

me·a·tal (mē-āt′l) *adj.* Relating to a meatus.

meato– *pref.* Meatus: *meatoscopy.*

me·at·o·plas·ty (mē-ăt′ə-plăs′tē) *n.* Reparative or reconstructive surgery of a meatus or canal.

me·a·tor·rha·phy (mē′ə-tôr′ə-fē) *n.* Suture of the wound made by performing a meatotomy.

me·a·tos·co·py (mē′ə-tŏs′kə-pē) *n.* The inspection of a meatus, especially of the urethra.

me·a·tot·o·my (mē′ə-tŏt′ə-mē) *n.* An incision made to enlarge a meatus, as of the urethra or ureter. Also called *porotomy.*

me·a·tus (mē-ā′təs) *n., pl.* **-tus·es** or **meatus** A body opening or passage, especially the external opening of a canal.

me·chan·i·cal (mǐ-kăn′ĭ-kəl) *adj.* **1.** Operated or produced by a mechanism or machine. **2.** Relating to, produced by, or dominated by physical forces. **3.** Interpreting and explaining the phenomena of the universe by referring to causally determined material forces; mechanistic.

mechanical alternation *n.* A disorder in which contractions of the heart are regular in time but are alternately stronger and weaker. Also called *alternation of heart.*

mechanical antidote *n.* A substance that prevents the absorption of a poison.

mechanical dysmenorrhea *n.* See **obstructive dysmenorrhea.**

mechanical ileus *n.* Obstruction of the bowel arising from a mechanical cause, such as volvulus, a gallstone, or adhesions.

mechanical jaundice *n.* See **obstructive jaundice.**

mechanical mixture *n.* A heterogeneous mixture of particles or masses distinguishable as such under the microscope or separable by filtration.

mechanical vector *n.* A vector that simply conveys pathogens to a susceptible individual and is not essential to the development of the organism.

mechanical ventilation *n.* A mode of assisted or controlled ventilation using mechanical devices that cycle automatically to generate airway pressure.

me·chan·ics (mǐ-kăn′ĭks) *n.* **1.** The branch of physics concerned with the analysis of the action of forces on matter or material systems. **2.** The design, construction, and use of machinery or of mechanical structures. **3.** The functional and technical aspects of an activity.

mech·a·nism (měk′ə-nĭz′əm) *n.* **1.** A machine or mechanical appliance. **2.** The arrangement of connected parts in a machine. **3.** A system of parts that operate or interact like those of a machine. **4.** An instrument or a process by which something is done or comes into being. **5.** The involuntary and consistent response of an organism to a given stimulus. **6.** A usually unconscious mental and emotional pattern that dominates behavior in a given situation or environment. **7.** The sequence of steps in a chemical reaction. **8.** The philosophical

doctrine that all natural phenomena are explicable by material causes and mechanical principles.

mech·a·nis·tic (měk′ə-nĭs′tĭk) *adj.* **1.** Mechanically determined. **2.** Of or relating to the philosophy of mechanism, especially one that tends to explain phenomena only by reference to physical or biological causes.

mech·a·no·re·cep·tor (měk′ə-nō-rĭ-sěp′tər) *n.* A specialized sensory end organ that responds to mechanical stimuli such as tension or pressure.

mech·a·no·ther·a·py (měk′ə-nō-thěr′ə-pē) *n.* Medical treatment by mechanical methods, such as massage. —**mech′a·no·ther′a·pist** *n.*

Meck·el (měk′əl), **Johann Friedrich** 1781–1833. German anatomist and embryologist known for his comprehensive descriptions of congenital defects.

Meckel scan *n.* A radiological scan of the gastric mucosa that is used to detect ectopic gastric mucosa in Meckel's diverticulum.

Meck·el's cartilage (měk′əlz) *n.* See **mandibular cartilage.**

Meckel's cavity *n.* The cavity between the two layers of the dura mater that encloses the roots of the trigeminal nerve and the trigeminal ganglion. Also called *trigeminal cavity.*

Meckel's diverticulum *n.* A diverticulum formed from the remains of an unobliterated yolk stalk, located on the ileum a short distance above the cecum and sometimes attached to the umbilicus.

Meckel syndrome *n.* A hereditary malformation syndrome characterized by sloping forehead, cleft palate, ocular anomalies, and polydactyly, resulting in death during the perinatal period. Also called *dysencephalia splanchnocystica.*

mec·li·zine (měk′lǐ-zēn′) *n.* An antihistaminic used in the prevention and treatment of nausea and motion sickness.

mec·lo·fen·a·mate sodium (měk′lō-fěn′ə-māt′) *n.* A nonsteroidal anti-inflammatory agent with analgesic and antipyretic actions.

me·co·nism (mē′kə-nĭz′əm) *n.* Opium addiction or poisoning.

me·co·ni·um (mǐ-kō′nē-əm) *n.* **1.** A dark green fecal material that accumulates in the fetal intestines and is discharged at or near the time of birth. **2.** See **opium.**

meconium aspiration *n.* Aspiration of amniotic fluid contaminated with meconium by a fetus in hypoxic distress.

meconium ileus *n.* Intestinal obstruction in a newborn child following the thickening of meconium resulting from a lack of trypsin and associated with cystic fibrosis of the pancreas.

meconium peritonitis *n.* Peritonitis caused by intestinal perforation in the fetus or newborn, and associated with congenital obstruction or fibrocystic disease of the pancreas.

med (měd) *adj.* Medical. Used informally. —*n.* A medication. Used informally, often in the plural.

med·e·vac (měd′ĭ-văk′) *n.* **1.** Air transport of persons to a place where they can receive medical or surgical care; medical evacuation. **2.** A helicopter or other aircraft used for such transport. —*v.* To transport a patient to a place where medical care is available.

Med·a·war (měd'ə-wər), **Peter Brian** 1915–1987. Brazilian-born British biologist. He shared a 1960 Nobel Prize for the discovery of acquired immunological tolerance.

me·di·a¹ (mē'dē-ə) *n.* A plural of **medium**.

me·di·a² (mē'dē-ə) *n.* The tunica media.

me·di·al (mē'dē-əl) *adj.* **1.** Relating to, situated in, or extending toward the middle; median. **2.** Being or relating to an average or a mean.

medial cord of brachial plexus *n.* A fasciculus formed by the anterior division of the inferior trunk, giving rise to the medial pectoral, the medial brachial cutaneous, the medial antebrachial cutaneous, the ulnar, and the medial root of the median nerves.

medial crest *n.* A ridge of bone on the posterior surface of the fibula separating the attachment of the posterior tibial muscle from that of the long flexor muscle of the great toe and the soleus muscle.

medial cuneiform bone *n.* The medial bone of the distal row of the tarsus and the largest of the three cuneiform bones, articulating with the intermediate cuneiform, navicular, and first and second metatarsal bones. Also called *first cuneiform bone*.

medial cutaneous nerve of arm *n.* A nerve that arises from the medial cord of the brachial plexus and supplies the skin of the medial side of the arm.

medial cutaneous nerve of calf *n.* A nerve that arises from the tibial nerve in the popliteal space, unites in the middle of the leg with the communicating branch of the common peroneal nerve to form the sural nerve, and is distributed to the skin of the distal and lateral surfaces of the leg and the ankle.

medial cutaneous nerve of forearm *n.* A nerve that arises from the medial cord of the brachial plexus and supplies the skin of the anterior and ulnar surfaces of the forearm.

medial forebrain bundle *n.* A fiber system running longitudinally through the lateral zone of the hypothalamus, connecting it with the midbrain tegmentum and various components of the limbic system.

medial geniculate body *n.* The medial group of a pair of prominent cell groups in the posteroinferior aspects of the thalamus, serving as the last of a series of processing stations along the auditory conduction pathway to the cerebral cortex.

medial ligament *n.* **1.** See **deltoid ligament**. **2.** The bundle of fibers strengthening the medial part of the articular capsule of the temporomandibular joint.

medial longitudinal fasciculus *n.* A longitudinal bundle of fibers extending from the upper border of the mesencephalon into the cervical segments of the spinal cord, composed largely of fibers from the vestibular nuclei ascending to the motor neurons innervating the external eye muscles, and descending to spinal cord segments innervating the musculature of the neck.

medial longitudinal stria *n.* A thin longitudinal band of nerve fibers accompanied by gray matter running along the surface of the corpus callosum on either side of the median line.

medial oc·cip·i·to·tem·po·ral gyrus (ŏk-sĭp'ĭ-tō-těm'-pər-əl, -těm'prəl) *n.* See **lingual gyrus**.

medial plantar nerve *n.* One of the two terminal branches of the tibial nerve running along the medial aspect of the sole to supply the abductor muscle of the big toe and the short flexor muscle of the toes and innervating the skin of the medial part of the foot and the medial three and one-half toes.

medial pterygoid muscle *n.* A muscle with origin from the pterygoid fossa of the sphenoid bone and the tuberosity of the maxilla, with insertion into the medial surface of the mandible, with nerve supply from the medial pterygoid branch of the mandibular division of the trigeminal nerve, and whose action raises the mandible and closes the jaw.

medial rectus muscle *n.* A muscle with origin from the fibrous ring surrounding the optic canal, with insertion into the medial part of the sclera of the eye, with nerve supply from the oculomotor nerve, and whose action directs the pupil medialward.

medial supraclavicular nerve *n.* One of several nerves arising from the cervical plexus that supply the skin over the upper medial part of the chest. Also called *anterior supraclavicular nerve*.

me·di·an (mē'dē-ən) *adj.* **1.** Relating to, located in, or extending toward the middle. **2.** Of, relating to, or situated in or near the plane that divides a bilaterally symmetrical animal into right and left halves; mesial. **3.** Of, relating to, or constituting the middle value in a distribution. —*n.* **1.** A median point, plane, line, or part. **2.** The middle value in a distribution, above and below which lie an equal number of values.

median artery *n.* An artery with its origin in the anterior interosseous artery and with distribution to the palm.

median bar of Mercier *n.* A band of fibromuscular tissue encircling the interureteric ridge of the urinary bladder, which occasionally can obstruct the urinary tract.

median groove of tongue *n.* A slight longitudinal depression that runs forward on the dorsal surface of the tongue. Also called *longitudinal raphe of tongue, median longitudinal raphe of tongue*.

median line *n.* **1.** Anterior median line. **2.** Posterior median line.

median longitudinal raphe of tongue *n.* See **median groove of tongue**.

median nerve *n.* A nerve that is formed by the union of the medial and lateral roots from the medial and lateral cords of the brachial plexus and supplies the muscular branches in the anterior region of the forearm and the muscular and cutaneous branches in the hand.

median plane *n.* A vertical plane along the midline of the body dividing the body into right and left halves. Also called *midsagittal plane*.

median rhinoscopy *n.* Examination of the roof of the nasal cavity and openings of the posterior ethmoidal cells and sphenoidal sinus using a long-bladed nasal speculum or a nasopharyngoscope.

median rhomboid glossitis *n.* A congenital disorder of the tongue characterized by a rhomboid or ovoid, sometimes elevated red area in the dorsal midline, just anterior to the vallate papillae, that lacks lingual papillae.

median sacral vein *n.* An unpaired vein that accompanies the middle sacral artery and empties into the left common iliac vein.

median vein *n.* An intermediate vein.

mediastinal emphysema *n.* A deflection of air, usually from a ruptured emphysematous bleb in the lung, into the mediastinal tissue.

mediastinal fibrosis *n.* The development of fibrous tissue in the upper mediastinum, causing obstruction of the superior vena cava.

mediastinal space *n.* See **mediastinum** (sense 2).

mediastinal vein *n.* Any of several small veins from the mediastinum emptying into the brachiocephalic vein or the superior vena cava.

me·di·as·ti·ni·tis (mē′dē-ăs′tə-nī′tĭs) *n.* Inflammation of the cellular tissue of the mediastinum.

me·di·as·ti·nog·ra·phy (mē′dē-ăs′tə-nŏg′rə-fē) *n.* Radiography of the mediastinum.

me·di·as·ti·no·per·i·car·di·tis (mē′dē-ăs′tə-nō-pĕr′ĭ-kär-dī′tĭs) *n.* Inflammation of the pericardium and of the surrounding mediastinal cellular tissue.

me·di·as·tin·o·scope (mē′dē-ăs-tĭn′ə-skōp′) *n.* An endoscope inserted through an incision above the sternum to examine the mediastinum.

me·di·as·ti·nos·co·py (mē′dē-ăs′tə-nŏs′kə-pē) *n.* Exploration of the mediastinum through a suprasternal incision.

me·di·as·ti·not·o·my (mē′dē-ăs′tə-nŏt′ə-mē) *n.* Incision into the mediastinum.

me·di·as·ti·num (mē′dē-ə-stī′nəm) *n.,* *pl.* **–na** (-nə) **1.** A septum between two parts of an organ or a cavity. **2.** The region in mammals between the pleural sacs, containing the heart and all of the thoracic viscera except the lungs. Also called *interpleural space, mediastinal space.* —**me′di·as·ti′nal** (-nəl) *adj.*

mediastinum testis *n.* A mass of connective tissue at the back of the testis that encloses the rete testis.

me·di·ate (mē′dē-āt′) *v.* To effect or convey as an intermediate agent or mechanism. —*adj.* (-ĭt) Being in a middle position.

mediate auscultation *n.* The use of a stethoscope to examine the internal sounds of a body.

mediate percussion *n.* Percussion effected by the intervention of a finger or a pleximeter between the striking finger or plexor and the part percussed.

med·ic (mĕd′ĭk) *n.* **1.** A member of a military medical corps. **2.** A physician or surgeon. **3.** A medical student or intern.

med·i·ca·ble (mĕd′ĭ-kə-bəl) *adj.* Potentially responsive to treatment with medicine; curable.

Med·i·caid *or* **med·i·caid** (mĕd′ĭ-kād′) *n.* A program in the United States, jointly funded by the states and the federal government, that reimburses hospitals and physicians for providing care to qualifying people who cannot finance their own medical expenses.

med·i·cal (mĕd′ĭ-kəl) *adj.* **1.** Of, relating to, or characterizing the study or practice of medicine. **2.** Requiring treatment by medicine. —*n.* A thorough physical examination.

medical assistant *n. Abbr.* **MA** A person trained to assist a physician or other medical provider in clinical and administrative procedures.

medical diathermy *n.* Diathermy in which the tissues are warmed but not destroyed.

medical examiner *n. Abbr.* **ME 1.** A physician officially authorized by a governmental unit to ascertain causes of deaths, especially those not occurring under natural circumstances. **2.** A physician who examines employees of a particular firm or applicants for life insurance.

medical genetics *n.* The study of the etiology, pathogenesis, and natural history of diseases and disorders that are at least partially genetic in origin.

med·i·ca·lize (mĕd′ĭ-kə-līz′) *v.* To characterize a behavior or condition as a disorder requiring medical treatment.

medical jurisprudence *n.* See **forensic medicine**.

medical law *n.* The branch of law that deals with the application of medical knowledge to legal problems.

medical psychology *n.* The branch of psychology concerned with the application of psychological principles to the practice of medicine.

medical record *n.* A chronological written account of a patient's examination and treatment that includes the patient's medical history and complaints, the physician's physical findings, the results of diagnostic tests and procedures, and medications and therapeutic procedures.

medical tran·scrip·tion·ist (trăn-skrĭp′shə-nĭst) *n.* A person who transcribes medical reports dictated by a physician concerning a patient's health care.

me·dic·a·ment (mĭ-dĭk′ə-mənt, mĕd′ĭ-kə-) *n.* An agent that promotes recovery from injury or ailment; medicine.

Med·i·care *or* **med·i·care** (mĕd′ĭ-kâr′) *n.* A program under the US Social Security Administration that reimburses hospitals and physicians for medical care provided to qualifying people over 65 years old.

med·i·cate (mĕd′ĭ-kāt′) *v.* **1.** To treat by medicine. **2.** To tincture or permeate with a medicinal substance.

med·i·ca·tion (mĕd′ĭ-kā′shən) *n.* **1.** A medicine; a medicament. **2.** The act or process of treating with medicine. **3.** Administration of medicine.

me·dic·i·nal (mĭ-dĭs′ə-nəl) *adj.* Of, relating to, or having the properties of medicine.

med·i·cine (mĕd′ĭ-sĭn) *n.* **1.** The science of diagnosing, treating, or preventing disease and other damage to the body or mind. **2.** The branch of this science encompassing treatment by drugs, diet, exercise, and other nonsurgical means. **3.** The practice of medicine. **4.** An agent, such as a drug, used to treat disease or injury.

med·i·co (mĕd′ĭ-kō′) *n.* **1.** A physician. **2.** A medical student.

medico– *pref.* Medical science: *medicolegal.*

med·i·co·chi·rur·gi·cal (mĕd′ĭ-kō-kī-rûr′jĭ-kəl) *adj.* Relating to medicine and surgery.

med·i·co·le·gal (mĕd′ĭ-kō-lē′gəl) *adj.* Of, relating to, or concerned with medicine and law.

Med·i·gap (mĕd′ĭgăp′) *n.* Private health insurance designed to supplement the coverage provided under governmental programs such as Medicare.

medio– *pref.* Middle: *mediocarpal.*

me·di·o·car·pal (mē′dē-ō-kär′pəl) *adj.* **1.** Of or relating to the central part of the carpus. **2.** Of or relating to the articulation between the two rows of carpal bones; carpocarpal.

me·di·o·dor·sal (mē′dē-ō-dôr′səl) *adj.* Relating to the median plane and the dorsal plane.

me·di·o·lat·er·al (mē′dē-ō-lăt′ər-əl) *adj.* Relating to the median plane and a side.

me·di·o·ne·cro·sis (mē′dē-ō-nə-krō′sĭs) *n.* Necrosis of the tunica media of a blood vessel.

me·di·o·tar·sal (mē′dē-ō-tär′səl) *adj.* Relating to the middle of the tarsus.

mediotarsal amputation *n.* See **Chopart's amputation.**

Med·i·ter·ra·ne·an anemia (měd′ĭ-tə-rā′nē-ən) *n.* See **thalassemia.**

Mediterranean exanthematous fever *n.* A disease occurring sporadically in the Mediterranean littoral marked by severe chills with abrupt rise of temperature, pains in the joints, tonsillitis, diarrhea, vomiting, and a rash of elevated nonconfluent macules beginning on the thighs and spreading to the entire body.

Mediterranean fever *n.* **1.** See **brucellosis. 2.** See **familial paroxysmal polyserositis.**

Mediterranean-hemoglobin E disease *n.* Thalassemia characterized by the presence of hemoglobin E in the blood.

me·di·um (mē′dē-əm) *n., pl.* **–di·ums** *or* **–di·a** (-dē-ə) **1.** Something, such as an intermediate course of action, that occupies a position or represents a condition midway between extremes. **2.** An intervening substance through which something else is transmitted or carried on. **3.** An agency by which something is accomplished, conveyed, or transferred. **4.** The substance, often nutritive, in which a specific organism lives and thrives. **5.** A culture medium. **6.** A filtering substance, such as filter paper. —*adj.* Occurring or being between two degrees, amounts, or quantities; intermediate.

me·di·us (mē′dē-əs) *adj.* Of, relating to, or being an anatomical structure that is between two other similar structures or that is midway in position; middle.

MEDLARS *abbr.* Medical Literature Analysis and Retrieval System (computerized index system of the US National Library of Medicine)

MEDLINE (měd′līn′) *n.* A system providing telephone linkage between a number of medical libraries in the United States and MEDLARS for rapid retrieval of medical bibliographies.

me·dor·rhe·a (mē′də-rē′ə, měd′ə-) *n.* See **gleet.**

Med·rol (měd′rôl′) A trademark for the drug methylprednisolone.

med·rox·y·pro·ges·ter·one acetate (mĭ-drŏk′sē-prō-jěs′tə-rōn′) *n.* A progestin used to treat menstrual disorders and in hormone replacement therapy, often in combination with estrogen.

me·dul·la (mĭ-dŭl′ə) *n., pl.* **–dul·las** *or* **–dul·lae** (-dŭl′ē) The inner core of certain organs or body structures, such as the marrow of bone. Also called *medullary substance.* —**me·dul′lar, med·ul·lar·y** (měd′l-ěr′ē, mə-dŭl′ə-rē) *adj.*

medulla ob·lon·ga·ta (ŏb′lŏng-gä′tə, -gä′tə) *n., pl.* **–ga·tas** *or* **–ga·tae** (-gä′tē, -gä′tē) The lowermost portion of the vertebrate brain, continuous with the spinal cord and responsible for the control of respiration, circulation, and other bodily functions.

medulla of adrenal gland *n.* Any of the anastomosing cords of cells located in the core of the adrenal gland that display a chromaffin reaction because of the presence of epinephrine and norepinephrine in their granules.

medulla of hair shaft *n.* The central axis of some hairs surrounded by the cortex.

medulla of kidney *n.* The inner darker portion of the parenchyma of the kidneys that consists of the renal pyramids.

medulla of lymph node *n.* The central portion of a lymph node consisting of cordlike masses of lymphocytes separated by lymph sinuses.

medullary artery of brain *n.* Any of the branches of the cortical arteries that penetrate to and supply the white matter of the cerebrum.

medullary carcinoma *n.* A malignant neoplasm consisting chiefly of epithelial cells.

medullary cavity *n.* The marrow cavity in the shaft of a long bone.

medullary center *n.* The mass of white matter composing the interior of the cerebral hemisphere.

medullary cone *n.* The tapering lower end of the spinal cord.

medullary groove *n.* See **neural groove.**

medullary membrane *n.* See **endosteum.**

medullary plate *n.* See **neural plate.**

medullary pyramid *n.* See **renal pyramid.**

medullary ray *n.* The center of the renal, cortical lobule, consisting of the ascending or descending limbs of the nephronic loop or of the collecting tubules. Also called *Ferrein's pyramid.*

medullary sheath *n.* See **myelin sheath.**

medullary space *n.* The marrow-filled central cavity together with the cellular intervals between the trabeculae of bone.

medullary sponge kidney *n.* A cystic disease of the renal pyramids characterized by calculus formation and hematuria but usually not with renal failure.

medullary stria of fourth ventricle *n.* Any of the slender fascicles of fibers extending transversely below the ependymal floor of the ventricle from the median sulcus to enter the inferior cerebellar peduncle. Also called *acoustic stria.*

medullary stria of thalamus *n.* A narrow compact bundle of fibers extending along the line of attachment of the roof of the third ventricle to the thalamus on each side and terminating posteriorly in the habenular nucleus.

medullary substance *n.* **1.** The fatty material present in the myelin sheath of nerve fibers. **2.** See **medulla.**

med·ul·lat·ed (měd′l-ā′tĭd) *adj.* **1.** Myelinated. **2.** Having a medulla.

medullated fiber *n.* See **myelinated fiber.**

med·ul·lec·to·my (měd′l-ěk′tə-mē) *n.* Surgical removal of a medullary substance or part.

med·ul·li·za·tion (měd′l-ĭ-zā′shən) *n.* Replacement of bone tissue by marrow, as in osteitis.

med·ul·lo·ar·thri·tis (měd′l-ō-är-thrī′tĭs, mĭ-dŭl′ō-) *n.* Inflammation of the cancelled articular extremity of a long bone.

med·ul·lo·blas·to·ma (měd′l-ō-blă-stō′mə, mĭ-dŭl′ō-)

n. A glioma consisting of neoplastic cells that resemble the undifferentiated cells of the primitive neural tube.

med·ul·lo·ep·i·the·li·o·ma (měd′l-ō-ěp′ə-thē′lē-ō′-mə, mǐ-dǔl′ō-) *n.* **1.** See **ependymoma. 2.** Malignant ciliary epithelioma.

Me·du·sa head (mǐ-dōō′sə, -zə) *n.* Dilated cutaneous veins radiating from the umbilicus. Also called *caput medusae, Cruveilhier's sign.*

mef·e·nam·ic acid (měf′ə-năm′ĭk) *n.* A crystalline compound that is used as an anti-inflammatory drug and as an analgesic.

mef·lo·quine (měf′lə-kwīn′, -kwēn′) *n.* A drug that is used mainly for the prevention and treatment of malaria resistant to chloroquine phosphate.

Me·fox·in (mə-fŏk′sĭn) A trademark for the drug cefoxitin sodium.

mega– *pref.* **1.** Large: *megacephaly.* **2.** One million (10^6): *megahertz.*

meg·a·bac·te·ri·um (měg′ə-băk-tîr′ē-əm) *n.* A bacterium of unusually large size.

meg·a·blad·der (měg′ə-blăd′ər) *n.* See **megalocystis.**

meg·a·ceph·a·ly (měg′ə-sĕf′ə-lē) *n.* See **macrocephaly.** —**meg′a·ce·phal′ic** (-sə-făl′ĭk), **meg′a·ceph′a·lous** (-sĕf′ə-lĕs) *adj.*

meg·a·co·lon (měg′ə-kō′lən) *n.* Extreme dilation and hypertrophy of the colon.

meg·a·cy·cle (měg′ə-sī′kəl) *n.* See **megahertz.**

meg·a·cys·tic syndrome (měg′ə-sĭs′tĭk) *n.* A syndrome characterized by a large thin-walled bladder, regurgitation of the urine into the ureters, and dilated ureters.

meg·a·cys·tis (měg′ə-sĭs′tĭs) *n.* See **megalocystis.**

meg·a·don·tism (měg′ə-dŏn′tĭz′əm) *n.* See **macrodontia.**

meg·a·dose (měg′ə-dōs′) *n.* An exceptionally large dose, as of a drug or vitamin.

meg·a·e·soph·a·gus (měg′ə-ĭ-sŏf′ə-gəs) *n.* Abnormal enlargement of the lower portion of the esophagus, as seen in patients with achalasia.

meg·a·gam·ete (měg′ə-găm′ēt′, -gə-mēt′) *n.* See **macrogamete.**

meg·a·hertz (měg′ə-hûrts′) *n. Abbr.* **MHz** One million cycles per second. Used especially as a radio frequency unit. Also called *megacycle.*

meg·a·kar·y·o·blast (měg′ə-kăr′ē-ə-blăst′) *n.* The precursor of a megakaryocyte.

meg·a·kar·y·o·cyte (měg′ə-kăr′ē-ə-sīt′) *n.* A large bone marrow cell with a lobulate nucleus that gives rise to blood platelets. Also called *megalokaryocyte.*

meg·a·kar·y·o·cyt·ic leukemia (měg′ə-kăr′ē-ō-sīt′ĭk) *n.* Myelopoietic disease characterized by the proliferation of megakaryocytes in the bone marrow and sometimes by the presence of a considerable number of megakaryocytes in the blood.

me·gal·gia (mě-găl′jə) *n.* Very severe pain.

megalo– or **megal–** *pref.* Large; of exaggerated size or greatness: *megalocephaly.*

meg·a·lo·blast (měg′ə-lō-blăst′) *n.* An abnormally large nucleated red blood cell found especially in pernicious anemia or in certain vitamin deficiencies. —**meg′a·lo·blas′tic** *adj.*

megaloblastic anemia *n.* Anemia in which there is a predominant number of megaloblasts and relatively

few normoblasts among the hyperplastic erythroid cells in the bone marrow.

meg·a·lo·car·di·a (měg′ə-lō-kär′dē-ə) *n.* See **cardiomegaly.**

meg·a·lo·ceph·a·ly (měg′ə-lō-sĕf′ə-lē) *n.* See **macrocephaly.** —**meg′a·lo·ce·phal′ic** (-sə-făl′ĭk), **meg′a·lo·ceph′a·lous** (-sĕf′ə-ləs) *adj.*

meg·a·lo·chei·ri·a or **meg·a·lo·chi·ri·a** (měg′ə-lō-kī′rē-ə) *n.* See **macrocheiria.**

meg·a·lo·cor·ne·a (měg′ə-lō-kôr′nē-ə) *n.* See **macrocornea.**

meg·a·lo·cys·tis (měg′ə-lō-sĭs′tĭs) *n.* An abnormally enlarged or distended bladder. Also called *megabladder, megacystis.*

meg·a·lo·cyte (měg′ə-lō-sīt′) *n.* A large nonnucleated red blood cell.

meg·a·lo·don·tia (měg′ə-lō-dŏn′shə) *n.* See **macrodontia.**

meg·a·lo·en·ceph·a·lon (měg′ə-lō-ĕn-sĕf′ə-lŏn′) *n.* An abnormally large brain.

meg·a·lo·en·ceph·a·ly (měg′ə-lō-ĕn-sĕf′ə-lē) *n.* Abnormal largeness of the brain. —**meg′a·lo·en′ce·phal′ic** (-ĕn′sə-făl′ĭk) *adj.*

meg·a·lo·en·ter·on (měg′ə-lō-ĕn′tə-rŏn′) *n.* An abnormal enlargement of the intestine. Also called *enteromegaly.*

meg·a·lo·gas·tri·a (měg′ə-lō-găs′trē-ə) *n.* Abnormally large size of the stomach.

meg·a·lo·glos·si·a (měg′ə-lō-glô′sē-ə) *n.* See **macroglossia.**

meg·a·lo·he·pat·i·a (měg′ə-lō-hə-păt′ē-ə) *n.* See **hepatomegaly.**

meg·a·lo·kar·y·o·cyte (měg′ə-lō-kăr′ē-ə-sīt′) *n.* See **megakaryocyte.**

meg·a·lo·ma·ni·a (měg′ə-lō-mā′nē-ə, -mān′yə) *n.* **1.** A psychopathological condition in which delusional fantasies of wealth, power, or omnipotence predominate. **2.** An obsession with grandiose or extravagant things or actions. —**meg′a·lo·ma′ni·ac′** *n.* —**meg′a·lo·ma·ni′a·cal** (-mə-nī′ə-kəl), **meg′a·lo·man′ic** (-măn′ĭk) *adj.*

meg·a·lo·me·li·a (měg′ə-lō-mē′lē-ə, -mēl′yə) *n.* See **macromelia.**

meg·a·lo·pe·nis (měg′ə-lō-pē′nĭs) *n.* See **macropenis.**

meg·a·loph·thal·mus (měg′ə-lŏf-thăl′məs) *n.* A developmental anomaly in which the eyes grow to an abnormally large size. Also called *macrophthalmia, megophthalmus.*

meg·a·lo·po·di·a (měg′ə-lō-pō′dē-ə) *n.* See **macropodia.**

meg·a·lo·sple·ni·a (měg′ə-lō-splē′nē-ə) *n.* See **splenomegaly.**

meg·a·lo·syn·dac·ty·ly (měg′ə-lō-sĭn-dăk′tə-lē) *n.* A condition in which the fingers or toes are webbed or fused and of large size.

meg·a·lo·u·re·ter (měg′ə-lō-yōō-rē′tər, -yŏŏr′ĭ-tər) *n.* A congenitally enlarged ureter without evidence of obstruction or infection.

–megaly *suff.* Enlargement: *splenomegaly.*

meg·a·rec·tum (měg′ə-rĕk′təm) *n.* Extreme dilation of the rectum.

meg·a·scop·ic (měg′ə-skŏp′ĭk) *adj.* Macroscopic.

meg·a·vi·ta·min (mĕg′ə-vī′tə-mĭn) *n.* A dose of a vitamin greatly exceeding the amount required to maintain health.

meg·a·volt (mĕg′ə-vōlt′) *n. Abbr.* **MV** One million volts.

meg·lu·mine (mĕg′loo-mēn) *n.* A crystalline base whose salts are used as radiopaque media.

meg·oph·thal·mus (mĕg′ŏf-thăl′məs) *n.* See **megalophthalmus.**

me·grim (mē′grĭm) *n.* See **migraine.**

mei·bo·mi·an (mī-bō′mē-ən) *adj.* Relating to or described by Heinrich Meibom, German physician and anatomist (1638-1700).

Meibomian gland *n.* Any of the various branched, modified, sebaceous glands situated in the tarsus of the eyelid, the secretions of which prevent the eyelids from sticking together. Also called *tarsal gland.*

mei·bo·mi·tis (mī′bō-mī′tĭs) *or* **mei·bo·mi·a·ni·tis** (mī-bō′mē-ə-nī′tĭs) *n.* Inflammation of the Meibomian glands.

meio– *pref.* Variant of **mio–.**

mei·o·sis (mī-ō′sĭs) *n., pl.* **–ses** (-sēz′) The special process of cell division in sexually reproducing organisms that results in the formation of gametes, consisting of two nuclear divisions in rapid succession that in turn result in the formation of four gametocytes, each containing half the number of chromosomes that is found in somatic cells. —**mei·ot·ic** (-ŏt′ĭk) *adj.* —**mei·ot·i·cal·ly** *adv.*

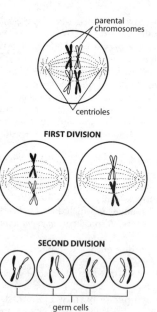

parental chromosomes

centrioles

FIRST DIVISION

SECOND DIVISION

germ cells

meiosis
light and dark chromosomes indicate chromosomes from two different individuals

Meiss·ner (mīs′nər), **Georg** 1829–1905. German physiologist and anatomist known for his microscopic investigations of the skin and the vestibular and cochlear nerves.

Meiss·ner's corpuscle (mīs′nərz) *n.* See **tactile corpuscle.**

meit·ner·i·um (mīt-nûr′ē-əm) *n. Symbol* **Mt** A radioactive synthetic element whose longest-lived isotopes have mass numbers of 266 and 268 with half-lives of 3.4 milliseconds and 70 milliseconds. Atomic number 109.

mel–[1] *pref.* Variant of **melo–**[1].

mel–[2] *pref.* Variant of **melo–**[2].

me·lag·ra (mē-lăg′rə) *n.* Rheumatic or muscular pains in the arms or legs.

me·lal·gia (mə-lăl′jə) *n.* Pain in a limb.

mel·an·cho·li·a (mĕl′ən-kō′lē-ə) *n.* A mental disorder characterized by depression, apathy, and withdrawal. —**mel·an·cho·li·ac** (-lē-ăk′) *adj. & n.*

melancholia at·ton·i·ta (ə-tŏn′ĭ-tə) *n.* The catatonic state in schizophrenia that is characterized by immobility and muscular rigidity. Also called *melancholia stuporosa.*

mel·an·chol·ic (mĕl′ən-kŏl′ĭk) *adj.* **1.** Affected with or being subject to melancholy. **2.** Of or relating to melancholia.

mel·an·chol·y (mĕl′ən-kŏl′ē) *n.* **1.** Sadness or depression of the spirits; gloom. **2.** Melancholia.

mel·a·ne·de·ma (mĕl′ə-nĭ-dē′mə) *n.* Dark brown or black granules of insoluble pigment in the blood.

me·lan·ic (mə-lăn′ĭk) *adj.* **1.** Of, relating to, or exhibiting melanism. **2.** Of, relating to, or affected with melanosis; melanotic.

mel·a·nif·er·ous (mĕl′ə-nĭf′ər-əs) *adj.* Containing melanin or other black pigment.

mel·a·nin (mĕl′ə-nĭn) *n.* Any of a group of naturally occurring dark pigments composed of granules of highly irregular polymers that usually contain nitrogen or sulfur atoms, especially the pigment found in skin, hair, fur, and feathers.

mel·a·nism (mĕl′ə-nĭz′əm) *n.* **1.** See **melanosis. 2.** Dark coloration of the skin, hair, fur, or feathers because of a high concentration of melanin.

melano– *or* **melan–** *pref.* Black; dark: *melanin.*

mel·a·no·am·e·lo·blas·to·ma (mĕl′ə-nō-ăm′ə-lō-blă-stō′mə) *n.* See **melanotic neuroectodermal tumor.**

mel·a·no·blast (mĕl′ə-nō-blăst′, mə-lăn′ə-) *n.* A precursor cell of a melanocyte or melanophore. —**mel′a·no·blas′tic** *adj.*

mel·a·no·blas·to·ma (mĕl′ə-nō-blă-stō′mə) *n.* See **melanoma.**

mel·a·no·car·ci·no·ma (mĕl′ə-nō-kär′sə-nō′mə) *n.* See **melanoma.**

mel·a·no·cyte (mĕl′ə-nō-sīt′) *n.* An epidermal cell capable of synthesizing melanin. —**mel′a·no·cyt′ic** (-sĭt′ĭk) *adj.*

melanocyte-stimulating hormone *n. Abbr.* **MSH** A hormone secreted by the pituitary gland that regulates skin color in humans and other vertebrates by stimulating melanin synthesis in melanocytes and melanin granule dispersal in melanophores. Also called *intermedin.*

mel·a·no·cy·to·ma (mĕl′ə-nō-sī-tō′mə) *n.* **1.** A benign neoplasm composed of melanocytes. **2.** A usually benign, deeply pigmented melanoma of the optic disk.

mel·a·no·der·ma (mĕl′ə-nō-dûr′mə) *n.* An abnormal darkening of the skin caused by deposition of excess melanin or of metallic substances.

mel·a·no·der·ma·ti·tis (mĕl′ə-nō-dûr′mə-tī′tĭs) *n.*

Dermatitis characterized by increased skin pigmentation due to the excessive deposit of melanin.

mel·a·no·der·mic (mĕl′ə-nō-dûr′mĭk) *adj.* Relating to or characterized by melanoderma.

me·lan·o·gen (mĕ-lăn′ə-jən, -jĕn′, mĕl′ə-nō-jĕn′) *n.* A colorless precursor of melanin.

mel·a·no·gen·e·sis (mĕl′ə-nō-jĕn′ĭ-sĭs) *n.* The formation of melanin by living cells.

mel·a·no·glos·si·a (mĕl′ə-nō-glô′sē-ə) *n.* See **black tongue**.

mel·a·noid (mĕl′ə-noid′) *adj.* **1.** Related to melanin; black-pigmented. **2.** Affected with melanosis. —*n.* A dark pigment that resembles melanin, formed from the glucosamines in chitin.

mel·a·no·leu·ko·der·ma (mĕl′ə-nō-loo′kə-dûr′mə) *n.* A marbled or mottled appearance of the skin.

melanoleukoderma col·li (kŏl′ī) *n.* See **syphilitic leukoderma**.

mel·a·no·ma (mĕl′ə-nō′mə) *n., pl.* **–mas** *or* **–ma·ta** (-mə-tə) A dark-pigmented, malignant, frequently widely metastasizing tumor arising from a melanocyte and occurring most commonly in the skin. Also called *malignant melanoma, melanoblastoma, melanocarcinoma, melanotic carcinoma.*

mel·a·no·ma·to·sis (mĕl′ə-nō′mə-tō′sĭs) *n.* A condition characterized by the occurrence of numerous widespread melanomas.

mel·a·no·nych·i·a (mĕl′ə-nō-nĭk′ē-ə) *n.* Black pigmentation of the nails.

mel·a·no·phage (mĕl′ə-nə-fāj′, mə-lăn′ə-) *n.* A histiocyte that contains phagocytized melanin.

mel·a·no·phore (mĕl′ə-nə-fôr′, mə-lăn′ə-) *n.* A pigment cell that contains melanin, especially as found in the skin of amphibians and reptiles.

mel·a·no·pla·ki·a (mĕl′ə-nō-plā′kē-ə, mə-lăn′ə-) *n.* The occurrence of pigmented patches on the tongue and buccal mucous membranes.

mel·a·no·sis (mĕl′ə-nō′sĭs) *n.* Abnormally dark pigmentation of the skin or other tissues, resulting from a disorder of pigment metabolism. Also called *melanism.* —**mel′a·not′ic** (-nŏt′ĭk) *adj.*

melanosis co·li (kō′lī) *n.* Melanosis of the mucosa of the large intestine, due to accumulation of pigment within macrophages in the lamina propria mucosae.

mel·a·no·some (mĕl′ə-nō-sōm′, mə-lăn′ə-) *n.* Any of the usually oval pigment granules that are produced by melanocytes.

melanotic carcinoma *n.* See **melanoma**.

melanotic neuroectodermal tumor *n.* A benign tumor commonly seen in the maxilla, containing melanin-pigmented cells. Also called *melanoameloblastoma, pigmented ameloblastoma.*

melanotic whitlow *n.* A melanoma beginning in the skin at the border of or beneath the nail.

mel·a·no·troph (mĕl′ə-nō-trŏf′, -trōf′) *n.* A cell of the pituitary gland that produces the hormone that stimulates melanocyte production.

mel·a·nu·ri·a (mĕl′ə-noor′ē-ə) *n.* The excretion of urine of a dark color, resulting from the presence of melanin or other pigments or from the action of coal tar derivatives.

mel·a·nu·ric (mĕl′ə-noor′ĭk) *adj.* Relating to or characterized by melanuria.

me·las·ma (mə-lăz′mə) *n.* **1.** A patchy or generalized dark pigmentation of the skin. **2.** See **chloasma**.

melasma u·ni·ver·sa·le (yoo′nə-vər-sä′lē) *n.* See **senile melanoderma**.

mel·a·to·nin (mĕl′ə-tō′nĭn) *n.* A hormone derived from serotonin and produced by the pineal gland that stimulates color change in the epidermis of amphibians and reptiles and that is believed to influence estrus in mammals.

me·le·na (mə-lē′nə) *n.* The passage of black tarlike stools containing blood that has been acted on by the intestinal juices.

Me·le·ney's gangrene (mə-lē′nēz) *n.* A form of gangrene of the skin and subcutaneous tissues, usually following an operation, caused by a synergistic interaction between microaerophilic nonhemolytic streptococci and aerobic hemolytic staphylococci; it produces extensive tissue necrosis with ulceration. Also called *Meleney's ulcer.*

mel·e·tin (mĕl′ĭ-tn, -tĭn) *n.* See **quercetin**.

mel·i·oi·do·sis (mĕl′ē-oi-dō′sĭs) *n.* An infectious disease, primarily affecting rodents in India and Southeast Asia but also communicable to humans, that is caused by the bacterium *Pseudomonas pseudomallei;* it produces a characteristic caseous nodule that breaks down into an abscess.

me·li·tis (mə-lī′tĭs) *n.* Inflammation of the cheek.

Mel·la·ril (mĕl′ə-rĭl) A trademark for the drug thioridazine.

melo–¹ *or* **mel–** *pref.* Limb: *melalgia.*

melo–² *or* **mel–** *pref.* Cheek: *meloplasty.*

mel·o·plas·ty (mĕl′ə-plăs′tē) *n.* Reparative or plastic surgery of the cheek.

mel·o·rhe·os·to·sis (mĕl′ə-rē′ŏs-tō′sĭs) *n.* Rheostosis confined to the long bones.

me·lo·tia (mə-lō′shə) *n.* Congenital displacement of the auricle of the ear.

me·man·tine hydrochloride (mə-măn′tēn) *n.* A drug used to treat moderate to severe symptoms of Alzheimer's disease, whose action is to inhibit NMDA receptors.

mem·ber (mĕm′bər) *n.* **1.** A distinct part of a whole. **2.** A part or an organ of a human or animal body, especially a limb.

mem·bra·na (mĕm-brā′nə) *n., pl.* **–nae** (-nē) A membrane, especially a biomembrane.

membrana ad·ven·ti·ti·a (ăd′vĕn-tĭsh′ē-ə) *n.* **1.** See **tunica adventitia**. **2.** See **decidua capsularis**.

mem·brane (mĕm′brān′) *n.* **1.** A thin pliable layer of tissue covering surfaces, enveloping a part, lining a cavity, or separating or connecting structures or organs. **2.** Cell membrane. **3.** A thin sheet of natural or synthetic material that is permeable to substances in solution.

membrane bone *n.* A bone developed within the membrane of a connective tissue.

membrane-coating granule *n.* See **keratinosome**.

membrane expansion theory *n.* The theory that adsorption of anesthetics into membranes alters the membrane function to produce anesthesia.

membrane potential *n.* The potential inside a cell membrane measured relative to the fluid just outside; it is negative under resting conditions and becomes positive during an action potential.

mem·bra·ni·form (mĕm-brā′nə-fôrm′) *adj.* Having the appearance or structure of a membrane.

mem·bra·no·car·ti·lag·i·nous (mĕm′brə-nō-kär′tl-ăj′ə-nəs) *adj.* **1.** Of, relating to, or being both membranous and cartilaginous. **2.** Developing from membrane and cartilage, as some bones.

mem·bra·noid (mĕm′brə-noid′) *adj.* Membraniform.

mem·bra·no·pro·lif·er·a·tive **glomerulonephritis** (mĕm′brə-nō-prə-lĭf′ə-rā′tĭv, -lĭf′ər-ə-, mĕm-brā′nō-) *n.* Chronic glomerulonephritis characterized by mesangial cell proliferation, increased lobular separation of glomeruli, thickening of glomerular capillary walls, and low serum levels of complement. Also called *lobular glomerulonephritis.*

mem·bra·nous (mĕm′brə-nəs) *adj.* **1.** Relating to, made of, or similar to a membrane. **2.** Characterized by the formation of a membrane or a layer similar to a membrane.

membranous ampulla *n.* A nearly spherical enlargement of one end of each of the three semicircular canals where they connect with the utricle.

membranous cataract *n.* A secondary cataract composed of the remains of the thickened lenticular capsule and the largely degenerated lens.

membranous dysmenorrhea *n.* Dysmenorrhea accompanied by exfoliation of the menstrual decidual membrane.

membranous glomerulonephritis *n.* Glomerulonephritis characterized histologically by diffuse thickening of glomerular capillary basement membranes and clinically by an insidious onset of the nephrotic syndrome and by failure of proteinuria to disappear. Also called *lipoid nephrosis.*

membranous labyrinth *n.* The group of fluid-filled membranous sacs of the inner ear that are associated with the senses of hearing and balance.

membranous laryngitis *n.* A form of laryngitis in which there is a pseudomembranous exudate on the vocal cords.

membranous ossification *n.* The development of bone tissue within connective tissue.

membranous rhinitis *n.* Chronic inflammation of the nasal mucous membrane accompanied by a fibrinous or pseudomembranous exudate. Also called *fibrinous rhinitis.*

mem·brum (mĕm′brəm) *n., pl.* **–bra** (-brə) Member. Used in anatomy.

mem·o·ry (mĕm′ə-rē) *n.* **1.** The mental faculty of retaining and recalling past experience based on the mental processes of learning, retention, recall, and recognition. **2.** Persistent modification of behavior resulting from experience. **3.** The capacity of a material, such as plastic or metal, to return to a previous shape after deformation. **4.** The capability of the immune system to produce a specific secondary response to an antigen it has previously encountered.

memory engram *n.* An engram.

memory trace *n.* An engram.

men– *pref.* Variant of **meno–**.

men·ac·me (mĕ-năk′mē) *n.* The period of a woman's life in which menstrual activity occurs.

men·a·di·ol di·ac·e·tate (mĕn′ə-dī′ôl′ dī-ăs′ĭ-tāt′, -ōl′) *n.* See **acetomenaphthane**.

men·a·di·one (mĕn′ə-dī′ōn′) *n.* A synthetic vitamin K derivative occurring as a yellow crystalline powder and used as a vitamin K supplement.

men·a·quin·one (mĕn′ə-kwĭn′ōn′, -kwī′nōn′) *n. Abbr.* **MK** See **vitamin K₂**.

me·nar·che (mə-när′kē) *n.* The first menstrual period, usually during puberty. —**me·nar′che·al** *adj.*

Men·del (mĕn′dl), **Gregor Johann** 1822–1884. Austrian botanist and founder of the science of genetics. He discovered Mendel's laws.

Mendel-Bechterew reflex *n.* See **Bechterew-Mendel reflex**.

men·de·le·vi·um (mĕn′də-lē′vē-əm) *n. Symbol* **Md** A synthetic radioactive element; its most stable isotope is Md 258 with a half-life of 56 days. Atomic number 101.

Men·de·li·an *or* **men·de·li·an** (mĕn-dē′lē-ən, -dĕl′yən) *adj.* Relating to or described by Gregor Mendel or his theories of genetics.

mendelian inheritance *n.* Inheritance that conforms to Mendel's laws.

Men·del·ism (mĕn′dl-ĭz′əm) *or* **Men·de·li·an·ism** (mĕn-dē′lē-ə-nĭz′əm) *n.* The theoretical principles of heredity formulated by Gregor Mendel; Mendel's laws.

Men·del's law (mĕn′dlz) *n.* **1.** One of two principles of heredity first formulated by Gregor Mendel, founded on his experiments with pea plants and stating that the members of a pair of homologous chromosomes segregate during meiosis and are distributed to different gametes. Also called *law of segregation.* **2.** The second of these two principles, stating that each member of a pair of homologous chromosomes segregates during meiosis independently of the members of other pairs, so that alleles carried on different chromosomes are distributed randomly to the gametes. Also called *law of independent assortment.*

Ménétrièr's disease (mā′nə-trē-ârz′, mā-nā-trē-āz′) *n.* Enlargement of the stomach caused by excessive enlargement of the gastric mucosa. Also called *hypertrophic gastritis.*

Mé·nière's disease (mān-yârz′) *n.* A pathological condition of the inner ear that is characterized by dizziness, ringing in the ears, and progressive loss of hearing. Also called *auditory vertigo, endolymphatic hydrops, labyrinthine vertigo.*

me·nin·ge·al (mə-nĭn′jē-əl) *adj.* Of, relating to, or affecting the meninges.

meningeal artery *n.* **1.** An artery with its origin in the anterior ethmoidal artery, with distribution to the meninges in the anterior cranial fossa; anterior meningeal artery. **2.** An artery with its origin in the maxillary artery, with branches to the petrosal, ganglionic, superior tympanic, frontal, and parietal arteries, with distribution to the parts mentioned and to the anterior and middle cranial fossae; middle meningeal artery. **3.** An artery with its origin in the ascending pharyngeal artery, with distribution to the dura mater of the posterior cranial fossa; posterior meningeal artery.

meningeal vein *n.* Any of several veins that accompany the meningeal arteries, communicate with the sinuses of the dura mater and diploic veins, and drain into the regional veins outside the cranial vault.

me·nin·ge·or·rha·phy (mə-nĭn'jē-ôr'ə-fē) *n.* Suture of the cranial or spinal meninges.

me·nin·gi·o·ma (mə-nĭn'jē-ō'mə) *n., pl.* **–mas** *or* **–ma·ta** (-mə-tə) A slow-growing tumor of the meninges often creating pressure and damaging the brain and adjacent tissues, occurring most often in adults.

men·in·gism (mĕn'ĭn-jĭz'əm, mə-nĭn'-) *or* **men·in·gis·mus** (mĕn'ĭn-jĭz'məs, mə-nĭn'-) *n.* A condition of meningeal irritation in which symptoms mimic those of meningitis but in which no inflammation is present, often occurring during febrile illnesses in children.

meningitic streak *n.* A line of redness following the drawing of the fingernail or of a pencil point across the skin, seen especially in cases of meningitis.

men·in·gi·tis (mĕn'ĭn-jī'tĭs) *n., pl.* **men·in·git·i·des** (-jĭt'ĭ-dēz') Inflammation of the meninges of the brain and the spinal cord, most often the result of a bacterial or viral infection and characterized by fever, vomiting, intense headache, and stiff neck. **—men'in·git'ic** (-jĭt'-ĭk) *adj.*

meningo– *or* **meningi–** *or* **mening–** *pref.* Meninges: *meningococcus.*

me·nin·go·cele (mə-nĭng'gə-sēl') *n.* Protrusion of the meninges of the brain or spinal cord through a defect in the skull or spinal column forming a cyst filled with cerebrospinal fluid.

meningococcal meningitis *n.* An acute infectious disease affecting children and young adults characterized by inflammation of the meninges of the brain and spinal cord, headache, vomiting, convulsions, stiff neck, light sensitivity, and purpuric eruptions, and caused by the meningococcus, *Neisseria meningitidis.* Also called *cerebrospinal meningitis.*

me·nin·go·coc·ce·mi·a (mə-nĭng'gō-kŏk-sē'mē-ə) *n.* The presence of meningococci in the blood.

me·nin·go·coc·cus (mə-nĭng'gə-kŏk'əs, -nĭn'jə-) *n., pl.* **–coc·ci** (-kŏk'sī, -kī) A bacterium (*Neisseria meningitidis*) that causes cerebrospinal meningitis. **—me·nin'go·coc'cal** (-kŏk'əl), **me·nin'go·coc'cic** (-kŏk'sĭk) *adj.*

me·nin·go·cor·ti·cal (mə-nĭng'gō-kôr'tĭ-kəl) *adj.* Relating to the meninges and the cortex of the brain.

me·nin·go·cyte (mə-nĭng'gə-sīt') *n.* A mesenchymal epithelial cell occurring in the subarachnoid space.

me·nin·go·en·ceph·a·li·tis (mə-nĭng'gō-ĕn-sĕf'ə-lī'tĭs) *n.* Inflammation of the brain and its membranes. Also called *cerebromeningitis, encephalomeningitis.*

me·nin·go·en·ceph·a·lo·cele (mə-nĭng'gō-ĕn-sĕf'ə-lō-sēl') *n.* The protrusion of the meninges and the brain through a congenital defect in the cranium. Also called *encephalomeningocele.*

me·nin·go·en·ceph·a·lo·my·e·li·tis (mə-nĭng'gō-ĕn-sĕf'ə-lō-mī'ə-lī'tĭs) *n.* Inflammation of the brain, the spinal cord, and their membranes.

me·nin·go·en·ceph·a·lop·a·thy (mə-nĭng'gō-ĕn-sĕf'-ə-lŏp'ə-thē) *n.* Any of various disorders affecting the meninges and the brain. Also called *encephalomeningopathy.*

me·nin·go·my·e·li·tis (mə-nĭng'gō-mī'ə-lī'tĭs) *n.* Inflammation of the spinal cord and its enveloping arachnoid and pia mater, and, less commonly, dura mater.

me·nin·go·my·e·lo·cele (mə-nĭng'gō-mī'ə-lə-sēl') *n.* See **myelomeningocele**.

me·nin·go·os·te·o·phle·bi·tis (mə-nĭng'gō-ŏs'tē-ō-flĭ-bī'tĭs) *n.* Inflammation of the veins located in the periosteum.

me·nin·go·ra·dic·u·lar (mə-nĭng'gō-rə-dĭk'yə-lər) *adj.* Relating to the meninges and the cranial or spinal nerve roots.

me·nin·go·ra·dic·u·li·tis (mə-nĭng'gō-rə-dĭk'yə-lī'tĭs) *n.* Inflammation of the meninges and the cranial or spinal nerve roots.

me·nin·gor·rha·chid·i·an (mə-nĭng'gō-rə-kĭd'ē-ən) *adj.* Relating to the spinal cord and its meninges.

me·nin·gor·rha·gia (mə-nĭng'gə-rā'jə) *n.* Hemorrhage into or beneath the cerebral or the spinal meninges.

men·in·go·sis (mĕn'ĭng-gō'sĭs) *n.* The membranous union of bones, as in the skull of a newborn.

me·nin·go·vas·cu·lar (mə-nĭng'gō-văs'kyə-lər) *adj.* **1.** Relating to the blood vessels in the meninges. **2.** Relating to the meninges and the blood vessels.

me·ninx (mē'nĭngks) *n., pl.* **me·nin·ges** (mə-nĭn'jēz) A membrane, especially one of the three membranes enclosing the brain and spinal cord.

men·is·cec·to·my (mĕn'ĭ-sĕk'tə-mē) *n.* Excision of a meniscus, usually from the knee joint.

men·is·ci·tis (mĕn'ĭ-sī'tĭs) *n.* Inflammation of a fibrocartilaginous meniscus.

me·nis·co·cyte (mə-nĭs'kə-sīt') *n.* See **sickle cell**.

me·nis·co·cy·to·sis (mə-nĭs'kō-sī-tō'sĭs) *n.* See **sickle cell anemia**.

me·nis·co·fem·o·ral ligament (mə-nĭs'kō-fĕm'ər-əl) *n.* Either of two bands, anterior and posterior, that extend upward from the lateral meniscus, pass before and behind the posterior cruciate ligament, and reach the medial condyle of the femur.

me·nis·cus (mə-nĭs'kəs) *n., pl.* **–nis·cus·es** *or* **–nis·ci** (-nĭs'ī, -kī, -kē) **1.** A body that is crescent-shaped. **2.** A concavo-convex lens. **3.** The curved upper surface of a nonturbulent liquid in a container that is concave if the liquid wets the walls and convex if it does not. **4.** A disk of cartilage that acts as a cushion between the ends of bones in a joint. **—me·nis'cal** (-kəl), **me·nis'cate'** (-kāt'), **me·nis'coid'** (-koid'), **men'is·coi'dal** (mĕn'ĭs-koid'l) *adj.*

Men·kes syndrome (mĕng'kəz) *n.* See **kinky-hair disease**.

meno– *or* **men–** *pref.* **1.** Menstruation: *menarche.* **2.** Menses: *menorrhagia.*

men·o·me·tror·rha·gia (mĕn'ō-mē'trə-rā'jə) *n.* Irregular or excessive bleeding during menstruation and between menstrual periods.

men·o·pause (mĕn'ə-pôz') *n.* The cessation of menstruation, occurring usually between the ages of 45 and 55. Also called *climacteric.* **—men'o·paus'al** *adj.*

men·or·rha·gia (mĕn'ə-rā'jə) *n.* See **hypermenorrhea**.

men·or·rhal·gia (mĕn'ə-răl'jə) *n.* See **dysmenorrhea**.

men·nos·che·sis (mə-nŏs'kĭ-sĭs, mĕn'ə-skē'sĭs) *n.* Suppression of menstruation.

me·nos·ta·sis (mə-nŏs'tə-sĭs) *n.* See **amenorrhea**.

men·o·stax·is (mĕn'ə-stăk'sĭs) *n.* See **hypermenorrhea**.

men·o·tro·pins (mĕn'ə-trō'pĭnz) *n.* A purified extract of postmenopausal urine primarily containing follicle-stimulating hormone.

men·ses (mĕn′sēz) *n*. The monthly flow of blood and cellular debris from the uterus that begins at puberty and ceases at menopause. Also called *catamenia, emmenia, menstrual period.*

men·stru·al (mĕn′strōō-əl) *or* **men·stru·ous** (-əs) *adj.* Of or relating to menstruation.

menstrual cup *n*. A rubber cup that is inserted into the vagina and placed over the cervix to collect menstrual flow.

menstrual cycle *n*. The recurring cycle of physiological changes in the uterus, ovaries, and other sexual structures that occur from the beginning of one menstrual period through the beginning of the next.

menstrual period *n*. See **menses**.

men·stru·ant (mĕn′strōō-ənt) *n*. A girl or woman who menstruates. —*adj.* Capable of menstruating.

men·stru·ate (mĕn′strōō-āt′) *v*. To undergo menstruation.

men·stru·a·tion (mĕn′strōō-ā′shən) *n*. The process or an instance of discharging the menses.

men·stru·um (mĕn′strōō-əm) *n.*, *pl.* **-stru·ums** *or* **-stru·a** (-strōō-ə) A solvent, especially one used in extracting compounds from plant and animal tissues and preparing drugs.

men·tal[1] (mĕn′tl) *adj*. **1.** Of or relating to the mind; intellectual. **2.** Of, relating to, or affected by a disorder of the mind. **3.** Intended for treatment of people affected with disorders of the mind.

men·tal[2] (mĕn′tl) *adj.* Of or relating to the chin.

mental age *n*. *Abbr.* **MA** A measure of mental development as determined by intelligence tests, generally restricted to children and expressed as the age at which that level is typically attained.

mental artery *n*. An artery that is the terminal branch of the inferior alveolar artery, with distribution to the chin.

mental deficiency *n*. See **mental retardation**.

mental disease *n*. See **mental illness**.

mental disorder *n*. See **mental illness**.

mental foramen *n*. The front opening of the mandibular canal on the body of the mandible alongside and above the tubercle of the chin.

mental health *n*. **1.** A state of emotional and psychological well-being in which an individual is able to use his or her cognitive and emotional capabilities, function in society, and meet the ordinary demands of everyday life. **2.** A branch of medicine that deals with the achievement and maintenance of psychological well-being.

mental hospital *n*. See **psychiatric hospital**.

mental hygiene *n*. The branch of psychiatry that deals with the science and practice of maintaining and restoring mental health, and of preventing mental disorder through education, early treatment, and public health measures.

mental illness *n*. Any of various psychiatric conditions that are usually characterized by impairment of an individual's normal cognitive, emotional, or behavioral functioning, and are caused by psychological or psychosocial factors. Also called *mental disease, mental disorder.*

mental image *n*. A mental picture of something not real or present that is produced by the memory or the imagination.

men·tal·i·ty (mĕn-tăl′ĭ-tē) *n*. The sum of a person's intellectual capabilities or endowment.

mental nerve *n*. A branch of the inferior alveolar nerve arising in the mandibular canal and passing through the mental foramen to the chin and the lower lip.

mental point *n*. See **pogonion**.

mental retardation *n*. Subnormal intellectual development or functioning that is the result of congenital causes, brain injury, or disease and is characterized by any of various deficiencies, ranging from impaired learning ability to social and vocational inadequacy. Also called *mental deficiency.*

mental scotoma *n*. See **blind spot** (sense 3).

mental spine *n*. A slight projection located in the middle line of the rear surface of the body of the lower jawbone that gives attachment below to the geniohyoid muscle and above to the genioglossus muscle. Also called *genial tubercle.*

mental symphysis *n*. The fibrocartilaginous union of the two halves of an infant's lower jawbone that ossifies during the first year.

men·thol (mĕn′thôl′) *n*. A white crystalline organic compound obtained from peppermint oil or synthesized and used as a mild topical anesthetic.

men·to·an·te·ri·or position (mĕn′tō-ăn-tîr′ē-ər) *n*. A cephalic presentation of the fetus with the chin pointing to either the right or left front quarter of the mother's pelvis.

men·to·plas·ty (mĕn′tə-plăs′tē) *n*. Surgical alteration of the chin. Also called *genioplasty.*

men·to·pos·te·ri·or position (mĕn′tō-pŏ-stîr′ē-ər) *n*. A cephalic presentation of the fetus with the chin pointing to either the right or left rear quarter of the mother's pelvis.

men·to·trans·verse position (mĕn′tō-trănz-vûrs′, -trăns-, -trănz′vûrs′, -trăns′-) *n*. A cephalic presentation of the fetus with the chin pointing to either the right or left iliac fossa of the mother's pelvis.

men·tum (mĕn′təm) *n.*, *pl.* **-ta** (-tə) The chin.

me·per·i·dine hydrochloride (mə-pĕr′ĭ-dēn′) *n*. A synthetic narcotic compound that is used as an analgesic and a sedative.

me·phit·ic (mə-fĭt′ĭk) *adj.* Having a foul odor; foul-smelling.

me·phi·tis (mə-fī′tĭs) *n*. **1.** An offensive smell; a stench. **2.** A poisonous or foul-smelling gas emitted from the earth.

Meph·y·ton (mĕf′ĭ-tən) A trademark for a drug preparation of vitamin K.

me·piv·a·caine hydrochloride (mə-pĭv′ə-kān′) *n*. A drug used for local anesthesia.

mep·ro·bam·ate (mĕp′rō-băm′āt′, mĕ-prō′bə-) *n*. A carbamate derivative used as a sedative and a muscle relaxant.

mEq *or* **meq** *abbr.* milliequivalent

mer- *pref.* Variant of **mero-**.

-mer *suff.* Variant of **-mere**.

me·ral·gia (mə-răl′jə) *n*. Pain in the thigh.

meralgia par·aes·thet·i·ca (păr′ĭs-thĕt′ĭ-kə) *n*. Paresthesia in the outer side of the lower thigh in the area of distribution of the lateral femoral cutaneous nerve. Also called *Bernhardt's disease.*

mer·bro·min (mər-brō′mĭn) *n.* A green crystalline organic compound that forms a red aqueous solution, used as a germicide and an antiseptic.

mer·cap·tan (mər-kăp′tăn′) *n.* Any of a class of organic compounds in which the oxygen of an alcohol has been replaced by sulfur and which have distinctive, often disagreeable, odors. Also called *thiol.*

mercapto– *pref.* Containing the univalent radical SH: *mercaptopurine.*

mer·cap·to·pu·rine (mər-kăp′tō-pyo͝or′ēn) *n.* A purine analog that acts as an antimetabolite by interfering with purine synthesis, used primarily in the treatment of acute leukemia.

mer·cap·tu·ric acid (mûr′kăp-to͝or′ĭk) *n.* A condensation product formed from the coupling of cysteine with aromatic compounds, formed as a conjugate in the liver and excreted in the urine.

Mer·cier's bar (mər-sē-āz′, měr-syāz′) *n.* See **interureteric fold.**

mer·cu·ri·al (mər-kyo͝or′ē-əl) *adj.* Containing or caused by the action of the element mercury. —*n.* A pharmacological or chemical preparation containing mercury.

mer·cu·ri·al·ism (mər-kyo͝or′ē-ə-lĭz′əm) *n.* See **mercury poisoning.**

mer·cu·ric (mər-kyo͝or′ĭk) *adj.* Relating to or containing mercury, especially with a valence of 2.

mercuric chloride *n.* A poisonous white crystalline compound used as an antiseptic and a disinfectant.

Mer·cu·ro·chrome (mər-kyo͝or′ə-krōm′) A trademark for a preparation of merbromin.

mer·cu·rous (mər-kyo͝or′əs, mûr′kyər-əs) *adj.* Relating to or containing mercury, especially with a valence of 1.

mercurous chloride *n.* See **calomel.**

mer·cu·ry (mûr′kyə-rē) *n. Symbol* **Hg** A silvery-white poisonous metallic element, liquid at room temperature, used in thermometers and various pharmaceuticals including antiseptics, diuretics, and antibacterials. Its radioisotope Hg-197 is used in diagnostic imaging of renal function and in brain scans. Atomic number 80. Also called *hydrargyrum.*

mercury poisoning *n.* Poisoning caused by mercury or a compound containing mercury, with the acute form characterized by stomach ulcers and renal tubule toxicity and the chronic form affecting the central nervous system and causing emotional instability. Also called *hydrargyria, mercurialism.*

mer·cy killing (mûr′sē) *n.* Euthanasia.

–mere *or* **–mer** *suff.* Part; segment: *blastomere, polymer.*

Me·rid·i·a (mə-rĭd′ē-ə) A trademark for the drug sibutramine.

me·rid·i·an (mə-rĭd′ē-ən) *n.* **1.** An imaginary line encircling a globular body at right angles to its equator and passing through its poles. **2.** Either half of such a great circle from pole to pole. **3.** Any of the longitudinal lines or pathways on the body along which the acupuncture points are distributed.

me·rid·i·o·nal (mə-rĭd′ē-ə-nəl) *adj.* Of or relating to meridians or a meridian.

meridional aberration *n.* An optical aberration produced in the plane of a single meridian of a lens.

Mer·kel's corpuscle (mûr′kəlz) *n.* See **tactile disk.**

mero– *or* **mer–** *pref.* **1.** Part; segment: *merogenesis.* **2.** Partial; partially: *meromelia.*

mer·o·blas·tic (měr′ə-blăs′tĭk) *adj.* Undergoing partial cleavage. Used of a fertilized egg.

mer·o·cele (mîr′ə-sēl′) *n.* See **femoral hernia.**

mer·o·crine (měr′ə-krĭn, -krīn′, -krēn′) *adj.* Of or relating to a gland whose secretory cells remain undamaged during secretion.

merocrine gland *n.* A gland whose secretory cells produce a secretion but are not destroyed or damaged during the process.

mer·o·di·a·stol·ic (měr′ō-dī′ə-stŏl′ĭk) *adj.* Of or relating to a part of the diastole of the heart.

mer·o·gen·e·sis (měr′ō-jěn′ĭ-sĭs) *n.* The process of reproducing by segmentation. —**mer′o·ge·net′ic** (-jə-nět′ĭk) *adj.*

me·rog·o·ny (mə-rŏg′ə-nē) *n.* **1.** Incomplete development of an ovum. **2.** See **schizogony.**

mer·o·me·li·a (měr′ō-mē′lē-ə, -mēl′yə) *n.* Congenital absence of part of a limb.

mer·o·mi·cro·so·mi·a (měr′ō-mī′krə-sō′mē-ə) *n.* Abnormal smallness of some portion of the body.

mer·o·my·o·sin (měr′ə-mī′ə-sĭn) *n.* Either of two protein subunits of a myosin molecule, obtained especially through the digestive action of trypsin.

me·ro·pi·a (mə-rō′pē-ə) *n.* Partial blindness.

mer·o·ra·chis·chi·sis *or* **mer·or·rha·chis·chi·sis** (měr′ō-rə-kĭs′kĭ-sĭs) *n.* The fissure of a portion of the spinal cord.

me·ros·mi·a (mə-rŏz′mē-ə) *n.* A partial loss of the sense of smell leading to an inability to perceive certain odors.

mer·o·sys·tol·ic (měr′ō-sĭ-stŏl′ĭk) *adj.* Of or relating to a part of the systole of the heart.

me·rot·o·my (mə-rŏt′ə-mē) *n.* Division into parts, especially of a cell.

mer·o·zo·ite (měr′ə-zō′īt) *n.* A protozoan cell that arises from the schizogony of a parent sporozoan and may enter either the asexual or sexual phase of the life cycle.

mer·o·zy·gote (měr′ə-zī′gōt′) *n.* An incomplete bacterial zygote containing only a fragment of the genome from one of its parent cells.

Mer·ri·field (měr′ə-fēld′), **R(obert) Bruce** Born 1921. American biochemist. He won a 1984 Nobel Prize for developing a method of synthesizing peptides and proteins from amino acids.

Mer·thi·o·late (mər-thī′ə-lāt′) A trademark for the compound thimerosal.

Merz·bach·er-Pelizaeus disease (mûrts′băk′ər-) *n.* A familial degenerative disease of the brain that is marked by progressive sclerosis of white matter of the frontal lobes, mental deficiency, and vasomotor disorders. Also called *aplasia axialis extracorticalis, hereditary cerebral leukodystrophy, Pelizaeus-Merzbacher disease.*

mes– *pref.* Variant of **meso–.**

me·sad (mē′zăd′, mē′săd′) *or* **me·si·ad** (mē′zē-ăd′, -sē-) *adv.* Toward the median plane of the body or of a part.

me·sal·a·mine (mə-săl′ə-mēn′) *n.* A salicylate used as an anti-inflammatory gastrointestinal agent for the treatment of ulcerative colitis, proctosigmoiditis, and proctitis.

mesangial nephritis *n.* Glomerulonephritis with an increase in glomerular mesangial cells or matrix.

mesangial proliferative glomerulonephritis *n.* Glomerulonephritis that is characterized clinically by the nephrotic syndrome and histologically by diffuse glomerular increases in endocapillary and mesangial cells and in mesangial matrix. Also called *diffuse mesangial proliferation.*

mes·an·gi·um (měz-ăn′jē-əm) *n.* The central part of the renal glomerulus between capillaries. —**mes·an′gi·al** *adj.*

mes·a·or·ti·tis (měz′ā-ôr-tī′tĭs) *n.* Inflammation of the middle layer of the aorta.

mes·ar·te·ri·tis (měz-är′tə-rī′tĭs) *n.* Inflammation of the middle layer of an artery.

me·sat·i·pel·lic (mě-săt′ə-pěl′ĭk) *or* **me·sat·i·pel·vic** (-pěl′vĭk) *adj.* Having a moderate size pelvis with a pelvic index between 90 and 95.

mesatipellic pelvis *n.* A pelvis in which the anteroposterior and transverse diameters are equal or in which the transverse diameter is not more than one centimeter longer than the anteroposterior diameter.

mes·ax·on (měz-ăk′sŏn′) *n.* The plasma membrane of the neurolemma that surrounds a nerve axon.

mes·ca·line (měs′kə-lēn′, -lĭn) *n.* An alkaloid drug obtained from buttons of a small cactus (*Lophophora williamsii)* that has hallucinatory effects.

mes·ec·to·derm (měz-ěk′tə-dûrm′) *n.* The part of the mesenchyme derived from ectoderm, especially from the embryonic neural crest from which the pigment cells, meninges, and most of the branchial cartilages develop.

mes·en·ce·phal·ic (měz′ěn-sə-făl′ĭk) *adj.* Of or relating to the mesencephalon.

mesencephalic flexure *n.* See **cephalic flexure.**

mesencephalic tegmentum *n.* A part of the mesencephalon consisting of white fibers running lengthwise through gray matter from the substantia nigra to the level of the cerebral aqueduct.

mes·en·ceph·a·li·tis (měz′ěn-sěf′ə-lī′tĭs) *n.* Inflammation of the mesencephalon.

mes·en·ceph·a·lon (měz′ěn-sěf′ə-lŏn′) *n.* The portion of the vertebrate brain that develops from the middle section of the embryonic brain. Also called *midbrain.*

mes·en·ceph·a·lot·o·my (měz′ěn-sěf′ə-lŏt′ə-mē) *n.* Surgical sectioning of any structure in the mesencephalon, especially of the pain-conducting tracts for the relief of unbearable pain.

mes·en·chyme (měz′ən-kīm′) *n.* The part of the embryonic mesoderm that consists of loosely packed, unspecialized cells that are set in a gelatinous ground substance, from which connective tissue, bone, cartilage, and the circulatory and lymphatic systems develop. —**mes·en′chy·mal** (měz-ěng′kə-məl, měz′-ən-kī′məl) *adj.*

mes·en·chy·mo·ma (měz′ən-kī-mō′mə, -kə-) *n., pl.* **–mas** *or* **–ma·ta** (-mə-tə) A neoplasm containing a mixture of cells resembling those of the mesenchyme and its derivatives other than fibrous tissue.

mesenteric artery *n.* **1.** An artery with its origin in the aorta, with branches to the left colic, sigmoid, and superior rectal arteries; inferior mesenteric artery. **2.** An artery with its origin in the aorta, with branches to the inferior pancreaticoduodenal, jejunal, ileal, ileocolic, appendicular, right colic, and middle colic arteries; superior mesenteric artery.

mesenteric ganglion *n.* **1.** The lowest of the sympathetic prevertebral ganglions located at the origin of the inferior mesenteric artery from the aorta of the heart and containing the sympathetic neurons innervating the descending and sigmoid colon; inferior mesenteric ganglion. **2.** A paired sympathetic ganglion at the origin of the superior mesenteric artery; superior mesenteric ganglion.

mes·en·ter·i·o·pex·y (měz′ən-těr′ē-ə-pěk′sē) *n.* Surgical fixation of a torn or incised mesentery. Also called *mesopexy.*

mes·en·ter·i·or·rha·phy (měz′ən-těr′ē-ôr′ə-fē) *n.* The surgical suture of the mesentery. Also called *mesorrhaphy.*

mes·en·ter·i·pli·ca·tion (měz′ən-těr′ə-plĭ-kā′shən) *n.* Surgical reduction of a mesentery by making one or more tucks in it.

mes·en·ter·i·tis (měz-ěn′tə-rī′tĭs) *n.* Inflammation of the mesentery.

mes·en·te·ri·um (měz′ən-tîr′ē-əm) *n., pl.* **–te·ri·a** (-tîr′ē-ə) Mesentery.

mes·en·ter·on (měz-ěn′tə-rŏn′) *n.* See **midgut** (sense 1).

mes·en·ter·y (měz′ən-těr′ē) *n.* **1.** A double layer of peritoneum attached to the abdominal wall and enclosing in its fold certain organs of the abdominal viscera. **2.** A fold of the peritoneum that connects the intestines to the dorsal abdominal wall, especially such a fold that envelops the jejunum and ileum. —**mes′en·ter′ic** *adj.*

me·si·ad (mē′zē-ăd′, -sē-) *adv.* Variant of **mesad.**

me·si·al (mē′zē-əl, -zhəl) *adj.* **1.** Of, in, near, or toward the middle. **2.** Situated toward the middle of the front of the jaw along the curve of the dental arch.

mesial angle *n.* The angle formed by the meeting of the mesial surface of a tooth with the labial, buccal, or lingual surface.

mesial occlusion *n.* Malocclusion in which the lower teeth articulate with the upper teeth in a position anterior to normal. Also called *mesioclusion.*

mesio– *pref.* Mesial: *mesiolabial.*

me·si·o·buc·cal (mē′zē-ō-bŭk′əl) *adj.* Of or relating to the mesial and the buccal surfaces of a tooth, especially the angle formed by the junction of these two surfaces.

me·si·o·cer·vi·cal (mē′zē-ō-sûr′vĭ-kəl) *adj.* **1.** Relating to the line angle of a tooth cavity preparation at the junction of the mesial and cervical walls. **2.** Relating to the area of a tooth at the junction of the mesial surface and the cervical region.

me·si·o·clu·sion (mē′zē-ə-kloo′zhən) *or* **me·si·o·oc·clu·sion** (mē′zē-ō-ə-kloo′zhən) *n.* See **mesial occlusion.**

me·si·o·dens (mē′zē-ə-děnz′) *n.* A supernumerary tooth located in the midline of the anterior maxillae between the maxillary central incisor teeth.

me·si·o·dis·tal (mē′zē-ō-dĭs′tǝl) *adj*. Of or relating to the mesial and distal surfaces of a tooth, especially the plane or diameter joining them.

me·si·o·gin·gi·val (mē′zē-ō-jĭn′jǝ-vǝl, -jĭn-jī′-) *adj*. Of or relating to the angle formed by the junction of the mesial surface with the gingival line of a tooth.

me·si·o·la·bi·al (mē′zē-ō-lā′bē-ǝl) *adj*. Of or relating to the mesial and the labial surfaces of a tooth, especially the angle formed by their junction.

me·si·o·lin·gual (mē′zē-ō-lĭng′gwǝl) *adj*. Of or relating to the mesial and the lingual surfaces of a tooth, especially the angle formed by their junction.

me·si·o·lin·guo·oc·clu·sal (mē′zē-ō-lĭng′gwō-ǝ-kloo′-zǝl) *adj*. Relating to the mesial, lingual, and occlusal surfaces of a tooth, especially the angle formed by their junction.

me·si·o·lin·guo·pul·pal (mē′zē-ō-lĭng′gwō-pŭl′pǝl) *adj*. Of or relating to the mesial, lingual, and pulpal surfaces in a tooth cavity preparation.

me·si·o·oc·clu·sal (mē′zē-ō-ǝ-kloo′zǝl) *adj*. Of or relating to the mesial and the occlusal surfaces of a tooth, especially the angle formed by the junction of these surfaces.

me·si·o·ver·sion (mē′zē-ō-vûr′zhǝn) *n*. Malposition of a tooth distal to its normal position and in a posterior direction following the curvature of the dental arch.

Mes·mer (měz′mǝr, měs′-), **Franz** or **Friedrich Anton** 1734–1815. Austrian physician who sought to treat disease through animal magnetism, an early therapeutic application of hypnotism.

mes·mer·ism (měz′mǝ-rĭz′ǝm, měs′-) *n*. **1.** A strong or spellbinding appeal; fascination. **2.** Hypnotic induction that is believed to involve animal magnetism. **3.** Hypnotism.

meso– or **mes–** *pref*. **1.** In the middle; middle: *mesoderm*. **2.** Intermediate: *mesomere*. **3.** Mesentery: *mesoileum*. **4.** Characterizing a superimposable isomer: meso-*2,3-dichlorobutane*.

mes·o·ap·pen·dix (měz′ō-ǝ-pěn′dĭks) *n*. The short mesentery of the appendix lying behind the terminal ileum.

mes·o·bi·lane (měz′ō-bī′lān′) *n*. A colorless compound resulting from the reduction of bilirubin in the tissues. Also called *mesobilirubinogen*.

mes·o·bil·i·ru·bin (měz′ō-bĭl′ĭ-roo′bĭn) *n*. A yellow crystalline compound formed by the reduction of bilirubin and occurring in the small intestine.

mes·o·bil·i·ru·bin·o·gen (měz′ō-bĭl′ĭ-roo-bĭn′ǝ-jǝn) *n*. See **mesobilane**.

mes·o·blast (měz′ǝ-blăst′) *n*. The middle germinal layer of an early embryo, consisting of undifferentiated cells destined to become the mesoderm. —**mes′o·blas′tic** *adj*.

mes·o·blas·te·ma (měz′ǝ-blă-stē′mǝ) *n*. The cells that constitute the early undifferentiated mesoderm. —**mes′o·blas·te′mic** (-stē′mĭk) *adj*.

mes·o·car·di·a (měz′ǝ-kär′dē-ǝ) *n*. An atypical central position of the heart in the chest, as in the embryo.

mes·o·car·di·um (měz′ǝ-kär′dē-ǝm) *n*., *pl*. **–di·a** (-dē-ǝ) Either of the two layers of the embryonic mesen-

tery supporting the embryonic heart in the pericardial cavity.

mes·o·ca·val shunt (měz′ǝ-kā′vǝl) *n*. Anastomosis or graft anastomosis of the side of the superior mesenteric vein to the proximal end of the divided inferior vena cava performed as a means of controlling portal hypertension.

mes·o·ce·cum (měz′ǝ-sē′kǝm) *n*. The part of the mesentery that is attached to the cecum. —**mes′o·ce′cal** (-kǝl) *adj*.

mes·o·ce·phal·ic (měz′ō-sǝ-făl′ĭk) *adj*. Having a head of medium breadth, with a cephalic index between 76 and 80.

mes·o·co·lon (měz′ǝ-kō′lǝn) *n*. The fold of peritoneum attaching the colon to the posterior abdominal wall. —**mes′o·col′ic** (-kŏl′ĭk, -kō′lĭk) *adj*.

mes·o·col·o·pex·y (měz′ǝ-kŏl′ǝ-pěk′sē, -kō′lǝ-) *n*. The surgical shortening of the mesocolon to suspend it or fix it in place. Also called *mesocoloplication*.

mes·o·cord (měz′ǝ-kôrd′) *n*. A fold of amnion that sometimes binds a segment of the umbilical cord to the placenta.

mes·o·derm (měz′ǝ-dûrm′) *n*. The middle embryonic germ layer, lying between the ectoderm and the endoderm, from which connective tissue, muscle, bone, and the urogenital and circulatory systems develop. —**mes′o·der′mic** *adj*.

mes·o·di·a·stol·ic (měz′ǝ-dī′ǝ-stŏl′ĭk) *adj*. Of or relating to the middle of the diastole of the heart.

mes·o·du·o·de·num (měz′ǝ-doo′ǝ-dē′nǝm, -doo-ŏd′-n-ǝm) *n*. The part of the mesentery that connects the duodenum to the wall of the embryonic abdominal cavity. —**mes′o·du′o·de′nal** *adj*.

mes·o·ep·i·did·y·mis (měz′ō-ěp′ĭ-dĭd′ǝ-mĭs) *n*. An occasional fold of the tunica vaginalis testis that binds the epididymis to the testis.

mes·o·gas·tri·um (měz′ǝ-găs′trē-ǝm) *n*., *pl*. **–tri·a** (-trē-ǝ) The portion of the embryonic mesentery that is attached to the early stomach. Also called *mesogaster*. —**mes′o·gas′tric** (-trĭk) *adj*.

mes·o·gen·ic (měz′ǝ-jěn′ĭk) *adj*. Of or relating to the capacity of a virus to lethally infect embryonic hosts after a short incubation period but that is incapable of infecting immature and adult hosts.

me·sog·li·a (mĭ-sŏg′lē-ǝ) *n*. Neuroglial cells of mesodermic origin. Also called *mesoglial cell*.

mes·o·glu·te·us (měz′ǝ-gloo′tē-ǝs, -gloo-tē′-) *n*. The gluteus medius muscle. —**mes′o·glu′te·al** *adj*.

mes·o·il·e·um (měz′ǝ-ĭl′ē-ǝm) *n*. The mesentery of the ileum.

mes·o·je·ju·num (měz′ō-jǝ-joo′nǝm) *n*. The mesentery of the jejunum.

mes·o·lym·pho·cyte (měz′ǝ-lĭm′fǝ-sīt′) *n*. A mononuclear leukocyte of medium size, probably a lymphocyte, having a deeply staining nucleus that is relatively smaller than that in most lymphocytes.

mes·o·me·li·a (měz′ǝ-mē′lē-ǝ, -mēl′yǝ) *n*. A condition in which the forearms and lower legs are abnormally short. —**mes′o·mel′ic** (-měl′ĭk) *adj*.

mesomelic dwarfism *n*. Dwarfism that is characterized by shortened forearms and lower legs.

mes·o·mere (měz′ə-mîr′) *n.* **1.** A blastomere of intermediate size that is larger than a micromere but smaller than a macromere. **2.** The middle zone of the mesoderm of a chordate embryo, from which excretory tissue develops.

mes·o·met·a·neph·ric carcinoma (měz′ə-mět′ə-něf′-rĭk) *n.* See **mesonephroma**.

mes·o·me·tri·um (měz′ə-mē′trē-əm) *n.* The part of the broad ligament of the uterus that is below the mesosalpinx.

mes·o·morph (měz′ə-môrf′) *n.* An individual characterized by a robust muscular body build in which tissues derived from the embryonic mesodermal layer predominate. —**mes′o·mor′phic** *adj.* —**mes′o·mor′-phism, mes′o·mor′phy** *n.*

mesonephric duct *n.* See **wolffian duct**.

mesonephric fold *n.* See **urogenital ridge**.

mesonephric ridge *n.* The embryonic urogenital ridge, from which the more medial gonadal ridge is later demarcated.

mes·o·ne·phro·ma (měz′ō-nə-frō′mə) *n.* Any of various rare tumors possibly derived from the mesonephros and occurring in the genital tract. Also called *mesometanephric carcinoma*.

mes·o·neph·ros (měz′ə-něf′rəs, -rŏs′) *n., pl.* **–neph·roi** (-něf′roi′) The second of the three excretory organs that develop in a vertebrate embryo, replaced by the metanephros in higher vertebrates. Also called *wolffian body*. —**mes′o·neph′ric** *adj.*

mes·o·neu·ri·tis (měz′ə-nŏŏ-rī′tĭs) *n.* Inflammation of a nerve or its connective tissue without involvement of its sheath.

mes·o·pex·y (měz′ə-pěk′sē) *n.* See **mesenteriopexy**.

mes·o·phil (měz′ə-fĭl′) *or* **mes·o·phile** (-fīl′) *n.* A microorganism with an optimum growth temperature that is between 20°C and 45°C. —**mes′o·phil′ic** (-fĭl′-ĭk) *adj.*

mes·o·phle·bi·tis (měz′ō-flĭ-bī′tĭs) *n.* Inflammation of the middle coat of a vein.

me·soph·ry·on (mə-zŏf′rē-ŏn′, -ən) *n.* See **glabella** (sense 2).

mes·o·por·phy·rin (měz′ō-pôr′fə-rĭn) *n.* Any of various porphyrin compounds produced from a protoporphyrin by the addition of hydrogen to the double bond of each of the vinyl groups.

me·sor·chi·um (mə-zôr′kē-əm) *n.* **1.** A fold of tunica vaginalis testis in the fetus supporting the mesonephros and the developing testis. **2.** A fold of tunica vaginalis testis in the adult between the testis and epididymis. —**me·sor′chi·al** *adj.*

mes·o·rec·tum (měz′ə-rěk′təm) *n.* The mesentery supporting the rectum.

me·sor·rha·phy (mə-zôr′ə-fē) *n.* See **mesenteriorrhaphy**.

mes·o·sal·pinx (měz′ō-săl′pĭngks) *n.* The part of the broad ligament of the uterus enclosing a fallopian tube.

mes·o·sig·moid (měz′ō-sĭg′moid′) *n.* The mesentery of the sigmoid flexure.

mes·o·sig·moid·i·tis (měz′ō-sĭg′moi-dī′tĭs) *n.* Inflammation of the mesosigmoid.

mes·o·sig·moi·do·pex·y (měz′ō-sĭg-moi′də-pěk′sē) *n.* The surgical fixation of the mesosigmoid.

mes·o·sys·tol·ic (měz′ə-sĭ-stŏl′ĭk) *adj.* Relating to the middle of the systole of the heart.

mes·o·ten·di·ne·um (měz′ō-těn-dĭn′ē-əm) *n.* Any of the synovial layers that pass from a tendon to the wall of a tendon sheath where tendons lie within osteofibrous canals. Also called *mesotendon*.

mes·o·the·li·o·ma (měz′ə-thē′lē-ō′mə) *n., pl.* **–mas** *or* **–ma·ta** (-mə-tə) A rare neoplasm derived from the lining cells of the pleura and peritoneum and growing as a thick sheet composed of spindle cells or fibrous tissue covering the viscera.

mes·o·the·li·um (měz′ə-thē′lē-əm) *n., pl.* **–li·a** (-lē-ə) The layer of flat cells of mesodermal origin that lines the embryonic body cavity and gives rise to the squamous cells of the peritoneum, pericardium, and pleura. —**mes′o·the′li·al** *adj.*

mes·o·var·i·um (měz′ō-vâr′ē-əm) *n., pl.* **–i·a** (-ē-ə) A short peritoneal fold connecting the anterior border of the ovary with the posterior layer of the broad ligament of the uterus.

mes·sen·ger RNA (měs′ən-jər) *n.* See **mRNA**.

mes·tra·nol (měs′trə-nôl′, -nōl′) *n.* A synthetic estrogen used in combination with a progestin in oral contraceptive preparations.

mes·y·late (měs′ə-lāt′) *n.* A salt or ester of methanesulfonic acid.

Met *abbr.* methionine

MET *abbr.* metabolic equivalent

meta– *or* **met–** *pref.* **1.** Later in time: *metestrus.* **2.** At a later stage of development: *metanephros.* **3.** Situated behind: *metacarpus.* **4.** Change; transformation: *metachromatism.* **5.** Alternation: *metagenesis.* **6.** Beyond; transcending; more comprehensive: *metapsychology.* **7.** At a higher state of development: *metazoan.* **8.** Having undergone metamorphosis: *metamyelocyte.* **9.** Derivative or related chemical substance: *metaprotein.* **10.** *Abbr.* **m–** Of or relating to one of three possible isomers of a benzene ring with two attached chemical groups, in which the carbon atoms with attached groups are separated by one unsubstituted carbon atom. Usually used in italic: meta-*dibromobenzene.*

me·tab·a·sis (mĭ-tăb′ə-sĭs) *n.* A change in the symptoms, course, or treatment of a disease.

met·a·bi·o·sis (mět′ə-bī-ō′sĭs) *n.* Dependence of one organism on another for the preparation of an environment in which it can live.

met·a·bi·sul·fite test (mět′ə-bī-sŭl′fīt′) *n.* A test for sickle-cell hemoglobin in which red blood cells are deoxygenated by the addition of sodium metabisulfite and the cells containing the defective hemoglobin assume a sickle shape.

met·a·bol·ic (mět′ə-bŏl′ĭk) *adj.* Of, relating to, or resulting from metabolism.

metabolic acidosis *n.* Decreased pH and bicarbonate concentration of the body fluids caused either by the accumulation of excess acids stronger than carbonic acid or by abnormal losses of bicarbonate from the body.

metabolic alkalosis *n.* An increase in the alkalinity of body fluids due to an increase in alkali intake or a decrease in acid concentration, as from vomiting.

metabolic coma *n.* A coma due to disorders of the neuronal mechanisms of energy transfer or due to impairment or deprivation of the energy sources.

metabolic craniopathy *n.* See **Morgagni's syndrome.**

metabolic equivalent *n. Abbr.* **MET** The energy expended while resting, usually calculated as the energy used to burn 3 to 4 milliliters of oxygen per kilogram of body weight per minute.

metabolic syndrome *n.* See **syndrome X.**

me·tab·o·lism (mĭ-tăb′ə-lĭz′əm) *n.* **1.** The complex of physical and chemical processes occurring within a living cell or organism that are necessary for the maintenance of life. In metabolism some substances are broken down to yield energy for vital processes while other substances, necessary for life, are synthesized. **2.** The functioning of a specific substance, such as water, within the living body.

me·tab·o·lite (mĭ-tăb′ə-līt′) *n.* **1.** A substance produced by metabolism. **2.** A substance necessary for or taking part in a particular metabolic process.

me·tab·o·lize (mĭ-tăb′ə-līz′) *v.* **1.** To subject to metabolism. **2.** To produce by metabolism. **3.** To undergo change by metabolism.

met·a·car·pal (mĕt′ə-kär′pəl) *adj.* Of or relating to the metacarpus. —*n.* Any of the five long bones that form the metacarpus and articulate with the bones of the distal row of the carpus and with the five proximal phalanges. —**met′a·car′pal·ly** *adv.*

metacarpal artery *n.* **1.** Any of four arteries on the dorsal surface of the carpus; dorsal metacarpal artery. **2.** Any of three arteries that spring from the deep palmar arch and anastomose with the dorsal metacarpal arteries; palmar metacarpal artery.

met·a·car·pec·to·my (mĕt′ə-kär-pĕk′tə-mē) *n.* Surgical excision of one or all of the metacarpals.

met·a·car·po·pha·lan·ge·al (mĕt′ə-kär′pō-fə-lăn′jē-əl, -fā-) *adj. Abbr.* **MCP** Of or relating to the metacarpus and the phalanges of the hand, especially to the articulations between them.

metacarpophalangeal joint *n.* Any of the spheroid joints between the heads of the metacarpal bones and the bases of the proximal phalanges.

met·a·car·pus (mĕt′ə-kär′pəs) *n., pl.* **-pi** (-pī) The part of the hand that includes the five bones between the fingers and the wrist.

met·a·cen·tric (mĕt′ə-sĕn′trĭk) *adj.* Having the centromere of a chromosome in the median position so that the arms are of equal length. —*n.* A metacentric chromosome.

metacentric chromosome *n.* A chromosome with a centrally placed centromere that divides the chromosome into two arms of about equal length.

met·a·cer·car·i·a (mĕt′ə-sər-kăr′ē-ə) *n., pl.* **-i·ae** (-ē-ē′) The encysted maturing stage of a trematode in its intermediate host prior to transfer to the definitive host, usually representing the organism's infectious stage.

met·a·chro·ma·sia (mĕt′ə-krō-mā′zhə) *n.* **1.** The characteristic of a cell or tissue component of taking on a color different from that of the dye with which it is stained. **2.** The property of certain dyes to stain different substances different colors.

met·a·chro·mat·ic (mĕt′ə-krō-măt′ĭk) *adj.* **1.** Of or relating to metachromasia. **2.** Relating to the property of certain chemical substances to appear as different colors depending upon the wavelength of light under which they are viewed.

metachromatic body *n.* A concentrated deposit of phosphate polymer, lipid, and nucleoprotein occurring in many bacteria, algae, fungi, and protozoa, and having staining properties different from those of the surrounding protoplasm.

metachromatic leukodystrophy *n.* An inherited metabolic disorder characterized by myelin loss, accumulation of metachromatic lipids in the white matter of the central and peripheral nervous systems, a marked excess of sulfatidates in white matter and in urine, progressive paralysis, and dementia.

metachromatic stain *n.* A stain that has the ability to produce different colors in various histological or cytological structures.

met·a·chro·ma·tism (mĕt′ə-krō′mə-tĭz′əm) *n.* Metachromasia.

met·a·chro·mo·phil (mĕt′ə-krō′mə-fĭl′) *or* **met·a·chro·mo·phile** (-fĭl′) *adj.* Metachromatic.

met·a·gen·e·sis (mĕt′ə-jĕn′ĭ-sĭs) *n.* See **alternation of generations.**

Met·a·gon·i·mus (mĕt′ə-gŏn′ə-məs) *n.* A genus of flukes that encyst on fish and infest humans and other fish-eating animals, including *Metagonimus yokogawai,* a common intestinal fluke in eastern Asia and the Balkan states, which causes diarrhea when ingested in its larval form in raw fish.

met·a·her·pet·ic keratitis (mĕt′ə-hər-pĕt′ĭk) *n.* Inflammation of the cornea in herpetic keratitis due to structural damage of the corneal tissue.

met·al (mĕt′l) *n.* **1.** Any of a category of electropositive elements that usually reflect light, are generally good conductors of heat and electricity, and can be melted or fused, hammered into thin sheets, or drawn into wires. Typical metals form salts with nonmetals, basic oxides with oxygen, and alloys with one another. **2.** An alloy of two or more metallic elements. **3.** An object made of metal.

metal fume fever *n.* An occupational disease caused by inhalation of particles and fumes of metallic oxides and characterized by malarialike symptoms.

metallo– *or* **metall–** *pref.* Metal: *metalloenzyme.*

me·tal·lo·en·zyme (mĭ-tăl′ō-ĕn′zīm) *n.* An enzyme having a metal, usually an ion, linked to its protein component.

me·tal·lo·por·phy·rin (mĭ-tăl′ō-pôr′fə-rĭn) *n.* A compound, such as heme, formed by the combination of a porphyrin with a metal.

me·tal·lo·pro·tein (mĭ-tăl′ō-prō′tēn′) *n.* A protein containing a metal ion within its structure.

me·tal·lo·thi·o·ne·in (mĭ-tăl′ō-thī′ə-nē′ĭn) *n.* A small metal-binding protein, rich in sulfur-containing amino acids, that is synthesized in the liver and kidney and important in ion transport.

met·a·mer (mĕt'ə-mər) *n.* **1.** A compound that contains the same number and type of atoms as other compounds but with a different distribution of radicals. **2.** A color that appears to the eye to be identical to another color but which in fact has a different spectral composition.

met·a·mere (mĕt'ə-mîr') *n.* Any of the homologous segments, lying in a longitudinal series, that compose the body of certain animals, such as lobsters. Also called *somite.* —**met'a·mer'ic** (-mĕr'ĭk) *adj.*

metameric nervous system *n.* The part of the nervous system innervating the body structures that develop in ontogeny from the segmentally arranged somites or from the branchial arches in the head.

me·tam·er·ism (mə-tăm'ə-rĭz'əm) *n.* The condition of having the body divided into metameres, exhibited in most animals only in the early embryonic stages of development.

met·a·mor·phop·si·a (mĕt'ə-môr-fŏp'sē-ə) *n.* A visual disorder in which images appear distorted in various ways.

met·a·mor·pho·sis (mĕt'ə-môr'fə-sĭs) *n., pl.* **-ses** (-sēz') **1.** A marked change in appearance, character, condition, or function. Also called *transformation.* **2.** A change in the form and often habits of an animal during normal development after the embryonic stage. Metamorphosis includes, in insects, the transformation of a maggot into an adult fly and a caterpillar into a butterfly and, in amphibians, the changing of a tadpole into a frog. **3.** A usually degenerative pathological change in the structure of a particular body tissue. —**met'a·mor·phot'ic** (-môr-fŏt'ĭk) *adj.*

Met·a·mu·cil (mĕt'ə-myoō'sĭl) A trademark for a therapeutic preparation containing psyllium.

met·a·my·el·o·cyte (mĕt'ə-mī'ə-lə-sīt') *n.* A transitional form of myelocyte having a nuclear construction intermediate between the mature myelocyte and the two-lobed granulocyte. Also called *juvenile cell.*

metanephric duct *n.* The slender tubular portion of the embryonic metanephric diverticulum that later forms the ureter.

met·a·neph·rine (mĕt'ə-nĕf'rĭn, -rēn') *n.* A catabolite of epinephrine excreted in the urine and found in some tissues.

met·a·neph·ro·gen·ic (mĕt'ə-nĕf'rə-jĕn'ĭk) *adj.* Capable of giving rise to the metanephroi.

met·a·neph·ros (mĕt'ə-nĕf'rəs, -rŏs') *n., pl.* **-roi** (-roi') The third and final excretory organ that develops in a vertebrate embryo. In birds, reptiles, and mammals it replaces the mesonephros as the functional excretory organ and develops into the adult kidney. —**met'a·neph'ric** (-rĭk) *adj.*

met·a·phase (mĕt'ə-fāz') *n.* The stage of mitosis and meiosis, following prophase and preceding anaphase, during which the chromosomes are aligned along the metaphase plate.

metaphase plate *n.* An imaginary plane perpendicular to the spindle fibers of a dividing cell, along which chromosomes align during metaphase.

met·a·phos·phor·ic acid (mĕt'ə-fŏs-fôr'ĭk) *n.* An inorganic compound used as a dehydrating agent and in dental cements.

metaphysial dysostosis *n.* A rare developmental abnormality of the skeleton in which the metaphyses of tubular bones expand as a result of the deposition of cartilage.

metaphysial dysplasia *n.* A disorder in which the metaphyses of long bones fail to produce normal new tubular structures and instead appear to be expanded and porous.

me·taph·y·sis (mĭ-tăf'ĭ-sĭs) *n., pl.* **-ses** (-sēz') The zone of growth between the epiphysis and diaphysis during development of a bone. —**met'a·phys'i·al** (mĕt'ə-fĭz'ē-əl) *adj.*

met·a·pla·sia (mĕt'ə-plā'zhə) *n.* **1.** Normal transformation of tissue from one type to another, as in the ossification of cartilage to form bone. **2.** Transformation of cells from a normal to an abnormal state.

met·a·plasm (mĕt'ə-plăz'əm) *n.* See **cell inclusion** (sense 1). —**met'a·plas'tic** (-plăs'tĭk) *adj.*

metaplastic anemia *n.* Pernicious anemia in which the various elements in the blood change into multisegmented, unusually large neutrophiles, immature myeloid cells, and distorted platelets.

metaplastic carcinoma *n.* Carcinoma occurring in the upper respiratory tract or alimentary tract or in the breast, and composed of spindle-shaped tumor cells.

metaplastic ossification *n.* The formation of bone in normally soft structures.

metaplastic polyp *n.* See **hyperplastic polyp.**

met·a·pro·ter·e·nol sulfate (mĕt'ə-prō-tĕr'ə-nôl) *n.* A bronchodilator used in the treatment of bronchial asthma. Also called *orciprenaline sulfate.*

met·a·psy·chol·o·gy (mĕt'ə-sī-kŏl'ə-jē) *n.* **1.** Philosophical inquiry supplementing the empirical science of psychology and dealing with aspects of the mind that cannot be evaluated on the basis of objective or empirical evidence. **2.** A comprehensive system of psychology involving several very different approaches to mental processes as described in the Freudian theory of the mind.

met·ar·te·ri·ole (mĕt'är-tîr'ē-ōl') *n.* Any of the small peripheral blood vessels that are structurally and anatomically intermediate between the arterioles and the true capillaries and that contain scattered groups of smooth muscle fibers in their walls.

met·a·ru·bri·cyte (mĕt'ə-roō'brĭ-sīt') *n.* An orthochromatic normoblast.

me·tas·ta·sis (mə-tăs'tə-sĭs) *n., pl.* **-ses** (-sēz') **1.** Transmission of pathogenic microorganisms or cancerous cells from an original site to one or more sites elsewhere in the body, usually by way of the blood vessels or lymphatics. **2.** A secondary cancerous growth formed by transmission of cancerous cells from a primary growth located elsewhere in the body. —**met'a·stat'ic** (mĕt'ə-stăt'ĭk) *adj.*

me·tas·ta·size (mə-tăs'tə-sīz') *v.* To be transmitted or transferred by or as if by metastasis.

metastatic abscess *n.* A secondary abscess formed at a distance from the primary abscess, as a result of the transport of pyogenic bacteria through the lymph or blood.

metastatic calcification *n.* Calcification of nonosseous viable tissue composed of cells that secrete acidic materials.

met·a·tar·sal (mĕt′ə-tär′səl) *adj.* Of or relating to the metatarsus. —*n.* Any of the five long bones that form the anterior portion of the foot and articulate posteriorly with the three cuneiform and the cuboid bones and anteriorly with the five proximal phalanges.

metatarsal artery *n.* **1.** Any of the three branches of the arcuate artery supplying the three lateral toes and the lateral side of the second toe through the dorsal digital artery; dorsal metatarsal artery. **2.** Any of the four branches of the plantar arch that divide into the plantar digital arteries to supply the toes; plantar metatarsal artery.

met·a·tar·sal·gia (mĕt′ə-tär-săl′jə) *n.* A cramping, burning pain that focuses in the region of the metatarsal bones of the foot.

met·a·tar·sec·to·my (mĕt′ə-tär-sĕk′tə-mē) *n.* Excision of the metatarsus.

met·a·tar·so·pha·lan·ge·al (mĕt′ə-tär′sō-fə-lăn′jē-əl, -fā-) *adj.* Of or relating to the metatarsal bones and the phalanges of the foot, especially the articulations between them.

metatarsophalangeal joint *n.* Any of the spheroid joints between the heads of the metatarsal bones and the bases of the proximal phalanges of the toes.

met·a·tar·sus (mĕt′ə-tär′səs) *n., pl.* **–si** (-sī, -sē) The middle part of the foot that forms the instep and includes the five bones between the toes and ankle.

metatarsus la·tus (lā′təs) *n.* A deformity of the foot caused by a sinking of the transverse arch.

metatarsus var·us (vâr′əs) *n.* A deformity of the foot in which the forepart of the foot is rotated and fixed on the long axis of the foot, so that the sole faces the midline of the body. Also called *intoe.*

met·a·thal·a·mus (mĕt′ə-thăl′ə-məs) *n.* The most caudal part of the thalamus, composed of the medial and lateral geniculate bodies.

me·tath·e·sis (mĭ-tăth′ĭ-sĭs) *n., pl.* **–ses** (-sēz′) Double decomposition of chemical compounds in which an element or radical of one compound exchanges places with another element or radical in another compound.

me·tath·e·size (mĭ-tăth′ĭ-sīz′) *v.* To subject to or undergo metathesis.

met·a·troph·ic (mĕt′ə-trŏf′ĭk, -trō′fĭk) *adj.* **1.** Of or relating to the ability to undertake anabolism. **2.** Of or relating to the ability to obtain nourishment from varied sources, as from nitrogenous and carbonaceous organic matter.

met·a·trop·ic dwarfism (mĕt′ə-trŏp′ĭk, -trō′pĭk) *n.* A congenital skeletal dysplasia in which the development of dwarfism changes with time; at birth the trunk lengthens relative to the limbs but later it begins to shorten.

Met·a·zo·a (mĕt′ə-zō′ə) *n.* A subdivision of the animal kingdom that includes all multicellular animal organisms having cells that are differentiated and form tissues and organs. —**met′a·zo′an** *adj. & n.*

met·a·zo·on·o·sis (mĕt′ə-zō-ŏn′ə-sĭs, -zō′ə-nō′-) *n.* A zoonosis that requires both a vertebrate and an invertebrate host for completion of the life cycle of the infective organism.

Metch·ni·koff (mĕch′nĭ-kôf′), **Elie** 1845–1916. Russian zoologist. He shared a 1908 Nobel Prize for the discovery of phagocytes and their role in the immune system.

met·en·ceph·a·lon (mĕt′ĕn-sĕf′ə-lŏn′) *n.* The anterior part of the embryonic hindbrain, which gives rise to the cerebellum and pons. —**met′en·ce·phal′ic** (-sə-făl′ĭk) *adj.*

met·en·keph·a·lin (mĕt′ĕn-kĕf′ə-lĭn) *n.* An enkephalin that has a terminal methionine residue and occurs naturally as one of two such pentapeptides that are formed in the brain.

me·te·or·ism (mē′tē-ə-rĭz′əm) *n.* See **tympanites.**

me·te·or·o·trop·ic (mē′tē-ôr′ə-trŏp′ĭk, -trō′pĭk) *adj.* Of or relating to diseases whose occurrences are affected by the weather.

me·ter (mē′tər) *n. Abbr.* **m** The standard unit of length in the International System of Units that is equivalent to 39.37 inches.

–meter *suff.* Measuring device: *refractometer.*

meter angle *n.* The unit of ocular convergence equal to the amount of convergence required to view binocularly an object at 1 meter and exerting 1 diopter of accommodation.

meter-candle *n.* See **lux.**

meter-kilogram-second system *n. Abbr.* **mks, MKS** A system of units using the meter, the kilogram, and the second as basic units of length, mass, and time.

met·es·trus (mĕ-tĕs′trəs) *n.* The period of sexual inactivity that follows estrus.

met·for·min (mĕt-fôr′mĭn) *n.* An oral antidiabetic agent that decreases glucose production by the liver and lowers plasma glucose levels.

meth (mĕth) *n.* Methamphetamine hydrochloride.

meth– *pref.* Methyl: *methane.*

meth·a·done hydrochloride (mĕth′ə-dōn′) *n.* A potent addictive synthetic narcotic drug used to alleviate pain and as a substitute narcotic in the treatment of heroin addiction.

meth·am·phet·a·mine hydrochloride (mĕth′ăm-fĕt′-ə-mēn′, -mĭn) *n.* A crystalline amine used as a central nervous system stimulant and in the treatment of obesity.

meth·ane (mĕth′ān′) *n.* An odorless, colorless, flammable gas that is the major constituent of natural gas and is used as a fuel and as an important source of hydrogen. Also called *marsh gas.*

meth·ane·sul·fon·ic acid (mĕth′ān-sŭl-fŏn′ĭk) *n.* A liquid soluble in water, alcohol, and ether used as a reaction catalyst.

meth·an·o·gen (mĕ-thăn′ə-jən, -jĕn′) *n.* Any of various anaerobic methane-producing bacteria belonging to the family Methanobacteriaceae.

meth·a·nol (mĕth′ə-nôl′, -nōl′) *n.* A colorless, toxic, flammable liquid used as an antifreeze, a general solvent, a fuel, and a denaturant for ethyl alcohol. Also called *carbinol, methyl alcohol, wood alcohol.*

meth·a·qua·lone (mĕth′ə-kwā′lōn′) *n.* A potentially habit-forming drug used as a sedative and hypnotic.

metHb *abbr.* methemoglobin

met·hem·al·bu·min (mĕt′hē-măl-byoō′mĭn) *n.* An abnormal albumin-heme complex formed in the blood during diseases that are characterized by extensive hemolysis.

met·hem·al·bu·mi·ne·mi·a (mĕt′hē-măl-byōō′mə-nē′mē-ə) *n.* Methemalbumin in the blood.

met·he·mo·glo·bin (mĕt-hē′mə-glō′bĭn) *n. Abbr.* **metHb** A brownish-red crystalline organic compound formed in the blood when hemoglobin is oxidated either by decomposition of the blood or by the action of various oxidizing drugs or toxic agents. It contains iron in the ferric state and cannot function as an oxygen carrier.

met·he·mo·glo·bi·ne·mi·a (mĕt′hē-mə-glō′bə-nē′mē-ə) *n.* Methemoglobin in the blood.

met·he·mo·glo·bi·nu·ri·a (mĕt′hē-mə-glō′bə-nŏŏr′ē-ə) *n.* Methemoglobin in the urine.

me·the·na·mine (mə-thē′nə-mēn′, -mĭn) *n.* An organic compound used as a urinary tract antiseptic.

meth·i·cil·lin (mĕth′ĭ-sĭl′ĭn) *n.* A synthetic antibiotic related to penicillin and most commonly used in treatment of infections caused by staphylococci that produce beta-lactamase.

me·thim·a·zole (mə-thĭm′ə-zōl′) *n.* A drug that inhibits the synthesis of thyroid hormone and is used to treat hyperthyroidism.

me·thi·o·nine (mə-thī′ə-nēn′) *n. Abbr.* **Met** A sulfur-containing essential amino acid obtained from various proteins or prepared synthetically and used as a dietary supplement and in pharmaceuticals.

meth·od (mĕth′əd) *n.* **1.** A means or manner of procedure, especially a regular and systematic way of accomplishing something. **2.** Orderly arrangement of parts or steps to accomplish an end. **3.** The procedures and techniques characteristic of a particular discipline or field of knowledge.

meth·o·trex·ate (mĕth′ə-trĕk′sāt′) *n. Abbr.* **MTX** A toxic antimetabolite that acts as a folic acid antagonist, used as an antineoplastic agent and in the treatment of rheumatoid arthritis and psoriasis. Also called *amethopterin*.

methoxy– *pref.* Containing the radical group, CH_3O: *methoxyflurane*.

me·thox·y·flu·rane (mə-thŏk′sē-flŏŏr′ān′) *n.* A potent, nonflammable, nonexplosive anesthetic administered by inhalation.

me·thox·yl (mə-thŏk′səl) *n.* The univalent radical, OCH_3.

meth·yl (mĕth′əl) *n.* The alkyl group, often a univalent radical, CH_3, derived from methane and occurring in many important organic compounds.

methyl alcohol *n.* See **methanol.**

meth·yl·ate (mĕth′ə-lāt′) *v.* **1.** To mix or combine with methyl alcohol. **2.** To combine with the methyl radical. —*n.* An organic compound in which the hydrogen of the hydroxyl group of methyl alcohol is replaced by a metal.

meth·yl·cel·lu·lose (mĕth′əl-sĕl′yə-lōs′, -lōz′) *n.* A powdery substance that swells in water to form a gel, is prepared by the methylation of natural cellulose, and is used as a food additive, a bulk-forming laxative, an emulsifier, and a thickener.

meth·yl·do·pa (mĕth′əl-dō′pə) *n.* A drug used in the treatment of high blood pressure.

meth·yl·ene (mĕth′ə-lēn′) *n.* A bivalent hydrocarbon radical, CH_2, that is a component of unsaturated hydrocarbons and is derived from methane by the removal of two hydrogen atoms.

methylene azure *n.* A dye used as a biological stain and formed by the oxidation of methylene blue.

methylene blue *n.* A basic aniline dye that forms a deep blue solution when dissolved in water and is used as a bacteriological stain and as an antidote for cyanide poisoning.

methyl green *n.* A basic dye used as a chromatin stain, as a differential stain for RNA and DNA, and as a tracking dye for DNA in electrophoresis.

meth·yl·ma·lo·nic aciduria (mĕth′əl-mə-lō′nĭk, -lŏn′-ik) *n.* A metabolic disorder resulting from an enzyme deficiency and characterized by the presence of excessive amounts of methylmalonic acid in the urine; it can be congenital or acquired because of a vitamin B_{12} deficiency.

meth·yl·mor·phine (mĕth′əl-môr′fēn′) *n.* See **codeine.**

meth·yl·ol (mĕth′ə-lôl) *n.* The monovalent radical, CH_2OH, present in primary alcohols. Also called *hydroxymethyl*.

meth·yl·pen·tose (mĕth′əl-pĕn′tōs′, -tōz′) *n.* A six-carbon monosaccharide having a methyl group on the sixth carbon.

meth·yl·phen·i·date (mĕth′əl-fĕn′ĭ-dāt′, -fē′nĭ-) *n.* A drug chemically related to amphetamine and that acts as a mild stimulant of the central nervous system, used especially in the form of its hydrochloride for the treatment of narcolepsy in adults and hyperkinetic disorders in children.

meth·yl·pred·nis·o·lone (mĕth′əl-prĕd-nĭs′ə-lōn′) *n.* An anti-inflammatory steroid administered to children and adolescents to relieve the pain induced by sickle cell anemia.

methyl salicylate *n.* The methyl ester of salicylic acid; an essential oil derived from birch or wintergreen or made synthetically, used as a counterirritant in ointments to treat muscle pain.

meth·yl·sul·fate (mĕth′əl-sŭl′fāt′) *n.* A colorless, oily, carcinogenic liquid used as a methylating agent.

meth·yl·tes·tos·ter·one (mĕth′əl-tĕs-tŏs′tə-rōn′) *n.* A synthetic methyl derivative of testosterone used in the treatment of male sex hormone deficiency.

meth·yl·trans·fer·ase (mĕth′əl-trăns′fə-rās′, -rāz′) *n.* Any of several enzymes that catalyze the transfer of methyl groups from one compound to another. Also called *transmethylase*.

methyl violet *n.* Any of several basic dyes, such as gentian violet, that are derivatives of pararosaniline and are used as histological and bacteriological stains.

metMb *abbr.* metmyoglobin

met·my·o·glo·bin (mĕt-mī′ə-glō′bĭn) *n. Abbr.* **metMb** Myoglobin in which the ferrous ion of the heme prosthetic group is oxidized.

met·o·clo·pra·mide (mĕt′ə-klō′prə-mīd′) *n.* A dopamine antagonist that facilitates muscular movement in the upper gastrointestinal tract and is usually used to treat nausea and gastroesophageal reflux.

me·ton·y·my (mə-tŏn′ə-mē) *n.* In schizophrenia, a language disturbance in which an inappropriate but related word is used in place of the correct one.

me·top·ic (mə-tŏp′ĭk) *adj.* Of or relating to the forehead or the anterior portion of the cranium.

metopic suture *n.* A persistent frontal suture.

met·o·pon (mĕt′ə-pŏn′) *n.* A narcotic drug derived from morphine and used in the form of its hydrochloride as an analgesic.

met·o·po·plas·ty (mĕt′ə-pō-plăs′tē, mə-tŏp′ə-plăs′tē) *n.* The surgical repair of the skin or the bone of the forehead.

me·to·pro·lol tartrate (mə-tō′prə-lôl′, -lōl′) *n.* A beta-blocker used primarily to treat hypertension and angina pectoris.

me·tox·e·ny (mə-tŏk′sə-nē) *n.* A change of host by a parasite; heteroecism. —**me·tox′e·nous** (-nəs) *adj.*

me·tra (mē′trə) *n., pl.* **–trae** (-trē) See **uterus.**

me·tral·gia (mĭ-trăl′jə) *n.* See **hysteralgia.**

me·tra·to·ni·a (mē′trə-tō′nē-ə) *n.* Lack of tone or flaccidity of the uterine walls following childbirth.

me·trat·ro·phy (mĭ-trăt′rə-fē) *or* **me·tra·tro·phi·a** (mē′-trə-trō′fē-ə) *n.* Atrophy of the uterus.

me·tri·a (mē′trē-ə) *n.* An inflammatory condition following childbirth, such as pelvic cellulitis.

met·ric (mĕt′rĭk) *adj.* Of or relating to the meter or the metric system.

–metrics *suff.* The application of statistics and mathematical analysis to a field of study: *biometrics.*

metric system *n.* A decimal system of units based on the meter as a unit length, the kilogram as a unit mass, and the second as a unit time.

me·tri·tis (mĭ-trī′tĭs) *n.* Inflammation of the uterus.

metro– *or* **metr–** *pref.* Uterus: *metritis.*

me·tro·cyte (mē′trə-sīt′) *n.* See **mother cell.**

me·tro·dyn·i·a (mē′trə-dĭn′ē-ə) *n.* See **hysteralgia.**

me·tro·fi·bro·ma (mē′trə-fī-brō′mə) *n.* A fibroma of the uterus.

me·tro·lym·phan·gi·tis (mē′trō-lĭm′făn-jī′tĭs) *n.* Inflammation of the uterine lymphatics.

me·tro·ma·la·cia (mē′trō-mə-lā′shə) *n.* The pathological softening of the uterine tissues.

me·tro·ni·da·zole (mĕt′rə-nī′də-zōl′) *n.* A synthetic antimicrobial drug used in the treatment of vaginal trichomoniasis and intestinal amebiasis.

me·tro·pa·ral·y·sis (mē′trō-pə-răl′ĭ-sĭs) *n.* Paralysis of the uterine muscle during or immediately after childbirth.

metropathia hem·or·rhag·i·ca (hĕm′ə-răj′ĭ-kə) *n.* Abnormal, excessive, often continuous, uterine bleeding due to persistence of the follicular phase of the menstrual cycle.

me·trop·a·thy (mĭ-trŏp′ə-thē)   *or*   **me·tro·path·i·a** (mē′trə-păth′ē-ə) *n.* A disease of the uterus. —**me′-tro·path′ic** *adj.*

me·tro·per·i·to·ni·tis (mē′trō-pĕr′ĭ-tn-ī′tĭs) *n.* Inflammation of the uterus and its peritoneal covering. Also called *perimetritis.*

me·tro·phle·bi·tis (mē′trō-flĭ-bī′tĭs) *n.* Inflammation of the uterine veins, usually following childbirth.

met·ro·plas·ty (mē′trə-plăs′tē) *n.* See **uteroplasty.**

me·tror·rha·gia (mē′trə-rā′jə) *n.* Bleeding from the uterus that is not associated with menstruation.

me·tror·rhe·a (mē′trə-rē′ə) *n.* A discharge, especially of mucus or pus, from the uterus.

me·tro·sal·pin·gi·tis (mē′trō-săl′pĭn-jī′tĭs) *n.* Inflammation of the uterus and of one or both fallopian tubes.

me·tro·sal·pin·gog·ra·phy (mē′trō-săl′pĭng-gŏg′rə-fē, -pĭn-) *n.* See **hysterosalpingography.**

me·tro·scope (mē′trə-skōp′) *n.* See **hysteroscope.**

me·tro·stax·is (mē′trə-stăk′sĭs) *n.* A slight but continuous uterine hemorrhage.

me·tro·ste·no·sis (mē′trō-stə-nō′sĭs) *n.* A narrowing of the uterine cavity.

–metry *suff.* The process or science of measuring: *micrometry.*

me·tyr·a·pone (mə-tîr′ə-pōn′) *n.* An inhibitor of the hydroxylation of adrenocortical steroids administered as a diagnostic aid in determining pituitary gland function.

mev *or* **Mev** *or* **MeV** *abbr.* million electron volts

Mev·a·cor (mĕv′ə-kôr′) A trademark for the drug lovastatin.

Mey·er·hof (mī′ər-hôf′), **Otto** 1884–1951. German-born American physiologist. He shared a 1922 Nobel Prize for his discovery of the relationship between consumption of oxygen and production of lactic acid in muscles.

Mey·nert's decussation (mī′nərts) *n.* See **tegmental decussation** (sense 1).

mg *abbr.* milligram

Mg The symbol for the element **magnesium.**

MHC *abbr.* major histocompatibility complex

mho (mō) *n., pl.* **mhos** A siemens.

MHz *abbr.* megahertz

MI *abbr.* myocardial infarction; mitral insufficiency

Mi·chae·lis constant (mĭ-kā′lĭs) *or* **Michaelis-Men·ten constant** (-mĕn′tən) *n.* A constant that is equal to the substrate concentration at which an enzyme reaction proceeds at half the maximum velocity.

Michaelis-Gut·mann body (-gŭt′mən, -gōōt′män) *n.* A rounded laminated body containing calcium and iron and found within macrophages in the bladder wall in malacoplakia.

Michaelis-Men·ten hypothesis (-mĕn′tən) *n.* The hypothesis that a complex is formed between an enzyme and its substrate; the complex then dissociates to yield free enzyme and the reaction products, with the rate of dissociation determining the overall rate of substrate-product conversion.

mi·con·a·zole nitrate (mĭ-kŏn′ə-zōl′) *n.* An antifungal used topically or parenterally.

mi·cra·cous·tic *or* **mi·cro·cous·tic** (mī′krə-kōō′stĭk) *adj.* 1. Of, relating to, or characterized by faint sounds. 2. Having the ability to magnify very faint sounds to make them audible.

mi·cren·ceph·a·ly (mī′krĕn-sĕf′ə-lē) *or* **mi·cro·en·ceph·a·ly** (mī′krō-ĕn-) *n.* The condition of having an abnormally small brain.

micro– *or* **micr–** *pref.* 1. Small: *microblast.* 2. Abnormally small: *microcephaly.* 3. Requiring or involving microscopy: *microsurgery.* 4. *Symbol* μ One-millionth (10^{-6}): *microliter.*

mi·cro·ab·scess (mī′krō-ăb′sĕs′) *n.* A very small circumscribed collection of white blood cells in solid tissues.

mi·cro·ad·e·no·ma (mī′krō-ăd′n-ō′mə) *n.* A very small pituitary adenoma thought to cause hypersecretion syndromes.

mi·cro·aer·o·phil (mī′krō-âr′ə-fĭl′) *or* **mi·cro·aer·o·phile** (-fĭl′) *n.* An aerobic bacterium that survives in environments having a lower concentration of oxygen than is present in air. —*adj.* Of, relating to, or behaving like such an organism. —**mi′cro·aer′o·phil′ic** (-fĭl′ĭk) *adj.*

mi·cro·a·nas·to·mo·sis (mī′krō-ə-năs′tə-mō′sĭs) *n.* Anastomosis of minute structures performed with the aid of a surgical microscope.

mi·cro·a·nat·o·my (mī′krō-ə-năt′ə-mē) *n.* See **histology.** —**mi′cro·a·nat′o·mist** *n.*

mi·cro·an·eu·rysm (mī′krō-ăn′yə-rĭz′əm) *n.* A focal dilation of the venous end of retinal capillaries occurring in diabetes mellitus, retinal vein obstruction, and absolute glaucoma.

mi·cro·an·gi·og·ra·phy (mī′krō-ăn′jē-ŏg′rə-fē) *n.* Radiography of the minute blood vessels of an organ obtained by injection of a contrast medium and enlargement of the resulting radiograph.

mic·ro·an·gi·o·path·ic hemolytic anemia (mī′krō-ăn′jē-ə-păth′ĭk) *n.* The fragmentation of red blood cells because of narrowing or obstruction of small blood vessels.

mi·cro·an·gi·op·a·thy (mī′krō-ăn′jē-ŏp′ə-thē) *n.* See **capillaropathy.** —**mi′cro·an′gi·o·path′ic** (-ə-păth′ĭk) *adj.*

mi·cro·As·trup method (mī′krō-ăs′trəp) *n.* An interpolation technique for acid-base measurement.

mi·crobe (mī′krōb′) *n.* A microorganism, especially a bacterium that causes disease; a minute life form. No longer in technical use. —**mi·cro′bi·al** (mī-krō′bē-əl) *adj.*

mi·cro·bi·cide (mī-krō′bĭ-sīd′) *n.* An agent destructive to microorganisms. —**mi·cro′bi·cid′al** (-sīd′l) *adj.*

mi·cro·bi·ol·o·gy (mī′krō-bī-ŏl′ə-jē) *n.* The branch of biology that deals with microorganisms and their effects on other living organisms. —**mi′cro·bi′o·log′ic** (-ə-lŏg′ĭk) *adj.* —**mi′cro·bi·ol′o·gist** *n.*

mi·cro·bi·o·ta (mī′krō-bī-ō′tə) *n.* The microorganisms that typically inhabit a bodily organ or part; flora.

mi·cro·blast (mī′krə-blăst′) *n.* A small nucleated red blood cell.

mi·cro·ble·phar·i·a (mī′krō-blĕ-făr′ē-ə) *or* **mi·cro·bleph·a·rism** (-blĕf′ə-rĭz′əm) *or* **mi·cro·bleph·a·ron** (-blĕf′ə-rŏn′) *n.* A rare developmental anomaly characterized by eyelids that are abnormally short.

mi·cro·bod·y (mī′krō-bŏd′ē) *n.* See **peroxisome.**

mi·cro·bra·chi·a (mī′krō-brā′kē-ə) *n.* Abnormal smallness of the arms.

mi·cro·car·di·a (mī′krō-kär′dē-ə) *n.* Abnormal smallness of the heart.

mi·cro·cen·trum (mī′krō-sĕn′trəm) *n.* See **centrosome.**

mi·cro·ceph·a·ly (mī′krō-sĕf′ə-lē) *n.* Abnormal smallness of the head. Also called *nanocephaly.* —**mi′cro·ce·phal′ic** (-sə-făl′ĭk) *adj.*

mi·cro·chei·li·a *or* **mi·cro·chi·li·a** (mī′krō-kī′lē-ə) *n.* Abnormal smallness of the lips.

mi·cro·chei·ri·a *or* **mi·cro·chi·ri·a** (mī′krō-kī′rē-ə) *n.* Abnormal smallness of the hands.

mi·cro·chem·is·try (mī′krō-kĕm′ĭ-strē) *n.* Chemistry that deals with minute quantities of materials, frequently less than one milligram in mass or one milliliter in volume.

mi·cro·cin·e·ma·tog·ra·phy (mī′krō-sĭn′ə-mə-tŏg′rə-fē) *n.* The use of motion pictures that are taken through magnifying lenses to study an organ or system in motion.

mi·cro·cir·cu·la·tion (mī′krō-sûr′kyə-lā′shən) *n.* The flow of blood or lymph through the smallest vessels of the body, especially as the venules, capillaries, and arterioles.

Mi·cro·coc·ca·ce·ae (mī′krō-kŏ-kā′sē-ē) *n.* A family of aerobic or facultatively anaerobic bacteria containing gram-positive spherical cells that occur singly or in pairs, tetrads, irregular masses, or chains, and that include free-living, saprophytic, parasitic, and pathogenic species.

mi·cro·coc·cus (mī′krō-kŏk′əs) *n., pl.* **–coc·ci** (-kŏk′-sī′, -kŏk′ī′) A bacterium of the genus *Micrococcus.* —**mi′cro·coc′cal** (-kŏk′əl) *adj.*

Micrococcus *n.* A genus of aerobic, gram-positive, spherical bacteria that occur singly, in pairs, or in irregular masses and are saprophytic or parasitic but not pathogenic.

mi·cro·co·lon (mī′krō-kō′lən) *n.* An abnormally small colon, often developing because of a decreased functional state.

mi·cro·co·ri·a (mī′krō-kôr′ē-ə) *n.* A congenital contraction of the pupil of the eye.

mi·cro·cor·ne·a (mī′krō-kôr′nē-ə) *n.* An abnormally thin and flat cornea.

mi·cro·cous·tic (mī′krə-kōō′stĭk) *adj.* Variant of **micracoustic.**

mi·cro·cu·rie (mī′krō-kyōōr′ē) *n. Abbr.* **μCi** A unit or quantity of radiation equivalent to one-millionth of a curie.

mi·cro·cyst (mī′krə-sĭst′) *n.* A minute cyst, often only observable microscopically.

mi·cro·cyte (mī′krə-sīt′) *n.* An abnormally small red blood cell that is less than five micrometers in diameter and may occur in certain forms of anemia. Also called *microerythrocyte.* —**mi′cro·cyt′ic** (mī′krə-sĭt′ĭk) *adj.*

mi·cro·cy·the·mi·a (mī′krō-sī-thē′mē-ə) *n.* See **microcytosis.**

microcytic anemia *n.* Anemia in which the average size of red blood cells is smaller than normal.

mi·cro·cy·to·sis (mī′krō-sī-tō′sĭs) *n.* The presence of microcytes in the blood. Also called *microcythemia.*

mi·cro·dac·ty·ly (mī′krō-dăk′tə-lē) *n.* Abnormal smallness or shortness of the fingers or toes.

mi·cro·dis·sec·tion (mī′krō-dĭ-sĕk′shən, -dī-) *n.* The dissection of tissues under magnification, usually by the precise manipulation of specialized needles.

mi·cro·don·tia (mī′krə-dŏn′shə) *n.* A condition of having one or more disproportionately small teeth.

mi·cro·drep·a·no·cyt·ic anemia (mī′krō-drĕp′ə-nō-sĭt′ĭk) *n.* Anemia, clinically resembling sickle cell anemia, in which individuals are heterozygous for both the sickle cell gene and a thalassemia gene. Also called *sickle cell-thalassemia disease.*

mi·cro·drep·a·no·cy·to·sis (mī′krō-drĕp′ə-nō-sī-tō′-sĭs, -drə-păn′ō-) *n.* A congenital chronic hemolytic anemia caused by the presence of sickle cell hemoglobin and thalassemia hemoglobin in the red blood cells.

mi·cro·e·lec·trode (mī′krō-ĭ-lĕk′trōd′) *n.* A very small electrode, often used to study electrical characteristics of living cells and tissues.

mi·cro·en·ceph·a·ly (mī′krō-ĕn-sĕf′ə-lē) *n.* Variant of micrencephaly.

mi·cro·e·ryth·ro·cyte (mī′krō-ĭ-rĭth′rə-sīt′) *n.* See microcyte.

mi·cro·ev·o·lu·tion (mī′krō-ĕv′ə-lōō′shən, -ē′və-) *n.* Evolution resulting from a succession of relatively small genetic variations that often cause the formation of new subspecies.

mi·cro·fi·bril (mī′krō-fī′brəl, -fĭb′rəl) *n.* An extremely small fibril.

mi·cro·fil·a·ment (mī′krō-fĭl′ə-mənt) *n.* Any of the minute fibers located throughout the cytoplasm of cells, composed of actin and functioning primarily in maintaining the structural integrity of a cell.

mi·cro·fil·a·re·mi·a (mī′krō-fĭl′ə-rē′mē-ə) *n.* Infection of the blood with microfilariae.

mi·cro·fi·lar·i·a (mī′krō-fə-lâr′ē-ə) *n., pl.* –i·ae (-ē-ē′) The minute larval form of a filarial worm. —**mi′cro·fi·lar′i·al** *adj.*

mi·cro·gam·ete (mī′krō-găm′ēt′, -gə-mēt′) *n.* The smaller of a pair of conjugating gametes, usually the male, in a heterogamous organism.

mi·cro·ga·me·to·cyte (mī′krō-gə-mē′tə-sīt′) *n.* A gametocyte that gives rise to microgametes.

mi·cro·gas·tri·a (mī′krō-găs′trē-ə) *n.* Abnormal smallness of the stomach.

mi·cro·ge·ni·a (mī′krō-jē′nē-ə) *n.* Abnormal smallness of the chin.

mi·cro·gen·i·tal·ism (mī′krō-jĕn′ĭ-tl-ĭz′əm) *n.* Abnormal smallness of the external genitalia.

mi·cro·glan·du·lar adenosis (mī′krō-glăn′jə-lər) *n.* A glandular disease of the breast in which irregular clusters of small tubules are present in adipose or fibrous tissues.

mi·crog·li·a (mī-krŏg′lē-ə) *n.* Any of the small neuroglial cells of the central nervous system having long processes and ameboid and phagocytic activity at sites of neural damage or inflammation. Also called *Hortega cell.*

mi·crog·li·a·cyte (mī-krŏg′lē-ə-sīt′) *n.* A cell, especially an embryonic cell, of the microglia.

mi·crog·li·o·ma (mī-krŏg′lē-ō′mə, mī′krō-glī-ō′mə) *n.* A brain neoplasm derived from microglial cells that is structurally similar to reticulum cell sarcoma.

mi·cro·glos·si·a (mī′krō-glŏ′sē-ə) *n.* Abnormal smallness of the tongue.

mi·cro·gna·thi·a (mī′krō-nā′thē-ə, mī′krŏg-nā′-) *n.* Abnormal smallness of the jaws, especially of the mandible.

mi·cro·gram (mī′krə-grăm′) *n. Abbr.* **μg, mcg** A unit of weight equal to one-millionth (10^{-6}) of a gram.

mi·cro·graph (mī′krə-grăf′) *n.* **1.** A drawing or photographic reproduction of an object as viewed through a microscope. **2.** An instrument for measuring minute movements by recording photographically corresponding movements registered by a diaphragm moving in unison with the original object.

mi·cro·gy·ri·a (mī′krō-jī′rē-ə) *n.* Abnormal smallness of the convolutions of the brain.

mi·cro·he·pat·i·a (mī′krō-hǐ-păt′ē-ə) *n.* Abnormal smallness of the liver.

mi·cro·in·ci·sion (mī′krō-ĭn-sĭzh′ən) *n.* The destruction of cellular organelles by laser beam. Also called *micropuncture.*

mi·cro·in·jec·tion (mī′krō-ĭn-jĕk′shən) *n.* Injection of minute amounts of a substance into a microscopic structure, such as a single cell.

mi·cro·in·va·sion (mī′krō-ĭn-vā′zhən) *n.* Invasion of in situ carcinoma into tissue that is immediately adjacent, being the earliest stage of malignant neoplastic invasion.

mi·cro·li·ter (mī′krō-lē′tər) *n.* A unit of volume equal to one-millionth (10^{-6}) of a liter.

mi·cro·lith (mī′krə-lĭth′) *n.* A minute calculus, usually multiple and resembling coarse sand.

mi·cro·li·thi·a·sis (mī′krō-lĭ-thī′ə-sĭs) *n.* The formation, presence, or discharge of minute calculi or gravel.

mi·cro·ma·nip·u·la·tion (mī′krō-mə-nĭp′yə-lā′shən) *n.* The manipulation of minute instruments and needles under a microscope in order to perform delicate procedures, such as microsurgery.

mi·cro·me·li·a (mī′krō-mē′lē-ə, -mĕl′yə) *n.* Abnormal shortness or smallness of limbs. Also called *nanomelia.* —**mi′cro·mel′ic** (-mĕl′ĭk, -mē′lĭk) *adj.*

micromelic dwarfism *n.* Dwarfism characterized by disproportionately short or small limbs.

mi·cro·mere (mī′krō-mîr′) *n.* A very small blastomere, as at the animal pole of certain eggs.

mi·cro·me·tas·ta·sis (mī′krō-mə-tăs′tə-sĭs) *n.* The spread of cancer cells from the primary site with the secondary tumors too small to be clinically detected. —**mi′cro·met′a·stat′ic** (-mĕt′ə-stăt′ĭk) *adj.*

mi·crom·e·ter[1] (mī-krŏm′ĭ-tər) *n.* A device for measuring very small distances, objects, or angles, especially one based on the rotation of a finely threaded screw, as in relation to a microscope.

mi·crom·e·ter[2] (mī′krō-mē′tər) *n. Abbr.* **μm** A unit of length equal to one thousandth (10^{-3}) of a millimeter or one millionth (10^{-6}) of a meter. Also called *micron.*

mi·crom·e·try (mī-krŏm′ĭ-trē) *n.* The measurement of minute objects with a micrometer.

micromicro– *pref. Symbol* **μμ** One-trillionth (10^{-12}): *micromicrogram.*

mi·cro·my·e·li·a (mī′krō-mī-ē′lē-ə) *n.* Abnormal smallness or shortness of the spinal cord.

mi·cro·my·e·lo·blast (mī′krō-mī′ə-lə-blăst′) *n.* A small myeloblast, often the predominant cell in myeloblastic leukemia.

mi·cro·my·e·lo·blas·tic leukemia (mī′krō-mī′ə-lə-blăs′tĭk) *n.* Granulocytic leukemia that is characterized by abnormal numbers of micromyeloblasts in the blood, bone marrow, and other tissues.

mi·cron *or* **mi·kron** (mī′krŏn′) *n., pl.* –crons *or* –cra (-krə) *or* –krons *or* –kra (-krə) *Abbr.* **μm** See micrometer[2].

mi·cro·nod·u·lar (mī′krō-nŏj′ə-lər) *adj.* Of or characterized by the presence of minute nodules.

mi·cro·nu·cle·us (mī′krō-nōō′klē-əs) *n.* **1.** A minute nucleus. **2.** The smaller of two nuclei in ciliate protozoans that contains genetic material and functions in reproduction.

mi·cro·nu·tri·ent (mī′krō-nōō′trē-ənt) *n.* A substance, such as a vitamin or mineral, that is essential in minute amounts for the proper growth and metabolism of a living organism.

mi·cro·nych·i·a (mī′krō-nĭk′ē-ə) *n.* Abnormal smallness of the fingernails or toenails.

mi·cro·or·gan·ism (mī′krō-ôr′gə-nĭz′əm) *n.* An organism of microscopic or submicroscopic size, especially a bacterium or protozoan.

mi·cro·pa·thol·o·gy (mī′krō-pă-thŏl′ə-jē) *n.* The microscopic study of disease changes.

mi·cro·pe·nis (mī′krō-pē′nĭs) *n.* An abnormally small penis. Also called *microphallus.*

mi·cro·phage (mī′krə-fāj′) *n.* A small phagocytic white blood cell.

mi·cro·pha·ki·a (mī′krō-fā′kē-ə) *n.* See **spherophakia.**

mi·cro·phal·lus (mī′krō-făl′əs) *n.* See **micropenis.**

mi·cro·pho·ni·a (mī′krō-fō′nē-ə) *or* **mi·croph·o·ny** (mī-krŏf′ə-nē) *n.* Weakness of voice.

mi·cro·pho·to·graph (mī′krō-fō′tə-grăf′) *n.* **1.** A photograph requiring magnification for viewing. **2.** See **photomicrograph.**

mi·croph·thal·mi·a (mī′krŏf-thăl′mē-ə) *n.* Abnormal smallness of the eye. Also called *microphthalmos, nanophthalmia, nanophthalmos.*

mi·cro·pi·pette (mī′krō-pī-pĕt′) *n.* **1.** A very small pipette used in microinjection. **2.** A pipette used to measure very small volumes of liquids.

mi·cro·pleth·ys·mog·ra·phy (mī′krō-plĕth′ĭz-mŏg′rə-fē) *n.* The technique of measuring and recording minute changes in the size of a limb or organ as a result of the volume of blood flowing into and out of it.

mi·cro·po·di·a (mī′krō-pō′dē-ə) *n.* Abnormal smallness of the feet.

mi·crop·si·a (mī-krŏp′sē-ə) *n.* A visual disorder in which objects appear much smaller than they actually are, possibly caused by a retinal disorder but often associated with hallucination or an unconscious attempt to shrink the world to a less threatening size.

mi·cro·punc·ture (mī′krō-pŭngk′chər) *n.* See **microincision.**

mi·cro·re·frac·tom·e·ter (mī′krō-rē′frăk-tŏm′ĭ-tər) *n.* A refractometer used in the study of blood cells.

mi·cro·res·pi·rom·e·ter (mī′krō-rĕs′pə-rŏm′ĭ-tər) *n.* An apparatus for measuring the utilization of oxygen by small numbers of isolated tissues or cells.

mi·cro·scope (mī′krə-skōp′) *n.* **1.** An optical instrument that uses a lens or a combination of lenses to produce magnified images of small objects, especially of objects too small to be seen by the unaided eye. **2.** An instrument, such as an electron microscope, that uses electronic, acoustic, or other processes to magnify objects.

mi·cro·scop·ic (mī′krə-skŏp′ĭk) *or* **mi·cro·scop·i·cal** (-ĭ-kəl) *adj.* **1.** Too small to be seen by the unaided eye but large enough to be studied under a microscope. **2.** Of, relating to, or concerned with a microscope. **3.** Being or characterized as exceedingly small; minute.

microscopic anatomy *n.* The study of the structure of cells, tissues, and organs of the body as seen with a microscope.

mi·cros·co·py (mī-krŏs′kə-pē) *n.* **1.** The study of microscopes. **2.** The use of microscopes. **3.** Investigation by means of a microscope.

mi·cro·sleep (mī′krə-slēp′) *n.* A period of sleep that lasts up to a few seconds, usually experienced by narcoleptics or by severely sleep-deprived people.

mi·cro·some (mī′krə-sōm′) *n.* A small particle in the cytoplasm of a cell, typically consisting of fragmented endoplasmic reticulum to which ribosomes are attached.

mi·cro·so·mi·a (mī′krə-sō′mē-ə) *n.* Abnormal smallness of the whole body, as in dwarfism. Also called *nanocormia.*

mi·cro·spec·tro·pho·tom·e·try (mī′krō-spĕk′trō-fō-tŏm′ĭ-trē) *n.* **1.** The technique of measuring the light that is absorbed, reflected, or emitted by a microscopic specimen at different wavelengths. **2.** Such a technique used to characterize and quantify nucleoproteins in single cells or cell organelles on the basis of their natural ultraviolet absorption spectra or following stoichiometric binding in selective cytochemical staining reactions.

mi·cro·spec·tro·scope (mī′krō-spĕk′trə-skōp′) *n.* A spectroscope used with a microscope for observing the spectra of microscopic objects.

mi·cro·sphe·ro·cy·to·sis (mī′krō-sfîr′ō-sī-tō′sĭs) *n.* A blood condition seen in hemolytic jaundice in which small spherocytes predominate and red blood cells are smaller and more globular than normal.

mi·cro·sphyg·my (mī′krō-sfĭg′mē) *n.* A weak pulse that is difficult to detect manually.

mi·cro·sple·ni·a (mī′krō-splē′nē-ə) *n.* Abnormal smallness of the spleen.

Mi·cros·po·rum (mī-krŏs′pər-əm, mī′krə-spôr′əm) *n.* A genus of pathogenic fungi that causes dermatophytosis in animals and humans.

mi·cro·steth·o·scope (mī′krō-stĕth′ə-skōp′) *n.* A stethoscope that amplifies the sounds heard.

mi·cro·sto·mi·a (mī′krō-stō′mē-ə) *n.* Abnormal smallness of the mouth.

mi·cro·sur·ger·y (mī′krō-sûr′jə-rē) *n.* Surgery on minute body structures or cells performed with the aid of a microscope and other specialized instruments, such as a micromanipulator.

mi·cro·su·ture (mī′krō-sōō′chər) *n.* Suture material having a tiny caliber and used in microsurgery.

mi·cro·sy·ringe (mī′krō-sə-rĭnj′, -sîr′ĭnj) *n.* A hypodermic syringe having a micrometer screw attached to the piston, thus allowing accurately measured minute quantities of fluid to be injected.

mi·cro·ti·a (mī-krō′shē-ə, -shə) *n.* Abnormal smallness of the auricle of the ear.

mi·cro·tome (mī′krə-tōm′) *n.* An instrument that is used to cut a specimen, as of organic tissue, into thin sections for microscopic examination. Also called *histotome.*

mi·crot·o·my (mī-krŏt′ə-mē) *n.* The preparation of specimens with a microtome. Also called *histotomy.* —**mi′cro·tom′ic** (mī′krə-tŏm′ĭk) *adj.*

mi·cro·tu·bule (mī′krō-tōō′byōōl) *n.* Any of the proteinaceous cylindrical hollow structures that are distributed throughout the cytoplasm of eukaryotic cells, providing structural support and assisting in cellular locomotion and transport.

mi·cro·vil·lus (mī′krō-vĭl′əs) *n., pl.* **–vil·li** (-vĭl′ī′) Any of the minute hairlike structures projecting from the surface of certain types of epithelial cells, especially those of the small intestine.

mi·cro·wave (mī′krə-wāv′, -krō-) *n.* A high-frequency electromagnetic wave, one millimeter to one meter in wavelength, intermediate between infrared and shortwave radio wavelengths. —*v.* To cook or heat using microwaves.

mi·crox·y·phil (mī-krŏk′sə-fĭl′) *n.* A multinuclear eosinophilic white blood cell.

mi·cro·zo·on (mī′krə-zō′ŏn′, -ən) *n., pl.* **–zo·a** (-zō′ə) A microscopic animal.

mi·crur·gi·cal (mī-krûr′jĭ-kəl) *adj.* Of or relating to procedures performed on minute structures under a microscope.

mic·tion (mĭk′shən) *n.* See **urination**.

mic·tu·rate (mĭk′chə-rāt′, mĭk′tə-) *v.* To urinate.

mic·tu·ri·tion (mĭk′chə-rĭsh′ən, -tə-) *n.* **1.** See **urination**. **2.** The desire to urinate. **3.** The frequency of urination.

MID *abbr.* minimal infecting dose

mid– *pref.* Middle: *midbrain*.

mi·daz·o·lam (mĭ-dăz′ə-lăm′) *n.* A colorless crystalline derivative of diazepam with sedative and anxiolytic properties, usually used in its hydrochloride form as an intravenous anesthetic.

mid·bod·y (mĭd′bŏd′ē) *n.* **1.** The anatomical middle region of the trunk of the body. **2.** One of several granules composed of microtubules that forms between daughter cells during the telophase of mitosis.

mid·brain (mĭd′brān′) *n.* See **mesencephalon**.

mid·dle age (mĭd′l) *n.* The time of human life between youth and old age, usually reckoned as the years between 40 and 60. Also called *midlife*.

middle artery of knee *n.* An artery with its origin in the popliteal artery and with distribution to the synovial membrane and cruciate ligaments of the knee joint.

middle cardiac vein *n.* A vein that begins at the apex of the heart and passes through the posterior interventricular sulcus to the coronary sinus.

middle cerebellar peduncle *n.* The largest of the three paired peduncles, composed mainly of fibers that originate from the pontine nuclei, cross the midline in the basilar part of the pons, and emerge on the opposite side as a massive bundle arching dorsally along the lateral side of the pontine tegmentum into the cerebellum.

middle cerebral vein *n.* **1.** A vein that accompanies the middle cerebral artery deep into the fissure of Sylvius and empties into the basal vein; deep middle cerebral vein. **2.** A large vein passing along the line of the fissure of Sylvius to join the cavernous sinus; superficial middle cerebral vein.

middle cervical cardiac nerve *n.* A bundle of fibers running downward from the middle cervical ganglion of the sympathetic trunk to join the cardiac plexus.

middle cluneal nerve *n.* Any of the terminal branches of the dorsal rami of the sacral nerves, supplying the skin of the midgluteal region.

middle colic vein *n.* A tributary of the superior mesenteric vein, accompanying the middle colic artery.

middle collateral artery *n.* An artery that is the posterior terminal branch of the deep brachial artery, anastomosing with the arteries that form the articular network of the elbow.

middle constrictor muscle of pharynx *n.* A muscle with its origin in the stylohyoid ligament and the hyoid bone, with insertion to the pharyngeal raphe in the posterior wall of the pharynx, with nerve supply from the pharyngeal plexus, and whose action narrows the pharynx in swallowing.

middle cuneiform bone *n.* See **intermediate cuneiform bone**.

middle ear *n.* The space located between the eardrum and the inner ear that contains the three auditory ossicles, which convey vibrations through the oval window to the cochlea. Also called *tympanic cavity, tympanum*.

middle lobe syndrome *n.* Atelectasis with chronic pneumonitis in the middle lobe of the right lung due to compression of the middle lobe bronchus, usually by enlarged lymph nodes.

middle meningeal vein *n.* Any of the veins that accompany the middle meningeal artery and empty into the pterygoid plexus.

middle rectal node *n.* A node along the middle rectal artery that receives afferents from the pararectal nodes and sends efferents to the internal iliac nodes.

middle rectal vein *n.* Any of the veins that pass from the rectal venous plexus to the hypogestric vein.

middle scalene muscle *n.* A muscle with origin from the costotransverse lamellae of the transverse processes of the second to the sixth cervical vertebrae, with insertion into the first rib posterior to the subclavian artery, with nerve supply from the cervical plexus, and whose action raises the first rib.

middle supraclavicular nerve *n.* See **intermediate supraclavicular nerve**.

middle temporal sulcus *n.* The sulcus between the middle and inferior temporal gyri.

middle temporal vein *n.* A vein that arises near the lateral angle of the eye and joins the superficial temporal veins to form the retromandibular vein.

middle thyroid vein *n.* Any of the veins that pass from the thyroid gland across the common carotid artery to empty into the internal jugular vein.

midge (mĭj) *n.* Any of various gnatlike flies, some species of which, such as the biting midges of the family Ceratopogonidae, serve as vectors for parasitic diseases.

midg·et (mĭj′ĭt) *n.* A person of extremely small stature who is otherwise normally proportioned. Now considered offensive.

mid·gut (mĭd′gŭt′) *n.* **1.** The middle section of the digestive tract in a vertebrate embryo from which the ileum, jejunum, and portions of the duodenum and colon develop. Also called *mesenteron*. **2.** The middle portion of the digestive tract of certain invertebrates, such as arthropods, that is lined with an enzyme-secreting tissue and that serves as the main site of digestion and absorption.

mid·lev·el provider (mĭd′lĕv′əl) *n.* A medical provider who is not a physician but is licensed to diagnose and treat patients under the supervision of a physician.

mid·life (mĭd′līf′) *n.* See **middle age.** —*adj.* Of, relating to, or characteristic of middle age.

midlife crisis *n.* A period of psychological doubt and anxiety that some people experience in middle age.

mid·line (mĭd′līn′) *n.* A medial line, especially the medial line or plane of the body.

midline myelotomy *n.* The surgical severing of the midline transverse fibers of the spinal cord. Also called *commissurotomy.*

mid·riff (mĭd′rĭf) *n.* See **diaphragm** (sense 1).

mid·sag·it·tal plane (mĭd-săj′ĭ-tl) *n.* See **median plane.**

mid·sec·tion (mĭd′sĕk′shən) *n.* A middle section, especially the midriff of the body.

mid·wife (mĭd′wīf′) *n., pl.* **–wives** (-wīvz′) A person, usually a woman, who is trained to assist women in childbirth. —*v.* To assist in the birth of a baby.

mid·wife·ry (mĭd-wĭf′ə-rē, mĭd′wĭf′rē, -wī′fə-rē) *n.* The techniques and practice of a midwife including childbirth assistance, the independent care of essentially normal healthy women and infants before, during, and after childbirth, and, in collaboration with medical personnel, the consultation, management, and referral of cases in which abnormalities develop.

Mie·scher (mē′shər), **Johann Friedrich** 1844–1895. Swiss physiologist who discovered (1869) nucleic acid.

Mie·scher's granulomatosis (mē′shərz) *n.* A variant of necrobiosis lipoidica. Also called *granulomatosis disciformis chronica et progressiva.*

mi·fep·ri·stone (mĭ-fĕp′rĭ-stōn) *n.* See **RU 486.**

mi·graine (mī′grān′) *n.* A severe recurring headache, usually affecting only one side of the head, that is characterized by sharp pain and is often accompanied by nausea, vomiting, and visual disturbances. Also called *hemicrania, megrim, sick headache.*

mi·grat·ing abscess (mī′grā′tĭng) *n.* See **wandering abscess.**

mi·gra·tion (mī-grā′shən) *n.* **1.** The moving from place to place, as of disease symptoms. **2.** See **diapedesis. 3.** The movement of a tooth or teeth out of normal position. **4.** The movement of one or more atoms from one position to another within a molecule. **5.** The movement of ions between electrodes during electrolysis.

migration inhibition test *n.* An in vitro method of testing for cellular immune response in which macrophages are placed in a capillary tube containing a specific antigen.

mi·kron (mī′krŏn′) *n.* Variant of **micron.**

Mi·ku·licz′ aphthae (mĭk′ə-lĭch′ĭz, mē′kōō-) *n.* See **aphthae majores.**

Mi·ku·licz disease (mĭk′ə-lĭch′, mē′kōō-) *n.* Benign swelling of the lacrimal glands and usually also of the salivary glands as a result of infiltration and replacement of the normal gland structure by lymphoid tissue.

Mikulicz drain *n.* A drain made of several strings of gauze placed into a wound and held together by a single layer of gauze.

Mikulicz operation *n.* Excision of the bowel in two stages: the diseased area is first exteriorized, enclosed by the abdomen around it, and excised; then the spur is cut and the stoma closed.

Mikulicz syndrome *n.* Enlargement of the lacrimal and salivary glands occurring as a complication of a disease other than Mikulicz disease, such as lymphosarcoma, leukemia, or uveoparotid fever.

Miles′ operation (mīlz) *n.* Resection of the abdomen and perineum in cases of carcinoma of the rectum.

mil·i·ar·i·a (mĭl′ē-âr′ē-ə) *n.* See **heat rash.**

miliaria ru·bra (rōō′brə) *n.* See **heat rash.**

mil·i·ar·y (mĭl′ē-ĕr′ē) *adj.* **1.** Having the appearance of grains derived from haylike millet grass. **2.** Characterized by the presence of small skin lesions that have the size and appearance of millet seeds.

miliary abscess *n.* Any of numerous minute collections of pus widely disseminated throughout an area or the whole body.

miliary embolism *n.* An obstruction occurring simultaneously in a number of capillaries.

miliary fever *n.* An infectious disease characterized by fever, profuse sweating, and the production of sudamina, occurring formerly in severe epidemics.

mi·lieu (mĭl-yōō′, mēl-yœ′) *n., pl.* **–lieus** *or* **–lieux** (-lyœ′) **1.** The totality of one's surroundings; an environment. **2.** The social setting of a mental patient.

milieu therapy *n.* Psychotherapy in which the milieu is arranged for the benefit of the patient.

mil·i·um (mĭl′ē-əm) *n., pl.* **–i·a** (-ē-ə) A small, white or yellowish cystlike mass just below the surface of the skin, caused by retention of the secretion of a sebaceous gland. Also called *pearly tubercle, whitehead.*

milk (mĭlk) *n.* **1.** A whitish liquid containing proteins, fats, lactose, and various vitamins and minerals that is produced by the mammary glands of all mature female mammals after they have given birth and serves as nourishment for their young. **2.** The milk of cows, goats, or other animals, used as food by humans. **3.** A liquid, such as coconut milk, milkweed sap, plant latex, or various medical emulsions, that is similar to milk in appearance. —*v.* **1.** To draw milk from the teat or udder of a female mammal. **2.** To press out, drain off, or remove by or as if by milking; strip.

milk-alkali syndrome *n.* A chronic disorder of the kidneys that resembles nephrosis and is induced by protracted therapy of peptic ulcer with alkalis and a high milk regimen; reversible in early stages.

milk crust *n.* Seborrhea of the scalp of an infant.

milk duct *n.* See **lactiferous duct.**

milk fever *n.* A slight elevation of temperature following childbirth, possibly due to the establishment of the secretion of milk.

milk leg *n.* A painful swelling of the leg occurring in women after childbirth as a result of clotting and inflammation of the femoral veins. Also called *phlegmasia alba dolens.*

milk line *n.* See **mammary ridge.**

milk of magnesia *n.* A milky white aqueous suspension of magnesium hydroxide used as an antacid and a laxative.

milk ring test *n.* See **abortus Bang ring test.**

milk sickness *n.* An acute, now rare disease characterized by trembling, vomiting, and severe intestinal pain, caused by eating dairy products or meat from a cow that has fed on white snakeroot.

milk spots *pl.n.* **1.** White plaques of hyalinized fibrous tissue situated in the epicardium and overlying the right ventricle of the heart where not covered by lung. **2.** White macroscopic areas in the omentum due to accumulation of macrophages and lymphocytes.

milk sugar *n.* See **lactose** (sense 1, 2).

milk tooth *n.* See **deciduous tooth.**

Mil·ler-Abbott tube (mĭl′ər-) *n.* A tube used for intestinal decompression.

milli– *pref.* One thousandth (10^{-3}): *millisecond.*

mil·li·am·pere (mĭl′ē-ăm′pîr) *n. Abbr.* **mA** A unit of current that is equal to one thousandth (10^{-3}) of an ampere.

mil·li·cu·rie (mĭl′ĭ-kyŏŏr′ē) *n. Abbr.* **mCi** A unit of radioactivity equal to one thousandth (10^{-3}) of a curie.

mil·li·e·quiv·a·lent (mĭl′ē-ĭ-kwĭv′ə-lənt) *n. Abbr.* **mEq** One thousandth (10^{-3}) of a gram equivalent of a chemical element, an ion, a radical, or a compound.

mil·li·gram (mĭl′ĭ-grăm′) *n. Abbr.* **mg** A metric unit of mass equal to one thousandth (10^{-3}) of a gram.

mil·li·li·ter (mĭl′ə-lē′tər) *n. Abbr.* **ml** A unit of volume equal to one thousandth (10^{-3}) of a liter, 1 cubic centimeter, or about 15 minims.

mil·li·me·ter (mĭl′ə-mē′tər) *n. Abbr.* **mm** A unit of length equal to one thousandth (10^{-3}) of a meter (0.0394 inch).

mil·li·mi·cron (mĭl′ə-mī′krŏn) *n. Abbr.* **mμ** A unit of length that is equal to one thousandth (10^{-3}) of a micrometer or one billionth (10^{-9}) of a meter; nanometer.

mil·li·mole (mĭl′ə-mōl′) *n. Abbr.* **mmol** One thousandth (10^{-3}) of a mole.

mil·li·os·mole (mĭl′ē-ŏz′mōl′, -ŏs′-) *n.* One thousandth (10^{-3}) of an osmole.

mil·li·sec·ond (mĭl′ĭ-sĕk′ənd) *n. Abbr.* **ms, msec** One thousandth (10^{-3}) of a second.

mil·li·volt (mĭl′ə-vōlt′) *n. Abbr.* **mV** A unit of potential difference equal to one thousandth (10^{-3}) of a volt.

mil·pho·sis (mĭl-fō′sĭs) *n.* Loss of the eyelashes. Also called *madarosis.*

Mil·roy's disease (mĭl′roiz′) *n.* Congenital hereditary lymphedema of the legs.

Mil·stein (mĭl′stēn′), **Cesar** 1927–2002. Argentinian-born British immunologist. He shared a 1984 Nobel Prize for developing a method of producing monoclonal antibodies.

Mil·town (mĭl′toun′) A trademark for the drug meprobamate.

mi·me·sis (mĭ-mē′sĭs, mī-) *n.* **1.** The appearance of symptoms of a disease not actually present, often caused by hysteria. **2.** Symptomatic imitation of one organic disease by another.

mi·met·ic (mĭ-mĕt′ĭk, mī-) *adj.* **1.** Of or exhibiting mimicry. **2.** Of or relating to mimesis. **—mi·met′i·cal·ly** *adv.*

mim·ic (mĭm′ĭk) *v.* **1.** To resemble closely; simulate. **2.** To take on the appearance of. **—mim′ic** *adj. & n.*

mim·ic·ry (mĭm′ĭ-krē) *n.* The resemblance of one organism to another or to an object in its surroundings for concealment and protection.

Min·a·ma·ta disease (mĭn′ə-mä′tə) *n.* A degenerative neurological disorder caused by poisoning with a mercury compound in seafood from waters contaminated with mercury, characterized by burning or tingling sensations, poor articulation of speech, and the loss of coordination and peripheral vision.

mind (mīnd) *n.* **1.** The human consciousness that originates in the brain and is manifested especially in thought, perception, emotion, will, memory, and imagination. **2.** The collective conscious and unconscious processes in a sentient organism that direct and influence mental and physical behavior.

mind-altering *adj.* Producing mood changes or distorted perceptions; hallucinogenic.

mind-bending *adj.* Intensely affecting the mind, especially to the extent of producing hallucinations.

mind-blowing *adj.* **1.** Producing hallucinatory effects. **2.** Intensely affecting the mind or emotions.

mind-body *adj.* Of, involving, or resulting from the connection between one's physical health and the state of one's mind or spirit.

mind-expanding *adj.* **1.** Producing intensified or distorted perceptions; psychedelic. **2.** Producing an increased perceptive awareness.

mind·scape (mīnd′skāp′) *n.* A mental or psychological scene or area of the imagination.

mind·set *or* **mind-set** (mīnd′sĕt′) *n.* **1.** A fixed mental attitude or disposition that predetermines a person's responses to and interpretations of situations. **2.** An inclination or a habit.

min·er·al (mĭn′ər-əl) *n.* **1.** A naturally occurring, homogeneous inorganic solid substance having a definite chemical composition and characteristic crystalline structure, color, and hardness. **2.** An inorganic element, such as calcium, iron, potassium, sodium, or zinc, that is essential to the nutrition of humans, animals, and plants.

min·er·al·o·cor·ti·coid (mĭn′ər-ə-lō-kôr′tĭ-koid′) *n.* Any of a group of steroid hormones that are secreted by the adrenal cortex and regulate the balance of water and electrolytes in the body.

mineral oil *n.* **1.** Any of various light hydrocarbon oils, especially a distillate of petroleum. **2.** A refined distillate of petroleum, used as a laxative.

mineral water *n.* Naturally occurring or prepared water that contains dissolved mineral salts, elements, or gases, and is often used therapeutically.

min·er's lung (mī′nərz) *n.* See **anthracosis.**

mini– *pref.* Small; miniature: *minilaparotomy.*

min·i·lap·a·rot·o·my (mĭn′ē-lăp′ə-rŏt′ə-mē) *n.* A method of female sterilization by surgical ligation of the fallopian tubes, performed through a small incision above the pubic symphysis.

min·im (mĭn′əm) *n.* **1.** In the United States, a unit of volume equal to $\frac{1}{60}$ of a fluid dram, or 0.0616 milliliters. **2.** In Great Britain, $\frac{1}{20}$ of a scruple, or 0.0592 milliliters. **3.** The smallest or the least of several similar structures.

min·i·mal brain dysfunction (mĭn′ə-məl) *n.* Attention deficit disorder. No longer in scientific use.

minimal dose *n.* The smallest quantity of a drug that will, or will likely, produce a physiological effect in an adult.

minimal infecting dose *n. Abbr.* **MID** The smallest quantity of infectious material regularly producing infection.

minimal lethal dose *n. Abbr.* **MLD** The smallest quantity of a toxic substance or infectious agent that is found to be lethal.

minimal reacting dose *n. Abbr.* **MRD** The smallest quantity of a toxic substance causing a reaction.

Min·i·press (mĭn'ə-prĕs') A trademark for the drug prazosin.

min·i·stroke (mĭn'ē-strōk') *n.* See **transient ischemic attack.**

Min·ne·so·ta mul·ti·pha·sic personality inventory test (mĭn'ĭ-sō'tə mŭl'tə-fā'zĭk, mŭl'tē-, -tī-) *n.* A psychological test for persons 16 or more years of age, consisting of a questionnaire containing statements to be agreed or disagreed with and coded in 14 personality scales.

Mi·no·cin (mĭ-nō'sĭn) A trademark for the drug minocycline.

min·o·cy·cline hydrochloride (mĭn'ə-sī'klēn', -klĭn) *n.* A broad-spectrum antibiotic that is derived from tetracycline.

mi·nor (mī'nər) *adj.* **1.** Lesser or smaller in amount, extent, or size. **2.** Lesser in seriousness or danger.

minor agglutinin *n.* See **group agglutinin.**

minor duodenal papilla *n.* A slight elevation marking the opening of the accessory pancreatic duct into the duodenum.

minor hysteria *n.* A mild form of hysteria that is characterized chiefly by subjective pains, nervousness, undue sensitiveness, and sometimes attacks of emotional excitement but without paralysis or other major symptoms.

minor salivary gland *n.* Any of the small salivary glands of the oral cavity, including the labial, buccal, molar, lingual, and palatine glands.

minor sublingual ducts *n.* See **ducts of Rivinus.**

Mi·not (mī'nət), **George Richards** 1885–1950. American physician. He shared a 1934 Nobel Prize for discovering that a diet of liver relieves anemia.

mi·nox·i·dil (mə-nŏk'sĭ-dĭl') *n.* A vasodilator that is administered orally to treat hypertension and topically to promote the regrowth of hair in male pattern baldness.

Min·te·zol (mĭn'tə-zōl') A trademark for the drug thiabendazole.

mi·nus cyclophoria (mī'nəs) *n.* See **incyclophoria.**

min·ute volume (mĭn'ĭt) *n.* The volume of any fluid or gas moved per minute.

mio– *or* **meio–** *pref.* **1.** Less; fewer: *miosphygmia.* **2.** Contraction: *miocardia.*

mi·o·car·di·a (mī'ō-kär'dē-ə) *n.* See **systole.** —**mi'o·car'di·al** *adj.*

mi·o·sis *or* **my·o·sis** (mī-ō'sĭs) *n., pl.* **–ses** (-sēz) **1.** The period of decline of a disease in which the intensity of the symptoms begins to diminish. **2.** Constriction of the pupil of the eye, resulting from a normal response to an increase in light or caused by certain drugs or pathological conditions.

mi·o·sphyg·mi·a (mī'ō-sfĭg'mē-ə) *n.* A condition in which pulse beats are fewer than heart beats.

mi·ot·ic (mī-ŏt'ĭk) *n.* A substance that causes constriction of the pupil of the eye. —*adj.* Characterized by, involving, or causing miosis.

mir·a·cle drug (mĭr'ə-kəl) *n.* A usually new drug that proves extraordinarily effective.

Mir·a·pex (mîr'ə-pĕks') A trademark for the drug pramipexole.

mire (mîr) *n.* Any of the test objects on the arm of a keratometer whose image, as reflected on the curved surface of the cornea, is used in calculating the amount of astigmatism.

mir·ror-im·age cell (mĭr'ər-ĭm'ĭj) *n.* **1.** A cell whose nuclei have identical features and are placed in the cytoplasm in similar fashion. **2.** A binucleate form of a Reed-Sternberg cell commonly found in Hodgkin's disease.

mirror speech *n.* A speech disorder in which the order of syllables in a word is reversed.

mir·ya·chit (mîr-yä'chĭt) *n.* A nervous disease observed in Siberia, similar to latah.

mis–[1] *pref.* Bad; badly; wrong; wrongly: *misdiagnosis.*

mis–[2] *pref.* Variant of **miso–.**

mis·an·thro·py (mĭs-ăn'thrə-pē, mĭz-) *n.* Hatred or mistrust of humankind. —**mis'an·throp'ic** (mĭs'ən-thrŏp'ĭk) *adj.* —**mis'an·thrope'** (mĭs'ən-thrōp') **mis·an'thro·pist** *n.*

mis·car·riage (mĭs'kăr'ĭj, mĭs-kăr'-) *n.* See **spontaneous abortion.**

mis·car·ry (mĭs'kăr'ē, mĭs-kăr'ē) *v.* To have a miscarriage; abort.

mis·ceg·e·na·tion (mĭ-sĕj'ə-nā'shən, mĭs'ĭ-jə-) *n.* Marriage or sexual relations between individuals of different races.

mis·ci·ble (mĭs'ə-bəl) *adj.* Capable of being and remaining mixed in all proportions. Used of liquids. —**mis'ci·bil'i·ty** *n.*

mis·di·ag·no·sis (mĭs-dī'əg-nō'sĭs) *n., pl.* **–ses** (-sēz) An incorrect diagnosis. —**mis·di'ag·nose'** *v.*

miso– *or* **mis–** *pref.* Hatred: *misogamy.*

mi·sog·a·my (mĭ-sŏg'ə-mē) *n.* Hatred of marriage. —**mis'o·gam'ic** (mĭs'ə-găm'ĭk) *adj.* —**mi·sog'a·mist** *n.*

mi·sog·y·ny (mĭ-sŏj'ə-nē) *n.* Hatred of women. —**mi·sog'y·nist** *n.* —**mi·sog'y·nis'tic** *adj.*

mis·o·pe·di·a (mĭs'ō-pē'dē-ə) *or* **mi·sop·e·dy** (mĭ-sŏp'ĭ-dē) *n.* Hatred of children.

missed abortion (mĭst) *n.* An abortion in which the fetus dies but is retained within the uterus for two months or longer.

missed labor *n.* A condition in which a pregnant woman experiences uterine contractions at the normal term, but the contractions soon stop, and the fetus is retained, usually lifeless, within the uterus for an indefinite period.

mis·sense (mĭs'sĕns') *n.* A section within a strand of messenger RNA containing a codon altered through mutation so that it codes for a different amino acid.

missense mutation *n.* A mutation in which a base change or substitution results in a codon that causes insertion of a different amino acid into the growing polypeptide chain, giving rise to an altered protein.

Mitch·ell (mĭch′əl), **Peter Dennis** 1920–1992. British biochemist. He won a 1978 Nobel Prize for contributions to the understanding of biological energy transfer.

Mitch·ell's disease (mĭch′əlz) *n.* See **erythromelalgia.**

mite (mīt) *n.* Any of numerous small or minute arachnids of the order Acarina, certain species of which are parasitic on animals and plants, infest stored food products, and in some cases transmit disease.

mite typhus *n.* See **scrub typhus.**

mith·ri·da·tism (mĭth′rĭ-dā′tĭz′əm) *n.* Tolerance or immunity to a poison acquired by taking gradually larger doses of it. —**mith′ri·dat′ic** (-dăt′ĭk) *adj.*

mi·ti·cide (mī′tĭ-sīd′) *n.* An agent that kills mites. —**mi′ti·cid′al** (-sīd′l) *adj.*

mit·i·gate (mĭt′ĭ-gāt′) *v.* To moderate in force or intensity. —**mit′i·ga′tion** *n.*

mi·to·chon·dri·on (mī′tə-kŏn′drē-ən) *n., pl.* –**dri·a** (-drē-ə) A spherical or elongated organelle in the cytoplasm of nearly all eukaryotic cells, containing genetic material and many enzymes important for cell metabolism, including those responsible for the conversion of food to usable energy. It consists of two membranes: an outer smooth membrane and an inner membrane arranged to form cristae. —**mi′to·chon′dri·al** (-drē-əl) *adj.*

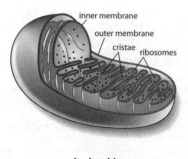

mitochondrion
cutaway view

mi·to·gen (mī′tə-jən) *n.* An agent that stimulates mitosis and lymphocyte transformation. —**mi′to·gen′ic** (mī′tə-jĕn′ĭk, mĭt′ə-) *adj.* —**mi′to·ge·nic′i·ty** (-jə-nĭs′-ĭ-tē) *n.*

mi·to·gen·e·sis (mī′tə-jĕn′ĭ-sĭs) *n.* Induction of mitosis in a cell.

mi·to·ge·net·ic (mī′tə-jə-nĕt′ĭk) *adj.* Relating to the factor or factors causing cell mitosis.

mi·to·my·cin (mī′tə-mī′sĭn) *n.* Any of a group of antibiotics produced by the soil actinomycete *Streptomyces caespitosus* that inhibit DNA synthesis and are used against bacteria and cancerous tumor cells.

mi·to·sis (mī-tō′sĭs) *n., pl.* –**ses** (-sēz) **1.** The process in cell division by which the nucleus divides, typically

in four stages (prophase, metaphase, anaphase, and telophase) resulting in two new nuclei, each of which has exactly the same chromosome and DNA content as the original cell. Also called *indirect nuclear division, karyokinesis, mitotic division.* **2.** The entire process of cell division including division of the nucleus and the cytoplasm. —**mi·tot·ic** (-tŏt′ĭk) *adj.* —**mi·tot′i·cal·ly** *adv.*

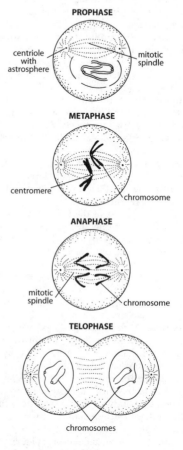

PROPHASE

centriole with astrosphere — mitotic spindle

METAPHASE

centromere — chromosome

ANAPHASE

mitotic spindle — chromosome

TELOPHASE

chromosomes

mitosis

mitotic figure *n.* The microscopic appearance of a cell undergoing mitosis.

mitotic rate *n.* The proportion of cells in a tissue that are undergoing mitosis, expressed as a mitotic index or, roughly, as the number of cells in mitosis in each microscopic high-power field in tissue sections.

mitotic spindle *n.* The fusiform figure characteristic of a dividing cell, consisting of microtubules, some of which become attached to each chromosome at its centromere and provide the mechanism for chromosomal movement. Also called *nuclear spindle.*

mi·to·xan·trone hydrochloride (mī′tō-zăn′trōn′) *n.* A synthetic antineoplastic drug used intravenously in the initial therapy for acute nonlymphocytic leukemia in adults.

mi·tral (mī′trəl) *adj.* **1.** Relating to a mitral valve. **2.** Shaped like a bishop's miter. Used of a structure resembling the shape of a headband or turban.

mitral atresia *n.* The congenital absence of the normal mitral valve orifice.

mitral cell *n.* Any of the large triangular nerve cells in the olfactory bulb.

mitral insufficiency *n.* *Abbr.* **MI** Incompetence of the mitral valve of the heart resulting in backflow of blood from the left ventricle to the left atrium. Also called *mitral regurgitation.*

mi·tral·i·za·tion (mī′trə-lĭ-zā′shən) *n.* A straightening of the left heart border in a chest x-ray because of increased prominence of the convexity formed by the main pulmonary artery and its left main branch or the left atrial appendage or both.

mitral murmur *n.* A murmur produced at the mitral valve. It can be either obstructive or regurgitant.

mitral orifice *n.* See **left ventricular opening.**

mitral regurgitation *n.* *Abbr.* **MR** See **mitral insufficiency.**

mitral stenosis *n.* *Abbr.* **MS** A narrowing of the mitral valve usually caused by rheumatic fever and resulting in an obstruction to the flow of blood from the left atrium to the left ventricle.

mitral valve *n.* A valve of the heart, composed of two triangular flaps, that is located between the left atrium and left ventricle and regulates blood flow between these chambers. Also called *bicuspid valve, left atrioventricular valve.*

mitral valve prolapse *n.* *Abbr.* **MVP** A condition in which there is excessive retrograde movement of the mitral valve into the left atrium during left ventricular systole, often allowing mitral regurgitation.

mit·tel·schmerz (mĭt′l-shmûrts′, -shmĕrts′) *n.* Abdominal pain occurring at the time of ovulation, resulting from irritation of the peritoneum by bleeding from the ovulation site. Also called *intermenstrual pain.*

mixed agglutination reaction (mĭkst) *n.* A test to identify isoantigens in which the aggregates formed by agglutination contain two different kinds of cells having common antigenic determinants. Also called *mixed agglutination test.*

mixed aphasia *n.* Motor and sensory aphasia.

mixed astigmatism *n.* Astigmatism in which one meridian is hyperopic while the one at a right angle to it is myopic.

mixed connective-tissue disease *n.* A disease of the connective tissues, combining features of systemic lupus erythematosus and systemic sclerosis or polymyositis and characterized by the presence of serum antibodies to nuclear ribonucleoprotein.

mixed expired gas *n.* One or more complete breaths of expired gas coming thoroughly mixed from the alveolar dead space and the alveoli of the lungs. Also called *expired gas.*

mixed gland *n.* **1.** A gland containing both serous and mucous secretory units. **2.** A gland having both exocrine and endocrine portions.

mixed lymphocyte culture test *n.* A test for histocompatibility of HL-A antigens in which donor and recipient lymphocytes are mixed in culture.

mixed nerve *n.* A nerve that contains both sensory and motor fibers.

mixed paralysis *n.* Motor and sensory paralysis.

mixed tumor *n.* A tumor composed of two or more types of tissue.

mix·ture (mĭks′chər) *n.* **1.** A composition of two or more substances that are not chemically combined with each other and are capable of being separated. **2.** A preparation consisting of a liquid holding an insoluble medicinal substance in suspension by means of some viscid material.

Mi·ya·ga·wa·nel·la (mē′yə-gä′wə-nĕl′ə) *n.* See **Chlamydia.**

MK *abbr.* menaquinone

mks system *or* **MKS system** *abbr.* meter-kilogram-second system

ml *abbr.* milliliter

MLD *or* **mld** *abbr.* minimal lethal dose

M line *n.* A fine dark band in the center of the H band in the myofibrils of striated muscle fibers. Also called *M band.*

mm *abbr.* millimeter

M-mode *n.* A diagnostic ultrasound presentation of the temporal changes in echoes in which the depth of echo-producing interfaces is displayed along one axis and time is displayed along the second axis, recording motion of the interfaces toward and away from the transducer.

mmol *abbr.* millimole

MMPI *abbr.* Minnesota Multiphasic Personality Inventory

MMR *abbr.* measles, mumps, rubella vaccine

Mn The symbol for the element **manganese.**

M′Nagh·ten rule (mĭk-nôt′n) *n.* An 1843 English rule used as a classic example of a test of criminal responsibility and stating that a defense based on a plea of insanity must prove that, at the time of the act, the accused individual was mentally ill, and was not aware of the nature and quality of the act, or, if aware, did not know the act was wrong.

mne·men·ic (nĭ-mĕn′ĭk) *or* **mne·mic** (nē′mĭk) *adj.* Relating to memory.

mne·mon·ic (nĭ-mŏn′ĭk) *adj.* Relating to, assisting, or intended to assist the memory. —*n.* A device, such as a formula or rhyme, used as an aid in remembering. —**mne·mon′i·cal·ly** *adv.*

mne·mon·ics (nĭ-mŏn′ĭks) *n.* A system to develop or improve the memory.

Mo The symbol for the element **molybdenum.**

mo·bi·lize (mō′bə-līz′) *v.* **1.** To make mobile or capable of movement. **2.** To restore the power of motion to a joint. **3.** To release into the body, as glycogen from the liver. —**mo′bi·li·za′tion** (-lĭ-zā′shən) *n.*

Mö·bi·us disease (mō′bē-əs, mœ′bē-ŏŏs) *n.* A periodic migraine headache accompanied by paralysis of the muscles that move the eyes.

Mö·bi·us′ sign (mō′bē-ə-sĭz, mœ′bē-ŏŏs) *n.* An indication of Graves' disease in which ocular convergence is impaired.

Möbius syndrome *n.* A developmental bilateral facial paralysis usually associated with oculomotor or other neurological disorders.

mo·dal·i·ty (mō-dăl′ĭ-tē) *n.* **1.** A therapeutic method or agent, such as surgery, chemotherapy, or electrotherapy, that involves the physical treatment of a disorder. **2.** Any of the various types of sensation, such as vision or hearing.

mode (mōd) *n.* **1.** The value or item occurring most frequently in a series of observations or statistical data. **2.** The number or range of numbers in a mathematical set that occurs the most frequently.

mod·el·ing (mŏd′l-ĭng) *n.* **1.** The acquisition of a new skill by observing and imitating that behavior being performed by another individual. **2.** In behavior modification, a treatment procedure in which the therapist models the target behavior which the learner is to imitate. **3.** A continuous process by which a bone is altered in size and shape during its growth by resorption and formation of bone at different sites and rates.

mod·i·fi·ca·tion (mŏd′ə-fĭ-kā′shən) *n.* Any of the changes in an organism that are caused by environment or activity and are not genetically transmissable to offspring.

mod·i·fied radical mastectomy (mŏd′ə-fīd′) *n.* Surgical removal of the entire breast and the lymphatic-bearing tissue in the armpit.

mo·di·o·lus (mō-dī′ə-ləs) *n., pl.* **–li** (-lī′) The central conical bony core of the cochlea of the ear.

mod·u·la·tion (mŏj′ə-lā′shən) *n.* **1.** The functional and morphological fluctuation of cells in response to changing environmental conditions. **2.** The variation of a property in an electromagnetic wave or signal, such as amplitude, frequency, or phase.

moi·e·ty (moi′ĭ-tē) *n.* One of two or more parts into which something may be divided, such as the various parts of a vitamin or molecule.

moist gangrene (moist) *n.* A form of gangrene in which the necrosed part is moist and soft.

moist rale *n.* A bubbling sound heard on auscultation, caused by the pressure of a fluid secretion in the bronchial tubes or in a cavity.

moist wart *n.* See **genital wart.**

Mo·ko·la virus (mə-kō′lə) *n.* A rabies-related virus of the genus *Lyssavirus* found most commonly in Africa and causing a fatal neurological disease in humans and cats.

mol (mōl) *n.* Variant of **mole**[3].

mo·lal (mō′ləl) *adj.* Of, relating to, or being a solution that contains one mole of solute in 1,000 grams of solvent.

mo·lal·i·ty (mō-lăl′ĭ-tē) *n.* The molal concentration of a solute, usually expressed as the number of moles of solute per 1,000 grams of solvent.

mo·lar[1] (mō′lər) *adj.* **1.** Relating to or being a solution that contains one mole of solute per liter of solution. **2.** Of, relating to, or characterizing the physical properties of a body of matter as a whole, especially the mass of a body, as opposed to the molecular or atomic properties. **3.** *Abbr.* **M** Of, relating to, or being a solution whose concentration is expressed as moles of solute per liter of solution. **4.** Containing one mole of a substance.

mo·lar[2] (mō′lər) *n.* A tooth having a crown with three, four, or five cusps on the grinding surface, a bifid root in the lower jaw, and three conical roots in the upper jaw. In permanent dentition, there are three on either side behind the premolars; in deciduous dentition, there are two on either side behind the canines. —*adj.* **1.** Relating to the molars. **2.** Capable of grinding.

molar absorption coefficient *n. Symbol* **ε** A spectrophotometric unit indicating the light a substance absorbs with respect to length, usually centimeters, and concentration, usually moles per liter.

mo·lar·i·ty (mō-lăr′ĭ-tē) *n. Abbr.* **M** The molar concentration of a solution, usually expressed as the number of moles of solute per liter of solution.

mold[1] (mōld) *n.* **1.** A shaped receptacle into which material is pressed or poured in making a cast. **2.** A frame around which something is formed or shaped. **3.** The shape of an artificial tooth or teeth. —*v.* **1.** To shape a mass of plastic material in or on a mold. **2.** To change in shape. Used especially of the adaptation of the fetal head to the pelvic canal. —**mold′a·ble** *adj.*

mold[2] (mōld) *n.* Any of various filamentous fungi, generally a circular colony having a woolly or furry appearance, that grow on the surface of organic matter and contribute to its disintegration.

mole[1] (mōl) *n.* A small congenital growth on the skin, usually slightly raised and dark and sometimes hairy, especially a pigmented nevus. Also called *nevus pigmentosus.*

mole[2] (mōl) *n.* **1.** A fleshy abnormal mass formed in the uterus by the degeneration or abortive development of an ovum. **2.** See **hydatidiform mole.**

mole[3] *or* **mol** (mōl) *n.* **1.** The amount of a substance that contains as many atoms, molecules, ions, or other elementary units as the number of atoms in 0.012 kilogram of carbon 12. The number is 6.0225×10^{23}, or Avogadro's number. Also called *gram molecule.* **2.** The mass in grams of this amount of a substance, numerically equal to the molecular weight of the substance. Also called *gram-molecular weight.*

mo·lec·u·lar (mə-lĕk′yə-lər) *adj.* Of, relating to, or consisting of molecules.

molecular biology *n.* The branch of biology that deals with the formation, structure, and activity of macromolecules essential to life, such as nucleic acids, and especially with their role in cell replication and the transmission of genetic information.

molecular disease *n.* A disease in which there is an abnormality in or a deficiency of a particular molecule, such as hemoglobin in sickle cell anemia.

molecular formula *n.* A chemical formula that shows the number and kinds of atoms in a molecule.

molecular genetics *n.* The branch of genetics that deals with hereditary transmission and variation on the molecular level.

molecular layer of cerebellar cortex *n.* The outer layer of the cortex of the cerebellum, containing the cell bodies and dendrites of Purkinje cells, the axons of the granule cells, and the cell bodies, dendrites, and axons of basket cells.

molecular medicine *n.* The branch of medicine that deals with the influence of gene expression on disease processes and with genetically based treatments, such as gene therapy.

molecular movement *n.* See **Brownian movement.**

molecular rotation *n.* The value equaling $\frac{1}{100}$ of the product of the specific rotation of an optically active compound and its molecular weight.

molecular surgery *n.* A technique used to increase the drug susceptibility of tumor cells by introducing gene segments into such cells so as to alter their drug resistance.

molecular weight *n.* *Abbr.* **mol wt, MW** The sum of the atomic weights of all the atoms in a molecule. Also called *formula weight.*

mol·e·cule (mŏl′ĭ-kyōōl′) *n.* The smallest particle into which an element or a compound can be divided without changing its chemical and physical properties; a group of atoms that is held together chemically.

mole fraction *n.* The ratio of the moles of one component of a system to the total moles of all components present.

mo·li·men (mə-lī′mən) *n.*, *pl.* **-lim·i·na** (-lĭm′ə-nə) Abnormal strain or tension associated with a normal physiological function, especially menstruation.

mol·li·ti·es (mə-lĭsh′ē-ēz) *n.* See **malacia.**

mol·lus·cous (mə-lŭs′kəs) *adj.* Of, relating to, or resembling molluscum.

mol·lus·cum (mə-lŭs′kəm) *n.*, *pl.* **-ca** (-kə) Any of various skin diseases marked by the occurrence of soft spherical tumors on the face or the body.

molluscum con·ta·gi·o·sum (kən-tā′jē-ō′səm) *n.* An infectious disease of the skin caused by a virus of the family Poxviridae and characterized by the appearance of small, pearly, umbilicated papular epithelial lesions containing many inclusion bodies.

Mo·lo·ney test (mə-lō′nē) *n.* A test to detect a high degree of sensitivity to diphtheria toxoid, in which diluted toxoid is given intradermally.

molt (mōlt) *v.* To shed periodically part or all of a coat or an outer covering, such as feathers, cuticle, or skin, which is then replaced by a new growth. —*n.* **1.** The act or process of molting. **2.** The material cast off during molting.

mol wt *abbr.* molecular weight

mo·lyb·de·num (mə-lĭb′də-nəm) *n.* *Symbol* **Mo** A hard metallic element that is an essential trace element in plant and animal nutrition. Atomic number 42.

mo·lyb·dic (mə-lĭb′dĭk) *adj.* Of, relating to, or containing molybdenum or a compound containing molybdenum, especially with a valence of 6.

mo·lyb·dous (mə-lĭb′dəs) *adj.* Of, relating to, or containing molybdenum or a compound containing molybdenum, especially with a valence of less than 6.

mon– *pref.* Variant of **mono–.**

mo·nad (mō′năd′) *n.* **1.** An atom or a radical with a valence of 1. **2.** A single-celled microorganism, especially a protozoan of the genus *Monas.* **3.** Any of the four chromatids of a tetrad that, after the first and second meiotic divisions, separate to become the chromosomal material in each of the four daughter cells. —**mo·nad′·ic** (mə-năd′ik), **mo·nad′i·cal** *adj.*

mon·ar·thric (mŏn-är′thrĭk) *adj.* Monarticular.

mon·ar·thri·tis (mŏn′är-thrī′tĭs) *n.* Arthritis of a single joint.

mon·ar·tic·u·lar (mŏn′är-tĭk′yə-lər) *adj.* Of or affecting a single joint.

mon·as·ter (mŏn-ăs′tər) *n.* The single-star formation of chromosomes that forms at the equatorial plate at the end of prophase in mitosis.

mon·ath·e·to·sis (mŏn′ăth-ĭ-tō′sĭs) *n.* Athetosis affecting only one hand or foot.

mon·a·tom·ic (mŏn′ə-tŏm′ĭk) *adj.* **1.** Occurring as single atoms. **2.** Having one replaceable atom or radical. **3.** Univalent. —**mon′a·tom′ic·al·ly** *adv.*

mon·au·ral (mŏn-ôr′əl) *adj.* Of or relating to sound reception by one ear. —**mon·au′ral·ly** *adv.*

monaural diplacusis *n.* A form of diplacusis in which one sound is perceived as two in the same ear.

Mönck·e·berg's arteriosclerosis (mœ̌ong′kə-bûrgz′, mĕng′kə-, mœng′kə-bĕrks′) *n.* Arteriosclerosis of the peripheral arteries, especially in the legs of older adults, characterized by deposition of calcium in the medial coat. Also called *Mönckeberg's calcification, Mönckeberg's sclerosis.*

Mon·di·ni dysplasia (mŏn-dē′nē) *n.* A congenital abnormality of the structures of the inner ear causing partial or complete hearing loss.

Mon·dor's disease (mŏn′dôrz′, môN-dôrz′) *n.* Thrombophlebitis of the thoracoepigastric vein of the breast and chest wall.

mo·ne·cious (mə-nē′shəs) *adj.* Variant of **monoecious.**

mon·es·thet·ic (mŏn′ĭs-thĕt′ĭk) *adj.* Relating to a single sense or sensation.

Mon·ge's disease (mŏn′hāz) *n.* See **chronic mountain sickness.**

Mon·go·li·an *or* **mon·go·li·an** (mŏng-gō′lē-ən, -gōl′-yən, mŏn-) *adj.* Relating to Down syndrome. No longer in technical use. Now considered offensive.

Mongolian fold *n.* Epicanthic fold. No longer in technical use.

mongolian spot *n.* Any of a number of dark-bluish or mulberry-colored spots on the lower back, observed in newborn infants, that enlarge for a short time after birth and then gradually recede. Also called *blue spot.*

mon·gol·ism *or* **Mon·gol·ism** (mŏng′gə-lĭz′əm, mŏn′-) *n.* Down syndrome. No longer in technical use.

Mon·gol·oid *or* **mon·gol·oid** (mŏng′gə-loid′, mŏn′-) *adj.* Of or relating to Down syndrome. Not in technical use. —*n.* A person affected with Down syndrome. No longer in technical use. Now considered offensive.

mo·nil·e·thrix (mə-nĭl′ə-thrĭks′) *n.* A condition in which the hair is brittle and shows a series of constrictions, resembling strings of spindle-shaped beads. Also called *beaded hair, moniliform hair.*

Mo·nil·i·a (mə-nĭl′ē-ə) *n.* A class of imperfect fungi that do not form asci or basidia, including pathogenic genera such as *Candida* and *Cryptococcus* and the medically important genus *Penicillium.*

mo·nil·i·al (mə-nĭl′ē-əl) *adj.* Of or caused by a fungus of the genus *Candida.*

mo·ni·li·a·sis (mō′nə-lī′ə-sĭs, mŏn′ə-) *n.* See **candidiasis.**

mo·nil·i·form (mə-nĭl′ə-fôrm′) *adj.* Having the shape of a string of beads.

moniliform hair *n.* See **monilethrix.**

Mo·nil·i·for·mis (mə-nĭl′ə-fôr′mĭs) *n.* A genus of acanthocephalan worms, including a species, *M.*

moniliformis, that is normally found in rats and is a rare parasite in humans.

mo·nil·i·id (mə-nĭl′ē-ĭd) *n.* A skin condition characterized by minute macular or papular lesions, occurring as an allergic reaction to infection with a fungus of the genus *Candida.*

Mon·i·stat (mŏn′ĭ-stăt′) A trademark for the drug miconazole nitrate.

mon·i·tor (mŏn′ĭ-tər) *n.* A usually electronic device used to record, regulate, or control a process or system.

Mo·niz (mō-nēz′, -nēsh′), **Antonio Caetano de Abreu Freire Egas** 1874–1955. Portuguese neurosurgeon. He shared a 1949 Nobel Prize for the development of prefrontal lobotomy as a radical treatment for severe psychoses.

monks·hood (mŭngks′ho͝od′) *n.* See **aconite.**

mono– *or* **mon–** *pref.* **1.** One; single; alone: *monomorphic.* **2.** Monomolecular; monatomic: *monolayer.* **3.** Containing one atom, molecule, or group: *monomer.*

mon·o (mŏn′ō) *n.* Infectious mononucleosis.

mon·o·ac·id (mŏn′ō-ăs′ĭd) *n.* An acid having one replaceable hydrogen atom.

mon·o·am·ide (mŏn′ō-ăm′īd′, -ĭd) *n.* An amide compound containing one amido group.

mon·o·am·ine (mŏn′ō-ăm′ēn, -ə-mēn′) *n.* An amine compound containing one amino group, especially a compound that functions as a neurotransmitter.

monoamine oxidase *n. Abbr.* **MAO** An enzyme in the cells of most tissues that catalyzes the oxidative deamination of monoamines such as serotonin.

monoamine oxidase inhibitor *n. Abbr.* **MAOI** Any of a class of antidepressant and hypotensive drugs that block the action of monoamine oxidase in the brain, thereby allowing the accumulation of monoamines such as norepinephrine.

mon·o·am·i·ner·gic (mŏn′ō-ăm′ə-nûr′jĭk) *adj.* Of or being nerve cells or fibers that transmit nerve impulses by monoamine neurotransmitters.

mon·o·am·ni·ot·ic twins (mŏn′ō-ăm′nē-ŏt′ĭk) *pl.n.* Identical twins within a common amnion.

mon·o·ba·sic (mŏn′ə-bā′sĭk) *adj.* **1.** Having only one hydrogen ion to donate to a base in an acid-base reaction. **2.** Having only one metal ion or positive radical.

monobasic acid *n.* An acid having only one hydrogen atom that can be displaced in a chemical reaction.

mon·o·blast (mŏn′ə-blăst′) *n.* An immature cell that develops into a monocyte.

mon·o·cho·re·a (mŏn′ō-kô-rē′ə) *n.* Chorea affecting the head alone or only one extremity.

mon·o·cho·ri·on·ic (mŏn′ō-kôr′ē-ŏn′ĭk) *or* **mon·o·cho·ri·al** (-kôr′ē-əl) *adj.* Having a single or common chorion. Used of monozygotic twins.

mon·o·chro·mat (mŏn′ə-krō′măt) *n.* A person with achromatopsia.

mon·o·chro·mat·ic (mŏn′ə-krō-măt′ĭk) *adj.* **1.** Having or appearing to have only one color. **2.** Of or relating to a pure spectral color of a single wavelength. **3.** Of or exhibiting achromatopsia. —**mon′o·chro·mat′i·cal·ly** *adv.*

monochromatic aberration *n.* Any of several defects in the optical image due to the nature of a lens, including spherical, coma, curvature, and distortion aberrations.

mon·o·chro·ma·tism (mŏn′ə-krō′mə-tĭz′əm) *n.* **1.** The state of having or exhibiting only one color. **2.** See **achromatopsia.**

mon·o·chro·mat·o·phil (mŏn′ə-krō-măt′ə-fĭl) *or* **mon·o·chro·mat·o·phile** (-fīl′) *adj.* Staining readily with only one kind of dye. —*n.* A cell or tissue staining readily with only one kind of dye.

mon·o·clo·nal (mŏn′ə-klō′nəl) *n.* Of or relating to a protein from a single clone of cells, all molecules of which are the same, as in the Bence-Jones protein.

monoclonal antibody *n.* Any of a class of highly specific antibodies produced by the clones of a single hybrid cell formed in the laboratory by the fusion of a B cell with a tumor cell and widely used in medical and biological research.

mon·o·crot·ic (mŏn′ō-krŏt′ĭk) *adj.* Of or being a pulse whose curve on the pulse tracing presents a smooth, single-crested curve that has no notch in the downward line.

mo·noc·ro·tism (mə-nŏk′rə-tĭz′əm) *n.* The state in which the pulse is monocrotic.

mo·noc·u·lar (mŏ-nŏk′yə-lər) *adj.* **1.** Having or affecting one eye only. **2.** Having a single eyepiece, as certain microscopes or other optical instruments.

monocular diplopia *n.* A form of double vision in which two objects are seen with the same eye, and that is caused by an opacity in the visual axis. Also called *monodiplopia.*

mon·o·cyte (mŏn′ə-sīt′) *n.* A large, circulating, phagocytic white blood cell that has a single well-defined nucleus and very fine granulation in the cytoplasm and that constitutes from 3 to 8 percent of the white blood cells in humans. —**mon′o·cyt′ic** (-sĭt′ĭk), **mon′o·cy′toid′** (-sī′toid′) *adj.*

monocytic leukemia *n.* Leukemia in which the blood contains large numbers of monocytes, characterized by swelling of the gums, oral ulcers, bleeding in the skin or mucous membranes, secondary infection, and an enlarged spleen.

monocytic leukocytosis *n.* See **monocytosis.**

mon·o·cy·to·pe·ni·a (mŏn′ə-sī′tə-pē′nē-ə) *n.* An abnormally low number of monocytes in the blood. Also called *monocytic leukopenia.*

mon·o·cy·to·sis (mŏn′ə-sī-tō′sĭs) *n.* An abnormal increase in the number of monocytes in the blood, occurring in infectious mononucleosis and certain bacterial infections such as tuberculosis. Also called *monocytic leukocytosis.*

Mo·nod (mô-nō′), **Jacques Lucien** 1910–1976. French biochemist. He shared a 1965 Nobel Prize for the study of regulatory activity in body cells.

mon·o·dac·ty·ly (mŏn′ō-dăk′tə-lē) *n.* The presence of a single finger on the hand or a single toe on the foot.

mon·o·der·mo·ma (mŏn′ō-dər-mō′mə) *n.* A neoplasm composed of tissues from a single germ layer.

mon·o·di·plo·pi·a (mŏn′ō-dĭ-plō′pē-ə) *n.* See **monocular diplopia.**

mo·noe·cious *or* **mo·ne·cious** (mə-nē′shəs) *adj.* **1.** Having unisexual reproductive organs or flowers, with the organs or flowers of both sexes carried on a single plant, as in corn. **2.** Hermaphroditic.

mon·o·ga·met·ic (mŏn′ō-gə-mĕt′ĭk) *adj.* Producing gametes that contain only one type of sex chromosome.

mo·nog·a·my (mə-nŏg′ə-mē) *n.* **1.** The practice or condition of being married to only one person at a time. **2.** The condition of having only one mate. —**mo·nog′a·mous** *adj.*

mon·o·gen·e·sis (mŏn′ə-jĕn′ĭ-sĭs) *n.* **1.** The theory that all living organisms are descended from a single cell or organism. **2.** The production of similar organisms in successive generations. **3.** Asexual reproduction, as by sporulation or parthenogenesis. **4.** The process of parasitizing a single host, in or on which the entire life cycle of the parasite is passed. —**mon′o·ge·net′ic** (-jə-nĕt′ĭk) *adj.*

mon·o·gen·ic (mŏn′ə-jĕn′ĭk) *adj.* **1.** Of or relating to monogenesis; monogenetic. **2.** Relating to monogenism. **3.** Of or regulated by one gene or one of a pair of allelic genes, as an inherited characteristic or a hereditary disease.

mo·nog·e·nism (mə-nŏj′ə-nĭz′əm) *n.* The theory that all human beings are descended from a single pair of ancestors.

mo·nog·e·nous (mə-nŏj′ə-nəs) *adj.* Asexually produced, as by fission, gemmation, or sporulation.

mon·o·hy·drate (mŏn′ō-hī′drāt′) *n.* A compound, such as calcium chloride monohydrate, that contains one molecule of water.

mon·o·hy·dric alcohol (mŏn′ō-hī′drĭk) *n.* An alcohol containing one hydroxyl group.

mon·o·lay·er (mŏn′ō-lā′ər) *n.* **1.** A film or layer one molecule thick formed at the interface between water and either oil or air by a substance such as a partially esterified fatty acid that contains both hydrophobic and hydrophilic groups in the same molecule. **2.** A confluent sheet of cells, one cell deep, growing on a surface in a cell culture.

mon·o·loc·u·lar (mŏn′ō-lŏk′yə-lər) *adj.* Having a single cavity or chamber.

mon·o·ma·ni·a (mŏn′ə-mā′nē-ə, -mān′yə) *n.* Pathological obsession with one idea or subject, as in paranoia. —**mon′o·ma′ni·ac′** (-mā′nē-ăk′) *n.* —**mon′o·ma·ni′a·cal** (-mə-nī′ə-kəl) *adj.*

mon·o·mel·ic (mŏn′ō-mĕl′ĭk) *adj.* Of or affecting a single limb.

mon·o·mer (mŏn′ə-mər) *n.* **1.** The molecular unit that joins with similar units to form a polymer. **2.** The protein structural unit of a virion capsid. **3.** The subunit of a protein composed of several such units loosely associated with one another.

mon·o·mer·ic (mŏn′ə-mĕr′ĭk) *adj.* **1.** Consisting of a single part. **2.** Of, relating to, or consisting of monomers. **3.** Of or relating to a hereditary disease or characteristic controlled by genes at a single locus.

mon·o·mo·lec·u·lar (mŏn′ō-mə-lĕk′yə-lər) *adj.* **1.** Of or relating to a single molecule. **2.** Relating to a single layer of molecules.

mon·o·mor·phic (mŏn′ō-môr′fĭk) *or* **mon·o·mor·phous** (-fəs) *adj.* **1.** Having only one form, as one crystal form. **2.** Having one or the same genotype, form, or structure through a series of developmental changes. —**mon′o·mor′phism** *n.*

mon·o·my·o·ple·gia (mŏn′ō-mī′ə-plē′jə) *n.* Paralysis limited to a single muscle.

mon·o·my·o·si·tis (mŏn′ō-mī′ə-sī′tĭs) *n.* Inflammation of a single muscle.

mon·o·neu·ral (mŏn′ō-noŏr′əl) *adj.* **1.** Having only one neuron. **2.** Supplied by a single nerve.

mon·o·neu·ral·gia (mŏn′ō-noŏ-răl′jə) *n.* Pain along the course of a single nerve.

mon·o·neu·ri·tis (mŏn′ō-noŏ-rī′tĭs) *n.* Inflammation of a single nerve.

mononeuritis mul·ti·plex (mŭl′tə-plĕks′) *n.* Inflammation of several separate nerves in unrelated portions of the body.

mon·o·neu·rop·a·thy (mŏn′ō-noŏ-rŏp′ə-thē) *n.* Disease involving a single nerve.

mon·o·nu·cle·ar (mŏn′ō-noŏ′klē-ər) *adj.* Having only one nucleus.

mononuclear phagocyte system *n.* *Abbr.* **MPS** A widely distributed collection of both free and fixed macrophages derived from bone marrow precursor cells by way of monocytes; their substantial phagocytic activity is mediated by immunoglobulin and by the serum complement system.

mon·o·nu·cle·o·sis (mŏn′ō-noŏ′klē-ō′sĭs) *n.* **1.** Abnormally large numbers of mononuclear white blood cells in the blood, especially forms that are not normal. **2.** Infectious mononucleosis.

mon·o·nu·cle·o·tide (mŏn′ō-noŏ′klē-ə-tīd′) *n.* A nucleotide consisting of one molecule each of a phosphoric acid, a sugar, and either a purine or a pyrimidine base.

mon·o·oc·tan·o·in (mŏn′ō-ŏk-tăn′ō-ĭn, -ŏk′tə-nō′ĭn) *n.* A semisynthetic esterified glycerol used as a solubilizing agent for radiolucent gallstones retained in the biliary tract after removal of the gallbladder.

mon·o·ox·y·gen·ase (mŏn′ō-ŏk′sĭ-jə-nās′, -nāz′) *n.* Any of a group of enzymes that catalyze both the addition of a single oxygen atom from molecular oxygen into a substrate and the reduction of a second oxygen atom in the substrate to water.

mon·o·pa·re·sis (mŏn′ō-pə-rē′sĭs, -păr′ĭ-sĭs) *n.* Paresis affecting a single extremity or part of one.

mon·o·par·es·the·sia (mŏn′ō-păr′ĭs-thē′zhə) *n.* Paresthesia affecting a single region only.

mo·nop·a·thy (mə-nŏp′ə-thē) *n.* **1.** A single uncomplicated disease. **2.** A local disease affecting only one organ or part. —**mon′o·path′ic** (mŏn′ə-păth′ĭk) *adj.*

mon·o·pha·sia (mŏn′ə-fā′zhə) *n.* A form of aphasia characterized by the inability to speak more than a single word or phrase.

mon·o·pha·sic (mŏn- ō-fā′zik) *adj.* **1.** Of or affected by monophasia. **2.** Having only one phase or stage. **3.** Of or being a disorder with a single phase.

mon·o·phe·nol (mŏn′ō-fē′nôl′, -nōl′) *n.* A compound containing one phenolic hydroxyl group.

monophenol oxidase *n.* A copper-containing enzyme that catalyzes the oxidation of monophenols such as tyrosine.

mon·o·pho·bi·a (mŏn′ō-fō′bē-ə) *n.* An abnormal fear of being alone.

mon·o·phos·phate (mŏn′ə-fŏs′fāt′) *n.* An ester of phosphoric acid containing one phosphate group.

mon·oph·thal·mos (mŏn'ŏf-thăl'mŏs') *or* **mon·oph·thal·mi·a** (-thăl'mē-ə) *n.* Congenital absence of one eye due to failure of outgrowth of the primary ocular vesicle, with absence of ocular tissues. —**mon'oph·thal'-mic** *adj.*

mon·o·phy·let·ic (mŏn'ō-fī-lĕt'ĭk) *adj.* 1. Descended or derived from one original stock or source. 2. Of or being the theory that all blood cells are derived from one common stem cell. —**mon'o·phy'le·tism** (-fī'lĭ-tĭz'əm) *n.*

mon·o·ple·gia (mŏn'ə-plē'jə) *n.* Paralysis of a single limb, muscle, or muscle group. —**mon'o·ple'gic** (-jĭk) *adj.*

mon·o·ploid (mŏn'ə-ploid') *adj.* Having a single set of chromosomes; haploid.

mon·o·po·di·a (mŏn'ə-pō'dē-ə) *n.* A congenital malformation characterized by only one foot being externally recognizable.

mon·o·po·lar cautery (mŏn'ə-pō'lər) *n.* Cauterization using high frequency electrical current passed from a single electrode where cauterization occurs; the patient's body serves as a ground.

mon·or·chism (mŏn-ôr'kĭz'əm) *or* **mon·or·chid·ism** (mŏn-ôr'kĭ-dĭz'əm) *n.* A condition in which only one testis is apparent, the other testis being absent or undescended.

mon·o·sac·cha·ride (mŏn'ə-săk'ə-rīd', -rĭd) *n.* A carbohydrate that cannot be decomposed to a simpler carbohydrate by hydrolysis, especially one of the hexoses. Also called *simple sugar.*

mon·o·so·di·um glutamate (mŏn'ə-sō'dē-əm) *n.* *Abbr.* **MSG** A white odorless crystalline compound that is a salt of glutamic acid; it is used as a flavor enhancer in foods, an application that may cause Chinese restaurant syndrome in sensitive people, and is used intravenously as an adjunct in treating encephalopathies associated with liver disease.

mon·o·some (mŏn'ə-sōm') *n.* 1. A chromosome having no homologue, especially an unpaired X-chromosome. 2. A single ribosome, especially one combined with a molecule of mRNA. —**mon'o·so'mic** (-sō'mĭk) *adj.* —**mon'o·so'my** *n.*

mon·o·so·mi·a (mŏn'ə-sō'mē-ə) *n.* In conjoined twins, the condition in which the trunks are completely merged although the heads remain separate.

mon·o·spasm (mŏn'ə-spăz'əm) *n.* A spasm that affects only one muscle or group of muscles or a single extremity.

mon·os·tot·ic (mŏn'ŏs-tŏt'ĭk) *adj.* Involving only a single bone.

mon·o·stra·tal (mŏn'ō-strāt'l) *adj.* Composed of a single layer.

mon·o·symp·to·mat·ic (mŏn'ō-sĭm'tə-măt'ĭk) *adj.* Of or being a disease or pathological condition manifested by only one marked symptom.

mon·o·syn·ap·tic (mŏn'ō-sə-năp'tĭk) *adj.* Having a single neural synapse.

mon·o·ther·a·py (mŏn'ō-thĕr'ə-pē) *n.* Treatment of a disorder with a single drug.

mon·o·ther·mi·a (mŏn'ō-thûr'mē-ə) *n.* Evenness of body temperature throughout the day.

mo·not·ri·chous (mə-nŏt'rĭ-kəs) *or* **mon·o·trich·ic** (mŏn'ə-trĭk'ĭk) *or* **mo·not·ri·chate** (mə-nŏt'rĭ-kĭt) *adj.* Having a single flagellum at only one pole or end. Used of certain bacteria.

mon·o·un·sat·u·rat·ed (mŏn'ō-ŭn-săch'ə-rā'tĭd) *adj.* Of or relating to long-chain carbon compounds, especially fatty acids, having one double bond per molecule. Foods containing monounsaturated fatty acids may decrease the level of LDL cholesterol in the blood.

mon·o·va·lent (mŏn'ə-vā'lənt) *adj.* 1. Able to form only one covalent or ionic bond. 2. Having a valence of one; univalent. 3. Of or relating to an antiserum containing an antibody or antibodies specific for one antigen. 4. Containing antigens from a single strain of a microorganism. 5. Having only one site of attachment. Used of an antibody or antigen. —**mon'o·va'-lence, mon'o·va'len·cy** *n.*

mo·nox·e·nous (mə-nŏk'sə-nəs) *adj.* Relating to monogenesis; monogenetic.

mon·ox·ide (mə-nŏk'sīd') *n.* An oxide with each molecule containing one oxygen atom.

mon·o·zy·got·ic (mŏn'ō-zī-gŏt'ĭk) *adj.* Derived from a single fertilized ovum or embryonic cell mass. Used especially of identical twins.

Mon·ro (mən-rō') Family of Scottish anatomists and educators, including **Alexander,** (1697–1767), a renowned professor of anatomy at Edinburgh University (from 1720), who helped establish Edinburgh as a center of medical training and his son **Alexander,** (1733–1817), who worked on methods of surgical anesthesia.

Mon·ro's foramen (mən-rōz') *n.* See **interventricular foramen.**

mons (mŏnz) *n.,* *pl.* **mon·tes** (mŏn'tēz) An anatomical prominence or slight elevation above the general level of the surface.

mons pu·bis (pyo͞o'bĭs) *n., pl.* **montes pubis** A rounded fleshy protuberance situated over the pubic bones that becomes covered with hair during puberty. Also called *pubis.*

mon·ster (mŏn'stər) *n.* 1. An animal, a plant, or other organism having structural defects or deformities. 2. A fetus or an infant that is grotesquely abnormal and usually not viable.

mons ve·ne·ris (vĕn'ər-ĭs) *n., pl.* **montes veneris** The female mons pubis.

Mon·ta·gnier (mŏn'tən-yā', môn-tä-nyā') **Luc** Born 1932. French virologist who was one of the first to identify the virus that causes AIDS and to develop a blood test for it.

mon·te·lu·kast (mŏn'tə-lo͞o'kăst) *n.* A leukotriene receptor antagonist that reduces the inflammatory response and is used to treat asthma.

mon·tic·u·lus (mŏn-tĭk'yə-ləs) *n., pl.* **–li** (-lī') 1. A slight rounded projection above a surface. 2. The central portion of the superior vermis, forming a projection on the surface of the cerebellum.

mood (mo͞od) *n.* A state of mind or emotion.

mood disorder *n.* Any of a group of psychiatric disorders, including depression and bipolar disorder, characterized by a pervasive disturbance of mood that is not caused by an organic abnormality. Also called *affective disorder.*

mood swing *n.* Alternation of a person's emotional state between periods of euphoria and depression.

mood·y (mōo′dē) *adj.* **1.** Given to frequent changes of mood; temperamental. **2.** Subject to periods of depression; sulky. **3.** Expressive of a mood, especially a sullen or gloomy mood.

moon face *or* **moon facies** (mōon) *n.* The round usually red face seen in Cushing's syndrome or in hyperadrenocorticalism.

Moore (mōor, môr), **Stanford** 1913–1982. American biochemist. He shared a 1972 Nobel Prize for pioneering studies of the enzyme ribonuclease.

MOPP (mŏp) *n.* A cancer chemotherapy drug consisting of Mustargen; Oncovin; procarbazine hydrochloride, an antineoplastic drug; and prednisone.

Mor·ax·el·la (môr′ăk-sĕl′ə) *n.* A genus of aerobic nonmotile bacteria, containing gram-negative cocci or short rods, that are parasitic on the mucous membranes of humans and other mammals; the type species, *M. lacunata,* causes conjunctivitis in humans.

mor·bid (môr′bĭd) *adj.* **1.** Relating to or caused by disease; pathological or diseased. **2.** Psychologically unhealthy or unwholesome.

mor·bid·i·ty (môr-bĭd′ĭ-tē) *n.* **1.** The quality of being morbid. **2.** A diseased state. **3.** The incidence or prevalence of a disease. **4.** Morbidity rate.

morbidity rate *n.* The proportion of patients with a particular disease during a given year per given unit of population.

morbid obesity *n.* The condition of weighing at least twice the ideal weight.

mor·bif·ic (môr-bĭf′ĭk) *adj.* Relating to or causing disease; pathogenic.

mor·bil·li (môr-bĭl′ī) *pl.n.* Measles; rubeola.

mor·bil·li·form (môr-bĭl′ə-fôrm′) *adj.* Resembling the dusky red eruption of measles.

Mor·bil·li·vi·rus (môr-bĭl′ĭ-vī′rəs) *n.* A genus of viruses of the family Paramyxoviridae that includes the causative agents of measles.

mor·bus (môr′bəs) *n., pl.* **-bi** (-bī) A disease.

mor·cel·la·tion (môr′sə-lā′shən) *n.* Division into and removal of small pieces, as of a tumor.

morcellation operation *n.* Vaginal hysterectomy in which the uterus is removed by lateral halves after being split.

mor·dant (môr′dnt) *adj.* Serving to fix colors in dyeing. —*n.* A reagent, such as tannic acid, that fixes dyes to cells, tissues, or other materials. —*v.* To treat with a mordant.

mor. dict. *abbr. Latin* more dicto (as directed)

Mor·ga·gni (môr-gä′nyē), **Giovanni Battista** 1682–1771. Italian anatomist considered to be the founder of pathological anatomy. By collecting case histories and performing postmortem examinations, he discovered relationships between disease and physiological changes and was the first to describe the anatomical structures that bear his name.

mor·ga·gni·an cyst (môr-gän′yē-ən) *n.* A fluid-filled cyst that is attached to the fimbriated end of the uterine tube or to the upper end of the testis and is a remnant of the embryonic mesonephric duct.

Mor·ga·gni's cataract (môr-gä′nyēz) *n.* A hypermature

cataract in which the lens becomes a soft sac of milky fluid with a dense nucleus at the bottom.

Morgagni's crypt *n.* See **anal sinus.**

Morgagni's disease *n.* See **Adams-Stokes syndrome.**

Morgagni's nodule *n.* See **nodule of semilunar valve.**

Morgagni's prolapse *n.* Chronic inflammation of the recessed areas in the wall of the larynx between the vestibular and vocal folds.

Morgagni's syndrome *n.* Hyperostosis frontalis interna accompanied by excessive hair growth and obesity, most commonly affecting women around menopause. Also called *metabolic craniopathy.*

mor·gan (môr′gən) *n. Abbr.* **M** A unit for expressing the relative distance between genes on a chromosome based on the frequency with which the genes cross over; one unit equals a theoretical crossover value of 100 percent between two loci.

Morgan, Thomas Hunt 1866–1945. American biologist. He won a 1933 Nobel Prize for establishing the chromosome theory of heredity by his studies of the fruit fly *Drosophila.*

Mor·gan's bacillus (môr′gənz) *n.* A gram-negative aerobic bacterium, *Proteus morganii,* that occurs in the intestinal tract of humans and is present in normal and diarrheal stools.

morgue (môrg) *n.* A place in which dead bodies are temporarily kept until identified and claimed or until arrangements for burial have been made.

mo·ri·a (môr′ē-ə) *n.* **1.** Dullness of mind; mental lethargy. **2.** A mental state characterized by frivolity, joviality, and the inability to be serious.

mor·i·bund (môr′ə-bŭnd′) *n.* At the point of death; dying. —**mor′i·bun′di·ty** (-bŭn′dĭ-tē) *n.*

morn·ing-af·ter pill (môr′nĭng-ăf′tər) *n.* A pill containing a drug, especially an estrogen or estrogen substitute such as diethylstilbestrol, that prevents implantation of a fertilized ovum and is therefore effective as a contraceptive after sexual intercourse.

morning sickness *n.* Nausea and vomiting upon rising in the morning, especially during early pregnancy. Also called *nausea gravidarum.*

mo·ron (môr′ŏn′) *n.* A person of mild mental retardation having a mental age of from 7 to 12 years and generally having communication and social skills enabling some degree of academic or vocational education. The term belongs to a classification system no longer in use and is now considered offensive. —**mo·ron′ic** (mə-rŏn′ĭk, mô-) *adj.* —**mo′ron′ism, mo·ron′i·ty** (mə-rŏn′ĭ-tē, mô-) *n.*

Mo·ro's reflex (môr′ōz) *n.* See **startle reflex** (sense 1).

–morph *suff.* Form; shape; structure: *endomorph.*

mor·phe·a (môr-fē′ə) *n.* A localized form of scleroderma characterized by hardened, slightly depressed patches of dermal fibrous tissue. Also called *circumscribed scleroderma, localized scleroderma.*

–morphic *suff.* Having a specified shape or form: *homomorphic.*

mor·phine (môr′fēn′) *n.* A bitter crystalline alkaloid extracted from opium, the soluble salts of which are used in medicine as an analgesic, a light anesthetic, or a sedative. Also called *morphia.*

mor·phin·ism (môr′fē-nĭz′əm) *n.* **1.** Addiction to morphine. **2.** A diseased condition caused by habitual or addictive use of morphine.

mor·phi·a (môr′fē-ə) *n.* See **morphine.**

–morphism *suff.* The condition or quality of having a specified form: *isomorphism.*

morpho– *or* **morph–** *pref.* Form; shape; structure: *morphogenesis.*

mor·pho·gen·e·sis (môr′fō-jĕn′ĭ-sĭs) *n.* Differentiation of cells and tissues in the early embryo which results in establishing the form and structure of the various organs and parts of the body. —**mor′pho·ge·net′ic** (-jə-nĕt′ĭk), **mor′pho·gen′ic** *adj.*

morphogenetic movement *n.* The movement of cells in the early embryo that change the shape or form of differentiating cells and tissues.

mor·phol·o·gy (môr-fŏl′ə-jē) *n.* **1.** The branch of biology that deals with the form and structure of organisms without consideration of function. **2.** The form and structure of an organism or one of its parts. —**mor′pho·log′i·cal** (-fə-lŏj′ĭ-kəl), **mor′pho·log′ic** *adj.* —**mor·phol′o·gist** *n.*

mor·phom·e·try (môr-fŏm′ĭ-trē) *n.* Measurement of the form of organisms or of their parts. —**mor′pho·met′ric** (môr′fə-mĕt′rĭk) *adj.*

mor·pho·sis (môr-fō′sĭs) *n.,* pl. **-ses** (-sēz) The manner in which an organism or any of its parts changes form or undergoes development.

–morphous *suff.* Having a specified shape or form: *polymorphous.*

Mor·quio's syndrome (môr′kē-ōz′) *n.* A hereditary disorder of mucopolysaccharide metabolism that is characterized by the presence of keratan sulfate in the urine and that results in short stature due to severe deformity of the spine and the thorax, long bones with irregular epiphyses, enlarged joints, flaccid ligaments, and a waddling gait. Also called *Morquio's disease, Morquio-Ulrich disease, type IV mucopolysaccharidosis.*

mors (môrz) *n.* Death.

mor. sol. *abbr. Latin* more solito (as customary)

mor·tal (môr′tl) *adj.* **1.** Liable or subject to death. **2.** Causing death; fatal.

mor·tal·i·ty (môr-tăl′ĭ-tē) *n.* **1.** The quality or condition of being mortal. **2.** Death rate.

mortality rate *n.* See **death rate.**

mor·tar (môr′tər) *n.* **1.** A vessel in which drugs or other substances are crushed or ground with a pestle. **2.** A machine in which materials are ground and blended or crushed.

mor·ti·fi·ca·tion (môr′tə-fĭ-kā′shən) *n.* Death or decay of one part of a living body; gangrene; necrosis.

mor·ti·fy (môr′tə-fī′) *v.* To undergo mortification; to become gangrenous or to necrotize.

mor·tise joint (môr′tĭs) *n.* See **ankle joint.**

Mor·ton (môr′tn), **William Thomas Green** 1819–1868. American dentist and pioneer anesthetist who in 1846 gave the first public demonstration of ether as an anesthetic in a surgical procedure.

Mor·ton's syndrome (môr′tnz) *n.* Congenital shortening of the first metatarsal with pain between the heads of two or more of the metatarsals, usually caused by irritation of the nerve between the heads of the metatarsals. Also called *Morton's neuralgia.*

mor·tu·ar·y (môr′chōō-ĕr′ē) *n.* A place, especially a funeral home, where dead bodies are kept before burial or cremation.

mor·u·la (môr′yə-lə, môr′ə-) *n.,* pl. **-lae** (-lē′) The spherical embryonic mass of blastomeres formed before the blastula and resulting from cleavage of the fertilized ovum. —**mor′u·lar** *adj.* —**mor′u·la′tion** (-lā′-shən) *n.*

Mor·u·la·vi·rus (môr′yə-lə-vī′rəs, môr′ə-) *n.* A genus of viruses of the family Microviridae that includes the phage group of bacterial viruses.

Mor·van's disease (môr′vənz, môr-vänz′) *n.* See **syringomyelia.**

mo·sa·ic (mō-zā′ĭk) *adj.* Patterned in small squares; tesselated. —*n.* An organism exhibiting mosaicism.

mosaic inheritance *n.* Inheritance in which the paternal influence is dominant in one group of cells and the maternal influence is dominant in another.

mo·sa·i·cism (mō-zā′ĭ-sĭz′əm) *n.* A condition in which tissues of genetically different types occur in the same organism.

mosaic wart *n.* A grouping of numerous, closely aggregated plantar warts on the sole of the foot.

mos·qui·to (mə-skē′tō) *n.,* pl. **-toes** *or* **-tos** Any of various two-winged insects of the family Culicidae, in which the female of most species has a long proboscis for sucking blood. Some species are vectors of diseases such as malaria and yellow fever.

mosquito forceps *or* **mosquito clamp** *n.* A small, straight or curved hemostatic forceps used to hold delicate tissue or compress a bleeding vessel.

Mosz·ko·wicz's test (mŏs′kə-wĭts′, -wĭt′sĭz) *n.* A test for arteriosclerosis in which a lower limb is made anemic by means of a tourniquet bandage, which is removed after 5 minutes; in cases of arteriosclerosis color returns slowly, sometimes requiring several minutes to suffuse the entire limb.

Mo·tais operation (mō-tā′, mō-tĕ′) *n.* Transplantation of the middle third of the tendon of the superior rectus muscle of the eyeball into the upper lid to supplement the action of the levator muscle in cases of ptosis.

moth·er (mŭth′ər) *n.* **1.** A woman who conceives, gives birth to, or raises and nurtures a child. **2.** A female parent of an animal. **3.** A structure, such as a mother cell, from which other similar bodies are formed.

mother cell *n.* A cell that divides to produce two or more daughter cells. Also called *metrocyte.*

mother cyst *n.* A cyst, especially a hydatid cyst, that encloses other cysts, occurring most frequently in the liver. Also called *parent cyst.*

mother yaw *n.* A large granulomatous lesion that may be the initial lesion in yaws and is most commonly present on the hand, leg, or foot. Also called *buba madre, frambesioma.*

mo·tile (mōt′l, mō′tīl′) *adj.* **1.** Moving or having the power to move spontaneously. **2.** Of or relating to mental imagery that arises primarily from sensations of bodily movement and position rather than from visual or auditory sensations. —**mo·til′i·ty** (mō-tĭl′ĭ-tē) *n.*

mo·tion (mō′shən) *n.* **1.** The act or process of changing position or place. **2.** The manner in which the body or a body part moves.

motion sickness *n.* Nausea and dizziness induced by motion, as in travel by aircraft, car, or ship. Also called *kinesia.*

mo·tive (mō′tĭv) *n.* An emotion, desire, physiological need, or similar impulse that acts as an incitement to action. Also called *learned drive.* —*adj.* Causing or able to cause motion.

mo·to·fa·cient (mō′tō-fā′shənt) *adj.* **1.** Causing motion. **2.** Of or being the second phase of muscular activity in which actual movement is produced.

mo·to·neu·ron (mō′tə-nŏŏr′ŏn′) *n.* A motor neuron.

mo·tor (mō′tər) *adj.* **1.** Causing or producing motion. **2.** Of or being nerves that carry impulses from the nerve centers to the muscles. **3.** Involving or relating to movements of the muscles. **4.** Of or relating to an organism's overt reaction to a stimulus.

motor aphasia *n.* Aphasia in which the power to communicate by writing, speaking, or using signs is lost. Also called *ataxic aphasia, Broca's aphasia, expressive aphasia.*

motor area *n.* See **motor cortex.**

motor ataxia *n.* Inability to perform coordinated muscular movements necessary for moving the body, as for walking.

motor cortex *n.* The region of the cerebral cortex influencing movements of the face, neck and trunk, and arm and leg. Also called *excitable area, motor area, Rolando's area.*

motor decussation *n.* See **pyramidal decussation.**

motor endplate *n.* The large and complex terminal formation by which the axon of a motor neuron establishes synaptic contact with a striated muscle fiber. Also called *motor plate.*

motor fiber *n.* Any of the fibers in a mixed nerve that transmit motor impulses.

motor image *n.* The cerebral image of possible body movements.

motor nerve *n.* An efferent nerve conveying an impulse that excites muscular contraction.

motor neuron *n.* A neuron that conveys impulses from the central nervous system to a muscle, gland, or other effector tissue.

motor neuron disease *n.* Any of various diseases of motor neurons, such as progressive muscular atrophy, amyotrophic lateral sclerosis, progressive bulbar paralysis, and primary lateral sclerosis.

motor nuclei *pl.n.* See **nuclei of origin.**

motor paralysis *n.* Loss of voluntary control of muscular contraction.

motor plate *n.* See **motor endplate.**

motor speech center *n.* See **Broca's center.**

motor unit *n.* A single somatic motor neuron and the group of muscle fibers innervated by it.

motor urgency *n.* Urgent desire to empty the urinary bladder due to overactive detrusor function.

Mo·trin (mō′trĭn) A trademark for the drug ibuprofen.

mot·tled enamel (mŏt′ld) *n.* Defective enamel formation, varying in appearance from small white opacities to yellow and black spotting, due to excessive fluoride ingestion during tooth formation.

mound·ing (moun′dĭng) *n.* See **myoedema.**

mount (mount) *v.* To prepare a specimen for microscopic examination, especially by positioning on a slide.

moun·tain sickness (moun′tən) *n.* Altitude sickness brought on by the diminished oxygen pressure at mountain elevations.

mouse-tooth forceps (mous′tŏŏth′) *n.* A forceps with one or two fine teeth at the tip of each blade that mesh with the tooth or teeth on the opposite blade.

mouth (mouth) *n., pl.* **mouths** (mouthz) **1.** The body opening through which an animal takes in food. **2.** The oral cavity. **3.** The opening to any cavity or canal in an organ or a bodily part.

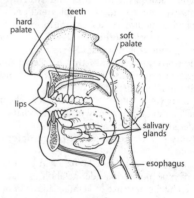

mouth

mouth-to-mouth resuscitation *n.* A technique used to resuscitate a person who has stopped breathing, in which the rescuer presses his or her mouth against that of the victim and, allowing for passive exhalation, forces air into the lungs every few seconds. Also called *mouth-to-mouth respiration.*

mouth·wash (mouth′wŏsh′) *n.* A medicated liquid for cleaning the mouth and treating diseased mucous membranes. Also called *collutory.*

mov·a·ble joint (mōō′və-bəl) *n.* **1.** A joint in which the opposing bony surfaces are covered with a layer of hyaline cartilage or fibrocartilage and in which some degree of free movement is possible. Also called *diarthrodial joint, diarthrosis, synarthrosis, synovial joint.* **2.** A joint, either a synchondrosis or a symphysis, in which the apposed bony surfaces are united by cartilage. Also called *amphiarthrosis, cartilaginous joint, synarthrodial joint, synarthrosis.*

movable testis *n.* A condition in which the testis tends to ascend to the upper part of the scrotum or into the inguinal canal.

move·ment (mōōv′mənt) *n.* **1.** The act or an instance of moving; a change in place or position. **2.** An evacuation of the bowels; defecation.

mox·a (mŏk′sə) *n.* A cone or cylinder of cotton wool or other combustible material, placed on the skin and ignited in order to produce counterirritation.

mox·i·bus·tion (mŏk′sĭ-bŭs′chən) *n.* The burning of moxa or other substances on the skin to treat diseases or to produce analgesia.

MPD *abbr.* maximal permissible dose; multiple personality disorder

M protein *n.* A surface protein present on strep bacteria that prevents white blood cells from engulfing and destroying the bacteria.

MPS *abbr.* mononuclear phagocyte system

MR *abbr.* mitral regurgitation

MRCP *abbr.* Member of the Royal College of Physicians

MRCS *abbr.* Member of the Royal College of Surgeons

MRD *or* **mrd** *abbr.* minimal reacting dose

MRI *abbr.* magnetic resonance imaging

mRNA (ĕm′är-ĕn-ā′) *n.* RNA, synthesized from a DNA template during transcription, that mediates the transfer of genetic information from the cell nucleus to ribosomes in the cytoplasm, where it serves as a template for protein synthesis. Also called *messenger RNA.*

ms *abbr.* millisecond

MS *abbr.* multiple sclerosis; mitral stenosis

msec *abbr.* millisecond

MSG *abbr.* monosodium glutamate

MSH *abbr.* melanocyte-stimulating hormone

Mt The symbol for the element **meitnerium.**

MTX *abbr.* methotrexate

mu (myo͞o, mo͞o) *n. Symbol* μ The 12th letter of the Greek alphabet. —*adj.* Of, relating to, or being a polypeptide chain that is one of five types of heavy chains present in immunoglobins.

Mu *abbr.* Mache unit

muc– *or* **muci–** *pref.* Variants of **muco–.**

mu·cif·er·ous (myo͞o-sĭf′ər-əs) *adj.* Muciparous.

mu·ci·form (myo͞o′sə-fôrm′) *adj.* Resembling mucus.

mu·ci·lage (myo͞o′sə-lĭj) *n.* A viscid preparation consisting of a solution of a plant-based gum in water and used in pharmacy as an excipient.

mu·ci·lag·i·nous (myo͞o′sə-lăj′ə-nəs) *adj.* Resembling mucilage; moist and sticky.

mu·cin (myo͞o′sĭn) *n.* Any of a group of glycoproteins found especially in the secretions of mucous membranes. —**mu′cin·ous** *adj.*

mu·cin·ase (myo͞o′sə-nās′, -nāz′) *n.* An enzyme, usually a hyaluronidase, that catalyzes the hydrolysis of mucopolysaccharide substances such as mucins. Also called *mucopolysaccharidase.*

mu·ci·ne·mi·a (myo͞o′sə-nē′mē-ə) *n.* Presence of mucin in blood. Also called *myxemia.*

mu·cin·o·gen (myo͞o-sĭn′ə-jən, -jĕn′) *n.* Any of various substances, such as glycoproteins, that form mucin through the imbibition of water.

mu·cin·oid (myo͞o′sə-noid′) *adj.* Resembling mucin.

mu·ci·no·sis (myo͞o′sə-nō′sĭs) *n.* A condition in which mucin is present in the skin in excessive amounts, or in abnormal distribution.

mucinous carcinoma *n.* An adenocarcinoma in which the neoplastic cells secrete significant amounts of mucin. Also called *colloid carcinoma.*

mu·cip·a·rous (myo͞o-sĭp′ə-rəs) *adj.* Secreting, producing, or containing mucus.

muciparous gland *n.* See **mucous gland.**

muco– *or* **muci–** *or* **muc–** *pref.* **1.** Mucus: *mucoprotein.* **2.** Mucosa: *mucin.*

mu·co·cele (myo͞o′kə-sēl′) *n.* **1.** A mucous polyp. **2.** A retention cyst of the lacrimal sac, paranasal sinuses, appendix, or gallbladder.

mu·co·cu·ta·ne·ous (myo͞o′kō-kyo͞o-tā′nē-əs) *adj.* Of or relating to the skin and a mucous membrane.

mucocutaneous junction *n.* The site of transition from skin to epithelium of a mucous membrane.

mucocutaneous leishmaniasis *n.* A chronic variable disease caused by *Leishmania braziliensis,* endemic in Central and South America, and characterized by lesions of the skin and mucous membranes, which heal but are followed after months or years by other often eroding lesions on the tongue and mucous membranes of the mouth and nose. Also called *American leishmaniasis, nasopharyngeal leishmaniasis, New World leishmaniasis.*

mucocutaneous lymph node syndrome *n.* A disease affecting young children, characterized by high fever, conjunctivitis, pharyngitis, enlargement of the cervical lymph nodes, bright red rashes on the hands and feet, and desquamation of fingers and toes. Also called *Kawasaki disease.*

mu·co·en·ter·i·tis (myo͞o′kō-ĕn′tə-rī′tĭs) *n.* **1.** Inflammation of the intestinal mucous membrane. **2.** See **mucomembranous enteritis.**

mu·co·ep·i·der·moid (myo͞o′kō-ĕp′ĭ-dûr′moid′) *adj.* Relating to a mixture of mucus-secreting and epithelial cells.

mu·coid (myo͞o′koid′) *n.* Any of various glycoproteins similar to the mucins, especially a mucoprotein. —*adj.* Of, containing, or resembling mucus.

mucoid degeneration *n.* The degeneration of connective tissue into a gelatinous or mucoid substance.

mu·co·lip·i·do·sis (myo͞o′kō-lĭp′ĭ-dō′sĭs) *n.* Any of a group of hereditary metabolic storage diseases resembling Hurler's syndrome but with normal urinary mucopolysaccharides.

mucolipidosis I *n.* Mucolipidosis having symptoms resembling those of Hurler's syndrome but milder, and with moderate mental retardation. Also called *lipomucopolysaccharidosis.*

mucolipidosis II *n.* Mucolipidosis characterized by symptoms resembling those of Hurler's syndrome but more severe, with normal levels of urinary mucopolysaccharides and the presence of inclusion bodies in cultured fibroblasts. Also called *inclusion cell disease.*

mucolipidosis III *n.* Mucolipidosis characterized by symptoms resembling those of Hurler's syndrome, but milder, with restricted joint mobility, short stature, mild mental retardation, and dysplastic skeletal changes.

mucolipidosis IV *n.* Mucolipidosis marked by psychomotor retardation, cloudy corneas, and retinal degeneration, with the presence of inclusion bodies in cultured fibroblasts.

mu·co·lyt·ic (myo͞o′kə-lĭt′ĭk) *adj.* Capable of dissolving, digesting, or liquefying mucus.

mu·co·mem·bra·nous (myo͞o′kō-mĕm′brə-nəs) *adj.* Relating to a mucous membrane.

mucomembranous enteritis *n.* A disease of the intestinal mucous membrane characterized by constipation or diarrhea, colic, and the passage of pseudomembranous shreds or incomplete casts of the intestine. Also called *mucoenteritis.*

mu·co·pep·tide (myōō′kō-pĕp′tīd) *n.* See **peptidoglycan.**

mu·co·per·i·os·te·al (myōō′kō-pĕr′ē-ŏs′tē-əl) *adj.* Relating to mucoperiosteum.

mu·co·per·i·os·te·um (myōō′kō-pĕr′ē-ŏs′tē-əm) *n.* Mucous membrane and periosteum so intimately united as to form nearly a single membrane.

mu·co·pol·y·sac·cha·ri·dase (myōō′kō-pŏl′ē-săk′ə-rī-dās′, -dāz′) *n.* See **mucinase.**

mu·co·pol·y·sac·cha·ride (myōō′kō-pŏl′ē-săk′ə-rīd′) *n.* Any of a group of polysaccharides with high molecular weight that contain amino sugars and often form complexes with proteins. Also called *galactosaminoglycan, glycosaminoglycan.*

mu·co·pol·y·sac·cha·ri·do·sis (myōō′kō-pŏl′ē-săk′ə-rī-dō′sĭs) *n.* Any of several inherited diseases of mucopolysaccharide metabolism characterized by the accumulation of mucopolysaccharides in the tissues and their excretion in urine, resulting in various defects of bone, cartilage, and connective tissue.

mu·co·pol·y·sac·cha·ri·du·ri·a (myōō′kō-pŏl′ē-săk′-ə-rī-dŏŏr′ē-ə) *n.* The excretion of mucopolysaccharides in the urine.

mu·co·pro·tein (myōō′kō-prō′tēn′) *n.* Any of a group of organic compounds, such as the mucins, that consist of a complex of proteins and mucopolysaccharides and are found in body tissues and fluids.

mu·co·pu·ru·lent (myōō′kō-pyŏŏr′ə-lənt) *adj.* Containing mucus and pus.

Mu·cor (myōō′kôr) *n.* A genus of fungi of the family Mucoraceae, several species of which are pathogenic to humans.

mu·cor·my·co·sis (myōō′kôr-mī-kō′sĭs) *n.* See **zygomycosis.**

mu·co·sa (myōō-kō′sə) *n., pl.* **–sas** *or* **–sae** (-sē) See **mucous membrane.** —**mu·co′sal** *adj.*

mu·co·san·guin·e·ous (myōō′kō-săng-gwĭn′ē-əs) *or* **mu·co·san·guin·o·lent** (-gwĭn′ə-lənt) *adj.* Containing blood and mucus.

mu·co·sec·to·my (myōō′kə-sĕk′tə-mē) *n.* Excision of the mucosa, usually of the rectum prior to ileoanal anastomosis for treatment of ulcerative colitis.

mu·co·se·rous (myōō′kō-sîr′əs) *adj.* Containing or producing both mucus and serum.

mucoserous cell *n.* A glandular cell whose histologic characteristics fall between those of serous and mucous cells.

mu·co·sul·fa·ti·do·sis (myōō′kō-sŭl′fə-tĭ-dō′sĭs) *n.* A condition caused by deficiency of sulfatase enzymes and steroid sulfatases and characterized by coarse facial features, ichthyosis, hepatosplenomegaly, and skeletal abnormalities.

mu·cous (myōō′kəs) *adj.* 1. Containing, producing, or secreting mucus. 2. Relating to, consisting of, or resembling mucus.

mucous cell *n.* A cell that secretes mucus.

mucous colitis *n.* A disease of the mucous membrane of the colon, characterized by colicky pain, constipation or diarrhea, and the passage of mucous or slimy pseudomembranous shreds and patches. Also called *myxomembranous colitis.*

mucous connective tissue *n.* A gelatinous type of connective tissue characteristically supporting the blood vessels of the umbilical cord.

mucous gland *n.* A gland that secretes mucus. Also called *muciparous gland.*

mucous membrane *n.* A membrane lining all body passages that communicate with the exterior, such as the respiratory, genitourinary, and alimentary tracts, and having cells and associated glands that secrete mucus. Also called *mucosa.*

mucous plug *n.* A mass of mucus and cells filling the cervical canal between menstrual periods or during pregnancy.

mu·co·vis·ci·do·sis (myōō′kō-vĭs′ĭ-dō′sĭs) *n.* See **cystic fibrosis.**

mu·cus (myōō′kəs) *n.* The viscous slippery substance that consists chiefly of mucin, water, cells, and inorganic salts and that is secreted as a protective lubricant coating by the cells and glands of the mucous membranes.

mud fever *n.* Leptospirosis caused by the spirochete, *Leptospira grippotyphosa.*

Muehr·cke's lines (mŏŏr′kəz, mür′-) *n.* Parallel white lines in the fingernails and toenails associated with hypoalbuminemia.

Muel·ler electronic tonometer (myōō′lər) *n.* A Schiötz tonometer to which is attached an electronic device for indicating the extent of corneal indentation.

Muir-Torre syndrome (myŏŏr′-) *n.* See **Torre's syndrome.**

mu·li·e·bri·a (myōō′lē-ē′brē-ə, -ĕb′rē-ə) *n.* The female genital organs.

Mul·ler (mŭl′ər), **Hermann Joseph** 1890–1967. American geneticist. He won a 1946 Nobel Prize for the study of the hereditary effect of x-rays on genes.

Mül·ler (mŭl′ər, myōō′lər, mü′-), **Johannes Peter** 1801–1858. German physiologist who studied the physiology of the nerves and sense organs and described (1825) the müllerian duct.

mül·le·ri·an (myōō-lîr′ē-ən, -lĕr′-) *adj.* Relating to or described by German anatomist and physiologist Johannes Peter Müller (1801-1858).

müllerian duct *or* **Mül·ler's duct** (mŭl′ərz, myōō′lərz, mü′-) *n.* Either of two embryonic tubes extending along the mesonephros that become the uterine tubes, uterus, and part of the vagina in the female and that form the prostatic utricle in the male. Also called *paramesonephric duct.*

mul·tan·gu·lar bone (mŭl′tăng′gyə-lər) *n.* 1. The trapezium bone. 2. The trapezoid bone.

multi– *pref.* 1. Many; much; multiple: *multiarticular.* 2. More than one: *multiparous.* 3. More than two: *multipolar.*

mul·ti·ar·tic·u·lar (mŭl′tē-är-tĭk′yə-lər, mŭl′tī-) *adj.* Relating to or involving many joints.

mul·ti·ax·i·al joint (mŭl′tē-ăk′sē-əl, -tī-) *n.* A joint in which movement occurs in a number of axes. Also called *polyaxial joint*.

mul·ti·cel·lu·lar (mŭl′tē-sĕl′yə-lər, -tī-) *adj*. Having or consisting of many cells. —**mul′ti·cel′lu·lar′i·ty** (-lăr′ĭ-tē) *n*.

mul·ti·cus·pid (mŭl′tē-kŭs′pĭd, -tī-) *n*. A molar tooth with three or more cusps or projections on the crown. —**mul′ti·cus′pi·date′** (-pĭ-dāt′) *adj*.

mul·ti·fac·to·ri·al inheritance (mŭl′tĭ-făk-tôr′ē-əl) *n*. Inheritance involving many factors, of which at least one is genetic but none is of overwhelming importance, as in the causation of a disease by multiple genetic and environmental factors.

mul·ti·fid (mŭl′tə-fĭd′) *adj*. Divided into many clefts or segments.

mul·tif·i·dus (mŭl-tĭf′ĭ-dəs) *n*. A muscle with origin from the sacrum, the sacroiliac ligament, the lumbar vertebrae, the thoracic vertebrae, and the last four cervical vertebrae, with insertion into the spinous processes of all the vertebrae up to and including the axis, with nerve supply from the dorsal branches of the spinal nerve, and whose action rotates the vertebral column.

mul·ti·fo·cal (mŭl′tĭ-fō′kəl) *adj*. Relating to or arising from many foci.

multifocal lens *n*. A lens with segments providing two or more powers.

mul·ti·form (mŭl′tə-fôrm′) *adj*. Occurring in or having many forms or shapes; polymorphic. —**mul′ti·for′mi·ty** (-fôr′mĭ-tē) *n*.

mul·ti·grav·i·da (mŭl′tĭ-grăv′ĭ-də) *n*. A pregnant woman with one or more previous pregnancies.

mul·ti·in·farct dementia (mŭl′tē-ĭn′färkt′, -ĭn-färkt′, mŭl′tī-) *n*. See **vascular dementia**.

mul·ti·in·fec·tion (mŭl′tē-ĭn-fĕk′shən, -tī-) *n*. A mixed infection with two or more varieties of microorganisms developing simultaneously.

mul·ti·la·mel·lar body (mŭl′tē-lə-mĕl′ər, -tī-) *n*. See **cytosome** (sense 2).

mul·ti·lo·bar (mŭl′tē-lō′bər, -bär′, -tī-) *or* **mul·ti·lo·bate** (-lō′bāt′) *or* **mul·ti·lobed** (-lōbd′) *adj*. Having many lobes.

mul·ti·lob·u·lar (mŭl′tĭ-lŏb′yə-lər) *adj*. Having many lobules.

mul·ti·lo·cal (mŭl′tē-lō′kəl, mŭl′tī-) *adj*. Of or relating to traits resulting from the effects of multiple genetic loci operating together and simultaneously.

mul·ti·loc·u·lar (mŭl′tĭ-lŏk′yə-lər) *adj*. Having or consisting of many small compartments or cavities.

multilocular cyst *n*. A cyst containing several compartments formed by membranous septa.

mul·ti·nod·u·lar (mŭl′tĭ-nŏj′ə-lər) *or* **mul·ti·nod·u·late** (-lāt′) *adj*. Having many nodules.

multinodular goiter *n*. Adenomatous goiter with several colloid nodules.

mul·ti·nu·cle·ar (mŭl′tē-no͞o′klē-ər, -tī-) *adj*. Multinucleate.

multinuclear leukocyte *n*. See **polymorphonuclear leukocyte**.

mul·ti·nu·cle·ate (mŭl′tē-no͞o′klē-ət, -tī-) *or* **mul·ti·nu·cle·at·ed** (-ā′tĭd) *adj*. Having two or more nuclei.

mul·tip·a·ra (mŭl-tĭp′ər-ə) *n., pl.* **–ras** *or* **–rae** (-rē) A woman who has given birth two or more times.

mul·ti·par·i·ty (mŭl′tĭ-păr′ĭ-tē) *n*. The condition of being a multipara.

mul·tip·a·rous (mŭl-tĭp′ər-əs) *adj*. **1.** Relating to a multipara. **2.** Giving birth to more than one offspring at a time.

mul·ti·ple chemical sensitivity (mŭl′tə-pəl) *n. Abbr.* **MCS** An allergic condition attributed to extreme sensitivity to various environmental chemicals, as in air, food, water, building materials, or fabrics. Also called *chemical sensitivity*.

multiple fission *n*. Division of the nucleus, simultaneously or successively, into a number of daughter nuclei, followed by division of the cell body into an equal number of parts, each containing a nucleus.

multiple fracture *n*. The simultaneous fracture of several bones.

multiple lentigines syndrome *n*. An inherited syndrome characterized by multiple lentigines and electrocardiographic abnormalities, and often by abnormal distance between the eyes, pulmonary stenosis, and retarded growth.

multiple mucosal neuroma syndrome *n*. A syndrome seen in young persons and characterized by multiple submucosal neuromas or neurofibromas of the tongue, lips, and eyelids, sometimes accompanied by tumors of the thyroid or adrenal medulla or by subcutaneous neurofibromatosis.

multiple myeloma *n*. A malignant proliferation of plasma cells in bone marrow causing numerous tumors and characterized by the presence of abnormal proteins in the blood.

multiple myositis *n*. The occurrence of multiple foci of acute inflammation in the muscular tissue and overlying skin in various parts of the body, accompanied by fever and other signs of systemic infection.

multiple neuritis *n*. See **polyneuritis**.

multiple neurofibroma *n*. See **neurofibromatosis**.

multiple personality disorder *n. Abbr.* **MPD** A dissociative disorder in which two or more distinct personalities exist in the same person, each of which prevails at a particular time. Also called *dissociative identity disorder*.

multiple pregnancy *n*. The state of bearing two or more fetuses simultaneously.

multiple puncture tuberculin test *n*. A tine test in which the tuberculin or purified protein is inserted under the skin by repeated punctures with several needles or prongs.

multiple sclerosis *n. Abbr.* **MS** A chronic degenerative disease of the central nervous system in which gradual destruction of myelin occurs in patches throughout the brain or spinal cord or both, interfering with the nerve pathways and causing muscular weakness, loss of coordination, and speech and visual disturbances. It occurs chiefly in young adults and is thought to be caused by a defect in the immune system that may be of genetic or viral origin.

multiple stain *n*. A mixture of several dyes, each having an independent selective action on one or more portions of the tissue specimen.

multiple symmetric lipomatosis *n.* The accumulation and progressive enlargement of collections of adipose tissue in the subcutaneous tissue of the head, neck, upper trunk, and upper portions of the upper extremities.

multiple vision *n.* See **polyopia.**

mul·ti·pli·ca·tion (mŭl′tə-plĭ-kā′shən) *n.* **1.** The act or process of multiplying or the condition of being multiplied. **2.** Propagation of plants and animals; procreation.

mul·ti·pli·ca·tive division (mŭl′tə-plĭk′ə-tĭv, mŭl′tə-plĭ-kā′tĭv) *n.* Reproduction by simultaneous division of a mother cell into daughter cells.

mul·ti·ply (mŭl′tə-plī′) *v.* **1.** To increase the amount, number, or degree of. **2.** To breed or propagate.

mul·ti·po·lar (mŭl′tĭ-pō′lər) *adj.* Having more than two poles. Used of a nerve cell that has branches that project from several points.

multipolar cell *n.* A neuron having several dendrites arising from the cell body.

multipolar neuron *n.* A neuron with one axon and three or more dendrites.

mul·ti·syn·ap·tic (mŭl′tē-sĭ-năp′tĭk, -tī-) *adj.* Having or relating to two or more synapses.

mul·ti·sys·tem·ic (mŭl′tĭ-sĭ-stĕm′ĭk, -stē′mĭk) *adj.* Relating to a disease or condition that affects many organ systems of the body.

mul·ti·va·lent (mŭl′tĭ-vā′lənt) *adj.* **1.** Polyvalent. **2.** Of or relating to the association of three or more homologous chromosomes during the first division of meiosis. **3.** Having several sites of attachment for an antibody or antigen. **4.** Having various meanings or values. —**mul′ti·va′lence** *n.*

multivalent vaccine *n.* See **polyvalent vaccine.**

mul·ti·vi·ta·min (mŭl′tə-vī′tə-mĭn) *adj.* Containing many vitamins. —*n.* A preparation containing many vitamins.

mum·mi·fi·ca·tion (mŭm′ə-fĭ-kā′shən) *n.* The shriveling of a dead and retained fetus.

mumps (mŭmps) *pl.n.* An acute inflammatory contagious disease caused by a paramyxovirus and characterized by swelling of the salivary glands, especially the parotids, and sometimes of the pancreas, ovaries, or testes. This disease, mainly affecting children, can be prevented by vaccination. Also called *epidemic parotitis.*

mumps skin test antigen *n.* A sterile suspension of killed mumps virus used to determine mumps susceptibility or to confirm a tentative diagnosis.

mumps virus *n.* A paramyxovirus that causes mumps, transmitted by infected salivary secretions. Also called *epidemic parotitis virus.*

mumps virus vaccine *n.* A vaccine containing live attenuated mumps virus prepared in chick embryo cell cultures, used to immunize against mumps.

Mun·chau·sen syndrome *or* **Munch·hau·sen syndrome** (mŭn′chou′zən, mŭnch′hou′-, münкн′hou′-) *n.* A psychological disorder characterized by the repeated fabrication of disease symptoms for the purpose of gaining medical attention.

Munchausen syndrome by proxy *n.* A psychological disorder in which a parent or other caregiver seeks attention from medical professionals by causing or fabricating disease symptoms in a child.

Mun·ro's microabscess (mən-rōz′) *n.* A microscopic collection of polymorphonuclear white blood cells found in the stratum corneum in psoriasis. Also called *Munro's abscess.*

mu·pir·o·cin calcium (myōō-pîr′ə-sĭn) *n.* An antibiotic that is produced by the bacterium *Pseudomonas fluorescens* and inhibits protein synthesis by streptococcal and staphylococcal bacteria. It is used locally in the treatment of bacterial skin infections, such as impetigo.

mu·ral (myŏŏr′əl) *adj.* Of or relating to the wall of any cavity.

mural endocarditis *n.* Endocarditis other than valvular, affecting the endocardium of the heart chamber walls. Also called *parietal endocarditis.*

mural thrombosis *n.* Formation of a thrombus in contact with the endocardial lining of a cardiac chamber or, if not occlusive, with a wall of a large blood vessel.

mural thrombus *n.* A thrombus formed on and attached to a diseased patch of endocardium.

mu·ram·i·dase (myōō-răm′ĭ-dās′, -dāz′) *n.* See **lysozyme.**

mu·re·in (myŏŏr′ē-ĭn, myŏŏr′ēn′) *n.* See **peptidoglycan.**

mu·ri·at·ic (myŏŏr′ē-ăt′ĭk) *adj.* Relating to brine.

mu·rine (myŏŏr′īn′) *adj.* Of, relating to, or transmitted by a member of the rodent family Muridae, including rats and mice.

murine typhus *n.* A comparatively mild, acute, endemic form of typhus caused by the microorganism *Rickettsia typhi,* transmitted from rats to humans by fleas and characterized by fever, headache, and muscular pain. Also called *endemic typhus.*

mur·mur (mûr′mər) *n.* An abnormal sound that is heard during the auscultation of the heart, lungs, or blood vessels.

Mur·phy (mûr′fē), **William Parry** 1892–1987. American physician. He shared a 1934 Nobel Prize for discovering that a diet of liver relieves anemia.

Murphy drip *n.* See **proctoclysis.**

Mur·ray (mûr′ē), **Joseph E.** Born 1919. American physician. He shared a 1990 Nobel Prize for developing techniques for bone marrow and kidney transplants.

Mus·ca (mŭs′kə) *n.* A genus of flies of the family Muscidae that includes *M. domestica,* the common housefly, a species involved in the transfer of numerous pathogens.

mus·cae vol·i·tan·tes (mŭs′ē vŏl′ĭ-tăn′tēz, mŭs′kē) *pl.n.* Floaters.

mus·ca·rine (mŭs′kə-rēn′) *n.* A highly toxic alkaloid related to the cholines and having neurologic effects, isolated from certain mushrooms, especially *Amanita muscaria.* —**mus′ca·rin′ic** (-rĭn′ĭk) *adj.*

mus·cle (mŭs′əl) *n.* **1.** A tissue consisting predominantly of contractile cells and classified as skeletal, cardiac, or smooth, the last lacking transverse striations characteristic of the first two. **2.** Any of the contractile organs of the body by which movements of the various organs and parts are effected, and whose fibers are usually attached at each extremity to a bone or other structure by a tendon.

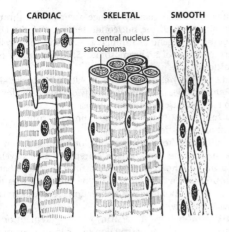

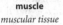

muscle
muscular tissue

mus·cle·bound *or* **mus·cle-bound** (mŭs′əl-bound′) *adj.* Having inelastic, overdeveloped muscles that function poorly together for concerted action.

muscle fiber *n.* A cylindrical multinucleate cell composed of myofibrils that contract when stimulated.

muscle hemoglobin *n.* See **myoglobin**.

muscle of antitragus *n.* A band of transverse muscular fibers located on the outer surface of the antitragus, that arise from the border of the notch between the tragus and antitragus, and that insert into the anthelix and the helix.

muscle of facial expression *n.* See **facial muscle**.

muscle of heart *n.* See **cardiac muscle**.

muscle of larynx *n.* Any of the intrinsic muscles that regulate the length, position, and tension of the vocal cords and adjust the size of the openings between the aryepiglottic folds, the ventricular folds, and the vocal folds.

muscle of tragus *n.* A band of vertical muscular fibers on the outer surface of the tragus of the ear.

muscle of uvula *n.* A muscle with origin from the posterior nasal spine, whose insertion forms the bulk of the uvula and whose action raises the uvula.

muscle plasma *n.* An alkaline fluid in muscle that coagulates spontaneously, separating into myosin and muscle serum.

muscle plate *n.* See **myotome** (sense 1).

muscle serum *n.* The fluid remaining after coagulation of muscle plasma and separation of myosin.

muscles of auditory ossicles *pl.n.* The stapedius muscle and the tensor muscle of the tympanic membrane considered as a unit.

muscles of eyeball *pl.n.* The muscles in the eye socket, comprising the four rectus muscles, the two oblique muscles, and the upper eyelid elevator muscle.

muscles of head *pl.n.* The muscles of facial expression, mastication, and the suboccipital muscles considered as a group.

muscles of mastication *pl.n.* The masseter, temporal, lateral pterygoid, and medial pterygoid muscles considered as a group.

muscle spasm *n.* Persistent increased tension and shortness in a muscle or group of muscles that cannot be released voluntarily.

muscle spindle *n.* A stretch receptor found in vertebrate muscle.

mus·cu·lar (mŭs′kyə-lər) *adj.* **1.** Of, relating to, or consisting of muscle. **2.** Having or characterized by well-developed muscles.

muscular anesthesia *n.* Loss of muscle sense, specifically, loss of the ability to determine the position of a limb or to distinguish differences in weight.

muscular asthenopia *n.* Asthenopia due to imbalance of the extrinsic ocular muscles.

muscular dystrophy *n. Abbr.* **MD 1.** Any of a group of progressive muscle disorders caused by a defect in one or more genes that control muscle function and characterized by gradual irreversible wasting of skeletal muscle. Also called *myodystrophy.* **2.** Pseudohypertrophic muscular dystrophy.

mus·cu·lar·is (mŭs′kyə-lâr′ĭs) *n.* The muscular coat of a hollow organ or tubular structure.

mus·cu·lar·i·ty (mŭs′kyə-lăr′ĭ-tē) *n.* The state or condition of having well-developed muscles.

muscular layer of mucosa *n.* The thin layer of smooth muscle found in most parts of the digestive tube, located outside the lamina propria mucosae and adjacent to the tela submucosa.

muscular relaxant *n.* An agent that relaxes striated muscle.

muscular system *n.* All the muscles of the body collectively, especially the voluntary skeletal muscles.

muscular triangle *n.* The triangle bounded by the sternocleidomastoid muscle, by the superior belly of the omohyoid muscle, and by the anterior midline of the neck, and occupied by the infrahyoid muscles.

mus·cu·la·ture (mŭs′kyə-lə-chŏŏr′) *n.* The arrangement of the muscles in a part or in the body as a whole.

mus·cu·lo·ap·o·neu·rot·ic (mŭs′kyə-lō-ăp′ə-nōō-rŏt′-ĭk) *adj.* Relating to a muscle and its aponeurosis of origin or insertion.

mus·cu·lo·cu·ta·ne·ous (mŭs′kyə-lō-kyōō-tā′nē-əs) *adj.* Of or supplying the muscle and the skin.

musculocutaneous nerve *n.* A nerve that arises from the lateral cord of the brachial plexus, and that passes through the coracobrachial muscle and then downward between the brachial and the biceps muscles, supplying these three muscles and being prolonged as the lateral cutaneous nerve of the forearm.

mus·cu·lo·mem·bra·nous (mŭs′kyə-lō-mĕm′brə-nəs) *adj.* Relating to both muscle and membrane.

mus·cu·lo·phren·ic artery (mŭs′kyə-lō-frĕn′ĭk) *n.* An artery with its origin in the lateral terminal branch of the internal thoracic artery, with distribution to the diaphragm and the intercostal muscles, and with anastomoses to the branches of the pericardiacophrenic and inferior phrenic.

musculophrenic vein *n.* Any of the veins that accompany the musculophrenic artery and drain blood from the upper abdominal wall, the lower intercostal spaces, and the diaphragm.

mus·cu·lo·skel·e·tal (mŭs′kyə-lō-skĕl′ĭ-tl) *adj.* Relating to or involving the muscles and the skeleton.

mus·cu·lo·spi·ral paralysis (mŭs′kyə-lō-spī′rəl) *n.* Paralysis of the muscles of the forearm due to injury of the radial nerve.

mus·cu·lo·ten·di·nous (mŭs′kyə-lō-tĕn′də-nəs) *adj.* Relating to both muscle and tendon.

musculotendinous cuff *n.* See rotator cuff.

mus·cu·lo·trop·ic (mŭs′kyə-lō-trŏp′ĭk, -trŏ′pĭk) *adj.* Of, affecting, acting upon, or attracted to muscular tissue.

mus·cu·lo·tu·bal canal (mŭs′kyə-lō-tōo′bəl) *n.* A canal beginning at the petrous portion of the temporal bone, passing to the tympanic cavity, and divided into one canal for the auditory tube and into another canal for the tensor muscle of the tympanic membrane.

mus·cu·lus (mŭs′kyə-ləs) *n., pl.* **-li** (-lī′) Muscle.

mu·si·co·ther·a·py (myōo′zĭ-cō-thĕr′ə-pē) *n.* The treatment of mental disorders by means of music.

Mus·set's sign (mōo-sāz′, mü-) *n.* An indication of aortic insufficiency in which the head rhythmically nods in synchrony with the heartbeat.

mus·si·ta·tion (mŭs′ĭ-tā′shən) *n.* Movement of the lips as if speaking but without sound.

mus·tard gas (mŭs′tərd) *n.* An oily, volatile liquid that is corrosive to the skin and mucous membranes, causes severe, sometimes fatal respiratory damage, and was used in World War I as a chemical warfare agent.

Mustard operation *n.* Correction of abnormal blood circulation that is due to the transposed great arteries by creating an intra-arterial baffle that partitions the atrium and directs the pulmonary venous blood through the right ventricular opening and the systemic venous blood through the mitral valve into the left ventricle.

mustard plaster *n.* A medicinal plaster made with a pastelike mixture of powdered black mustard, flour, and water, used especially as a counterirritant.

mu·ta·cism (myōo′tə-sĭz′əm) *n.* See mytacism.

mu·ta·gen (myōo′tə-jən, -jĕn′) *n.* An agent, such as ultraviolet light or a radioactive element, that can induce or increase the frequency of mutation in an organism. —**mu′ta·gen′ic** *adj.* —**mu′ta·gen′i·cal·ly** *adv.* —**mu′ta·ge·nic′i·ty** (-jə-nĭs′ĭ-tē) *n.*

mu·ta·gen·e·sis (myōo′tə-jĕn′ĭ-sĭs) *n., pl.* **-ses** (-sēz′) The formation or development of a mutation.

mu·ta·gen·ize (myōo′tə-jĕn′īz) *v.* To cause mutation in a cell or an organism.

mu·tant (myōot′nt) *n.* An organism possessing one or more genes that have undergone mutation. —*adj.* Resulting from or undergoing mutation.

mutant gene *n.* A gene that has lost, gained, or exchanged some of the material it received from its parent, resulting in a permanent transmissible change in its function.

mu·tase (myōo′tās, -tāz) *n.* Any enzyme that catalyzes the rearrangement of atoms within a molecule, especially one that causes the transfer of a phosphate group from one carbon atom to another.

mu·ta·tion (myōo-tā′shən) *n.* 1. The act or process of being altered or changed. 2. An alteration or change, as in nature, form, or quality. 3. A sudden structural change within a gene or chromosome of an organism resulting in the creation of a new character or trait not found in the parental type. 4. The process by which

such a sudden structural change occurs, either through an alteration in the nucleotide sequence of the DNA coding for a gene or through a change in the physical arrangement of a chromosome. 5. A mutant. —**mu·ta′tion·al** *adj.*

mute (myōot) *adj.* Unable or unwilling to speak. —*n.* One who does not have the faculty of speech. No longer in technical use; considered offensive.

mu·tein (myōo′tēn′, -tē-ĭn) *n.* A protein arising as a result of a mutation.

mu·ti·lat·ing keratoderma (myōot′l-ā′tĭng) *n.* An inherited keratoderma of the extremities that develops during childhood and is characterized by fibrous bands around the middle phalanx of the fingers or toes that may cause spontaneous amputation. Also called *Vohwinkel syndrome.*

mu·ti·la·tion (myōot′l-ā′shən) *n.* Disfigurement or injury by removal or destruction of a conspicuous or essential part of the body. —**mu′ti·late′** *v.*

mut·ism (myōo′tĭz′əm) *n.* Absence of the faculty of speech.

mu·ton (myōo′tŏn′) *n.* The smallest unit of a chromosome in which alteration can be effective in causing a mutation.

mu·tu·al·ism (myōo′chōo-ə-lĭz′əm) *n.* A symbiotic relationship in which both species benefit. —**mu′tu·al·is′tic** *adj.*

mu·tu·al·ist (myōo′chōo-ə-lĭst) *n.* See symbion.

mu·tu·al resistance (myōo′chōo-əl) *n.* See antagonism.

mV *abbr.* millivolt

MV *abbr.* megavolt

MVA *abbr.* motor vehicle accident

MVP *abbr.* mitral valve prolapse

MW *abbr.* molecular weight

My *abbr.* myopia

my– *pref.* Variant of **myo–**.

my·al·gia (mī-ăl′jə) *n.* Muscular pain or tenderness, especially when diffuse and nonspecific. Also called *myodynia.* —**my·al′gic** (-jĭk) *adj.*

My·am·bu·tol (mī-ăm′byə-tôl′, - tōl′) A trademark for the drug ethambutol.

my·as·the·ni·a (mī′əs-thē′nē-ə) *n.* 1. Abnormal muscular weakness or fatigue. 2. Myasthenia gravis. —**my′as·then′ic** (-thĕn′ĭk) *adj.*

myasthenia grav·is (grăv′ĭs) *n.* A disease characterized by progressive fatigue and generalized weakness of the skeletal muscles, especially those of the face, neck, arms, and legs, caused by impaired transmission of nerve impulses following an autoimmune attack on acetylcholine receptors. Also called *Goldflam disease.*

myasthenic facies *n.* The facial expression in myasthenia gravis, consisting of drooping of the eyelids and corners of the mouth and weakness of the facial muscles.

my·a·to·ni·a (mī′ə-tō′nē-ə) *or* **my·at·o·ny** (mī-ăt′n-ē) *n.* Lack of muscle tone. Also called *amyotonia.*

myatonia con·gen·i·ta (kən-jĕn′ĭ-tə) *n.* See amyotonia congenita.

my·at·ro·phy (mī-ăt′rə-fē) *n.* Variant of myoatrophy.

My·ce·lex (mī′sə-lĕks′) A trademark for the drug clotrimazole.

my·ce·li·um (mī-sē′lē-əm) *n., pl.* **-li·a** (-lē-ə) The vegetative part of a fungus, which consists of a mass of branching, threadlike hyphae. —**my·ce′li·al, my·ce′li·an** *adj.*

my·cete (mī′sēt′) *n.* A fungus.

–**mycete** *suff.* Fungus: *actinomycete.*

my·ce·tism (mī′sĭ-tĭz′əm) *or* **my·ce·tis·mus** (mī′sĭ-tĭz′-məs) *n.* Mushroom poisoning.

myceto– *or* **mycet–** *pref.* Fungus: *mycetogenic.*

my·ce·to·ge·net·ic (mī-sē′tō-jə-nĕt′ĭk, mī′sĭ-tō-) *or* **my·ce·to·gen·ic** (-jĕn′ĭk) *adj.* Caused by fungi.

my·ce·to·ma (mī′sĭ-tō′mə) *n.* **1.** A chronic, slowly progressing bacterial or fungal infection usually of the foot or leg, characterized by nodules that discharge an oily pus. Also called *Madura boil.* **2.** A tumor that is produced by filamentous fungi. —**my′ce·to′ma·tous** (-tō′mə-təs, -tŏm′ə-) *adj.*

my·cid (mī′sĭd) *n.* An allergic reaction to a remote focus of mycotic infection.

–**mycin** *suff.* A substance derived from a bacterium in the order Actinomycetales: *erythromycin.*

myco– *or* **myc–** *pref.* Fungus: *mycology.*

my·co·bac·te·ri·o·sis (mī′kō-băk-tîr′ē-ō′sĭs) *n.* Infection with mycobacteria.

my·co·bac·te·ri·um (mī′kō-băk-tîr′ē-əm) *n.* Any of various slender rod-shaped aerobic bacteria of the genus *Mycobacterium,* which includes the bacteria that cause tuberculosis and leprosy.

Mycobacterium *n.* A genus of aerobic, nonmotile bacteria containing gram-positive rods and including both parasitic and saprophytic species.

Mycobacterium bal·ne·i (băl′nē-ī′) *n. Mycobacterium marinum.*

Mycobacterium kan·sas·i·i (kăn-zăs′ē-ī′) *n.* A bacterium that causes a pulmonary disease that resembles tuberculosis.

Mycobacterium lep·rae (lĕp′rē) *n.* Hansen's bacillus.

Mycobacterium ma·ri·num (mə-rī′nəm) *n.* A bacterium that causes swimming pool granuloma.

Mycobacterium phle·i (flē′ī) *n.* Timothy hay bacillus.

Mycobacterium scrof·u·la·ce·um (skrŏf′yə-lā′sē-əm) *n.* A bacterium frequently associated with cervical adenitis in children.

Mycobacterium tuberculosis *n.* Tubercic bacillus.

my·co·der·ma·ti·tis (mī′kō-dûr′mə-tī′tĭs) *n.* A skin eruption of mycotic origin.

my·col·o·gy (mī-kŏl′ə-jē) *n.* The branch of science dealing with the study of fungi. —**my·col′o·gist** *n.*

my·co·phage (mī′kə-fāj′) *n.* A virus that infects fungi.

my·co·plas·ma (mī′kō-plăz′mə) *n., pl.* **-mas** *or* **-ma·ta** (-mə-tə) A microorganism of the genus *Mycoplasma.* Also called *pleuropneumonia-like organism.* —**my′co·plas′mal** *adj.*

Mycoplasma *n.* A genus of nonmotile parasitic pathogenic microorganisms whose members lack a true cell wall, are gram-negative, and require sterols such as cholesterol for growth.

Mycoplasma hom·i·nis (hŏm′ə-nĭs) *n.* A microorganism that is found in the genital tract and anal canal of humans.

mycoplasmal pneumonia *n.* See **primary atypical pneumonia.**

Mycoplasma my·coi·des (mī-koi′dēz) *n.* A microorganism that causes pleuropneumonia in cattle and goats.

Mycoplasma pha·ryn·gis (fə-rĭn′jĭs) *n.* A microorganism occurring in humans as a commensal between the soft palate and the epiglottis.

Mycoplasma pneu·mo·ni·ae (nōō-mō′nē-ē) *n.* A microorganism causing primary atypical pneumonia in humans.

My·co·plas·ma·ta·les (mī′kō-plăz′mə-tā′lēz) *n.* An order of gram-negative nonmotile microorganisms that do not possess a true cell wall but are instead enclosed by a three-layered membrane and include pathogenic and saprophytic species, such as the pleuropneumonia-like organisms.

my·co·sis (mī-kō′sĭs) *n., pl.* **-ses** (-sēz) **1.** A disease caused by fungi. **2.** A fungal infection in or on a part of the body.

mycosis fun·goi·des (fŭng-goi′dēz) *n.* A chronic progressive lymphoma arising in the skin and initially simulating an inflammatory dermatosis.

My·co·stat·in (mī′kə-stăt′n) A trademark for the drug nystatin.

my·cot·ic (mī-kŏt′ĭk) *adj.* **1.** Relating to mycosis. **2.** Relating to a fungus.

mycotic aneurysm *n.* An aneurysm caused by the growth of fungi within the vessel wall, usually following impaction of a septic embolus.

my·co·tox·i·co·sis (mī′kō-tŏk′sĭ-kō′sĭs) *n.* Poisoning caused by ingestion of a mycotoxin.

my·co·tox·in (mī′kō-tŏk′sĭn) *n.* A toxin produced by a fungus.

my·co·vi·rus (mī′kō-vī′rəs) *n.* A virus that infects fungi.

my·dri·a·sis (mĭ-drī′ə-sĭs) *n.* Prolonged abnormal dilation of the pupil of the eye induced by a drug or caused by disease.

myd·ri·at·ic (mĭd′rē-ăt′ĭk) *adj.* Causing dilation of the pupils. —*n.* A mydriatic drug.

my·ec·to·my (mī-ĕk′tə-mē) *n.* Excision of a portion of muscle.

my·ec·to·py (mī-ĕk′tə-pē) *or* **my·ec·to·pi·a** (mī′ĭk-tō′pē-ə) *n.* Dislocation of a muscle.

myel– *pref.* Variant of **myelo–.**

my·el·ap·o·plex·y (mī′ə-lăp′ə-plĕk′sē) *n.* See **hematomyelia.**

my·e·la·te·li·a (mī′ə-lə-tē′lē-ə) *n.* A developmental defect of the spinal cord.

my·e·le·mi·a (mī′ə-lē′mē-ə) *n.* See **myelocytosis.**

my·e·len·ceph·a·lon (mī′ə-lĕn-sĕf′ə-lŏn′) *n.* The posterior portion of the embryonic hindbrain, from which the medulla oblongata develops. —**my′e·len·ce·phal′ic** (-sə-făl′ĭk) *adj.*

my·e·lin (mī′ə-lĭn) *or* **my·e·line** (-lĭn, -lēn′) *n.* **1.** A white fatty material composed chiefly of alternating layers of lipids and lipoproteins that encloses the axons of myelinated nerve fibers. **2.** Droplets of lipid formed during autolysis and postmortem decomposition. —**my′e·lin′ic** *adj.*

my·e·li·nat·ed (mī′ə-lə-nā′tĭd) *adj.* Having a myelin sheath.

myelinated fiber *n.* An axon enveloped by a myelin sheath. Also called *medullated fiber.*

my·e·li·na·tion (mī′ə-lə-nā′shən) *or* **my·e·li·ni·za·tion** (-nĭ-zā′shən) *n.* The acquisition, development, or formation of a myelin sheath around a nerve fiber.

my·e·li·nol·y·sis (mī′ə-lə-nŏl′ĭ-sĭs) *n.* Dissolution of the myelin sheaths of nerve fibers.

myelin sheath *n.* The insulating envelope of myelin that surrounds the core of a nerve fiber or axon and that facilitates the transmission of nerve impulses, formed from the cell membrane of the Schwann cell in the peripheral nervous system and from oligodendroglia cells. Also called *medullary sheath.*

my·e·li·tis (mī′ə-lī′tĭs) *n.* **1.** Inflammation of the spinal cord. **2.** Inflammation of the bone marrow. —**my′e·lit′ic** (-lĭt′ĭk) *adj.*

myelo– *or* **myel–** *pref.* **1.** Spinal cord: *myelitis.* **2.** Bone marrow: *myeloma.*

my·e·lo·blast (mī′ə-lə-blăst′) *n.* An immature cell of the bone marrow that is the precursor of a myelocyte. Also called *premyelocyte.*

my·e·lo·blas·te·mi·a (mī′ə-lō-blă-stē′mē-ə) *n.* The presence of myeloblasts in the circulating blood.

my·e·lo·blas·tic leukemia (mī′ə-lə-blăs′tĭk) *n.* A form of granulocytic leukemia characterized by abnormal numbers of myeloblasts in the blood and in various tissues.

my·e·lo·blas·to·ma (mī′ə-lō-blă-stō′mə) *n.* A malignant tumor consisting of myeloblasts.

my·e·lo·blas·to·sis (mī′ə-lō-blă-stō′sĭs) *n.* The presence of unusually large numbers of myeloblasts in the tissues or blood.

my·e·lo·cele (mī′ə-lə-sēl′) *n.* **1.** Protrusion of the spinal cord in cases of spina bifida. **2.** The central canal of the spinal cord.

my·e·lo·cyst (mī′ə-lə-sĭst′) *n.* A cyst that develops from a rudimentary medullary canal in the central nervous system.

my·e·lo·cys·to·cele (mī′ə-lō-sĭs′tə-sēl′) *n.* Spina bifida containing spinal cord substance.

my·e·lo·cyte (mī′ə-lə-sīt′) *n.* **1.** A large cell of the bone marrow that is a precursor of the mature granulocytes of the blood. **2.** A nerve cell of the gray matter of the brain or spinal cord. —**my′e·lo·cyt′ic** (-sĭt′ĭk) *adj.*

my·e·lo·cy·the·mi·a (mī′ə-lō-sī-thē′mē-ə) *n.* Myelocytes in the blood, especially in persistently large numbers.

myelocytic leukemia *n.* See **myelogenous leukemia.**

my·e·lo·cy·to·ma (mī′ə-lō-sī-tō′mə) *n.,* *pl.* **–mas** *or* **–ma·ta** (-mə-tə) A nodular, circumscribed, relatively dense accumulation of myelocytes.

my·e·lo·cy·to·sis (mī′ə-lō-sī-tō′sĭs) *n.* The occurrence of abnormally large numbers of myelocytes in the tissues or blood. Also called *myelemia.*

my·e·lo·dys·pla·sia (mī′ə-lō-dĭs-plā′zhə) *n.* Abnormal development of the spinal cord.

my·e·lo·fi·bro·sis (mī′ə-lō-fī-brō′sĭs) *n.* Fibrosis of the bone marrow associated with myeloid metaplasia, leukoerythroblastosis, and thrombocytopenia. Also called *myelosclerosis.*

my·e·lo·gen·e·sis (mī′ə-lō-jĕn′ĭ-sĭs) *n.* The development of bone marrow.

my·e·lo·ge·net·ic (mī′ə-lō-jə-nĕt′ĭk) *or* **my·e·lo·gen·ic** (-jĕn′ĭk) *adj.* **1.** Of or relating to myelogenesis. **2.** Myelogenous.

my·e·log·e·nous (mī-ə-lŏj′ə-nəs) *adj.* Produced by or originating in the bone marrow.

myelogenous leukemia *or* **myelogenic leukemia** *n.* Leukemia characterized by proliferation of myeloid tissue in areas such as bone marrow and the spleen and by the abnormal increase of granulocytes, myelocytes, and myeloblasts in tissues and in blood. Also called *granulocytic leukemia, myelocytic leukemia, myeloid leukemia.*

my·e·lo·gone (mī′ə-lə-gōn′) *or* **my·e·lo·go·ni·um** (mī′ə-lə-gō′nē-əm) *n.* An immature white blood cell of the bone marrow characterized by a relatively large, fairly deeply stained, finely reticulated nucleus that contains palely stained nucleoli, and by a scant amount of rimlike, nongranular, moderately basophilic cytoplasm.

my·e·lo·gram (mī′ə-lə-grăm′) *n.* An x-ray of the spinal cord after injection of air or a radiopaque substance into the subarachnoid space. —**my′e·log′ra·phy** (-lŏg′rə-fē) *n.*

my·e·loid (mī′ə-loid′) *adj.* **1.** Of, relating to, or derived from the bone marrow. **2.** Of or relating to the spinal cord.

myeloid leukemia *n.* See **myelogenous leukemia.**

myeloid metaplasia *n.* A syndrome characterized by anemia, enlargement of the spleen, and the presence of nucleated red blood cells and immature granulocytes in the blood, and accompanied by extramedullary hematopoiesis in the spleen and liver.

my·e·loi·do·sis (mī′ə-loi-dō′sĭs) *n.* Hyperplastic development of myeloid tissue.

myeloid sarcoma *n.* See **granulocytic sarcoma.**

myeloid series *n.* The various stages of cell development such as those seen in the granulocytic and erythrocytic series.

myeloid tissue *n.* Bone marrow consisting of the developmental and adult stages of red blood cells, granulocytes, and megakaryocytes in a stroma of reticular cells and fibers, with sinusoidal vascular channels.

my·e·lo·li·po·ma (mī′ə-lō-lĭ-pō′mə, -lī-) *n.* A benign tumor of the adrenal gland composed of adipose tissue, lymphocytes, and hemopoietic cells.

my·e·lo·ma (mī′ə-lō′mə) *n.,* *pl.* **–mas** *or* **–ma·ta** (-mə-tə) A tumor composed of cells derived from hemopoietic tissues of the bone marrow.

my·e·lo·ma·la·cia (mī′ə-lō-mə-lā′shə) *n.* Softening of the spinal cord.

my·e·lo·ma·to·sis (mī′ə-lō′mə-tō′sĭs) *n.* The occurrence of myelomas throughout the body.

my·e·lo·me·nin·go·cele (mī′ə-lō-mə-nĭng′gə-sēl′) *n.* Protrusion of the spinal membranes and spinal cord through a defect in the vertebral column. Also called *meningomyelocele.*

my·e·lo·mere (mī′ə-lə-mîr′) *n.* A neuromere of the spinal cord.

my·e·lo·neu·ri·tis (mī′ə-lō-nŏŏ-rī′tĭs) *n.* See **neuromyelitis.**

my·e·lon·ic (mī′ə-lŏn′ĭk) *adj.* Of or relating to the spinal cord.

my·e·lo·path·ic (mī′ə-lō-păth′ĭk) *adj.* Of or relating to myelopathy.

my·e·lop·a·thy (mī′ə-lŏp′ə-thē) *n.* Disturbance or disease of the spinal cord.

my·e·lop·e·tal (mī′ə-lŏp′ĭ-tl) *adj.* Directed toward the spinal cord. Used of nerve impulses.

myelophthisic anemia *n.* See **leukoerythroblastosis.**

my·e·loph·thi·sis (mī'ə-lŏf'thĭ-sĭs, -lō-tī'-) *n.* **1.** Wasting or atrophy of the spinal cord. **2.** Replacement of hemopoietic tissue in the bone marrow by abnormal tissue, usually fibrous tissue or malignant tumors. Also called *panmyelophthisis.* —**my'e·lo·phthis'ic** (mī'ə-lō-tĭz'ĭk, -tī'zĭk) *adj.*

my·e·lo·plast (mī'ə-lə-plăst') *n.* Any of the various cells that occur in the bone marrow and that form white blood cells, especially those cells in an early stage of development.

my·e·lo·poi·e·sis (mī'ə-lō-poi-ē'sĭs) *n.* The formation of bone marrow or of blood cells derived from bone marrow. —**my'e·lo·poi·et'ic** (-ĕt'ĭk) *adj.*

my·e·lo·pro·lif·er·a·tive (mī'ə-lō-prə-lĭf'ə-rā'tĭv) *adj.* Relating to or characterized by unusual proliferation of myelopoietic tissue.

myeloproliferative syndrome *n.* Any of a group of conditions resulting from a disorder in the rate of formation of cells of the bone marrow and including chronic granulocytic leukemia, erythremia, myelofibrosis, panmyelosis, and erythroleukemia.

my·e·lo·ra·dic·u·li·tis (mī'ə-lō-rə-dĭk'yə-lī'tĭs) *n.* An inflammation of the spinal cord and nerve roots.

my·e·lo·ra·dic·u·lo·dys·pla·sia (mī'ə-lō-rə-dĭk'yə-lō-dĭs-plā'zhə) *n.* Congenital maldevelopment of the spinal cord and spinal nerve roots.

my·e·lo·ra·dic·u·lop·a·thy (mī'ə-lō-rə-dĭk'yə-lŏp'ə-thē) *n.* Disease of the spinal cord and spinal nerve roots. Also called *radiculomyelopathy.*

my·e·lor·rha·gia (mī'ə-lō-rā'jə) *n.* See **hematomyelia.**

my·e·lor·rha·phy (mī'ə-lôr'ə-fē) *n.* Suture of a wound of the spinal cord.

my·e·lo·sar·co·ma (mī'ə-lō-sär-kō'mə) *n.* A malignant tumor derived from bone marrow or from one of its cellular elements.

my·e·lo·sar·co·ma·to·sis (mī'ə-lō-sär-kō'mə-tō'sĭs) *n.* The occurrence of myelosarcomas at various sites throughout the body.

my·e·lo·scle·ro·sis (mī'ə-lō-sklə-rō'sĭs) *n.* See **myelofibrosis.**

my·e·lo·sis (mī'ə-lō'sĭs) *n., pl.* **-ses** (-sēz) **1.** Abnormal proliferation of bone marrow tissue. **2.** Abnormal proliferation of medullary tissue in the spinal cord.

my·e·lo·to·mog·ra·phy (mī'ə-lō-tō-mŏg'rə-fē) *n.* Tomographic depiction of the spinal subarachnoid space following injection of a contrast medium.

my·e·lot·o·my (mī'ə-lŏt'ə-mē) *n.* Incision of the spinal cord.

my·e·lo·tox·ic (mī'ə-lō-tŏk'sĭk) *adj.* **1.** Inhibitory, depressant, or destructive to a component of bone marrow. **2.** Relating to, derived from, or having the features of diseased bone marrow.

my·en·ter·ic (mī'ĕn-tĕr'ĭk) *adj.* Relating to or characterizing the myenteron.

myenteric plexus *n.* A plexus of unmyelinated fibers and postganglionic autonomic cell bodies lying in the muscular coat of the esophagus, stomach, and intestines, and communicating with the subserous and submucous plexuses.

my·en·ter·on (mī-ĕn'tə-rŏn') *n.* The muscular coat of the intestine.

my·es·the·sia (mī'ĭs-thē'zhə) *n.* The sensation felt in a muscle when it is contracting. Also called *kinesthetic sense.*

my·ia·sis (mī'ə-sĭs, mī-ī'ə-sĭs) *n., pl.* **-ses** (-sēz) **1.** Infestation of tissue by fly larvae. **2.** A disease resulting from such infestation.

My·lan·ta (mī-lăn'tə) A trademark for a preparation containing simethicone, aluminum hydroxide, and magnesium hydroxide that is used as an antacid and antiflatulent.

My·li·con (mī'lĭ-kŏn') A trademark for the drug simethicone.

my·lo·hy·oid (mī'lō-hī'oid') *adj.* Relating to the region of the molar teeth of the lower jaw and the hyoid bone.

mylohyoid muscle *n.* A muscle with origin from the mylohyoid line of the mandible, with insertion into the upper border of the hyoid bone and the raphe separating the muscle from its fellow, with nerve supply from the mylohyoid nerve, and whose action elevates the floor of the mouth and tongue and depresses the jaw when the hyoid is fixed.

mylohyoid nerve *n.* A small branch of the inferior alveolar nerve that is distributed to the anterior belly of the digastric muscle and to the mylohyoid muscle.

myo– *or* **my–** *pref.* Muscle: *myograph.*

my·o·ar·chi·tec·ton·ic (mī'ō-är'kĭ-tĕk-tŏn'ĭk) *adj.* Relating to the structural arrangement of muscle or fibers.

my·o·at·ro·phy (mī'ō-ăt'rə-fē) *or* **my·at·ro·phy** (mī-ăt'rə-fē) *n.* Muscular atrophy.

my·o·blast (mī'ə-blăst') *n.* A primitive muscle cell having the potential to develop into a muscle fiber. Also called *sarcoblast.*

my·o·blas·tic (mī'ə-blăs'tĭk) *adj.* Relating to a myoblast or to the formation of muscle cells.

my·o·blas·to·ma (mī'ō-blă-stō'mə) *n.* A tumor composed of immature muscle cells.

my·o·bra·di·a (mī'ə-brā'dē-ə) *n.* Sluggish reaction of muscle following stimulation.

myocardial bridge *n.* A bridge of cardiac muscle fibers extending over the epicardial aspect of a coronary artery.

myocardial depressant factor *n. Abbr.* **MDF** A toxic factor in shock that impairs cardiac contractility.

myocardial infarction *n. Abbr.* **MI** Necrosis of a region of the myocardium caused by an interruption in the supply of blood to the heart, usually as a result of occlusion of a coronary artery. Also called *cardiac infarction.*

myocardial insufficiency *n.* See **heart failure** (sense 1).

my·o·car·di·o·graph (mī'ō-kär'dē-ə-grăf') *n.* An instrument for making tracings of the movements of the heart muscle.

my·o·car·di·op·a·thy (mī'ō-kär'dē-ŏp'ə-thē) *n.* See **cardiomyopathy.**

my·o·car·di·or·ra·phy (mī'ō-cär'dē-ôr'ə-fē) *n.* Suture of the myocardium.

my·o·car·di·tis (mī'ō-kär-dī'tĭs) *n.* See **carditis.**

my·o·car·di·um (mī'ō-kär'dē-əm) *n., pl.* **–di·a** (-dē-ə) The middle layer of the heart, consisting of cardiac muscle. —**my'o·car'di·al** *adj.*

my·o·car·do·sis (mī'ō-kär-dō'sĭs) *n.* **1.** Symptomatic signs of cardiac disease without any discoverable pathological lesion. **2.** Any of various degenerative conditions of the heart muscle, except myofibrosis.

my·o·cele (mī′ə-sēl′) *n.* Protrusion of muscle substance through an opening in its sheath.

my·o·cel·lu·li·tis (mī′ō-sĕl′yə-lī′tĭs) *n.* Inflammation of muscle and cellular tissue.

my·o·ce·ro·sis (mī′ō-sə-rō′sĭs) *n.* Waxy degeneration of the muscles.

My·o·chry·sine (mī′ō-krī′sĭn) A trademark for the drug gold sodium thiomalate.

my·o·clo·ni·a (mī′ə-klō′nē-ə) *n.* Any of various disorders characterized by myoclonus.

myoclonic astatic epilepsy *n.* A form of petit mal occurring in children with neurologic disabilities and mental retardation and characterized by atonic seizures and tonic-clonic attacks that generally are not halted by medication.

my·oc·lo·nus (mī-ŏk′lə-nəs) *n.* A sudden shocklike twitching of muscles or parts of muscles without any rhythm or pattern, occurring in various brain disorders. —**my′o·clon′ic** (mī′ə-klŏn′ĭk) *adj.*

myoclonus epilepsy *n.* A familial epilepsy beginning in childhood or adolescence and characterized by progressive mental deterioration, by the abrupt or continuous clonus of parts or groups of muscles, and, histologically, by the presence of Lafora bodies in parts of the central nervous system. Also called *Lafora body disease, Lafora's disease.*

myoclonus mul·ti·plex (mŭl′tə-plĕks′) *n.* A disorder characterized by rapid contractions occurring simultaneously or consecutively in various unrelated muscles. Also called *Friedreich's disease, paramyoclonus, polyclonia, polymyoclonus.*

my·o·cyte (mī′ə-sīt′) *n.* A muscle cell.

my·o·cy·tol·y·sis (mī′ō-sī-tŏl′ĭ-sĭs) *n.* The dissolution of muscle fiber.

myocytolysis of heart *n.* Local loss of myocardial syncytium as a result of a metabolic imbalance, insufficient in intensity or duration to cause stromal injury or to elicit an inflammatory reaction.

my·o·cy·to·ma (mī′ō-sī-tō′mə) *n., pl.* –**mas** *or* –**ma·ta** (-mə-tə) A benign tumor derived from muscle.

my·o·de·mi·a (mī′ō-dē′mē-ə) *n.* Fatty degeneration of muscle.

my·o·dyn·i·a (mī′ō-dĭn′ē-ə) *n.* See **myalgia**.

my·o·dys·to·ny (mī′ō-dĭs′tə-nē) *n.* A condition of slow relaxation interrupted by a succession of slight contractions following electrical stimulation of a muscle.

my·o·dys·tro·phy (mī′ō-dĭs′trə-fē) *n.* See **muscular dystrophy**.

my·o·e·de·ma (mī′ō-ĭ-dē′mə) *n.* Localized contraction of a degenerating muscle, occurring at the point of a sharp blow. Also called *idiomuscular contraction, mounding.*

my·o·e·las·tic (mī′ō-ĭ-lăs′tĭk) *adj.* Of or relating to closely associated smooth muscle fibers and elastic connective tissue.

my·o·e·lec·tric (mī′ō-ĭ-lĕk′trĭk) *adj.* Of or relating to the electrical properties of muscle tissue from which impulses may be amplified, used especially in the control or operation of prosthetic devices.

my·o·en·do·car·di·tis (mī′ō-ĕn′dō-kär-dī′tĭs) *n.* Inflammation of the endocardium and of the muscular wall of the heart.

my·o·ep·i·the·li·o·ma (mī′ō-ĕp′ə-thē′lē-ō′mə) *n.* A benign tumor of myoepithelial cells.

my·o·ep·i·the·li·um (mī′ō-ĕp′ə-thē′lē-əm) *n.* Contractile spindle-shaped cells arranged longitudinally or obliquely around sweat glands and around the secretory alveoli of the mammary gland. —**my′o·ep′i·the′-li·al** *adj.*

my·o·fa·cial pain-dysfunction syndrome (mī′ō-fā′-shəl) *n.* See **temporomandibular joint syndrome**.

my·o·fas·ci·al (mī′ō-făsh′ē-əl) *adj.* Of or relating to the fascia surrounding and separating muscle tissue.

my·o·fas·ci·tis (mī′ō-fă-sī′tĭs) *n.* See **myositis fibrosa**.

my·o·fi·bril (mī′ə-fī′brəl, -fĭb′rəl) *n.* One of the threadlike longitudinal fibrils occurring in a skeletal or cardiac muscle fiber. Also called *sarcostyle.*

my·o·fi·bro·blast (mī′ō-fī′brə-blăst′) *n.* A fibroblast having some of the characteristics of smooth muscle cells, such as contractile properties.

my·o·fi·bro·ma (mī′ō-fī-brō′mə) *n.* A benign tumor that consists chiefly of fibrous connective tissue, with variable numbers of muscle cells forming portions of the tumor.

my·o·fi·bro·sis (mī′ō-fī-brō′sĭs) *n.* Chronic myositis with diffuse hyperplasia of the interstitial connective tissue pressing upon and causing atrophy of the muscular tissue.

my·o·fi·bro·si·tis (mī′ō-fī′brə-sī′tĭs) *n.* See **perimysitis**.

my·o·fil·a·ment (mī′ə-fĭl′ə-mənt) *n.* Any of the ultramicroscopic filaments, made up of actin and myosin, that are the structural units of a myofibril.

my·o·gen·e·sis (mī′ə-jĕn′ĭ-sĭs) *n.* The formation of muscle cells or fibers.

my·o·gen·ic (mī′ə-jĕn′ĭk) *or* **my·o·ge·net·ic** (mī′ō-jə-nĕt′ĭk) *adj.* **1.** Giving rise to or forming muscular tissue. **2.** Of muscular origin.

my·og·e·nous (mī-ŏj′ə-nəs) *adj.* Relating to the origin of muscle cells or fibers; myogenic.

my·o·glo·bin (mī′ə-glō′bĭn) *n. Abbr.* **Mb** The oxygen-transporting protein of muscle, resembling blood hemoglobin in function but with only one heme as part of the molecule and with one-fourth the molecular weight. Also called *muscle hemoglobin.*

my·o·glo·bi·nu·ri·a (mī′ə-glō′bə-nŏŏr′ē-ə) *n.* Excretion of myoglobin in the urine.

my·o·glob·u·lin (mī′ō-glŏb′yə-lĭn) *n.* Globulin present in muscle tissue.

my·o·glob·u·li·nu·ri·a (mī′ō-glŏb′yə-lə-nŏŏr′ē-ə) *n.* Excretion of myoglobulin in the urine.

my·o·gram (mī′ə-grăm′) *n.* The tracing of muscular contractions made by a myograph. —**my′o·graph′** (-grăf′) *n.* —**my·o·graph′ic** *adj.* —**my·og′ra·phy** (mī-ŏg′rə-fē) *n.*

my·oid (mī′oid′) *adj.* Resembling muscle.

myoid cell *n.* See **peritubular contractile cell**.

my·o·in·o·si·tol (mī′ō-ĭ-nō′sĭ-tôl′, -tōl′, -ĭ-nō′-) *n.* A form of inositol that is a component of the vitamin B complex and occurs widely in microorganisms, higher plants, and animals.

my·o·kin·e·sim·e·ter (mī′ō-kĭn′ĭ-sĭm′ĭ-tər, -kī′nĭ-) *n.* A device for registering the duration and the extent of contraction of muscles in response to electric stimulation.

my·o·ky·mi·a (mī′ō-kī′mē-ə, -kĭm′ē-ə) *n.* A benign condition, often familial, characterized by irregular twitching of groups of muscle fibers giving a rippling appearance to the overlying skin. Also called *kymatism.*

my·o·li·po·ma (mī′ō-lĭ-pō′mə, -lī-) *n.* A benign tumor that consists chiefly of fat cells, with variable numbers of muscle cells forming portions of the tumor.

my·ol·o·gy (mī-ŏl′ə-jē) *n.* The scientific study of muscles. —**my′o·log′ic** (mī′ə-lŏj′ĭk) *adj.* —**my·ol′o·gist** *n.*

my·ol·y·sis (mī-ŏl′ĭ-sĭs) *n.* The dissolution or liquefaction of muscular tissue.

my·o·ma (mī-ō′mə) *n., pl.* –**mas** *or* –**ma·ta** (-mə-tə) A benign tumor of muscular tissue. —**my·o′ma·tous** (-ō′mə-təs, -ŏm′ə-) *adj.*

my·o·ma·la·cia (mī′ō-mə-lā′shə) *n.* Pathological softening of muscular tissue.

my·o·mec·to·my (mī′ə-mĕk′tə-mē) *n.* Surgical removal of a myoma, especially of a uterine myoma.

my·o·mel·a·no·sis (mī′ō-mĕl′ə-nō′sĭs) *n.* Abnormal dark pigmentation of muscular tissue.

my·o·mere (mī′ə-mîr′) *n.* The segment within a metamere that develops into skeletal muscle.

my·om·e·ter (mī-ŏm′ĭ-tər) *n.* An instrument for measuring the extent of a muscular contraction.

my·o·me·tri·al (mī′ō-mē′trē-əl) *adj.* Of or relating to the myometrium.

my·o·me·tri·tis (mī′ō-mĭ-trī′tĭs) *n.* Inflammation of the muscular wall of the uterus.

my·o·me·tri·um (mī′ō-mē′trē-əm) *n.* The muscular wall of the uterus.

my·o·ne·cro·sis (mī′ō-nə-krō′sĭs) *n.* Necrosis of muscle.

my·o·neme (mī′ə-nēm′) *n.* A muscle fibril.

my·o·neu·ral (mī′ə-nŏŏr′əl) *adj.* Of or relating to both muscles and nerves, especially to nerve endings in muscle tissue.

myoneural blockade *n.* Inhibition of nerve impulse transmission at myoneural junctions by a drug such as curare.

my·o·neu·ral·gia (mī′ō-nŏŏ-răl′jə) *n.* Neuralgic pain in a muscle.

myoneural junction *n.* The synaptic connection of the axon of a motor neuron with a muscle fiber.

my·o·pal·mus (mī′ə-păl′məs) *n.* The twitching of a muscle.

my·o·pa·ral·y·sis (mī′ō-pə-răl′ĭ-sĭs) *n.* Paralysis of the muscles.

my·o·pa·re·sis (mī′ō-pə-rē′sĭs, -păr′ĭ-) *n.* Slight muscular paralysis.

my·op·a·thy (mī-ŏp′ə-thē) *n.* Any of various abnormal conditions or diseases of the muscular tissues, especially one involving skeletal muscle. —**my′o·path′ic** (mī′ə-păth′ĭk) *adj.*

my·ope (mī′ōp′) *n.* One who is affected by myopia.

my·o·per·i·car·di·tis (mī′ō-pĕr′ĭ-kär-dī′tĭs) *n.* Inflammation of the muscular wall of the heart and of the enveloping pericardium.

my·o·pi·a (mī-ō′pē-ə) *n. Abbr.* **M, My** A visual defect in which distant objects appear blurred because their images are focused in front of the retina rather than on it; nearsightedness; shortsightedness. —**my·op′ic** (-ŏp′ĭk, -ō′pĭk) *adj.*

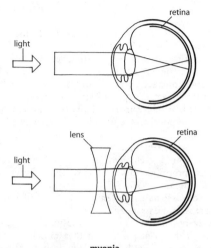

myopia
Top: *myopic vision*
Bottom: *corrected vision*

myopic astigmatism *n.* Astigmatism in which one meridian is myopic while the one at a right angle to it is without refractive error.

myopic crescent *n.* A white or grayish white crescent-shaped area in the fundus of the eye caused by atrophy of the choroid.

my·o·plasm (mī′ə-plăz′əm) *n.* The contractile portion of the muscle cell.

my·o·plas·tic (mī′ə-plăs′tĭk) *adj.* **1.** Of or relating to plastic surgery of the muscles. **2.** Of or relating to the use of muscular tissue in correcting defects.

my·o·plas·ty (mī′ə-plăs′tē) *n.* Plastic surgery of muscular tissue.

my·or·rha·phy (mī-ôr′ə-fē) *n.* Suture of a muscle.

my·or·rhex·is (mī′ə-rĕk′sĭs) *n.* Tearing of a muscle.

my·o·sal·pinx (mī′ō-săl′pĭngks) *n.* The muscular tunic of the uterine tube.

my·o·sar·co·ma (mī′ō-sär-kō′mə) *n.* A malignant tumor derived from muscular tissue.

my·o·scle·ro·sis (mī′ō-sklə-rō′sĭs) *n.* Chronic myositis with hyperplasia of the interstitial connective tissue.

my·o·sin (mī′ə-sĭn) *n.* The commonest protein in muscle cells, a globulin responsible for the elastic and contractile properties of muscle and combining with actin to form actomyosin.

myosin filament *n.* One of the contractile elements in skeletal, cardiac, and smooth muscle fibers.

my·o·sit·ic (mī′ə-sĭt′ĭk) *adj.* Of or relating to myositis.

my·o·si·tis (mī′ə-sī′tĭs) *n.* Inflammation of a muscle, especially a voluntary muscle, characterized by pain, tenderness, and sometimes spasm in the affected area. Also called *initis.*

myositis fi·bro·sa (fī-brō′sə) *n.* The induration of a muscle through an interstitial growth of fibrous tissue. Also called *myofascitis.*

myositis os·sif·i·cans (ŏ-sĭf′ĭ-kănz′) *n.* Ossification or the deposit of bone in muscle tissue, causing pain and swelling.

my·o·spasm (mī′ə-spăz′əm) *n.* Spasmodic contraction of a muscle.

my·o·tac·tic (mī′ə-tăk′tĭk) *adj.* Relating to the muscular sense of touch.

my·ot·a·sis (mī-ŏt′ə-sĭs) *n.* Stretching of a muscle. —**my′o·tat′ic** (mī′ə-tăt′ĭk) *adj.*

myotatic contraction *n.* A contraction of a skeletal muscle that occurs as part of a myotatic reflex.

myotatic irritability *n.* The ability of a muscle to contract in response to the stimulus produced by a sudden stretching.

myotatic reflex *n.* Tonic contraction of the muscles in response to a stretching force, due to stimulation of muscle proprioceptors. Also called *deep tendon reflex, stretch reflex.*

my·o·ten·o·si·tis (mī′ō-tĕn′ə-sī′tĭs) *n.* Inflammation of a muscle and its tendon.

my·o·te·not·o·my (mī′ō-tĕ-nŏt′ə-mē) *n.* Cutting through the principal tendon of a muscle, with partial or complete division of the muscle itself. Also called *tenomyotomy.*

my·o·tome (mī′ə-tōm′) *n.* **1.** The segment of a somite in a vertebrate embryo that differentiates into skeletal muscle. Also called *muscle plate.* **2.** A muscle or group of muscles derived from one somite and innervated by a single segment of a spinal nerve. **3.** A knife for dividing muscle.

my·ot·o·my (mī-ŏt′ə-mē) *n.* **1.** Dissection of the muscles. **2.** Surgical division of a muscle.

my·o·to·ni·a (mī′ə-tō′nē-ə) *n.* Delayed relaxation of a muscle after an initial contraction. —**my′o·ton′ic** (-tŏn′ĭk) *adj.*

myotonia a·troph·i·ca (ə-trŏf′ĭ-kə) *n.* See **myotonic dystrophy.**

myotonia con·gen·i·ta (kən-jĕn′ĭ-tə) *n.* A hereditary disease characterized by tonic spasm or temporary rigidity of certain muscles after an attempt has been made to move them. Also called *Thomsen's disease.*

myotonic dystrophy *n.* A chronic, slowly progressing, inherited disease that usually manifests its first symptoms when individuals reach their 30s, characterized by a wasting of the muscles, failing vision, opacity of the lens of the eyes, ptosis, slurred speech, and general muscular weakness. Also called *myotonia atrophica, Steinert's disease.*

my·ot·o·noid (mī-ŏt′n-oid′) *adj.* Of or relating to a muscular reaction characterized by slow contraction or relaxation.

my·ot·o·nus (mī-ŏt′n-əs) *n.* A tonic spasm or temporary rigidity of a muscle or group of muscles.

my·ot·o·ny (mī-ŏt′n-ē) *n.* Muscular tonus or tension.

my·ot·ro·phy (mī-ŏt′rə-fē) *n.* Nutrition of muscular tissue.

my·o·tube (mī′ə-tōōb′) *n.* A developing skeletal muscle fiber with a tubular appearance.

my·o·tu·bu·lar myopathy (mī′ō-tōō′byə-lər) *n.* See centronuclear myopathy.

my·rin·ga (mə-rĭng′gə) *n.* See **eardrum.**

myr·in·gec·to·my (mĭr′ĭn-jĕk′tə-mē) *n.* The excision of the tympanic membrane of the ear. Also called *myringodectomy.*

myr·in·gi·tis (mĭr′ĭn-jī′tĭs) *n.* Inflammation of the tympanic membrane. Also called *tympanitis.*

myringo– or **myring–** *pref.* Tympanic membrane: *myringoplasty.*

my·rin·go·dec·to·my (mə-rĭng′gō-dĕk′tə-mē) *n.* See **myringectomy.**

my·rin·go·plas·ty (mə-rĭng′gə-plăs′tē) *n.* Surgical repair of a damaged tympanic membrane.

my·rin·go·sta·pe·di·o·pex·y (mə-rĭng′gō-stā-pē′dē-ə-pĕk′sē) *n.* Tympanoplasty in which the tympanic membrane is functionally connected with the stapes.

myr·in·got·o·my (mĭr′ĭng-gŏt′ə-mē) *n.* Surgical puncture of the tympanic membrane, as for the removal of fluid or the drainage of pus. Also called *tympanostomy, tympanotomy.*

my·rinx (mī′rĭngks′, mĭr′ĭngks′) *n.* See **eardrum.**

myr·me·ci·a (mĭr-mē′shē-ə) *n.* Verruca in which the lesion has a domed configuration.

my·so·phil·i·a (mī′sə-fĭl′ē-ə) *n.* A pathological interest in dirt and filth, sometimes with sexual manifestations.

my·so·pho·bi·a (mī′sə-fō′bē-ə) *n.* An abnormal fear of dirt or contamination.

my·o·sis (mī-ō′sĭs) *n.* Variant of **miosis.**

my·ta·cism (mī′tə-sĭz′əm) *n.* Stammering in which the letter *m* is frequently substituted for other consonants. Also called *mutacism.*

myx·ad·e·no·ma (mĭk-săd′n-ō′mə) *n.* An adenoma having the structure of a mucous gland.

myx·as·the·ni·a (mĭk′săs-thē′nē-ə) *n.* Faulty secretion of mucus.

myx·e·de·ma (mĭk′sĭ-dē′mə) *n.* A disease that is caused by decreased activity of the thyroid gland in adults and is characterized by dry skin, swellings around the lips and nose, mental deterioration, and a subnormal basal metabolic rate. —**myx′e·dem′a·tous** (-dĕm′ə-təs, -dē′mə-), **myx′e·dem′ic** (-dĕm′ĭk) *adj.*

myx·e·mi·a (mĭk-sē′mē-ə) *n.* See **mucinemia.**

myxo– or **myx–** *pref.* Mucus: *myxoma.*

myx·o·chon·dro·fi·bro·sar·co·ma (mĭk′sō-kŏn′drō-fī′brō-sär-kō′mə) *n.* A fibrosarcoma in which there are intimately associated foci of cartilaginous and myxomatous tissue.

myx·o·chon·dro·ma (mĭk′sō-kŏn-drō′mə) *n.* A chondroma in which the stroma resembles primitive mesenchymal tissue.

myx·o·cyte (mĭk′sə-sīt′) *n.* One of the stellate or polyhedral cells present in mucous tissue.

myx·o·fi·bro·ma (mĭk′sō-fī-brō′mə) *n.* A benign tumor of fibrous connective tissue in which focal or diffuse degenerative changes result in portions that resemble primitive mesenchymal tissue. Also called *fibroma myxomatodes.*

myx·o·fi·bro·sar·co·ma (mĭk′sō-fī′brō-sär-kō′mə) *n.* A fibrosarcoma in which degenerative change or growth of less differentiated anaplastic cells results in portions that resemble primitive mesenchymal tissue.

myx·oid (mĭk′soid′) *adj.* Containing or resembling mucus; mucoid.

myxoid cyst *n.* See **ganglion** (sense 1).

myx·o·li·po·ma (mĭk′sō-lĭ-pō′mə, -lī-) *n.* A lipoma in which degenerative changes result in portions that resemble mucoid mesenchymal tissue.

myx·o·ma (mĭk-sō′mə) *n., pl.* **–mas** *or* **–ma·ta** (-mə-tə) A benign tumor composed of connective tissue embedded in mucus. —**myx·o′ma·tous** (-sō′mə-təs, -sŏm′ə-) *adj.*

myx·o·ma·to·sis (mĭk-sō′mə-tō′sĭs) *n.* **1.** A condition characterized by the growth of many myxomas. **2.** A highly infectious, usually fatal disease of rabbits that is caused by a pox virus and is characterized by many skin tumors similar to myxomas.

myx·o·mem·bra·nous colitis (mĭk′sō-měm′brə-nəs) *n.* See **mucous colitis**.

myx·o·pap·il·lar·y ependymoma (mĭk′sō-păp′ə-lĕr′ē, -pə-pĭl′ə-rē) *n.* A slow-growing ependymoma of the terminal filum occurring most often in young adults and consisting of cuboidal cells surrounding a mucinous vascular core.

myx·o·pap·il·lo·ma (mĭk′sō-păp′ə-lō′mə) *n.* A papilloma in which the stroma resembles primitive mesenchymal tissue.

myx·o·poi·e·sis (mĭk′sō-poi-ē′sĭs) *n.* The production of mucus.

myx·or·rhe·a (mĭk′sə-rē′ə) *n.* See **blennorrhea** (sense 1).

myx·o·sar·co·ma (mĭk′sō-sär-kō′mə) *n.* A sarcoma characterized by immature, relatively undifferentiated cells that grow rapidly and invade extensively, resulting in tissue that resembles primitive mesenchymal tissue.

myx·o·vi·rus (mĭk′sə-vī′rəs) *n.* Formerly, any of a group of RNA-containing viruses with an affinity for mucins, now included in the families of Orthomyxoviridae and Paramyxoviridae. These viruses include the influenza virus, parainfluenza virus, respiratory syncytial virus, and measles virus.

N

ν The Greek letter *nu.* Entries beginning with this character are alphabetized under **nu.**

n *abbr.* refractive index

N¹ The symbol for the element **nitrogen.**

N² *abbr.* newton

Na The symbol for the element **sodium.**

NA *abbr.* Nomina Anatomica (official system for anatomical nomenclature)

nab·i·lone (năb′ə-lōn′) *n.* A synthetic cannabinoid used in the treatment of nausea and vomiting associated with cancer chemotherapy.

na·bo·thi·an cyst (nə-bō′thē-ən) *n.* A retention cyst that develops when a mucous gland of the uterine cervix is obstructed. Also called *nabothian follicle.*

na·cre·ous (nā′krē-əs) *adj.* Resembling mother-of-pearl; lustrous.

NAD¹ (ĕn′ā-dē′) *n.* Nicotinamide adenine dinucleotide; a coenzyme occurring in most living cells and used as an oxidizing or reducing agent in various metabolic processes.

NAD² *abbr.* no apparent distress; no appreciable disease

NAD⁺ *n.* The oxidized form of NAD.

NADH (ĕn′ā-dē-āch′) *n.* The reduced form of NAD.

na·do·lol (nā-dō′lōl) *n.* A beta-blocker drug used primarily to treat angina pectoris.

NADP (ĕn-ā′dē-pē′) *n.* Nicotinamide adenine dinucleotide phosphate; a coenzyme occurring in most living cells and utilized similarly to NAD but interacting with different metabolites.

NADP⁺ *n.* The oxidized form of NADP.

NADPH (ĕn′ā-dē′pē-āch′) *n.* The reduced form of NADP.

Nae·ge·li syndrome (nā′gə-lē) *n.* An inherited disorder characterized by reticular skin pigmentation, diminished sweating, the absence of teeth, and hyperkeratosis of the palms and soles.

naf·cil·lin sodium (năf′sĭl′ĭn) *n.* An intravenous antibiotic used to treat staphylococcal infections.

Naff·zi·ger operation (năf′zĭ-gər) *n.* Removal of the lateral and superior orbital walls for the relief of severe exophthalmos.

Naffziger syndrome *n.* See **scalenus anterior syndrome.**

naf·ti·fine hydrochloride (năf′tə-fēn′) *n.* A broad-spectrum antifungal agent used in the topical treatment of tinea infections.

Nä·ge·le obliquity (nā′gə-lē′, nĕg′ə-lə) *n.* Inclination of the fetal head in cases of flat pelvis so that the anterior parietal bone presents to the birth canal. Also called *anterior asynclitism.*

Nä·ge·le's pelvis (nā′gə-lēz′, nĕg′ə-ləz) *n.* An obliquely contracted pelvis marked by the arrested development of one lateral half of the sacrum and by deviation of the pubic symphysis to the opposite side.

Nägele's rule *n.* A rule used as a means of estimating date of delivery by counting back three months from the first day of the last menstrual period and adding seven days.

nail (nāl) *n.* **1.** A fingernail or toenail. **2.** A slender rod used in operations to fasten together the divided extremities of a broken bone.

nail bed *n.* The formative layer of cells at the base of the fingernail or toenail; the matrix. Also called *keratogenous membrane, matrix unguis.*

nail fold *n.* A fold of hard skin overlapping the base and sides of a fingernail or toenail.

nail-patella syndrome *n.* See **onychoosteodysplasia.**

nail pit *n.* One of the small depressions on the surface of the nail plate caused by defective nail formation.

nail skin *n.* See **perionychium.**

na·ive *or* **na·ïve** (nä-ēv′) *or* **na·if** *or* **na·ïf** (-ēf′) *adj.* **1.** Lacking worldliness and sophistication. **2.** Simple and credulous as a child. **3.** Not previously subjected to experiments. **4.** Not having previously taken or received a particular drug. —*n.* One who is artless, credulous, or uncritical.

na·ked virus (nā′kĭd) *n.* A virus without an enclosing envelope, consisting only of a nucleocapsid.

nal·bu·phine hydrochloride (năl-byōō′fēn′) *n.* A synthetic opioid analgesic that has both agonist and antagonist narcotic properties.

na·li·dix·ic acid (nā′lĭ-dĭk′sĭk) *n.* A compound used in the treatment of infections of the genital and urinary tracts caused by gram-negative bacteria.

nal·ox·one hydrochloride (năl′ək-sōn′, nə-lŏk′sōn) *n.* A drug used as an antagonist to narcotic drugs such as morphine.

nal·trex·one (năl-trĕk′sōn) *n.* An endorphin and narcotic antagonist. It is devoid of pharmacologic action when administered in the absence of narcotics.

Na·men·da (nə-mĕn′də) A trademark for the drug memantine hydrochloride.

NAME syndrome (nām) *n.* See **LAMB syndrome.**

NANB hepatitis *abbr.* non-A, non-B hepatitis

na·nism (nā′nĭz′əm, năn′ĭz′-) *n.* See **dwarfism.**

nano– *pref.* **1.** Extremely small: *nanoid.* **2.** One-billionth (10^{-9}): *nanometer.*

nan·o·ceph·a·ly (năn′ō-sĕf′ə-lē) *n.* See **microcephaly.** —**nan′o·ce·phal′ic** (năn′ō-sə-fāl′ĭk), **nan′o·ceph′a·lous** (-sĕf′ə-ləs) *adj.*

nan·o·cor·mi·a (năn′ə-kôr′mē-ə) *n.* See **microsomia.**

nan·o·gram (năn′ə-grăm′) *n. Abbr.* **ng** One billionth (10^{-9}) of a gram.

nan·oid (năn′oid′) *adj.* Dwarflike.

nan·o·me·li·a (năn′ə-mē′lē-ə, -mēl′yə) *n.* See **micromelia.**

nan·o·me·ter (năn′ə-mē′tər) *n. Abbr.* **nm** One billionth (10^{-9}) of a meter.

nan·oph·thal·mi·a (năn′ŏf-thăl′mē-ə) *n.* See **microphthalmia.**

nan·oph·thal·mos (năn′ŏf-thăl′mŏs′) *n.* See **microphthalmia.**

Na·no·phy·e·tus sal·min·co·la (nā′nō-fī-ē′təs săl-mĭng′kə-lə) *n.* A parasitic fish-borne fluke that infests mammals that eat fish. Also called *Troglotrema salmincola.*

na·nous (nā′nəs, năn′əs) *adj.* Dwarfish.

na·nus (nā′nəs, năn′əs) *n.* A dwarf.

nape (nāp, năp) *n.* The back of the neck.

naph·tha (năf′thə, năp′-) *n.* Any of several highly volatile, flammable liquid mixtures of hydrocarbons distilled from petroleum, coal tar, or natural gas and used as solvents and in making various chemicals.

naph·tha·lene *or* **naph·tha·line** (năf′thə-lēn′, năp′-) *or* **naph·tha·lin** (-lĭn) *n.* A toxic carcinogenic hydrocarbon derived from coal tar or petroleum and used as a solvent. —**naph′tha·len′ic** (-lĕn′ĭk) *adj.*

naph·thol (năf′thôl′, -thōl′, năp′-) *or* **naph·tol** (-tôl, -tōl) *n.* An organic compound occurring in two isomeric forms, alpha-naphthol and beta-naphthol. Also called *naphthalenol.*

naphthol yellow S *n.* An acid dye used as a stain for basic proteins in microspectrophotometry.

Nap·ro·syn (năp′rə-sĭn′) A trademark for the drug naproxen.

na·prox·en (nə-prŏk′sən) *n.* A drug used to reduce inflammation and pain, especially in the treatment of arthritis.

nap·sy·late (năp′sə-lāt′) *n.* A sulfonate form of napthalene, used in the preparation of various pharmaceuticals.

Nar·can (när′kăn′) A trademark for the drug naloxone hydrochloride.

nar·cis·sism (när′sĭ-sĭz′əm) *or* **nar·cism** (när′sĭz′əm) *n.* **1.** Excessive love or admiration of oneself or. **2.** A psychological condition characterized by self-preoccupation, lack of empathy, and unconscious deficits in self-esteem. **3.** Erotic pleasure derived from contemplation or admiration of one's own body or self, especially as a fixation on or a regression to an infantile stage of development. **4.** The attribute of the human psyche characterized by admiration of oneself but within normal limits. —**nar′cis·sist** *n.* —**nar′cis·sis′tic** *adj.*

narco- *pref.* **1.** Numbness; stupor; lethargy: *narcolepsy.* **2.** Narcotic: *narcoanalysis.*

nar·co·a·nal·y·sis (när′kō-ə-năl′ĭ-sĭs) *n.,* *pl.* **-ses** (-sēz′) Psychotherapy conducted while the patient is in a sleeplike state induced by barbiturates or other drugs, especially as a means of releasing repressed feelings or thoughts. Also called *narcosynthesis.* —**nar′co·an′a·lyt′ic** (-ăn′ə-lĭt′ĭk) *adj.*

nar·co·hyp·ni·a (när′kō-hĭp′nē-ə) *n.* General numbness sometimes experienced upon waking.

nar·co·hyp·no·sis (när′kō-hĭp-nō′sĭs) *n.* Stupor or deep sleep induced by hypnosis.

nar·co·lep·sy (när′kə-lĕp′sē) *n.* A disorder characterized by sudden and uncontrollable, though often brief, attacks of deep sleep, sometimes accompanied by paralysis and hallucinations. Also called *hypnolepsy.* —**nar′co·lep′tic** (-lĕp′tĭk) *adj. & n.*

nar·co·ma (när-kō′mə) *n.* Stupor induced by a narcotic.

nar·co·sis (när-kō′sĭs) *n.,* *pl.* **-ses** (-sēz) General and nonspecific reversible depression of neuronal excitability, produced by a physical or chemical agent, usually resulting in stupor rather than in anesthesia.

nar·co·syn·the·sis (när′kō-sĭn′thĭ-sĭs) *n.* See **narcoanalysis.**

nar·co·ther·a·py (när′kō-thĕr′ə-pē) *n.* Psychotherapy conducted while the patient is under the influence of a sedative or narcotic drug.

nar·cot·ic (när-kŏt′ĭk) *n.* A drug derived from opium or opiumlike compounds, with potent analgesic effects associated with significant alteration of mood and behavior, and with the potential for dependence and tolerance following repeated administration. —*adj.* Capable of inducing a state of stuporous analgesia.

narcotic blockade *n.* The use of drugs to inhibit the effects of narcotic substances.

narcotic reversal *n.* The termination of the action of narcotics by the administration of antagonists, such as naloxone hydrochloride.

nar·co·tism (när′kə-tĭz′əm) *n.* **1.** Addiction to narcotics such as opium, heroin, or morphine. **2.** Narcosis.

nar·co·tize (när′kə-tīz′) *v.* To place under the influence of a narcotic. —**nar′co·ti·za′tion** (-tĭ-zā′shən) *n.*

Nar·dil (när′dĭl′) A trademark for the drug phenelzine.

nar·is (nâr′ĭs) *n.,* *pl.* **-es** (-ēz) The anterior opening on either side of the nasal cavity.

nar·row-an·gle glaucoma (năr′ō-ăng′gəl) *n.* See **angle-closure glaucoma.**

Na·sa·cort (nā′zə-kôrt′) A trademark for the drug triamcinolone.

na·sal (nā′zəl) *adj.* Of, in, or relating to the nose.

nasal bone *n.* An elongated rectangular bone that forms the bridge of the nose.

nasal capsule *n.* The cartilage surrounding the developing nasal cavity of an embryo.

nasal cavity *n.* The cavity on either side of the nasal septum, extending from the nares to the pharynx, and lying between the floor of the cranium and the roof of the mouth.

nasal concha *n.* See **ethmoidal crest** (sense 1, 2).

nasal crest *n.* The midline ridge in the floor of the nasal cavity to which the vomer is attached.

Na·sal·crom (nā′zəl-krŏm′) A trademark for the drug cromolyn sodium.

Na·sa·lide (nā′zə-līd′) A trademark for the drug flunisolide.

nasal meatus *n.* Any of three passages, designated inferior, middle, and superior, in the nasal cavity that are formed by the projection of the ethmoidal crests.

nasal muscle *n.* A muscle whose transverse part arises from the maxilla on each side and passes across the bridge of the nose, and whose alar part arises from the maxilla and attaches to the ala of the nose, with nerve supply from the facial nerve, and whose action dilates the nostrils.

nasal pit *n.* One of a pair of depressions formed in the developing face and giving rise to the rostral portion of the nasal meatus. Also called *olfactory pit.*

nasal point *n.* See **nasion.**

nasal reflex *n.* Sneezing caused by irritation of the nasal mucous membrane.

nasal septum *n.* The wall dividing the nasal cavity into halves, composed of a central supporting skeleton covered by a mucous membrane.

nasal spine of frontal bone *n.* A projection from the center of the nasal part of the frontal bone.

nas·cent (năs′ənt, nā′sənt) *adj.* **1.** Coming into existence; emerging. **2.** Of or relating to the state of a chemical element at the moment it is set free from one of its compounds. —**nas′cen·cy** *n.*

na·si·on (nā′zē-ŏn′) *n.* The point on the skull corresponding to the middle of the nasofrontal suture. Also called *nasal point.*

naso– *pref.* Nose: *nasopharynx.*

na·so·an·tral (nā′zō-ăn′trəl) *adj.* Relating to the nose and the maxillary sinus.

na·so·cil·i·ar·y nerve (nā′zō-sĭl′ē-ĕr′ē) *n.* A branch of the ophthalmic nerve that serves to supply the mucous membrane of the nose, the tip of the nose, and the conjunctiva.

na·so·fron·tal (nā′zō-frŭn′təl) *adj.* Relating to the nose and the forehead, or to the nasal cavity and the frontal sinuses.

nasofrontal vein *n.* A vein located in the anterior medial part of the eye socket, connecting an ophthalmic vein with the angular vein.

na·so·gas·tric (nā′zō-găs′trĭk) *adj. Abbr.* **NG** Relating to or involving the nasal passages and the stomach.

nasogastric tube *n.* A tube that is passed through the nasal passages and into the stomach.

na·so·la·bi·al (nā′zō-lā′bē-əl) *adj.* Relating to the nose and the upper lip.

nasolabial node *n.* Any of the lymph nodes near the junction of the superior labial and facial arteries.

na·so·lac·ri·mal (nā′zō-lăk′rə-məl) *adj.* Relating to the nasal bones and the lacrimal bones, or to the nasal cavity and the lacrimal ducts.

nasolacrimal canal *n.* The bony canal that is formed by the maxilla, lacrimal bone, and inferior concha and transmits the nasolacrimal duct.

nasolacrimal duct *n.* The passage leading downward from the lacrimal sac on each side of the nose, through which tears are conducted into the nasal cavity.

na·so·o·ral (nā′zō-ôr′əl) *adj.* Relating to the nose and the mouth.

na·so·pal·a·tine (nā′zō-păl′ə-tīn′) *adj.* Relating to the nose and the palate.

nasopalatine nerve *n.* A branch from the pterygopalatine ganglion, supplying the mucous membrane of the hard palate.

nasopharyngeal leishmaniasis *n.* See **mucocutaneous leishmaniasis.**

na·so·phar·yn·gi·tis (nā′zō-făr′ĭn-jī′tĭs) *n.* Inflammation of the nasal passages and of the upper part of the pharynx.

na·so·pha·ryn·go·la·ryn·go·scope (nā′zō-fə-rĭng′gō-lə-rĭng′gə-skōp′, -lə-rĭn′jə-) *n.* An endoscope that is used to visualize the upper airways and the pharynx. —**na′so·phar′yn·gos′co·py** (-făr′ĭn-gŏs′kə-pē, -făr′ĭng-) *n.*

na·so·phar·ynx (nā′zō-făr′ĭngks) *n.* The part of the pharynx above the soft palate that is continuous with the nasal passages. Also called *epipharynx.* —**na′so·pha·ryn′geal** (-fə-rĭn′jəl, -făr′ən-jē′əl) *adj.*

na·so·scope (nā′zə-skōp′) *n.* An instrument for examining the nasal passages; a rhinoscope.

na·so·si·nu·si·tis (nā′zō-sī′nə-sī′tĭs) *n.* Inflammation of the nasal cavities and the accessory sinuses.

na·so·tra·che·al tube (nā′zō-trā′kē-əl) *n.* An endotracheal tube inserted through the nasal passages.

Nas·se's law (năs′ĭz) *n.* The law that states that hemophilia affects only boys but is transmitted through females.

na·sus (nā′səs, -zəs) *n.* The nose.

na·tal (nāt′l) *adj.* **1.** Of, relating to, or accompanying birth. **2.** Of or relating to the buttocks.

na·tal·i·ty (nā-tăl′ĭ-tē) *n.* The ratio of births to the general population; the birth rate.

na·tes (nā′tēz) *pl.n.* The buttocks.

Na·thans (nā′thənz), **Daniel** 1928–1999. American microbiologist. He shared a 1978 Nobel Prize for the discovery of restriction enzymes and their application to molecular genetics.

na·ti·mor·tal·i·ty (nā′tə-môr-tăl′ĭ-tē) *n.* The proportion of fetal and neonatal deaths to the general natality; the perinatal death rate.

Na·tion·al Formulary (năsh′ə-nəl) *n. Abbr.* **NF** An official compendium providing standards and specifications to evaluate the quality of pharmaceuticals and therapeutic agents.

na·tive (nā′tĭv) *adj.* **1.** Originating, growing, or produced in a certain place or region; indigenous. **2.** Occurring in nature pure or uncombined with other substances.

native immunity *n.* See **innate immunity.**

na·tre·mi·a (nā-trē′mē-ə) *n.* The presence of sodium in the blood.

na·trif·er·ic (nā-trĭf′ər-ĭk) *adj.* Tending to increase sodium transport.

na·tri·um (nā′trē-əm) *n.* Sodium.

na·tri·u·re·sis (nā′trə-yŏŏ-rē′sĭs) *n.* Excretion of excessive amounts of sodium in the urine.

na·tri·u·ret·ic (nā′trə-yŏŏ-rĕt′ĭk) *adj.* Relating to or characterized by natriuresis. —*n.* A chemical compound that may be used to inhibit the tubular reabsorption of ions from glomerular filtrate, especially sodium ions, thereby resulting in greater amounts of that ion in the urine.

nat·u·ral antibody (năch′ər-əl, năch′rəl) *n.* See **normal antibody.**

natural childbirth *n.* A method of childbirth in which medical intervention is minimized and the mother often practices relaxation and breathing techniques to control pain and ease delivery.

natural dye *n.* A dye obtained from animals or plants.

natural history *n.* **1.** The study and description of organisms and natural objects, especially their origins, evolution, and interrelationships. **2.** A collection of facts about the development of a natural process or object.

natural immunity *n.* See **innate immunity.**

natural killer cell *n. Abbr.* **NK cell** A killer cell that is activated by double-stranded RNA and fights off viral infections and tumors.

natural mutation *n.* See **spontaneous mutation.**

natural selection *n.* The process in nature by which, according to Darwin's theory of evolution, only the organisms best adapted to their environment tend to survive and transmit their genetic characters in increasing numbers to succeeding generations while those less adapted tend to be eliminated.

na·tur·op·a·thy (nā′chə-rŏp′ə-thē) *n.* A system of therapeutics in which surgery and prescription medications are avoided, and preparations such as vitamins, nutritional supplements, and herbs are used to treat and prevent disease. —**na′tur·o·path′** (nā′chər-ə-păth′, nə-chŏŏr′-) *n.* —**na′tur·o·path′ic** *adj.*

nau·se·a (nô′zē-ə, -zhə, -sē-ə, -shə) *n.* A feeling of sickness characterized by gastrointestinal distress and an urge to vomit.

nausea grav·i·dar·um (grăv′ĭ-dâr′əm) *n.* See **morning sickness**.

nau·se·ant (nô′zē-ənt, -zhē-, -sē-, -shē-) *adj.* Inducing nausea or vomiting. —**nau′se·ant** *n.*

nau·se·ate (nô′zē-āt′, -zhē-, -sē-, -shē-) *v.* To feel or cause to feel nausea.

nau·se·at·ed (nô′zē-ā′tĭd, -zhē-, -sē-, -shē-) *adj.* Affected with nausea.

nau·seous (nô′shəs, -zē-əs) *adj.* **1.** Causing nausea. **2.** Affected with nausea. —**nau′seous·ly** *adv.*

Nav·ane (năv′ān′) A trademark for the drug thiothixene.

na·vel (nā′vəl) *n.* The mark on the surface of the abdomen that indicates where the umbilical cord was attached to the fetus during gestation. Also called *belly-button, umbilicus.*

na·vic·u·lar (nə-vĭk′yə-lər) *n.* **1.** A comma-shaped bone of the wrist that is located in the first row of carpals. **2.** A concave bone of the foot, located between the talus and the metatarsals. Also called *scaphoid.* —*adj.* Shaped like a boat.

navicular abdomen *n.* A condition in which the anterior abdominal wall is sunken, having a concave rather than a convex contour. Also called *scaphoid abdomen.*

navicular fossa of urethra *n.* The terminal portion of the urethra in the glans penis.

navicular fossa of vestibule of vagina *n.* See **fossa of vestibule of vagina**.

Nb The symbol for the element **niobium**.

NBT test (ĕn′bē-tē′) *n.* See **nitroblue tetrazolium test**.

Nd The symbol for the element **neodymium**.

Ne The symbol for the element **neon**.

near point (nîr) *n.* The nearest point of distinct vision.

near·sight·ed (nîr′sī′tĭd) *adj.* Unable to see distant objects clearly; myopic.

near·sight·ed·ness (nîr′sī′tĭd-nĭs) *n.* Myopia.

ne·ar·thro·sis (nē′är-thrō′sĭs) *or* **ne·o·ar·thro·sis** (nē′-ō-) *n.* **1.** A pseudarthrosis arising in an ununited fracture. **2.** A new joint resulting from a total joint replacement operation.

neb·u·la (nĕb′yə-lə) *n., pl.* **-las** *or* **-lae** (-lē′) **1.** A faint, foglike opacity of the cornea. **2.** A class of oily preparations for use in a nebulizer.

neb·u·liz·er (nĕb′yə-lī′zər) *n.* A device used to reduce liquid to an extremely fine cloud, especially for delivering medication to the deep part of the respiratory tract.

Ne·ca·tor (nĭ-kā′tər) *n.* A genus of nematode hookworms that includes certain intestinal parasites.

ne·ca·to·ri·a·sis (nĭ-kā′tə-rī′ə-sĭs) *n.* Infestation with the hookworm *Necator americanus,* whose adults attach to villi in the small intestine and suck blood, causing anemia.

neck (nĕk) *n.* **1.** The part of the body joining the head to the shoulders or trunk. **2.** A narrow or constricted part of a structure, as of a bone or organ, that joins its parts; a cervix. **3.** The part of a tooth between the crown and the root.

ne·crec·to·my (nĭ-krĕk′tə-mē) *n.* Surgical removal of necrosed tissue.

necro– *or* **necr–** *pref.* **1.** Dead body; corpse: *necrophilia.* **2.** Death: *necrobiosis.*

nec·ro·bi·o·sis (nĕk′rō-bī-ō′sĭs) *n.* **1.** Physiological or normal death of cells or tissues as a result of changes associated with development, aging, or use. **2.** Necrosis of a small area of tissue. Also called *bionecrosis.* —**nec′-ro·bi·ot′ic** (-ŏt′ĭk) *adj.*

necrobiosis li·poi·di·ca (lĭ-poi′dĭ-kə) *n.* A condition, occasionally associated with diabetes, in which shiny atrophic lesions develop on the legs. Also called *necrobiosis lipoidica diabeticorum.*

necrobiotic xanthogranuloma *n.* A cutaneous and subcutaneous xanthogranuloma with focal necroses that manifest as multiple large, sometimes ulcerated nodules, especially around the eyes; it is associated with paraproteinemia.

nec·ro·cy·to·sis (nĕk′rō-sī-tō′sĭs) *n.* The abnormal or pathological death of cells.

nec·ro·gen·ic (nĕk′rə-jĕn′ĭk) *or* **ne·crog·e·nous** (nə-krŏj′ə-nəs) *adj.* Relating to, living in, or having origin in dead matter.

necrogenic wart *n.* See **postmortem wart**.

ne·crol·o·gy (nə-krŏl′ə-jē) *n.* The science of the collection, classification, and interpretation of mortality statistics. —**ne·crol′o·gist** *n.*

ne·crol·y·sis (nĕ-krŏl′ĭ-sĭs) *n.* Necrosis and loosening of tissue.

nec·ro·ma·ni·a (nĕk′rə-mā′nē-ə, -mān′yə) *n.* **1.** An abnormal tendency to dwell with longing on death. **2.** See **necrophilia** (sense 1).

nec·roph·a·gous (nə-krŏf′ə-gəs) *adj.* **1.** Feeding on carrion or corpses. **2.** Necrophilous.

nec·ro·phil·i·a (nĕk′rə-fĭl′ē-ə) *n.* **1.** An abnormal fondness for being in the presence of dead bodies. Also called *necromania.* **2.** Sexual contact with or erotic desire for dead bodies. —**nec′ro·phil′i·ac′** (-ē-ăk′) *adj. & n.*

nec·roph·i·lous (nə-krŏf′ə-ləs) *adj.* Having a preference for dead tissue. Used of certain bacteria.

nec·ro·pho·bi·a (nĕk′rə-fō′bē-ə) *n.* An abnormal fear of death or corpses. —**nec′ro·pho′bic** *adj.*

nec·rop·sy (nĕk′rŏp′sē, -rəp-) *n.* See **autopsy**.

ne·crose (nĕ-krōs′, -krōz′, nĕk′rōs′, -rōz′) *v.* To undergo or cause to undergo necrosis.

ne·cro·sis (nə-krō′sĭs) *n., pl.* **-ses** (-sēz′) Death of cells or tissues through injury or disease, especially in a localized area of the body. —**ne·crot′ic** (-krŏt′ĭk) *adj.*

nec·ro·sper·mi·a (nĕk′rə-spûr′mē-ə) *n.* A condition in which there are dead or immobile spermatozoa in the semen.

necrotic cirrhosis *n.* See **postnecrotic cirrhosis**.

necrotic inflammation *n.* Inflammation characterized by rapid necrosis throughout the affected tissue.

necrotic pulp *n.* Dental pulp that is necrotic as a result of trauma, chemical action, or infection, and that produces no response to thermal stimulation. Also called *dead pulp, devitalized pulp, nonvital pulp.*

nec·ro·tize (nĕk′rə-tīz′) *v.* To undergo necrosis or cause to necrose.

ne·cro·tiz·ing enterocolitis (nĕk′rə-tī′zĭng) *n.* Extensive ulceration and necrosis of the ileum and colon in premature infants in the neonatal period.

necrotizing fasciitis *n.* Tissue death such as that associated with group A streptococcus infection.

necrotizing sialometaplasia *n.* Squamous metaplasia of the salivary gland ducts and lobules with ischemic necrosis of the salivary gland lobules, occurring most frequently in the hard palate.

necrotizing ulcerative gingivitis *n.* *Abbr.* **NUG** See trench mouth.

ne·crot·o·my (nə-krŏt′ə-mē) *n.* **1.** Excision of dead tissue. **2.** Dissection of a dead body.

ne·doc·ro·mil sodium (nə-dŏk′rə-mĭl′) *n.* A anti-inflammatory drug used in inhaler form to treat mild-to-moderate asthma.

nee·dle (nēd′l) *n.* **1.** A slender, usually sharp-pointed instrument used for puncturing tissues, suturing, or passing a ligature around an artery. **2.** A hollow, slender, sharp-pointed instrument used for injection or aspiration. —*v.* To separate tissues by means of one or two needles in the dissection of small parts.

needle bath *n.* Water projected against the body in very fine sprays from many jets.

needle biopsy *n.* Removal of a specimen for biopsy by aspirating it through a needle or trocar that pierces the skin or the external surface of an organ and continues into the underlying tissue to be examined. Also called *aspiration biopsy.*

needle-holder *n.* An instrument for grasping a needle used in suturing. Also called *needle forceps.*

nee·dling (nēd′l-ĭng) *n.* Dissection of a soft or secondary cataract.

ne·fa·zo·done (nə-fā′zə-dōn′, -făz′ə-) *n.* An oral antidepressant with a chemical structure unrelated to SSRIs, tricyclics, or monoamine oxidase inhibitors, thought to inhibit neuronal uptake of serotonin and norepinephrine.

ne·ga·tion (nĭ-gā′shən) *n.* A denial, contradiction, or negative statement.

neg·a·tive (nĕg′ə-tĭv) *adj.* **1.** Expressing, containing, or consisting of a negation, refusal, or denial. **2.** Marked by failure of response or absence of a reaction. **3.** Not indicating the presence of microorganisms, disease, or a specific condition. **4.** Moving or turning away from a stimulus, such as light. **5.** Relating to or designating an electric charge of the same sign as that of an electron.

negative accommodation *n.* Adjustment of the lens for distant vision by relaxation of the ciliary muscles of the eye.

negative base excess *n.* A measure of metabolic acidosis based on the amount of strong alkali that would have to be added per unit volume of whole blood to titrate it to pH 7.4 while at a specified temperature and carbon dioxide pressure.

negative convergence *n.* The outward divergence of the visual axes when the eyes are not required to be convergent, as when looking at the far point of normal vision or during sleep.

negative declination *n.* See intorsion (sense 2).

negative end-expiratory pressure *n.* A subatmospheric pressure that develops at the airway at the end of expiration.

negative feedback *n.* Feedback that reduces the output of a system.

negative pressure *n.* Pressure that is less than ambient temperature.

negative scotoma *n.* A scotoma that is not ordinarily perceived and is detected only on examination of the visual field.

negative stain *n.* A stain forming an opaque or colored background to an object that appears translucent or colorless.

negative-strand virus *n.* An RNA virus whose genome is complementary to mRNA and that carries RNA polymerases necessary for the synthesis of mRNA.

negative transfer *n.* Interference of previous learning in the process of learning something new.

neg·a·tiv·ism (nĕg′ə-tĭ-vĭz′əm) *n.* A tendency to do the opposite of what one is requested to do, or to resist stubbornly for no apparent reason. —**neg′a·tiv·ist** *n.* —**neg′a·tiv·is′tic** *adj.*

neg·a·tron (nĕg′ə-trŏn′) *n.* **1.** See electron. **2.** An electron with a negative charge, as contrasted with a positron.

Ne·gri body (nā′grē) *n.* An eosinophilic inclusion body found in the cytoplasm of certain nerve cells containing the rabies virus.

Neis·ser (nī′sər), **Albert Ludwig Sigesmund** 1855–1916. German bacteriologist and physician who discovered (1879) the gonococcal bacterium that causes gonorrhea.

Neis·se·ri·a (nī-sîr′ē-ə) *n.* A genus of aerobic to facultatively anaerobic bacteria containing gram-negative cocci and including the causative agents of gonorrhea and meningitis.

Neisseria gon·or·rhoe·ae (gŏn′ə-rē′ē) *n.* Gonococcus.

Neisseria men·in·git·i·dis (mĕn′ĭn-jĭt′ĭ-dĭs) *n.* The bacteria that is the causative agent of cerebrospinal meningitis; meningococcus.

Né·la·ton catheter (nā-lə-tŏn′, -tôɴ′) *n.* A flexible catheter made of soft rubber.

Né·la·ton's line (nā-lə-tŏnz′, -tôɴz′) *n.* A line drawn from the anterior superior iliac spine to the tuberosity of the ischium.

nel·fin·a·vir (nĕl-fĭn′ə-vîr) *n.* A protease-inhibiting drug usually used in combination with other drugs to suppress the replication of HIV.

Nel·son syndrome (nĕl′sən) *n.* A syndrome characterized by hyperpigmentation of the skin and enlargement of the sella turcica and caused by the development of a pituitary tumor following adrenalectomy for Cushing's syndrome. Also called *postadrenalectomy syndrome.*

nem (něm) *n.* A nutritional unit described as 1 gram of breast milk of specific nutritional components having a caloric value equivalent to $\frac{2}{3}$ calorie.

nem·a·line myopathy (něm′ə-līn′, -lĭn) *n.* Congenital, nonprogressive muscle weakness most evident in the proximal muscles, with characteristic threadlike rods seen in some muscle cells.

nemato– *or* **nemat–** *pref.* Thread; threadlike: *nematocyst.*

nem·a·to·cide (něm′ə-tĭ-sīd′, nə-măt′ĭ-) *or* **nem·a·ti·cide** *n.* A substance or preparation used to kill nematodes. —**nem′a·to·cid′al** (-sīd′l) *adj.*

nem·a·to·cyst (něm′ə-tə-sĭst′, nə-măt′ə-) *n.* A capsule within specialized cells of certain coelenterates containing a barbed, threadlike tube that delivers a paralyzing sting.

Nem·a·to·da (něm′ə-tō′də) *n.* A phylum of worms including species parasitic in humans and plants as well as free-living nonparasitic species in soil or water. It includes the intestinal roundworms and filarial roundworms.

nem·a·tode (něm′ə-tōd′) *n.* A parasitic worm of the class Nematoda. Also called *roundworm.*

nem·a·to·di·a·sis (něm′ə-tō-dī′ə-sĭs) *n.* Infection with nematode parasites.

nem·a·toid (něm′ə-toid′) *adj.* Relating to nematodes.

Nem·bu·tal (něm′byə-tôl′) A trademark for the drug pentobarbital sodium.

neo– *pref.* **1.** New; recent: *neonatal.* **2.** New and different: *Neo-Freudian.* **3.** New and abnormal: *neoplasm.*

ne·o·an·ti·gen (nē′ō-ăn′tĭ-jən) *n.* See **tumor antigen.**

ne·o·ar·thro·sis (nē′ō-är-thrō′sĭs) *n.* Variant of **near-throsis.**

ne·o·blas·tic (nē′ə-blăs′tĭk) *adj.* Developing in or characteristic of new tissue.

ne·o·cer·e·bel·lum (nē′ō-sĕr′ə-bĕl′əm) *n.* The large lateral portion of the cerebellar hemisphere receiving its dominant input from afferent nerves originating from all parts of the cerebral cortex.

ne·o·cor·tex (nē′ō-kôr′tĕks′) *n.* See **isocortex.**

ne·o·cys·tos·to·my (nē′ō-sĭ-stŏs′tə-mē) *n.* A surgical procedure in which the ureter or a segment of the ileum is implanted into the bladder.

Ne·o-Dar·win·ism (nē′ō-där′wə-nĭz′əm) *n.* Darwinism as modified by the findings of modern genetics.

ne·o·dym·i·um (nē′ō-dĭm′ē-əm) *n. Symbol* **Nd** A rare-earth element used for coloring glass. Atomic number 60.

Ne·o-Freud·i·an (nē′ō-froi′dē-ən) *adj.* Of, relating to, or characterizing any psychoanalytic system based on but modifying Freudian doctrine by emphasizing social factors, interpersonal relations, or other cultural influences in personality development or in causation of the neuroses.

ne·o·gen·e·sis (nē′ō-jĕn′ĭ-sĭs) *n.* Regeneration of tissue. —**ne′o·ge·net′ic** (-jə-nĕt′ĭk) *adj.*

ne·o·ki·net·ic (nē′ō-kə-nĕt′ĭk, -kī-) *adj.* Relating to the nervous motor system that controls voluntary muscular movements.

ne·ol·o·gism (nē-ŏl′ə-jĭz′əm) *n.* A meaningless word used by a psychotic.

ne·o·mem·brane (nē′ō-mĕm′brān′) *n.* See **false membrane.**

ne·o·my·cin (nē′ə-mī′sĭn) *n.* A broad-spectrum antibiotic derived from strains of the actinomycete *Streptomyces fradiae* and used in its sulfate form as an intestinal antiseptic in surgery.

ne·on (nē′ŏn′) *n. Symbol* **Ne** A rare inert colorless gaseous element that occurs in air and glows reddish orange in an electric discharge. Atomic number 10.

ne·o·na·tal (nē′ō-nāt′l) *adj.* Of or relating to the first 28 days of an infant's life.

neonatal anemia *n.* See **erythroblastosis fetalis.**

neonatal hepatitis *n.* Hepatitis of unknown cause characterized by the onset of obstructive jaundice in the first few weeks of life and marked by hepatocyte degeneration and the appearance of multinucleated giant cells in the liver.

neonatal herpes *n.* A herpesvirus type two infection transmitted to the newborn during passage through an infected birth canal.

neonatal medicine *n.* See **neonatology.**

neonatal mortality rate *n.* The ratio of the number of deaths in the first 28 days of life to the number of live births occurring in the same population during the same period of time.

neonatal tetany *n.* A continuous general muscular hypertonicity in newborns and young infants. Also called *tetanism.*

ne·o·nate (nē′ə-nāt′) *n.* A neonatal infant.

ne·o·na·tol·o·gy (nē′ō-nā-tŏl′ə-jē) *n.* The branch of pediatrics that deals with the diseases and care of newborns. Also called *neonatal medicine.* —**ne′o·na·tol′o·gist** *n.*

ne·o·pal·li·um (nē′ō-păl′ē-əm) *n., pl.* **–pal·li·ums** *or* **–pal·li·a** (-păl′ē-ə) See **isocortex.**

ne·o·pla·sia (nē′ō-plā′zhə) *n.* The pathological process that results in the formation and growth of a neoplasm.

ne·o·plasm (nē′ə-plăz′əm) *n.* An abnormal new growth of tissue that grows by cellular proliferation more rapidly than normal, continues to grow after the stimuli that initiated the new growth cease, shows partial or complete lack of structural organization and functional coordination with the normal tissue, and usually forms a distinct mass of tissue which may be either benign or malignant. —**ne′o·plas′tic** (-plăs′tĭk) *adj.*

ne·op·ter·in (nē-ŏp′tər-ĭn) *n.* A pteridine present in body fluids, elevated levels of which result from immune system activation, malignant disease, allograft rejection, and viral infections, especially in AIDS.

ne·o·stig·mine (nē′ō-stĭg′mēn, -mĭn) *n.* A drug that inhibits acetylcholinesterase, used in its bromide form orally and its methylsulfate form parenterally to treat myasthenia gravis.

ne·o·stri·a·tum (nē′ō-strī-ā′təm) *n.* The caudate nucleus and putamen considered as one, and distinguished from the globus pallidus.

Neo-Synephrine (nē′ō-sĭ-nĕf′rĭn) A trademark for an over-the-counter nasal decongestant containing the hydrochloride form of either phenylephrine or oxymetazoline.

ne·ot·e·ny (nē-ŏt′n-ē) *n.* The attainment of sexual maturity by an organism still in its larval stage.

ne·o·thal·a·mus (nē′ō-thăl′ə-məs) *n.* The portion of the thalamus projecting to the isocortex.

ne·o·type (nē′ə-tīp′) *n.* A new specimen selected to replace a holotype that has been lost or destroyed.

ne·o·vas·cu·lar·i·za·tion (nē′ō-văs′kyə-lər-ĭ-zā′shən) *n.* **1.** Proliferation of blood vessels in tissue not normally containing them. **2.** Proliferation of blood vessels of a different kind than usual in tissue.

neph·e·lometer (něf′ə-lŏm′ĭ-tər) *n.* An apparatus used to measure the size and concentration of particles in a liquid by determining the amount of light scattered by the liquid. —**neph′e·lo·met′ric** (-lō-mět′rĭk) *adj.* —**neph′e·lom′e·try** *n.*

nephr– *pref.* Variant of **nephro–**.

ne·phral·gia (nə-frăl′jə) *n.* Pain in the kidney.

ne·phrec·ta·sis (nə-frĕk′tə-sĭs) *n.* Dilation or distention of the pelvis of the kidney.

ne·phrec·to·my (nə-frĕk′tə-mē) *n.* Surgical removal of a kidney.

neph·rel·co·sis (něf′rĕl-kō′sĭs) *n.* A condition in which the mucous membrane of the pelvis or calices of the kidney ulceration.

neph·ric (něf′rĭk) *adj.* Relating to or connected with a kidney.

ne·phrid·i·um (nə-frĭd′ē-əm) *n.,* *pl.* **–i·a** (-ē-ə) The embryonic excretory organ from which the kidney develops.

ne·phrit·ic (nə-frĭt′ĭk) *adj.* Of, relating to, or affected with nephritis.

nephritic syndrome *n.* A syndrome comprising the clinical symptoms of nephritis, hematuria, hypertension, and renal failure.

ne·phri·tis (nə-frī′tĭs) *n.,* *pl.* **–phri·tis·es** *or* **–phrit·i·des** (-frĭt′ĭ-dēz′) Acute or chronic inflammation of the kidneys.

neph·ri·to·gen·ic (něf′rĭ-tə-jěn′ĭk, nə-frĭt′ə-) *adj.* Causing nephritis.

nephro– *or* **nephr–** *pref.* Kidney; kidneylike structure: *nephrotomy.*

neph·ro·blas·to·ma (něf′rō-blă-stō′mə) *n.* See **Wilms' tumor**.

neph·ro·cal·ci·no·sis (něf′rō-kăl′sə-nō′sĭs) *n.* Renal lithiasis characterized by diffusely scattered foci of calcification in the kidneys.

neph·ro·cap·sec·to·my (něf′rō-kăp-sěk′tə-mē) *n.* Excision of the capsule of the kidney.

neph·ro·car·di·ac (něf′rō-kär′dē-ăk′) *adj.* Of, relating to, or involving the heart and the kidneys.

neph·ro·cele (něf′rə-sēl′) *n.* Hernial displacement of a kidney.

neph·ro·cys·to·sis (něf′rō-sĭ-stō′sĭs) *n.* The formation of renal cysts.

neph·ro·ge·net·ic (něf′rō-jə-nět′ĭk) *or* **neph·ro·gen·ic** (-jěn′ĭk) *adj.* Giving rise to kidney tissue.

nephrogenic diabetes insipidus *n.* Diabetes insipidus caused by an inability of the kidney tubules to respond to antidiuretic hormone and reabsorb water.

ne·phrog·e·nous (nə-frŏj′ə-nəs) *adj.* Arising from kidney tissue.

neph·ro·gram (něf′rə-grăm′) *n.* A radiograph of the kidney following the intravenous injection of a radiopaque substance. —**ne·phrog′ra·phy** (nə-frŏg′rə-fē) *n.*

neph·roid (něf′roid′) *adj.* Resembling a kidney; kidney-shaped.

neph·ro·lith (něf′rə-lĭth′) *n.* See **kidney stone**.

neph·ro·li·thi·a·sis (něf′rō-lĭ-thī′ə-sĭs) *n.* Calculi in the kidneys.

neph·ro·li·thot·o·my (něf′rō-lĭ-thŏt′ə-mē) *n.* Incision into the kidney for the removal of a calculus.

ne·phrol·o·gy (nə-frŏl′ə-jē) *n.* The medical science that deals with the kidneys, especially their functions or diseases. —**ne·phrol′o·gist** *n.*

ne·phrol·y·sis (nə-frŏl′ĭ-sĭs) *n.* **1.** The operation of freeing of the kidney from inflammatory adhesions, with preservation of the capsule. **2.** The destruction of renal cells. —**neph′ro·lyt′ic** (něf′rə-lĭt′ĭk) *adj.*

ne·phro·ma (nə-frō′mə) *n.,* *pl.* **–mas** *or* **–ma·ta** (-mə-tə) A tumor arising from renal tissue.

neph·ro·meg·a·ly (něf′rō-měg′ə-lē) *n.* Extreme hypertrophy of one or both kidneys.

neph·ron (něf′rŏn) *n.* The functional unit of the kidney, consisting of the renal corpuscle, the proximal and distal convoluted tubules, and the nephronic loop.

ne·phron·ic loop (ně-frŏn′ĭk) *n.* The U-shaped part of the nephron extending from the proximal to the distal convoluted tubules; it consists of descending and ascending limbs. Also called *Henle's loop, loop of Henle.*

ne·phrop·a·thy (nə-frŏp′ə-thē) *n.* A disease of the kidney. Also called *renopathy.* —**neph′ro·path′ic** (něf′rə-păth′ĭk) *adj.*

neph·ro·pex·y (něf′rə-pěk′sē) *n.* Surgical fixation of a floating or mobile kidney.

neph·roph·thi·sis (něf-rŏf′thī-sĭs) *n.* **1.** Suppurative nephritis with wasting of the substance of the kidney. **2.** Tuberculosis of the kidney.

neph·rop·to·sis (něf′rŏp-tō′sĭs) *n.* Prolapse of the kidney.

neph·ro·py·e·li·tis (něf′rō-pī′ə-lī′tĭs) *n.* See **pyelonephritis**.

neph·ro·py·e·lo·plas·ty (něf′rō-pī′ə-lə-plăs′tē) *n.* Plastic surgery of the kidney and renal pelvis.

neph·ro·py·o·sis (něf′rō-pī-ō′sĭs) *n.* Suppuration of the kidney.

neph·ror·rha·phy (něf-rôr′ə-fē) *n.* Suture of the kidney.

neph·ro·scle·ro·sis (něf′rō-sklə-rō′sĭs) *n.* Induration of the kidney from overgrowth and contraction of the interstitial connective tissue. —**neph′ro·scle·rot′ic** (-rŏt′ĭk) *adj.*

ne·phro·sis (nə-frō′sĭs) *n.,* *pl.* **–ses** (-sēz) **1.** Disease of the kidneys marked by degeneration of renal tubular epithelium. **2.** See **nephrotic syndrome**. —**ne·phrot′ic** (-frŏt′ĭk) *adj.*

ne·phros·to·gram (nə-frŏs′tə-grăm′) *n.* A radiograph of the kidney after a contrast agent has been administered through a nephrostomy tube. —**ne·phros′to·my** *n.*

ne·phrot·ic syndrome (nə-frŏt′ĭk) *n.* A clinical state marked by edema, albuminuria, decreased plasma albumin, doubly refractile bodies in the urine, and usually increased blood cholesterol. It results from increased permeability of the glomerular capillary basement membranes. Also called *nephrosis*.

neph·ro·to·mo·gram (nĕf′rō-tō′mə-grăm′) *n.* A sectional radiograph of the kidneys following intravenous administration of contrast material to improve visualization of the renal parenchyma. —**neph′ro·to·mog′ra·phy** (-tō-mŏg′rə-fē) *n.*

ne·phrot·o·my (nə-frŏt′ə-mē) *n.* An incision into the kidney.

neph·ro·tox·ic·i·ty (nĕf′rō-tŏk-sĭs′ĭ-tē) *n.* The quality or state of being toxic to kidney cells.

neph·ro·tox·in (nĕf′rō-tŏk′sĭn) *n.* A cytotoxin specific for cells of the kidney. —**neph′ro·tox′ic** *adj.*

neph·ro·troph·ic (nĕf′rə-trŏf′ĭk, -trō′fĭk) *or* **neph·ro·trop·ic** (-trŏp′ĭk, -trō′pĭk) *adj.* Renotrophic.

neph·ro·tu·ber·cu·lo·sis (nĕf′rō-tōō-bûr′kyə-lō′sĭs) *n.* Tuberculosis of the kidney.

neph·ro·u·re·ter·ec·to·my (nĕf′rō-yōō-rē′tə-rĕk′tə-mē) *n.* The surgical removal of a kidney and its ureter.

neph·ro·u·re·ter·o·cys·tec·to·my (nĕf′rō-yōō-rē′tə-rō-sĭ-stĕk′tə-mē) *n.* Surgical removal of a kidney, ureter, and part or all of the bladder.

nep·tu·ni·um (nĕp-tōō′nē-əm) *n. Symbol* **Np** A metallic radioactive element found in trace quantities in uranium ores or synthesized; its longest-lived isotope is Np 237 with a half-life of 2.1 million years. Atomic number 93.

nerve (nûrv) *n.* **1.** Any of the cordlike bundles of nervous tissue made up of myelinated or unmyelinated nerve fibers and held together by a connective tissue sheath through which sensory stimuli and motor impulses pass between the brain or other parts of the central nervous system and the eyes, glands, muscles, and other parts of the body. **2.** The sensitive tissue in the pulp of a tooth. **3. nerves** Nervous agitation caused by fear, anxiety, or stress.

nerve avulsion *n.* The forcible disengagement of a portion of a nerve to produce paralysis.

nerve block *n.* Interruption of the passage of impulses through a neuron by the injection of alcohol or an anesthetic.

nerve block anesthesia *n.* Conduction anesthesia in which a local anesthetic is injected about the peripheral nerves.

nerve cell *n.* **1.** See **neuron. 2.** The body of a neuron without its axon and dendrites.

nerve conduction *n.* The transmission of an impulse along a nerve fiber.

nerve decompression *n.* The relief of pressure on a nerve trunk by the excision of constricting bands or the widening of the bony canal.

nerve fiber *n.* A threadlike process of a neuron, especially the axon that conducts nerve impulses.

nerve gas *n.* Any of various poisonous gases that interfere with the functioning of nerves by inhibiting cholinesterase.

nerve graft *n.* A graft in which a healthy nerve is used to replace a portion of a defective one.

nerve growth factor *n. Abbr.* **NGF** A protein that stimulates the growth of sympathetic and sensory nerve cells.

nerve growth factor antiserum *n.* An antiserum containing antibodies against nerve growth factor.

nerve impulse *n.* A wave of physical and chemical excitation that moves along a nerve fiber in response to a stimulus.

nerve of pterygoid canal *n.* The nerve that constitutes the motor and sympathetic roots of the pterygopalatine ganglion and runs through the pterygoid canal to the pterygopalatine fossa.

nerve of tensor muscle of soft palate *n.* A branch of the mandibular nerve passing through the otic ganglion and supplying the tensor muscle of the soft palate.

nerve of tensor tympani muscle *n.* A branch of the mandibular nerve passing through the otic ganglion and supplying the tensor muscle of the tympanic membrane.

nerve plexus *n.* A plexus formed by nerves interlaced with numerous communicating branches.

nerve root·let (rōot′lĭt, rōot′-) *n.* See **root filament.**

nerve tissue *n.* A highly differentiated tissue composed of nerve cells, nerve fibers, dendrites, and neuroglia.

nerve to stapedius muscle *n.* A branch of the facial nerve arising in the facial canal and innervating the stapedius muscle.

nerve trunk *n.* The main stem of a nerve, consisting of a bundle of nerve fibers bound together by a tough sheath of connective tissue.

ner·vi·mo·tor (nûr′və-mō′tər) *adj.* Relating to a motor nerve.

ner·von (nûr′vŏn′) *n.* A crystalline cerebroside in brain tissue.

ner·von·ic acid (nûr-vŏn′ĭk) *n.* An unsaturated fatty acid that forms by hydrolysis in cerebrosides such as nervon.

nerv·ous (nûr′vəs) *adj.* **1.** Of or relating to the nerves or nervous system. **2.** Stemming from or affecting the nerves or nervous system, as a disease. **3.** Easily agitated or distressed.

nervous bladder *n.* A urinary bladder condition in which there is a need to urinate frequently but a failure to empty the bladder completely.

nervous breakdown *n.* A severe or incapacitating emotional disorder, especially when occurring suddenly and marked by depression.

nervous indigestion *n.* Indigestion caused by stress or by an emotion such as anxiety.

nervous lobe *n.* The bulbous part of the neurohypophysis attached to the hypothalamus by the infundibulum and composed of pituicytes, blood vessels, and terminals of nerve fibers from the supraoptic and paraventricular nuclei.

nervous system *n.* The system of cells, tissues, and organs that regulates the body's responses to internal and external stimuli. In vertebrates it consists of the brain, spinal cord, nerves, ganglia, and parts of the receptor and effector organs.

ner·vus (nûr′vəs) *n., pl.* **-vi** (-vī) A nerve.

Nes·a·caine (nĕs′ə-kān′) A trademark for the drug chloroprocaine hydrochloride.

net·tle rash (nĕt′l) *n.* See **urticaria.**

net·work (nĕt′wûrk′) *n.* **1.** A fabric or structure in which cords, threads, or wires cross at regular intervals. **2.** A body structure resembling such a fabric or structure.

Neu·feld capsular swelling (noi′fĕlt) *n.* An increase in the opacity and visibility of the capsule of encapsulated organisms resulting from exposure to specific, agglutinating, anticapsular antibodies. Also called *Neufeld reaction, quellung reaction.*

neur– *pref.* Variant of neuro–.

neu·ral (noor′əl) *adj.* **1.** Of or relating to a nerve or the nervous system. **2.** Of, relating to, or located on the same side of the body as the spinal cord; dorsal.

neural arch *n.* See **vertebral arch.**

neural crest *n.* A band of neuroectodermal cells that lie dorsolateral to the developing spinal cord, where they separate into clusters of cells that develop into dorsal-root ganglion cells, autonomic ganglion cells, chromaffin cells of the adrenal medulla, neurolemma cells, or integumentary pigment cells.

neural crest syndrome *n.* A syndrome consisting of loss of pain sensibility, autonomic dysfunction, pupillary abnormalities, neurogenic anhidrosis, vasomotor instability, aplasia of dental enamel, meningeal thickening, hyperflexion, and albinism.

neural fold *n.* The elevated margins of the embryonic neural groove.

neu·ral·gia (noo-răl′jə) *n.* Sharp, severe paroxysmal pain extending along a nerve or group of nerves. Also called *neurodynia.* —**neu·ral′gic** *adj.*

neuralgia fa·ci·a·lis ve·ra (fā′shē-ā′lĭs vîr′ə) *n.* See **geniculate neuralgia.**

neural groove *n.* The gutterlike groove formed in the midline of the embryo's dorsal surface by the progressive elevation of the lateral margins of the neural plate, resulting in the formation of the neural tube. Also called *medullary groove.*

neural plate *n.* The thickened dorsal plate of ectoderm that differentiates into the neural tube and neural crest. Also called *medullary plate.*

neural spine *n.* The middle point of the vertebral arch, represented by the spinous process.

neural tube *n.* A dorsal tubular structure in the vertebrate embryo that develops into the brain and spinal cord.

neu·ra·min·ic acid (noor′ə-mĭn′ĭk) *n.* An aldol condensation product of mannosamine and pyruvic acid and the parent acid of sialic acids.

neu·ra·min·i·dase (noor′ə-mĭn′ĭ-dās′, -dāz′) *n.* An enzyme that catalyzes the hydrolysis of terminal acylneuraminic residues from oligosaccharides, glycoproteins, and glycolipids. It is present as a surface antigen in myxoviruses. Also called *sialidase.*

neu·ran·a·gen·e·sis (noor′ăn-ə-jĕn′ĭ-sĭs) *n.* Regeneration of a nerve.

neu·ra·poph·y·sis (noor′ə-pŏf′ĭ-sĭs) *n.* See **lamina of vertebral arch.**

neu·ra·prax·i·a (noor′ə-prăk′sē-ə) *n.* Injury to a nerve resulting in paralysis without degeneration and followed by rapid and complete recovery of function.

neu·ras·the·ni·a (noor′əs-thē′nē-ə) *n.* A complex of symptoms characterized by chronic fatigue and weakness, loss of memory, and generalized aches and pains. —**neu′ras·then′ic** (-thĕn′ĭk) *adj.*

neu·rax·is (noo-răk′sĭs) *n.* The axial unpaired part of the central nervous system, composed of the spinal cord, rhombencephalon, mesencephalon, and diencephalon.

neu·rec·ta·sis (noo-rĕk′tə-sĭs) *or* **neu·rec·ta·sia** (noor′-ĭk-tā′zhə) *n.* The surgical operation of stretching of a nerve or a nerve trunk. Also called *neurotony.*

neu·rec·to·my (noo-rĕk′tə-mē) *n.* Surgical removal of a nerve or part of a nerve.

neu·rec·to·pi·a (noor′ĭk-tō′pē-ə) *or* **neu·rec·to·py** (noo-rĕk′tə-pē) *n.* **1.** Dislocation of a nerve trunk. **2.** A condition in which a nerve follows an anomalous course.

neu·rer·gic (noo-rûr′jĭk) *adj.* Relating to the activity of a nerve.

neu·rex·er·e·sis (noor′ĕk-sĕr′ĭ-sĭs) *n.* Surgical extraction of a nerve.

neu·ri·lem·ma *or* **neu·ro·lem·ma** (noor′ə-lĕm′ə) *n.* The delicate membranous covering that forms the myelin sheath around the axons of peripheral nerves. Also called *sheath of Schwann.*

neurilemma cell *or* **neurolemma cell** *n.* See **Schwann cell.**

neu·ri·le·mo·ma *or* **neu·ri·lem·mo·ma** (noor′ə-lə-mō′-mə) *n.* A benign, encapsulated neoplasm that originates from a neurilemma. Also called *neurinoma, schwannoma.*

neu·ri·mo·tor (noor′ə-mō′tər) *adj.* Of or relating to a motor nerve.

neu·ri·no·ma (noor′ə-nō′mə) *n.* See **neurilemoma.**

neuritic plaque *n.* See **senile plaque.**

neu·ri·tis (noo-rī′tĭs) *n.* The inflammation of a nerve or group of nerves that is characterized by pain, loss of reflexes, and atrophy of the affected muscles. —**neu·rit′ic** (-rĭt′ĭk) *adj.*

neuro– *or* **neur–** *pref.* **1.** Nerve: *neuroblast.* **2.** Neural: *neuropathology.*

neu·ro·a·nas·to·mo·sis (noor′ō-ə-năs′tə-mō′sĭs) *n.* Surgical formation of a junction between nerves.

neu·ro·a·nat·o·my (noor′ō-ə-năt′ə-mē) *n.* **1.** The branch of anatomy that deals with the nervous system. **2.** The neural structure of an organ or part. —**neu′ro·an′a·tom′i·cal** (-ăn′ə-tŏm′ĭ-kəl) *adj.*

neu·ro·ar·throp·a·thy (noor′ō-är-thrŏp′ə-thē) *n.* A joint disorder caused by loss of sensation in the joints.

neu·ro·ax·on·al (noor′ō-ăk′sə-nəl, -ăk-sŏn′əl) *adj.* Of, relating to, or being the axon of a neuron.

neu·ro·bi·ol·o·gy (noor′ō-bī-ŏl′ə-jē) *n.* The biological study of the nervous system. —**neu′ro·bi′o·log′i·cal** (-bī′ə-lŏj′ĭ-kəl) *adj.*

neu·ro·blast (noor′ə-blăst′) *n.* An embryonic cell from which a nerve cell develops.

neu·ro·blas·to·ma (noor′ō-blă-stō′mə) *n.* A malignant tumor composed of neuroblasts, originating in the autonomic nervous system or the adrenal medulla and occurring most commonly in infants and young children.

neu·ro·car·di·ac (noor′ō-kär′dē-ăk′) *adj.* Relating to the nerve supply of the heart.

neu·ro·chem·is·try (nŏŏr′ō-kĕm′ĭ-strē) *n.* The study of the chemical composition and processes of the nervous system and the effects of chemicals on it. —**neu′-ro·chem′i·cal** (-kəl) *adj.*

neu·ro·cho·ri·o·ret·i·ni·tis (nŏŏr′ō-kôr′ē-ō-rĕt′n-ī′tĭs) *n.* Inflammation of the choroid coat of the eye, the retina, and the optic nerve.

neu·ro·cho·roid·i·tis (nŏŏr′ō-kôr′oi-dī′tĭs) *n.* Inflammation of the choroid coat of the eye and the optic nerve.

neu·ro·cir·cu·la·to·ry asthenia (nŏŏr′ō-sûr′kyə-lə-tôr′ē) *n.* A former designation for a syndrome that is characterized by increased susceptibility to fatigue, dyspnea, rapid pulse, precordial pain, and anxiety, and is observed especially in soldiers on active duty. Also called *DaCosta's syndrome, effort syndrome, irritable heart, soldier's heart.*

neu·roc·la·dism (nŏŏ-rŏk′lə-dĭz′əm) *n.* The growth of axons from one segment of a cut nerve to bridge the gap to the other segment.

neu·ro·cra·ni·um (nŏŏr′ō-krā′nē-əm) *n.* The part of the skull enclosing the brain.

neu·ro·cris·top·a·thy (nŏŏr′ō-krĭ-stŏp′ə-thē) *n.* Maldevelopment or neoplasia of tissues originating in the neural crest.

neu·ro·cyte (nŏŏr′ə-sīt′) *n.* See **neuron.**

neu·ro·cy·tol·y·sis (nŏŏr′ō-sī-tŏl′ĭ-sĭs) *n.* Destruction of nerve cells.

neu·ro·cy·to·ma (nŏŏr′ō-sī-tō′mə) *n.* See **ganglioneuroma.**

neu·ro·de·gen·er·a·tive (nŏŏr′ō-dĭ-jĕn′ər-ə-tĭv) *adj.* Of, relating to, or being a progressive loss of neurologic functions.

neu·ro·den·drite (nŏŏr′ō-dĕn′drīt′) *n.* See **dendrite.**

neu·ro·den·dron (nŏŏr′ō-dĕn′drŏn′) *n.* See **dendrite.**

neu·ro·der·ma·ti·tis (nŏŏr′ō-dûr′mə-tī′tĭs) *n.* A chronic skin disorder characterized by localized or disseminated lichenified skin lesions that itch severely. It is possibly a psychogenic disorder. Also called *neurodermatosis.*

neu·ro·dy·nam·ic (nŏŏr′ō-dī-năm′ĭk) *adj.* Of, relating to, or characterized by nervous energy.

neu·ro·dyn·i·a (nŏŏr′ō-dĭn′ē-ə) *n.* See **neuralgia.**

neu·ro·ec·to·derm (nŏŏr′ō-ĕk′tə-dûrm′) *n.* The region of embryonic ectoderm that develops into the brain and spinal cord as well as into the nervous tissue of the peripheral nervous system. —**neu′ro·ec′to·der′mal** *adj.*

neu·ro·en·ceph·a·lo·my·e·lop·a·thy (nŏŏr′ō-ĕn-sĕf′ə-lō-mī′ə-lŏp′ə-thē) *n.* Disease of the brain, spinal cord, and nervous tissue.

neu·ro·en·do·crine (nŏŏr′ō-ĕn′də-krĭn, -krēn′, -krīn′) *adj.* 1. Of, relating to, or involving the interaction between the nervous system and the hormones of the endocrine glands. 2. Of or relating to the cells that release a hormone into the blood in response to a neural stimulus.

neu·ro·en·do·cri·nol·o·gy (nŏŏr′ō-ĕn′də-krə-nŏl′ə-jē) *n.* The study of the interaction between the nervous system and the endocrine glands.

neu·ro·ep·i·the·li·um (nŏŏr′ō-ĕp′ə-thē′lē-əm) *n.* 1. The part of the embryonic ectoderm that develops into the nervous system. 2. The highly specialized epithelial cells of sensory organs such as the eye and nose. —**neu′ro·ep′i·the′li·al** *adj.*

neu·ro·fi·bril (nŏŏr′ə-fī′brəl, -fĭb′rəl) *n.* Any of the long, thin, microscopic fibrils that run through the body of a neuron and extend into the axon and dendrites, giving the neuron support and shape. —**neu′ro·fi′bril·lar** (-brə-lər) *adj.*

neu·ro·fi·bro·ma (nŏŏr′ō-fī-brō′mə) *n.* A moderately firm, benign, nonencapsulated tumor that results from the disorderly proliferation of Schwann cells and that includes portions of nerve fibers. Also called *fibroneuroma, schwannoma.*

neu·ro·fi·bro·ma·to·sis (nŏŏr′ō-fī-brō′mə-tō′sĭs) *n.* A genetic disease characterized by multiple neurofibromas and pigmented spots on the skin, sometimes accompanied by bone deformity and a predisposition to cancers, especially of the brain. Also called *multiple neurofibroma, neuromatosis, Recklinghausen's disease, von Recklinghausen's disease.*

neu·ro·fil·a·ment (nŏŏr′ə-fĭl′ə-mənt) *n.* Any of the long fine threads that make up a neurofibril.

neu·ro·gan·gli·on (nŏŏr′ō-găng′glē-ən) *n.* See **ganglion** (sense 1).

neu·ro·gen·e·sis (nŏŏr′ə-jĕn′ĭ-sĭs) *n.* Formation of nervous tissue.

neu·ro·ge·net·ic (nŏŏr′ō-jə-nĕt′ĭk) *adj.* Variant of **neurogenic.**

neu·ro·ge·net·ics (nŏŏr′ō-jə-nĕt′ĭks) *n.* The study of genetic factors that contribute to development of neurological disorders.

neu·ro·gen·ic (nŏŏr′ə-jĕn′ĭk) *or* **neu·ro·ge·net·ic** (-jə-nĕt′ĭk) *adj.* 1. Originating in the nerves or nervous tissue. 2. Caused or affected by the nerves or nervous system.

neurogenic bladder *n.* Defective functioning of the urinary bladder due to impaired nerve supply.

neu·rog·e·nous (nŏŏ-rŏj′ə-nəs) *adj.* Originating in the nerves or the nervous tissue.

neu·rog·li·a (nŏŏ-rŏg′lē-ə, nŏŏr′ə-glē′ə, -glī′-) *n.* The supportive tissue of the nervous system, including the network of branched cells in the central nervous system (astrocytes, microglia, and oligodendrocytes) and the supporting cells of the peripheral nervous system (Schwann cells and satellite cells). Also called *glia, reticulum.* —**neu·rog′li·al** *adj.*

neu·rog·li·a·cyte (nŏŏ-rŏg′lē-ə-sīt′) *n.* Any of the cells of the neuroglia; a glial cell.

neu·rog·li·o·ma·to·sis (nŏŏ-rŏg′lē-ō′mə-tō′sĭs) *n.* See **gliomatosis.**

neu·ro·gram (nŏŏr′ə-grăm′) *n.* See **engram.**

neu·ro·his·tol·o·gy (nŏŏr′ō-hĭ-stŏl′ə-jē) *n.* The branch of histology that deals with the nervous system.

neu·ro·hor·mone (nŏŏr′ō-hôr′mōn) *n.* A hormone secreted by or acting on a part of the nervous system.

neu·ro·hy·poph·y·sis (nŏŏr′ō-hī-pŏf′ĭ-sĭs, -hī-) *n., pl.* **-ses** (-sēz′) The posterior portion of the pituitary gland, having a rich supply of nerve fibers and releasing oxytocin and vasopressin. Also called *posterior lobe of hypophysis.*

neu·roid (nŏŏr′oid′) *adj.* Relating to or resembling a nerve; nervelike.

neu·ro·lem·ma (nŏŏr'ə-lĕm'ə) *n.* Variant of **neuri-lemma**.

neurolemma cell *n.* Variant of **neurilemma cell**.

neu·ro·lep·tan·al·ge·sia (nŏŏr'ō-lĕp'tăn-əl-jē'zhə) *n.* An intense analgesic and amnesic state produced by the combination of narcotic analgesics and neuroleptic drugs.

neu·ro·lep·tan·es·the·sia (nŏŏr'ō-lĕp'tăn-ĭs-thē'zhə) *n.* General anesthesia induced by the intravenous administration of neuroleptic drugs in combination with inhalation of a weak anesthetic.

neu·ro·lep·tic (nŏŏr'ə-lĕp'tĭk) *n.* A tranquilizing drug, especially one used in treating mental disorders. —*adj.* Having a tranquilizing effect.

neuroleptic malignant syndrome *n.* Hyperthermia in reaction to the use of neuroleptic drugs, accompanied by extrapyramidal and autonomic disturbances that may be fatal.

neu·rol·o·gy (nŏŏ-rŏl'ə-jē) *n.* The branch of medical science that deals with the nervous system and disorders affecting it. —**neu·rol'o·gist** *n.*

neu·rol·y·sin (nŏŏ-rŏl'ĭ-sĭn, nŏŏr'ə-lī'sĭn) *n.* A substance that destroys ganglion and cortical cells. Also called *neurotoxin.*

neu·rol·y·sis (nŏŏ-rŏl'ĭ-sĭs) *n.* **1.** The breaking down or destruction of nerve tissue, especially as a result of disease. **2.** The surgical freeing of a nerve from inflammatory adhesions. —**neu'ro·lyt'ic** (nŏŏr'ə-lĭt'ĭk, nyŏŏr'-) *adj.*

neu·ro·ma (nŏŏ-rō'mə) *n., pl.* **–mas** *or* **–ma·ta** (-mə-tə) A neoplasm derived from nerve tissue.

neuroma cu·tis (kyŏŏ'tĭs) *n.* Neurofibroma of the skin.

neu·ro·ma·la·cia (nŏŏr'ō-mə-lā'shə) *n.* Softening of nerve tissue as a result of disease.

neuroma tel·an·gi·ec·to·des (tĕl-ăn'jē-ĭk-tō'dēz) *n.* A neurofibroma having numerous blood vessels.

neu·ro·ma·to·sis (nŏŏr'ō-mə-tō'sĭs) *n.* See **neurofibro-matosis**.

neu·ro·mere (nŏŏr'ə-mîr') *n.* Any of the segments of the neural tube that constitute the embryonic brain. Also called *encephalomere.*

neu·ro·mus·cu·lar (nŏŏr'ō-mŭs'kyə-lər) *adj.* **1.** Of, relating to, or affecting both nerves and muscles. **2.** Having the characteristics of both nervous and muscular tissue.

neuromuscular blocking agent *n.* Any of various compounds, such as curare, that compete with neurotransmitters for nerve cell receptor sites, thus preventing the contraction of skeletal muscles.

neuromuscular spindle *n.* A spindle-shaped end organ in skeletal muscle in which afferent nerve fibers terminate and which is sensitive to passive stretching of the muscle enclosing it.

neuromuscular system *n.* The muscles of the body together with the nerves supplying them.

neu·ro·my·as·the·ni·a (nŏŏr'ō-mī'əs-thē'nē-ə) *n.* Muscular weakness, usually of emotional origin.

neu·ro·my·e·li·tis (nŏŏr'ō-mī'ə-lī'tĭs) *n.* Neuritis combined with inflammation of the spinal cord. Also called *myeloneuritis.*

neuromyelitis op·ti·ca (ŏp'tĭ-kə) *n.* A demyelinating disorder associated with transverse myelopathy and optic neuritis. Also called *Devic's disease.*

neu·ro·my·op·a·thy (nŏŏr'ō-mī-ŏp'ə-thē) *n.* A disorder or disease affecting nerves and associated muscle tissue.

neu·ro·my·o·si·tis (nŏŏr'ō-mī'ə-sī'tĭs) *n.* Neuritis with inflammation of the related muscles. No longer in technical use.

neu·ron (nŏŏr'ŏn') *or* **neu·rone** (-ōn') *n.* Any of the impulse-conducting cells that constitute the brain, spinal column, and nerves, consisting of a nucleated cell body with one or more dendrites and a single axon. Also called *nerve cell, neurocyte.*

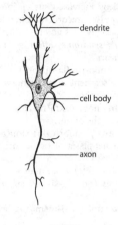

neuron

neu·ro·nal (nŏŏr'ə-nəl, nŏŏ-rō'nəl) *adj.* Relating to a neuron.

neu·ro·ne·vus (nŏŏr'ō-nē'vəs) *n.* Any of various intradermal nevi containing nests of hyalinized nevus cells that resemble nerve bundles.

neu·ro·nop·a·thy (nŏŏr'ə-nŏp'ə-thē) *n.* A disorder of a neuron.

neu·ron·o·phage (nŏŏ-rŏn'ə-fāj') *n.* A phagocyte that ingests neurons.

neu·ron·o·pha·gia (nŏŏr'ŏn-ə-fā'jə) *or* **neu·ro·noph·a·gy** (nŏŏr'ə-nŏf'ə-jē) *n.* Destruction of nerve cells by phagocytes.

Neu·ron·tin (nŏŏ-rŏn'tn) A trademark for the drug gabapentin.

neu·ro·on·col·o·gy (nŏŏr'ōg-ŏn-kŏl'ə-jē) *n.* The branch of medical science dealing with tumors of the nervous system.

neuro-oncology surgery *n.* Brain surgery that employs various techniques, such as sterotaxis, to locate, dislodge, and remove tumors.

neu·ro·oph·thal·mol·o·gy (nŏŏr'ō-ŏf'thəl-mŏl'ə-jē, -thăl-, -ŏp'-) *n.* The branch of medical science dealing with the relationship of the eyes to the central nervous system.

neu·ro·o·tol·o·gy (nŏŏr'ō-ō-tŏl'ə-jē) *n.* The branch of medical science dealing with the neurologic study of the ear.

neu·ro·pap·il·li·tis (nŏŏr'ō-păp'ə-lī'tĭs) *n.* See **optic neuritis**.

neu·ro·pa·ral·y·sis (nŏŏr'ō-pə-răl'ĭ-sĭs) *n.* Paralysis that results from a disease of the nerve that supplies the affected part. —**neu′ro·par′a·lyt′ic** (-păr′ə-lĭt′ĭk) *adj.*

neuroparalytic keratitis *n.* Ulceration of the cornea associated with trigeminal paralysis.

neuropathic arthropathy *n.* See **neuropathic joint.**

neuropathic bladder *n.* See **autonomic neurogenic bladder.**

neuropathic joint *n.* A destructive joint disease caused by diminished proprioceptive sensation that results in repeated subliminal injury. Also called *neuropathic arthropathy.*

neu·ro·path·o·gen·e·sis (no͝or′ō-păth′ə-jĕn′ĭ-sĭs) *n.* The origin or development of a disease of the nervous system.

neu·ro·pa·thol·o·gy (no͝or′ō-pə-thŏl′ə-jē) *n.* The study of diseases of the nervous system. —**neu′ro·path′o·log′i·cal** *adj.*

neu·rop·a·thy (no͝o-rŏp′ə-thē) *n.* A disease or abnormality of the nervous system, especially one affecting the cranial or spinal nerves. —**neu′ro·path′ic** (no͝or′ə-păth′ĭk) *adj.*

neu·ro·pep·tide (no͝or′ō-pĕp′tīd′) *n.* Any of various peptides found in neural tissue, such as endorphins and enkephalins.

neu·ro·phar·ma·col·o·gy (no͝or′ō-fär′mə-kŏl′ə-jē) *n.* The study of the action of drugs on the nervous system.

neu·ro·phy·sin (no͝or′ə-fī′sĭn) *n.* Any of several proteins synthesized in the hypothalamus that transport and store hormones.

neu·ro·phys·i·ol·o·gy (no͝or′ō-fĭz′ē-ŏl′ə-jē) *n.* The branch of physiology that deals with the functions of the nervous system.

neu·ro·pil (no͝or′ə-pĭl′) *or* **neu·ro·pile** (-pīl′) *n.* The complex net of axonal, dendritic, and glial branchings that forms the bulk of the central nervous system gray matter of the brain and in which the nerve cell bodies are embedded.

neu·ro·plasm (no͝or′ə-plăz′əm) *n.* The protoplasm of a neuron.

neu·ro·plas·ty (no͝or′ə-plăs′tē) *n.* Surgery to repair or restore nerve tissue.

neu·ro·ple·gic (no͝or′ə-plē′jĭk) *adj.* Of or relating to paralysis resulting from disease affecting the nervous system.

neu·ro·po·di·a (no͝or′ə-pō′dē-ə) *pl.n.* See **axon terminals.**

neu·ro·pore (no͝or′ə-pôr′) *n.* Either the anterior or posterior opening leading from the central canal of the embryonic neural tube to the exterior.

neu·ro·psy·chi·a·try (no͝or′ō-sĭ-kī′ə-trē, -sī-) *n.* The medical science dealing with both organic and psychic disorders of the nervous system.

neu·ro·psy·chol·o·gy (no͝or′ō-sī-kŏl′ə-jē) *n.* The science that deals with the interrelationships between neurology and psychology.

neu·ro·psy·chop·a·thy (no͝or′ō-sī-kŏp′ə-thē) *n.* An emotional illness that is neurologic, or functional, or both, in origin.

neu·ro·ra·di·ol·o·gy (no͝or′ō-rā′dē-ŏl′ə-jē) *n.* **1.** The branch of radiology that deals with the nervous system. **2.** The use of x-rays in the diagnosis and treatment of nervous system disorders.

neu·ro·ret·i·ni·tis (no͝or′ō-rĕt′n-ī′tĭs) *n.* Inflammation of the retina and optic nerve.

neu·ror·rha·phy (no͝o-rôr′ə-fē) *n.* The surgical suturing of a divided nerve. Also called *neurosuture.*

neu·ro·sar·co·clei·sis (no͝or′ō-sär′kō-klī′sĭs) *n.* Surgical procedure to relieve neuralgia in which a nerve traversing a wall of an osseous canal is transplanted into soft tissue.

neu·ro·sar·coi·do·sis (no͝or′ō-sär′koi-dō′sĭs) *n.* A granulomatous disease of unknown cause involving the central nervous system, usually with concomitant systemic involvement.

neu·ro·sci·ence (no͝or′ō-sī′əns) *n.* Any of the sciences, such as neuroanatomy and neurobiology, that deal with the nervous system.

neu·ro·se·cre·tion (no͝or′ō-sĭ-krē′shən) *n.* **1.** The secretion of substances, such as hormones, by neurons. **2.** A substance that is secreted by neurons. —**neu′ro·se·cre′to·ry** (-krē′tə-rē) *adj.*

neu·ro·sen·so·ry (no͝or′ō-sĕn′sə-rē) *adj.* Of or relating to the sensory activity or functions of the nervous system.

neu·ro·sis (no͝o-rō′sĭs) *n., pl.* **-ses** (-sēz) A psychological state characterized by excessive anxiety or insecurity, compensated for by various defense mechanisms and lacking evidence of neurologic or other organic disease. No longer used in psychiatric diagnosis.

neu·ro·splanch·nic (no͝or′ō-splăngk′nĭk) *adj.* Neurovisceral.

Neu·ros·po·ra (no͝o-rŏs′pər-ə) *n.* A genus of ascomycetous fungi used extensively for research in genetics and cellular biochemistry.

neu·ro·sthe·ni·a (no͝or′ō-sthē′nē-ə) *n.* A condition in which neurons respond with abnormal force or rapidity to slight stimuli.

neu·ro·sur·ger·y (no͝or′ō-sûr′jə-rē) *n.* Surgery on any part of the nervous system. —**neu′ro·sur′geon** (-jən) *n.* —**neu′ro·sur′gi·cal** (-jĭ-kəl) *adj.*

neu·ro·su·ture (no͝or′ō-so͞o′chər) *n.* See **neurorrhaphy.**

neu·ro·syph·i·lis (no͝or′ō-sĭf′ə-lĭs) *n.* Nervous system manifestations of syphilis including tabes dorsalis and general paresis.

neu·ro·ten·di·nous (no͝or′ō-tĕn′də-nəs) *adj.* Of or relating to a nerve and a tendon.

neurotendinous spindle *n.* See **Golgi tendon organ.**

neu·ro·ten·sin (no͝or′ō-tĕn′sĭn) *n.* A 13-amino acid peptide found in the brain and spinal cord that affects pituitary hormone release and gastrointestinal functions.

neu·ro·the·ke·o·ma (no͝or′ō-thē′kē-ō′mə) *n.* A benign myxoma originating in cutaneous nerve sheath.

neu·rot·ic (no͝o-rŏt′ĭk) *adj.* Of, relating to, derived from, or affected with a neurosis. —*n.* A person suffering from a neurosis.

neu·ro·ti·za·tion (no͝or′ə-tĭ-zā′shən) *n.* **1.** The development of nerve tissue. **2.** The regeneration of a nerve.

neu·rot·me·sis (no͝or′ŏt-mē′sĭs) *n.* The condition in which there is complete division of a nerve.

neu·rot·o·my (no͝o-rŏt′ə-mē) *n.* Surgical division of a nerve.

neurotonic pupil *n.* A pupil that does not dilate after a light source that caused it to contract is reduced or removed.

neu·rot·o·ny (nŏo-rŏt′n-ē) *n.* See **neurectasis.** —**neu′-ro·ton′ic** (nŏor′ə-tŏn′ĭk) *adj.*

neu·ro·tox·in (nŏor′ō-tŏk′sĭn) *n.* See **neurolysin.** —**neu′ro·tox′ic** *adj.*

neu·ro·trans·mit·ter (nŏor′ō-trănz′mĭt-ər, -trăns′-) *n.* Any of the various chemical substances, such as acetylcholine, that transmit nerve impulses across a synapse.

neu·ro·trip·sy (nŏor′ə-trĭp′sē) *n.* The surgical crushing of a nerve.

neu·rot·ro·phy (nŏo-rŏt′rə-fē) *n.* The nutrition and metabolism of tissues under the influence of nerves. —**neu′ro·troph′ic** (nŏor′ə-trŏf′ĭk, -trō′fĭk) *adj.*

neu·rot·ro·py (nŏo-rŏt′rə-pē) *or* **neu·rot·ro·pism** (-pĭz′əm) *n.* The tendency to affect, be attracted to, or attack nervous tissue. —**neu′ro·trop′ic** (nŏor′ə-trŏp′-ĭk, -trō′pĭk) *adj.*

neu·ro·tu·bule (nŏor′ō-tōo′byōol) *n.* An elongated microtubule occurring in the cell body, dendrites, axon, and in some synaptic endings of neurons.

neu·ro·vac·cine (nŏor′ō-văk-sēn′ -văk′sēn′) *n.* A vaccine virus, such as that in the smallpox vaccine, of known strength cultivated in vivo in the brains of rabbits.

neu·ro·vas·cu·lar (nŏor′ō-văs′kyə-lər) *adj.* Of or relating to both nerves and blood vessels.

neu·ro·vi·rus (nŏor′ō-vī′rəs) *n.* A vaccine virus modified by passage into, and growth in, nervous tissue.

neu·ro·vis·cer·al (nŏor′ō-vĭs′ər-əl) *adj.* Of or relating to innervation of the internal organs by the autonomic nervous system.

neu·ru·la (nŏor′ə-lə, -yə-lə) *n., pl.* **-lae** (-lē′) An early stage of embryonic development in which neurulation begins.

neu·ru·la·tion (nŏor′ə-lā′shən, -yə-lā′-) *n.* The formation of the embryonic neural plate and its transformation into the neural tube.

neu·ter (nŏo′tər) *adj.* **1.** Having undeveloped or imperfectly developed sexual organs. **2.** Sexually undeveloped. —*n.* A castrated animal. —*v.* To castrate or spay.

neu·tral (nŏo′trəl) *adj.* **1.** Belonging to neither kind; not one thing or the other; indifferent. **2.** Of or relating to a solution or compound that is neither acidic nor alkaline. **3.** Of or relating to a compound that does not ionize in solution. **4.** Of or relating to a particle, object, or system that has a net electric charge of zero.

neu·tral·i·za·tion (nŏo′trə-lĭ-zā′shən) *n.* **1.** A reaction between an acid and a base that yields a salt and water. **2.** The rendering ineffective of an action or substance, such as a drug. **3.** The change of an acid solution to neutral by titration of an alkaline solution. **4.** The change of an alkaline solution to neutral by titration of an acid solution.

neutralization plate *n.* A metal plate used for the internal fixation of a long bone fracture to neutralize the forces producing displacement.

neutralization test *n.* See **protection test.**

neu·tral·iz·ing antibody (nŏo′trə-lī′zĭng) *n.* An antibody that reacts with an infectious agent, usually a virus, and destroys or inhibits its infectiveness and virulence.

neutral mutation *n.* A mutation with a negligible impact on genetic fitness.

neutral stain *n.* A compound of an acid and a basic dye that can produce staining effects that differ from those produced by either dye alone.

neu·tri·no (nŏo-trē′nō) *n., pl.* **-nos** Any of three electrically neutral subatomic particles in the lepton family.

neutro– *or* **neutr–** *pref.* Neutral: *neutrophil.*

neu·tron (nŏo′trŏn′) *n.* An electrically neutral subatomic particle in the baryon family, having a mass 1,839 times that of the electron, stable when bound in an atomic nucleus, and having a mean lifetime of approximately 1.0×10^3 seconds as a free particle. It and the proton form nearly the entire mass of atomic nuclei.

neu·tro·pe·ni·a (nŏo′trə-pē′nē-ə) *n.* The presence of abnormally small numbers of neutrophils in the blood. Also called *neutrophilic leukopenia.*

neu·tro·phil (nŏo′trə-fĭl′) *or* **neu·tro·phile** (-fĭl′) *n.* **1.** A neutrophil cell, especially an abundant type of granular white blood cell that is highly destructive of microorganisms. **2.** A cell or tissue that manifests no special affinity for acid or basic dyes. —*adj.* Not stained strongly or definitely by either acid or basic dyes but stained readily by neutral dyes. Used especially of white blood cells. —**neu′tro·phile′** (-fĭl′), **neu′tro·phil′ic** (-fĭl′ĭk) *adj.*

neu·tro·phil·i·a (nŏo′trə-fĭl′ē-ə) *n.* An increase of neutrophilic white blood cells in blood or tissues.

neu·tro·phil·ic leukocyte (nŏo′trə-fĭl′ĭk) *n.* A highly phagocytic, polymorphonuclear white blood cell containing granules that do not stain deeply with acid or basic dyes.

neutrophilic leukopenia *n.* See **neutropenia.**

neu·tro·tax·is (nŏo′trə-tăk′sĭs) *n.* A response designated as attractive, repulsive, or neutral, shown by neutrophilic white blood cells when stimulated by a substance.

ne·vir·a·pine (nə-vîr′ə-pēn′, -pĭn) *n.* A non-nucleoside analog that is used as an antiviral drug in treating HIV infection.

ne·void (nē′void′) *adj.* Resembling a nevus.

nevoid elephantiasis *n.* The congenital enlargement and obstruction of lymph vessels causing a thickening of skin on all or a part of an extremity on one side of the body.

ne·vose (nē′vōs′, -vōz′) *or* **ne·vous** (-vəs) *adj.* **1.** Having nevi. **2.** Nevoid.

ne·vo·xan·tho·en·do·the·li·o·ma (nē′vō-zăn′thō-ĕn′dō-thē′lē-ō′mə) *n.* See **juvenile xanthogranuloma.**

ne·vus (nē′vəs) *n., pl.* **-vi** (-vī′) **1.** A congenital circumscribed growth or mark on the skin, such as a mole or birthmark, colored by hyperpigmentation or increased vascularity. **2.** A benign localized overgrowth of melanin-forming cells arising in the skin early in life.

nevus cell *n.* A cell of a pigmented cutaneous nevus whose absence of dendrites differentiates from a melanocyte.

nevus flam·me·us (flăm′ē-əs) *n.* See **port-wine stain.**

nevus pig·men·to·sus (pĭg′mən-tō′səs, -měn-) *n.* See **mole**[1].

nevus se·ba·ce·us (sə-bā′sē-əs) *n.* Congenital hyperplasia of the sebaceous glands with papillary acanthosis of the epidermis.

nevus spi·lus (spī′ləs) *n.* A flat mole.

nevus u·ni·us lat·er·is (yōō-nī′əs lăt′ər-ĭs, yōō′nē-əs) *n.* A congenital linear nevus limited to one side of the body or to portions of the extremities on one side of the body.

nevus vas·cu·lar·is (văs′kyə-lâr′ĭs) *or* **nevus vas·cu·lo·sus** (-lō′səs) *n.* A congenital red-colored nevus that is irregular in shape and that is caused by an overgrowth of the cutaneous capillaries.

new·born (nōō′bôrn′) *adj.* Very recently born. —*n.* A neonate.

New Hamp·shire rule (nōō′ hămp′shər, hăm′-) *n.* An 1871 US rule used as a test of criminal responsibility and stating that criminal intent is not involved if the criminal act was due to insanity.

new·ton (nōōt′n) *n. Abbr.* **N** In the meter-kilogram-second system, the unit of force required to accelerate a mass of one kilogram one meter per second per second, equal to 100,000 dynes.

new·to·ni·an constant of gravitation (nōō-tō′nē-ən) *n. Abbr.* **G** See **gravitational constant.**

newton-meter *n.* A unit of the meter-kilogram-second system equal to the energy expended, or work done, by a force of one newton acting through a distance of one meter and equal to one joule.

New World leishmaniasis *n.* See **mucocutaneous leishmaniasis.**

Nex·i·um (něk′sē-əm) A trademark for the drug esomeprazole magnesium.

nex·us (něk′səs) *n., pl.* **nexus** *or* **–us·es** See **gap junction.**

Neze·lof type of thymic alymphoplasia (něz′lôf) *n.* See **cellular immunodeficiency.**

NF *abbr.* National Formulary

ng *abbr.* nanogram

NG *abbr.* nasogastric

NGF *abbr.* nerve growth factor

NGU *abbr.* nongonococcal urethritis

Ni The symbol for the element **nickel.**

ni·a·cin (nī′ə-sĭn) *n.* A crystalline acid that is a component of the vitamin B complex and is used to treat and prevent pellagra. Also called *nicotinic acid.*

ni·a·cin·a·mide (nī′ə-sĭn′ə-mīd′) *n.* See **nicotinamide.**

nib (nĭb) *n.* The smooth or serrated portion of a dental instrument that comes into contact with restorative material being condensed.

ni·car·di·pine (nī-kär′də-pēn′) *n.* A calcium channel blocker drug used to treat hypertension.

niche (nĭch, nēsh) *n.* **1.** An eroded or ulcerated area detected by contrast radiography. **2.** The function or position of an organism or population within an ecological community. **3.** The particular area within a habitat occupied by an organism.

nick·el (nĭk′əl) *n. Symbol* **Ni** A silvery hard ductile metallic element used in alloys and in corrosion-resistant surfaces. Atomic number 28.

nick·ing (nĭk′ĭng) *n.* A localized constriction in blood vessels of the retina of the eye.

Ni·co·las-Fa·vre disease (nē′kō-lə-făv′ər, nē-kō-lä′fä′-vrə) *n.* See **venereal lymphogranuloma.**

Ni·colle (nē-kôl′), **Charles Jean Henri** 1866–1936. French bacteriologist. He won a 1928 Nobel Prize for discovering the carrier of typhus.

Nic·o·rette (nĭk′ə-rĕt′) A trademark for an over-the-counter preparation of chewing gum containing nicotine, used to treat nicotine dependence.

nicotin– *pref.* **1.** Nicotine: *nicotinic.* **2.** Nicotinic acid: *nicotinamide.*

nic·o·tin·a·mide (nĭk′ə-tĭn′ə-mīd, -tē′nə-) *n.* The biologically active amide of niacin having similar vitamin activity and used in the prevention and treatment of pellagra. Also called *niacinamide.*

nicotinamide adenine dinucleotide *n.* NAD

nicotinamide adenine dinucleotide phosphate *n.* NADP.

nic·o·tine (nĭk′ə-tēn′) *n.* A colorless, poisonous alkaloid derived from the tobacco plant and used as an insecticide. It is the substance in tobacco to which smokers can become addicted.

nic·o·tin·ic (nĭk′ə-tĭn′ĭk, -tē′nĭk) *adj.* **1.** Of or relating to nicotine. **2.** Of or relating to niacin.

nicotinic acid *n.* See **niacin.**

nic·o·tin·ism (nĭk′ə-tē-nĭz′əm) *n.* Nicotine poisoning caused by excessive use of tobacco and characterized by depression of the central and autonomic nervous systems.

Nic·o·trol (nĭk′ə-trôl′) A trademark for a preparation that contains nicotine, is used to treat nicotine dependence, and is available as an inhaler, nasal spray, and skin patch.

nic·ti·ta·tion (nĭk′tĭ-tā′shən) *n.* Winking.

NICU *abbr.* neonatal intensive-care unit

ni·dal (nīd′l) *adj.* Of, relating to, or characteristic of a nidus.

ni·date (nī′dāt) *v.* To become implanted in the uterus. Used of an early embryo.

ni·da·tion (nī-dā′shən) *n.* The implantation of the early embryo in the uterine mucosa.

NIDDM *abbr.* non-insulin-dependent diabetes mellitus

ni·dus (nī′dəs) *n., pl.* **–dus·es** *or* **–di** (-dī) **1.** A central point or focus of bacterial growth in a living organism. **2.** A nest, especially one for the eggs of insects, spiders, pathogenic organisms, or small animals. **3.** A cavity where spores develop. **4.** A point or place at which something originates, accumulates, or develops, as the center around which calculi form.

nidus a·vis (ā′vĭs) *n.* A deep depression on each side of the inferior surface of the cerebellum in which the cerebellar tonsil rests. Also called *nidus hirundinus.*

Nie·mann-Pick cell (nē′män′-) *n.* A rounded or polygonal mononuclear cell with indistinctly or palely staining, foamlike cytoplasm that contains numerous droplets of sphingomyelin; it is characteristic of Niemann-Pick disease. Also called *Pick cell.*

Niemann-Pick disease *n.* An inherited disorder of lipid metabolism characterized by gastrointestinal disturbances and enlargement and abnormalities of blood-forming organs; it occurs primarily in infants of eastern European Jewish descent and it leads to early death. Also called *Pick's disease*[2], *sphingomyelin lipidosis.*

ni·fed·i·pine (nī-fĕd′ə-pēn′) *n.* A coronary vasodilator and calcium-channel blocking agent that reduces calcium ions available to heart and smooth muscle, used in the treatment of angina pectoris.

night-blind (nīt′blīnd′) *adj.* Affected with nyctalopia.

night blindness *n.* See **nyctalopia.**

Night·in·gale (nīt′n-gāl′), **Florence** 1820–1910. British nurse who organized (1854) and directed a unit of field nurses during the Crimean War and is considered the founder of modern nursing.

night·mare (nīt′mâr′) *n.* **1.** A dream arousing feelings of intense fear, horror, and distress. **2.** An event or experience that is intensely distressing.

night palsy *n.* A temporary numbness and paresis of an extremity that is caused by its compression during sleep.

night terrors *n.* A state of intense fear and agitation, usually occurring in children, that causes the person to wake up screaming with fear and to remain distressed during a period of semiconsciousness.

night vision *n.* Vision occurring in dim light.

ni·gra (nī′grə) *n.* See **substantia nigra.**

ni·gri·ti·es (nī-grĭsh′ē-ēz′) *n.* Black pigmentation, usually of the tongue.

nigrosine (nī′grə-sēn′, -sĭn′) *or* **ni·gro·sin** (-sĭn) *n.* Any of a class of aniline dyes that vary from blue to black and are used as stains for nervous tissue and as a negative stain for bacteria and spirochetes.

ni·gro·stri·a·tal (nī′grō-strī-āt′l) *adj.* Of or relating to the efferent connection of the substantia nigra with the striate body.

NIH *abbr.* National Institutes of Health

ni·hil·ism (nī′ə-lĭz′əm, nē′-) *n.* **1.** The belief that destruction of existing political or social institutions is necessary for future improvement. **2.** A delusion, experienced in some mental disorders, that the world or one's mind, body, or self does not exist.

Ni·kol·sky's sign (nĭ-kŏl′skēz) *n.* An indication of pemphigus vulgaris in which apparently normal epidermis may be separated at the basal layer and rubbed off when pressed with a sliding motion.

nin·hy·drin (nĭn-hī′drĭn) *n.* A poisonous crystalline oxidizing agent used as an analytic reagent.

ninhydrin reaction *n.* A test for proteins, peptones, peptides, and amino acids possessing free carboxyl and alpha-amino groups in which ninhydrin reacts with such compounds to produce a blue color.

ninth cranial nerve (nīnth) *n.* See **glossopharyngeal nerve.**

ni·o·bi·um (nī-ō′bē-əm) *n.* *Symbol* **Nb** A soft ductile metallic element that is used in steel alloys and superconductors. Atomic number 41.

Nip·ah virus (nĭp′ə) *n.* A single-stranded RNA virus that is transmitted from animals and causes fever and myalgias that can progress to encephalitis in humans.

nip·ple (nĭp′əl) *n.* The projection at the apex of the mammary gland, on the surface of which the lactiferous ducts open, surrounded by the circular pigmented areola. Also called *mamilla, papilla mammae, teat, thelium.*

nipple line *n.* See **mamillary line.**

nipple shield *n.* A cap or dome placed over the nipple of the breast to protect it during nursing.

Nir·en·berg (nîr′ĭn-bûrg′), **Marshall Warren** Born 1927. American biochemist. He shared a 1968 Nobel Prize for the study of genetic codes.

Nissl substance (nĭs′l) *n.* Material consisting of granular endoplasmic reticulum and ribosomes and occurring in nerve cell bodies and dendrites. Also called *Nissl body, Nissl granule.*

nit (nĭt) *n.* The egg or young of a parasitic insect, such as a louse.

ni·trate (nī′trāt′, -trĭt) *n.* **1.** The univalent radical NO_3. **2.** A compound containing such a radical, such as a salt or ester of nitric acid. —*v.* To treat with nitric acid or a nitrate, usually to change an organic compound into a nitrate.

ni·tric acid (nī′trĭk) *n.* A transparent, colorless to yellowish, fuming corrosive liquid that is a highly reactive oxidizing agent.

ni·tri·da·tion (nī′trĭ-dā′shən) *n.* The formation of nitrogen compounds through the action of ammonia.

ni·tride (nī′trīd′) *n.* A compound containing nitrogen with another more electropositive element, such as phosphorus or a metal.

ni·tri·fi·ca·tion (nī′trə-fĭ-kā′shən) *n.* **1.** The oxidation of an ammonia compound into nitric acid, nitrous acid, or any nitrate or nitrite, especially by the action of bacteria. **2.** The treatment or combination of a substance with nitrogen or compounds containing nitrogen.

ni·trile *or* **ni·tril** (nī′trəl) *n.* An organic cyanide containing a CN group.

nitrilo– *pref.* Containing trivalent nitrogen bonded to three identical groups: *nitrilotriacetic acid.*

ni·trite (nī′trīt′) *n.* **1.** The univalent radical NO_2. **2.** A compound containing such a radical, such as a salt or ester of nitrous acid.

ni·tri·tu·ri·a (nī′trĭ-tŏŏr′ē-ə) *n.* The presence of nitrites or nitrates, or both, in the urine.

nitro– *or* **nitr–** *pref.* **1.** Nitrate; nitrogen: *nitrogenase.* **2.** Containing the univalent radical NO_2: *nitrous.*

ni·tro·blue tet·ra·zo·li·um test (nī′trō-blōō′ tĕt′rə-zō′lē-əm) *n.* A test to detect the phagocytic ability of polymorphonuclear white blood cells. Also called *NBT test.*

ni·tro·cel·lu·lose (nī′trō-sĕl′yə-lōs′, -lōz′) *n.* See **cellulose nitrate.**

ni·tro dye (nī′trō) *n.* Any of a group of acidic dyes often used in staining cytoplasm.

ni·tro·fu·ran (nī′trō-fyŏŏr′ăn′, -fyŏō-răn′) *n.* Any of several drugs derived from furan that are used to inhibit bacterial growth.

ni·tro·fur·an·to·in (nī′trō-fyŏō-răn′tō-ĭn) *n.* A derivative of nitrofuran used in the treatment of bacterial infections of the urinary tract.

ni·tro·gen (nī′trə-jən) *n.* *Symbol* **N** A nonmetallic element that constitutes nearly four fifths of the air by volume, occurring as a colorless, odorless, almost inert diatomic gas, N_2, in various minerals and in all proteins. Atomic number 7.

ni·trog·e·nase (nī-trŏj′ə-nās′, -nāz′, nī′trə-jə-) *n.* An enzyme of certain bacteria that activates the conversion of nitrogen to ammonia.

nitrogen balance *n.* The difference between the amount

of nitrogen taken into the body and the amount excreted or lost.

nitrogen cycle *n.* **1.** The circulation of nitrogen in nature, consisting of a cycle of chemical reactions in which atmospheric nitrogen is compounded, dissolved in rain, and deposited in the soil, where it is assimilated and metabolized by bacteria and plants, eventually returning to the atmosphere by bacterial decomposition of organic matter. **2.** See **carbon-nitrogen cycle.**

nitrogen distribution *n.* See **nitrogen partition.**

nitrogen equivalent *n.* The nitrogen content of protein, used in calculating the grams of protein metabolized by the body as a function of the grams of nitrogen excreted in the urine.

nitrogen lag *n.* The length of time between ingestion of a given protein and the urinary excretion of the amount of nitrogen equal to that in the protein.

nitrogen mustard *n.* Any of various toxic blistering compounds analogous to mustard gas but containing nitrogen rather than sulfur, sometimes used to control or check the growth of neoplastic cells.

nitrogen narcosis *n.* **1.** Narcosis produced by nitrogenous materials such as those occurring in certain forms of uremia and hepatic coma. **2.** A stuporous condition variously characterized by disorientation, euphoria, and loss of judgment and skill, attributed to nitrogen entering the blood during breathing of normal air at increased pressure, as occurs with deep-sea divers. Also called *rapture of the deep.*

ni·trog·e·nous (nī-trŏj′ə-nəs) *adj.* Relating to or containing nitrogen.

nitrogen partition *n.* The determination of the distribution of nitrogen in the urine among the various constituents. Also called *nitrogen distribution.*

ni·tro·glyc·er·in *or* **ni·tro·glyc·er·ine** (nī′trō-glĭs′ər-ĭn, -trə-) *n.* A thick, pale yellow liquid that is explosive on concussion or exposure to sudden heat, used as a vasodilator in medicine.

ni·tro·prus·side test (nī′trō-prŭs′īd′) *n.* A test for cystinuria in which sodium cyanide and then nitroprusside are added to urine.

ni·tros·a·mine (nī-trō′sə-mēn′, nī′trōs-ăm′ēn) *n.* Any of a class of organic compounds present in various foods and other products and found to be carcinogenic and mutagenic in laboratory animals.

nitroso– *pref.* Nitrosyl: *nitrosobenzene.*

ni·tro·syl (nī′trə-sĭl) *n.* The univalent radical NO.

ni·trous (nī′trəs) *adj.* Of, derived from, or containing nitrogen, especially in a valence state lower than that in a comparable nitric compound.

nitrous acid *n.* A weak inorganic acid existing only in solution or in the form of its salts.

nitrous oxide *n.* A colorless sweet-tasting gas used as a mild anesthetic in dentistry and surgery.

ni·tryl (nī′trəl) *n.* The univalent radical NO_2.

Nix (nĭks) A trademark for the drug permethrin.

ni·zat·i·dine (nī-zăt′ĭ-dēn′) *n.* A histamine antagonist used in the treatment of active duodenal ulcers.

Ni·zo·ral (nī′zə-răl′) A trademark for a preparation of ketoconazole.

NKA *abbr.* no known allergies

NK cell *abbr.* natural killer cell

NKDA *abbr.* no known drug allergies

NLD *abbr.* nonverbal learning disorder

nm *abbr.* nanometer

NMDA receptor (ĕn′ĕm′dē′ā′) *n.* A brain receptor activated by the amino acid glutamate, which when excessively stimulated may cause cognitive defects in Alzheimer's disease. Also called *N-methyl-D-aspartate receptor.*

NMR *abbr.* nuclear magnetic resonance

No The symbol for the element **nobelium.**

no·bel·i·um (nō-bĕl′ē-əm) *n. Symbol* **No** A radioactive synthetic element in the actinide series; its longest-lived isotope is No 259 with a half-life of 58 minutes. Atomic number 102.

no·ble gas (nō′bəl) *n.* Any of the elements in Group O of the periodic table, including helium, neon, argon, krypton, xenon, and radon, which are monatomic and with limited exceptions chemically inert. Also called *inert gas.*

No·car·di·a (nō-kär′dē-ə) *n.* A genus of aerobic, grampositive, primarily saprophytic actinomycetes that are transitional between bacteria and fungi and that form filaments that fragment to single nonmotile microorganisms, including some species that may be pathogenic to humans and other animals.

Nocardia as·ter·oi·des (ăs′tə-roi′dēz) *n.* A species of *Nocardia* that causes nocardiosis.

Nocardia ca·vi·ae (kā′vē-ē′) *n.* A species of *Nocardia* that causes mycetoma in humans.

Nocardia far·ci·ni·ca (fär-sĭ′nĭ-kə) *n.* A species of *Nocardia* that sometimes causes systemic nocardiosis.

no·car·di·o·sis (nō-kär′dē-ō′sĭs) *n.* A generalized disease in humans that is caused by *Nocardia asteroides* or occasionally by *N. farcinica* and that is characterized by pulmonary lesions that may be subclinical or chronic and may spread to other organs of the body, especially the brain.

noci– *pref.* Injury; pain; painful stimulus: *nociperception.*

no·ci·cep·tive (nō′sĭ-sĕp′tĭv) *adj.* **1.** Causing pain. Used of a stimulus. **2.** Caused by or responding to a painful stimulus.

nociceptive reflex *n.* A reflex elicited by a painful stimulus.

no·ci·cep·tor (nō′sĭ-sĕp′tər) *n.* A sensory receptor that responds to pain.

no·ci·fen·sor (nō′sĭ-fĕn′sər) *n.* **1.** A process or mechanism that acts to protect the body from injury. **2.** A system of nerves in the skin and mucous membranes that react to adjacent injury by causing vasodilation.

no·ci·in·flu·ence (nō′sē-ĭn′floō-əns) *n.* An injurious or harmful influence.

no·ci·per·cep·tion (nō′sĭ-pər-sĕp′shən) *n.* The perception of injurious stimuli, as by nerve centers.

no code *n.* An order given by a physician to refrain from initiating a code blue for a patient undergoing cardiac arrest.

noct– *pref.* Night: *nocturia.*

noc·tam·bu·lism (nŏk-tăm′byə-lĭz′əm) *n.* See **sleepwalking.**

noct. maneq. *abbr. Latin* nocte maneque (at night and in the morning)

noc·tu·ri·a (nŏk-tŏŏr′ē-ə) *n.* Urination at night, especially if excessive.

noc·tur·nal (nŏk-tûr′nəl) *adj.* **1.** Of, relating to, or occurring in the night. **2.** Most active at night.

nocturnal emission *n.* An involuntary ejaculation of semen during sleep.

nocturnal enuresis *n.* See **bed-wetting.**

nocturnal myoclonus *n.* Frequently repeated muscular jerks at the moment of dropping off to sleep.

nod·al (nōd′l) *adj.* Of, relating to, resembling, being, or situated near or at a node.

nodal bradycardia *n.* See **atrioventricular nodal rhythm.**

nodal escape *n.* Cardiologic escape in which the atrioventricular node serves as pacemaker.

nodal extrasystole *n.* See **atrioventricular nodal extrasystole.**

nodal point *n.* One of the two points in a compound optical system, located so that a light ray directed through the first point will leave the system through the second point, parallel to its original direction. Also called *axial point.*

nodal rhythm *n.* See **atrioventricular nodal rhythm.**

nod·ding spasm (nŏd′ĭng) *n.* **1.** A falling of the head onto the chest that is most commonly seen in infants and is caused by the loss of tone in the neck muscles, as in epilepsy, or by tonic spasm of anterior neck muscles. **2.** A nodding of the head caused by a clonic spasm of the sternocleidomastoid muscle. Also called *salaam convulsion.*

node (nōd) *n.* **1.** A knob, knot, protuberance, or swelling. **2.** A protuberant growth or swelling in a tissue. **3.** A knuckle or finger joint.

node of Cloquet *n.* One of the deep inguinal lymph nodes located in or adjacent to the femoral canal and which is sometimes mistaken for a femoral hernia when enlarged.

no·dose (nō′dōs′) *adj.* Having many nodes or knotlike swellings. —**no·dos′i·ty** (-dŏs′ĭ-tē) *n.*

nodose rheumatism *n.* Acute or subacute articular rheumatism accompanied by the formation of nodules on the tendons, ligaments, and periosteum in the area of the affected joints.

no·dous (nō′dəs) *adj.* Having many nodes; nodose.

nodular amyloidosis *n.* Amyloidosis in which amyloid occurs as small masses or nodules beneath the skin or mucous membranes. Also called *amyloid tumor, focal amyloidosis.*

nodular fasciitis *n.* A tumorlike proliferation of fibroblasts with mild inflammatory exudation occurring in a fascia. Also called *proliferative fasciitis.*

nodular leprosy *n.* See **tuberculoid leprosy.**

nodular lymphoma *n.* Malignant lymphoma characterized by nodules resembling normal lymph nodes but consisting of undifferentiated cells that are similar to lymphocytes or contain variable numbers of larger histiocytelike cells. Also called *Brill-Symmers disease, follicular lymphoma.*

nodular non·sup·pu·ra·tive panniculitis (nŏn-sŭp′-yə-rā′tĭv) *n.* Panniculitis having no known cause and characterized by recurring attacks of fever and the formation of tender subcutaneous nodules on the trunk

and legs. Also called *Christian's disease, Weber-Christian disease.*

nod·u·la·tion (nŏj′ə-lā′shən) *n.* The formation or presence of nodules.

nod·ule (nŏj′ōol) *n.* **1.** A small node. **2.** A small mass of tissue or aggregation of cells. —**nod′u·lar** (nŏj′ə-lər), **nod′u·lose′** (-lōs′), **nod′u·lous** (-ləs) *adj.*

nodule of semilunar valve *n.* A nodule located at the center of the free border of each semilunar valve at the beginning of the pulmonary artery and aorta. Also called *Arantius' nodule, Bianchi's nodule, Morgagni's nodule.*

nod·u·lus (nŏj′ə-ləs) *n., pl.* **-li** (-lī′) **1.** A small node; nodule. **2.** The posterior extremity of the lower part of the vermis of the cerebellum.

no·dus (nō′dəs) *n., pl.* **-di** (-dī) A circumscribed mass of tissue; a node.

nodus lym·phat·i·cus (lĭm-făt′ĭ-kəs) *n.* Lymph node.

No·gu·chi (nō-gōō′chē), **Hideyo** 1876–1928. Japanese-born American bacteriologist who discovered the cause of syphilis and yellow fever and who worked to develop treatments for them.

noise pollution (noiz) *n.* An annoying or physiologically damaging environmental noise level.

Nol·va·dex (nōl′və-dĕks′) A trademark for the drug tamoxifen.

no·ma (nō′mə) *n.* A severe, often gangrenous inflammation of the lips and cheek or of the female genitals that often occurs following an infectious disease and is found most often in children in poor hygienic or malnourished condition. Also called *stomatonecrosis.*

no·men·cla·ture (nō′mən-klā′chər, nō-mĕn′klə-) *n.* A system of names used in a science, as of anatomical structures or biological organisms.

nom·i·nal aphasia (nŏm′ə-nəl) *n.* Aphasia that is characterized by the impaired ability to recall the names of persons and things. Also called *anomia, anomic aphasia.*

nom·o·graph (nŏm′ə-grăf′, nō′mə-) *or* **nom·o·gram** (-grăm′) *n.* A graph consisting of three coplanar curves, each curve graduated for a different variable so that a straight line cutting all three curves intersects the related values of each variable. —**nom′o·graph′ic** *adj.* —**no·mog′ra·phy** (nō-mŏg′rə-fē) *n.*

nom·o·top·ic (nŏm′ə-tŏp′ĭk, nō′mə-) *adj.* Relating to or occurring at the usual or normal place.

non– *pref.* Not: *noninvasive.*

non·ab·sorb·a·ble suture (nŏn′əb-zôr′bə-bəl) *n.* A surgical suture made from a material unaffected by the biological activities of the body tissues, and therefore permanent unless removed.

non·al·co·hol·ic (nŏn′ăl-kə-hô′lĭk) *adj.* A beverage usually containing less than 0.5 percent alcohol by volume.

non-A, non-B hepatitis (nŏn-ā′nŏn-bē′) *n. Abbr.* **NANB hepatitis** Hepatitis that is caused by a virus that is antigenically different from hepatitis viruses A and B.

non·bac·te·ri·al verrucous endocarditis (nŏn′băk-tîr′ē-əl) *n.* See **Libman-Sacks endocarditis.**

non·ca·lor·ic (nŏn′kə-lôr′ĭk) *adj.* Having few or no calories.

non·chro·maf·fin paraganglioma (nŏn-krō′mə-fĭn) *n.* See **chemodectoma.**

non·chro·mo·som·al (nŏn′krō-mə-sō′məl) *adj.* Not situated on or involving a chromosome.

non·com·mu·ni·cat·ing hydrocephalus (nŏn′kə-myōō′nĭ-kā′tĭng) *n.* A form of hydrocephalus in which the ventricles of the brain are blocked and cerebrospinal fluid cannot pass to the subarachnoid space. Also called *obstructive hydrocephalus.*

non·com·pet·i·tive inhibition (nŏn′kəm-pĕt′ĭ-tĭv) *n.* Enzyme inhibition in which the inhibiting compound does not compete with the natural substrate for the active site on the enzyme but inhibits reaction by combining with the enzyme-substrate complex after the complex is formed.

non com·pos men·tis (nŏn kŏm′pəs mĕn′tĭs) *adj.* Not of sound mind and hence not legally responsible; mentally incompetent.

non·con·ju·ga·tive plasmid (nŏn-kŏn′jə-gā′tĭv) *n.* A plasmid that cannot move to another bacterium during conjugation but requires mediation by a conjugative plasmid.

non·de·po·lar·iz·ing block (nŏn′dē-pō′lə-rī′zĭng) *n.* A paralysis of skeletal muscle unaccompanied by changes in polarity of the motor end plate, as occurs following administration of tubocurarine chloride.

nondepolarizing neuromuscular blocking agent *n.* A compound that paralyzes skeletal muscle by inhibiting the release of neurotransmitters at the neuromuscular junction.

non·di·rec·tive (nŏn′dĭ-rĕk′tĭv, -dī-) *adj.* Of, relating to, or being a psychotherapeutic or counseling technique in which the therapist takes an unobtrusive role in order to encourage free expression.

non·dis·junc·tion (nŏn′dĭs-jŭngk′shən) *n.* The failure of one or more pairs of chromosomes to separate at the miotic stage of karyokinesis, with the result that both chromosomes are carried to one daughter cell and none to the other. —**non′dis·junc′tion·al** *adj.*

non·e·lec·tro·lyte (nŏn′ĭ-lĕk′trə-līt′) *n.* A substance whose molecules in solution do not dissociate to ions and thus do not conduct an electric current.

non·es·sen·tial (nŏn′ĭ-sĕn′shəl) *adj.* Being a substance required for normal functioning but not needed in the diet because the body can synthesize it.

nonessential amino acid *n.* An alpha-amino acid that is required for protein synthesis and can be synthesized by humans.

non·fa·mil·ial hyperlipoproteinemia (nŏn′fə-mĭl′yəl) *n.* See **acquired hyperlipoproteinemia.**

non·fat (nŏn′făt′) *adj.* Lacking fat solids or having the fat content removed.

non·fen·es·trat·ed forceps (nŏn-fĕn′ĭ-strā′tĭd) *n.* An obstetrical forceps without openings in the blades, thus facilitating rotation of the head.

non·flam·ma·ble (nŏn-flăm′ə-bəl) *adj.* Not flammable, especially not readily ignited and not rapidly burned.

non·gon·o·coc·cal urethritis (nŏn′gŏn-ə-kŏk′əl) *n.* *Abbr.* **NGU** Inflammation of the urethra similar to that of gonorrhea but usually caused by infection with the rickettsia *Chlamydia trachomatis* and occurring mostly in males.

non-Hodg·kin's lymphoma (nŏn-hŏj′kĭnz) *n.* Any of various malignant lymphomas characterized by the absence of Reed-Sternberg cells.

non·i·den·ti·cal (nŏn′ĭ-dĕn′tĭ-kəl) *adj.* **1.** Not being the same; different. **2.** Fraternal, as of twins.

non·im·mune fetal hydrops (nŏn′ĭ-myoōn′) *n.* A combination of edema and ascites in a fetus not affected by erythroblastosis fetalis.

nonimmune serum *n.* Serum that does not contain antibodies to a given antigen.

non·im·mu·ni·ty (nŏn′ĭ-myoō′nĭ-tē) *n.* See **aphylaxis.**

non·in·su·lin·de·pend·ent diabetes mellitus (nŏn-ĭn′sə-lĭn-dĭ-pĕn′dənt) *n. Abbr.* **NIDDM** See **diabetes mellitus** (sense 2).

non·in·va·sive (nŏn′ĭn-vā′sĭv) *adj.* **1.** Not penetrating the body, as by incision. Used especially of a diagnostic procedure. **2.** Not invading healthy tissue.

non·i·so·lat·ed proteinuria (nŏn-ī′sə-lā′tĭd) *n.* Proteinuria associated with other abnormalities.

non·la·mel·lar bone (nŏn′lə-mĕl′ər) *n.* See **woven bone.**

non·lead·ed (nŏn-lĕd′ĭd) *adj.* Containing no lead; lead-free.

non·lip·id histiocytosis (nŏn-lĭp′ĭd, -lī′pĭd) *n.* An acute, progressive, usually fatal disease occurring in infants and young children and marked by a purpuric rash, excessive tissue proliferation without lipid storage in the reticuloendothelial system, enlargement of the lymph nodes, liver, and spleen, and invasion of the spleen, liver, and bone marrow by histiocytes. Also called *Letterer-Siwe disease.*

non·med·ul·lat·ed fiber (nŏn-mĕd′l-ā′tĭd) *n.* See **unmyelinated fiber.**

non·nu·cle·o·side analogue (nŏn-noō′klē-ə-sīd′) *n.* Any of a structurally diverse group of antiviral agents, including delavirdine and nevirapine, that inhibit the enzyme reverse transcriptase and are used to treat HIV.

non·ob·struc·tive jaundice (nŏn′əb-strŭk′tĭv) *n.* Jaundice in which the main biliary passages of the liver are not obstructed, as in hemolytic jaundice.

non·os·te·o·gen·ic fibroma (nŏn′ŏs-tē-ə-jĕn′ĭk) *n.* See **fibrous cortical defect.**

non·ox·y·nol-9 (nŏn-ŏk′sə-nôl′-, -nôl′-) *n.* A spermicide that is widely used in contraceptive creams, foams, and lubricants.

non·pen·e·trance (nŏn-pĕn′ĭ-trəns) *n.* **1.** The state in which a genetic trait although present in the appropriate genotype fails to manifest itself in the phenotype. **2.** The obscuring of genetic traits by nongenetic mechanisms.

non·pen·e·trant trait (nŏn-pĕn′ĭ-trənt) *n.* A genetic trait that is not manifested phenotypically because of factors outside its own locus.

non·pen·e·trat·ing wound (nŏn-pĕn′ĭ-trā′tĭng) *n.* A wound, especially to the thorax or abdomen, produced without disruption of the surface of the body.

non·per·sis·tent (nŏn′pər-sĭs′tənt) *adj.* Having a short life or existence under natural conditions.

non·pre·scrip·tion (nŏn′prĭ-skrĭp′shən) *adj.* Sold legally without the prescription of a physician; over-the-counter.

non·pro·pri·e·tary name (nŏn′prə-prī′ĭ-tĕr′ē) *n.* A short name of a chemical, drug, or other substance not subject to trademark rights but recognized by government agencies and other organizations.

non·pro·tein nitrogen (nŏn-prō′tēn′) *n. Abbr.* **NPN** The nitrogen content of substances other than protein in blood, tissues, and waste materials.

non·rap·id eye movement (nŏn-răp′ĭd) *n. Abbr.* **NREM** Slow oscillation of the eyes during the portion of the sleep cycle when no dreaming occurs.

non·re·breath·ing anesthesia (nŏn′rē-brē′thĭng) *n.* A technique for inhalation anesthesia in which valves exhaust all exhaled air from the circuit.

non·re·sis·tant (nŏn′rĭ-zĭs′tənt) *adj.* **1.** Not resistant, especially to a disease or environmental factor, such as heat or moisture. **2.** Submissively obedient.

non·se·cre·tor (nŏn′sĭ-krē′tər) *n.* An individual whose saliva does not contain antigens of the ABO blood group.

non·self (nŏn-sĕlf′) *n.* That which the immune system identifies as foreign to the body.

non·sense triplet (nŏn′sĕns′, -səns) *n.* A codon that causes the premature termination of a growing polypeptide chain, thus producing incomplete protein fragments.

non·sex·u·al generation (nŏn-sĕk′shoo-əl) *n.* See **asexual generation.**

non·spe·cif·ic immunity (nŏn′spĭ-sĭf′ĭk) *n.* See **innate immunity.**

nonspecific protein *n.* A protein substance that elicits an immunological response not mediated by a specific antigen-antibody reaction.

nonspecific urethritis *n.* Urethritis not resulting from gonococcal or other identifiable infectious agents.

non·ste·roi·dal (nŏn′stĭ-roid′l, -stĕ-) *or* **non·ster·oid** (nŏn-stîr′oid, -stĕr′-) *adj.* Not being or containing a steroid. —*n.* A drug or other substance not containing a steroid.

non·stress test (nŏn′strĕs′) *n.* An ultrasound examination of a fetus that measures fetal well-being by correlating fetal movement with changes in fetal heartbeat.

non·throm·bo·cy·to·pe·nic purpura (nŏn′thrŏm-bō-sī′tə-pē′nĭk) *n.* Purpura that is not accompanied by a decrease of platelets in the blood. Also called *purpura simplex.*

non·tox·ic goiter (nŏn-tŏk′sĭk) *n.* Goiter not accompanied by hyperthyroidism.

non·trop·i·cal sprue (nŏn-trŏp′ĭ-kəl) *n.* See **celiac disease.**

non·un·ion (nŏn-yoon′yən) *n.* The failure of a fractured bone to heal normally.

non·va·lent (nŏn-vā′lənt) *adj.* Not capable of forming chemical compounds; having no valency.

non·ver·bal learning disorder (nŏn-vûr′bəl) *n. Abbr.* **NLD** A neurological disorder of the right cerebral hemisphere in which the processing of nonverbal and visual-spatial information is impaired, leading to deficits in balance and coordination, pattern recognition, mathematical ability, and visual memory.

non·vi·a·ble (nŏn-vī′ə-bəl) *adj.* Not capable of living or developing independently. Used especially of an embryo or fetus.

non·vi·tal pulp (nŏn-vīt′l) *n.* See **necrotic pulp.**

Noo·nan's syndrome (noo′nənz) *n.* An inherited condition characterized by congenital heart disease, pulmonary stenosis, webbed neck, and pigeon breast. Also called *male Turner's syndrome.*

nor– *pref.* A precursor compound that differs from its successor by the absence of a radical group, usually methyl: *norepinephrine.*

nor·a·dren·a·lin (nôr′ə-drĕn′ə-lĭn) *n.* See **norepinephrine.**

nor·ad·ren·er·gic (nôr′ăd-rə-nûr′jĭk) *adj.* Stimulated by or releasing norepinephrine.

nor·ep·i·neph·rine (nôr′ĕp-ə-nĕf′rĭn) *n.* A substance, both a hormone and neurotransmitter, secreted by the adrenal medulla and the nerve endings of the sympathetic nervous system to cause vasoconstriction and increases in heart rate, blood pressure, and the sugar level of the blood. Also called *levarterenol, noradrenalin.*

nor·eth·an·dro·lone (nôr′ĕth-ăn′drə-lōn′) *n.* An androgenic steroid chemically and pharmacologically similar to testosterone.

nor·eth·in·drone (nôr-ĕth′ĭn-drōn′) *n.* A progestational agent with some estrogenic and androgenic activity that is used as a substitute for progesterone and, in combination with an estrogen, as an oral contraceptive.

nor·flox·a·cin (nôr-flŏk′sə-sĭn) *n.* An oral antibiotic of the fluoroquinolone class.

nor·ges·trel (nôr-jĕs′trəl) *n.* A synthetic progestogen used in combination with estrogen as an oral contraceptive.

nor·leu·cine (nôr-loo′sēn′) *n.* A crystalline alpha-amino acid that is isomeric to leucine and isoleucine but not found in proteins and formed in the deamination of lysine. Also called *caprine.*

nor·ma (nôr′mə) *n., pl.* **–mae** (-mē) A line or pattern defining the contour of a part, especially of various aspects of the cranium.

nor·mal (nôr′məl) *adj.* **1.** Conforming with, adhering to, or constituting a norm, standard, pattern, level, or type; typical. **2.** Functioning or occurring in a natural way; lacking observable abnormalities or deficiencies. **3.** Occurring naturally and not because of disease, inoculation, or any experimental treatment. Used of immunity. **4.** Of, relating to, or being a solution having one gram equivalent weight of solute per liter of solution. **5.** Of, relating to, or being an aliphatic hydrocarbon having a straight and unbranched chain of carbon atoms. **6.** Of, relating to, or characterized by average intelligence or development. —*n.* The usual or the expected state, form, amount, or degree.

normal antibody *n.* An antibody that has been induced without known exposure to the specific antigen, usually the result of naturally occurring contact. Also called *natural antibody.*

normal antitoxin *n.* A serum that has the capacity to neutralize an equivalent quantity of normal toxin solution.

normal human plasma *n.* Sterile plasma obtained by pooling the liquid portion of whole blood to which has been added a solution of potassium or sodium citrate, or both, from eight or more healthy adult humans and by exposing it to ultraviolet light to destroy bacterial and viral contaminants.

normal human serum albumin *n.* A sterile preparation of serum albumin obtained by fractionating blood plasma proteins from healthy persons and used as a transfusion material.

normal occlusion *n.* The normal arrangement of teeth and their supporting structures that approaches an ideal or standard arrangement.

normal opsonin *n.* Opsonin normally present in the blood and not the product of stimulation by a known specific antigen.

normal pressure hydrocephalus *n.* A hydrocephalic condition in which the spinal fluid pressure remains normal, resulting from the inability of the arachnoid granulations to absorb cerebrospinal fluid, and characterized by progressive dementia. Also called *occult hydrocephalus.*

normal serum *n.* A nonimmune serum, especially serum from an individual prior to immunization.

normal values *pl.n.* A set of laboratory test values used to characterize apparently healthy individuals, now replaced by reference values.

nor·met·a·neph·rine (nôr′mĕt-ə-nĕf′rĭn) *n.* A catabolite of norepinephrine found, together with metanephrine, in the urine and in some tissues.

normo– *pref.* Normal: *normochromia.*

nor·mo·blast (nôr′mə-blăst′) *n.* A nucleated red blood cell, the immediate precursor of a normal red blood cell in humans.

nor·mo·cap·ni·a (nôr′mə-kăp′nē-ə) *n.* A state of normal arterial carbon dioxide pressure.

nor·mo·chro·mi·a (nôr′mō-krō′mē-ə) *n.* Normal blood color because of a normal amount of hemoglobin in the red blood cells.

nor·mo·chro·mic anemia (nôr′mō-krō′mĭk) *n.* Anemia in which the concentration of hemoglobin in the red blood cells is within the normal range.

nor·mo·cyte (nôr′mə-sīt′) *n.* A red blood cell having normal size, shape, or color.

nor·mo·cyt·ic anemia (nôr′mō-sĭt′ĭk) *n.* Anemia in which the red blood cells are normal in size.

nor·mo·cy·to·sis (nôr′mō-sī-tō′sĭs) *n.* A state of the blood in which the erythrocytes are normal in size and hemoglobin content.

Nor·mo·dyne (nôr′mə-dīn′) A trademark for the drug labetalol hydrochloride.

nor·mo·gly·ce·mi·a (nôr′mō-glī-sē′mē-ə) *n.* See **euglycemia.** —**nor′mo·gly·ce′mic** *adj.*

nor·mo·ka·le·mi·a (nôr′mō-kā-lē′mē-ə) *n.* A normal level of potassium in the blood.

nor·mo·ka·le·mic periodic paralysis (nôr′mō-kā-lē′mĭk) *n.* An inherited form of periodic paralysis in which the serum potassium concentration is within normal limits during attacks. Onset usually occurs between the ages of 2 and 5 years, often associated with severe quadriplegia.

nor·mo·ten·sive (nôr′mō-tĕn′sĭv) *adj.* Of or relating to a normal arterial blood pressure; normotonic.

nor·mo·ther·mi·a (nôr′mō-thûr′mē-ə) *n.* **1.** A condition of normal body temperature. **2.** An environmental temperature that does not cause more or less activity of body cells. —**nor′mo·ther′mic** *adj.*

nor·mo·ton·ic (nôr′mō-tŏn′ĭk) *adj.* **1.** Of or relating to normal muscular tone. **2.** Normotensive.

nor·mo·vo·le·mi·a (nôr′mō-vŏ-lē′mē-ə) *n.* A normal blood volume.

nor·o·vi·rus (nôr′ō-vī′rəs) *n.* A single-stranded RNA virus in the genus *Norovirus* of the family Caliciviridae, formerly called Norwalk virus, that causes acute gastroenteritis.

No·rox·in (nə-rŏk′sĭn) A trademark for the drug norfloxacin.

Nor·plant (nôr′plănt′) A trademark used for the drug levonorgestrel when it is implanted under the skin.

Nor·pra·min (nôr′prə-mĭn) A trademark for the drug desipramine hydrochloride.

Nor·rie's disease (nôr′ēz) *n.* A rare sex-linked blindness characterized by tissue masses on the retina or vitreous body, iris atrophication, and cataracts.

North American blastomycosis (nôrth) *n.* Blastomycosis. No longer in technical use.

North·ern blot analysis (nôr′thərn) *n.* An electrophoretic procedure used to separate and identify RNA fragments.

Nor·throp (nôr′thrəp), **John Howard** 1891–1987. American biochemist. He shared a 1946 Nobel Prize for discovering methods of producing pure enzymes and virus proteins.

nor·trip·ty·line hydrochloride (nôr-trĭp′tə-lēn′) *n.* A tricyclic compound used as an antidepressant.

Nor·vir (nôr′vîr′) A trademark for the drug ritonavir.

Nor·walk virus (nôr′wôk′) *n.* A norovirus.

nos·ca·pine (nŏs′kə-pēn′) *n.* An alkaloid occurring in opium that suppresses the cough reflex and is used as an antitussive.

nose (nōz) *n.* The part of the human face or the forward part of the head of other vertebrates that contains the nostrils and organs of smell and forms the beginning of the respiratory tract.

nose·bleed (nōz′blēd′) *n.* A nasal hemorrhage; bleeding from the nose.

nose job *n.* Rhinoplasty, especially one performed for cosmetic purposes. Used informally.

nose·piece (nōz′pēs′) *n.* The part of a microscope, often rotatable, to which one or more objective lenses are attached.

noso– *pref.* Disease: *nosology.*

nos·o·co·mi·al (nŏs′ə-kō′mē-əl) *adj.* **1.** Of or relating to a hospital. **2.** Of or being a secondary disorder associated with being treated in a hospital but unrelated to the patient's primary condition.

nos·o·gen·e·sis (nŏs′ō-jĕn′ĭ-sĭs) *or* **no·sog·e·ny** (nō-sŏj′ə-nē) *n.* See **pathogenesis.**

nos·o·gen·ic (nŏs′ə-jĕn′ĭk) *adj.* Pathogenic.

no·sog·ra·phy (nō-sŏg′rə-fē, -zŏg′-) *n.* The systematic description of diseases.

no·sol·o·gy (nō-sŏl′ə-jē, -zŏl′-) *n.* **1.** The branch of medicine that deals with the classification of diseases. Also called *nosonomy, nosotaxy.* **2.** A classification of diseases. —**no·so·log′i·cal** (-sə-lŏj′ĭ-kəl), **no′so·log′ic** (-ĭk) adj. —**no·sol′o·gist** n.

nos·o·ma·ni·a (nŏs′ə-mā′nē-ə, -mān′yə) n. An unfounded abnormal belief that one is suffering from some special disease.

no·son·o·my (nō-sŏn′ə-mē) n. See **nosology.**

nos·o·phil·i·a (nŏs′ə-fĭl′ē-ə) n. A desire to be ill; love of sickness.

nos·o·pho·bi·a (nŏs′ə-fō′bē-ə) n. An inordinate fear of disease.

nos·o·poi·et·ic (nŏs′ə-poi-ĕt′ĭk) adj. Pathogenic.

Nos·o·psyl·lus (nŏs′ə-sĭl′əs) n. A genus of fleas commonly found on rodents including N. fasciatus, the northern rat flea, which infrequently transmits the plague bacillus to humans.

nos·o·tax·y (nŏs′ə-tăk′sē) n. See **nosology.**

nos·tal·gia (nŏ-stăl′jə, nə-) n. **1.** A bittersweet longing for things, persons, or situations of the past. **2.** The condition of being homesick; homesickness. —**nos·tal′gic** (-jĭk) adj.

nos·tril (nŏs′trəl) n. A naris.

nos·trum (nŏs′trəm) n. A medicine whose effectiveness is unproved and whose ingredients are usually secret; a quack remedy.

no·tan·ce·pha·li·a (nō′tăn-sə-fā′lē-ə, -fāl′yə) n. A fetal malformation characterized by absence of the lower posterior region of the skull.

no·tan·en·ce·pha·li·a (nō′tăn-ĕn-sə-fā′lē-ə, -fāl′yə) n. A malformation marked by defective development or absence of the cerebellum.

notch (nŏch) n. **1.** An indentation at the edge of a structure; an incisure. **2.** An upstroke or peak on a pulse tracing.

no·ten·ceph·a·lo·cele (nō′tĕn-sĕf′ə-lō-sēl′) n. A malformation in the back part of the cranium with protrusion of brain substance.

no·ti·fi·a·ble disease (nō′tə-fī′ə-bəl) n. A disease that must be reported to public health authorities at the time it is diagnosed because it is potentially dangerous to human or animal health. Also called reportable disease.

no·to·chord (nō′tə-kôrd′) n. **1.** A flexible rodlike structure that forms the main support of the body in the lowest chordates; a primitive backbone. **2.** A similar structure in embryos of higher vertebrates, from which the spinal column develops. —**no′to·chord′al** adj.

nour·ish (nûr′ĭsh) v. To provide with food or other substances necessary for sustaining life and growth.

nour·ish·ment (nûr′ĭsh-mənt) n. Something that nourishes; food.

no·vo·bi·o·cin (nō′və-bī′ə-sĭn) n. An antibiotic produced by the actinomycete Streptomyces nivens and used to treat infections by gram-positive bacteria.

No·vo·cain (nō′və-kān′) A trademark used for an anesthetic preparation of procaine.

No·vo·lin (nō′və-lĭn′) A trademark for a drug preparation of insulin.

nox·ious (nŏk′shəs) adj. Harmful to living things; injurious to health.

Np The symbol for the element **neptunium.**

NP abbr. nurse practitioner; neuropsychiatry

NPN abbr. nonprotein nitrogen

NPO abbr. Latin nil per os (nothing by mouth)

NREM abbr. non-rapid eye movement

nRNA (ĕn′är-ĕn-ā′) n. RNA that is found in the nucleus either in association with the chromosomes or in the nucleoplasm. Also called nuclear RNA.

NSAID (ĕn′sād′) n. A nonsteroidal anti-inflammatory drug, such as aspirin or ibuprofen.

NSR abbr. normal sinus rhythm

nu (nōō, nyōō) n. Symbol ν The 13th letter of the Greek alphabet.

Nu·bain (nōō′bān′) A trademark for the drug nalbuphine hydrochloride.

nu·cha (nōō′kə) n. The back of the neck; the nape. —**nu′chal** adj.

nuchal ligament n. A band at the back of the neck, extending cranially from the occipital bone to the rear border of the great foramen and caudally to the seventh cervical spinous process.

nuchal plane n. The external surface of the squamous part of the occipital bone giving attachment to the muscles of the back of the neck.

nuchal translucency n. A radiologic sign that appears as a translucent spot on a fetal sonogram and indicates subcutaneous fluid in the nuchal region of a fetus. It can be measured in early pregnancy to assess the risk of chromosomal abnormalities, especially Down syndrome.

nucle– pref. Variant of **nucleo–.**

nu·cle·ar (nōō′klē-ər) adj. **1.** Of or forming a nucleus. **2.** Of or relating to atomic nuclei.

nuclear cataract n. A cataract involving only the inner dense portion of the lens.

nuclear envelope n. See **nuclear membrane.**

nuclear family n. A family unit consisting of a mother and father and their progeny.

nuclear hyaloplasm n. See **karyolymph.**

nuclear inclusion body n. Either of two types of usually acidophilic inclusion bodies: granular or hyaline, as in herpes simplex, and circumscribed, as in poliomyelitis. Also called nucleoid.

nuclear jaundice n. See **kernicterus.**

nuclear magnetic resonance n. Abbr. **NMR** The absorption of electromagnetic radiation of a specific frequency by an atomic nucleus that is placed in a strong magnetic field, used especially in spectroscopic studies of molecular structure and in medicine to measure rates of metabolism.

nuclear medicine n. The branch of medicine that deals with the use of radionuclides in the diagnosis and treatment of disease.

nuclear membrane n. The double-layered membrane enclosing the nucleus of a cell. Also called nuclear envelope.

nuclear ophthalmoplegia n. Ophthalmoplegia that is due to a lesion of the nuclei of origin of the eye's motor nerves.

nuclear pore n. An octagonal opening where the inner and outer membranes of the nuclear envelope are continuous.

nuclear RNA n. See **nRNA.**

nuclear spindle n. See **mitotic spindle.**

nuclear stain n. A stain selective for cell nuclei, usually based on the binding of a basic dye to DNA or to nucleohistone.

nuclear transfer *n.* The transfer of the nucleus of one cell to another cell whose nucleus has been removed.

nu·cle·ase (nōō′klē-ās′, -āz′) *n.* Any of several enzymes, such as endonuclease and exonuclease, that hydrolize nucleic acids.

nu·cle·ate (nōō′klē-āt′, -ĭt) *adj.* Nucleated. —*v.* (-āt′) **1.** To form into a nucleus. **2.** To serve or act as a nucleus for. **3.** To provide a nucleus for. —*n.* A salt of a nucleic acid.

nu·cle·at·ed (nōō′klē-ā′tĭd) *adj.* Having a nucleus or nuclei.

nu·cle·a·tion (nōō′klē-ā′shən) *n.* **1.** The beginning of chemical or physical changes at discrete points in a system, such as the formation of crystals in a liquid. **2.** The formation of cell nuclei.

nu·cle·i (nōō′klē-ī′) *n.* Plural of **nucleus.**

nu·cle·ic acid (nōō-klē′ĭk, -klā′-) *n.* Any of a group of complex compounds found in all living cells and viruses, composed of purines, pyrimidines, carbohydrates, and phosphoric acid. Nucleic acids in the form of DNA and RNA control cellular function and heredity.

nucleic-acid probe *n.* A nucleic-acid fragment that is complementary to another nucleic-acid sequence and thus, when labeled in some manner, as with a radioisotope, can be used to identify complementary segments present in the nucleic-acid sequences of various microorganisms.

nu·cle·i·form (nōō′klē-ə-fôrm′, nōō-klē′-) *adj.* Shaped like or resembling a nucleus.

nu·cle·in (nōō′klē-ĭn) *n.* Any of the substances present in the nucleus of a cell, consisting chiefly of proteins, phosphoric acids, and nucleic acids.

nuclei ner·vi ves·tib·u·lo·coch·le·ar·is (nûr′vī vĕ-stĭb′yə-lō-kŏk′lē-âr′ĭs) *pl.n.* The combined cochlear and vestibular nuclei.

nuclei of origin *pl.n.* Collections of motor neurons forming a column continuous in the spinal cord but discontinuous in the medulla and pons and giving origin to the spinal and cranial motor nerves. Also called *motor nuclei.*

nucleo– *or* **nucle–** *pref.* **1.** Nucleus: *nucleon; nucleoplasm.* **2.** Nucleic acid: *nucleoprotein.*

nu·cle·o·cap·sid (nōō′klē-ō-kăp′sĭd) *n.* The basic structure of a virus, consisting of a core of nucleic acid enclosed in a protein coat.

nu·cle·of·u·gal (nōō′klē-ŏf′yə-gəl, -ŏf′ə-) *adj.* **1.** Moving within the cell body in a direction away from the nucleus. **2.** Moving in a direction away from a nerve nucleus. Used of nerve impulse.

nu·cle·o·his·tone (nōō′klē-ō-hĭs′tōn′) *n.* A nucleoprotein whose protein part is a histone.

nu·cle·oid (nōō′klē-oid′) *n.* **1.** See **nucleus** (sense 2). **2.** See **nuclear inclusion body.** —*adj.* Resembling a nucleolus.

nucleolar satellite *n.* A small dot of chromatin found adjacent to the nucleolus in the nerve cells of females.

nu·cle·o·late (nōō′klē-ə-lāt′) *or* **nu·cle·o·lat·ed** (-lā′tĭd) *adj.* Having a nucleolus or nucleoli.

nu·cle·o·li·form (nōō-klē′ə-lə-fôrm′, nōō′klē-ō′-) *adj.* Resembling a nucleolus.

nu·cle·o·loid (nōō-klē′ə-loid′) *adj.* Resembling a nucleolus.

nu·cle·o·lo·ne·ma (nōō-klē′ə-lō-nē′mə) *n.* The irregular network of fine ribonucleoprotein granules or microfilaments forming most of the nucleolus.

nu·cle·o·lus (nōō-klē′ə-ləs) *n.*, *pl.* **–li** (-lī′) A small, typically round granular body composed of protein and RNA in the nucleus of a cell, usually associated with a specific chromosomal site and involved in ribosomal RNA synthesis and the formation of ribosomes. —**nu·cle′o·lar** (-lər) *adj.*

nu·cle·on (nōō′klē-ŏn′) *n.* A proton or neutron, especially as part of an atomic nucleus. —**nu′cle·on′ic** *adj.*

nu·cle·op·e·tal (nōō′klē-ŏp′ĭ-tl) *adj.* **1.** Moving within the cell body in a direction toward the nucleus. **2.** Moving in a direction toward a nerve nucleus. Used of a nerve impulse.

nu·cle·o·phile (nōō′klē-ə-fīl′) *or* **nu·cle·o·phil** (-fīl′) *n.* A chemical compound or group that is attracted to nuclei and tends to donate or share electrons. —**nu′cle·o·phil′ic** (-fīl′ĭk) *adj.*

nu·cle·o·plasm (nōō′klē-ə-plăz′əm) *n.* Protoplasm of a cell nucleus. Also called *karyoplasm.*

nu·cle·o·pro·tein (nōō′klē-ō-prō′tēn′) *n.* Any of a group of substances found in the nuclei of all living cells and in viruses and composed of a protein and a nucleic acid.

nu·cle·or·rhex·is (nōō′klē-ə-rĕk′sĭs) *n.* Fragmentation of a cell nucleus.

nu·cle·o·si·dase (nōō′klē-ə-sī′dās′, -dāz′, -klē-ō′sī-) *n.* Any of various enzymes that catalyze the hydrolysis of nucleosides, releasing their purine or pyrimidine base.

nu·cle·o·side (nōō′klē-ə-sīd′) *n.* Any of various compounds consisting of a sugar, usually ribose or deoxyribose, and a purine or pyrimidine base, especially a compound obtained by hydrolysis of a nucleic acid, such as adenosine or guanine.

nucleoside analogue *n.* Any of a group of antiviral drugs that inhibit the viral enzyme reverse transcriptase and are used in the treatment of HIV infection.

nu·cle·o·some (nōō′klē-ə-sōm′) *n.* Any of the repeating subunits of chromatin, consisting of a DNA chain coiled around a core of histones. —**nu′cle·o·som′al** (-sō′məl) *adj.*

nu·cle·o·ti·dase (nōō′klē-ə-tī′dās, -dāz) *n.* An enzyme that catalyzes the hydrolysis of a nucleotide to a nucleoside and phosphoric acid.

nu·cle·o·tide (nōō′klē-ə-tīd′) *n.* Any of various compounds consisting of a nucleoside combined with a phosphate group and forming the basic constituent of DNA and RNA.

nu·cle·o·ti·dyl·trans·fer·ase (nōō′klē-ə-tīd′l-trăns′fə-rās′, -rāz′) *n.* Any of various enzymes that catalyze the transfer of nucleotide residues from nucleoside diphosphates or triphosphates into dimer or polymer forms.

nu·cle·o·tox·in (nōō′klē-ə-tŏk′sĭn) *n.* A toxin acting upon the cell nuclei.

nu·cle·us (nōō′klē-əs) *n.*, *pl.* **–cle·us·es** *or* **–cle·i** (-klē-ī′) **1.** A large, membrane-bound, usually spherical protoplasmic structure within a living cell, containing the cell's hereditary material and controlling its metabolism, growth, and reproduction. Also called *karyon.* **2.** A membraneless structure in microorganisms that contains genetic material but does not itself replicate. Also called *nucleoid.* **3.** A group of specialized nerve cells or a localized mass of gray matter in the brain or spinal cord. **4.** The substance around which a urinary or other calculus forms. **5.** The positively charged central region of an atom that is composed of protons and neutrons and that contains almost all of the mass of the atom. **6.** A group of atoms bound in a structure, such as a benzene ring, that is resistant to alteration in chemical reactions.

nucleus fas·tig·i·i (fă-stĭj′ē-ī′, -stī′jē-) *n.* The most medial of the deep cerebellar nuclei, near the midline in the white matter underneath the vermis of the cerebellar cortex, receiving axons of Purkinje cells and fibers from the vestibular nerve and nuclei.

nucleus grac·i·lis (grăs′ə-lĭs) *n.* The medial of the three nuclei of the dorsal spinal column, receiving dorsal root fibers conveying sensory innervation of the leg.

nucleus of solitary tract *n.* A slender cell column that extends through the dorsal part of the medulla oblongata, is the visceral sensory nucleus of the brainstem, and receives the afferent fibers of the vagus, glossopharyngeal, and facial nerves via the solitary tract.

nu·clide (nōō′klīd′) *n.* A type of atom specified by its atomic number, atomic mass, and energy state, such as carbon 14. —**nu·clid·ic** (nōō-klĭd′ĭk) *adj.*

NUG *abbr.* necrotizing ulcerative gingivitis

null cell *n.* See **killer cell.**

nul·li·grav·i·da (nŭl′ĭ-grăv′ĭ-də) *n.* A woman who has never conceived a child.

nul·lip·a·ra (nə-lĭp′ər-ə) *n.* A woman who has never given birth. —**nul·lip·a·rous** (-rəs) *adj.*

numb (nŭm) *adj.* **1.** Being unable or only partially able to feel sensation or pain; deadened or anesthetized. **2.** Being emotionally unresponsive; indifferent. —*v.* To make or become numb.

num·ber (nŭm′bər) *n.* **1.** A symbol expressive of a certain value or of a specific quantity determined by count. **2.** The place of any unit in a series.

num·mu·lar (nŭm′yə-lər) *adj.* **1.** Shaped like a coin; disk-shaped. Used especially of the thick mucous or mucopurulent sputum in certain respiratory diseases because of the discoid shape assumed when it is flattened on the bottom of a sputum mug containing water or transparent disinfectant. **2.** Arranged like stacks of coins. Used of red blood corpuscles in rouleaux formation.

Nu·prin (nōō′prĭn) A trademark for the drug ibuprofen.

nurse (nûrs) *n.* **1.** A person trained to care for the sick or disabled, especially one educated in the scientific basis of human response to health problems and trained to assist a physician. **2.** A wet nurse. **3.** An individual who cares for an infant or young child. —*v.* **1.** To serve as a nurse. **2.** To provide or take nourishment from the breast; suckle.

nurse anesthetist *n.* A person who, after completing the basic education of a nurse, is further trained in the supervised administration of anesthetics.

nurse·maid's elbow (nûrs′mādz′) *n.* See **Malgaigne's luxation.**

nurse-midwife *n.* A person formally educated and certified to practice in the two disciplines of nursing and midwifery. —**nurse-midwifery** *n.*

nurse practitioner *n. Abbr.* **NP** A registered nurse with special training for providing primary health care, including many tasks customarily performed by a physician.

nurse's aide (nûr′sĭz) *n.* A person who assists nurses at a hospital or other medical facility in tasks requiring little or no formal training or education.

nurs·ing (nûr′sĭng) *n.* **1.** The profession of a nurse. **2.** The tasks performed or care provided by a nurse. **3.** The act or practice of breast-feeding.

nursing home *n.* See **skilled nursing facility.**

nu·ta·tion (nōō-tā′shən) *n.* The act of nodding the head, especially involuntarily.

nu·tra·ceu·ti·cal (nōō′trə-sōō′tĭ-kəl) *n.* A food or naturally occurring food supplement thought to have a beneficial effect on human health.

nu·tri·ent (nōō′trē-ənt) *n.* A source of nourishment, especially an ingredient in a food.

nutrient artery *n.* An artery of variable origin that supplies the medullary cavity of a long bone.

nutrient artery of femur *n.* Either of two arteries, superior and inferior, arising from the first and third perforating arteries, respectively, or sometimes from the second and the fourth arteries.

nutrient artery of fibula *n.* An artery with its origin in the peroneal artery, with distribution to the fibula.

nutrient artery of humerus *n.* An artery with its origin in the deep brachial artery and with distribution to the medullary cavity of the humerus.

nutrient canal *n.* A canal in the shaft of a long bone or in other locations in irregular bones through which the nutrient artery enters.

nutrient foramen *n.* The external opening of the nutrient canal in a bone.

nutrient vessel *n.* A nutrient artery.

nu·tri·ment (nōō′trə-mənt) *n.* **1.** A source of nourishment; food. **2.** An agent that promotes growth or development.

nu·tri·tion (nōō-trĭsh′ən) *n.* **1.** The process by which living organisms obtain food and use it for growth, metabolism, and repair. Its stages include ingestion, digestion, absorption, transport, assimilation, and excretion. **2.** The science that deals with food and nourishment, including dietary guidelines, food composition, and the roles that various nutrients have in maintaining health. —**nu·tri′tion·al** *adj.*

nu·tri·tion·ist (nōō-trĭsh′ə-nĭst) *n.* One who is trained or is an expert in the field of nutrition.

nu·tri·tion·ist's calorie (nōō-trĭsh′ə-nĭsts) *n.* See **calorie** (sense 1).

nu·tri·tious (nōō-trĭsh′əs) *adj.* Providing nourishment; nourishing.

nu·tri·tive (nōō′trĭ-tĭv) *adj.* **1.** Of or relating to nutrition. **2.** Nutritious; nourishing.

nutritive equilibrium *n.* A balance between intake and excretion of nutritive material, with no gain or loss in weight. Also called *physiologic equilibrium.*

nu·tri·ture (nōō′trə-chōōr′, -chər) *n.* **1.** The state of the nutrition of the body. **2.** Nutritional status, especially with regard to a specific nutrient.

nyc·tal·gia (nĭk-tăl′jə) *n.* Night pain, especially the bone pains of syphilis occurring at night.

nyc·ta·lo·pi·a (nĭk′tə-lō′pē-ə) *n.* A condition of the eyes in which vision is normal in daylight or other strong light but is abnormally weak or completely lost at night or in dim light and that results from vitamin A deficiency, disease, or hereditary factors. Also called *night blindness.* —**nyc′ta·lo′pic** (-lō′pĭk, -lŏp′ĭk) *adj.*

nyc·ter·ine (nĭk′tə-rīn′, -rēn′, -tər-ĭn′) *adj.* **1.** Occurring at night. **2.** Dark; obscure.

nyc·ter·o·hem·er·al (nĭk′tə-rō-hĕm′ər-əl) *adj.* Both daily and nightly.

nycto– *or* **nyct–** *pref.* Night: *nyctophobia.*

nyc·to·phil·i·a (nĭk′tə-fĭl′ē-ə) *n.* A preference for the night or darkness. Also called *scotophilia.*

nyc·to·pho·bi·a (nĭk′tə-fō′bē-ə) *n.* An abnormal fear of night or of the dark. Also called *scotophobia.*

nym·pha (nĭm′fə) *n., pl.* **–phae** (-fē) Either of the labia minora. —**nym′phal** *adj.*

nym·phec·to·my (nĭm-fĕk′tə-mē) *n.* Surgical removal of one or both of the labia minora.

nym·phi·tis (nĭm-fī′tĭs) *n.* Inflammation of the labia minora.

nympho– *or* **nymph–** *pref.* **1.** Nymphae: *nymphitis.* **2.** Sexual desire: *nymphomania.*

nym·pho·ma·ni·a (nĭm′fə-mā′nē-ə, -mān′yə) *n.* A disorder in which a woman exhibits extreme or obsessive desire for sexual stimulation or gratification. —**nym′-pho·ma′ni·ac′** (-nē-ăk′) *adj. & n.* —**nym′pho·ma·ni′a·cal** (-mə-nī′ə-kəl) *adj.*

nym·phon·cus (nĭm-fŏng′kəs) *n.* A swelling or hypertrophy of one or both labia minora.

nym·phot·o·my (nĭm-fŏt′ə-mē) *n.* An incision into the labia minora or into the clitoris.

nys·tag·mi·form (nĭ-stăg′mə-fôrm′) *adj.* Nystagmoid.

nys·tag·mo·graph (nĭ-stăg′mə-grăf′) *n.* An apparatus for measuring the amplitude and velocity of ocular movements in nystagmus by measuring the change in the resting potential of the eye as the eye moves. —**nys′tag·mog′ra·phy** (nĭs′tăg-mŏg′rə-fē) *n.*

nys·tag·mus (nĭ-stăg′məs) *n.* A rapid, involuntary oscillatory motion of the eyeball. —**nys·tag′mic** (-mĭk), **nys·tag′moid′** (-moid′) *adj.*

nys·ta·tin (nĭs′tə-tĭn) *n.* An antibiotic produced by the actinomycete *Streptomyces noursei* and used especially in the treatment of fungal infections.

Nys·ten's law (nē-stănz′) *n.* The principle that rigor mortis first affects the muscles of the head and then spreads toward the hands and feet.

Ny·tol (nī′tôl′) A trademark for the drug diphenhydramine.

nyx·is (nĭk′sĭs) *n.* A pricking or puncture; paracentesis.

O

o The Greek letter *omicron.* Entries beginning with this character are alphabetized under **omicron.**

ω, Ω **1.** The Greek letter *omega.* Entries beginning with this character are alphabetized under **omega.** **2.** *Symbol* Ω The symbol for **ohm.**

O¹ The symbol for the element **oxygen.**

O² *abbr.* oculus

o– *abbr.* ortho– (often italic)

–o– Used as a connective to join word elements: *acidophilic.*

OA *abbr.* osteoarthritis

O agglutinin (ō) *n.* An agglutinin that reacts with, and is formed as the result of stimulation by, the relatively thermostable antigens present in the cell bodies of microorganisms.

O antigen *n.* A somatic antigen of nonmotile bacteria.

oat cell (ōt) *n.* A short, bluntly spindle-shaped, anaplastic cell containing a relatively large, hyperchromatic nucleus and observed in some carcinomas.

oat cell carcinoma *n.* A highly malignant carcinoma, especially of the lungs, composed of small ovoid undifferentiated cells. Also called *small cell carcinoma.*

OB *abbr.* obstetrics

ob·dor·mi·tion (ŏb′dôr-mĭsh′ən) *n.* Numbness of an extremity due to pressure on the sensory nerve.

o·be·li·on (ō-bē′lē-ŏn′) *n.* A craniometric point on the sagittal suture between the parietal foramina near the lambdoid suture. —**o·be′li·ac′** (-ăk′) *adj.*

o·bese (ō-bēs′) *adj.* Extremely fat; very overweight.

o·be·si·ty (ō-bē′sĭ-tē) *n.* The condition of being obese; increased body weight caused by excessive accumulation of fat.

o·bex (ō′bĕks′) *n.* The point on the midline of the dorsal surface of the medulla oblongata that marks the caudal angle of the rhomboid fossa.

ob-gyn *or* **OB-GYN** (ō′bē-jē′wī-ĕn′) *n.* **1.** The combined practice or field of obstetrics and gynecology. **2.** An obstetrician-gynecologist.

ob·ject choice (ŏb′jĭkt, -jĕkt′) *n.* In psychoanalytic theory, the object, usually a person, upon which an individual's psychic energy is centered.

ob·jec·tive (əb-jĕk′tĭv) *n.* The lens or lenses in the lower end of a microscope or other optical instrument that first receives light rays from the object being examined and forms its image. —*adj.* **1.** Based on observable phenomena; presented factually. **2.** Indicating a symptom or condition perceived as a sign of disease by someone other than the person affected.

objective sensation *n.* A sensation caused by some material object.

objective symptom *n.* A symptom evident to the observer; a sign.

object relationship *n.* The emotional bond between an individual and another person.

ob·li·gate (ŏb′lĭ-gĭt, -gāt′) *adj.* Able to exist or survive only in a particular environment or by assuming a particular role.

obligate aerobe *n.* An organism, such as a bacterium, that can live only in the presence of oxygen.

obligate anaerobe *n.* An organism, such as a bacterium, that can live only in the absence of oxygen.

obligate parasite *n.* An organism that cannot lead an independent nonparasitic existence.

o·blique (ō-blēk′, ə-blēk′) *adj.* Situated in a slanting position; not transverse or longitudinal.

oblique diameter *n.* The diameter of the pelvic inlet from the sacroiliac joint of one side to the opposite iliopectineal eminence.

oblique fracture *n.* A fracture in which the line of break runs obliquely to the axis of the bone.

oblique lie *n.* An anatomical relationship in which the fetal axis crosses the maternal axis at an angle other than a right angle.

oblique vein of left atrium *n.* A tributary of the coronary sinus, located on the posterior wall of the left atrium and developed from a branch of the common cardinal vein.

o·bliq·ui·ty (ō-blĭk′wĭ-tē, ə-blĭk′-) *n.* See **asynclitism.**

o·blit·er·ate (ə-blĭt′ə-rāt′, ō-blĭt′-) *v.* **1.** To remove an organ or another body part completely, as by surgery, disease, or radiation. **2.** To blot out, especially through filling of a natural space by fibrosis or inflammation. —**o·blit′er·a′tion** *n.*

o·blit·er·at·ing endarteritis (ə-blĭt′ə-rā′tĭng, ō-blĭt′-) *n.* An extreme degree of proliferating endarteritis that closes the lumen of the artery. Also called *obliterating arteritis.*

o·blit·er·a·tive bronchitis (ə-blĭt′ə-rā′tĭv, -ər-ə-tĭv, ō-blĭt′-) *n.* Fibrinous bronchitis in which the exudate is not expectorated but becomes organized, obliterating the affected portion of the bronchial tubes.

ob·lon·ga·ta (ŏb′lŏng-gä′tə, -gä′tə) *n.* The medulla oblongata.

OBS *abbr.* organic brain syndrome

ob·ses·sion (əb-sĕsh′ən, ŏb-) *n.* **1.** Compulsive preoccupation with an idea or an unwanted feeling or emotion, often accompanied by symptoms of anxiety. **2.** A compulsive, often unreasonable idea or emotion. —**ob·ses′sion·al** *adj.*

ob·ses·sive (əb-sĕs′ĭv, ŏb-) *adj.* Of, characteristic of, or causing an obsession. —**ob·ses′sive** *n.*

obsessive-compulsive *adj.* Having a tendency to dwell on unwanted thoughts or perform certain repetitious rituals, especially as a defense against anxiety from unconscious conflicts. —*n.* A person who exhibits obsessive-compulsive behavior.

obsessive-compulsive disorder *n. Abbr.* **OCD** A psychiatric disorder characterized by the persistent intrusion of repetitive, unwanted thoughts, sometimes accompanied by compulsive actions, that the individual is unable to prevent and that interfere with normal functioning.

ob·stet·ric (ŏb-stĕt′rĭk, əb-) *or* **ob·stet·ri·cal** (-rĭ-kəl) *adj.* Of or relating to the profession of obstetrics or the care of women during and after pregnancy.

obstetrical binder *n.* A garment covering the abdomen and providing support after childbirth.

obstetrical forceps *n.* Forceps used for grasping and pulling on or rotating the fetal head. The blades are introduced individually into the vaginal canal and joined after being placed in correct position.

obstetrical hand *n.* See **accoucheur's hand.**

obstetrical paralysis *n.* See **birth palsy.**

obstetric conjugate *n.* The shortest pelvic diameter through which the fetal head must pass during birth, measured from the promontory of the sacrum to a point a few millimeters from the top of the pubic symphysis.

obstetric conjugate of outlet *n.* The conjugate of outlet when the coccyx has been displaced backward.

ob·ste·tri·cian (ŏb′stĭ-trĭsh′ən) *n.* A physician who specializes in obstetrics.

obstetrician-gynecologist *n.* A physician who specializes in obstetrics and gynecology.

ob·stet·rics (ŏb-stĕt′rĭks, əb-) *n. Abbr.* **OB** The branch of medicine that deals with the care of women during pregnancy, childbirth, and the recuperative period following delivery.

ob·sti·nate (ŏb′stə-nĭt) *adj.* **1.** Stubbornly adhering to an attitude, opinion, or course of action. **2.** Difficult to alleviate or cure.

ob·sti·pa·tion (ŏb′stə-pā′shən) *n.* Intestinal obstruction; severe constipation.

ob·struct (əb-strŭkt′, ŏb-) *v.* To block or close a body passage so as to hinder or interrupt a flow. —**ob·struc′tive** *adj.*

ob·struct·ed testis (əb-strŭk′tĭd) *n.* A testis whose descent has been prevented by fascial bands at the inguinal canal or at the upper scrotum.

ob·struc·tion (əb-strŭk′shən, ŏb-) *n.* **1.** The blocking of a body passage, as by clogging or stricture. **2.** The state of being obstructed. **3.** Something, such as a mass or stricture, that obstructs.

obstructive apnea *n.* Apnea that results from obstructed air passages or from inadequate respiratory muscle activity.

obstructive dysmenorrhea *n.* Dysmenorrhea caused by an obstruction to the escape of the menstrual blood. Also called *mechanical dysmenorrhea.*

obstructive hydrocephalus *n.* See **noncommunicating hydrocephalus.**

obstructive jaundice *n.* Jaundice resulting from obstruction of the flow of bile from the liver to the duodenum. Also called *mechanical jaundice.*

obstructive murmur *n.* A murmur caused by a narrowing of one of the valvular orifices.

obstructive thrombus *n.* A thrombus due to obstruction in the vessel from compression or other cause.

ob·stru·ent (ŏb′strōō-ənt) *adj.* Obstructing or closing the natural passages of the body. —*n.* An obstruent medicine or agent.

ob·tund (ŏb-tŭnd′) *v.* To dull or blunt, especially sensation or pain. —**ob·tund′ent** *adj.*

ob·tu·rate (ŏb′tə-rāt′) *v.* To close or obstruct. —**ob′tu·ra′tion** *n.*

ob·tu·ra·ting embolism (ŏb′tə-rā′tĭng) *n.* The complete blockage of a blood vessel by an embolism.

ob·tu·ra·tor (ŏb′tə-rā′tər) *n.* **1.** A structure, such as the soft palate, that closes an opening in the body. **2.** A prosthetic device that serves to close an opening or cleft, especially in the palate. **3.** A stylus or removable plug used during the insertion of many tubular instruments.

obturator artery *n.* An artery with origin in the internal iliac artery, with distribution to the ilium, pubis, obturator and adductor muscles and with pubic, acetabular, anterior, and posterior branches.

obturator canal *n.* An opening through which the obturator nerve and vessels pass from the pelvic cavity into the thigh.

obturator crest *n.* A ridge that extends from the pubic tubercle to the acetabular notch, giving attachment to the pubofemoral ligament of the hip joint.

obturator foramen *n.* A large oval or irregularly triangular aperture in the hipbone.

obturator hernia *n.* A hernia through the obturator foramen.

obturator nerve *n.* A nerve that arises from the second, third, and fourth lumbar nerves in the psoas muscle, enters the thigh through the obturator canal, and supplies the muscles and skin on the medial side of the thigh.

obturator vein *n.* A vein that is formed by a union of tributaries draining the hip joint and the muscles of the upper and back part of the thigh, enters the pelvis by the obturator canal, and empties into the internal iliac vein.

ob·tuse (ŏb-tōōs′, əb-) *adj.* **1.** Lacking quickness of perception or intellect. **2.** Not sharp or acute; blunt.

ob·tu·sion (ŏb-tōō′zhən) *n.* The dulling or deadening of awareness or sensibility.

oc·cip·i·tal (ŏk-sĭp′ĭ-tl) *adj.* Of or relating to the occipital bone. —*n.* The occipital bone.

occipital artery *n.* **1.** An artery with origin in the external carotid artery, and with sternocleidomastoid, muscular, meningeal, auricular, occipital, mastoid, and descending branches. **2.** An artery that is one of the terminal branches of the posterior cerebral artery and supplies lateral portions of the temporal lobe; lateral occipital artery. **3.** An artery that is one of the terminal branches of the posterior cerebral artery, with distribution by several branches to the corpus callosum and portions of the occipital lobe, including the visual cortex; medial occipital artery.

occipital bone *n.* A bone at the lower and posterior part of the skull, consisting of basilar, condylar, and squamous parts and enclosing the foramen magnum.

oc·cip·i·tal·i·za·tion (ŏk-sĭp′ĭ-tl-ĭ-zā′shən) *n.* Bony ankylosis between the atlas and the occipital bone.

occipital lobe *n.* The posterior lobe of each cerebral hemisphere, having the shape of a three-sided pyramid and containing the visual center of the brain.

occipital pole *n.* The most posterior promontory of each cerebral hemisphere.

occipital sinus *n.* An unpaired dural sinus commencing at the confluence of the sinuses and passing downward to the great foramen.

occipital vein *n.* **1.** A vein that drains the occipital region and empties into the internal jugular vein or the suboccipital plexus. **2.** Any of the superficial veins draining the occipital cortex and emptying into the superior sagittal and transverse sinus.

occipito– *pref.* Occiput; occipital: *occipitofrontal.*

oc·cip·i·to·an·te·ri·or position (ŏk-sĭp′ĭ-tō-ăn-tîr′ē-ər) *n.* A cephalic presentation of the fetus with the occiput turned toward either the right or left front quarter of the mother's pelvis.

oc·cip·i·to·fa·cial (ŏk-sĭp′ĭ-tō-fā′shəl) *adj.* Of or relating to the occiput and the face.

oc·cip·i·to·fron·tal (ŏk-sĭp′ĭ-tō-frŭn′tl) *adj.* **1.** Of or relating to the occiput and the forehead. **2.** Of or relating to the occipital and frontal lobes of the cerebral cortex.

occipitofrontal diameter *n.* The diameter of the fetal head from the external occipital protuberance to the most prominent point of the frontal bone in the midline.

occipitofrontal muscle *n.* A part of the epicranial muscle, of which the occipital belly arises from the occipital bone and inserts into the galea aponeurotica, and the frontal belly arises from the galea and inserts into the skin of the eyebrow and nose, with nerve supply from the facial nerve, and whose action moves the scalp.

oc·cip·i·to·men·tal (ŏk-sĭp′ĭ-tō-měn′tl) *adj.* Of or relating to the occiput and the chin.

occipitomental diameter *n.* The diameter of the fetal head from the external occipital protuberance to the midpoint of the chin.

oc·cip·i·to·pos·te·ri·or position (ŏk-sĭp′ĭ-tō-pŏ-stîr′ē-ər, -pō-) *n.* A cephalic presentation of the fetus with the occiput turned toward either the right or left rear quarter of the mother's pelvis.

oc·cip·i·to·trans·verse position (ŏk-sĭp′ĭ-tō-trănz-vûrs′, -trăns-, -trănz′vûrs′, -trăns′-) *n.* A cephalic presentation of the fetus in which the occiput is turned toward either the right or left iliac fossa of the mother's pelvis.

oc·ci·put (ŏk′sə-pŭt′, -pət) *n., pl.* **–puts** or **oc·cip·i·ta** (ŏk-sĭp′ĭ-tə) The back part of the head or skull.

oc·clude (ə-klōōd′) *v.* **1.** To cause to become closed; obstruct. **2.** To prevent the passage of. **3.** To bring together the upper and lower teeth in proper alignment for chewing. **4.** To enclose a virus, as in an inclusion body. **5.** In chemistry, to absorb and retain gases and other substances. —**oc·clud′ent** *adj.*

oc·clu·sal (ə-klōō′zəl) *adj.* **1.** Of or relating to occlusion or closure. **2.** Of or relating to the contacting surfaces of opposing teeth, especially the biting or chewing surfaces.

occlusal analysis *n.* A study of the relationships of the occlusal surfaces of opposing teeth, including the effect these relationships have on related structures. Also called *bite analysis.*

occlusal equilibration *n.* The modification of the chewing and biting surfaces of teeth by grinding.

occlusal force *n.* The force exerted on opposing teeth when the jaws are closed or tightened.

occlusal imbalance *n.* An inharmonious functional relationship between the teeth of the maxilla and those of the mandible.

occlusal position *n.* The relationship of the mandible and maxillae when the jaws are closed and the teeth are in contact.

oc·clu·sion (ə-klōō′zhən) *n.* **1.** The act of occluding or the state of being occluded. **2.** An obstruction or closure of a body passage. **3.** Any contact between the cutting or chewing surfaces of opposing teeth. **4.** The alignment of the teeth of the upper and lower jaws when brought together. **5.** The absorption of a gas or other substance, as by a metal. **6.** The inclusion of one substance within another.

occlusion of pupil *n.* An opaque membrane closing the pupillary area.

oc·clu·sive (ə-klōō′zĭv) *adj.* **1.** Occluding or tending to occlude. **2.** Of or being a bandage or dressing that closes a wound and keeps it from the air.

occlusive dressing *n.* A dressing that seals a wound from air or bacteria.

occlusive ileus *n.* Complete mechanical blocking of the lumen of the intestine.

occlusive meningitis *n.* Leptomeningitis causing occlusion of the spinal fluid pathways.

oc·cult (ə-kŭlt′, ŏk′ŭlt′) *adj.* **1.** Hidden; concealed. **2.** Detectable only by microscopic examination or by chemical analysis. **3.** Not accompanied by readily detectable signs or symptoms.

occult blood *n.* Blood that is present in amounts too small to be seen and can be detected only by chemical analysis or microscopic examination.

occult fracture *n.* A fracture that does not appear in x-rays, although the bone shows new bone formation within three or four weeks of fracture.

occult hydrocephalus *n.* See **normal pressure hydrocephalus.**

oc·cu·pa·tion·al dermatitis (ŏk′yə-pā′shə-nəl) *n.* Contact dermatitis caused by an allergic reaction to or irritation from substances normally encountered in an occupation.

occupational disease *n.* A pathological condition resulting from a toxic agent, hazard, or repetitive operation encountered during the usual performance of one's occupation.

occupational medicine *n.* The branch of medicine that deals with the prevention and treatment of diseases and injuries occurring at work or in specific occupations.

occupational therapy *n. Abbr.* **OT** The use of productive or creative activity in the treatment or rehabilitation of physically or emotionally disabled people. —**occupational therapist** *n.*

OCD *abbr.* obsessive-compulsive disorder

O·cho·a (ō-chō′ə), **Severo** 1905–1993. Spanish-born American biochemist. He shared a 1959 Nobel Prize for work on the biological synthesis of nucleic acids.

o·chrom·e·ter (ō-krŏm′ĭ-tər) *n.* An instrument for

determining the capillary blood pressure by measuring the force necessary to blanch the skin of a finger.

o·chro·no·sis (ō′krə-nō′sĭs) *n.* A condition observed in certain patients with alkaptonuria and marked by pigmentation of cartilage and sometimes of other tissues. —**o′chro·not′ic** (-nŏt′ĭk) *adj.*

oc·tan (ŏk′tăn′) *adj.* Occurring every eighth day. Used of a recurring fever.

octo– *or* **oct–** *or* **octa–** *pref.* Eight: *octan.*

oc·to·ge·nar·i·an (ŏk′tə-jə-nâr′ē-ən) *adj.* Being between 80 and 90 years of age. —*n.* A person between 80 and 90 years of age.

oc·u·lar (ŏk′yə-lər) *adj.* **1.** Of or relating to the eye or the sense of sight. **2.** Resembling the eye in form or function. —*n.* The eyepiece of a microscope.

ocular humor *n.* Either of the two humors of the eye, the aqueous humor or the vitreous humor.

ocular hypertelorism *n.* Extreme width between the eyes due to an enlarged sphenoid bone, sometimes associated with other congenital deformities and mental retardation. Also called *Greig's syndrome.*

oc·u·lar·ist (ŏk′yə-lər-ĭst) *n.* One skilled in the design, fabrication, and fitting of artificial eyes and in the making of prostheses associated with the appearance or function of the eyes.

ocular larva migrans *n.* Visceral larva migrans involving the eyes, primarily of older children, and marked by decreased visual acuity and strabismus.

ocular myopathy *n.* A progressive muscular dystrophy of the external ocular muscles that begins with the gradual onset of ptosis.

ocular tension *n.* Resistance of the tunics of the eye to deformation, estimated digitally or measured by a tonometer.

ocular vertigo *n.* Vertigo due to refractive errors or imbalance of the extrinsic muscles of the eye.

ocular vesicle *n.* Either of the paired evaginations of the forebrain of the embryo from which the sensory and pigment layers of the retina of the eye develop. Also called *optic vesicle.*

oc·u·list (ŏk′yə-lĭst) *n.* **1.** A physician who specializes in treating diseases of the eyes; an ophthalmologist. **2.** An optometrist.

oculo– *pref.* Eye; ocular: *oculomotor.*

oc·u·lo·au·ric·u·lo·ver·te·bral dysplasia (ŏk′yə-lō-ô-rĭk′yə-lō-vûr′tə-brəl, -vər-tē′brəl) *n.* A complex of syndromes characterized by cysts on the eyeball, swellings around the auricle of the ear, an abnormally small jaw, and vertebral anomalies.

oc·u·lo·cer·e·bro·re·nal syndrome (ŏk′yə-lō-sĕr′ə-brō-rē′nəl, -sə-rē′brō-) *n.* A sex-linked disorder characterized by hydrophthalmia, cataracts, mental retardation, aminoaciduria, reduced renal ammonia production, and vitamin D-resistant rickets. Also called *Lowe's syndrome, Lowe-Terrey-MacLachlan syndrome.*

oc·u·lo·cu·ta·ne·ous (ŏk′yə-lō-kyōō-tā′nē-əs) *adj.* Of or relating to the eyes and skin.

oc·u·lo·den·to·dig·i·tal dysplasia (ŏk′yə-lō-dĕn′tō-dĭj′ĭ-tl) *n.* A complex of disorders characterized by anomalies of the eye or its iris, malformed and malpositioned teeth, and anomalies of the fingers including webbing, permanently bent joints, or missing digits.

oc·u·lo·der·mal melanosis (ŏk′yə-lō-dûr′məl) *n.* Pigmentation of the conjunctiva and skin around the eye, usually limited to one side of the face. Also called *Ota's nevus.*

oc·u·lo·fa·cial (ŏk′yə-lō-fā′shəl) *adj.* Of or relating to the eyes and face.

oc·u·log·ra·phy (ŏk′yə-lŏg′rə-fē) *n.* A method of recording eye position and eye movements.

oc·u·lo·gy·ri·a (ŏk′yə-lō-jī′rē-ə) *n.* The limits of rotation of the eyeballs.

oc·u·lo·gy·ric (ŏk′yə-lō-jī′rĭk) *adj.* Of or relating to the turning of the eyeballs in the sockets.

oculogyric crisis *n.* A spasmodic movement of the eyeballs into a fixed position, usually upward, that persists for several minutes or hours.

oc·u·lo·mo·tor (ŏk′yə-lō-mō′tər) *adj.* **1.** Relating to or causing movements of the eyeball. **2.** Of or relating to the oculomotor nerve.

oculomotor nerve *n.* A nerve originating in the midbrain below the cerebral aqueduct, supplying all the extrinsic muscles of the eye except the lateral rectus and the superior oblique muscles, and supplying the elevator muscle of the upper eyelid, the ciliary muscle, and the sphincter muscle of the pupil. Also called *third cranial nerve.*

oculomotor nucleus *n.* The group of motor neurons that innervate the external eye muscles except the lateral rectus and the superior oblique muscles and lie in the midbrain near the midline in the most ventral part of the central gray substance.

oc·u·lo·na·sal (ŏk′yə-lō-nā′zəl) *adj.* Of or relating to the eyes and nose.

oc·u·lo·pleth·ys·mog·ra·phy (ŏk′yə-lō-plĕth′ĭz-mŏg′rə-fē) *n.* Indirect measurement of the hemodynamic significance of internal carotid artery stenosis or occlusion.

oc·u·lo·pneu·mo·pleth·ys·mog·ra·phy (ŏk′yə-lō-nōō′mō-plĕth′ĭz-mŏg′rə-fē) *n.* A method of bilateral measurement of ophthalmic artery pressure that reflects pressure and flow in the internal carotid artery.

oc·u·lo·pu·pil·lar·y (ŏk′yə-lō-pyōō′pə-lĕr′ē) *adj.* Of or relating to the pupil of the eye.

oc·u·lo·ver·te·bral dysplasia (ŏk′yə-lō-vûr′tə-brəl, -vər-tē′brəl) *n.* A complex of disorders marked by anomalies or defects of the eye and its orbit, dysplasia of the maxilla, an enlarged mouth with poorly aligned and malformed teeth and jaws, vertebral malformations, and branched hypoplastic ribs.

oc·u·lo·zy·go·mat·ic (ŏk′yə-lō-zī′gə-măt′ĭk, -zĭg′ə-) *adj.* Of or relating to the orbit of the eye, or to its margin, and the zygomatic bone.

oc·u·lus (ŏk′yə-ləs) *n., pl.* **-li** (-lī′) *Abbr.* **O** Eye.

ocy– *pref.* Variant of **oxy–.**

OD *abbr.* Doctor of Optometry; *Latin* oculus dexter (right eye); overdose

–ode *suff.* Way; path: *electrode.*

o·don·tal·gia (ō′dŏn-tăl′jə) *n.* See **toothache.** —**o′don·tal′gic** *adj.*

o·don·tec·to·my (ō′dŏn-tĕk′tə-mē) *n.* Removal of teeth by the bending back of a mucoperiosteal flap and excision of bone from around the root before the application of force to remove the tooth.

–odontia *suff.* The form, condition, or manner of treating the teeth: *orthodontia*.

odonto– *or* **odont–** *pref.* Tooth: *odontoid*.

o·don·to·blast (ō-dŏn′tə-blăst′) *n.* One of the cells forming the outer surface of dental pulp that produces tooth dentin. —**o·don′to·blas′tic** *adj.*

odontoblastic layer *n.* A layer of connective tissue cells at the periphery of the dental pulp of the tooth.

o·don·to·blas·to·ma (ō-dŏn′tə-blă-stō′mə) *n.* **1.** A tumor composed of neoplastic epithelial and mesenchymal cells that may differentiate into cells able to produce calcified tooth substances. **2.** An odontoma in its early formative stage.

o·don·to·clast (ō-dŏn′tə-klăst′) *n.* A cell that may produce resorption of the roots of deciduous teeth.

o·don·to·gen·e·sis (ō-dŏn′tə-jĕn′ĭ-sĭs) *n.* The formation and development of teeth. Also called *odontogeny, odontosis*.

odontogenesis im·per·fec·ta (ĭm′pər-fĕk′tə) *n.* An odontogenic developmental anomaly characterized by deficient formation of enamel and dentin causing the affected teeth to exhibit a marked reduction in radiopacity so that unusually large pulp chambers with thin enamel and dentin are seen.

o·don·to·gen·ic (ō-dŏn′tə-jĕn′ĭk) *adj.* **1.** Of or relating to the formation and development of teeth. **2.** Arising in tissues that form the teeth, as a tumor.

odontogenic cyst *n.* A cyst originating in tissue that forms teeth.

o·don·tog·e·ny (ō′dŏn-tŏj′ə-nē) *n.* See **odontogenesis**.

o·don·toid (ō-dŏn′toid′) *adj.* **1.** Shaped like a tooth. **2.** Of or relating to the odontoid process.

odontoid process *n.* A small, toothlike, upward projection from the second vertebra of the neck around which the first vertebra rotates.

odontoid process of epistropheus *n.* See **dens** (sense 2).

o·don·tol·o·gy (ō′dŏn-tŏl′ə-jē) *n.* The study of the structure, development, and abnormalities of the teeth. —**o·don′to·log′i·cal** (-tə-lŏj′ĭ-kəl) *adj.*

o·don·tol·y·sis (ō′dŏn-tŏl′ĭ-sĭs) *n.* See **erosion** (sense 2).

o·don·to·ma (ō′dŏn-tō′mə) *n., pl.* **–mas** *or* **–ma·ta** (-mə-tə) **1.** A tumor of odontogenic origin. **2.** A developmental anomaly of odontogenic origin, resembling a hard tumor and composed of enamel, dentin, cementum, and pulp tissue.

o·don·to·neu·ral·gia (ō-dŏn′tō-nōō-răl′jə) *n.* Facial neuralgia caused by a decayed tooth.

o·don·ton·o·my (ō′dŏn-tŏn′ə-mē) *n.* The nomenclature of dental structures and tissues.

o·don·top·a·thy (ō′dŏn-tŏp′ə-thē) *n.* A disease of the teeth or of their sockets.

o·don·to·sis (ō′dŏn-tō′sĭs) *n.* See **odontogenesis**.

o·don·tot·o·my (ō′dŏn-tŏt′ə-mē) *n.* The act or procedure of cutting into the crown of a tooth.

o·dor (ō′dər) *n.* **1.** The property or quality of a thing that affects, stimulates, or is perceived by the sense of smell. **2.** A sensation, stimulation, or perception of the sense of smell.

o·dyn·a·cu·sis (ō-dĭn′ə-kōō′sĭs, -kyōō′-) *n.* Hypersensitivity of the organ of hearing, so that noises cause actual pain.

odyno– *pref.* Pain; painful: *odynacusis*.

o·dy·nom·e·ter (ō′də-nŏm′ĭ-tər) *n.* See **algesiometer**.

o·dyn·o·pha·gia (ō-dĭn′ə-fā′jə) *n.* See **dysphagia**.

o·dyn·o·pho·ni·a (ō-dĭn′ə-fō′nē-ə) *n.* Pain caused by using the voice.

oe– For words beginning with *oe–* that are not found here, see under *e–*.

oed·i·pal *or* **Oed·i·pal** (ĕd′ə-pəl, ē′də-) *adj.* Of or characteristic of the Oedipus complex.

oedipal phase *n.* In psychoanalytic theory, the stage in psychosexual development, usually occurring between the ages of 3 and 7, characterized by manifestation of the Oedipal complex.

oed·i·pism (ĕd′ə-pĭz′əm, ē′də-) *n.* **1.** Self-infliction of injury to the eyes. **2.** Manifestation of the Oedipus complex.

Oed·i·pus complex (ĕd′ə-pəs, ē′də-) *n.* In psychoanalytic theory, a subconscious sexual desire in a child, especially a male child, for the parent of the opposite sex, usually accompanied by hostility to the parent of the same sex.

oer·sted (ûr′stĕd′) *n.* The centimeter-gram-second electromagnetic unit of magnetic intensity, equal to the magnetic intensity one centimeter from a unit magnetic pole.

oe·soph·a·gus (ĭ-sŏf′ə-gəs) *n.* Variant of **esophagus**.

oes·trid (ĕs′trĭd) *n.* A botfly of the family Oestridae.

oes·tro·gen (ĕs′trə-jən) *n.* Variant of **estrogen**.

oes·trus (ĕs′trəs) *n.* Variant of **estrus**.

of·fi·cial (ə-fĭsh′əl) *adj.* Authorized by or contained in the *US Pharmacopoeia* or *National Formulary*. Used of drugs.

official formula *n.* A chemical formula for a pharmaceutical or compound, especially one contained in the *US Pharmacopoeia* or the *National Formulary*.

of·fic·i·nal (ə-fĭs′ə-nəl, ŏf′ĭ-sī′nəl) *adj.* **1.** Readily available in pharmacies; not requiring special preparation. **2.** Recognized by a pharmacopoeia. —*n.* An official drug.

off·spring (ôf′sprĭng′) *n.* **1.** The progeny or descendants of a person, animal, or plant considered as a group. **2.** A child of particular parentage.

o·flox·a·cin (ə-flŏk′sə-sĭn) *n.* An antibiotic of the fluoroquinolone class.

O·gen (ō′jən) A trademark for a drug containing estropipate.

O·gi·no-Knaus rule (ō-gē′nō-knous′) *n.* The rule of contraception stating that the time in the menstrual period when conception is most likely to occur is approximately midway between two menstrual periods, with conception being least likely just before or just after menstruation. It is the basis of the rhythm method of contraception.

O·gu·chi's disease (ō-gōō′chēz) *n.* An inherited nonprogressive form of night blindness.

ohm (ōm) *n. Symbol* Ω A unit of electrical resistance equal to that of a conductor in which a current of one ampere is produced by a potential of one volt across its terminals.

oh·ne Hauch (ō′nä houch′, hоuкн′) *n.* **1.** The nonspreading growth of nonflagellated bacteria on agar media. **2.** Somatic agglutination.

oi– For words beginning with *oi-* that are not found here, see under *e-*.

–oic *suff.* Containing a carboxyl group or one of its derivatives: *caproic acid.*

–oid *suff.* Resembling; one that resembles: *cancroid.*

o·id·i·o·my·cin (ō-ĭd′ē-ō-mī′sĭn) *n.* **1.** An antigen used to demonstrate cutaneous hypersensitivity in patients infected with one of the Candida species of fungi. **2.** One of a series of antigens used to demonstrate an immunocompromised patient's capacity to react to any cutaneous antigen.

oil (oil) *n.* Any of numerous mineral, vegetable, and synthetic substances and animal and vegetable fats that are generally slippery, combustible, viscous, liquid or liquefiable at room temperatures, soluble in various organic solvents such as ether but not in water, and used in a great variety of products, especially lubricants and fuels.

oil gland *n.* A gland, such as a sebaceous gland, that secretes an oily substance.

oint·ment (oint′mənt) *n.* A highly viscous or semisolid preparation usually containing medicinal substances and intended for external application.

OKT cell (ō′kā-tē′) *n.* Ortho-Kung T cell

–ol[1] *suff.* An alcohol or phenol: *glycerol.*

–ol[2] *suff.* Variant of *–ole.*

o·lan·za·pine (ə-lăn′zə-pēn′) *n.* A psychotropic drug that is used orally and intramuscularly in the treatment of schizophrenia, bipolar disorder, and acute psychosis.

Old World leishmaniasis (ōld) *n.* See **cutaneous leishmaniasis.**

–ole *or* **–ol** *suff.* **1.** A usually heterocyclic chemical compound containing a five-membered ring: *pyrrole.* **2.** A chemical compound, especially an ether, that does not contain hydroxyl: *indole.*

o·le·ag·i·nous (ō′lē-ăj′ə-nəs) *adj.* Oily; greasy.

o·le·ate (ō′lē-āt′) *n.* **1.** A salt or ester of oleic acid. **2.** A pharmacopeial preparation consisting of a combination or solution of an alkaloid or metallic base in oleic acid.

o·lec·ra·non (ō-lĕk′rə-nŏn′) *n.* The large process on the upper end of the ulna that projects behind the elbow joint and forms the point of the elbow. —**o·lec′ra·nal** (-nəl), **o′le·cra′ni·al** (ō′lĭ-krā′nē-əl), **o′le·cra′ni·an** (-nē-ən) *adj.*

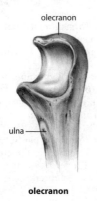

olecranon

ulna

olecranon

o·le·fin (ō′lə-fĭn) *n.* Any of a group of unsaturated open chain hydrocarbons possessing one or more double bonds, the simplest of which is ethylene.

o·le·ic acid (ō-lē′ĭk) *n.* An organic acid that is prepared from fats and is used in the preparation of oleates and lotions.

oleo– *or* **ole–** *pref.* Oil: *oleic acid.*

ol·fac·tion (ŏl-făk′shən, ōl-) *n.* The sense of smell.

ol·fac·to·ry (ŏl-făk′tə-rē, -trē, ōl-) *adj.* Of, relating to, or contributing to the sense of smell.

olfactory anesthesia *n.* See **anosmia.**

olfactory bulb *n.* The bulblike distal end of the olfactory lobe where the olfactory nerves begin.

olfactory epithelium *n.* Pseudostratified epithelium that contains olfactory, receptor, and nerve cells whose axons connect with the olfactory bulb of the brain.

olfactory foramen *n.* Any of the openings in the cribriform plate of the ethmoid bone, transmitting the olfactory nerves.

olfactory gland *n.* Any of the branched tubuloalveolar glands situated in the mucous membrane of the olfactory region of the nasal cavity that produce mucus to moisten the olfactory epithelium and dissolve odor-containing gases. Also called *Bowman's gland.*

olfactory groove *n.* The sagittal groove on the lower or orbital surface of each frontal lobe of the cerebrum, demarcating the straight gyrus from the orbital gyri. Also called *olfactory sulcus.*

olfactory membrane *n.* The portion of the nasal mucosa having olfactory receptor cells and olfactory glands.

olfactory nerve *n.* Any of numerous olfactory filaments in the olfactory portion of the nasal mucosa that enter the olfactory bulb, where they terminate in synaptic contact with mitral cells, tufted cells, and granule cells. Also called *first cranial nerve.*

olfactory pit *n.* See **nasal pit.**

olfactory receptor cell *n.* Any of the specialized, nucleated cells of the mucous membrane of the nose that serve as the receptors for smell.

olfactory sulcus *n.* See **olfactory groove.**

ol·i·ge·mi·a (ŏl′ĭ-gē′mē-ə) *n.* A deficiency in the amount of blood in the body. Also called *hyphemia, hypovolemia.* —**ol′i·ge′mic** (-gē′mĭk) *adj.*

oligo– *or* **olig–** *pref.* Few: *oligosaccharide.*

ol·i·go·am·ni·os (ŏl′ĭ-gō-ăm′nē-ŏs′) *n.* A deficiency in the amount of amniotic fluid. Also called *oligohydramnios.*

ol·i·go·cys·tic (ŏl′ĭ-gō-sĭs′tĭk) *adj.* Consisting of an atypically small number of cysts.

ol·i·go·dac·ty·ly (ŏl′ĭ-gō-dăk′tə-lē) *or* **ol·i·go·dac·tyl·i·a** (-dăk-tĭl′ē-ə) *n.* The presence of fewer than five fingers or toes on a hand or foot.

ol·i·go·den·dri·a (ŏl′ĭ-gō-dĕn′drē-ə) *n.* See **oligodendroglia.**

ol·i·go·den·dro·cyte (ŏl′ĭ-gō-dĕn′drə-sīt′) *n.* One of the cells comprising the oligodendroglia.

ol·i·go·den·drog·li·a (ŏl′ĭ-gō-dĕn-drŏg′lē-ə) *n.* Neuroglia consisting of cells similar to but smaller than astrocytes, found in the central nervous system and associated with the formation of myelin. Also called *oligodendria.*

oligodendroglia cell *n.* A form of oligodendrocyte that is a component of central nervous system tissue and that may contribute to formation of the myelin sheath around axons of neurons.

ol·i·go·den·dro·gli·o·ma (ŏl′ĭ-gō-dĕn′drō-glē-ō′mə, -glī-) *n.* A relatively rare and slow-growing glioma characterized by numerous small, round or ovoid oligodendroglial cells uniformly distributed in a sparse fibrillary stroma.

ol·i·go·dip·si·a (ŏl′ĭ-gō-dĭp′sē-ə) *n.* Abnormal absence of thirst.

ol·i·go·don·tia (ŏl′ĭ-gō-dŏn′shə) *n.* **1.** Presence of less than a full complement of teeth. **2.** See **hypodontia.**

ol·i·go·dy·nam·ic (ŏl′ĭ-gō-dī-năm′ĭk) *adj.* Active or effective in very small quantities, as certain germicides or heavy-metal toxins.

ol·i·go·ga·lac·ti·a (ŏl′ĭ-gō-gə-lăk′tē-ə, -shē-ə) *n.* Slight or deficient secretion of milk from the mammary glands.

ol·i·go·hy·dram·ni·os (ŏl′ĭ-gō-hī-drăm′nē-ŏs′) *n.* See **oligoamnios.**

ol·i·go·hy·dru·ri·a (ŏl′ĭ-gō-hī-drŏŏr′ē-ə) *n.* Excretion of abnormally small quantities of urine, as occurs in dehydration.

ol·i·go·men·or·rhe·a (ŏl′ĭ-gō-mĕn′ə-rē′ə) *n.* Abnormally slight or infrequent menstrual flow.

ol·i·go·mor·phic (ŏl′ĭ-gō-môr′fĭk) *adj.* Having or passing through few changes of form.

ol·i·go·nu·cle·o·tide (ŏl′ĭ-gō-nōō′klē-ə-tīd) *n.* A polymeric chain of two to ten nucleotides.

ol·i·gop·ne·a (ŏl′ĭ-gŏp-nē′ə, -gŏp′nē-ə) *n.* Abnormally infrequent respiration.

ol·i·go·pty·a·lism (ŏl′ĭ-gō-tī′ə-lĭz′əm, -gŏp-tī′-) *n.* A slight or scanty secretion of saliva.

ol·i·go·ri·a (ŏl′ĭ-gôr′ē-ə) *n.* An abnormal lack of interest in one's surroundings or relationships, as occurs in depression.

ol·i·go·sac·cha·ride (ŏl′ĭ-gō-săk′ə-rīd′) *n.* A carbohydrate that consists of a relatively small number of monosaccharides.

ol·i·go·sper·mi·a (ŏl′ĭ-gō-spûr′mē-ə) *n.* A subnormal concentration of spermatozoa in the ejaculated semen. Also called *oligozoospermia.*

ol·i·go·sy·nap·tic (ŏl′ĭ-gō-sĭ-năp′tĭk) *adj.* Of or being neural conduction pathways that are made up of a sequence of only a few nerve cells and thus are interrupted by only a few synaptic junctions.

ol·i·go·tro·phi·a (ŏl′ĭ-gō-trō′fē-ə) *or* **ol·i·got·ro·phy** (-gŏt′rə-fē) *n.* Inadequate or deficient nutrition.

ol·i·go·zo·o·sper·mi·a (ŏl′ĭ-gō-zō′ə-spûr′mē-ə) *n.* See **oligospermia.**

ol·i·gu·ri·a (ŏl′ĭ-gyŏŏr′ē-ə) *n.* Abnormally slight or infrequent urination.

o·li·va (ō-lī′və) *n., pl.* **–vae** (-vē) See **olivary body.**

ol·i·var·y (ŏl′ə-vĕr′ē) *adj.* **1.** Of or relating to the olivary body. **2.** Relating to or shaped like an olive.

olivary body *n.* A smooth oval prominence of the ventrolateral surface of the medulla oblongata lateral to the pyramidal tract, corresponding to the olivary nucleus. Also called *oliva, olive.*

olivary nucleus *n.* A dense aggregate of small nerve cells arranged in a folded lamina, corresponding in position to the olivary body, and projecting to all parts of the contralateral half of the cerebellar cortex; inferior olivary nucleus.

ol·ive (ŏl′ĭv) *n.* See **olivary body.**

ol·i·vif·u·gal (ŏl′ə-vĭf′yə-gəl) *adj.* In a direction away from the olivary body.

ol·i·vip·e·tal (ŏl′ə-vĭp′ĭ-tl) *adj.* In a direction toward the olivary body.

ol·i·vo·pon·to·cer·e·bel·lar (ŏl′ə-vō-pŏn′tō-sĕr′ə-bĕl′ər) *adj.* Relating to the olivary nucleus, the pons, and the cerebellum.

olivopontocerebellar atrophy *n.* A progressive neurologic disease marked by loss of neurons in the cerebellar cortex, the pons, and the olivary nucleus.

Ol·lier's disease (ŏl′ē-āz′, ô-lyāz′) *n.* See **enchondromatosis.**

Ollier-Thiersch graft (-tîrsh′) *n.* A thin split-skin graft, usually in small pieces.

OM *abbr.* otitis media

–oma *suff.* Tumor: *lipoma.*

o·ma·liz·u·mab (ō′mə-lĭz′yə-măb′) *n.* A monoclonal antibody used as a parenteral drug to treat severe asthma.

o·me·ga (ō-mĕg′ə, ō-mē′gə, ō-mā′-) *n. Symbol* ω, Ω The 24th letter of the Greek alphabet. —*adj.* Of or characterizing a chemical group or position at the end of a molecular chain, such as omega-oxidation.

omega-3 fatty acid *n.* Any of various polyunsaturated fatty acids that are found primarily in fish, fish oils, vegetable oils, and leafy green vegetables, and that seem to reduce the risk of stroke and heart attack.

omega-oxidation theory *n.* The theory that the oxidation of fatty acids commences at the omega methyl group with beta-oxidation and then proceeds from both ends of the fatty acid chain.

O·menn's syndrome (ō′mĕnz′) *n.* A rapidly fatal familial immunodeficiency disease characterized by widespread reddening of the skin, diarrhea, repeated infections, enlargement of the liver and spleen, and leukocytosis.

o·men·tal (ō-mĕn′tl) *adj.* Relating to the omentum.

omental bursa *n.* An isolated portion of the peritoneal cavity lying dorsal to the stomach and opening into the general peritoneal cavity at the epiploic foramen. Also called *lesser peritoneal cavity.*

omental graft *n.* A segment of omentum, with its supplying blood vessels, transplanted as a free flap to a distant area.

o·men·tec·to·my (ō′mĕn-tĕk′tə-mē) *n.* Resection or excision of the omentum.

o·men·ti·tis (ō′mĕn-tī′tĭs) *n.* Peritonitis involving the omentum.

omento– *or* **oment–** *pref.* Omentum: *omentectomy.*

o·men·to·pex·y (ō-mĕn′ə-pĕk′sē) *n.* **1.** Suture of the greater omentum to the abdominal wall. **2.** Suture of the omentum to another organ to increase arterial circulation. Also called *omentofixation.*

o·men·to·plas·ty (ō-mĕn′tə-plăs′tē) *n.* A surgical procedure in which a portion of the greater omentum is used to cover or fill a defect, augment arterial or portal venous circulation, absorb effusions, or increase lymphatic drainage.

o·men·tor·rha·phy (ō'měn-tôr'ə-fē) *n.* Suture of an opening in the omentum.

o·men·tu·lum (ō-měn'tyə-ləm, -chə-) *n.* See **lesser omentum.**

o·men·tum (ō-měn'təm) *n., pl.* **–tums** or **–ta** (-tə) One of the folds of the peritoneum that connect the stomach with other abdominal organs, especially the greater omentum or the lesser omentum.

o·mep·ra·zole (ō-měp'rə-zōl') *n.* A drug of the proton pump inhibitor class.

om·i·cron (ŏm'ĭ-krŏn', ō'mĭ-) *n. Symbol* **o** The 15th letter of the Greek alphabet.

omn. hor. *abbr. Latin* omni hora (every hour)

Om·ni·cef (ŏm'nĭ-sĕf') A trademark for the drug cefdinir.

om·ni·fo·cal lens (ŏm'nə-fō'kəl) *n.* A lens that corrects for near and distant vision whose section for near vision is a continuously variable curve.

om·ni·vore (ŏm'nə-vôr') *n.* An omnivorous person or animal.

omo– *pref.* Shoulder: *omohyoid.*

o·mo·cla·vic·u·lar triangle (ō'mō-klə-vĭk'yə-lər) *n.* See **subclavian triangle.**

o·mo·hy·oid (ō'mō-hī'oid') *n.* A muscle having two bellies attached to an intermediate tendon, with origin by the inferior belly from the upper border of the scapula, with insertion by the superior belly into the hyoid bone, with nerve supply from the upper cervical nerve through the cervical ansa, and whose action depresses the hyoid bone.

om·pha·lec·to·my (ŏm'fə-lĕk'tə-mē) *n.* Excision of the navel or of a tumor connected with it.

om·pha·lel·co·sis (ŏm'fə-lĕl-kō'sĭs) *n.* Ulceration at the navel.

om·phal·ic (ŏm-făl'ĭk) *adj.* Of or relating to the navel; umbilical.

om·pha·li·tis (ŏm'fə-lī'tĭs) *n.* Inflammation of the navel and surrounding parts.

omphalo– or **omphal–** *pref.* Umbilicus; navel: *omphalectomy.*

om·pha·lo·an·gi·op·a·gous twins (ŏm'fə-lō-ăn'jē-ŏp'ə-gəs) *pl.n.* See **allantoidoangiopagous twins.**

om·phal·o·cele (ŏm-făl'ə-sēl', ŏm'fə-lō-) *n.* Congenital herniation of viscera into the base of the umbilical cord. Also called *exomphalos.*

om·pha·lo·en·ter·ic (ŏm'fə-lō-ĕn-tĕr'ĭk) *adj.* Relating to the navel and the intestine.

om·pha·lo·mes·en·ter·ic (ŏm'fə-lō-měz'ən-tĕr'ĭk, -měs'-) *adj.* Relating to the navel and the mesentery.

omphalomesenteric duct *n.* See **yolk stalk.**

om·pha·lo·phle·bi·tis (ŏm'fə-lō-flĭ-bī'tĭs) *n.* Inflammation of the umbilical veins.

om·pha·lor·rha·gia (ŏm'fə-lō-rā'jə) *n.* Bleeding from the navel.

om·pha·lor·rhe·a (ŏm'fə-lō-rē'ə) *n.* A serous discharge from the navel.

om·pha·lor·rhex·is (ŏm'fə-lō-rĕk'sĭs) *n.* Rupture of the umbilical cord during childbirth.

om·pha·los (ŏm'fə-lŏs', -ləs) *n., pl.* **-li** (-lī') The navel.

om·pha·lo·site (ŏm'fə-lə-sīt', ŏm-făl'ə-) *n.* The underdeveloped member of unequal monochorionic twins that derives its blood supply from the placenta of the autosite and is not capable of independent existence or separation from the placenta.

om·pha·lo·spi·nous (ŏm'fə-lō-spī'nəs) *adj.* Of or being a line connecting the navel and the anterior superior spine of the ilium.

om·pha·lot·o·my (ŏm'fə-lŏt'ə-mē) *n.* Cutting of the umbilical cord at birth.

OMS *abbr.* organic mental syndrome

–on¹ *suff.* **1.** A subatomic particle: *neutron.* **2.** A unit: *photon.* **3.** A basic hereditary unit: *codon.*

–on² *suff.* Inert gas: *radon.*

–on³ *suff.* A chemical compound that is not a ketone or a compound that contains oxygen in a carbonyl group: *parathion.*

o·nan·ism (ō'nə-nĭz'əm) *n.* **1.** See **coitus interruptus.** **2.** Masturbation.

On·cho·cer·ca (ŏng'kō-sûr'kə) *n.* A genus of elongated filariform nematodes that inhabit the connective tissue of their hosts, usually within firm nodules in which they are coiled and entangled.

on·cho·cer·ci·a·sis (ŏng'kō-sər-kī'ə-sĭs) or **on·cho·cer·co·sis** (-sər-kō'sĭs) *n.* A disease occurring in tropical Africa and Central America, transmitted by black flies and caused by infestation with filariform nematodes of the genus *Onchocerca,* especially *O. volvulus,* and characterized by nodular swellings on the skin and lesions of the eyes. Also called *river blindness, volvulosis.*

onco– *pref.* **1.** Tumor: *oncology.* **2.** Mass; swelling: *oncolysis.*

on·co·cyte (ŏng'kə-sīt') *n.* A large granular acidophilic tumor cell having numerous mitochondria.

on·co·cyt·ic hepatocellular tumor (ŏng'kə-sĭt'ĭk) *n.* A tumor in which malignant hepatocytes are intersected by fibrous lamellated bands.

on·co·cy·to·ma (ŏng'kō-sī-tō'mə) *n., pl.* **-mas** or **-ma·ta** (-mə-tə) A glandular tumor that is chiefly composed of oncocytes, occurring most often in the salivary glands.

on·co·fe·tal (ŏng'kō-fēt'l) *adj.* Of or relating to substances associated with tumor formation and present in fetal tissue.

oncofetal antigen *n.* One of the tumor-associated antigens present in fetal tissue but not in normal adult tissue, such as alpha-fetoprotein and carcinoembryonic antigen.

oncofetal marker *n.* A tumor marker produced by tumor tissue and by fetal tissue of the same type as the tumor, but not by normal adult tissue from which the tumor arises.

on·co·gene (ŏng'kə-jēn) *n.* A gene that causes the transformation of normal cells into cancerous tumor cells, especially a viral gene that transforms a host cell into a tumor cell.

on·co·gen·e·sis (ŏng'kō-jĕn'ĭ-sĭs) *n.* The formation and development of tumors.

on·co·gen·ic (ŏng'kō-jĕn'ĭk) or **on·cog·e·nous** (ŏng-kŏj'ə-nəs) *adj.* Causing or tending to cause the formation and development of tumors. —**on'co·ge·nic'i·ty** (-jə-nĭs'ĭ-tē) *n.*

oncogenic virus *n.* A virus capable of inducing the formation of tumors. Also called *tumor virus.*

on·col·o·gy (ŏng-kŏl′ə-jē) *n.* The branch of medicine dealing with the physical, chemical, and biological properties of tumors, including study of their development, diagnosis, treatment, and prevention. —**on′co·log′i·cal** (-kə-lŏj′ĭ-kəl), **on′co·log′ic** (-lŏj′ĭk) *adj.* —**on·col′o·gist** *n.*

on·col·y·sis (ŏn-kŏl′ĭ-sĭs, ŏng-) *n.* **1.** The destruction of a tumor or tumor cells. **2.** The reduction of any swelling or mass. —**on′co·lyt′ic** (ŏng′kə-lĭt′ĭk) *adj.*

on·co·plas·tic carcinoma (ŏng′kō-plăs′tĭk) *n.* An undifferentiated carcinoma showing no microscopic evidence of origin from a specific epithelial tissue.

on·cor·na·vi·rus (ŏng-kôr′nə-vī′rəs) *n.* A virus of the subfamily Oncovirinae; an RNA tumor virus. Also called *oncovirus.*

on·co·sis (ŏng-kō′sĭs) *n.* **1.** Formation of a tumor or tumors. **2.** A condition characterized by swelling.

on·cot·ic (ŏng-kŏt′ĭk) *adj.* **1.** Of or relating to the formation of tumors. **2.** Of or caused by a condition of swelling.

on·cot·o·my (ŏng-kŏt′ə-mē) *n.* Surgical incision of an abscess, cyst, or tumor.

on·co·trop·ic (ŏng′kə-trŏp′ĭk, -trō′pĭk) *adj.* Having a special affinity for tumors or tumor cells.

On·co·vin (ŏng′kə-vĭn) A trademark for vincristine sulfate.

On·co·vir·i·nae (ŏng′kō-vĭr′ə-nē) *n.* A subfamily of retroviruses that contain single-stranded RNA and produce tumors in birds and mammals.

on·co·vi·rus (ŏng′kō-vī′rəs) *n.* See **oncornavirus.**

–one *suff.* **1.** A ketone: *acetone.* **2.** A compound that contains oxygen, especially in a carbonyl radical: *lactone.*

1,3-di·phos·pho·glyc·er·ate (-dī-fŏs′fō-glĭs′ə-rāt′) *n.* A diphosphate of glyceric acid that is an important intermediate in glycolysis, fermentation, and photosynthesis.

1,4-alpha-glucan branching enzyme *n.* An enzyme in muscles that catalyzes the breakdown of alpha-1,4 linkages in glycogen and the formation of alpha-1,6 linkages, thus creating branches in glycogen and increasing its solubility; brancher enzyme.

o·nei·ric (ō-nī′rĭk) *adj.* **1.** Of, relating to, or suggestive of dreams. **2.** Of, relating to, or characterizing the clinical state of oneirophrenia.

o·nei·rism (ō-nī′rĭz′əm) *n.* An abnormal state of consciousness in which dreamlike, often disturbing illusions are experienced while awake.

o·nei·ro·dyn·i·a (ō-nī′rō-dĭn′ē-ə) *n.* Intense mental disturbance or distress associated with dreaming.

o·nei·ro·phre·ni·a (ō-nī′rə-frē′nē-ə, -frĕn′ē-ə) *n.* A mental state that is characterized by hallucinations and other disturbances and is associated with prolonged deprivation of sleep, sensory isolation, or psychoactive drugs.

o·nei·ros·co·py (ō′nī-rŏs′kə-pē) *n.* See **dream analysis.**

–onium *suff.* Containing a positively charged radical: *carbonium.*

on·lay (ŏn′lā′) *n.* **1.** A cast restoration, usually made of gold, that is attached to the occlusal surface of a tooth. **2.** A bone graft applied to the exterior surface of the bone.

on-off phenomenon (ŏn′ôf′) *n.* A state in the treatment of Parkinson's disease with dopa in which the individual exhibits a rapid fluctuation of akinetic and choreoathetotic movements.

on·o·mat·o·ma·ni·a (ŏn′ə-măt′ə-mā′nē-ə, -măn′yə) *n.* An abnormal concentration on certain words and their supposed significance or on the effort to recall a particular word.

on·o·mat·o·pho·bi·a (ŏn′ə-măt′ə-fō′bē-ə) *n.* An abnormal dread of certain words or names because of their supposed significance.

on·set (ŏn′sĕt′) *n.* A beginning; a start, as of a cold.

onto– *or* **ont–** *pref.* Organism; being: *ontogeny.*

on·to·gen·e·sis (ŏn′tō-jĕn′ĭ-sĭs) *n.* See **ontogeny.**

on·to·ge·net·ic (ŏn′tō-jə-nĕt′ĭk) *adj.* Of or relating to ontogeny.

on·tog·e·ny (ŏn-tŏj′ə-nē) *n.* The origin and development of an individual organism from embryo to adult. Also called *ontogenesis.*

On·uf's nucleus (ŏn′əfs) *n.* A nucleus of small somatic motor neurons that are located in the ventral horn of the spinal cord at the level of the second sacral vertebra and innervate the vesicorectal sphincters.

on·y·chal·gia (ŏn′ĭ-kăl′jə) *n.* Pain in the fingernails or toenails.

on·y·cha·tro·phi·a (ŏn′ĭ-kə-trō′fē-ə) *or* **on·y·chat·ro·phy** (-kăt′rə-fē) *n.* Atrophy of the fingernails or toenails.

on·y·chaux·is (ŏn′ĭ-kôk′sĭs) *n.* Marked overgrowth of the fingernails or toenails.

on·y·chec·to·my (ŏn′ĭ-kĕk′tə-mē) *n.* Surgical removal of a toenail or fingernail.

o·nych·i·a (ō-nĭk′ē-ə) *n.* Inflammation of the fingernail or toenail matrix. Also called *onychitis.*

onycho– *or* **onych–** *pref.* Fingernail or toenail: *onychopathy.*

on·y·choc·la·sis (ŏn′ĭ-kŏk′lə-sĭs) *n.* Breaking of the fingernails or toenails.

on·y·cho·dys·tro·phy (ŏn′ĭ-kō-dĭs′trə-fē) *n.* Dystrophic changes in fingernails or toenails, such as malformation or discoloration, occurring as a congenital defect or due to illness or injury.

on·y·cho·graph (ŏn′ĭ-kō-grăf′, ō-nĭk′ə-grăf′, ŏ-nĭk′-) *n.* An instrument for recording the capillary blood pressure as shown by the circulation under a fingernail or toenail.

on·y·cho·gry·po·sis (ŏn′ĭ-kō-grə-pō′sĭs) *or* **on·y·cho·gry·pho·sis** (-grə-fō′sĭs) *n.* Enlargement of the fingernails or toenails accompanied by increased thickening and curvature.

on·y·cho·het·er·o·to·pi·a (ŏn′ĭ-kō-hĕt′ər-ə-tō′pē-ə) *n.* Abnormal placement of a fingernail or toenail.

on·y·choid (ŏn′ĭ-koid′) *adj.* Resembling a fingernail or toenail in structure or form.

on·y·chol·y·sis (ŏn′ĭ-kŏl′ĭ-sĭs) *n.* The separation or loosening of a fingernail or toenail from its nail bed.

on·y·cho·ma (ŏn′ĭ-kō′mə) *n.* A tumor arising from the nail bed of a fingernail or toenail.

on·y·cho·ma·de·sis (ŏn′ĭ-kō′mə-dē′sĭs) *n.* Complete shedding of a fingernail or toenail, usually associated with a systemic illness.

on·y·cho·ma·la·cia (ŏn′ĭ-kō′mə-lā′shə) *n.* Abnormal softness of the fingernails or toenails.

on·y·cho·my·co·sis (ŏn′ĭ-kō-mī-kō′sĭs) *n.* A fungal infection of the fingernails or toenails that results in thickening, roughness, and splitting of the nails. It is usually caused by *Trichophyton rubrum* or *T. mentagrophytes*. Also called *tinea unguium*.

on·y·cho·os·te·o·dys·pla·sia (ŏn′ĭ-kō-ŏs′tē-ō-dĭs-plā′zhə) *n.* A hereditary skeletal disorder characterized by defects in the nails, hypoplasia of the patella and iliac horns, and renal abnormalities. Also called *nail-patella syndrome*.

on·y·chop·a·thy (ŏn′ĭ-kŏp′ə-thē) *n.* A disease of the fingernails or toenails. Also called *onychosis.* —**on′y·cho·path′ic** (-kō-păth′ĭk) *adj.*

on·y·choph·a·gy (ŏn′ĭ-kŏf′ə-jē) *or* **on·y·cho·pha·gia** (-kō-fā′jə) *n.* The habit of nail biting.

on·y·cho·plas·ty (ŏn′ĭ-kō-plăs′tē) *n.* A corrective or plastic operation on the matrix of a fingernail or toenail.

on·y·chor·rhex·is (ŏn′ĭ-kə-rĕk′sĭs) *n.* Abnormal brittleness of the fingernails or toenails with splitting of the free edge.

on·y·cho·schiz·i·a (ŏn′ĭ-kō-skĭz′ē-ə) *n.* Splitting of the fingernails or toenails in layers.

on·y·cho·sis (ŏn′ĭ-kō′sĭs) *n.* See **onychopathy**.

on·y·chot·il·lo·ma·ni·a (ŏn′ĭ-kŏt′l-ō-mā′nē-ə, -mān′-yə, ŏn′ĭ-kō-tĭl′ə-) *n.* A tendency to pick at the fingernails or toenails.

on·y·chot·o·my (ŏn′ĭ-kŏt′ə-mē) *n.* Incision into a toenail or fingernail.

on·yx (ŏn′ĭks) *n.* **1.** See **unguis**. **2.** A collection of pus in the anterior chamber of the eye.

oo– *pref.* Egg; ovum: *oogenesis.*

o·o·cyst (ō′ə-sĭst′) *n.* A thick-walled structure in which sporozoan zygotes develop and that serves to transfer them to new hosts.

o·o·cyte (ō′ə-sīt′) *n.* A cell from which an egg or ovum develops by meiosis; a female gametocyte.

o·o·gam·ete (ō′ə-găm′ēt′, -gə-mēt′) *n.* A female gamete, especially the larger of two gametes produced by an oogamous species.

o·og·a·mous (ō-ŏg′ə-məs) *adj.* Characterized by or having small motile male gametes and large nonmotile female gametes.

o·o·gen·e·sis (ō′ə-jĕn′ĭ-sĭs) *n.* The formation and the development of the ovum. Also called *ovigenesis.* —**o′o·ge·net′ic** (-jə-nĕt′ĭk) *adj.*

o·o·go·ni·um (ō′ə-gō′nē-əm) *n., pl.* **–ni·ums** *or* **–ni·a** (-nē-ə) The primitive egg mother cell from which the oocytes develop. —**o′o·go′ni·al** (-nē-əl) *adj.*

o·o·ki·ne·sis (ō′ə-kə-nē′sĭs, -kī-) *n.* The chromosomal movements of the egg that take place during maturation and fertilization.

o·o·ki·nete (ō′ə-kə-nēt′, -kī′nēt′) *n.* The motile zygote of the malarial organism that penetrates the mosquito stomach to form an oocyst under the outer gut lining.

o·o·lem·ma (ō′ə-lĕm′ə) *n.* See **zona pellucida**.

o·o·pho·rec·to·my (ō′ə-fə-rĕk′tə-mē) *n.* See **ovariectomy**.

o·o·pho·ri·tis (ō′ə-fə-rī′tĭs) *n.* Inflammation of an ovary. Also called *ovaritis.*

oophoro– *or* **oophor–** *pref.* Ovary: *oophoropexy.*

o·oph·o·ro·cys·tec·to·my (ō-ŏf′ə-rō-sĭ-stĕk′tə-mē) *n.* Excision of an ovarian cyst.

o·oph·o·ro·cys·to·sis (ō-ŏf′ə-rō-sĭ-stō′sĭs) *n.* Ovarian cyst formation.

o·oph·o·ro·hys·ter·ec·to·my (ō-ŏf′ə-rō-hĭs′tə-rĕk′tə-mē) *n.* See **ovariohysterectomy**.

o·oph·o·ron (ō-ŏf′ə-rŏn′) *n.* See **ovary**.

o·oph·o·ro·pex·y (ō-ŏf′ə-rə-pĕk′sē) *n.* Surgical fixation or suspension of an ovary.

o·oph·o·ro·plas·ty (ō-ŏf′ə-rə-plăs′tē) *n.* Plastic surgery on an ovary.

o·oph·o·ros·to·my (ō-ŏf′ə-rŏs′tə-mē) *n.* See **ovariostomy**.

o·oph·o·rot·o·my (ō-ŏf′ə-rŏt′ə-mē) *n.* See **ovariotomy** (sense 2).

o·o·plasm (ō′ə-plăz′əm) *n.* The protoplasmic portion of the ovum.

o·o·sphere (ō′ə-sfîr′) *n.* A large nonmotile female gamete or egg cell, formed in an oogonium and ready for fertilization.

o·o·spore (ō′ə-spôr′) *n.* A fertilized female cell or zygote, especially one with thick chitinous walls, developed from a fertilized oosphere.

o·o·tid (ō′ə-tĭd′) *n.* The nearly mature ovum after the first maturation division has been completed and the second initiated.

o·pac·i·fi·ca·tion (ō-păs′ə-fĭ-kā′shən) *n.* **1.** The process of making something opaque. **2.** The formation of opacities.

o·pac·i·ty (ō-păs′ĭ-tē) *n.* **1.** The quality or state of being opaque. **2.** An opaque or nontransparent area, as of the cornea.

o·pal·es·cent (ō′pə-lĕs′ənt) *adj.* Resembling an opal in the display of various colors, often used to describe certain bacterial cultures.

o·paque (ō-pāk′) *adj.* Impenetrable by light; neither transparent nor translucent.

o·pen-an·gle glaucoma (ō′pən-ăng′gəl) *n.* Primary glaucoma in which the aqueous humor has free access to the trabecular reticulum. Also called *simple glaucoma.*

open biopsy *n.* Incision or excision of a region from which a biopsy is taken.

open bite *n.* See **apertognathia**.

open chain compound *n.* See **acyclic compound**.

open chest massage *n.* Cardiac massage in which the heart is compressed with the hand inside the thoracic cavity.

open circuit method *n.* A method for measuring oxygen consumption and carbon-dioxide production by collecting expired gas over a given period of time, measuring its volume, and determining its composition.

open comedo *n.* See **blackhead**.

open dislocation *n.* A dislocation complicated by a wound opening from the surface down to the affected joint. Also called *compound dislocation.*

open drainage *n.* The admittance of air into a wound or cavity to facilitate drainage.

open drop anesthesia *n.* Inhalation anesthesia using the open drop technique.

open drop technique *n.* A technique for producing inhalation anesthesia in which drops of a liquid anesthetic, such as ether, are placed on a gauze mask or cone applied over the mouth and nose.

open flap *n.* See **flat flap.**

open fracture *n.* A fracture in which broken bone fragments lacerate soft tissue and protrude through an open wound in the skin. Also called *compound fracture.*

open heart surgery *n.* Surgery in which the thoracic cavity is opened to expose the heart and the blood is recirculated and oxygenated through a heart-lung machine.

open hospital *n.* A hospital in which physicians who are not members of the attending and consulting staff may admit and treat patients.

o·pen·ing (ō′pə-nǐng) *n.* **1.** The act or an instance of becoming unobstructed or of being made to open. **2.** An open space that serves as a passage or gap. **3.** A breach or aperture.

opening snap *n.* A sharp, high-pitched click in early diastole, associated with the opening of the abnormal valve in cases of mitral stenosis.

open pneumothorax *n.* A free communication between the exterior and the pleural space either via the lung or through the chest wall, as through an open wound. Also called *blowing wound, sucking wound.*

open reduction *n.* Reduction of a fractured bone by manipulation after incision into skin and muscle over the site of the fracture.

open tuberculosis *n.* **1.** A tuberculous ulceration or other form of tuberculosis in which tubercle bacilli are present in the excretions or secretions. **2.** Pulmonary tuberculosis, especially with cavitation.

open wound *n.* A wound in which the injured tissues are exposed to the air.

op·er·a·ble (ŏp′ər-ə-bəl, ŏp′rə-) *adj.* Being treatable by surgical operation with a reasonable degree of safety and chance of success. —**op′er·a·bil′i·ty** *n.*

op·er·ant (ŏp′ər-ənt) *adj.* **1.** Operating to produce effects; effective. **2.** Of, relating to, or being a response that occurs spontaneously and is identified by its reinforcing or inhibiting effects. —*n.* In operant conditioning, a behavior or specific response chosen by the experimenter or therapist. Also called *target response.*

operant conditioning *n.* A process of behavior modification in which a subject is encouraged to behave in a desired manner through positive or negative reinforcement, so that the subject comes to associate the pleasure or displeasure of the reinforcement with the behavior.

op·er·ate (ŏp′ə-rāt′) *v.* To perform surgery.

op·er·at·ing microscope (ŏp′ə-rā′tǐng) *n.* See **surgical microscope.**

operating room *n. Abbr.* **OR** A room equipped for performing surgical operations.

op·er·a·tion (ŏp′ə-rā′shən) *n.* **1.** A surgical procedure, usually using instruments, for remedying an injury, ailment, defect, or dysfunction. **2.** The act, manner, or process of functioning.

op·er·a·tive (ŏp′ər-ə-tǐv, -ə-rā′tǐv, ŏp′rə-) *adj.* **1.** Of, relating to, or resulting from a surgical operation. **2.** Functioning effectively; efficient.

op·er·a·tor (ŏp′ə-rā′tər) *n.* An operator gene.

operator gene *n.* A gene that interacts with a specific repressor to control the functioning of the adjacent structural genes.

o·per·cu·li·tis (ō-pûr′kyə-lī′tǐs) *n.* See **pericoronitis.**

o·per·cu·lum (ō-pûr′kyə-ləm) *n., pl.* **–lums** or **–la** (-lə) **1.** Something resembling a lid or cover. **2.** The portions of the frontal, parietal, and temporal lobes covering the insula. **3.** The mucus sealing the endocervical canal of the uterus after conception. **4.** The attached flap in cases of torn retinal detachment. **5.** The mucosal flap partially or completely covering an unerupted tooth. —**o·per′cu·lar** (-lər) *adj.*

op·er·on (ŏp′ə-rŏn′) *n.* A unit of gene activity consisting of a sequence of genetic material that functions in a coordinated manner to control the production of mRNA and that consists of an operator gene, a promoter, and two or more structural genes.

o·phi·a·sis (ō-fī′ə-sǐs) *n.* Alopecia areata in which the loss of hair occurs in bands partially or completely encircling the head.

o·phri·tis (ŏ-frī′tǐs) *or* **oph·ry·i·tis** (ŏf′rē-ī′tǐs) *n.* Dermatitis in the region of the eyebrows.

oph·ry·on (ŏf′rē-ŏn′, ō′frē-) *n.* The point on the midline of the forehead just above the glabella.

oph·ry·o·sis (ŏf′rē-ō′sǐs) *n.* Spasmodic wrinkling of the eyebrow.

oph·thal·mal·gia (ŏf′thəl-măl′jə) *n.* Pain in the eyeball.

oph·thal·mi·a (ŏf-thăl′mē-ə, ŏp-) *n.* **1.** Severe, often purulent conjunctivitis. **2.** Inflammation of the deep eye structures. Also called *ophthalmitis.*

ophthalmia ne·o·na·to·rum (nē′ō-nā-tôr′əm) *n.* Any of various forms of conjunctivitis in newborns, usually contracted during birth from passage through the infected birth canal of the mother. Also called *infantile purulent conjunctivitis.*

oph·thal·mic (ŏf-thăl′mǐk, ŏp-) *adj.* Of or relating to the eye; ocular.

ophthalmic artery *n.* An artery with origin in the internal carotid artery that passes through the optic foramen and that branches to the central artery of the retina and to the ciliary, meningeal, lacrimal, conjunctival, episcleral, supraorbital, ethmoidal, palpebral, nasal, and supratrochlear arteries.

ophthalmic nerve *n.* The ophthalmic branch of the trigeminal nerve, whose frontal, lacrimal, and nasociliary branches supply sensation to the eye socket and its contents, the anterior part of the nasal cavity, and the skin of the nose and forehead.

ophthalmic solution *n.* A sterile solution that is free from foreign particles and is compounded and dispensed for eyedrops.

oph·thal·mi·tis (ŏf′thəl-mī′tǐs, ŏp′-) *n.* See **ophthalmia** (sense 2).

ophthalmo– *or* **ophthalm–** *pref.* Eye; eyeball: *ophthalmoscope.*

oph·thal·mo·di·aph·a·no·scope (ŏf-thăl′mō-dī-ăf′ə-nə-skōp′, ŏp-) *n.* An instrument for viewing the interior of the eye by transmitted light.

oph·thal·mo·dy·na·mom·e·ter (ŏf-thăl′mō-dī′nə-mŏm′ĭ-tər, ŏp-) *n.* **1.** An instrument for determining the near point of convergence of the eyes. **2.** An instrument that measures the blood pressure in the retinal vessels. —**oph·thal′mo·dy′na·mom′e·try** *n.*

oph·thal·mog·ra·phy (ŏf′thəl-mŏg′rə-fē, -thăl-, ŏp′-) *n.* The recording of movements the eye makes during reading by photographing a mark on the cornea or by making a tracing of light reflexes. —**oph·thal′mo·graph′** (ŏf-thăl′mə-grăf′, ŏp-) *n.*

oph·thal·mo·lith (ŏf-thăl′mə-lĭth′, ŏp-) *n.* See **dacryolith.**

oph·thal·mol·o·gist (ŏf′thəl-mŏl′ə-jĭst, -thăl-, ŏp′-) *n.* A physician who specializes in ophthalmology.

oph·thal·mol·o·gy (ŏf′thəl-mŏl′ə-jē, -thăl-, ŏp′-) *n.* The branch of medicine that deals with the anatomy, functions, pathology, and treatment of the eye. —**oph·thal′mo·log′ic** (-thăl′mə-lŏj′ĭk), **oph·thal′mo·log′i·cal** (-ĭ-kəl) *adj.*

oph·thal·mo·ma·la·cia (ŏf-thăl′mō-mə-lā′shə, ŏp-) *n.* Abnormal softening of the eyeball.

oph·thal·mo·man·dib·u·lo·mel·ic dysplasia (ŏf-thăl′mō-măn-dĭb′yə-lō-mĕl′ĭk, ŏp-) *n.* An inherited disorder that is characterized by corneal clouding and multiple abnormalities of the mandible and limbs.

oph·thal·mom·e·ter (ŏf′thəl-mŏm′ĭ-tər, -thăl-, ŏp′-) *n.* See **keratometer.**

oph·thal·mo·my·co·sis (ŏf-thăl′mō-mī-kō′sĭs, ŏp-) *n.* Any of various diseases of the eye or its appendages caused by a fungus.

oph·thal·mo·my·i·tis (ŏf-thăl′mō-mī-ī′tĭs, ŏp-) *n.* Inflammation of the extrinsic muscles of the eye.

oph·thal·mop·a·thy (ŏf′thəl-mŏp′ə-thē, -thăl-, ŏp′-) *n.* A disease of the eyes.

oph·thal·mo·ple·gia (ŏf-thăl′mō-plē′jə, ŏp-) *n.* Paralysis of one or more of the muscles of the eye. —**oph·thal′mo·ple′gic** *adj.*

oph·thal·mo·scope (ŏf-thăl′mə-skōp′, ŏp-) *n.* An instrument for examining the interior structures of the eye, especially the retina, consisting essentially of a mirror that reflects light into the eye and a central hole through which the eye is examined.

oph·thal·mos·co·py (ŏf′thəl-mŏs′kə-pē, -thăl-, ŏp′-) *n.* Examination of the interior of the eye through the pupil with an ophthalmoscope. —**oph·thal′mo·scop′ic** (-thăl′mə-skŏp′ĭk), **oph·thal′mo·scop′i·cal** (-ĭ-kəl) *adj.*

oph·thal·mo·vas·cu·lar (ŏf-thăl′mō-văs′kyə-lər, ŏp-) *adj.* Relating to the blood vessels of the eye.

–opia *suff.* A visual condition or defect of a specified kind: *anisometropia.*

o·pi·ate (ō′pē-ĭt, -āt′) *n.* **1.** Any of various sedative narcotics that contain opium or one or more of its natural or synthetic derivatives. **2.** A drug, hormone, or other chemical substance that has sedative or narcotic effects similar to those containing opium or its derivatives. Also called *opioid.* —*adj.* **1.** Of or containing opium or any of its derivatives. **2.** Resembling opium or its derivatives in activity. **3.** Inducing sleep or sedation; soporific. —*v.* (-āt′) To subject to the action of an opiate. —**o′pi·ate** (-ĭt, -āt′) *adj.*

opiate receptor *n.* Any of various cell membrane receptors that can bind with morphine and other opiates; concentrations of such receptors are especially high in regions of the brain having pain-related functions.

o·pi·oid (ō′pē-oid′) *n.* See **opiate** (sense 2). —*adj.* Opiate. —**o′pi·oid′** *adj.*

o·pi·o·mel·a·no·cor·tin (ō′pē-ō-mĕl′ə-nō-kôr′tĭn) *n.* A linear polypeptide of the pituitary gland that contains the nucleotide sequences of endorphins and various pituitary hormones.

o·pis·the·nar (ə-pĭs′thə-när′) *n.* The back of the hand.

o·pis·thi·on (ə-pĭs′thē-ŏn′) *n.* The middle point on the rear margin of the great foramen.

opistho– *pref.* Back; backward: *opisthotonos.*

op·is·thor·chi·a·sis (ŏp′ĭs-thôr-kī′ə-sĭs, ō-pĭs′thôr-) *n.* Infection of the biliary tract with trematodes of the genus *Opisthorchis,* caused by ingesting raw or inadequately cooked fish infected with the parasites.

Op·is·thor·chis (ŏp′ĭs-thôr′kĭs, ō′pĭs-) *n.* A genus of trematodes found in the bile ducts or gallbladder of fish-eating mammals, birds, and fish.

Opisthorchis fe·lin·e·us (fē-lĭn′ē-əs, -lī′nē-) *n.* A trematode that causes opisthorchiasis and is frequently found in Eastern Europe, Siberia, India, Japan, and Southeast Asia.

Opisthorchis viv·er·ri·ni (vĭv′ə-rī′nī) *n.* A trematode that causes opisthorchiasis and is commonly found in Thailand.

op·is·thot·o·nos (ŏp′ĭs-thŏt′n-əs) *n.* A tetanic spasm in which the head and feet are drawn backward and the spine arches forward. —**o·pis′tho·ton′ic** (ə-pĭs′thə-tŏn′ĭk) *adj.*

o·pi·um (ō′pē-əm) *n.* A bitter, yellowish-brown, strongly addictive narcotic drug prepared from the dried juice of unripe pods of the opium poppy and containing alkaloids such as morphine, codeine, and papaverine. Also called *meconium.*

opium poppy *n.* A plant native to Turkey and adjacent areas, having grayish-green leaves and variously colored flowers and cultivated as a source of opium.

Op·pen·heim's disease (ŏp′ən-hīmz′) *n.* See **amyotonia congenita.**

Oppenheim's syndrome *n.* See **amyotonia congenita.**

op·por·tun·is·tic (ŏp′ər-tōō-nĭs′tĭk) *adj.* **1.** Of or relating to an organism capable of causing disease only in a host whose resistance is lowered. **2.** Of or relating to a disease caused by an opportunistic organism.

opportunistic infection *n.* An infection by a microorganism that normally does not cause disease but becomes pathogenic when the body's immune system is impaired and unable to fight off infection, as in AIDS and certain other diseases.

op·pos·er muscle of little finger (ə-pō′zər) *n.* A muscle with origin from the hamate bone and flexor retinaculum, with insertion into the shaft of the fifth metacarpal bone, with nerve supply from the ulnar nerve, and whose action draws the ulnar side of the hand toward the center of the palm.

opposer muscle of thumb *n.* A muscle with origin from the trapezium bone and the flexor retinaculum, with insertion into the first metacarpal bone, with nerve supply from the median nerve, and whose action allows the thumb to move in a direction in contrast to that of the other fingers.

op·po·si·tion·al disorder (ŏp′ə-zĭsh′ə-nəl) *n.* A behavioral disorder in which an individual, usually between the ages of 3 and 18, exhibits a persistent pattern of disobedient and intentionally provocative opposition to authority figures. It is characterized by consistently negativistic behaviors such as temper tantrums, violation of rules, argumentativeness, and dawdling.

op·sin (ŏp′sĭn) *n.* A protein of the retina, especially the protein constituent of rhodopsin, that makes up one of the visual pigments.

op·sin·o·gen (ŏp-sĭn′ə-jən, -jĕn′) *n.* A substance that stimulates the formation of opsonin. Also called *opsogen.*

op·si·u·ri·a (ŏp′sĭ-yŏŏr′ē-ə) *n.* A more rapid excretion of urine during fasting than after a full meal.

op·so·clo·nus (ŏp′sō-klō′nəs) *n.* Rapid, irregular, nonrhythmic movements of the eye in horizontal and vertical directions.

op·so·gen (ŏp′sə-jən, -jĕn′) *n.* See **opsinogen.**

op·so·ma·ni·a (ŏp′sə-mā′nē-ə, -mān′yə) *n.* An intense longing for a particular kind of food, or for highly seasoned food.

op·son·ic (ŏp-sŏn′ĭk) *adj.* Of, relating to, or produced by opsonins.

opsonic index *n.* The ratio of the amount of opsonin in the blood of a person with an infectious disease to the amount of opsonin in the blood sample of a healthy person.

op·so·nin (ŏp′sə-nĭn) *n.* An antibody in blood serum that causes bacteria or other foreign cells to become more susceptible to the action of phagocytes.

op·so·ni·za·tion (ŏp′sə-nĭ-zā′shən) *n.* The process by which bacteria are altered by opsonins so as to become more readily and more efficiently engulfed by phagocytes.

op·so·nize (ŏp′sə-nīz′) *v.* To make bacteria or other cells more susceptible to the action of phagocytes.

op·so·no·cy·to·pha·gic (ŏp′sə-nō-sī′tə-fā′jĭk, -făj′ĭk) *adj.* Relating to the increased efficiency with which white blood cells devour bacteria in blood that contains opsonin.

op·so·nom·e·try (ŏp′sə-nŏm′ĭ-trē) *n.* The measurement of the opsonic index or of the opsonocytophagic activity.

–opsy *suff.* Examination: *biopsy.*

opt– *pref.* Variant of **opto–.**

op·tes·the·sia (ŏp′tĭs-thē′zhə) *n.* Visual sensibility to light stimuli.

op·tic (ŏp′tĭk) *or* **op·ti·cal** (ŏp′tĭ-kəl) *adj.* **1.** Of or relating to the eye or vision. **2.** Of or relating to the science of optics or optical equipment.

optical aberration *n.* The failure of light rays from a point source to form a perfect image after passing through an optical system.

optical activity *n.* The property of an asymmetrical molecule in solution to rotate the plane of polarized light either clockwise or counterclockwise.

optical allachesthesia *n.* See **visual allesthesia.**

optical density *n.* See **absorbance.**

optical image *n.* An image formed by the refraction or reflection of light.

optical isomerism *n.* Stereoisomerism involving the arrangement of substituents about an asymmetric carbon atom or atoms so that the various isomers differ in how they rotate a plane of polarized light.

optical rotation *n.* The change or rotation in the plane of polarization that occurs when polarized light is passed through an optically active substance.

optic axis *n.* The line connecting the anterior and the posterior poles of the eye.

optic canal *n.* The short canal through the lesser wing of the sphenoid bone at the apex of the eye socket through which the optic nerve and the ophthalmic artery pass. Also called *optic foramen.*

optic capsule *n.* The embryonic structure from which the sclera of the eye develops.

optic center *n.* The point in the lens of the eye where light rays cross as they move from the cornea to the retina.

optic chiasm *n.* A flattened quadrangular body that is the point of crossing of the fibers of the optic nerves. Also called *optic decussation.*

optic cup *n.* A two-walled cuplike depression, formed by invagination of the optic vesicle, that develops into the pigmented and sensory layers of the retina. Also called *eyecup.*

optic decussation *n.* See **optic chiasm.**

optic disk *n.* The small, circular, optically insensitive region in the retina containing no rods or cones, where fibers of the optic nerve emerge from the eyeball. Also called *blind spot, optic papilla.*

optic foramen *n.* See **optic canal.**

op·ti·cian (ŏp-tĭsh′ən) *n.* A person who practices opticianry.

op·ti·cian·ry (ŏp-tĭsh′ən-rē) *n.* The professional practice of filling prescriptions for ophthalmic lenses that includes dispensing eyeglasses and fitting contact lenses.

optic lobe *n.* Either of two lobes of the dorsal mesencephalon, containing primary visual centers.

optic nerve *n.* A nerve that originates from the retina and passes out of the eye socket to the chiasm, where part of its fibers cross to the opposite side and pass to the geniculate bodies and anterior quadrigeminal body. Also called *second cranial nerve.*

optic neuritis *n.* Inflammation of the optic nerve. Also called *neuropapillitis, retrobulbar neuritis.*

optico– *pref.* Optic; optic nerve: *opticopupillary.*

op·ti·co·cil·i·ar·y (ŏp′tĭ-kō-sĭl′ē-ĕr′ē) *adj.* Relating to the optic and the ciliary nerves.

op·ti·co·ki·net·ic nystagmus (ŏp′tĭ-kō-kə-nĕt′ĭk, -kī-) *n.* A nystagmus induced by looking at moving visual stimuli.

op·ti·co·pu·pil·lar·y (ŏp′tĭ-kō-pyŏŏ′pə-lĕr′ē) *adj.* Relating to the optic nerve and the pupil.

optic papilla *n.* See **optic disk.**

optic radiation *n.* The massive fanlike fiber system

passing from the lateral geniculate body of the thalamus to the visual cortex.

op·tics (ŏp′tĭks) *n.* The science concerned with the properties of light, its refraction and absorption, and the refracting media of the eye.

optic tract *n.* A continuation of the optic nerve beyond its hemidecussation in the optic chiasm.

optic vesicle *n.* See **ocular vesicle**.

op·ti·mum dose (ŏp′tə-məm) *n.* The quantity of a radiological or pharmacological substance that will produce the desired effect without any unfavorable effects.

opto– *or* **opt–** *pref.* Eye; vision: *optometry.*

op·to·ki·net·ic (ŏp′tō-kə-nĕt′ĭk, -kī-) *adj.* Relating to the occurrence of twitchings or movements of the eye when moving objects are viewed.

op·tom·e·ter (ŏp-tŏm′ĭ-tər) *n.* An instrument for determining the refraction of the eye.

op·tom·e·try (ŏp-tŏm′ĭ-trē) *n.* The health care profession concerned with examination, diagnosis, and treatment of the eyes and related structures, and with determination and correction of vision problems using lenses and other optical aids. **—op·tom′e·trist** *n.*

op·to·my·om·e·ter (ŏp′tō-mī-ŏm′ĭ-tər) *n.* An instrument for determining the relative power of the extrinsic muscles of the eye.

OPV *abbr.* oral poliovirus vaccine

OR *abbr.* operating room

o·ra (ôr′ə) *n.,* *pl.* **o·rae** (ôr′ē) An edge or margin.

o·rad (ôr′ăd′) *adj.* **1.** In a direction toward the mouth. **2.** Situated nearer the mouth in relation to a specific reference point.

o·ral (ôr′əl) *adj.* **1.** Of or relating to the mouth. **2.** Used in or taken through the mouth. **3.** Of or relating to the first stage of psychosexual development in psychoanalytic theory, in which the mouth is the focus of exploration and pleasure. **—o′ral·ly** *adv.*

oral biology *n.* The study of the biological phenomena associated with the mouth in health and in disease.

oral cavity *n.* The part of the mouth behind the teeth and gums that is bounded above by the hard and soft palates and below by the tongue and the mucous membrane connecting it with the inner part of the mandible.

oral contraceptive *n.* A pill, typically containing estrogen or progesterone, that prevents conception or pregnancy. Also called *birth control pill.*

oral hygiene *n.* See **dental hygiene**.

o·ral·i·ty (ôr-ăl′ĭ-tē) *n.* The psychic organization derived from and characteristic of the oral stage of psychosexual development.

oral lactose tolerance test *n.* A test for deficiency of the enzyme lactase, which metabolizes lactose into glucose, in which plasma glucose levels are measured after a quantity of lactose has been ingested.

oral pathology *n.* The branch of dentistry concerned with the diseases of oral and paraoral structures, including oral soft tissues and mucous membranes and the teeth, jaws, and salivary glands.

oral phase *n.* In psychoanalytic theory, the first stage in psychosexual development, from birth to about 18 months, when the mouth is the focus of the infant's needs, expression, gratification, and pleasurable erotic experiences.

oral poliovirus vaccine *n.* *Abbr.* **OPV** See **poliovirus vaccine** (sense 2).

oral rehydration therapy *n.* Treatment for diarrhea-related dehydration in which an electrolyte solution containing fluids and vital ions is administered.

oral surgery *n.* The branch of dentistry concerned with the surgical and adjunctive treatment of diseases, injuries, and deformities of the oral and maxillofacial region.

O·rap (ôr′ăp′) A trademark for the drug pimozide.

or·bic·u·lar (ôr-bĭk′yə-lər) *adj.* Circular.

or·bic·u·lar·e (ôr-bĭk′yə-lâr′ē) *n.* See **lenticular process of incus**.

orbicular muscle of eye *n.* A muscle consisting of three parts: the orbital or external part, the palpebral or internal part, and the lacrimal part. The nerve supply of all three parts is from the facial nerve; the action of all three parts closes the eye and wrinkles the forehead vertically.

orbicular muscle of mouth *n.* A muscle with origin from the septum of the nose, by the superior incisive bundle from the incisor fossa of the maxilla, and the lower jaw on each side of the symphysis; the fibers surround the mouth between the skin and the mucous membrane of lips and cheeks and are blended with other muscles; with nerve supply from the facial nerve, and whose action closes the lips.

orbicular zone *n.* The fibers of the articular capsule of the hip joint encircling the neck of the femur. Also called *zonular band.*

or·bit (ôr′bĭt) *n.* See **orbital cavity**.

or·bi·ta (ôr′bĭ-tə) *n.,* *pl.* **–tae** (-tē′) Orbit.

or·bit·al (ôr′bĭ-tl) *adj.* Relating to an orbit.

orbital cavity *n.* The bony cavity containing the eyeball and its associated muscles, vessels, and nerves. Also called *eye socket, orbit.*

or·bi·ta·le (ôr′bĭ-tā′lē) *n.* The lowermost point in the lower margin of the bony orbit that may be felt under the skin.

orbital gyrus *n.* Any of the small, irregular convolutions on the concave inferior surface of each frontal lobe of the cerebrum.

orbital muscle *n.* A rudimentary nonstriated muscle, crossing the infraorbital groove and the sphenomaxillary fissure and united with the periosteum of the eye socket.

orbital plane *n.* The orbital surface of the maxilla that lies perpendicular to the Frankfort plane at the orbitale.

orbital process *n.* The anterior and larger of the two processes at the upper extremity of the vertical plate of the palatine bone, articulating with the upper jawbone and the ethmoid and sphenoid bones.

or·bi·tog·ra·phy (ôr′bĭ-tŏg′rə-fē) *n.* A diagnostic technique for radiographic evaluation in suspected blowout fracture of the orbit.

or·bi·to·na·sal (ôr′bĭ-tō-nā′zəl) *adj.* Relating to the orbit and the nose or nasal cavity.

or·bi·to·nom·e·ter (ôr′bĭ-tə-nŏm′ĭ-tər) *n.* An instrument for measuring the resistance of the eyeball as it is pressed backward into its socket. —or′bi·to·nom′e·try *n.*

or·bi·tot·o·my (ôr′bĭ-tŏt′ə-mē) *n.* An incision into the orbit.

Or·bi·vi·rus (ôr′bə-vī′rəs) *n.* A genus of reoviruses that includes the Colorado tick fever virus of humans and certain viruses formerly included with the arboviruses.

or·ce·in (ôr′sē-ĭn) *n.* A natural dye derived from orcinol and used in various histologic staining methods as a purple dye complex.

or·chi·al·gia (ôr′kē-ăl′jə) *n.* Testicular pain. Also called *didymalgia, testalgia.*

or·chid·ic (ôr-kĭd′ĭk) *adj.* Relating to the testis.

or·chi·di·tis (ôr′kĭ-dī′tĭs) *n.* Variant of **orchitis**.

orchido– *or* orchid– *pref.* Testis: *orchidectomy*.

or·chi·dom·e·ter (ôr′kĭ-dŏm′ĭ-tər) *n.* 1. A caliper used to measure the size of testes. 2. A set of sized models of testes that are used for comparison of testicular development.

or·chi·ec·to·my (ôr′kē-ĕk′tə-mē) *or* or·chi·dec·to·my (-kĭ-dĕk′-) *n.* Surgical removal of one or both testes. Also called *testectomy*.

or·chi·ep·i·did·y·mi·tis (ôr′kē-ĕp′ĭ-dĭd′ə-mī′tĭs) *n.* Inflammation of the testis and epididymis.

orchio– *or* orchi– *pref.* Testis: *orchiotomy*.

or·chi·o·cele (ôr′kē-ə-sēl′) *n.* 1. A tumor of the testis. 2. A testis retained in the inguinal canal.

or·chi·op·a·thy (ôr′kē-ŏp′ə-thē) *n.* Disease of a testis.

or·chi·o·pex·y (ôr′kē-ə-pĕk′sē) *n.* Surgical freeing of an undescended testicle with implantation into the scrotum. Also called *cryptorchidopexy*.

or·chi·o·plas·ty (ôr′kē-ə-plăs′tē) *n.* Plastic surgery of the testis.

or·chi·ot·o·my (ôr′kē-ŏt′ə-mē) *n.* An incision into a testis.

or·chis (ôr′kĭs) *n.* See **testis**.

or·chi·tis (ôr-kī′tĭs) *or* or·chi·di·tis (ôr′kĭ-dī′tĭs) *n.* Inflammation of the testis. Also called *didymitis, testitis.* —or·chit′ic (ôr-kĭt′ĭk) *adj.*

or·ci·pren·a·line sulfate (ôr′sə-prĕn′ə-lēn′, -līn′, -lĭn) *n.* See **metaproterenol sulfate**.

or·der (ôr′dər) *n.* A taxonomic category of organisms ranking above a family and below a class.

or·der·ly (ôr′dər-lē) *n.* An attendant in a hospital.

or·di·nate (ôr′dn-ĭt, -āt′) *n.* The plane Cartesian coordinate representing the distance from a specified point to the *x*-axis, measured parallel to the *y*-axis.

o·rex·i·gen·ic (ə-rĕk′sə-jĕn′ĭk) *adj.* Having a stimulating effect on the appetite.

or·gan (ôr′gən) *n.* A differentiated part of the body that performs a specific function.

organ– *pref.* Variant of **organo–**.

organ culture *n.* 1. The maintenance or growth of tissues, organ primordia, or the parts or whole of an organ in vitro in such a way as to allow differentiation or preservation of the architecture or function. 2. A culture of such tissue or such an organ.

or·gan·elle (ôr′gə-nĕl′) *n.* A differentiated structure within a cell, such as a mitochondrion, vacuole, or microsome, that performs a specific function. Also called *organoid*.

or·gan·ic (ôr-găn′ĭk) *adj.* 1. Of, relating to, or affecting organs or an organ of the body. 2. Of or designating carbon compounds. 3. Of, relating to, or derived from living organisms. 4. Of, marked by, or involving the use of fertilizers or pesticides that are strictly of animal or vegetable origin. 5. Raised or conducted without the use of drugs, hormones, or synthetic chemicals. —or′gan·ic′i·ty (ôr′gə-nĭs′ĭ-tē) *n.*

organic acid *n.* Any of various acids containing one or more carbon-containing radicals.

organic brain syndrome *n. Abbr.* **OBS** Any of a group of acute or chronic syndromes involving temporary or permanent impairment of brain function caused by trauma, infection, toxin, tumor, or tissue sclerosis, and causing mild-to-severe impairment of memory, orientation, judgment, intellectual functions, and emotional adjustment. Also called *organic mental syndrome*.

organic chemistry *n.* The chemistry of compounds containing carbon.

organic compound *n.* A compound containing hydrocarbon groups.

organic contracture *n.* Contracture that is usually due to fibrosis within the muscle and persists whether the individual is conscious or unconscious.

organic disease *n.* A disease in which there is a structural change to some tissue or organ of the body.

organic evolution *n.* See **biologic evolution**.

or·gan·i·cism (ôr-găn′ĭ-sĭz′əm) *n.* 1. The theory that all disease is associated with structural alterations of organs. 2. The theory that the total organization of an organism, rather than the functioning of individual organs, is the principal or exclusive determinant of every life process.

organic mental disorder *n.* Any of a group of mental disturbances resulting from temporary or permanent brain dysfunction caused by organic factors such as alcohol, metabolic disorders, and aging.

organic mental syndrome *n. Abbr.* **OMS** See **organic brain syndrome**.

organic murmur *n.* A murmur caused by an organic lesion.

organic vertigo *n.* Vertigo that is caused by a lesion of the brain.

or·gan·ism (ôr′gə-nĭz′əm) *n.* An individual form of life, such as a plant, animal, bacterium, protist, or fungus; a body made up of organs, organelles, or other parts that work together to carry on the various processes of life. —or′gan·is′mal (-nĭz′məl), or′gan·is′mic (-mĭk) *adj.*

or·gan·i·za·tion (ôr′gə-nĭ-zā′shən) *n.* 1. The act or process of organizing. 2. The state or manner of being organized. 3. Something that has been organized or made into an ordered whole. 4. Something made up of elements with varied functions that contribute to the whole and to collective functions. 5. A structure through which individuals cooperate systematically to conduct business. 6. The conversion of coagulated blood, exudate, or dead tissue into fibrous tissue.

or·gan·ize (ôr′gə-nīz′) *v.* 1. To put together into an orderly, functional, structured whole. 2. To arrange in a coherent form.

or·gan·iz·er (ôr′gə-nī′zər) *n.* **1.** One that organizes. **2.** A group of cells that induces differentiation of cells in the embryo and controls the growth and development of adjacent parts through the action of an evocator. Also called *inductor.*

organo– *or* **organ–** *pref.* **1.** Organ: *organotrophic.* **2.** Organic: *organomercurial.*

or·gan·o·chlo·rine (ôr-găn′ə-klôr′ēn′, -ĭn) *n.* Any of various hydrocarbon pesticides, such as DDT, that contain chlorine.

organ of Corti *n.* A specialized structure located on the inner surface of the basilar membrane of the cochlea containing hair cells that transmit sound vibrations to the nerve fibers. Also called *spiral organ.*

or·gan·o·gel (ôr-găn′ə-jĕl′) *n.* A hydrogel with an organic liquid, not water, as the dispersion means.

or·gan·o·gen·e·sis (ôr′gə-nō-jĕn′ĭ-sĭs, ôr-găn′ə-) *n.* The formation and development of the organs of living things. Also called *organogeny.* —**or′gan·o·ge·net′ic** (-jə-nĕt′ĭk) *adj.*

or·gan·og·ra·phy (ôr′gə-nŏg′rə-fē) *n.* Scientific description of the organs of living things.

or·gan·oid (ôr′gə-noid′) *adj.* Resembling an organ. —*n.* See **organelle.**

organoid tumor *n.* A tumor that is glandular in origin and that contains epithelium, connective tissue, and other tissue structures that give it a complex structure similar to an organ.

or·gan·o·lep·tic (ôr′gə-nō-lĕp′tĭk, ôr-găn′ə-) *adj.* **1.** Of or relating to perception by a sensory organ. **2.** Involving the use of sense organs.

or·gan·ol·o·gy (ôr′gə-nŏl′ə-jē) *n.* The branch of biology that deals with the structure and function of organs. —**or′gan·o·log′ic** (ôr′gə-nə-lŏj′ĭk, ôr-găn′ə-), **or′gan·o·log′i·cal** (-ĭ-kəl) *adj.*

or·ga·no·ma (ôr′gə-nō′mə) *n.* A neoplasm that has identifiable types of organ tissue.

or·gan·o·meg·a·ly (ôr′gə-nō-mĕg′ə-lē, ôr-găn′ə-) *n.* See **visceromegaly.**

or·gan·o·mer·cu·ri·al (ôr-găn′ō-mər-kyoŏr′ē-əl) *n.* An organic compound that contains mercury. —**or·gan′o·mer·cu′ri·al** *adj.*

or·gan·o·me·tal·lic (ôr′găn′ō-mə-tăl′ĭk) *adj.* Of, relating to, or constituting an organic compound containing a metal, especially one in which a metal atom is bonded directly to a carbon atom.

or·ga·non (ôr′gə-nŏn′) *or* **or·ga·num** (-nəm) *n., pl.* **–nons** *or* **–nums** *or* **–na** (-nə) **1.** An organ. **2.** A set of principles for use in scientific investigation.

or·gan·o·phos·phate (ôr′găn′ə-fŏs′fāt) *n.* Any of several organic compounds containing phosphorus, some of which are used as fertilizers and pesticides.

or·gan·o·ther·a·py (ôr′gə-nō-thĕr′ə-pē, ôr-găn′ō-) *n.* The treatment of disease with preparations derived from animal endocrine organs or glandular extracts such as insulin and thyroxin. —**or′gan·o·ther′a·peu′tic** (-thĕr′ə-pyoō′tĭk) *adj.*

or·gan·o·troph·ic (ôr′gə-nō-trŏf′ĭk, -trō′fĭk, ôr-găn′ə-) *adj.* Relating to the nourishment of an organ.

or·gan·ot·ro·pism (ôr′gə-nŏt′rə-pĭz′əm) *n.* The attraction of chemical compounds or microorganisms to tissues or organs of the body. —**or′gan·o·trop′ic** (ôr′-gə-nō-trŏp′ĭk, -trō′pĭk, ôr-găn′ə-) *adj.*

organ-specific *adj.* Of, relating to, or being a serum produced by the injection of the cells from a certain organ or tissue from one animal into another, with the result that the serum destroys the cells of the corresponding organ.

organ-specific antigen *n.* A heterogenetic antigen that is specific to a particular organ, whether of a single species or of many species. Also called *tissue-specific antigen.*

or·gasm (ôr′găz′əm) *n.* The highest point of sexual excitement, marked by strong feelings of pleasure and marked normally by ejaculation of semen by the male and by vaginal contractions within the female. Also called *climax.* —**or·gas′mic** (ôr-găz′mĭk) *adj.*

o·ri·ent (ôr′ē-ənt, -ĕnt′) *v.* **1.** To locate or place in a particular relation to the points of the compass. **2.** To align or position with respect to a point or system of reference. **3.** To make familiar with or adjusted to facts, principles, or a situation.

o·ri·en·tate (ôr′ē-ən-tāt′) *v.* To orient.

o·ri·en·ta·tion (ôr′ē-ən-tā′shən) *n.* **1.** The act of orienting or the state of being oriented. **2.** Location or position relative to the points of the compass. **3.** The relative position of one atom with respect to another to which it is connected. **4.** Sexual orientation. **5.** Introductory instruction concerning a new situation. **6.** Awareness of the objective world in relation to one's self.

o·ri·en·ting reflex (ôr′ē-ĕn′tĭng) *n.* An aspect of responding to environmental stimuli in which an organism's initial response to a change or novel stimulus makes the organism more sensitive to the stimulation, as when the pupil of the eye dilates in response to dim light. Also called *orienting response.*

orienting response *n.* See **orienting reflex.**

or·i·fice (ôr′ə-fĭs) *n.* An opening, especially to a cavity or passage of the body; a mouth or vent. —**or′i·fi′cial** (-fĭsh′əl) *adj.*

or·i·fi·ci·um (ôr′ə-fĭsh′ē-əm) *n.* An orifice.

o·rig·a·num oil (ə-rĭg′ə-nəm) *n.* A volatile oil obtained from various species of plants of the genus *Origanum,* used as a rubefacient, as a constituent in veterinary liniments, and in microscopic techniques.

or·i·gin (ôr′ə-jĭn) *n.* **1.** The point at which something comes into existence or from which it derives or is derived. **2.** The fact of originating; rise or derivation. **3.** The point of attachment of a muscle that remains relatively fixed during contraction. **4.** The starting point of a cranial or spinal nerve.

o·rig·i·nate (ə-rĭj′ə-nāt′) *v.* **1.** To bring into being; create. **2.** To come into being; start.

Or·i·nase (ôr′ĭ-nās′) A trademark for the drug tolbutamide.

Or·mond′s disease (ôr′mŏndz′) *n.* See **idiopathic retroperitoneal fibrosis.**

Orn *abbr.* ornithine

or·ni·thine (ôr′nə-thēn′) *n. Abbr.* **Orn** An amino acid formed by the hydrolysis of arginine and important in the formation of urea.

or·ni·thi·nu·ri·a (ôr′nə-thĭ-no͞or′ē-ə) *n.* Excessive amounts of ornithine in the urine.

Or·ni·thod·o·ros (ôr′nə-thŏd′ə-rəs) *n.* A genus of soft ticks, several species of which are vectors of pathogens of various relapsing fevers.

or·ni·tho·sis (ôr′nə-thō′sĭs) *n.* A disease of birds caused by *Chlamydia psittaci* and contracted by humans through contact with infected birds.

oro– *pref.* Mouth: *oronasal.*

o·ro·dig·i·to·fa·cial (ôr′ō-dĭj′ĭ-tō-fā′shəl) *adj.* Relating to the mouth, fingers, and face.

orodigitofacial dysostosis *n.* An inherited syndrome that is lethal in males and is characterized by various defects of the oral cavity, face, and hands. Also called *orofaciodigital syndrome.*

o·ro·fa·cial (ôr′ō-fā′shəl) *adj.* Relating to the mouth and face.

o·ro·fa·ci·o·dig·i·tal syndrome (ôr′ō-fā′shē-ō-dĭj′ĭ-tl) *n.* See **orodigitofacial dysostosis.**

o·ro·lin·gual (ôr′ō-lĭng′gwəl) *adj.* Of or relating to the mouth and tongue.

o·ro·na·sal (ôr′ō-nā′zəl) *adj.* Relating to the mouth and nose.

o·ro·pha·ryn·go·lar·yn·gi·tis (ôr′ō-fə-rĭng′gō-lăr′ĭn-jī′tĭs) *n.* Inflammation of the mucosa of the upper respiratory tract, as from inhalation or ingestion of chemical or physical agents.

o·ro·phar·ynx (ôr′ō-făr′ĭngks) *n.* The pharynx between the soft palate and the epiglottis. —**o′ro·pha·ryn′ge·al** (-fə-rĭn′jē-əl, -jəl, -făr′ĭn-jē′əl) *adj.*

o·ro·so·mu·coid (ôr′ə-sō-myo͞o′koid′) *n.* A glycoprotein in blood plasma.

o·ro·tate (ôr′ə-tāt′) *n.* A salt or ester of orotic acid.

o·rot·ic acid (ô-rŏt′ĭk) *n.* An important intermediate in the formation of pyrimidine nucleotides.

orotic aciduria *n.* An inherited disorder of pyrimidine metabolism characterized by megaloblastic anemia, leukopenia, retarded growth, and the excretion of orotic acid in the urine.

o·ro·tra·che·al tube (ôr′ō-trā′kē-əl) *n.* An endotracheal tube inserted through the mouth.

O·ro·ya fever (ə-roi′ə, ô-rô′yä) *n.* An acute endemic disease of the central Andes caused by the bacterium *Bartonella bacilliformis* and marked by high fever, rheumatic pains, albuminuria, and progressive severe anemia. Also called *Carrión's disease.*

or·phan disease (ôr′fən) *n.* A disease that is so rare that it is not considered commercially viable to develop drugs to treat it.

orphan drug *n.* Any of various drugs or biologicals that may be useful in treating disease but are not considered to be commercially viable.

orphan virus *n.* Any of various viruses, such as enteric orphan viruses, that may not be specifically associated with disease but may exhibit pathogenicity.

or·ther·ga·sia (ôr′thər-gā′zhə) *n.* Normal intellectual and emotional adjustment.

or·the·sis (ôr-thē′sĭs) *n.* An orthopedic brace, splints, or appliance.

or·thet·ics (ôr-thĕt′ĭks) *n.* See **orthotics.** —**or·thet′ic** *adj.*

ortho– *or* **orth–** *pref.* **1.** Straight; upright; vertical: *orthotropic.* **2.** Correct; correction: *orthopsychiatry.* **3.** Hydrated form of an acid or of its salts: *orthoboric acid.* **4.** Diatomic molecules in which the nuclei have the same direction of spin: *orthohydrogen.* **5.** *Abbr.* **o–** Of or relating to one of three possible isomers of a benzene ring with adjacent carbon atoms having attached chemical groups: ortho-*dibromobenzene.*

or·tho·cho·re·a (ôr′thō-kô-rē′ə, -kə-) *n.* A form of chorea in which the spasms occur chiefly when the patient is in an erect posture.

or·tho·chro·mat·ic (ôr′thə-krō-măt′ĭk) *adj.* Staining with the same color as that of the dye used. Used of a cell or tissue.

or·tho·cy·to·sis (ôr′thō-sī-tō′sĭs) *n.* A condition in which all cellular elements in the blood are mature forms.

or·tho·don··tia (ôr′thə-dŏn′shə) *n.* See **orthodontics.**

or·tho·don·tics (ôr′thə-dŏn′tĭks) *n.* The dental specialty and practice of preventing and correcting irregularities of the teeth, as by the use of braces. Also called *orthodontia, orthodonture.* —**or′tho·don′tic** *adj.* —**or′tho·don′tist** *n.*

or·tho·don·tist (ôr′thə-dŏn′tĭst) *n.* A person who specializes in orthodontics.

or·tho·don·ture (ôr′thə-dŏn′chər) *n.* See **orthodontics.**

or·tho·dox sleep (ôr′thə-dŏks′) *n.* Sleep characterized by a slow alpha rhythm and the absence of REM.

or·tho·drom·ic (ôr′thə-drŏm′ĭk) *adj.* Conducting impulses in the normal direction. Used of a nerve cell.

or·tho·gna·thi·a (ôr′thō-nā′thē-ə, -năth′-, ôr′thŏg′-) *n.* The study of the causes and treatment of conditions related to malposition of the jawbones.

or·tho·gnath·ic (ôr′thō-năth′ĭk, ôr′thəg-) *or* **or·thog·na·thous** (ôr-thŏg′nə-thəs) *adj.* **1.** Relating to orthognathia. **2.** Having a jaw that does not project forward.

or·tho·grade (ôr′thə-grād′) *adj.* Walking or standing erect.

orthograde degeneration *n.* See **wallerian degeneration.**

or·tho·ker·a·tol·o·gy (ôr′thō-kĕr′ə-tŏl′ə-jē) *n.* A method of improving unaided vision by molding the cornea with contact lenses.

or·tho·ker·a·to·sis (ôr′thō-kĕr′ə-tō′sĭs) *n.* The formation of an anuclear keratin layer.

Or·tho-Kung T cell (ôr′thō-kŭng′) *n.* Any of various classes of cells recognizable to monoclonal antibodies of T cell antigens. Also called *OKT cell.*

or·tho·me·chan·i·cal (ôr′thō-mĭ-kăn′ĭ-kəl) *adj.* Of or relating to a physical orthopedic device such as a brace, prosthesis, or orthotic appliance.

or·thom·e·ter (ôr-thŏm′ĭ-tər) *n.* An instrument for determining the degree of protrusion or retraction of the eyeballs.

or·tho·mo·lec·u·lar (ôr′thō-mə-lĕk′yə-lər) *adj.* Of, relating to, or being a theory holding that mental diseases or abnormalities result from various chemical imbalances or deficiencies and can be cured by restoring proper levels of chemical substances, such as vitamins and minerals, in the body.

Or·tho·myx·o·vir·i·dae (ôr′thō-mĭk′sō-vîr′ĭ-dē) *n.* A family of myxoviruses that includes the various types of influenza viruses.

Ortho-Novum (ôr′thō-nō′vəm) A trademark for any of several oral contraceptives that contain norethindrone and either ethinyl estradiol or mestranol.

or·tho·pe·dics *or* **or·tho·pae·dics** (ôr′thə-pē′dĭks) *n.* The branch of medicine that deals with the prevention and correction of injuries or disorders of the skeletal system and associated muscles, joints, and ligaments, often by surgery. —**or′tho·pe′dic** *adj.*

or·tho·pe·dist *or* **or·tho·pae·dist** (ôr′thə-pē′dĭst) *n.* A specialist in orthopedics.

or·tho·per·cus·sion (ôr′thō-pər-kŭsh′ən) *n.* Very light percussion of the chest, used to determine the size of the heart.

or·tho·pho·ri·a (ôr′thə-fôr′ē-ə) *n.* The normal condition of balance between the muscles of the eyes that permits the lines of sight to meet at an object being looked at. —**or′tho·phor′ic** (-fôr′ĭk) *adj.*

or·tho·phos·phor·ic acid (ôr′thō-fŏs-fôr′ĭk) *n.* See **phosphoric acid.**

or·thop·ne·a (ôr′thŏp-nē′ə, ôr-thŏp′nē-ə) *n.* Discomfort in breathing that is relieved by sitting or standing in an erect position.

or·thop·ne·ic (ôr′thŏp-nē′ĭk) *adj.* Relating to or suffering from orthopnea.

Or·tho·pox·vi·rus (ôr′thō-pŏks′vī′rəs) *n.* A genus of poxviruses that includes the viruses that cause smallpox and cowpox.

or·tho·psy·chi·a·try (ôr′thō-sĭ-kī′ə-trē, -sī-) *n.* The psychiatric study, treatment, and prevention of emotional and behavioral problems, especially of those that arise during early development.

or·thop·tics (ôr-thŏp′tĭks) *n.* The study and treatment of defective binocular vision, of defects in the action of the ocular muscles, or of faulty visual habits. —**or·thop′tic** *adj.*

or·tho·scope (ôr′thə-skōp′) *n.* An instrument used to examine the eye that eliminates corneal refraction by means of a layer of water.

or·tho·scop·ic (ôr′thə-skŏp′ĭk) *adj.* **1.** Of or relating to an orthoscope. **2.** Having normal vision; free from visual distortion. **3.** Giving an undistorted image. Used of an optical instrument.

or·thos·co·py (ôr-thŏs′kə-pē) *n.* Examination of the eye with an orthoscope.

or·tho·sis (ôr-thō′sĭs) *n., pl.* **–ses** (-sēz) An external orthopedic appliance that prevents or assists the movement of the spine or limbs.

or·tho·stat·ic (ôr′thə-stăt′ĭk) *adj.* Relating to or caused by standing upright, as hypertension.

orthostatic hypotension *n.* A form of low blood pressure precipitated by moving from a lying or sitting position to standing up straight. Also called *postural hypotension.*

orthostatic proteinuria *n.* Nonpathological proteinuria usually occurring between the ages of 10 and 20, and manifested when the individual stands erect but disappears when the person lies down.

or·thot·ic (ôr-thŏt′ĭk) *adj.* Of or relating to orthotics.

—*n.* An orthopedic appliance designed to straighten or support a body part.

or·thot·ics (ôr-thŏt′ĭks) *n.* The science that deals with the use of specialized mechanical devices to support or to supplement weakened or abnormal joints or limbs. Also called *orthetics.*

or·thot·ist (ôr-thŏt′ĭst, ôr′thə-tĭst) *n.* A specialist in orthotics.

or·thot·o·nos *or* **or·thot·o·nus** (ôr-thŏt′n-əs) *n.* A form of tetanic spasm in which the neck, limbs, and body are held fixed in a straight line.

or·tho·top·ic (ôr′thə-tŏp′ĭk) *adj.* In the normal or usual position.

or·tho·trop·ic (ôr′thə-trŏp′ĭk, -trō′pĭk) *adj.* Tending to grow or form along a vertical axis. —**or·thot′ro·pism** (ôr-thŏt′rə-pĭz′əm) *n.*

os[1] (ŏs) *n., pl.* **o·ra** (ôr′ə) **1.** An opening into a hollow organ or canal. **2.** The oral cavity; mouth.

os[2] (ŏs) *n., pl.* **os·sa** (ŏs′ə) Bone.

Os The symbol for the element **osmium.**

OS *abbr. Latin* oculus sinister (left eye)

os·che·al (ŏs′kē-əl) *adj.* Relating to the scrotum.

os·che·i·tis (ŏs′kē-ī′tĭs) *n.* An inflammation of the scrotum.

oscheo– *or* **osche–** *pref.* Scrotum: *oscheohydrocele.*

os·che·o·hy·dro·cele (ŏs′kē-ō-hī′drə-sēl′) *n.* See **scrotal hernia.**

os·che·o·plas·ty (ŏs′kē-ə-plăs′tē) *n.* See **scrotoplasty.**

os·cil·late (ŏs′ə-lāt′) *v.* **1.** To swing back and forth with a steady, uninterrupted rhythm. **2.** To vary between alternate extremes, usually within a definable period of time. —**os′cil·la′tor** *n.* —**os′cil·la·to′ry** (-lə-tôr′ē) *adj.*

os·cil·lat·ing vision (ŏs′ə-lā′tĭng) *n.* See **oscillopsia.**

os·cil·la·tion (ŏs′ə-lā′shən) *n.* **1.** The act of oscillating. **2.** The state of being oscillated. **3.** A single oscillatory cycle. **4.** A stage in inflammation in which the accumulation of white blood cells in the small vessels arrests the passage of blood, thus causing a to-and-fro movement of the blood at each cardiac contraction. —**os′cil·la′tion·al** *adj.*

oscillatory potential *n.* The variable voltage in the positive deflection of the electroretinogram of the dark-adapted eye arising from amacrine cells.

os·cil·lo·gram (ə-sĭl′ə-grăm′) *n.* **1.** The graph traced by an oscillograph. **2.** An instantaneous oscilloscope trace or photograph.

os·cil·lo·graph (ə-sĭl′ə-grăf′) *n.* An instrument that records oscillations, as of an electric current and voltage. —**os·cil′lo·graph′ic** *adj.* —**os′cil·log′ra·phy** (ŏs′ə-lŏg′rə-fē) *n.*

os·cil·lom·e·ter (ŏs′ə-lŏm′ĭ-tər) *n.* An apparatus for measuring oscillations, especially those of the bloodstream in sphygmometry. —**os′cil·lo·met′ric** (ŏs′ə-lō-mĕt′tĭk) *adj.*

os·cil·lom·e·try (ŏs′ə-lŏm′ĭ-trē) *n.* The measurement of oscillations by means of an oscillometer.

os·cil·lop·si·a (ŏs′ə-lŏp′sē-ə) *n.* The sensation that viewed objects are moving or wavering back and forth. Also called *oscillating vision.*

os·cil·lo·scope (ə-sĭl′ə-skōp′) *n.* An electronic instrument that produces an instantaneous trace on the screen that corresponds to oscillations of voltage and current. —**os·cil·lo·scop·ic** (-skŏp′ĭk) *adj.*

os coc·cy·gis (kŏk′sə-jĭs, kŏk-sī′jĭs) *n.* The coccyx.

os cox·ae (kŏk′sē) *n.* The hipbone.

os·cu·lum (ŏs′kyə-ləm) *n.,* *pl.* **–la** (-lə) A pore or a minute opening.

–ose[1] *suff.* Possessing; having the characteristics of; full of: *ramose.*

–ose[2] *suff.* **1.** Carbohydrate: *fructose.* **2.** Product of protein hydrolysis: *proteose.*

Os·good-Schlatter disease (ŏs′good′-, ŏz′-) *n.* Osteochondrosis of the tibial tubercle. Also called *Schlatter-Osgood disease.*

OSHA (ō′shə) *n.* Occupational Safety and Health Administration, a branch of the US Department of Labor responsible for establishing and enforcing safety and health standards in the workplace.

os in·ter·met·a·tar·se·um (ĭn′tər-mĕt′ə-tär′sē-əm) *n.* A supernumerary bone at the base of the first metatarsal bone or between the first and second metatarsal bones, usually fused with one or the other or with the medial cuneiform bone.

–osis *suff.* **1.** Condition; process; action: *osmosis.* **2.** Diseased or abnormal condition: *proptosis.* **3.** Increase; formation: *leukocytosis.*

Os·ler (ŏs′lər, ŏz′-), Sir **William** 1849–1919. Canadian-born British physician who wrote *The Principles and Practice of Medicine* (1892), the definitive textbook of medicine for his time and one that has been frequently revised and translated. He was also known as an advocate for humane values in the world.

Os·ler node (ŏs′lər, ŏz′-) *n.* A small, raised, and tender cutaneous lesion that is characteristic of subacute bacterial endocarditis, usually appearing in the pads of fingers or toes.

Os·ler's disease (ŏs′lərz, ŏz′-) *n.* See **erythremia.**

Osler's sign *n.* An indication of acute bacterial endocarditis in which small, circumscribed, painful erythematous swellings appear in the skin and the subcutaneous tissues of the hands and feet.

Osler-Vaquez disease *n.* See **erythremia.**

os·mate (ŏz′māt′) *n.* A salt of osmic acid.

os·mat·ic (ŏz-măt′ĭk) *adj.* Having or characterized by a well-developed sense of smell.

os·mic acid (ŏz′mĭk) *n.* A crystalline oxide of osmium that is a volatile caustic and strong oxidizing agent, the aqueous solution of which is used as a stain for fat and myelin and as a general fixative for electron microscopy.

os·mics (ŏz′mĭks) *n.* The science that deals with smells and the olfactory sense.

os·mi·dro·sis (ŏz′mĭ-drō′sĭs) *n.* See **bromidrosis.**

os·mi·o·phil·ic (ŏz′mē-ə-fĭl′ĭk) *adj.* Readily stained with osmic acid.

os·mi·um (ŏz′mē-əm) *n. Symbol* **Os** A hard metallic element, found in small amounts in osmiridium and platinum ores. Atomic number 76.

osmo-[1] *or* **osm–** *pref.* Smell; odor: *osmidrosis.*

osmo-[2] *or* **osm–** *pref.* Osmosis: *osmolarity.*

os·mo·lal·i·ty (ŏz′mō-lăl′ĭ-tē, ŏs′-) *n.* The concentration of an osmotic solution, usually expressed in terms of osmoles.

os·mo·lar·i·ty (ŏz′mō-lăr′ĭ-tē, ŏs′-) *n.* The osmotic concentration of a solution expressed as osmoles of solute per liter of solution.

os·mole (ŏz′mōl′, ŏs′-) *n.* The molecular weight of a solute, in grams, divided by the number of ions or particles into which it dissociates in solution. —**os·mo′lar** (ŏz-mō′lər, ŏs-) *adj.*

os·mo·re·cep·tor[1] (ŏz′mō-rĭ-sĕp′tər, ŏs′-) *n.* A receptor in the central nervous system, probably the hypothalamus, that responds to changes in the osmotic pressure of the blood.

os·mo·re·cep·tor[2] (ŏz′mō-rĭ-sĕp′tər, ŏs′-) *n.* A receptor that receives olfactory stimuli.

os·mo·reg·u·la·tion (ŏz′mə-rĕg′yə-lā′shən, ŏs′-) *n.* The maintenance of an optimal constant osmotic pressure in the body of a living organism. —**os′mo·reg′u·la·to′ry** (-lə-tôr′ē) *adj.*

os·mose (ŏz′mōs′, ŏs′-) *v.* To diffuse or cause to diffuse by osmosis.

os·mo·sis (ŏz-mō′sĭs, ŏs-) *n.,* *pl.* **–ses** (-sēz) **1.** Diffusion of fluid through a semipermeable membrane until there is an equal concentration of fluid on both sides of the membrane. **2.** The tendency of fluids to diffuse in such a manner. —**os·mot′ic** (-mŏt′ĭk) *adj.* —**os·mot′i·cal·ly** *adv.*

osmotic pressure *n.* The pressure exerted by the flow of water through a semipermeable membrane separating two solutions with different concentrations of solute.

osmotic shock *n.* The rupture of bacterial or other cells in a solution following a sudden reduction in osmotic pressure; it is sometimes induced to release cellular components for biochemical analysis.

os·phre·sis (ŏs-frē′sĭs) *n.* The sense of smell.

os·phret·ic (ŏs-frĕt′ĭk) *adj.* Relating to the sense of smell.

os·se·in *or* **os·se·ine** (ŏs′ē-ĭn) *n.* The collagen component of bone. Also called **ostein.**

osseo– *pref.* Bone: *osseocartilaginous.*

os·se·o·car·ti·lag·i·nous (ŏs′ē-ō-kär′tl-ăj′ə-nəs) *adj.* Relating to or composed of bone and cartilage.

os·se·o·mu·cin (ŏs′ē-ō-myoo′sĭn) *n.* The ground substance of bony tissue.

os·se·ous (ŏs′ē-əs) *adj.* Composed of, containing, or resembling bone; bony.

osseous ampulla *n.* A circumscribed dilation of one extremity of each of the three bony semicircular canals in the inner ear.

osseous hydatid cyst *n.* A hydatid cyst found in the long bones or the pelvic arch that grows in an uncontrolled fashion, breaking the bone and eventually spreading to new sites.

osseous labyrinth *n.* A series of cavities that are located in the petrous portion of the temporal bone, consisting of the cochlea, the vestibule, and the semicircular canals, and lodging the membranous labyrinth. Also called *bony labyrinth.*

osseous lacuna *n.* A cavity in bony tissue occupied by an osteocyte.

ossi– *pref.* Bone: *ossiferous.*

os·si·cle (ŏs′ĭ-kəl) *n.* A small bone, especially one of the three bones of the middle ear that are articulated in a manner that forms a chain for transmitting sound from the tympanic membrane to the oval window. Also called *bonelet*. —**os·sic′u·lar** (ŏ-sĭk′yə-lər), **os·sic′u·late** (-lĭt) *adj.*

os·sic·u·lec·to·my (ŏ-sĭk′yə-lĕk′tə-mē) *n.* Surgical removal of the ossicles of the middle ear.

os·si·cu·lot·o·my (ŏ-sĭk′yə-lŏt′ə-mē) *n.* Surgical division of an ossicle of the middle ear or of a fibrous band causing ankylosis between two ossicles.

os·sic·u·lum (ŏ-sĭk′yə-ləm) *n.*, *pl.* **–la** (-lə) A small bone; an ossicle.

os·sif·er·ous (ŏ-sĭf′ər-əs) *adj.* Containing or producing bone.

os·sif·ic (ŏ-sĭf′ĭk) *adj.* Of, forming, or developing into bone.

os·si·fi·ca·tion (ŏs′ə-fĭ-kā′shən) *n.* **1.** The natural process of bone formation. **2.** The hardening or calcification of soft tissue into a bonelike material. **3.** A mass or deposit of such material.

os·si·fy (ŏs′ə-fī′) *v.* To change into bone.

os·te·al (ŏs′tē-əl) *adj.* **1.** Bony; osseous. **2.** Relating to bone or to the skeleton.

os·te·al·gia (ŏs′tē-ăl′jə) *n.* A pain in a bone. —**os′te·al′gic** (-jĭk) *adj.*

os·tec·to·my (ŏs-tĕk′tə-mē) *n.* **1.** Surgical removal of a bone or of part of a bone. **2.** In dentistry, resection of supporting osseous structures to eliminate periodontal pockets.

os·te·in *or* **os·te·ine** (ŏs′tē-ĭn) *n.* See **ossein**.

os·te·i·tis (ŏs′tē-ī′tĭs) *or* **os·ti·tis** (ŏ-stī′tĭs) *n.* Inflammation of bone or bony tissue.

osteitis de·for·mans (dē-fôr′mănz′) *n.* See **Paget's disease** (sense 1).

osteitis fi·bro·sa cys·ti·ca (fī-brō′sə sĭs′tĭ-kə) *n.* The resorption and replacement of calcified bone with fibrous tissue caused by hyperparathyroidism or similar conditions that affect the concentration of mineral salts such as calcium and phosphorus. Also called *Recklinghausen's disease of bone*.

osteitis fun·go·sa (fŭng-gō′sə) *n.* Chronic osteitis in which the Haversian canals are dilated and filled with granulation tissue.

os·tem·py·e·sis (ŏs′tĕm-pī-ē′sĭs) *n.* Suppuration in a bone.

osteo– *or* **oste–** *pref.* Bone: *osteoarthritis.*

os·te·o·an·a·gen·e·sis (ŏs′tē-ō-ăn′ə-jĕn′ĭ-sĭs) *n.* The regeneration of bone tissue.

os·te·o·ar·thri·tis (ŏs′tē-ō-är-thrī′tĭs) *n. Abbr.* **OA** A form of arthritis, occurring mainly in older persons, that is characterized by chronic degeneration of the cartilage of the joints. Also called *degenerative joint disease, hypertrophic arthritis, osteoarthrosis*. —**os′te·o·ar·thrit′ic** (-thrĭt′ĭk) *adj.*

os·te·o·ar·throp·a·thy (ŏs′tē-ō-är-thrŏp′ə-thē) *n.* A disorder affecting bones and joints.

os·te·o·ar·thro·sis (ŏs′tē-ō-är-thrō′sĭs) *n.* See **osteoarthritis**.

os·te·o·blast (ŏs′tē-ə-blăst′) *n.* A cell from which bone develops; a bone-forming cell. —**os′te·o·blas′tic** *adj.*

os·te·o·blas·to·ma (ŏs′tē-ō-blă-stō′mə) *n.* A benign tumor of bone characterized by areas of osteoid and calcified tissue.

os·te·o·car·ti·lag·i·nous (ŏs′tē-ō-kär′tl-ăj′ə-nəs) *adj.* Relating to or composed of bone and cartilage.

os·te·o·chon·dri·tis (ŏs′tē-ō-kŏn-drī′tĭs) *n.* Inflammation of a bone along with its cartilage.

osteochondritis de·for·mans ju·ve·ni·lis (dē-fôr′mănz′ jōō′və-nī′lĭs) *n.* Osteochondrosis of the upper end of the femur. Also called *Calvé-Perthes disease, coxa plana, Legg-Calvé-Perthes disease, Perthes disease*.

osteochondritis deformans juvenilis dor·si (dôr′sī) *n.* See **Scheuermann's disease**.

osteochondritis dis·se·cans (dĭs′ĭ-kănz′) *n.* Separation of a portion of joint cartilage and of underlying bone, usually involving the knee.

os·te·o·chon·dro·dys·tro·phy (ŏs′tē-ō-kŏn′drə-dĭs′trə-fē) *or* **os·te·o·chon·dro·dys·tro·phi·a** (-dĭs-trō′fē-ə) *n.* See **chondroosteodystrophy**.

os·te·o·chon·dro·ma (ŏs′tē-ō-kŏn-drō′mə) *n.* A benign cartilaginous neoplasm that consists of a pedicle of normal bone covered with a rim of proliferating cartilage cells.

os·te·o·chon·dro·ma·to·sis (ŏs′tē-ō-kŏn′drō-mə-tō′sĭs) *n.* See **hereditary multiple exostoses**.

os·te·o·chon·dro·sar·co·ma (ŏs′tē-ō-kŏn′drō-sär-kō′mə) *n.* A chondrosarcoma arising in bone.

os·te·o·chon·dro·sis (ŏs′tē-ō-kŏn-drō′sĭs) *n.* Any of a group of disorders involving one or more centers of ossification of the bones in children and characterized by degeneration or aseptic necrosis followed by reossification.

os·te·oc·la·sis (ŏs′tē-ŏk′lə-sĭs) *n., pl.* **–ses** (-sēz′) **1.** The process of dissolution and resorption of bony tissue. **2.** Surgical fracture of a bone that is performed to correct a deformity. Also called *diaclasis*.

os·te·o·clast (ŏs′tē-ə-klăst′) *n.* **1.** A large multinucleate cell found in growing bone that resorbs bony tissue, as in the formation of canals and cavities. Also called *osteophage*. **2.** An instrument used in surgical osteoclasis. —**os′te·o·clas′tic** *adj.*

osteoclast-activating factor *n.* A lymphokine that stimulates bone resorption and inhibits bone collagen synthesis.

os·te·o·clas·to·ma (ŏs′tē-ō-klă-stō′mə) *n.* See **giant cell tumor of bone**.

os·te·o·cra·ni·um (ŏs′tē-ō-krā′nē-əm) *n.* The fetal cranium after ossification of the membranous cranium has advanced to firmness.

os·te·o·cys·to·ma (ŏs′tē-ō-sĭ-stō′mə) *n.* See **solitary bone cyst**.

os·te·o·cyte (ŏs′tē-ə-sīt′) *n.* A branched cell embedded in the matrix of bone tissue.

os·te·o·den·tin (ŏs′tē-ō-děn′tĭn) *n.* Dentin that resembles bone in structure.

os·te·o·der·ma·to·poi·ki·lo·sis (ŏs′tē-ō-dûr′mə-tō-poi′kə-lō′sĭs) *n.* Osteopoikilosis with skin lesions on the back of the thighs and buttocks. Also called *Buschke-Ollendorf syndrome*.

os·te·o·der·mi·a (ŏs′tē-ō-dûr′mē-ə) *n.* See **osteosis cutis**.

os·te·o·di·as·ta·sis (ŏs′tē-ō-dī-ăs′tə-sĭs) *n.* The separation of two adjacent bones, as of the cranium.

os·te·o·dyn·i·a (ŏs′tē-ō-dĭn′ē-ə) *n.* Pain in a bone.

os·te·o·dys·tro·phy (ŏs′tē-ō-dĭs′trə-fē) *n.* Defective formation of bone. Also called *osteodystrophia.*

os·te·o·ec·ta·sia (ŏs′tē-ō-ĭk-tā′zhə) *n.* Bowing of the bones, particularly of the legs.

os·te·o·fi·bro·ma (ŏs′tē-ō-fī-brō′mə) *n.* A benign bone tumor, consisting chiefly of dense fibrous connective tissue and bone.

os·te·o·fi·bro·sis (ŏs′tē-ō-fī-brō′sĭs) *n.* Fibrosis of bone, mainly involving bone marrow.

os·te·o·gen (ŏs′tē-ə-jən, -jĕn′) *n.* The substance forming the inner layer of the periosteum, from which new bone is formed.

os·te·o·gen·e·sis (ŏs′tē-ə-jĕn′ĭ-sĭs) *n.* Formation and development of bony tissue. Also called *osteogeny.*

osteogenesis im·per·fec·ta (ĭm′pər-fĕk′tə) *n.* A hereditary disease marked by abnormal fragility and plasticity of bone, with deformity of long bones, a bluish discoloration of the sclerae, recurring fractures resulting from minimal trauma, and often otosclerosis. Also called *brittle bones.*

osteogenetic fiber *n.* Any of the fibers in the osteogenetic layer.

osteogenetic layer *n.* The inner bone-forming layer of the periosteum.

os·te·o·gen·ic (ŏs′tē-ə-jĕn′ĭk) *or* **os·te·o·ge·net·ic** (-ō-jə-nĕt′ĭk) *adj.* Of, relating to, or characteristic of osteogenesis.

osteogenic sarcoma *n.* See **osteosarcoma.**

os·te·og·e·nous (ŏs′tē-ŏj′ə-nəs) *adj.* Osteogenic.

os·te·og·e·ny (ŏs′tē-ŏj′ə-nē) *n.* See **osteogenesis.**

os·te·o·hal·i·ste·re·sis (ŏs′tē-ō-hăl′ĭ-stə-rē′sĭs, -hă-lĭs′tə-) *n.* A loss or deficiency of the mineral constituents of bone resulting in softening of the bones.

os·te·oid (ŏs′tē-oid′) *adj.* Resembling bone. —*n.* The bone matrix, especially before calcification.

osteoid osteoma *n.* A painful benign tumor usually originating in one of the bones of the lower extremities and characterized by a nidus composed of vascularized connective tissue and osteoid material and surrounded by a large zone of thickened bone.

os·te·o·lip·o·chon·dro·ma (ŏs′tē-ō-lĭp′ō-kŏn-drō′mə) *n.* A benign tumor of cartilaginous tissue containing bony tissue and fat cells.

os·te·ol·o·gy (ŏs′tē-ŏl′ə-jē) *n.* The branch of anatomy that deals with the structure and function of bones. —**os′te·o·log′i·cal** (-ə-lŏj′ĭ-kəl) *adj.*

os·te·ol·y·sis (ŏs′tē-ŏl′ĭ-sĭs) *n.* Dissolution or degeneration of bone tissue resulting from disease. —**os′te·o·lyt′ic** (-ə-lĭt′ĭk) *adj.*

os·te·o·ma (ŏs′tē-ō′mə) *n.,* *pl.* **–mas** *or* **–ma·ta** (-mə-tə) A benign tumor composed of bony tissue, often developing on the skull.

os·te·o·ma·la·cia (ŏs′tē-ō-mə-lā′shə) *n.* A bone disease characterized by bone demineralization due to deficiency or impaired metabolism of vitamin D or phosphates. Also called *adult rickets, late rickets.*

os·te·o·ma·la·cic (ŏs′tē-ō-mə-lā′sĭk) *adj.* Of, relating to, or characterized by osteomalacia.

osteomalacic pelvis *n.* A pelvic deformity in osteomalacia in which the pressure of the trunk on the sacrum and lateral pressure of the femoral heads produce a three-cornered pelvic aperture while the pubic bone becomes beak-shaped. Also called *beaked pelvis.*

osteoma med·ul·lar·e (mĕd′ə-lâr′ē) *n.* An osteoma containing spaces filled with various elements of bone marrow.

osteoma spon·gi·o·sum (spŏn′jē-ō′səm, spŭn′-) *n.* A spongy osteoma primarily of cancellous bone tissue.

os·te·o·ma·toid (ŏs′tē-ō′mə-toid′) *n.* An abnormal nodule or small overgrowth of bone, usually occurring bilaterally and symmetrically in juxtaepiphysial regions.

os·te·o·mere (ŏs′tē-ə-mîr′) *n.* One of a series of similar bone segments, such as a vertebrae.

os·te·o·my·e·li·tis (ŏs′tē-ō-mī′ə-lī′tĭs) *n.* Inflammation of bone and bone marrow. Also called *central osteitis.*

os·te·o·my·e·lo·dys·pla·sia (ŏs′tē-ō-mī′ə-lō-dĭs-plā′zhə) *n.* A disease characterized by enlargement of the marrow cavities of the bones, thinning of the osseous tissue, large thin-walled vascular spaces, leukopenia, and irregular fever.

os·te·on (ŏs′tē-ŏn′) *or* **os·te·one** (-ōn′) *n.* A central canal and the concentric osseous lamellae encircling it, occurring in compact bone. Also called *haversian system.*

os·te·o·ne·cro·sis (ŏs′tē-ō-nə-krō′sĭs) *n.* Necrosis of bone.

os·te·o·path (ŏs′tē-ə-păth′) *or* **os·te·op·a·thist** (ŏs′tē-ŏp′ə-thĭst) *n.* A physician practicing osteopathy.

os·te·o·path·i·a (ŏs′tē-ə-păth′ē-ə) *n.* See **osteopathy** (sense 2).

osteopathia con·den·sans (kən-dĕn′sănz′) *n.* See **osteopoikilosis.**

osteopathia stri·a·ta (strī-ā′tə) *pl.n.* Linear striations, visible by radiographic examination, in the metaphyses of long or flat bones.

osteopathic medicine *n.* See **osteopathy** (sense 1).

osteopathic physician *n.* An osteopath.

os·te·op·a·thy (ŏs′tē-ŏp′ə-thē) *n.* **1.** A system of medicine based on the theory that disturbances in the musculoskeletal system affect other bodily parts and cause many disorders that can be corrected by various manipulative techniques used in conjunction with conventional therapeutic procedures. Also called *osteopathic medicine.* **2.** A disease of a bone. Also called *osteopathia.* —**os′te·o·path′ic** (-ə-păth′ĭk) *adj.*

os·te·o·pe·ni·a (ŏs′tē-ə-pē′nē-ə) *n.* A condition of bone in which there is a generalized reduction in bone mass that is less severe than that in osteoporosis, caused by the resorption of bone at a rate that exceeds bone synthesis.

os·te·o·per·i·os·ti·tis (ŏs′tē-ō-pĕr′ē-ŏs-tī′tĭs) *n.* Inflammation of the periosteum and the underlying bone.

os·te·o·pe·tro·sis (ŏs′tē-ō-pĕ-trō′sĭs) *n.* An inherited disorder in which bone and cartilage, especially in long bones, become dense and hardened to an extent that marrow is obliterated, and anemia, spleen and liver enlargement, blindness, and progressive deafness occur; it begins in infancy and sometimes results in early death. Also called *Albers-Schönberg disease, marble bone disease, marble bones.* —**os′te·o·pe·trot′ic** (-trŏt′ĭk) *adj.*

os·te·o·phage (ŏs′tē-ə-fāj′) *n.* See **osteoclast** (sense 1).

os·te·o·phle·bi·tis (ŏs′tē-ō-flĭ-bī′tĭs) *n.* Inflammation of the veins of a bone.

os·te·o·phyte (ŏs′tē-ə-fīt′) *n.* A small abnormal bony outgrowth. Also called *osteophyma.*

os·te·o·plas·tic (ŏs′tē-ə-plăs′tĭk) *adj.* **1.** Of or relating to osteoplasty. **2.** Relating to or functioning in bone formation.

os·te·o·plas·ty (ŏs′tē-ə-plăs′tē) *n.* **1.** Surgical repair or alteration of bone. Also called *bone grafting.* **2.** In dentistry, surgical resection of bony structures to form or correct the contour of the gums.

os·te·o·poi·ki·lo·sis (ŏs′tē-ō-poi′kə-lō′sĭs) *n.* An inherited condition characterized by bones that are mottled because of widespread small foci of compact bone in the spongy bone. Also called *osteopathia condensans.*

os·te·o·pon·tin (ŏs′tē-ō-pŏn′tn) *n.* A phosphorylated glycoprotein that is abundant in bone mineral matrix and accelerates bone regeneration and remodeling. It is also produced in other tissues and plays a role in the regulation and progression of many diseases, as by enhancing the invasive and proteolytic capabilities of tumor cells.

os·te·o·po·ro·sis (ŏs′tē-ō-pə-rō′sĭs) *n., pl.* **–ses** (-sēz) A disease characterized by decrease in bone mass and density, occurring especially in postmenopausal women, resulting in a predisposition to fractures and bone deformities such as vertebral collapse. —**os′te·o· po·rot′ic** (-rŏt′ĭk) *adj.*

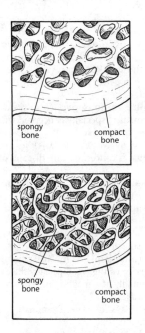

osteoporosis
Top: *detail of normal femur*
Bottom: *detail of osteoporotic femur*

os·te·o·pro·gen·i·tor cell (ŏs′tē-ō-prō-jĕn′ĭ-tər) *n.* A mesenchymal cell that differentiates into an osteoblast. Also called *preosteoblast.*

os·te·o·ra·di·o·ne·cro·sis (ŏs′tē-ō-rā′dē-ō-nə-krō′sĭs) *n.* Necrosis of bone caused by exposure to ionizing radiation.

os·te·or·rha·phy (ŏs′tē-ôr′ə-fē) *n.* The surgical suturing or joining of fragments of broken bone, usually by wiring them together. Also called *osteosuture.*

os·te·o·sar·co·ma (ŏs′tē-ō-sär-kō′mə) *n.* A malignant bone tumor. Also called *osteogenic sarcoma.*

os·te·o·scle·ro·sis (ŏs′tē-ō-sklə-rō′sĭs) *n.* Abnormal hardening of bone or bone marrow. —**os′te·o·scle· rot′ic** (-rŏt′ĭk) *adj.*

osteosclerosis con·gen·i·ta (kən-jĕn′ĭ-tə) *n.* See **achondroplasia.**

os·te·o·sis (ŏs′tē-ō′sĭs) *or* **os·to·sis** (ŏ-stō′sĭs) *n.* The formation of bony tissue, especially over connective or other tissue.

osteosis cu·tis (kyōō′tĭs) *n.* Bone formation in the skin and tissue by osseous metaplasia of calcium deposits. Also called *osteodermia.*

os·te·o·su·ture (ŏs′tē-ō-sōō′chər) *n.* See **osteorrhaphy.**

os·te·o·syn·the·sis (ŏs′tē-ō-sĭn′thĭ-sĭs) *n.* The process of mechanically bringing the ends of a fractured bone close together, as by wiring together or attaching to a metal plate.

os·te·o·throm·bo·sis (ŏs′tē-ō-thrŏm-bō′sĭs) *n.* Thrombosis in one or more of the veins of a bone.

os·te·o·tome (ŏs′tē-ə-tōm′) *n.* A chisel-like instrument for cutting bone.

os·te·ot·o·my (ŏs′tē-ŏt′ə-mē) *n.* Surgical division or sectioning of bone.

os·te·o·tribe (ŏs′tē-ə-trīb′) *n.* An instrument for filing or abrading away necrosed or carious bone.

os·te·o·trite (ŏs′tē-ə-trīt′) *n.* An instrument, resembling a dental bur, for grinding away carious bone.

os·ti·tis (ŏ-stī′tĭs) *n.* Variant of **osteitis.**

os·ti·um (ŏs′tē-əm) *n., pl.* **–ti·a** (-tē-ə) A small opening or orifice, as in a body organ. —**os′ti·al** *adj.*

ostium ab·dom·i·na·le tu·bae u·ter·i·nae (ăb-dŏm′-ə-nā′lē tōō′bē yōō′tə-rī′nē) *n.* The fimbriated or ovarian extremity of an oviduct.

ostium of uterus *n.* The opening of the uterus into the vagina.

ostium u·ter·i·num tu·bae (yōō′tə-rī′nəm tōō′bē) *n.* The uterine opening of the oviduct.

os·to·mate (ŏs′tə-māt′) *n.* One who has undergone an ostomy.

os·to·my (ŏs′tə-mē) *n.* Surgical construction of an artificial excretory opening, such as a colostomy.

os·to·sis (ŏ-stō′sĭs) *n.* Variant of **osteosis.**

Ost·wald's solubility coefficient (ōst′wôldz′, ôst′välts) *n. Symbol* **λ** The quantity of solvent needed to dissolve a quantity of gas at a given temperature and pressure.

OT *abbr.* occupational therapy

ot– *pref.* Variant of **oto–.**

o·tal·gia (ō-tăl′jə) *n.* Pain in the ear; earache. —**o·tal′· gic** *adj.*

O·ta's nevus (ō′təz) *n.* See **oculodermal melanosis.**

OTC *abbr.* over-the-counter

ot·he·ma·to·ma (ōt′hē-mə-tō′mə) *n.* A purplish rounded hard swelling of the external ear.

ot·hem·or·rha·gia (ōt′hĕm-ə-rā′jə) *n.* Hemorrhage from the ear.

oth·er-di·rect·ed (ŭth′ər-dĭ-rĕk′tĭd, -dī-) *adj.* Directed or guided chiefly by external standards as opposed to one's own standards or values.

o·tic (ō′tĭk, ŏt′ĭk) *adj.* Of, relating to, or located near the ear; auricular.

–otic *suff.* **1.** Of, relating to, or characterized by a specified condition or process: *anabiotic.* **2.** Having a specified disease or abnormal condition: *epizootic.* **3.** Characterized by an increase or formation of a specified kind: *leukocytotic.*

otic capsule *n.* The embryonic cartilage capsule that surrounds the inner ear mechanism and develops into bony tissue.

otic ganglion *n.* An autonomic ganglion situated just below the oval foramen medial to the mandibular nerve, with distribution of the postganglionic fibers to the parotid gland. Also called *otoganglion.*

otic vesicle *n.* See **auditory vesicle.**

otitic meningitis *n.* Infection of the meninges occurring as a result of mastoiditis or otitis media.

o·ti·tis (ō-tī′tĭs) *n.* Inflammation of the ear. —**o·tit′ic** (ō-tĭt′ĭk) *adj.*

otitis ex·ter·na (ĭk-stûr′nə) *n.* Inflammation of the external auditory canal.

otitis externa cir·cum·scrip·ta (sûr′kəm-skrĭp′tə) *n.* Furunculosis of the external auditory canal. Also called *otitis furunculosa.*

otitis externa dif·fu·sa (dĭ-fyoō′sə) *n.* Inflammation of the external auditory meatus.

otitis fu·run·cu·lo·sa (fə-rŭng′kyə-lō′sə) *n.* See **otitis externa circumscripta.**

otitis in·ter·na (ĭn-tûr′nə) *n.* See **labyrinthitis.**

otitis me·di·a (mē′dē-ə) *n. Abbr.* **OM** Inflammation of the middle ear, occurring commonly in children as a result of infection and often causing pain and temporary hearing loss.

otitis my·cot·i·ca (mī-kŏt′ĭ-kə) *n.* A fungous growth in the external auditory canal, often of a species of *Aspergillus.*

oto– *or* **ot–** *pref.* Ear: *otology.*

o·to·an·tri·tis (ō′tō-ăn-trī′tĭs) *n.* Inflammation of the mastoid antrum.

O·to·bi·us (ō-tō′bē-əs) *n.* A genus of argasid ticks common in the southwest United States and Mexico whose nymphs may attack human ears.

o·to·ceph·a·ly (ō′tō-sĕf′ə-lē) *n.* A congenital malformation of the head characterized by a markedly diminished or absent lower jaw and the joining or close approach of the ears on the front of the neck below the face.

o·to·clei·sis (ō′tō-klī′sĭs) *n.* The closing of the auditory tube of the ear either by a new growth or accumulation of cerumen.

o·to·co·ni·um (ō′tə-kō′nē-əm) *n., pl.* **–ni·a** (-nē-ə) See **statoconium.**

o·to·cra·ni·um (ō′tō-krā′nē-əm) *n.* The bony case of the internal and middle ear consisting of the petrous portion of the temporal bone. —**o′to·cra′ni·al** *adj.*

o·to·cyst (ō′tə-sĭst′) *n.* The structure formed by invagination of the embryonic ectodermal tissue that develops into the inner ear. —**o′to·cys′tic** *adj.*

o·to·dyn·i·a (ō′tə-dĭn′ē-ə) *n.* Pain in the ear; earache.

o·to·en·ceph·a·li·tis (ō′tō-ĕn-sĕf′ə-lī′tĭs) *n.* Inflammation of the brain caused by the extension of an infection from an inflamed middle ear.

o·to·gan·gli·on (ō′tō-găng′glē-ən) *n.* See **otic ganglion.**

o·to·gen·ic (ō′tə-jĕn′ĭk) *or* **o·tog·e·nous** (ō-tŏj′ə-nəs) *adj.* Of or originating within the ear, especially from inflammation of the ear.

o·to·lar·yn·gol·o·gy (ō′tō-lăr′ĭn-gŏl′ə-jē) *n.* The branch of medicine that deals with diagnosis and treatment of diseases of the ear, larynx, and upper respiratory tract. —**o′to·lar′yn·gol′o·gist** *n.*

o·to·lith (ō′tə-lĭth′) *n.* **1.** Any of numerous minute calcareous particles found in the inner ear of certain lower vertebrates and in the statocysts of many invertebrates. **2.** See **otosteon.** —**o′to·lith′ic** *adj.*

o·tol·o·gy (ō-tŏl′ə-jē) *n.* The branch of medicine that deals with the ear. —**o′to·log′ic** (ō′tə-lŏj′ĭk) *adj.* —**o·tol′o·gist** *n.*

o·to·mu·cor·my·co·sis (ō′tō-myoō′kôr-mī-kō′sĭs) *n.* An infection of the ear caused by fungi of the Mucoraceae family.

o·to·my·co·sis (ō′tō-mī-kō′sĭs) *n.* A fungal infection of the external auditory canal.

o·top·a·thy (ō-tŏp′ə-thē) *n.* A disease of the ear.

o·to·pha·ryn·geal (ō′tō-fə-rĭn′jəl, -făr′ĭn-jē′əl) *adj.* Of, relating to, or characterizing the middle ear and the pharynx.

o·to·plas·ty (ō′tə-plăs′tē) *n.* The surgical repair, restoration, or alteration of the auricle of the ear.

o·to·pol·y·pus (ō′tō-pŏl′ə-pəs) *n.* A polyp in the external auditory canal, usually arising from the middle ear.

o·to·py·or·rhe·a (ō′tō-pī′ə-rē′ə) *n.* Chronic otitis media resulting in perforation of the eardrum and a purulent discharge.

o·to·rhi·no·lar·yn·gol·o·gy (ō′tō-rī′nō-lăr′ĭn-gŏl′ə-jē) *n.* The medical specialty concerned with diseases of the ear, nose, and throat.

o·to·rhi·nol·o·gy (ō′tō-rī′nŏl′ə-jē) *n.* The branch of medicine that is concerned with diseases of the ear and nose.

o·tor·rha·gia (ō′tə-rā′jē-ə) *n.* Bleeding from the external auditory canal of the ear.

o·tor·rhe·a (ō′tə-rē′ə) *n.* A discharge from the ear.

o·to·scle·ro·sis (ō′tō-sklə-rō′sĭs) *n.* A formation of spongy bone about the stapes and the oval window of the ear, causing progressive deafness.

o·to·scope (ō′tə-skōp′) *n.* An instrument for examining the interior of the ear, especially the eardrum, consisting essentially of a magnifying lens and a light. Also called *auriscope.*

o·tos·co·py (ō-tŏs′kə-pē) *n.* Examination of the ear by means of an otoscope.

ot·os·te·al (ō-tŏs′tē-əl) *adj.* Of or relating to the small bones of the middle ear.

ot·os·te·on (ō-tŏs′tē-ŏn′) *n.* **1.** Any of the small bones of the middle ear. **2.** A calcareous concretion in the inner ear that is larger than a statoconium. Also called *otolith.*

o·tot·o·my (ō-tŏt′ə-mē) *n.* Incision of the ear.

o·to·tox·ic (ō′tə-tŏk′sĭk) *adj.* Having a toxic effect on the ear, especially on its nerve supply.

Ot·to pelvis (ŏt′ō, ôt′ō) *n.* An inward bulging of the acetabulum causing the prominence of the femur to be reduced.

OU *abbr. Latin* oculus uterque (either eye, each eye)

oua·ba·in (wä-bä′ĭn) *n.* A white poisonous glycoside extracted from the seeds of the African trees *Strophanthus gratus* and *Acokanthera ouabaio* and used as a heart stimulant.

ounce (ouns) *n. Abbr.* **oz, oz. 1.** A unit of weight in the US Customary System, an avoirdupois unit equal to 437.5 grains or 28.35 grams. **2.** A unit of apothecary weight equal to 480 grains or 31.10 grams. **3.** A fluid ounce.

–ous *suff.* **1.** Possessing; full of; characterized by: *filamentous.* **2.** Having a valence lower than that of a specified element in compounds or ions named with adjectives ending in *-ic: ferrous.*

out·er ear (ou′tər) *n.* See **external ear.**

out-of-body *adj.* Of, relating to, or marked by the psychological sensation of perceiving oneself from an external perspective, as though the mind or soul has left the body and is acting of its own volition.

out·pa·tient (out′pā′shənt) *n.* A patient who is admitted to a hospital or clinic for treatment that does not require an overnight stay.

out·put (out′pŏŏt′) *n.* The amount produced, ejected, or excreted by an entity during a specified time.

ov– *pref.* Variant of **ovi–.**

o·val amputation (ō′vəl) *n.* Amputation in which flaps are constructed by oval incisions through the skin and muscle.

ov·al·bu·min (ŏv′əl-byōō′mĭn, ō′vəl-) *n.* See **egg albumin.**

oval foramen *n.* **1.** The oval opening in the septum between the right and left atria of the fetal heart. **2.** A large oval opening in the greater wing of the sphenoid bone, transmitting the mandibular nerve and a small meningeal artery.

oval fossa *n.* **1.** An oval depression on the lower part of the septum of the right atrium. Its floor corresponds to a septum of the fetal heart. **2.** See **hiatus saphenus.**

o·va·lo·cyte (ō′və-lō-sīt′, ō-văl′ə-) *n.* See **elliptocyte.**

o·va·lo·cy·to·sis (ō′və-lō-sī-tō′sĭs, ō-văl′ə-) *n.* See **elliptocytosis.**

oval window *n.* An oval opening located on the medial wall of the tympanic cavity, leading into the vestibule, to which the base of the stapes is connected and through which the ossicles of the ear transmit the sound vibrations to the cochlea. Also called *fenestra of vestibule.*

o·var·i·al·gia (ō-vâr′ē-ăl′jə) *n.* A pain in the ovary.

ovarian artery *n.* An artery with its origin in the aorta, with distribution to the ureter, ovary, ovarian ligament, and uterine tube, and with anastomosis to the uterine artery.

ovarian cycle *n.* The normal sex cycle that includes development of an ovarian follicle, rupture of the follicle, discharge of the ovum, and formation and regression of a corpus luteum.

ovarian cyst *n.* A cystic tumor of the ovary, which is usually benign.

ovarian follicle *n.* A cavity in the ovary containing a maturing ovum surrounded by its encasing cells.

ovarian fossa *n.* The depression in the parietal peritoneum of the pelvis in which the ovary is situated.

ovarian pregnancy *n.* An ectopic pregnancy developing in an ovarian follicle. Also called *ovariocyesis.*

o·var·i·ec·to·my (ō-vâr′ē-ĕk′tə-mē) *n.* The surgical removal of one ovary or of both ovaries. Also called *oophorectomy.*

ovario– *or* **ovari–** *pref.* Ovary: *ovariocele.*

o·var·i·o·cele (ō-vâr′ē-ə-sēl′) *n.* A hernia of an ovary.

o·var·i·o·cen·te·sis (ō-vâr′ē-ō-sĕn-tē′sĭs) *n.* Puncture of an ovary or ovarian cyst.

o·var·i·o·cy·e·sis (ō-vâr′ē-ō-sī-ē′sĭs) *n.* See **ovarian pregnancy.**

o·var·i·o·hys·ter·ec·to·my (ō-vâr′ē-ō-hĭs′tə-rĕk′tə-mē) *n.* The surgical removal of one or both ovaries and the uterus. Also called *oophorohysterectomy.*

o·var·i·or·rhex·is (ō-vâr′ē-ə-rĕk′sĭs) *n.* Rupture of an ovary.

o·var·i·o·sal·pin·gec·to·my (ō-vâr′ē-ō-săl′pĭn-jĕk′tə-mē) *n.* Surgical removal of an ovary and the corresponding oviduct.

o·var·i·o·sal·pin·gi·tis (ō-vâr′ē-ō-săl′pĭn-jī′tĭs) *n.* Inflammation that involves an ovary and the corresponding oviduct.

o·var·i·os·to·my (ō-vâr′ē-ŏs′tə-mē) *n.* Surgical formation of a temporary fistula to drain an ovarian cyst. Also called *oophorostomy.*

o·var·i·ot·o·my (ō-vâr′ē-ŏt′ə-mē) *n.* **1.** Ovariectomy. **2.** Incision into an ovary, as to perform a biopsy. Also called *oophorotomy.*

o·va·ri·tis (ō′və-rī′tĭs) *n.* See **oophoritis.**

ovar·i·um (ō- vâr′ē- ŭm) *n., pl.* **–i·a** (-ē- ə) One of the paired female reproductive organs that produce ova; an ovary.

o·va·ry (ō′və-rē) *n.* One of the paired female reproductive organs that produce ova and certain sex hormones, including estrogen. Also called *oophoron.* **—o·var′i·an** (ō-vâr′ē-ən) *adj.*

o·ver·anx·ious disorder (ō′vər-ăngk′shəs, -ăng′shəs) *n.* A generalized and persistent anxiety in children or adults that is not the result of separation or recent stress and is characterized by self-consciousness and obsessive concern over past behavior, future events, personal health, and competence in athletics, social, or academic arenas.

o·ver·bite (ō′vər-bīt′) *n.* A malocclusion of the teeth in which the front upper incisor and canine teeth project over the lower. Also called *vertical overlap.*

o·ver·com·pen·sa·tion (ō′vər-kŏm′pən-sā′shən) *n.* Excessive compensation, especially the exertion of effort beyond what is needed to compensate for a physical or psychological characteristic or defect.

o·ver·cor·rec·tion (ō′vər-kə-rĕk′shən) *n.* An adjustment that surpasses a set criterion, especially of a desired behavior.

o·ver·den·ture (ō′vər-dĕn′chər) *n.* See **overlay denture.**

o·ver·de·ter·mi·na·tion (ō′vər-dĭ-tûr′mə-nā′shən) *n.* In psychoanalytic theory, the concept that multiple causes collaborate to produce a single behavior, emotion, mental symptom, or dream.

o·ver·dom·i·nance (ō′vər-dŏm′ə-nəns) *n.* The condition in which a heterozygote has a phenotype that is more pronounced or better adapted than that of either homozygote. —**o′ver·dom′i·nant** *adj.*

o·ver·dose (ō′vər-dōs′) *n.* An excessive dose, especially of a narcotic.

o·ver·eat (ō′vər-ēt′) *v.* To eat to excess, especially habitually.

o·ver·ex·press (ō′vər-ĭk-sprĕs′) *v.* To produce in excess, as does the genetic material of cancer cells.

o·ver·feed (ō′vər-fēd′) *v.* To feed or eat too often or too much.

o·ver·hy·drate (ō′vər-hī′drāt) *v.* To cause to take excessive fluids into the body, as through intravenous injection.

o·ver·jet (ō′vər-jĕt′) *or* **o·ver·jut** (-jŭt′) *n.* See **horizontal overlap.**

o·ver·lap (ō′vər-lăp′) *n.* **1.** A part or portion of a structure that extends or projects over another. **2.** The suturing of one layer of tissue above or under another layer to provide additional strength, often used in dental surgery. —*v.* (ō′vər-lăp′) **1.** To lie over and partly cover something. **2.** To perform a surgical overlap.

o·ver·lay denture (ō′vər-lā′) *n.* A complete denture supported by both soft tissue and natural teeth that have been altered to accept the denture. Also called *overdenture.*

o·ver·med·i·cate (ō′vər-mĕd′ĭ-kāt′) *v.* To medicate a patient excessively.

o·ver·pre·scribe (ō′vər-prĭ-skrīb′) *v.* To prescribe medication excessively.

o·ver·re·act (ō′vər-rē-ăkt′) *v.* To react with unnecessary or inappropriate force, emotional display, or violence.

o·ver·rid·ing (ō′vər-rī′dĭng) *adj.* **1.** First in priority; more important than all others. **2.** Of or relating to a fracture in which the broken ends of the bone slip past each other and are held in the overlap position by contracted muscles. **3.** Of or relating to a fetal head that is palpable above the pubic symphysis because of the disproportion between the size of the fetal head and the size of the maternal pelvis.

o·ver·sexed (ō′vər-sĕkst′) *adj.* Having or showing an excessive sexual appetite or interest in sex.

o·ver·shoot (ō′vər-shōōt′) *n.* A change from steady state in response to a sudden change in some factor, as in electric potential or polarity when a cell or tissue is stimulated.

o·ver·stretch (ō′vər-strĕch′) *v.* **1.** To stretch one's body or muscles to the point of strain or injury. **2.** To stretch or extend over.

o·ver-the-count·er (ō′vər-thə-koun′tər) *adj. Abbr.* **OTC** That can be sold legally without a doctor's prescription.

o·ver·win·ter·ing (ō′vər-wĭn′tər-ĭng) *n.* The persistence of an infectious agent in its vector for an extended period, as in the cooler winter months, during which the vector has no opportunity to be reinfected or to infect another host.

ovi– *or* **ovo–** *or* **ov–** *pref.* Egg; ovum: *oviferous.*

o·vi·cid·al (ō′vĭ-sīd′l) *adj.* Relating to or causing death of an ovum.

o·vi·duct (ō′vĭ-dŭkt′) *n.* See **fallopian tube.** —**o′vi·duc′tal, o′vi·du′cal** (-dōō′kəl) *adj.*

o·vif·er·ous (ō-vĭf′ər-əs) *adj.* Bearing or producing ova.

o·vi·form (ō′və-fôrm′) *adj.* Shaped like an egg; ovoid.

o·vi·gen·e·sis (ō′və-jĕn′ĭ-sĭs) *n.* See **oogenesis.** —**o′vi·ge·net′ic** (-jə-nĕt′ĭk) *adj.*

o·vi·sac (ō′vĭ-săk′) *n.* An egg-containing capsule, such as a Graafian follicle.

o·void (ō′void′) *or* **o·voi·dal** (ō-void′l) *n.* Something that is shaped like an egg. —*adj.* Shaped like an egg; oviform.

o·vo·plasm (ō′və-plăz′əm) *n.* The cytoplasm of an unfertilized ovum.

o·vo·tes·tis (ō′vō-tĕs′tĭs) *n., pl.* **–tes** (-tēz′) A hermaphroditic reproductive organ that produces both sperm and eggs, found in certain gastropods.

ovular membrane *n.* See **vitelline membrane** (sense 1).

o·vu·late (ō′vyə-lāt′, ŏv′yə-) *v.* To produce ova; discharge eggs from the ovary.

o·vu·la·tion (ō′vyə-lā′shən, ŏv′yə-) *n.* The discharge of an ovum from the ovary.

o·vu·la·to·ry (ō′vyə-lə-tôr′ē, ŏv′yə-) *adj.* Of, relating to, or characterizing ovulation.

o·vule (ō′vyōōl, ŏv′yōōl) *n.* **1.** A small or immature ovum of a mammal. **2.** A small egglike structure. Also called *ovulum.* —**o′vu·lar** (ō′vyə-lər, ŏv′yə-), **o′vu·lar′y** (-lĕr′ē) *adj.*

o·vu·lo·cy·clic (ō′vyə-lō-sī′klĭk, -sĭk′lĭk, ŏv′yə-) *adj.* Relating to a phenomenon associated with and recurring at a certain time within the ovulatory cycle.

o·vu·lum (ō′vyə-ləm, ŏv′yə-) *n.* See **ovule** (sense 2).

o·vum (ō′vəm) *n., pl.* **o·va** (ō′və) The female reproductive cell or gamete; egg.

Ow·ren's disease (ō′rĕnz′) *n.* See **parahemophilia.**

ox–¹ *pref.* Variant of **oxo–.**

ox–² *pref.* Variant of **oxy–.**

ox·a·cil·lin sodium (ŏk′sə-sĭl′ĭn) *n.* A semisynthetic penicillin effective against penicillin-resistant infections, especially those of staphylococci.

ox·a·late (ŏk′sə-lāt′) *n.* A salt or ester of oxalic acid.

oxalate calculus *n.* A hard urinary calculus composed of calcium oxalate; it can be smooth or covered with minute sharp spines.

ox·a·le·mi·a (ŏk′sə-lē′mē-ə) *n.* An excess of oxalates in the blood.

ox·al·ic acid (ŏk-săl′ĭk) *n.* A poisonous crystalline organic acid found in many plants and used as an agent in chemical reduction.

ox·a·lo·a·ce·tic acid (ŏk′sə-lō-ə-sē′tĭk, ŏk-săl′ō-) *or* **ox·al·a·ce·tic acid** (ŏk-sĕl′ə-sē′tĭk, ŏk′sə-lə-) *n.* A colorless crystalline dicarboxylic acid that is formed by oxidation of malic acid in the Krebs cycle and by transamination from aspartic acid. It is important in the metabolism of carbohydrates and in the synthesis of amino acids.

ox·a·lo·sis (ŏk′sə-lō′sĭs) *n.* The widespread deposition of calcium oxalate crystals in the kidneys, bones, arterial media, and myocardium, with increased urinary excretion of oxalate.

ox·a·lo·suc·cin·ic acid (ŏk′sə-lō-sək-sĭn′ĭk, ŏk-săl′ō-) *n.* A product of the dehydrogenation of isocitric acid and an intermediate in the Krebs cycle. Also called *oxalourea.*

ox·a·lu·ri·a (ŏk′sə-lŏŏr′ē-ə) *n.* The excretion of an excess of oxalic acid or oxalates, especially calcium oxalate, in the urine.

ox·az·e·pam (ŏk-săz′ə-păm′) *n.* A tranquilizing drug related to benzodiazepine and used especially in the treatment of insomnia and alcohol withdrawal.

ox·i·dant (ŏk′sĭ-dənt) *n.* See **oxidizer.**

ox·i·dase (ŏk′sĭ-dās′, -dāz′) *n.* Any of a group of enzymes that catalyze oxidation, especially an enzyme that reacts with molecular oxygen to catalyze the oxidation of a substrate.

ox·i·da·tion (ŏk′sĭ-dā′shən) *n.* **1.** The combination of a substance with oxygen. **2.** A reaction in which the atoms in an element lose electrons and the valence of the element is correspondingly increased.

oxidation-reduction *n.* A chemical reaction in which an atom or ion loses electrons to another atom or ion. Also called *redox.*

ox·i·da·tive (ŏk′sĭ-dā′tĭv) *adj.* Of, relating to, or characterized by oxidation.

oxidative phosphorylation *n.* The formation of ATP from the energy released by the oxidation of various substrates, especially the organic acids involved in the Krebs cycle.

ox·ide (ŏk′sīd′) *n.* A binary compound of an element or radical with oxygen.

ox·i·dize (ŏk′sĭ-dīz′) *v.* **1.** To combine with oxygen; change into an oxide. **2.** To increase the positive charge or valence of an element by removing electrons.

ox·i·dized cellulose (ŏk′sĭ-dīzd′) *n.* Partially oxidized cellulose in the form of an absorbable gauze used to stanch blood flow during surgical procedures in which ligation is not feasible.

oxidized glutathione *n.* The form of glutathione that acts in cells as a hydrogen acceptor and forms disulfide linkages.

ox·i·diz·er (ŏk′sĭ-dī′zər) *n.* A substance that oxidizes another substance; an oxidizing agent. Also called *oxidant.*

ox·i·do·re·duc·tase (ŏk′sĭ-dō-rĭ-dŭk′tās′, -tāz′) *n.* An enzyme that catalyzes an oxidation-reduction.

ox·ime (ŏk′sēm) *n.* Any of a group of compounds formed by treating aldehydes or ketones with a nitrogen-containing reducing agent.

ox·im·e·ter (ŏk-sĭm′ĭ-tər) *n.* Pulse oximeter.

oxo– *or* **ox–** *pref.* Oxygen: *oxosuccinic acid.*

ox·o·lin·ic acid (ŏk′sə-lĭn′ĭk) *n.* An antibacterial agent used in the treatment of urinary tract infections.

oxy– *or* **ox–** *pref.* Oxygen, especially additional oxygen: *oxygenation.*

ox·y·bar·bi·tu·rate (ŏk′sē-bär-bĭch′ər-ĭt, -ə-rāt′, -bär′-bĭ-tŏŏr′ĭt, -āt′) *n.* Any of various barbiturates that act as hypnotics and contain an oxygen atom.

ox·y·bu·ty·nin chloride (ŏk′sē-byŏŏt′n-ĭn) *n.* An anticholinergic drug used to treat incontinence and other urinary symptoms.

ox·y·ceph·a·ly (ŏk′sē-sĕf′ə-lē) *n.* A congenital abnormality of the skull in which the top of the head assumes a conical or pointed shape because of premature closing of the lambdoid and coronal sutures. Also called *acrocephaly.* —**ox′y·ce·phal′ic** (-sə-făl′ĭk), **ox′y·ceph′·a·lous** (-sĕf′ə-ləs) *adj.*

ox·y·chro·mat·ic (ŏk′sē-krō-măt′ĭk) *adj.* Of or relating to an acidophil.

ox·y·co·done (ŏk′sĭ-kō′dōn′) *n.* A narcotic alkaloid related to codeine, used as an analgesic and sedative chiefly in the form of its hydrochloride salt.

Ox·y·con·tin (ŏk′sē-kŏn′tn) A trademark for the drug oxycodone.

ox·y·es·the·sia (ŏk′sē-ĭs-thē′zhə) *n.* See **hyperesthesia.**

ox·y·gen (ŏk′sĭ-jən) *n. Symbol* **O** **1.** An element constituting 21 percent of the atmosphere by volume that occurs as a diatomic gas, O_2, combines with most elements, is essential for plant and animal respiration, and is required for nearly all combustion. Atomic number 8. **2.** A medicinal gas used therapeutically for oxygen supplementation, containing not less than 99.0 percent, by volume, of O_2.

oxygen affinity hypoxia *n.* Hypoxia due to the reduced ability of hemoglobin to release oxygen.

ox·y·gen·ase (ŏk′sĭ-jə-nās′, -nāz′) *n.* An enzyme that catalyzes the incorporation of molecular oxygen into its substrate. Also called *direct oxidase.*

ox·y·gen·ate (ŏk′sĭ-jə-nāt′) *or* **ox·y·gen·ize** (-jə-nīz′) *v.* To treat, combine, or infuse with oxygen.

oxygenated hemoglobin *n.* See **oxyhemoglobin.**

ox·y·gen·a·tion (ŏk′sĭ-jə-nā′shən) *n.* The addition of oxygen to a chemical substance or physical system.

oxygen capacity *n.* The amount of oxygen that a quantity of blood is able to absorb.

oxygen consumption *n.* An expression of the rate at which oxygen is used by tissues, usually given in microliters of oxygen consumed in 1 hour by 1 milligram dry weight of tissue.

oxygen debt *n.* The amount of extra oxygen required by muscle tissue to oxidize lactic acid and replenish depleted ATP and phosphocreatine following vigorous exercise.

oxygen deficit *n.* The difference between oxygen uptake of the body during early stages of exercise and during a similar duration in a steady state of exercise, sometimes considered as the formation of oxygen debt.

oxygen demand *n.* Biochemical oxygen demand.

oxygen-deprivation theory of narcosis *n.* The theory that narcotics inhibit oxidation and that this inhibition narcotizes the cell.

oxygen mask *n.* A masklike device that is placed over the mouth and nose and through which oxygen is supplied from an attached storage tank.

oxygen tent *n.* A canopy placed over the head and shoulders or over the entire body of a patient to provide oxygen at a higher level than normal.

oxygen toxicity *n.* A condition resulting from breathing high partial pressures of oxygen, characterized by visual and hearing abnormalities, unusual fatigue, muscular twitching, anxiety, confusion, incoordination, and convulsions.

ox·y·geu·sia (ŏk′sĭ-gyŏŏ′zhə, -jŏŏ′-) *n.* See **hypergeusia.**

ox·y·heme (ŏk′sĭ-hēm′) *n.* See **hematin.**

ox·y·he·mo·chro·mo·gen (ŏk′sē-hē′mə-krō′mə-jən) *n.* See **hematin.**

ox·y·he·mo·glo·bin (ŏk′sē-hē′mə-glō′bĭn) *n.* Hemoglobin in combination with oxygen, present in arterial blood. Also called *oxygenated hemoglobin.*

ox·y·me·taz·o·line (ŏk′sē-mĭ-tăz′ə-lēn′, -mĕt′ə-zō-) *n.* A vasoconstricting drug that is used topically in the form of its hydrochloride to reduce nasal congestion.

ox·y·my·o·glo·bin (ŏk′sē-mī′ə-glō′bĭn) *n.* A pigment formed by the oxidation of myoglobin.

ox·yn·tic (ŏk-sĭn′tĭk) *adj.* Forming or secreting acid, as the parietal cells of gastric glands.

oxyntic cell *n.* See **parietal cell.**

ox·y·phil (ŏk′sĭ-fĭl′) *or* **ox·y·phile** (-fīl′) *n.* **1.** See **eosinophil** (sense 1). **2.** See **oxyphil cell.** —**ox′y·phil′ic** (-fĭl′ĭk) *adj.*

oxyphil cell *n.* A cell in the parathyroid gland that stains easily with acid dyes. Also called *oxyphil.*

oxyphilic leukocyte *n.* See **eosinophil** (sense 1).

ox·y·pho·ni·a (ŏk′sĭ-fō′nē-ə) *n.* Shrillness or high pitch of the voice.

ox·y·pol·y·gel·a·tin (ŏk′sē-pŏl′ē-jĕl′ə-tn) *n.* An oxidized polymerized gelatin used as a plasma extender in transfusions.

ox·yt·a·lan (ŏk-sĭt′ə-lăn′) *n.* A type of connective tissue fiber distinct from collagen or elastic fibers and found in the periodontal membrane and gums.

ox·y·tet·ra·cy·cline (ŏk′sē-tĕt′rə-sī′klĭn, -klēn′) *n.* A broad-spectrum antibiotic derived from the actinomycete *Streptomyces rimosus* and used to treat a variety of bacterial infections.

ox·y·to·cia (ŏk′sĭ-tō′shə) *n.* An unusually rapid childbirth.

ox·y·to·cic (ŏk′sĭ-tō′sĭk) *adj.* Hastening or facilitating childbirth, especially by stimulating contractions of the uterus. Used of a drug. —*n.* An oxytocic drug.

ox·y·to·cin (ŏk′sĭ-tō′sĭn) *n.* A short polypeptide hormone that is released from the posterior lobe of the pituitary gland, stimulates the contraction of smooth muscle of the uterus during labor, and facilitates release of milk from the breast during nursing.

ox·y·u·ri·a·sis (ŏk′sē-yōō-rī′ə-sĭs) *n.* Infestation with parasitic nematodes of the family *Oxyuridae.*

ox·y·u·ri·cide (ŏk′sĭ-yōōr′ĭ-sīd′) *n.* An agent that destroys pinworms.

Ox·y·u·ri·dae (ŏk′sĭ-yōōr′ĭ-dē) *n.* A family of parasitic nematodes found in the large intestine of vertebrates and in the intestine of invertebrates.

Ox·y·u·ris (ŏk′sĭ-yōōr′ĭs) *n.* A genus of nematodes that contains certain species parasitic in the large intestine of humans.

–oyl *suff.* An organic acid radical: *fumaroyl.*

oz *or* **oz.** *abbr.* ounce

o·ze·na (ō-zē′nə) *n.* A chronic disease of the nose characterized by intranasal crusting, atrophy, and a fetid odor.

o·zone (ō′zōn′) *n.* A blue gaseous allotrope of oxygen formed naturally from diatomic oxygen by electric discharge or exposure to ultraviolet radiation. It is an unstable, powerfully bleaching, poisonous oxidizing agent with a pungent irritating odor, used to deodorize air, purify water, treat industrial wastes, and as a bleach.

o·zo·sto·mi·a (ō′zə-stō′mē-ə) *n.* Foul-smelling breath; halitosis.

P

π   The Greek letter *pi*. Entries beginning with this character are alphabetized under **pi**.

φ   The Greek letter *phi*. Entries beginning with this character are alphabetized under **phi**.

ψ   The Greek letter *psi*. Entries beginning with this character are alphabetized under **psi**.

P   The symbol for the element **phosphorus**.

p– *abbr.* para–

p53 (pē′fĭf′tē-thrē′) *n.* A protein that is the product of a tumor suppressor gene, regulates cell growth and proliferation, and prevents unrestrained cell division after chromosomal damage, as from ultraviolet or ionizing radiation. The absence of p53 as a result of a gene mutation increases the risk of developing various cancers.

Pa   The symbol for the element **protactinium**.

PA *abbr.* physician's assistant; posteroanterior; pulmonary artery

PABA (pä′bə) *n.* Para-aminobenzoic acid; a crystalline para form of aminobenzoic acid that is part of the vitamin B complex, required by many organisms for the formation of folic acids, and widely used in sunscreens to absorb ultraviolet light. Also called *vitamin Bₓ*.

PAC *abbr.* premature atrial contraction

pac·chi·o·ni·an (păk′ē-ō′nē-ən) *adj.* Relating to or described by Italian anatomist Antonio Pacchioni (1665–1726).

pacchionian body *n.* See **arachnoid granulation**.

pacchionian depression *n.* Any of various small pits on the inner surface of the skull along the sagittal sinus that contain arachnoid granulations.

pace·fol·low·er (pās′fŏl′ō-ər) *n.* A cell in excitable tissue that responds to stimuli from a pacemaker.

pace·mak·er (pās′mā′kər) *n.* **1.** A part of the body, such as the specialized mass of cardiac muscle fibers of the sinoatrial node, that sets the pace or rhythm of physiological activity. **2.** Any of several usually miniaturized and surgically implanted electronic devices used to stimulate or regulate contractions of the heart muscle. **3.** A substance whose rate or reaction sets the pace for a series of chain reactions. **4.** The rate-limiting reaction itself. —**pace′mak′ing** *adj. & n.*

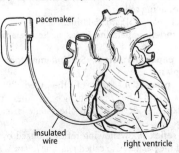

pacemaker
fixed-rate artificial pacemaker

pachy– *pref.* Thick: *pachyderma*.

pach·y·bleph·a·ron (păk′ē-blĕf′ə-rŏn′) *n.* Thickening of the tarsal border of the eyelid.

pach·y·ceph·a·ly (păk′ē-sĕf′ə-lē) *n.* Abnormal thickness of the skull. —**pach′y·ce·phal′ic** (păk′ē-sə-făl′ĭk) *adj.*

pach·y·chei·li·a *or* **pach·y·chi·li·a** (păk′ĭ-kī′lē-ə) *n.* Swelling or abnormal thickness of the lips.

pach·y·chro·mat·ic (păk′ē-krō-măt′ĭk) *adj.* Having coarse chromatin threads.

pach·y·dac·ty·ly (păk′ē-dăk′tə-lē) *n.* Abnormal enlargement of the fingers or toes.

pach·y·der·ma (păk′ĭ-dûr′mə) *n.* Abnormally thick skin.

pachyderma la·ryn·gis (lə-rĭn′jĭs) *n.* A circumscribed connective tissue hyperplasia at the posterior commissure of the larynx.

pachyderma lym·phan·gi·ec·tat·i·ca (lĭm-făn′jē-ĭk-tăt′ĭ-kə) *n.* Elephantiasis due to lymph stasis.

pach·y·der·ma·to·cele (păk′ĭ-dûr′mə-tə-sēl′, -dûr-măt′ə-) *n.* **1.** See **cutis laxa**. **2.** A neurofibroma of extremely large size.

pachyderma ve·si·cae (vĭ-sī′kē′, -sē′-) *n.* Elephantiasis with lymph vesicles on the skin surface.

pach·y·der·mo·per·i·os·to·sis (păk′ĭ-dûr′mō-pĕr′ē-ŏ-stō′sĭs) *n.* A hereditary syndrome characterized by clubbing of the digits, periostosis of the long bones, and coarsening of the facial features, with thickening, furrowing, and oiliness of the skin of the face and forehead.

pach·y·glos·si·a (păk′ĭ-glŏs′ē-ə) *n.* See **macroglossia**.

pach·y·gy·ri·a (păk′ĭ-jī′rē-ə) *n.* Unusually thick convolutions of the cerebral cortex.

pach·y·lep·to·men·in·gi·tis (păk′ē-lĕp′tō-mĕn′ĭn-jī′tĭs) *n.* Inflammation of the membranes of the brain or spinal cord.

pach·y·men·in·gi·tis (păk′ē-mĕn′ĭn-jī′tĭs) *n.* A condition in which the dura mater becomes inflamed. Also called *perimeningitis*.

pach·y·me·nin·gop·a·thy (păk′ē-mĕn′ĭng-gŏp′ə-thē) *n.* Disease of the dura mater.

pach·y·me·ninx (păk′ē-mē′nĭngks) *n.* See **dura mater**.

pa·chyn·sis (pă-kĭn′sĭs) *n.* A pathological thickening of a bodily organ, tissue, or structure. —**pa·chyn′tic** *adj.*

pach·y·o·nych·i·a (păk′ē-ō-nĭk′ē-ə) *n.* Abnormal thickness of the fingernails or toenails.

pachyonychia con·gen·i·ta (kən-jĕn′ĭ-tə) *n.* A hereditary syndrome marked by abnormal thickness and elevation of the nail plates, palmar and plantar hyperkeratosis, and a whitish and glazed tongue due to papillary atrophy. Also called *Jadassohn-Lewandowsky syndrome*.

pach·y·per·i·os·ti·tis (păk′ĭ-pĕr′ē-ŏ-stō′sĭs) *n.* Proliferative thickening of the periosteum caused by inflammation.

pach·y·per·i·to·ni·tis (păk′ē-pĕr′ĭ-tn-ī′tĭs) *n.* Inflammation of the peritoneum with thickening of the membrane.

pach·y·pleu·ri·tis (păk′ē-ploo-rī′tĭs) *n.* Inflammation of the pleura with thickening of the membrane.

pach·y·sal·pin·gi·tis (păk′ē-săl′pĭn-jī′tĭs) *n.* See **chronic interstitial salpingitis.**

pach·y·sal·pin·go·o·va·ri·tis (păk′ē-săl-pĭng′gō-ō′və-rī′tĭs) *n.* Chronic parenchymatous inflammation of the ovary and fallopian tube.

pach·y·so·mi·a (păk′ĭ-sō′mē-ə) *n.* Pathological thickening of the soft parts of the body, especially as occurring in acromegaly.

pach·y·tene (păk′ĭ-tēn′) *n.* The third stage of the prophase of meiosis during which the homologous chromosomes become short and thick and divide into four distinct chromatids.

pach·y·vag·i·nal·i·tis (păk′ē-văj′ə-nə-lī′tĭs) *n.* Chronic inflammation, with thickening, of the tunica vaginalis testis.

pach·y·vag·i·ni·tis (păk′ē-văj′ə-nī′tĭs) *n.* Chronic vaginitis with thickening and hardening of the vaginal walls.

pa·cif·a·rin (pə-sĭf′ər-ĭn) *n.* Any of various bacterial products that, introduced in small amounts, protect an organism from an infection or disease without killing the infectious agent.

pac·ing catheter (pā′sĭng) *n.* A cardiac catheter having one or two electrodes at its tip that, when connected to a pulse generator and positioned in the right atrium or ventricle, artificially pace the heart.

Pa·ci·ni (pə-chē′nē, pä-), **Filippo** 1812–1883. Italian anatomist who described the microscopic structure of the lamellated corpuscle.

pacinian corpuscle *n.* See **lamellated corpuscle.**

pack (păk) *v.* **1.** To fill, stuff, plug, or tampon. **2.** To enwrap or envelop the body in a sheet, blanket, or other covering. **3.** To apply a dressing or covering to a surgical site. —*n.* **1.** The swathing of a patient or body part in hot, cold, wet, or dry materials, such as cloth towels, sheets, or blankets. **2.** The materials so used. **3.** An ice pack; an ice bag.

packed-cell volume (păkt′-) *n.* The volume of blood cells in a sample of blood after it has been centrifuged.

pack·er (păk′ər) *n.* **1.** An instrument for tamponing. **2.** See **plugger.**

pack·ing (păk′ĭng) *n.* **1.** The insertion of gauze or other material into a body cavity or wound for therapeutic purposes. **2.** The material so used; a pack.

pac·li·tax·el (păk′lĭ-tăk′səl) *n.* An anticancer drug derived from the bark of the Pacific yew tree and used to treat refractory ovarian and breast cancer.

pad (păd) *n.* **1.** A soft material forming a cushion, used in applying or relieving pressure on a part, or in filling a depression so that dressings can fit snugly. **2.** A fatty mass of tissue acting as a cushion in the body, such as the fleshy underside of a finger or toe.

paed– *pref.* Variant of **pedo–.**

paedo– *pref.* Variant of **pedo–.**

pae·do·morph or **pe·do·morph** (pē′də-môrf′) *n.* An organism that retains juvenile characteristics in the adult form.

pae·do·mor·phism or **pe·do·mor·phism** (pē′də-môr′-fĭz′əm) *n.* **1.** Retention of juvenile characteristics in the adult, occurring in mammals. **2.** Description of adult behavior in terms appropriate to child behavior. —**pae′do·mor′phic** (-fĭk) *adj.*

pae·do·mor·pho·sis or **pe·do·mor·pho·sis** (pē′də-môr′fə-sĭs) *n., pl.* **–ses** (-sēz′) Phylogenetic change in which juvenile characteristics are retained in the adult form of an organism.

PAF *abbr.* platelet-aggregating factor

Pag·et (păj′ĭt), Sir **James** 1814–1899. British surgeon and pathologist who discovered (1834) the parasitic worm that causes trichinosis, described (1874) Paget's disease of the breast, and identified (1877) osteitis deformans.

Pag·et's cell (păj′ĭts) *n.* Any of the large, epithelial cells with clear cytoplasm associated with Paget's disease of the breast or an apocrine gland cancer.

Paget's disease *n.* **1.** A disease, occurring chiefly in old age, in which the bones become enlarged and weakened, often resulting in fracture or deformation. Also called *osteitis deformans.* **2.** A breast cancer affecting the areola and nipple. **3.** A skin cancer arising from apocrine sweat glands.

Paget-von Schröt·ter syndrome (-vŏn shrĕt′ər, -fôn shrœ′tər) *n.* See **thrombose par effort.**

pa·go·pha·gia (pā′gō-fā′jə) *n.* A craving to eat ice, often associated with iron-deficiency anemia.

–pagus *suff.* Conjoined twins: *ectopagus.*

PAH *abbr. para*-aminohippuric acid.

pain (pān) *n.* **1.** An unpleasant sensation occurring in varying degrees of severity as a consequence of injury, disease, or emotional disorder. **2.** One of the uterine contractions occurring in childbirth.

pain-pleasure principle *n.* See **pleasure principle.**

paint (pānt) *n.* A solution or suspension of one or more medicaments applied to the skin with a brush or large applicator. —*v.* To apply medicine to; swab.

paint·er's colic (pān′tərz) *n.* Chronic intestinal pains and constipation caused by lead poisoning.

pair bond (pâr) *n.* The temporary or permanent association formed between a female and male animal during courtship and mating.

Pa·la·de (pə-lä′dē), **George Emil** Born 1912. Russian-born American biologist. He shared a 1974 Nobel Prize for contributions to the understanding of the components of living cells.

pal·a·tal (păl′ə-təl) *adj.* Palatine.

palatal index or **palatine index** *n.* See **palatomaxillary index.**

palatal papillomatosis *n.* See **inflammatory papillary hyperplasia.**

palatal process *n.* Any of the medially directed shelves from the oral surface of the embryonic maxillae that develop into the palate after midline fusion.

palatal reflex *n.* Swallowing reflex induced by stimulation of the palate. Also called *palatine reflex.*

pal·ate (păl′ĭt) *n.* The bony and muscular partition between the oral and nasal cavities; the roof of the mouth.

pal·a·tine (pălʹə-tīnʹ) *adj.* Of or relating to the palate.
palatine artery *n.* **1.** An artery with origin in the facial artery, with distribution to the lateral walls of the pharynx, tonsils, auditory tubes, and soft palate; and with anastomoses to a branch of the facial, lingual, and descending palatine arteries; ascending palatine artery. **2.** An artery with origin in the maxillary artery, with distribution to the soft palate, gums, and bones and mucous membrane of the hard palate; and with anastomoses to the sphenopalatine, palatine, pharyngeal, and tonsillar branches of the facial arteries; descending palatine artery. **3.** An artery that is the anterior branch of the descending palatine artery, supplying the gums and mucous membrane of the hard palate; major palatine artery. **4.** An artery that is of the descending palatine artery in the greater palatine canal, with distribution to the soft palate and tonsils; minor palatine artery.
palatine bone *n.* An irregularly shaped bone posterior to the maxilla, which forms part of the nasal cavity, the eye socket, and the hard palate.
palatine crest *n.* A transverse ridge near the posterior border of the bony palate, located on the inferior surface of the horizontal lamina of the palatine bone.
palatine process *n.* Either of a pair of horizontal plates of the upper jawbone that form the front portion of the roof of the mouth.
palatine reflex *n.* See **palatal reflex.**
palatine ridge *n.* A low narrow elevation in the center of the hard palate, extending rearward over the length of the mucosa of the hard palate.
palatine spine *n.* Any of the longitudinal ridges along the palatine grooves on the lower surface of the palatine process of the upper jawbone.
palatine tonsil *n.* See **tonsil** (sense 2).
palatine vein *n.* A vein that drains the palatine regions and empties into the facial vein.
pal·a·ti·tis (pălʹə-tīʹtĭs) *n.* Inflammation of the palate.
palato– *pref.* Palate: *palatoplasty.*
pal·a·to·glos·sal (pălʹə-tō-glôʹsəl) *adj.* Relating to the palate and the tongue.
palatoglossal arch *n.* Either of two ridges or folds of mucous membrane passing from the soft palate to the side of the tongue and enclosing the palatoglossus muscle.
pal·a·to·glos·sus (pălʹə-tō-glôʹsəs) *n.* A muscle with insertion into the side of the tongue, with nerve supply from the pharyngeal plexus, and whose action raises the back of the tongue and narrows the fauces.
pal·a·tog·na·thous (pălʹə-tŏgʹnə-thəs) *adj.* Having a cleft palate.
pal·a·to·max·il·lar·y (pălʹə-tō-măkʹsə-lĕrʹē) *adj.* Relating to the palate and the maxilla.
palatomaxillary index *n.* A number indicating the relation between the dental arch and palate, equal to the palatomaxillary width multiplied by 100 and divided by the palatomaxillary length. Also called *palatal index.*
pal·a·to·na·sal (pălʹə-tō-nāʹzəl) *adj.* Relating to the palate and the nasal cavity.
pal·a·to·pha·ryn·geal (pălʹə-tō-fə-rĭnʹjəl, -fărʹĭn-jēʹəl) *adj.* Relating to the palate and the pharynx.

palatopharyngeal arch *n.* Either of two ridges or folds of mucous membrane passing from the soft palate to the wall of the pharynx and enclosing the palatopharyngeal muscle.
palatopharyngeal muscle *n.* A muscle that forms the posterior pillar of the fauces, with origin from the soft palate, with insertion into the posterior border of the thyroid cartilage and the aponeurosis of the pharynx, with nerve supply from the pharyngeal plexus, and whose action narrows the fauces, depresses the soft palate, and elevates the pharynx and the larynx.
pal·a·to·phar·yn·gor·rha·phy (pălʹə-tō-fărʹĭng-gôrʹə-fē) *n.* See **staphylopharyngorrhaphy.**
pal·a·to·plas·ty (pălʹə-tə-plăsʹtē) *n.* Surgery of the palate to restore form and function. Also called *uranoplasty.*
pal·a·to·ple·gia (pălʹə-tō-plēʹjə) *n.* Paralysis of the muscle of the soft palate.
pal·a·tor·rha·phy (pălʹə-tôrʹə-fē) *n.* Suture of a cleft palate. Also called *staphylorrhaphy, uranorrhaphy.*
pal·a·tos·chi·sis (pălʹə-tŏsʹkĭ-sĭs) *n.* See **cleft palate.**
pa·la·tum (pə-lāʹtəm) *n., pl.* **–ta** (-tə) The palate.
paleo– *or* **pale–** *pref.* **1.** Ancient; prehistoric; old: *paleopathology.* **2.** Early; primitive: *paleokinetic.*
pa·le·o·cer·e·bel·lum (pāʹlē-ō-sĕrʹə-bĕlʹəm) *n.* The phylogenetically old part of the cerebellum that includes most of the vermis as well as the adjacent medial zone of the cerebellar hemispheres rostral to the primary fissure. Also called *spinocerebellum.*
pa·le·o·cor·tex (pāʹlē-ō-kôrʹtĕks) *n.* The phylogenetically oldest part of the cortical mantle of the cerebral hemisphere, represented by the olfactory cortex.
pa·le·o·e·col·o·gy (pāʹlē-ō-ĭ-kŏlʹə-jē) *n.* The branch of ecology that deals with the interaction between ancient organisms and their environment.
pa·le·o·ki·net·ic (pāʹlē-ō-kə-nĕtʹĭk, -kī-) *adj.* Of or relating to the primitive motor mechanisms underlying muscular reflexes.
pa·le·o·pa·thol·o·gy (pāʹlē-ō-pă-thŏlʹə-jē) *n.* The study of disease in prehistoric times as revealed in archaeologic artifacts.
pa·le·o·stri·a·tum (pāʹlē-ō-strī-āʹtəm) *n.* The phylogenetically old part of the striate body, corresponding to the globus pallidus. —**paʹle·o·stri·aʹtal** (-ātʹl) *adj.*
pa·le·o·thal·a·mus (pāʹlē-ō-thălʹə-məs) *n.* The intralaminar nuclei, believed to be the components of the thalamus to develop earliest in evolution.
pal·i·ki·ne·sia (pălʹĭ-kə-nēʹzhə, -kī-) *n.* Involuntary repetition of movements.
pal·i·la·li·a (pălʹĭ-lāʹlē-ə) *n.* See **paliphrasia.**
pal·in·drome (pălʹĭn-drōmʹ) *n.* A segment of double-stranded DNA in which the nucleotide sequence of one strand reads in reverse order to that of the complementary strand. —**pal·in·droʹmic** (-drōʹmĭk, -drŏmʹĭk) *adj.*
pal·in·dro·mi·a (pălʹĭn-drōʹmē-ə) *n.* A relapse or recurrence of a disease.
pal·in·dro·mic (pălʹĭn-drōʹmĭk, -drŏmʹĭk) *adj.* Relapsing; recurring.
pal·in·gen·e·sis (pălʹĭn-jĕnʹĭ-sĭs) *n.* The repetition by a single organism of various stages in the evolution of its species during embryonic development.

pal·i·nop·si·a (păl′ə-nŏp′sē-ə) *n.* Abnormally recurring visual imagery.

pal·i·phra·sia (păl′ə-frā′zhə) *n.* Involuntary repetition of words or sentences in talking. Also called *palilalia.*

pal·la·di·um (pə-lā′dē-əm) *n. Symbol* **Pd** A soft ductile metallic element occurring naturally with platinum, especially in gold, nickel, and copper ores, and used as a catalyst in hydrogenation and in dentistry. Atomic number 46.

pall·an·es·the·sia (păl′ăn-ĭs-thē′zhə) *n.* The inability to perceive vibration. Also called *apallesthesia.*

pall·es·the·sia (păl′ĭs-thē′zhə) *n.* The perception of vibration. —**pall′es·thet′ic** (-thĕt′ĭk) *adj.*

pal·li·al (păl′ē-əl) *adj.* Of or relating to the cerebral cortex.

pal·li·ate (păl′ē-āt′) *v.* To reduce the severity of; to relieve somewhat.

pal·li·a·tive (păl′ē-ā′tĭv, păl′ē-ə-tĭv) *adj.* Relieving or soothing the symptoms of a disease or disorder without effecting a cure.

palliative treatment *n.* Treatment to alleviate symptoms without curing the disease.

pal·li·dal (păl′ĭ-dl) *adj.* Relating to the globus pallidus.

pal·li·dec·to·my (păl′ĭ-dĕk′tə-mē) *n.* Excision or destruction of the globus pallidus.

pal·li·do·an·sot·o·my (păl′ĭ-dō-ăn-sŏt′ə-mē) *n.* The production of lesions in the globus pallidus and the lenticular ansa, usually by stereotaxy, in order to stop involuntary movements or to relieve muscular rigidity.

pal·li·dot·o·my (păl′ĭ-dŏt′ə-mē) *n.* A lesion-producing surgical procedure on the globus pallidus to relieve involuntary movements or muscular rigidity.

pal·li·dum (păl′ĭ-dəm) *n.* See **globus pallidus.**

pal·li·um (păl′ē-əm) *n., pl.* **–li·ums** *or* **–li·a** (-lē-ə) The mantle of gray matter with the underlying white substance. Also called *brain mantle, mantle.*

pal·lor (păl′ər) *n.* Paleness, as of the skin.

palm (päm) *n.* The inner surface of the hand that extends from the wrist to the base of the fingers.

pal·ma (păl′mə, päl′-) *n., pl.* **–mae** (-mē) The palm.

pal·mar (păl′mər, päl′-, pä′mər) *adj.* Of, relating to, or corresponding to the palm of the hand.

palmar arch *n.* **1.** The deep arterial arch located below the long flexor tendons in the hand, formed by the radial artery in conjunction with the deep palmar branch of the ulnar artery. **2.** The superficial arterial arch in the hand located above the long flexor tendons, formed principally by the ulnar artery and usually completed by a communication with the superficial palmar branch of the radial artery.

palmar digital artery *n.* **1.** Any of the three arteries arising from the superficial palmar arch and running to the interdigital clefts where each divides into the two proper palmar digital arteries; common palmar digital artery. **2.** Any of the arteries that pass along the side of each finger; proper palmar digital artery; collateral digital artery.

palmar digital vein *n.* Any of the veins that form paired accompanying veins along the proper and common digital arteries and empty into the superficial palmar venous arch.

palmar fibromatosis *n.* Nodular fibroblastic proliferation in the palm of one or both hands, preceding or associated with Dupuytren's contracture.

palmar interosseous muscle *n.* Any of three muscles, the first with its origin from the second metacarpal, and the second and the third with origin from the fourth and fifth metacarpals; the first with insertion into the index finger, and the second and the third with insertion into the ring and little fingers; with nerve supply from the ulnar nerve, and whose action adducts the fingers toward the axis of the middle finger.

palmar metacarpal vein *n.* Any of the veins that empty into the deep venous arch, from which the radial and ulnar veins arise.

pal·mate (păl′māt′, păl′māt, pä′māt′) *or* **pal·mat·ed** (-mā′tĭd) *adj.* Having a shape similar to that of a hand with the fingers extended.

palmate fold *n.* Either of two longitudinal ridges, anterior and posterior, in the mucous membrane lining the uterine cervix.

pal·mic (păl′mĭk) *adj.* Relating to a palmus; pulsating or throbbing.

pal·mit·ic acid (păl-mĭt′ĭk, päl-, pä-mĭt′-) *n.* A saturated fatty acid occurring in palm oil and other fats. Also called *hexadecanoic acid.*

pal·mi·to·le·ic acid (păl′mĭ-tō-lē′ĭk, päl′-, pä′-) *n.* An unsaturated fatty acid that is a common constituent of the glycerides of human adipose tissue.

pal·mo·plan·tar keratoderma (păl′mō-plăn′tər, -tär′, päl′mō-, pä′mō-) *n.* An inherited disorder in which diffuse or patchy areas of hypertrophy occur symmetrically and bilaterally on the horny layer of the epidermis on the palms and soles.

pal·mus (păl′məs) *n., pl.* **–mi** (-mī) A rhythmical fibrillary contraction in a muscle.

pal·pa·ble (păl′pə-bəl) *n.* **1.** Perceptible to touch; capable of being palpated. **2.** Evident; obvious.

pal·pate (păl′pāt′) *v.* To examine by feeling and pressing with the palms of the hands and the fingers. —**pal·pa′tion** *n.* —**pal′pa·tor′y** (-pə-tôr′ē) *adj.*

palpatory percussion *n.* Finger percussion in which the resistance of the tissues under the finger as well as the sound elicited are used in aiding diagnosis.

pal·pe·bra (păl′pə-brə, păl-pē′-) *n., pl.* **–pe·bras** *or* **–pe·brae** (-pə-brē′, -pē′brē) See **eyelid.** —**pal′pe·bral** (păl′pə-brəl, păl-pē′brəl, -pĕb′rəl) *adj.*

palpebral artery *n.* Any of the lateral and medial sets of the branches of the ophthalmic artery supplying the upper and lower eyelids.

palpebral fissure *n.* The longitudinal opening between the upper and lower eyelids.

pal·pe·bro·na·sal fold (păl′pə-brō-nā′zəl) *n.* See **epicanthic fold.**

pal·pi·ta·tion (păl′pĭ-tā′shən) *n.* Perceptible forcible pulsation of the heart, usually with an increase in frequency or force, with or without irregularity in rhythm.

pal·sy (pôl′zē) *n.* Complete or partial muscle paralysis, often accompanied by loss of sensation and uncontrollable body movements or tremors.

pal·u·dism (păl′yə-dĭz′əm) *n.* See **malaria.**

p·a·mi·no·hip·pu·ric acid clearance (pē′ə-mē′nō-hə-pyo͞or′ĭk) *n.* A test to determine renal plasma flow using *p*-aminohippuric acid which, if injected intravenously to achieve low plasma concentrations, is almost totally cleared by the kidneys.

pam·pin·i·form (păm-pĭn′ə-fôrm′) *adj.* Having the shape of a tendril.

pampiniform plexus *n.* A plexus that is formed, in the male, by veins from the testicle and the epididymis, lies in front of the vas deferens, and forms part of the spermatic cord; in the female, the plexus is formed by the ovarian veins between the layers of the broad ligament.

pan– *pref.* **1.** All: *panagglutinins.* **2.** General; whole: *panimmunity.*

pan·a·ce·a (păn′ə-sē′ə) *n.* A remedy claimed to be curative of all problems or disorders; a cure-all.

pan·ac·i·nar emphysema (păn-ăs′ĭ-nər, -när′) *n.* See panlobular emphysema.

Pan·a·dol (păn′ə-dôl′, -dŏl′) A trademark for the drug acetaminophen.

pan·ag·glu·ti·nin (păn′ə-glo͞ot′n-ĭn) *n.* An agglutinin that reacts with all human red blood cells.

pan·an·gi·i·tis (păn′ăn-jē-ī′tĭs) *n.* Inflammation involving all of the tissue layers of a blood vessel.

pan·ar·thri·tis (păn′är-thrī′tĭs) *n.* **1.** Inflammation involving all the tissues of a joint. **2.** Inflammation of all the joints of the body.

pan·at·ro·phy (păn-ăt′rə-fē) *n.* **1.** Atrophy of all the parts of a structure. **2.** General atrophy of the body.

pan·cake kidney (păn′kāk′) *n.* A disk-shaped organ produced by congenital fusion of both poles of the embryonic kidneys.

pan·car·di·tis (păn′kär-dī′tĭs) *n.* Diffuse inflammation of the heart.

Pan·coast's operation (păn′kōsts′) *n.* Division of the trigeminal nerve at the oval foramen.

Pan·coast syndrome (păn′kōst′) *n.* A syndrome characterized by pain and tingling of the arm, constriction of the pupil, and paralysis of the elevator muscle of the upper eyelid, caused by pressure on the brachial plexus resulting from invasion of a malignant tumor in the apex of the lung.

pan·co·lec·to·my (păn′kə-lĕk′tə-mē) *n.* Surgical removal of the entire colon.

pan·cre·as (păng′krē-əs) *n., pl.* **pan·cre·a·ta** (păng-krē′ə-tə) A lobulated gland without a capsule, extending from the concavity of the duodenum to the spleen, consisting of a flattened head within the duodenal concavity, an elongated three-sided body extending across the abdomen, and a tail touching the spleen, and secreting insulin and glucagon internally and pancreatic juice externally into the intestine. —**pan′cre·at′ic** (păng′krē-ăt′ĭk) *adj.*

pancreat– *pref.* Variant of pancreato–.

pan·cre·a·tal·gia (păng′krē-ə-tăl′jə) *n.* Pain arising from, or felt in or near, the pancreas.

pan·cre·a·tec·to·my (păng′krē-ə-tĕk′tə-mē) *n.* Excision of the pancreas.

pancreatic artery *n.* **1.** An artery with origin in the splenic artery and with distribution to the head and body of the pancreas; dorsal pancreatic artery. **2.** An

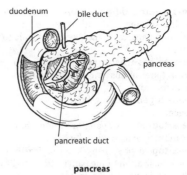

duodenum bile duct

pancreas

pancreatic duct

pancreas
cutaway view

artery with origin in the dorsal pancreatic artery and with distribution to the body and tail of the pancreas; inferior pancreatic artery. **3.** An artery with origin in the splenic artery and with distribution to the tail of the pancreas; great pancreatic artery.

pancreatic digestion *n.* Digestion in the intestine by the enzymes of the pancreatic juice.

pancreatic duct *n.* The excretory duct of the pancreas, extending through the gland from tail to head, where it empties into the duodenum. Also called *Wirsung's canal.*

pancreatic juice *n.* A clear, alkaline secretion of the pancreas containing enzymes that aid in the digestion of proteins, carbohydrates, and fats.

pancreatico– *pref.* Pancreas: *pancreaticoduodenal.*

pan·cre·at·i·co·du·o·de·nal (păng′krē-ăt′ĭ-kō-do͞o′ə-dē′nəl, -do͞o-ŏd′n-əl) *adj.* Relating to the pancreas and the duodenum.

pancreaticoduodenal artery *n.* **1.** Either of two arteries, anterior and posterior, with origin in the superior mesenteric artery and with distribution to the head of the pancreas and to the duodenum; inferior pancreaticoduodenal artery. **2.** Either of two arteries, anterior and superior, with origin in the gastroduodenal artery and with distribution to the head of the pancreas, the duodenum, and the common bile duct; superior pancreaticoduodenal artery.

pancreaticoduodenal vein *n.* Any of the veins that accompany the superior and inferior pancreaticoduodenal arteries and empty into the superior mesenteric or portal veins.

pancreatic vein *n.* Any of the veins draining the pancreas and emptying into the splenic and superior mesenteric veins.

pan·cre·a·tin (păng′krē-ə-tĭn, păng-krē′ə-tĭn) *n.* A mixture of pancreatic juice enzymes, such as amylase, lipase, and trypsin, extracted from animals such as cattle or hogs and used as a digestive aid.

pan·cre·a·ti·tis (păng′krē-ə-tī′tĭs) *n.* Inflammation of the pancreas.

pancreato– *or* **pancreat–** *pref.* Pancreas: *pancreatolith.*

pan·cre·a·to·du·o·de·nec·to·my (păng′krē-ə-tō-do͞o′-ō-dn-ĕk′tə-mē, -do͞o-ŏd′n-ĕk′-) *n.* Excision of all or part of the pancreas together with the duodenum. Also called *Whipple's operation.*

pan·cre·a·to·du·o·de·nos·to·my (păng'krē-ə-tō-dōō'ə-dn-ŏs'tə-mē, -dōō-ŏd'n-ŏs'-) *n.* Surgical anastomosis of a pancreatic duct, cyst, or fistula to the duodenum.

pan·cre·a·to·gas·tros·to·my (păng'krē-ə-tō-gă-strŏs'tə-mē) *n.* Surgical anastomosis of a pancreatic cyst or fistula to the stomach.

pan·cre·a·to·gen·ic (păng'krē-ə-tō-jĕn'ĭk) *adj.* Pancreatogenous.

pan·cre·a·tog·en·ous (păng'krē-ə-tŏj'ə-nəs) *adj.* Of pancreatic origin; formed in the pancreas.

pan·cre·a·tog·ra·phy (păng'krē-ə-tŏg'rə-fē) *n.* Radiographic visualization of the pancreatic ducts after injection of radiopaque material into the collecting system.

pan·cre·a·to·je·ju·nos·to·my (păng'krē-ə-tō-jə-jōō'nŏs'tə-mē, -jē'jōō-, -jĕj'ōō-) *n.* The surgical formation of an artificial opening between the jejunum and a pancreatic duct, cyst, or fistula.

pan·cre·at·o·lith (păng'krē-ăt'ə-lĭth') *n.* A concretion in the pancreatic duct.

pan·cre·a·to·li·thec·to·my (păng'krē-ə-tō-lĭ-thĕk'tə-mē, -ăt'ō-) *n.* See pancreatolithotomy.

pan·cre·a·to·li·thi·a·sis (păng'krē-ə-tō-lĭ-thī'ə-sĭs, -ăt'ō-) *n.* Concretions in the pancreatic duct system.

pan·cre·a·to·li·thot·o·my (păng'krē-ə-tō-lĭ-thŏt'ə-mē, -ăt'ō-) *n.* Surgical removal of a pancreatic concretion. Also called *pancreatolithectomy.*

pan·cre·a·tol·y·sis (păng'krē-ə-tŏl'ĭ-sĭs) *n.* Destruction of pancreatic tissue. —**pan'cre·at·o·lyt'ic** (-ăt'ə-lĭt'ĭk) *adj.*

pan·cre·a·top·a·thy (păng'krē-ə-tŏp'ə-thē) *n.* Disease of the pancreas.

pan·cre·a·tot·o·my (păng'krē-ə-tŏt'ə-mē) *n.* Incision of the pancreas.

pan·cre·a·trop·ic (păng'krē-ə-trŏp'ĭk, -trō'pĭk) *adj.* Exerting an action on the pancreas.

pan·cre·lip·ase (păng'krĭ-lĭp'ās', -lī'pās') *n.* A lipolytic concentrate of pancreatic enzymes standardized for lipase content and used as an enzyme substitute when pancreatic enzymes are insufficient.

pan·cre·o·zy·min (păng'krē-ō-zī'mĭn) *n.* See cholecystokinin.

pan·cy·to·pe·ni·a (păn'sī-tə-pē'nē-ə) *n.* A pronounced reduction in all of the formed elements of the blood.

pan·dem·ic (păn-dĕm'ĭk) *adj.* Epidemic over a wide geographic area. —*n.* A pandemic disease.

Pan·der (păn'dər), **Christian Heinrich** 1794–1865. Russian-born German anatomist and pioneer embryologist. With Karl Ernst von Baer he discovered the distinct structural layers of the chick embryo.

pan·en·ceph·a·li·tis (păn'ĕn-sĕf'ə-lī'tĭs) *n.* Encephalitis that affects both the gray and white matter of the brain, resulting in progressive loss of mental and motor functions.

pan·en·do·scope (păn-ĕn'də-skōp') *n.* An illuminated instrument for inspecting the interior of the urethra as well as the bladder.

pan·es·the·sia (păn'ĭs-thē'zhə) *n.* The sum of all the sensations experienced by a person at one time.

Pa·neth's granular cell (pä'näts, -nĕts) *n.* Any of the coarsely granular secretory cells located in the intestinal glands of the small intestine and appendix.

pang (păng) *n.* A sudden sharp spasm of pain.

pan·hy·po·pi·tu·i·ta·rism (păn'hī-pō-pĭ-tōō'ĭ-tə-rĭz'-əm) *n.* A state in which secretion of the anterior pituitary hormones is inadequate or absent as a result of destruction of the anterior pituitary gland.

pan·ic (păn'ĭk) *n.* A sudden overpowering feeling of terror. —**pan'ic** *v.*

panic attack *n.* The sudden onset of intense anxiety, characterized by feelings of intense fear and apprehension and accompanied by palpitations, shortness of breath, sweating, and trembling. Also called *anxiety attack.*

panic disorder *n.* An anxiety disorder characterized by the occurrence of intense episodes of extreme anxiety and accompanying symptoms such as shortness of breath, chest pain, sweating, and dizziness.

pan·im·mu·ni·ty (păn'ĭ-myōō'nĭ-tē) *n.* General immunity to all infectious diseases.

pan·lob·u·lar emphysema (păn-lŏb'yə-lər) *n.* Emphysema affecting all parts of the lobules. Also called *panacinar emphysema.*

pan·mic·tic (păn-mĭk'tĭk) *adj.* Relating to panmixia.

pan·mix·i·a (păn-mĭk'sē-ə) *or* **pan·mix·is** (-mĭk'sĭs) *n.* Random mating within a breeding population.

pan·my·e·loph·thi·sis (păn'mī-ə-lŏf'thĭ-sĭs, -lō-tī'-) *n.* See myelophthisis (sense 2).

pan·my·e·lo·sis (păn'mī-ə-lō'sĭs) *n.* Myeloid metaplasia with abnormal immature blood cells in the spleen and liver, associated with myelofibrosis.

Pan·ner's disease (păn'ərz) *n.* Osteochondrosis of the capitellum of the humerus.

pan·nic·u·lar hernia (pă-nĭk'yə-lər) *n.* An escape of subcutaneous fat through a gap in a fascia or in an aponeurosis. Also called *fatty hernia.*

pan·nic·u·lec·to·my (pə-nĭk'yə-lĕk'tə-mē) *n.* Excision of superficial fat of the abdomen.

pan·nic·u·li·tis (pə-nĭk'yə-lī'tĭs) *n.* Inflammation of the subcutaneous fat, especially of the abdominal wall.

pan·nic·u·lus (pə-nĭk'yə-ləs) *n., pl.* **–li** (-lī') A sheet or layer of tissue.

panniculus ad·i·po·sus (ăd'ə-pō'səs) *n.* The superficial fascia that contains a fatty deposit in its areolar substance.

panniculus car·no·sus (kär-nō'səs) *n.* The platysma.

pan·nus (păn'əs) *n., pl.* **pan·ni** (păn'ī) **1.** A membrane of granulation tissue covering the normal surface of the articular cartilages in rheumatoid arthritis. **2.** A membrane of granulation tissue covering the normal surface of the cornea in trachoma.

pan·oph·thal·mi·a (păn'ŏf-thăl'mē-ə, -ŏp-) *or* **pan·oph·thal·mi·tis** (-thəl-mī'tĭs) *n.* Purulent inflammation of all parts of the eye.

pan·o·ram·ic radiograph (păn'ə-răm'ĭk) *n.* A radiograph of the maxilla and mandible extending from the left to right glenoid fossa.

panoramic x-ray film *n.* A dental x-ray film that gives a panoramic view of the entire upper and lower dental arch and the temporomandibular joint.

pan·o·ti·tis (păn'ō-tī'tĭs) *n.* Inflammation of the entire ear.

pan·si·nus·i·tis (păn'sī-nə-sī'tĭs) *n.* Inflammation of all paranasal sinuses on one or both sides.

pan·sys·tol·ic (păn′sĭ-stŏl′ĭk) *adj.* Relating to or lasting throughout the systole of a heartbeat.

pansystolic murmur *n.* A murmur extending through the entire systolic interval, from the first to the second sound.

pant (pănt) *v.* To breathe rapidly and shallowly.

pan·tal·gia (păn-tăl′jə) *n.* Pain involving the entire body.

pan·to·mo·gram (păn-tō′mə-grăm′) *n.* A panoramic radiographic record of the maxillary and mandibular dental arches and of their associated structures. —**pan·to′mo·graph′** (-grăf′) *n.* —**pan′to·mog′ra·phy** (-mŏg′rə-fē) *n.*

pan·to·pra·zole sodium (păn-tō′prə-zōl′) *n.* A proton pump inhibitor drug used primarily to treat erosive esophagitis and hypersecretory conditions such as Zollinger-Ellison syndrome.

pan·to·then·ate (păn′tə-thĕn′āt′, păn-tŏth′ə-nāt′) *n.* A salt or ester of pantothenic acid.

pan·to·then·ic acid (păn′tə-thĕn′ĭk) *n.* An oily acid that is widely found in plant and animal tissues, is a component of CoA and a part of the vitamin B$_2$ complex, and functions as a growth factor.

pap (păp) *n.* Soft or semiliquid food, as for infants.

pa·pa·in (pə-pā′ĭn, -pī′ĭn) *or* **pa·pa·in·ase** (-ə-nās′, -nāz′) *n.* An enzyme, or a crude extract containing it, that digests protein, catalyzes the hydrolysis or transfer of esters, amides, or other chemical groups containing sulfur, and is used as a digestive aid.

Pa·pa·ni·co·laou smear (pä′pə-nē′kə-lou′, păp′ə-nĭk′-ə-lou′) *n.* See **Pap smear.**

Papanicolaou stain *n.* A multichromatic stain used principally on exfoliated cytologic specimens, giving great transparency and detail, and important in cancer screening, especially of smears of the female genital tract.

Papanicolaou test *n.* See **Pap smear.**

pa·pav·er·ine (pə-păv′ə-rēn′, -ər-ĭn) *n.* A nonaddictive opium derivative used medicinally to relieve spasms of smooth muscle.

pa·per chromatography (pā′pər) *n.* A form of partition chromatography in which the moving phase is a liquid and the stationary phase is paper.

paper mill worker's disease *n.* An inflammation of alveoli of the lung that is caused by an allergic reaction to airborne spores of a fungi found in moldy wood pulp.

pa·pil·la (pə-pĭl′ə) *n., pl.* **–pil·lae** (-pĭl′ē) **1.** A small nipplelike projection, such as a protuberance on the skin, at the root of a hair or feather, or at the base of a developing tooth. **2.** One of the small, round or cone-shaped protuberances on the top of the tongue that contain taste buds. **3.** A pimple or pustule. —**pap′-il·lar′y** (păp′ə-lĕr′ē, pə-pĭl′ə-rē) *adj.* —**pap′il·late′** (păp′ə-lāt′, pə-pĭl′ĭt) *adj.* —**pap·il·lose** (păp′ə-lōs′, pə-pĭl′ōs′) *adj.*

papilla mam·mae (măm′ē) *n.* See **nipple.**

papilla of corium *n.* See **dermal papilla.**

papillary adenocarcinoma *n.* An adenocarcinoma containing fingerlike processes of vascular connective tissue covered by neoplastic epithelium, projecting into cysts or the cavity of glands or follicles.

papillary adenoma of large intestine *n.* See **villous adenoma.**

papillary carcinoma *n.* A malignant neoplasm characterized by the formation of many irregular, fingerlike projections of fibrous stroma covered with a layer of neoplastic epithelial cells.

papillary cystadenoma *n.* An adenoma of the epididymis or collecting ducts and rete of the testis.

papillary cystadenoma lym·pho·ma·to·sum (lĭm′fō-mə-tō′səm) *n.* See **adenolymphoma.**

papillary cystic adenoma *n.* A tumor in which the lumens of the acini are frequently distended by fluid and the neoplastic epithelial elements tend to form irregular fingerlike projections.

papillary duct *n.* The principal straight excretory duct in the kidney medulla and papillae whose openings form the cribriform area.

papillary hidradenoma *n.* A solitary cystic or papillary tumor occurring usually in the labia majora. Also called *apocrine adenoma.*

papillary muscle *n.* Any of the group of myocardial bundles that terminate in the tendinous cords that attach to the cusps of the atrioventricular valves.

papillary stasis *n.* See **papilledema.**

papillary tumor *n.* See **papilloma.**

pap·il·lec·to·my (păp′ə-lĕk′tə-mē) *n.* Surgical removal of any papilla.

pap·il·le·de·ma (păp′ə-lĭ-dē′mə, pə-pĭl′ĭ-) *n.* Edema of the optic disk. Also called *choked disk, papillary stasis.*

pa·pil·li·form (pə-pĭl′ə-fôrm′) *adj.* Resembling or shaped like a papilla.

pap·il·li·tis (păp′ə-lī′tĭs) *n.* **1.** Inflammation of the optic disk. **2.** Inflammation of a renal papilla.

papillo– *pref.* Papilla; papillary: *papilloadenocystoma.*

pap·il·lo·ad·e·no·cys·to·ma (păp′ə-lō-ăd′n-ō-sĭ-stō′mə) *n.* A benign epithelial tumor characterized by glands or glandlike structures, cysts, and fingerlike projections of neoplastic cells covering a core of fibrous connective tissue.

pap·il·lo·car·ci·no·ma (păp′ə-lō-kär′sə-nō′mə) *n.* **1.** A papilloma that has become malignant. **2.** A carcinoma that is characterized by papillary, fingerlike projections of neoplastic cells with cores of fibrous stroma as a supporting structure.

pap·il·lo·ma (păp′ə-lō′mə) *n., pl.* **–mas** *or* **–ma·ta** (-mə-tə) A benign epithelial tumor projecting from the surrounding surface. Also called *papillary tumor, villoma.* —**pap′il·lo′ma·tous** (-təs) *adj.*

pap·il·lo·ma·to·sis (păp′ə-lō′mə-tō′sĭs) *n.* **1.** The development of numerous papillomas. **2.** Papillary projections of the epidermis forming a microscopically undulating surface.

pap·il·lo·ma·tous (pap-i-lō′mă-tŭs) *adj.* Relating to a papilloma.

papilloma virus *n.* A DNA virus of the genus *Papillomavirus.*

Pap·il·lo·ma·vi·rus (păp′ə-lō′mə-vī′rəs) *n.* A genus of DNA-containing viruses including the papilloma and wart viruses of humans and other animals.

pap·il·lo·ret·i·ni·tis (păp′ə-lō-rĕt′n-ī′tĭs) *n.* Papillitis with extension of the inflammation to neighboring parts of the retina. Also called *retinopapillitis.*

pap·il·lot·o·my (păp′ə-lŏt′ə-mē) *n.* Incision into the major duodenal papilla.

Pa·po·va·vir·i·dae (pə-pō′və-vîr′ĭ-dē′) *n.* A family of small antigenically distinct viruses, comprising the genera *Papillomavirus* and *Polyomavirus,* that replicate in nuclei of infected cells.

pa·po·va·vi·rus (pə-pō′və-vī′rəs) *n.* A virus of the family Papovaviridae.

Pap·pen·hei·mer body (păp′ən-hī′mər) *n.* A phagosome containing ferruginous granules, found in red blood cells in sideroblastic anemia, hemolytic anemia, and sickle cell anemia.

Pap smear (păp) *n.* A screening test, especially for cervical cancer, in which a smear of cells exfoliated or scraped from the cervix or vagina is treated with Papanicolaou stain and examined under a microscope for pathological changes. Also called *Papanicolaou smear, Papanicolaou test, Pap test.*

PAP technique (păp) *n.* An enzymatic antigen detection technique in which an unlabeled antibody peroxidase reacts with both the rabbit antihorseradish peroxidase antibody and with free horseradish peroxidase to form a soluble complex of peroxidase antiperoxidase, or PAP.

Pap test *n.* See Pap smear.

papular acrodermatitis of childhood *n.* See Gianotti-Crosti syndrome.

papular mucinosis *n.* See lichen myxedematosus.

papular tuberculid *n.* A form of cutaneous tuberculosis characterized by a generalized papular eruption in young patients with active infection, thought to be caused by an allergic reaction to the tubercle bacillus. Also called *lichen scrofulosorum.*

papular urticaria *n.* See lichen urticatus.

pap·u·la·tion (păp′yə-lā′shən) *n.* The formation of papules.

pap·ule (păp′yōol) *n., pl.* **–ules** *or* **–u·lae** (-yə-lē′) A small, solid, usually inflammatory elevation of the skin that does not contain pus. —**pap′u·lar** (-yə-lər) *adj.*

papulo– *pref.* Papule: *papulosquamous.*

pap·u·lo·er·y·them·a·tous (păp′yə-lō-ĕr′ə-thĕm′ə-təs, -thē′mə-) *adj.* Relating to an eruption of papules on an erythematous surface.

pap·u·lo·ne·crot·ic tuberculid (păp′yə-lō-nə-krŏt′ĭk) *n.* A chronic form of cutaneous tuberculosis caused by an allergic reaction to the tubercle bacillus, characterized by dusky-red papules primarily on the extremities that become crusty and ulcerated.

pap·u·lo·pus·tu·lar (păp′yə-lō-pŭs′chə-lər) *adj.* Relating to an eruption composed of papules and pustules.

pap·u·lo·sis (păp′yə-lō′sĭs) *n.* The occurrence of numerous widespread papules.

pap·u·lo·squa·mous (păp′yə-lō-skwā′məs, -skwä′-) *adj.* Relating to an eruption composed of papules and scales.

pap·u·lo·ve·sic·u·lar (păp′yə-lō-vĕ-sĭk′yə-lər) *adj.* Relating to an eruption composed of papules and vesicles.

pap·y·ra·ceous (păp′ə-rā′shəs) *adj.* Resembling parchment or paper.

par (pär) *n., pl.* **pa·ri·a** (pä′rē-ə) A pair; specifically, a pair of cranial nerves.

par·a (păr′ə) *n.* A woman who has given birth to an infant or infants.

para– *or* **par–** *pref.* **1.** Beside; near; alongside: *paranucleus.* **2.** Beyond: *parapsychology.* **3.** Incorrect; abnormal: *paradipsia.* **4.** Similar to; resembling: *paratyphoid.* **5.** Subsidiary; assistant: *paramedical.* **6.** Isomeric; polymeric: *paraldehyde.* **7.** A diatomic molecule in which the nuclei have opposite spin directions: *parahydrogen.* **8.** *Abbr.* **p–** Of or relating to one of three possible isomers of a benzene ring with two attached chemical groups in which the carbon atoms with attached groups are separated by two unsubstituted carbon atoms. Usually in italic: para-*bromoiodobenzene.*

–para *suff.* A woman who has given birth to a specified number of children: *multipara.*

par·a·a·mi·no·ben·zo·ic acid (păr′ə-ə-mē′nō-bĕn-zō′ĭk, -ăm′ə-) *n.* PABA.

par·a·a·mi·no·hip·pu·ric acid (păr′ə-ə-mē′nō-hə-pyŏor′ĭk) *n. Abbr.* **PAH** The glycine amide of para-aminobenzoic acid used in renal function tests.

par·a·a·mi·no·sal·i·cyl·ic acid (păr′ə-ə-mē′nō-săl′ĭ-sĭl′ĭk) *n. Abbr.* **PAS, PASA** A bacteriostatic agent used against tubercle bacilli.

par·a·a·or·tic body (păr′ə-ā-ôr′tĭk) *n.* A small mass of chromaffin tissue found near the sympathetic ganglia along the abdominal aorta.

par·a·bal·lism (păr′ə-băl′ĭz′əm) *n.* Severe jerking movements of both legs.

par·a·bas·al body (păr′ə-bā′səl, -zəl) *n.* A structure near the nucleus in certain parasitic flagellates.

par·a·bi·o·sis (păr′ə-bī-ō′sĭs) *n.* **1.** The fusion of whole eggs or embryos, as occurs in conjoined twins. **2.** Surgical joining of the vascular systems of two organisms. —**par·a·bi·ot·ic** (-ŏt′ĭk) *adj.*

par·a·blast (păr′ə-blăst′) *n.* The nutritive yolk of a meroblastic egg.

par·a·blep·si·a (păr′ə-blĕp′sē-ə) *n.* Abnormality of the vision, as in visual illusions or hallucinations.

par·a·bu·li·a (păr′ə-bōo′lē-ə, -byōo′-) *n.* Abnormality of volition or will, as when one impulse is checked and replaced by another.

par·a·ca·sein (păr′ə-kā′sēn′, -sē-ĭn) *n.* A compound produced by the action of rennin upon casein.

Par·a·cel·sus (păr′ə-sĕl′səs), **Philippus Aureolus** 1493–1541. German-Swiss alchemist and physician who introduced the concept of disease to medicine. He held that illness was the result of external agents attacking the body rather than imbalances within the body and advocated the use of chemicals against disease-causing agents.

par·a·ce·nes·the·sia (păr′ə-sē′nĭs-thē′zhə) *n.* A deterioration in one's sense of bodily well-being.

par·a·cen·te·sis (păr′ə-sĕn-tē′sĭs) *n.* Surgical puncture or tapping of a fluid-filled body cavity, especially the abdomen, with a hollow needle or trochar to withdraw fluid. —**par·a·cen·tet·ic** (-tĕt′ĭk) *adj.*

par·a·cen·tral fissure (păr′ə-sĕn′trəl) *n.* A curved fissure on the medial surface of the cerebral hemisphere, bounding the paracentral gyrus and separating it from the precuneus and the cingulate gyrus.

par·a·cer·vi·cal (păr′ə-sûr′vĭ-kəl) *adj.* Adjacent to the uterine cervix.

par·a·cer·vix (păr′ə-sûr′vĭks) *n.* The connective tissue of the pelvic floor, extending laterally from the fibrous subserous coat of the uterine cervix and between the layers of the broad ligament.

par·ac·et·al·de·hyde (păr-ăs′ĭ-tăl′də-hīd′) *n.* See **paraldehyde.**

par·a·chol·er·a (păr′ə-kŏl′ər-ə) *n.* A disease clinically resembling Asiatic cholera, but due to an organism different from *Vibrio cholerae.*

par·a·chord·al (păr′ə-kôr′dl) *adj.* Alongside the anterior portion of the notochord in the embryo. Used of the cartilaginous bars on either side that enter into the formation of the base of the skull.

par·a·chro·ma (păr′ə-krō′mə) *n.* Abnormal coloration of the skin. Also called *parachromatosis.*

par·a·chro·ma·top·si·a (păr′ə-krō′mə-tŏp′sē-ə) *n.* See **dichromatism** (sense 2).

par·a·chro·ma·to·sis (păr′ə-krō′mə-tō′sĭs) *n.* See **parachroma.**

par·a·chute mitral valve (păr′ə-shoot′) *n.* A congenital deformity of the mitral valve in which there is only one papillary muscle present.

parachute reflex *n.* See **startle reflex** (sense 1).

par·a·coc·cid·i·oi·dal granuloma (păr′ə-kŏk-sĭd′ē-oid′l) *n.* See **paracoccidioidomycosis.**

par·a·coc·cid·i·oi·do·my·co·sis (păr′ə-kŏk-sĭd′ē-oi′-dō-mī-kō′sĭs) *n.* A chronic mycosis caused by *Paracoccidioides brasiliensis,* characterized by primary lesions of the lungs with dissemination to many internal organs, by conspicuous ulcerative granulomas of the mucous membranes of the cheeks and nose with extensions to the skin, and by generalized lymphangitis. Also called *Almeida's disease, Lutz-Splendore-Almeida disease, paracoccidioidal granuloma, South American blastomycosis.*

par·a·co·li·tis (păr′ə-kə-lī′tĭs) *n.* Inflammation of the peritoneal coat of the colon.

par·a·crine (păr′ə-krĭn) *adj.* Relating to the release of locally acting substances from endocrine cells.

par·a·cu·sis (păr′ə-koo′sĭs, -kyoo′-) *or* **par·a·cu·sia** (-zhə) *n.* **1.** Impaired hearing. **2.** An auditory illusion or hallucination.

par·a·cys·tic (păr′ə-sĭs′tĭk) *adj.* Alongside or near the urinary bladder.

par·a·cys·ti·tis (păr′ə-sĭ-stī′tĭs) *n.* Inflammation of the connective tissue and other structures surrounding the urinary bladder.

par·a·did·y·mis (păr′ə-dĭd′ə-mĭs) *n.* A small body, sometimes attached to the front of the lower part of the spermatic cord, above the head of the epididymis, composed of the remnants of tubules of the mesonephros. Also called *parepididymis.*

par·a·dip·si·a (păr′ə-dĭp′sē-ə) *n.* An abnormal craving for fluids without relation to bodily need.

par·a·dox (păr′ə-dŏks′) *n.* That which is apparently, though not actually, inconsistent with or opposed to the known facts in any case. —**par′a·dox′i·cal** *adj.*

paradoxical contraction *n.* A contraction of the shin muscles in response to sudden backward flexing of the foot, as during a physical examination.

paradoxical diaphragm phenomenon *n.* A phenomenon occurring in pyopneumothorax, hydropneu-

mothorax, and some cases of injury in which the diaphragm on the affected side rises during inspiration and falls during expiration.

paradoxical embolism *n.* The obstruction of a systemic artery by an embolus that originates in the venous system and reaches the arterial system through a septal defect or an open oval foramen of the heart.

paradoxical pulse *n.* An exaggeration of the normal variation in the pulse during respiration, in which the pulse becomes weaker as one inhales and stronger as one exhales; it is characteristic of constrictive pericarditis or pericardial effusion.

paradoxical reflex *n.* A reflex in which the usual response is reversed or does not conform to the pattern characteristic of the particular reflex.

paradoxical respiration *n.* The deflation of the lung during inspiration and inflation during expiration.

paradoxical sleep *n.* See REM sleep.

par·aes·the·sia (păr′ĭs-thē′zhə) *n.* Variant of **paresthesia.**

par·af·fi·no·ma (păr′ə-fə-nō′mə) *n.* A tumefaction, usually a granuloma, caused by the prosthetic or therapeutic injection of paraffin.

par·a·fol·lic·u·lar cell (păr′ə-fə-lĭk′yə-lər) *n.* Any of the cells rich in mitochondria occurring in the thyroid epithelium, especially around the follicle.

par·a·gan·gli·o·ma (păr′ə-găng′glē-ō′mə) *n.* A tumor usually derived from the chromoceptor or chromaffin tissue of a paraganglion or the medulla of the adrenal gland.

par·a·gan·gli·on (păr′ə-găng′glē-ən) *n.,* *pl.* **–gli·a** (-glē-ə) A small round body containing chromaffin cells, found near the aorta and in the kidney, liver, heart, and gonads. Also called *chromaffin body.*

par·a·geu·sia (păr′ə-gyoo′zhə, -joo′-) *n.* A disordered or abnormal sense of taste.

par·a·gon·i·mi·a·sis (păr′ə-gŏn′ə-mī′ə-sĭs) *n.* Infestation with a worm of the genus *Paragonimus,* especially *P. westermani.*

Par·a·gon·i·mus (păr′ə-gŏn′ə-məs) *n.* A genus of lung flukes parasitic in humans and other mammals that feed upon crustaceans.

Paragonimus wes·ter·man·i (wĕs′tər-măn′ī) *n.* A lung fluke that causes paragonimiasis in humans.

par·a·gram·ma·tism (păr′ə-grăm′ə-tĭz′əm) *n.* See **paraphasia.**

par·a·graph·i·a (păr′ə-grăf′ē-ə) *n.* **1.** The loss of the ability to write from dictation, although the words are understood. **2.** Writing one word when another is intended.

par·a·he·mo·phil·i·a (păr′ə-hē′mə-fĭl′ē-ə, -fēl′yə) *n.* A congenital deficiency of factor V characterized by abnormally slow blood coagulation. Also called *Owren's disease.*

par·a·hip·po·cam·pal gyrus (păr′ə-hĭp′ə-kăm′pəl) *n.* A long convolution located on the medial surface of the temporal lobe of the brain and forming the lower part of the gyrus fornicatus. Also called *hippocampal gyrus.*

par·a·hor·mone (păr′ə-hôr′mōn′) *n.* A substance that is produced from ordinary metabolism and acts like a hormone in influencing the activity of a distant organ.

par·a·in·flu·en·za 1 virus (păr′ə-ĭn′floo-ĕn′zə) *n.* A paramyxovirus that causes acute laryngotracheitis in children and, sometimes, in adults. Also called *hemadsorption virus type 2.*

parainfluenza 2 virus *n.* A paramyxovirus associated with acute laryngotracheitis and croup in young children and minor upper respiratory infections in adults. Also called *croup-associated virus.*

parainfluenza 3 virus *n.* A paramyxovirus associated with pharyngitis, bronchiolitis, and pneumonia in children and with respiratory infections in adults. Also called *hemadsorption virus type 1.*

parainfluenza 4 virus *n.* A paramyxovirus associated with minor respiratory illness in children.

parainfluenza 5 virus *n.* A paramyxovirus that is pathogenic in monkeys but has no known pathogenic effects in humans; it includes the simian viruses.

parainfluenza virus *n.* Any of five types of viruses of the genus *Paramyxovirus* that are associated with various respiratory infections, especially in children.

par·a·ker·a·to·sis (păr′ə-kĕr′ə-tō′sĭs) *n.* Retention of nuclei in the cells of the stratum corneum of the epidermis, as in psoriasis.

par·a·ki·ne·sia (păr′ə-kə-nē′zhə, -kī-) *or* **par·a·ki·ne·sis** (-sĭs) *n.* An abnormality of motor function.

par·a·la·li·a (păr′ə-lā′lē-ə) *n.* A speech defect, especially one in which one sound is habitually substituted for another.

par·al·de·hyde (pə-răl′də-hīd′) *n.* A potent hypnotic and sedative suitable for oral, rectal, intravenous, and intramuscular administration. Also called *paracetaldehyde.*

par·a·lex·i·a (păr′ə-lĕk′sē-ə) *n.* Misapprehension in the reading of written or printed words and substitution of other meaningless words for them.

par·al·ge·si·a (păr′ăl-jē′zē-ə, -zhə) *n.* A disorder or abnormality of the sense of pain.

par·al·lax (păr′ə-lăks′) *n.* The apparent displacement of an object that is caused by a change in the position from which it is viewed. —**par′al·lac′tic** (-lăk′tĭk) *adj.*

parallax test *n.* Measurement of the deviation in strabismus by the alternate cover test, combined with neutralization of the deviation using prisms.

par·al·ler·gic (păr′ə-lûr′jĭk) *adj.* Relating to an allergic state in which the body, after being sensitized with a specific allergen, becomes predisposed to nonspecific stimuli.

par·a·lo·gi·a (păr′ə-lō′jē-ə) *n.* False reasoning; self-deception.

pa·ral·y·sis (pə-răl′ĭ-sĭs) *n., pl.* **–ses** (-sēz′) **1.** Loss of power of voluntary movement in a muscle through injury or through disease of its nerve supply. **2.** Loss of sensation over a region of the body.

paralysis ag·i·tans (ăj′ĭ-tănz′) *n.* See **Parkinson's disease.**

par·a·lyt·ic (păr′ə-lĭt′ĭk) *adj.* **1.** Of or relating to paralysis. **2.** Affected with paralysis. —*n.* A person affected with paralysis.

paralytic abasia *n.* Abasia due to paralysis of the leg muscles.

paralytic dementia *n.* See **general paresis.**

paralytic ileus *n.* Nonmechanical obstruction of the bowel from paralysis of the bowel wall, usually as a result of localized or generalized peritonitis or shock. Also called *adynamic ileus, enteroplegia.*

par·a·ly·zant (păr′ə-lī′zənt, pə-răl′ĭ-zənt) *adj.* Causing paralysis. —*n.* An agent, such as curare, that causes paralysis.

par·a·lyze (păr′ə-līz′) *v.* To affect with paralysis; cause to be paralytic.

par·a·mas·ti·tis (păr′ə-mă-stī′tĭs) *n.* See **submammary mastitis.**

Par·a·me·ci·um (păr′ə-mē′shē-əm, -sē-əm) *n.* A genus of freshwater ciliate protozoans, characteristically slipper-shaped and covered with cilia, and commonly used for genetic research and other studies.

par·a·med·ic (păr′ə-mĕd′ĭk) *n.* A person who is trained to give emergency medical treatment or assist medical professionals.

par·a·med·i·cal (păr′ə-mĕd′ĭ-kəl) *adj.* **1.** Of, relating to, or being a person trained to give emergency medical treatment or assist medical professionals. **2.** Relating to the medical profession in an adjunctive capacity, especially to the allied health fields.

par·a·me·ni·a (păr′ə-mē′nē-ə) *n.* A disorder or irregularity of menstruation.

par·a·mes·o·neph·ric duct (păr′ə-mĕz′ə-nĕf′rĭk) *n.* See **müllerian duct.**

pa·ram·e·ter (pə-răm′ĭ-tər) *n.* **1.** One of a set of measurable factors, such as temperature and pressure, that define a system and determine its behavior and are varied in an experiment. **2.** A factor that determines a range of variations; a boundary. **3.** A statistical quantity, such as a mean or standard deviation of a total population, that is calculated from data and describes a characteristic of the population as opposed to a sample from the population. **4.** A psychoanalytic tactic, other than interpretation, used by the analyst to further the patient's progress. **5.** A factor that restricts what is possible or what results. Not in technical use. **6.** A distinguishing characteristic or feature. Not in technical use. —**par′a·met′ric** (păr′ə-mĕt′rĭk) *adj.*

par·a·me·tri·tis (păr′ə-mĭ-trī′tĭs) *n.* Inflammation of the cellular tissue adjacent to the uterus. Also called *pelvic cellulitis.*

par·a·me·tri·um (păr′ə-mē′trē-əm) *n., pl.* **–tri·a** (-trē-ə) The connective tissue of the pelvic floor extending laterally from the fibrous subserous coat of the supracervical portion of the uterus, and between the layers of the broad ligament. —**par′a·me′tri·al, par′a·me′tric** (-mē′trĭk) *adj.*

par·a·mim·i·a (păr′ə-mĭm′ē-ə) *n.* The use of inappropriate or incorrect gestures in speaking.

par·am·ne·sia (păr′ăm-nē′zhə) *n.* A distortion of memory in which fantasy and objective experience are confused.

par·a·mor·phine (păr′ə-môr′fēn′) *n.* See **thebaine.**

par·am·y·loid (pă-răm′ə-loid′) *n.* A variety of amyloid deposit found in the lymph nodes in certain chronic nonspecific inflammations and in primary localized amyloidosis.

par·am·y·loi·do·sis (pa-răm′ə-loi-dō′sĭs) *n.* A condition resulting from the abnormal accumulation of amyloidlike proteins in tissues.

par·a·my·oc·lo·nus (păr′ə-mī-ŏk′lə-nəs) *n.* See **myoclonus multiplex**.

par·a·my·o·to·ni·a (păr′ə-mī′ə-tō′nē-ə) *n.* An atypical form of myotonia.

Par·a·myx·o·vir·i·dae (păr′ə-mĭk′sə-vîr′ĭ-dē′) *n.* A family of RNA-containing viruses similar in morphology to the influenza viruses.

par·a·myx·o·vi·rus (păr′ə-mĭk′sə-vī′rəs) *n.* A member of the genus *Paramyxovirus*.

Paramyxovirus *n.* A genus of viruses that contain RNA and are similar to but larger and more variable in size than the related myxovirus; it includes the Sendai virus, the parainfluenza viruses, and the viruses that cause measles and mumps.

par·a·na·sal sinus (păr′ə-nā′zəl) *n.* Any of the paired cavities, designated frontal, sphenoidal, maxillary, and ethmoidal, located in the bones of the face and lined by a mucous membrane continuous with that of the nasal cavity.

par·a·ne·o·pla·sia (păr′ə-nē′ō-plā′zhə) *n.* Hormonal, neurological, hematological, and other clinical and biochemical disturbances associated with malignant neoplasms but not directly related to invasion by the primary tumor or its metastases. —**par′a·ne′o·plas′tic** (-plăs′tĭk) *adj.*

paraneoplastic syndrome *n.* A syndrome directly resulting from a malignant neoplasm but not from the presence of tumor cells in the affected parts.

par·a·neph·ros (păr′ə-nĕf′rŏs′) *n., pl.* -**neph·roi** (-nĕf′roi′) See **adrenal gland**. —**par′a·neph′ric** (-nĕf′rĭk) *adj.*

par·a·noi·a (păr′ə-noi′ə) *n.* **1.** A psychotic disorder characterized by systematized delusions, especially of persecution or grandeur, in the absence of other personality disorders. **2.** Extreme, irrational distrust of others.

par·a·noi·ac (păr′ə-noi′ăk′, -noi′ĭk) *n.* A paranoid. —*adj.* Of, relating to, or resembling paranoia.

par·a·noid (păr′ə-noid′) *adj.* Relating to, characteristic of, or affected with paranoia. —*n.* One affected with paranoia.

paranoid personality *n.* A personality disorder characterized by unwarranted mistrust and suspicion, hypersensitivity to the words or actions of others, and rigidity of emotions or behavior.

paranoid schizophrenia *n.* Schizophrenia characterized predominantly by megalomania and delusions of persecution.

par·a·no·mi·a (păr′ə-nō′mē-ə) *n.* Aphasia in which objects are called by the wrong names.

par·a·nu·cle·ar (păr′ə-nōō′klē-ər) *adj.* Outside of, but near, the nucleus.

par·a·nu·cle·ate (păr′ə-nōō′klē-ĭt, -āt′) *adj.* Relating to or having a paranucleus.

par·a·nu·cle·us (păr′ə-nōō′klē-əs) *n.* An accessory nucleus or small mass of chromatin lying near the nucleus.

par·a·op·er·a·tive (păr′ə-ŏp′ər-ə-tĭv, -ə-rā′tĭv, -ŏp′rə-) *adj.* Relating to the accessories and preparation necessary to perform a surgical procedure.

par·a·pa·re·sis (păr′ə-pə-rē′sĭs, -păr′ĭ-sĭs) *n.* Partial paralysis of the lower extremities. —**par′a·pa·ret′ic** (-rĕt′ĭk) *adj.*

par·a·per·i·to·ne·al hernia (păr′ə-pĕr′ĭ-tn-ē′əl) *n.* A vesical hernia in which only a part of the protruded organ is covered by the peritoneum of the sac.

par·a·pha·sia (păr′ə-fā′zhə) *or* **par·a·phra·sia** (-frā′zhə) *n.* Aphasia in which one loses the power of speaking correctly, substitutes one word for another, and jumbles words and sentences in such a way as to make speech unintelligible. Also called *paragrammatism.* —**par′a·pha′sic** (-fā′zĭk) *adj.*

pa·ra·phi·a (pə-rā′fē-ə) *n.* A disorder of the sense of touch. Also called *parapsia.*

par·a·phil·i·a (păr′ə-fĭl′ē-ə, -fēl′yə) *n.* A psychosexual disorder in which sexual gratification is obtained through highly unusual practices that are harmful or humiliating to others or socially repugnant, such as voyeurism or pedophilia.

par·a·phi·mo·sis (păr′ə-fī-mō′sĭs) *n.* **1.** Constriction of the glans penis by a phimotic foreskin, which has been retracted behind the corona. Also called *capistration.* **2.** Retraction of the lid behind a protruding eyeball.

par·a·ple·gia (păr′ə-plē′jə, -jē-ə) *n.* Complete paralysis of the lower half of the body including both legs, usually caused by damage to the spinal cord. —**par′a·ple′gic** (-plē′jĭk) *adj. & n.*

par·a·prax·i·a (păr′ə-prăk′sē-ə) *or* **par·a·prax·is** (păr′-ə-prăk′sĭs) *n.* Defective performance of purposive acts, such as a slip of the tongue, thought to reveal a subconscious motive.

par·a·pro·tein (păr′ə-prō′tēn′) *n.* An abnormal plasma protein, such as a macroglobulin, cryoglobulin, or myeloma protein.

par·a·pro·tein·e·mi·a (păr′ə-prō′tē-nē′mē-ə) *n.* Abnormal proteins in the blood.

pa·rap·si·a (pə-răp′sē-ə) *n.* See **paraphia.**

par·a·pso·ri·a·sis (păr′ə-sə-rī′ə-sĭs) *n.* A chronic dermatosis of unknown origin, with erythematous, papular, and scaling lesions appearing in persistent and often enlarging plaques.

par·a·psy·chol·o·gy (păr′ə-sī-kŏl′ə-jē) *n.* The study of extrasensory perception, such as telepathy, psychokinesis, and clairvoyance. —**par′a·psy′cho·log′i·cal** (-sī′kə-lŏj′ĭ-kəl) *adj.*

par·a·quat (păr′ə-kwŏt′) *n.* A colorless compound or related yellow compound used as a herbicide.

par·a·re·flex·i·a (păr′ə-rĭ-flĕk′sē-ə) *n.* A condition characterized by abnormal reflexes.

par·a·ro·san·i·lin (păr′ə-rō-zăn′ə-lĭn) *n.* A red biological stain used to detect cellular DNA, mucopolysaccharides, and proteins.

par·ar·rhyth·mi·a (păr′ə-rĭth′mē-ə) *n.* A cardiac dysrhythmia in which two independent rhythms coexist, but not as a result of A-V block.

par·a·si·noi·dal (păr′ə-sī-noid′l) *adj.* Near a sinus, especially a cerebral sinus.

parasinoidal sinus *n.* Any of the lateral expansions of the superior sagittal sinus of the dura mater.

par·a·site (păr′ə-sīt′) *n.* **1.** An organism that grows, feeds, and is sheltered on or in a different organism while contributing nothing to the survival of its host. **2.** In conjoined twins, the usually incomplete twin that derives its support from the more nearly normal fetus.

par·a·si·te·mi·a (păr′ə-sī-tē′mē-ə) *n.* The presence of parasites in the blood.

par·a·sit·ic (păr′ə-sĭt′ĭk) *or* **par·a·sit·i·cal** (-ĭ-kəl) *adj.* **1.** Of, relating to, or characteristic of a parasite. **2.** Caused by a parasite.

parasitic cyst *n.* A cyst, such as a hydatid cyst, formed by the larva of a parasite.

par·a·sit·i·cide (păr′ə-sĭt′ĭ-sīd′) *n.* An agent or preparation used to destroy parasites. —*adj.* Destructive to parasites. —**par′a·sit′i·cid′al** (-sīd′l) *adj.*

parasitic melanoderma *n.* Darkening or discoloration of the skin caused by chronic scratching of the bites of the body louse. Also called *vagabond's disease, vagrant's disease.*

par·a·sit·ism (păr′ə-sĭ-tĭz′əm, -sī-) *n.* A symbiotic relationship in which one species, the parasite, benefits at the expense of the other, the host.

par·a·sit·ize (păr′ə-sĭ-tīz′, -sī-) *v.* To live on or in a host as a parasite.

par·a·si·to·gen·ic (păr′ə-sī′tə-jĕn′ĭk) *adj.* **1.** Caused by a parasite. **2.** Favoring parasitism.

par·a·si·tol·o·gy (păr′ə-sĭ-tŏl′ə-jē, -sī-) *n.* The study of parasites and parasitism. —**par′a·si′to·log′ic** (-sī′tə-lŏj′ĭk), **par′a·si′to·log′i·cal** (-ĭ-kəl) *adj.*

par·a·si·to·sis (păr′ə-sĭ-tō′sĭs, -sī-) *n., pl.* **-ses** (-sēz) Infestation with parasites.

par·a·si·tot·ro·pism (păr′ə-sī-tŏt′rə-pĭz′əm) *n.* The affinity of particular drugs or other agents for parasites rather than for their hosts. —**par′a·si′to·trop′ic** (-sī′tə-trŏp′ĭk, -trō′pĭk) *adj.*

par·a·som·ni·a (păr′ə-sŏm′nē-ə) *n.* Any of various sleep dysfunctions, such as somnambulism.

par·a·spa·di·as (păr′ə-spā′dē-əs) *or* **par·a·spa·di·a** (-dē-ə) *n.* A congenital defect of the penis in which the urethra opens to one side of the normal opening.

par·a·sta·sis (păr′ə-stā′sĭs, pə-răs′tə-sĭs) *n.* **1.** The relationship among causal mechanisms that can compensate for, or mask defects in, each other. **2.** In genetics, a relationship between non-alleles considered to be a form of epistasis.

par·a·sym·pa·thet·ic (păr′ə-sĭm′pə-thĕt′ĭk) *adj.* Of, relating to, or affecting the parasympathetic nervous system. —**par′a·sym′pa·thet′i·cal·ly** *adv.*

parasympathetic ganglion *n.* Any of the ganglia of the autonomic nervous system composed of cholinergic neurons receiving afferent fibers originating from preganglionic visceral motor neurons in either the brainstem or the middle sacral segments of the spinal cord.

parasympathetic nerve *n.* One of the nerves of the parasympathetic nervous system.

parasympathetic nervous system *n.* The part of the autonomic nervous system originating in the brainstem and the lower part of the spinal cord that, in general, inhibits or opposes the physiological effects of the sympathetic nervous system, as in tending to stimulate digestive secretions or slow the heart.

par·a·sym·pa·tho·lyt·ic (păr′ə-sĭm′pə-thō-lĭt′ĭk) *adj.* Blocking the effects of the parasympathetic nervous system.

par·a·sym·pa·tho·mi·met·ic (păr′ə-sĭm′pə-thō-mĭ-mĕt′ĭk, -mī-) *adj.* Having an action resembling that caused by stimulation of the parasympathetic nervous system.

par·a·sy·nap·sis (păr′ə-sĭ-năp′sĭs) *n.* Side-to-side union of homologous chromosomes in the process of reduction.

par·a·syn·o·vi·tis (păr′ə-sĭn′ə-vī′tĭs, -sī′nə-) *n.* Inflammation of the tissues immediately adjacent to a joint.

par·a·sys·to·le (păr′ə-sĭs′tə-lē) *n.* An arrhythmia characterized by a second automatic rhythm existing simultaneously with normal sinus rhythm.

par·a·tax·ic distortion (păr′ə-tăk′sĭk) *n.* An attitude toward a person based on a distorted evaluation, usually due to identifying that person with emotionally significant individuals from the past.

par·a·te·ne·sis (păr′ə-tə-nē′sĭs) *n.* The passage of a parasite by one or a series of hosts with no effect on the completion of the life cycle of the parasite.

par·a·ten·ic host (păr′ə-tĕn′ĭk) *n.* An intermediate host whose presence may be required for the completion of a parasite's life cycle but in which no development of the parasite occurs.

par·a·ten·on (păr′ə-tĕn′ən, -ŏn′) *n.* The fatty or synovial material between a tendon and its sheath.

par·a·ter·mi·nal gyrus (păr′ə-tûr′mə-nəl) *n.* See **subcallosal gyrus.**

par·a·thi·on (păr′ə-thī′ŏn) *n.* A highly poisonous organic phosphate insecticide that is an irreversible inhibitor of cholinesterase.

par·a·thy·rin (păr′ə-thī′rĭn) *n.* See **parathyroid hormone.**

par·a·thy·roid (păr′ə-thī′roid) *adj.* **1.** Adjacent to the thyroid gland. **2.** Of, relating to, or obtained from the parathyroid glands. —*n.* **1.** Either of the parathyroid glands. **2.** A parathyroid hormone.

par·a·thy·roid·ec·to·my (păr′ə-thī′roi-dĕk′tə-mē) *n.* Excision of the parathyroid glands.

parathyroid gland *n.* Any of usually four small kidney-shaped glands that lie in pairs near or within the posterior surface of the thyroid gland and secrete a hormone necessary for the metabolism of calcium and phosphorus.

parathyroid hormone *n. Abbr.* **PTH** A peptide hormone produced by the parathyroid glands that regulates the amount of calcium in the body. Also called *parathyrin.*

parathyroid tetany *n.* Tetany following surgical injury to or excision of the parathyroid glands. Also called *parathyroprival tetany.*

par·a·thy·ro·trop·ic (păr′ə-thī′rō-trŏp′ĭk, -trō′pĭk) *or* **par·a·thy·ro·troph·ic** (-trŏf′ĭk, -trō′fĭk) *adj.* Influencing the activity or growth of the parathyroid glands.

par·a·troph·ic (păr′ə-trŏf′ĭk, -trō′fĭk) *adj.* Deriving sustenance from living organic material.

par·a·ty·phoid (păr′ə-tī′foid′) *adj.* Resembling typhoid.

par·a·ty·phoid fever (păr′ə-tī′foid′) *n.* An acute intestinal disease, similar to typhoid fever but less severe, caused by food contaminated with bacteria of the genus *Salmonella.* Also called *enteric fever.*

par·a·um·bil·i·cal vein (păr′ə-ŭm-bĭl′ĭ-kəl) *n.* Any of the small veins that arise from cutaneous veins about the umbilicus and terminate as accessory portal veins.

par·a·u·re·thral duct (păr′ə-yōo-rē′thrəl) *n.* Any of the inconstant ducts along the female urethra that convey the mucoid secretion of the paraurethral glands to the vestibule.

paraurethral gland *n.* Any of several small mucus glands that deliver secretions into the female urethra near its opening.

par·a·vag·i·ni·tis (păr′ə-văj′ə-nī′tĭs) *n.* Inflammation of the connective tissue alongside the vagina.

par·a·ven·tric·u·lar nucleus (păr′ə-věn-trĭk′yə-lər) *n.* A triangular group of large neurons in the periventricular zone of the front half of the hypothalamus, functionally associated with the rear lobe of the pituitary gland.

par·a·ver·te·bral (păr′ə-vûr′tə-brəl, -vər-tē′brəl) *adj.* Located along a vertebra or the vertebral column.

paravertebral ganglion *n.* See **ganglion of sympathetic trunk.**

par·ax·i·al (pă-răk′sē-əl) *adj.* Located alongside of the axis of a body or part.

par·ax·on (pă-răk′sŏn′) *n.* A collateral branch of an axon.

Pa·ré (pä-rā′), **Ambroise** 1517?–1590. French surgeon who made numerous improvements to operating methods, including the ligature of arteries rather than cauterization.

par·e·gor·ic (păr′ə-gôr′ĭk) *n.* A camphorated tincture of opium, taken internally for the relief of diarrhea and intestinal pain.

pa·ren·chy·ma (pə-rĕng′kə-mə) *n.* The distinguishing cells of a gland or organ, contained in and supported by the stroma. —**pa·ren′chy·mal, par′en·chym′a·tous** (păr′ĕn-kĭm′ə-təs) *adj.*

pa·ren·chy·ma·ti·tis (pə-rĕng′kə-mə-tī′tĭs) *n.* Inflammation of the parenchyma of a gland or organ.

parenchymatous degeneration *n.* See **cloudy swelling.**

parenchymatous goiter *n.* Goiter in which there is an increase in the follicles with proliferation of the epithelium. Also called *follicular goiter.*

parenchymatous hemorrhage *n.* Bleeding into the substance of an organ.

parenchymatous keratitis *n.* A chronic inflammation of the cornea characterized by cellular infiltration of its middle and posterior layers. Also called *interstitial keratitis.*

parenchymatous neuritis *n.* Inflammation of nervous tissue, especially the axons and myelin.

par·ent (pâr′ənt) *n.* 1. One who begets, gives birth to, or nurtures and raises a child; a father or mother. 2. An ancestor; a progenitor. 3. An organism that produces or generates offspring. —*v.* 1. To act as a parent to; to rear and nurture. 2. To cause to come into existence; to serve as a source for; originate.

pa·ren·tal (pə-rĕn′tl) *adj.* 1. Of, relating to, or characteristic of a parent. 2. Of or designating the generation of organisms from which hybrid offspring are produced.

parental generation *n.* The generation of individuals of different genotypes that are mated, usually for scientific purposes, to produce hybrids.

parent cyst *n.* See **mother cyst.**

par·en·ter·al (pă-rĕn′tər-əl) *adj.* 1. Located outside the alimentary canal. 2. Taken into the body or administered in a manner other than through the digestive tract, as by intravenous or intramuscular injection. —**par·en′ter·al·ly** *adv.*

par·en·ter·ic fever (păr′ən-tĕr′ĭk) *n.* Any of a group of fevers clinically resembling typhoid and paratyphoid fevers but caused by different bacteria.

par·ep·i·did·y·mis (pă-rĕp′ĭ-dĭd′ə-mĭs) *n.* See **paradidymis.**

pa·re·sis (pə-rē′sĭs, păr′ĭ-sĭs) *n., pl.* **–ses** (-sēz) 1. Slight or partial paralysis. 2. General paresis. —**pa·ret′ic** (pə-rĕt′ĭk) *adj. & n.*

par·es·the·sia *or* **par·aes·the·sia** (păr′ĭs-thē′zhə) *n.* A skin sensation, such as burning, prickling, itching, or tingling, with no apparent physical cause. —**par′es·thet′ic** (-thĕt′ĭk) *adj.*

pa·reu·ni·a (pə-rōo′nē-ə, păr-yōo′-) *n.* Sexual intercourse.

pa·ri·es (pâr′ē-ēz′) *n., pl.* **pa·ri·e·tes** (pə-rī′ĭ-tēz′) A wall of a body part, organ, or cavity, as of the chest or abdomen. Often used in the plural.

pa·ri·e·tal (pə-rī′ĭ-tl) *adj.* 1. Relating to or forming the wall of any cavity. 2. Of or relating to either of the parietal bones.

parietal bone *n.* Either of two irregularly quadrilateral bones between the frontal and occipital bones that together form the sides and top of the skull.

parietal cell *n.* A cell of the gastric glands that secretes hydrochloric acid. Also called *acid cell, oxyntic cell.*

parietal emissary vein *n.* A vein that connects the superior sagittal sinus with tributaries of the superficial temporal vein and with other scalp veins.

parietal endocarditis *n.* See **mural endocarditis.**

parietal fistula *n.* A blind or complete fistula opening on the wall of the thorax or the abdomen.

parietal foramen *n.* An opening in the parietal bone near the sagittal margin to the rear.

parietal hernia *n.* A hernia in which only a portion of the wall of the intestine is involved. Also called *Richter's hernia, Littre's hernia.*

parietal lobe *n.* The middle portion of each cerebral hemisphere, separated from the frontal lobe by the central sulcus, from the temporal lobe by the lateral sulcus, and from the occipital lobe only partially by the parieto-occipital sulcus on its medial aspect.

parietal node *n.* Any of the lymph nodes draining the walls of the abdomen or the pelvis.

parietal thrombus *n.* An arterial thrombus adhering to one side of the wall of the vessel.

parietal wall *n.* The internal body wall that is formed from the somatopleure.

parieto– *pref.* Paries: *parietography.*

pa·ri·e·tog·ra·phy (pə-rī′ĭ-tŏg′rə-fē) *n.* Radiographic imaging of the walls of an organ.

pa·ri·e·to·oc·cip·i·tal sulcus (pə-rī′ĭ-tō-ŏk-sĭp′ĭ-tl) *n.* A deep fissure on the medial surface of the cerebral cortex, marking the border between the parietal lobe and the cuneus of the occipital lobe. Also called *parieto-occipital fissure.*

Pa·ri·naud's oc·u·lo·glan·du·lar syndrome (pä-rē-nōz′ ŏk′yə-lō-glăn′jə-lər) *n.* Conjunctival granuloma in one eye accompanied by swelling of the lymph nodes in front of the auricle of the ear, seen in tularemia, chancre, and tuberculosis.

Parinaud's ophthalmoplegia *n.* Paralysis of the ocular muscles in which the eyes look upward.

par·i·ty (păr′ĭ-tē) *n.* The state of having given birth to an infant or infants.

Par·kin·son (pär′kĭn-sən), **James** 1755–1824. British physician who gave (1817) a comprehensive description of paralysis agitans, or Parkinson's disease, and was the first to recognize (1812) perforation of the appendix as a cause of death in appendicitis.

par·kin·so·ni·an (pär′kĭn-sō′nē-ən) *adj.* Relating to Parkinsonism.

Par·kin·son·ism *or* **par·kin·son·ism** (pär′kĭn-sə-nĭz′əm) *n.* **1.** Any of a group of nervous disorders similar to Parkinson's disease, marked by muscular rigidity, tremor, and impaired motor control and often having a specific cause, such as the use of certain drugs or frequent exposure to toxic chemicals. Also called *Parkinson's syndrome.* **2.** Parkinson's disease.

Par·kin·son's disease (pär′kĭn-sənz) *n.* A progressive nervous disease occurring most often after the age of 50, associated with the destruction of brain cells that produce dopamine, and characterized by muscular tremor, slowing of movement, partial facial paralysis, peculiarity of gait and posture, and weakness. Also called *paralysis agitans.*

Parkinson's facies *n.* The expressionless or masklike features characteristic of Parkinsonism. Also called *masklike face.*

Parkinson's syndrome *n.* See **Parkinsonism.**

Par·lo·del (pär′lə-dĕl′) A trademark for the drug bromocriptine.

par·om·phal·o·cele (păr′ŏm-făl′ə-sēl′, -ŏm′fə-lō-) *n.* **1.** A tumor near the navel. **2.** A hernia through a defect in the abdominal wall near the navel.

par·o·nych·i·a (păr′ə-nĭk′ē-ə) *n.* Inflammation of the tissue surrounding a nail. —**par′o·nych′i·al** *adj.*

par·o·oph·o·ron (păr′ō-ŏf′ə-rŏn′) *n.* Any of the scattered rudimentary tubules located in the broad ligament between the epoophoron and the uterus. Also called *parovarium.*

par·oph·thal·mi·a (păr′ŏf-thăl′mē-ə, -ŏp-) *n.* Inflammation of the tissues surrounding the eye.

par·op·si·a (păr-ŏp′sē-ə) *or* **par·op·sis** (-sĭs) *n.* Disorientation of the perception of direction in hemianopsia caused by occipital lesions.

par·or·chid·i·um (păr′ôr-kĭd′ē-əm) *n.* See **ectopic testis.**

par·o·rex·i·a (păr′ə-rĕk′sē-ə) *n.* Abnormal or inappropriate appetite, especially a craving for items unsuitable as food; pica.

pa·ros·mi·a (pə-rŏz′mē-ə) *n.* A distortion of the sense of smell, as in smelling odors that are not present.

par·os·te·o·sis (păr-ŏs′tē-ō′sĭs) *or* **par·os·to·sis** (păr′ŏs-tō′sĭs) *n.* **1.** Development of bone in an unusual location, as in the skin. **2.** Abnormal or defective ossification.

pa·rot·ic (pə-rŏt′ĭk) *adj.* Near or beside the ear.

pa·rot·id (pə-rŏt′ĭd) *adj.* **1.** Situated near the ear. **2.** Of or relating to a parotid gland. —*n.* A parotid gland.

parotid duct *n.* The duct of the parotid gland opening from the cheek into the vestibule of the mouth opposite the neck of the upper second molar tooth. Also called *Steno's duct, Stensen's duct.*

pa·rot·i·dec·to·my (pə-rŏt′ĭ-dĕk′tə-mē) *n.* Surgical removal of a parotid gland.

parotid gland *n.* Either of a pair of major salivary glands situated below and in front of each ear and opening into the parotid duct; the largest of the major salivary glands.

parotid notch *n.* The space between the ramus of the mandible and the mastoid process of the temporal bone of the skull.

parotid papilla *n.* The projection at the opening of the parotid duct.

parotid vein *n.* Any of the parotid branches of the facial vein that drain part of the parotid gland and empty into the retromandibular vein.

par·o·ti·tis (păr′ə-tī′tĭs) *or* **pa·rot·i·di·tis** (pə-rŏt′ĭ-dī′tĭs) *n.* Inflammation of the parotid glands, as in mumps. —**par′o·tit′ic** (-tĭt′ĭk) *adj.*

par·ous (păr′əs, pâr′-) *adj.* Having given birth one or more times.

–parous *suff.* Giving birth to; producing: *multiparous.*

par·o·var·i·um (păr′ō-vâr′ē-əm) *n.* See **paroophoron.** —**par′o·var′i·an** *adj.*

par·ox·e·tine (pă-rŏk′sĭ-tēn′) *n.* A selective serotonin reuptake inhibitor used as an oral antidepressant.

par·ox·ysm (păr′ək-sĭz′əm) *n.* **1.** A sharp spasm or fit; a convulsion. **2.** A sudden onset of a symptom or disease, especially one with recurrent manifestations, such as the chills and fever of malaria. —**par′ox·ys′mal** (-ək-sĭz′məl) *adj.*

paroxysmal nocturnal dyspnea *n. Abbr.* **PND** Acute dyspnea caused by the lung congestion and edema that results from partial heart failure and occurring suddenly at night, usually an hour or two after the individual has fallen asleep.

paroxysmal nocturnal hemoglobinuria *n.* An infrequent disorder the onset of which usually occurs in the third or fourth decades of life and is characterized by periods of hemolytic anemia, hemoglobinuria primarily at night, pallor, bronzing of the skin, moderate splenomegaly, and red blood cells that are macrocytic and vary considerably in size. Also called *Marchiafava-Micheli syndrome.*

paroxysmal tachycardia *n.* Recurrent attacks of tachycardia, having abrupt onset and termination and originating from an ectopic focus.

paroxysmal trepidant abasia *n.* Abasia due to spastic stiffening of the legs.

par·rot fever (păr′ət) *n.* See **psittacosis.**

Par·rot's disease (pă-rōz′, pä-) *n.* Pseudoparalysis of one or more of the extremities occurring in infants in whom congenital exposure to syphilis has caused inflammation of an epiphysis.

Par·ry's disease (păr′ēz) *n.* See **Graves' disease.**

pars (pärs) *n., pl.* **par·tes** (pär′tēz) A part or portion of a structure, especially of an anatomical structure.

pars a·mor·pha (ə-môr′fə) *n*. The part of the nucleolus that occupies irregular spaces in the nucleolonema and contains finely filamentous matter.

pars gran·u·lo·sa (grăn′yə-lō′sə) *n*. The granular and filamentous part of the nucleolonema.

pars pla·na (plā′nə) *n*. See **ciliary disk**.

pars-pla·ni·tis (pärz′plā-nī′tĭs) *n*. A clinical syndrome characterized by inflammation of the peripheral retina of the eye or of the ciliary disk, exudation into the overlying vitreous base, and edema of the optic disk and adjacent retina.

pars tym·pan·i·ca (tĭm-păn′ĭ-kə) *n*. The tympanic portion of the temporal bone, forming the greater part of the wall of the external acoustic meatus.

part (pärt) *n*. **1.** A portion, division, piece, or segment of a whole. **2.** Any of several equal portions or fractions that can constitute a whole or into which a whole can be divided. **3.** An organ, member, or other division of an organism. **4.** An anatomical part; pars. **5. parts** The external genitalia.

part. aeq. *abbr. Latin* partes aequales, partibus aequalibus (equal parts or amounts, in equal parts or amounts)

par·the·no·gen·e·sis (pär′thə-nō-jĕn′ĭ-sĭs) *n*. A form of reproduction in which an unfertilized egg develops into a new individual, occurring commonly among insects and certain other arthropods. —**par′the·no·ge·net′ic** (-jə-nĕt′ĭk) *adj*.

par·the·nog·e·none (pär′thə-nŏj′ə-nōn′) *n*. An organism produced by parthenogenesis.

par·tial agglutinin (pär′shəl) *n*. See **group agglutinin**.

partial antigen *n*. See **hapten**.

partial-birth abortion *n*. A late-term abortion, especially one in which a viable fetus is partially delivered through the cervix before being extracted. Not in technical use.

partial denture *n*. A removable or fixed dental prosthesis that restores one or more, but less than all, of the natural teeth or associated parts and is supported by the teeth or the soft tissue. Also called *bridgework*.

partial ophthalmoplegia *n*. Ophthalmoplegia involving only one or two of the extrinsic or intrinsic ocular muscles.

partial pressure *n*. The pressure that one component of a mixture of gases would exert if it were alone in a container.

partial seizure *n*. See **focal seizure**.

partial-thickness flap *n*. See **split-thickness flap**.

partial-thickness graft *n*. See **split-thickness graft**.

partial volume *n*. The actual volume occupied by one species of molecule or particle in a solution.

par·ti·cle (pär′tĭ-kəl) *n*. **1.** A very small piece or part. **2.** An elementary particle. **3.** A subatomic particle.

par·tic·u·late (pər-tĭk′yə-lĭt, -lāt′, pär-) *adj*. Of or occurring in the form of fine particles. —*n*. A particulate substance.

par·ti·tion (pär-tĭsh′ən) *n*. **1.** The act or process of dividing something into parts. **2.** The state of being so divided. **3.** A wall, septum, or other separating membrane in an organism.

partition chromatography *n*. Separation of similar substances by repeated extraction by two immiscible liquids.

par·tu·ri·ent (pär-tŏor′ē-ənt) *adj*. **1.** Of or relating to giving birth. **2.** About to bring forth young; being in labor.

parturient canal *n*. See **birth canal**.

par·tu·ri·fa·cient (pär-tŏor′ə-fā′shənt) *n*. Inducing or accelerating childbirth; oxytocic. —*n*. A drug facilitating childbirth.

par·tu·ri·om·e·ter (pär-tŏor′ē-ŏm′ĭ-tər) *n*. A device for determining the force of the uterine contractions in childbirth.

par·tu·ri·tion (pär′tŏo-rĭsh′ən, pär′chə-) *n*. The process of labor and delivery in the birth of a child.

part. vic. *abbr. Latin* partitis vicibus (in divided parts, amounts, or doses)

par·vi·cel·lu·lar (pär′vĭ-sĕl′yə-lər) *adj*. Relating to or composed of cells of small size.

par·vo (pär′vō) *n*. A parvovirus.

Par·vo·vir·i·dae (pär′vō-vîr′ĭ-dē′) *n*. A family of small viruses containing single-stranded DNA; replication and assembly occur in the nucleus of infected cells.

par·vo·vi·rus (pär′vō-vī′rəs) *n*. Any of a group of small viruses of the genus *Parvovirus* that cause disease in many vertebrates, especially mammals such as dogs and cattle.

PAS or **PASA** *abbr. para*-aminosalicylic acid; periodic acid-Schiff

pas·cal (pă-skăl′, pä-skäl′) *n*. A unit of pressure equal to one newton per square meter.

Pas·cal's law (pă-skälz′, pä-skälz′) *n*. The principle that fluids at rest transmit pressure equally in every direction.

Pa·schen body (päsh′ən, pä′shən) *n*. A particle of virus observed in relatively large numbers in squamous cells of the skin in smallpox or vaccinia.

pass (păs) *v*. **1.** To go across; go through. **2.** To cause to move into a certain position. **3.** To cease to exist; die. **4.** To be voided from the body.

pas·sage (păs′ĭj) *n*. **1.** A movement from one place to another. **2.** The process of passing from one condition or stage to another. **3.** A path, channel, or duct through, over, or along which something may pass. **4.** An act of emptying, as of the bowels. **5.** The process of passing or maintaining a group of microorganisms or cells through a series of hosts or cultures.

Pas·sa·vant's cushion (păs′ə-vănts′) *n*. A prominence on the posterior wall of the nasal pharynx formed by contraction of the superior constrictor of the pharynx during swallowing.

pas·sive (păs′ĭv) *n*. **1.** Accepting or submitting without resistance or objection. **2.** Of or being an inactive or submissive role in a relationship, especially a sexual relationship. **3.** Chemically unreactive except under special or extreme conditions; inert.

passive-aggressive personality *n*. A personality disorder in which aggressive feelings are manifested in passive ways, especially through stubbornness, procrastination, and inefficiency so as to resist adequate social and occupational performance.

passive anaphylaxis *n*. An anaphylactic response in a nonsensitized individual caused by inoculation with serum from a sensitized individual. Also called *antiserum anaphylaxis*.

passive clot *n.* A clot that is formed in an aneurysmal sac following the cessation of circulation through the aneurysm.

passive congestion *n.* Congestion in a part of the body caused by the obstruction or slowing of drainage of venous blood.

passive hemagglutination *n.* Passive agglutination in which red blood cells are used to adsorb soluble antigen onto their surfaces; the red blood cells then agglutinate in the presence of antiserum specific for the adsorbed antigen. Also called *indirect hemagglutination test.*

passive hyperemia *n.* Hyperemia resulting from an obstruction in the flow of blood from a body part. Also called *venous hyperemia.*

passive immunity *n.* Immunity acquired by the transfer of antibodies from another individual, as through injection or placental transfer to a fetus.

passive movement *n.* Movement of a joint without participation or effort on the part of the subject.

passive smoke *n.* See **secondhand smoke.**

passive transfer *n.* The transfer of skin-sensitizing antibodies from the blood of an allergic individual to that of a nonallergic individual in order to test for an allergic reaction to specific allergens.

passive tremor *n.* A tremor occurring at rest, and diminishing or ceasing during voluntary movement.

pas·siv·ism (păs′ə-vĭz′əm) *n.* **1.** Passive character, attitude, or behavior. **2.** A pattern or attitude of submissiveness, especially in sexual relations.

paste (pāst) *n.* A smooth semisolid mixture, soft enough to flow slowly and not retain its shape.

Pas·teur (păs-tûr′, pä-stœr′), **Louis** 1822–1895. French chemist who founded modern microbiology, invented pasteurization, and developed vaccines for anthrax, rabies, and chicken cholera.

Pas·teu·rel·la (păs′chə-rĕl′ə, păs′tə-) *n.* A genus of aerobic to facultatively anaerobic, nonmotile bacteria of the family Pastuerellaceae containing small gram-negative rods; they are parasites of humans and other animals.

Pasteurella mul·to·ci·da (mŭl′tō-sī′də) *n.* A bacterium that causes fowl cholera and hemorrhagic septicemia in warm-blooded animals.

Pasteurella pes·tis (pĕs′tĭs) *n.* See **Yersinia pestis.**

Pasteurella pseudotuberculosis *n.* See **Yersinia pseudotuberculosis.**

Pasteurella tu·la·ren·sis (tōō′lə-rĕn′sĭs) *n.* *Francisella tularensis.*

pas·teu·rel·lo·sis (păs′chər-ə-lō′sĭs, păs′tər-) *n.* Infection with bacteria of the genus *Pasteurella.*

pas·teur·i·za·tion (păs′chər-ĭ-zā′shən, păs′tər-) *n.* **1.** The process of heating a beverage, such as milk or beer, to a specific temperature for a specific period of time in order to kill microorganisms that could cause disease, spoilage, or undesired fermentation. **2.** The process of destroying most microorganisms in certain foods, such as fish or clam meat, by irradiating them with gamma rays or other radiation to prevent spoilage.

pas·teur·ize (păs′chə-rīz′, păs′tə-) *v.* To treat by pasteurization.

Pasteur treatment *n.* A treatment for infection by the rabies virus in which a series of increasingly strong inoculations with attenuated virus is given to stimulate antibody production during the incubation period of the disease.

pas·tille *or* **pas·til** (pă-stēl′) *n.* **1.** A small medicated or flavored tablet; a troche. **2.** A tablet containing aromatic substances that is burned to fumigate or deodorize the air.

patch (păch) *n.* **1.** A small circumscribed area differing from the surrounding surface. **2.** A dressing or covering applied to protect a wound or sore. **3.** A transdermal patch.

patch test *n.* A test for allergic sensitivity in which a suspected allergen is applied to the skin on a small surgical pad for a period of time to determine if an allergic response is present.

pa·tel·la (pə-tĕl′ə) *n.,* *pl.* **–tel·lae** (-tĕl′ē) **1.** A flat triangular bone located in the combined tendon of the extensors of the leg and covering the front surface of the knee joint. Also called *kneecap.* **2.** A pan-shaped anatomical formation. **—pa·tel′lar, pa·tel′late** (-tĕl′ĭt, -āt′) *adj.*

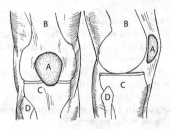

patella
anterior (left) *and lateral views of a knee joint:*
A. patella, B. femur, C. tibia, D. fibula

patellar fossa of vitreous *n.* The saucer-shaped depression of the vitreous humor formed by the posterior convexity of the lens of the eye.

patellar ligament *n.* A strong flattened fibrous band adjoining the margins of the patella to the tuberosity of the tibia.

patellar reflex *n.* A reflex contraction of the quadriceps muscle resulting in a sudden involuntary extension of the leg, produced by a sharp tap to the tendon below the patella. Also called *knee jerk, knee-jerk reflex, knee reflex, quadriceps reflex.*

pat·el·lec·to·my (păt′l-ĕk′tə-mē) *n.* Excision of the patella.

pa·tel·li·form (pə-tĕl′ə-fôrm′) *adj.* Shaped like the patella; pan-shaped.

pa·ten·cy (pāt′n-sē) *n.* The state or quality of being open, expanded, or unblocked.

pat·ent (păt′nt) *n.* **1.** A grant made by a government that confers upon the creator of an invention the sole right to make, use, and sell that invention for a set period of time. **2.** An invention protected by such a grant. *—adj.* **1.** Of, relating to, or being a nonprescription drug or other medical preparation that is often protected by a trademark. **2.** (pāt′nt) Not blocked; open. **3.** (pāt′nt) Spreading open; expanded. **—v. 1.** To obtain a patent on or for something, such as an invention. **2.** To invent, originate, or be the proprietor of an idea. **3.** To grant a patent to someone or for something.

pa·tent ductus ar·te·ri·o·sus (pāt′nt; är-tîr′ē-ō′səs) *n. Abbr.* **PDA** A congenital cardiac defect caused by failure of the ductus arteriosus to close at birth.

pat·ent medicine (păt′nt) *n.* A nonprescription drug or other medical preparation that is often protected by a trademark.

pa·ter·nal (pə-tûr′nəl) *adj.* **1.** Relating to or characteristic of a father or fatherhood. **2.** Received or inherited from a father. **3.** Related through one's father.

pa·ter·ni·ty (pə-tûr′nĭ-tē) *n.* **1.** The state of being a father; fatherhood. **2.** Descent on a father's side; paternal descent.

paternity test *n.* A test using blood group identification of a mother, child, and putative father to establish the probability of paternity.

–path *suff.* **1.** A practitioner of a specified kind of medical treatment: *naturopath.* **2.** One affected by a specified kind of disorder: *sociopath.*

path·er·ga·sia (păth′ər-gā′zhə) *n.* A physiological or anatomical defect that limits normal emotional adjustment.

path·er·gy (păth′ər-jē) *n.* An abnormal reaction to an allergen; it may be either subnormal or abnormally severe.

path·find·er (păth′fīn′dər) *n.* A filiform bougie for introduction through a narrow stricture as a guide for the passage of a larger instrument.

patho– *or* **path–** *pref.* Disease; suffering: *pathogen.*

path·o·bi·ol·o·gy (păth′ō-bī-ŏl′ə-jē) *n.* The study or practice of pathology with greater emphasis on the biological than on the medical aspects.

path·o·clis·is (păth′ə-klĭs′ĭs) *n.* **1.** A specific tendency toward a sensitivity to a particular toxin or toxins. **2.** A tendency for toxins to attack certain organs.

path·o·gen (păth′ə-jən) *n.* An agent that causes disease, especially a living microorganism such as a bacterium, virus, or fungus.

path·o·gen·e·sis (păth′ə-jěn′ĭ-sĭs) *or* **pa·thog·e·ny** (pə-thŏj′ə-nē) *n.* The development of a disease or morbid condition. Also called *nosogenesis.*

path·o·gen·ic (păth′ə-jěn′ĭk) *or* **path·o·ge·net·ic** (-jə-nĕt′ĭk) *adj.* **1.** Having the capability to cause disease. **2.** Producing disease. **3.** Relating to pathogenesis. —**path′o·ge·nic′i·ty** (-jə-nĭs′ĭ-tē) *n.*

pathogenic occlusion *n.* An occlusal relationship of the teeth capable of producing pathological changes in the supporting tissues.

pa·thog·no·mon·ic (pə-thŏg′nə-mŏn′ĭk, păth′əg-nō-) *adj.* Characteristic or symptomatic of a particular disease or condition.

pathognomonic symptom *n.* A symptom that is a definitive indication of a certain disease or condition.

pa·thog·ra·phy (pə-thŏg′rə-fē) *n.* The retrospective study, often by a physician, of the possible influence and effects of disease on the life and work of a historical personage or group.

path·o·log·i·cal (păth′ə-lŏj′ĭ-kəl) *or* **path·o·log·ic** (-ĭk) *adj.* **1.** Of or relating to pathology. **2.** Relating to or caused by disease. —**path′o·log′i·cal·ly** *adv.*

pathological anatomy *n.* See **anatomical pathology.**

pathologic calcification *n.* **1.** The presence of calculi in excretory or secretory passages. **2.** The calcification of tissues other than bone and teeth.

pathologic fracture *n.* A bone fracture occurring at a site weakened by disease, especially by a neoplasm or bone necrosis.

pathologic myopia *n.* Progressive myopia marked by changes in the fundus of the eye, posterior staphyloma, and subnormal corrected visual acuity.

pathologic retraction ring *n.* A constriction of the junction between the thinned lower uterine segment and the thick retracted upper uterine segment caused by obstructed labor; a sign of impending rupture of the uterus. Also called *Bandl's ring.*

pa·thol·o·gist (pă-thŏl′ə-jĭst) *n.* A specialist in pathology who practices chiefly in the laboratory as a consultant to clinical colleagues.

pa·thol·o·gy (pă-thŏl′ə-jē) *n.* **1.** The medical science concerned with all aspects of disease with an emphasis on the essential nature, causes, and development of abnormal conditions, as well as with the structural and functional changes that result from disease processes. **2.** The anatomical or functional manifestations of a disease.

path·o·mi·me·sis (păth′ō-mĭ-mē′sĭs, -mī-) *n.* Mimicry of the symptoms or effects of a disease, whether intentional or unconscious.

path·o·phys·i·ol·o·gy (păth′ō-fĭz′ē-ŏl′ə-jē) *n.* **1.** The functional changes associated with or resulting from disease or injury. **2.** The study of such changes. Also called *physiopathology.* —**path′o·phys′i·o·log′ic** (-ə-lŏj′ĭk), **path′o·phys′i·o·log′i·cal** (-ĭ-kəl) *adj.* —**path′o·phys′i·ol′o·gist** *n.*

pa·tho·sis (pă-thō′sĭs) *n., pl.* **–ses** (-sēz′) **1.** A state of disease. **2.** A diseased condition. **3.** A disease entity.

path·way (păth′wā′) *n.* **1.** A course usually followed by a body part or process. **2.** A chain of nerve fibers along which impulses normally travel. **3.** A sequence of enzymatic or other reactions by which one biological material is converted to another.

–pathy *suff.* **1.** Disease: *neuropathy.* **2.** A system of treating disease: *homeopathy.*

pa·tient (pā′shənt) *n.* One who receives medical attention, care, or treatment.

Pat·rick's test (păt′rĭks) *n.* A test in which the joint is stressed, used to determine the presence of sacroiliac disease.

pat·ri·lin·e·al (păt′rə-lĭn′ē-əl) *adj.* Relating to, based on, or tracing ancestral descent through the paternal line.

pat·ro·cli·nous (păt′rə-klī′nəs) *or* **pat·ri·cli·nous** (-rĭ-) *adj.* Having inherited traits that more closely resemble the father's side than the mother's side.

pat·terned alopecia (păt′ərnd) *n.* See **male pattern baldness.**

pat·tern·ing (păt′ər-nĭng) *n.* A method of physical therapy in which a rigid pattern of exercises is imposed to stimulate weak or paralyzed nerves and muscles to act on their own.

pat·tern sensitive epilepsy (păt′ərn) *n.* A form of reflex epilepsy precipitated by seeing certain patterns.

pat·u·lin (păch′ə-lĭn) *n.* A toxic antibiotic that is derived from the metabolites of certain fungi, such as *Aspergillus, Penicillium,* and *Gymnoascus,* and has carcinogenic activity.

pat·u·lous (păch′ə-ləs) *adj.* Freely open or exposed; patent.

pau·ci·bac·il·lar·y (pô′sə-băs′ə-lĕr′ē, -bə-sĭl′ə-rē) *adj.* Having or made up of few bacilli.

pau·ci·sy·nap·tic (pô′sē-sĭ-năp′tĭk) *adj.* Oligosynaptic.

Pau·ling (pô′lĭng), **Linus Carl** 1901–1994. American chemist. He won a 1954 Nobel Prize for work on the nature of chemical bonding and the 1962 Nobel Peace Prize for his efforts toward disarmament.

paunch (pônch, pänch) *n.* The belly, especially a protruding one; a potbelly.

paunch·y (pôn′chē, pän′-) *adj.* Having a potbelly.

pause (pôz) *n.* A temporary stop or cessation.

Pau·tri·er's microabscess (pō-trē-āz′) *n.* A microscopic lesion in the epidermis, seen in mycosis fungoides. Also called *Pautrier's abscess.*

Pav·lov (păv′lôf′, -lŏv′, päv′ləf), **Ivan Petrovich** 1849–1936. Russian physiologist known for his discovery of the conditioned response. He won a 1904 Nobel Prize for his research on the nature of digestion.

Pav·lo·vi·an conditioning (păv-lō′vē-ən, -lô′-) *n.* A process of behavior modification by which a subject comes to respond in a desired manner to a previously neutral stimulus that has been repeatedly presented along with an unconditioned stimulus that elicits the desired response.

pa·vor noc·tur·nus (pā′vər nŏk-tûr′nəs, pā′vôr′) *n.* Night-terrors.

Pax·il (păk′sĭl) A trademark for the drug paroxetine.

Payne operation (pān) *n.* A jejunoileal bypass for treating morbid obesity.

Payr's sign (pīrz) *n.* An indication of thrombophlebitis in which pain results when the sole of the foot receives pressure.

Pb The symbol for the element **lead**².

PBG *abbr.* porphobilinogen

PBI *abbr.* protein-bound iodine

p.c. *abbr. Latin* post cibum (after meals)

PCB (pē′sē-bē′) *n.* Polychlorinated biphenyl; any of a family of industrial compounds produced by chlorination of biphenyl, noted primarily as an environmental pollutant that accumulates in animal tissue with resultant pathogenic and teratogenic effects.

PCL *abbr.* posterior cruciate ligament

PCOD *abbr.* polycystic ovary disease

PCP *abbr.* phencyclidine; primary care physician

PCR *abbr.* polymerase chain reaction

PCT *abbr.* porphyria cutanea tarda

Pd The symbol for the element **palladium**.

PD *abbr.* prism diopter

PDA *abbr.* patent ductus arteriosus; personal digital assistant

PDLL *abbr.* poorly differentiated lymphocytic lymphoma

PDR A trademark for Physicians' Desk Reference, a group of reference books containing drug listings, especially one for prescription drugs.

PE *abbr.* physical examination; pulmonary embolism

peak expiratory flow (pēk) *n.* The maximum flow of air at the outset of forced expiration, which is reduced in proportion to the severity of airway obstruction, as in asthma.

peak flow meter *n.* A portable instrument that detects minute decreases in air flow and that is used by people with asthma to monitor small changes in breathing capacity.

pearl (pûrl) *n.* **1.** A small sphere of thin glass containing amyl nitrite or other volatile fluid, designed to be crushed, as in a handkerchief, so that its contents can be inhaled. **2.** Any of a number of small tough masses of mucus occurring in the sputum in asthma.

pearl tumor *n.* See **cholesteatoma**.

pearl·y tubercle (pûr′lē) *n.* See **milium**.

peau d'o·range (pō′ dô-räNzh′) *n.* A swollen pitted skin surface overlying carcinoma of the breast in which there is both stromal infiltration and lymphatic obstruction with edema.

pec (pĕk) *n.* A pectoral muscle. Often used in the plural.

pec·cant (pĕk′ənt) *adj.* Producing disease.

Pec·quet (pĕ-kā′), **Jean** 1622–1674. French anatomist who first described (1647) the thoracic duct.

pec·ten (pĕk′tən) *n., pl.* **–tens** *or* **–ti·nes** (-tə-nēz′) A body structure or an organ resembling a comb.

pecten band *n.* A fibrous induration of the anal pecten that results from a passive congestion or chronic inflammation.

pec·te·ni·tis (pĕk′tə-nī′tĭs) *n.* Inflammation of the sphincter muscle of the anus.

pec·te·no·sis (pĕk′tə-nō′sĭs) *n.* Exaggerated enlargement of the anal pecten.

pec·tin (pĕk′tĭn) *n.* Any of a group of water-soluble colloidal carbohydrates of high molecular weight found in ripe fruits, such as apples, plums, and grapefruit, and used to jell various foods, drugs, and cosmetics.

pec·ti·nate (pĕk′tə-nāt′) *or* **pec·ti·nat·ed** (-nā′tĭd) *adj.* Having projections resembling the teeth of a comb; comblike. —**pec′ti·na′tion** *n.*

pectinate line *n.* See **anocutaneous line**.

pectinate muscle *n.* Any of the prominent ridges of atrial myocardium located on the inner surfaces of much of the right atrium and of both auricles.

pectinate zone *n.* The outer region of the basal layer of the cochlear duct of the ear.

pec·tin·e·al (pĕk-tĭn′ē-əl) *adj.* **1.** Of or relating to the pubic bone. **2.** Relating to any comblike structure.

pectineal ligament *n.* A thick, strong fibrous band that passes laterally from the lacunar ligament along the pectineal line of the pubis.

pectineal line of pubis *n.* The continuation on the superior pubic ramus of the terminal line, forming a sharp ridge.

pectineal muscle *n.* A muscle with origin from the crest of the pubis, with insertion into the pectineal line of the femur, with nerve supply from the obturator and femoral nerves, and whose action adducts the thigh and assists in flexion.

pec·tin·i·form (pĕk-tĭn′ə-fôrm′) *adj.* Pectinate.

pec·to·ral (pĕk′tər-əl) *adj.* **1.** Relating to or situated in the breast or chest. **2.** Useful in relieving disorders of the chest or respiratory tract. —*n.* A muscle of the chest, esp. the pectoralis major.

pectoral girdle *n.* A bony or cartilaginous structure in vertebrates, attached to and supporting the forelimbs. Also called *pectoral arch.*

pec·to·ral·is major (pĕk′tə-răl′ĭs) *n.* A muscle with origin from the clavicle, the anterior surface of the episternum, the sternum, the cartilages of the first to the sixth ribs, and the aponeurosis of the external oblique abdominal muscle; with insertion into the greater tubercle of the humerus, with nerve supply from the anterior thoracic nerve, and whose action adducts the arm and rotates it medially.

pectoralis minor *n.* A muscle with origin from the third to the fifth ribs, with insertion into the coracoid process of the scapula, with nerve supply from the anterior thoracic nerve, and whose action lowers the scapula or raises the ribs.

pectoral muscle *n.* Either of two muscles in the chest, the pectoralis major or the pectoralis minor.

pectoral nerve *n.* Either of two nerves, designated medial and lateral, that arise from the brachial plexus and pass to the pectoral muscles.

pectoral vein *n.* Any of the veins draining the pectoral muscles and emptying into the subclavian vein.

pec·to·ril·o·quy (pĕk′tə-rĭl′ə-kwē) *n.* Transmission of the voice sound through the pulmonary structures so that it is unusually audible on auscultation of the chest, indicating either consolidation of the lung parenchyma or the presence of a large cavity.

pec·tus (pĕk′təs) *n., pl.* **pec·to·ra** (pĕk′tə-rə) The chest, especially the anterior wall; breast; thorax.

pectus car·i·na·tum (kăr′ə-nā′təm) *n.* See **pigeon breast.**

pectus ex·ca·va·tum (ĕk′skə-vā′təm) *n.* See **funnel chest.**

pectus re·cur·va·tum (rē′kûr-vā′təm) *n.* See **funnel chest.**

ped– *pref.* Variant of **pedo–.**

ped·al (pĕd′l, pēd′l) *adj.* Of or relating to a foot or footlike part.

ped·er·ast (pĕd′ə-răst′) *n.* A man who has sexual relations, especially anal intercourse, with a boy. **—ped′er·as′ty** *n.*

pe·de·sis (pĭ-dē′sĭs) *n., pl.* **–ses** (-sēz) See **Brownian movement.**

pe·di·at·ric (pē′dē-ăt′rĭk) *adj.* Of or relating to pediatrics.

pe·di·a·tri·cian (pē′dē-ə-trĭsh′ən) *or* **pe·di·at·rist** (-ăt′rĭst) *n.* A specialist in pediatrics.

pe·di·at·rics (pē′dē-ăt′rĭks) *n.* The branch of medicine that deals with the development and care of infants and children and the treatment of their diseases.

ped·i·cel (pĕd′ĭ-səl, -sĕl′) *n.* **1.** A small stalk, part, or organ, especially one serving as a support. **2.** The secondary process of a podocyte that helps form the visceral capsule of a renal corpuscle. Also called *footplate, foot process.* **—ped′i·cel′lar** (-sĕl′ər) *adj.*

ped·i·cel·late (pĕd′ĭ-sĕl′ĭt, -āt′) *adj.* Having or supported by a pedicel or pedicle.

ped·i·cel·la·tion (pĕd′ĭ-sə-lā′shən) *n.* Formation of a pedicel, pedicle, or peduncle.

ped·i·cle (pĕd′ĭ-kəl) *n.* **1.** A constricted portion or stalk. **2.** A slender stalk by which the base of a nonsessile tumor is attached to normal tissue. Also called *peduncle.* **3.** A stalk through which a skin flap receives its blood supply until the skin flap is transferred to its intended site of attachment.

pedicle flap *n.* A surgical flap sustained by a blood-carrying stem from the donor site during transfer.

pe·dic·u·lar (pə-dĭk′yə-lər) *adj.* Of, relating to, or caused by lice.

pe·dic·u·late (pə-dĭk′yə-lĭt, -lāt′) *adj.* Having a pedicle or peduncle; not sessile; pedunculate.

pe·dic·u·la·tion (pə-dĭk′yə-lā′shən) *n.* Infestation with lice.

pe·dic·u·li·cide (pə-dĭk′yə-lĭ-sīd′) *n.* An agent used to destroy lice.

pe·dic·u·lo·sis (pə-dĭk′yə-lō′sĭs) *n.* The state of being infested with lice. **—pe·dic′u·lous** (-ləs) *adj.*

pe·dic·u·lus (pə-dĭk′yə-ləs) *n., pl.* **–li** (-lī′) A pedicle.

Pediculus *n.* A genus of parasitic lice of the family Pediculidae that live in the hair and that includes species that infest the human scalp and body.

ped·i·gree (pĕd′ĭ-grē′) *n.* An ancestral line of descent, especially as diagrammed on a chart, to show ancestral history and to analyze Mendelian inheritance of certain traits including familial diseases.

pedigree analysis *n.* The study of an inherited trait in a group of related individuals to determine the pattern and characteristics of the trait, including its mode of inheritance, age of onset, and phenotypic variability.

pedo– *or* **ped–** *or* **paed–** *or* **paedo–** *pref.* Child; children: *pedodontics.*

pe·do·don·tia (pē′də-dŏn′shə) *n.* Pedodontics.

pe·do·don·tics (pē′də-dŏn′tĭks) *n.* The branch of dentistry that deals with the care and treatment of children's teeth. **—pe′do·don′tist** (-dŏn′tĭst) *n.*

ped·o·dy·na·mom·e·ter (pĕd′ō-dī′nə-mŏm′ĭ-tər) *n.* An instrument for measuring the strength of the leg muscles.

pe·dol·o·gy (pē-dŏl′ə-jē) *n.* The study of the physical, mental, and social development and characteristics of children.

pe·do·morph (pē′də-môrf′) *n.* Variant of **paedomorph.**

pe·do·mor·phism (pē′də-môr′fĭz′əm) *n.* Variant of **paedomorphism.**

pe·do·mor·pho·sis (pē′də-môr′fə-sĭs) *n.* Variant of **paedomorphosis.**

ped·o·phil·i·a (pĕd′ə-fĭl′ē-ə, pē′də-) *n.* The act or fantasy on the part of an adult of engaging in sexual activity with a child or children. **—ped′o·phile′** (-fīl′) *n.* **—ped′o·phil′i·ac′** (-fĭl′ē-ăk′) *adj. & n.*

pe·dor·thics (pĭ-dôr′thĭks) *n.* The art concerned with the design, manufacture, fit, and modification of foot appliances as prescribed for relief of painful or disabling conditions of the foot.

pe·dun·cle (pĭ-dŭng′kəl, pē′dŭng′kəl) *n.* **1.** See **pedicle** (sense 1). **2.** See **pedunculus** (sense 2). **—pe·dun′cu·lar** (pĭ-dŭng′kyə-lər) *adj.*

peduncle of corpus callosum *n.* See **subcallosal gyrus.**

peduncular ansa *n.* A complex nerve fiber bundle connecting the anterior part of the temporal lobe with the mediodorsal nucleus of the thalamus.

pe·dun·cu·late (pĭ-dŭng′kyə-lĭt, -lāt′) *or* **pe·dun·cu·lat·ed** (-lā′tĭd) *adj.* Having a peduncle.

pe·dun·cu·lot·o·my (pĭ-dŭng′kyə-lŏt′ə-mē) *n.* Total or partial surgical section of the cerebral peduncle.

pe·dun·cu·lus (pĭ-dŭng′kyə-ləs) *n.*, *pl.* **-li** (-lī′) **1.** An anatomical stalk or stem, such as the stalklike base to which a tumor is attached to normal tissue. **2.** Any of several stalklike connecting structures in the brain, composed either of white matter or of white and gray matter. Also called *peduncle*.

pedunculus of pineal body *n.* See **habenula** (sense 3).

PEEP *abbr.* positive end-expiratory pressure

peep·ing Tom (pē′pĭng) *n.* A person who gets pleasure, especially sexual pleasure, from secretly watching others; a voyeur.

peg-and-sock·et joint (pĕg′ənd-sŏk′ĭt) *n.* See **gomphosis**.

pegged tooth (pĕgd) *n.* A conical tooth whose sides converge from the neck at the gums to the incisal region.

Pel-Ebstein disease (pĕl′-) *n.* Hodgkin's disease that includes periodic fevers.

Pel-Ebstein fever *n.* The remittent fever common in Hodgkin's disease.

Pel·ger-Hu·ët nuclear anomaly (pĕl′gər-hyōō′ĭt) *n.* Congenital inhibition of lobulation of the nuclei of neutrophilic white blood cells.

pe·li·o·sis (pē′lē-ō′sĭs, pĕl′ē-) *n.* See **purpura**.

peliosis hep·a·tis (hĕp′ə-tĭs) *n.* The presence of blood-filled cavities in the liver.

Pe·li·zae·us-Merzbacher disease (pĕl′ĭ-zā′əs-, pā′lē-tsä′ōŏs-) *n.* See **Merzbacher-Pelizaeus disease**.

pel·lag·ra (pə-lăg′rə, -lā′grə, -lä′-) *n.* A disease caused by a deficiency of niacin and protein in the diet and characterized by skin eruptions, digestive and nervous system disturbances, and eventual mental deterioration. —**pel·lag′rous** *adj.*

pel·lag·rin (pə-lăg′rĭn, -lā′grĭn, -lä′-) *n.* A person affected with pellagra.

Pel·le·gri·ni's disease (pĕl′ĭ-grē′nēz) *n.* **1.** A calcification in the medial collateral ligament, usually due to trauma. Also called *Pellegrini-Stieda disease*. **2.** A bony growth at the internal condyle of the femur.

pel·let (pĕl′ĭt) *n.* **1.** A small pill; a pilule. **2.** A small rod-shaped or ovoid mass, as of compressed steroid hormones, intended for subcutaneous implantation in body tissues to provide timed release over an extended period of time.

pel·li·cle (pĕl′ĭ-kəl) *n.* A thin skin or film on the surface of a liquid. —**pel·lic′u·lar** (pə-lĭk′yə-lər) *adj.*

pel·lu·cid (pə-lōō′sĭd) *adj.* Admitting the passage of light; transparent or translucent.

pel·ta·tion (pĕl-tā′shən) *n.* Protection provided by inoculation with an antiserum or vaccine.

pelvi– *pref.* Variant of **pelvio–**.

pel·vic (pĕl′vĭk) *adj.* Of, relating to, or near the pelvis.

pelvic arch *n.* See **pelvic girdle**.

pelvic axis *n.* A hypothetical line curving through the center point of the pelvic plane of outlet, the pelvic plane of least dimension, the pelvic plane of greatest dimension, and the pelvic plane of inlet. Also called *plane of pelvic canal*.

pelvic cavity *n.* The space bounded by the bones of the pelvis and pelvic girdle.

pelvic cellulitis *n.* See **parametritis**.

pelvic diaphragm *n.* The paired coccygeal muscle and elevator muscle of the anus with the fascia above and below them.

pelvic direction *n.* The curved line denoting the direction of the axis of the canal of the pelvis.

pel·vi·ceph·a·log·ra·phy (pĕl′vĭ-sĕf′ə-lŏg′rə-fē) *n.* Radiographic measurement of the birth canal and of the fetal head.

pel·vi·ceph·a·lom·e·try (pĕl′vĭ-sĕf′ə-lŏm′ĭ-trē) *n.* Measurement of the pelvic diameters in relation to those of the fetal head.

pelvic fascia *n.* The fascia covering the muscles that pass from the interior of the pelvis to the thigh, the pelvic organs, and the vessels and nerves in the subperitoneal space.

pelvic ganglion *n.* Any of the parasympathetic ganglia on either side of the pelvic plexus.

pelvic girdle *n.* A bony or cartilaginous structure in vertebrates, attached to and supporting the hind limbs or fins. Also called *pelvic arch*.

pelvic inflammatory disease *n. Abbr.* **PID** Inflammation of the female genital tract, especially of the fallopian tubes, caused by any of several microorganisms, chiefly chlamydia and gonococci, and characterized by severe abdominal pain, high fever, vaginal discharge, and in some cases destruction of tissue that can result in sterility.

pelvic limb *n.* See **lower extremity**.

pelvic peritonitis *n.* Inflammation of the peritoneum surrounding the uterus and the fallopian tubes. Also called *pelviperitonitis*.

pelvic plane of greatest dimensions *n.* The plane extending from the middle of the posterior surface of the pubic symphysis to the junction of the second and third sacral vertebrae, passing laterally through the ischial bones over the middle of the acetabulum.

pelvic plane of inlet *n.* A plane that passes in front through the pubic symphysis and the pubic crest on either side, laterally by the iliopectineal lines, and in the rear by the promontory of the sacrum and is the upper opening of the small pelvis.

pelvic plane of least dimensions *n.* The plane that extends from the end of the sacrum to the lower border of the pubic symphysis, bounded posteriorly by the end of the sacrum, laterally by the ischial spines, and anteriorly by the lower border of the pubic symphysis.

pelvic plane of outlet *n.* An imaginary plane that passes in front through the pubic arch, laterally by the rami of the ischium and the sacrotuberous ligament on either side, and in the rear by these ligaments and the tip of the coccyx and is the lower opening of the small pelvis.

pelvic pole *n.* The breech end of the fetus.

pelvic splanchnic nerve *n.* Any of the branches from the second, third, and fourth sacral nerves that join the inferior hypogastric plexus, carrying parasympathetic and sensory fibers.

pelvic version *n.* Version in which a transverse or an oblique presentation is converted into a pelvic presentation by manipulating the buttocks of the fetus.

pel·vi·fix·a·tion (pĕl′və-fĭk-sā′shən) *n.* Surgical attachment of a floating pelvic organ to the wall of the cavity.

pel·vi·li·thot·o·my (pĕl′və-lĭ-thŏt′ə-mē) *n.* Surgical

removal of a renal calculus through an incision in the renal pelvis. Also called *pyelolithotomy.*

pel·vim·e·ter (pĕl-vĭm′ĭ-tər) *n.* An instrument shaped like calipers and used for measuring the dimensions of the pelvis.

pel·vim·e·try (pĕl-vĭm′ĭ-trē) *n.* Measurement of the dimensions and capacity of the pelvis, especially of the adult female pelvis.

pelvio– *or* **pelvi–***or* **pelvo–** *pref.* Pelvis: *pelviotomy.*

pel·vi·o·plas·ty (pĕl′vē-ə-plăs′tē) *n.* Symphysiotomy or pubiotomy for enlargement of the pelvic outlet.

pel·vi·ot·o·my (pĕl′vē-ŏt′ə-mē) *or* **pel·vit·o·my** (pĕl-vĭt′ə-mē) *n.* **1.** See **symphysiotomy. 2.** See **pubiotomy. 3.** See **pyelotomy.**

pel·vi·per·i·to·ni·tis (pĕl′və-pĕr′ĭ-tn-ī′tĭs) *n.* See **pelvic peritonitis.**

pel·vis (pĕl′vĭs) *n., pl.* **–vis·es** *or* **–ves** (-vēz) **1.** A basin-shaped structure of the vertebrate skeleton, composed of the innominate bones on the sides, the pubis in front, and the sacrum and coccyx behind, that rests on the lower limbs and supports the spinal column. **2.** The cavity formed by this structure. **3.** A basinlike or cup-shaped anatomical cavity.

pelvis jus·to major (jŭs′tō) *n.* A gynecoid pelvis having greater than normal measurements in all diameters.

pelvis justo minor *n.* A gynecoid pelvis with smaller than normal measurements in all diameters.

pelvis major *n.* See **large pelvis.**

pelvis minor *n.* See **small pelvis.**

pel·vi·ver·te·bral angle (pĕl′və-vûr′tə-brəl, -vər-tē′brəl) *n.* The angle formed by the pelvis with the general axis of the trunk or spine.

pel·vo·spon·dy·li·tis os·sif·i·cans (spŏn′dl-ī′tĭs ŏ-sĭf′ĭ-kănz′) *n.* Deposit of bony substance between the vertebrae of the sacrum.

pem·o·line (pĕm′ə-lēn′) *n.* A white, crystalline synthetic compound that is used as a mild stimulant of the central nervous system, especially in the treatment of depression.

pem·phi·goid (pĕm′fĭ-goid′) *adj.* Resembling pemphigus. **—***n.* A disease resembling pemphigus except as being nonacantholytic and generally benign.

pem·phi·gus (pĕm′fĭ-gəs, pĕm-fī′gəs) *n.* Any of several acute or chronic skin diseases characterized by groups of itching blisters. **—pem′phi·gous** *adj.*

pemphigus er·y·the·ma·to·sus (ĕr′ə-thē′mə-tō′səs, -thĕm′ə-) *n.* A skin eruption marked by scaling blisters and patches on scalp, face, and trunk.

pemphigus fo·li·a·ce·us (fō′lē-ā′shē-əs, -sē-əs) *n.* Chronic pemphigus in which extensive scaling dermatitis, with no perceptible blistering, may be present in addition to the bullae.

pemphigus gan·gre·no·sus (găng′grə-nō′səs) *n.* See **impetigo neonatorum.**

pemphigus veg·e·tans (vĕj′ĭ-tănz′) *n.* **1.** Pemphigus vulgaris in which verrucous lesions develop on the eroded surfaces left by ruptured bullae and new bullae continue to form. **2.** Chronic benign pemphigus with lesions commonly in the armpits and the perineum. Also called *Hallopeau's disease.*

pemphigus vul·gar·is (vŭl-gâr′ĭs) *n.* Pemphigus occurring in middle age, in which cutaneous flaccid

acantholytic suprabasal bullae and oral mucosal erosions are first localized but become generalized after a few months, forming blisters that break easily and are slow to heal.

pen·du·lar nystagmus (pĕn′jə-lər, -də-) *n.* A nystagmus that in most positions of gaze has oscillations of equal speed and amplitude, usually arising from a visual disturbance.

pen·e·trance (pĕn′ĭ-trəns) *n.* The frequency, under given environmental conditions, with which a specific genotype is expressed by those individuals that possess it, usually given as a percentage.

pen·e·trant gene (pĕn′ĭ-trənt) *n.* A gene that causes a trait in a specified genotype to be expressed.

pen·e·trat·ing wound (pĕn′ĭ-trā′tĭng) *n.* A wound accompanied by disruption of the body surface that extends into the underlying tissue or into a body cavity.

pen·e·trom·e·ter (pĕn′ĭ-trŏm′ĭ-tər) *or* **pen·e·tram·e·ter** (-trăm′ĭ-tər) *n.* **1.** A device for measuring penetrating power of radiation, especially x-rays. **2.** A device for measuring the penetrability of semisolids.

–penia *suff.* Lack; deficiency: *leukopenia.*

pen·i·cil·la·mine (pĕn′ĭ-sĭl′ə-mēn′) *n.* A degradation product of penicillin that is used as a chelating agent and in the treatment of rheumatoid arthritis and copper poisoning.

pen·i·cil·lin (pĕn′ĭ-sĭl′ĭn) *n.* Any of a group of broad-spectrum antibiotic drugs obtained from penicillium molds or produced synthetically, most active against gram-positive bacteria and used in the treatment of various infections and diseases.

pen·i·cil·li·nase (pĕn′ĭ-sĭl′ĭ-nās′, -nāz′) *n.* See **beta-lactamase.**

penicillin G *n.* The most commonly used penicillin compound, used primarily in the form of its stable salts. Also called *benzylpenicillin.*

penicillin V *n.* A semisynthetic oral penicillin compound that is very stable even in high humidity and that resists destruction by gastric juice.

pen·i·cil·li·um (pĕn′ĭ-sĭl′ē-əm) *n., pl.* **–cil·li·ums** *or* **–cil·li·a** (-sĭl′ē-ə) Any of various bluish-green fungi of the genus *Penicillium* that grow as molds on decaying fruits and ripening cheese and are used in the production of penicillin.

Penicillium *n.* A genus of fungi of the class Ascomycetes, some species of which yield several antibiotic substances and biologics.

pen·i·cil·lus (pĕn′ĭ-sĭl′əs) *n., pl.* **–cil·li** (-sĭl′ī) **1.** Any of the tufts formed by the repeated subdivision of the minute arterial twigs in the spleen. **2.** Any of the complex systems of branches bearing organs that produce conida organs in fungi of the *Penicillium.*

pe·nile (pē′nīl′, -nəl) *adj.* Of or relating to the penis.

pe·nis (pē′nĭs) *n., pl.* **–nis·es** *or* **–nes** (-nēz) The male organ of copulation and of urinary excretion, formed by three columns of erectile tissue, two arranged laterally on the dorsum and one medianiy below; the extremity is formed by an expansion of the corpus spongiosum, covered by a free fold of skin.

pe·nis·chi·sis (pē-nĭs′kĭ-sĭs) *n.* A fissure of the penis resulting in an abnormal urethral opening, as in epispadias, hypospadias, or paraspadias.

pe·ni·tis (pē-nī′tĭs) *n.* Inflammation of the penis. Also called *phallitis.*

pen·nate (pĕn′āt′) *adj.* **1.** Having feathers or wings. **2.** Resembling a feather.

pen·ni·form (pĕn′ə-fôrm′) *adj.* Shaped like or resembling a feather.

penta– *or* **pent–** *pref.* **1.** Five: *pentameter.* **2.** Containing five atoms, molecules, or groups: *pentose.*

pen·ta·me·tho·ni·um bromide (pĕn′tə-mĕ-thō′nē-əm) *n.* A ganglionic blocking agent used as an antihypertensive.

pen·ta·pi·per·i·um meth·yl·sul·fate (pĕn′tə-pī-pĕr′ē-əm mĕth′əl-sŭl′fāt′) *n.* An anticholinergic agent used especially in the treatment of peptic ulcer.

pen·ta·quine (pĕn′tə-kwēn′, -kwĭn) *or* **pen·ta·quin** (-kwĭn) *n.* A synthetic drug used with quinine in the prevention or treatment of malaria.

pen·taz·o·cine hydrochloride (pĕn-tăz′ə-sēn′) *n.* A synthetic narcotic drug used as a nonaddictive analgesic, often in place of morphine.

pen·tet·ic acid (pĕn-tĕt′ĭk) *n.* Diethylenetriamine penta-acetic acid; a chelating agent, especially for iron but also showing an affinity for heavy metals that is used in the treatment of iron-storage disease and poisoning from heavy and radioactive metals.

pen·to·bar·bi·tal sodium (pĕn′tə-bär′bĭ-tôl′, -tăl′) *n.* A white crystalline or powdery barbiturate used as a hypnotic, sedative, and anticonvulsive drug. Also called *pentobarbitone.*

pen·to·bar·bi·tone (pĕn′tə-bär′bĭ-tōn′) *n.* See **pentobarbital sodium.**

pen·tose (pĕn′tōs′, -tōz′) *n.* Any of a class of monosaccharides having five carbon atoms per molecule and including ribose and several other sugars.

pentose phosphate pathway *n.* A secondary pathway for the metabolism of glucose in tissues other than skeletal muscle, in which five-carbon sugars are synthesized and NADPH is produced in the cytoplasm outside the mitochondria. Also called *Dickens shunt.*

pen·to·su·ri·a (pĕn′tō-sŏŏr′ē-ə) *n.* The excretion of one or more pentoses in the urine.

Pen·to·thal (pĕn′tə-thôl′) A trademark for the drug thiopental sodium.

pen·tox·if·yl·line (pĕn′tŏk-sĭf′ə-lēn′, -lĭn, pĕn-tŏk′sə-fĭl′ēn′, -ĭn) *n.* A bitter-tasting compound that decreases blood viscosity and improves blood flow, used in the treatment of intermittent claudication.

pen·tyl (pĕn′təl) *n.* See **amyl.**

pe·o·til·lo·ma·ni·a (pē′ō-tĭl′ə-mā′nē-ə) *n.* A nervous tic consisting of a constant pulling of the penis.

Pep·cid (pĕp′sĭd) A trademark for the drug famotidine.

pep·lo·mer (pĕp′lə-mər) *n.* A subunit of the peplos of a virion.

pep·los (pĕp′ləs, -lŏs′) *n., pl.* **–los·es** The coat or envelope of lipoprotein material that surrounds certain virions.

pep pill *n.* A tablet or capsule containing a stimulant drug, especially an amphetamine.

pep·sin *or* **pep·sine** (pĕp′sĭn) *n.* **1.** Any of various digestive enzymes found in gastric juice that catalyze the hydrolysis of proteins to peptides. **2.** A substance

containing pepsin, obtained from the stomachs of hogs and calves and used as a digestive aid.

pepsin A *n.* The principal digestive enzyme of gastric juice that is formed from pepsinogen and catalyzes the hydrolysis of peptide bonds to form proteoses and peptones.

pep·sin·o·gen (pĕp-sĭn′ə-jən) *n.* The inactive precursor to pepsin, formed in the chief cells of the mucous membrane of the stomach and converted to pepsin by hydrochloric acid during digestion. Also called *propepsin.*

pep·tic (pĕp′tĭk) *adj.* **1.** Relating to or assisting digestion. **2.** Associated with the action of digestive secretions. **3.** Of or involving pepsin. **4.** Capable of digesting. —*n.* A digestive agent.

peptic cell *n.* See **zymogenic cell.**

peptic digestion *n.* See **gastric digestion.**

peptic esophagitis *n.* See **reflux esophagitis.**

peptic ulcer *n.* An ulcer of the upper digestive tract, usually in the stomach or duodenum, where the mucous membrane is exposed to gastric secretions.

pep·ti·dase (pĕp′tĭ-dās′, -dāz′) *n.* An enzyme that catalyzes the hydrolysis of peptides into amino acids.

pep·tide (pĕp′tīd′) *n.* Any of various natural or synthetic compounds containing two or more amino acids linked by the carboxyl group of one amino acid and the amino group of another. —**pep·tid′ic** (-tĭd′ĭk) *adj.*

peptide bond *n.* The chemical bond formed between the carboxyl groups and amino groups of neighboring amino acids, constituting the primary linkage of all protein structures.

pep·ti·der·gic (pĕp′tĭ-dûr′jĭk) *adj.* Of or being nerve cells or fibers that may use small peptide molecules as their neurotransmitters.

pep·ti·do·gly·can (pĕp′tĭ-dō-glī′kən, -kăn′) *n.* A polymer found in the cell walls of prokaryotes that consists of polysaccharide and peptide chains in a strong molecular network. Also called *mucopeptide, murein.*

pep·ti·doid (pĕp′tĭ-doid′) *n.* A compound formed by the condensation of two amino acids, with the linkage involving at least one group that is not a carboxyl or an amino group.

pep·ti·do·lyt·ic (pĕp′tĭ-dō-lĭt′ĭk) *adj.* **1.** Of or relating to the cleavage of peptides. **2.** Causing the digestion of peptides.

Pep·to-Bis·mol (pĕp′tō-bĭz′môl) A trademark for a preparation of bismuth subsalicylate.

pep·to·gen·ic (pĕp′tə-jĕn′ĭk) *or* **pep·tog·e·nous** (pĕp-tŏj′ə-nəs) *adj.* **1.** Producing pepsin or peptones. **2.** Promoting digestion.

pep·tol·y·sis (pĕp-tŏl′ĭ-sĭs) *n.* The hydrolysis of peptones.

pep·to·lyt·ic (pĕp′tə-lĭt′ĭk) *adj.* **1.** Of or relating to peptolysis. **2.** Of or being an enzyme or other agent that hydrolyzes peptones.

pep·tone (pĕp′tōn′) *n.* Any of various soluble compounds that do not coagulate, are obtained by acid or enzyme hydrolysis of natural protein, and are used as nutrients in culture media. —**pep·ton′ic** (-tŏn′ĭk) *adj.*

pep·to·nize (pĕp′tə-nīz′) *v.* **1.** To convert protein into a soluble peptone by enzymatic action. **2.** To dissolve food by means of a proteolytic enzyme. **3.** To combine with peptone. —**pep′to·ni·za′tion** (-nĭ-zā′shən) *n.*

per– *pref.* **1.** Thoroughly; completely; intensely: *perfuse.* **2.** Containing an element in its highest oxidation state: *perchloric acid.* **3.** Containing a large or the largest possible proportion of an element: *peroxide.* **4.** Containing the peroxy group: *peracid.*

per·ac·id (pûr′ăs′ĭd) *n.* **1.** Any of various acids containing the peroxy group. **2.** An inorganic acid, such as perchloric acid, containing the largest proportion of oxygen in a series of related acids.

per·a·cute (pûr′ə-kyo͞ot′) *adj.* Very acute. Used of a disease.

per a·num (pər ā′nəm) *adv.* Through or by way of the anus, as in the administration of medication.

per·ceive (pər-sēv′) *v.* **1.** To become aware of directly through any of the senses, especially sight or hearing. **2.** To achieve understanding of; apprehend. —**per·ceiv′a·ble** *adj.*

per·cept (pûr′sĕpt′) *n.* **1.** The object of perception. **2.** A mental impression of something perceived by the senses, viewed as the basic component in the formation of concepts. **3.** In clinical psychology, a single unit of perceptual report, such as one of the responses to an inkblot in the Rorschach test.

per·cep·tion (pər-sĕp′shən) *n.* **1.** The process, act, or faculty of perceiving. **2.** Recognition and interpretation of sensory stimuli based chiefly on memory.

per·cep·tive (pər-sĕp′tĭv) *adj.* **1.** Of or relating to perception. **2.** Having the ability to perceive. **3.** Keenly discerning. —**per′cep·tiv′i·ty** (pûr′sĕp-tĭv′ĭ-tē) *n.*

per·cep·tu·al (pər-sĕp′cho͞o-əl) *adj.* Of, based on, or involving perception.

per·chlo·rate (pər-klôr′āt′) *n.* A salt or ester of perchloric acid.

per·chlo·ric acid (pər-klôr′ĭk) *n.* A clear colorless liquid that is the highest in oxygen content of the series of chlorine acids and is a powerful oxidant used as a catalyst.

Per·co·cet (pûr′kə-sĕt′) A trademark for a drug containing oxycodone and acetaminophen.

Per·co·dan (pûr′kə-dăn′) A trademark for the drug oxycodone.

per·co·late (pûr′kə-lāt′) *v.* **1.** To cause a liquid to pass slowly through a porous substance or small holes; filter. **2.** To drain or seep through. **3.** To cause a solvent liquid to pass through a mixture, such as a powdered drug, so as to extract the soluble portion. —*n.* (-lĭt, -lāt′) A liquid that has been percolated. —**per′co·la′tion** *n.*

per con·tig·u·um (pər kən-tĭg′yo͞o-əm) *adv.* By or through contiguity, as in the spread of infection or inflammation between adjacent structures.

per con·tin·u·um (pər kən-tĭn′yo͞o-əm) *adv.* By or through continuity, as in the spread of infection or inflammation from one part to another through continuous tissue.

per·cuss (pər-kŭs′) *v.* To strike or tap firmly; perform percussion.

per·cus·sion (pər-kŭsh′ən) *n.* A method of medical diagnosis in which various areas of the body, especially the chest, back, and abdomen, are tapped with the

finger or a plexor to determine by resonance the condition of internal organs.

per·cus·sor (pər-kŭs′ər) *n.* See **plexor.**

per·cu·ta·ne·ous (pûr′kyo͞o-tā′nē-əs) *adj.* Passed, done, or effected through the unbroken skin.

percutaneous transluminal coronary angioplasty *n.* *Abbr.* **PTCA** A procedure for enlarging a narrowed arterial lumen by peripheral introduction of a balloon-tip catheter followed by dilation of the lumen as the inflated catheter tip is withdrawn.

per·en·ceph·a·ly (pûr′ĕn-sĕf′ə-lē) *n.* A condition marked by cerebral cysts.

per·fect fungus (pûr′fĭkt) *n.* A fungus known to have both sexual and asexual stages in its life cycle.

per·fec·tion·ism (pər-fĕk′shə-nĭz′əm) *n.* A tendency to set rigid high standards of personal performance. —**per·fec′tion·ist** *adj. & n.*

perfect stage *n.* The sexual phase in the life cycle of a fungus in which spores are produced following nuclear fusion.

per·fo·rate (pûr′fə-rāt′) *v.* **1.** To make a hole or holes in, as from injury, disease, or medical procedure. **2.** To pass into or through (a body structure or tissue). —*adj.* (pûr′fər-ĭt, -fə-rāt′) Having been perforated.

per·fo·ra·ted (pûr′fə-rā′tĭd) *adj.* Pierced with one or more holes.

perforated layer of sclera *n.* The perforated portion of the sclera through which the fibers of the optic nerve pass.

perforated substance *n.* Either of the two perforated substances of the brain, designated anterior and posterior. Also called *perforated space.*

perforated ulcer *n.* An ulcer extending through the wall of an organ.

per·fo·ra·ting abscess (pûr′fə-rā′tĭng) *n.* An abscess that penetrates tissue barriers and enters adjacent areas.

perforating artery *n.* An artery with its origin in the deep artery of the thigh, with distribution as three or four vessels that pass through the great adductor muscle to the posterior and lateral parts of the thigh.

perforating fiber *n.* Any of the bundles of collagen fibers that pass into the outer circumferential lamellae of bone or into the cementum of teeth.

perforating vein *n.* Any of the veins that accompany the perforating arteries, drain the lateral vastus and the hamstring muscles, and terminate in the deep femoral vein.

perforating wound *n.* A wound having an entrance and an exit.

per·fo·ra·tion (pûr′fə-rā′shən) *n.* **1.** The act of perforating or the state of being perforated. **2.** An abnormal opening in a hollow organ or viscus, as one made by rupture or injury.

per·fuse (pər-fyo͞oz′) *v.* **1.** To pour or diffuse a liquid over or through something. **2.** To force blood or other fluid to flow from the artery through the vascular bed of a tissue or to flow through the lumen of a hollow structure. —**per·fu′sive** (pər-fyo͞o′sĭv) *adj.*

per·fu·sion (pər-fyo͞o′zhən) *n.* **1.** The act of perfusing. **2.** The injection of fluid into a blood vessel in order to reach an organ or tissues, usually to supply nutrients and oxygen.

per·go·lide mesylate (pĕr′gə-līd′) *n.* An ergot derivative with dopaminergic properties.

Per·go·nal (pûr′gə-nôl′) A trademark for the drug menotropins.

peri– *pref.* **1.** Around; about; enclosing: *perimysium.* **2.** Near: *perinatal.*

Per·i·ac·tin (pĕr′ē-ăk′tĭn) A trademark for the drug cyproheptadine hydrochloride.

per·i·ad·e·ni·tis (pĕr′ē-ăd′n-ī′tĭs) *n.* Inflammation of the tissues surrounding a gland.

periadenitis mu·co·sa ne·crot·i·ca re·cur·rens (myōō-kō′sə nĭ-krŏt′ĭ-kə rĭ-kûr′ĕnz′) *n.* Recurrent aphthous stomatitis, marked by attacks of lesions that begin as small, firm nodules which then enlarge, ulcerate, and heal by scar formation, leaving numerous atrophied scars on the oral mucosa. Also called *Sutton's disease.*

per·i·an·gi·i·tis (pĕr′ē-ăn′jē-ī′tĭs) *n.* Inflammation of the adventitia or the tissues surrounding a blood vessel or lymphatic vessel. Also called *perivasculitis.*

per·i·a·or·ti·tis (pĕr′ē-ā′ôr-tī′tĭs) *n.* Inflammation of the adventitia of the aorta and of the tissues surrounding it.

per·i·ap·i·cal (pĕr′ē-ā′pĭ-kəl, -ăp′ĭ-) *adj.* **1.** At or around the apex of a root of a tooth. **2.** Of or being the periodontal membrane and adjacent bone.

periapical ce·men·tal dysplasia (sĭ-mĕn′tl) *n.* A benign, painless condition of the jaws that occurs almost exclusively in middle-aged black females and is characterized by multiple lesions that usually involve vital mandibular anterior teeth, surround the root apices, and become opaque as they mature.

periapical curettage *n.* **1.** The removal of a cyst or granuloma from its pathological bony crypt by using a curette. **2.** The removal of tooth fragments, pieces of dead bone, or debris from a tooth socket by using a curette.

periapical granuloma *n.* A growing mass of granulation tissue surrounding the apex of a nonvital tooth and arising in response to necrosis of the tooth pulp. Also called *apical granuloma, dental granuloma.*

periapical periodontal cyst *n.* A cyst about the root of a dead tooth, usually caused by dental caries or disease of the pulp. Also called *radicular cyst.*

periapical radiograph *n.* A radiograph showing tooth apices and surrounding structures in a particular intraoral area.

per·i·ap·pen·di·ce·al abscess (pĕr′ē-ə-pĕn′dĭ-sē′əl) *n.* See **appendiceal abscess.**

per·i·ap·pen·di·ci·tis (pĕr′ē-ə-pĕn′dĭ-sī′tĭs) *n.* An inflammation of the tissue that surrounds the vermiform appendix.

per·i·aq·ue·duc·tal (pĕr′ē-ăk′wĭ-dŭk′təl) *adj.* Situated around the aqueduct of the brain.

per·i·ar·te·ri·al plexus (pĕr′ē-är-tîr′ē-əl) *n.* An autonomic plexus that accompanies an artery.

periarterial sympathectomy *n.* Sympathectomy that is achieved by decortication of the arteries.

per·i·ar·te·ri·tis (pĕr′ē-är′tə-rī′tĭs) *n.* Inflammation of the outer coat of an artery.

periarteritis no·do·sa (nō-dō′sə) *n.* See **polyarteritis nodosa.**

per·i·ar·thri·tis (pĕr′ē-är-thrī′tĭs) *n.* Inflammation of the tissues surrounding a joint.

per·i·ar·tic·u·lar (pĕr′ē-är-tĭk′yə-lər) *adj.* Surrounding a joint.

periarticular abscess *n.* An abscess surrounding a joint but not usually affecting it.

per·i·ax·il·lar·y (pĕr′ē-ăk′sə-lĕr′ē) *adj.* Surrounding or adjacent to the armpit.

per·i·bron·chi·al (pĕr′ə-brŏng′kē-əl) *adj.* Of, relating to, or surrounding a bronchus or the bronchi.

per·i·bron·chi·o·lar (pĕr′ə-brŏng′kē-ō′lər) *adj.* Of, relating to, or surrounding the bronchioles.

per·i·bron·chi·o·li·tis (pĕr′ə-brŏng′kē-ō-lī′tĭs) *n.* Inflammation of tissues surrounding bronchioles.

per·i·bron·chi·tis (pĕr′ə-brŏn-kī′tĭs, brŏng-) *n.* Inflammation of the tissues surrounding the bronchi or bronchial tubes.

per·i·car·di·ac (pĕr′ĭ-kär′dē-ăk′) *or* **per·i·car·di·al** (-əl) *adj.* **1.** Surrounding or adjacent to the heart. **2.** Of or relating to the pericardium.

per·i·car·di·a·co·phren·ic artery (pĕr′ĭ-kär-dī′ə-kō-frĕn′ĭk) *n.* An artery with its origin in the internal thoracic artery, with distribution to the pericardium, diaphragm, and pleura; and with anastomoses to the phrenic arteries and branches of the internal thoracic artery.

pericardiacophrenic vein *n.* Any of the veins that accompany the pericardiacophrenic artery and empty into the brachiocephalic vein or the superior vena cava.

per·i·car·di·al cavity (pĕr′ĭ-kär′dē-əl) *n.* The fluid-filled space between the two layers of the pericardium.

pericardial decompression *n.* See **cardiac decompression.**

pericardial fremitus *n.* The vibration in the chest wall produced by the friction of opposing roughened surfaces of the pericardium.

pericardial friction sound *n.* An oscillating creaking sound sometimes heard on auscultation, caused by the rubbing together of inflamed pericardial surfaces as the heart contracts and relaxes. Also called *pericardial rub.*

pericardial murmur *n.* A friction sound, synchronous with the heart movements, heard in certain cases of pericarditis.

pericardial rub *n.* See **pericardial friction sound.**

pericardial vein *n.* Any of several small veins from the pericardium that empty into the brachiocephalic vein or the superior vena cava.

per·i·car·di·ec·to·my (pĕr′ĭ-kär′dē-ĕk′tə-mē) *n.* Excision of a portion of the pericardium.

per·i·car·di·o·cen·te·sis (pĕr′ĭ-kär′dē-ō-sĕn-tē′sĭs) *n.* Paracentesis of the pericardium.

per·i·car·di·o·per·i·to·ne·al (pĕr′ĭ-kär′dē-ō-pĕr′ĭ-tn-ē′əl) *adj.* Relating to the pericardial and peritoneal cavities.

per·i·car·di·o·phren·ic (pĕr′ĭ-kär′dē-ə-frĕn′ĭk) *adj.* Relating to the pericardium and the diaphragm.

per·i·car·di·o·pleu·ral (pĕr′ĭ-kär′dē-ō-plŏor′əl) *adj.* Relating to the pericardial and pleural cavities.

per·i·car·di·or·rha·phy (pĕr′ĭ-kär′dē-ôr′ə-fē) *n.* Suture of the pericardium.

per·i·car·di·os·to·my (pĕr′ĭ-kär′dē-ŏs′tə-mē) *n.* Surgical construction of an opening into the pericardium.

per·i·car·di·ot·o·my (pĕr′ĭ-kär′dē-ŏt′ə-mē) *n.* Incision into the pericardium.

per·i·car·di·tis (pĕr′ĭ-kär-dī′tĭs) *n.* Inflammation of the pericardium.

pericarditis o·blit·er·ans (ə-blĭt′ə-rănz′) *n.* Inflammation of the pericardium leading to adhesion of the two layers, thus obliterating the sac.

per·i·car·di·um (pĕr′ĭ-kär′dē-əm) *n., pl.* **–di·a** (-dē-ə) The fibroserous sac enclosing the heart and the roots of the great vessels, consisting of two layers: the visceral layer or epicardium, immediately surrounding the heart; and the outer parietal layer, which forms the sac and is lined with a serous membrane. Also called *heart sac, theca cordis.* —**per′i·car′di·al** (-dē-əl), **per′i·car′di·ac′** (-dē-ăk′) *adj.*

per·i·ce·men·ti·tis (pĕr′ĭ-sē′mĕn-tī′tĭs) *n.* Periodontitis. No longer in technical use.

per·i·cho·lan·gi·tis (pĕr′ĭ-kō′lăn-jī′tĭs) *n.* Inflammation of the tissues surrounding the bile ducts.

per·i·chon·dral bone (pĕr′ĭ-kŏn′drəl) *n.* A collar or cuff of osseous tissue that forms in the perichondrium of the cartilage in the development of a long bone.

per·i·chon·dri·tis (pĕr′ĭ-kŏn-drī′tĭs) *n.* Inflammation of the perichondrium.

per·i·chon·dri·um (pĕr′ĭ-kŏn′drē-əm) *n., pl.* **–dri·a** (-drē-ə) The dense irregular fibrous membrane of connective tissue covering the surface of cartilage except at the endings of joints. —**per′i·chon′dri·al** (-drē-əl) *adj.*

per·i·chrome (pĕr′ĭ-krōm′) *adj.* Of or being a nerve cell in which the chromophil substance is scattered throughout the cytoplasm.

per·i·co·li·tis (pĕr′ĭ-kə-lī′tĭs) *or* **per·i·co·lon·i·tis** (-kō′lə-nī′tĭs) *n.* Inflammation of the connective tissue or of the peritoneum surrounding the colon. Also called *serocolitis.*

per·i·col·pi·tis (pĕr′ĭ-kŏl-pī′tĭs) *n.* See **perivaginitis.**

per·i·cor·o·ni·tis (pĕr′ĭ-kôr′ə-nī′tĭs) *n.* Inflammation of the gingiva surrounding the crown of a tooth. Also called *operculitis.*

per·i·cra·ni·tis (pĕr′ĭ-krā-nī′tĭs) *n.* Inflammation of the pericranium.

per·i·cra·ni·um (pĕr′ĭ-krā′nē-əm) *n., pl.* **–ni·a** (-nē-ə) The external periosteum that covers the outer surface of the skull. —**per′i·cra′ni·al** *adj.*

per·i·cys·tic (pĕr′ĭ-sĭs′tĭk) *adj.* **1.** Surrounding or adjacent to the urinary bladder or the gallbladder. **2.** Surrounding a cyst.

per·i·cys·ti·tis (pĕr′ĭ-sĭ-stī′tĭs) *n.* Inflammation of the tissues surrounding the urinary bladder.

per·i·cyte (pĕr′ĭ-sīt′) *n.* A slender, relatively undifferentiated, connective tissue cell that occurs about capillaries or other small blood vessels. Also called *adventitial cell.*

per·i·cyt·ic venule (pĕr′ĭ-sĭt′ĭk) *n.* See **postcapillary venule.**

per·i·den·tal membrane (pĕr′ĭ-dĕn′tl) *n.* See **periodontium.**

per·i·derm (pĕr′ĭ-dûrm′) *or* **per·i·der·ma** (pĕr′ĭ-dûr′mə) *n.* The outermost layer of the epidermis of an embryo or fetus up to the sixth month of gestation. Also called *epitrichium.*

per·i·des·mi·tis (pĕr′ĭ-dĕz-mī′tĭs) *n.* Inflammation of the connective tissue surrounding a ligament.

per·i·des·mi·um (pĕr′ĭ-dĕz′mē-əm) *n.* The connective tissue membrane surrounding a ligament.

per·i·did·y·mis (pĕr′ĭ-dĭd′ə-mĭs) *n.* The thick fibrous membrane forming the outer coat of the testis.

per·i·did·y·mi·tis (pĕr′ĭ-dĭd′ə-mī′tĭs) *n.* Inflammation of the perididymis.

per·i·di·ver·tic·u·li·tis (pĕr′ĭ-dī′vûr-tĭk′yə-lī′tĭs) *n.* Inflammation of the tissues surrounding an intestinal diverticulum.

per·i·du·o·de·ni·tis (pĕr′ĭ-dōō′ō-dn-ī′tĭs, -dōō-ŏd′n-ī′-) *n.* Inflammation of the tissues surrounding the duodenum.

per·i·en·ceph·a·li·tis (pĕr′ē-ĕn-sĕf′ə-lī′tĭs) *n.* Inflammation of the cerebral membranes, especially of the pia mater.

per·i·en·ter·i·tis (pĕr′ē-ĕn′tə-rī′tĭs) *n.* Inflammation of the peritoneal coat of the intestine. Also called *seroenteritis.*

per·i·e·soph·a·gi·tis (pĕr′ē-ĭ-sŏf′ə-jī′tĭs) *n.* Inflammation of the tissues surrounding the esophagus.

per·i·fol·lic·u·li·tis (pĕr′ə-fə-lĭk′yə-lī′tĭs) *n.* Inflammatory infiltrate surrounding the hair follicles, usually occurring in conjunction with folliculitis.

per·i·gas·tri·tis (pĕr′ĭ-gă-strī′tĭs) *n.* Inflammation of the peritoneal coat of the stomach.

per·i·glot·tis (pĕr′ĭ-glŏt′ĭs) *n.* The mucous membrane of the tongue.

per·i·hep·a·ti·tis (pĕr′ə-hĕp′ə-tī′tĭs) *n.* Inflammation of the serous or peritoneal covering of the liver.

per·i·in·farc·tion block (pĕr′ē-ĭn-färk′shən) *n.* An electrocardiographic abnormality that is associated with an old myocardial infarct and is caused by delayed activation of the myocardium in the region of the infarct.

per·i·je·ju·ni·tis (pĕr′ē-jə-jōō′nī′tĭs, -ə-jē′jōō-, -jĕj′ōō-) *n.* Inflammation of the tissues surrounding the jejunum.

per·i·kar·y·on (pĕr′ĭ-kăr′ē-ŏn, -ən) *n., pl.* **–kar·y·a** (-kăr′ē-ə) **1.** The cytoplasm of a cell, exclusive of its nucleus. **2.** The cell body of a neuron. **3.** The body of the odontoblast exclusive of the dentinal fiber.

per·i·lab·y·rin·thi·tis (pĕr′ə-lăb′ə-rĭn-thī′tĭs) *n.* Inflammation of the parts about the labyrinth of the ear.

per·i·lar·yn·gi·tis (pĕr′ə-lăr′ĭn-jī′tĭs) *n.* Inflammation of the tissues around the larynx.

per·i·lymph (pĕr′ə-lĭmf′) *n.* The fluid in the space between the membranous and bony labyrinths of the inner ear.

per·i·lym·phan·gi·tis (pĕr′ə-lĭm′făn-jī′tĭs) *n.* Inflammation of tissues surrounding a lymphatic vessel.

per·i·lym·phat·ic (pĕr′ə-lĭm-făt′ĭk) *adj.* **1.** Of or relating to the perilymph. **2.** Surrounding or adjacent to a lymphatic node or vessel.

perilymphatic duct *n.* A fine canal connecting the perilymphatic space of the cochlea with the subarachnoid space. Also called *cochlear aqueduct.*

perilymphatic space *n.* The space between the bony and membranous portions of the inner ear.

per·i·men·in·gi·tis (pĕr′ə-mĕn′ĭn-jī′tĭs) *n.* See **pachymeningitis.**

per·i·men·o·pause (pĕr′ə-mĕn′ə-pôz′) *n.* The period of a woman's life characterized by physiological changes associated with the end of reproductive capacity and terminating with the completion of menopause. Also called *climacteric.*

pe·rim·e·ter (pə-rĭm′ĭ-tər) *n.* **1.** The outer limits of an area; circumference. **2.** An instrument used to measure field of vision.

per·i·met·ric (pĕr′ə-mĕt′rĭk) *adj.* **1.** Of, relating to, or surrounding the uterus. **2.** Of or relating to the perimetrium. **3.** Of or relating to the circumference of any part or area. **4.** Of or relating to perimetry.

per·i·me·tri·tis (pĕr′ə-mĭ-trī′tĭs) *n.* See **metroperitonitis.** —**per′i·me·trit′ic** (-trĭt′ĭc) *adj.*

per·i·me·tri·um (pĕr′ə-mē′trē-əm) *n., pl.* **-tri·a** (-trē-ə) The serous peritoneal coat of the uterus.

pe·rim·e·try (pə-rĭm′ĭ-trē) *n.* The determination of the limits of the visual field.

per·i·my·e·li·tis (pĕr′ə-mī′ə-lī′tĭs) *n.* See **endosteitis.**

per·i·my·o·si·tis (pĕr′ə-mī′ə-sī′tĭs) *n.* Inflammation of the loose cellular tissue surrounding a muscle. Also called *perimysiitis.*

per·i·mys·i·i·tis (pĕr′ə-mĭs′ē-ī′tĭs, -mĭz′-) *or* **per·i·my·si·tis** (-mĭ-sī′tĭs, -zī′-) *n.* **1.** Inflammation of the perimysium. Also called *myofibrositis.* **2.** See **perimyositis.**

per·i·my·si·um (pĕr′ə-mĭzh′ē-əm, -mĭz′ē-əm) *n., pl.* **-my·si·a** (-ē-ə) The fibrous sheath enveloping each of the primary bundles of skeletal muscle fibers. —**per′i·my′si·al** *adj.*

per·i·na·tal (pĕr′ə-nāt′l) *adj.* Of, relating to, or being the period around childbirth, especially the five months before and one month after birth. —**per′i·na′tal·ly** *adv.*

perinatal medicine *n.* The branch of medicine concerned with the care of the mother and fetus during pregnancy, labor, and delivery.

per·i·na·tol·o·gy (pĕr′ə-nā-tŏl′ə-jē) *n.* The subspecialty of obstetrics concerned with the care of mothers, fetuses, and infants during the perinatal period. —**per′i·na·tol′o·gist** *n.*

perineal artery *n.* An artery with its origin in the internal pudendal artery, with distribution to the superficial structures of the perineum, and with anastomosis to the external pudendal arteries.

perineal hernia *n.* A hernia protruding through the pelvic diaphragm. Also called *perineocele.*

perineal nerve *n.* Any of the superficial terminal branches of the pudendal nerve, supplying most of the muscles and the skin of the perineum.

perineal section *n.* An incision through the perineum, especially external urethrotomy.

perineal space *n.* Either of two perineal spaces, designated deep and superficial.

perineo– *pref.* Perineum: *perineotomy.*

per·i·ne·o·cele (pĕr′ə-nē′ə-sēl′) *n.* See **perineal hernia.**

per·i·ne·o·plas·ty (pĕr′ə-nē′ə-plăs′tē) *n.* Reparative or plastic surgery of the perineum.

per·i·ne·or·rha·phy (pĕr′ə-nē-ôr′ə-fē) *n.* Suture of the perineum.

per·i·ne·o·scro·tal (pĕr′ə-nē′ə-skrōt′l) *adj.* Relating to the perineum and the scrotum.

per·i·ne·os·to·my (pĕr′ə-nē-ŏs′tə-mē) *n.* Urethrostomy through an incision in the perineum.

per·i·ne·ot·o·my (pĕr′ə-nē-ŏt′ə-mē) *n.* Incision into the perineum, as in external urethrotomy or lithotomy or to facilitate childbirth.

per·i·ne·o·vag·i·nal (pĕr′ə-nē-ə-văj′ə-nəl) *adj.* Relating to the perineum and the vagina.

per·i·ne·phri·tis (pĕr′ə-nə-frī′tĭs) *n.* Inflammation of the tissues surrounding a kidney.

per·i·neph·ri·um (pĕr′ə-nĕf′rē-əm) *n., pl.* **-ri·a** (-rē-ə) The connective and fatty tissues surrounding a kidney. —**per′i·neph′ral** (-frəl), **per′i·neph′ri·al** (-rē-əl), **per′i·neph′ric** (-rĭk) *adj.*

per·i·ne·um (pĕr′ə-nē′əm) *n., pl.* **-ne·a** (-nē′ə) **1.** The portion of the body in the pelvis occupied by urogenital passages and the rectum, bounded in front by the pubic arch, in the back by the coccyx, and laterally by part of the hipbone. **2.** The region between the scrotum and the anus in males, and between the posterior vulva junction and the anus in females. —**per′i·ne′al** (-nē′əl) *adj.*

per·i·neu·ral anesthesia (pĕr′ə-no͝or′əl) *n.* Injection of an anesthetic agent about a nerve.

per·i·neu·ri·tis (pĕr′ə-no͝o-rī′tĭs) *n.* Inflammation of the perineurium.

per·i·neu·ri·um (pĕr′ə-no͝or′ē-əm) *n., pl.* **-neu·ri·a** (-ē-ə) The sheath of connective tissue enclosing a bundle of nerve fibers. —**per′i·neu′ri·al** *adj.*

pe·ri·od (pîr′ē-əd) *n.* **1.** An interval of time characterized by the occurrence of a certain condition, event, or phenomenon. **2.** One of the stages of a disease. **3.** A menstrual period. **4.** A sequence of elements arranged in order of increasing atomic number.

pe·ri·od·ic (pîr′ē-ŏd′ĭk) *adj.* **1.** Having or marked by repeated cycles. **2.** Recurring at regular intervals.

per·i·od·ic acid (pûr′ī-ŏd′ĭk) *n.* A white, crystalline inorganic acid that contains iodine and is used as an oxidizer.

per·i·od·ic acid-Schiff (pûr′ī-ŏd′ĭk) *adj. Abbr.* **PAS** Of, relating to, or being a reaction that tests for polysaccharides and related substances through the treatment of tissue sections with periodic acid stain and Schiff's reagent.

pe·ri·od·ic disease (pîr′ē-ŏd′ĭk) *n.* A disease for which symptoms tend to recur at regular intervals.

pe·ri·o·dic·i·ty (pîr′ē-ə-dĭs′ĭ-tē) *n.* **1.** The quality or state of being periodic; recurrence at regular intervals. **2.** The tendency of chemical elements to have similar properties when arranged according to their atomic number. **3.** The position of an element in the periodic table.

periodic law *n.* The principle that properties of elements recur periodically as atomic numbers increase.

periodic neutropenia *n.* Neutropenia recurring at regular intervals, associated with various types of infectious diseases. Also called *cyclic neutropenia.*

periodic paralysis *n.* A group of diseases marked by episodes of muscular weakness or flaccid paralysis without loss of consciousness, speech, or sensation.

periodic table *n.* A tabular arrangement of the elements according to their atomic numbers so that elements with similar chemical properties are in the same column.

per·i·o·don·tal (pĕr'ē-ə-dŏn'tl) *adj.* **1.** Surrounding or encasing a tooth. **2.** Relating to or affecting tissues and structures surrounding and supporting the teeth.

periodontal ligament *n.* The connective tissue surrounding the root of a tooth and attaching it to its bony socket. Also called *alveolodental ligament, periodontal membrane.*

periodontal membrane fiber *n.* Any of the collagen fibers that run from the cementum to the alveolar bone and suspend a tooth in its socket.

per·i·o·don·tics (pĕr'ē-ə-dŏn'tĭks) *n.* The branch of dentistry concerned with the care and treatment of the tissues surrounding and supporting the teeth. Also called *periodontia.* —**per'i·o·don'tic** *adj.* —**per'i·o·don'tist** *n.*

per·i·o·don·tist (pĕr'ē-ə-dŏn'tĭst) *n.* A dentist who specializes in periodontics.

per·i·o·don·ti·tis (pĕr'ē-ō'dŏn-tī'tĭs) *n.* Disease of the periodontium characterized by inflammation of the gums, resorption of the alveolar bone, and degeneration of the periodontal membrane.

per·i·o·don·ti·um (pĕr'ē-ə-dŏn'shē-əm) *n., pl.* **–tia** (-shə, -shē-ə) The tissues that surround and support the teeth, including the gums, cementum, periodontal ligament, and alveolar and supporting bone. Also called *alveolodental membrane, peridental membrane.*

per·i·o·don·to·cla·sia (pĕr'ē-ō-dŏn'tə-klā'zhə) *n.* Pathological destruction of the periodontium. No longer in technical use.

per·i·o·don·to·sis (pĕr'ē-ō'dŏn-tō'sĭs) *n.* A degenerative disease of the periodontal ligament and tooth sockets, characterized by looseness and migration of teeth.

per·i·o·nych·i·a (pĕr'ē-ə-nĭk'ē-ə) *n.* Inflammation of the perionychium.

per·i·o·nych·i·um (pĕr'ē-ə-nĭk'ē-əm) *n., pl.* **–i·a** (-ē-ə) The border of epidermal tissue surrounding a fingernail or toenail. Also called *nail skin.*

per·i·o·o·pho·ri·tis (pĕr'ē-ō'ə-fə-rī'tĭs) *n.* Inflammation of the peritoneal covering of the ovary. Also called *periovaritis.*

per·i·o·oph·o·ro·sal·pin·gi·tis (pĕr'ē-ō-ŏf'ə-rō-săl'pĭn-jī'tĭs) *n.* Inflammation of the peritoneum and other tissues surrounding the ovary and oviduct.

per·i·op·er·a·tive (pĕr'ē-ŏp'ər-ə-tĭv, -ə-rā'tĭv, -ŏp'rə-) *adj.* Occurring during a surgical operation.

per·i·or·bit (pĕr'ē-ôr'bĭt) *n.* The periosteum of the orbit. Also called *orbital fascia.*

per·i·or·bit·al (pĕr'ē-ôr'bĭ-tl) *adj.* **1.** Situated around the orbit of the eye. **2.** Of, relating to, or characterizing the periorbit.

per·i·or·chi·tis (pĕr'ē-ôr-kī'tĭs) *n.* Inflammation of the tunica vaginalis testis.

periosteal bud *n.* A vascular connective tissue bud from the perichondrium that enters the cartilage of a developing long bone and contributes to the formation of a center for ossification.

periosteal graft *n.* A graft of periosteum, usually placed on bare bone.

periosteo– *pref.* Periosteum: *periosteotomy.*

per·i·os·te·o·ma (pĕr'ē-ŏs'tē-ō'mə) *n.* A neoplasm derived from the periosteum of a bone. Also called *periosteophyte.*

per·i·os·te·o·my·e·li·tis (pĕr'ē-ŏs'tē-ō-mī'ə-lī'tĭs) *n.* Inflammation of the entire bone, including the periosteum and the marrow.

per·i·os·te·o·phyte (pĕr'ē-ŏs'tē-ə-fīt') *n.* See **periosteoma.**

per·i·os·te·o·plas·tic amputation (pĕr'ē-ŏs'tē-ə-plăs'tĭk) *n.* See **subperiosteal amputation.**

per·i·os·te·o·sis (pĕr'ē-ŏs'tē-ō'sĭs) *or* **per·i·os·to·sis** (-ŏ-stō'sĭs) *n.* Formation of a periosteoma.

per·i·os·te·ot·o·my (pĕr'ē-ŏs'tē-ŏt'ə-mē) *n.* Incision of the periosteum.

per·i·os·te·um (pĕr'ē-ŏs'tē-əm) *n., pl.* **–te·a** (-tē-ə) The thick fibrous membrane covering the entire surface of a bone except its articular cartilage and serving as an attachment for muscles and tendons. —**per'i·os'te·al** (-tē-əl) *adj.*

per·i·os·ti·tis (pĕr'ē-ŏ-stī'tĭs) *or* **per·i·os·te·i·tis** (-ŏs'tē-ī'tĭs) *n.* Inflammation of the periosteum.

per·i·o·tic (pĕr'ē-ō'tĭk) *adj.* **1.** Situated around the ear. **2.** Of or relating to the bones immediately around the inner ear.

per·i·o·va·ri·tis (pĕr'ē-ō'və-rī'tĭs) *n.* See **perioophoritis.**

per·i·pach·y·men·in·gi·tis (pĕr'ə-păk'ē-mĕn'ĭn-jī'tĭs) *n.* A condition in which the parietal layer of the dura mater becomes inflamed.

per·i·pan·cre·a·ti·tis (pĕr'ə-păng'krē-ə-tī'tĭs) *n.* Inflammation of the peritoneal covering of the pancreas.

pe·riph·er·ad (pə-rĭf'ə-răd') *adj.* Toward the periphery.

pe·riph·er·al (pə-rĭf'ər-əl) *adj.* **1.** Related to, located in, or constituting an outer boundary or periphery. **2.** Perceived or perceiving near the outer edges of the retina. **3.** Of or relating to the surface or outer part of a body or organ; external. **4.** Of, relating to, or being part of the peripheral nervous system.

peripheral dysostosis *n.* Dysostosis of the metacarpals and metatarsals that may be hereditary and is accompanied by variable facial features.

peripheral motor neuron *n.* See **postganglionic motor neuron.**

peripheral nervous system *n.* The part of the vertebrate nervous system constituting the nerves outside the central nervous system and including the cranial nerves, the spinal nerves, and the sympathetic and parasympathetic nervous systems.

peripheral ossifying fibroma *n.* A gingival fibroma derived from cells of the periodontal ligament and usually developing in response to local irritants such as plaque and calculus on associated teeth.

peripheral scotoma *n.* A scotoma outside of the central 30 degrees of the visual field.

peripheral vascular disease *n. Abbr.* **PVD** Any of various diseases, especiallly arteriosclerosis, occuring in blood vessels outside the heart and the brain.

peripheral vision *n.* Vision produced by light rays falling on areas of the retina beyond the macula. Also called *indirect vision.*

pe·riph·er·y (pə-rĭf'ə-rē) *n.* **1.** The outermost part or region within a precise boundary; the part away from center. **2.** The outer surface of a solid.

per·i·phle·bi·tis (pĕr'ə-flĭ-bī'tĭs) *n.* Inflammation of the outer coat of a vein or of tissues surrounding it.

per·i·po·ri·tis (pĕr′ə-pə-rī′tĭs) *n.* A skin condition characterized by miliary papules and papulovesicles accompanied by infection with staphylococcal bacteria, occurring most frequently in infants.

per·i·proc·ti·tis (pĕr′ə-prŏk-tī′tĭs) *n.* Inflammation of the areolar tissue about the rectum. Also called *perirectitis.*

per·i·pros·ta·ti·tis (pĕr′ə-prŏs′tə-tī′tĭs) *n.* Inflammation of the tissues surrounding the prostate.

per·i·py·le·phle·bi·tis (pĕr′ə-pī′lə-flĭ-bī′tĭs) *n.* Inflammation of the tissues around the portal vein.

per·i·rec·ti·tis (pĕr′ə-rĕk-tī′tĭs) *n.* See **periproctitis.**

per·i·rhi·zo·cla·sia (pĕr′ə-rī′zə-klā′zhə) *n.* Inflammatory destruction of tissues directly surrounding the root of a tooth including the cementum and the adjacent layers of alveolar bone.

per·i·sal·pin·gi·tis (pĕr′ĭ-săl′pĭn-jī′tĭs) *n.* Inflammation of the peritoneal covering of the fallopian tube.

per·i·sal·pinx (pĕr′ĭ-săl′pĭngks) *n.* The peritoneal covering of the uterine tube.

per·i·scop·ic (pĕr′ĭ-skŏp′ĭk) *adj.* Of, relating to, or permitting the observation of objects from positions in or out of the direct line of sight.

per·i·sig·moid·i·tis (pĕr′ĭ-sĭg′moi-dī′tĭs) *n.* Inflammation of the connective tissues surrounding the sigmoid flexure of the colon.

per·i·sper·ma·ti·tis (pĕr′ĭ-spûr′mə-tī′tĭs) *n.* Inflammation of the tissues surrounding the spermatic cord of the scrotum.

per·i·splanch·ni·tis (pĕr′ĭ-splăngk-nī′tĭs) *n.* Inflammation surrounding any visceral organ.

per·i·sple·ni·tis (pĕr′ĭ-splĭ-nī′tĭs) *n.* Inflammation of the peritoneal covering of the spleen.

per·i·spon·dy·li·tis (pĕr′ĭ-spŏn′dl-ī′tĭs) *n.* Inflammation of the tissues about a vertebra.

per·i·stal·sis (pĕr′ĭ-stôl′sĭs, -stăl′-) *n., pl.* **-ses** (-sēz) The wavelike muscular contractions of the intestine or other tubular structure that propel the contents onward by alternate contraction and relaxation. Also called *vermicular movement.* **—per′i·stal′tic** (-stôl′tĭk, -stăl′-) *adj.*

pe·ris·to·le (pə-rĭs′tə-lē) *n.* The tonic contractions of the walls of the stomach about its contents. **—per′i·stol′ic** (pĕr′ĭ-stŏl′ĭk) *adj.*

per·i·tec·to·my (pĕr′ĭ-tĕk′tə-mē) *n.* The removal of a pericorneal strip of the conjunctiva to correct pannus. Also called *peritomy.*

per·i·ten·din·e·um (pĕr′ĭ-tĕn-dĭn′ē-əm) *n., pl.* **-e·a** (-ē-ə) Any of the fibrous sheaths surrounding the primary bundles of fibers in a tendon.

per·i·ten·di·ni·tis (pĕr′ĭ-tĕn′də-nī′tĭs) *n.* Inflammation of the sheath of a tendon. Also called *peritenontitis.*

per·i·the·li·um (pĕr′ə-thē′lē-əm) *n., pl.* **-li·a** (-lē-ə) The connective tissue surrounding small blood vessels and capillaries.

per·i·thy·roid·i·tis (pĕr′ə-thī′roi-dī′tĭs) *n.* Inflammation of the capsule or tissues surrounding the thyroid gland.

pe·rit·o·my (pə-rĭt′ə-mē) *n.* 1. See **peritectomy.** 2. See **circumcision.**

peritoneal cavity *n.* The potential space between the parietal and visceral layers of the peritoneum.

peritoneal dialysis *n.* The removal of soluble substances and water from the body by transfer across the peritoneum, utilizing a solution which is intermittently introduced into and removed from the peritoneal cavity.

per·i·to·ne·al·gia (pĕr′ĭ-tn-ē-ăl′jə) *n.* Pain in the peritoneum.

peritoneo- *pref.* Peritoneum: *peritoneoscopy.*

per·i·to·ne·o·cen·te·sis (pĕr′ĭ-tn-ē′ō-sĕn-tē′sĭs) *n.* 1. Paracentesis of the peritoneal cavity. 2. Paracentesis of the abdominal cavity; abdominocentesis.

per·i·to·ne·oc·ly·sis (pĕr′ĭ-tn-ē-ŏk′lĭ-sĭs, -ē′ə-klī′sĭs) *n.* Irrigation of the abdominal cavity.

per·i·to·ne·op·a·thy (pĕr′ĭ-tn-ē-ŏp′ə-thē) *n.* Disease of the peritoneum.

per·i·to·ne·o·per·i·car·di·al (pĕr′ĭ-tn-ē′ō-pĕr′ĭ-kär′dē-əl) *adj.* Of or relating to the peritoneum and the pericardium.

per·i·to·ne·o·pex·y (pĕr′ĭ-tn-ē′ə-pĕk′sē) *n.* Surgical suspension or fixation of the peritoneum.

per·i·to·ne·o·plas·ty (pĕr′ĭ-tn-ē′ə-plăs′tē) *n.* The surgical loosening of adhesions in the abdominal viscera and the covering of the resultant raw surfaces with peritoneum to prevent recurrence.

per·i·to·ne·o·scope (pĕr′ĭ-tn-ē′ə-skōp′) *n.* See **laparoscope.**

per·i·to·ne·os·co·py (pĕr′ĭ-tn-ē-ŏs′kə-pē) *n.* Internal examination of the peritoneum with a peritoneoscope passed through an incision in the abdominal wall. Also called *celioscopy, ventroscopy.*

per·i·to·ne·ot·o·my (pĕr′ĭ-tn-ē-ŏt′ə-mē) *n.* Incision of the peritoneum.

per·i·to·ne·o·ve·nous shunt (pĕr′ĭ-tn-ē′ō-vē′nəs) *n.* A shunt between the peritoneal cavity and the venous system, usually by means of a catheter.

per·i·to·ne·um *or* **per·i·to·nae·um** (pĕr′ĭ-tn-ē′əm) *n., pl.* **-to·ne·a** *or* **-to·nae·a** (-tn-ē′ə) The serous sac consisting of mesothelium and a thin layer of irregular connective tissue that lines the abdominal cavity, covers most of the viscera contained therein, and itself forms two cavities, the peritoneal and the omental bursa, which are connected by the epiploic foramen. **—per′i·to·ne′al** *adj.*

per·i·to·ni·tis (pĕr′ĭ-tn-ī′tĭs) *n.* Inflammation of the peritoneum.

peritonitis de·for·mans (dē-fôr′mănz′) *n.* Chronic peritonitis in which thickening of the intestinal mesentery and the contracting of adhesions may cause the membrane to shorten and the intestines to kink and retract.

per·i·ton·sil·lar abscess (pĕr′ĭ-tŏn′sə-lər) *n.* An abscess formed usually above and behind the tonsil, due to extension of infection beyond the tonsillar capsule. Also called *quinsy.*

per·i·ton·sil·li·tis (pĕr′ĭ-tŏn′sə-lī′tĭs) *n.* Inflammation of the connective tissue above and behind the tonsil.

pe·rit·ri·chal (pə-rĭt′rĭ-kəl) *or* **pe·rit·ri·chate** (-kāt′) *adj.* Having flagella uniformly distributed over the surface. Used of bacteria.

pe·rit·ri·chous (pə-rĭt′rĭ-kəs) *adj.* 1. Of, relating to, or having cilia or other appendicular organs projecting from the periphery of a cell. 2. Peritrichal.

per·i·tu·bu·lar contractile cell (pĕr′ĭ-too′byə-lər) *n.*

Any of various flattened cells that surround seminiferous tubules. Also called *myoid cell.*

per·i·u·re·ter·i·tis (pĕr′ē-yŏ͞o-rē′tə-rī′tĭs, -yŏ͞or′ĭ-tə-) *n.* Inflammation of the tissues surrounding a ureter.

per·i·u·re·thri·tis (pĕr′ē-yŏ͞or′ĭ-thrī′tĭs) *n.* Inflammation of the tissues surrounding the urethra.

per·i·u·ter·ine (pĕr′ē-yŏ͞o′tər-ĭn, -tə-rīn′) *adj.* Of, relating to, or surrounding the uterus.

per·i·vag·i·ni·tis (pĕr′ə-văj′ə-nī′tĭs) *n.* Inflammation of the connective tissue around the vagina. Also called *pericolpitis.*

per·i·vas·cu·lar fibrous capsule (pĕr′ə-văs′kyə-lər) *n.* A layer of connective tissue ensheathing the hepatic artery, portal vein, and bile ducts as they ramify within the liver. Also called *Glisson's capsule.*

per·i·vas·cu·li·tis (pĕr′ə-văs′kyə-lī′tĭs) *n.* See **periangiitis.**

per·i·ves·i·cal (pĕr′ə-věs′ĭ-kəl) *adj.* Pericystic.

per·i·vis·cer·al (pĕr′ə-vĭs′ər-əl) *adj.* Surrounding the viscera.

per·i·vis·cer·i·tis (pĕr′ə-vĭs′ə-rī′tĭs) *n.* Inflammation of the tissues surrounding a viscus.

per·lèche (pər-lĕsh′, pĕr-) *n.* See **angular cheilitis.**

per·ma·nent cartilage (pûr′mə-nənt) *n.* Cartilage that remains as such and does not become converted into bone.

permanent dentition *n.* See **secondary dentition.**

permanent tooth *n.* Any of the teeth of the secondary dentition. Also called *second tooth.*

per·man·ga·nate (pər-măng′gə-nāt′) *n.* Any of the salts of permanganic acid, all of which are strong oxidizing agents.

per·man·gan·ic acid (pûr′măn-găn′ĭk, -măng-) *n.* An unstable inorganic acid existing only in dilute solution. Its purple aqueous solution is used as an oxidizing agent.

Per·max (pûr′măks′) A trademark for the drug pergolide mesylate.

per·me·a·bil·i·ty (pûr′mē-ə-bĭl′ĭ-tē) *n.* **1.** The property or condition of being permeable. **2.** The rate of flow of a liquid or gas through a porous material.

per·me·a·ble (pûr′mē-ə-bəl) *adj.* That can be permeated or penetrated, especially by liquids or gases.

per·me·ase (pûr′mē-ās′) *n.* An enzyme that promotes the passage of a substance across a cell membrane.

per·me·ate (pûr′mē-āt′) *v.* **1.** To spread or flow throughout; pervade. **2.** To pass through the openings or interstices of, as a liquid through a membrane. —*n.* (-ĭt, -āt′) One that can permeate. —**per′me·ant** (-ənt), **per′me·a′tive** (-ā′tĭv) *adj.*

per·me·a·tion (pûr′mē-ā′shən) *n.* The process of spreading through or penetrating, as in the extension of a malignant neoplasm by continuous proliferation of the cells along the blood or lymph vessels.

per·meth·rin (pər-mĕth′rĭn) *n.* A topical insecticide used to treat head lice and nits, scabies, and various species of ticks.

per·ni·cious (pər-nĭsh′əs) *adj.* Tending to cause death or serious injury; deadly.

pernicious anemia *n.* A severe form of anemia most often affecting older adults, caused by failure of the stomach to absorb vitamin B_{12} and characterized by abnormally large red blood cells, gastrointestinal disturbances, and lesions of the spinal cord. Also called *Addison's anemia, malignant anemia.*

pernicious vomiting *n.* Uncontrollable vomiting.

pero– *pref.* Malformed; defective: *perodactyly.*

pe·ro·dac·ty·ly (pîr′ə-dăk′tə-lē) *n.* A congenital condition characterized by deformed fingers or toes.

pe·ro·me·li·a (pîr′ə-mē′lē-ə, -mēl′yə) *n.* Severe congenital malformations of the limbs.

per·o·ne·al (pĕr′ə-nē′əl) *adj.* Of or relating to the fibula or to the outer portion of the leg.

peroneal artery *n.* An artery with its origin in the posterior tibial artery, with distribution to the soleus muscle, the long flexor muscle of the big toe, the muscles of the fibula, the inferior tibiofibular articulation, and the ankle joint; and with anastomoses to the lateral malleolar, lateral tarsal, and lateral plantar arteries, and to the dorsal artery of the foot. Also called *fibular artery.*

peroneal brev·is (brĕv′ĭs) *n.* A muscle with origin from the lower two thirds of the lateral surface of the fibula, with insertion into the base of the fifth metatarsal bone, with nerve supply from the peroneal nerve, and whose action everts the foot. Also called *fibularis brevis.*

peroneal long·us (lŏn′gəs) *n.* A muscle with origin from the fibula and the tibia, with insertion to the medial cuneiform bone and the base of the first metatarsal, with nerve supply from the peroneal nerve, and whose action causes plantar flexion and eversion of the foot. Also called *fibularis longus.*

peroneal muscle *n.* Either of two muscles of the lower leg, the peroneal longus or the peroneal brevis.

peroneal muscular atrophy *n.* A hereditary form of muscular atrophy characterized by progressive wasting of the distal muscles of the extremities, usually affecting the legs before the arms. Also called *Charcot-Marie-Tooth disease.*

peroneal vein *n.* Any of the veins that accompany the peroneal artery and enter the popliteal vein. Also called *fibular vein.*

per·o·ral (pər-ôr′əl) *adj.* Performed or administered through or by way of the mouth.

per os (pər ŏs) *adv.* By way of the mouth, as in the administration of medication.

per·ox·i·dase (pə-rŏk′sĭ-dās′, -dāz′) *n.* Any of a group of enzymes that occur especially in plant cells and catalyze the oxidation of a substance by a peroxide.

per·ox·ide (pə-rŏk′sīd′) *n.* **1.** A compound, such as sodium peroxide, that contains a peroxy group and yields hydrogen peroxide when treated with an acid. **2.** Hydrogen peroxide.

per·ox·i·some (pə-rŏk′sĭ-sōm′) *n.* A cell organelle containing enzymes, such as catalase and oxidase, that catalyze the production and breakdown of hydrogen peroxide. Also called *microbody.*

per·ox·y (pə-rŏk′sē) *adj.* Containing the bivalent group O_2.

per·phen·a·zine (pər-fĕn′ə-zēn′) *n.* A crystalline compound used as a tranquilizer especially in the treatment of psychosis and to prevent or alleviate nausea and vomiting.

per·rec·tum (pər rĕk′təm) *adv.* By way of the rectum, as in the administration of medication.

per·salt (pûr′sôlt′) *n.* A salt containing the greatest proportion possible of the peroxy group.

per·sev·er·a·tion (pər-sĕv′ə-rā′shən) *n.* **1.** Uncontrollable repetition of a particular response, such as a word, phrase, or gesture, despite the absence or cessation of a stimulus, usually caused by brain injury or other organic disorder. **2.** The tendency to continue or repeat an act or activity after the cessation of the original stimulus.

per·sist·ence (pər-sĭs′təns) *n.* **1.** Continuance of an effect after the cause is removed. **2.** Continuance of a part or organ, rather than having it disappear in an early stage of development.

per·sist·ent anterior hyperplastic primary vitreous body (pər-sĭs′tənt) *n.* A unilateral congenital abnormality of the eye occurring in full-term infants and characterized by a retrolental fibrovascular membrane, leukokoria, microphthalmos, shallow anterior chamber, and elongated ciliary processes.

persistent chronic hepatitis *n.* Benign chronic hepatitis that may follow acute hepatitis A or B, or may complicate bowel diseases.

persistent posterior hyperplastic primary vitreous body *n.* A unilateral congenital anomaly of the eye in full-term infants that is associated with a congenital retinal fold and a vitreous membranous stalk containing remnants of the hyaloid artery.

persistent trun·cus ar·te·ri·o·sus (trŭng′kəs är-tîr′ē-ō′səs) *n.* A congenital cardiovascular deformity resulting from the failure of the septum between the aorta and pulmonary trunk to develop and characterized by a common arterial trunk opening out of both ventricles with the pulmonary arteries branching from the ascending common trunk.

per·son (pûr′sən) *n.* **1.** A living human. **2.** The composite of characteristics that make up an individual personality; the self. **3.** The living body of a human. **4.** Physique and general appearance.

per·so·na (pər-sō′nə) *n., pl.* **–nas** *or* **–nae** (-nē) The role that one assumes or displays in public or society; one's public image or personality, as distinguished from the inner self.

per·son·al care (pûr′sə-nəl) *n.* The occupation of attending to the physical needs of people who are disabled or otherwise unable to take care of themselves, including tasks such as bathing, management of bodily functions, and cooking.

personal equation *n.* A constant but slight error in judgment, perceptual response, or action that is specific to an individual and is so constant that it is usually possible to allow for it when assessing that person's statements or conclusions, thus arriving at approximate exactness.

per·son·al·i·ty (pûr′sə-năl′ĭ-tē) *n.* **1.** The quality or condition of being a person. **2.** The totality of qualities and traits, as of character or behavior, that are peculiar to a specific person. **3.** The pattern of collective character, behavioral, temperamental, emotional, and mental traits of a person. **4.** Distinctive qualities of a person, especially those personal characteristics that make one socially appealing.

personality disorder *n.* Any of a group of disorders in which patterns of perceiving, relating to, and thinking about one's self and one's environment interfere with the long-term functioning of an individual, often manifested in deviant behavior and lifestyle.

personality formation *n.* The organization and structure of the components of a person's character or personality.

personality inventory *n.* A questionnaire that is scored to yield a profile of the particular traits or characteristics that make up the respondent's personality.

personality profile *n.* **1.** A method of presenting the results of psychological testing in graphic form. **2.** A brief description of the personality of an individual.

personality test *n.* A test, usually involving a standardized series of questions or tasks, used to describe or evaluate a subject's personality traits.

per·spi·ra·tion (pûr′spə-rā′shən) *n.* **1.** The fluid, consisting of water with small amounts of urea and salts, that is excreted through the pores of the skin by the sweat glands. **2.** The act or process of excreting this fluid through the pores of the skin. —**per·spir′a·to′ry** (pər-spīr′ə-tôr′ē, pûr′spər-ə-) *adj.*

per·spire (pər-spīr′) *v.* To excrete perspiration through the pores of the skin.

Pert (pûrt), **Candace Beebe** Born 1946. American biochemist noted for her study of brain chemicals and the locations of their receptors.

Per·thes disease (pĕr′tēz, -tĕs) *n.* See **osteochondritis deformans juvenilis.**

per tu·bam (pər tōō′bəm) *adv.* Through a tube, as in the administration of food, liquids, or medication.

per·tus·sis (pər-tŭs′ĭs) *n.* See **whooping cough.**

pertussis immune globulin *n.* A sterile solution of globulins derived from the plasma of adult human donors who have been immunized against and have formed antibodies to pertussis, used in the prevention and treatment of pertussis.

pertussis vaccine *n.* A vaccine containing inactivated *Bordetella pertussis* bacteria, often used in the diphtheria, tetanus toxoids, and pertussis vaccine to immunize against whooping cough. Also called *whooping cough vaccine.*

Per·utz (pə-rōōts′, pĕr′əts), **Max Ferdinand** 1914–2002. Austrian-born English biochemist. He shared a 1962 Nobel Prize for determining the molecular structure of blood components.

Pe·ru·vi·an wart (pə-rōō′vē-ən) *n.* A soft conical or pedunculated papule that erupts in groups as a manifestation of the second stage of bartonellosis. Also called *verruca peruana, verruca peruviana.*

per·va·sive developmental disorder (pər-vā′sĭv) *n.* Any of several disorders, such as autism and Asperger's syndrome, characterized by severe deficits in many areas of development, including social interaction and communication, or by the presence of repetitive, stereotyped behaviors. Such disorders are usually evident in the first years of life and are often associated with some degree of mental retardation.

per·ver·sion (pər-vûr′zhən) *n.* A practice or act, especially one that is sexual in nature, considered abnormal or deviant.

per·vert·ed (pər-vûr′tĭd) *adj.* **1.** Deviating from what is considered normal or correct. **2.** Of, relating to, or practicing sexual perversion.

per vi·as na·tu·ra·les (pər vī′əs năch′ə-rā′lēz) *adv.* Through the natural passages, as in a vaginal delivery of a child.

per·vi·ous (pûr′vē-əs) *adj.* Open to passage or entrance; permeable.

pes (pās) *n., pl.* **pe·des** (pěd′ās′) **1.** The foot. **2.** A foot-like or basal structure or part. **3.** Talipes.

pes an·se·ri·nus (ăn′sə-rī′nəs) *n.* **1.** The tendinous expansions of the sartorius, gracilis, and semitendinous muscles at the medial border of the tuberosity of the tibia. **2.** See **intraparotid plexus.**

pes hip·po·cam·pi (hĭp′ə-kăm′pī) *n.* The anterior thickened extremity of the hippocampus.

pes·sa·ry (pěs′ə-rē) *n.* **1.** Any of various devices worn in the vagina to support or correct the position of the uterus or rectum. **2.** A contraceptive diaphragm. **3.** A medicated vaginal suppository.

pest (pěst) *n.* **1.** An injurious plant or animal, especially one harmful to humans. **2.** A deadly epidemic disease; a pestilence.

pest house *n.* A hospital for patients affected with plague or other infectious disease.

pes·ti·cide (pěs′tĭ-sīd′) *n.* A chemical used to kill pests, especially insects.

pes·tif·er·ous (pě-stĭf′ər-əs) *adj.* **1.** Producing or breeding infectious disease. **2.** Infected with or contaminated by an epidemic disease.

pes·ti·lence (pěs′tə-ləns) *n.* **1.** A usually fatal epidemic disease, especially bubonic plague. **2.** An epidemic of such a disease.

pes·ti·len·tial (pěs′tə-lěn′shəl) *adj.* Of, relating to, or tending to produce a pestilence.

pes·tle (pěs′əl, pěs′təl) *n.* A club-shaped, hand-held tool for grinding or mashing substances in a mortar.

pes var·us (vâr′əs) *n.* See **talipes varus.**

PET *abbr.* positron emission tomography

peta– *pref.* One quadrillion (10^{15}): *petagram.*

–petal *suff.* Moving toward: *basipetal.*

pe·te·chi·a (pə-tē′kē-ə) *n., pl.* **–chi·ae** (-kē-ī′) A small purplish spot on a body surface, such as the skin or a mucous membrane, caused by a minute hemorrhage and often seen in typhus. —**pe·te′chi·al** *adj.*

petechial hemorrhage *n.* Capillary hemorrhage into the skin, forming petechiae. Also called *punctate hemorrhage.*

Pe·ters′ ovum (pē′tərz, pā′tərs) *n.* A fertilized ovum that is 13 to 14 days into its development.

pet·i·o·late (pět′ē-ə-lāt′, pět′ē-ō′lĭt) *or* **pet·i·o·lat·ed** (pět′ē-ə-lā′tĭd) *or* **pet·i·oled** (pět′ē-ōld′) *adj.* Having a petiole.

pet·i·ole (pět′ē-ōl′) *n.* A stem or pedicle.

pet·it mal (pět′ē mäl′, măl′) *n.* A form of epilepsy, occurring most often in adolescents and children, characterized by frequent but transient lapses of consciousness and only rare spasms or falling. Also called *absence, petit mal epilepsy.*

Pe·tit′s lumbar triangle (pə-tēz′) *n.* See **lumbar triangle.**

pe·tri dish (pē′trē) *n.* A shallow circular dish with a loose-fitting cover, used to culture bacteria or other microorganisms.

pet·ri·fac·tion (pět′rə-făk′shən) *or* **pet·ri·fi·ca·tion** (-fĭ-kā′shən) *n.* A process of fossilization in which dissolved minerals replace organic matter.

pé·tris·sage (pā-trē-säzh′) *n.* A manipulation in massage in which the muscles are kneaded.

petro– *or* **petri–** *or* **petr–** *pref.* Rock; stone; stone-like hardness: *petrous.*

pet·roc·ip·i·tal (pět′rŏk-sĭp′ĭ-tl) *adj.* Of or relating to the petrous portion of the temporal bone and to the occipital bone of the skull.

pet·ro·la·tum (pět′rə-lā′təm) *n.* See **petroleum jelly.**

pe·tro·le·um ben·zin (pə-trō′lē-əm běn′zĭn) *n.* See **benzine** (sense 1).

petroleum jelly *n.* A colorless-to-amber semisolid mixture of hydrocarbons obtained from petroleum and used in medicinal ointments. Also called *petrolatum.*

pet·ro·mas·toid (pět′rə-măs′toid′) *adj.* Of or relating to the petrous and the mastoid portions of the temporal bone of the skull.

pe·tro·sa (pə-trō′sə) *n., pl.* **–sae** (-sē) The petrous portion of the temporal bone.

pe·tro·sal (pə-trō′səl) *adj.* Relating to or located near the petrous portion of the temporal bone.

pet·ro·si·tis (pět′rə-sī′tĭs) *n.* Inflammation of the petrous portion of the temporal bone and its air cells.

pet·ro·sphe·noid (pět′rə-sfē′noid′) *adj.* Of or relating to the petrous portion of the temporal bone and to the sphenoid bone of the skull.

pet·ro·squa·mo·sal (pět′rō-skwə-mō′səl) *or* **pet·ro·squa·mous** (-skwā′məs, -skwä′-) *adj.* Of or relating to the petrous and the squamous portions of the temporal bone of the skull.

pet·ro·tym·pan·ic fissure (pět′rō-tĭm-păn′ĭk) *n.* A fissure between the tympanic and petrous portions of the temporal bone. Also called *glaserian fissure.*

pet·rous (pět′rəs) *adj.* **1.** Of stony hardness. **2.** Of or relating to the dense hard portion of the temporal bone that forms a protective case for the inner ear.

petrous ganglion *n.* The lower of two sensory ganglions on the glossopharyngeal nerve as it traverses the jugular foramen. Also called *inferior ganglion of glossopharyngeal nerve.*

PET scan (pět) *n.* A cross-sectional image produced by a PET scanner.

PET scanner *n.* A device that produces cross-sectional x-rays of metabolic processes by means of positron emission tomography. —**PET scanning** *n.*

Pet·ten·kof·fer (pět′n-kô′fər), **Max Josef von** 1818–1901. German chemist noted for his work in the fields of hygiene and disease prevention. He theorized that clean water, adequate ventilation, and effective sewage disposal would prevent the spread of disease.

Peutz-Jeghers syndrome (poōts′-, poets′-) *n.* Inherited polyposis of the intestinal tract, characterized by multiple harmartomas, especially of the jejunum, and associated with melanin spots on the lips, buccal mucosa, and fingers. Also called *Jeghers-Peutz syndrome.*

pex·is (pěk′sĭs) *n.* **1.** Fixation by means of surgery. **2.** The fixation of substances in tissues, such as for histologic examination.

–pexy *suff.* Surgical fixation of an organ: *hysteropexy.*

Pey·er's patches *or* **Pey·er's glands** (pī′ərz) *pl.n.* See **aggregated lymphatic follicles.**

Pey·ro·nie's disease (pā-rō-nēz′) *n.* A disease of unknown cause in which patches or strands of dense fibrous tissue surround the cavernous body of the penis, causing deformity and painful erection.

PFB (pē′ĕf-bē′) *n.* Pseudofolliculitis.

Pfeif·fer's bacillus (fī′fərz, pfī′-) *n.* See **Haemophilus influenzae.**

Pfeiffer syndrome *n.* See **type V acrocephalosyndactyly.**

Pflü·ger (floō′gər, pflü′-), **Eduard Friedrich Wilhelm** 1829–1910. German physiologist noted for his work on the sensory function of the spinal cord.

PFT *abbr.* pulmonary function test

pg *abbr.* picogram

pH (pē′āch′) *n.* A measure of the acidity or alkalinity of a solution, numerically equal to 7 for neutral solutions, increasing with increasing alkalinity and decreasing with increasing acidity. The pH scale commonly in use ranges from 0 to 14.

PH *abbr.* public health

PHA *abbr.* phytohemagglutinin

phaco– or **phako–** *pref.* **1.** Lens: *phacomalacia.* **2.** Lens-shaped: *phacoma.*

phac·o·an·a·phy·lax·is (făk′ō-ăn′ə-fə-lăk′sĭs) *n.* Hypersensitivity to protein of the lens of the eye.

phac·o·cele (făk′ə-sēl′) *n.* Hernia of the lens of the eye.

phac·o·cys·tec·to·my (făk′ō-sĭ-stĕk′tə-mē) *n.* Surgical removal of a portion of the capsule of the lens of the eye.

phac·o·e·mul·si·fi·ca·tion (făk′ō-ĭ-mŭl′sə-fĭ-kā′shən) *n.* Removal of a cataract by emulsifying the lens ultrasonically.

phac·o·er·y·sis (făk′ō-ĕr′ĭ-sĭs) *n.* Extraction of a cataract of the lens of the eye using suction.

phac·o·gen·ic glaucoma (făk′ō-jĕn′ĭk) *n.* See **phacomorphic glaucoma.**

phac·oid (făk′oid′) *adj.* Having the shape of a lentil; lens-shaped.

pha·col·y·sis (fă-kŏl′ĭ-sĭs) *n.* The surgical breakdown and removal of the lens of the eye. —**phac′o·lyt′ic** (făk′ə-lĭt′ĭk) *adj.*

pha·co·ma or **pha·ko·ma** (fă-kō′mə) *n., pl.* **-mas** or **-ma·ta** (-mə-tə) A hamartoma found in phacomatosis.

phac·o·ma·la·cia (făk′ō-mə-lā′shə) *n.* Softening of the lens of the eye.

phac·o·ma·to·sis or **phak·o·ma·to·sis** (făk′ō-mə-tō′-sĭs) *n.* Any of a group of congenital and hereditary diseases characterized by the development of hamartomas in various tissues and including neurofibromatosis, Lindau's disease, Sturge-Weber syndrome, and tuberous sclerosis.

phac·o·mor·phic glaucoma (făk′ō-môr′fĭk) *n.* Secondary glaucoma caused either by excessive size or by spherical shape of the lens. Also called *phacogenic glaucoma.*

phac·o·scope (făk′ə-skōp′) *n.* An instrument used to observe changes in the crystalline lens during accommodation.

phaeo– *pref.* Variant of **pheo–.**

phae·o·hy·pho·my·co·sis (fē′ō-hī′fō-mī-kō′sĭs) *n.* Any of a group of superficial and deep infections caused by dematiaceous fungi that form hyphae and yeastlike cells in tissue.

phage (fāj) *n.* See **bacteriophage.**

–phage *suff.* One that eats: *macrophage.*

phag·e·de·na (făj′ĭ-dē′nə) *n.* A cutaneous ulcer that rapidly spreads peripherally, destroying tissues as it increases in size. Also called *phagedenic ulcer.* —**phag′e·den′ic** (-dĕn′ĭk) *adj.*

phage display *n.* A technique using recombinant DNA technology to create bacteriophages with a desired peptide embedded in the surface of their protein shells. Agonists and antagonists of the target peptide can then be identified experimentally, enabling the engineering of antibodies and development of new drugs.

–phagia or **–phagy** *suff.* The eating of a specified substance or in a specified manner: *dysphagia.*

phago– *pref.* Eating; consuming: *phagocyte.*

phag·o·cyte (făg′ə-sīt′) *n.* A cell, such as a white blood cell, that engulfs and absorbs waste material, harmful microorganisms, or other foreign bodies in the bloodstream and tissues.

phag·o·cyt·ic (făg′ə-sĭt′ĭk) *adj.* **1.** Of or relating to phagocytes. **2.** Of, relating to, or characterized by phagocytosis.

phagocytic index *n.* The average number of bacteria observed in the cytoplasm of neutrophils after a mixture of blood serum, bacteria, and neutrophils has been incubated.

phagocytic pneumonocyte *n.* An alveolar phagocyte containing hemosiderin, carbon, or other foreign particles.

phag·o·cy·tin (făg′ə-sīt′n) *n.* A labile bacteriocide isolated from polymorphonuclear white blood cells.

phag·o·cy·tize (făg′ə-sī-tīz′, -sī′-) *v.* To ingest by phagocytosis; phagocytose.

phag·o·cy·tol·y·sis (făg′ə-sī-tŏl′ĭ-sĭs) *n.* The destruction of phagocytes or white blood cells that occurs during the process of blood coagulation or as the result of the introduction of certain antagonistic foreign substances into the body. —**phag′o·cy′to·lyt′ic** (făg′ə-sī′tə-lĭt′ĭk) *adj.*

phag·o·cy·tose (făg′ə-sī-tōs′, -tōz′, -sī′tōs, -tōz) *v.* To phagocytize.

phag·o·cy·to·sis (făg′ə-sī-tō′sĭs) *n.* The engulfing and ingestion of bacteria or other foreign bodies by phagocytes. —**phag′o·cy·tot′ic** (-tŏt′ĭk) *adj.*

phag·o·ly·so·some (făg′ə-lī′sə-sōm′) *n.* A cellular body that is formed by the union of a phagosome or ingested particle with a lysosome that contains hydrolytic enzymes.

phag·o·some (făg′ə-sōm′) *n.* A membrane-bound vesicle formed in a cell by an inward folding of the cell membrane to hold foreign matter taken into the cell by phagocytosis.

–phagy *suff.* Variant of **–phagia.**

pha·kic eye (fā′kĭk) *n.* An eye containing the natural lens.

phako– *pref.* Variant of **phaco–.**

pha·ko·ma (fă-kō′mə) *n.* Variant of **phacoma.**

phak·o·ma·to·sis (făk′ō-mə-tō′sĭs) *n.* Variant of **phacomatosis.**

pha·lan·ge·al (fə-lăn′jəl, fā-) or **pha·lan·gal** (-lăng′gəl) or **pha·lan·ge·an** (-lăn′jē-ən) *adj.* Of or relating to a phalanx or phalanges.

phalangeal cell *n.* Any of the supporting cells of the spiral organ, attached to the basement membrane and forming rows that support the hair cells. Also called *Deiters' cell.*

phalangeal joint *n.* See **digital joint.**

phal·an·gec·to·my (făl′ən-jĕk′tə-mē) *n.* Excision of one or more phalanges of the hand or foot.

pha·lanx (fā′lăngks′, făl′ăngks′) *n., pl.* **pha·lanx·es** *or* **pha·lan·ges** (fə-lăn′jēz, fā-) Any of the long bones of the fingers or toes, numbering 14 for each hand or foot: two for the thumb or big toe, and three each for the other four digits.

phal·lec·to·my (fă-lĕk′tə-mē) *n.* Surgical removal of the penis.

phal·lic (făl′ĭk) *adj.* **1.** Of, relating to, or resembling a phallus. **2.** Of or relating to the third stage of psychosexual development in psychoanalytic theory during which the genital organs first become the focus of sexual feeling.

phallic phase *n.* In psychoanalytic theory, the stage in psychosexual development, usually occurring between the ages of 3 and 7, when a child's interest and curiosity are centered around the genital organs and masturbation is the primary source of pleasurable experiences.

phal·li·tis (fă-lī′tĭs) *n.* See **penitis.**

phallo– *or* **phall–** *pref.* Penis: *phalloplasty.*

phal·lo·camp·sis (făl′ō-kămp′sĭs) *n.* Curvature of the penis when erect.

phal·lo·dyn·i·a (făl′ō-dĭn′ē-ə) *n.* Pain in the penis.

phal·loi·din (fă-loid′n) *n.* A heat-stable, toxic, cyclic peptide produced by *Amanita phalloides* that acts by binding actin and causes vomiting, convulsions, diarrhea, asthenia, and death.

phal·lo·plas·ty (făl′ə-plăs′tē) *n.* Reparative or plastic surgery of the penis.

phal·lot·o·my (fă-lŏt′ə-mē) *n.* Incision into the penis.

phal·lus (făl′əs) *n., pl.* **phal·lus·es** *or* **phal·li** (făl′ī′) **1.** The penis. **2.** The sexually undifferentiated tissue in an embryo that becomes the penis or clitoris. **3.** The immature penis considered in psychoanalysis as the libidinal object of infantile sexuality in the male.

–phane *or* **–phan** *suff.* A substance resembling something specified: *tryptophan.*

phan·ta·sia (făn-tā′zhə) *n.* See **fantasy.**

phan·tasm (făn′tăz′əm) *n.* **1.** Something apparently seen but having no physical reality; an apparition. **2.** An illusory mental image.

phan·tas·ma·go·ri·a (făn-tăz′mə-gôr′ē-ə) *or* **phan·tas·ma·go·ry** (făn-tăz′mə-gôr′ē) *n., pl.* **–ri·as** *or* **–ries** A fantastic sequence of haphazardly associative imagery, as seen in dreams or fever.

phan·tom *or* **fan·tom** (făn′təm) *n.* **1.** Something apparently seen, heard, or sensed, but having no physical reality. **2.** An image that appears only in the mind; an illusion. **3.** A model, especially a transparent one, of the human body or of any of its parts. —*adj.* **1.** Resembling, characteristic of, or being a phantom; illusive. **2.** Fictitious; nonexistent.

phantom corpuscle *n.* See **achromocyte.**

phantom limb *n.* The sensation that an amputated limb is still attached, often associated with painful paresthesia. Also called *pseudesthesia.*

phantom limb pain *n.* Pain or discomfort felt by an amputee in the area of the missing limb.

phantom tumor *n.* An accumulation of fluid in the interlobar spaces of the lung occurring as a result of congestive heart failure and appearing radiologically as a neoplasm.

phar·ma·ceu·ti·cal (fär′mə-sōō′tĭ-kəl) *or* **phar·ma·ceu·tic** (-tĭk) *adj.* Of or relating to pharmacy or pharmacists. —*n.* A pharmaceutical product or preparation.

phar·ma·ceu·tics (fär′mə-sōō′tĭks) *n.* **1.** The science of preparing and dispensing drugs. **2.** Pharmaceutical preparations; medicinal drugs.

phar·ma·cist (fär′mə-sĭst) *n.* One who prepares and dispenses drugs; a druggist.

pharmaco– *pref.* Drug; medicine: *pharmacology.*

phar·ma·co·di·ag·no·sis (fär′mə-kō-dī′əg-nō′sĭs) *n.* The use of drugs in the diagnosis of disease.

phar·ma·co·dy·nam·ics (fär′mə-kō′dī-năm′ĭks) *n.* The study of the action or effects of drugs on living organisms. —**phar′ma·co′dy·nam′ic** *adj.*

phar·ma·co·ge·net·ics (fär′mə-kō-jə-nĕt′ĭks) *n.* The study of genetic factors that influence an organism's reaction to a drug. Also called *pharmacogenomics.*

phar·ma·cog·no·sy (fär′mə-kŏg′nə-sē) *n.* The branch of pharmacology that deals with drugs in their crude or natural state.

phar·ma·co·ki·net·ics (fär′mə-kō-kə-nĕt′ĭks, -kī-) *n.* **1.** The process by which a drug is absorbed, distributed, metabolized, and eliminated by the body. **2.** The study of this process. —**phar′ma·co·ki·net′ic** *adj.*

phar·ma·col·o·gy (fär′mə-kŏl′ə-jē) *n.* **1.** The science of drugs, including their composition, uses, and effects. **2.** The characteristics or properties of a drug, especially those that make it medically effective. —**phar′ma·co·log′ic** (-kə-lŏj′ĭk) *adj.*

phar·ma·co·pe·ial (fär′mə-kə-pē′əl) *adj.* **1.** Of or relating to a pharmacopoeia. **2.** Relating to a drug in the list of the United States Pharmacopoeia or similar pharmacopoeia.

pharmacopeial gel *n.* A suspension in water of an insoluble hydrated drug in which the particle size approaches or attains colloidal dimensions.

phar·ma·co·poe·ia *or* **phar·ma·co·pe·ia** (fär′mə-kə-pē′ə) *n.* **1.** A book containing an official list of medicinal drugs together with articles on their preparation and use. **2.** A collection or stock of drugs.

phar·ma·co·psy·cho·sis (fär′mə-kō-sī-kō′sĭs) *n.* A psychosis caused by taking a drug.

phar·ma·co·ther·a·py (fär′mə-kō-thĕr′ə-pē) *n.* Treatment of disease through the use of drugs.

phar·ma·cy (fär′mə-sē) *n.* **1.** The art of preparing and dispensing drugs. **2.** A place where drugs are sold; a drugstore. Also called *apothecary.*

PharmD *abbr. Latin* Pharmaciae Doctor (Doctor of Pharmacy)

pharm·ing (fär′mĭng) *n.* The production of pharmaceuticals from genetically altered plants or animals.

pharyng– *pref.* Variant of **pharyngo–.**

phar·yn·gal·gia (făr′ĭn-găl′jə, făr′ĭng-) *n.* Pain in the pharynx. Also called *pharyngodynia.*

pha·ryn·geal (fə-rĭn′jəl, făr′ĭn-jē′əl) *or* **pha·ryn·gal** (fə-rĭng′gəl) *adj.* Of, relating to, located in, or coming from the pharynx.

pharyngeal arch *n.* See **branchial arch.**

pharyngeal bursa *n.* A cystic remnant of the notochord sometimes found in the posterior wall of the nasopharynx at the lower end of the pharyngeal tonsil. Also called *Luschka's bursa.*

pharyngeal calculus *n.* See **pharyngolith.**

pharyngeal opening of auditory tube *n.* An opening in the upper nasopharynx behind the posterior extremity of the inferior concha on each side.

pharyngeal pouch *n.* Any of the paired evaginations of embryonic pharyngeal endoderm that give rise to epithelial tissues and organs such as the thymus and thyroid glands. Also called *branchial pouch.*

pharyngeal reflex *n.* **1.** See **swallowing reflex. 2.** See **vomiting reflex.**

pharyngeal tonsil *n.* A collection of aggregated lymphoid nodules that occur on the posterior wall and roof of the nasopharynx, hypertrophy of which constitutes adenoids.

pharyngeal vein *n.* Any of the veins from the pharyngeal plexus that empty into the internal jugular vein.

phar·yn·gec·to·my (făr′ĭn-jĕk′tə-mē) *n.* Surgical removal of all or part of the pharynx.

phar·yn·gem·phrax·is (făr′ĭn-jĕm-frăk′sĭs) *n.* Obstruction of the pharynx.

phar·yn·gis·mus (făr′ĭn-jĭz′məs) *n.* A spasm of the muscles of the pharynx. Also called *pharyngospasm.*

phar·yn·gi·tis (făr′ĭn-jī′tĭs) *n.* Inflammation of the pharynx. —**phar′yn·git′ic** (-jĭt′ĭk) *adj.*

pharyngo– *or* **pharyng–** *pref.* Pharynx: *pharyngoscope.*

pha·ryn·go·cele (fə-rĭng′gə-sēl′) *n.* Protrusion of mucous membrane through the wall of the pharynx; hernia of the pharynx.

pha·ryn·go·con·junc·ti·val fever (fə-rĭng′gō-kŏn′jŭngk-tī′vəl) *n.* An epidemic disease caused by an adenovirus and characterized by fever, pharyngitis, and conjunctivitis.

pha·ryn·go·dyn·i·a (fə-rĭng′gō-dĭn′ē-ə) *n.* See **pharyngalgia.**

pha·ryn·go·ep·i·glot·tic (fə-rĭng′gō-ĕp′ĭ-glŏt′ĭk) *or* **pha·ryn·go·ep·i·glot·tid·e·an** (-glŏ-tĭd′ē-ən) *adj.* Of or relating to the pharynx and the epiglottis.

pha·ryn·go·e·soph·a·ge·al (fə-rĭng′gō-ĭ-sŏf′ə-jē′əl) *adj.* Of or relating to the pharynx and the esophagus.

pharyngoesophageal diverticulum *n.* A diverticulum of the posterior pharyngeal wall opening just behind the cricoid cartilage.

pha·ryn·go·glos·sal (fə-rĭng′gō-glŏs′səl) *adj.* Of or relating to the pharynx and the tongue.

pha·ryn·go·ker·a·to·sis (fə-rĭng′gō-kĕr′ə-tō′sĭs) *n.* A thickening of the lining of the lymphoid follicles of the pharynx and the formation of a pseudomembranous exudate.

pha·ryn·go·la·ryn·geal (fə-rĭng′gō-lə-rĭn′jəl, -lăr′ĭn-jē′əl) *adj.* Of or relating to the pharynx and the larynx.

pha·ryn·go·lar·yn·gi·tis (fə-rĭng′gō-lăr′ĭn-jī′tĭs) *n.* Inflammation of the pharynx and the larynx.

pha·ryn·go·lith (fə-rĭng′gə-lĭth′) *n.* A concretion occurring in the pharynx. Also called *pharyngeal calculus.*

phar·yn·gol·o·gy (făr′ĭn-gŏl′ə-jē, făr′ĭng-) *n.* The medical study of the pharynx and its diseases.

pha·ryn·go·my·co·sis (fə-rĭng′gō-mī-kō′sĭs) *n.* A fungal infection affecting the mucous membrane of the pharynx.

pha·ryn·go·na·sal (fə-rĭng′gō-nā′zəl) *adj.* Of or relating to the pharynx and the nasal cavity.

phar·yn·gop·a·thy (făr′ĭn-gŏp′ə-thē, făr′ĭng-) *n.* Disease of the pharynx.

pha·ryn·go·pe·ris·to·le (fə-rĭng′gō-pə-rĭs′tə-lē) *n.* A narrowing of the lumen of the pharynx.

pha·ryn·go·plas·ty (fə-rĭng′gə-plăs′tē) *n.* Plastic surgery of the pharynx.

pha·ryn·go·ple·gia (fə-rĭng′gō-plē′jə) *n.* Paralysis of the muscles of the pharynx.

pha·ryn·go·rhi·ni·tis (fə-rĭng′gō-rī-nī′tĭs) *n.* Inflammation of the mucous membrane of the pharynx and the nasal cavity.

pha·ryn·go·scle·ro·ma (fə-rĭng′gō-sklə-rō′mə) *n.* A scleroma in the mucous membrane of the pharynx.

pha·ryn·go·scope (fə-rĭng′gə-skōp′) *n.* An instrument used in examining the pharynx. —**phar′yn·gos′co·py** (făr′ĭn-gŏs′kə-pē, făr′ĭng-) *n.*

pha·ryn·go·spasm (fə-rĭng′gō-spăz′əm) *n.* See **pharyngismus.**

pha·ryn·go·ste·no·sis (fə-rĭng′gō-stə-nō′sĭs) *n.* Stricture of the pharynx.

phar·yn·got·o·my (făr′ĭn-gŏt′ə-mē, făr′ĭng-) *n.* Incision of the pharynx.

phar·ynx (făr′ĭngks) *n., pl.* **phar·ynx·es** *or* **pha·ryng·es** (fə-rĭn′jēz) The upper section of the alimentary canal that extends from the mouth and nasal cavities to the larynx.

phase (fāz) *n.* **1.** A characteristic form, appearance, or stage of development that occurs in a cycle or that distinguishes some individuals of a group. **2.** A discrete homogeneous part of a material system that is mechanically separable from the rest, as is ice from water. **3.** Any of the forms or states, solid, liquid, gas, or plasma, in which matter can exist, depending on temperature and pressure. **4.** A particular stage in a periodic process or phenomenon such as a wave form or time pattern. —*v.* To introduce, one stage at a time.

phase I block *n.* Inhibition of nerve impulse transmission across the myoneural junction associated with depolarization of the motor end plate, as in the muscle paralysis produced by succinylcholine.

phase II block *n.* Inhibition of nerve impulse transmission across the myoneural junction unaccompanied by depolarization of the motor end plate, as in the muscle paralysis produced by tubocurarine.

phase contrast microscope *n.* A microscope that uses the differences in the phase of light transmitted or reflected by a specimen to form distinct, contrasting images of different parts of the specimen. Also called *phase microscope.*

–phasia *suff.* A speech disorder of a specified kind: *dysphasia.*

phas·mid (făz′mĭd) *n.* Either of a pair of caudal chemoreceptors occurring in nematodes of the class, Secernentea.

PhD *abbr.* *Latin* Philosophiae Doctor (Doctor of Philosophy)

Phe *abbr.* phenylalanine

Phem·is·ter graft (fĕm′ĭ-stər) *n.* An autogenous bone graft applied on the outside of an injured bone, used in treating delayed union of a fracture.

phe·na·caine (fē′nə-kān′, fĕn′ə-) *n.* A white crystalline compound used in the form of its hydrochloride as a local anesthetic in ophthalmology.

phe·nac·e·tu·ric acid (fə-năs′ĭ-toŏr′ĭk) *or* **phen·yl·ac·e·tu·ric acid** (fĕn′əl-ăs′ĭ-) *n.* The end product of the metabolism of phenylated fatty acids containing even numbers of carbon atoms.

phe·nan·threne (fə-năn′thrēn′) *n.* A colorless crystalline hydrocarbon obtained by fractional distillation of coal-tar oils and used in drugs.

phe·nate (fē′nāt′) *n.* A salt or ester of phenol.

phen·a·zo·pyr·i·dine hydrochloride (fĕn′ə-zō-pĭr′ĭ-dēn′) *n.* An oral analgesic used to treat urinary tract pain and urgency.

phen·cy·cli·dine (fĕn-sī′klĭ-dēn′, -dĭn, -sĭk′lĭ-) *n. Abbr.* **PCP** A drug used as an anesthetic in veterinary medicine and illegally as a hallucinogen.

phen·el·zine (fĕn′əl-zēn′) *n.* A monoamine oxidase inhibitor used especially in the form of its sulfate as an antidepressant.

phe·nic acid (fē′nĭk, fĕn′ĭk) *n.* See **phenol** (sense 1).

pheno– *or* **phen–** *pref.* **1.** Showing; displaying: *phenotype.* **2.** Relating to or derived from benzene: *phenol.* **3.** Containing phenyl: *phenothiazine.*

phe·no·bar·bi·tal (fē′nō-bär′bĭ-tôl′, -tăl′) *n.* A crystalline barbiturate used as a sedative, hypnotic, and anticonvulsant.

phe·no·bar·bi·tone (fē′nō-bär′bĭ-tōn′) *n.* Phenobarbital.

phe·no·cop·y (fē′nə-kŏp′ē) *n.* **1.** An environmentally induced, nonhereditary variation in an organism, closely resembling a genetically determined trait. **2.** An individual exhibiting such a variation.

phe·no·de·vi·ant (fē′nō-dē′vē-ənt) *n.* An individual with a phenotype significantly different from that of the population to which it belongs.

phe·nol (fē′nôl′, -nōl′) *n.* **1.** A caustic, poisonous, white crystalline compound derived from benzene and used in pharmaceuticals and in dilute form as an antiseptic. Also called *carbolic acid, phenic acid.* **2.** Any of a class of aromatic organic compounds having at least one hydroxyl group attached directly to the benzene ring.

phe·no·late (fē′nə-lāt′) *n.* A salt of phenol. Also called *phenoxide.*

phenol coefficient *n.* See **Rideal-Walker coefficient.**

phe·no·lic (fĭ-nō′lĭk, -nŏl′ĭk) *adj.* Of, relating to, containing, or derived from phenol. —*n.* Any of various synthetic thermosetting resins, obtained by the reaction of phenols with simple aldehydes and used as adhesives.

phe·nol·phthal·ein (fē′nōl-thăl′ēn′, -thăl′ē-ĭn, -thā′lēn′, -thā′lē-ĭn) *n.* A white or pale yellow crystalline powder used as an acid-base indicator and a laxative.

phenol red *n.* A bright to dark red, water-soluble crystalline dye used as an acid-base indicator and to test kidney function and renal blood flow. Also called *phenolsulfonphthalein.*

phe·nol·sul·fon·phthal·ein (fē′nōl-sŭl′fōn-thăl′ēn′, -thăl′ē-ĭn, -thā′lēn′, -thā′lē-ĭn, -sŭl′fōn-) *n. Abbr.* **PSP** See **phenol red.**

phe·nom·e·non (fĭ-nŏm′ə-nŏn′, -nən) *n.* **1.** *pl.* **–na** (-nə) An occurrence, circumstance, or fact that is perceptible by the senses, especially one in relation to a disease. **2.** *pl.* **–nons** An unusual, significant, or unaccountable fact or occurrence; a marvel.

phe·no·thi·a·zine (fē′nō-thī′ə-zēn′) *n.* **1.** A yellow organic compound used in veterinary anthelmintics. Also called *thiodiphenylamine.* **2.** Any of a group of drugs derived from this compound and used as tranquilizers in the treatment of psychiatric disorders, such as schizophrenia.

phe·no·type (fē′nə-tīp′) *n.* **1.** The observable physical or biochemical characteristics of an organism, as determined by both genetic makeup and environmental influences. **2.** The expression of a specific trait, such as stature or blood type, based on genetic and environmental influences. **3.** An individual or group of organisms exhibiting a particular phenotype. —**phe′no·typ′ic** (-tĭp′ĭk) *adj.*

phenotypic value *n.* The metrical quantity of some trait associated with a particular phenotype.

phe·nox·ide (fĭ-nŏk′sīd′) *n.* See **phenolate.**

phe·nox·y·ben·za·mine (fē-nŏk′sē-bĕn′zə-mēn′) *n.* A long-acting alpha-blocker used in the form of its hydrochloride as a vasodilator in the treatment of peripheral vascular diseases.

phe·no·zy·gous (fē′nə-zī′gəs) *adj.* Having a narrow cranium as compared with the width of the face, so that when the skull is viewed from above, the zygomatic arches are visible.

phen·pro·ba·mate (fĕn-prō′bə-māt′) *n.* A skeletal muscle relaxant that also has antianxiety action. Also called *proformiphen.*

phen·ter·mine (fĕn′tər-mēn′) *n.* An oily liquid whose crystalline hydrochloride form was formerly used in the treatment of obesity.

phen·yl (fĕn′il) *n.* The univalent radical of phenol.

phen·yl·a·ce·tic acid (fĕn′əl-ə-sē′tĭk, fē′nəl-) *n.* An abnormal product of phenylalanine catabolism that appears in the urine in phenylketonuria.

phen·yl·ac·e·tu·ric acid (fĕn′əl-ăs′ĭ-toŏr′ĭk) *n.* Variant of **phenaceturic acid.**

phen·yl·al·a·ni·nase (fĕn′əl-ăl′ə-nĭ-nās′, -nāz′, fē′nəl-) *n.* See **phenylalanine 4-monooxygenase.**

phen·yl·al·a·nine (fĕn′əl-ăl′ə-nēn′, fē′nəl-) *n. Abbr.* **Phe** An essential amino acid that occurs as a constituent of many proteins and is normally converted to tyrosine in the body.

phenylalanine 4-monooxygenase *n.* An enzyme that catalyzes the oxidation of phenylalanine to tyrosine. Also called *phenylalaninase.*

phen·yl·bu·ta·zone (fĕn′əl-byoō′tə-zōn′, fē′nəl-) *n.* A white or light yellow compound that is used as an anti-inflammatory and analgesic drug in the treatment of arthritis, bursitis, and gout.

phen·yl·eph·rine (fĕn′əl-ĕf′rēn, fē′nəl-) *n.* An adrenergic drug that is a powerful vasoconstrictor and is used to relieve nasal congestion, dilate the pupils, and maintain blood pressure during anesthesia.

phen·yl·eth·yl alcohol (fĕn′əl-ĕth′əl, fē′nəl-) *n.* An antibacterial agent that is the natural constituent of certain volatile oils.

phen·yl·ke·to·nu·ri·a (fĕn′əl-kēt′n-ŏŏr′ē-ə, fē′nəl-) *n. Abbr.* **PKU** A genetic disorder in which the body lacks the enzyme necessary to metabolize phenylalanine to tyrosine. Left untreated, the disorder can cause brain damage and progressive mental retardation as a result of the accumulation of phenylalanine and its breakdown products.

phen·yl·lac·tic acid (fĕn′əl-lăk′tĭk, fē′nəl-) *n.* A product of phenylalanine catabolism that occurs in the urine in phenylketonuria.

phen·yl·pro·pa·nol·a·mine (fĕn′əl-prō′pə-nŏl′ə-mēn′, fē′nəl-) *n.* An adrenergic drug that acts as a vasoconstrictor and is used as a nasal decongestant, a bronchodilator, an appetite suppressant, and a mild stimulant.

phen·y·to·in (fĕn′ĭ-tō′ĭn, fə-nĭt′ō-) *n.* An anticonvulsant drug chemically related to the barbiturates and used most commonly in the treatment of epilepsy.

pheo– *or* **phaeo–** *pref.* Dusky, gray, or dun: *pheochrome.*

phe·o·chrome (fē′ə-krōm′) *adj.* Staining darkly with chromic salts.

phe·o·chro·mo·cyte (fē′ō-krō′mə-sīt′) *n.* A chromaffin cell of a sympathetic paraganglion, of a pheochromocytoma, or of the medulla of an adrenal gland.

phe·o·chro·mo·cy·to·ma (fē′ō-krō′mō-sī-tō′mə) *n., pl.* **–mas** *or* **–ma·ta** (-mə-tə) A usually benign tumor of the adrenal medulla or the sympathetic nervous system in which the affected cells secrete increased amounts of epinephrine or norepinephrine.

phe·re·sis (fə-rē′sĭs, fĕr′ĭ-) *n.* Apheresis.

pher·o·mone (fĕr′ə-mōn′) *n.* A chemical that is secreted by an animal, especially an insect, and that influences the behavior or development of others of the same species.

PhG *abbr.* Graduate in Pharmacy

phi *n. Symbol* **φ** The 21st letter of the Greek alphabet.

Phi·a·loph·o·ra (fī′ə-lŏf′ər-ə) *n.* A genus of fungi including several species that cause chromomycosis and mycetoma.

Phil·a·del·phi·a chromosome (fĭl′ə-dĕl′fē-ə) *n.* An abnormal minute chromosome found in white blood cells in many cases of chronic myelocytic leukemia.

–phile *or* **–phil** *suff.* **1.** One that loves or has a strong affinity or preference for: *thermophile.* **2.** Loving; having a strong affinity or preference for: *basophil.*

–philia *suff.* **1.** Tendency toward: *hemophilia.* **2.** Abnormal attraction to: *necrophilia.*

–philiac *suff.* **1.** One that has a tendency toward: *hemophiliac.* **2.** One that has an abnormal attraction to: *necrophiliac.*

Phil·lips catheter (fĭl′ĭps) *n.* A urethral catheter with a woven filiform guide.

–philous *or* **–philic** *suff.* Having a strong affinity or preference for; loving: *necrophilous.*

phil·trum (fĭl′trəm) *n., pl.* **–tra** (-trə) The vertical indentation in the midline of the upper lip. Also called *infranasal depression.*

phi·mo·sis (fī-mō′sĭs, fĭ-) *n., pl.* **–ses** (-sēz) An abnormal constriction of the foreskin that prevents it from being drawn back to uncover the glans penis.

phi·mot·ic (fī-mŏt′ĭk, fĭ-) *adj.* Relating to phimosis.

phleb·ar·ter·i·ec·ta·si·a (flĕb′är-tîr′ē-ĭk-tā′zhə) *n.* See vasodilation.

phleb·ec·ta·si·a (flĕb′ĭk-tā′zhə) *n.* Dilation of the veins. Also called *venectasia.*

phle·bec·to·my (flĭ-bĕk′tə-mē) *n.* Excision of a segment of a vein. Also called *venectomy.*

phleb·em·phrax·is (flĕb′ĕm-frăk′sĭs) *n.* Venous thrombosis.

phle·bis·mus (flĭ-bĭz′məs) *n.* Venous congestion and phlebectasia.

phle·bi·tis (flĭ-bī′tĭs) *n.* Inflammation of a vein. **—phle·bit′ic** (-bĭt′ĭk) *adj.*

phlebo– *or* **phleb–** *pref.* Vein: *phlebotomy.*

phle·boc·ly·sis (flĭ-bŏk′lĭ-sĭs, flĕb′ə-klī′sĭs) *n.* Intravenous injection of an isotonic solution of dextrose or other substances.

phleb·o·gram (flĕb′ə-grăm′) *n.* A graphic tracing of the jugular venous pulse. Also called *venogram.*

phleb·o·graph (flĕb′ə-grăf′) *n.* An instrument for making a graphic recording of the venous pulse. Also called *venous sphygmograph.*

phle·bog·ra·phy (flĭ-bŏg′rə-fē) *n.* The process of recording the venous pulse. Also called *venography.*

phleb·o·lith (flĕb′ə-lĭth′) *n.* A calcareous deposit in a venous wall or thrombus.

phleb·o·li·thi·a·sis (flĕb′ō-lĭ-thī′ə-sĭs) *n.* The formation of phleboliths.

phleb·o·ma·nom·e·ter (flĕb′ō-mă-nŏm′ĭ-tər) *n.* A manometer for measuring venous blood pressure.

phleb·o·phle·bos·to·my (flĕb′ō-flĭ-bŏs′tə-mē) *n.* See venovenostomy.

phleb·o·plas·ty (flĕb′ə-plăs′tē) *n.* Surgical repair of a vein.

phleb·or·rha·gia (flĕb′ə-rā′jə) *n.* Venous hemorrhage.

phle·bor·rha·phy (flĭ-bôr′ə-fē) *n.* The surgical suturing of a vein.

phleb·or·rhex·is (flĕb′ə-rĕk′sĭs) *n.* Rupture of a vein.

phleb·o·scle·ro·sis (flĕb′ō-sklə-rō′sĭs) *n.* The thickening or hardening of the walls of a vein. Also called *venosclerosis.*

phle·bos·ta·sis (flĭ-bŏs′tə-sĭs) *n.* **1.** The abnormally slow motion of blood in the veins, usually with venous distention. **2.** The compression of the proximal veins of an extremity by use of tourniquets. Also called *venostasis.*

phleb·o·ste·no·sis (flĕb′ō-stə-nō′sĭs) *n.* Narrowing of the lumen of a vein.

phleb·o·throm·bo·sis (flĕb′ō-thrŏm-bō′sĭs) *n.* Thrombosis in a vein without primary inflammation.

phle·bot·o·mist (flĭ-bŏt′ə-mĭst) *n.* **1.** One who practices phlebotomy. **2.** One who draws blood for analysis or transfusion.

Phle·bot·o·mus (flĭ-bŏt′ə-məs) *n.* A genus of very small midges or bloodsucking sand flies that includes various species that are vectors of kala azar, cutaneous leishmaniasis, and phlebotomus fever.

phlebotomus fever *n.* An infectious but not contagious denguelike disease occurring in the Balkan Peninsula and other parts of southern Europe, caused by an arbovirus introduced by the bite of the sand fly *Phlebotomus papatasi.* Also called *sandfly fever.*

phlebotomus fever virus *n.* An arbovirus transmitted by sand flies and causing phlebotomus fever.

phle·bot·o·my (flĭ-bŏt′ə-mē) *n.* The act or practice of opening a vein by incision or puncture to remove blood. Also called *venesection, venotomy.*

phlegm (flĕm) *n.* **1.** Thick, sticky, stringy mucus secreted by the mucous membrane of the respiratory tract, as during a cold or other respiratory infection. **2.** One of the four humors of ancient and medieval physiology, thought to cause sluggishness, apathy, and evenness of temper. —**phlegm′y** *adj.*

phleg·ma·sia (flĕg-mā′zhə) *n.* Inflammation, especially when acute and severe.

phlegmasia al·ba do·lens (ăl′bə dō′lĕnz′) *n.* See **milk leg.**

phlegmasia ce·ru·le·a do·lens (sə-rōō′lē-ə dō′lĕnz′) *n.* Thrombosis of the veins of a limb characterized by sudden severe pain, swelling, cyanosis, and edema, followed by circulatory collapse and shock.

phleg·mat·ic (flĕg-măt′ĭk) *or* **phleg·mat·i·cal** (-ĭ-kəl) *adj.* **1.** Of or relating to phlegm. **2.** Having or suggesting a calm, sluggish temperament; unemotional.

phleg·mon (flĕg′mŏn′) *n.* Acute suppurative inflammation affecting the subcutaneous connective tissue. —**phleg′mon·ous** (-mə-nəs) *adj.*

phlegmonous abscess *n.* An abscess characterized by an intense local inflammatory reaction that produces hardening and thickening of the affected area.

phlegmonous gastritis *n.* Gastritis marked by severe inflammation, chiefly of the submucous coat, with purulent infiltration of the stomach wall.

phlegmonous mastitis *n.* Abscess or cellulitis of the breast.

phlo·ro·glu·cin·ol (flôr′ə-glōō′sə-nôl′, -nōl′) *n.* A white, slightly sweet, crystalline compound used as an antispasmodic, analytical reagent, and decalcifier of bone specimens for microscopic examination. Also called *phloroglucin.*

phlyc·te·na *or* **phlyc·tae·na** (flĭk-tē′nə) *n.,* *pl.* **-nae** (-nē) A small blister or vesicle, especially one of multiple blisters caused by a mild burn. —**phlyc′ten′ar** (flĭk′tĕn′ər) *adj.*

phlyc·te·noid (flĭk′tə-noid′) *adj.* Resembling a phlyctena.

phlyc·ten·u·la (flĭk-tĕn′yə-lə) *n.,* *pl.* **-lae** (-lē) A small red nodule of lymphoid cells, with an ulcerated apex, occurring in the conjunctiva of the eye. Also called *phlyctenule.* —**phlyc′ten′u·lar** (-lər) *adj.*

phlyctenular keratitis *n.* Inflammation of the corneal conjunctiva and formation of small red nodules of lymphoid tissue near the corneoscleral limbus.

phlyc·ten·ule (flĭk′tĕn′yōōl, -tə-nyōōl′) *n.* See **phlyctenula.**

phlyc·ten·u·lo·sis (flĭk-tĕn′yə-lō′sĭs) *n.* A nodular hypersensitive disease of the corneal and conjunctival epithelium of the eye caused by an endogenous toxin.

–phobe *suff.* One that fears or is averse to a specified thing: *xenophobe.*

pho·bi·a (fō′bē-ə) *n.* **1.** A persistent, abnormal, or irrational fear of a specific thing or situation that compels one to avoid the feared stimulus. **2.** A strong fear, dislike, or aversion.

–phobia *suff.* An intense, abnormal, or illogical fear of a specified thing: *claustrophobia.*

pho·bic (fō′bĭk) *adj.* Of, relating to, arising from, or having a phobia. —*n.* One who has a phobia.

–phobic *or* **–phobous** *suff.* **1.** Having a fear of or aversion for: *photophobic.* **2.** Lacking an affinity for: *lyophobic.*

pho·bo·pho·bi·a (fō′bə-fō′bē-ə) *n.* A morbid dread or fear of developing a phobia.

pho·co·me·li·a (fō′kō-mē′lē-ə, -mēl′yə) *n.* A birth defect in which the upper portion of a limb is absent or poorly developed, so that the hand or foot attaches to the body by a short, flipperlike stump. —**pho′co·me′lic** (-mē′lĭk) *adj.*

phocomelic dwarf *n.* A dwarf in whom the shafts of the long bones are extremely short or in whom the intermediate parts of the limbs are absent.

phon– *pref.* Variant of **phono–.**

pho·nal (fō′nəl) *adj.* **1.** Of, relating to, or being sound. **2.** Of, relating to, or characterizing the voice.

pho·nas·the·ni·a (fō′năs-thē′nē-ə) *n.* Difficult or abnormal voice production characterized by enunciation that is too high, too loud, or too hard.

pho·nate (fō′nāt′) *v.* To utter speech sounds; vocalize.

pho·na·tion (fō-nā′shən) *n.* The utterance of sounds through the use of the vocal cords; vocalization. —**pho′na·to′ry** (fō′nə-tôr′ē) *adj.*

pho·neme (fō′nēm′) *n.* The smallest phonetic unit in a language that is capable of conveying a distinction in meaning, as the *m* of *mat* and the *b* of *bat* in English.

pho·nen·do·scope (fō-nĕn′də-skōp′) *n.* A stethoscope that intensifies auscultatory sounds.

pho·net·ic (fə-nĕt′ĭk) *adj.* **1.** Of or relating to phonetics. **2.** Representing the sounds of speech with a set of distinct symbols, each designating a single sound.

pho·net·ics (fə-nĕt′ĭks) *n.* The branch of linguistics that deals with the sounds of speech and their production, combination, description, and representation by written symbols.

pho·ni·at·rics (fō′nē-ăt′rĭks) *n.* The scientific study of speech and speech habits.

phon·ic (fŏn′ĭk) *adj.* Of, relating to, or having the nature of sound, especially speech sounds.

phono– *or* **phon–** *pref.* Sound; voice; speech: *phonometer.*

pho·no·an·gi·og·ra·phy (fō′nō-ăn′jē-ŏg′rə-fē) *n.* The recording and analysis of the frequency-intensity components of the bruit of turbulent arterial blood flow that are audible through an atherosclerotic stenotic lesion.

pho·no·car·di·o·graph (fō′nə-kär′dē-ə-grăf′) *n.* A device consisting of microphones and recording equipment used to monitor and record heart sounds and murmurs. —**pho′no·car′di·og′ra·phy** (-ŏg′rə-fē) *n.*

pho·no·cath·e·ter (fō′nō-kăth′ĭ-tər) *n.* A cardiac catheter with a miniature microphone in its tip used in recording sounds and murmurs from within the heart and large blood vessels.

pho·no·gram (fō′nə-grăm′) *n*. **1.** A graphic tracing depicting the duration and intensity of a sound. **2.** A character or symbol, as in a phonetic alphabet, representing a word or phoneme in speech.

pho·nom·e·ter (fə-nŏm′ĭ-tər, fō-) *n*. An instrument used to measure the pitch and intensity of sounds.

pho·no·my·oc·lo·nus (fō′nō-mī-ŏk′lə-nəs) *n*. A condition characterized by fibrillary contractions of a muscle that can be heard on auscultation even though they are not visible.

pho·nop·a·thy (fə-nŏp′ə-thē, fō-) *n*. Any of various diseases of the vocal organs that affect speech.

pho·no·pho·tog·ra·phy (fō′nō-fə-tŏg′rə-fē) *n*. The process of graphically recording the movements that sound waves impart to a diaphragm.

pho·nop·si·a (fə-nŏp′sē-ə, fō-) *n*. A condition in which hearing certain sounds elicits a subjective sensation of color.

pho·no·re·cep·tion (fō′nō-rĭ-sĕp′shən) *n*. Perception of or response to sound waves.

pho·no·re·cep·tor (fō′nō-rĭ-sĕp′tər) *n*. A receptor for sound stimuli.

pho·no·re·no·gram (fō′nō-rē′nə-grăm′) *n*. A sound recording of the renal arterial pulse produced by means of a phonocatheter placed in the renal pelvis.

–phony *suff*. Sound: *microphony.*

–phore *suff*. Bearer; carrier: *chromatophore.*

pho·re·sis (fə-rē′sĭs, fôr′ĭ-) *n*. See **electrophoresis** (sense 1).

–phoresis *suff*. Transmission: *electrophoresis.*

phor·e·sy (fôr′ĭ-sē) *n*. A symbiotic relationship, especially among arthropods and some fishes, in which one organism transports another organism of a different species.

pho·ri·a (fôr′ē-ə) *n*. The relative directions of the eyes during binocular fixation on a given object in the absence of an adequate fusion stimulus.

phoro– or **phor–** *pref*. Movement; direction; phoria: *phoro-optometer.*

pho·ro·op·tom·e·ter (fôr′ō-ŏp-tŏm′ĭ-tər) *n*. An instrument for determining phorias, ductions, and refractive states of the eyes.

pho·rop·ter (fə-rŏp′tər) *n*. A device containing different lenses used for refraction of the eye during sight testing.

phos– *pref*. Light: *phosgene.*

phos·gene (fŏs′jēn′, fŏz′-) *n*. A colorless volatile liquid or gas used as a poison gas and in making dyes.

phosph– *pref*. Variant of **phospho-**.

phos·pha·tase (fŏs′fə-tās′, -tāz′) *n*. Any of numerous enzymes that catalyze the hydrolysis of esters of phosphoric acid and are important in the absorption and metabolism of carbohydrates, nucleotides, and phospholipids and in the calcification of bone.

phos·phate (fŏs′fāt′) *n*. A salt or ester of phosphoric acid. —*adj*. Containing the trivalent radical PO_4.

phosphate diabetes *n*. A condition marked by excessive phosphate in the urine due to an inability of the renal tubules to reabsorb it.

phos·pha·te·mi·a (fŏs′fə-tē′mē-ə) *n*. An abnormally high concentration of inorganic phosphates in the blood.

phos·phat·ic (fŏs-făt′ĭk) *adj*. Relating to or containing phosphate.

phos·pha·tide (fŏs′fə-tīd′) *n*. See **phospholipid**.

phos·pha·ti·dyl·cho·line (fŏs′fə-tīd′l-kō′lēn′) *n*. A phospholipid that is a major component of cellular membranes and functions in the transport of lipoproteins in tissues.

phos·pha·ti·dyl·glyc·er·ol (fŏs′fə-tīd′l-glĭs′ə-rôl′, -rōl′) *n*. A phosphatidic acid that is a constituent in human amniotic fluid and is used as an indicator of fetal lung maturity when present in the last trimester of gestation.

phos·pha·tu·ri·a (fŏs′fə-tŏŏr′ē-ə) *n*. An excess of phosphates in the urine.

phos·phene (fŏs′fēn′) *n*. A sensation of light caused by excitation of the retina by mechanical or electrical means rather than by light, as when the eyeballs are pressed through closed lids.

phos·phide (fŏs′fīd′) or **phos·phid** (-fĭd) *n*. A compound of phosphorus and a more electropositive element or radical.

phos·phite (fŏs′fīt′) *n*. A salt or ester of phosphorous acid.

phospho– or **phosph–** *pref*. **1.** Phosphorus: *phosphide.* **2.** Phosphate: *phospholipid.*

phos·pho·am·i·dase (fŏs′fō-ăm′ĭ-dās′, -dāz′) *n*. An enzyme that catalyzes the hydrolysis of phosphorus-nitrogen bonds, especially the hydrolysis of phosphocreatine to creatine and phosphoric acid.

phos·pho·am·ide (fŏs′fō-ăm′īd′) *n*. Any of the various amides of phosphoric acid and their salts or esters.

phos·pho·cho·line (fŏs′fō-kō′lēn′) *n*. An intermediate in the synthesis of phosphatidylcholine in tissues.

phos·pho·cre·a·tine (fŏs′fō-krē′ə-tēn′) or **phos·pho·cre·a·tin** (-tĭn) *n*. An organic compound found in muscle tissue and capable of storing and providing energy for muscular contraction. Also called *creatine phosphate.*

phos·pho·di·es·ter·ase (fŏs′fō-dī-ĕs′tə-rās′, -rāz′) *n*. Any of a class of enzymes that catalyze the cleaving of phosphodiester bonds, such as those between nucleotides in nucleic acids, to produce smaller nucleotide units or mononucleotides but not inorganic phosphate.

phos·pho·di·es·ter·ase inhibitor (fŏs′fō-dī-ĕs′tə-rās′, -rāz′) *n*. Any of a class of drugs that suppress the enzyme phosphodiesterase, increasing the production of cyclic GMP, which facilitates vasodilation, causing erection in males.

phos·pho·di·es·ter bond (fŏs′fō-dī-ĕs′tər) *n*. The covalent chemical bond that holds together the polynucleotide chains of RNA and DNA by joining a specific carbon in the phosphate group in a sugar having five carbons, such as ribose, to a specific carbon in the hydroxyl group of the five-carbon sugar in the adjacent nucleotide.

phos·pho·e·nol·py·ru·vic acid (fŏs′fō-ē′nôl-pī-rōō′-vĭk, -pĭ-) *n*. The phosphoric ester of the enol form of pyruvic acid that is an intermediate in the conversion of glucose to pyruvic acid.

phos·pho·glyc·er·ide (fŏs′fō-glĭs′ə-rīd′) *n*. A phospholipid containing glycerol phosphate.

phos·pho·hex·ose isomerase deficiency (fŏs'fō-hĕk'sōs') *n.* See **glucosephosphate isomerase deficiency.**

phos·pho·lip·ase (fŏs'fō-lĭp'ās', -lī'pās') *n.* An enzyme that catalyzes the hydrolysis of a phospholipid. Also called *lecithinase.*

phos·pho·lip·id (fŏs'fō-lĭp'ĭd) *n.* Any of various phosphorous-containing lipids that are composed mainly of fatty acids, a phosphate group, and a simple organic molecule. Also called *phosphatide.*

phos·pho·mu·tase (fŏs'fō-myoo'tās, -tāz) *n.* Any of various enzymes associated with intramolecular transfer catalysis because the donor is regenerated.

phos·pho·ne·cro·sis (fŏs'fō-nə-krō'sĭs) *n.* Necrosis of the osseous tissue of the jaw as a result of phosphorus poisoning.

phos·pho·pro·tein (fŏs'fō-prō'tēn') *n.* Any of a group of proteins, such as casein, containing chemically bound phosphoric acid.

phosphor– *pref.* Variant of **phosphoro–.**

phos·pho·res·cence (fŏs'fə-rĕs'əns) *n.* **1.** Persistent emission of light following exposure to and removal of incident radiation. **2.** Emission of light without burning or by very slow burning without appreciable heat, as from the slow oxidation of phosphorous. —**phos'pho·res'cent** *adj.*

phos·pho·ri·bo·i·som·er·ase (fŏs'fō-rī'bō-ī-sŏm'ə-rās, -rāz') *n.* See **ribose 5-phosphate isomerase.**

phos·phor·ic (fŏs-fôr'ĭk) *adj.* Of, relating to, or containing phosphorus, especially with a valence of 5 or a valence higher than that of a comparable phosphorous compound.

phosphoric acid *n.* A clear colorless liquid used in pharmaceuticals. Also called *orthophosphoric acid.*

phos·pho·rism (fŏs'fə-rĭz'əm) *n.* Chronic phosphorus poisoning.

phosphoro– *or* **phosphor–** *pref.* **1.** Phosphorus: *phosphorous acid.* **2.** Phosphorescent: *phosphorogen.*

phos·pho·rol·y·sis (fŏs'fə-rŏl'ĭ-sĭs) *n.* The splitting of a bond by the addition of phosphoric acid to a compound, analogous to hydrolysis.

phos·pho·rous (fŏs'fər-əs, fŏs-fôr'əs) *adj.* Of, relating to, or containing phosphorus, especially with a valence of 3 or a valence lower than that of a comparable phosphoric compound.

phos·pho·rus (fŏs'fər-əs) *n. Symbol* **P 1.** A highly reactive poisonous nonmetallic element occurring naturally in phosphates, such as hydroxyapatite, and an essential constituent of protoplasm, nerve tissue, and bone. Its radioisotope is used to localize and treat cancers and peritoneal or pleural effusions caused by metastatic disease, to determine blood volume, to study peripheral vascular disease, and to treat blood diseases such as polycythemia vera, chronic myelocytic leukemia, and chronic lymphocytic leukemia. Atomic number 15. **2.** A phosphorescent substance.

phosphorus-32 *n.* A radioactive beta-emitting isotope of phosphorus having a half-life of 14.3 days and used as a tracer in studies of the metabolism of nucleic acids and phospholipids, and also used in the treatment of certain diseases of the osseous and hematopoietic systems.

phos·pho·ryl·ase (fŏs'fər-ə-lās', -lāz') *n.* An enzyme that catalyzes the production of glucose phosphate from glycogen and inorganic phosphate.

phosphorylase phosphatase *n.* An enzyme that catalyzes the conversion of phosphatase by splitting it into halves with the subsequent release of four phosphates. Also called *phosphorylase-rupturing enzyme, PR enzyme.*

phosphorylase-rupturing enzyme *n.* See **phosphorylase phosphatase.**

phos·pho·ryl·a·tion (fŏs'fər-ə-lā'shən) *n.* The addition of phosphate to an organic compound through the action of a phosphorylase or kinase.

phos·pho·sug·ar (fŏs'fō-shoog'ər) *n.* A sugar containing an alcohol group esterified with phosphoric acid.

phos·pho·trans·fer·ase (fŏs'fō-trăns'fə-rās', -rāz') *n.* Any of a class of enzymes, including the kinases, that catalyze the transfer of phosphorus-containing groups from one compound to another. Also called *transphosphatase.*

phos·pho·tri·ose isomerase (fŏs'fō-trī'ōs') *n.* See **triosephosphate isomerase.**

pho·tal·gia (fō-tăl'jə) *n.* Pain caused by light. Also called *photodynia.*

pho·tic (fō'tĭk) *adj.* **1.** Of or relating to light. **2.** Penetrated by or receiving light. **3.** Designating or relating to the layer of a body of water that is penetrated by sufficient sunlight for photosynthesis.

pho·tism (fō'tĭz'əm) *n.* The production of a sensation of light or color by a stimulus to another sense organ, such as that of hearing or touch.

photo– *or* **phot–** *pref.* **1.** Light; radiant energy: *photosynthesis.* **2.** Photographic: *photofluorography.*

pho·to·ag·ing (fō'tō-ā'jĭng) *n.* **1.** The process by which skin is changed or damaged as a result of exposure to ultraviolet radiation in sunlight and other sources. **2.** The long-term effects of this process on the skin, as wrinkles, discoloration, or susceptibility to cancer.

pho·to·bi·ol·o·gy (fō'tō-bī-ŏl'ə-jē) *n.* The study of the effects of light on living organisms and biological processes. —**pho'to·bi'o·log'ic** (-bī'ə-lŏj'ĭk), **pho'to·bi'o·log'i·cal** (-ĭ-kəl) *adj.*

pho·to·bi·ot·ic (fō'tō-bī-ŏt'ĭk) *adj.* Depending on light for life and growth.

pho·to·cat·a·lyst (fō'tō-kăt'l-ĭst) *n.* A substance that helps bring about a light-catalyzed reaction, such as chlorophyll in photosynthesis.

photochemical smog *n.* Air pollution produced by the action of sunlight on hydrocarbons, nitrogen oxides, and other pollutants.

pho·to·chem·is·try (fō'tō-kĕm'ĭ-strē) *n.* The branch of chemistry that deals with the effects of light on chemical systems. —**pho'to·chem'i·cal** (-ĭ-kəl) *adj.*

pho·to·che·mo·ther·a·py (fō'tō-kē'mō-thĕr'ə-pē, -kĕm'ō-) *n.* See **photoradiation.**

pho·to·chro·mic lens (fō'tə-krō'mĭk) *n.* A light-sensitive eyeglass lens that automatically darkens in sunlight and clears in reduced light.

pho·to·co·ag·u·la·tion (fō'tō-kō-ăg'yə-lā'shən) *n.* Surgical coagulation of tissue by means of intense light energy, such as a laser, that is performed to destroy abnormal tissues or to form adhesive scars, especially in ophthalmology. —**pho′to·co·ag′u·late′** v.

pho·to·co·ag·u·la·tor (fō′tō-kō-ăg′yə-lā′tər) n. An apparatus used in photocoagulation.

pho·to·de·grad·a·ble (fō′tō-dĭ-grā′də-bəl) adj. Capable of being chemically broken down by light.

pho·to·der·ma·ti·tis (fō′tō-dûr′mə-tī′tĭs) n. Dermatitis caused by exposure to ultraviolet light.

pho·to·dis·tri·bu·tion (fō′tō-dĭs′trə-byōō′shən) n. The areas on the skin that receive the greatest exposure to sunlight and are involved in eruptions due to photosensitivity.

pho·to·dy·nam·ic (fō′tō-dī-năm′ĭk) adj. **1.** Of or relating to the energy of light. **2.** Enhancing the effects of or inducing a toxic reaction to light, especially to ultraviolet light.

pho·to·dy·nam·ics (fō′tō-dī-năm′ĭks) n. The science that deals with the activating effects of light on living organisms.

photodynamic therapy n. A type of phototherapy in which a nontoxic light-sensitive compound that has been injected into a patient is exposed selectively to light, whereupon it becomes toxic to targeted malignant and other diseased cells.

pho·to·dyn·i·a (fō′tə-dĭn′ē-ə) n. See **photalgia**.

pho·to·e·lec·tric (fō′tō-ĭ-lĕk′trĭk) or **pho·to·e·lec·tri·cal** (-trĭ-kəl) adj. Of or relating to the electric effects, especially increased conductivity, caused by light.

pho·to·fluor·o·gram (fō′tə-floor′ə-grăm′, -flôr′-) n. A photograph made by photofluorography.

pho·to·fluo·rog·ra·phy (fō′tō-floo-rŏg′rə-fē, -flô-) n. The photographic record of x-ray images produced by a fluoroscope. Also called *fluorography*. —**pho′to·fluor′o·graph′ic** (-floor′ə-grăf′ĭk, -flôr′-) adj.

pho·to·gas·tro·scope (fō′tō-găs′trə-skōp′) n. An instrument for taking photographs of the interior of the stomach.

pho·to·gene (fō′tə-jēn′) n. See **afterimage**.

pho·to·gen·ic (fō′tə-jĕn′ĭk) adj. **1.** Producing or emitting light; phosphorescent. **2.** Caused or produced by light, as a seizure.

photogenic epilepsy n. A form of reflex epilepsy in which seizures are provoked by a flickering light.

pho·to·in·ac·ti·va·tion (fō′tō-ĭn-ăk′tə-vā′shən) n. Inactivation, as of a substance, by light.

pho·to·lu·mi·nes·cent (fō′tō-loo′mə-nĕs′ənt) adj. Having the ability to become luminescent upon exposure to visible light. —**pho′to·lu′mi·nes′cence** n.

pho·tol·y·sis (fō-tŏl′ĭ-sĭs) n. Chemical decomposition induced by light or other radiant energy. —**pho′to·lyt′ic** (-tə-lĭt′ĭk) adj.

pho·to·mi·cro·graph (fō′tō-mī′krə-grăf′) n. A photograph made through a microscope. Also called *microphotograph*. —v. To photograph an object through a microscope. —**pho′to·mi′cro·graph′ic** adj. —**pho′to·mi·crog′ra·phy** (-mī-krŏg′rə-fē) n.

pho·to·my·oc·lo·nus (fō′tō-mī-ŏk′lə-nəs) n. Clonic muscular spasms in response to visual stimuli.

pho·ton (fō′tŏn′) n. The quantum of electromagnetic energy, generally regarded as a discrete particle having zero mass, no electric charge, and an indefinitely long lifetime. —**pho·ton′ic** adj.

pho·to·patch test (fō′tō-păch′) n. A test for contact

photosensitization in which a patch containing the suspected sensitizer is applied to the skin for 48 hours; if there is no reaction, the area is exposed to a reddening dose of ultraviolet light; if the reaction is then positive, a more severe reaction develops at the patch site than in surrounding skin.

pho·to·per·cep·tive (fō′tō-pər-sĕp′tĭv) adj. Capable of receiving and perceiving light.

pho·to·pe·ri·od (fō′tō-pîr′ē-əd) n. The duration of an organism's daily exposure to light, considered especially with regard to the effect of such exposure on growth and development. —**pho′to·pe′ri·od′ic** (-ŏd′ĭk), **pho′to·pe′ri·od′i·cal** (-ĭ-kəl) adj.

pho·to·pe·ri·od·ism (fō′tō-pîr′ē-ə-dĭz′əm) or **pho·to·pe·ri·o·dic·i·ty** (-pîr′ē-ə-dĭs′ĭ-tē) n. The response of an organism to changes in its photoperiod, especially as indicated by vital processes.

pho·to·pho·bi·a (fō′tə-fō′bē-ə) n. **1.** An abnormal sensitivity to or intolerance of light, especially by the eyes, as may be caused by eye inflammation, lack of pigmentation in the iris, or various diseases. **2.** An abnormal or irrational fear of light.

pho·to·pho·bic (fō′tə-fō′bĭk) adj. **1.** Exhibiting photophobia. **2.** Avoiding light. **3.** Growing best in the absence of light.

pho·toph·thal·mi·a (fō′tŏf-thăl′mē-ə, -ŏp-) n. An inflammatory reaction of the external parts of the eye caused by intense light, as in snow blindness.

pho·to·pi·a (fō-tō′pē-ə) n. Vision in bright light, mediated by cone cells of the retina; daylight vision. Also called *photopic vision*. —**pho·to′pic** (-tō′pĭk, -tŏp′ĭk) adj.

photopic adaptation n. See **light adaptation**.

photopic eye n. See **light-adapted eye**.

photopic vision n. See **photopia**.

pho·top·si·a (fō-tŏp′sē-ə) n. The sensation of seeing lights, sparks, or colors caused by retinal or cerebral disease. Also called *photopsy*.

pho·top·sin (fō-tŏp′sĭn) n. The protein component of the pigment iodopsin in the cones of the retina of the eye.

pho·top·sy (fō-tŏp′sē) n. See **photopsia**.

pho·to·ptar·mo·sis (fō′tō-tär-mō′sĭs) n. Reflex sneezing in response to bright light striking the retina.

pho·to·ra·di·a·tion (fō′tō-rā′dē-ā′shən) n. A treatment for cancer in which an individual is injected with a photosensitizing agent and the cancerous tissue is exposed to visible light, often by means of a fiberoptic probe. Also called *photochemotherapy*.

photoradiation therapy n. Photoradiation.

pho·to·re·ac·tion (fō′tō-rē-ăk′shən) n. A photochemical reaction.

pho·to·re·ac·ti·va·tion (fō′tō-rē-ăk′tə-vā′shən) n. The activation by light of something previously inactive or inactivated.

pho·to·re·cep·tion (fō′tō-rĭ-sĕp′shən) n. The detection, absorption, and use of light, as for vision in animals or phototropism and photosynthesis in plants. —**pho′to·re·cep′tive** (-tĭv) adj.

pho·to·re·cep·tor (fō′tō-rĭ-sĕp′tər) n. A nerve ending, cell, or group of cells specialized to sense or receive light.

photoreceptor cell n. **1.** Any of the rod cells present in the retina of the eye. **2.** Any of the cone cells present in the retina.

pho·to·ret·i·nop·a·thy (fō′tō-rĕt′n-ŏp′ə-thē) *n.* A macular burn from excessive exposure to sunlight or other intense light, causing reduced visual acuity. Also called *photoretinitis*.

pho·to·scan (fō′tə-skăn′) *n.* See **scintigram**.

pho·to·sen·si·tive (fō′tō-sĕn′sĭ-tĭv) *adj.* **1.** Sensitive or responsive to light or other radiant energy. **2.** Abnormally sensitive or reactive to light.

pho·to·sen·si·tiv·i·ty (fō′tō-sĕn′sĭ-tĭv′ĭ-tē) *n.* **1.** Sensitivity or responsiveness to light. **2.** An abnormally heightened response, especially of the skin, to sunlight or ultraviolet radiation, caused by certain disorders or chemicals and characterized by a toxic or allergic reaction.

pho·to·sen·si·ti·za·tion (fō′tō-sĕn′sĭ-tĭ-zā′shən) *n.* The act or process of inducing photosensitivity.

pho·to·sen·si·tize (fō′tō-sĕn′sĭ-tīz′) *v.* To make an organism, cell, or substance photosensitive.

pho·to·sta·ble (fō′tō-stā′bəl) *adj.* Unchanged upon exposure to light.

pho·to·steth·o·scope (fō′tō-stĕth′ə-skōp′) *n.* A device that converts sound into flashes of light, used for continuous observation of the fetal heart.

pho·to·syn·thate (fō′tō-sĭn′thāt) *n.* A chemical product of photosynthesis.

pho·to·syn·the·sis (fō′tō-sĭn′thĭ-sĭs) *n.* The process in green plants and certain other organisms by which cells containing chlorophyll by which carbohydrates are synthesized from carbon dioxide and a source of hydrogen, such as water, using light as an energy source. —**pho′·to·syn·thet′ic** (-sĭn-thĕt′ĭk) *adj.*

pho·to·syn·the·size (fō′tō-sĭn′thĭ-sīz′) *v.* To synthesize by the process of photosynthesis.

pho·to·tax·is (fō′tō-tăk′sĭs) *n.* The movement of an organism or cell toward or away from a source of light. —**pho′to·tac′tic** (-tăk′tĭk) *adj.*

pho·to·ther·a·py (fō′tō-thĕr′ə-pē) *n.* The treatment of a disorder, especially of the skin, by exposure to light, including ultraviolet and infrared radiation. Also called *light treatment*.

pho·tot·o·nus (fō-tŏt′n-əs) *n.* The state of being sensitive to or irritated by light. —**pho′to·ton′ic** (fō′tə-tŏn′ĭk) *adj.*

pho·to·tox·ic (fō′tō-tŏk′sĭk) *adj.* Rendering the skin susceptible to damage by light. Used of certain medications. —**pho′to·tox·ic′i·ty** (-tŏk-sĭs′ĭ-tē) *n.*

pho·tot·ro·pism (fō-tŏt′rə-pĭz′əm) *n.* Growth or movement of a sessile organism toward or away from a light source. —**pho′to·tro′pic** (fō′tə-trō′pĭk, -trŏp′-ĭk) *adj.*

pho·tu·ri·a (fō-tŏŏr′ē-ə) *n.* The passage of phosphorescent urine.

phren– *pref.* Variant of **phreno–**.

phre·nal·gia (frə-năl′jə) *n.* Pain in the diaphragm.

phren·em·phrax·is (frĕn′ĕm-frăk′sĭs) *n.* See **phreniclasia**.

phreni– *pref.* Variant of **phreno–**.

–phrenia *suff.* Mental disorder: *schizophrenia*.

phren·ic (frĕn′ĭk, frē′nĭk) *adj.* **1.** Of or relating to the mind. **2.** Of or relating to the diaphragm.

phrenic artery *n.* **1.** An artery having its origin as the first paired branch from the abdominal aorta inferior to the diaphragm and with distribution to the diaphragm; inferior phrenic artery. **2.** Either of a pair of small arteries given off from the thoracic aorta just superior to the diaphragm and with distribution over the upper surface of the diaphragm; superior phrenic artery.

phren·i·cec·to·my (frĕn′ĭ-sĕk′tə-mē) *n.* Excision of a portion of the phrenic nerve. Also called *phrenicoexeresis*.

phrenic ganglion *n.* Any of several small autonomic ganglions contained in the plexuses accompanying the inferior phrenic arteries.

phren·i·cla·sia (frĕn′ĭ-klā′zhə) *n.* Surgical crushing of a section of the phrenic nerve as a substitute for phrenicotomy. Also called *phrenemphraxis, phrenicotripsy*.

phrenic nerve *n.* A nerve that arises mainly from the fourth cervical nerve and is primarily the motor nerve of the diaphragm but also sends sensory fibers to the pericardium.

phren·i·co·col·ic ligament (frĕn′ĭ-kō-kŏl′ĭk, -kō′lĭk) *n.* A triangular fold of peritoneum attached to the left flexure of the colon and to the diaphragm, on which the inferior extremity of the spleen rests.

phren·i·co·ex·er·e·sis (frĕn′ĭ-kō-ĕk-sĕr′ĭ-sĭs) *n.* See **phrenicectomy**.

phren·i·co·pleu·ral fascia (frĕn′ĭ-kō-plŏŏr′əl) *n.* The thin layer of endothoracic fascia between the diaphragmatic pleura and the diaphragm.

phren·i·cot·o·my (frĕn′ĭ-kŏt′ə-mē) *n.* Surgical division of the phrenic nerve to cause paralysis of the diaphragm on one side.

phren·i·co·trip·sy (frĕn′ĭ-kō-trĭp′sē) *n.* See **phreniclasia**.

phre·ni·tis (frĭ-nī′tĭs) *n.* **1.** Inflammation of the diaphragm. **2.** Encephalitis. No longer in technical use. —**phre·nit′ic** (-nĭt′ĭk) *adj.*

phreno– *or* **phren–** *or* **phreni–** *pref.* **1.** Mind: *phrenoplegia*. **2.** Diaphragm: *phrenogastric*.

phren·o·car·di·a (frĕn′ə-kär′dē-ə) *n.* Precordial pain and dyspnea of psychogenic origin.

phren·o·col·ic (frĕn′ō-kŏl′ĭk, -kō′lĭk) *adj.* Relating to the diaphragm and the colon.

phren·o·col·o·pex·y (frĕn′ō-kŏl′ə-pĕk′sē, -kō′lə-) *n.* Suture of a prolapsed transverse colon to the diaphragm.

phren·o·gas·tric (frĕn′ō-găs′trĭk) *adj.* Relating to the diaphragm and stomach.

phren·o·he·pat·ic (frĕn′ō-hĭ-păt′ĭk) *adj.* Relating to the diaphragm and liver.

phre·nol·o·gy (frĭ-nŏl′ə-jē) *n.* The study of the shape and protuberances of the skull, based on the now discredited belief that they reveal character and mental capacity.

phren·o·ple·gia (frĕn′ə-plē′jə) *n.* Paralysis of the diaphragm.

phren·op·to·si·a (frĕn′ŏp-tō′sē-ə, -zē-ə) *n.* Abnormal downward displacement of the diaphragm.

phren·o·sin (frĕn′ə-sĭn) *n.* A cerebroside abundant in white matter of the brain and composed of cerebronic acid, galactose, and sphingosine.

phryn·o·der·ma (frĭn′ə-dûr′mə) *n.* A follicular hyperkeratotic eruption that is associated with vitamin A deficiency.

PHS *abbr.* Public Health Service

phthal·ein *or* **phthal·eine** (thăl′ēn′, thăl′ē-ĭn, thā′lēn′, thā′lē-ĭn) *n.* Any of a group of chemical compounds formed by a reaction of phthalic anhydride with a phenol, from which certain synthetic dyes are derived.

phthal·ic (thăl′ĭk, fthăl′-) *adj.* **1.** Relating to or derived from naphthalene. **2.** Relating to phthalic acid.

phthalic acid *n.* A colorless crystalline organic acid prepared from naphthalene and used in the synthesis of dyes and other organic compounds.

phthalic anhydride *n.* A white crystalline compound prepared by oxidizing naphthalene and used in the manufacture of phthaleins and other dyes.

phthal·o·cy·a·nine (thăl′ō-sī′ə-nēn′) *n.* Any of several stable, light-fast, blue or green organic pigments used in enamels and plastics.

phthi·ri·a·sis (thĭ-rī′ə-sĭs, thī-) *n.* Infestation with lice, especially crab lice; pediculosis.

phthiriasis pu·bis (pyōō′bĭs) *n.* Infestation of the pubic hair and sometimes the eyelashes with crab lice.

Phthir·us (thĭr′əs, thī′rəs) *n.* Pthirus.

phthi·sis (thī′sĭs, tī′-) *or* **phthis·ic** (tĭz′ĭk, thĭz′-) *n.* **1.** A disease characterized by the wasting away or atrophy of the body or part of the body. **2.** Tuberculosis of the lungs. No longer in technical use.

phyco– *pref.* Seaweed; algae: *phycomycete.*

phy·co·my·cete (fī′kō-mī′sēt′, -mī-sēt′) *n.* Any of various fungi that resemble algae and that include certain molds and mildews. —**phy′co·my·ce′tous** *adj.*

phy·co·my·co·sis (fī′kō-mī-kō′sĭs) *n.* See **zygomycosis.**

phy·lax·is (fī-lăk′sĭs) *n.* Protection against infection.

phylo– *pref.* Tribe, race, or phylum: *phylogenesis.*

phy·lo·gen·e·sis (fī′lō-jĕn′ĭ-sĭs) *n.* See **phylogeny** (sense 1).

phy·lo·ge·net·ic (fī′lō-jə-nĕt′ĭk) *adj.* **1.** Of or relating to phylogeny or phylogenetics. **2.** Relating to or based on evolutionary development or history.

phy·lo·ge·net·ics (fī′lō-jə-nĕt′ĭks) *n.* The study of phylogeny.

phy·log·e·ny (fī-lŏj′ə-nē) *n.* **1.** The evolutionary development and history of a species or higher taxonomic grouping of organisms. Also called *phylogenesis.* **2.** The evolutionary development of an organ or other part of an organism. —**phy′lo·gen′ic** (-jĕn′ĭk) *adj.*

phy·lum (fī′ləm) *n.,* *pl.* **-la** (-lə) A taxonomic category that is a primary division of a kingdom and ranks above a class in size.

phy·ma (fī′mə) *n.* A nodule or small rounded tumor of the skin.

phy·ma·to·sis (fī′mə-tō′sĭs) *n.* The occurrence or growth of phymas in the skin.

phys. *abbr.* physical; physician; physiological; physiology

phys– *pref.* Variant of **physio–.**

phy·sal·i·form (fī-săl′ə-fôrm′, fĭ-) *adj.* Resembling a bubble or bubbles.

phys·a·lis (fĭs′ə-lĭs) *n.* A vacuole in a giant cell of certain malignant neoplasms, such as chondromas.

phys·e·al (fĭz′ē-əl) *adj.* Relating to the area of bone that separates the metaphysis and the epiphysis, in which the cartilage grows.

phys. ed. *or* **phys ed** *abbr.* physical education

physi– *pref.* Variant of **physio–.**

phys·i·at·rics (fĭz′ē-ăt′rĭks) *n.* **1.** See **physical medicine.** **2.** See **physical therapy.**

phys·i·at·rist (fĭz′ē-ăt′rĭst, fĭ-zī′ə-trĭst) *n.* **1.** A physician who specializes in physical medicine. **2.** A health care professional who administers physical therapy; a physical therapist.

phys·i·at·ry (fĭz′ē-ăt′rē, fĭ-zī′ə-trē) *n.* See **physical medicine.**

phys·ic (fĭz′ĭk) *n.* A medicine or drug, especially a cathartic.

phys·i·cal (fĭz′ĭ-kəl) *adj.* *Abbr.* **phys.** **1.** Of or relating to the body as distinguished from the mind or spirit. **2.** Involving or characterized by vigorous bodily activity. **3.** Of or relating to material things. **4.** Of or relating to matter and energy or the sciences dealing with them, especially physics. —*n.* A physical examination. —**phys′i·cal′i·ty** (-kăl′ĭ-tē) *adj.*

physical allergy *n.* Hypersensitivity caused by exposure to various physical factors such as heat, cold, light, or mechanical irritation.

physical chemistry *n.* Scientific analysis of the properties and behavior of chemical systems primarily by physical theory and technique.

physical diagnosis *n.* Diagnosis based on a physical examination of a patient.

physical education *n.* *Abbr.* **phys. ed., phys ed** Education in the care and development of the human body, stressing athletics and including hygiene.

physical examination *n.* *Abbr.* **PE** A medical examination to determine a person's health or physical fitness, especially for a specified activity or service.

physical half-life *n.* See **half-life** (sense 1).

physical medicine *n.* The branch of medicine that deals with the diagnosis, treatment, and prevention of disease and disability by physical means such as manipulation, massage, and exercise, often with the aid of mechanical devices and with the application of heat, cold, electricity, radiation, or water. Also called *physiatrics, physiatry.*

physical mixture *n.* A homogeneous mixture separable by a process such as distillation but not by filtration.

physical sign *n.* Any of various signs that are elicited by auscultation, percussion, or palpation.

physical therapy *n.* *Abbr.* **PT** The treatment of physical dysfunction or injury by the use of therapeutic exercise and the application of modalities that are intended to restore or facilitate normal function or development. Also called *physiatrics, physiotherapy.* —**physical therapist** *n.*

phy·si·cian (fĭ-zĭsh′ən) *n.* *Abbr.* **phys. 1.** *Abbr.* **phys.** A person licensed to practice medicine; a medical doctor. **2.** A person who practices general medicine as distinct from surgery.

phy·si·cian's assistant (fĭ-zĭsh′ənz) *n.,* *pl.* **physicians′ assistants** *Abbr.* **PA** A person trained and licensed to provide basic medical services, usually under the supervision of a physician.

phys·i·co·chem·i·cal (fĭz′ĭ-kō-kĕm′ĭ-kəl) *adj.* **1.** Relating to both physical and chemical properties. **2.** Relating to physical chemistry.

phys·ics (fĭz′ĭks) *n.* **1.** *Abbr.* **phys.** The science of matter and energy and of interactions between the two, grouped in traditional fields such as acoustics, optics, mechanics, thermodynamics, and electromagnetism, as well as in modern extensions including atomic and nuclear physics, cryogenics, solid-state physics, particle physics, and plasma physics. **2.** Physical properties, interactions, processes, or laws.

physio– *or* **physi–** *or* **phys–** *pref.* **1.** Nature; natural: *physiognomy.* **2.** Physical: *physiotherapy.*

phys·i·o·gen·ic (fĭz′ē-ō-jĕn′ĭk) *adj.* Relating to or caused by physiological activity.

phys·i·og·no·my (fĭz′ē-ŏg′nə-mē, -ŏn′ə-mē) *n.* **1.** Facial features, especially when considered as an indicator of character or as a factor in diagnosis. **2.** Estimation of one's character and mental qualities by a study of the face and general bodily carriage.

phys·i·o·log·i·cal (fĭz′ē-ə-lŏj′ĭ-kəl) *or* **phys·i·o·log·ic** (-ĭk) *adj. Abbr.* **phys. 1.** Of or relating to physiology. **2.** Being in accord with or characteristic of the normal functioning of a living organism. **3.** Relating to the action of a drug when given to a healthy person, as distinguished from its therapeutic action.

physiological anatomy *n.* The study of organs with respect to their functions. Also called *functional anatomy.*

physiological dead space *n.* The sum of anatomical and alveolar dead space.

physiological drive *n.* A drive that stems from the biological needs of an organism. Also called *primary drive.*

physiological psychology *n.* See **psychophysiology.**

physiological saline *n.* A sterile solution of sodium chloride that is isotonic to body fluids, used to maintain living tissue temporarily and as a solvent for parenterally administered drugs.

physiological sphincter *n.* A sphincter not recognizable in surgical specimens by dissection or histological techniques.

physiologic antidote *n.* A substance that produces systemic effects opposing those of a given poison.

physiologic congestion *n.* See **functional congestion.**

physiologic cup *n.* A funnel-shaped depression in the optic disk.

physiologic dwarf *n.* An undersized person whose development has been symmetrical and at a normal rate, but less extensive than normal.

physiologic equilibrium *n.* See **nutritive equilibrium.**

physiologic excavation *n.* See **excavation of optic disk.**

physiologic hypertrophy *n.* A temporary increase in size of an organ or part to provide for a natural increase of function such as occurs in the walls of the uterus and in the mammary glands during pregnancy. Also called *functional hypertrophy.*

physiologic jaundice *n.* Mild jaundice of newborns caused mainly by functional immaturity of the liver. Also called *physiologic icterus.*

physiologic leukocytosis *n.* Leukocytosis not directly related to a pathological condition but instead occurring in apparently normal conditions.

physiologic occlusion *n.* Occlusion of the teeth in harmony with the functions of the masticatory system.

physiologic rest position *n.* The habitual postural position of the mandible when at rest in the upright position and the condyles are in a neutral unstrained position in the mandibular fossae. Also called *postural position.*

physiologic retraction ring *n.* A ridge on the inner uterine surface at the boundary between the upper and lower uterine segments that occurs in the course of normal labor.

physiologic scotoma *n.* See **blind spot** (sense 1).

physiologic unit *n.* The smallest division of an organ that will perform its specific function.

phys·i·ol·o·gy (fĭz′ē-ŏl′ə-jē) *n. Abbr.* **phys. 1.** The biological study of the functions of living organisms and their parts. **2.** All the functions of a living organism or any of its parts. —**phys′i·ol′o·gist** *n.*

phys·i·o·pa·thol·o·gy (fĭz′ē-ō-pə-thŏl′ə-jē) *n.* See **pathophysiology.**

phys·i·o·ther·a·py (fĭz′ē-ō-thĕr′ə-pē) *n.* See **physical therapy.** —**phys′i·o·ther′a·peu′tic** (-thĕr′ə-pyōō′tĭk) *adj.* —**phys′i·o·ther′a·pist** *n.*

phy·sique (fĭ-zēk′) *n.* The body considered with reference to its proportions, muscular development, and appearance.

physo– *pref.* Swelling or distention caused by air or gas: *physometra.*

phy·so·cele (fī′sə-sēl′) *n.* **1.** A swelling filled with gas. **2.** A hernial sac distended with gas.

phy·so·me·tra (fī′sə-mē′trə) *n.* Distention of the uterine cavity with air or gas.

phy·so·py·o·sal·pinx (fī′sō-pī′ə-săl′pĭngks) *n.* Pyosalpinx accompanied by the formation of gas in the affected fallopian tube.

phy·tan·ic acid (fī-tăn′ĭk) *n.* An acid derived from phytol that inhibits the oxidation of palmitic acid and accumulates in the serum and tissues of patients with Refsum's disease.

–phyte *suff.* **1.** A plant with a specified character or habitat: *saprophyte.* **2.** A pathological growth: *osteophyte.*

phyto– *or* **phyt–** *pref.* Plant: *phytohormones.*

phy·to·ag·glu·ti·nin (fī′tō-ə-glōōt′n-ĭn) *n.* A lectin that causes agglutination of red blood cells or white blood cells.

phy·to·be·zoar (fī′tō-bē′zôr′) *n.* See **food ball.**

phy·to·chem·i·cal (fī′tō-kĕm′ĭ-kəl) *n.* A nonnutritive bioactive plant substance, such as a flavonoid or carotenoid, considered to have a beneficial effect on human health.

phy·to·der·ma·ti·tis (fī′tō-dûr′mə-tī′tĭs) *n.* Dermatitis caused by various mechanisms including mechanical and chemical injury, allergy, or photosensitization at skin sites previously exposed to plants.

phy·to·es·tro·gen (fī′tō-ĕs′trə-jən) *n.* Any of a group of substances, including isoflavones, that are derived from plants and have biological effects on animals similar to those of estrogen.

phy·to·he·mag·glu·ti·nin (fī′tō-hē′mə-glōōt′n-ĭn) *n. Abbr.* **PHA** A hemagglutinin extracted from a plant. Also called *phytolectin.*

phy·toid (fī′toid′) *adj.* Resembling a plant.

phy·tol (fī′tôl′) *n.* A liquid alcohol used in the synthesis of vitamins E and K.

phy·to·lec·tin (fī′tō-lĕk′tĭn) *n.* See **phytohemagglutinin.**

phy·to·mi·to·gen (fī′tō-mī′tə-jən, -jĕn′) *n.* A mitogenetic lectin causing lymphocyte transformation accompanied by mitotic proliferation of the resulting blast cells identical to that produced by antigenic stimulation.

phy·to·nu·tri·ent (fī′tō-nōō′trē-ənt) *n*. A substance derived from plants, such as a pigment, that is beneficial to health, especially one that is neither a vitamin nor a mineral.

phy·to·phlyc·to·der·ma·ti·tis (fī′tō-flĭk′tō-dûr′mə-tī′tĭs) *n*. See **meadow dermatitis**.

phy·to·pho·to·der·ma·ti·tis (fī′tō-fō′tō-dûr′mə-tī′tĭs) *n*. See **meadow dermatitis**.

phy·to·tox·ic (fī′tō-tŏk′sĭk) *adj*. **1**. Poisonous to plants. **2**. Of or relating to a phytotoxin. —**phy′to·tox·ic′i·ty** (-tŏk-sĭs′ĭ-tē) *n*.

phy·to·tox·in (fī′tō-tŏk′sĭn) *n*. A toxin produced by a plant.

pi (pī) *n., pl.* **pis** *Symbol* **π** The 16th letter of the Greek alphabet.

pI (pē′ī′) *n*. The pH value for the isoelectric point of a given substance in solution.

pi·a (pī′ə, pē′ə) *n*. The pia mater. —**pi′al** *adj*.

pi·a·a·rach·ni·tis (pī′ə-ə-răk-nī′tĭs, pē′ə-) *n*. See **leptomeningitis**.

pi·a·a·rach·noid (pī′ə-ə-răk′noid′, pē′ə-) *or* **pi·a·rach·noid** (pī′ə-răk′-, pē′-) *n*. See **leptomeninges**.

Pia·get (pē′ə-zhā′, pyä-), **Jean** 1896–1980. Swiss child psychologist noted for his studies of intellectual and cognitive development in children.

pia ma·ter (pī′ə mā′tər, pē′ə mä′tər) *n*. The fine vascular membrane that closely envelops the brain and spinal cord under the arachnoid and the dura mater.

pi·an (pē-ăn′, pyän) *n*. See **yaws**.

pi·ca (pī′kə) *n*. An abnormal craving or appetite for nonfood substances, such as dirt, paint, or clay.

Pick cell (pĭk) *n*. See **Niemann-Pick cell**.

Pick's atrophy (pĭks) *n*. Circumscribed atrophy of the cerebral cortex.

Pick's disease[1] *n*. A condition occurring as a result of constrictive pericarditis and characterized by inflammation of one or more serous membranes including the peritoneum and the pleura, chronic congestive enlargement of the liver, and persistent or recurrent buildup of serous fluid.

Pick's disease[2] *n*. See **Niemann-Pick disease**.

pick·wick·i·an syndrome (pĭk-wĭk′ē-ən) *n*. A syndrome characterized by extreme obesity, hypoventilation, and general debility.

pico– *pref*. **1**. One-trillionth (10^{-12}): *picogram*. **2**. Very small: *picornavirus*.

pi·co·gram (pē′kə-grăm′, pī′-) *n. Abbr.* **pg** One-trillionth (10^{-12}) of a gram.

pi·co·me·ter (pē′kə-mē′tər, pī′-) *n. Abbr.* **pm** One-trillionth (10^{-12}) of a meter.

Pi·cor·na·vir·i·dae (pē-kôr′nə-vîr′ĭ-dē) *n*. A family of very small nonenveloped viruses having a core of single-stranded RNA and including the polioviruses, coxsackieviruses, and echoviruses.

pi·cor·na·vi·rus (pē-kôr′nə-vī′rəs, pĭ-) *n*. A virus of the family Picornaviridae.

pic·rate (pĭk′rāt′) *n*. A salt or ester of picric acid.

pic·ric acid (pĭk′rĭk) *n*. A poisonous, explosive, yellow, crystalline acid used as an application in burns, eczema, erysipelas, and pruritus and in the manufacture of dyes and explosives.

picro– *or* **picr–** *pref*. **1**. Bitter: *picrotoxin*. **2**. Picric acid: *picrate*.

pic·ro·car·mine stain (pĭk′rō-kär′mĭn, -mīn′) *n*. A red crystalline water-soluble powder that produces excellent staining of keratohyaline granules.

pic·ro·tox·in (pĭk′rə-tŏk′sĭn) *n*. A bitter crystalline compound derived from the seed of an East Indian woody vine and used as a stimulant, especially in treating barbiturate poisoning.

PID *abbr*. pelvic inflammatory disease

pie·bald·ness (pī′bôld′nĭs) *n*. A skin disorder that is characterized by pigmentless patches of scalp hair that give the hair a streaked appearance. Also called *piebaldism*.

pie·bald skin (pī′bôld′) *n*. See **leukoderma**.

pi·e·dra (pē-ā′drə) *n*. A fungal disease of the hair marked by small black or white nodular masses.

Pierre Ro·bin syndrome (pyĕr′ rô-băɴ′) *n*. Abnormal smallness of the jaw and tongue, often accompanied by cleft palate and bilateral eye defects such as myopia, congenital glaucoma, and retinal detachment.

pi·e·zo·gen·ic pedal papule (pī-ē′zō-jĕn′ĭk) *n*. Papules of the heel induced by pressure, occurring probably as a result of the herniation of fat tissue due to degeneration of dermal collagen.

PIF *abbr*. prolactin-inhibiting factor

pi·geon breast (pĭj′ən) *n*. A chest deformity marked by a projecting sternum, often occurring as a result of infantile rickets. Also called *chicken breast, pectus carinatum*.

pigeon-toed *adj*. Having the toes turned inward.

pig·ment (pĭg′mənt) *n*. **1**. A substance used as coloring. **2**. Dry coloring matter, usually an insoluble powder to be mixed with water, oil, or another base to produce paint and similar products. **3**. A substance that produces a characteristic color in tissue. **4**. A medicinal preparation applied to the skin like paint. —*v*. To color with pigment.

pig·men·tar·y (pĭg′mən-tĕr′ē) *adj*. Of or relating to a pigment.

pigmentary retinopathy *n*. See **retinitis pigmentosa**.

pig·men·ta·tion (pĭg′mən-tā′shən) *n*. **1**. Coloration of tissues by pigment. **2**. Deposition of pigment by cells.

pigment cell *n*. See **chromatophore**.

pig·ment·ed (pĭg′mən-tĭd) *adj*. Colored as the result of a deposit of pigment.

pigmented ameloblastoma *n*. See **melanotic neuroectodermal tumor**.

pigmented vil·lo·nod·u·lar synovitis (vĭl′ō-nŏj′ə-lər) *n*. Diffuse outgrowths of the synovial membrane of a joint, usually the knee.

pig·men·to·ly·sin (pĭg′mən-tŏl′ĭ-sĭn) *n*. An antibody that causes destruction of pigment.

pig·men·tum ni·grum (pĭg-mĕn′təm nī′grəm) *n*. Melanin of the choroid coat of the eye.

pi·lar (pī′lər) *or* **pi·la·ry** (pī′lə-rē) *adj*. Of, relating to, or covered with hair.

pilar cyst *n*. See **sebaceous cyst**.

pilar tumor of scalp *n*. A benign solitary tumor occurring on the scalp in elderly women.

Pi·la·tes (pĭ-lä′tēz) A trademark for a system of conditioning exercises often performed on specialized apparatus.

pile (pīl) *n.* A hemorrhoid.

pi·le·ous (pī′lē-əs) *adj.* Hairy.

pileous gland *n.* A sebaceous gland emptying into a hair follicle.

piles (pīlz) *pl.n.* See **hemorrhoid** (sense 2).

pi·lif·er·ous (pī-lĭf′ər-əs) *adj.* Bearing or producing hair.

pi·li·form (pī′lə-fôrm′, pĭl′ə-) *adj.* Having the form of a hair.

pi·li tor·ti (pī′lī′ tôr′tī) *n.* See **twisted hairs.**

pill (pĭl) *n.* **1.** A small pellet or tablet of medicine, often coated, taken by swallowing whole or by chewing. **2.** An oral contraceptive.

pil·lar (pĭl′ər) *n.* A structure or part that provides support and resembles a column or pillar.

pillars of fauces *pl.n.* The palatoglossal arch and palatopharyngeal arch.

pillars of fornix *pl.n.* The column of fornix and the crus of fornix.

pil·low splint (pĭl′ō) *n.* A splint that is inflatable or that is made from unusually bulky fabric.

pill-rolling *n.* A circular movement or tremor of the tips of the thumb and the index finger when brought together, seen in Parkinson's disease.

pilo– *pref.* Hair: *pilomotor.*

pi·lo·be·zoar (pī′lō-bē′zôr′) *n.* See **hairball.**

pi·lo·car·pine (pī′lō-kär′pēn′) *n.* A colorless or yellow poisonous compound used to induce sweating, promote salivation, and treat glaucoma.

pi·lo·cys·tic (pī′lō-sĭs′tĭk) *adj.* Containing hair. Used of dermoid cysts.

pi·lo·e·rec·tion (pī′lō-ĭ-rĕk′shən) *n.* Erection of hair.

pi·loid (pī′loid′) *adj.* Resembling hair; hairlike.

pi·lo·jec·tion (pī′lə-jĕk′shən) *n.* The process of shooting a stiff mammalian hair into a saccular aneurysm in the brain to produce thrombosis, used in treating the aneurysm.

pi·lo·ma·trix·o·ma (pī′lō-mā′trĭk-sō′mə) *n.* A benign, often calcified tumor of the skin and the tissue just below the skin, often occurring as a single lesion on the face or upper extremities. Also called *Malherbe's calcifying epithelioma.*

pi·lo·mo·tor (pī′lə-mō′tər) *adj.* Moving the hair. Used of the erector muscles of hairs in the skin and the postganglionic sympathetic nerve fibers that innervate them.

pilomotor reflex *n.* Contraction of the smooth muscle of the skin caused by mild application of a tactile stimulus or by local cooling and resulting in goose bumps.

pi·lo·ni·dal (pī′lə-nīd′l) *adj.* Of or relating to a growth of hair in a dermoid cyst or in the deeper layers of the skin.

pilonidal sinus *n.* A fistula or pit in the sacral region, communicating with the exterior and containing hair that may act as a foreign body and produce chronic inflammation. Also called *pilonidal fistula.*

pi·lose (pī′lōs) *or* **pi·lous** (-ləs) *adj.* Covered with fine, soft hair.

pi·lo·se·ba·ceous (pī′lō-sĭ-bā′shəs) *adj.* Relating to the hair follicles and sebaceous glands.

Piltz sign (pĭlts) *n.* See **tonic pupil.**

pil·ule (pĭl′yōōl) *n.* A small pill or pellet.

pi·lus (pī′ləs) *n.,* *pl.* **–li** (-lī′) **1.** A hair. **2.** A fine filamentous appendage, somewhat analogous to the flagellum, that occurs on some bacteria. Also called *fimbria.*

pilus in·car·na·tus (ĭn′kär-nā′təs) *n.* An ingrown hair.

pi·mel·ic acid (pĭ-mĕl′ĭk) *n.* A crystalline intermediate formed in the oxidation of oleic acid. Also called *heptanedioic acid.*

pimelo– *pref.* Fat; fatty: *pimelopterygium.*

pim·e·lo·pter·y·gi·um (pĭm′ə-lō-tə-rĭj′ē-əm) *n.* A pterygium containing fat.

pim·o·zide (pĭm′ə-zīd′) *n.* An antipsychotic drug used to treat chronic schizophrenia and in the management of Tourette's syndrome.

pim·ple (pĭm′pəl) *n.* A small red swelling of the skin, usually caused by acne.

pin (pĭn) *n.* **1.** A thin rod for securing the ends of fractured bones. **2.** A peg for fixing the crown to the root of a tooth. —*v.* To fasten or secure with a pin or pins.

Pi·nard's maneuver (pē-närz′) *n.* A method for delivering a fetus in breech position in which one leg is bent and passed along the thigh of the other leg as the foot of the bent leg is brought down and out.

pince·ment (păns-mäN′, păns-) *n.* A pinching manipulation in massage.

pin·cer nail (pĭn′sər) *n.* Transverse overcurvature of the nail that increases distally, causing the lateral borders of the nail to pinch the soft tissue.

pinch graft (pĭnch) *n.* A graft made with small bits of partial-thickness or full-thickness skin.

Pin·cus (pĭng′kəs, pĭn′-), **Gregory Goodwin** 1903–1967. American physiologist. Through his studies of natural hormones that inhibit ovulation in mammals, he developed the first effective oral contraceptive, which was first tested in 1954.

pin·do·lol (pĭn′də-lôl′, -lōl′) *n.* A beta-blocker used in the treatment of hypertension.

pin·e·al (pĭn′ē-əl, pī′nē-) *adj.* **1.** Having the form of a pine cone. **2.** Of or relating to the pineal body.

pineal body *n.* A small, unpaired, flattened glandular structure lying in the depression between the two superior colliculi of the brain and secreting the hormone melatonin. Also called *conarium, epiphysis, pineal gland.*

pin·e·al·ec·to·my (pĭn′ē-ə-lĕk′tə-mē, pī′nē-) *n.* Surgical removal of the pineal body.

pineal gland *n.* See **pineal body.**

pin·e·a·lo·cyte (pĭn′ē-ə-lō-sīt′, pī′nē-, pĭ-nē′-, pī-nē′-) *n.* A cell of the pineal body having long processes ending in bulbous expansions.

pin·e·a·lo·ma (pĭn′ē-ə-lō′mə, pī′nē-) *n.,* *pl.* **–mas** *or* **–ma·ta** (-mə-tə) A neoplasm derived from the pineal body and characterized by large, round, or polygonal cells with large nuclei and small cells that resemble lymphocytes.

pineal stalk *n.* The attachment of the pineal body to the roof of the third ventricle, containing the pineal recess of the third ventricle.

Pi·nel (pē-nĕl′), **Philippe** 1745–1826. French physician and pioneer of psychiatry who made reforms that led to more humane treatment for the mentally ill and began the classification of a number of mental disorders.

pin·e·o·blas·to·ma (pĭn′ē-ō-blă-stō′mə) *n.* A pinealoma having poorly differentiated cells.

pine tar (pīn) *n.* A viscous or semisolid brown-to-black substance produced by distillation of pine wood and used as an expectorant and antiseptic.

pin·guec·u·la (pĭng-gwĕk′yə-lə) *or* **pin·guic·u·la** (-gwĭk′-) *n.* **1.** A yellowish spot that is sometimes observed on either side of the cornea in older individuals. **2.** A thickening of the connective tissue of the conjunctiva.

pin·hole pupil (pĭn′hōl′) *n.* An extremely contracted pupil of the eye.

pin·i·form (pĭn′ə-fôrm′, pī′nə-) *adj.* Having the form of a pine cone.

pink disease *n.* See **acrodynia** (sense 1).

pink·eye (pĭngk′ī′) *n.* See **acute contagious conjunctivitis.**

pink·ie *or* **pink·y** (pĭng′kē) *n.* The little finger.

pin·na (pĭn′ə) *n.,* *pl.* **pin·nae** (pĭn′ē) See **auricle** (sense ?). —**pin′nal** *adj.*

pin·o·cyte (pĭn′ə-sīt′, pī′nə-) *n.* A cell that exhibits pinocytosis.

pin·o·cy·to·sis (pĭn′ə-sĭ-tō′sĭs, -sī-, pī′nə-) *n.* Introduction of fluids into a cell by invagination of the cell membrane, followed by formation of vesicles within the cells. —**pin′o·cy·tot′ic** (-tŏt′ĭk) *adj.*

pin·o·some (pĭn′ə-sōm′, pī′nə-) *n.* A fluid-filled vacuole formed by pinocytosis.

Pins′ syndrome (pĭns) *n.* Diminution of vocal fremitus and of the vesicular murmur accompanied by a slight distant blowing sound, heard in the posteroinferior region of the chest on the left side in cases of pericardial effusion.

pint (pīnt) *n.* **1.** A unit of volume or capacity in the US Customary System, used in liquid measure, equal to 16 fluid ounces, 28.875 cubic inches, or .473 liter. **2.** A unit of volume or capacity in the US Customary System, used in dry measure, equal to $\frac{1}{2}$ quart or 0.551 liter.

pin·ta (pĭn′tə, pēn′tä) *n.* A contagious skin disease prevalent in tropical America, caused by the spirochete *Treponema carateum* and characterized by thickening and spotty discoloration of the skin.

pin·worm (pĭn′wûrm′) *n.* Any of various small nematode worms of the family Oxyuridae that are parasitic on mammals, especially *Enterobius vermicularis,* a species that infests the human intestines and rectum. Also called *seatworm, threadworm.*

PIP *abbr.* proximal interphalangeal joint

pi·per·a·cil·lin sodium (pī-pĕr′ə-sĭl′ĭn) *n.* A semisynthetic broad-spectrum antibiotic related to penicillin and active against a variety of gram-positive and gram-negative bacteria.

pi·per·a·zine (pī-pĕr′ə-zēn′, pĭ-) *n.* A colorless crystalline compound used as a hardener for epoxy resins, an antihistamine, and an anthelmintic.

pi·per·i·dine (pī-pĕr′ĭ-dēn′, pĭ-) *n.* A strongly basic, colorless liquid from which certain phenothiazine antipsychotics are derived.

pi·pette *or* **pi·pet** (pī-pĕt′) *n.* A narrow, usually calibrated glass tube into which small amounts of liquid are suctioned for transfer or measurement.

Pip·ra·cil (pĭp′rə-sĭl′) A trademark for the drug piperacillin sodium.

pir·bu·ter·ol (pĭr-byōō′tə-rôl′, -rōl′) *n.* An analog of albuterol that acts as a bronchodilator and is used in the treatment of asthma.

pir·i·form (pĭr′ə-fôrm′, pī′rə-) *adj.* Shaped like a pear.

piriform muscle *n.* A muscle with origin from the margins of the pelvic sacral foramina and the sciatic notch of the ilium, with insertion into the great trochanter, with nerve supply from the sciatic plexus, and whose action rotates the thigh laterally.

Pir·o·plas·ma (pĭr′ə-plăz′mə, pī′rə-) *n.* Babesia.

pir·o·plas·mo·sis (pĭr′ə-plăz-mō′sĭs) *n.* See **babesiosis.**

pi·rox·i·cam o·la·mine (pĭ-rŏk′sĭ-kăm′ ô′lə-mēn′) *n.* A nonsteroidal anti-inflammatory agent with analgesic and antipyretic actions.

pi·si·form (pī′sə-fôrm′) *adj.* Resembling a pea in size or shape. —*n.* Pisiform bone.

pisiform bone *n.* A small bone in the proximal row of the wrist, lying on the anterior surface of the triquetrum bone, with which alone it articulates.

pit (pĭt) *n.* **1.** A natural hollow or depression in the body or an organ. **2.** A pockmark. **3.** A sharp-pointed depression in the enamel surface of a tooth, caused by faulty or incomplete calcification or formed by the confluent point of two or more lobes of enamel. —*v.* **1.** To mark with cavities, depressions, or scars. **2.** To retain an impression after being indented. Used of the skin.

pitch wart (pĭch) *n.* A precancerous keratotic epidermal tumor that is common among individuals who work with pitch and coal tar derivatives.

pith (pĭth) *n.* **1.** The soft inner substance of a hair. **2.** Spinal cord or bone marrow. No longer in technical use. —*v.* To sever or destroy the spinal cord of a vertebrate animal, usually by means of a needle inserted into the vertebral canal.

pith·e·coid (pĭth′ĭ-koid′, pī-thē′koid′) *adj.* Resembling or relating to the apes, especially the anthropoid apes.

Pi·to·cin (pĭ-tō′sĭn) A trademark for preparations of oxytocin.

pit of stomach *n.* See **epigastric fossa.**

Pi·tres·sin (pĭ-trĕs′ĭn) A trademark for a drug preparation of vasopressin.

pit·ted keratolysis (pĭt′ĭd) *n.* A noninflammatory bacterial infection of the soles, and occasionally the palms, that produces depressions in the horny layer of the epidermis, usually at weight-bearing sites.

pit·ting (pĭt′ĭng) *n.* The formation of well-defined, relatively deep depressions in a surface.

pitting edema *n.* Edema that retains for a time the indentation produced by pressure.

Pitts·burgh pneumonia (pĭts′bûrg′) *n.* Legionnaires' disease caused by *Legionella micdadei.*

pi·tu·i·cyte (pĭ-tōō′ĭ-sīt′) *n.* A small branching cell of the posterior lobe of the pituitary gland.

pi·tu·i·cy·to·ma (pĭ-tōō′ĭ-sī-tō′mə) *n.* A gliogenous neoplasm derived from pituicytes and marked by cells with long branching processes that form a complex network of cytoplasmic material.

pi·tu·i·ta·rism (pĭ-tōō′ĭ-tə-rĭz′əm) *n.* Pituitary dysfunction.

pi·tu·i·tar·y (pĭ-tōō′ĭ-tĕr′ē) *n.* **1.** The pituitary gland. **2.** An extract from the anterior or posterior lobes of the pituitary gland, prepared for therapeutic use. —*adj.*

1. Of or relating to the pituitary gland. **2.** Of or secreting phlegm or mucus; mucous.

pituitary basophil adenoma *n.* A tumor of the basophilic cells of the anterior pituitary gland, associated with Cushing's syndrome.

pituitary basophilism *n.* See **Cushing's syndrome.**

pituitary cachexia *n.* See **Simmonds disease.**

pituitary dwarfism *n.* A rare form of dwarfism caused by the absence of a functional anterior pituitary gland. Also called *Lorain-Lévi syndrome.*

pituitary fossa *n.* A depression of the sphenoid bone housing the pituitary gland. Also called *hypophysial fossa.*

pituitary gigantism *n.* A rare form of gigantism caused by hypersecretion of pituitary growth hormone, usually the result of a pituitary adenoma.

pituitary gland *n.* A small, oval endocrine gland attached to the base of the vertebrate brain and consisting of an anterior and posterior lobe, the secretions of which control the other endocrine glands and influence growth, metabolism, and maturation. Also called *hypophysis, master gland.*

pituitary gonadotropic hormone *n.* See **anterior pituitary gonadotropin.**

pituitary growth hormone *n.* See **growth hormone.**

pituitary myxedema *n.* Myxedema resulting from inadequate secretion of thyrotropic hormone.

pit·y·ri·a·sis (pĭt′ĭ-rī′ə-sĭs) *n., pl.* **-ses** (-sēz′) Any of various skin diseases of humans and animals, characterized by epidermal shedding of flaky scales. —**pit′y·ri′a·sic** (-sĭk) *adj.*

pityriasis al·ba (ăl′bə) *n.* See **seborrheic dermatitis.**

pityriasis lin·guae (lĭng′gwē) *n.* See **geographical tongue.**

pityriasis ro·se·a (rō′sē-ə, -zē-ə) *n.* A self-limited eruption of macules or papules involving principally the trunk and extremities.

pityriasis ru·bra (rōō′brə) *n.* See **exfoliative dermatitis.**

pityriasis rubra pi·lar·is (pĭ-lâr′ĭs) *n.* A chronic eruption of the hair follicles, which become firm, red, surmounted with horny plugs, and often form scaly patches.

pityriasis ver·si·col·or (vûr′sĭ-kŭl′ər) *n.* See **tinea versicolor.**

pit·y·roid (pĭt′ĭ-roid′) *adj.* Furfuraceous.

Pit·y·ros·po·rum (pĭt′ĭ-rŏs′pər-əm, pĭt′ĭ-rō-spôr′əm) *n.* A genus of fungi that includes one species that can cause tinea versicolor and another that is found primarily on the face and scalp and appears in dandruff and seborrheic dermatitis.

piv·ot joint (pĭv′ət) *n.* See **trochoid joint.**

pix·el (pĭk′səl) *n.* The smallest image-forming unit of a video display.

pK (pē′kā′) *n.* **1.** The negative logarithm of the dissociation constant of an electrolyte. **2.** A value equal to the pH at which equal concentrations of the acidic and basic forms of a substance are present.

PK *abbr.* psychokinesis

PKU *abbr.* phenylketonuria

pla·ce·bo (plə-sē′bō) *n., pl.* **-bos** or **-boes 1.** A substance containing no medication and prescribed or given to reinforce a patient's expectation to get well.

2. An inactive substance or preparation used as a control in an experiment or test to determine the effectiveness of a medicinal drug.

placebo effect *n.* A beneficial effect in a patient following a particular treatment that arises from the patient's expectations concerning the treatment rather than from the treatment itself.

pla·cen·ta (plə-sĕn′tə) *n., pl.* **-tas** or **-tae** (-tē) The membranous vascular organ in female mammals that permits metabolic interchange between fetus and mother. It develops during pregnancy from the chorion of the embryo and the decidua basalis of the maternal uterus and permits the absorption of oxygen and nutritive materials into the fetal blood and the release of carbon dioxide and nitrogenous waste from it, without the direct mixing of maternal and fetal blood. It is expelled following birth. —**pla·cen′tal** *adj.*

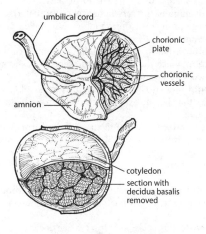

placenta
Top: *full-term placenta seen from fetal side*
Bottom: *full-term placenta seen from maternal side*

placenta ac·cre·ta (ə-krē′tə) *n.* Abnormal adherence of the chorionic villi to the myometrium, associated with partial or complete absence of the decidua basalis and the stratum spongiosum.

placenta cir·cum·val·la·ta (sûr′kəm-və-lā′tə) *n.* A cup-shaped placenta having raised edges and a thick, white, opaque ring around its periphery.

placenta fen·es·tra·ta (fĕn′ĭ-strā′tə) *n.* A placenta in which there are areas of thinning, sometimes involving the lack of placental tissue in some areas.

placenta in·cre·ta (ĭn-krē′tə) *n.* Placenta accreta in which chorionic villi invade the myometrium.

placental barrier *n.* The semipermeable layer of tissue in the placenta that serves as a selective membrane to substances passing from maternal to fetal blood.

placental circulation *n.* Circulation of blood through the placenta during intrauterine life, serving fetal needs for aeration, absorption, and excretion.

placental dystocia *n.* The retention or difficult passage of the placenta following delivery.

placental growth hormone *n.* See **human placental lactogen.**

placental lobe *n.* The unit of the human placenta, incompletely separated by septa, that contains the fetal cotyledon or cotyledons and the surrounding blood-filled intervillous space.

placental membrane *n.* The semipermeable layer of tissue separating maternal blood from fetal blood in the placenta.

placental presentation *n.* See **placenta previa**.

placental souffle *n.* See **uterine souffle**.

placenta mar·gi·na·ta (mär′jə-nā′tə) *n.* A placenta having raised edges that are less elevated than those of placenta circumvallata.

placenta mem·bra·na·ce·a (mĕm′brə-nā′sē-ə) *n.* An abnormally thin placenta covering an unusually large area of the uterus.

placenta pre·vi·a (prē′vē-ə) *n.* A condition in which the placenta is implanted in the lower segment of the uterus so that it is adjacent to or obstructs the internal opening of the cervix. It may cause maternal hemorrhage prior to or during labor. Also called *placental presentation.*

placenta re·flex·a (rĭ-flĕk′sə) *n.* An anomaly of the placenta in which the margin is thickened so as to appear turned back upon itself.

placenta spu·ri·a (spyŏor′ē-ə) *n.* A mass of placental tissue that has no vascular connection with the main placenta.

plac·en·ta·tion (plăs′ən-tā′shən) *n.* **1.** Formation of a placenta in the uterus. **2.** The type or structure of a placenta.

plac·en·ti·tis (plăs′ən-tī′tĭs) *n.* Inflammation of the placenta.

plac·en·tog·ra·phy (plăs′ən-tŏg′rə-fē) *n.* Radiography of the placenta following injection of a radiopaque substance.

plac·en·to·ma (plăs′ən-tō′mə) *n.* See **deciduoma**.

Pla·ci·do's disk (plä-sē′dōz) *n.* See **keratoscope**.

plac·ode (plăk′ōd′) *n.* An area of thickening in the embryonic epithelial layer from which some organ or structure later develops.

pla·fond (plə-fŏn′, plä-fôn′) *n.* An anatomical part that is farthest from the midline of the body, especially the articular surface of the distal end of the tibia.

plagio– *pref.* Slanting; inclining: *plagiocephaly.*

pla·gi·o·ceph·a·ly (plā′jē-ō-sĕf′ə-lē) *n.* An asymmetrical deformity of the skull due to premature closure of the lambdoid and coronal sutures on one side. —**pla′·gi·o·ce·phal′ic** (-sə-făl′ĭk) *adj.*

plague (plāg) *n.* **1.** A highly infectious, usually fatal, epidemic disease; a pestilence. **2.** A highly fatal infectious disease caused by the bacterium *Yersinia pestis*, transmitted primarily by the bite of a rat flea, and occurring in bubonic, pneumonic, and septicemic forms.

plague vaccine *n.* A vaccine prepared from live, killed, or attenuated *Yersinia pestis* used to immunize against bubonic plague.

plain film (plān) *n.* An x-ray taken without the use of a contrast medium.

Plan B (plăn) A trademark for a drug that contains levonorgestrel and is a morning-after pill.

Planck's constant (plăngks) *n. Symbol* **h** The constant of proportionality relating the energy of a photon to the frequency of that photon. Its value is approximately 6.626×10^{-34} joule-second.

plane (plān) *n.* **1.** A surface containing all the straight lines that connect any two points on it. **2.** A flat or level surface. **3.** An imaginary surface formed by extension through any axis of the body or through two definite points on the body.

plane joint *n.* A synovial joint in which the opposing surfaces are nearly planes and in which there is only a slight, gliding motion. Also called *arthrodia, arthrodial joint, gliding joint.*

plane of pelvic canal *n.* See **pelvic axis**.

plane suture *n.* A simple, firm apposition of two smooth surfaces of bones, with no overlap. Also called *harmonic suture.*

pla·nig·ra·phy (plə-nĭg′rə-fē) *n.* See **tomography**.

plan·ing (plā′nĭng) *n.* See **dermabrasion**.

Planned Parenthood (plănd) A service mark used for an organization that provides family planning services.

plano– *or* **plani–** *or* **plan–** *pref.* Flat: *planocellular.*

pla·no·cel·lu·lar (plā′nō-sĕl′yə-lər) *adj.* Relating to or composed of flat cells.

pla·no·con·cave (plā′nō-kŏn-kāv′, -kŏn′kāv′) *adj.* Flat on one side and concave on the other.

planoconcave lens *n.* A lens that is flat on one side and concave on the other.

pla·no·con·vex (plā′nō-kŏn-vĕks′, -kŏn′vĕks′) *n.* Flat on one side and convex on the other.

planoconvex lens *n.* A lens that is flat on one side and convex on the other.

pla·nog·ra·phy (plə-nŏg′rə-fē, plā-) *n.* See **tomography**.

pla·no·val·gus (plā′nō-văl′gəs) *n.* A condition in which the longitudinal arch of the foot is flattened and turned outward.

plan·ta (plăn′tə) *n., pl.* **–tae** (-tē) The sole.

plan·tal·gia (plăn-tăl′jə) *n.* Pain on the sole over the fascia of the plantar muscle.

plan·tar (plăn′tər, -tär′) *adj.* Of, relating to, or occurring on the sole.

plantar arch *n.* The arterial arch formed by the lateral plantar artery running across the bases of the metatarsal bones and joining the dorsal artery of the foot.

plantar artery *n.* **1.** An artery that is the larger of two branches of the posterior tibial artery, forms the plantar arch and supplies the sole and the plantar surfaces of the toes; with anastomoses to the medial plantar artery and the dorsal artery of the foot; lateral plantar artery. **2.** An artery that is a branch of the posterior tibial artery, with distribution to the medial side of the sole, and with anastomoses to the dorsal artery of the foot and the lateral plantar artery; medial plantar artery.

plantar digital artery *n.* **1.** Any of four arteries arising from a superficial plantar arch and uniting with the plantar metatarsal arteries; common plantar digital artery. **2.** Any of the arteries that are the digital branches of the plantar metatarsal arteries; proper plantar digital artery.

plantar digital vein *n.* Any of the veins that arise in the toes and pass back to form the four metatarsal veins.

plantar fasciitis *n.* Inflammation of the fascia on the plantar surface of the foot, usually at the attachment to the heel, often making it painful to walk.

plantar fibromatosis *n.* Nodular fibroblastic proliferation in the sole of one or both feet, rarely associated with contracture.

plantar interosseous muscle *n.* Any of three muscles with origin from the third, fourth, and fifth metatarsal bones, with insertion to the proximal phalanx of the same toes, with nerve supply from the lateral plantar nerve, and whose action adducts the three lateral toes.

plantar metatarsal vein *n.* Any of the veins that are formed from the plantar digital veins and empty into the medial and lateral plantar veins.

plantar muscle *n.* A muscle with origin from the femur, with insertion to the tendon and the deep fascia of the ankle, with nerve supply from the tibial nerve, and whose action causes the plantar flexion of the foot.

plantar nerve *n.* Either of two branches of the tibial nerve that innervate the foot, with the smaller lateral one supplying the deep muscles of the foot and the lateral skin of the sole and fourth and fifth toes, and the larger medial one supplying muscles on the medial aspect of the foot and the skin of the first four toes and the medial two-thirds of the sole.

plantar quadrate muscle *n.* A muscle with origin by two heads from the lateral and medial borders of the calcaneus, with insertion into the tendons of the long flexor muscle of the toes, with nerve supply from the lateral plantar nerve, and whose action assists the long flexor muscle. Also called *quadrate muscle of sole.*

plantar reflex *n.* Contraction of the toes in response to tactile stimulation of the ball of the foot.

plantar wart *n.* A wart occurring on the sole. Also called *verruca plantaris.*

plan·ti·grade (plăn′tĭ-grād′) *adj.* Walking with the entire sole on the ground, as humans do.

pla·num (plā′nəm) *n., pl.* **-na** (-nə) A plane or flat surface.

plaque (plăk) *n.* **1.** A small disk-shaped formation or growth; a patch. **2.** A deposit of fatty material on the inner lining of an arterial wall, characteristic of atherosclerosis. **3.** Dental plaque. **4.** A clear, often round patch of lysed cells in an otherwise opaque layer of a bacteria or cell culture. **5.** A scaly patch formed on the skin by psoriasis. **6.** A sharply defined zone of demyelination characteristic of multiple sclerosis.

–plasia *or* **–plasy** *suff.* Growth; development: *achondroplasia.*

plasm (plăz′əm) *n.* Germ plasm.

plasm– *pref.* Variant of **plasmo–**.

–plasm *suff.* Material forming cells or tissue: *cytoplasm.*

plas·ma (plăz′mə) *or* **plasm** (plăz′əm) *n.* **1.** The clear, yellowish fluid portion of blood, lymph, or intramuscular fluid in which cells are suspended. **2.** Cell-free, sterilized blood plasma, used in transfusions. **3.** Protoplasm or cytoplasm. —**plas·mat·ic** (plăz-măt′ĭk), **plas′mic** (-mĭk) *adj.*

plasma– *pref.* Plasma: *plasmacrit.*

plasma accelerator globulin *n.* See **factor V**.

plas·ma·blast (plăz′mə-blăst′) *n.* The stem cell of a plasma cell.

plasma cell *n.* An antibody-producing lymphocyte

derived from a B cell upon reaction with a specific antigen. Also called *plasmacyte.*

plasma cell leukemia *n.* A disease characterized by leukocytosis and other symptoms suggestive of leukemia and associated with diffuse infiltration and aggregation of plasma cells in the spleen, liver, bone marrow, and lymph nodes and by significant numbers of plasma cells in the blood.

plasma cell mastitis *n.* A condition of the breast characterized by tumorlike indurated masses containing numerous plasma cells.

plasma cell myeloma *n.* A malignant plasmacytoma of bone.

plas·ma·crit (plăz′mə-krĭt′) *n.* The percentage of the volume of blood occupied by plasma.

plasmacrit test *n.* A serologic screening method used as an aid in the diagnosis of syphilis.

plas·ma·cyte *or* **plas·mo·cyte** (plăz′mə-sīt′) *n.* See **plasma cell.**

plas·ma·cy·to·ma (plăz′mə-sī-tō′mə) *n., pl.* **–mas** *or* **–ma·ta** (-mə-tə) A discrete, usually solitary mass of neoplastic plasma cells in bone or in one of various extramedullary sites.

plas·ma·cy·to·sis (plăz′mə-sī-tō′sĭs) *n.* **1.** Plasma cells in the blood. **2.** An unusually large proportion of plasma cells in tissues or exudates.

plasma fibronectin *n.* An adhesive plasma glycoprotein that functions as an opsonin.

plas·ma·gel (plăz′mə-jĕl′) *n.* A jellylike state of cytoplasm, characteristically occurring in the pseudopod of the amoeba.

plas·ma·gene (plăz′mə-jēn′) *n.* A self-replicating hereditary structure thought to exist in cytoplasm and function in a manner analogous to, but independent of, chromosomal genes.

plas·ma·lem·ma (plăz′mə-lĕm′ə) *n.* See **cell membrane.**

plas·mal·o·gen (plăz-măl′ə-jən, -jĕn′) *n.* Any of various glycerophospholipids in which a fatty acid group is replaced by a fatty aldehyde group.

plasma membrane *n.* See **cell membrane.**

plas·ma·phe·re·sis (plăz′mə-fə-rē′sĭs, -fĕr′ə-) *n.* A process in which plasma is taken from donated blood and the remaining components, mostly red blood cells, are returned to the donor.

plas·ma·phe·ret·ic (plăz′mə-fə-rĕt′ĭk) *adj.* Relating to plasmapheresis.

plasma protein *n.* Any of the various dissolved proteins of blood plasma, including antibodies and blood-clotting proteins, that act by holding fluid in blood vessels by osmosis.

plasma renin activity *n. Abbr.* **PRA** The estimation of renin in plasma by measuring the rate of formation of angiotensin I or II.

plasma thromboplastin antecedent *n. Abbr.* **PTA** See **factor XI.**

plas·mid (plăz′mĭd) *n.* A circular, double-stranded unit of DNA that replicates within a cell independently of the chromosomal DNA and is most often found in bacteria; it is used in recombinant DNA research to transfer genes between cells. Also called *extrachromosomal element.*

plas·min (plăz′mĭn) *n.* An enzyme that hydrolyzes peptides and esters of arginine and histidine and converts fibrin to soluble products. Also called *fibrinase, fibrinolysin.*

plas·min·o·gen (plăz-mĭn′ə-jən) *n.* The inactive precursor to plasmin that is found in body fluids and blood plasma. Also called *profibrinolysin.*

plasminogen activator *n.* See **urokinase.**

plasmo– *or* **plasm–** *pref.* Plasma: *plasmin.*

plas·mo·cyte (plăz′mə-sīt′) *n.* Variant of **plasmacyte.**

plas·mo·di·al (plăz-mō′dē-əl) *adj.* Relating to a plasmodium or a species of the genus *Plasmodium.*

plas·mo·di·um (plăz-mō′dē-əm) *n., pl.* **–di·a** (-dē-ə) **1.** A multinucleate mass of cytoplasm formed by the aggregation of a number of amoeboid cells, as that characteristic of the vegetative phase of the slime molds. **2.** A protozoan of the genus *Plasmodium,* which includes the parasites that cause malaria.

Plasmodium *n.* A genus of protozoans that are parasites of the red blood cells of vertebrates and include the causative agents of malaria.

Plasmodium fal·cip·a·rum (făl-sĭp′ə-rəm) *n.* A protozoan that causes falciparum malaria.

Plasmodium ma·lar·i·ae (mə-lâr′ē-ē) *n.* A protozoan that causes quartan malaria.

Plasmodium o·va·le (ō-vā′lē) *n.* A protozoan that is the agent of the least common form of human malaria, which is characterized by fimbriated red blood cells that often have an oval shape.

Plasmodium vi·vax (vī′văks′) *n.* A protozoan that is the most common malarial parasite of humans, causing vivax malaria.

plas·mog·a·my (plăz-mŏg′ə-mē) *n.* Fusion of two or more cells or protoplasts without fusion of the nuclei, as occurs in higher terrestrial fungi.

plas·mol·y·sis (plăz-mŏl′ĭ-sĭs) *n., pl.* **–ses** (-sēz′) Shrinkage or contraction of the protoplasm away from the wall of a living plant or bacterial cell, caused by loss of water through osmosis. —**plas′mo·lyt′ic** (plăz′mə-lĭt′ĭk) *adj.*

plas·mo·lyze (plăz′mə-līz′) *v.* To subject to or undergo plasmolysis.

plas·mon (plăz′mŏn′) *n.* The aggregate of cytoplasmic or extranuclear genetic material in an organism.

plas·mor·rhex·is (plăz′mə-rĕk′sĭs) *n.* The splitting open of a cell from pressure of the protoplasm.

plas·mos·chi·sis (plăz-mŏs′kĭ-sĭs) *n.* The splitting of protoplasm into fragments.

plas·mo·trop·ic (plăz′mə-trŏp′ĭk, -trō′pĭk) *adj.* Relating to or manifesting plasmotropism.

plas·mot·ro·pism (plăz-mŏt′rə-pĭz′əm) *n.* A condition in which the bone marrow, spleen, and liver contain strongly hemolytic bodies that cause the destruction of the red blood cells, which are not affected while in the blood.

plas·ter (plăs′tər) *n.* **1.** Plaster of Paris. **2.** A pastelike mixture applied to a part of the body for healing or cosmetic purposes.

plaster bandage *n.* A roller bandage impregnated with plaster of Paris and applied moist to make a rigid dressing for a fracture or diseased joint.

plaster cast *n.* See **cast** (sense 2).

plaster of Par·is (păr′ĭs) *n.* Any of a group of gypsum cements, essentially hemihydrated calcium sulfate, a white powder that forms a paste when mixed with water and hardens into a solid, used in making casts and molds.

plas·tic (plăs′tĭk) *adj.* **1.** Capable of being shaped or formed. **2.** Easily influenced; impressionable. **3.** Capable of building tissue; formative. —*n.* Any of various organic compounds produced by polymerization, capable of being molded, extruded, cast into various shapes and films, or drawn into filaments used as textile fibers. —**plas·tic′i·ty** (plăs-tĭs′ĭ-tē) *n.*

–plastic *suff.* Forming; growing; changing; developing: *neoplastic.*

plas·tic·i·ty (plăs-tĭs′ĭ-tē) *n.* The ability to change and adapt, especially the ability of the central nervous system to acquire alternative pathways for sensory perception or motor skills.

plastic lymph *n.* See **inflammatory lymph.**

plastic pleurisy *n.* See **dry pleurisy.**

plastic surgery *n.* Surgery to remodel, repair, or restore body parts, especially by the transfer of tissue.

plas·tid (plăs′tĭd) *n.* **1.** Any of several pigmented cytoplasmic organelles found in plant cells and other organisms, having various physiological functions, such as the synthesis and storage of food. Also called *trophoplast.* **2.** One of the granules of foreign or differentiated matter, food particles, or waste material in cells.

–plasty *suff.* Molding or forming surgically; plastic surgery: *dermatoplasty.*

–plasy *suff.* Variant of **–plasia.**

plate (plāt) *n.* **1.** A smooth, flat, relatively thin, rigid body of uniform thickness. **2.** A thin flat layer, part, or structure. **3.** A thin metallic or plastic support fitted to the gums to anchor artificial teeth. **4.** A metal bar applied to a fractured bone in order to maintain the ends in apposition. **5.** The agar layer within a Petri dish or similar vessel. **6.** A sheet of glass or metal that is light-sensitive and on which a photographic image can be recorded. —*v.* To form a very thin layer of a bacterial culture by streaking it on the surface of agar to isolate individual organisms from which a colonial clone will develop.

pla·teau pulse (plă-tō′) *n.* The slow, sustained pulse of aortic stenosis, producing a prolonged flat-topped curve in the sphygmogram.

plate culture *n.* A culture or culture medium contained in a flat transparent dish and used chiefly for growing microorganisms.

plate·let (plāt′lĭt) *n.* A minute, irregularly shaped, disklike cytoplasmic body found in blood plasma that promotes blood clotting and has no definite nucleus, no DNA, and no hemoglobin. Also called *blood platelet, thrombocyte.*

platelet-aggregating factor *n. Abbr.* **PAF** A substance released from rabbit basophilic white blood cells that causes aggregation of platelets and is involved in the deposition of immune complexes. Also called *platelet-activating factor.*

platelet aggregation test *n.* A test of the ability of platelets to adhere to one another and form a hemostatic plug.

platelet-derived growth factor *n.* A substance in platelets that is mitogenic for cells at the site of a wound, causing endothelial proliferation.

platelet factor 3 *n.* A phospholipid lipoprotein blood coagulation factor derived from platelets that acts with certain plasma thromboplastin factors to convert prothrombin to thrombin.

plate·let·phe·re·sis (plāt′lĭt-fə-rē′sĭs, -fĕr′ə-) *n.* A process in which platelets are removed from donated blood and the remaining components are returned to the donor.

platelet tissue factor *n.* See **thromboplastin.**

Plat·i·nol (plăt′ə-nôl′, -nŏl′) A trademark for the drug cisplatin.

plat·i·num (plăt′n-əm) *n. Symbol* **Pt** A ductile malleable metallic element usually occurring mixed with other metals such as iridium, osmium, or nickel and used as a catalyst and in dentistry. Atomic number 78.

platy– *pref.* Flat: *platyhelminth.*

plat·y·ba·sia (plăt′ĭ-bā′zhə) *n.* A developmental anomaly of the skull in which the base of the posterior cranial fossa bulges upward.

plat·y·ceph·a·ly (plăt′ĭ-sĕf′ə-lē) *n.* Flatness of the skull in which the vertical cranial index is below 70.

plat·y·hel·minth (plăt′ĭ-hĕl′mĭnth) *n.* See **flatworm.**

Plat·y·hel·min·thes (plăt′ĭ-hĕl-mĭn′thēz) *n.* A phylum of flatworms having a flat, bilaterally symmetric body and no body cavity and including the tapeworms and flukes.

plat·y·pel·lic pelvis (plăt′ĭ-pĕl′ĭk) *n.* A flat oval pelvis in which the transverse diameter is longer than the anteroposterior diameter.

pla·typ·ne·a (plă-tĭp′nē-ə) *n.* Difficulty in breathing when erect, relieved by lying down.

pla·tys·ma (plə-tĭz′mə) *n., pl.* **–mas** *or* **–ma·ta** (-mə-tə) A platelike muscle in the neck extending to the lower face with origin from the subcutaneous layer and fascia covering the greater pectoral and deltoid muscles at the level of the first or second rib, with insertion to the mandible, the risorius muscle and platysma of the opposite side, with nerve supply from a branch of the facial nerve, and whose action depresses the lower lip and wrinkles the skin of the neck and the upper chest.

plat·y·spon·dyl·i·a (plăt′ĭ-spŏn-dĭl′ē-ə) *or* **plat·y·spon·dyl·i·sis** (-dĭl′ĭ-sĭs) *n.* Flatness of the vertebral bodies.

play therapy (plā) *n.* A form of psychotherapy used with children to help them express or act out their experiences, feelings, and problems by playing with dolls, toys, and other play material, under the guidance or observation of a therapist.

pleas·ure principle (plĕzh′ər) *n.* In psychoanalysis, the tendency or drive to achieve pleasure and avoid pain as the chief motivating force in behavior. Also called *pain-pleasure principle.*

pled·get (plĕj′ĭt) *n.* A small, flat absorbent pad used to medicate, drain, or protect a wound or sore.

–plegia *suff.* Paralysis: *monoplegia.*

pleiotropic gene *n.* A gene that causes a number of distinct but seemingly unrelated phenotypic effects. Also called *polyphenic gene.*

plei·ot·ro·pism (plī-ŏt′rə-pĭz′əm) *or* **plei·ot·ro·py** (-pē) *n.* The control by a single gene of several distinct and seemingly unrelated phenotypic effects. —**plei′o·trop′ic** (plī′ə-trŏp′ĭk, -trō′pĭk) *adj.*

pleo– *or* **pleio–** *pref.* More: *pleocytosis.*

ple·o·cy·to·sis (plē′ō-sī-tō′sĭs) *n.* The presence of a greater number of cells than normal, as in the cerebrospinal fluid.

ple·o·mas·ti·a (plē′ə-măs′tē-ə) *n.* See **polymastia.**

pleomorphic lipoma *n.* See **atypical lipoma.**

ple·o·mor·phism (plē′ə-môr′fĭz′əm) *n.* **1.** See **polymorphism. 2.** The occurrence of two or more structural forms during a life cycle, especially of certain plants. —**ple′o·mor′phic** (-fĭk), **ple′o·mor′phous** (-fəs) *adj.*

ple·o·nasm (plē′ə-năz′əm) *n.* An excess in the number or size of parts.

ple·on·os·te·o·sis (plē′ŏn-ŏs′tē-ō′sĭs) *n.* Excessive ossification of bone.

ple·ro·cer·coid (plîr′ō-sûr′koid′) *n.* The infective larva of some tapeworms, characterized by its solid elongated body.

ples·sim·e·ter (plĕ-sĭm′ĭ-tər) *n.* Variant of **pleximeter.**

ples·sor (plĕs′ər) *n.* Variant of **plexor.**

pleth·o·ra (plĕth′ər-ə) *n.* **1.** An excess of blood in the circulatory system or in one organ or area. **2.** An excess of any of the body fluids. —**ple·thor′ic** (plĕ-thôr′ĭk) *adj.*

ple·thys·mo·gram (plĕ-thĭz′mə-grăm′) *n.* A record or tracing produced by a plethysmograph.

ple·thys·mo·graph (plĕ-thĭz′mə-grăf′) *n.* An instrument that measures variations in the size of an organ or body part on the basis of the amount of blood passing through or present in the part. —**ple·thys′mo·graph′ic** *adj.*

pleth·ys·mom·e·try (plĕth′ĭz-mŏm′ĭ-trē) *n.* Measurement of the fullness of a hollow organ.

pleur– *pref.* Variant of **pleuro–.**

pleu·ra (ploŏr′ə) *n., pl.* **pleu·rae** (ploŏr′ē) The thin serous membrane that envelops each lung and folds back to make a lining for the chest cavity. —**pleu′ral** *adj.*

pleural cavity *n.* The potential space between the parietal and visceral layers of the pleura. Also called *pleural space.*

pleural effusion *n.* An exudate of fluid into the pleural cavity.

pleural fluid *n.* The thin film of serous fluid between the visceral and parietal pleurae.

pleural fremitus *n.* The vibration in the chest wall produced by the rubbing together of the roughened opposing surfaces of the pleura.

pleu·ral·gia (ploŏ-răl′jə) *n.* See **pleurodynia** (sense 2).

pleural ring *n.* See **annular ring.**

pleural space *n.* See **pleural cavity.**

pleu·ra·poph·y·sis (ploŏr′ə-pŏf′ĭ-sĭs) *n.* A rib or corresponding process on a cervical or lumbar vertebra.

pleu·rec·to·my (ploŏ-rĕk′tə-mē) *n.* Excision of the pleura.

pleu·ri·sy (ploŏr′ĭ-sē) *n.* An inflammation of the pleura, usually occurring because of complications of a disease such as pneumonia, and accompanied by accumulation of fluid in the pleural cavity, chills, fever, and painful breathing and coughing. Also called *pleuritis.*

pleu·rit·ic (plo͞o-rĭt′ĭk) *adj.* Of or relating to pleurisy.

pleuritic rub *n.* A sound heard on auscultation that is produced by the rubbing together of the roughened surfaces of the costal and visceral pleurae.

pleu·ri·tis (plo͞o-rī′tĭs) *n.* See **pleurisy.**

pleuro– *or* **pleur–** *pref.* 1. Side; lateral: *pleurocentrum.* 2. Pleura; pleural: *pleurotomy.*

pleu·ro·cele (plo͞or′ə-sēl′) *n.* See **pneumonocele.**

pleu·ro·cen·te·sis (plo͞or′ō-sĕn-tē′sĭs) *n.* See **thoracentesis.**

pleu·ro·cen·trum (plo͞or′ə-sĕn′trəm) *n.* One of the lateral halves of the body of a vertebra.

pleu·roc·ly·sis (plo͞o-rŏk′lĭ-sĭs) *n.* Washing out of the pleural cavity.

pleu·rod·e·sis (plo͞o-rŏd′ĭ-sĭs) *n.* The surgical creation of a fibrous adhesion between the visceral and parietal layers of the pleura, thus obliterating the pleural cavity.

pleu·ro·dyn·i·a (plo͞or′ə-dĭn′ē-ə) *n.* 1. Pleuritic pain in the chest. 2. Paroxysmal pain and soreness of the muscles between the ribs, usually due to muscular rheumatism. Also called *pleuralgia.* 3. Epidemic pleurodynia.

pleu·ro·e·soph·a·ge·al muscle (plo͞or′ō-ĭ-sŏf′ə-jē′əl) *n.* Any of the muscular fasciculi that arise from the mediastinal pleura and reinforce the musculature of the esophagus.

pleu·ro·gen·ic (plo͞or′ə-jĕn′ĭk) *or* **pleu·rog·e·nous** (plo͞o-rŏj′ə-nəs) *adj.* Of pleural origin; beginning in the pleura.

pleu·rog·ra·phy (plo͞o-rŏg′rə-fē) *n.* Radiography of the pleural cavity.

pleu·ro·hep·a·ti·tis (plo͞or′ō-hĕp′ə-tī′tĭs) *n.* Hepatitis with extension of the inflammation to the neighboring portion of the pleura.

pleu·ro·lith (plo͞or′ə-lĭth′) *n.* A concretion in the pleural cavity.

pleu·rol·y·sis (plo͞o-rŏl′ĭ-sĭs) *n.* Surgical division of pleural adhesions.

pleu·ro·per·i·car·di·al (plo͞or′ō-pĕr′ĭ-kär′dē-əl) *adj.* Relating to the pleura and the pericardium.

pleu·ro·per·i·car·di·tis (plo͞or′ō-pĕr′ĭ-kär-dī′tĭs) *n.* Inflammation of the pericardium and the pleura.

pleu·ro·per·i·to·ne·al (plo͞or′ō-pĕr′ĭ-tn-ē′əl) *adj.* Relating to the pleura and the peritoneum.

pleu·ro·pneu·mo·nia (plo͞or′ō-no͞o-mōn′yə) *n.* Inflammation of the pleura and lungs; pneumonia aggravated by pleurisy.

pleu·ro·pneu·mon·ia·like organism (plo͞or′ō-no͞o-mōn′yə-līk) *n. Abbr.* **PPLO** See **mycoplasma.**

pleu·ro·pul·mo·nar·y (plo͞or′ō-po͞ol′mə-nĕr′ē, -pŭl′-) *adj.* Relating to the pleura and the lungs.

pleu·rot·o·my (plo͞o-rŏt′ə-mē) *n.* See **thoracotomy.**

pleu·ro·vis·cer·al (plo͞or′ō-vĭs′ər-əl) *adj.* Visceropleural.

plex·al (plĕk′səl) *adj.* Relating to a plexus.

plex·ec·to·my (plĕk-sĕk′tə-mē) *n.* The excision of a plexus.

plex·i·form (plĕk′sə-fôrm′) *adj.* Resembling or forming a plexus; weblike.

plexiform neurofibroma *n.* A neurofibroma in which Schwann cells proliferate inside the nerve sheath, producing an irregularly thickened, distorted, tortuous structure. Also called *plexiform neuroma.*

plex·im·e·ter (plĕk-sĭm′ĭ-tər) *or* **ples·sim·e·ter** (plĕ-sĭm′-) *or* **plex·om·e·ter** (plĕk-sŏm′-) *n.* A small thin plate held against the body and struck with a plexor in diagnosis by percussion.

plex·i·tis (plĕk-sī′tĭs) *n.* Inflammation of a plexus.

plex·o·gen·ic (plĕk′sə-jĕn′ĭk) *adj.* Giving rise to weblike or plexiform structures.

plex·or (plĕk′sər) *or* **ples·sor** (plĕs′ər) *n.* A small, usually rubber-headed hammer used alone or with a pleximeter in examination or diagnosis by percussion. Also called *percussor.*

plex·us (plĕk′səs) *n., pl.* **plexus** *or* **–us·es** 1. A structure in the form of a network, especially of nerves, blood vessels, or lymphatics. 2. A combination of interlaced parts; a network.

plexus thyroideus impar *n.* A venous plexus located in front of the lower portion of the trachea, forms from anastomoses between the inferior thyroid veins, and terminates in the inferior thyroid vein.

pli·ca (plī′kə) *n., pl.* **–cae** (-kē) 1. A fold or ridge, as of skin or membrane. 2. See **false membrane.** —**pli′cal** *adj.*

pli·cate (plī′kāt′) *or* **pli·cat·ed** (-kā′tĭd) *adj.* Arranged in folds like those of a fan; pleated.

pli·ca·tion (plī-kā′shən) *n.* 1. An operation for reducing the size of a hollow structure by taking folds or tucks in its walls. 2. The state of being folded.

pli·cot·o·my (plī-kŏt′ə-mē) *n.* Surgical division of the posterior fold of the tympanic membrane.

–ploid *suff.* Having or being a number of chromosomes that has a specified relationship to, or is a multiple of, the basic number of chromosomes of a group: *heteroploid.*

ploi·dy (ploi′dē) *n.* A multiple of the basic number of chromosomes in a cell.

plom·bage (pləm-bäzh′, plôm-) *n.* The use of an inert material to fill an abnormal cavity in the body.

PLSS *abbr.* portable life-support system

plug (plŭg) *n.* A dense mass of material filling a hole or closing an orifice. —*v.* To fill tightly with a plug.

plug·ger (plŭg′ər) *n.* A dental instrument used for condensing material in a cavity. Also called *packer.*

plum·bic (plŭm′bĭk) *adj.* Of, relating to, or containing lead, especially with a valence of four.

plum·bism (plŭm′bĭz′əm) *n.* Chronic lead poisoning.

plum·bum (plŭm′bəm) *n.* The metallic element lead.

Plum·mer-Vin·son syndrome (plŭm′ər-vĭn′sən) *n.* Difficulty in swallowing caused by degeneration of the muscle of the esophagus, atrophy of the papillae of the tongue, and hypochromic anemia.

pluri– *pref.* More than one; several: *pluriglandular.*

plu·ri·glan·du·lar (plo͞or′ĭ-glăn′jə-lər) *adj.* Of or relating to several glands or their secretions.

plu·rip·o·tent (plo͞o-rĭp′ə-tənt) *or* **plu·ri·po·ten·tial** (plo͞or′ĭ-pə-tĕn′shəl) *adj.* 1. Capable of affecting more than one organ or tissue. 2. Not fixed as to potential development. Used of an embryonic cell.

plus cyclophoria (plŭs) *n.* See **excyclophoria.**

plu·to·ni·um (plo͞o-tō′nē-əm) *n. Symbol* **Pu** A naturally radioactive, metallic transuranic element, occurring in uranium ores or produced artificially by neutron bombardment of uranium, used in radionuclide batteries in pacemakers. Its longest-lived isotope is Pu 244 with a half-life of 77 million years. Atomic number 94.

pm *abbr.* picometer

Pm The symbol for the element **promethium**.

PM *abbr.* postmortem

PMDD *abbr.* premenstrual dysphoric disorder

PMH *abbr.* past medical history

P-mi·tra·le (-mī-trā′lē) *n.* An electrocardiographic syndrome consisting of broad, notched P waves in many leads with a prominent late negative component to the P wave.

PMN *abbr.* polymorphonuclear leukocyte

PMS *abbr.* premenstrual syndrome

PND *abbr.* paroxysmal nocturnal dyspnea

–pnea *suff.* Breath; respiration: *dyspnea.*

pneum– *pref.* Variant of **pneumo–**.

pneu·mar·thro·gram (nōō-mär′thrə-grăm′) *n.* A radiograph produced by pneumarthrography.

pneu·mar·throg·ra·phy (nōō′mär-thrŏg′rə-fē) *or* **pneu·mo·ar·throg·ra·phy** (nōō′mō-är-) *n.* Radiographic examination of a joint following the introduction of air, with or without another contrast medium.

pneu·mar·thro·sis (nōō′mär-thrō′sĭs) *n.* The presence of air in a joint.

pneu·mat·ic (nōō-măt′ĭk) *adj.* **1.** Of or relating to air or other gases. **2.** Relating to respiration. **3.** Relating to a structure that is filled with air.

pneumatic bone *n.* A bone that is hollow or contains many air cells, such as the mastoid process of the temporal bone. Also called *hollow bone.*

pneu·ma·ti·za·tion (nōō′mə-tĭ-zā′shən) *n.* The development of air cells or cavities, such as those of the mastoid and ethmoidal bones.

pneumato– *or* **pneumat–** *pref.* **1.** Air; gas: *pneumatocardia.* **2.** Breath; respiration: *pneumatograph.*

pneu·ma·to·car·di·a (nōō′mə-tō-kär′dē-ə) *n.* Air bubbles or gas in the blood of the heart.

pneu·ma·to·cele (nōō′mə-tō-sēl′, nōō-măt′ə-) *n.* **1.** A emphysematous or gaseous swelling. **2.** See **pneumonocele**. **3.** A thin-walled cavity formed within the lung, characteristic of staphylococcus pneumonia.

pneu·ma·tom·e·ter (nōō′mə-tŏm′ĭ-tər) *n.* An instrument for measuring the force or volume of inspiration or expiration in the lungs.

pneu·ma·tor·rha·chis (nōō′mə-tôr′ə-kĭs) *n.* See **pneumorrhachis**.

pneu·ma·to·sis (nōō′mə-tō′sĭs) *n.* Abnormal accumulation of gas in any tissue or other part of the body.

pneumatosis cys·toi·des in·tes·ti·na·lis (sĭ-stoi′dēz ĭn-tĕs′tə-nā′lĭs) *n.* See **intestinal emphysema**.

pneu·ma·tu·ri·a (nōō′mə-tŏŏr′ē-ə) *n.* Passage of gas or air from the urethra during or after urination.

pneu·mec·to·my (nōō-mĕk′tə-mē) *n.* Variant of **pneumonectomy**.

pneumo– *or* **pneum–** *pref.* **1.** Air; gas: *pneumothorax.* **2.** Pulmonary: *pneumoconiosis.* **3.** Respiration: *pneumograph.* **4.** Pneumonia: *pneumococcus.*

pneu·mo·an·gi·og·ra·phy (nōō′mō-ăn′jē-ŏg′rə-fē) *n.* The radiographic study of the pulmonary and the bronchial blood vessels.

pneu·mo·ar·throg·ra·phy (nōō′mō-är-thrŏg′rə-fē) *n.* Variant of **pneumarthrography**.

pneu·mo·ba·cil·lus (nōō′mō-bə-sĭl′əs) *n.*, *pl.* **-cil·li** (-sĭl′ī′) A nonmotile, gram-negative bacterium *(Klebsiella pneumoniae)* that causes a severe form of pneumonia and is associated with other respiratory infections.

pneu·mo·car·di·al (nōō′mə-kär′dē-əl) *adj.* Cardiopulmonary.

pneu·mo·cele (nōō′mə-sēl′) *n.* See **pneumonocele**.

pneu·mo·cen·te·sis (nōō′mō-sĕn-tē′sĭs) *n.* Variant of **pneumonocentesis**.

pneu·mo·ceph·a·lus (nōō′mō-sĕf′ə-ləs) *n.* The presence of air or gas within the cranial cavity.

pneu·mo·coc·cal vaccine (nōō′mə-kŏk′əl) *n.* A vaccine that contains purified capsular polysaccharide antigen from the most common infectious types of *Streptococcus pneumoniae,* used to immunize against pneumonococcal disease.

pneu·mo·coc·ce·mi·a (nōō′mō-kŏk-sē′mē-ə) *n.* The presence of pneumococci in the blood.

pneu·mo·coc·ci·dal (nōō′mə-kŏk-sīd′l) *adj.* Destructive to pneumococci.

pneu·mo·coc·co·sis (nōō′mə-kŏ-kō′sĭs) *n.* Infection with pneumococci.

pneu·mo·coc·co·su·ri·a (nōō′mə-kŏk′ə-sōōr′ē-ə) *n.* The presence of pneumococci or of their capsular substance in the urine.

pneu·mo·coc·cus (nōō′mə-kŏk′əs) *n.*, *pl.* **-coc·ci** (-kŏk′sī′, -kŏk′ī′) A nonmotile, gram-positive bacterium *(Streptococcus pneumoniae)* that is the most common cause of bacterial pneumonia and is associated with meningitis and other infectious diseases. —**pneu′mo·coc′cal** (-kŏk′əl) *adj.*

pneu·mo·co·ni·o·sis (nōō′mō-kō′nē-ō′sĭs) *n.*, *pl.* **-ses** (-sēz) A disease of the lungs, such as asbestosis or silicosis, caused by long-term inhalation of particulate matter, especially mineral or metallic dust.

pneu·mo·cra·ni·um (nōō′mō-krā′nē-əm) *n.* The presence of air between the cranium and the dura mater.

pneu·mo·cys·tis (nōō′mə-sĭs′tĭs) *n.* A pneumonia caused by the parasitic protozoan *Pneumocystis carinii* and affecting primarily individuals with an immunodeficiency disease, such as AIDS.

Pneumocystis ca·ri·ni·i (kə-rī′nē-ī′) *n.* A parasite transitional between a fungus and protozoan, frequently occurring as aggregate forms existing within rounded cystlike structures. It is the causative agent of pneumocystosis.

pneu·mo·cys·tog·ra·phy (nōō′mō-sĭ-stŏg′rə-fē) *n.* Radiography of the bladder following the injection of air.

pneu·mo·cys·to·sis (nōō′mō-sĭ-stō′sĭs) *n.* Pneumonia that results from infection with *Pneumocystis carinii,* occurs frequently among immunologically compromised individuals, and is characterized by alveoli filled with a network of acidophilic material that enmeshes the organisms. Also called *interstitial plasma cell pneumonia.*

pneu·mo·der·ma (nōō′mə-dûr′mə) *n.* See **subcutaneous emphysema**.

pneu·mo·dy·nam·ics (nōō′mō-dī-năm′ĭks) *n.* The mechanics of respiration.

pneu·mo·en·ceph·a·log·ra·phy (nōō′mō-ĕn-sĕf′ə-lŏg′rə-fē) *n.* Radiographic visualization of the cerebral ventricles and subarachnoid spaces after the injection of air or gas. —**pneu′mo·en·ceph′a·lo·gram′** (-ə-lə-grăm′, -ə-lō-) *n.*

pneu·mo·gas·tric (nōō′mō-găs′trĭk) *adj.* Relating to the lungs and the stomach.

pneumogastric nerve *n.* See **vagus nerve.**

pneu·mo·gram (nōō′mə-grăm′) *n.* A radiograph of an organ inflated with air.

pneu·mog·ra·phy (nōō-mŏg′rə-fē) *n.* Radiography of the lungs. —**pneu′mo·graph′** (nōō′mə-grăf′), **pneu·mat′o·graph′** (nōō-măt′ə-grăf′) *n.*

pneu·mo·he·mo·per·i·car·di·um (nōō′mō-hē′mō-pĕr′ĭ-kär′dē-əm) *n.* See **hemopneumopericardium.**

pneu·mo·he·mo·tho·rax (nōō′mō-hē′mə-thôr′ăks′) *n.* See **hemopneumothorax.**

pneu·mo·hy·dro·me·tra (nōō′mō-hī′drō-mē′trə) *n.* The presence of gas and serum in the uterine cavity.

pneu·mo·hy·dro·per·i·car·di·um (nōō′mō-hī′drō-pĕr′ĭ-kär′dē-əm) *n.* See **hydropneumopericardium.**

pneu·mo·hy·dro·per·i·to·ne·um (nōō′mō-hī′drō-pĕr′ĭ-tn-ē′əm) *n.* See **hydropneumoperitoneum.**

pneu·mo·hy·dro·tho·rax (nōō′mō-hī′drə-thôr′ăks′) *n.* See **hydropneumothorax.**

pneu·mo·lith (nōō′mə-lĭth′) *n.* A calculus in the lung.

pneu·mo·li·thi·a·sis (nōō′mō-lĭ-thī′ə-sĭs) *n.* The formation of calculi in the lungs.

pneu·mo·me·di·as·ti·num (nōō′mō-mē′dē-ə-stī′-nəm) *n.* The escape of air into the mediastinal tissues, usually from interstitial emphysema or from a ruptured pulmonary bleb.

pneu·mo·my·e·log·ra·phy (nōō′mō-mī′ə-lŏg′rə-fē) *n.* Radiographic examination of the spinal canal after the injection of air or gas.

pneu·mo·nec·to·my (nōō′mə-nĕk′tə-mē) *or* **pneu·mec·to·my** (nōō-mĕk′tə-mē) *n.* Surgical removal of all or part of a lung.

pneu·mo·nia (nōō-mōn′yə) *n.* An acute or chronic disease marked by inflammation of the lungs and caused by viruses, bacteria, or other microorganisms and sometimes by physical and chemical irritants.

pneu·mon·ic (nōō-mŏn′ĭk) *adj.* **1.** Relating to, affected by, or similar to pneumonia. **2.** Of, affecting, or relating to the lungs; pulmonary.

pneumonic plague *n.* A frequently fatal form of bubonic plague in which the lungs are infected and the disease is transmissible by coughing.

pneu·mo·ni·tis (nōō′mə-nī′tĭs) *n.* Inflammation of lung tissue. Also called *pulmonitis.*

pneumono– *or* **pneumon–** *pref.* Lung; pulmonary: *pneumonotomy.*

pneu·mo·no·cele (nōō′mə-nō-sēl′, nōō-mŏn′ə-) *n.* Protrusion of a portion of the lung through a defect in the chest wall. Also called *pleurocele, pneumatocele, pneumocele.*

pneu·mo·no·cen·te·sis (nōō′mə-nō-sĕn-tē′sĭs) *or* **pneu·mo·cen·te·sis** (nōō′mō-) *n.* Paracentesis of the lung.

pneu·mo·no·coc·cal (nōō′mə-nō-kŏk′əl) *adj.* Relating to or associated with *Streptococcus pneumoniae.*

pneu·mo·no·cyte (nōō′mə-nō-sīt′, nōō-mŏn′ə-) *n.* Any of the cells lining the alveoli in the respiratory part of the lung.

pneu·mo·no·pex·y (nōō′mə-nō-pĕk′sē, nōō-mō′nə-) *n.* Surgical fixation of the lung by suturing the costal and pulmonary pleurae or by causing their adhesion.

pneu·mo·nor·rha·phy (nōō′mə-nôr′ə-fē) *n.* Suture of the lung.

pneu·mo·not·o·my (nōō′mə-nŏt′ə-mē) *n.* Incision of the lung. Also called *pneumotomy.*

pneu·mo·or·bi·tog·ra·phy (nōō′mō-ôr′bĭ-tŏg′rə-fē) *n.* Radiographic visualization of the eye socket after the injection of a gas.

pneu·mo·per·i·car·di·um (nōō′mō-pĕr′ĭ-kär′dē-əm) *n.* The presence of gas in the pericardial sac.

pneu·mo·per·i·to·ne·um (nōō′mō-pĕr′ĭ-tn-ē′əm) *n.* The presence of air or gas in the peritoneal cavity as a result of disease or for the treatment of certain conditions.

pneu·mo·per·i·to·ni·tis (nōō′mō-pĕr′ĭ-tn-ī′tĭs) *n.* Inflammation of the peritoneum, with an accumulation of gas in the peritoneal cavity.

pneu·mo·pleu·ri·tis (nōō′mō-plŏo-rī′tĭs) *n.* Pleurisy with the presence of air or gas in the pleural cavity.

pneu·mo·py·e·log·ra·phy (nōō′mō-pī′ə-lŏg′rə-fē) *n.* Radiographic examination of the kidney after a gas has been injected into the kidney pelvis.

pneu·mo·py·o·tho·rax (nōō′mō-pī′ə-thôr′ăks′) *n.* See **pyopneumothorax.**

pneu·mo·ra·di·og·ra·phy (nōō′mō-rā′dē-ŏg′rə-fē) *n.* Radiographic study of an organ or part after air has been injected into it.

pneu·mo·ret·ro·per·i·to·ne·um (nōō′mō-rĕt′rō-pĕr′-ĭ-tn-ē′əm) *n.* Escape of air into the retroperitoneal tissues.

pneu·mor·rha·chis (nōō′mə-rā′kĭs, nōō-môr′ə-kĭs) *n.* The presence of gas in the spinal canal. Also called *pneumatorrhachis.*

pneu·mo·tach·o·gram (nōō′mə-tăk′ə-grăm′) *n.* A record produced by a pneumotachograph.

pneu·mo·tach·o·graph (nōō′mə-tăk′ə-grăf′) *n.* An apparatus for recording the rate of airflow to and from the lungs. Also called *pneumotachometer.*

pneu·mo·tho·rax (nōō′mō-thôr′ăks′) *n.* Accumulation of air or gas in the pleural cavity, occurring as a result of disease or injury or as a treatment of tuberculosis and other lung diseases.

pneu·mot·o·my (nōō-mŏt′ə-mē) *n.* See **pneumono·tomy.**

PNPB *abbr.* positive-negative pressure breathing

Po The symbol for the element **polonium.**

PO *abbr. Latin* per os (by mouth)

pock (pŏk) *n.* **1.** The characteristic pustular cutaneous lesion of smallpox. **2.** A pockmark.

pock·et (pŏk′ĭt) *n.* **1.** In anatomy, a cul-de-sac or pouchlike cavity. **2.** A diseased space between the inflamed gum and the surface of a tooth. **3.** A collection of pus in a nearly closed sac. —*v.* **1.** To enclose within a confined space. **2.** To approach the surface at a localized spot, as with the thinned-out wall of an abscess which is about to rupture.

pock·et·ed calculus (pŏk′ĭ-tĭd) *n*. See **encysted calculus**.

pock·mark (pŏk′märk′) *n*. A pitlike scar that is left on the skin by smallpox or another eruptive disease. —**pock′marked′** *adj*.

po·dag·ra (pə-dăg′rə) *n*. Gout, especially of the big toe. —**po·dag′ral, po·dag′ric** *adj*.

po·dal·gia (pō-dăl′jə) *n*. Pain in the foot. Also called *pododynia, tarsalgia*.

po·dal·ic (pō-dăl′ĭk) *adj*. Of or relating to the foot.

podalic version *n*. Version resulting in delivery of the fetus by the feet.

pod·ar·thri·tis (pŏd′är-thrī′tĭs) *n*. Inflammation of any of the tarsal or metatarsal joints.

pod·e·de·ma (pŏd′ĭ-dē′mə) *n*. Edema of the feet and ankles.

podiatric medicine *n*. See **podiatry**.

po·di·a·try (pə-dī′ə-trē) *n*. The branch of medicine concerned with the diagnosis and medical, surgical, mechanical, physical, and adjunctive treatment of the diseases, injuries, and defects of the foot. Also called *chiropody, podiatric medicine*. —**po′di·at′ric** (pō′dē-ăt′-rĭk) *adj*. —**po·di′a·trist** *n*.

podo– *or* **pod–** *pref*. Foot; foot-shaped: *pododynia*.

pod·o·cyte (pŏd′ə-sīt′) *n*. An epithelial cell of the renal glomerulus, attached to the outer surface of the glomerular capillary basement membrane by cytoplasmic foot processes.

pod·o·dy·na·mom·e·ter (pŏd′ō-dī′nə-mŏm′ĭ-tər) *n*. An instrument for measuring the strength of the muscles of the foot or leg.

pod·o·dyn·i·a (pŏd′ə-dĭn′ē-ə) *n*. See **podalgia**.

pod·o·gram (pŏd′ə-grăm′) *n*. An imprint or outline tracing of the sole.

pod·o·mech·a·no·ther·a·py (pŏd′ō-mĕk′ə-nō-thĕr′ə-pē) *n*. The treatment of foot conditions with mechanical devices such as arch supports.

pod·o·phyl·lin (pŏd′ə-fĭl′ĭn) *n*. A bitter-tasting resin obtained from the dried root of the May apple and used in medicine as a cathartic and caustic.

pod·o·phyl·lo·tox·in (pŏd′ə-fĭl′ə-tŏk′sĭn) *n*. A toxic polycyclic substance having cathartic properties and antineoplastic activity.

POEMS syndrome (pō′əmz) *n*. A condition characterized by polyneuropathy, organomegaly, endocrinopathy, monoclonal gammopathy, and skin changes.

po·go·ni·a·sis (pō′gə-nī′ə-sĭs) *n*. **1.** Growth of a beard on a woman. **2.** Excessive facial hairiness in men.

po·go·ni·on (pə-gō′nē-ən) *n*. The most anterior point of the chin on the mandible in the midline. Also called *mental point*.

–poiesis *suff*. Production; creation; formation: *hemopoiesis*.

–poietic *suff*. Productive; formative: *galactopoietic*.

poikilo– *pref*. Irregular or variable: *poikilocyte*.

poi·ki·lo·blast (poi′kə-lə-blăst′, poi-kĭl′ə-) *n*. A nucleated red blood cell of irregular shape.

poi·ki·lo·cyte (poi′kə-lə-sīt′, poi-kĭl′ə-) *n*. A red blood cell of irregular shape.

poi·ki·lo·cy·to·sis (poi′kə-lō-sī-tō′sĭs) *n*. The presence of poikilocytes in the peripheral blood. Also called *poikilocythemia*.

poi·ki·lo·der·ma (poi′kə-lō-dûr′mə) *n*. A variegated hyperpigmentation and telangiectasia of the skin, followed by atrophy.

poi·ki·lo·therm (poi′kə-lə-thûrm′, poi-kĭl′ə-) *n*. An organism, such as a fish or reptile, having a body temperature that varies with the temperature of its surroundings; an ectotherm.

poi·ki·lo·ther·mic (poi′kə-lō-thûr′mĭk) *or* **poi·ki·lo·ther·mal** (-məl) *or* **poi·ki·lo·ther·mous** (-məs) *adj*. **1.** Of or relating to an organism having a body temperature that varies with the temperature of its surroundings; cold-blooded. **2.** Capable of existing and growing in media of varying temperatures. —**poi′ki·lo·ther′mi·a, poi′ki·lo·ther′mism** *n*.

point (point) *n*. **1.** A sharp or tapered end. **2.** A slight projection. **3.** A stage or condition reached. —*v*. To become ready to open, as an abscess or boil.

point A *n*. See **subspinale**.

point angle *n*. The junction of three surfaces, as of the crown of a tooth or the walls of a cavity.

point B *n*. See **supramentale**.

poin·ted wart (poin′tĭd) *n*. See **genital wart**.

point epidemic *n*. An epidemic in which several cases of a disease occur within a few days or hours due to exposure to a common source of infection such as food or water.

poin·til·lage (pwăn-tē-yäzh′) *n*. A massage manipulation with the tips of the fingers.

point mutation *n*. A mutation that involves a single nucleotide and may consist of loss of a nucleotide, substitution of one nucleotide for another, or the insertion of an additional nucleotide.

point of fixation *n*. The point on the retina at which the light rays coming directly from an object are focused. Also called *fixation point*.

point of ossification *n*. The site of earliest bone formation via accumulation of osteoblasts within connective tissue or of earliest destruction of cartilage before onset of ossification.

point source *n*. A source, especially of pollution or radiation, occupying a very small area and having a concentrated output.

point-system test types *pl.n*. A near vision test chart containing test types that are multiples of a point ($\frac{1}{72}$ inch), lower-case letters being one-half the designated point size.

poise (poiz, pwäz) *n*. A centimeter-gram-second unit of dynamic viscosity equal to one dyne-second per square centimeter.

Poi·seuille's law (pwä-zœ′yēz) *n*. The principle that the volume of a homogeneous fluid passing per unit time through a capillary tube is directly proportional to the pressure difference between its ends and to the fourth power of its internal radius, and inversely proportional to its length and to the viscosity of the fluid.

Poiseuille's space *n*. See **still layer**.

poi·son (poi′zən) *n*. **1.** A substance taken internally or applied externally that is injurious to health or dangerous to life. **2.** A chemical substance that inhibits another substance or a reaction. —*v*. To kill or harm with poison.

poison gas *n.* A gas or vapor used especially in chemical warfare to injure, disable, or kill upon inhalation or contact.

poi·son·ing (poi′zə-nĭng) *n.* **1.** The state of being poisoned. **2.** The administration of a poison.

poison ivy *n.* A North American shrub or vine that has compound leaves with three leaflets, small green flowers, and whitish berries and that causes a rash on contact. Also called *poison oak*.

poison oak *n.* **1.** Either of two shrubs, *Rhus toxicodendron* of the southeast United States or *R. diversiloba* of western North America, related to poison ivy and causing a rash on contact. **2.** See **poison ivy.**

poi·son·ous (poi′zə-nəs) *adj.* Relating to or caused by a poison.

poison sumac *n.* A swamp shrub of the southeast United States, having compound leaves and greenish-white berries and causing an itching rash on contact with the skin.

pok·er spine (pō′kər) *n.* Stiff spine resulting from widespread joint immobility or overwhelming muscle spasm.

po·lar (pō′lər) *adj.* **1.** Of or relating to a pole. **2.** Having poles. Used of certain nerve cells having one or more processes.

polar body *n.* Either of two small cells formed by the ovum during its maturation, the first usually released just before ovulation and the second not until after the ovum has been discharged from the ovary and penetrated by a sperm cell.

polar cataract *n.* A capsular cataract limited to the anterior or posterior polar region of the lens.

po·lar·i·ty (pō-lăr′ĭ-tē, pə-) *n.* **1.** The property of having two opposite poles, such as those possessed by a magnet, or of having opposite properties or characteristics. **2.** The direction or orientation of positivity relative to negativity.

po·lar·i·za·tion (pō′lər-ĭ-zā′shən) *n.* **1.** The production or condition of polarity. **2.** A process or state in which rays of light exhibit different properties in different directions, especially the state in which all the vibration takes place in one plane. **3.** The partial or complete polar separation of positive and negative electric charge in a nuclear, atomic, molecular, or chemical system. **4.** The coating of an electrode with a thick layer of hydrogen bubbles, with the result that the flow of current is weakened or arrested. **5.** The development of differences in potential between two points in living tissues, as between the inside and outside of the cell wall.

po·lar·ized light (pō′lə-rīzd′) *n.* Light that is reflected or transmitted through certain media so that all vibrations are restricted to a single plane.

polar star *n.* See **daughter star.**

pole (pōl) *n.* **1.** Either of the two points at the extremities of the axis of an organ or body. **2.** Either extremity of an axis through a sphere. **3.** Either of two oppositely charged terminals, as in an electric cell.

po·lice·man (pə-lēs′mən) *n.* An instrument, usually a rubber-tipped rod, for removing solid particles from a glass container.

pol·i·clin·ic (pŏl′ē-klĭn′ĭk) *n.* The department of a hospital or health care facility that treats outpatients.

po·li·o (pō′lē-ō′) *n.* Poliomyelitis.

polio– *pref.* **1.** Gray: *poliosis.* **2.** Gray matter: *polioclastic.*

po·li·o·clas·tic (pō′lē-ō-klăs′tĭk) *adj.* Destructive to the gray matter of the nervous system.

po·li·o·dys·tro·phi·a (pō′lē-ō-dĭ-strō′fē-ə) *n.* See **poliodystrophy.**

poliodystrophia cer·e·bri pro·gres·si·va in·fan·ta·lis (sĕr′ə-brī prō′grĭ-sī′və ĭn-făn′tə-lĭs) *n.* Progressive cerebral poliodystrophy.

po·li·o·dys·tro·phy (pō′lē-ō-dĭs′trə-fē) *n.* Wasting of the gray matter of the nervous system. Also called *poliodystrophia.*

po·li·o·en·ceph·a·li·tis (pō′lē-ō-ĕn-sĕf′ə-lī′tĭs) *n.* An acute infectious inflammation of the brain's gray matter, either of the cortex or of the central nuclei.

po·li·o·en·ceph·a·lo·me·nin·go·my·e·li·tis (pō′lē-ō-ĕn-sĕf′ə-lō-mə-nĭng′gō-mī′ə-lī′tĭs) *n.* Inflammation of the gray matter of the brain and spinal cord and of their meningeal covering.

po·li·o·en·ceph·a·lo·my·e·li·tis (pō′lē-ō-ĕn-sĕf′ə-lō-mī′ə-lī′tĭs) *n.* See **poliomyeloencephalitis.**

po·li·o·en·ceph·a·lop·a·thy (pō′lē-ō-ĕn-sĕf′ə-lŏp′ə-thē) *n.* Disease of the gray matter of the brain.

po·li·o·my·e·li·tis (pō′lē-ō-mī′ə-lī′tĭs) *n.* A highly infectious viral disease that chiefly affects children and, in its acute forms, causes inflammation of motor neurons of the spinal cord and brainstem, leading to paralysis, muscular atrophy, and often deformity. Also called *infantile paralysis.*

poliomyelitis immune globulin *n.* A sterile solution of globulins containing antibodies normally present in adult blood that is used as a passive immunological agent to confer temporary protection against paralytic polio and to attenuate or prevent poliomyelitis, measles, and infectious hepatitis.

poliomyelitis virus *n.* The picornavirus that causes poliomyelitis. Serologic types 1, 2, and 3 are recognized, type 1 being responsible for most cases of paralytic poliomyelitis and most epidemics. Also called *poliovirus, poliovirus hominis.*

po·li·o·my·e·lo·en·ceph·a·li·tis (pō′lē-ō-mī′ə-lō-ĕn-sĕf′ə-lī′tĭs) *n.* Acute anterior poliomyelitis with encephalitis. Also called *polioencephalomyelitis.*

po·li·o·my·e·lop·a·thy (pō′lē-ō-mī′ə-lŏp′ə-thē) *n.* Disease of the gray matter of the spinal cord.

po·li·o·sis (pō′lē-ō′sĭs) *n.* An absence or lessening of melanin in hair of the scalp, brows, or lashes.

po·li·o·vi·rus (pō′lē-ō-vī′rəs) *n.* See **poliomyelitis virus.**

poliovirus hom·i·nis (hŏm′ə-nĭs) *n.* See **poliomyelitis virus.**

poliovirus vaccine *or* **poliomyelitis vaccine** *n.* **1.** An aqueous suspension of inactivated strains of poliomyelitis virus given by injection, now largely replaced by the oral vaccine. Also called *inactivated poliovirus vaccine.* **2.** An aqueous suspension of live attenuated strains of poliomyelitis virus, given orally for active immunization against poliomyelitis. Also called *oral poliovirus vaccine.*

Po·lit·zer bag (pō′lĭt-sər) *n.* A pear-shaped rubber bag used to force air through the eustachian tube.

po·lit·zer·i·za·tion (pō′lĭt-sər-ĭ-zā′shən, pŏl′ĭt-) *n.* Inflation of the auditory tube and middle ear with a Politzer bag.

pol·len (pŏl′ən) *n.* Microspores of seed plants carried by wind or insects prior to fertilization.

pollen count *n.* The average number of pollen grains, usually of ragweed, in a cubic yard or other standard volume of air over a 24-hour period at a specified time and place.

pol·lex (pŏl′ĕks′) *n., pl.* **pol·li·ces** (pŏl′ĭ-sēz′) The thumb.

pol·li·ci·za·tion (pŏl′ĭ-sĭ-zā′shən) *n.* Surgical construction of a substitute thumb.

pol·li·no·sis *or* **pol·le·no·sis** (pŏl′ə-nō′sĭs) *n.* Hay fever caused by an allergic reaction to pollen.

pol·lut·ant (pə-lōōt′nt) *n.* Something that pollutes, especially a waste material that contaminates air, soil, or water.

pol·lute (pə-lōōt′) *v.* **1.** To make unfit for or harmful to living things, especially by the addition of waste matter; contaminate. **2.** To make less suitable for an activity, especially by the introduction of unwanted factors. —**pol·lut′er** *n.*

pol·lu·tion (pə-lōō′shən) *n.* **1.** The act or process of polluting or the state of being polluted, especially the contamination of soil, water, or the atmosphere by the discharge of harmful substances. **2.** A pollutant or group of pollutants.

po·lo·ni·um (pə-lō′nē-əm) *n. Symbol* **Po** A naturally radioactive metallic element, occurring in minute quantities in uranium ores; its most readily available isotope is Po 210, with a half-life of 138.39 days. Atomic number 84.

poly– *pref.* **1.** More than one; many; much: *polyatomic.* **2.** More than usual; excessive; abnormal: *polydipsia.* **3.** Polymer; polymeric: *polyethylene.*

pol·y·a·cryl·a·mide gel (pŏl′ē-ə-krĭl′ə-mīd′) *n.* A hydrated polymer consisting of a long chain of amide groups, used as a medium for substances that undergo gel electrophoresis.

polyacrylamide gel electrophoresis *n.* A technique for determining the molecular weight of proteins, in which proteins that have been coated in an anionic detergent undergo electrophoresis in a polyacrylamide gel.

pol·y·ad·e·ni·tis (pŏl′ē-ăd′n-ī′tĭs) *n.* Inflammation of many lymph nodes.

pol·y·ad·e·nop·a·thy (pŏl′ē-ăd′n-ŏp′ə-thē) *or* **pol·y·ad·e·no·sis** (-ō′sĭs) *n.* A disorder affecting many lymph nodes.

pol·y·ad·e·nyl·ic acid (pŏl′ē-ăd′n-ĭl′ĭk) *n.* A polymer of adenylic acid attached to mRNA that stabilizes the molecule before transport from the nucleus into the cytoplasm.

pol·y·a·mine (pŏl′ē-ə-mēn′, -ăm′ēn) *n.* Any of a group of organic compounds that contain two or more amino groups.

pol·y·an·gi·i·tis (pŏl′ē-ăn′jē-ī′tĭs) *n.* Inflammation of more than one type of blood vessel.

pol·y·an·i·on (pŏl′ē-ăn′ī′ən) *n.* Any of multiple anionic sites on proteoglycans in the renal glomeruli that restrict filtration of anionic molecules and facilitate filtration of cationic proteins.

pol·y·ar·te·ri·tis (pŏl′ē-är′tə-rī′tĭs) *n.* Simultaneous inflammation of a number of arteries.

polyarteritis no·do·sa (nō-dō′sə) *n.* Systemic inflammation and necrosis occurring in medium-sized or small arteries. Also called *Kussmaul's disease, periarteritis nodosa.*

pol·y·ar·thric (pŏl′ē-är′thrĭk) *adj.* Multiarticular.

pol·y·ar·thri·tis (pŏl′ē-är-thrī′tĭs) *n.* Simultaneous inflammation of several joints.

polyarthritis rheu·mat·i·ca a·cu·ta (rōō-măt′ĭ-kə ə-kyōō′tə) *n.* Acute articular or inflammatory rheumatism, associated with rheumatic fever.

pol·y·ar·tic·u·lar (pŏl′ē-är-tĭk′yə-lər) *adj.* Multiarticular.

pol·y·ax·i·al joint (pŏl′ē-ăk′sē-əl) *n.* See **multiaxial joint.**

pol·y·ba·sic (pŏl′ē-bā′sĭk) *adj.* Of or relating to an acid that has two or more hydrogen atoms that can be replaced by basic atoms or radicals.

polybasic acid *n.* An acid having two or more hydrogen atoms that can be displaced.

pol·y·blast (pŏl′ē-blăst′) *n.* One of a group of ameboid, mononucleated, phagocytic cells found in inflammatory exudates.

pol·y·chlo·rin·at·ed biphenyl (pŏl′ē-klôr′ə-nā′tĭd) *n.* PCB

pol·y·chon·dri·tis (pŏl′ē-kŏn-drī′tĭs) *n.* Simultaneous inflammation of many cartilages.

pol·y·chro·ma·sia (pŏl′ē-krō-mā′zhə) *n.* See **polychromatophilia.**

pol·y·chro·mat·ic (pŏl′ē-krō-măt′ĭk) *or* **pol·y·chro·mic** (-krō′mĭk) *or* **pol·y·chro·mous** (-krō′məs) *adj.* Having or exhibiting many colors.

pol·y·chro·mat·o·phil (pŏl′ē-krō-măt′ə-fĭl′, -krō′mə-tə-) *n.* A young or degenerated red blood cell staining with acid, neutral, or basic dyes. Also called *polychromatic cell, polychromatocyte.* —*adj.* Staining readily with acid, neutral, or basic dyes.

pol·y·chro·mat·o·phil·i·a (pŏl′ē-krō-măt′ə-fĭl′ē-ə, -krō′mə-tō-) *or* **pol·y·chro·mo·phil·i·a** (-krō′mə-) *n.* Affinity for more than one type of stain, especially for both basic and acid stains. Also called *polychromasia.* —**pol′y·chro·mat′o·phil′ic** (-fĭl′ĭk), **pol′y·chro·mat′o·phile′** (-fīl′) *adj.*

pol·y·chro·me·mi·a (pŏl′ē-krō-mē′mē-ə) *n.* An increase in the total amount of hemoglobin in the blood.

pol·y·clin·ic (pŏl′ē-klĭn′ĭk) *n.* A clinic, hospital, or health care facility that treats various types of diseases and injuries.

pol·y·clone (pŏl′ē-klōn′) *n.* A clone descended from one or more small groups of cells, especially ones of genetically different origins. —**pol′y·clo′nal** *adj.* —**pol′y·clo′nal·ly** *adv.*

pol·y·clo·ni·a (pŏl′ē-klō′nē-ə) *n.* See **myoclonus multiplex.**

pol·y·co·ri·a (pŏl′ē-kôr′ē-ə) *n.* Two or more pupils in one iris.

pol·y·crot·ic (pŏl′ē-krŏt′ĭk) *adj.* Relating to or marked by polycrotism.

po·lyc·ro·tism (pə-lĭk′rə-tĭz′əm) *n.* A condition in which the sphygmographic tracing shows several upward breaks in the descending wave.

pol·y·cy·e·sis (pŏl′ē-sī-ē′sĭs) *n.* Multiple pregnancy.

pol·y·cys·tic (pŏl′ē-sĭs′tĭk) *adj.* Having or containing many cysts.

polycystic kidney *n.* An inherited progressive disease characterized by formation of multiple cysts of varying size scattered diffusely throughout both kidneys and resulting in destruction of the kidney parenchyma, hypertension, bloody urine, and uremia. Also called *polycystic disease of kidneys.*

polycystic liver *n.* Gradual cystic dilation of intralobular bile ducts that fail to involute in embryologic development of the liver.

polycystic ovary disease *n. Abbr.* **PCOD** Sclerocystic disease of the ovary, characterized by enlarged ovaries, hirsutism, obesity, menstrual irregularity, and hyperinsulinism. Also called *Stein-Leventhal syndrome.*

pol·y·cy·the·mi·a (pŏl′ē-sī-thē′mē-ə) *n.* A condition characterized by an abnormal increase in the number of red blood cells in the blood. Also called *erythrocythemia, hypercythemia, hypererythrocythemia, hyperglobulia.*

polycythemia hy·per·ton·i·ca (hī′pər-tŏn′ĭ-kə) *n.* Polycythemia associated with hypertension, but without splenomegaly.

polycythemia ru·bra (rōō′brə) *n.* See **erythremia.**

polycythemia ve·ra (vîr′ə) *n.* See **erythremia.**

pol·y·dac·tyl (pŏl′ē-dăk′təl) or **pol·y·dac·ty·lous** (-tə-ləs) *adj.* Having more than the normal number of digits on a hand or foot.

pol·y·dac·ty·ly (pŏl′ē-dăk′tə-lē) or **pol·y·dac·tyl·ism** (-tə-lĭz′əm) *n.* A condition characterized by the presence of more than five digits on a hand or foot. Also called *hyperdactyly.*

pol·y·dip·si·a (pŏl′ē-dĭp′sē-ə) *n.* Excessive or abnormal thirst. —**pol′y·dip′sic** *adj.*

pol·y·dys·pla·sia (pŏl′ē-dĭs-plā′zhə) *n.* Abnormal development in several types of tissue.

pol·y·e·lec·tro·lyte (pŏl′ē-ĭ-lĕk′trə-līt′) *n.* An electrolyte, such as a protein or polysaccharide, having a high molecular weight.

pol·y·em·bry·o·ny (pŏl′ē-ĕm′brē-ə-nē, -ĕm-brī′-) *n.* Development of more than one embryo from a single egg or ovule.

pol·y·en·do·crine deficiency syndrome (pŏl′ē-ĕn′də-krĭn, -krēn′, -krīn′) *n.* Pathological dysfunction of several endocrine glands. Also called *polyglandular deficiency syndrome.*

pol·y·e·no·ic acid (pŏl′ē-ē-nō′ĭk) *n.* Any of various fatty acids having more than one double bond in the carbon chain, as in linoleic acid.

pol·y·er·gic (pŏl′ē-ûr′jĭk) *adj.* Capable of acting in several different ways.

pol·y·es·the·sia (pŏl′ē-ĭs-thē′zhə) *n.* A disorder of sensation in which a single touch or other stimulus is felt as several.

pol·y·es·trous (pŏl′ē-ĕs′trəs) *adj.* Ovulating more than once a year.

pol·y·eth·yl·ene glycol (pŏl′ē-ĕth′ə-lēn′) *n.* Any of a family of high molecular weight compounds that can be liquid or waxlike in consistency, are soluble in water and in many organic solvents, and are used in detergents and as emulsifiers and plasticizers.

pol·y·ga·lac·ti·a (pŏl′ē-gə-lăk′tē-ə, -shē-ə) *n.* Excessive secretion of breast milk, especially at the weaning period.

pol·y·ga·lac·tu·ro·nase (pŏl′ē-gə-lăk′tər-ə-nās′, -năz′, -găl′ăk-tōor′-) *n.* An enzyme that catalyzes the hydrolysis of specific linkages in galacturonides and other polysaccharides.

pol·y·gene (pŏl′ē-jēn′) *n.* One of a group of nonallelic genes acting together to produce quantitative variations of a particular character.

pol·y·gen·ic (pŏl′ē-jĕn′ĭk) *adj.* Relating to a characteristic or disease controlled by the interaction of genes at more than one locus.

pol·y·glan·du·lar (pŏl′ē-glăn′jə-lər) *adj.* Pluriglandular.

polyglandular deficiency syndrome *n.* See **polyendocrine deficiency syndrome.**

pol·y·graph (pŏl′ē-grăf′) *n.* An instrument that simultaneously records changes in physiological processes such as heartbeat, blood pressure, and respiration.

pol·y·gy·ri·a (pŏl′ĭ-jī′rē-ə) *n.* An excessive number of convolutions in the brain.

pol·y·hi·dro·sis (pŏl′ē-hī-drō′sĭs, -hĭ-) or **pol·y·i·dro·sis** (pŏl′ē-ĭ-) *n.* See **hyperhidrosis.**

pol·y·hy·dram·ni·os (pŏl′ē-hī-drăm′nē-ŏs′) *n.* See **hydramnios.**

pol·y·hy·dric (pŏl′ē-hī′drĭk) *adj.* Containing more than one hydroxyl group.

poly I:C (pŏl′ē ī′sē′) *n.* A synthetic chemical that resembles the RNA of infectious viruses and is used to stimulate the production of interferon by the immune system.

pol·y·lep·tic (pŏl′ē-lĕp′tĭk) *adj.* Occurring in many paroxysms, as malaria or epilepsy.

pol·y·mas·ti·a (pŏl′ē-măs′tē-ə) *n.* A condition in which more than two breasts are present. Also called *hypermastia, pleomastia.*

pol·y·me·li·a (pŏl′ə-mē′lē-ə, -mēl′yə) *n.* The presence of more than the normal number of limbs or parts of limbs.

pol·y·men·or·rhe·a (pŏl′ē-mĕn′ə-rē′ə) *n.* The occurrence of menstrual cycles at frequency that is higher than normal.

pol·y·mer (pŏl′ə-mər) *n.* Any of numerous compounds of usually high molecular weight and consisting of up to millions of repeated linked units, each a relatively light and simple molecule.

pol·y·mer·ase (pŏl′ə-mə-rās′, -rāz′) *n.* Any of various enzymes that catalyze polymerization, especially those that catalyze the synthesis of polynucleotides of DNA or RNA using an existing strand of DNA or RNA as a template.

polymerase chain reaction *n. Abbr.* **PCR** A technique for amplifying DNA sequences in vitro by separating the DNA into two strands and incubating it with oligonucleotide primers and DNA polymerase. A specific sequence of DNA can be amplified by as many as one billion times.

polymer fume fever *n.* A condition marked by fever, pain in the chest, and cough caused by the inhalation of fumes given off by the plastic polytetrafluorethylene when heated.

pol·y·me·ri·a (pŏl′ə-mîr′ē-ə) *n.* An excessive number of parts, limbs, or organs of the body.

pol·y·mer·ic (pŏl′ə-měr′ĭk) *adj.* **1.** Having the properties of a polymer. **2.** Of or relating to polymeria.

po·lym·er·i·za·tion (pə-lĭm′ər-ĭ-zā′shən, pŏl′ə-mər-) *n.* **1.** The bonding of two or more monomers to form a polymer. **2.** A chemical process that effects this bonding.

pol·y·mer·ize (pŏl′ə-mə-rīz′, pə-lĭm′ə-) *v.* To undergo or subject to polymerization.

polymorphic reticulosis *n.* See **lymphomatoid granulomatosis.**

pol·y·mor·phism (pŏl′ē-môr′fĭz′əm) *n.* **1.** The occurrence of different forms, stages, or types in individual organisms or in organisms of the same species, independent of sexual variations. **2.** Crystallization of a compound in at least two distinct forms. Also called *pleomorphism.* —**pol′y·mor′phic, pol′y·mor′phous** *adj.*

pol·y·mor·pho·cel·lu·lar (pŏl′ē-môr′fə-sěl′yə-lər) *adj.* Relating to or formed of cells of several different kinds.

pol·y·mor·pho·nu·cle·ar (pŏl′ē-môr′fə-nōo′klē-ər) *adj.* Having a lobed nucleus. Used especially of neutrophilic white blood cells.

polymorphonuclear leukocyte *n. Abbr.* **PMN** A white blood cell, usually neutrophilic, having a nucleus that is divided into lobes connected by strands of chromatin. Also called *multinuclear leukocyte.*

polymorphous perverse *adj.* Characterized by or displaying sexual tendencies that have no specific direction, as in an infant or young child, but that may evolve into acts that are regarded as perversions in adults.

pol·y·my·al·gia (pŏl′ē-mī-ăl′jə) *n.* Pain in several muscle groups.

pol·y·my·oc·lo·nus (pŏl′ē-mī-ŏk′lə-nəs) *n.* See **myoclonus multiplex.**

pol·y·my·o·si·tis (pŏl′ē-mī′ə-sī′tĭs) *n.* Inflammation of several voluntary muscles simultaneously.

pol·y·myx·in (pŏl′ē-mĭk′sĭn) *n.* Any of various mainly toxic antibiotics derived from strains of the soil bacterium *Bacillus polymyxa* and used to treat various infections with gram-negative bacteria.

pol·y·ne·sic (pŏl′ē-nē′sĭk) *adj.* Occurring in many separate foci.

pol·y·neu·ral (pŏl′ē-nōor′əl) *adj.* Relating to, supplied by, or affecting several nerves.

pol·y·neu·ral·gia (pŏl′ē-nōo-răl′jə) *n.* Simultaneous neuralgia of several nerves.

polyneuritic psychosis *n.* See **Korsakoff's syndrome.**

pol·y·neu·ri·tis (pŏl′ē-nōo-rī′tĭs) *n.* Inflammation of several nerves at one time, marked by paralysis, pain, and muscle wasting. Also called *multiple neuritis.* —**pol′y·neu·rit′ic** (-rĭt′ĭk) *adj.*

pol·y·neu·rop·a·thy (pŏl′ē-nōo-rŏp′ə-thē) *n.* A generalized disorder of peripheral nerves.

pol·y·nu·cle·ar (pŏl′ē-nōo′klē-ər) *or* **pol·y·nu·cle·ate** (-klē-ĭt) *or* **pol·y·nu·cle·at·ed** (-klē-ā′tĭd) *adj.* Multinuclear.

pol·y·nu·cle·o·tid·ase (pŏl′ē-nōo′klē-ə-tī′dās, -dāz) *n.* Any of the enzymes catalyzing the hydrolysis of polynucleotides to oligonucleotides or mononucleotides.

pol·y·nu·cle·o·tide (pŏl′ē-nōo′klē-ə-tīd′) *n.* A linear polymer containing an indefinite, usually large number of nucleotides linked from one ribose or deoxyribose to another by phosphoric residues.

pol·y·o·don·tia (pŏl′ē-ō-dŏn′shə) *n.* The presence of supernumerary teeth.

pol·y·on·co·sis (pŏl′ē-ŏng-kō′sĭs) *n.* The formation of multiple tumors.

pol·y·o·nych·i·a (pŏl′ē-ō-nĭk′ē-ə) *n.* The presence of supernumerary nails on the fingers or toes.

pol·y·o·pi·a (pŏl′ē-ō′pē-ə) *n.* The perception of several visual images of one object. Also called *multiple vision.*

pol·y·or·chism (pŏl′ē-ôr′kĭz′əm) *or* **pol·y·or·chi·dism** (-ôr′kĭ-dĭz′əm) *n.* The presence of supernumerary testes.

pol·y·os·tot·ic (pŏl′ē-ŏs-tŏt′ĭk) *adj.* Involving more than one bone.

pol·y·o·ti·a (pŏl′ē-ō′shē-ə) *n.* The presence of an extra auricle on one or both sides of the head.

pol·y·o·vu·lar (pŏl′ē-ō′vyə-lər, -ŏv′yə-) *adj.* Containing more than one ovum.

pol·y·o·vu·la·to·ry (pŏl′ē-ō′vyə-lə-tôr′ē, -ŏv′yə-) *n.* Discharging several ova in one ovulatory cycle.

pol·yp (pŏl′ĭp) *n.* A usually nonmalignant growth of tissue protruding from the mucous lining of an organ such as the nose, bladder, or intestine, often causing obstruction. Also called *polypus.* —**pol′yp·oid′** *adj.*

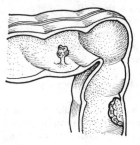

polyp
in a sigmoid colon:
peduncular (left) and sessile polyps

pol·yp·ec·to·my (pŏl′ə-pěk′tə-mē) *n.* Excision of a polyp.

pol·y·pep·tide (pŏl′ē-pěp′tīd′) *n.* A peptide containing many amino acids, typically between 10 and 100.

pol·y·pha·gia (pŏl′ē-fā′jə) *n.* Excessive eating; gluttony.

pol·y·pha·lan·gism (pŏl′ē-fə-lăn′jĭz′əm, -fā-) *n.* See **hyperphalangism.**

pol·y·phar·ma·cy (pŏl′ē-fär′mə-sē) *n.* The mixing of many drugs in one prescription.

pol·y·phe·nic gene (pŏl′ē-fē′nĭk) *n.* See **pleiotropic gene.**

pol·y·pho·bi·a (pŏl′ĭ-fō′bē-ə) *n.* An abnormal fear of many things; a condition marked by the presence of many phobias.

pol·y·phra·sia (pŏl′ĭ-frā′zhə) *n.* Extreme talkativeness.

pol·y·phy·let·ic (pŏl′ē-fī-lĕt′ĭk) *adj.* **1.** Descended or derived from more than one ancestral stock or source. **2.** Of or being the theory that blood cells are derived from several different stem cells, depending on the particular blood cell type. —**pol′y·phy′le·tism** (-fī′lĭ-tĭz′-əm) *n.*

pol·y·plas·tic (pŏl′ē-plăs′tĭk) *adj.* **1.** Formed of several different structures. **2.** Capable of assuming several forms.

pol·y·ple·gia (pŏl′ē-plē′jə) *n.* Paralysis of several muscles.

pol·y·ploid (pŏl′ē-ploid′) *adj.* Having extra sets of chromosomes. —*n.* An organism with more than two sets of chromosomes. —**pol′y·ploi′dy** *n.*

pol·yp·ne·a (pŏl′ĭp-nē′ə) *n.* See **tachypnea.**

pol·yp·oid (pŏl′ə-poid′) *adj.* Resembling a polyp.

po·lyp·or·ous (pō-lĭp′ər-əs, pə-) *adj.* Having many small perforations; cribriform.

pol·y·po·si·a (pŏl′ē-pō′zē-ə) *n.* Sustained excessive consumption of fluids.

pol·yp·o·sis (pŏl′ə-pō′sĭs) *n.* The presence of several polyps.

pol·y·pous (pŏl′ə-pəs) *adj.* Relating to, resembling, or characterized by the presence of a polyp or polyps.

polypous gastritis *n.* Chronic gastritis in which there is irregular atrophy of the mucous membrane with knobby or polypoid projections.

pol·y·ptych·i·al (pŏl′ē-tĭk′ē-əl, -tī′kē-əl) *adj.* Folded or arranged so as to form more than one layer.

pol·y·pus (pŏl′ə-pəs) *n., pl.* **-pi** (-pī′) See **polyp.**

pol·y·ra·dic·u·li·tis (pŏl′ē-rə-dĭk′yə-lī′tĭs) *n.* Inflammation of the nerve roots.

pol·y·ra·dic·u·lo·neu·rop·a·thy (pŏl′ē-rə-dĭk′yə-lō-nōō-rŏp′ə-thē) *n.* See **acute idiopathic polyneuritis.**

pol·y·ri·bo·some (pŏl′ē-rī′bə-sōm′) *n.* A cluster of ribosomes connected by a strand of mRNA and functioning as a unit in protein synthesis. Also called *polysome.*

pol·y·sac·cha·ride (pŏl′ē-săk′ə-rīd′) *or* **pol·y·sac·cha·rid** (-rĭd) *or* **pol·y·sac·cha·rose** (-rōs′, -rōz′) *n.* Any of a class of carbohydrates, such as starch and cellulose, consisting of a number of monosaccharides joined by glycosidic bonds. Also called *glycan.*

pol·y·se·ro·si·tis (pŏl′ē-sîr′ō-sī′tĭs) *n.* Chronic inflammation of several serous membranes with effusions in serous cavities resulting in fibrous thickening of the serosa and constrictive pericarditis. Also called *Concato's disease.*

pol·y·si·nus·i·tis (pŏl′ē-sī′nə-sī′tĭs) *n.* Simultaneous inflammation of two or more sinuses.

pol·y·some (pŏl′ē-sōm′) *n.* See **polyribosome.**

pol·y·so·mi·a (pŏl′ē-sō′mē-ə) *n.* A fetal malformation involving two or more imperfect and partially fused bodies.

pol·y·so·mic (pŏl′ē-sō′mĭk) *adj.* Having an extra copy of one or more chromosomes. —*n.* A polysomic organism or cell.

pol·y·som·no·gram (pŏl′ē-sŏm′nə-grăm′) *n.* The record obtained in polysomnography.

pol·y·som·nog·ra·phy (pŏl′ē-sŏm-nŏg′rə-fē) *n.* Simultaneous and continuous monitoring of normal and abnormal physiological activity during sleep.

pol·y·so·my (pŏl′ē-sō′mē) *n.* The state of a cell nucleus in which a specific chromosome is represented more than twice.

pol·y·sor·bate (pŏl′ē-sôr′bāt′) *n.* Any of a class of emulsifiers used in some pharmaceuticals.

pol·y·sper·mi·a (pŏl′ē-spûr′mē-ə) *n.* **1.** A secretion of spermatozoa that is abnormally profuse. **2.** See **polyspermy.**

pol·y·sper·my (pŏl′ē-spûr′mē) *n.* The entrance of more than one spermatozoon into the ovum. Also called *polyspermia.*

pol·y·stich·i·a (pŏl′ē-stĭk′ē-ə) *n.* An abnormal arrangement of the eyelashes in two or more rows.

po·lys·ti·chous (pə-lĭs′tĭ-kəs) *adj.* Arranged in two or more rows.

pol·y·sym·brach·y·dac·ty·ly (pŏl′ē-sĭm-brăk′ē-dăk′-tə-lē) *n.* A congenital malformation of the hand and foot in which the shortened digits are syndactylous and polydactylous.

pol·y·syn·ap·tic (pŏl′ē-sĭ-năp′tĭk) *adj.* Of or involving neural conduction pathways formed by a chain of many synaptically connected nerve cells.

pol·y·syn·dac·ty·ly (pŏl′ē-sĭn-dăk′tə-lē) *n.* A congenital condition in which multiple fingers or toes are webbed.

pol·y·ten·di·ni·tis (pŏl′ē-tĕn′də-nī′tĭs) *n.* Inflammation of several tendons at the same time.

pol·y·the·li·a (pŏl′ē-thē′lē-ə, -thēl′yə) *n.* The presence of supernumerary nipples on the breast or elsewhere. Also called *hyperthelia.*

pol·y·to·mog·ra·phy (pŏl′ē-tō-mŏg′rə-fē) *n.* Tomography of several sectional planes of the body using a machine specifically designed to effect complex motion.

pol·y·trich·i·a (pŏl′ē-trĭk′ē-ə) *n.* Excessive hairiness.

pol·y·typ·ic (pŏl′ē-tĭp′ĭk) *or* **pol·y·typ·i·cal** (-ĭ-kəl) *adj.* Having several variant forms, especially subspecies or varieties.

pol·y·un·sat·u·rat·ed (pŏl′ē-ŭn-săch′ə-rā′tĭd) *adj.* Of or relating to long-chain carbon compounds, especially fatty acids, having two or more double bonds per molecule. Foods containing polyunsaturated fatty acids help reduce the level of LDL cholesterol in the blood.

pol·y·u·ri·a (pŏl′ē-yŏŏr′ē-ə) *n.* Excessive passage of urine, as in diabetes. Also called *hydruria.*

pol·y·va·lent (pŏl′ē-vā′lənt) *adj.* **1.** Acting against or interacting with more than one kind of antigen, antibody, toxin, or microorganism. **2.** Having more than one chemical valence. —**pol′y·va′lence, pol′y·va′len·cy** *n.*

polyvalent allergy *n.* Hypersensitivity that occurs simultaneously to several specific antigens.

polyvalent serum *n.* An antiserum obtained from an animal that has been inoculated with several species or strains of a bacterium.

polyvalent vaccine *n.* A vaccine prepared from cultures of two or more strains of the same species of microorganism or virus. Also called *multivalent vaccine.*

pol·y·vi·nyl (pŏl'ē-vī'nəl) *adj.* Of, relating to, or characterizing a polymerized thermoplastic vinyl, such as polyvinyl chloride.

polyvinyl chloride *n. Abbr.* **PVC** A common thermoplastic vinyl that is used in a variety of manufactured products.

po·made acne (pō-mād', -mäd', pŏ-) *n.* Acne caused by repeated application of hair ointments that block the release of sebum from hair follicles, seen most commonly on the forehead and temples of young African Americans.

Pom·er·oy's operation (pŏm'ə-roiz') *n.* Excision of a ligated portion of the fallopian tubes.

POMP (pē'ō-ĕm-pē') *n.* A drug that is used in cancer chemotherapy and is composed of purinethol (6-mercaptopurine), Oncovin (vincristine sulfate), methotrexate, and prednisone.

Pom·pe's disease (pŏm'pəz) *n.* See **type 2 glycogenosis.**

pom·pho·lyx (pŏm'fə-līks') *n.* See **dyshidrosis.**

pons (pŏnz) *n., pl.* **pon·tes** (pŏn'tēz) **1.** The part of the brainstem that is intermediate between the medulla oblongata and the mesencephalon and is composed of a ventral part and the tegmentum. **2.** A bridgelike formation connecting two disjoined parts of a structure or organ.

pons Va·ro·li·i (və-rō'lē-ī') *n.* A band of nerve fibers on the ventral surface of the brainstem that links the medulla oblongata and the cerebellum with upper portions of the brain.

pon·tic (pŏn'tĭk) *n.* An artificial tooth on a fixed partial denture.

pon·tile (pŏn'tīl') *or* **pon·tine** (-tīn', -tēn') *adj.* Of or relating to a pons.

pontine angle tumor *n.* A tumor that grows in the proximal portion of the acoustic nerve, especially in the angle formed by the cerebellum and the lateral pons.

pontine flexure *n.* The dorsally concave curvature of the embryonic rhombencephalon. Also called *basicranial flexure, transverse rhombencephalic flexure.*

pontine nuclei *pl.n.* The very large mass of gray matter filling the pons and serving as a major way station in impulse conduction from the cerebral cortex of one hemisphere to the posterior lobe of the opposite cerebellar hemisphere.

pon·to·med·ul·lar·y groove (pŏn'tō-mĕd'l-ĕr'ē, -mə-dŭl'ə-rē) *n.* The transverse groove on the ventral aspect of the brainstem that demarcates the pons from the medulla oblongata and from which emerge the sixth, seventh, and eighth cranial nerves.

pool (po͞ol) *n.* A collection of blood in any region of the body due to dilation and retardation of the circulation in capillaries and veins.

pooled serum (po͞old) *n.* Serum obtained from a number of individuals and mixed together. Also called *pooled blood serum.*

poor·ly differentiated lymphocytic lymphoma (po͞or'lē) *n. Abbr.* **PDLL** A B-cell lymphoma with nodu-

lar or diffuse lymph node or bone marrow involvement by large lymphoid cells.

pop·les (pŏp'lēz) *n., pl.* **pop·li·tes** (pŏp'lĭ-tēz) The back part of the knee.

pop·lit·e·al (pŏp-lĭt'ē-əl, pŏp'lĭ-tē'əl) *adj.* Relating to the poples.

popliteal artery *n.* An artery that is the continuation of the femoral artery in the popliteal space, bifurcating into the anterior and posterior tibial arteries, with branches to the lateral and medial superior genicular, middle genicular, lateral and medial inferior genicular, and sural arteries.

popliteal entrapment syndrome *n.* A crush syndrome resulting from compression of the popliteal artery and impairment of its blood flow by structures of the popliteal space.

popliteal ligament *n.* **1.** A broad fibrous band attached to the lateral condyle of the femur and passing medially and downward in the posterior part of the capsule of the knee joint; arcuate popliteal ligament. **2.** A fibrous band that extends across the back of the knee from the insertion of the semimembranosus on the medial condyle of the tibia to the lateral condyle of the femur; oblique popliteal ligament; slanting popliteal ligament.

popliteal muscle *n.* A muscle with origin from the lateral condyle of the femur, with insertion into the posterior surface of the tibia, with nerve supply from the tibial nerve, and whose action flexes the leg and rotates it medially.

popliteal vein *n.* A vein that arises at the lower border of the popliteal muscle by union of the anterior and posterior tibial veins and enters the great adductor muscle to become the femoral vein.

pop·per (pŏp'ər) *n.* An ampule of amyl nitrite or butyl nitrite used as a stimulant drug.

pop·py (pŏp'ē) *n.* **1.** Any of numerous plants of the genus *Papaver*, having showy red, orange, or white flowers, a milky juice, and capsules that dehisce through terminal pores. **2.** An extract from the sap of unripe poppy seedpods, used in medicine and narcotics.

pop·u·la·tion (pŏp'yə-lā'shən) *n.* **1.** The total number of people inhabiting a specific area. **2.** The set of individuals, items, or data from which a statistical sample is taken. **3.** All the organisms that constitute a specific group or occur in a specified habitat.

population genetics *n.* The branch of genetics that deals with the genetic makeup of populations.

POR *abbr.* problem-oriented record

pore (pôr) *n.* **1.** A minute opening in an animal or plant tissue. **2.** One of the minute openings of the sweat glands of the skin.

por·en·ce·pha·li·a (pôr'ĕn-sə-fā'lē-ə, -fāl'yə) *n.* See **porencephaly.**

por·en·ceph·a·li·tis (pôr'ĕn-sĕf'ə-lī'tĭs) *n.* Chronic inflammation of the brain with the formation of cavities in the brain substance.

por·en·ceph·a·ly (pôr'ĕn-sĕf'ə-lē) *n.* Occurrence of cavities in the brain substance, usually communicating with the lateral ventricles. Also called *poren-*

cephalia. —**por'en·ce·phal'ic** (-ĕn'sə-făl'ĭk), **por'en·ceph'a·lous** (-sĕf'ə-ləs) *adj.*

po·ri·on (pôr'ē-ŏn') *n.*, *pl.* **po·ri·a** (pôr'ē-ə) The central point on the upper margin of the external auditory meatus.

po·ro·cele (pôr'ə-sēl) *n.* A hernia with indurated coverings.

po·ro·ker·a·to·sis (pôr'ō-kĕr'ə-tō'sĭs) *n.* A rare dermatosis marked by thickening of the stratum corneum together with progressive centrifugal atrophy.

po·ro·ma (pə-rō'mə, pô-) *n.* 1. See **callosity.** 2. See **exostosis.** 3. Induration following inflammation of subcutaneous connective tissue. 4. A benign tumor lining the skin openings of sweat glands.

po·ro·sis (pə-rō'sĭs, pô-) *n.*, *pl.* **-ses** (-sēz) A porous condition, as of the bones.

po·ros·i·ty (pə-rŏs'ĭ-tē, pô-) *n.* 1. The state or property of being porous. 2. A structure or part that is porous. 3. A cavity or perforation.

po·rot·o·my (pə-rŏt'ə-mē, pô-) *n.* See **meatotomy.**

po·rous (pôr'əs) *adj.* 1. Full of or having pores. 2. Admitting the passage of gas or liquid through pores. —**po'rous·ness** *n.*

por·phin (pôr'fĭn) *or* **por·phine** (-fēn') *n.* The unsubstituted heterocyclic ring consisting of four pyrrole rings; it is the basic unit of the porphyrins.

por·pho·bi·lin (pôr'fō-bī'lĭn) *n.* An intermediate in the synthesis of porphyrins and heme.

por·pho·bi·lin·o·gen (pôr'fō-bī-lĭn'ə-jən, -jĕn') *n.* *Abbr.* **PBG** A porphyrin precursor found in large quantities in the urine in cases of acute or congenital porphyria.

por·phyr·i·a (pôr-fîr'ē-ə) *n.* Any of several disorders of porphyrin metabolism, usually hereditary, characterized by large amounts of porphyrins in the blood and urine.

porphyria cu·ta·ne·a tar·da (kyŏō-tā'nē-ə tär'də) *n.* *Abbr.* **PCT** Porphyria characterized by liver dysfunction and photosensitive cutaneous lesions, with hyperpigmentation and scleroderma-like changes in skin, neurologic manifestations, and porphyrinuria. Also called *symptomatic porphyria.*

por·phy·rin (pôr'fə-rĭn) *n.* Any of various heterocyclic compounds, derived from pyrrole, that occur universally in protoplasm, contain a central metal atom, and provide the foundation structure for hemoglobin, chlorophyll, and certain enzymes.

por·phy·rin·o·gen (pôr'fə-rĭn'ə-jən, -jĕn') *n.* Any of the intermediates in the biosynthesis of heme.

por·phy·ri·nu·ri·a (pôr'fə-rə-nŏŏr'ē-ə) *n.* The excretion of abnormal concentrations of porphyrins and related compounds in the urine. Also called *purpurinuria.*

por·ri·go (pə-rī'gō) *n.* Any of various diseases of the scalp.

por·ta (pôr'tə) *n.*, *pl.* **-tae** (-tē) 1. See **hilum.** 2. See **interventricular foramen.**

por·ta·ca·val (pôr'tə-kā'vəl) *adj.* Relating to the portal vein and the inferior vena cava.

portacaval shunt *n.* Any of various communications between the portal vein and the general circulation, especially a surgical anastomosis between the portal vein and the vena cava.

por·tal (pôr'tl) *adj.* 1. Of or relating to a porta or hilum. 2. Of or relating to the portal vein or the portal system. 3. Of or relating to a point of entrance to an organ, especially the transverse fissure of the liver, through which the blood vessels enter. —*n.* 1. The portal vein. 2. The point of entry into the body of a pathogenic microorganism.

portal canal *n.* Any of the various spaces in the liver that contain connective tissue and the branchings of the bile ducts, portal vein, hepatic artery, nerves, and lymphatics.

portal circulation *n.* Circulation of blood to the liver from the small intestine via the portal vein.

portal cirrhosis *n.* See **Laënnec's cirrhosis.**

portal fissure *n.* A transverse fissure on the visceral surface of the liver between the caudate and quadrate lobes, lodging the portal vein, hepatic artery, hepatic nerve plexus, hepatic ducts, and lymphatic vessels. Also called *caudal transverse fissure.*

portal hypertension *n.* Hypertension in the portal system as seen in cirrhosis of the liver and other conditions causing obstruction to the portal vein.

portal lobule of liver *n.* A polygonal mass of liver tissue that at its center has a portal canal and at its periphery several central hepatic veins.

portal system *n.* A system of vessels in which blood, after passing through one capillary bed, is conveyed through a second capillary network.

portal-systemic encephalopathy *n.* Encephalopathy associated with cirrhosis of the liver, attributed to the passage of toxic nitrogenous substances from the portal to the systemic circulation. Also called *hepatic encephalopathy.*

portal vein *n.* A wide short vein that is formed by the superior mesenteric and splenic veins behind the pancreas, ascends in front of the inferior vena cava, and divides into right and left branches that ramify within the liver. Also called *hepatic portal vein.*

Por·ter (pôr'tər), **Rodney Robert** 1917–1985. British biochemist. He shared a 1972 Nobel Prize for his research on the chemical structure and nature of antibodies.

Por·ter's sign (pôr'tərz) *n.* An indication of aneurysm of the aortic arch marked by pulsation of the trachea when the cricoid cartilage of the larynx is drawn upward with the thumb and forefinger while the individual sits with the head thrown back and mouth closed.

por·ti·o (pôr'shē-ō', -tē-ō') *n.*, *pl.* **-ti·o·nes** (-shē-ō'nēz, -tē-) A part or segment, as of an organ.

portio su·pra·vag·i·na·lis (sŏō'prə-văj'ə-nā'lĭs) *n.* The part of the cervix of the uterus lying above the attachment of the vagina.

portio vag·i·na·lis (văj'ə-nā'lĭs) *n.* The part of the cervix of the uterus within the vagina.

porto– *pref.* Portal: *portosystemic.*

por·to·bil·i·o·ar·te·ri·al (pôr'tō-bĭl'ē-ō-är-tîr'ē-əl) *adj.* Relating to the portal vein, the biliary ducts, and the hepatic artery.

por·to·en·ter·os·to·my (pôr'tō-ĕn'tə-rŏs'tə-mē) *n.* A surgical procedure for the treatment of biliary atresia in which a Roux-en-Y anastomosis is connected to the hepatic end of the divided extravascular portal structures, including the rudimentary bile ducts. Also called *Kasai operation.*

por·to·gram (pôr′tə-grăm′) *n.* A radiographic image obtained by portography.

por·tog·ra·phy (pôr-tŏg′rə-fē) *n.* X-ray visualization of the portal circulation using radiopaque material introduced into the spleen or into the portal vein.

por·to·sys·tem·ic (pôr′tō-sĭ-stĕm′ĭk) *adj.* Relating to connections between the portal and systemic venous systems.

port-wine stain (pôrt′wīn′) *n.* A purplish area of the skin, usually on the head and neck, appearing at birth and caused by an overgrowth of the cutaneous capillaries. Also called *nevus flammeus, port-wine mark.*

po·rus (pôr′əs) *n., pl.* **po·ri** (pôr′ī) A pore, meatus, or foramen.

po·si·tion (pə-zĭsh′ən) *n.* **1.** A place occupied. **2.** A bodily attitude or posture, especially a posture assumed by a patient to facilitate the performance of diagnostic, surgical, or therapeutic procedures. **3.** The relation of an arbitrarily chosen portion of the fetus to the right or left side of the mother. —**position** *v.* —**po·si′tion·al** *adj.*

positional nystagmus *n.* A nystagmus occurring only when the head is in a particular position.

position effect *n.* Variation in the expression of a gene that results from changes in the gene's position along a chromosome.

position sense *n.* See **posture sense.**

pos·i·tive (pŏz′ĭ-tĭv) *adj.* **1.** Characterized by or displaying certainty, acceptance, or affirmation. **2.** Indicating the presence of a particular disease, condition, or organism. **3.** Indicating or characterized by response or motion toward the source of a stimulus, such as light. **4.** Relating to or designating electric charge of a sign opposite to that of an electron. —**pos′i·tiv′i·ty** *n.*

positive accommodation *n.* Accommodation for near vision by contraction of the ciliary muscles of the eye.

positive convergence *n.* The inward deviation of the visual axes.

positive declination *n.* See **extorsion** (sense 2).

positive electron *n.* See **positron.**

positive end-expiratory pressure *n. Abbr.* **PEEP** A technique used in respiratory therapy in which pressure is maintained in the airway so that the lungs empty less completely in expiration.

positive-negative pressure breathing *n. Abbr.* **PNPB** Inflation of the lungs with positive pressure and deflation with negative pressure as through the action of an automatic ventilator.

positive scotoma *n.* A scotoma that is perceived as a black spot within the field of vision.

positive stain *n.* Direct binding of a dye with a tissue component to produce contrast.

pos·i·tron (pŏz′ĭ-trŏn′) *n.* A positively charged particle of the same mass and magnitude of charge as an electron. Also called *antielectron, positive electron.*

positron emission tomography *n. Abbr.* **PET** Tomography in which a computer-generated image of local metabolic and physiological functions in tissues is produced through the detection of gamma rays that are emitted when introduced radionuclides decay and release positrons.

po·sol·o·gy (pə-sŏl′ə-jē, pō-) *n.* The medical or pharmacological study of the dosages of medicines and drugs. —**po′so·log′ic** (pō′sə-lŏj′ĭk) *adj.*

post– *pref.* **1.** After; later: *postpartum.* **2.** Behind; posterior to: *postaxial.*

post·ad·re·nal·ec·to·my syndrome (pōst′ə-drē′nə-lĕk′tə-mē) *n.* See **Nelson syndrome.**

post·ax·i·al (pōst-ăk′sē-əl) *adj.* **1.** Posterior to the axis of the body or to the axis of a limb in the anatomical position. **2.** Of or being the portion of a limb bud lying caudal to the axis of the limb.

post·bra·chi·al (pōst-brā′kē-əl, -brăk′ē-) *adj.* On or in the posterior part of the upper arm.

post·cap·il·lar·y venule (pōst-kăp′ə-lĕr′ē) *n.* Microvasculature that is sensitive to histamines and is the site of extravasation of blood cells. Also called *pericytic venule.*

post·ca·va (pōst-kā′və) *n.* See **inferior vena cava.** —**post·ca′val** *adj.*

post·cen·tral area (pōst-sĕn′trəl) *n.* The cortex of the postcentral gyrus

postcentral gyrus *n.* The anterior convolution of the parietal lobe, bounded in front by the central sulcus and in back by the interparietal sulcus.

postcentral sulcus *n.* The sulcus that demarcates the postcentral gyrus from the superior and inferior parietal lobules.

post·ci·bal (pōst-sī′bəl) *adj.* Following a meal; postprandial.

post·co·i·tal (pōst-kō′ĭ-tl, -kō-ēt′l) *adj.* Following coitus. —**post·co′i·tal·ly** *adv.*

post·co·i·tus (pōst-kō′ĭ-təs, -kō-ē′-) *n.* The period immediately after coitus.

post·com·mis·sur·ot·o·my syndrome (pōst-kŏm′ə-shoō-rŏt′ə-mē, -soō-) *n.* A syndrome of uncertain cause appearing within a few weeks after an operation on a cardiac valve, characterized by fever, chest pain, pericardial rub or effusion, and pleural rub or effusion.

post·cor·di·al (pōst-kôr′dē-əl) *adj.* Posterior to the heart.

post·cos·tal anastomosis (pōst-kŏs′tl) *n.* The longitudinal connection of the seven intersegmental arteries in an embryo that gives rise to the vertebral artery.

post·cra·ni·al (pōst-krā′nē-əl) *adj.* **1.** Situated behind the cranium. **2.** Consisting of the parts or structures behind the cranium.

post·cu·bi·tal (pōst-kyoō′bĭ-tl) *adj.* On or in the posterior or dorsal part of the forearm.

post·duct·al (pōst-dŭk′təl) *adj.* Relating to that part of the aorta distal to the aortic opening of the arterial canal.

post·em·bry·on·ic (pōst′ĕm-brē-ŏn′ĭk) *adj.* Following the embryonic stage of development.

pos·te·ri·or (pŏ-stîr′ē-ər, pō-) *adj.* **1.** Located behind a part or toward the rear of a structure. **2.** Relating to the caudal end of the body in quadrupeds or the dorsal side in humans. **3.** Near the tail or caudal end of certain embryos.

posterior ampullar nerve *n.* A branch of the vestibular part of the eighth cranial nerve that supplies the ampullary crest of the posterior semicircular duct of the ear.

posterior asynclitism *n.* See **Litzmann obliquity**.

posterior auricular nerve *n.* A branch of the facial nerve, which supplies the posterior auricular and intrinsic muscles of the auricle and, through its occipital branch, innervates the occipital belly of the occipitofrontal muscle.

posterior auricular vein *n.* A tributary to the external jugular vein, draining the region behind the ear.

posterior cardinal vein *n.* Any of the major drainage channels from the caudal part of an embryo.

posterior cerebral commissure *n.* A thin band of white matter crossing from side to side beneath the habenula of the pineal body and over the entrance to the cerebral aqueduct and largely composed of fibers connecting mesoencephalic regions.

posterior chamber of eye *n.* The ringlike space filled with aqueous humor between the iris, the crystalline lens, and the ciliary body.

posterior column of spinal cord *n.* The dorsolateral ridge of gray matter in each lateral half of the spinal cord. Also called *dorsal column of spinal cord*.

posterior condyloid foramen *n.* See **condylar canal**.

posterior cord of brachial plexus *n.* A fasciculus formed by the posterior divisions of the upper, middle, and lower trunks and giving rise to the subscapular, thoracodorsal, axillary, and radial nerves.

posterior cruciate ligament *n.* *Abbr.* **PCL** The cruciate ligament of the knee that crosses from the posterior intercondylar area of the tibia to the anterior part of the medial condyle of the femur.

posterior cutaneous nerve of arm *n.* A branch of the radial nerve supplying the skin of the posterior surface of the arm.

posterior cutaneous nerve of forearm *n.* A branch of the radial nerve supplying the skin of the dorsal surface of the forearm.

posterior cutaneous nerve of thigh *n.* A nerve that arises from the first three sacral nerves and supplies the skin of the posterior surface of the thigh and of the popliteal region.

posterior embryotoxon *n.* A congenital defect of the eye characterized by an enlarged anterior limiting ring.

posterior ethmoidal nerve *n.* The posterior branch of the nasociliary nerve.

posterior facial vein *n.* See **retromandibular vein**.

posterior focal point *n.* The point on the retina where parallel light rays entering the eye are focused.

posterior funiculus *n.* The large wedge-shaped fiber bundle composed largely of dorsal root fibers.

posterior horn *n.* **1.** The occipital division of the lateral ventricle of the brain, extending backward into the occipital lobe. Also called *dorsal horn*. **2.** The posterior gray column of the spinal cord in cross section. Also called *dorsal horn*.

posterior intercostal vein *n.* Any of the veins draining the intercostal spaces posteriorly.

posterior interosseous nerve *n.* The deep terminal branch of the radial nerve, supplying the supinator and all the extensor muscles in the forearm.

posterior labial nerve *n.* Any of the terminal branches of the perineal nerve, supplying the skin of the posterior portion of the labia majora and the vestibule of the vagina.

posterior labial vein *n.* Any of the veins that pass from the labia majora to the internal pudendal veins.

posterior lacrimal crest *n.* A vertical ridge on the orbital surface of the lacrimal bone that together with the anterior lacrimal crest bounds the fossa for the lacrimal sac.

posterior lateral nasal artery *n.* Any of the arteries that are branches of the sphenopalatine artery and supply the posterior parts of the conchae and the lateral nasal wall.

posterior limiting ring *n.* A circular bundle of the sclera of the eye at the level of the termination of the deep trabeculae. Also called *Schwalbe's ring*.

posterior lobe of hypophysis *n.* See **neurohypophysis**.

posterior median fissure *n.* See **posterior median sulcus**.

posterior median line *n.* The line of intersection of the midsagittal plane with the posterior surface of the body.

posterior median sulcus *n.* The longitudinal groove marking the posterior midline of the medulla oblongata and continuous below with the posterior median sulcus of the spinal cord. Also called *posterior median fissure*.

posterior nasal spine *n.* The sharp posterior extremity of the nasal crest.

posterior palatine foramen *n.* See **greater palatine foramen**.

posterior perforated substance *n.* The bottom of the interpeduncular fossa at the base of the mesencephalon, containing openings for the passage of perforating branches of cerebral arteries.

posterior pyramid of medulla *n.* See **fasciculus gracilis**.

posterior rhinoscopy *n.* Examination of the nasopharynx and posterior portion of the nasal cavity using a rhinoscope or a nasopharyngoscope.

posterior root *n.* See **dorsal root**.

posterior scalene muscle *n.* A muscle with origin from the fourth to the sixth cervical vertebrae, with insertion into the second rib, with nerve supply from the cervical and brachial plexuses, and whose action elevates the second rib.

posterior scleritis *n.* Scleritis that exhibits a tendency to extend posteriorly to the sheath of eyeball and to cause chemosis.

posterior scrotal nerve *n.* Any of several terminal branches of the perineal nerve supplying the skin of the rear portion of the scrotum.

posterior scrotal vein *n.* Any of the veins passing from the scrotum to the internal pudendal veins.

posterior septal artery of nose *n.* A branch of the sphenopalatine artery, supplying the nasal septum and accompanying the nasopalatine nerve.

posterior spinocerebellar tract *n.* A compact bundle of heavily myelinated fibers that is located at the periphery of the dorsal half of the lateral funiculus of the spinal cord, consists of thick fibers originating in the thoracic nucleus on the same side of the cord, terminates in the vermis, and conveys proprioceptive information.

posterior staphyloma *n.* A bulging of a weakened sclera at the posterior of the eyeball resulting from loss of the choroid lining.

posterior supraclavicular nerve *n.* See **lateral supraclavicular nerve.**

posterior synechia *n.* Adhesion of the iris to the capsule of the lens.

posterior tibial muscle *n.* A muscle with origin from the posterior surface of the tibia, the head and shaft of the fibula, and the posterior surface of the interosseous membrane; with insertion into the navicular, the three cuneiform, the cuboid, and the second, third, and fourth metatarsal bones; with nerve supply from the tibial nerve, and whose action causes the plantar flexion and inversion of the foot.

posterior tibial vein *n.* One of two veins that accompany the posterior tibial artery and terminate into the popliteal vein.

posterior vein of left ventricle *n.* A vein that arises on the diaphragmatic surface of the heart near the apex, runs to the left and parallel to the posterior interventricular sulcus, and empties in the coronary sinus.

posterior vein of septum pel·lu·ci·dum (pə-lōo′sĭ-dəm) *n.* A vein that drains the rear part of the septum pellucidum.

postero– *pref.* Posterior: *posterosuperior.*

pos·ter·o·an·te·ri·or (pŏs′tə-rō-ăn-tîr′ē-ər) *adj. Abbr.* **PA 1.** Relating to both back and front. **2.** In x-ray imaging, taken or viewed from back to front through the body.

pos·ter·o·ex·ter·nal (pŏs′tə-rō-ĭk-stûr′nəl) *adj.* In back and to the outer side.

pos·ter·o·in·fe·ri·or (pŏs′tə-rō-ĭn-fîr′ē-ər) *adj.* In back and below.

pos·ter·o·in·ter·nal (pŏs′tə-rō-ĭn-tûr′nəl) *adj.* In back and to the inner side.

pos·ter·o·lat·er·al (pŏs′tə-rō-lăt′ər-əl) *adj.* In back and away from the middle line.

posterolateral groove *n.* A longitudinal furrow located on either side of the posterior median sulcus of the spinal cord and medulla oblongata and marking the line of entrance of the posterior nerve roots.

pos·ter·o·me·di·al (pŏs′tə-rō-mē′dē-əl) *adj.* In back and toward the middle line.

pos·ter·o·me·di·an (pŏs′tə-rō-mē′dē-ən) *adj.* In back and in the central line.

pos·ter·o·su·pe·ri·or (pŏs′tə-rō-sōo-pîr′ē-ər) *adj.* In back and above.

post·es·trus (pōst-ĕs′trəs) *or* **post·es·trum** (-trəm) *n.* The period in the estrus cycle following estrus, characterized by the growth of the corpus luteum and physiological changes related to the production of progesterone.

post·ex·tra·sys·tol·ic pause (pōst′ĕk-strə-sĭ-stŏl′ĭk) *n.* The somewhat prolonged cycle in the heartbeat immediately following an extrasystole.

postextrasystolic T wave *n.* The T wave of the sinus beat immediately following an extrasystole.

post·fron·tal (pōst-frŭn′tl) *adj.* **1.** At the back of the frontal bone; behind the forehead. **2.** Toward the rear of the frontal lobe.

post·gan·gli·on·ic (pōst′găng-glē-ŏn′ĭk) *adj.* Located posterior or distal to a ganglion.

postganglionic motor neuron *n.* A motor neuron that forms a synapse with one or more preganglionic motor neurons, is located outside the central nervous system, and has its unmyelinated axon ending in smooth muscle, cardiac muscle, or a gland. Also called *ganglionic motor neuron, peripheral motor neuron.*

post·gas·trec·to·my syndrome (pōst′gă-strĕk′tə-mē) *n.* See **dumping syndrome.**

post·hep·a·tit·ic cirrhosis (pōst′hĕp-ə-tĭt′ĭk) *n.* See **active chronic hepatitis.**

pos·thi·o·plas·ty (pŏs′thē-ə-plăs′tē) *n.* Reparative or plastic surgery of the prepuce.

pos·thi·tis (pŏs-thī′tĭs) *n.* Inflammation of the prepuce.

pos·tho·lith (pŏs′thə-lĭth′) *n.* A calculus occurring beneath the foreskin.

post·hyp·not·ic (pōst′hĭp-nŏt′ĭk) *adj.* Following hypnotism.

posthypnotic suggestion *n.* A suggestion made to a hypnotized person that specifies an action to be performed after awakening, often in response to a cue.

post·hy·po·gly·ce·mic hyperglycemia (pōst′hī-pō-glī-sē′mĭk) *n.* See **Somogyi effect.**

post·ic·tal (pōst-ĭk′təl) *adj.* Following a seizure.

post·ma·ture (pōst′mə-chŏor′, -tŏor′) *adj.* Remaining in the uterus longer than the normal gestational period.

post·men·o·paus·al (pōst′mĕn-ə-pô′zəl) *adj.* Of or occurring in the time following menopause.

post·men·stru·al (pōst-mĕn′strōo-əl) *adj.* Of or occurring in the time following menstruation.

post·mor·tem (pōst-môr′təm) *adj.* Relating to or occurring during the period after death. —*n.* See **autopsy.**

postmortem delivery *n.* The extraction of a fetus after its mother has died.

postmortem examination *n.* See **autopsy.**

postmortem livedo *n.* A purple coloration of the skin, except in areas of contact pressure, appearing within one half to two hours after death, as a result of gravitational movement of blood within the vessels. Also called *postmortem lividity.*

postmortem rigidity *n.* See **rigor mortis.**

postmortem wart *n.* A tuberculous warty growth that can occur on the hand of an individual who performs postmortem examinations. Also called *anatomical wart, dissection tubercle, necrogenic wart, verruca necrogenica.*

post·na·sal (pōst-nā′zəl) *adj.* **1.** Located or occurring posterior to the nose or the nasal cavity. **2.** Relating to the posterior portion of the nasal cavity.

postnasal drip *n.* The chronic secretion of mucus from the posterior nasal cavities.

post·na·tal (pōst-nāt′l) *adj.* Of or occurring after birth, especially in the period immediately after birth.

post·ne·crot·ic cirrhosis (pōst′nə-krŏt′ĭk) *n.* Cirrhosis characterized by necrosis involving whole lobules, with the collapse of the reticular framework to form large scars; it may follow viral or toxic necrosis, or develop as a result of dietary deficiencies. Also called *necrotic cirrhosis.*

post·op *or* **post·op** (pōst′ŏp′) *adj.* Postoperative. Used informally.

post·op·er·a·tive (pōst-ŏp′ər-ə-tĭv, -ŏp′rə-, -ŏp′ə-rā′-) *adj.* Happening or done after a surgical operation.

post·o·ral (pōst-ôr′əl) *adj.* Situated behind or at the back of the mouth.

postoral arch *n.* Any of the series of branchial arches caudal to the mouth.

post·or·bit·al (pōst-ôr′bĭ-tl) *adj.* Situated behind the socket of the eye.

post·o·vu·la·to·ry (pōst-ō′vyə-lə-tôr′ē, -ŏv′yə-) *adj.* Of or occurring in the period shortly after ovulation.

post·par·tum (pōst-pär′təm) *adj.* Of or occurring in the period shortly after childbirth.

postpartum hemorrhage *n.* Hemorrhage from the birth canal in excess of 500 milliliters during the first 24 hours after birth.

postpartum pituitary necrosis syndrome *n.* See **Sheehan's syndrome.**

postpartum psychosis *n.* An acute mental disorder occurring in the mother following childbirth.

postpartum tetanus *n.* See **puerperal tetanus.**

post·per·fu·sion lung (pōst′pər-fyoo′zhən) *n.* A condition in which abnormal pulmonary function develops in individuals who have undergone cardiac surgery involving the use of an extracorporeal circulation system.

post·per·i·car·di·ot·o·my syndrome (pōst-pĕr′ĭ-kär′dē-ŏt′ə-mē) *n.* The occurrence of the symptoms of pericarditis, with or without fever and often in repeated episodes, after cardiac surgery.

post·po·li·o syndrome (pōst-pō′lē-ō′) *n.* A condition occurring most often in individuals who contracted severe cases of polio before age 10 and characterized by fatigue, exhaustion, muscle weakness, painful joints, and occasionally difficult breathing.

post·pran·di·al (pōst-prăn′dē-əl) *adj.* Following a meal, especially dinner. —**post·pran′di·al·ly** *adv.*

postprandial lipemia *n.* See **alimentary lipemia.**

post·pu·ber·al (pōst-pyoo′bər-əl) *or* **post·pu·ber·tal** (-bər-tl) *adj.* Postpubescent.

post·pu·bes·cent (pōst′pyoo-bĕs′ənt) *adj.* Occurring after puberty.

post·sphyg·mic (pōst-sfĭg′mĭk) *adj.* Occurring after the pulse wave.

postsphygmic interval *n.* The interval in the cardiac cycle following the sphygmic interval to the opening of the atrioventricular valves. Also called *postsphygmic period.*

post·syn·ap·tic (pōst′sĭ-năp′tĭk) *adj.* Situated behind or occurring after a synapse.

postsynaptic membrane *n.* The part of the cell membrane of a neuron or muscle fiber with which an axon terminal forms a synapse.

post-term infant (pōst′tûrm′) *n.* An infant born after the 42nd week of gestation.

post·tib·i·al (pōst-tĭb′ē-əl) *adj.* On or in the posterior portion of the leg.

post·trans·fu·sion (pōst′trăns-fyoo′zhən) *adj.* Occurring after or as a consequence of blood transfusion.

post·trau·mat·ic (pōst′-trô-măt′ĭk, -trou-) *adj.* Following or resulting from injury or trauma.

posttraumatic epilepsy *n.* A convulsive epileptic seizure that occurs as a result of a head injury.

posttraumatic neck syndrome *n.* A syndrome characterized by pain, tenderness, tight neck musculature, vasomotor instability, and other symptoms, such as dizziness and blurred vision, resulting from injury to the neck.

posttraumatic stress disorder *n. Abbr.* **PTSD** An anxiety disorder affecting individuals who have experienced or witnessed profoundly traumatic events, such as torture, rape, military combat, or a natural disaster, characterized by recurrent flashbacks of the traumatic event, nightmares, anxiety, fatigue, forgetfulness, and social withdrawal. Also called *posttraumatic stress syndrome.*

posttraumatic syndrome *n.* A syndrome characterized by headache, dizziness, neurasthenia, hypersensitivity to stimuli, and diminished concentration, caused by injury to the head.

pos·tu·late (pŏs′chə-lāt′) *v.* To assume or assert the truth or necessity of, especially as a basis of an argument. —*n.* An unproved assertion or assumption, especially a statement offered as the basis of a theory. —**pos′tu·la′tion** *n.*

pos·tur·al (pŏs′chər-əl) *adj.* Relating to or involving posture.

postural contraction *n.* The maintenance of muscular tension sufficient to maintain posture.

postural drainage *n.* A therapeutic technique for drainage, used in bronchiectasis and lung abscess, in which the patient is placed head downward so that the trachea is down and below the affected area.

postural hypotension *n.* See **orthostatic hypotension.**

postural position *n.* See **physiologic rest position.**

postural proteinuria *n.* Proteinuria associated with body position, such as orthostatic proteinuria.

postural syncope *n.* A syncope that occurs upon assuming an upright position and is caused by inadequate blood flow to the brain resulting from failure of normal vasoconstrictive mechanisms.

postural vertigo *n.* Vertigo that occurs with a change of position, usually when moving from a lying or sitting to a standing position.

pos·ture (pŏs′chər) *n.* **1.** A position of the body or of body parts. **2.** A characteristic or prescribed way of bearing one's body; carriage.

posture sense *n.* The ability to recognize the position in which a limb is passively placed without visual perception. Also called *position sense.*

post·vac·ci·nal encephalitis (pōst-văk′sə-nəl, -văk-sē′-) *n.* Demyelinating encephalitis following vaccination.

post·val·var (pōst-văl′vər) *or* **post·val·vu·lar** (-văl′vyə-lər) *adj.* Relating to a position distal to the pulmonary or aortic valves.

post·ver·te·bral (pōst-vûr′tə-brəl, pōst′vər-tē′-) *adj.* Situated behind the vertebrae.

po·ta·ble (pō′tə-bəl) *adj.* Fit to drink; drinkable.

pot·ash (pŏt′ăsh′) *n.* **1.** Any of several compounds containing potassium, especially soluble compounds such as potassium oxide and various potassium sulfates, used chiefly in fertilizers. **2.** See **potassium carbonate. 3.** See **potassium hydroxide.**

po·tas·si·um (pə-tăs′ē-əm) *n. Symbol* **K** A soft, highly or explosively reactive metallic element that occurs in nature only in compounds and is found in or converted to a wide variety of salts used especially in fertilizers and soaps. Its radioisotopes are used in various diagnostic studies, including myocardial scans, detection and localization of tumors, determination of intracellular fluid space, and determination of renal blood flow. Atomic number 19. Also called *kalium.* —**po·tas′-sic** *adj.*

potassium-40 *n.* A naturally occurring beta-emitting radioactive isotope of potassium having a half-life of 1.3 billion years; it is the chief source of natural radioactivity of living tissue.

potassium-42 *n.* An artificially produced beta-emitting isotope of potassium having a half-life of 12.36 hours; it is used as a radioactive tracer in studies of potassium distribution in bodily fluids.

potassium-43 *n.* An artificially produced beta-emitting isotope of potassium having a half-life of 22 hours; it is used as a radioactive tracer in myocardial perfusion studies.

potassium bicarbonate *n.* A compound in the form of a white powder or colorless crystals, used in baking powder and as an antacid medicine.

potassium bitartrate *n.* A white, acid, crystalline solid or powder used as a component of laxatives.

potassium bromide *n.* A white crystalline solid or powder used as a sedative.

potassium carbonate *n.* A transparent, white, deliquescent, granular powder used in making soaps. Also called *potash.*

potassium chlorate *n.* A poisonous crystalline compound used as an oxidizing agent and disinfectant.

potassium chloride *n.* A colorless crystalline solid or powder, KCl, used in various pharmaceutical preparations to correct potassium deficiency.

potassium hydroxide *n.* A caustic white solid used as a bleach and in the manufacture of soaps, dyes, and many potassium compounds. Also called *potash.*

potassium iodide *n.* A white crystalline compound used as a source of iodine to treat thyrotoxic crisis and to prevent thyroid cancer in the event of overexposure to nuclear radiation. It is also used as an expectorant and antifungal.

potassium permanganate *n.* A dark purple crystalline compound used as an oxidizing agent and disinfectant and in deodorizers and dyes.

potassium sodium tartrate *n.* A colorless efflorescent crystalline compound used as a laxative. Also called *Rochelle salt, Seignette's salt.*

pot·bel·ly (pŏt′bĕl′ē) *n.* A protruding abdominal region.

po·ten·cy (pōt′n-sē) *n.* **1.** The quality or condition of being potent. **2.** The pharmacological activity of a compound.

po·tent (pōt′nt) *adj.* **1.** Exerting or capable of exerting strong physiological or chemical effects. **2.** Able to perform sexual intercourse. Used of a male.

po·ten·tial (pə-tĕn′shəl) *adj.* Capable of being but not yet in existence; latent. —*n.* **1.** The inherent ability or capacity for growth, development, or coming into being. **2.** The work required to bring a unit electric charge, magnetic pole, or mass from an infinitely distant position to a designated point in a static electric, magnetic, or gravitational field, respectively. **3.** The potential energy of a unit charge at any point in an electric circuit measured with respect to a specified reference point in the circuit or to ground; voltage.

potential cautery *n.* An agent, such as potassium hydroxide, that causes the formation of an eschar by chemical means. Also called *virtual cautery.*

potential energy *n.* The energy that exists in a body as a result of its position or condition rather than of its motion.

po·ten·ti·ate (pə-tĕn′shē-āt′) *v.* **1.** To make potent or powerful. **2.** To enhance or increase the effect of a drug. **3.** To promote or strengthen a biochemical or physiological action or effect. —**po·ten′ti·a′tion** *n.*

po·tion (pō′shən) *n.* A liquid medicinal dose or drink.

Pott (pŏt), **Percivall** 1714–1788. British surgeon who helped replace the extensive use of escharotics and cautery in surgical procedures with more humane methods and described various pathologic conditions, including Pott's fracture.

Pot·ter's facies (pŏt′ərz) *n.* The facial appearance characteristic of bilateral renal agenesis and other severe renal malformations, consisting of ocular hypertelorism, low-set ears, receding chin, and flattening of the nose.

Potter's syndrome *n.* A combination of birth defects characterized by the absence of one or both kidneys, underdeveloped lungs, and Potter's facies, and resulting in neonatal respiratory distress, circulatory abnormalities, acidosis, cyanosis, edema, and death.

Pott's abscess (pŏts) *n.* A tuberculous abscess of the spine.

Pott's disease *n.* See **tuberculous spondylitis.**

Pott's fracture *n.* A fracture of the lower part of the fibula and of the bony prominence near the ankle joint, causing the foot to turn out.

Potts' operation *n.* Direct side-to-side anastomosis between the aorta and the pulmonary artery as a palliative procedure in congenital malformation of the heart.

pouch (pouch) *n.* A pocketlike space in the body.

pou·drage (poo-dräzh′) *n.* The surgical application of powder, such as the dusting of opposing pleural surfaces with a slightly irritating powder in order to secure adhesion.

poul·tice (pōl′tĭs) *n.* A soft moist adhesive mass, as of meal or clay, that is usually heated, spread on cloth, and applied to warm, moisten, or stimulate an aching or inflamed part of the body. Also called *cataplasm.* —**poul′tice** *v.*

pound (pound) *n.* **1.** A unit of weight that is the basis of the avoirdupois system, equal to 16 ounces or 453.592 grams. **2.** A unit of apothecary weight equal to 12 ounces or 373.242 grams.

Pou·part's ligament (poo-pärz′) *n.* See **inguinal ligament.**

Poupart's line *n.* An imaginary perpendicular line passing through the center of the inguinal ligament on either side.

po·vi·done (pō′vĭ-dōn′) *n.* A polymer used as a vehicle for drugs, especially iodine.

povidone iodine *n.* A topical preparation containing povidone and iodine, used for antisepsis of the skin.

Pow·as·san encephalitis (pə-wä′sən) *n.* An acute disease of children varying clinically from undifferentiated febrile illness to encephalitis, caused by a tickborne virus.

pow·der (pou′dər) *n.* **1.** A dry mass of pulverized or finely dispersed solid particles. **2.** Any of various medicinal or cosmetic preparations in the form of powder. **3.** A single dose of a powdered drug.

pow·er (pou′ər) *n.* **1.** The capacity to perform or act effectively. **2.** Strength or force that is exerted or that is capable of being exerted. **3.** The amount of work done per unit time. **4.** A measure of the magnification of an optical instrument, such as a microscope or telescope.

pox (pŏks) *n.* **1.** A disease such as chickenpox or smallpox, characterized by purulent skin eruptions that may leave pockmarks. **2.** Syphilis.

Pox·vir·i·dae (pŏks-vîr′ĭ-dē′) *n.* A family of large complex DNA viruses, including the vaccinia and variola viruses, that are pathogenic to humans and animals and have an affinity for skin tissue.

pox·vi·rus (pŏks′vī′rəs) *n.* A virus of the family Poxviridae.

PP *abbr.* pyrophosphate

ppb *abbr.* parts per billion

PPCA *abbr.* proserum prothrombin conversion accelerator

PPD *abbr.* purified protein derivative of tuberculin

PPLO *abbr.* pleuropneumonialike organism

ppm *abbr.* parts per million

PPO *abbr.* preferred provider organization

PPPPPP *abbr.* pain, pallor, paresthesia, pulselessness, paralysis, and prostration (symptom complex of acute arterial occlusion)

ppt *abbr.* parts per thousand; parts per trillion

P-pul·mo·na·le (-pool′mə-nā′lē, -pŭl′-) *n.* An electrocardiographic syndrome marked by tall, narrow, peaked P waves, presumed to be characteristic of cor pulmonale.

Pr The symbol for the element **praseodymium**.

PRA *abbr.* plasma renin activity

prac·ti·cal nurse (prăk′tĭ-kəl) *n.* **1.** A licensed practical nurse. **2.** A person who has had practical experience in nursing care but who is not a graduate of a degree program in nursing.

prac·tice (prăk′tĭs) *v.* To engage in the profession of medicine or one of the allied health professions. —*n.* **1.** The exercise of the profession of medicine. **2.** The business of a practicing physician or group of physicians, including facilities and customary patients.

prac·ti·tion·er (prăk-tĭsh′ə-nər) *n.* One who practices medicine or an allied health profession.

Pra·der-Wil·li syndrome (prä′dər-wĭl′ē, prä′dər-vĭl′ē) *n.* A congenital syndrome of unknown cause characterized by short stature, mental retardation, excessive eating and obesity, and sexual infantilism.

prag·mat·ag·no·si·a (prăg′mə-tăg-nō′zē-ə, -zhə) *n.* Loss of the power of recognizing objects.

prag·mat·am·ne·sia (prăg′mə-tăm-nē′zhə) *n.* Loss of the memory of the appearance of objects.

prag·ma·tism (prăg′mə-tĭz′əm) *n.* A way of approaching situations or solving problems that emphasizes practical applications and consequences. —**prag·mat′·ic** (-măt′ĭk) *adj.* —**prag′ma·tist** *n.*

Prague maneuver (präg) *n.* A method for delivering a fetus in breech position in which the infant's shoulders are grasped from below by one hand while the other hand supports the legs.

Prague pelvis *n.* See **spondylolisthetic pelvis.**

pram·i·pex·ole (prăm′ĭ-pĕk′sōl′) *n.* A dopamine agonist used to treat Parkinson's disease.

pran·di·al (prăn′dē-əl) *adj.* Of or relating to a meal.

pra·se·o·dym·i·um (prā′zē-ō-dĭm′ē-əm, prä′sē-) *n.* *Symbol* **Pr** A soft malleable ductile rare-earth element that develops a characteristic green tarnish in air and is used to color glass and ceramics yellow and in metallic alloy. Atomic number 59.

Praus·nitz-Küst·ner reaction (prous′nĭts-küst′nər) *n.* A reaction based on passive transfer of allergic sensitivity in which serum from an allergic individual is injected into cutaneous sites on a normal individual and the injected sites are then exposed to antigens to which the donor is allergic; the cutaneous sites show a characteristic wheal-and-flare reaction.

Prav·a·chol (prăv′ə-kōl′) A trademark for the drug pravastatin.

prav·a·stat·in (prăv′ə-stăt′n) *n.* A statin drug used to treat hyperlipidemia.

Prax·ag·o·ras (prăk-săg′ər-əs) 4th century BC. Greek physician who was the first to distinguish between arteries and veins.

prax·e·ol·o·gy *or* **prax·i·ol·o·gy** (prăk′sē-ŏl′ə-jē) *n.* The study of human conduct.

pra·zi·quan·tel (prā′zĭ-kwän′tĕl′) *n.* A synthetic heterocyclic broad-spectrum anthelmintic agent effective against parasitic schistosome species as well as most other trematodes and adult cestodes.

pra·zo·sin (prā′zō-sĭn) *n.* A crystalline vasodilator used in the form of its hydrochloride as a treatment for hypertension.

pre– *pref.* **1.** Earlier; before; prior to: *prenatal.* **2.** Anterior; in front of: *preaxial.*

pre·ad·o·les·cence (prē′ăd-l-ĕs′əns) *n.* The period of childhood just preceding the onset of puberty, often designated as between the ages of 10 and 12 in girls and 11 and 13 in boys.

pre·a·dult (prē′ə-dŭlt′) *adj.* Of or relating to the period preceding adulthood or the adult stage of the life cycle.

pre·ag·o·nal (prē-ăg′ə-nəl) *adj.* Immediately preceding death.

pre·an·es·thet·ic (prē′ăn-ĭs-thĕt′ĭk) *adj.* Before anesthesia.

pre·an·ti·sep·tic (prē′ăn-tĭ-sĕp′tĭk) *adj.* Of or being the period in the history of medicine and surgery before the adoption of the principles of antisepsis.

pre·a·sep·tic (prē′ə-sĕp′tĭk, -ā-sĕp′-) *adj.* Of or being the period in the history of medicine and surgery when the principles of asepsis were not yet known or adopted.

pre·au·to·mat·ic pause (prē′ô-tə-măt′ĭk) *n.* A temporary pause in cardiac activity before an escape in an artificial pacemaker.

pre·ax·i·al (prē-ăk′sē-əl) *adj.* **1.** Situated in front of or superior to the median axis of the body or a body part. **2.** Of or being the portion of a limb bud lying cranial to the axis of the limb. —**pre·ax′i·al·ly** *adv.*

pre·can·cer (prē′kăn′sər) *n.* A lesion from which a malignant tumor is presumed to develop in a significant number of instances and that may or may not be recognizable clinically or by microscopic changes in the affected tissue.

pre·can·cer·ous (prē-kăn′sər-əs) *adj.* Of, relating to, or being a condition or lesion that typically precedes or develops into a cancer.

pre·cap·il·lar·y (prē-kăp′ə-lĕr′ē) *adj.* Preceding a capillary. Used of an arteriole or venule.

pre·car·ti·lage (prē-kär′tl-ĭj) *n.* A closely packed aggregation of mesenchymal cells just prior to their differentiation into embryonic cartilage.

pre·ca·va (prē-kā′və, -kä′-) *n., pl.* **–vae** (-vē) See **superior vena cava.** —**pre·ca′val** *adj.*

pre·cen·tral area (prē-sĕn′trəl) *n.* The cortex of the precentral gyrus.

precentral cerebellar vein *n.* An unpaired vein that originates in the precentral cerebellar fissure, passes before and above the culmen, and ends in the great cerebral vein.

precentral gyrus *n.* The posterior convolution of the frontal lobe, bounded in back by the central sulcus and in front by the precentral sulcus.

precentral sulcus *n.* An interrupted fissure anterior to and generally parallel with the central sulcus, marking the anterior border of the precentral gyrus.

pre·cep·tor (prĭ-sĕp′tər, prē′sĕp′tər) *n.* An expert or specialist, such as a physician, who gives practical experience and training to a student, especially of medicine or nursing.

pre·cep·tor·ship (prĭ-sĕp′tər-shĭp′) *n.* A period of practical experience and training for a student, especially of medicine or nursing, that is supervised by an expert or specialist in a particular field.

pre·cip·i·ta·ble (prĭ-sĭp′ĭ-tə-bəl) *adj.* Capable of being precipitated.

pre·cip·i·tant (prĭ-sĭp′ĭ-tənt) *n.* A substance that causes a precipitate to form when it is added to a solution.

pre·cip·i·tate (prĭ-sĭp′ĭ-tāt′, -tĭt) *n.* **1.** A solid or solid phase separated from a solution. **2.** A punctate opacity on the posterior surface of the cornea developing from inflammatory cells in the vitreous body. Also called *punctate keratitis.* —*v.* (-tāt′) **1.** To cause a solid substance to be separated from a solution. **2.** To be separated from a solution as a solid.

precipitate labor *n.* Labor that results in rapid expulsion of the fetus.

pre·cip·i·ta·tion (prĭ-sĭp′ĭ-tā′shən) *n.* The process of separating a substance from a solution as a solid.

pre·cip·i·tin (prĭ-sĭp′ĭ-tĭn) *n.* An antibody that under suitable conditions combines with and causes a specific soluble antigen to precipitate.

pre·cip·i·tin·o·gen (prĭ-sĭp′ĭ-tĭn′ə-jən) *n.* An antigen that stimulates the formation of specific precipitin

when injected into an animal body; a precipitable soluble antigen.

precipitin test *n.* A serologic test in which antibody reacts with a specific soluble antigen to form a precipitate. Also called *precipitin reaction.*

pre·clin·i·cal (prē-klĭn′ĭ-kəl) *adj.* **1.** Of or relating to the period of a disease before the appearance of symptoms. **2.** Of or being a period in medical education before the student is involved with patients and clinical work.

pre·co·cious (prĭ-kō′shəs) *adj.* Showing unusually early development or maturity. —**pre·coc′ity** (-kŏs′ĭ-tē), **pre·co′cious·ness** *n.*

precocious puberty *n.* A condition in which the changes associated with puberty begin at an unexpectedly early age, often caused by a pathological process involving a glandular secretion of estrogens or androgens.

pre·cog·ni·tion (prē′kŏg-nĭsh′ən) *n.* Knowledge of something in advance of its occurrence, especially by extrasensory perception. —**pre·cog′ni·tive** *adj.*

pre·col·lag·e·nous fiber (prē′kə-lăj′ə-nəs) *n.* An immature argyrophilic fiber.

pre·con·cep·tu·al stage (prē′kən-sĕp′chōō-əl) *n.* The stage of development in an infant's life in which sensorimotor activity predominates.

pre·con·scious (prē-kŏn′shəs) *n.* See **foreconscious.**

pre·con·vul·sive (prē′kən-vŭl′sĭv) *adj.* Of, relating to, or being the stage in an epileptic paroxysm preceding convulsions.

pre·cor·di·a (prē-kôr′dē-ə) *pl.n.* The precordium.

precordial lead (lēd) *n.* **1.** A lead of an electrocardiograph that has one electrode placed in any of six standard positions on the chest and another electrode placed on a limb. **2.** A record obtained from such a lead. Also called *chest lead.*

pre·cor·di·um (prē-kôr′dē-əm) *n.* The part of the body comprising the epigastrium and anterior surface of the lower thorax. —**pre·cor′di·al** *adj.*

pre·cos·tal anastomosis (prē-kŏs′tl) *n.* The longitudinal connection of intersegmental arteries in an embryo that gives rise to the thyrocervical and costocervical trunks.

pre·cu·ne·us (prē-kyōō′nē-əs) *n., pl.* **–ne·i** (-nē-ī′) A division of the medial surface of each cerebral hemisphere between the cuneus and the paracentral lobule. Also called *quadrate lobe.* —**pre·cu′ne·ate** (-āt′, -ĭt) *adj.*

pre·cur·sor (prĭ-kûr′sər, prē′kûr′sər) *n.* **1.** One that precedes and indicates something to come. **2.** One that precedes another; a forerunner or predecessor. **3.** A biochemical substance, such as an intermediate compound in a chain of enzymatic reactions, that gives rise to a more stable or definitive product.

pre·cur·so·ry cartilage (prĭ-kûr′sə-rē) *n.* See **temporary cartilage.**

pre·de·cid·u·al (prē′dĭ-sĭj′ōō-əl) *adj.* Of or relating to the premenstrual or secretory phase of the menstrual cycle.

pre·den·tin (prē-dĕn′tən) *n.* The organic fibrillar matrix of the dentin before its calcification.

pre·di·a·be·tes (prē′dī-ə-bē′tĭs, -tēz) *n.* The condition of having a hereditary tendency or high probability for developing diabetes mellitus, although neither symptoms nor test results confirm the presence of the disease.

pre·di·as·to·le (prē-dī-ăs′tə-lē) *n.* The interval in the cardiac rhythm immediately preceding diastole. Also called *late systole.* —**pre′di·as·tol′ic** (-dī-ə-stŏl′ĭk) *adj.*

pre·dic·tive value (prĭ-dĭk′tĭv) *n.* The likelihood that a positive test result indicates disease or that a negative test result excludes disease.

pre·di·gest (prē′dī-jĕst′, -dĭ-) *v.* To subject food to partial digestion, usually through an enzymatic or chemical process, before being eaten. —**pre′di·ges′tion** *n.*

pre·dis·pose (prē′dĭ-spōz′) *v.* To make susceptible, as to a disease.

pre·dis·po·si·tion (prē′dĭs-pə-zĭsh′ən) *n.* 1. The state of being predisposed. 2. A condition of special susceptibility, as to a disease.

pred·nis·o·lone (prĕd-nĭs′ə-lōn′) *n.* A synthetic steroid similar to hydrocortisone and used in various compounds as an anti-inflammatory, immunosuppressive, antiallergic, and anticancer drug.

pred·ni·sone (prĕd′nĭ-sōn′, -zōn′) *n.* A synthetic steroid similar to cortisone that is used as an antiallergic, immunosuppressive, and anticancer drug and as an anti-inflammatory agent in the treatment of rheumatoid arthritis.

pre·duct·al (prē-dŭk′təl) *adj.* Of or relating to the part of the aorta proximal to the aortic opening of the arterial canal.

pre·e·clamp·si·a (prē′ĭ-klămp′sē-ə) *n.* A disorder occurring during late pregnancy or immediately following parturition, characterized by hypertension, edema, and proteinuria. —**pre′e·clamp′tic** (-tĭk) *adj.*

pre·e·jec·tion period (prē′ĭ-jĕk′shən) *n.* The interval in the electrocardiogram between the onset of the QRS complex and cardiac ejection.

pre·em·bry·o (prē-ĕm′brē-ō′) *n.* A fertilized ovum up to 14 days old, before uterine implantation.

pree·mie *or* **pre·mie** (prē′mē) *n.* A prematurely born infant.

pre·ex·ci·ta·tion (prē′ĕk-sī-tā′shən) *n.* Premature activation of part of the ventricular myocardium by an impulse that travels by an anomalous path and so avoids physiological delay in the atrioventricular junction.

preexcitation syndrome *n.* See **Wolff-Parkinson-White syndrome.**

pre·ferred provider organization (prĭ′fûrd′) *n. Abbr.* **PPO** A medical insurance plan in which members receive more coverage if they choose health care providers approved by or affiliated with the plan.

pre·fron·tal (prē-frŭn′tl) *adj.* 1. Of, relating to, or situated in the anterior part of the frontal lobe. 2. Situated anterior to the frontal bone.

prefrontal area *n.* See **frontal cortex.**

prefrontal lobotomy *n.* A lobotomy in which the white fibers that connect the thalamus to the prefrontal and frontal lobes of the brain are severed, performed as a treatment for intense anxiety or violent behavior.

pre·gan·gli·on·ic (prē-găng′glē-ŏn′ĭk) *adj.* Situated proximal to or preceding a ganglion, especially a ganglion of the autonomic nervous system.

preganglionic motor neuron *n.* A motor neuron having a cell body located in the brain or spinal cord and a myelinated axon that travels out of the central nervous system as part of a cranial or spinal nerve before separating and extending into the autonomic ganglion.

Pregl (prā′gəl), **Fritz** 1869–1930. Austrian chemist. He won a 1923 Nobel Prize for his development of a method of analyzing organic substances weighing one milligram or less.

preg·nan·cy (prĕg′nən-sē) *n.* 1. The condition of a woman or female mammal from conception until birth; the condition of being pregnant. 2. The period during which a woman or female mammal is pregnant. Also called *cyesis.*

pregnancy gingivitis *n.* Inflammatory changes in the gum tissue appearing during pregnancy.

preg·nane (prĕg′nān′) *n.* A crystalline steroid hydrocarbon that is the parent compound of corticosteroids and progesterones.

preg·nane·di·ol (prĕg′nān-dī′ôl) *n.* A steroid metabolite of progesterone that is biologically inactive; a form of the compound occurs in the urine of pregnant women.

preg·nane·di·one (prĕg′nān-dī′ōn) *n.* An unsoluble metabolite of progesterone formed in relatively small quantities and occurring in either of two isomeric configurations: alpha or beta.

preg·nane·tri·ol (prĕg′nān-trī′ôl) *n.* A urinary metabolite of 17-alpha-hydroxyprogesterone and a precursor in the biosynthesis of cortisol; its excretion increases in certain diseases of the adrenal cortex and following administration of corticotropin.

preg·nant (prĕg′nənt) *adj.* Carrying developing offspring within the body.

pre·hen·sile (prē-hĕn′səl, -sīl′) *adj.* Adapted for seizing, grasping, or holding, especially by wrapping around an object. —**pre′hen·sil′i·ty** (-sīl′ĭ-tē) *n.*

pre·hen·sion (prē-hĕn′shən) *n.* The act of grasping or seizing.

pre·hor·mone (prē-hôr′mōn′) *n.* A glandular secretory product that is a precursor of a hormone but has little or no inherent biological potency itself.

pre·ic·tal (prē-ĭk′təl) *adj.* Occurring before a convulsion or stroke.

pre·im·plan·ta·tion diagnosis (prē-ĭm′plăn-tā′shən) *n.* A procedure in which embryos generated using in vitro fertilization techniques can be screened for the presence of the gene for a particular characteristic or defect prior to uterine implantation.

pre·load (prē′lōd′) *n.* The load to which a muscle is subjected before shortening.

Pre·log (prĕl′ōg′), **Vladimir** 1906–1998. Bosnian-born Swiss chemist. He shared a 1975 Nobel Prize for research on the structure of biological molecules.

pre·log·i·cal thinking (prē-lŏj′ĭ-kəl) *n.* A form of concrete thinking characteristic of children, to which schizophrenic persons are sometimes said to regress.

Prelone (prē′lōn′) A trademark for the drug prednisolone.

pre·ma·lig·nant (prē′mə-lĭg′nənt) *adj.* Precancerous.

Prem·a·rin (prĕm′ə-rĭn′) A trademark for a drug preparation of conjugated estrogens.

pre·ma·ture (prē′mə-chŏŏr′, -tŏŏr′) *adj.* **1.** Occurring or developing before the usual or expected time. **2.** Born after a gestation period of less than the normal time, especially, in human infants, after a period of less than 37 weeks. —**pre′ma·tu′ri·ty** *n.*

premature atrial contraction *n. Abbr.* **PAC** An ectopic heartbeat that originates in the atria and precedes a typical atrial contraction.

premature birth *n.* The birth of an infant after the period of viability but before full term.

premature delivery *n.* The birth of a premature baby.

premature ejaculation *n.* During sexual intercourse, more rapid achievement of climax and ejaculation in the male than he or his partner wishes. Also called *prospermia.*

premature labor *n.* The onset of labor before the 37th completed week of pregnancy.

premature-senility syndrome *n.* See **progeria.**

premature systole *n.* See **extrasystole.**

premature ventricular contraction *n. Abbr.* **PVC** An extrasystole involving the ventricles of the heart, sometimes producing accompanying palpitations.

pre·max·il·la (prē′măk-sĭl′ə) *n.* Either of two bones located in front of and between the maxillary bones in the upper jaw of vertebrates.

pre·max·il·lar·y bone (prē-măk′sə-lĕr′ē) *n.* See **incisive bone.**

pre·med (prē′mĕd′) *adj.* Premedical.

pre·med·i·cal (prē-mĕd′ĭ-kəl) *adj.* Preparing for or relating to the studies that prepare one for the study of medicine.

pre·med·i·ca·tion (prē′mĕd-ĭ-kā′shən) *n.* **1.** Administration of drugs prior to anesthesia to allay apprehension, produce sedation, and facilitate the administration of anesthesia to the patient. **2.** A drug or drugs used for such purposes.

pre·me·no·paus·al (prē′mĕn-ə-pô′zəl) *adj.* Of or relating to the years or the stage of life immediately before the onset of menopause.

pre·men·stru·al (prē-mĕn′strŏŏ-əl) *adj.* Of or occurring in the period just before menstruation.

premenstrual dysphoric disorder *n. Abbr.* **PMDD** A severe form of premenstrual syndrome, characterized by affective symptoms causing significant disturbances in relationships or social adaptation, with symptoms ceasing shortly after the onset of menstrual bleeding.

premenstrual syndrome *n. Abbr.* **PMS** A group of symptoms, including abdominal bloating, breast tenderness, headache, fatigue, irritability, and depression, that occur in many women from 2 to 14 days before the onset of menstruation. Also called *premenstrual tension.*

pre·men·stru·um (prē-mĕn′strŏŏ-əm) *n.* The period just preceding menstruation.

pre·mie (prē′mē) *n.* Variant of **preemie.**

pre·mo·lar (prē-mō′lər) *n.* Any of eight bicuspid teeth located in pairs on each side of the upper and lower jaws behind the canines and in front of the molars. Also called *bicuspid.*

pre·mon·o·cyte (prē-mŏn′ə-sīt′) *n.* An immature monocyte not normally present in the blood. Also called *promonocyte.*

pre·mor·bid (prē-môr′bĭd) *adj.* Preceding the occurrence of disease.

Prem·pro (prĕm′prō′) A trademark for a drug combination of conjugated estrogens and medroxyprogesterone acetate, used for postmenopausal hormone replacement therapy.

pre·mu·ni·tion (prē′myŏŏ-nĭsh′ən) *n.* See **infection immunity.** —**pre·mune′** (prē-myŏŏn′) *adj.* —**pre·mu′ni·tive** *adj.*

pre·my·e·lo·blast (prē-mī′ə-lə-blăst′) *n.* The earliest recognizable precursor of the myeloblast.

pre·my·e·lo·cyte (prē-mī′ə-lə-sīt′) *n.* See **myeloblast.**

pre·na·tal (prē-nāt′l) *adj.* Preceding birth. Also called *antenatal.*

pre·ne·o·plas·tic (prē′nē-ə-plăs′tĭk) *adj.* Preceding the formation of a benign or malignant neoplasm.

PR enzyme (pē′är′) *n.* See **phosphorylase phosphatase.**

pre-op *or* **pre·op** (prē′ŏp′) *adj.* Preoperative. Used informally.

pre·op·er·a·tive (prē-ŏp′ər-ə-tĭv, -ŏp′rə-, -ŏp′ə-rā′-) *adj.* Preceding a surgical operation.

pre·o·ral (prē-ôr′əl) *adj.* Situated or located in front of the mouth.

pre·os·te·o·blast (prē-ŏs′tē-ə-blăst′) *n.* See **osteoprogenitor cell.**

pre·ox·y·gen·a·tion (prē′ŏk-sĭ-jə-nā′shən) *n.* Administration of pure oxygen prior to induction of general anesthesia in order to eliminate nitrogen from the lungs and body tissues.

prep (prĕp) *v.* To prepare for a medical examination or surgical procedure.

prep·a·ra·tion (prĕp′ə-rā′shən) *n.* A substance, such as a medicine, prepared for a particular purpose.

pre·pa·tel·lar bursitis (prē′pə-tĕl′ər) *n.* See **housemaid's knee.**

pre·pat·ent period (prē-păt′nt, -pāt′nt) *n.* The interval between infection of an individual by a parasitic organism and the first ability to detect from that host a diagnostic stage of the organism.

pre·po·ten·tial (prē′pə-tĕn′shəl) *n.* The slow depolarization of a cell membrane that occurs between action potentials.

pre·psy·chot·ic (prē′sī-kŏt′ĭk) *adj.* **1.** Relating to the period prior to the onset of psychosis. **2.** Of or being a mental state or condition having the potential to elicit a psychotic episode.

pre·pu·ber·al (prē-pyŏŏ′bər-əl)*or* **pre·pu·ber·tal** (-bər-təl) *adj.* Before puberty; prepubescent.

pre·pu·ber·ty (prē-pyŏŏ′bər-tē) *n.* The period of life immediately before puberty, often marked by accelerated physical growth.

pre·pu·bes·cence (prē′pyŏŏ-bĕs′əns) *n.* Prepuberty.

pre·pu·bes·cent (prē′pyŏŏ-bĕs′ənt) *adj.* Of or characteristic of prepuberty. —*n.* A prepubescent child.

pre·puce (prē′pyŏŏs′) *n.* **1.** See **foreskin. 2.** A loose fold of skin covering the glans clitoridis.

pre·pu·tial (prē-pyŏŏ′shəl) *adj.* Of or relating to the prepuce.

preputial gland *n.* Any of the small sebaceous glands of the corona of the penis and the inner surface of the prepuce that secrete smegma.

pre·pu·ti·ot·o·my (prē-pyoo'shē-ŏt'ə-mē) *n.* Incision of the prepuce.

pre·pu·ti·um (prē-pyoo'shē-əm) *n.,* pl. **–ti·a** (-shē-ə) The prepuce.

pre·py·lo·ric vein (prē'pī-lôr'ĭk, -pĭ-) *n.* A tributary of the right gastric vein that passes anteriorly to the pylorus at its junction with the duodenum.

pre·sa·cral neurectomy (prē-sā'krəl) *n.* Surgical removal of the presacral plexus to relieve severe dysmenorrhea. Also called *Cotte's operation, presacral sympathectomy.*

pres·by·a·cu·sis (prĕz'bē-ə-kyoo'sĭs) *or* **pres·by·a·cu·sia** (-zhə) *n.* Hearing loss occurring as part of the aging process. Also called *presbycusis.*

pres·by·at·rics (prĕz'bē-ăt'rĭks) *n.* See **geriatrics.**

pres·by·cu·sis (prĕz'bĭ-kyoo'sĭs) *n.* See **presbyacusis.**

presbyo– *or* **presby–** *pref.* Old age: *presbyopia.*

pres·by·ope (prĕz'bē-ōp') *n.* A person affected with presbyopia.

pres·by·o·pi·a (prĕz'bē-ō'pē-ə) *n.* Inability of the eye to focus sharply on nearby objects, resulting from loss of elasticity of the crystalline lens with advancing age. —**pres'by·op'ic** (-ŏp'ĭk, -ō'pĭk) *adj.*

pre·scribe (prĭ-skrīb') *v.* To give directions, either orally or in writing, for the preparation and administration of a remedy to be used in the treatment of a disease.

pre·scrip·tion (prĭ-skrĭp'shən) *n.* **1.** An order, especially by a physician, for the preparation and administration of a medicine, therapeutic regimen, assistive or corrective device, or other treatment. **2.** A prescribed medicine.

pres·ence of mind (prĕz'əns) *n.* The ability to think and act calmly and efficiently, especially in an emergency situation.

pre·se·nile (prē-sē'nīl', -sĕn'īl') *adj.* **1.** Of or characteristic of the period prior to the usual onset of senility. **2.** Affected with presenility.

presenile dementia *n.* **1.** Any of various forms of dementia developing before old age. **2.** Alzheimer's disease. No longer in technical use.

pre·se·nil·i·ty (prē'sĭ-nĭl'ĭ-tē) *n.* The condition of one affected with the physical and mental characteristics of old age at an abnormally young age.

pre·sent (prĭ-zĕnt') *v.* **1.** To appear or be felt first during birth. Used of the part of the fetus that proceeds first through the birth canal. **2.** To place oneself in the presence of a doctor or other medical provider as a patient with a complaint or condition. **3.** To manifest a symptom. **4.** To attach or be capable of attaching to a cell surface, especially for detection by other molecules.

pres·en·ta·tion (prĕz'ən-tā'shən, prē'zən-) *n.* **1.** The act of presenting. **2.** The position of the fetus in the uterus at the beginning of labor, described in terms of the part that emerges or is felt first. **3.** The part of the fetal body in advance during birth.

pre·sent·a·tive (prĭ-zĕn'tə-tĭv) *n.* **1.** Having the capacity or function of bringing an idea or image to mind. **2.** Perceived or capable of being perceived directly rather than through association. **3.** Having the ability to so perceive.

pre·ser·va·tive (prĭ-zûr'və-tĭv) *n.* A substance added to food products or to organic solutions to prevent decomposition due to chemical change or bacterial action.

pre·so·mite (prē-sō'mīt') *adj.* Relating to the embryonic stage before the appearance of somites.

pre·sphyg·mic (prē-sfĭg'mĭk) *adj.* Of or being the brief interval following the filling of the ventricles of the heart with blood and preceding the pulse beat.

presphygmic interval *n.* The brief period at the beginning of the ventricular systole during which the pressure rises before the semilunar valves open. Also called *presphygmic period.*

pres·sor (prĕs'ôr', -ər) *adj.* **1.** Producing increased blood pressure. **2.** Causing constriction of the blood vessels.

pressor base *n.* **1.** Any of several products of intestinal putrefaction believed to cause hypertension when absorbed. Also called *pressor amine.* **2.** An alkaline substance that raises blood pressure.

pres·so·re·cep·tive (prĕs'ō-rĭ-sĕp'tĭv) *adj.* Capable of receiving as stimuli changes in pressure, especially changes of blood pressure.

pres·so·re·cep·tor (prĕs'ō-rĭ-sĕp'tər) *n.* See **baroreceptor.**

pressor fiber *n.* Any of the sensory nerve fibers that cause vasoconstriction and a rise in blood pressure on stimulation.

pressor nerve *n.* An afferent nerve that when stimulated causes the constriction of a blood vessel, thereby raising the blood pressure.

pres·so·sen·si·tive (prĕs'ō-sĕn'sĭ-tĭv) *adj.* Pressoreceptive.

pres·sure (prĕsh'ər) *n.* **1.** The act of pressing or condition of being pressed. **2.** A stress or force acting in any direction against resistance. **3.** Force applied uniformly over a surface, measured as force per unit of area.

pressure dressing *n.* A dressing that exerts pressure on the area covered to prevent the collection of fluids in the underlying tissues, usually used after skin grafting and in the treatment of burns.

pressure epiphysis *n.* A secondary center of ossification that forms at the articular end of a long bone.

pressure paralysis *n.* Paralysis due to compression of a nerve or nerve trunk or the spinal cord.

pressure point *n.* **1.** Any of the various locations on the body where pressure may be applied to control bleeding. **2.** A point that is extremely sensitive to the application of pressure.

pressure reversal *n.* Cessation of anesthesia by hyperbaric pressure.

pressure sense *n.* The ability to discriminate various degrees of pressure on the surface of one's body.

pressure sore *n.* See **bedsore.**

pressure-volume index *n.* A method of evaluating the dynamics of cerebrospinal fluid.

pre·ster·num (prē-stûr'nəm) *n.* See **episternum.**

presumed ocular histoplasmosis (prĭ-zoomd') *n.* Hemorrhagic chorioretinitis of the macular region associated with chorioretinal atrophy.

pre·sup·pu·ra·tive (prē-sŭp'yə-rā'tĭv) *adj.* Of or being an early stage of inflammation prior to the formation of pus.

pre·syn·ap·tic (prē′sĭ-năp′tĭk) *adj*. Relating to the area on the proximal side of a synaptic gap.

presynaptic membrane *n*. The part of the cell membrane of an axon terminal that faces the cell membrane of the neuron or muscle fiber with which the axon terminal establishes a synapse.

pre·sys·to·le (prē-sĭs′tə-lē) *n*. The interval in the cardiac rhythm immediately preceding systole. —**pre′sys·tol′ic** (-sĭ-stŏl′ĭk) *adj*.

presystolic gallop *n*. A gallop rhythm in which an abnormal fourth heart sound occurs in late diastole.

presystolic murmur *n*. A murmur heard at the end of ventricular diastole, during atrial systole, usually due to obstruction at an atrioventricular orifice.

presystolic thrill *n*. A thrill sometimes felt on palpation over the apex of the heart, immediately before the ventricular contraction.

pre·tar·sal (prē-tär′səl) *adj*. Of, relating to, or being the front or lower portion of the tarsus.

pre·teen (prē′tēn′) *adj*. **1.** Relating to or designed for children especially between the ages of 10 and 12. **2.** Being a child especially between the ages of 10 and 12; preadolescent. —*n*. A preteen boy or girl.

pre·term (prē′tûrm′, prē-tûrm′) *adj*. Occurring or appearing before the expected time at the end of a full-term pregnancy. —*n*. An infant born prematurely.

preterm infant *n*. An infant born before the 37th week of gestation.

pre·tib·i·al fever (prē-tĭb′ē-əl) *n*. A mild disease caused by *Leptospira autumalis* and characterized by fever, splenomegaly, and a rash on the front of the legs. Also called *Fort Bragg fever.*

pretibial myxedema *n*. See **circumscribed myxedema**.

Prev·a·cid (prĕv′ə-sĭd′) A trademark for the drug lansoprazole.

prev·a·lence (prĕv′ə-ləns) *n*. The total number of cases of a disease in a given population at a specific time.

pre·ven·tive (prĭ-vĕn′tĭv) *or* **pre·ven·ta·tive** (-tə-tĭv) *adj*. Preventing or slowing the course of an illness or disease; prophylactic. —*n*. A preventive agent or treatment.

preventive dentistry *n*. The branch of dentistry that deals with the preservation of healthy teeth and gums and the prevention of dental caries and oral disease.

preventive medicine *n*. The branch of medical science concerned with the prevention of disease and the promotion of physical and mental health through the study of the etiology and epidemiology of disease processes.

preventive treatment *n*. See **prophylactic treatment**.

pre·ver·te·bral ganglia (prē-vûr′tə-brəl, prē′vər-tē′brəl) *n*. Any of the sympathetic ganglions lying in front of the vertebral column, including the celiac, aorticorenal, and the superior and inferior mesenteric ganglions.

pre·vi·us (prē′vē-əs) *adj*. Of or relating to the blockage of passages in childbirth; obstructing.

PRF *abbr.* prolactin-releasing factor

pri·a·pic (prī-ā′pĭk, -ăp′ĭk) *or* **pri·a·pe·an** (prī′ə-pē′ən) *adj*. **1.** Of, relating to, or resembling a phallus; phallic. **2.** Relating to or excessively concerned with masculinity.

pri·a·pism (prī′ə-pĭz′əm) *n*. Persistent, usually painful erection of the penis, especially as a consequence of disease and not related to sexual arousal.

Price-Jones curve (prīs′jōnz′) *n*. A curve indicating the distribution of red blood cells with respect to the length of their diameters.

prick·le cell (prĭk′əl) *n*. An epidermal cell that, as a histological artifact, develops numerous intercellular bridges that give it a prickly appearance.

prickle cell layer *n*. The layer of polyhedral cells in the epidermis. Also called *spinous layer.*

prick·ly heat (prĭk′lē) *n*. See **heat rash**.

pril·o·caine (prĭl′ō-kān′) *n*. A local anesthetic used in its hydrochloride form for nerve blocks and in combination with lidocaine for topical use.

Pri·lo·sec (prī′lō-sĕk′) A trademark for the drug omeprazole.

pri·mal (prī′məl) *adj*. **1.** Being first in time; original. **2.** Of first or central importance; primary. —**pri·mal′i·ty** (-măl′ĭ-tē) *n*.

primal scene *n*. In psychoanalysis, the actual or imagined observation by a child of sexual intercourse, particularly between the parents.

primal therapy *n*. A method of psychotherapy that encourages patients to identify and relive early traumatic experiences and to release anger and other painful emotions by aggressive behaviors such as screaming.

pri·mar·y (prī′mĕr′ē, -mə-rē) *adj*. **1.** Being first or highest in importance; principal. **2.** Occurring first in time or sequence; earliest. **3.** Preliminary to a later stage of development; primordial; embryonic. **4.** Immediate; direct. **5.** Of, relating to, or being a sequence of amino acids in a protein.

primary adhesion *n*. See **healing by first intention**.

primary adrenocortical insufficiency *n*. Adrenocortical insufficiency caused by disease, destruction, or surgical removal of the adrenal cortices.

primary alcohol *n*. An alcohol containing the univalent organic radical CH_2OH.

primary aldosteronism *n*. Aldosteronism due to a tumor on the adrenal gland that causes excessive secretion of aldosterone. Also called *Conn's syndrome, idiopathic aldosteronism.*

primary amenorrhea *n*. Amenorrhea in which menstruation has never occurred.

primary amyloidosis *n*. A rare form of amyloidosis that is sometimes hereditary and is characterized by amyloid deposits in the heart, tongue, gastrointestinal tract, and skeletal muscle.

primary anesthetic *n*. The compound that contributes most to loss of sensation when a mixture of anesthetics is administered.

primary atelectasis *n*. Failure of the lungs to expand after birth, as in stillborn infants or in liveborn infants who die before respiration is established. Also called *anectasis.*

primary atypical pneumonia *n*. An acute systemic disease with involvement of the lungs, caused by *Mycoplasma pneumoniae* and marked by high fever and cough. Also called *atypical pneumonia, mycoplasmal pneumonia.*

primary brain vesicle *n*. See **cerebral vesicle**.

primary care *n.* The initial medical care given by a health care provider to a patient, especially as part of regular, ambulatory care, and sometimes followed by referral to other medical providers.

primary care physician *n. Abbr.* **PCP** A physician, such as a family practitioner or internist who is chosen by an individual to provide continuous medical care, trained to treat a wide variety of health-related problems, and responsible for referral to specialists as needed.

primary cataract *n.* A cataract occurring independently of any other disease of the eye.

primary coccidioidomycosis *n.* A disease caused by the inhalation of the conidia of *Coccidioides immitis* and producing symptoms that resemble pneumonia or pulmonary tuberculosis. Also called *desert fever.*

primary complex *n.* The typical lesions of primary pulmonary tuberculosis, consisting of a small peripheral focus of infection, with hilar or paratracheal lymph node involvement.

primary dentin *n.* Dentin that forms until the root is completed.

primary dentition *n.* **1.** The first set of teeth, 20 in all, that usually erupt between the sixth and 28th months. **2.** The eruption of the first set of teeth. Also called *deciduous dentition.*

primary deviation *n.* The deviation of an eye with a paralyzed muscle when the healthy eye focuses on an object.

primary digestion *n.* Digestion in the alimentary canal.

primary disease *n.* A disease arising spontaneously and not associated with or caused by a previous disease or injury.

primary drive *n.* See **physiological drive.**

primary dysmenorrhea *n.* Dysmenorrhea resulting from a functional disturbance and not to inflammation, growths, or anatomical factors. Also called *essential dysmenorrhea.*

primary fissure of cerebellum *n.* A deep V-shaped fissure that marks the upper surface of the cerebellum and separates the anterior lobe from the rest of the cerebellum.

primary gain *n.* Alleviation of anxiety that results from conversion of emotional conflict into demonstrably organic illnesses.

primary hemochromatosis *n.* A specific inherited metabolic defect characterized by increased absorption and accumulation of iron in the body tissues.

primary hemorrhage *n.* Hemorrhage immediately following an injury or operation.

primary herpetic stomatitis *n.* First infection of oral tissues with herpes simplex virus, characterized by gum inflammation, vesicles, and ulcers.

primary hyperoxaluria and oxalosis *n.* An inherited metabolic disorder characterized by the excretion of large amounts of oxalate in the urine and accompanied by nephrocalcinosis, nephrolithiasis, and extrarenal oxalosis.

primary lysosome *n.* A cytoplasmic body that is produced at the Golgi complex where hydrolytic enzymes are incorporated.

primary nondisjunction *n.* Nondisjunction occurring in a previously normal cell.

primary oocyte *n.* An oocyte that is in its growth phase and is at a stage that is prior to the completion of the first maturation division.

primary ovarian follicle *n.* An immature ovarian follicle in which the developing oocyte is surrounded by a layer or layers of cuboidal or columnar follicular cells.

primary pentosuria *n.* See **essential pentosuria.**

primary process *n.* In psychoanalysis, the mental process directly related to the functions of the id and characteristic of unconscious mental activity, marked by unorganized, illogical thinking and by the tendency to seek immediate discharge and gratification of instinctual demands.

primary pulmonary lobule *n.* A unit of pulmonary tissue that includes a bronchiole, alveolar ducts, sacs, and alveoli. Also called *respiratory lobule.*

primary reaction *n.* See **vaccinia** (sense 2).

primary sex characteristic *n.* Any of various anatomical structures, such as the testes or ovaries, concerned directly with reproduction.

primary spermatocyte *n.* The spermatocyte arising by a growth phase from a spermatogonium.

primary syphilis *n.* The first stage of syphilis, marked by formation of a painless chancre at the point of infection and by hardening and swelling of adjacent lymph nodes.

primary tooth *n.* See **deciduous tooth.**

primary tuberculosis *n.* Tuberculosis caused by infection with tubercle bacilli and characterized by the formation of a primary complex in the lungs consisting of a small peripheral pulmonary focus and hilar or paratracheal lymph node involvement; it may cavitate and heal with scarring or progress.

primary union *n.* See **healing by first intention.**

pri·mate (prī′māt′) *n.* A mammal of the order Primates, which includes the anthropoids and prosimians, that is characterized by refined development of the hands and feet, a shortened snout, and a large brain. —**pri·ma′tial** (-mā′shəl) *adj.*

prim·er (prī′mər) *n.* A segment of DNA or RNA that is complementary to a given DNA sequence and that is needed to initiate replication by DNA polymerase.

pri·mi·grav·i·da (prī′mĭ-grăv′ĭ-də) *n.* A woman in her first pregnancy.

pri·mip·a·ra (prī-mĭp′ər-ə) *n., pl.* **–a·ras** *or* **–a·rae** (-ə-rē′) **1.** A woman who is pregnant for the first time. **2.** A woman who has given birth for the first time to an infant or infants, alive or stillborn. —**pri′mi·par′i·ty** (-mĭ-păr′ĭ-tē) *n.* —**pri·mip′a·rous** *adj.*

prim·i·tive (prĭm′ĭ-tĭv) *adj.* **1.** Primary; basic. **2.** Of or being an earliest or original stage. **3.** Being little evolved from an early ancestral type.

primitive costal arch *n.* Any of the arches formed from the costal processes or elements that give rise to the ribs in the thoracic region of the embryonic vertebral column.

primitive furrow *n.* The groove in the primitive streak of the embryonic disk.

primitive node *n.* A knotlike thickening at the anterior end of the primitive streak of the blastoderm at the point of origin of the embryonic head. Also called *Hensen's node, primitive knot.*

primitive streak *n.* An ectodermal ridge in the midline at the caudal end of the embryonic disk from which the intraembryonic mesoderm arises.

pri·mor·di·al (prī-môr′dē-əl) *adj.* **1.** Being or happening first in sequence of time; primary; original. **2.** Belonging to or characteristic of the earliest stage of development of an organism or part. **3.** Relating to a primordium.

primordial ovarian follicle *n.* An ovarian follicle in which the primordial oocyte is surrounded by a single layer of flattened follicular cells.

pri·mor·di·um (prī-môr′dē-əm) *n., pl.* **–di·a** (-dē-ə) An aggregation of cells in the embryo indicating the first trace of an organ or structure.

prin·ceps (prĭn′sĕps′) *adj.* Principal; main. Used in anatomy to distinguish several arteries.

prin·ci·pal artery of thumb (prĭn′sə-pəl) *n.* An artery with origin in the radial artery, with distribution to the palmar surface and sides of the thumb, and with anastomoses to the arteries on the dorsum of the thumb.

principal optic axis *n.* A line extending through the center of a lens at a right angle to the lens surface.

principal point *n.* One of the two points in an optical system where the axis is cut by the two principal planes. Lines drawn from these to corresponding points on the object and the image will be parallel.

prin·ci·ple (prĭn′sə-pəl) *n.* **1.** A basic truth, law, or assumption. **2.** A rule or law concerning the functioning of natural phenomena or mechanical processes. **3.** One of the elements composing a chemical compound, especially one that gives some special quality or effect. **4.** The essential ingredient in a drug.

Prin·gle's disease (prĭng′gəlz) *n.* See **adenoma sebaceum.**

Prin·i·vil (prĭn′ə-vĭl′) A trademark for the drug lisinopril.

P-R interval *n.* The time elapsing between the beginning of the P wave and the beginning of the QRS complex in an electrocardiogram; it corresponds to the atriocarotid interval of the venous pulse.

Prinz·met·al's angina (prĭnz′mĕt′lz, prĭnts′-) *n.* Angina pectoris marked by pain that is not precipitated by cardiac work, is usually of longer duration, and is usually more severe. Also called *angina inversa.*

pri·on (prē′ŏn) *n.* A microscopic protein particle similar to a virus but lacking nucleic acid, possibly the infectious agent responsible for scrapie and other degenerative diseases of the nervous system.

prism (prĭz′əm) *n.* **1.** A solid figure whose bases or ends have the same size and shape and are parallel to one another, and each of whose sides is a parallelogram. **2.** A transparent body of this form, often of glass and usually with triangular ends, used for separating white light passed through it into a spectrum or for reflecting beams of light. **3.** Such a body used in testing or correcting imbalance of the extrinsic ocular muscles. —**pris·mat·ic** (-măt′ĭk) *adj.*

prism bar *n.* A graduated series of prisms mounted on a frame and used in ocular diagnosis.

prism diopter *n. Abbr.* **PD** The unit measuring the deflection of light passing through a prism equal to a deflection of 1 centimeter at a distance of 1 meter.

pris·on fever (prĭz′ən) *n.* See **typhus.**

pri·vate duty nurse (prī′vĭt) *n.* A nurse who is not a member of a hospital staff but is called upon to take special care of an individual patient.

private parts *pl.n.* The external organs of sex and excretion.

priv·i·leged site (prĭv′ə-lĭjd, prĭv′lĭjd) *n.* An area in the body lacking lymphatic drainage, such as the cornea of the eye, in which rejection of foreign tissue grafts does not occur.

PRL *abbr.* prolactin

p.r.n. *or* **PRN** *abbr. Latin* pro re nata (as the situation demands)

Pro *abbr.* proline

pro– *pref.* **1.** Earlier; before; prior to: *progenitor.* **2.** Rudimentary: *pronucleus.* **3.** Anterior; in front of: *procephalic.*

pro·ac·cel·er·in (prō′ăk-sĕl′ər-ĭn) *n.* See **factor V.**

pro·ac·ro·so·mal granule (prō′ăk-rə-sō′məl) *n.* One of the small carbohydrate-rich granules appearing in vesicles of the Golgi complex of spermatids and coalescing to form an acrosomal granule.

pro·ac·ti·va·tor (prō-ăk′tĭ-vā′tər) *n.* A substance that, when enzymatically split, yields a fragment capable of activating another substance or process.

pro·bac·te·ri·o·phage (prō′băk-tîr′ē-ə-fāj′) *n.* See **prophage.**

pro·band (prō′bănd′) *n.* An individual or member of a family being studied in a genetic investigation. Also called *index case, propositus.*

pro·bang (prō′băng′) *n.* A long, slender, flexible rod having a tuft or sponge at the end, used chiefly to remove foreign bodies from or apply medication to the larynx or esophagus.

probe (prōb) *n.* **1.** A slender, flexible surgical instrument with a blunt bulbous tip, used to explore a wound or body cavity. **2.** A substance, such as DNA, that is radioactively labeled or otherwise marked and used to detect or identify another substance in a sample. —*v.* To explore a wound or body cavity with a probe.

pro·ben·e·cid (prō-bĕn′ĭ-sĭd) *n.* A uricosuric drug derived from benzoic acid and used chiefly in the treatment of gout.

probe syringe *n.* A syringe with a slender elongated tip that may also be used as a probe, as in treatment of diseases of the lacrimal passages.

pro·bi·o·sis (prō′bī-ō′sĭs) *n.* An association of two organisms that enhances the life processes of both. —**pro·bi·ot·ic** (-bī-ŏt′ĭk) *adj.*

pro·bi·ot·ic (prō′bī-ŏt′ĭk) *n.* A dietary supplement containing live bacteria or yeast that supplements normal gastrointestinal flora, especially after depletion of flora caused by infection or ingestion of an antibiotic drug.

prob·lem·o·ri·ent·ed record (prŏb′ləm-ôr′ē-ĕn′tĭd) *n. Abbr.* **POR** A system of record keeping in which a list of the patient's problems is created and relevant medical history, physical findings, laboratory data, medications, and treatments are listed under the appropriate medical problem.

pro·caine (prō′kān′) *n.* A white crystalline powder that is used in its hydrochloride form as a local anesthetic.

pro·cap·sid (prō-kăp′sĭd) *n.* A protein shell lacking a virus genome.

pro·car·ba·zine (prō-kär′bə-zēn) *n.* A potent antineoplastic used in the treatment of advanced Hodgkin's disease.

pro·car·box·y·pep·ti·dase (prō′kär-bŏk′sē-pĕp′tĭ-dās′, -dāz′) *n.* The inactive precursor of a carboxypeptidase.

Pro·car·di·a (prō-kär′dē-ə) A trademark for the drug nifedipine.

pro·car·y·ote (prō-kăr′ē-ōt′) *n.* Variant of **prokaryote.** —**pro′car·y·ot′ic** (-ŏt′ĭk) *adj.*

pro·ce·dure (prə-sē′jər) *n.* **1.** A series of steps taken to accomplish an end. **2.** A surgical operation or technique.

pro·cen·tri·ole (prō-sĕn′trē-ōl′) *n.* The early phase in development of centrioles or basal bodies from the centrosphere.

pro·ce·phal·ic (prō′sə-făl′ĭk) *adj.* Relating to or located on or near the front of the head.

pro·cer·coid (prō-sûr′koid) *n.* The first stage in the aquatic life cycle of certain tapeworms following ingestion of the newly hatched larva by a copepod.

pro·ce·rus muscle (prō-sîr′əs) *n.* A muscle with origin from the membrane covering the bridge of the nose, with insertion into the frontal bone, with nerve supply from a branch of the facial nerve, and whose action assists the frontal bone.

proc·ess (prŏs′ĕs′, prō′sĕs′) *n., pl.* **proc·ess·es** (prŏs′-ĕs′ĭz, prō′sĕs′-, prŏs′ĭ-sēz′, prō′sĭ-) **1.** A series of actions, changes, or functions bringing about a result. **2.** Advance or progress, as of a disease. **3.** An outgrowth of tissue; a projecting part, as of a bone. —**proc′ess** *adj.* —**proc′ess** *v.*

process schizophrenia *n.* A severe form of schizophrenia in which chronic and progressive organic brain changes are considered the primary cause, and for which prognosis is poor.

pro·chlor·per·a·zine (prō′klôr-pâr′ə-zēn′) *n.* A phenothiazine drug used in the treatment of schizophrenia and nonpsychotic anxiety and as an antiemetic.

pro·chon·dral (prō-kŏn′drəl) *adj.* Of or relating to a stage of embryonic development that precedes formation of cartilage.

pro·chy·mo·sin (prō-kī′mə-sĭn) *n.* The precursor of chymosin. Also called *prorennin, renninogen.*

pro·ci·den·tia (prō′sĭ-dĕn′shə, prŏs′ĭ-) *n.* A sinking or prolapse of an organ or part.

pro·co·ag·u·lant (prō′kō-ăg′yə-lənt) *n.* **1.** The precursor of various blood factors necessary for coagulation. **2.** An agent that promotes blood coagulation.

pro·col·la·gen (prō-kŏl′ə-jən) *n.* The soluble precursor of collagen possibly formed by fibroblasts in the process of collagen synthesis.

pro·con·ver·tin (prō′kən-vûr′tn) *n.* See **factor VII.**

pro·cre·ate (prō′krē-āt′) *v.* **1.** To beget and conceive offspring; to reproduce. **2.** To produce or create; originate. —**pro′cre·a′tion** *n.*

pro·cre·a·tive (prō′krē-ā′tĭv) *adj.* **1.** Capable of reproducing; generative. **2.** Of or directed to procreation.

Pro·crit (prō′krĭt′) A trademark for the drug epoetin alfa.

proc·tal·gia (prŏk-tăl′jə) *n.* Pain at the anus or in the rectum. Also called *proctodynia, rectalgia.*

proc·ta·tre·sia (prŏk′tə-trē′zhə, -zhē-ə) *n.* See **anal atresia.**

proc·tec·ta·sia (prŏk′tĭk-tā′zhə) *n.* Dilation of the anus or rectum.

proc·tec·to·my (prŏk-tĕk′tə-mē) *n.* Surgical resection of the rectum. Also called *rectectomy.*

proc·teu·ryn·ter (prŏk′tyŏŏ-rĭn′tər) *n.* An inflatable bag used to dilate the rectum.

proc·ti·tis (prŏk-tī′tĭs) *n.* Inflammation of the rectum or anus. Also called *rectitis.*

procto– *or* **proct–** *pref.* Anus or rectum: *proctalgia.*

proc·to·cele (prŏk′tə-sēl′) *n.* **1.** Prolapse of the rectum. Also called *rectocele.* **2.** Herniation of the rectum. Also called *rectocele.*

proc·toc·ly·sis (prŏk-tŏk′lĭ-sĭs) *n., pl.* **–ses** (-sēz′) The slow, continuous, drop-by-drop administration of saline solution into the rectum and sigmoid colon. Also called *Murphy drip.*

proc·to·coc·cy·pex·y (prŏk′tō-kŏk′sə-pĕk′sē) *n.* Surgical fixation of a prolapsed rectum to the tissues anterior to the coccyx. Also called *rectococcypexy.*

proc·to·co·lec·to·my (prŏk′tō-kə-lĕk′tə-mē) *n.* The surgical removal of the rectum and all or part of the colon.

proc·to·co·lon·os·co·py (prŏk′tō-kō′lə-nŏs′kə-pē) *n.* Inspection of the interior of the rectum and the lower colon.

proc·to·col·po·plas·ty (prŏk′tō-kŏl′pə-plăs′tē) *n.* Surgical closure of a rectovaginal fistula.

proc·to·cys·to·plas·ty (prŏk′tō-sĭs′tə-plăs′tē) *n.* Surgical closure of a rectovesical fistula.

proc·to·cys·tot·o·my (prŏk′tō-sĭ-stŏt′ə-mē) *n.* Incision into the bladder from the rectum.

proc·to·de·al (prŏk′tə-dē′əl) *adj.* Of or relating to the proctodeum.

proc·to·de·um *or* **proc·to·dae·um** (prŏk′tə-dē′əm) *n., pl.* **–de·ums** *or* **–de·a** (-dē-ə) *or* **–dae·ums** *or* **–dae·a** (-dē-ə) An inward fold on the surface of the embryonic ectoderm that develops into part of the anal passage. Also called *anal pit.*

proc·to·dyn·i·a (prŏk′tə-dĭn′ē-ə) *n.* See **proctalgia.**

proc·tol·o·gy (prŏk-tŏl′ə-jē) *n.* The branch of medicine that deals with the diagnosis and treatment of disorders of the colon, rectum, and anus. —**proc′to·log′ic** (-tə-lŏj′ĭk) *adj.* —**proc·tol′o·gist** *n.*

proc·to·pa·ral·y·sis (prŏk′tō-pə-răl′ĭ-sĭs) *n.* Paralysis of the anus.

proc·to·pex·y (prŏk′tə-pĕk′sē) *n.* Surgical fixation of a prolapsed rectum. Also called *rectopexy.*

proc·to·plas·ty (prŏk′tə-plăs′tē) *n.* Reparative or plastic surgery of the anus or of the rectum. Also called *rectoplasty.*

proc·to·ple·gia (prŏk′tə-plē′jə) *n.* Paralysis of the anus and the rectum resulting from paraplegia.

proc·top·to·si·a (prŏk′tŏp-tō′sē-ə) *or* **proc·top·to·sis** (-tō′sĭs) *n.* Prolapse of the rectum and the anus.

proc·tor·rha·phy (prŏk-tôr′ə-fē) *n.* Surgical suturing of a lacerated rectum or anus.

proc·tor·rhe·a (prŏk′tə-rē′ə) *n.* A mucoserous discharge from the rectum.

proc·to·scope (prŏk′tə-skōp′) *n.* An instrument for examining the rectum consisting of a tube or speculum equipped with a light. Also called *rectoscope.* —**proc·tos′co·py** (-tŏs′kə-pē) *n.*

proc·to·sig·moid·ec·to·my (prŏk′tō-sĭg′moi-dĕk′tə-mē) *n.* The excision of the rectum and the sigmoid colon.

proc·to·sig·moid·i·tis (prŏk′tō-sĭg′moi-dī′tĭs) *n.* Inflammation of the sigmoid colon and the rectum.

proc·to·sig·moid·os·co·py (prŏk′tō-sĭg′moi-dŏs′kə-pē) *n.* Direct inspection of the rectum and the sigmoid colon using a sigmoidoscope.

proc·to·spasm (prŏk′tə-spăz′əm) *n.* **1.** Spasmodic stricture of the anus. **2.** Spasmodic contraction of the rectum.

proc·to·ste·no·sis (prŏk′tō-stə-nō′sĭs) *n.* Stricture of the rectum or the anus. Also called *rectostenosis.*

proc·tos·to·my (prŏk-tŏs′tə-mē) *n.* Surgical formation of an artificial opening into the rectum. Also called *rectostomy.*

proc·tot·o·my (prŏk-tŏt′ə-mē) *n.* Incision into the rectum. Also called *rectotomy.*

proc·to·tre·sia (prŏk′tə-trē′zhə) *n.* Surgical correction of an imperforate anus.

proc·to·val·vot·o·my (prŏk′tō-văl-vŏt′ə-mē) *n.* Incision of the rectal valves.

pro·cum·bent (prō-kŭm′bənt) *adj.* Lying face down; prone.

pro·cur·sive epilepsy (prō-kûr′sĭv) *n.* A psychomotor seizure initiated by twirling or running.

prodromal stage *n.* See **incubative stage.**

pro·drome (prō′drōm′) *n., pl.* **–dromes** *or* **–dro·ma·ta** (-drō′mə-tə) An early symptom indicating the onset of an attack or disease. —**pro·dro′mal** (-drō′məl), **pro·drom′ic** (-drŏm′ĭk) *adj.*

pro·drug (prō′drŭg′) *n.* A class of drugs, initially in inactive form, that are converted into active form in the body by normal metabolic processes.

pro·duc·er (prə-dōō′sər, prō-) *n.* A photosynthetic green plant or chemosynthetic bacterium, constituting the first trophic level in a food chain; an autotrophic organism.

prod·uct (prŏd′əkt) *n.* **1.** Something produced by human or mechanical effort or by a natural process. **2.** A substance resulting from a chemical reaction.

pro·duc·tive (prə-dŭk′tĭv, prō-) *adj.* **1.** Producing or capable of producing mucus or sputum. **2.** Forming new tissue, as of an inflammation.

productive cough *n.* A cough that expels mucus or sputum from the respiratory tract.

pro·en·zyme (prō-ĕn′zīm′) *n.* The inactive or nearly inactive precursor of an enzyme, converted into an active enzyme by proteolysis. Also called *zymogen.*

pro·e·ryth·ro·blast (prō′ĭ-rĭth′rə-blăst′) *n.* See **pronor-moblast.**

pro·e·ryth·ro·cyte (prō′ĭ-rĭth′rə-sīt′) *n.* An immature nucleated red blood cell.

pro·es·tro·gen (prō-ĕs′trə-jən) *n.* A precursor of estrogen that becomes an active hormone only after it has been metabolized.

pro·es·trus (prō-ĕs′trəs) *n.* The period immediately before estrus in most female mammals, characterized by development of the endometrium and ovarian follicles.

pro·fi·bri·nol·y·sin (prō′fī-brə-nŏl′ĭ-sĭn) *n.* See **plasminogen.**

pro·file (prō′fīl′) *n.* **1.** A side view of an object or structure, especially of the human head. **2.** A formal summary or analysis of data, often in the form of a graph or table, representing distinctive features or characteristics.

pro·for·mi·phen (prō-fôr′mə-fĕn′) *n.* See **phenprobamate.**

pro·gas·trin (prō-găs′trĭn) *n.* A precursor of gastrin secreted by glands in the mucous membrane of the stomach.

pro·gen·i·tor (prō-jĕn′ĭ-tər) *n.* **1.** A direct ancestor. **2.** An originator of a line of descent.

prog·e·ny (prŏj′ə-nē) *n., pl.* **progeny** *or* **–nies 1.** One born of, begotten by, or derived from another; an offspring or descendant. **2.** Offspring or descendants considered as a group.

pro·ge·ri·a (prō-jîr′ē-ə) *n.* A rare congenital childhood disorder marked by gross retardation of growth after the first year and by rapid onset of the physical changes typical of old age, usually resulting in death before age 20. Also called *Hutchinson-Gilford syndrome, premature-senility syndrome.*

pro·ge·roid (prō-jîr′oid′) *adj.* Resembling old age.

pro·ges·ta·tion·al (prō′jĕs-tā′shə-nəl) *adj.* **1.** Of or relating to the phase of the menstrual cycle immediately following ovulation, characterized by secretion of progesterone. **2.** Of or relating to progesterone and its actions. **3.** Having actions similar to progesterone. Used of a drug.

pro·ges·ter·one (prō-jĕs′tə-rōn′) *n.* **1.** A steroid hormone secreted by the corpus luteum and by the placenta, that acts to prepare the uterus for implantation of the fertilized ovum, to maintain pregnancy, and to promote development of the mammary glands. Also called *corpus luteum hormone, luteohormone, progestational hormone.* **2.** A drug prepared from natural or synthetic progesterone, used in oral contraceptives, hormone replacement therapy, and in the treatment of menstrual and other gynecologic disorders.

pro·ges·tin (prō-jĕs′tĭn) *n.* **1.** A natural or synthetic progestational substance that mimics some or all of the actions of progesterone. **2.** A crude hormone of the corpus luteum from which progesterone can be isolated in pure form. No longer in technical use.

pro·ges·to·gen (prō-jĕs′tə-jən) *n.* Any of various substances having progestational effects; a progestin.

pro·glos·sis (prō-glô′sĭs) *n.* The tip of the tongue.

pro·glot·tid (prō-glŏt′ĭd)*or* **pro·glot·tis** (-glŏt′ĭs) *n., pl.* **–glot·tids** *or* **–glot·ti·des** (-glŏt′ĭ-dēz′) One of the segments of a tapeworm, containing both male and female reproductive organs. Also called *proglottis.*

prog·na·thous (prŏg′nə-thəs, prŏg-nā′-) *or* **prog·nath·ic** (prŏg-năth′ĭk, -nā′thĭk) *adj.* Having jaws that project forward to a marked degree. —**prog′na·thism** (-nə-thĭz′əm) *n.*

prog·no·sis (prŏg-nō′sĭs) *n., pl.* **–ses** (-sēz) **1.** A prediction of the probable course and outcome of a disease.

2. The likelihood of recovery from a disease. —**prog'-nos·ti'cian** (-nŏs-tĭsh'ən) *n.*

prog·nos·tic (prŏg-nŏs'tĭk) *adj.* **1.** Of, relating to, or useful in prognosis. **2.** Of or relating to prediction; predictive. —*n.* **1.** A sign or symptom indicating the future course of a disease. **2.** A sign of a future happening; a portent.

prog·nos·ti·cate (prŏg-nŏs'tĭ-kāt') *v.* To predict according to present indications or signs; foretell.

Pro·graf (prō'grăf') A trademark for the drug tacrolimus.

pro·grammed cell death (prō'grămd') *n.* See **apoptosis.**

pro·gress (prə-grĕs') *v.* **1.** To move forward; advance. **2.** To increase in scope or severity, as of a disease taking an unfavorable course.

pro·gres·sive (prə-grĕs'ĭv) *adj.* **1.** Moving forward; advancing. **2.** Proceeding in steps; continuing steadily by increments, as of a course of treatment. **3.** Tending to become more severe or wider in scope, as of a disease or paralysis.

progressive bulbar paralysis *n.* The progressive atrophy and paralysis of the muscles of the tongue, lips, palate, pharynx, and larynx due to atrophic degeneration of the innervating neurons. Also called *bulbar paralysis, Duchenne's disease, Erb's disease.*

progressive cataract *n.* A cataract in which the entire lens gradually becomes opaque.

progressive cerebral poliodystrophy *n.* A familial spastic paralysis of the extremities occurring in infants and young children in which seizures, blindness, and deafness develop during the first year of life, accompanied by progressive destruction and degeneration of neurons of the cerebral cortex. Also called *Alpers' disease, Christensen-Krabbe disease.*

progressive lipodystrophy *n.* A condition characterized by a complete loss of the subcutaneous fat of the upper torso, arms, neck, and face, sometimes with an increase of fat in the tissues about and below the pelvis. Also called *Barraquer's disease.*

progressive muscular atrophy *n.* Atrophy of the cells of the anterior cornua of the spinal cord, resulting in the progressive wasting and paralysis of the muscles of the extremities and trunk. Also called *Aran-Duchenne disease, Cruveilhier's disease, Duchenne-Aran disease.*

progressive ophthalmoplegia *n.* Progressive upper bulbar palsy, due to degeneration of the nuclei of the motor nerves of the eye.

progressive pigmentary dermatosis *n.* A chronic skin disorder resulting from hemorrhages into the skin, chiefly on the legs of young men, and characterized by purple patches that spread and turn brown. Also called *Schamberg's disease.*

progressive staining *n.* A procedure in which stain is applied until the desired intensity of tissue coloration is attained.

progressive systemic sclerosis *n.* A systemic disease marked by formation of hyalinized and thickened collagenous fibrous tissue, with thickening and adhesion of skin to underlying tissues, especially of the hands and face. Also called *scleroderma.*

progressive vaccinia *n.* A severe or even fatal form of vaccinia occurring as a complication of smallpox vaccination chiefly in persons with an immunologic deficiency or dyscrasia, characterized by progressive enlargement of the initial and secondary lesions.

pro·hor·mone (prō-hôr'mōn') *n.* An intraglandular precursor of a hormone.

pro·in·su·lin (prō-ĭn'sə-lĭn) *n.* A single-chain polypeptide that is the precursor of insulin, converted into insulin by enzymatic action.

proj·ect (prŏj'kt', -ĭkt) *n.* **1.** A plan or proposal; a scheme. **2.** An undertaking requiring concerted effort. —*v.* (prə-jĕkt') **1.** To extend forward or out; jut out. **2.** To cause an image to appear on a surface. **3.** In psychology, to externalize and attribute something, such as an emotion, to someone or something else.

pro·jec·tile vomiting (prə-jĕk'təl, -tīl') *n.* Expulsion of the contents of the stomach with great force.

pro·jec·tion (prə-jĕk'shən) *n.* **1.** The act of projecting or the condition of being projected. **2.** The attribution of one's own attitudes, feelings, or suppositions to others. **3.** The attribution of one's own attitudes, feelings, or desires to someone or something as a naive or unconscious defense against anxiety or guilt. **4.** The localization of visual impressions to a point in space relative to the person who is doing the viewing: straight ahead, right, left, above, or below. **5.** Any of the systems of nerve fibers by which a group of nerve cells discharges its nerve impulses to one or more other cell groups.

projection fiber *n.* Any of the nerve fibers connecting the cerebral cortex with other centers in the brain or spinal cord.

pro·jec·tive test (prə-jĕk'tĭv) *n.* A psychological test in which a subject's responses to ambiguous or unstructured stimuli, such as a series of cartoons or incomplete sentences, are analyzed to determine personality traits, feelings, or attitudes.

pro·kar·y·ote *or* **pro·car·y·ote** (prō-kăr'ē-ōt') *n.* An organism of the kingdom Prokaryotae, constituting the bacteria and cyanobacteria, characterized by the absence of a nuclear membrane and by DNA that is not organized into chromosomes. —**pro·kar'y·ot'ic** (-ŏt'-ĭk) *adj.*

pro·la·bi·um (prō-lā'bē-əm) *n.* The exposed part of the lip, especially the small elevation at the termination of the philtrum.

pro·lac·tin (prō-lăk'tĭn) *n.* *Abbr.* **PRL** A pituitary hormone that stimulates and maintains the secretion of milk. Also called *lactogenic hormone, lactotropin, luteotropic hormone, luteotropin.*

prolactin-inhibiting factor *n.* *Abbr.* **PIF** A substance of hypothalamic origin capable of inhibiting the synthesis and release of prolactin. Also called *prolactin-inhibiting hormone, prolactostatin.*

prolactin-producing adenoma *n.* A small, usually encapsulated, pituitary tumor composed of prolactin-producing cells, which causes symptoms of Forbes-Albright syndrome in women and impotence in men. Also called *prolactinoma.*

prolactin-releasing factor *or* **prolactin-releasing hormone** *n.* *Abbr.* **PRF** See **prolactoliberin.**

pro·lac·to·lib·er·in (prō-lăk'tō-lĭb'ər-ĭn) *n.* A substance of hypothalamic origin that stimulates the release of prolactin. Also called *prolactin-releasing factor.*

pro·lac·to·stat·in (prō-lăk'tō-stăt'n) *n.* See **prolactin-inhibiting factor.**

pro·la·mine *or* **pro·la·min** (prō'lə-mĭn, -mēn') *n.* Any of a class of simple proteins found in the seeds of wheat, rye, and other grains that are insoluble in water and neutral salt solutions but are soluble in dilute acids and alkalis.

pro·lan (prō'lăn') *n.* **1.** Human chorionic gonadotropin. No longer in scientific use. **2.** Either of two hormones of the pituitary gland, luteinizing hormone and follicle-stimulating hormone. No longer in scientific use.

pro·lapse (prō-lăps') *v.* To fall or slip out of place, as of an organ or part. —*n.* **pro·lap·sus** (prō-lăp'səs) The falling down or slipping out of place of an organ or part, such as the uterus.

prolapse of umbilical cord *n.* A condition in which part of the umbilical cord appears before the fetus during delivery, possibly leading to fetal death due to compression of the cord between the presenting part of the fetus and the maternal pelvis.

prolapse of uterus *n.* Displacement of the uterus downward due to laxity and atony of the muscles and fascia of the pelvic floor. Also called *falling of womb.*

pro·lep·sis (prō-lĕp'sĭs) *n., pl.* **-ses** (-sēz) The return of paroxysms of a recurrent disease at intervals that progressively become shorter. —**pro·lep'tic** (-lĕp'tĭk) *adj.*

pro·leu·ko·cyte (prō-lōo'kə-sīt') *n.* See **leukoblast.**

pro·li·dase (prō'lĭ-dās', -dāz') *n.* See **proline dipeptidase.**

pro·lif·er·ate (prə-lĭf'ə-rāt') *v.* To grow or multiply by rapidly producing new tissue, parts, cells, or offspring.

pro·lif·er·at·ing endarteritis (prə-lĭf'ə-rā'tĭng) *n.* Chronic endarteritis accompanied by a marked increase of fibrous tissue in the inner lining of the artery.

proliferating systematized angioendotheliomatosis *n.* A rare generalized cutaneous and visceral intracapillary proliferation of endothelial cells that is accompanied by vascular thrombosis and obstruction.

pro·lif·er·a·tion (prə-lĭf'ə-rā'shən) *n.* The growth and reproduction of similar cells.

pro·lif·er·a·tive (prə-lĭf'ə-rā'tĭv) *or* **pro·lif·er·ous** (-ər-əs) *adj.* Tending to proliferate.

proliferative fasciitis *n.* See **nodular fasciitis.**

proliferative gingivitis *n.* See **hyperplastic gingivitis.**

proliferative inflammation *n.* Inflammation characterized by a proliferation of tissue cells.

proliferative retinopathy *n.* Neovascularization of the retina extending into the vitreous body. Also called *retinitis proliferans.*

pro·lig·er·ous (prō-lĭj'ər-əs) *adj.* Of or relating to the production of offspring; germinating.

pro·li·nase (prō'lə-nās', -nāz') *n.* See **prolyl dipeptidase.**

pro·line (prō'lēn') *n. Abbr.* **Pro** An amino acid that is found in most proteins and is a major constituent of collagen.

proline dipeptidase *n.* An enzyme that catalyzes the cleavage of bonds between aminoacyl and proline groups. Also called *prolidase.*

proline im·i·no·pep·ti·dase (ĭm'ə-nō-pĕp'tĭ-dās', -dāz') *n.* An enzyme that catalyzes the hydrolysis of proline residues at specific terminal positions in peptides.

Pro·lix·in (prō-lĭk'sĭn) A trademark for the drug fluphenazine.

pro·lyl (prō'lĭl') *n.* The univalent acid radical, C_4H_8NCO, of proline.

prolyl dipeptidase *n.* An enzyme that catalyzes the cleavage of certain prolyl-amino acid bonds. Also called *prolinase.*

pro·mas·ti·gote (prō-măs'tĭ-gōt') *n.* The flagellate stage of a trypanosomatid protozoan, as that of any of the *Leishmania* parasites.

pro·meg·a·lo·blast (prō-mĕg'ə-lō-blăst') *n.* The first of four maturation stages of the megaloblast.

pro·met·a·phase (prō-mĕt'ə-fāz') *n.* The stage of mitosis or meiosis in which the nuclear membrane disintegrates, the centrioles reach the poles of the cell, and the chromosomes continue to contract.

pro·me·thi·um (prə-mē'thē-əm) *n. Symbol* **Pm** A radioactive rare-earth element prepared by fission of uranium. Pm 145 is the longest-lived isotope with a half-life of 17.7 years. Atomic number 61.

prom·i·nence (prŏm'ə-nəns) *n.* **1.** The quality or condition of being prominent. **2.** A small projection or protuberance.

prom·i·nent (prŏm'ə-nənt) *adj.* **1.** Projecting outward or upward; protuberant. **2.** Immediately noticeable; conspicuous.

prominent heel *n.* A condition marked by a tender swelling on the heel caused by a thickening of the periosteum or fibrous tissue covering the back of the calcaneus.

pro·mon·o·cyte (prō-mŏn'ə-sīt') *n.* See **premonocyte.**

prom·on·to·ry (prŏm'ən-tôr'ē) *n.* A projecting part.

pro·mot·er (prə-mō'tər) *n.* **1.** A substance that increases the activity of a catalyst. **2.** A DNA molecule to which RNA polymerase binds, initiating the transcription of mRNA. **3.** A chemical that may promote carcinogenicity or mutagenicity.

pro·mot·ing agent (prə-mō'tĭng) *n.* A noncarcinogenic substance that enhances tumor production in a tissue previously exposed to subcarcinogenic doses of a carcinogen. Also called *initiating agent.*

pro·mo·tion (prə-mō'shən) *n.* The stimulation of the progress or growth of a tumor following initiation by a promoter.

pro·my·e·lo·cyte (prō-mī'ə-lə-sīt') *n.* A cell containing a few granules formed in the transition from myeloblast to myelocyte during the development of a granulocyte; it is the predominant cell type seen in granulocytic leukemia. Also called *granular leukoblast, progranulocyte.*

pro·na·si·on (prō-nā'zē-ŏn') *n.* The point of the angle between the septum of the nose and the surface of the upper lip.

pro·nate (prō'nāt') *v.* **1.** To turn or rotate the hand or forearm so that the palm faces down or back. **2.** To turn or rotate the sole of the foot by abduction and eversion so that the inner edge of the sole bears the body's weight. **3.** To turn or rotate a limb so that the inner surface faces down or back. Used of a vertebrate animal. **4.** To place in a prone position.

pro·na·tion (prō-nā′shən) *n.* **1.** The act of pronating. **2.** The condition of being pronated, especially the condition of having flat feet.

pro·na·tor (prō′nā′tər) *n.* A muscle that effects or assists in pronation.

prone (prōn) *adj.* **1.** Lying with the front or face downward. **2.** Having a tendency; inclined. —*adv.* In a prone manner.

pro·neph·ros (prō-něf′rəs, -rŏs′) *n., pl.* **–roi** (-roi) *or* **–ra** (-rə) A kidneylike organ, being either part of the most anterior pair of three pairs of organs in a vertebrate embryo, usually disappearing early in embryonic development.

pro·nor·mo·blast (prō-nôr′mə-blăst′) *n.* The first of four stages in development of the normoblast. Also called *proerythroblast, rubriblast.*

pro·nu·cle·us (prō-nōō′klē-əs) *n.* **1.** One of two nuclei undergoing fusion in karyogamy. **2.** The haploid nucleus of a sperm or egg before fusion of the nuclei in fertilization.

pro·o·tic (prō-ō′tĭk, -ŏt′ĭk) *adj.* Occurring or located in front of the ear.

prop·a·gate (prŏp′ə-gāt′) *v.* **1.** To cause an organism to multiply or breed. **2.** To breed offspring. **3.** To transmit characteristics from one generation to another. **4.** To cause to move in some direction or through a medium, such as a wave or nerve impulse.

prop·a·ga·tion (prŏp′ə-gā′shən) *n.* **1.** Multiplication or increase, as by natural reproduction. **2.** The act or process of propagating, especially the process by which an impulse is transmitted along a nerve fiber.

prop·a·ga·tive (prŏp′ə-gā′tĭv) *adj.* **1.** Of, relating to, or involved in propagation. **2.** Relating to the germ cells of an animal or plant as distinguished from the somatic cells.

pro·pane (prō′pān′) *n.* A colorless hydrocarbon found in natural gas and petroleum and widely used as a fuel.

pro·pa·no·ic acid (prō′pə-nō′ĭk) *n.* See **propionic acid.**

pro·pa·nol (prō′pə-nôl′, -nōl′) *n.* See **propyl alcohol.**

Pro·pe·cia (prə-pē′shə) A trademark for the drug finasteride.

pro·pene (prō′pēn′) *n.* See **propylene.**

pro·pep·sin (prō-pĕp′sĭn) *n.* See **pepsinogen.**

pro·per·din (prō-pûr′dn) *n.* A natural protein in human blood serum that participates in the body's immune response by working in conjunction with the complement system.

properdin factor A *n.* A component of the properdin system that is a hydrazine-sensitive form of beta-globulin and the third component of complement.

properdin factor B *n.* A normal serum protein and a component of the properdin system.

properdin factor D *n.* A normal serum alpha-globulin required in the properdin system.

properdin factor E *n.* A serum protein required for activation of the third component of complement.

properdin system *n.* An alternative system by which, in

the absence of antibodies bound to immunoglobulins and components of complement, the immunological cascade occurs, with the activation of critical components of complement aided by the stabilizing properties of properdin.

prop·er fasciculus (prŏp′ər) *n.* Any of several ascending and descending association fiber systems of the spinal cord that lie deep in the funiculi adjacent to the gray matter. Also called *ground bundle.*

proper palmar digital nerve *n.* Any of ten palmar nerves of the digits of the hand derived from the common palmar digital nerves. Each nerve supplies a palmar quadrant of a digit and a part of the dorsal surface of the distal phalanx.

proper plantar digital nerve *n.* Any of ten nerves derived from the common plantar digital nerves. Each nerve supplies a plantar quadrant of a toe and part of the dorsal surface of the distal phalanx.

proper substance of cornea *n.* Transparent connective tissue, between the layers of which are spaces containing corneal cells.

proper substance of sclera *n.* Dense, white, fibrous tissue arranged in interlacing bundles, forming the main mass of the sclera.

pro·phage (prō′fāj′) *n.* The latent form of a bacteriophage in which viral genes are incorporated into bacterial chromosomes disrupting the bacterial cell. Also called *probacteriophage.*

pro·phase (prō′fāz′) *n.* **1.** The first stage of mitosis, during which the chromosomes condense and become visible, the nuclear membrane breaks down, and the spindle apparatus forms at opposite poles of the cell. **2.** The first stage of meiosis, during which the DNA replicates, homologous chromosomes undergo synapsis, chiasmata form, and the chromosomes contract. —**pro·pha·sic** (-fā′zĭk) *adj.*

pro·phy·lac·tic (prō′fə-lăk′tĭk, prŏf′ə-) *n.* **1.** A prophylactic agent, device, or measure, such as a vaccine or drug. **2.** A contraceptive device, especially a condom. —*adj.* Acting to defend against or prevent something, especially disease; protective.

prophylactic treatment *n.* The institution of measures to protect a person from a disease to which he or she has been, or may be, exposed. Also called *preventive treatment.*

pro·phy·lax·is (prō′fə-lăk′sĭs, prŏf′ə-) *n., pl.* **–lax·es** (-lăk′sēz′) Prevention of or protective treatment for disease.

pro·pi·o·ma·zine (prō′pē-ō′mə-zēn′) *n.* A drug used intramuscularly or intravenously as a sedative prior to the administration of anesthesia.

pro·pi·o·nate (prō′pē-ə-nāt′) *n.* A salt or ester of propionic acid.

Pro·pi·on·i·bac·te·ri·um (prō′pē-ŏn′ə-băk-tîr′ē-əm) *n.* A genus of saphrophytic nonmotile gram-positive bacteria, usually anaerobic, that occur in dairy products, on the skin, and in the intestinal tract; certain species may be pathogenic.

pro·pi·on·ic acid (prō′pē-ŏn′ĭk) *n.* A fatty acid found naturally in sweat and as a product of bacterial fermentation, used as a mold inhibitor in bread. Also called *propanoic acid.*

pro·pi·on·ic·ac·i·de·mi·a (prō′pē-ŏn′ĭ-kăs′ĭ-dē′mē-ə) *n.* An abnormally high concentration of propionic acid in the blood, caused by the deficiency of an enzyme and characterized by vomiting, lethargy, ketoacidosis, and leukopenia.

pro·plas·tid (prō-plăs′tĭd) *n.* A cytoplasmic organelle from which a plastid develops.

pro·pos·i·tus (prō-pŏz′ĭ-təs) *n., pl.* **–ti** (-tī′) **1.** See proband. **2.** A premise; an argument.

pro·pox·y·phene hydrochloride (prō-pŏk′sə-fēn′) *n.* An analgesic drug chemically related to methadone.

pro·pran·o·lol (prō-prăn′ə-lôl′, -lōl′) *n.* A beta-blocker used to treat hypertension, angina pectoris, and cardiac arrhythmia.

pro·pri·e·tar·y (prə-prī′ĭ-tĕr′ē) *adj.* **1.** Exclusively owned, as of a hospital. **2.** Owned by an individual or corporation under a trademark or patent, as of a drug. —*n.* A proprietary medicine.

proprietary hospital *n.* A hospital operated as a profit-making business and owned by a corporation, investment group, or by physicians who use it primarily for their own patients.

proprietary medicine *n.* A medicinal compound whose formula and often mode of manufacture are owned by an individual or corporation under a trademark or patent.

proprietary name *n.* The patented brand name or trademark under which a manufacturer markets a product.

pro·pri·o·cep·tion (prō′prē-ō-sĕp′shən) *n.* The unconscious perception of movement and spatial orientation arising from stimuli within the body itself.

proprioceptive mechanism *n.* The mechanism controlling position and movement, by which one is able to adjust muscular movements accurately and to maintain one's balance.

proprioceptive reflex *n.* A reflex induced by stimulation of proprioceptors.

pro·pri·o·cep·tor (prō′prē-ō-sĕp′tər) *n.* A sensory receptor, commonly found in muscles, tendons, joints, and the inner ear, that detects the motion or position of the body or a limb by responding to stimuli within the organism. —**pro′pri·o·cep′tive** *adj.*

prop·to·sis (prŏp-tō′sĭs) *n., pl.* **–ses** (-sēz) Forward displacement of an organ, especially an eyeball. —**prop·tot·ic** (-tŏt′ĭk) *adj.*

pro·pul·sion (prə-pŭl′shən) *n.* **1.** A driving or propelling force. **2.** The leaning or falling forward characteristic of the festination of Parkinsonism.

pro·pyl (prō′pĭl) *n.* A univalent organic radical, $CH_3CH_2CH_2$, derived from propane.

propyl alcohol *n.* A clear colorless liquid used as a solvent and as an antiseptic. Also called *propanol.*

pro·pyl·ene (prō′pə-lēn′) *n.* A flammable gas derived from processing petroleum hydrocarbon and used in organic synthesis. Also called *propene.*

pro·pyl·i·o·done (prō′pəl-ī′ə-dōn′) *n.* A radiopaque material used for bronchography.

pro·pyl·thi·o·u·ra·cil (prō′pəl-thī′ō-yŏŏr′ə-sĭl′) *n. Abbr.* **PTU** An agent that inhibits the synthesis of thyroid hormones and is used in the treatment of hyperthyroidism.

pro rat. aet. *abbr. Latin* pro ratione aetatis (according to age, as for a patient)

pro·ren·nin (prō-rĕn′ĭn) *n.* See prochymosin.

pro·ru·bri·cyte (prō-rōō′brĭ-sīt′) *n.* A basophilic normoblast.

Pros·car (prŏs′kär′) A trademark for the drug finasteride.

pro·se·cre·tin (prō′sĭ-krēt′n) *n.* The inactive precursor of secretin.

pro·sect (prō-sĕkt′) *v.* To dissect a cadaver or any part of the body for an anatomical demonstration.

pro·sec·tor (prō-sĕk′tər) *n.* An individual who dissects cadavers for anatomical instruction or pathological examination.

pros·en·ceph·a·lon (prŏs′ĕn-sĕf′ə-lŏn′) *n.* **1.** The most anterior of the three primary regions of the embryonic brain, from which the telencephalon and diencephalon develop. **2.** The segment of the adult brain that develops from the embryonic forebrain and includes the cerebrum, thalamus, and hypothalamus. —**pros′en·ce·phal′ic** (-sə-făl′ĭk) *adj.*

pro·se·rum prothrombin conversion accelerator (prō-sîr′əm) *n. Abbr.* **PPCA** See factor VIII.

pros·o·dem·ic (prŏs′ə-dĕm′ĭk) *adj.* Of or relating to a disease that is transmitted directly from person to person.

Pro·Som (prō′sŏm′) A trademark for the drug estazolam.

pros·o·pag·no·sia (prŏs′ə-păg-nō′zhə, -zē-ə) *n.* An inability or difficulty in recognizing familiar faces; it may be congenital or result from injury or disease of the brain.

pros·o·pal·gia (prŏs′ə-păl′jə) *n.* See trigeminal neuralgia. —**pros′o·pal′gic** (-jĭk) *adj.*

pros·o·pec·ta·sia (prŏs′ə-pĭk-tā′zhə) *n.* Enlargement of the face, as in acromegaly.

pros·o·pla·sia (prŏs′ə-plā′zhə) *n.* Progressive transformation to a higher level of function or complexity, such as the change the cells of the salivary ducts go through to become secreting cells.

prosopo– *or* **prosop–** *pref.* Face: *prosopospasm.*

pros·o·po·di·ple·gia (prŏs′ə-pō-dī-plē′jə) *n.* Paralysis affecting both sides of the face.

pros·o·po·neu·ral·gia (prŏs′ə-pō-nŏŏ-răl′jə) *n.* See trigeminal neuralgia.

pros·o·po·ple·gia (prŏs′ə-pō-plē′jə) *n.* See facial palsy. —**pros′o·po·ple′gic** (-jĭk) *adj.*

pros·o·pos·chi·sis (prŏs′ə-pŏs′kĭ-sĭs) *n.* A congenital facial cleft extending from the mouth to the orbit of the eye.

pros·o·po·spasm (prŏs′ə-pō-spăz′əm) *n.* See facial tic.

pros·per·mi·a (prō-spûr′mē-ə) *n.* See premature ejaculation.

pros·ta·cy·clin (prŏs′tə-sī′klĭn) *n.* A prostaglandin produced in the walls of blood vessels that acts as a vasodilator and inhibits platelet aggregation.

pros·ta·glan·din (prŏs′tə-glăn′dĭn) *n.* Any of a group of hormonelike substances produced in various tissues that are derived from amino acids and mediate a range of physiological functions, such as metabolism and nerve transmission.

pros·ta·no·ic acid (prŏs′tə-nō′ĭk) *n.* A 20-carbon acid skeleton that serves as the structural basis for the prostaglandins.

Pros·taph·lin (prŏs-tăf′lĭn) A trademark for the drug oxacillin sodium.

prostat– *pref.* Variant of **prostato–**.

pros·ta·tal·gia (prŏs′tə-tăl′jə) *n.* Pain in the prostate gland. Also called *prostatodynia*.

pros·tate (prŏs′tāt′) *n.* The prostate gland. —*adj.* Of or relating to the prostate gland. —**pro·stat′ic** (prŏ-stăt′-ĭk) *adj.*

pros·ta·tec·to·my (prŏs′tə-tĕk′tə-mē) *n.* Surgical removal of all or part of the prostate gland.

prostate gland *n.* A chestnut-shaped body that surrounds the beginning of the male urethra at the base of the bladder, consists of two lobes connected anteriorly by an isthmus and posteriorly by a middle lobe lying above and between the ejaculatory ducts, controls the release of urine from the bladder, and whose milky fluid secretion is discharged into the urethra during semen emission.

prostate-specific antigen *n. Abbr.* **PSA** A protease secreted by the epithelial cells of the prostate gland. Serum levels are elevated in patients with benign prostatic hyperplasia and prostate cancer.

prostatic ductule *n.* Any of the minute canals that receive the prostatic secretion and that discharge it through openings on either side of the urethral crest. Also called *prostatic duct.*

prostatic fluid *n.* A whitish secretion that is one of the constituents of semen.

prostatic massage *n.* **1.** The expression of prostatic secretions by applying pressure on the prostate with a finger in the rectum. **2.** The emptying of prostatic sini and ducts by repeated downward compression maneuvers, used in the treatment of inflammatory conditions of the prostate.

prostatic sinus *n.* The groove on either side of the urethral crest in the prostatic part of the urethra.

prostatic utricle *n.* A minute pouch in the prostate opening on the summit of the seminal colliculus that consists of the remains of the fused caudal ends of the paramesonephric ducts. Also called *masculine uterus.*

pros·ta·tism (prŏs′tə-tĭz′əm) *n.* A disorder characterized by decreased force of urination and dysuria, usually resulting from enlargement of the prostate gland.

pros·ta·ti·tis (prŏs′tə-tī′tĭs) *n.* Inflammation of the prostate gland. —**pros·ta·tit′ic** (-tĭt′ĭk) *adj.*

prostato– *or* **prostat–** *pref.* Prostate gland: *prostatectomy.*

pros·ta·to·cys·ti·tis (prŏs′tə-tō-sĭ-stī′tĭs) *n.* Inflammation of the prostate and the bladder.

pros·ta·to·cys·tot·o·my (prŏs′tə-tō-sĭ-stŏt′ə-mē) *n.* Incision through the prostate and the bladder wall with drainage through the perineum.

pros·ta·to·dyn·i·a (prŏs′tə-tō-dĭn′ē-ə) *n.* See **prosta-talgia.**

pros·tat·o·lith (prŏ-stăt′ə-lĭth′) *n.* A concretion in the prostate gland.

pros·ta·to·li·thot·o·my (prŏs′tə-tō-lĭ-thŏt′ə-mē) *n.* Incision of the prostate for removal of a calculus.

pros·ta·to·meg·a·ly (prŏs′tə-tō-mĕg′ə-lē) *n.* Enlargement of the prostate gland.

pros·ta·tor·rhe·a (prŏs′tə-tō-rē′ə) *n.* An abnormal discharge of prostatic fluid.

pros·ta·tot·o·my (prŏs′tə-tŏt′ə-mē) *n.* Incision into the prostate.

pros·ta·to·ve·sic·u·lec·to·my (prŏs′tə-tō-vĕ-sĭk′yə-lĕk′tə-mē) *n.* Surgical removal of the prostate gland and the seminal vesicles.

pros·ta·to·ve·sic·u·li·tis (prŏs′tə-tō-vĕ-sĭk′yə-lī′tĭs) *n.* Inflammation of the prostate gland and the seminal vesicles.

pros·the·sis (prŏs-thē′sĭs) *n., pl.* **–ses** (-sēz) **1.** An artificial device used to replace a missing body part, such as a limb or heart valve. **2.** Replacement of a missing body part with such a device.

pros·thet·ic (prŏs-thĕt′ĭk) *adj.* **1.** Serving as or relating to a prosthesis. **2.** Of or relating to prosthetics.

prosthetic group *n.* The nonprotein component of a conjugated protein, as the heme in hemoglobin.

pros·thet·ics (prŏs-thĕt′ĭks) *n.* The branch of medicine or surgery that deals with the production and application of artificial body parts. —**pros′the·tist** (prŏs′thĭ-tĭst) *n.*

pros·thi·on (prŏs′thē-ŏn′) *n.* The most anterior point on the maxillary alveolar process, between the central incisor teeth. Also called *alveolar point.*

pros·tho·don·tics (prŏs′thə-dŏn′tĭks) *n.* The branch of dentistry that deals with the replacement of missing teeth and related mouth or jaw structures by artificial devices. —**pros′tho·don′tist** *n.*

Pros·tig·min (prŏs-tĭg′mĭn) A trademark for the drug neostigmine in its bromide and methylsulfate forms.

pros·tra·tion (prŏ-strā′shən) *n.* Total exhaustion or weakness; collapse.

prot– *pref.* Variant of **proto–**.

pro·tac·tin·i·um (prō′tăk-tĭn′ē-əm) *n. Symbol* **Pa** A rare, extremely toxic radioactive element having 13 known isotopes, the most stable of which is Pa 231 with a half-life of 32,700 years. Atomic number 91.

pro·ta·mine (prō′tə-mēn′, -mĭn) *or* **pro·ta·min** (-mĭn) *n.* Any of a group of simple proteins found in fish sperm that are strongly basic, are soluble in water, are not coagulated by heat, and yield chiefly arginine upon hydrolysis. In purified form, they are used in a long-acting formulation of insulin and to neutralize the anticoagulant effects of heparin.

pro·ta·no·pi·a (prō′tə-nō′pē-ə) *n.* A form of color-blindness characterized by defective perception of red and confusion of red with green or bluish green.

prote– *pref.* Variant of **proteo–**.

pro·te·an (prō′tē-ən, prō-tē′-) *adj.* Readily taking on varied shapes, forms, or meanings.

pro·te·ase (prō′tē-ās′, -āz′) *n.* Any of various enzymes, including the proteinases and peptidases, that catalyze the hydrolytic breakdown of proteins.

protease inhibitor *n.* An anti-HIV drug that blocks the action of the enzyme protease, which is needed for viral replication.

pro·tec·tion test (prə-tĕk′shən) *n.* A test to determine the antimicrobial activity of a serum by inoculating a susceptible animal with a mixture of the serum and the virus or other microbe being tested. Also called *neutral-ization test.*

pro·tec·tive laryngeal reflex (prə-těk′tĭv) *n.* Closure of the glottis to prevent entry of foreign substances into the respiratory tract.

pro·te·id (prō′tē-ĭd) *n.* A protein. No longer in scientific use.

pro·tein (prō′tēn′) *n.* Any of a group of complex organic macromolecules that contain carbon, hydrogen, oxygen, nitrogen, and usually sulfur and are composed of chains of alpha-amino acids. Proteins are fundamental components of all living cells and include many substances, such as enzymes, hormones, and antibodies, that are necessary to the functioning of an organism. They are essential in the diet of animals for the growth and repair of tissue and can be obtained from foods such as meat, fish, eggs, milk, and legumes. —**pro′tein·a′ceous** (prōt′n-ā′shəs, prō′tē-nā′-) *adj.*

pro·tein·ase (prōt′n-ās′, -āz′) *n.* A protease that begins the hydrolytic breakdown of proteins usually by splitting them into polypeptide chains.

protein-bound iodine *n. Abbr.* **PBI** Thyroid hormone consisting of one or more of the iodothyronines bound to one or more of the serum proteins.

protein-bound iodine test *n.* A test to determine thyroid function in which serum protein-bound iodine is measured.

protein C *n.* A vitamin K–dependent plasma protein that enzymatically cleaves activated forms of factors V and VIII, thus inhibiting the coagulation of blood and interfering with the regulation of intravascular clot formation.

protein channel *n.* See **channel** (sense 2).

protein hydrolysate *n.* A sterile solution of amino acids and peptides prepared from a protein by acid or enzymatic hydrolysis and used intravenously for the maintenance of positive nitrogen balance in severe illness, after surgery of the alimentary tract, in the diets of infants allergic to milk, or as a high-protein dietary supplement.

protein-losing enteropathy *n.* Increased enteric loss of serum protein, especially albumin, causing hypoproteinemia.

protein metabolism *n.* Decomposition and synthesis of proteins in tissue. Also called *proteometabolism.*

pro·tein·oid (prōt′n-oid′) *n.* A proteinlike polypeptide formed abiotically from amino acid mixtures in the presence of heat, it may resemble early evolutionary forms of protein.

pro·tein·o·sis (prō′tē-nō′sĭs) *n.* A condition characterized by disordered protein formation and distribution, especially as manifested by the deposition of abnormal proteins in tissues.

protein S *n.* A vitamin K–dependent antithrombotic protein that functions as a cofactor with activated protein C.

pro·tein·u·ri·a (prōt′n-ŏŏr′ē-ə, prō′tē-nŏŏr′-) *n.* **1.** Excessive amounts of protein in the urine. **2.** See **albuminuria.**

proteo– or **prote–** *pref.* Protein: *proteolysis.*

pro·te·o·clas·tic (prō′tē-ō-klăs′tĭk) *adj.* Of, relating to, or causing proteolysis; proteolytic.

pro·te·o·gly·can (prō′tē-ō-glī′kăn′, -kən) *n.* Any of various mucopolysaccharides that are bound to protein

chains in covalent complexes and occur in the extracellular matrix of connective tissue.

pro·te·o·lip·id (prō′tē-ō-lĭp′ĭd, -lī′pĭd) *n.* Any of a class of lipid-soluble proteins.

pro·te·ol·y·sis (prō′tē-ŏl′ĭ-sĭs) *n.* The hydrolytic breakdown of proteins into simpler, soluble substances, as occurs in digestion.

pro·te·o·lyt·ic (prō′tē-ə-lĭt′ĭk) *adj.* Relating to, characterized by, or promoting proteolysis.

pro·te·ome (prō′tē-ōm′) *n.* The complete set of proteins that are produced by the genes of an organism.

pro·te·o·me·tab·o·lism (prō′tē-ō-mĭ-tăb′ə-lĭz′əm) *n.* See **protein metabolism.** —**pro′te·o·met′a·bol′ic** (-mět′ə-bŏl′ĭk) *adj.*

pro·te·o·mics (prō′tē-ō′mĭks) *n.* The analysis of the expression, localization, functions, and interactions of the proteins produced by the genes of an organism.

pro·te·ose (prō′tē-ōs′, -ōz′) *n.* Any of various water-soluble compounds that are produced during digestion by the hydrolytic breakdown of proteins.

Pro·te·us (prō′tē-əs) *n.* A genus of gram-negative, rod-shaped aerobic bacteria of the family Enterobacteriaceae that includes certain species associated with human enteritis and urinary tract infections.

Proteus mor·gan·i·i (môr-găn′ē-ī′) *n.* Morgan's bacillus.

Proteus vul·gar·is (vŭl-gâr′ĭs) *n.* A bacterium found in putrefying materials and in abscesses; it includes strains that agglutinate in typhus serum and are therefore used in diagnosis of typhus.

pro·throm·bin (prō-thrŏm′bĭn) *n.* A glycoprotein formed by and stored in the liver and present in the blood plasma that is converted to thrombin in the presence of thromboplastin and calcium ion during blood clotting. Also called *factor II.*

prothrombin accelerator *n.* See **factor V.**

pro·throm·bin·ase (prō-thrŏm′bə-nās′, -nāz′) *n.* An enzyme that catalyzes the hydrolysis of prothrombin to thrombin. Also called *factor X, Stuart factor.*

prothrombin test *n.* A method for determining prothrombin concentrations in blood based on the clotting time of oxalated blood plasma in the presence of thromboplastin and calcium chloride. Also called *Quick's test.*

pro·tist (prō′tĭst) *n.* A unicellular, eukaryotic organism belonging to the former taxonomic kingdom Protista.

Pro·tis·ta (prō-tĭs′tə) *n.* A former taxonomic kingdom made up of eukaryotic, unicellular organisms. Members of Protista now belong to the kingdom Protoctista, a new classification in most modern taxonomic systems.

pro·ti·um (prō′tē-əm, prō′shē-) *n.* See **hydrogen-1.**

proto– or **prot–** *pref.* **1.** First in time: *prototype.* **2.** First formed; primitive; original: *protoplast.* **3.** Having the least amount of a specified element or radical: *protoporphyrin.*

pro·to·col (prō′tə-kôl′, -kōl′) *n.* The plan for a course of medical treatment or for a scientific experiment.

pro·toc·tist (prō′tək-tĭst) *n.* A eukaryotic, unicellular organism belonging to the kingdom Protoctista, which includes protozoa, slime molds, and certain algae.

Pro·toc·tis·ta (prō′tək-tĭs′tə) *n.* A taxonomic kingdom consisting of unicellular protists and their descendant multicellular organisms, considered as a separate taxonomic kingdom in most modern classification systems.

pro·to·di·a·stol·ic (prō′tō-dī′ə-stŏl′ĭk) *adj.* Of or relating to the beginning of cardiac diastole.

protodiastolic gallop *n.* A gallop rhythm in which an abnormal third heart sound occurs in early diastole.

pro·to·du·o·de·num (prō′tō-dōō′ə-dē′nəm, -dōō-ŏd′-n-əm) *n.* The first part of the duodenum extending from the gastroduodenal pylorus to the major duodenal papilla and containing the duodenal glands.

pro·ton (prō′tŏn′) *n.* A stable, positively charged subatomic particle in the baryon family having a mass 1,836 times that of the electron.

Pro·ton·ix (prō-tŏn′ĭks) A trademark for the drug pantoprazole.

pro·to·on·co·gene (prō′tō-ŏng′kə-jēn′) *n.* A normal gene that has the potential to transform itself into an oncogene.

proton pump inhibitor *n.* A class of drugs that inhibit gastric acid secretion by interfering with the movement of hydrogen ions across cell membranes and are used mainly to treat peptic ulcers, gastroesophageal reflux disease, and esophagitis.

pro·to·path·ic (prō′tə-păth′ĭk) *adj.* Sensing pain, pressure, heat, or cold in a nonspecific manner, usually without localizing the stimulus. Used especially of certain sensory nerves.

protopathic sensibility *n.* Sensibility to low level and poorly localized stimulations of pain and temperature.

Pro·top·ic (prō-tŏp′ĭk) A trademark for the drug tacrolimus.

pro·to·plasm (prō′tə-plăz′əm) *n.* The complex, semifluid, translucent substance that constitutes the living matter of plant and animal cells and manifests the essential life functions of a cell. Composed of proteins, fats, and other molecules suspended in water, it includes the nucleus and cytoplasm. —**pro′to·plas′mic** (-plăz′mĭk) *adj.*

protoplasmic astrocyte *n.* An astrocyte found in the gray matter of the brain, having few fibrils and numerous branching processes.

pro·to·plast (prō′tə-plăst′) *n.* **1.** The living material of a plant or bacterial cell, including the protoplasm and plasma membrane after the cell wall has been removed. **2.** One that is the first made or formed; a prototype.

pro·to·por·phyr·i·a (prō′tō-pôr-fîr′ē-ə) *n.* Enhanced fecal excretion of protoporphyrin.

pro·to·por·phy·rin (prō′tō-pôr′fə-rĭn) *n.* A metal-free porphyrin that combines with iron to form the heme of iron-containing proteins.

protoporphyrin IX *n.* A porphyrin derivative that combines with ferrous iron to form the heme of hemoglobin and with ferric or ferrous iron to form the prosthetic groups of substances such as myoglobin, catalase, and the cytochromes.

pro·to·spasm (prō′tə-spăz′əm) *n.* A spasm beginning in one limb or one muscle that gradually becomes more generalized.

pro·to·troph (prō′tə-trŏf′, -trōf′) *n.* A bacterial strain that has the same nutritional requirements as the wild type strain from which it was derived. —**pro′to·troph′ic** (-trŏf′ĭk, -trō′fĭk) *adj.*

pro·to·type (prō′tə-tīp′) *n.* A primitive or ancestral form or species.

pro·to·ver·te·bra (prō′tō-vûr′tə-brə) *n.* **1.** A mesodermal somite. No longer in technical use. **2.** The caudal half of a sclerotome that is the primordium of the vertebral centrum. Also called *provertebra*.

pro·to·zo·a (prō′tə-zō′ə) *n.* Plural of **protozoan**.

pro·to·zo·an (prō′tə-zō′ən) *or* **pro·to·zo·on** (-ŏn′) *n.,* *pl.* **-zo·a** (-zō′ə) *or* **-zo·ans** *or* **-zo·a** *or* **-zo·ons** Any of a group of single-celled, usually microscopic, eukaryotic organisms, such as amoebas, ciliates, flagellates, and sporozoans. —**pro′to·zo′an, pro′to·zo′al, pro′to·zo′ic** *adj.*

pro·to·zo·i·a·sis (prō′tə-zō-ī′ə-sĭs) *n.* Infection with protozoa.

pro·to·zo·i·cide (prō′tə-zō′ĭ-sīd′) *n.* An agent destructive to protozoa.

pro·to·zo·ol·o·gy (prō′tə-zō-ŏl′ə-jē) *n.* The biological study of protozoa.

pro·to·zo·o·phage (prō′tə-zō′ə-fāj′) *n.* A phagocyte that ingests protozoa.

pro·tract (prō-trăkt′) *v.* To extend or protrude a body part.

pro·trac·tile (prō-trăk′təl, -tīl′) *or* **pro·tract·i·ble** (-tə-bəl) *adj.* That can be protracted; extensible, as of a limb.

pro·trac·tion (prō-trăk′shən) *n.* Extension of teeth or other maxillary or mandibular structures into a position anterior to the normal position.

pro·trac·tor (prō-trăk′tər) *n.* A muscle that extends a limb or other part.

pro·trude (prō-trōōd′) *v.* **1.** To push or thrust outward. **2.** To jut out; project.

pro·trud·ed disk (prō-trōō′dĭd) *n.* See **herniated disk**.

pro·tru·sion (prō-trōō′zhən) *n.* **1.** The act of protruding. **2.** The state of being protruded. **3.** A position of the mandible forward from centric relation.

pro·tru·sive occlusion (prō-trōō′sĭv) *n.* Occlusion that results when the lower jaw is protruded forward from its centric position.

pro·tu·ber·ance (prō-tōō′bər-əns) *n.* **1.** Something, such as a bulge, knob, or swelling, that protrudes. **2.** The condition of being protuberant.

pro·tu·ber·ant (prō-tōō′bər-ənt) *adj.* Swelling outward; bulging.

protuberant abdomen *n.* Unusual or prominent convexity of the abdomen, due to excessive subcutaneous fat, poor muscle tone, or an increase in the contents of the abdomen.

proud flesh (proud) *n.* The swollen flesh that surrounds a healing wound, caused by excessive granulation.

Pro·ven·til (prō-vĕn′tĭl, prō′vĕn′tl) A trademark for albuterol.

Pro·ver·a (prō-vĕr′ə) A trademark for a preparation of medroxyprogesterone acetate.

pro·ver·te·bra (prō-vûr′tə-brə) *n.* See **protovertebra**.

Prov·i·den·ci·a (prŏv′ĭ-dĕn′sē-ə) *n.* A genus of motile, peritrichous, nonsporeforming, aerobic or facultatively anaerobic bacteria containing gram-negative rods; it includes the species that can occur in urinary tract infections.

pro·vi·rus (prō′vī′rəs, prō-vī′-) *n., pl.* **–rus·es** The precursor or latent form of a virus that is capable of being integrated into the genetic material of a host cell and being replicated with it.

pro·vi·ta·min (prō-vī′tə-mĭn) *n.* A vitamin precursor that is converted to its active form through normal metabolic processes.

provitamin A *n.* Any of the carotenoids that are precursors of vitamin A and exhibit qualitatively the biological activity of beta-carotene; they are present in fish-liver oils, egg yolk, milk products, green-leaf or yellow vegetables, and fruits.

provitamin D₂ *n.* A substance, such as ergosterol, that can give rise to vitamin D_2.

prox·i·mad (prŏk′sə-măd′) *adv.* Toward a proximal part.

prox·i·mal (prŏk′sə-məl) *adj.* Nearer to a point of reference such as an origin, a point of attachment, or the midline of the body.

prox·i·mate (prŏk′sə-mĭt) *adj.* Closely related in space, time, or order; very near; proximal.

proximo– *pref.* Proximal: *proximoataxia.*

prox·i·mo·a·tax·i·a (prŏk′sə-mō-ə-tăk′sē-ə) *n.* Lack of muscular coordination in the proximal portions of the extremities.

Pro·zac (prō′zăk′) A trademark for fluoxetine hydrochloride.

pro·zone (prō′zōn′) *n.* The phenomenon in which mixtures of specific antigen and antibody do not agglutinate or precipitate visibly because of an excess of either antibody or antigen.

prune-belly syndrome *n.* See **abdominal muscle deficiency syndrome.**

pru·ri·go (proō-rī′gō) *n.* A chronic skin disease having various causes, marked by the eruption of pale, dome-shaped papules that itch severely. —**pru·rig′i·nous** (-rĭj′ə-nəs) *adj.*

prurigo mi·tis (mī′tĭs) *n.* A mild form of a chronic dermatitis characterized by recurring, intensely itching papules and nodules.

prurigo nod·u·lar·is (nŏj′ə-lâr′ĭs) *n.* An eruption of hard nodules in the skin, accompanied by intense itching.

prurigo sim·plex (sĭm′plĕks′) *n.* A mild form of prurigo marked by a tendency to relapse.

pru·ri·tus (proō-rī′təs) *n.* Severe itching, often of undamaged skin. —**pru·rit′ic** (-rĭt′ĭk) *adj.*

pruritus a·ni (ā′nī) *n.* Itching of varying intensity localized at the anus.

pruritus vul·vae (vŭl′vē) *n.* Itching of the external female genitalia.

Prus·sian blue (prŭsh′ən) *n.* See **Berlin blue.**

prus·sic acid (prŭs′ĭk) *n.* See **hydrocyanic acid.**

PSA *abbr.* prostate-specific antigen

psam·mo·car·ci·no·ma (săm′ō-kär′sə-nō′mə) *n.* A carcinoma containing calcified foci that resemble psammoma bodies. No longer in technical use.

psam·mo·ma (să-mō′mə) *n., pl.* **–mas** or **–ma·ta** (-mə-tə) Psammomatous meningioma. No longer in technical use.

psammoma body *n.* **1.** A mineralized body occurring in the meninges, choroid plexus, and in certain meningiomas. **2.** See **brain sand. 3.** See **calcospherite.**

psam·mo·ma·tous meningioma (sə-mō′mə-təs) *n.* A firm fibrous neoplasm of meninges of the brain and spinal cord characterized by psammona bodies. Also called *sand tumor.*

psam·mous (săm′əs) *adj.* Sandy.

pseud·a·graph·i·a (soō′də-grăf′ē-ə) *or* **pseu·do·a·graph·i·a** (soō′dō-ā-grăf′e-ə, -ə-grăf′-) *n.* Partial agraphia in which one cannot produce original writing but can copy correctly.

pseud·al·les·che·ri·a·sis (soō′də-lĕs′kə-rī′ə-sĭs) *n.* Any of various clinical disorders resulting from infection with the fungus *Pseudallescheria boydii* that include pulmonary colonization, fungemia, and invasive pneumonitis as well as mycotic keratitis, endophthalmitis, endocarditis, meningitis, sinusitis, brain abscesses, cutaneous and subcutaneous infections, and disseminated systemic infections.

pseud·an·ky·lo·sis (soō′dăng-kə-lō′sĭs) *n.* See **fibrous ankylosis.**

pseud·ar·thro·sis (soō′där-thrō′sĭs) *or* **pseu·do·ar·thro·sis** (soō′dō-är-) *n.* See **false joint.**

pseud·es·the·sia (soō′dĭs-thē′zhə) *or* **pseu·do·es·the·sia** (soō′dō-ĭs-) *n.* **1.** A subjective sensation not arising from an external stimulus. **2.** See **phantom limb.**

pseudo– *or* **pseud–** *pref.* **1.** False; deceptive; sham: *pseudohematuria.* **2.** Apparently similar: *pseudomyxoma.*

pseu·do·ac·an·tho·sis ni·gri·cans (soō′dō-ăk′ăn-thō′sĭs nī′grĭ-kănz′, nĭg′rĭ-) *n.* Acanthosis nigricans occurring secondary to maceration of the skin from excessive sweating, or in obese adults who have dark complexions, or in association with endocrine disorders.

pseu·do·ai·nhum (soō′dō-ī-nyoōm′) *n.* Nonspontaneous amputation of a digit, caused by a variety of disorders.

pseu·do·al·lele (soō′dō-ə-lēl′) *n.* A gene exhibiting pseudoallelism. —**pseu′do·al·le·lic** (-lē′lĭk, -lĕl′ĭk) *adj.*

pseu·do·al·le·lism (soō′dō-ə-lē′lĭz′əm, -lĕl′ĭz′-) *n.* The state in which two or more genes appear to occupy the same locus under certain conditions but can be shown to occupy closely linked loci under other conditions.

pseu·do·a·ne·mi·a (soō′dō-ə-nē′mē-ə) *n.* Pallor of the skin and mucous membranes without the blood signs of anemia. Also called *false anemia.*

pseu·do·an·eu·rysm (soō′dō-ăn′yə-rĭz′əm) *n.* A dilation of an artery with actual disruption of one or more layers of its walls, rather than with expansion of all wall layers. Also called *false aneurysm.*

pseu·do·ap·pen·di·ci·tis (soō′dō-ə-pĕn′dĭ-sī′tĭs) *n.* A complex of symptoms simulating appendicitis without inflammation of the appendix.

pseu·do·bul·bar (soō′dō-bŭl′bər, -bär′) *adj.* Appearing to be due to a bulbar lesion.

pseudobulbar paralysis *n.* Paralysis of the lips and tongue, with uncontrolled laughing or crying and difficulty in speaking and swallowing. It simulates progressive bulbar paralysis, and is due to cerebral lesions with bilateral involvement of the upper motor neurons.

pseu·do·car·ti·lage (sōō′dō-kär′tl-ĭj) *n.* See **chondroid tissue** (sense 1). —**pseu′do·car′ti·lag′i·nous** (-kär′tl-ăj′ə-nəs) *adj.*

pseu·do·cast (sōō′də-kăst′) *n.* An elongated ribbonlike mucous thread occurring in the urine, having poorly defined edges and pointed or split ends and resembling a urinary cast.

pseu·do·chan·cre (sōō′dō-shăng′kər) *n.* A nonspecific indurated sore resembling a chancre, usually located on the penis.

pseu·do·cho·lin·es·ter·ase deficiency (sōō′dō-kō′lə-něs′tə-rās′, -rāz′) *n.* An inheritable disorder manifested by exaggerated responses to drugs ordinarily hydrolyzed by serum pseudocholinesterase.

pseu·do·cho·re·a (sōō′dō-kô-rē′ə) *n.* A spasmodic disease or generalized tic resembling chorea.

pseu·do·chro·mes·the·sia (sōō′dō-krō′mĭs-thē′zhə) *n.* **1.** A form of synesthesia in which printed vowels or vowel sounds produce imaginary sensations of color. **2.** See **color hearing.**

pseu·do·chrom·hi·dro·sis (sōō′dō-krōm′hĭ-drō′sĭs, -hī-) *n.* A condition characterized by pigment on the skin that appears to be colored sweat but is actually local sites of active pigment-forming bacteria.

pseu·do·cir·rho·sis (sōō′dō-sĭ-rō′sĭs) *n.* See **cardiac cirrhosis.**

pseu·do·co·arc·ta·tion (sōō′dō-kō′ärk-tā′shən) *n.* Distortion, often with slight narrowing, of the aortic arch at the level of insertion of the arterial ligament.

pseu·do·col·loid (sōō′dō-kŏl′oid′) *n.* A colloidlike or mucoid substance found at sites such as ovarian cysts and Fordyce's spots.

pseu·do·cox·al·gia (sōō′dō-kŏk-săl′jə) *n.* See **transient synovitis.**

pseu·do·croup (sōō′dō-krōōp′, sōō′dō-krōōp′) *n.* See **laryngismus stridulus.**

pseu·do·cryp·tor·chism (sōō′dō-krĭp-tôr′kĭz′əm) *n.* A condition in which the testes descend to the scrotum but move up and down, rising high in the inguinal canal at one time and descending to the scrotum at another.

pseu·do·cy·e·sis (sōō′dō-sī-ē′sĭs) *n.* See **false pregnancy.**

pseu·do·cyl·in·droid (sōō′dō-sĭl′ən-droid′) *n.* A shred of mucus or other substance in the urine resembling a renal cast.

pseu·do·cyst (sōō′dō-sĭst′) *n.* **1.** An abnormal sac that resembles a cyst but has no membranous lining. Also called *adventitious cyst, false cyst.* **2.** A cyst whose wall is formed by a host cell and not by a parasite. **3.** A cyst consisting of a host cell enclosing a mass of *Toxoplasma* parasites, usually found in the brain.

pseu·do·de·men·tia (sōō′dō-dĭ-měn′shə) *n.* A condition of exaggerated indifference to one's surroundings without actual mental impairment.

pseu·do·diph·the·ri·a (sōō′dō-dĭf-thîr′ē-ə, -dĭp-) *n.* See **diphtheroid** (sense 1).

pseu·do·e·de·ma (sōō′dō-ĭ-dē′mə) *n.* A puffiness of the skin that is not the result of an accumulation of fluid.

pseu·do·e·phed·rine (sōō′dō-ĭ-fĕd′rĭn, -ĕf′ĭ-drēn′) *n.*

An isomer of ephedrine, used in its hydrochloride form as a nasal decongestant.

pseu·do·fol·lic·u·li·tis (sōō′dō-fə-lĭk′yə-lī′tĭs) *n.* Follicular papules or pustules resulting from close shaving or plucking of very curly hair and caused by the tips of hairs growing into the follicle wall or reentering the skin adjacent to the follicle.

pseu·do·frac·ture (sōō′dō-frăk′chər) *n.* A condition in which an x-ray shows formation of new bone with thickening of periosteum at the injury site.

pseu·do·gan·gli·on (sōō′dō-găng′glē-ən) *n.* A localized thickening of a nerve trunk having the appearance of a ganglion.

pseu·do·gene (sōō′də-jēn′) *n.* A segment of DNA resembling a gene but lacking a genetic function.

pseu·do·geu·ses·the·sia (sōō′dō-gyōō′zĭs-thē′zhə, -jōō′zĭs-) *n.* See **color taste.**

pseu·do·geu·sia (sōō′dō-gyōō′zhə, -jōō′-) *n.* A taste sensation that is not produced by an external stimulus.

pseu·do·gout (sōō′dō-gout′) *n.* See **articular chondrocalcinosis.**

pseu·do·he·ma·tu·ri·a (sōō′dō-hē′mə-tŏŏr′ē-ə) *n.* Redness of the urine caused by certain foods or drugs. Also called *false hematuria.*

pseu·do·her·maph·ro·dite (sōō′dō-hər-măf′rə-dīt′) *n.* A person exhibiting pseudohermaphroditism.

pseu·do·her·maph·ro·dit·ism (sōō′dō-hər-măf′rə-dī-tĭz′əm) *n.* A state in which an individual possesses the internal reproductive organs of one sex while exhibiting some of the external physical characteristics of the opposite sex. Also called *false hermaphroditism.*

pseu·do·her·ni·a (sōō′dō-hûr′nē-ə) *n.* Inflammation of the scrotal tissues or of an inguinal gland, simulating a strangulated hernia.

pseu·do·hy·per·par·a·thy·roid·ism (sōō′dō-hī′pər-păr′ə-thī′roi-dĭz′əm) *n.* Hypercalcemia occurring in association with a malignant neoplasm but without skeletal metastases or primary hyperparathyroidism, possibly caused by the formation of parathyroid hormone by nonparathyroid tumor tissue.

pseudohypertrophic muscular dystrophy *n.* The most common form of muscular dystrophy, in which fat and fibrous tissue infiltrate muscle tissue, causing eventual weakening of the respiratory muscles and the myocardium. The disease, which almost exclusively affects males, begins in early childhood and usually causes death before adulthood. Also called *childhood muscular dystrophy, Duchenne's disease, Duchenne's dystrophy, pseudohypertrophic muscular paralysis.*

pseu·do·hy·per·tro·phy (sōō′dō-hī-pûr′trə-fē) *n.* Increase at the site of an organ or part that is the result of an increase in the size or number of some other tissue, not of the specific functional elements. —**pseu′do·hy′per·tro′phic** (-trō′fĭk, -trŏf′ĭk) *adj.*

pseu·do·hy·po·na·tre·mi·a (sōō′dō-hī′pō-nə-trē′mē-ə) *n.* A low serum sodium concentration resulting from volume displacement by massive hyperlipidemia or hyperproteinemia, or by hyperglycemia.

pseu·do·hy·po·par·a·thy·roid·ism (sōō′dō-hī′pō-păr′ə-thī′roi-dĭz′əm) *n.* A sex-linked disorder resembling hypoparathyroidism, but which is unresponsive to treatment with parathyroid hormone; it is characterized by short stature, round face, achondroplasia, calcification of basal ganglia, true ectopic bone in fascial planes and skin, mental deficiency, hypocalcemia, hyperphosphatemia, and parathyroid tissue that is hyperplastic. Also called *Seabright bantam syndrome.*

pseu·do·ic·ter·us (soo′dō-ĭk′tər-əs) *n.* Discoloration of the skin not caused by bile pigments, as in Addison's disease. Also called *pseudojaundice.*

pseu·do·i·so·chro·mat·ic (soo′dō-ī′sə-krō-măt′ĭk) *adj.* Being apparently of the same color, as of certain charts used in testing colorblindness.

pseu·do·jaun·dice (soo′dō-jôn′dĭs, -jän′-) *n.* See **pseudoicterus.**

pseu·do·lo·gi·a (soo′də-lō′jē-ə) *n.* Pathological lying in speech or writing.

pseudologia fan·tas·ti·ca (făn-tăs′tĭ-kə) *n.* An elaborate and often fantastic account of exploits that is false but that the teller believes to be true.

pseu·do·ma·lig·nan·cy (soo′dō-mə-lĭg′nən-sē) *n.* A benign tumor that appears, clinically or histologically, to be a malignant neoplasm.

pseu·do·ma·ni·a (soo′dō-mā′nē-ə, -mān′yə) *n.* **1.** Feigned insanity. **2.** A mental disorder in which the individual alleges to have committed a crime, but has not. **3.** The pathological impulse to falsify or lie.

pseu·do·mem·brane (soo′dō-měm′brān′) *n.* See **false membrane.**

pseu·do·mem·bra·nous (soo′dō-měm′brə-nəs) *adj.* Relating to or marked by a false membrane.

pseudomembranous bronchitis *n.* See **fibrinous bronchitis.**

pseudomembranous enterocolitis *n.* Enterocolitis with the formation and passage of pseudomembranous material in the stools; it commonly follows prolonged antibiotic therapy. Also called *pseudomembranous colitis, pseudomembranous enteritis.*

pseudomembranous gastritis *n.* Gastritis characterized by the formation of a false membrane.

pseudomembranous inflammation *n.* A form of exudative inflammation characterized by the formation of a false membrane on a mucosal surface.

pseu·do·mo·nad (soo′də-mō′năd′) *n.* A member of the genus *Pseudomonas.*

Pseu·do·mo·nas (soo′də-mō′nəs, soo-dŏm′ə-nəs) *n.* A phylum of gram-negative, rod-shaped, mostly aerobic flagellated bacteria, commonly found in soil, water, and decaying matter and including some species that are plant and animal pathogens.

pseu·do·myx·o·ma (soo′dō-mĭk-sō′mə) *n.* A gelatinous mass resembling a myxoma but composed of epithelial mucus.

pseudomyxoma per·i·to·ne·i (pĕr′ĭ-tn-ē′ī) *n.* The accumulation of mucoid or mucinous material in the peritoneal cavity, either as a result of rupture of a mucocele of the appendix or of rupture of a benign or malignant cystic neoplasm of the ovary.

pseu·do·ne·o·plasm (soo′dō-nē′ə-plăz′əm) *n.* See **pseudotumor** (sense 2).

pseu·do·neu·ri·tis (soo′dō-noo-rī′tĭs) *n.* Congenital reddish appearance of the optic disk simulating optic neuritis.

pseu·do·neu·ro·gen·ic bladder (soo′dō-noor′ə-jĕn′-ĭk) *n.* Incoordination of the detrusor and sphincter muscles having psychologic basis.

pseu·do·pap·il·le·de·ma (soo′dō-păp′ə-lĭ-dē′mə, -pə-pĭl′ĭ-) *n.* Apparent swelling of the optic disk that occurs in hyperopia and drusen of the optic nerve.

pseu·do·pa·ral·y·sis (soo′dō-pə-răl′ĭ-sĭs) *n.* A voluntary restriction or inhibition of motion because of pain, incoordination, or other cause, not due to actual muscular paralysis. Also called *pseudoparesis.*

pseu·do·par·a·ple·gia (soo′dō-păr′ə-plē′jə) *n.* Apparent paralysis in the lower extremities, in which the tendon and skin reflexes and the electrical reactions are normal.

pseu·do·pa·re·sis (soo′dō-pə-rē′sĭs, -păr′ĭ-sĭs) *n.* See **pseudoparalysis.**

pseu·do·pe·lade (soo′dō-pĕ-läd′) *n.* A scarring type of alopecia, usually occurring in small areas and preceded by folliculitis.

pseu·do·plate·let (soo′dō-plāt′lĭt) *n.* Any of the various fragments of neutrophils that may be mistaken for platelets, especially in peripheral blood smears of leukemic patients.

pseu·do·pod (soo′də-pŏd′) *n.* A temporary projection of the cytoplasm of certain cells or of certain unicellular organisms, especially amoebas, that serves in locomotion and phagocytosis.

pseu·do·po·di·um (soo′də-pō′dē-əm) *n., pl.* –po·di·a (-pō′dē-ə) A pseudopod.

pseu·do·pol·yp (soo′dō-pŏl′ĭp) *n.* A projecting mass of granulation tissue, such as the masses that may develop in ulcerative colitis.

pseu·do·preg·nan·cy (soo′dō-prĕg′nən-sē) *n.* **1.** See **false pregnancy. 2.** A condition resembling pregnancy that occurs in some mammals, marked by persistence of the corpus luteum and usually following infertile copulation.

pseu·do·pseu·do·hy·po·par·a·thy·roid·ism (soo′dō-soo′dō-hī′pō-păr′ə-thī′roi-dĭz′əm) *n.* An inherited disorder that closely simulates the symptoms but not the consequences of pseudohypoparathyroidism, thus it has mild or no manifestations of hypoparathyroidism or tetanic convulsions.

pseu·dop·si·a (soo-dŏp′sē-ə) *n.* Visual hallucinations, illusions, or false perceptions.

pseu·do·pte·ryg·i·um (soo′dō-tə-rĭj′ē-əm) *n.* A pterygium of irregular shape that may appear at any part of the corneal margin of the eye and that occurs following diphtheria, a burn, or other injury of the conjunctiva.

pseu·dop·to·sis (soo′dŏp-tō′sĭs, soo′dō-tō′-) *n.* A condition resembling ptosis and due to blepharophimosis, blepharochalasis, or some other abnormality. Also called *false blepharoptosis.*

pseu·do·re·ac·tion (soo′dō-rē-ăk′shən) *n.* A reaction not caused by the substances used in a given test but rather by impurities or other materials in the test medium; a false reaction.

pseu·do·rick·ets (soo′dō-rĭk′ĭts) *n.* See **renal rickets.**

pseu·do·ro·sette (soo′dō-rō-zĕt′) *n.* The radial arrangement of neoplastic cells around a small blood vessel.

pseu·do·sar·co·ma (soo′dō-sär-kō′mə) *n.* A bulky polyploid malignant tumor of the esophagus composed of spindle cells with a focus of squamous cell carcinoma.

pseu·do·scar·la·ti·na (soo′dō-skär′lə-tē′nə) *n.* Erythema with fever resulting from causes other than infection with *Streptococcus pyogenes.*

pseu·do·scle·ro·sis (soo′dō-sklə-rō′sĭs) *n.* The cerebral changes caused by hepatolenticular degeneration. Also called *Strümpell-Westphal disease, Westphal-Strümpell disease.*

pseu·dos·mi·a (soo-dŏz′mē-ə) *n.* Subjective sensation of an odor that is not present.

pseu·do·stra·bis·mus (soo′dō-strə-bĭz′məs) *n.* The appearance of strabismus caused by epicanthus, abnormality in interorbital distance, or corneal light reflex not corresponding to the center of the pupil.

pseu·do·strat·i·fied epithelium (soo′dō-străt′ə-fīd′) *n.* Epithelium made up of cells that reach the basement membrane and appear to be stratified because their nuclei are at different levels.

pseu·do·trun·cus ar·te·ri·o·sus (soo′dō-trŭng′kəs är-tîr′ē-ō′səs) *n.* A congenital cardiovascular deformity characterized by atresia of the pulmonic valve and the lack of a main pulmonary artery with the lungs being supplied with blood either through an arterial duct or via bronchial arteries arising from the aorta.

pseu·do·tu·ber·cu·lo·sis (soo′dō-tōō-bûr′kyə-lō′sĭs) *n.* Any of several diseases characterized by granulomas that resemble tubercular nodules but that are not caused by the tubercle bacillus.

pseu·do·tu·mor (soo′dō-tōō′mər) *n.* **1.** A nonneoplastic enlargement that resembles a true neoplasm. **2.** A circumscribed fibrous exudate of inflammatory origin. Also called *pseudoneoplasm.* **3.** A condition characterized by cerebral edema with narrowed small ventricles but with increased intracranial pressure and frequently with papilledema, commonly associated with obesity in females between the ages of 13 and 40.

pseu·do-Tur·ner's syndrome (soo′dō-tûr′nərz) *n.* A syndrome characterized by short stature and a webbed neck, often associated with mental retardation and congential heart disease. Also called *Bonnevie-Ullrich syndrome.*

pseu·do·xan·tho·ma e·las·ti·cum (soo′dō-zăn-thō′mə ĭ-lăs′tĭ-kəm) *n.* See **elastoma.**

psi (sī, psī) *n. Symbol* ψ The 23rd letter of the Greek alphabet.

psil·o·cin (sĭl′ə-sĭn, sī′lə-) *n.* A potent hallucinogenic compound related to psilocybin.

psil·o·cy·bin (sĭl′ə-sī′bĭn, sī′lə-) *n.* A hallucinogenic compound obtained from the mushroom *Psilocybe mexicana.*

psi·lo·sis (sī-lō′sĭs) *n.* **1.** A falling out of hair. **2.** See **sprue** (sense 1).

P-sin·is·tro·car·di·a·le (pē′sĭn′ĭ-strō-kär′dē-ā′lē) *n.* An electrocardiographic syndrome characteristic of overloading of the left atrium of the heart.

psi phenomenon *n.* A phenomenon that includes both psychokinesis and extrasensory perception.

psit·ta·cine (sĭt′ə-sīn′) *adj.* **1.** Relating to, resembling, or characteristic of parrots. **2.** Of or belonging to the family Psittacidae, which includes the parrots, macaws, and parakeets.

psit·ta·co·sis (sĭt′ə-kō′sĭs) *n.* An infectious disease of parrots and related birds caused by the bacterium *Chlamydia psittaci* and communicable to humans, producing high fever, severe headache, and symptoms similar to pneumonia.

pso·as abscess (sō′əs) *n.* An abscess originating in tuberculous spondylitis and extending through the iliopsoas muscle to the inguinal region.

psoas major *n.* See **greater psoas muscle.**

psoas minor *n.* See **smaller psoas muscle.**

pso·ra·len (sôr′ə-lən) *n.* Any of a group of chemical compounds found naturally in certain plants that are used in the treatment of psoriasis and vitiligo.

pso·rel·co·sis (sôr′əl-kō′sĭs) *n.* Ulceration of the skin resulting from scabies.

pso·ri·a·si·form (sə-rī′ə-sə-fôrm′) *adj.* Resembling psoriasis.

pso·ri·a·sis (sə-rī′ə-sĭs) *n.* A noncontagious inflammatory skin disease characterized by recurring reddish patches covered with silvery scales.

pso·ri·at·ic (sôr′ē-ăt′ĭk) *or* **pso·ri·a·sic** (sə-rī′ə-sĭk) *adj.* Of, relating to, or characteristic of psoriasis.

psoriatic arthritis *n.* Combined psoriasis and arthritis, often affecting the interphalangeal joints.

psych– *pref.* Variant of **psycho–.**

psy·chal·gia (sī-kăl′jə) *n.* **1.** Psychological or emotional pain or distress that accompanies a mental effort, especially in depression. **2.** Physical pain that is possibly of psychological origin.

psy·cha·tax·i·a (sī′kə-tăk′sē-ə) *n.* The inability to fix one's attention or to make a sustained mental effort.

psy·che (sī′kē) *n.* The mind functioning as the center of thought, emotion, and behavior and consciously or unconsciously mediating the body's responses to the social and physical environment.

psy·che·del·ic (sī′kĭ-dĕl′ĭk) *adj.* Of, characterized by, or generating hallucinations, distortions of perception, altered states of awareness, and occasionally states resembling psychosis. —*n.* A drug, such as LSD or mescaline, that produces such effects.

psy·chi·at·ric (sī′kē-ăt′rĭk) *adj.* Of or relating to psychiatry.

psychiatric hospital *n.* A hospital for the care and treatment of patients affected with acute or chronic mental illness. Also called *mental hospital.*

psy·chi·a·trist (sĭ-kī′ə-trĭst, sī-) *n.* A physician who specializes in psychiatry.

psy·chi·a·try (sĭ-kī′ə-trē, sī-) *n.* The branch of medicine that deals with the diagnosis, treatment, and prevention of mental and emotional disorders.

psy·chic (sī′kĭk) *adj.* **1.** Of, relating to, affecting, or influenced by the human mind or psyche; mental. **2.** Capable of extraordinary mental processes, such as extrasensory perception and mental telepathy. **3.** Of or relating to such mental processes. —*n.* A person apparently responsive to psychic forces.

psychic trauma *n.* An upsetting experience precipitating or aggravating an emotional or mental disorder.

psy·cho (sī′kō) *n.* A psychopath. —*adj.* Crazy; insane.

psycho– *or* **psych–** *pref.* **1.** Mind; mental: *psychogenic.* **2.** Mental activities or processes: *psychomotor.* **3.** Psychology; psychological: *psychosocial.*

psy·cho·a·cous·tics (sī′kō-ə-kōō′stĭks) *n.* The scientific study of the perception of sound.

psy·cho·ac·tive (sī′kō-ăk′tĭv) *adj.* Affecting the mind or mental processes. Used of a drug.

psy·cho·a·nal·y·sis (sī′kō-ə-năl′ĭ-sĭs) *n., pl.* **-ses** (-sēz′) **1.** The method of psychological therapy originated by Sigmund Freud in which free association, dream interpretation, and analysis of resistance and transference are used to explore repressed or unconscious impulses, anxieties, and internal conflicts. Also called *psychoanalytic therapy.* **2.** The theory of personality developed by Freud that focuses on repression and unconscious forces and includes the concepts of infantile sexuality, resistance, transference, and division of the psyche into the id, ego, and superego. **3.** Psychotherapy incorporating this method and theory. —**psy′cho·an′a·lyt′ic** (-ăn′ə-lĭt′ĭk), **psy′cho·an′a·lyt′·i·cal** (-ĭ-kəl) *adj.*

psy·cho·an·a·lyst (sī′kō-ăn′ə-lĭst) *n.* A psychotherapist, usually a psychiatrist or a clinical psychologist, who is trained in psychoanalysis and employs its methods in treating emotional disorders.

psychoanalytic psychiatry *n.* The branch of psychiatry that applies the principles of psychoanalysis to the diagnosis and treatment of mental illness. Also called *dynamic psychiatry.*

psychoanalytic therapy *n.* See **psychoanalysis.**

psy·cho·an·a·lyze (sī′kō-ăn′ə-līz′) *v.* To treat using psychoanalysis.

psy·cho·bab·ble (sī′kō-băb′əl) *n.* Psychological jargon, especially that of psychotherapy.

psy·cho·bi·ol·o·gy (sī′kō-bī-ŏl′ə-jē) *n.* **1.** The study of the biological foundations of the mind, emotions, and mental processes. Also called *biopsychology.* **2.** The school of psychiatry that interprets personality, behavior, and mental illness in terms of adaptive responses to biological, social, cultural, and environmental factors. —**psy′cho·bi′o·log′ic** (-bī′ə-lŏj′ĭk), **psy′cho·bi′o·log′·i·cal** (-ĭ-kəl) *adj.*

psy·cho·chem·i·cal (sī′kō-kĕm′ĭ-kəl) *n.* A psychoactive drug or substance. —*adj.* Of or relating to psychochemicals.

psy·cho·chem·is·try (sī′kō-kĕm′ĭ-strē) *n.* The study of chemicals that have psychological effects.

psy·cho·di·ag·no·sis (sī′kō-dī′əg-nō′sĭs) *n.* **1.** Any of various methods used to discover the factors that underlie behavior, especially maladjusted or abnormal behavior. **2.** The branch of clinical psychology that emphasizes the use of psychological tests and techniques for assessing mental illness.

psy·cho·dra·ma (sī′kə-drä′mə) *n.* **1.** A psychotherapeutic and analytic technique in which people are assigned roles to be played spontaneously within a dramatic context devised by a therapist. **2.** A dramatization in which this technique is employed. —**psy′cho·dra·mat′ic** (-drə-măt′ĭk) *adj.*

psy·cho·dy·nam·ics (sī′kō-dī-năm′ĭks, -dĭ-) *n.* **1.** The interaction of various conscious and unconscious mental or emotional processes, especially as they influence personality, behavior, and attitudes. **2.** The study of personality and behavior in terms of such processes.

psy·cho·gen·e·sis (sī′kə-jĕn′ĭ-sĭs) *n.* **1.** The origin and development of psychological processes, personality, or behavior. **2.** Development of a physical disorder or illness resulting from psychic, rather than physiological, factors. —**psy′cho·ge·net′ic** (-jə-nĕt′ĭk) *adj.*

psy·cho·gen·ic deafness (sī′kə-jĕn′ĭk) *n.* Hearing loss or impairment caused by a mental or emotional disorder or trauma and having no evidence of an organic cause. Also called *functional deafness.*

psychogenic pain disorder *n.* A disorder characterized by severe prolonged pain for which there is psychological involvement rather than a physical basis.

psychogenic purpura *n.* See **autoerythrocyte sensitization syndrome.**

psychogenic vomiting *n.* Vomiting associated with emotional distress and anxiety but not causing weight loss, occurring usually during meals.

psy·cho·graph (sī′kə-grăf′) *n.* A graphic representation or chart of the personality traits of an individual or group. —**psy′cho·graph′ic** *adj.*

psy·cho·ki·ne·sis (sī′kō-kĭ-nē′sĭs, -kī-) *n., pl.* **-ses** (-sēz) *Abbr.* **PK 1.** An uncontrolled, maniacal outburst, resulting from defective inhibition. **2.** The production or control of motion, especially in inanimate and remote objects, purportedly by the exercise of psychic powers. —**psy′cho·ki·net′ic** (-kĭ-nĕt′ĭk, -kī-) *adj.*

psy·cho·lep·sy (sī′kə-lĕp′sē) *n.* A condition characterized by sudden mood changes accompanied by feelings of hopelessness and lethargy.

psy·cho·lin·guis·tics (sī′kō-lĭng-gwĭs′tĭks) *n.* The study of the influence of psychological factors on the development, use, and interpretation of language. —**psy′cho·lin·guis′tic** *adj.*

psy·cho·log·i·cal (sī′kə-lŏj′ĭ-kəl) *or* **psy·cho·log·ic** (-lŏj′ĭk) *adj.* **1.** Of or relating to psychology. **2.** Of, relating to, or arising from the mind or emotions. **3.** Influencing or intended to influence the mind or emotions.

psychological moment *n.* The time at which the mental state of a person is most likely to produce a desired response.

psy·chol·o·gist (sī-kŏl′ə-jĭst) *n.* A person trained and educated to perform psychological research, testing, and therapy.

psy·chol·o·gize (sī-kŏl′ə-jīz′) *v.* **1.** To explain behavior in psychological terms. **2.** To investigate, reason, or speculate in psychological terms.

psy·chol·o·gy (sī-kŏl′ə-jē) *n.* **1.** The science that deals with mental processes and behavior. **2.** The emotional and behavioral characteristics of an individual, group, or activity.

psy·cho·met·rics (sī′kə-mĕt′rĭks) *n.* The branch of psychology that deals with the design, administration, and interpretation of quantitative tests for the measurement of psychological variables such as intelligence, aptitude, and personality traits. Also called *psychometry.* —**psy′·cho·met′ric, psy′cho·met′ri·cal** *adj.*

psy·cho·mo·tor (sī′kō-mō′tər) *adj.* **1.** Of or relating to movement or muscular activity associated with mental processes. **2.** Relating to the combination of psychic and motor events, including disturbances.

psychomotor epilepsy *n.* An epileptic seizure often associated with temporal lobe disease and characterized by complex sensory, motor, and psychic symptoms such as impaired consciousness with amnesia, emotional outbursts, automatic behavior, and abnormal acts. Also called *psychomotor seizure, temporal lobe epilepsy.*

psy·cho·neu·ro·im·mu·nol·o·gy (sī′kō-noŏr′ō-ĭm′yə-nŏl′ə-jē) *n.* The study of the interaction of behavioral, neural, and endocrine factors and the functioning of the immune system.

psy·cho·neu·ro·sis (sī′kō-noŏ-rō′sĭs) *n.,* pl. **-ses** (-sēz) Neurosis. —**psy′cho·neu·rot′ic** (-rŏt′ĭk) *adj.*

psy·cho·path (sī′kə-păth′) *n.* A person with an antisocial personality disorder, especially one manifested in perverted, criminal, or amoral behavior.

psy·cho·path·ic (sī′kə-păth′ĭk) *adj.* **1.** Of, relating to, or characterized by psychopathy. **2.** Relating to or affected with an antisocial personality disorder that is usually characterized by aggressive, perverted, criminal, or amoral behavior.

psy·cho·pa·thol·o·gy (sī′kō-pə-thŏl′ə-jē) *n.* **1.** The study of the origin, development, and manifestations of mental or behavioral disorders. **2.** The manifestation of a mental or behavioral disorder.

psy·chop·a·thy (sī-kŏp′ə-thē) *n.* Mental disorder, especially when manifested by antisocial behavior.

psy·cho·phar·ma·ceu·ti·cal (sī′kō-fär′mə-soō′tĭ-kəl) *n.* A drug used in treating an emotional disorder.

psy·cho·phar·ma·col·o·gy (sī′kō-fär′mə-kŏl′ə-jē) *n.* The branch of pharmacology dealing with the study of the actions and the effects of psychoactive drugs. —**psy′cho·phar′ma·co·log′ic** (-kə-lŏj′ĭk), **psy′cho·phar′ma·co·log′i·cal** (-ĭ-kəl) *adj.*

psy·cho·phys·i·cal (sī′kō-fĭz′ĭ-kəl) *adj.* **1.** Of or relating to psychophysics. **2.** Psychosomatic.

psy·cho·phys·ics (sī′kō-fĭz′ĭks) *n.* The branch of psychology that deals with the relationships between physical stimuli and sensory response.

psy·cho·phys·i·o·log·ic disorder (sī′kō-fĭz′ē-ə-lŏj′ĭk) *n.* See **psychosomatic disorder.**

psy·cho·phys·i·ol·o·gy (sī′kō-fĭz′ē-ŏl′ə-jē) *n.* The study of correlations between the mind, behavior, and bodily mechanisms. Also called *physiological psychology.* —**psy′cho·phys′i·o·log′i·cal** (-ə-lŏj′ĭ-kəl), **psy′cho·phys′i·o·log′ic** (-ĭk) *adj.*

psy·cho·sen·so·ry (sī′kō-sĕn′sə-rē) *adj.* Of or relating to the mental perception and interpretation of sensory stimuli.

psy·cho·sex·u·al (sī′kō-sĕk′shoō-əl) *adj.* Of or relating to the mental and emotional aspects of sexuality.

psychosexual development *n.* In Freudian psychoanalytic theory, the influence that sexual growth has on personality development from birth to adult life, with the phases of sexual maturation designated as oral, anal, phallic, latency, and genital.

psychosexual dysfunction *n.* A disturbance of sexual functioning, such as impotence, premature ejaculation, or anorgasmy, that may be caused by one's mental and emotional difficulties concerning sexuality rather than physical disorders.

psy·cho·sis (sī-kō′sĭs) *n.,* pl. **-ses** (-sēz) A severe mental disorder, with or without organic damage, characterized by derangement of personality and loss of contact with reality and causing deterioration of normal social functioning.

psy·cho·so·cial (sī′kō-sō′shəl) *adj.* Involving aspects of both social and psychological behavior.

psy·cho·so·mat·ic (sī′kō-sō-măt′ĭk) *adj.* **1.** Of or relating to a disorder having physical symptoms but originating from mental or emotional causes. **2.** Relating to or concerned with the influence of the mind on the body, especially with respect to disease.

psychosomatic disorder *n.* A disorder characterized by physical symptoms resulting from psychological factors, usually involving a system of the body such as the gastrointestinal or genitourinary system. Also called *psychophysiologic disorder.*

psychosomatic medicine *n.* The branch of medicine that studies and treats disorders in which physical symptoms are influenced by psychological factors.

psy·cho·so·mi·met·ic (sī-kō′sō-mĭ-mĕt′ĭk, -mī-) *adj.* Psychotomimetic.

psy·cho·stim·u·lant (sī′kō-stĭm′yə-lənt) *n.* A drug having antidepressant or mood-elevating properties.

psy·cho·sur·ger·y (sī′kō-sûr′jə-rē) *n.* Brain surgery used to treat severe, intractable mental or behavioral disorders. —**psy′cho·sur′geon** (-sûr′jən) *n.*

psy·cho·ther·a·peu·tics (sī′kō-thĕr′ə-pyoō′tĭks) *n.* See **psychotherapy.**

psy·cho·ther·a·pist (sī′kō-thĕr′ə-pĭst) *n.* An individual, such as a psychiatrist, psychologist, psychiatric nurse, or psychiatric social worker, who practices psychotherapy.

psy·cho·ther·a·py (sī′kō-thĕr′ə-pē) *n.* The treatment of mental and emotional disorders through the use of psychological techniques designed to encourage communication of conflicts and insight into problems, with the goal being personality growth and behavior modification. Also called *psychotherapeutics.* —**psy′cho·ther′a·peu′tic** (-pyoō′tĭk) *adj.*

psy·chot·ic (sī-kŏt′ĭk) *adj.* Of, relating to, or affected by psychosis. —*n.* A person affected by psychosis.

psy·chot·o·gen·ic (sī-kŏt′ə-jĕn′ĭk) *adj.* Inducing psychosis, as a hallucinogenic drug.

psy·chot·o·mi·met·ic (sī-kŏt′ō-mə-mĕt′ĭk, -mī-) *adj.* Tending to induce hallucinations, delusions, or other symptoms of a psychosis. Used of a drug. —*n.* A psychotomimetic drug, such as LSD.

psy·cho·tro·pic (sī′kə-trō′pĭk, -trŏp′ĭk) *adj.* Having an altering effect on perception or behavior. Used especially of a drug. —*n.* A psychotropic drug or other agent.

psychro– *pref.* Cold: *psychrophilic.*

psy·chro·al·gia (sī′krō-ăl′jə) *n.* A painful sensation of cold.

psy·chrom·e·ter (sī-krŏm′ĭ-tər) *n.* An instrument that uses the difference in readings between thermometers specialized to measure the moisture content or relative humidity of air.

psy·chrom·e·try (sī-krŏm′ĭ-trē) *n.* The calculation of

relative humidity and water-vapor pressures from temperature and barometric pressure. Also called *hygrometry.*

psy·chro·phile (sī′krə-fīl′) *or* **psy·chro·phil** (-fīl) *n.* An organism that grows best at a low temperature.

psy·chro·phil·ic (sī′krō-fīl′ĭk) *adj.* Thriving at relatively low temperatures. Used of certain bacteria.

psy·chro·phore (sī′krə-fôr′) *n.* A catheter having two tubes through which cold water is circulated to apply cold to a canal or cavity.

psyl·li·um (sĭl′ē-əm) *n.* **1.** An annual Eurasian plant having opposite leaves and small flowers borne in dense spikes. **2.** The seeds of this plant, widely used as a mild bulk laxative and sometimes added to foods as a dietary source of soluble fiber.

Pt The symbol for the element **platinum.**

PT *abbr.* physical therapy

PTA *abbr.* plasma thromboplastin antecedent

PTCA *abbr.* percutaneous transluminal coronary angioplasty

pter·i·on (tĕr′ē-ŏn′, tîr′-) *n.* The junction of the greater wing of the sphenoid bone and the squamous temporal, the frontal, and the parietal bones.

ptero– *or* **pter–** *pref.* Wing; feather: *pterion.*

pter·op·ter·in (tĕr-ŏp′tər-ĭn) *n.* A crystalline conjugate of folic acid containing three molecules of glutamic acid instead of one and having the general properties of a polypeptide. Also called *pteroyltriglutamic acid.*

pter·o·yl·glu·tam·ic acid (tĕr′ō-ĭl-glōo-tăm′ĭk) *n.* Folic acid.

pter·o·yl·tri·glu·tam·ic acid (tĕr′ō-ĭl-trī′glōo-tăm′ĭk) *n.* See **pteropterin.**

pte·ryg·i·um (tə-rĭj′ē-əm) *n.,* *pl.* **–i·ums** *or* **–i·a** (-ē-ə) An abnormal mass of tissue arising from the conjunctiva of the inner corner of the eye that obstructs vision by growing over the cornea. —**pte·ryg′i·al** *adj.*

pterygo– *pref.* Pterygoid; pterygoid process: *pterygomandibular.*

pter·y·goid (tĕr′ĭ-goid′) *adj.* **1.** Of, relating to, or located in the region of the sphenoid bone. **2.** Resembling a wing; winglike. —*n.* Either of two processes descending from the body of the sphenoid bone.

pterygoid canal *n.* An opening through the pterygoid process of the sphenoid bone through which an artery, vein, and nerve pass.

pterygoid nerve *n.* Either of two motor branches of the mandibular nerve, designated lateral and medial, supplying the lateral and medial pterygoid muscles.

pterygoid process *n.* A long process of the sphenoid bone extending downward from the junction of its body and great wing.

pter·y·go·man·dib·u·lar (tĕr′ĭ-gō-măn-dĭb′yə-lər) *adj.* Of or relating to the pterygoid process and the mandible.

pter·y·go·max·il·lar·y (tĕr′ĭ-gō-măk′sə-lĕr′ē) *adj.* Relating to the pterygoid process and the maxilla.

pter·y·go·pal·a·tine (tĕr′ĭ-gō-păl′ə-tīn′) *adj.* Relating to the pterygoid process and the palatine bone.

pterygopalatine canal *n.* The canal that is formed between the maxilla and palatine bones and transmits the descending palatine artery and the greater palatine nerve.

pterygopalatine ganglion *n.* A small parasympathetic ganglion in the upper pterygopalatine fossa whose postsynaptic fibers supply the lacrimal and nasal glands. Also called *sphenopalatine ganglion.*

pterygopalatine nerve *n.* Either of two short sensory branches of the maxillary nerve in the pterygopalatine fossa, which pass through the pterygopalatine ganglion without synapse.

PTH *abbr.* parathyroid hormone

Pthir·us (thîr′əs, thī′rəs) *n.* A genus of parasitic lice of the family Pediculidae, formerly grouped in the genus *Pediculus,* the main species of which is the crab louse.

pti·lo·sis (tī-lō′sĭs) *n.* Loss of the eyelashes.

ptis·an (tĭz′ən, tĭ-zăn′) *n.* A medicinal infusion, such as sweetened barley water.

pto·maine (tō′mān′, tō-mān′) *n.* A basic nitrogenous organic compound produced by bacterial putrefaction of protein.

ptomaine poisoning *n.* Food poisoning, erroneously believed to be the result of ptomaine ingestion. Not in technical use.

ptosed (tōzd) *adj.* Ptotic.

pto·sis (tō′sĭs) *n.,* *pl.* **-ses** (-sēz) Abnormal lowering or drooping of an organ or part, especially a drooping of the upper eyelid caused by muscle weakness or paralysis.

–ptosis *suff.* Downward displacement or position: *blepharoptosis.*

ptot·ic (tŏt′ĭk) *adj.* Relating to or characterized by ptosis.

PTSD *abbr.* posttraumatic stress disorder

PTU *abbr.* propylthiouracil

pty·al·a·gogue (tī-ăl′ə-gŏg′) *n.* See **sialagogue.**

pty·a·lec·ta·sis (tī′ə-lĕk′tə-sĭs) *n.* See **sialectasis.**

pty·a·lin (tī′ə-lĭn) *n.* An amylase present in saliva that catalyzes the hydrolysis of starch into maltose and dextrin.

pty·a·lism (tī′ə-lĭz′əm) *n.* Excessive flow of saliva. Also called *hypersalivation, salivation, sialism, sialismus, sialorrhea, sialosis.*

ptyalo– *or* **ptyal–** *pref.* Saliva; salivary glands: *ptyalocele.*

pty·a·lo·cele (tī′ə-lō-sēl′) *n.* See **ranula.**

Pu The symbol for the element **plutonium.**

pu·bar·che (pyōo-bär′kē) *n.* The onset of puberty, particularly as manifested by the appearance of pubic hair.

pu·ber·al (pyōo′bər-əl)*or* **pu·ber·tal** (-bər-tl) *adj.* Of or relating to puberty.

pu·ber·ty (pyōo′bər-tē) *n.* The stage of adolescence in which an individual becomes physiologically capable of sexual reproduction.

pu·bes (pyōo′bēz) *n.,* *pl.* **pubes** **1.** The lower part of the abdomen, especially the region surrounding the external genitalia. **2.** The hair that appears on this region at puberty.

pu·bes·cence (pyōo-bĕs′əns) *n.* **1.** The state of being pubescent. **2.** The attainment or onset of puberty. **3.** The presence of downy or fine short hair.

pu·bes·cent (pyōo-bĕs′ənt) *adj.* **1.** Reaching or having reached puberty. **2.** Covered with fine short hairs.

pu·bic (pyōo′bĭk) *adj.* **1.** Of, relating to, or located in the region of the pubis or the pubes. **2.** Relating to the pubic region of the abdomen.

pubic angle *n.* See **subpubic angle.**

pubic arch *n.* The arch formed by the inferior rami of the pubic bones.

pubic bone *n.* The forward portion of either of the hipbones, at the juncture forming the front arch of the pelvis. Also called *pubis.*

pubic crest *n.* The rough anterior border of the body of the pubis that is continuous laterally with the pubic tubercle.

pubic region *n.* The lowest of the three median regions of the abdomen, which lies below the umbilical region and between the inguinal regions. Also called *hypogastrium.*

pubic symphysis *n.* The firm fibrocartilaginous joint between the two pubic bones.

pu·bi·ot·o·my (pyŏŏ′bē-ŏt′ə-mē) *n.* Surgical severance of the pubic bone a few centimeters lateral to the symphysis, especially to increase the capacity of a contracted pelvis sufficiently to permit the passage of a fetus during childbirth. Also called *pelviotomy.*

pu·bis (pyŏŏ′bĭs) *n.,* *pl.* **-bes** (-bēz) **1.** See **pubic bone. 2.** The hair of the pubic region just above the external genitals. **3.** A pubic hair. **4.** See **mons pubis.**

pub·lic health (pŭb′lĭk) *n. Abbr.* **PH** The science and practice of protecting and improving the health of a community, as by preventive medicine, health education, control of communicable diseases, application of sanitary measures, and monitoring of environmental hazards.

pubo– *pref.* Pubis; pubic: *puborectal.*

pu·bo·coc·cy·ge·us (pyŏŏ′bō-kŏk-sĭj′ē-əs) *n.* A muscle formed of the fibers of the elevator muscle of the anus, arising from the pelvic surface of the body of the pubis, and attaching to the coccyx.

pu·bo·pros·tat·ic (pyŏŏ′bō-prŏ-stăt′ĭk) *adj.* Relating to the pubic bone and the prostate gland.

puboprostatic muscle *n.* The smooth muscle fibers within the puboprostatic ligament.

pu·bo·rec·tal (pyŏŏ′bō-rĕk′təl) *adj.* Relating to the pubis and rectum.

puborectal muscle *n.* The part of the elevator muscle of the anus that passes from the body of the pubis around the anus to form a muscular sling at the level of the anorectal junction. The puborectal muscle relaxes during defecation.

pu·bo·vag·i·nal muscle (pyŏŏ′bō-văj′ə-nəl) *n.* The most medial muscular fibers of the elevator muscle of the anus, extending from the pubis into the lateral walls of the vagina.

pu·bo·ves·i·cal (pyŏŏ′bō-vĕs′ĭ-kəl) *adj.* Relating to the pubic bone and the urinary bladder.

pubovesical muscle *n.* Smooth muscle fibers within the female pubovesical ligament.

PUD *abbr.* peptic ulcer disease

pudendal artery *n.* **1.** An artery with distribution to the corpus cavernosum of the penis; internal pudendal artery. **2.** An artery with origin in the femoral artery; with distribution to the skin over the pubis, penis, scrotum, or labia majora; and with anastomoses to the dorsal artery of the penis or of the clitoris and to the posterior scrotal or labial arteries; external pudendal artery.

pudendal canal *n.* The space within the obturator fascia lining the lateral wall of the ischiorectal fossa that transmits the pudendal vessels and nerves. Also called *Alcock's canal.*

pudendal nerve *n.* A nerve that is formed by fibers from the second, third, and fourth sacral nerves, passes through the greater sciatic foramen, and accompanies the internal pudendal artery to terminate as the dorsal nerve of the penis or of the clitoris.

pu·den·dum (pyŏŏ-dĕn′dəm) *n.,* *pl.* **-da** (-də) The human external genitalia, especially of a woman. —**pu·den′dal** (-dĕn′dəl) *adj.*

pu·dic (pyŏŏ′dĭk) *adj.* Of or relating to the external human genitalia.

pu·er·il·ism (pyŏŏ′ər-ə-lĭz′əm, pyŏŏr′ə-) *n.* Childish behavior in an adult, especially as a symptom of mental illness.

pu·er·per·a (pyŏŏ-ûr′pər-ə) *n.,* *pl.* **-per·ae** (-pər-ē′) A woman who has just given birth.

pu·er·per·al (pyŏŏ-ûr′pər-əl) *adj.* Relating to, connected with, or occurring during childbirth or the period immediately following childbirth.

puerperal eclampsia *n.* Convulsions and coma that are associated with hypertension, edema, or proteinuria, occurring in a woman immediately following childbirth.

puerperal fever *n.* An illness caused by infection of the endometrium following childbirth or an abortion, marked by fever and septicemia and usually caused by unsterile technique. Also called *childbed fever.*

puerperal metritis *n.* Inflammation of the uterus following childbirth. Also called *lochiometritis.*

puerperal septicemia *n.* Severe septicemia resulting from an obstetric delivery or procedure.

puerperal tetanus *n.* Tetanus occurring during the puerperium, caused by obstetric infection. Also called *postpartum tetanus.*

pu·er·per·ant (pyŏŏ-ûr′pər-ənt) *adj.* Puerperal. —*n.* A woman who has just given birth.

pu·er·pe·ri·um (pyŏŏ′ər-pîr′ē-əm) *n.,* *pl.* **-pe·ri·a** (-pîr′ē-ə) **1.** The state of a woman during childbirth or immediately thereafter. **2.** The approximate six-week period lasting from childbirth to the return of normal uterine size.

PUFA *abbr.* polyunsaturated fatty acid

Pu·lex (pyŏŏ′lĕks′) *n.* A genus of fleas including *Pulex irritans,* the common flea that infests humans.

pu·lic·i·cide (pyŏŏ-lĭs′ĭ-sīd′) *or* **pu·li·cide** (pyŏŏ′lĭ-sīd′) *n.* A chemical agent destructive to fleas.

pul·mo (pŏŏl′mō, pŭl′-) *n.,* *pl.* **pul·mo·nes** (pŏŏl-mō′nēz, pŭl-) A lung.

pulmo– *pref.* Lung; pulmonary: *pulmoaortic.*

pul·mo·a·or·tic (pŏŏl′mō-ā-ôr′tĭk, pŭl′-) *adj.* Relating to the pulmonary artery and the aorta.

pulmon– *pref.* Variant of **pulmono–.**

pul·mo·nar·y (pŏŏl′mə-nĕr′ē, pŭl′-) *adj.* Of, relating to, or affecting the lungs.

pulmonary adenomatosis *n.* A neoplastic disease in which the alveoli and distal branches of the bronchi are filled with mucus, characterized by abundant production of sputum, chills, fever, cough, dyspnea, and pleuritic pain.

pulmonary alveolar proteinosis *n.* A chronic progressive lung disease of adults characterized by alveolar accumulation of granular proteinaceous material and little inflammatory cellular exudate.

pulmonary artery *n. Abbr.* **PA 1.** An artery that enters the hilus of the right lung, with branches distributed with the bronchi; right pulmonary artery. **2.** An artery that enters the hilus of the left lung, with branches distributed with the bronchi; left pulmonary artery.

pulmonary atresia *n.* The congenital absence of the normal valvular orifice into the pulmonary artery.

pulmonary capillary wedge pressure *n.* An indirect indication of left atrial pressure obtained by wedging a catheter into a small pulmonary artery tightly enough to block flow from behind and thus to sample the pressure beyond.

pulmonary circulation *n.* The passage of blood from the right ventricle through the pulmonary artery to the lungs and back through the pulmonary veins to the left atrium.

pulmonary dysmaturity syndrome *n.* A respiratory disorder occurring in premature infants incapable of normal pulmonary ventilation; the lungs contain widespread focal emphysematous blebs and the parenchyma has thickened alveolar walls. Also called *Wilson-Mikity syndrome.*

pulmonary edema *n.* Edema of the lungs usually due to mitral stenosis or left ventricular failure.

pulmonary embolism *n. Abbr.* **PE** The obstruction of pulmonary arteries, usually by detached fragments of a clot from a leg or pelvic vein.

pulmonary emphysema *n.* See **emphysema** (sense 1).

pulmonary function test *n. Abbr.* **PFT** Any of several breathing tests that measure the function of the lungs, including the rate of air flow and the volume of exhaled air, performed to assess lung function and to detect the presence of respiratory disease.

pulmonary hamartoma *n.* A hamartoma of the lung, producing a coin lesion that is composed primarily of cartilage and bronchial epithelium. Also called *adenochondroma.*

pulmonary hypertension *n.* Hypertension in the pulmonary circulation; it may be primary or secondary to pulmonary or cardiac disease.

pulmonary insufficiency *n.* Valvular insufficiency involving the pulmonary valve.

pulmonary ligament *n.* The reflection of the pleura from the mediastinum to the lung, continuing as a two-layered fold below the root of the lung.

pulmonary murmur *or* **pulmonic murmur** *n.* An obstructive or regurgitant murmur produced at the pulmonary orifice of the heart.

pulmonary opening *n.* The opening of the pulmonary trunk from the right ventricle that is guarded by the pulmonary valve.

pulmonary plexus *n.* Either of two autonomic plexuses, designated anterior and posterior, at the hilus of each lung, formed by branches of the vagus nerve and of the sympathetic and bronchial nerves, and from which branches accompany the bronchi and arteries into the lung.

pulmonary stenosis *n.* Narrowing of the opening into the pulmonary artery from the right ventricle.

pulmonary trunk *n.* An arterial trunk with origin from the right ventricle of the heart, and dividing into the right and left pulmonary arteries, which enter the corresponding lungs and branch with the bronchi.

pulmonary tuberculosis *n.* Tuberculosis of the lungs.

pulmonary valve *n.* A valve with semilunar cusps at the entrance to the pulmonary trunk from the right ventricle of the heart.

pulmonary vein *n.* A vein that carries oxygenated blood from the lungs to the left atrium of the heart.

pulmonary ventilation *n.* The total volume of gas per minute inspired or expired.

pul·mon·ic (pŏŏl-mŏn′ĭk, pŭl-) *adj.* Of or relating to the lungs; pulmonary.

pul·mo·ni·tis (pŏŏl′mə-nī′tĭs, pŭl′-) *n.* See **pneumonitis.**

pulmono– *or* **pulmon–** *pref.* Lung; pulmonary: *pulmonitis.*

pul·mo·nol·o·gist (pŏŏl′mə-nŏl′ə-jĭst, pŭl′-) *n.* A physician who specializes in the diagnosis and treatment of respiratory disorders.

pul·mo·nol·o·gy (pŏŏl′mə-nŏl′ə-jē, pŭl′-) *n.* The branch of medicine that deals with diseases of the respiratory system.

pul·mo·tor (pŏŏl′mō′tər, pŭl′-) *n.* A device used to inflate and deflate the lungs during resuscitation.

pulp (pŭlp) *n.* **1.** A soft, moist, shapeless mass of matter. **2.** Dental pulp. **3.** The soft, moist part of fruit. —**pulp′ous** (pŭl′pəs), **pulp′y** *adj.*

pulp amputation *n.* See **pulpotomy.**

pulp calcification *n.* Calcified nodules or amorphous deposits in the pulp of a tooth.

pulp canal *n.* See **root canal** (sense 1).

pulp cavity *n.* The central hollow of a tooth containing the dental pulp and including the root canal.

pulp chamber *n.* The portion of the pulp cavity that is contained in the crown or body of a tooth.

pul·pec·to·my (pŭl-pĕk′tə-mē) *n.* Removal of the dental pulp, including that in the roots.

pulp horn *n.* An elongation of the pulp of the tooth that extends toward the cusp.

pul·pi·fac·tion (pŭl′pə-făk′shən) *n.* Reduction of tissue to a pulpy condition.

pul·pi·tis (pŭl-pī′tĭs) *n.* Inflammation of dental pulp.

pulp nodule *n.* See **pulp stone.**

pul·pot·o·my (pŭl-pŏt′ə-mē) *n.* Surgical removal of a portion of the dental pulp, usually of the coronal portion. Also called *pulp amputation.*

pulp stone *n.* A calcified mass of dentin within the dental pulp. Also called *denticle, pulp nodule.*

pulp test *n.* See **vitality test.**

pulpy nucleus *n.* The soft central fibrocartilaginous portion of the intervertebral disk.

pul·sate (pŭl′sāt′) *v.* To expand and contract rhythmically; beat.

pul·sa·tile (pŭl′sə-təl, -tīl′) *adj.* Undergoing pulsation.

pul·sa·tion (pŭl-sā′shən) *n.* **1.** The act of pulsating. **2.** A single beat, throb, or vibration.

pulse (pŭls) *n.* The rhythmical dilation of arteries produced when blood is pumped outward by regular contractions of the heart, especially as palpated at the wrist or in the neck.

pulse deficit *n.* The difference between the heart rate and the palpable pulse, as is often seen in atrial fibrillation.

pulse generator *n.* A device that produces an electrical discharge at regular intervals, which can be modified as needed, as in an electronic pacemaker.

pulse·less disease (pŭls′lĭs) *n.* A progressive inflammatory disease that causes the arteries arising from the aortic arch to collapse, making it impossible to detect a pulse in the arms and neck, and resulting in a variety of symptoms associated with ischemia, such as temporary loss of consciousness. Also called *Takayasu's disease, Takayasu's syndrome.*

pulse oximeter *n.* A device, usually attached to the earlobe or fingertip, that measures the oxygen saturation of arterial blood. —**pulse oximetry** *n.*

pulse pressure *n.* The variation in blood pressure occurring in an artery during the cardiac cycle; the difference between systolic and diastolic pressures.

pulse rate *n.* The rate of the pulse as observed in an artery, expressed as beats per minute.

pulse therapy *n.* A short, intensive administration of pharmacotherapy, usually given at intervals such as weekly or monthly, often used in treating cancer.

pulse wave *n.* The progressive increase of pressure radiating through the arteries that occurs with each contraction of the left ventricle of the heart.

pul·sion (pŭl′shən) *n.* A swelling or pushing outward.

pulsion diverticulum *n.* A diverticulum formed by pressure from within a hollow organ, often causing herniation of the mucous membrane through the muscular layer.

pul·sus (pŭl′səs) *n.* A pulse.

pulsus alternans *n.* See **alternating pulse.**

pulsus cel·er (sĕl′ər) *n.* A pulse beat swift to rise and fall.

pulsus dif·fer·ens (dĭf′ə-rĕnz′) *n.* A condition in which the pulses in the two radial arteries differ in strength.

pulsus rar·us (râr′əs) *n.* A pulse beat slow to rise and fall. Also called *pulsus tardus.*

pul·ta·ceous (pŭl-tā′shəs) *adj.* Resembling pulp; pulpy.

pul·vi·nar (pŭl-vī′nər) *n.* The posterior extremity of the thalamus, forming a cushionlike prominence over the posterior aspect of the internal capsule.

pum·ice (pŭm′ĭs) *n.* A light, porous, glassy lava, used as an abrasive.

pump (pŭmp) *n.* **1.** A machine or device for raising, compressing, or transferring fluids. **2.** A molecular mechanism for the active transport of ions or molecules across a cell membrane. —*v.* **1.** To raise or cause to flow by means of a pump. **2.** To transport ions or molecules against a concentration gradient by the expenditure of chemically stored energy.

pump lung *n.* See **shock lung.**

pump-ox·y·gen·a·tor (pŭmp-ŏk′sĭ-jə-nā′tər) *n.* A mechanical device that can substitute for both the heart and lungs during open-heart surgery.

punch biopsy (pŭnch) *n.* Removal of a small cylindrical biopsy specimen by means of an instrument that either directly pierces the tissue or enters through the skin or a small incision in the skin.

punch-drunk *adj.* Showing signs of brain damage caused by repeated blows to the head. Used especially of a boxer.

punch-drunk syndrome *n.* A condition seen in boxers and alcoholics, caused by repeated cerebral concussions and characterized by weakness in the lower limbs, unsteadiness of gait, slowness of muscular movements, hand tremors, hesitancy of speech, and mental dullness.

punch graft *n.* A small graft of the full thickness of the scalp, removed with a circular punch and transplanted in large numbers to a bald area to grow hair.

punc·tate (pŭngk′tāt′) *adj.* Having tiny spots, points, or depressions.

punctate hemorrhage *n.* See **petechial hemorrhage.**

punctate hyalosis *n.* A form of hyalosis characterized by minute opacities in the vitreous humor.

punctate keratitis *n.* See **precipitate** (sense 2).

punctate keratoderma *n.* An inherited disorder in which horny papules, often with central craters, develop on the palms, soles, and fingers.

punc·ti·form (pŭngk′tə-fôrm′) *adj.* Very small but not microscopic.

punc·tum (pŭngk′təm) *n., pl.* **–ta** (-tə) **1.** The tip of a sharp anatomical process. **2.** A minute round spot differing in color or appearance from the surrounding tissues; a point.

punctum ce·cum (sē′kəm) *n.* See **blind spot** (sense 2).

punctum vas·cu·lo·sum (văs′kyə-lō′səm) *n.* One of the minute dots seen on a brain section, due to small drops of blood at the cut extremities of arteries.

punc·ture (pŭngk′chər) *v.* To pierce with a pointed object, as with a needle. —*n.* A hole or depression made by a sharp object. Also called *centesis.*

puncture wound *n.* A wound that is deeper than it is wide, produced by a narrow pointed object.

PUO *abbr.* pyrexia of unknown (or uncertain) origin (used of fevers before diagnosis is determined)

pu·pil (pyoo′pəl) *n.* The apparently black circular opening in the center of the iris of the eye, through which light passes to the retina. —**pu′pi·lar** *adj.*

pu·pil·lar·y (pyoo′pə-lĕr′ē) *adj.* Of or affecting the pupil of the eye.

pupillary distance *n.* The distance between the center of each pupil, used in fitting eyeglass frames and lenses.

pupillary membrane *n.* The thin central portion of the iridopupillary lamina occluding the pupil in fetal life.

pupillary reflex *n.* A reflex resulting in change in the diameter of the pupil of the eye.

pupillary-skin reflex *n.* Dilation of the pupil following scratching of the skin of the neck. Also called *ciliospinal reflex.*

pupillary zone *n.* The central region of the anterior surface of the iris of the eye.

pupillo– *pref.* Pupil: *pupillometry.*

pu·pil·lom·e·ter (pyoo′pə-lŏm′ĭ-tər) *n.* An instrument for measuring the diameter of the pupil of the eye.

pu·pil·lom·e·try (pyoo′pə-lŏm′ĭ-trē) *n.* Measurement of the pupil of the eye.

pu·pil·lo·ple·gia (pyoo′pə-lō-plē′jə) *n.* A condition characterized by the slow reaction of the pupil to light stimuli.

pu·pil·los·co·py (pyo͞o′pə-lŏs′kə-pē) *n.* See **retinoscopy**.

pu·pil·lo·sta·tom·e·ter (pyo͞o′pə-lō-stă-tŏm′ĭ-tər) *n.* An instrument for measuring the distance between the centers of the pupils.

pu·pil·lo·ton·ic pseudostrabismus (pyo͞o′pə-lō-tŏn′ĭk) *n.* See **Holmes-Adie syndrome**.

PUPPP (pē′yo͞o-pē′pē-pē′) *n.* Pruritic urticarial papules and plaques of pregnancy; an intensely itching and occasionally vesicular eruption of the trunk and arms appearing in the third trimester of pregnancy. Spontaneous healing occurs within ten days of term.

pur·blind (pûr′blīnd′) *adj.* **1.** Having poor vision; nearly or partly blind. **2.** Slow in understanding or discernment; dull.

pure (pyo͞or) *adj.* **1.** Having a homogeneous or uniform composition; not mixed. **2.** Free from adulterants or impurities. **3.** Produced by self-fertilization or continual inbreeding; homozygous.

pure absence *n.* See **simple absence**.

pureblood (pyo͞or′blŭd′) *or* **pure·blood·ed** (-blŭd′ĭd) *adj.* Of unmixed ancestry; purebred.

pure culture *n.* A culture consisting of the descendants of a single cell.

pur·ga·tion (pûr-gā′shən) *n.* Evacuation of the bowels through the use of a purgative medicine.

pur·ga·tive (pûr′gə-tĭv) *n.* An agent used for purging the bowels. —*adj.* Tending to cause evacuation of the bowels. —**pur′ga·tive** *adj.*

purge (pûrj) *v.* To cause evacuation of the bowels. —*n.* **1.** The act or process of purging. **2.** Something that purges, especially a medicinal purgative.

pu·ri·fied protein derivative of tuberculin (pyo͞or′ə-fīd′) *n. Abbr.* **PPD** Purified tuberculin containing the active protein fraction.

pu·rine (pyo͞or′ēn′) *n.* **1.** A colorless crystalline organic base that is the parent compound of various biologically important derivatives. **2.** Any of a group of organic compounds that are derived from or are structurally related to purine, including uric acid, caffeine, adenine, and guanine.

Pu·rine·thol (pyo͞o-rēn′thôl) A trademark for the drug mercaptopurine.

Pur·kin·je cell (pər-kĭn′jē, po͞or′kĭn-yĕ) *n.* Any of numerous neurons of the cerebral cortex having large flask-shaped cell bodies with massive dendrites and one slender axon. Also called *Purkinje corpuscle*.

Purkinje fiber *n.* Any of the specialized cardiac muscle fibers, part of the impulse-conducting network of the heart, that rapidly transmit impulses from the atrioventricular node to the ventricles.

Purkinje layer *n.* The layer of Purkinje cells between the molecular and the granular layers of the cerebellar cortex. Also called *ganglionic layer of cerebellar cortex*.

Pur·kin·je's figures (pər-kĭn′jēz, po͞or′kĭn-yĕz) *n.* Shadows of the retinal vessels, seen as dark lines on a reddish field when a light enters the eye through the sclera in a dark room.

Purkinje shift *n.* The change in the eye's region of maximal visual acuity as a function of availability of light; in the light-adapted eye the region is in the yellow range whereas in the dark-adapted eye the region is in the green range of the color spectrum.

pur·pu·ra (pûr′pə-rə, -pyə-) *n.* A condition characterized by hemorrhages in the skin and mucous membranes that result in the appearance of purplish spots or patches. Also called *peliosis*.

purpura an·nu·lar·is tel·an·gi·ec·to·des (ăn′yə-lâr′ĭs tĕl-ăn′jē-ĭk-tō′dēz) *n.* Ring-shaped skin lesions primarily of the lower extremities that are made up of minute telangiectases or minute purple-red spots filled with blood hemosiderin deposits. Also called *Majocchi's disease*.

purpura ful·mi·nans (fŭl′mə-nănz′) *n.* A severe and fatal form of idiopathic thrombocytopenic purpura that occurs especially in children, usually following an infectious illness, and that is characterized by low blood pressure, fever, and disseminated intravascular coagulation.

purpura hem·or·rhag·i·ca (hĕm′ə-răj′ĭ-kə) *n.* See **idiopathic thrombocytopenic purpura**.

purpura se·ni·lis (sə-nī′lĭs) *n.* The occurrence of petechiae and ecchymoses on the legs in old and disabled persons.

purpura sim·plex (sĭm′plĕks′) *n.* See **nonthrombocytopenic purpura**.

pur·pu·ric (pûr-pyo͞or′ĭk) *adj.* Relating to or affected with purpura.

pur·pu·rin (pûr′pyə-rĭn′) *n.* A reddish crystalline compound used as a biological stain.

pur·pu·ri·nu·ri·a (pûr′pyə-rə-no͞or′ē-ə) *n.* See **porphyrinuria**.

pursed lips breathing (pûrst) *n.* A technique, used by patients with chronic obstructive pulmonary disease, in which air is inhaled slowly through the nose and mouth and exhaled slowly through pursed lips.

purse-string instrument (pûrs′strĭng′) *n.* An intestinal clamp with jaws at an angle to the handle, used in performing a purse-string suture of the bowel.

purse-string suture *n.* A continuous circular suture that is pulled together to invert or close an opening.

pu·ru·lence (pyo͞or′ə-ləns) *n.* **1.** The condition of containing or discharging pus. **2.** Pus.

pu·ru·lent (pyo͞or′ə-lənt) *adj.* Containing, discharging, or causing the production of pus.

purulent inflammation *n.* An acute form of exudative inflammation in which the enzymes produced by white blood cells cause liquefaction of the affected tissues, resulting in the formation of pus. Also called *suppurative inflammation*.

purulent ophthalmia *n.* Purulent conjunctivitis, usually of gonorrheal origin.

purulent pleurisy *n.* Pleurisy accompanied by empyema.

purulent rhinitis *n.* Chronic rhinitis in which pus formation is excessive.

purulent synovitis *n.* See **suppurative arthritis**.

pu·ru·loid (pyo͞or′ə-loid′) *adj.* Resembling pus.

pus (pŭs) *n.* A generally viscous, yellowish-white fluid formed in infected tissue, consisting of white blood cells, cellular debris, and necrotic tissue.

pus·sy (pŭs′ē) *adj.* Containing or resembling pus.

pus·tu·lant (pŭs′chə-lənt) *adj.* Causing the formation of pustules.

pus·tu·lar (pŭs′chə-lər) *adj.* Of, relating to, or consisting of pustules.

pus·tu·late (pŭs′chə-lāt′) *v.* To form or cause to form pustules.

pus·tu·la·tion (pŭs′chə-lā′shən) *n.* The formation or appearance of pustules.

pus·tule (pŭs′chool, pŭs′tyool) *n.* **1.** A small inflamed skin swelling that is filled with pus; a pimple. **2.** A small swelling similar to a blister or pimple.

pus·tu·lo·sis (pŭs′chə-lō′sĭs) *n.* An eruption of pustules.

pustulosis pal·mar·is et plan·tar·is (păl-mâr′ĭs ĕt′-plăn-târ′ĭs) *n.* See **acrodermatitis continua.**

pu·ta·men (pyoo-tā′mən) *n.* The outer, larger, and darker gray of the three portions into which the lentiform nucleus of the brain is divided.

Put·nam-Da·na syndrome (pŭt′nəm-dā′nə) *n.* See **subacute combined degeneration of spinal cord.**

pu·tre·fac·tion (pyoo′trə-făk′shən) *n.* **1.** Decomposition of organic matter, especially protein, by microorganisms, resulting in production of foul-smelling matter. **2.** Putrefied matter. **3.** The condition of being putrefied.

pu·tre·fac·tive (pyoo′trə-făk′tĭv) *adj.* **1.** Bringing about putrefaction. **2.** Of, relating to, or characterized by putrefaction.

pu·tre·fy (pyoo′trə-fī′) *v.* **1.** To become decayed or cause to decay and have a foul odor. **2.** To make or become gangrenous.

pu·tres·cence (pyoo-trĕs′əns) *n.* **1.** A putrescent character or condition. **2.** Putrid matter.

pu·tres·cent (pyoo-trĕs′ənt) *adj.* **1.** Becoming putrid; putrefying. **2.** Of or relating to putrefaction.

pu·tres·ci·ble (pyoo-trĕs′ə-bəl) *adj.* Subject to putrefaction.

pu·tres·cine (pyoo-trĕs′ēn) *n.* A crystalline, slightly poisonous, colorless, foul-smelling ptomaine produced by the decarboxylation of ornithine, especially in decaying animal tissue.

pu·trid (pyoo′trĭd) *adj.* **1.** Decomposed; foul-smelling; rotten. **2.** Proceeding from, relating to, or exhibiting putrefaction.

Put·ti-Platt operation (poo′tē-plăt′) *n.* A surgical procedure to correct recurrent dislocation of a shoulder joint.

PUVA (poo′və, pyoo′-) *n.* Psoralen and ultraviolet light; a treatment for psoriasis combining the oral administration of psoralen with subsequent exposure to long wavelength ultraviolet light.

PVC *abbr.* polyvinyl chloride; premature ventricular contraction

PVD *abbr.* peripheral vascular disease

P wave *n.* A deflection in an electrocardiogram indicating depolarization of the atria.

py– *pref.* Variant of **pyo–.**

py·ar·thro·sis (pī′är-thrō′sĭs) *n.* See **suppurative arthritis.**

py·e·lec·ta·sis (pī′ə-lĕk′tə-sĭs) or **py·e·lec·ta·si·a** (pī′ə-lĭk-tā′zē-ə, -zhə) *n.* Dilation of the pelvis of the kidney.

py·e·li·tis (pī′ə-lī′tĭs) *n.* Acute inflammation of the pelvis of the kidney, caused by bacterial infection. **—py′e·lit′ic** (-lĭt′ĭk) *adj.*

pyelo– or **pyel–** *pref.* Renal pelvis: *pyeloplasty.*

py·e·lo·cal·i·ce·al (pī′ə-lō-kăl′ĭ-sē′əl) *adj.* Relating to the renal pelvis and the calices.

py·e·lo·cal·i·ec·ta·sis (pī′ə-lō-kăl′ē-ĕk′tə-sĭs, -kā′lē-) *n.* See **calicectasis.**

py·e·lo·cys·ti·tis (pī′ə-lō-sĭ-stī′tĭs) *n.* Inflammation of the renal pelvis and the urinary bladder.

py·e·lo·fluo·ros·co·py (pī′ə-lō-floo-rŏs′kə-pē, -flô-) *n.* Fluoroscopic examination of the renal pelves.

py·e·lo·gram (pī′ə-lə-grăm′) *n.* An x-ray obtained by pyelography.

py·e·log·ra·phy (pī′ə-lŏg′rə-fē) *n.* X-ray photography of the pelvis of the kidney and associated structures after injection with a radiopaque dye. Also called *pyeloureterography, ureteropyelography.*

py·e·lo·li·thot·o·my (pī′ə-lō-lĭ-thŏt′ə-mē) *n.* See **pelvilithotomy.**

py·e·lo·ne·phri·tis (pī′ə-lō-nə-frī′tĭs) *n.* Inflammation of the kidney and its pelvis, caused by bacterial infection. Also called *nephropyelitis.* **—py′e·lo·ne·phrit′ic** (-frĭt′ĭk) *adj.*

py·e·lo·ne·phro·sis (pī′ə-lō-nə-frō′sĭs) *n.* Disease of the pelvis of the kidney.

py·e·lo·plas·ty (pī′ə-lə-plăs′tē) *n.* Plastic or reconstructive surgery of the pelvis of the kidney to correct an obstruction.

py·e·lo·pli·ca·tion (pī′ə-lō-plĭ-kā′shən) *n.* A surgical procedure of taking tucks in the wall of the renal pelvis, formerly performed to treat hydronephrosis.

py·e·los·co·py (pī′ə-lŏs′kə-pē) *n.* Fluoroscopic observation of the pelvis and the calices of the kidney following injection of a contrast medium through the ureter.

py·e·los·to·my (pī′ə-lŏs′tə-mē) *n.* Surgical formation of an opening into the pelvis of the kidney to allow drainage of urine.

py·e·lot·o·my (pī′ə-lŏt′ə-mē) *n.* Incision into the pelvis of the kidney. Also called *pelviotomy.*

py·e·lo·u·re·ter·ec·ta·sis (pī′ə-lō-yoo-rē′tə-rĕk′tə-sĭs, -yoor′ĭ-tə-) *n.* Dilation of the pelvis of the kidney and the ureter.

py·e·lo·u·re·ter·og·ra·phy (pī′ə-lō-yoo-rē′tə-rŏg′rə-fē, -yoor′ĭ-) *n.* See **pyelography.**

py·e·lo·ve·nous (pī′ə-lō-vē′nəs) *adj.* Of or relating to the pelvis of the kidney and the renal veins.

py·em·e·sis (pī-ĕm′ĭ-sĭs) *n.* The vomiting of pus.

py·e·mi·a (pī-ē′mē-ə) *n.* Septicemia caused by pyogenic microorganisms in the blood, often resulting in the formation of multiple abscesses. Also called *pyohemia.* **—py·e′mic** *adj.*

pyemic abscess *n.* A hematogenous abscess resulting from pyemia, septicemia, or bacteremia. Also called *septicemic abscess.*

pyemic embolism *n.* The obstruction of an artery by an embolus detached from a pus-filled clot. Also called *infective embolism.*

Py·e·mo·tes trit·i·ci (pī′ə-mō′tēz trĭt′ĭ-sī′) *n.* A species of mites that cause acarodermatitis.

py·en·ceph·a·lus (pī′ĕn-sĕf′ə-ləs) *n.* See **pyocephalus.**

py·e·sis (pī-ē′sĭs) *n.* See **suppuration.**

pyg·ma·lion·ism (pĭg-māl′yə-nĭz′əm, -mā′lē-ə-) *n.* The state of being in love with an object of one's own creation.

pyg·my (pĭg′mē) *n.* **1.** An individual of unusually small size. **2. Pygmy** A member of any of various peoples, especially found in equatorial Africa and parts of southeast Asia, having an average height less than 5 feet. —*adj.* Unusually or atypically small.

pyk·nic (pĭk′nĭk) *adj.* Having a short, stocky physique.

pykno– or **pykn–** *pref.* Thick, dense, or compact: *pyknomorphous.*

pyk·no·dys·os·to·sis (pĭk′nō-dĭs′ŏs-tō′sĭs) *n.* An inherited disorder characterized by short stature, delayed closure of the fontanelles, and hypoplasia of the terminal phalanges.

pyk·no·mor·phous (pĭk′nō-môr′fəs) *adj.* Staining deeply because the stainable material is closely packed. Used of cells and tissue.

pyk·no·sis (pĭk-nō′sĭs) *n.* A condensation and reduction in the size of a cell or cell nucleus, usually associated with hyperchromatosis.

pyk·not·ic (pĭk-nŏt′ĭk) *adj.* Relating to or characterized by pyknosis.

py·lem·phrax·is (pī′lĕm-frăk′sĭs) *n.* Obstruction of the portal vein.

py·le·phle·bec·ta·sis (pī′lə-flĭ-bĕk′tə-sĭs) *n.* Dilation of the portal vein.

py·le·phle·bi·tis (pī′lə-flĭ-bī′tĭs) *n.* Inflammation of the portal vein or any of its branches.

py·le·throm·bo·phle·bi·tis (pī′lə-thrŏm′bō-flĭ-bī′tĭs) *n.* Inflammation of the portal vein accompanied by the formation of a thrombus.

py·le·throm·bo·sis (pī′lə-thrŏm-bō′sĭs) *n.* Thrombosis of the portal vein or of its branches.

pylor– *pref.* Variant of **pyloro–**.

py·lo·rec·to·my (pī′lə-rĕk′tə-mē) *n.* Surgical removal of the pylorus. Also called *gastropylorectomy, pylorogastrectomy.*

py·lor·ic (pī-lôr′ĭk, -pĭ-) *adj.* Relating to the pylorus.

pyloric antrum *n.* The bulging part of the lower end of the stomach between the body of the stomach and the pyloric canal.

pyloric canal *n.* The aboral segment of the stomach that succeeds the antrum and ends at the gastroduodenal junction.

pyloric cap *n.* See **duodenal cap** (sense 2).

pyloric gland *n.* Any of several coiled, tubular, mucus-secreting glands situated in the mucus membrane near the pyloric end of the stomach.

pyloric orifice *n.* The opening between the stomach and the upper part of the duodenum.

pyloric sphincter *n.* A thickening of the layer of the gastric musculature encircling the gastroduodenal junction. Also called *sphincter muscle of pylorus.*

pyloric stenosis *n.* Narrowing of the gastric pylorus, especially by congenital muscular hypertrophy or by scarring resulting from a peptic ulcer.

pyloric valve *n.* A fold of mucous membrane at the gastroduodenal junction, enclosing the pylorus.

pyloric vein *n.* A vein that receives veins from both surfaces of the upper portion of the stomach, runs to the right along the lesser curvature, and empties into the portal vein. Also called *right gastric vein.*

py·lo·ri·ste·no·sis (pī-lôr′ĭ-stə-nō′sĭs, pĭ-) or **py·lo·ro·ste·no·sis** (pī-lôr′ō-) *n.* Stricture or narrowing of the orifice of the pylorus.

pyloro– or **pylor–** *pref.* Pylorus: *pylorospasm.*

py·lo·ro·di·o·sis (pī-lôr′ō-dī-ō′sĭs) *n.* Surgical dilation of the pylorus.

py·lo·ro·du·o·de·ni·tis (pī-lôr′ō-dōō′ō-də-nī′tĭs, -dōō-ŏd′n-ī′-) *n.* Inflammation of the duodenum and the pyloric orifice.

py·lo·ro·gas·trec·to·my (pī-lôr′ō-gă-strĕk′tə-mē) *n.* See **pylorectomy**.

py·lo·ro·my·ot·o·my (pī-lôr′ō-mī-ŏt′ə-mē) *n.* Longitudinal incision through the anterior wall of the pyloric canal to the level of the submucosa, performed as a treatment for hypertrophic pyloric stenosis. Also called *Fredet-Ramstedt operation, Ramstedt operation.*

py·lo·ro·plas·ty (pī-lôr′ə-plăs′tē) *n.* The surgical widening of the pyloric canal to facilitate emptying of gastric contents into the duodenum; it is commonly performed in conjunction with truncal vagectomy to treat peptic ulcer.

py·lo·ro·spasm (pī-lôr′ə-spăz′əm) *n.* Spasmodic contraction of the pylorus.

py·lo·ros·to·my (pī′lə-rŏs′tə-mē) *n.* Surgical formation of a fistula from the abdominal surface into the stomach near the pylorus.

py·lo·rot·o·my (pī′lə-rŏt′ə-mē) *n.* Incision of the pylorus.

py·lo·rus (pī-lôr′əs) *n., pl.* **-lo·ri** (-lôr′ī′) **1.** The passage at the lower end of the stomach that opens into the duodenum. **2.** A muscular or myovascular structure that opens or closes an orifice or lumen of an organ.

pyo– or **py–** *pref.* Pus: *pyoderma.*

py·o·cele (pī′ə-sēl′) *n.* An accumulation of pus in a body cavity, such as the scrotum.

py·o·ceph·a·lus (pī′ō-sĕf′ə-ləs) *n.* The presence of purulent fluid in the brain. Also called *pyencephalus.*

py·o·che·zi·a (pī′ō-kē′zē-ə) *n.* A discharge of pus from the bowel.

py·o·coc·cus (pī′ō-kŏk′əs) *n.* A coccus that causes suppuration, especially *Streptococcus pyogenes.*

py·o·col·po·cele (pī′ō-kŏl′pə-sēl′) *n.* A vaginal tumor or cyst containing pus.

py·o·col·pos (pī′ō-kŏl′pŏs′) *n.* An accumulation of pus in the vagina.

py·o·cy·an·ic (pī′ō-sī-ăn′ĭk) *adj.* Of or relating to blue pus or the bacterium that causes it.

py·o·cy·a·no·gen·ic (pī′ō-sī′ə-nə-jĕn′ĭk) *adj.* Producing blue pus.

py·o·cyst (pī′ə-sĭst′) *n.* A cyst that contains pus.

py·o·der·ma (pī′ə-dûr′mə) *n.* A pyogenic skin disease. —**py′o·der′mic** *adj.*

pyoderma gan·gre·no·sum (găng′grə-nō′səm) *n.* A chronic skin disease, usually of the trunk, characterized by large spreading ulcers.

py·o·gen·e·sis (pī′ə-jĕn′ĭ-sĭs) *n.* Formation of pus.

py·o·gen·ic (pī′ə-jĕn′ĭk) *adj.* **1.** Producing pus. **2.** Of, relating to, or characterized by pyogenesis.

pyogenic granuloma *n.* A small rounded mass of inflamed, highly vascular granulation tissue on the skin, frequently having an ulcerated surface.

py·o·he·mi·a (pī′ə-hē′mē-ə) *n.* See **pyemia**.

py·o·he·mo·tho·rax (pī′ō-hē′mə-thôr′ăks′) *n.* The presence of pus and blood in the pleural cavity.

py·oid (pī′oid) *adj.* Of or resembling pus.

py·o·lab·y·rin·thi·tis (pī′ō-lăb′ə-rĭn-thī′tĭs) *n.* Suppurative inflammation of the labyrinth of the ear.

py·o·me·tra (pī′ə-mē′trə) *n.* An accumulation of pus in the uterine cavity.

py·o·me·tri·tis (pī′ō-mĭ-trī′tĭs) *n.* Suppurative inflammation of the uterus.

py·o·my·o·si·tis (pī′ō-mī′ə-sī′tĭs) *n.* Suppurative inflammation of muscle tissue characterized by abscesses, carbuncles, or infected sinuses.

py·o·ne·phri·tis (pī′ō-nə-frī′tĭs) *n.* Suppurative inflammation of the kidney.

py·o·neph·ro·li·thi·a·sis (pī′ō-nĕf′rō-lĭ-thī′ə-sĭs) *n.* The presence of pus and calculi in the kidney.

py·o·ne·phro·sis (pī′ō-nə-frō′sĭs) *n.* Distention of the pelvis and calices of the kidney, accompanied by suppuration and associated with obstruction.

py·o·o·var·i·um (pī′ō-ō-vâr′ē-əm) *n.* An ovarian abscess.

py·o·per·i·car·di·tis (pī′ō-pĕr′ĭ-kär-dī′tĭs) *n.* Suppurative inflammation of the pericardium.

py·o·per·i·car·di·um (pī′ō-pĕr′ĭ-kär′dē-əm) *n.* An accumulation of pus in the pericardial sac.

py·o·per·i·to·ne·um (pī′ō-pĕr′ĭ-tn-ē′əm) *n.* An accumulation of pus in the peritoneal cavity.

py·o·per·i·to·ni·tis (pī′ō-pĕr′ĭ-tn-ī′tĭs) *n.* Suppurative inflammation of the peritoneum.

py·oph·thal·mi·tis (pī′ŏf-thəl-mī′tĭs, -ŏp-) *n.* Suppurative inflammation of the eye.

py·o·phy·so·me·tra (pī′ō-fī′sə-mē′trə) *n.* The presence of pus and gas in the uterine cavity.

py·o·pneu·mo·cho·le·cys·ti·tis (pī′ō-nōō′mō-kō′lĭ-sĭ-stī′tĭs) *n.* The presence of pus and gas in an inflamed gallbladder, caused by gas-producing microorganisms or by the entry of air from the duodenum through the biliary ducts.

py·o·pneu·mo·hep·a·ti·tis (pī′ō-nōō′mō-hĕp′ə-tī′tĭs) *n.* The presence of pus and air in the liver, usually in association with an abscess.

py·o·pneu·mo·per·i·car·di·um (pī′ō-nōō′mō-pĕr′ĭ-kär′dē-əm) *n.* The presence of pus and gas in the pericardial sac.

py·o·pneu·mo·per·i·to·ne·um (pī′ō-nōō′mō-pĕr′ĭ-tn-ē′əm) *n.* The presence of pus and gas in the peritoneal cavity.

py·o·pneu·mo·per·i·to·ni·tis (pī′ō-nōō′mō-pĕr′ĭ-tn-ī′tĭs) *n.* Suppurative peritonitis accompanied by gas produced by gas-forming microorganisms or introduced from a ruptured bowel.

py·o·pneu·mo·tho·rax (pī′ō-nōō′mō-thôr′ăks′) *n.* The presence of gas and pus in the pleural cavity. Also called *pneumopyothorax.*

py·o·poi·e·sis (pī′ō-poi-ē′sĭs) *n.* See **suppuration.**

py·o·poi·et·ic (pī′ō-poi-ĕt′ĭk) *adj.* Producing pus.

py·op·ty·sis (pī-ŏp′tĭ-sĭs) *n.* The spitting of pus.

py·o·py·e·lec·ta·sis (pī′ō-pī′ə-lĕk′tə-sĭs) *n.* Dilation of the pelvis of the kidney as a result of suppurative inflammation.

py·or·rhe·a (pī′ə-rē′ə) *n.* **1.** Purulent inflammation of the gums and tooth sockets, often leading to loosening of the teeth. **2.** A discharge of pus.

py·o·sal·pin·gi·tis (pī′ō-săl′pĭn-jī′tĭs) *n.* Suppurative inflammation of the fallopian tube.

py·o·sal·pin·go·o·o·pho·ri·tis (pī′ō-săl-pĭng′gō-ō′ə-fə-rī′tĭs) *n.* Suppurative inflammation of the fallopian tube and the ovary.

py·o·sal·pinx (pī′ə-săl′pĭngks) *n.* Distention of a fallopian tube with pus.

py·o·sis (pī-ō′sĭs) *n.* See **suppuration.**

py·o·stat·ic (pī′ə-stăt′ĭk) *adj.* Arresting the formation of pus.

py·o·tho·rax (pī′ə-thôr′ăks′) *n.* Empyema in a plural cavity.

py·o·u·ra·chus (pī′ō-yŏŏr′ə-kəs) *n.* An accumulation of pus in the urachus of a fetus.

py·o·u·re·ter (pī′ō-yŏŏ-rē′tər, -yŏŏr′ĭ-tər) *n.* Distention of a ureter with pus.

pyr– *pref.* Variant of **pyro–.**

pyr·a·mid (pĭr′ə-mĭd) *n.* **1.** A solid figure with a polygonal base and triangular faces that meet at a common point. **2.** A structure or part shaped like a pyramid. —**py·ram′i·dal** (pĭ-răm′ĭ-dl) *adj.*

pyramidal bone *n.* See **triquetrum.**

pyramidal cataract *n.* A cone-shaped anterior polar cataract.

pyramidal cell *n.* Any of the large, triangular-shaped neurons in the cerebral cortex having one large apical dendrite and several smaller dendrites at the base.

pyramidal decussation *n.* Crossing of the bundles of the pyramidal tracts at the lower border of the medulla oblongata. Also called *motor decussation.*

pyramidal fracture *n.* A fracture of the midfacial bones, especially the upper jawbone, in which the principal fracture lines meet at a point above the nasal bones, forming a triangular section that is detached from the skull. Also called *LeFort II fracture.*

pyramidal muscle *n.* A muscle with origin from the crest of the pubis, with insertion into the lower portion of the linea alba, with nerve supply from the last thoracic nerve, and whose action makes the linea alba tense.

pyramidal muscle of auricle *n.* An occasional prolongation of the fibers of the muscle of the tragus to the spine of the helix.

pyramidal radiation *n.* The white fibers passing from the cortex of the brain to the pyramidal tract.

pyramidal tract *n.* A massive bundle of fibers that originates from the motor cortex and the postcentral gyrus and emerges on the ventral surface of the medulla oblongata. Most of the fibers cross to the opposite side in the pyramidal decussation and descend the length of the spinal cord to innervate muscles of the extremities.

pyramid of light *n.* A triangular area of reflected light at the lower part of the eardrum seen on examination of the ear.

pyramid of medulla oblongata *n.* An elongated white prominence on the ventral surface of the medulla oblongata on either side along the anterior median fissure, corresponding to the pyramidal tract. Also called *anterior pyramid.*

pyramid of tympanum *n.* A hollow conical projection behind the vestibular window in the middle ear, containing the stapedius muscle.

pyramid sign *n.* Any of the various signs indicating a pathological condition of the pyramidal tracts, such as Babinski's sign.

pyr·a·mine (pĭr′ə-mēn′) *or* **pyr·a·min** (-mĭn) *n.* See **toxopyrimidine.**

py·ra·nose (pī′rə-nōs′, -nōz′) *n.* A cyclic form of a sugar in which an oxygen bridges two carbon atoms, thus forming a ring containing five carbon atoms and an oxygen atom.

py·raz·o·lone (pĭ-răz′ə-lōn′) *n.* A class of nonsteroidal anti-inflammatory agents, such as phenylbutazone, used in the treatment of arthritis.

py·ret·ic (pī-rĕt′ĭk) *adj.* Relating to, producing, or affected by fever.

pyreto– *pref.* Fever: *pyretogenesis.*

py·re·to·gen·e·sis (pī′rĭ-tō-jĕn′ĭ-sĭs, pĭr′ĭ-) *n.* The origin and mode of production of fever. —**py′re·to·ge·net′ic** (-jə-nĕt′ĭk) *adj.*

py·re·to·gen·ic (pī′rĭ-tō-jĕn′ĭk, pĭr′ĭ-) *or* **pyr·e·tog·e·nous** (pī′rĭ-tŏj′ə-nəs, pĭr′ĭ-) *adj.* Pyrogenic.

py·rex·i·a (pī-rĕk′sē-ə) *n.* See **fever** (sense **?**). —**py·rex′-i·al, py·rex′ic** *adj.*

pyr·i·dine (pĭr′ĭ-dēn′) *n.* A flammable, colorless or yellowish liquid base that results from the dry distillation of organic matter containing nitrogen, has a penetrating odor, and is used in analytical chemistry and in the manufacture of various drugs and vitamins. —**py·rid′-ic** (pĭ-rĭd′ĭk) *adj.*

Py·rid·i·um (pĭ-rĭd′ē-əm) A trademark for the drug phenazopyridine hydrochloride.

pyr·i·dox·al (pĭr′ĭ-dŏk′səl) *n.* An aldehyde that is one of several active forms of pyridoxine and is important in amino acid synthesis.

pyridoxal 5-phosphate *n.* The phosphate form of pyridoxal that is a coenzyme belonging to the vitamin B$_6$ group and is essential to many reactions in tissue, such as amino acid decarboxylations.

pyr·i·dox·a·mine (pĭr′ĭ-dŏk′sə-mēn′) *n.* A crystalline amine that is one of several active forms of pyridoxine and is important in protein metabolism.

pyr·i·dox·ine (pĭr′ĭ-dŏk′sēn, -sĭn) *or* **pyr·i·dox·in** (-dŏk′sĭn) *n.* A pyridine derivative occurring especially in cereals, yeast, liver, and fish and serving as a coenzyme in amino acid synthesis.

py·ri·meth·a·mine (pī′rə-mĕth′ə-mēn′, -mĭn) *n.* A potent folic acid antagonist used as a prophylactic antimalarial agent against *Plasmodium falciparum* and in the treatment of toxoplasmosis.

py·rim·i·dine (pī-rĭm′ĭ-dēn′, pĭ-) *n.* 1. A crystalline organic base that is the parent substance of various biologically important derivatives. 2. Any of several basic compounds derived from or structurally related to pyrimidine, especially the nucleic acid constituents uracil, cytosine, and thymine.

pyro– *or* **pyr–** *pref.* 1. Fire; heat: *pyrophobia.* 2. Relating to the action of fire or heat: *pyrolysis.* 3. Fever: *pyrogen.* 4. Derived from an acid by the loss of a water molecule: *pyrophosphoric acid.*

py·ro·cat·e·chol (pī′rō-kăt′ĭ-kôl′, -kōl′) *n.* A biologically important organic phenol, having two hydroxyl groups attached to the benzene ring; used as a topical antiseptic. Also called *catechol.*

py·ro·gal·lol (pī′rō-găl′ôl′, -ōl′, -gô′lôl′, -lōl′) *n.* A white, toxic crystalline phenol used as a photographic developer and to treat certain skin diseases. Also called *pyrogallic acid.*

py·ro·gen (pī′rə-jən) *n.* A substance that produces a fever.

py·ro·gen·ic (pī′rō-jĕn′ĭk) *or* **py·rog·e·nous** (pī-rŏj′ə-nəs) *adj.* 1. Producing or produced by fever. 2. Caused by or generating heat. —**py′ro·ge·nic′i·ty** (-rō-jə-nĭs′-ĭ-tē) *n.*

py·ro·glob·u·lin (pī′rō-glŏb′yə-lĭn) *n.* Any of various immunoglobulins that coagulate when heated, usually associated with multiple myeloma or macroglobulinemia.

py·rol·y·sis (pī-rŏl′ĭ-sĭs) *n.* Decomposition or transformation of a chemical compound caused by heat.

py·ro·ma·ni·a (pī′rō-mā′nē-ə, -mān′yə) *n.* An uncontrollable impulse to start fires. —**py′ro·ma′ni·ac′** (-mā′nē-ăk′) *adj. & n.*

py·ro·nine (pī′rə-nēn′) *or* **py·ro·nin** (-nĭn) *n.* Any of several xanthene dyes that are ferric chloride complexes and are used in combination with methyl green to stain for RNA, DNA, and bacteria, and as a tracking dye for RNA in electrophoresis.

py·ro·pho·bi·a (pī′rə-fō′bē-ə) *n.* A fear of fire.

py·ro·phos·pha·tase (pī′rə-fŏs′fə-tās′, -tāz′) *n.* Any of various enzymes that selectively cleave a pyrophosphate situated between two phosphoric groups, leaving one phosphoric group on each of the two fragments.

py·ro·phos·phate (pī′rə-fŏs′fāt′) *n. Abbr.* **PP** A salt or ester of pyrophosphoric acid.

py·ro·phos·phor·ic acid (pī′rō-fŏs-fôr′ĭk) *n.* A syrupy viscous liquid used as a catalyst, in organic chemical synthesis, and, in its salt forms, as medicines.

py·ro·sis (pī-rō′sĭs) *n.* See **heartburn**.

py·rot·ic (pī-rŏt′ĭk) *adj.* 1. Of, relating to, or affected with heartburn. 2. Caustic.

py·rox·y·lin (pī-rŏk′sə-lĭn) *n.* A highly flammable cellulose nitrate used in the manufacture of collodion, plastics, and lacquers. Also called *trinitrocellulose.*

pyr·role (pîr′ōl′) *n.* A five-membered heterocyclic ring compound that has an odor similar to chloroform and is the parent compound of hemoglobin, chlorophyll, and other complex, biologically active substances. Also called *imidole.* —**pyr·ro′lic** (pĭ-rō′lĭk) *adj.*

pyr·rol·i·dine (pĭ-rŏl′ĭ-dēn′) *n.* A nearly colorless liquid pyrrole to which four hydrogen atoms have been added. It has an ammonialike odor and is the structural basis of proline and hydroxyproline.

py·ru·vate (pī-rōō′vāt, pĭ-) *n.* A salt or ester of pyruvic acid.

pyruvate kinase deficiency *n.* An inherited disorder in which essentially no pyruvate kinase is formed, characterized by hemolytic anemia.

py·ru·vic acid (pī-rōō′vĭk, pĭ-) *n.* A colorless organic liquid formed as a fundamental intermediate in protein and carbohydrate metabolism.

py·u·ri·a (pī-yŏor′ē-ə) *n.* The presence of pus in the urine, usually a sign of urinary tract infection.

Q

Q-band·ing stain (kyo͞o′băn′dĭng) *n.* A fluorescent stain for chromosomes, useful in identifying the Y-chromosome and certain DNA polymorphisms.

q.d. *abbr. Latin* quaque die (every day)

Q fever *n.* An infectious disease caused by the rickettsia *Coxiella burnetii*, characterized by fever, malaise, and muscular pains.

q.h. *abbr. Latin* quaque hora (every hour)

Qi *or* **qi** (chē) *n.* Variants of **chi**².

q.i.d. *abbr. Latin* quater in die (four times a day)

Qi Gong (chē gông, gŏng) *n.* A Chinese system of pre-scribed physical exercises or movements performed in a meditative state.

q.l. *abbr. Latin* quantum libet (as much as desired)

QRS complex *n.* The principal deflection in the electro-cardiogram, representing ventricular depolarization.

q.s. *abbr. Latin* quantum satis (as much as is enough); quantum sufficiat (as much as shall suffice)

qt *or* **qt.** *abbr.* quart

Q-T interval *n.* The time elapsing from the beginning of the QRS complex to the end of the T wave in an electrocardiogram, representing the total duration of electrical activity of the ventricles.

Quaa·lude (kwā′lo͞od′) A trademark formerly used for the drug methaqualone.

quack (kwăk) *n.* **1.** An untrained person who pretends to be a physician and dispenses medical advice and treatment. **2.** A charlatan. —**quack′er·y** *n.*

quad·rant (kwŏd′rənt) *n.* **1.** A circular arc of 90 degrees; one fourth of the circumference of a circle. **2.** A quarter portion of any roughly circular anatomical area such as the abdomen, measuring along imaginary axes at right angles to each other. —**quad·ran′tic** (kwŏ-drăn′tĭk) *adj.*

quadrantic hemianopsia *n.* Loss of vision in a quarter section of the visual field of one or both eyes. Also called *quadrantanopsia.*

quad·rate (kwŏd′rāt′, -rĭt) *adj.* Having four sides and four angles; square or rectangular.

quadrate foramen *n.* See **foramen of vena cava.**

quadrate lobe *n.* **1.** A lobe on the inferior surface of the liver between the fossa for the gallbladder and the fissure for the round ligament. **2.** See **precuneus.**

quadrate muscle of loins *n.* See **lumbar quadrate muscle.**

quadrate muscle of sole *n.* See **plantar quadrate muscle.**

quadrate muscle of thigh *n.* A muscle with origin from the lateral border of the tuberosity of the ischium, with insertion into the intertrochanteric crest, with nerve supply from the sacral plexus, and whose action rotates the thigh laterally.

quadrate muscle of upper lip *n.* A muscle composed of three heads usually described as three muscles: the elevator muscle of the upper lip and wing of the nose, the elevator muscle of the upper lip, and the lesser zygomatic muscle.

quadrate pronator muscle *n.* A muscle with origin from the anterior surface of the ulna, with insertion into the anterior surface of the radius, with nerve supply from the anterior interosseous nerve, and whose action pronates the forearm.

quadri– *or* **quadr–** *pref.* **1.** Four: *quadriplegia.* **2.** Square: *quadrate.*

quad·ri·ba·sic (kwŏd′rə-bā′sĭk) *adj.* Of or relating to an acid having four hydrogen atoms that are replaceable by atoms or radicals that are basic.

quad·ri·ceps (kwŏd′rĭ-sĕps′) *n.* The large four-part extensor muscle at the front of the thigh. —*adj.* Having four heads, said of certain muscles.

quadriceps muscle of thigh *n.* A muscle with origin by four heads: the rectus muscle of the thigh, the lateral vastus muscle, the intermediate vastus muscle, and the medial vastus muscle; with insertion into the patella and by a ligament to the tuberosity of the tibia, with nerve supply from the femoral nerve, and whose action extends the leg and flexes the thigh by action of the rectus muscle of the thigh.

quadriceps reflex *n.* See **patellar reflex.**

quad·ri·gem·i·nal (kwŏd′rə-jĕm′ə-nəl) *adj.* Consisting of four parts; fourfold.

quadrigeminal body *n.* Either of the eminences that together form the lamina tecti mesencephali and are designated inferior and anterior.

quadrigeminal rhythm *n.* A cardiac dysrhythmia in which heartbeats occur in groups of four, usually one sinus beat followed by three extrasystolic beats.

quad·ri·gem·i·num (kwŏd′rə-jĕm′ə-nəm) *n.* One of the quadrigeminal bodies of the mesencephalon.

quad·ri·pa·re·sis (kwŏd′rə-pə-rē′sĭs, -păr′ĭ-sĭs) *n.* See **tetraparesis.**

quad·ri·ped·al extensor reflex (kwŏd′rə-pĕd′l, -pēd′l) *n.* Extension of the arm on the affected side in hemiplegia when the patient is positioned to be on all fours. Also called *Brain's reflex.*

quad·ri·ple·gia (kwŏd′rə-plē′jə) *n.* Paralysis of all four limbs. Also called *tetraplegia.* —**quad′ri·ple′gic** *adj., n.*

quad·ri·va·lent (kwŏd′rə-vā′lənt) *adj.* **1.** Having four valences. **2.** Having a valence of four; tetravalent.

quad·ru·plet (kwŏ-dro͞o′plĭt, -drŭp′lĭt, kwŏd′rə-plĭt) *n.* One of four offspring born in a single birth.

qual·i·ta·tive analysis (kwŏl′ĭ-tā′tĭv) *n.* The testing of a substance or mixture to determine the characteristics of its chemical constituents.

qual·i·ty assurance (kwŏl′ĭ-tē) *n.* A system for evaluating performance, as in the delivery of services or the quality of products provided to consumers, customers, or patients.

quan·ti·ta·tive analysis (kwŏn′tĭ-tā′tĭv) *n.* The testing of a substance or mixture to determine the amounts and proportions of its chemical constituents.

quantitative trait *n.* A phenotype that is influenced by multiple genes.

quan·tum (kwŏn′təm) *n., pl.* **–ta** (-tə) **1.** The smallest amount of a physical quantity that can exist independently, especially a discrete quantity of electromagnetic radiation. **2.** This amount of energy regarded as a unit. **3.** A quantity or an amount.

quar·an·tine (kwôr′ən-tēn′) *n.* **1.** A period of time during which a vehicle, person, or material suspected of carrying a contagious disease is detained at a port of entry under enforced isolation to prevent disease from entering a country. **2.** A place for such detention. **3.** Enforced isolation or restriction of free movement that is imposed to prevent the spread of contagious disease. **4.** A condition of enforced isolation. **5.** A period of 40 days. *—v.* To isolate in or as if in quarantine.

quart (kwôrt) *n.* *Abbr.* **q., qt, qt. 1.** A unit of volume or capacity in the US Customary System, used in liquid measure, equal to 2 pints or 32 ounces (0.946 liter). **2.** A unit of volume or capacity in the US Customary System, used in dry measure, equal to 1.101 liters.

quar·tan (kwôrt′n) *adj.* Recurring every fourth day, counting inclusively, or every 72 hours. Used of a fever.

quartan malaria *n.* See **malariae malaria**.

quartz (kwôrts) *n.* A very hard crystalline form of silicon dioxide used in chemical apparatus and in optical and electric instruments.

qua·si·dom·i·nance (kwā′zī-dŏm′ə-nəns, -sī-, kwä′zē-, -sē-) *n.* The appearance of a recessive trait in generation after generation of a population as a result of repeated consanguineous matings; false dominance.

qua·ter·nar·y (kwŏt′ər-nĕr′ē, kwə-tûr′nə-rē) *adj.* **1.** Consisting of four; in fours. **2.** Relating to an atom bonded to four carbon atoms.

quea·sy *or* **quea·zy** (kwē′zē) *adj.* **1.** Experiencing nausea. **2.** Easily nauseated. **3.** Causing nausea; sickening.

Queck·en·stedt-Stookey test (kwĕk′ən-stĕd′-, kvĕk′-ən-shtĕt′-) *n.* A test to detect the blockage of subarachnoid channels in which the jugular vein is compressed; when there is blockage, compression causes little or no increase in the pressure of the spinal fluid.

quel·lung reaction (kwĕl′əng, kvĕl′ŏong) *n.* See **Neufeld capsular swelling**.

quench·ing (kwĕn′chĭng) *n.* **1.** The process of extinguishing, removing, or diminishing a physical property such as heat or light. **2.** The shifting of the energy spectrum from a true to a lower energy that occurs in liquid scintillation counting of beta emissions; caused by interfering materials in the counting solution, including foreign chemicals.

quer·ce·tin (kwûr′sĭ-tĭn) *n.* A yellow powdered crystalline compound produced synthetically or occurring as a glycoside in the rind and bark of numerous plants, used medicinally to treat abnormal capillary fragility. Also called *meletin*.

Ques·tran (kwĕs′trən) A trademark for the drug cholestyramine.

quet·i·a·pine fumarate (kwĕt′ī-ə-pēn′) *n.* An oral antipsychotic drug that acts as an antagonist of multiple neurotransmitters including serotonin and norepi-

nephrine, used in the treatment of schizophrenia.

quick (kwĭk) *n.* Sensitive or raw exposed flesh, as under the fingernails. *—adj.* **1.** Pregnant. **2.** Alive.

quick-cure resin *n.* See **autopolymer resin**.

quick·en (kwĭk′ən) *v.* To reach the stage of pregnancy when the fetus can be felt to move.

quick·en·ing (kwĭk′ə-nĭng) *n.* The initial signs of fetal life felt by the mother as a result of fetal movement.

Quick's test (kwĭks) *n.* See **prothrombin test**.

qui·et lung (kwī′ĭt) *n.* The deliberate collapsing of a lung during thoracic operations to facilitate surgical procedure by absence of movement.

quin·a·crine hydrochloride (kwĭn′ə-krēn′, -krĭn) *n.* The dihydrochloride form of an acridine derivative that is used as an antimalarial, an anthelmintic, and especially as a stain for Y chromatin in fluorescent microscopy.

Quin·a·glute (kwĭn′ə-glōot′) A trademark for the drug quinidine in its gluconate form.

quin·a·pril hydrochloride (kwĭn′ə-prĭl) *n.* An ACE inhibitor drug used to treat hypertension and congestive heart failure.

Quinck·e's disease (kwĭn′kēz, kwĭng′-, kvĭn′kəz) *n.* See **angioneurotic edema**.

Quincke's pulse *n.* Capillary pulsation, as shown by alternate reddening and blanching of the nailbed with each heartbeat; it is a sign of arteriolar dilation and aortic insufficiency. Also called *Quincke's sign*.

quin·i·dine (kwĭn′ĭ-dēn′) *n.* A colorless crystalline alkaloid that is a stereoisomer of quinine and is used as a treatment for malaria and cardiac arrhythmias.

qui·nine (kwī′nīn′) *n.* **1.** A bitter colorless amorphous powder or crystalline alkaloid derived from certain cinchona barks and used to treat malaria. **2.** Any of various compounds or salts of quinine.

qui·noi·dine (kwĭ-noi′dēn′, -dĭn) *n.* A brownish-black mixture of alkaloids remaining after extraction of crystalline alkaloids from cinchona bark, used as a quinine substitute.

quin·o·line (kwĭn′ə-lēn′, -lĭn) *n.* An aromatic organic base synthesized or obtained from coal tar and used as a food preservative and in making antiseptics.

quin·o·lone (kwĭn′ə-lōn′) *n.* Any of a class of synthetic broad-spectrum antibacterial drugs derived from quinoline compounds.

qui·none (kwĭ-nōn′, kwĭn′ōn′) *n.* Any of a class of aromatic compounds found widely in plants, especially the crystalline form used in making dyes.

quin·o·noid (kwĭn′ə-noid′, kwĭ-nō′-) *adj.* Containing or resembling quinone.

quin·sy (kwĭn′zē) *n.* See **peritonsillar abscess**.

quin·tan (kwĭn′tən) *adj.* Recurring every fifth day. Used of a fever.

quin·tu·plet (kwĭn-tŭp′lĭt, -tōo′plĭt, kwĭn′tə-plĭt) *n.* One of five offspring born in a single birth.

quo·tid·i·an (kwō-tĭd′ē-ən) *adj.* Recurring daily. Used especially of attacks of malaria.

quo·tient (kwō′shənt) *n.* The number obtained by dividing one quantity by another.

Q wave *n.* The initial downward deflection of the QRS complex in an electrocardiogram.

R

ρ The Greek letter *rho*. Entries beginning with this character are alphabetized under **rho.**

r *abbr.* racemic

R *abbr.* right; radical (usually an alkyl or aryl group); respiration; respiratory exchange ratio; *or* **r** roentgen

℞ *or* **R** *abbr. Latin* recipe (take)

Ra The symbol for the element **radium.**

RA *abbr.* rheumatoid arthritis

rab·bet·ing (răb′ĭ-tĭng) *n.* The making of congruous stepwise cuts on apposing bone surfaces for firmly holding together a fractured bone.

rab·id (răb′ĭd) *adj.* Of or affected by rabies.

ra·bies (rā′bēz) *n.* An infectious, highly fatal viral disease of warm blooded animals that attacks the central nervous system; symptoms include excitement, aggressiveness, and dementia, followed by paralysis and death. —**ra′bi·et′ic** (-ĕt′ĭk) *adj.*

rabies immune globulin *n.* Specific immune globulin from human donors who are immunized against rabies.

rabies vaccine *n.* **1.** A vaccine introduced by Pasteur as a method of treatment for the bite of a rabid animal, consisting of 23 daily injections of virus that are increased serially from noninfective doses to doses containing fully infective fixed virus. **2.** A similar vaccine prepared from rabies virus that is grown in duck embryos and then inactivated, requiring fewer injections; it has largely replaced the vaccine introduced by Pasteur.

rabies virus *n.* A rather large, bullet-shaped virus of the genus *Lyssavirus* that causes rabies.

rac·coon eyes (ră-kōōn′) *n.* The appearance produced by subconjunctival hemorrhages.

race (rās) *n.* **1.** A local geographic or global human population distinguished as a more or less distinct group by genetically transmitted physical characteristics. **2.** A population of organisms differing from others of the same species in the frequency of hereditary traits; a subspecies. **3.** A breed or strain, as of domestic animals.

ra·ce·mase (rā′sə-mās′, -māz′, răs′ə-) *n.* An enzyme that catalyzes racemization.

ra·ce·mate (rā′sə-māt′, răs′ə-) *n.* **1.** A racemic compound. **2.** The salt or ester of such a compound.

ra·ceme (rā-sēm′, rə-) *n.* An optically inactive chemical compound.

ra·ce·mic (rā-sē′mĭk, -sĕm′ĭk, rə-) *adj. Abbr.* **r** Of or relating to a chemical compound that contains equal quantities of dextrorotatory and levorotatory forms and therefore does not rotate the plane of incident polarized light.

ra·ce·mi·za·tion (rā′sə-mĭ-zā′shən, răs′ə-) *n.* Conversion of an optically active substance to a raceme.

rac·e·mose (răs′ə-mōs′) *adj.* Having or growing in a branching manner that resembles a bunch of grapes. Used of glands.

racemose aneurysm *n.* See **cirsoid aneurysm.**

race walking *n.* The sport of walking for speed, the rules of which require the racer to maintain continual foot contact with the ground and to keep the supporting leg straight at the knee when that leg is directly below the body.

ra·chi·al (rā′kē-əl) *adj.* Rachidial.

ra·chi·cen·te·sis (rā′kĭ-sĕn-tē′sĭs) *n.* See **lumbar puncture.**

ra·chid·i·al (rā-kĭd′ē-əl, rə-) *or* **ra·chid·i·an** (-ē-ən) *adj.* Relating to the vertebral column; spinal.

ra·chi·graph (rā′kĭ-grăf′) *n.* A graph for recording the curves of the vertebrae.

ra·chil·y·sis (rā-kĭl′ĭ-sĭs, rə-) *n.* Forcible correction of lateral curvature of the spine by lateral pressure against the convexity of the curve.

rachio– *or* **rachi–** *pref.* Spine; spinal: *rachiometer.*

ra·chi·o·cen·te·sis (rā′kē-ō-sĕn-tē′sĭs) *n.* See **lumbar puncture.**

ra·chi·om·e·ter (rā′kē-ŏm′ĭ-tər) *n.* An instrument that is used for measuring the curvature of the spinal column.

ra·chi·ot·o·my (rā′kē-ŏt′ə-mē) *n.* See **laminectomy.**

ra·chis (rā′kĭs) *n., pl.* **ra·chis·es** *or* **rach·i·des** (răk′ĭ-dēz′, rā′kĭ-) See **spinal column.**

ra·chis·chi·sis (rə-kĭs′kĭ-sĭs) *n.* See **spondyloschisis.**

rachitic pelvis *n.* A contracted and deformed pelvis, most commonly a flat pelvis, resulting from rachitic softening of the bones in early life.

rachitic rosary *n.* A row of beadlike prominences at the junction of a rib and its cartilage, often seen in rachitic children. Also called *beading of ribs.*

ra·chi·tis (rə-kī′tĭs) *n.* See **rickets.** —**ra·chit′ic** (-kĭt′ĭk) *adj.*

rach·i·to·gen·ic (răk′ĭ-tō-jĕn′ĭk) *adj.* Producing or causing rickets.

ra·cial (rā′shəl) *adj.* **1.** Of, relating to, or characteristic of race or races. **2.** Arising from or based on differences among human racial groups. —**ra′cial·ly** *adv.*

rack·et amputation (răk′ĭt) *n.* A circular or slightly oval amputation in which a long incision is made in the axis of the limb.

rad¹ (răd) *n.* A unit of energy absorbed from ionizing radiation, equal to 100 ergs per gram or 0.01 joule per kilogram of irradiated material.

rad² *abbr.* radian

ra·dar·ky·mog·ra·phy (rā′där-kī-mŏg′rə-fē) *n.* Video tracking of heart motion by means of image intensification and closed circuit television during fluoroscopy, enabling cardiac motion to be measured by reproducible linear graphic tracing.

ra·dec·to·my (rā-dĕk′tə-mē) *or* **ra·di·ec·to·my** (rā′dē-ĕk′tə-mē) *or* **ra·di·sec·to·my** (rā′dĭ-sĕk′tə-mē) *n.* See **root amputation.**

radi– *pref.* Variant of **radio–.**

ra·di·a·bil·i·ty (rā′dē-ə-bĭl′ĭ-tē) *n.* The property of being radiable.

ra·di·a·ble (rā′dē-ə-bəl) *adj.* Capable of being penetrated or examined by rays, especially x-rays.

ra·di·ad (rā′dē-ăd′) *adv.* In a direction toward the radial side.

ra·di·al (rā′dē-əl) *adj.* **1.** Of, relating to, or near the radius or forearm. **2.** Moving or directed along a radius. **3.** Radiating from or converging to a common center. —**ra′di·al·ly** *adv.*

radial artery *n.* **1.** An artery with its origin in the brachial artery and with branches to the radial recurrent, dorsal metacarpal, and dorsal digital arteries, the principal artery of the thumb, the palmar metacarpal, and muscular and carpal arteries. **2.** Radial index artery.

radial collateral artery *n.* An artery that is the anterior terminal branch of the deep brachial artery, anastomosing with the radial recurrent artery.

radial extensor muscle of wrist *n.* **1.** A muscle with its origin from the humerus, with insertion to the third metacarpal bone, with nerve supply from the radial nerve, and whose action extends and abducts the wrist toward the radius; short radial extensor muscle of wrist. **2.** A muscle with its origin from the humerus, with insertion to the second metacarpal bone, with nerve supply from the radial nerve, and whose action extends and abducts the wrist toward the radius; long radial extensor muscle of wrist.

radial flexor muscle of wrist *n.* A muscle with its origin from the humerus, with insertion to the second and third metacarpal bones, with nerve supply from the median nerve, and whose action flexes and abducts the wrist toward the radius.

radial growth phase *n.* The early pattern of growth of cutaneous malignant melanoma in which tumor cells spread laterally into the epidermis.

radial index artery *n.* An artery with its origin in the radial artery and with distribution to the radial side of the index finger.

radial keratotomy *n.* Surgical modification of corneal curvature to correct myopia by making symmetrical incisions into but not through the cornea.

radial nerve *n.* A nerve that arises from the posterior cord of the brachial plexus and divides into two terminal branches, designated superficial and deep, that supply muscular and cutaneous branches to the dorsal aspect of the arm and forearm.

radial vein *n.* Any of several veins continuing the palmar metacarpal veins on the lateral side and accompanying the radial artery.

ra·di·an (rā′dē-ən) *n. Abbr.* **rad** A unit of angular measure equal to the angle subtended at the center of a circle by an arc equal in length to the radius of the circle.

ra·di·ance (rā′dē-əns) *or* **ra·di·an·cy** (-ən-sē) *n.* **1.** The quality or state of being radiant. **2.** The radiant energy emitted per unit time in a specified direction by a unit area of an emitting surface.

ra·di·ant (rā′dē-ənt) *adj.* **1.** Emitting heat or light. **2.** Consisting of or emitted as radiation. —*n.* A point from which light radiates to the eye.

ra·di·ate (rā′dē-āt′) *v.* **1.** To spread out in all directions from a center. **2.** To emit or be emitted as radiation. —**ra′di·a′tive** *adj.*

radiate crown *n.* A fan-shaped fiber mass on the white matter of the cerebral cortex, composed of the widely radiating fibers of the internal capsule.

radiate ligament of rib *n.* The ligament connecting the head of each rib to the bodies of the two vertebrae with which the head articulates. Also called *stellate ligament.*

ra·di·a·tion (rā′dē-ā′shən) *n.* **1.** The act or condition of diverging in all directions from a center. **2.** The emission and propagation of energy in the form of rays or waves. **3.** The energy radiated or transmitted in the form of rays, waves, or particles. **4.** A stream of particles or electromagnetic waves that is emitted by the atoms and molecules of a radioactive substance as a result of nuclear decay. **5.** Radiotherapy. **6.** The radial arrangement of anatomical or histological parts. **7.** The spread of a group of organisms into new habitats.

radiation biology *n.* The study of the biological effects of ionizing radiation on living systems.

radiation dermatitis *n.* See **radiodermatitis.**

radiation of corpus callosum *n.* The radiation of the fibers of the corpus callosum in the medullary center of each cerebral hemisphere.

radiation oncology *n.* The branch of radiology that deals with the use of ionizing radiation to treat cancers.

radiation sickness *n.* Illness induced by ionizing radiation, ranging in severity from nausea, vomiting, headache, and diarrhea to loss of hair and teeth, reduction in red and white blood cell counts, extensive hemorrhaging, sterility, and death.

radiation therapy *n.* Radiotherapy.

rad·i·cal (răd′ĭ-kəl) *n. Abbr.* **R 1.** A group of elements or atoms usually passing intact from one compound to another but generally incapable of prolonged existence in a free state. **2.** A free radical. —*adj.* **1.** Of or being medical treatment by extreme, drastic, or innovative measures. **2.** Designed to act on or eliminate the root or cause of a pathological process.

radical hysterectomy *n.* Complete surgical removal of the uterus, upper vagina, and parametrium.

radical mastectomy *n.* Surgical removal of the entire breast, the pectoral muscles, the lymphatic-bearing tissue in the armpit, and other neighboring tissues. Also called *Halsted's operation.*

rad·i·cle (răd′ĭ-kəl) *n.* A small structure, such as a fibril of a nerve, that resembles a root.

rad·i·cot·o·my (răd′ĭ-kŏt′ə-mē) *n.* See **rhizotomy.**

ra·dic·u·la (rə-dĭk′yə-lə) *n., pl* **-lae** (-lē′) A spinal nerve root.

ra·dic·u·lal·gia (rə-dĭk′yə-lăl′jə) *n.* Neuralgia caused by irritation to the sensory root of a spinal nerve.

ra·dic·u·lar (rə-dĭk′yə-lər) *adj.* **1.** Relating to a radicle. **2.** Relating to the root of a tooth.

radicular cyst *n.* See **periapical periodontal cyst.**

radicular odontoma *n.* An odontoma positioned on or near the root of a tooth.

ra·dic·u·lec·to·my (rə-dĭk′yə-lĕk′tə-mē) *n.* See **rhizotomy.**

ra·dic·u·li·tis (rə-dĭk′yə-lī′tĭs) *n.* **1.** Inflammation of the intradural portion of a spinal nerve root prior to its entrance into the intervertebral foramen. **2.** Inflammation of the portion of a spinal nerve root between the intervertebral foramen and the nerve plexus.

radiculo– *or* **radicul–** *pref.* Root; rootlike: *radiculitis; radiculopathy.*

ra·dic·u·lo·gan·gli·o·ni·tis (rə-dĭk′yə-lō-găng′glē-ə-nī′tĭs) *n.* See **acute idiopathic polyneuritis.**

ra·dic·u·lo·me·nin·go·my·e·li·tis (rə-dĭk′yə-lō-mə-nĭng′gō-mī′ə-lī′tĭs) *n.* See **rhizomeningomyelitis.**

ra·dic·u·lo·my·e·lop·a·thy (rə-dĭk′yə-lō-mī′ə-lŏp′ə-thē) *n.* See **myeloradiculopathy.**

ra·dic·u·lo·neu·rop·a·thy (rə-dĭk′yə-lō-nŏŏ-rŏp′ə-thē) *n.* Disease of the spinal nerves and nerve roots.

ra·dic·u·lop·a·thy (rə-dĭk′yə-lŏp′ə-thē) *n.* Disease of the spinal nerve roots.

ra·di·ec·to·my (rā′dē-ĕk′tə-mē) *n.* Variant of **radectomy.**

radio– *or* **radi–** *pref.* **1.** Radiation; radiant energy: *radiometer.* **2.** Radioactive: *radiochemistry.* **3.** Radius: *radiobicipital.*

ra·di·o·ac·tive (rā′dē-ō-ăk′tĭv) *adj.* Of or exhibiting radioactivity.

radioactive constant *n.* See **decay constant.**

radioactive iodine *n.* Any of the radioisotopes of iodine, especially I^{131}, I^{125}, or I^{123}, used as tracers in biology and medicine.

radioactive isotope *n.* An isotope having an unstable nucleus that decomposes spontaneously by emission of a nuclear electron or helium nucleus and radiation, thus achieving a stable nuclear composition.

ra·di·o·ac·tiv·i·ty (rā′dē-ō-ăk-tĭv′ĭ-tē) *n.* **1.** Spontaneous emission of radiation, either directly from unstable atomic nuclei or as a consequence of a nuclear reaction. **2.** The radiation, including alpha particles, nucleons, electrons, and gamma rays, emitted by a radioactive substance.

ra·di·o·al·ler·go·sor·bent test (rā′dē-ō-ăl′ər-gō-zôr′bənt) *n. Abbr.* **RAST** A radioimmunoassay test to detect certain types of immunoglobulin-bound allergens responsible for tissue hypersensitivity.

ra·di·o·au·to·graph (rā′dē-ō-ô′tə-grăf′) *n.* See **autoradiograph.**

ra·di·o·bi·cip·i·tal (rā′dē-ō-bī-sĭp′ĭ-tl) *adj.* Of or relating to the radius and the biceps muscle.

ra·di·o·bi·ol·o·gy (rā′dē-ō-bī-ŏl′ə-jē) *n.* The study of the effects of radiation on living organisms.

ra·di·o·car·pal (rā′dē-ō-kär′pəl) *adj.* **1.** Of or relating to the radius and the bones of the carpus. **2.** Of or located on the radial or lateral side of the carpus.

radiocarpal joint *n.* See **wrist joint.**

ra·di·o·chem·is·try (rā′dē-ō-kĕm′ĭ-strē) *n.* The branch of chemistry dealing with radioactive materials. —**ra′di·o·chem′i·cal** (-ĭ-kəl) *adj.*

ra·di·o·cin·e·ma·tog·ra·phy (rā′dē-ō-sĭn′ə-mə-tŏg′rə-fē) *n.* The cinematic recording of the movements of organs during examination by radiography.

ra·di·o·cur·a·ble (rā′dē-ō-kyŏŏr′ə-bəl) *adj.* Curable by irradiation.

ra·di·o·dense (rā′dē-ō-dĕns′) *adj.* Radiopaque.

ra·di·o·den·si·ty (rā′dē-ō-dĕn′sĭ-tē) *n.* Radiopacity.

ra·di·o·der·ma·ti·tis (rā′dē-ō-dûr′mə-tī′tĭs) *n.* Dermatitis due to exposure to ionizing radiation. Also called *radiation dermatitis.*

ra·di·o·di·ag·no·sis (rā′dē-ō-dī′əg-nō′sĭs) *n.* Diagnosis by means of x-rays.

ra·di·o frequency (rā′dē-ō) *n.* A frequency that lies in the range within which radio waves may be transmitted, from about 10 kilohertz per second to about 300,000 megahertz.

ra·di·o·gold colloid (rā′dē-ō-gōld′) *n.* A colloidal dispersion of a radioactive isotope of gold that emits a negative beta particle and a gamma ray for each atom of gold present, used for irradiating closed serous cavities and for liver scans.

ra·di·o·gram (rā′dē-ō-grăm′) *n.* A radiograph.

ra·di·o·graph (rā′dē-ō-grăf′) *n.* An image produced on a radiosensitive surface, such as a photographic film, by radiation other than visible light, as by x-rays passed through an object.

ra·di·og·ra·phy (rā′dē-ŏg′rə-fē) *n.* The process by which radiographs are made.

ra·di·o·im·mu·ni·ty (rā′dē-ō-ĭ-myŏŏ′nĭ-tē) *n.* Reduced sensitivity to radiation.

ra·di·o·im·mu·no·as·say (rā′dē-ō-ĭm′yə-nō-ăs′ā, -ĭ-myŏŏ′-) *n. Abbr.* **RIA** The immunoassay of a substance, such as a hormone or an enzyme that has been radiolabeled.

ra·di·o·im·mu·no·dif·fu·sion (rā′dē-ō-ĭm′yə-nō-dĭ-fyŏŏ′zhən, -ĭ-myŏŏ′-) *n.* A method for the study of antigen-antibody reactions by gel diffusion using a radioisotope-labeled antigen or antibody.

ra·di·o·im·mu·no·e·lec·tro·pho·re·sis (rā′dē-ō-ĭm′yə-nō-ĭ-lĕk′trə-fə-rē′sĭs, -ĭ-myŏŏ′-) *n.* Immunoelectrophoresis in which the antigen or antibody is labeled with a radioisotope.

ra·di·o·im·mu·nol·o·gy (rā′dē-ō-ĭm′yə-nŏl′ə-jē) *n.* The study of immunity by radiolabeling and other radiological methods. —**ra′di·o·im′mu·no·log′i·cal** (-nə-lŏj′ĭ-kəl) *adj.*

ra·di·o·im·mu·no·pre·cip·i·ta·tion (rā′dē-ō-ĭm′yə-nō-prĭ-sĭp′ĭ-tā′shən, -ĭ-myŏŏ′-) *n.* Immunoprecipitation that uses a radioisotope-labeled antibody or an antigen.

ra·di·o·i·o·dine (rā′dē-ō-ī′ə-dīn′) *n.* A radioactive isotope of iodine widely used as a tracer.

ra·di·o·i·so·tope (rā′dē-ō-ī′sə-tōp′) *n.* A naturally or artificially produced radioactive isotope.

ra·di·o·la·bel (rā′dē-ō-lā′bəl) *v.* To tag a hormone, enzyme, or other substance with a radiotracer. —*n.* A radiotracer.

ra·di·o·le·sion (rā′dē-ō-lē′zhən) *n.* A lesion produced by ionizing radiation.

ra·di·o·li·gand (rā′dē-ō-lī′gənd, -lĭg′ənd) *n.* A molecule with a radionuclide tracer attached, usually used for radioimmunoassay procedures.

radiological anatomy *n.* The study of the body and its organs and tissues using x-ray imaging.

ra·di·ol·o·gy (rā′dē-ŏl′ə-jē) *n.* **1.** The branch of medicine that makes diagnostic images of anatomic structures through the use of electromagnetic radiation or sound waves and that treats disease through the use of radioactive compounds. Radiological imaging techniques include x-rays, CAT scans, PET scans, MRIs, and ultrasonograms. **2.** The use of radiation for the scientific examination of material structures; radioscopy. —**ra·di·o·log·i·cal** (-ə-lŏj′ĭ-kəl), **ra·di·o·log·ic** (-lŏj′ĭk) *adj.* —**ra·di·ol·o·gist** *n.*

ra·di·o·lu·cent (rā′dē-ō-lōō′sənt) *adj.* Characterized by allowing passage of x-rays or other radiation; not radiopaque. —**ra·di·o·lu·cen·cy** *n.*

ra·di·ol·y·sis (rā′dē-ŏl′ĭ-sĭs) *n., pl* **-ses** (-sēz) Molecular decomposition of a substance as a result of radiation. —**ra·di·o·lyt·ic** (-ə-lĭt′ĭk) *adj.*

ra·di·om·e·ter (rā′dē-ŏm′ĭ-tər) *n.* **1.** A device that measures the intensity of radiant energy, consisting of a partially evacuated glass bulb containing lightweight vertical vanes, each blackened on one side, suspended radially about a central vertical axis to permit their revolution about the axis as a result of incident radiation. **2.** An instrument that detects electromagnetic radiation. **3.** A device for determining the penetrative power of x-rays. —**ra·di·om·e·try** (-trē) *n.*

ra·di·o·mi·met·ic (rā′dē-ō-mĭ-mĕt′ĭk) *adj.* Affecting living tissue as does radiation.

ra·di·o·ne·cro·sis (rā′dē-ō-nə-krō′sĭs) *n.* Necrosis due to excessive exposure to radiation.

ra·di·o·neu·ri·tis (rā′dē-ō-nōō-rī′tĭs) *n.* Neuritis due to excessive exposure to radiation.

ra·di·o·nu·clide (rā′dē-ō-nōō′klīd′) *n.* A nuclide that has artificial or natural origin and that exhibits radioactivity.

ra·di·o·pac·i·ty (rā′dē-ō-păs′ĭ-tē) *n.* The quality or state of being radiopaque.

ra·di·o·paque (rā′dē-ō-pāk′) *adj.* Relatively impenetrable by x-rays or other forms of radiation.

ra·di·o·pa·thol·o·gy (rā′dē-ō-pă-thŏl′ə-jē) *n.* A branch of radiology or pathology dealing with effects of radioactive substances on cells and tissues.

ra·di·o·pel·vim·e·try (rā′dē-ō-pĕl-vĭm′ĭ-trē) *n.* Measurement of the pelvis by radiography.

ra·di·o·phar·ma·ceu·ti·cal (rā′dē-ō-fär′mə-sōō′tĭ-kəl) *n.* A radioactive compound used in diagnosis or therapy. —**ra·di·o·phar·ma·ceu·ti·cal** *adj.*

ra·di·o·phy·lax·is (rā′dē-ō-fə-lăk′sĭs) *n.* The lessened effect of a dose of radiation when administered after a previous smaller dose.

ra·di·o·pro·tec·tion (rā′dē-ō-prə-tĕk′shən) *n.* Protection against the harmful effects of radiation. —**ra·di·o·pro·tec·tive** *adj.*

ra·di·o·re·cep·tor (rā′dē-ō-rĭ-sĕp′tər) *n.* A receptor that normally responds to radiant energy such as light or heat.

ra·di·o·re·sis·tant (rā′dē-ō-rĭ-zĭs′tənt) *adj.* Not susceptible to destruction by exposure to radiation in the usual dosage range. Used of cells and tissues.

ra·di·os·co·py (rā′dē-ŏs′kə-pē) *n.* See **fluoroscopy.**

ra·di·o·sen·si·tive (rā′dē-ō-sĕn′sĭ-tĭv) *adj.* Sensitive to the action of radiation. Used especially of living structures. —**ra·di·o·sen·si·tiv·i·ty** *n.*

radiosurgery (rā′dē-ō-sûr′jə-rē) *n.* The use of ionizing radiation, either from an external source (such as an

X-ray machine) or an implant, to destroy diseased tissue, especially cancers.

ra·di·o·te·lem·e·try (rā′dē-ō-tə-lĕm′ĭ-trē) *n.* **1.** Telemetry. **2.** Biotelemetry.

ra·di·o·ther·a·peu·tic (rā′dē-ō-thĕr′ə-pyōō′tĭk) *adj.* Relating to radiotherapy or to radiotherapeutics.

ra·di·o·ther·a·peu·tics (rā′dē-ō-thĕr′ə-pyōō′tĭks) *n.* The study and use of ionizing radiation for therapeutic purposes.

ra·di·o·ther·a·py (rā′dē-ō-thĕr′ə-pē) *n.* Treatment of disease with radiation, especially by selective irradiation with x-rays or other ionizing radiation and by ingestion of radioisotopes. —**ra·di·o·ther·a·pist** *n.*

ra·di·o·ther·my (rā′dē-ō-thûr′mē) *n.* Diathermy using heat from radiant sources.

ra·di·o·tox·e·mi·a (rā′dē-ō-tŏk-sē′mē-ə) *n.* Radiation sickness caused by the products of disintegration produced by the action of x-rays or other forms of radiation and by the depletion of certain cells and enzyme systems.

ra·di·o·tox·ic (rā′dē-ō-tŏk′sĭk) *adj.* Of or being a radioactive substance that is toxic to living cells or tissues. —**ra·di·o·tox·ic·i·ty** (-tŏk-sĭs′ĭ-tē) *n.*

ra·di·o·trac·er (rā′dē-ō-trā′sər) *n.* A radioactive isotope used as tracer.

ra·di·o·trans·par·ent (rā′dē-ō-trăns-pâr′ənt) *adj.* Allowing transmission of radiant energy.

ra·di·o·trop·ic (rā′dē-ō-trŏp′ĭk, -trō′pĭk) *adj.* Moving or reacting in response to radiation. —**ra·di·ot·ro·pism** (-ŏt′rə-pĭz′əm) *n.*

ra·di·sec·to·my (rā′dĭ-sĕk′tə-mē) *n.* Variant of **radectomy.**

ra·di·um (rā′dē-əm) *n. Symbol* **Ra** A luminescent, highly radioactive metallic element found in minute amounts in uranium ores, used as a neutron source for some research purposes, and formerly used in cancer radiotherapy; its most stable isotope is Ra 226 with a half-life of 1,622 years. Atomic number 88.

radium therapy *n.* The use of radium in radiotherapy.

ra·di·us (rā′dē-əs) *n., pl.* **–di·us·es** *or* **–di·i** (-dē-ī′) **1.** A line segment that joins the center of a circle with any point on its circumference. **2.** A long, prismatic, slightly curved bone, the shorter and thicker of the two forearm bones, located laterally to the ulna.

ra·dix (rā′dĭks) *n., pl.* **ra·dix·es** *or* **rad·i·ces** (răd′ĭ-sēz′, rā′dĭ-) The primary or beginning portion of a part or organ, as of a nerve at its origin from the brainstem or spinal cord.

ra·don (rā′dŏn) *n. Symbol* **Rn** A radioactive, largely inert gaseous element formed by the radioactive decay of radium and used as a radiation source in radiotherapy and research; its most stable isotope is Rn 222 with a half-life of 3.82 days. Atomic number 86.

rag·weed (răg′wēd′) *n.* Any of various weeds of the genus *Ambrosia* having small greenish unisexual flower heads and producing abundant pollen that is one of the chief causes of hay fever.

rale *or* **râle** (räl) *n.* An abnormal or pathological respiratory sound heard on auscultation.

ra·lox·i·fene (rə-lŏk′sĭ-fēn′) *n.* A selective estrogen receptor modulator that acts as both an estrogen agonist and antagonist. It is usually used to treat and prevent osteoporosis in postmenopausal women.

ra·mal (rā′məl) *adj.* Of or relating to a ramus.

Ra·maz·zi·ni (rä′mät-tsē′nē), **Bernardino** 1633–1714. Italian physician who was a pioneer in the field of occupational medicine. In 1700 he published the first systematic study connecting the environmental hazards of specific professions to disease, such as lead exposure in potters and painters.

ram·i·fi·ca·tion (răm′ə-fĭ-kā′shən) *n.* A branching shape or arrangement.

ram·i·fy (răm′ə-fī′) *v.* To branch.

ram·i·sec·tion (răm′ĭ-sĕk′shən) *n.* Surgical section of the communicating branches of the sympathetic nervous system.

ra·mi·tis (rä-mī′tĭs) *n.* Inflammation of a ramus.

Ra·mon (rä-môn′), **Gaston Léon** 1886–1963. French bacteriologist who in 1936 discovered a method of producing toxoids, leading to the development of vaccinations against diphtheria and tetanus.

Ra·mòn y Ca·jal (rä-môn′ ē kä-häl′), **Santiago** 1852–1934. Spanish histologist. He shared a 1906 Nobel Prize for research on the nervous system.

ra·mose (rā′mōs′, rə-mōs′) *or* **ra·mous** (rā′məs) *adj.* Having many branches; branching.

Ram·say Hunt's syndrome (răm′zē hŭnts′) *n.* Hunt's syndrome.

Ram·stedt operation (răm′stĕt, räm′shtĕt) *n.* See **pyloromyotomy.**

ram·u·lus (răm′yə-ləs) *n., pl.* **–li** (-lī′) **1.** A small branch or twig. **2.** Any of the terminal divisions of a nerve or blood vessel.

ra·mus (rā′məs) *n., pl.* **–mi** (-mī′) **1.** Any of the primary divisions of a nerve or blood vessel. **2.** A part of an irregularly shaped bone that is thicker than a process and forms an angle with the main body, especially the ascending part of the lower jaw that makes a joint at the temple. **3.** Any of the primary divisions of a cerebral sulcus.

ran·cid (răn′sĭd) *adj.* Having the disagreeable odor or taste of decomposing oils or fats.

ran·dom mating (răn′dəm) *n.* A population mating system in which every female gamete has an equal opportunity to be fertilized by every male gamete.

range (rānj) *n.* In statistics, the difference or interval between the smallest and largest values in a frequency distribution.

range of accommodation *n.* The distance between one object that is viewed with minimal refractivity of the eye and another object that is viewed with maximal accommodation.

ra·nine (rā′nīn′) *adj.* **1.** Relating to or characteristic of frogs. **2.** Relating to the tongue undersurface.

ranine artery *n.* An artery that is the termination of the lingual artery, with distribution to the muscles and mucous membrane of the undersurface of the tongue; deep artery of tongue.

ra·nit·i·dine (rə-nĭt′ĭ-dēn′) *n.* An antagonist for one of two types of histamine receptors occurring on the surfaces of cells, especially gastric cells, that acts by inhibiting gastric acid secretion and is used in the treatment of duodenal ulcers.

ran·u·la (răn′yə-lə) *n.* A cyst on the underside of the tongue or the mouth floor caused by an obstructed salivary gland duct. Also called *ptyalocele, sialocele, sublingual cyst.* —**ran′u·lar** (-lər) *adj.*

ranula pan·cre·at·i·ca (păng′krē-ăt′ĭ-kə) *n.* A cystic tumor caused by obstruction of the pancreatic duct.

Ran·vier (rän-vyā′), **Louis Antoine** 1835–1922. French histologist noted for his studies of nerve endings and skin structure.

Ran·vier's node (rän′vyāz, rän-vyāz′, rän-) *n.* A short interval in the myelin sheath of a nerve fiber, occurring between every two successive segments of the myelin sheath.

Ra·oult's law (rä-ōōlz′) *n.* The principle that the vapor pressure of a solution is equal to the vapor pressure of the pure solvent multiplied by the mole fraction of the solvent in the solution.

Rap·a·mune (răp′ə-myōōn′) A trademark for the drug sirolimus.

rape (rāp) *n.* The crime of forcing another person to submit to sex acts, especially sexual intercourse. —*v.* To commit rape on. —**rap′ist** *n.*

ra·phe *or* **rha·phe** (rā′fē) *n., pl.* **–phae** (-fē′) A seamlike line or ridge between two similar parts of a body organ, as in the scrotum.

raphe nucleus *n.* Any of the various unpaired nerve cell groups that are located in and along the median plane of the mesencephalic and rhombencephalic tegmenta that include neurons with serotonin-carrying axons that extend to the hypothalamus, septum, hippocampus, and cingulate gyrus.

raphe of penis *n.* The continuation of the raphe of the scrotum onto the underside of the penis.

raphe of perineum *n.* The central anteroposterior line of the perineum, most marked in the male, continuous with the raphe of the scrotum.

raphe of scrotum *n.* A central cordlike line running over the scrotum from the anus to the root of the penis, marking the position of the scrotal septum.

rap·id canities (răp′ĭd) *n.* The whitening of hair overnight or in the period of a few days.

rapid eye movement *n. Abbr.* **REM** The rapid periodic jerky movement of the eyes during certain stages of the sleep cycle when dreaming takes place.

rapid plasma reagin test *n.* Any of a group of serologic tests for syphilis. Also called *RPR test.*

Rap·o·port test (răp′ə-pôrt′) *n.* A test used to evaluate suspected renovascular hypertension.

rap·port (ră-pôr′, rə-) *n.* Relationship, especially one of mutual trust or emotional affinity.

rap·ture of the deep (răp′chər) *n.* See **nitrogen narcosis.**

rare earth *n.* See **lanthanide.**

rare-earth element *n.* See **lanthanide.**

rar·e·fac·tion (râr′ə-făk′shən) *n.* A decrease in density and pressure in a medium, such as air, caused by the passage of a sound wave.

RAS *abbr.* reticular activating system

rash (răsh) *n.* A skin eruption.

ras·pa·to·ry (răs′pə-tôr′ē) *n.* An instrument used for scraping bone. Also called *rugine, scalprum.*

ras protein (răs) *n.* A protein that typically promotes cell division when a growth factor is present on the cell surface. Abnormal ras proteins, caused by genetic mutations, stimulate cell division and proliferation in the absence of a growth factor and facilitate the development of various cancers.

RAST *abbr.* radioallergosorbent test

rat (răt) *n.* Any of various long-tailed rodents of the genus *Rattus* and related genera, including certain strains used in scientific research and certain species that are vectors for various diseases.

rat-bite fever *n.* Headache, fever, lymphangitis, and lymphadenitis following the bite of a rat or other rodent, due either to a spirillum or to *Streptobacillus moniliformis.*

rate (rāt) *n.* **1.** A quantity measured with respect to another measured quantity. **2.** A measure of a part with respect to a whole; a proportion.

Rath·ke (rät′kə), **Martin Heinrich** 1793–1860. German biologist who discovered gill slits and branchial arches in bird and mammal embryos.

ra·tio (rā′shō, rā′shē-ō′) *n., pl.* **–tios 1.** Relation in degree or number between two similar things. **2.** The relation between two quantities expressed as the quotient of one divided by the other.

ra·tion·al (răsh′ə-nəl) *adj.* **1.** Having or exercising the ability to reason. **2.** Influenced by reasoning rather than by emotion. **3.** Of sound mind; sane. **4.** Based on scientific knowledge or theory rather than practical observation.

ra·tion·al·ize (răsh′ə-nə-līz′) *v.* **1.** To make rational. **2.** To devise self-satisfying but false or inconsistent reasons for one's behavior, especially as an unconscious defense mechanism through which irrational acts or feelings are made to appear rational to oneself. —**ra′-tion·al·i·za′tion** (-lĭ-zā′shən) *n.*

rational therapy *n.* Psychotherapy based on the premise that a lack of information or illogical thought patterns basically cause the patient's difficulties.

RAV *abbr.* Rous-associated virus

raw (rô) *adj.* **1.** Having subcutaneous tissue exposed. **2.** Inflamed; sore.

raw·boned (rô′bōnd′) *adj.* Having a lean, gaunt frame with prominent bones.

ray (rā) *n.* **1.** A narrow beam of light or other electromagnetic radiation. **2.** A narrow beam of particles, as a cathode. **3.** A structure or part having the form of a straight line extending from a point.

Ray, John 1627–1705. English naturalist who was the first to use anatomy to distinguish between specific plants and animals. He established the species as the basic classification of living things.

Ray·naud's disease (rā-nōz′, rĕ-) *n.* A circulatory disorder that affects the hands and feet, caused by insufficient blood supply to these parts and resulting in cyanosis, numbness, pain, and, in extreme cases, gangrene. Also called *Raynaud's syndrome.*

Raynaud's phenomenon *n.* Sensitivity of the hands to cold due to spasms of the digital arteries, resulting in blanching and numbness of the fingers.

Raynaud's syndrome *n.* See **Raynaud's disease.**

Rb The symbol for the element **rubidium.**

R-banding stain *n.* A stain method in which chromosomes are heated in a phosphate buffer, then treated with Giemsa stain to produce a banding pattern that is the reverse of that produced in G-banding.

RBBB *abbr.* right bundle branch block

RBC *or* **rbc** *abbr.* red blood cell

RCP *abbr.* Royal College of Physicians

RCS *abbr.* Royal College of Surgeons

RD *abbr.* reaction of degeneration; Registered Dietician

RDA *abbr.* recommended daily allowance

RDH *abbr.* Registered Dental Hygienist

RDS *abbr.* respiratory distress syndrome

Re The symbol for the element **rhenium.**

RE *abbr.* right extremity

re– *pref.* **1.** Again; anew: *rebreathing.* **2.** Backward; back: *recurvation.*

re·act (rē-ăkt′) *v.* **1.** To act in response to a stimulus. **2.** To undergo a chemical reaction.

re·ac·tant (rē-ăk′tənt) *n.* A substance participating in a chemical reaction, especially a directly reacting substance present at the start of the reaction.

re·ac·tion (rē-ăk′shən) *n.* **1.** A response of an organism or living tissue to a stimulus. **2.** The state resulting from such a response. **3.** A chemical change or transformation in which a substance decomposes, combines with other substances, or interchanges constituents with other substances. **4.** The response of cells or tissues to an antigen, as in a test for immunization. **5.** A pattern of behavior constituting a mental disorder or personality type.

reaction formation *n.* A defense mechanism by which an objectionable impulse is expressed in an opposite or contrasting attitude or behavior.

reaction of degeneration *n. Abbr.* **DR, RD** The electrical reaction in a degenerated nerve and in the muscles it supplies.

reaction time *n.* The interval between the presentation of a stimulus and the response to it.

re·ac·ti·vate (rē-ăk′tə-vāt′) *v.* **1.** To make active again. **2.** To restore the ability to function or the effectiveness of. —**re·ac′ti·va′tion** *n.*

re·ac·tive (rē-ăk′tĭv) *adj.* **1.** Tending to be responsive or to react to a stimulus. **2.** Characterized by reaction. **3.** Tending to participate readily in chemical reactions.

re·ac·tive depression (rē-ăk′tĭv) *n.* Depression precipitated by something intensely sad or distressing.

reactive hyperemia *n.* Hyperemia in a part resulting from the restoration of its temporarily blocked blood flow.

reactive schizophrenia *n.* A severe form of schizophrenia that is distinguished from process schizophrenia by its more acute onset, greater correlation with environmental stress, and better prognosis.

re·ac·tiv·i·ty (rē′ăk-tĭv′ĭ-tē) *n.* **1.** The property of reacting. **2.** The process of reacting.

read·through (rēd′throō′) *n.* Transcription of a nucleic acid sequence beyond its normal termination sequence.

re·a·gent (rē-ā′jənt) *n.* A substance used in a chemical reaction to detect, measure, examine, or produce other substances.

re·a·gin (rē-ā′jĭn) *n.* **1.** An antibody found in the blood of individuals having a genetic predisposition to allergies such as asthma and hay fever. **2.** A substance present in the blood of individuals having a positive serological test for syphilis. —**re′a·gin′ic** (rē′ə-jĭn′ĭk) *adj.*

reaginic antibody *n.* See **homocytotropic antibody.**

re·al·i·ty (rē-ăl′ĭ-tē) *n.* **1.** The quality or state of being actual or true. **2.** The totality of all things possessing actuality, existence, or essence. **3.** That which exists objectively and in fact.

reality awareness *n.* The ability to distinguish external objects as being different from oneself.

reality principle *n.* In psychoanalysis, awareness of and adjustment to environmental demands in a manner that moderates the pleasure principle and assures ultimate satisfaction of instinctual needs.

reality testing *n.* In psychoanalytic theory, the ego function by which the objective or real world and one's relationship to it are evaluated and appreciated by the self.

real-time ultrasound *n.* The use of a rapid succession of individual B-mode images to produce a moving video display.

ream·er (rē′mər) *n.* A rotating tool used to shape or enlarge holes.

re·bound phenomenon (rē′bound′, rĭ-bound′) *n.* See **Stewart-Holmes sign.**

rebound tenderness *n.* Pain or tenderness that occurs upon sudden release of pressure, especially abdominal pressure.

re·breath·ing (rē-brē′thĭng) *n.* The partial or complete inhalation of previously exhaled gases.

rebreathing anesthesia *n.* An inhalation anesthesia technique in which a portion or all exhaled gases are inhaled after carbon dioxide has been removed by the anesthetic apparatus.

rebreathing technique *n.* Use of a breathing or anesthesia circuit in which exhaled air is afterwards inhaled either with or without absorption of CO_2 from the exhaled air.

re·cal·ci·fi·ca·tion (rē-kăl′sə-fĭ-kā′shən) *n.* The restoration of lost calcium salts to body tissues.

re·call (rĭ-kôl′) *v.* To remember; recollect. —*n.* (rē′kôl′) The ability to remember information or experiences.

re·can·a·li·za·tion (rē-kăn′ə-lĭ-zā′shən) *n.* **1.** The restoration of the lumen of a blood vessel following thrombotic occlusion by restoration of the channel or by the formation of new channels. **2.** Spontaneous restoration of the lumen of an occluded duct or tube.

re·ca·pit·u·la·tion theory (rē′kə-pĭch′ə-lā′shən) *n.* See **biogenetic law.**

re·cep·tive aphasia (rĭ-sĕp′tĭv) *n.* See **sensory aphasia.**

re·cep·tor (rĭ-sĕp′tər) *n.* **1.** A specialized cell or group of nerve endings that responds to sensory stimuli. **2.** A molecular structure or site on the surface or interior of a cell that binds with substances such as hormones, antigens, drugs, or neurotransmitters.

receptor protein *n.* An intracellular protein or protein fraction having a high specific affinity for binding agents known to stimulate cellular activity, such as a steroid hormone or cyclic AMP.

re·cess (rē′sĕs′, rĭ-sĕs′) *n.* A small hollow or an indented area.

re·ces·sion (rĭ-sĕsh′ən) *n.* The withdrawal or retreating of tissue from its normal position.

re·ces·sive (rĭ-sĕs′ĭv) *adj.* **1.** Tending to go backward or recede. **2.** Of, relating to, or being an allele that does not produce a characteristic effect when present with a dominant allele. **3.** Of, relating to, or being a trait expressed only when the determining allele is present in the homozygous condition. —*n.* **1.** A recessive allele or trait. **2.** An organism having a recessive trait.

recessive character *n.* See **recessive trait.**

recessive gene *n.* A gene that is phenotypically expressed in the homozygous state but has its expression masked in the presence of a dominant gene.

recessive inheritance *n.* Inheritance in which a trait is recessive.

recessive trait *n.* An inherited character determined by a recessive gene. Also called *recessive character.*

re·cid·i·vism (rĭ-sĭd′ə-vĭz′əm) *n.* **1.** A tendency to lapse into a previous pattern of behavior, especially a pattern of criminal habits. **2.** The relapse of a disease or symptom. Also called *recidivation.*

re·cid·i·vist (rĭ-sĭd′ə-vĭst) *n.* A person who relapses, especially by returning to criminal behavior.

rec·i·pe (rĕs′ə-pē′) *n.* **1.** The heading that is used to indicate a medical prescription, usually ℞ **2.** A medical prescription.

re·cip·i·ent (rĭ-sĭp′ē-ənt) *adj.* Functioning as a receiver; receptive. —*n.* One who receives blood, tissue, or an organ from a donor.

re·cip·ro·cal (rĭ-sĭp′rə-kəl) *adj.* **1.** Of or relating to a neuromuscular phenomenon in which the excitation of one group of muscles is accompanied by the inhibition of another. **2.** Of or being a pair of crosses in which the male parent in one cross is of the same genotype or phenotype as the female parent in the other cross.

reciprocal transfusion *n.* An attempt to confer immunity by transfusing blood taken from a donor just recovered from an infectious disease into a recipient suffering from the same disease, at the same time transfusing an equal amount from the sick to the well person.

reciprocal translocation *n.* Translocation without demonstrable loss of genetic material.

Reck·ling·hau·sen's disease (rĕk′lĭng-hou′zənz) *n.* See **neurofibromatosis.**

Recklinghausen's disease of bone *n.* See **osteitis fibrosa cystica.**

Recklinghausen's tumor *n.* See **adenomatoid tumor.**

rec·li·na·tion (rĕk′lə-nā′shən) *n.* Surgical turning of a cataractous lens into the vitreous chamber to remove it from the line of vision.

rec·og·ni·tion (rĕk′əg-nĭsh′ən) *n.* **1.** An awareness that something perceived has been perceived before. **2.** The ability of one molecule to attach itself to another molecule having a complementary shape, as in enzyme-substrate interactions.

recognition factor *n.* Any of the factors that allow polymorphonuclear neutrophil leukocytes to recognize target antigens.

re·com·bi·nant (rē-kŏm′bə-nənt) *n.* **1.** An organism or a cell in which genetic recombination has taken place. **2.** Genetic material produced by splicing genes. —*adj.* **1.** Formed by or showing recombination, as a chromosome. **2.** Relating to recombinant DNA.

recombinant DNA *n.* Genetically engineered DNA prepared by transplanting or splicing one or more segments of DNA into the chromosomes of an organism from a different species. Such DNA becomes part of the host's genetic makeup and is replicated.

re·com·bi·nase (rē-kŏm′bə-nās′, -nāz′) *n.* An enzyme that catalyzes genetic recombination.

re·com·bi·na·tion (rē′kŏm-bə-nā′shən) *n.* The natural formation in offspring of genetic combinations not present in parents by the processes of crossing over or independent assortment.

re·com·bine (rē′kəm-bīn′) *v.* To undergo or cause genetic recombination; form new combinations.

rec·om·mend·ed daily allowance (rĕk′ə-mĕn′dĭd) *n.* *Abbr.* **RDA** The amounts of nutrients and calories an individual is recommended to consume daily, especially the amounts of vitamins and minerals recommended by the Food and Nutrition Board of the National Research Council.

re·con (rē′kŏn′) *n.* The smallest genetic unit capable of recombination.

re·con·struc·tive mammaplasty (rē′kən-strŭk′tĭv) *n.* The making of a simulated breast by plastic surgery for replacement of one that has been removed.

reconstructive surgery *n.* Plastic surgery.

re·cord (rĭ-kôrd′) *v.* **1.** To set down for preservation in writing or other permanent form. **2.** To register or indicate. —*n.* **rec·ord** (rĕk′ərd) **1.** An account, as of information or facts, set down especially in writing as a means of preserving knowledge. **2.** A medical record. **3.** In dentistry, a registration of desired jaw relations in a plastic material or on a device so that such relations may be transferred to an articulator. **4.** The known history of performance, activities, or achievement. **5.** A collection of related, often adjacent items of computer data, treated as a unit.

re·cov·ered memory (rĭ-kŭv′ərd) *n.* A memory that has been restored from the unconscious to the conscious mind, especially one of a traumatic childhood event.

re·cov·er·y room (rĭ-kŭv′ə-rē) *n.* A hospital room equipped for the care and observation of patients immediately following surgery.

rec·re·a·tion·al drug (rĕk′rē-ā′shə-nəl) *n.* A drug used nonmedically for personal enjoyment.

re·cru·des·cence (rē′krōō-dĕs′əns) *n.* A recurrence of a pathological process or its symptoms after a period of improvement or quiescence. —**re′cru·desce′** *v.* —**re′·cru·des′cent** *adj.*

recrudescent typhus *n.* See **Brill-Zinsser disease.**

re·cruit·ment (rĭ-krōōt′mənt) *n.* **1.** An abnormal disproportionate sensation of loudness felt in response to sounds of increasing intensity. **2.** The activation of additional motor neurons in response to sustained stimulation of a given receptor or afferent nerve.

rect– *pref.* Variant of **recto–.**

rec·tal (rĕk′təl) *adj.* Of, relating to, or situated near the rectum.

rectal ampulla *n.* A dilated portion of the rectum just above the anal canal.

rectal anesthesia *n.* General anesthesia following instillation of liquid anesthetics into the rectum.

rectal artery *n.* **1.** An artery with its origin in the internal pudendal artery, with distribution to the anal canal, the muscles and skin of the anal region, and the skin of the buttocks; inferior rectal artery. **2.** An artery with its origin in the internal iliac artery, with distribution to the middle portion of the rectum; middle rectal artery. **3.** An artery with its origin in the inferior mesenteric artery, with distribution to the upper part of the rectum; superior rectal artery.

rectal column *n.* See **anal column.**

rec·tal·gia (rĕk-tăl′jə) *n.* See **proctalgia.**

rectal sinus *n.* See **anal sinus.**

rec·tec·to·my (rĕk-tĕk′tə-mē) *n.* See **proctectomy.**

rec·ti·fy (rĕk′tə-fī′) *v.* **1.** To set right; correct. **2.** To refine or purify, especially by distillation.

rec·ti·tis (rĕk-tī′tĭs) *n.* See **proctitis.**

recto– *or* **rect–** *pref.* Rectum: *rectoscope.*

rec·to·cele (rĕk′tə-sēl′) *n.* See **proctocele.**

rec·to·coc·cyg·e·al muscle (rĕk′tō-kŏk-sĭj′ē-əl) *n.* A band of smooth muscle fibers passing from the posterior surface of the rectum to the anterior surface of the second or third coccygeal segment.

rec·to·coc·cy·pex·y (rĕk′tō-kŏk′sə-pĕk′sē) *n.* See **proctococcypexy.**

rec·to·pex·y (rĕk′tə-pĕk′sē) *n.* See **proctopexy.**

rec·to·plas·ty (rĕk′tə-plăs′tē) *n.* See **proctoplasty.**

rec·to·scope (rĕk′tə-skōp′) *n.* See **proctoscope.**

rec·to·sig·moid (rĕk′tō-sĭg′moid′) *n.* **1.** The rectum and the sigmoid colon considered as a unit. **2.** The junction of the rectum and the sigmoid colon.

rec·to·ste·no·sis (rĕk′tō-stə-nō′sĭs) *n.* See **proctostenosis.**

rec·tos·to·my (rĕk-tŏs′tə-mē) *n.* See **proctostomy.**

rec·tot·o·my (rĕk-tŏt′ə-mē) *n.* See **proctotomy.**

rec·to·u·re·thral muscle (rĕk′tō-yōō-rē′thrəl) *n.* Smooth muscle fibers that pass forward from the longitudinal muscle layer of the rectum to the spongy membrane just beyond the bulb of the penis.

rec·to·u·ter·ine (rĕk′tō-yōō′tər-ĭn, -tə-rīn′) *adj.* Relating to the rectum and the uterus.

rectouterine fold *n.* A fold of the peritoneum that contains the rectouterine muscle, passes from the rectum to the base of the broad ligament on either side, and forms the lateral boundary of the rectouterine pouch. Also called *Douglas's fold.*

rectouterine muscle *n.* A band of fibrous tissue and smooth muscle fibers on either side of the uterine cervix and the rectum in the rectouterine fold.

rectouterine pouch *n.* A pocket formed by the deflection of the peritoneum from the rectum to the uterus. Also called *Douglas cul-de-sac, Douglas pouch.*

rec·to·vag·i·nal septum (rĕk′tō-văj′ə-nəl) *n.* The fascial layer between the vagina and the lower part of the rectum.

rec·to·ves·i·cal muscle (rĕk′tō-vĕs′ĭ-kəl) *n.* Smooth muscle fibers in the folds in the male that extend backward from the sides of the bladder on either side of the rectum to the sacrum.

rectovesical pouch *n.* A pocket formed by the deflection of the peritoneum from the rectum to the male bladder.

rectovesical septum *n.* A fascial layer extending from the central tendon of the perineum to the peritoneum between the prostate and the rectum.

rec·tum (rĕk′təm) *n., pl.* **–tums** *or* **–ta** (-tə) The terminal portion of the large intestine, extending from the sigmoid flexure to the anal canal.

rec·tus abdominis (rĕk′təs) *n.* A muscle with origin from the pubis, with insertion into the xiphoid process and the fifth to seventh costal cartilages, and whose action flexes the vertebral column and draws the chest downward.

rectus femoris *n.* A muscle with origin from the ilium and the acetabulum, with insertion into a tendon of the quadriceps muscle of the thigh.

rectus lat·e·ra·lis (lăt′ə-rā′lĭs, -răl′ĭs) *n.* See **lateral rectus muscle.**

re·cum·bent (rĭ-kŭm′bənt) *adj.* Lying down, especially in a position of comfort; reclining. —**re·cum′bence, re·cum′ben·cy** *n.*

re·cu·per·ate (rĭ-kōō′pə-rāt′) *v.* To return to health or strength; recover.

re·cur (rĭ-kûr′) *v.* **1.** To happen, come up, or show up again or repeatedly. **2.** To return to one's attention or memory.

re·cur·rence (rĭ-kûr′əns) *n.* **1.** A return of symptoms as part of the natural progress of a disease, as in relapsing fever. **2.** See **relapse.**

recurrence risk *n.* Risk that a disease will occur elsewhere in a pedigree, given that at least one member of the pedigree exhibits the disease.

re·cur·rent (rĭ-kûr′ənt) *adj.* **1.** Occurring or appearing again or repeatedly. **2.** Turning in a reverse direction. Used of blood vessels and nerves.

recurrent aphthous ulcers *pl.n.* See **canker sore.**

recurrent artery *n.* **1.** An artery with its origin in the radial artery that ascends around the lateral side of the elbow joint; radial recurrent artery. **2.** An artery that is a branch of the anterior tibial artery and ascends to supply the front and sides of the knee joint; anterior tibial recurrent artery. **3.** An artery that is a branch of the posterior tibial artery, and ascends anterior to the popliteal muscle, and sends a small branch to the tibiofibular joint; posterior tibial recurrent artery. **4.** An artery with its origin in the ulnar artery, with distribution into anterior and posterior branches, and passing medially in front of and behind the elbow joint; recurrent ulnar artery.

recurrent canker sores *pl.n.* See **recurrent ulcerative stomatitis.**

recurrent fever *n.* See **relapsing fever.**

recurrent herpetic stomatitis *n.* Reactivation of herpes simplex virus in the oral tissues, characterized by vesicles and ulceration.

recurrent laryngeal nerve *n.* A branch of the vagus nerve that supplies the cardiac, tracheal and esophageal branches and terminates as the inferior laryngeal nerve.

recurrent ulcerative stomatitis *n.* An oral disease characterized by recurrent appearance of single or multiple painful ulcers having a grayish-yellow coating and surrounded by a narrow zone of inflammation. Also called *recurrent canker sores.*

recurring digital fibroma of childhood *n.* Any of several fibrous flesh-colored nodules on the the tips of the fingers and toes of infants and young children,

composed of spindle cells containing cytoplasmic inclusions. Also called *infantile digital fibromatosis.*

re·cur·va·tion (rē′kər-vā′shən) *n.* A backward bending or flexure. —**re·cur′vate′** (rĭ-kûr′vāt′, -vĭt) *adj.*

red blood cell (rĕd) *n. Abbr.* **RBC, rbc** A disk-shaped, biconcave cell in the blood that contains hemoglobin, lacks a nucleus, and transports oxygen and carbon dioxide to and from the tissues. Also called *erythrocyte, red cell, red corpuscle.*

red bone marrow *n.* Bone marrow characterized by meshes of the reticular network that contain the developmental stages of red blood cells, white blood cells, and megakaryocytes.

red bug *or* **redbug** *n.* See **chigger** (sense 1).

red cell *n.* See **red blood cell.**

red corpuscle *n.* See **red blood cell.**

Red Crescent *n.* **1.** A branch of the Red Cross organization operating in a Muslim country. **2.** The crescent-shaped emblem of such a branch.

Red Cross *n.* **1.** An international organization that cares for the wounded, sick, and homeless in wartime according to the terms of the Geneva Convention of 1864, and now also during and following natural disasters. **2.** A national branch of the Red Cross. **3.** The Red Cross emblem of this organization, a Geneva cross or a red Greek cross on a white background.

red hepatization *n.* The first stage of hepatization of lung tissue in pneumonia, in which the exudate is blood-stained.

red induration *n.* A condition observed in the lungs in which there is an advanced degree of acute passive congestion, acute pneumonitis, or a similar pathologic process.

red infarct *n.* See **hemorrhagic infarct.**

red·in·te·gra·tion (rĕd-ĭn′tĭ-grā′shən, rĭ-dĭn′-) *n.* **1.** The restoration of a lost or injured part. **2.** Evocation of a particular state of mind resulting from the recurrence of one of the elements that made up the original experience.

red muscle *n.* A muscle in which small dark fibers predominate and in which myoglobin and mitochondria are abundant.

red neuralgia *n.* See **erythromelalgia.**

red nucleus *n.* A large, well defined, somewhat elongated cell mass of reddish-gray hue that is located in the mesencephalic tegmentum, receives a massive projection from the contralateral half of the cerebellum, receives an additional projection from the ipsilateral motor cortex, and whose efferent connections are with the contralateral half of the rhombencephalic reticular formation and spinal cord.

re·dox (rē′dŏks′) *n.* See **oxidation-reduction.**

red pulp *n.* See **splenic pulp.**

red reflex *n.* See **light reflex** (sense 2).

re·duce (rĭ-dōōs′) *v.* **1.** To bring down, as in extent, amount, or degree; diminish. **2.** To lose weight, as by dieting. **3.** To restore a fractured or displaced body part to a normal condition or position. **4.** To decrease the valence of an atom by adding electrons. **5.** To remove oxygen from a compound. **6.** To add hydrogen to a compound. —**re·duc′i·ble** *adj.*

re·duced glutathione (rĭ-dōōsd′) *n.* The form of

glutathione that acts as a hydrogen donor during cellular oxidation-reduction reactions.

reduced hematin *n.* See heme.

reduced hemoglobin *n.* Hemoglobin in red blood cells after the oxygen of oxyhemoglobin is released in the tissues.

reducible hernia *n.* A hernia in which the contents of the sac can be returned to their normal location by manipulation.

re·duc·ing agent (rĭ-do͞o′sĭng) *n.* A substance that chemically reduces other substances, especially by donating an electron or electrons.

re·duc·tant (rĭ-dŭk′tənt) *n.* A reducing agent.

re·duc·tase (rĭ-dŭk′tās′, -tāz′) *n.* An enzyme that promotes reduction of an organic compound.

re·duc·tion (rĭ-dŭk′shən) *n.* **1.** The act, process, or result of reducing. **2.** The amount by which something is lessened or diminished. **3.** Restoration of an injured or dislocated part to its normal anatomical relation by surgery or manipulation. **4.** The first meiotic division, in which the chromosome number is reduced. Also called *reduction division, reduction of chromosomes.* **5.** A decrease in positive valence or an increase in negative valence by the gaining of electrons. **6.** A reaction in which hydrogen is combined with a compound. **7.** A reaction in which oxygen is removed from a compound. —**re·duc′tion·al** *adj.*

reduction deformity *n.* A congenital deformity in which a body part, especially a limb, is shorter than normal or missing.

reduction division *n.* See **reduction** (sense 4).

reduction mammaplasty *n.* Plastic surgery on the breast to reduce its size and often to improve its shape and position.

reduction of chromosomes *n.* See **reduction** (sense 4).

re·du·pli·ca·tion (rĭ-do͞o′plĭ-kā′shən) *n.* **1.** A redoubling. **2.** A duplication or doubling, as of the sounds of the heart in certain diseased states. **3.** The abnormal presence of two parts instead of a single part. **4.** A fold or duplicature. —**re·du′pli·cate′** *v.*

re·du·vi·id (rĭ-do͞o′vē-ĭd) *n.* A member of the family Reduviidae; an assassin bug.

Re·du·vi·i·dae (rĕ′do͞o-vī′ĭ-dē′, rĕj′o͞o-) *n.* A family of predatory insects comprising the assassin bugs, which attack humans and other animals. It includes the subfamily Triatominae, the kissing or cone-nose bugs, whose type genus *Triatoma* includes vectors of *Trypanosoma cruzi.*

Re·dux (rē′dŭks′) A trademark for the drug dexfenfluramine hydrochloride.

Reed (rēd), **Walter** 1851–1902. American surgeon who led the commission that proved experimentally that yellow fever is transmitted by mosquitoes.

Reed-Sternberg cell *n.* A giant binucleated or multinucleated acidophilic cell in the tissues in Hodgkin's disease. Also called *Sternberg-Reed cell.*

reef·er (rē′fər) *n.* Marijuana, especially a marijuana cigarette.

reef·ing (rē′fĭng) *n.* Surgical reduction of the extent of a tissue by folding it and securing with sutures.

re·en·try (rē-ĕn′trē) *n.* Return of the same impulse into an area of heart muscle that it has recently activated

but that is now no longer refractory, as in reciprocal rhythm.

ref·er·ence values (rĕf′ər-əns, rĕf′rəns) *pl.n.* A set of laboratory test values obtained from an individual or from a group in a defined state of health.

re·ferred pain (rĭ-fûrd′) *n.* Pain that is felt in a part of the body at a distance from its area of origin.

referred sensation *n.* A sensation felt in a place other than the site at which a stimulus was applied. Also called *reflex sensation.*

re·fine (rĭ-fīn′) *v.* To reduce to a pure state; purify.

re·flect (rĭ-flĕkt′) *v.* **1.** To bend back. **2.** To throw or bend back light, heat, or sound from a surface. **3.** To think seriously. **4.** To send back a motor impulse in response to a sensory stimulus.

re·flec·tion (rĭ-flĕk′shən) *n.* **1.** The act of reflecting or the state of being reflected. **2.** Something, such as light, radiant heat, sound, or an image, that is reflected. **3.** The folding of a membrane from the wall of a cavity over an organ and back to the wall. **4.** The folds so made. **5.** Mental concentration; careful consideration. **6.** A thought or an opinion resulting from such consideration. —**re·flec′tion·al** *adj.*

reflection coefficient *n. Symbol* **σ** A measure of the relative permeability of a particular membrane to a particular solute.

re·flec·tive (rĭ-flĕk′tĭv) *adj.* **1.** Of, relating to, produced by, or resulting from reflection. **2.** Capable of or producing reflection. **3.** Characterized by or given to meditation or contemplation; thoughtful.

re·flec·tor (rĭ-flĕk′tər) *n.* A surface that reflects light, heat, or sound.

re·flex (rē′flĕks′) *n.* **1.** An involuntary physiological response to a stimulus. **2.** An unlearned or instinctive response to a stimulus. **3.** Something, such as light or heat, that is reflected. —*adj.* **1.** Being an involuntary action or response, such as a sneeze, blink, or hiccup. **2.** Bent, turned, or thrown back; reflected. —*v.* (rĭ-flĕks′) **1.** To cause to undergo a reflex process. **2.** To reflect.

reflex arc *n.* The route followed by nerve impulses to produce a reflex act, from the periphery through the afferent nerve to the nervous system, and thence through the efferent nerve to the effector organ.

reflex cough *n.* A cough caused by irritation in some distant part, such as the ear or the stomach.

reflex epilepsy *n.* A form of epilepsy in which the seizures are induced by sensory stimuli such as music, movement, sudden noise, reading, and touching or seeing an object.

reflex inhibition *n.* A decrease in reflex activity caused by sensory stimuli.

reflex ligament *n.* A triangular fibrous band extending from the aponeurosis of an abdominal muscle to the pubic tubercle on the opposite side.

reflex neurogenic bladder *n.* An abnormal condition of urinary bladder function in which the bladder is cut off from upper motor neuron control but with the lower motor neuron reflex arc still intact.

re·flex·o·gen·ic (rĭ-flĕk′sə-jĕn′ĭk) *or* **re·flex·og·e·nous** (rē′flĕk-sŏj′ə-nəs) *adj.* Causing a reflex.

re·flex·o·graph (rĭ-flĕk′sə-grăf′) *n.* An instrument for graphically recording a reflex.

re·flex·ol·o·gy (rē′flĕk-sŏl′ə-jē) *n.* **1.** The study of reflex responses, especially as they affect behavior. **2.** A method of massage that relieves nervous tension through the application of finger pressure, especially to the feet.

re·flex·om·e·ter (rē′flĕk-sŏm′ĭ-tər) *n.* An instrument for measuring the force necessary to excite a reflex.

reflex sensation *n.* See **referred sensation.**

reflex symptom *n.* A disturbance of sensation or of function occurring at a remote location from the diseased area.

re·flux (rē′flŭks′) *n.* **1.** A flowing back. **2.** The process of refluxing. —*v.* To boil a liquid in a vessel attached to a condenser so that the vapors continuously condense for reboiling.

reflux esophagitis *n.* Inflammation of the lower esophagus from regurgitation of acid gastric contents, characterized by substernal pain and usually due to malfunction of the lower esophageal sphincter. Also called *peptic esophagitis.*

reflux otitis media *n.* Otitis media caused by nasopharyngeal secretions passing through the eustachian tube of the ear.

re·fract (rĭ-frăkt′) *v.* **1.** To deflect something, especially light, from a straight path by refraction. **2.** To determine the refraction of an eye or a lens.

re·frac·tion (rĭ-frăk′shən) *n.* **1.** The turning or bending of any wave, such as a light or sound wave, when it passes from one medium into another of different density. **2.** The ability of the eye to bend light so that an image is focused on the retina. **3.** Determination of the refractive characteristics of the eye and often the correction of refractive defects with lenses. Also called *refringence.* —**re·frac′tion·al, re·frac′tive** *adj.*

re·frac·tion·ist (rĭ-frăk′shə-nĭst) *n.* A person trained to measure the refraction of the eye and to determine the proper corrective lenses.

refractive index *n. Abbr.* **n** The ratio of the speed of light in air or in a vacuum to the speed of light in another medium.

refractive keratotomy *n.* Surgical modification of corneal curvature by incising the cornea to minimize hyperopia, myopia, or astigmatism.

re·frac·tom·e·ter (rē′frăk-tŏm′ĭ-tər) *n.* Any of several instruments used to measure the refractive index of a substance.

re·frac·tom·e·try (rē′frăk-tŏm′ĭ-trē) *n.* **1.** Measurement of the refractive index of a substance with a refractometer. **2.** Use of a refractometer in determining the refractive error of the eye.

re·frac·to·ry (rĭ-frăk′tə-rē) *adj.* **1.** Resistant to treatment, as a disease. **2.** Unresponsive to stimuli, as a muscle or nerve fiber.

refractory anemia *n.* Any of a group of anemic conditions that is not associated with another disease and that is marked by a persistent, frequently advanced anemia that can only be successfully treated through blood transfusions.

refractory period *n.* The period that follows effective stimulation, during which excitable tissue fails to respond to a stimulus of threshold intensity.

refractory state *n.* Subnormal excitability of a muscle or nerve immediately following a response to previous excitation.

re·frac·ture (rē-frăk′chər) *n.* The breaking of a bone that has united after a previous fracture.

re·fresh (rĭ-frĕsh′) *v.* **1.** To cause to recuperate; revive. **2.** To renew by stimulation. **3.** To pare or scrape the edges of a wound to promote healing.

re·frig·er·ant (rĭ-frĭj′ər-ənt) *adj.* **1.** Cooling or freezing; refrigerating. **2.** Reducing fever. —*n.* **1.** A substance, such as air, ammonia, water, or carbon dioxide, used to provide cooling either as the working substance of a refrigerator or by direct absorption of heat. **2.** An agent used to reduce fever.

re·frig·er·a·tion (rĭ-frĭj′ə-rā′shən) *n.* **1.** The act or process of cooling a substance. **2.** The act or process of preserving by cooling. **3.** The reducing of a fever. —**re·frig′er·ate′** *v.*

refrigeration anesthesia *n.* See **cryoanesthesia.**

re·frin·gence (rĭ-frĭn′jəns) *n.* See **refraction.**

re·frin·gent (rĭ-frĭn′jənt) *adj.* Of, relating to, or producing refraction; refractive.

Ref·sum's disease (rĕf′səmz) *n.* A rare inherited metabolic disorder characterized by a buildup of phytanic acid in tissues and a manifestation of such conditions as retinitis pigmentosa, polyneuritis, deafness, and nystagmus.

re·fu·sion (rĭ-fyoō′zhən) *n.* The return of blood to circulation following its temporary stoppage by the ligature of a limb.

re·gen·er·a·tion (rĭ-jĕn′ə-rā′shən) *n.* Regrowth of lost or destroyed parts or organs.

re·gen·er·a·tive polyp (rĭ-jĕn′ə-rā′tĭv, -ər-ə-tĭv) *n.* A hyperplastic polyp of the gastric mucosa.

re·gime (rā-zhēm′, rĭ-) *n.* A regulated system, as of diet and exercise; a regimen.

reg·i·men (rĕj′ə-mən, -mĕn′) *n.* **1.** A regulated system, as of diet, therapy, or exercise, intended to promote health or achieve another beneficial effect. **2.** A course of intense physical training.

re·gion (rē′jən) *n.* **1.** An area of the body having natural or arbitrary boundaries. **2.** A portion of the body having a special nervous or vascular supply. **3.** A part of an organ with a special function.

re·gion·al (rē′jə-nəl) *adj.* Of or affecting a region of the body.

regional anatomy *n.* The study of regions of the body. Also called *topographic anatomy.*

regional anesthesia *n.* Anesthesia characterized by the loss of sensation in a circumscribed region of the body, produced by the application of a regional anesthetic, usually by injection.

regional anesthetic *n.* Any of various anesthetic drugs, usually administered by local injection, that produce regional anesthesia.

regional enteritis *n.* See **Crohn's disease.**

regional hypothermia *n.* Perfusion with cold blood or local refrigeration to cool an organ that has been subjected to ischemia in order to reduce its metabolic requirements.

regional ileitis *n.* See **Crohn's disease.**

region of back *n.* Any of the topographical divisions of the back of the trunk, including the vertebral, sacral, scapular, infrascapular, and lumbar regions.

region of chest *n.* Any of the topographical divisions of the chest, including the presternal, pectoral, mammary, inframammary, and axillary regions.

region of face *n.* Any of the topographical divisions of the face, including the nasal, oral, mental, orbital, infraorbital, buccal, and zygomatic regions.

region of head *n.* Any of the topographical divisions of the cranium in relation to the bones of the cranial vault, including the frontal, parietal, occipital, and temporal regions.

region of inferior limb *n.* Any of the topographical divisions of the lower limb, including the buttock, thigh, knee, leg, ankle, and foot regions.

region of superior limb *n.* Any of the topographical divisions of the upper limb, including the deltoid muscle, arm, elbow, forearm, and hand regions.

reg·is·tered nurse (rĕj′ĭ-stərd) *n. Abbr.* **RN** A nurse who has graduated from an accredited school of nursing and has been registered and licensed to practice by a state authority.

reg·is·trar (rĕj′ĭ-strär′, rĕj′ĭ-strär′) *n.* An admitting officer in a hospital.

Reg·lan (rĕg′lăn′) A trademark for the drug metoclopramide.

re·gres·sion (rĭ-grĕsh′ən) *n.* **1.** A subsidence of the symptoms of a disease. **2.** A relapse of symptoms. **3.** Reversion to an earlier or less mature pattern of feeling or behavior. **4.** Relapse to a less perfect or developed state. **5.** The return of a population to an earlier or less complex physical type in successive generations. **6.** The relationship between the mean value of a random variable and the corresponding values of one or more independent variables.

re·gres·sive (rĭ-grĕs′ĭv) *adj.* **1.** Having a tendency to return or to revert. **2.** Characterized by regression. —**re·gres′sive·ness** *n.*

regressive staining *n.* A type of staining in which tissues are overstained and excess dye then removed selectively until the desired intensity is obtained.

reg·u·lar astigmatism (rĕg′yə-lər) *n.* Astigmatism in which the curvature in each meridian is equal throughout its course, and the meridians of greatest and least curvature are at right angles to each other.

reg·u·late (rĕg′yə-lāt′) *v.* **1.** To control or direct according to rule, principle, or law. **2.** To adjust to a particular specification or requirement. **3.** To adjust a mechanism for accurate and proper functioning. **4.** To put or maintain in order. —**reg′u·la′tive, reg′u·la·to′ry** (-lə-tôr′ē) *adj.* —**reg′u·la′tor** *n.*

reg·u·la·tion (rĕg′yə-lā′shən) *n.* **1.** The act of regulating or the state of being regulated. **2.** A principle, rule, or law designed to control or govern conduct. **3.** A governmental order having the force of law. **4.** The capacity of an embryo to continue normal development following injury to or alteration of a structure.

regulator gene (rĕg′yə-lā′tər) *n.* A gene that causes the production of a protein that represses the activity of another gene in an operon.

regulatory sequence *n.* A DNA sequence responsible for regulating gene expression.

re·gur·gi·tant murmur (rē-gûr′jĭ-tənt) *n.* A murmur due to leakage or backward flow at one of the valvular orifices of the heart.

re·gur·gi·tate (rē-gûr′jĭ-tāt′) *v.* **1.** To rush or surge back. **2.** To cause to pour back, especially to cast up partially digested food. —**re·gur′gi·tant** (-tənt) *adj.* —**re·gur′gi·ta′tion** *n.*

regurgitation jaundice *n.* Jaundice caused by biliary obstruction so that bile pigment secreted by the hepatic cells is reabsorbed into the bloodstream.

re·hab (rē′hăb′) *n.* Rehabilitation.

re·ha·bil·i·tant (rē′hə-bĭl′ĭ-tənt) *n.* One who is undergoing rehabilitation, as for a disability.

re·ha·bil·i·tate (rē′hə-bĭl′ĭ-tāt′) *v.* **1.** To restore to good health or useful life, as through therapy and education. **2.** To restore to good condition, operation, or capacity. —**re′ha·bil′i·ta′tion** *n.* —**re′ha·bil′i·ta′tive** *adj.*

re·hears·al (rĭ-hûr′səl) *n.* The process of repeating information, such as a name or a list of words, in order to remember it. —**re·hearse′** *v.*

re·hy·drate (rē-hī′drāt′) *v.* **1.** To cause rehydration of something. **2.** To replenish the body fluids of an individual.

re·hy·dra·tion (rē′hī-drā′shən) *n.* **1.** The restoration of fluid to a dehydrated substance. **2.** The replenishment of bodily fluids.

Reich·stein (rīk′stīn′, rīкн′shtīn′), **Tadeus** 1897–1996. Polish-born Swiss chemist. He shared a 1950 Nobel Prize for discoveries concerning the hormones of the adrenal cortex.

Rei·fen·stein's syndrome (rī′fən-stīnz′) *n.* A familial form of male pseudohermaphroditism characterized by ambiguous genitalia or hypospadias, postpubertal, abnormally large breasts, and infertility associated with sclerosis of the seminal tubules.

re·im·plan·ta·tion (rē′ĭm-plăn-tā′shən) *n.* See **replantation.**

re·in·fec·tion (rē′ĭn-fĕk′shən) *n.* A second infection that follows recovery from a previous infection by the same causative agent.

re·in·force (rē′ĭn-fôrs′) *v.* **1.** To give more force or effectiveness to something; strengthen. **2.** To reward an individual, especially an experimental subject, with a reinforcer subsequent to a desired response or performance. **3.** To stimulate a response by means of a reinforcer.

re·in·force·ment (rē′ĭn-fôrs′mənt) *n.* **1.** The act or process of reinforcing. **2.** Something that reinforces. **3.** The occurrence or experimental introduction of an unconditioned stimulus along with a conditioned stimulus. **4.** The strengthening of a conditioned response by such means. **5.** An event, a circumstance, or a condition that increases the likelihood that a given response will recur in a situation like that in which the reinforcing condition originally occurred.

re·in·forc·er (rē′ĭn-fôr′sər) *n.* A stimulus, such as a reward, that in operant conditioning maintains or strengthens a desired response.

re·in·ner·va·tion (rē′ĭn-ər-vā′shən) *n.* Restoration of nerve control of a paralyzed muscle or organ by means of the regrowth of nerve fibers, either spontaneously or after anastomosis.

reins (rānz) *pl.n.* The kidneys, loins, or lower back.

re·in·te·gra·tion (rē′ĭn-tĭ-grā′shən) *n.* **1.** Restoration to a condition of integration or unity. **2.** The return to well-adjusted functioning following mental illness. —**re·in′te·grate′** *v.* —**re·in′te·gra′tive** *adj.*

Reis·seis·sen′s muscles (rī′sī′sənz) *pl.n.* Microscopic smooth muscle fibers in small bronchial tubes.

Reiss·ner′s membrane (rīs′nərz) *n.* See **vestibular membrane.**

Reit·er′s syndrome (rī′tərz) *n.* A triad of disorders that can appear consecutively or concurrently and include inflammation of the urethra, the iris and ciliary body, and the joints. Also called *Reiter′s disease.*

re·ject (rĭ-jĕkt′) *v.* **1.** To refuse to accept, submit to, believe, or use something. **2.** To discard as defective or useless; throw away. **3.** To spit out or vomit. **4.** To resist immunologically introduction of a transplanted organ or tissue; fail to accept in one's body.

re·jec·tion (rĭ-jĕk′shən) *n.* **1.** The act of rejecting or the state of being rejected. **2.** The failure of a recipient's body to accept a transplanted tissue or organ as the result of immunological incompatability; immunological resistance to foreign tissue.

re·lapse (rĭ-lăps′) *v.* **1.** To regress after partial recovery from illness. **2.** To slip back into bad ways; backslide. **3.** To fall or slide back into a former state. —*n.* (rē′lăps, rĭ-lăps′) A falling back into a former state, especially the return of symptoms following an apparent recovery. Also called *recurrence.*

re·laps·ing fever (rĭ-lăp′sĭng) *n.* An acute infectious disease caused by a strain of *Borrelia* transmitted by lice or ticks and marked by recurring febrile attacks lasting about six days and separated from one other by apyretic intervals of about the same length. Also called *recurrent fever.*

relapsing polychondritis *n.* A degenerative disease of cartilage characterized by the collapse of the ears, the cartilaginous portion of the nose, and the tracheobronchial tree.

re·la·tion (rĭ-lā′shən) *n.* **1.** A logical or natural association between two or more things; relevance of one to another; connection. **2.** The connection of people by blood or marriage; kinship. **3.** A person connected to another by blood or marriage; a relative. **4.** The positional relationship of the teeth or other structures in the mouth.

re·la·tion·ship (rĭ-lā′shən-shĭp′) *n.* **1.** The condition or fact of being related; connection or association. **2.** Connection by blood or marriage; kinship.

rel·a·tive accommodation (rĕl′ə-tĭv) *n.* The quantity of accommodation required for binocular vision for any distance or for any degree of convergence.

relative humidity *n.* The ratio of the amount of water vapor in the air at a specific temperature to the maximum amount that the air could hold at that temperature, expressed as a percentage.

relative leukocytosis *n.* An increased proportion of one or more types of white blood cells in the blood without an actual increase in the total number of white blood cells.

relative polycythemia *n.* A relative increase in the number of red blood cells as a result of loss of the fluid portion of the blood.

relative scotoma *n.* A scotoma in which the visual impairment is not complete.

relative specificity *n.* The specificity of a medical screening test as determined by comparison with an established test of the same type.

re·lax (rĭ-lăks′) *v.* **1.** To make or become lax or loose. **2.** To relieve or become relieved from tension or strain.

re·lax·ant (rĭ-lăk′sənt) *n.* Something, such as a drug or therapeutic treatment, that relaxes or relieves muscular or nervous tension. —*adj.* Tending to relax or to relieve tension.

relaxant reversal *n.* The termination of the action of nondepolarizing neuromuscular relaxants by the administration of acetylcholinesterase inhibitors.

re·lax·a·tion (rē′lăk-sā′shən) *n.* **1.** The act of relaxing or the state of being relaxed. **2.** Refreshment of body or mind. **3.** A loosening or slackening. **4.** The lengthening of inactive muscle or muscle fibers.

relaxation suture *n.* A suture that is arranged so that it may be loosened if the tension of the wound becomes excessive.

re·lax·in (rĭ-lăk′sĭn) *n.* A female hormone secreted by the corpus luteum that helps soften the cervix and relax the pelvic ligaments in childbirth.

re·learn·ing (rē-lûr′nĭng) *n.* The process of regaining a skill or ability that has been partially or entirely lost. —**re·learn′** *v.*

re·leas·ing factor (rĭ-lē′sĭng) *n. Abbr.* **RF** A substance of hypothalamic origin capable of accelerating the secretion of a given hormone by the anterior lobe of pituitary gland. Also called *releasing hormone.*

Re·len·za (rĭ-lĕn′zə) A trademark for the drug zanamavir.

rel·ict (rĕl′ĭkt, rĭ-lĭkt′) *n.* Something that has survived; a remnant.

re·lieve (rĭ-lēv′) *v.* **1.** To cause a lessening or alleviation of something, such as pain, tension, or a symptom. **2.** To free an individual from pain, anxiety, or distress. —**re·liev′a·ble** *adj.*

Rel·pax (rĕl′păks′) A trademark for the drug eletriptan hydrobromide.

rem (rĕm) *n.* The amount of ionizing radiation required to produce the same biological effect as one rad of high-penetration x-rays.

REM *abbr.* rapid eye movement

Re·mak (rā′măk, -mäk), **Robert** 1815–1865. German physician who in 1842 discovered and named the three primary germ layers of the embryo. He also studied the nervous system extensively and pioneered the use of electrotherapy in the treatment of neurological disorders.

Re·mak′s sign (rā′măks, -mäks) *n.* An indication of tabes dorsalis and polyneuritis in which there is a dissociation of the sensations of touch and of pain.

rem·e·dy (rĕm′ĭ-dē) *n.* Something, such as medicine or therapy, that relieves pain, cures disease, or corrects a disorder. —*v.* To relieve or cure a disease or disorder.

re·mem·ber (rĭ-mĕm′bər) *v.* **1.** To recall to the mind; think of again. **2.** To retain in the memory. **3.** To return to an original shape or form after being deformed or altered.

re·min·er·al·i·za·tion (rē-mĭn′ər-ə-lĭ-zā′shən) *n.* The restoration of lost mineral constituents to the body, especially to bone.

re·mis·sion (rĭ-mĭsh′ən) *n.* **1.** Abatement or subsiding of the symptoms of a disease. **2.** The period during which the symptoms of a disease abate or subside.

re·mit (rĭ-mĭt′) *v.* **1.** To diminish; abate. **2.** To transmit money.

re·mit·tent (rĭ-mĭt′nt) *adj.* Characterized by temporary abatement in severity. Used especially of diseases. —**re·mit′tence, re·mit′ten·cy** *n.*

re·mod·el·ing (rē-mŏd′l-ĭng) *n.* A cyclical process by which bone maintains a dynamic steady state through resorption and formation of a small amount of bone at the same site.

re·mov·a·ble partial denture (rĭ-mōō′və-bəl) *n.* A partial denture that supplies teeth and associated structures on a partially toothless jaw and can be easily removed.

REM sleep (rĕm) *n.* A stage in the normal sleep cycle during which dreams occur and the body undergoes various physiological changes, including rapid eye movement, loss of reflexes, and increased pulse rate and brain activity. Also called *paradoxical sleep.*

ren (rĕn) *n., pl.* **re·nes** (rē′nēz) A kidney.

re·nal (rē′nəl) *adj.* Of or in the region of the kidneys.

renal artery *n.* An artery with its origin in the aorta and with distribution to the kidney.

renal carcinosarcoma *n.* See **Wilms′ tumor.**

renal cast *n.* Any of various casts that are formed in the renal tubule and found in the urine and consist of materials such as albumin, cells, and blood.

renal clearance *n.* The volume of plasma that is completely cleared of a specific compound per unit time, measured as a test of kidney function.

renal column *n.* Any of the prolongations of cortical substance separating the renal pyramids.

renal corpuscle *n.* A tuft of glomerular capillaries with the Bowman's capsule that encloses it. Also called *malpighian corpuscle.*

renal cortex *n.* The part of the kidney containing the glomeruli and the proximal and distal convoluted tubules.

renal cortical lobule *n.* A subdivision of the kidney, consisting of the medullary ray and the labyrinth, containing renal corpuscles and convoluted tubules.

renal failure *n.* Acute or chronic malfunction of the kidneys resulting from any of a number of causes, including infection, trauma, toxins, hemodynamic abnormalities, and autoimmune disease, and often resulting in systemic symptoms, especially edema, hypertension, metabolic acidosis, and uremia.

renal fascia *n.* The condensation of the fibroareolar tissue and fat surrounding and ensheathing the kidney. Also called *Gerota's capsule.*

renal ganglion *n.* Any of the small scattered sympathetic ganglions along the renal plexus.

renal glycosuria *n.* Recurring or persistent glycosuria with blood levels in the normal range, resulting from the failure of renal tubules to reabsorb glucose at a normal rate from the glomerular filtrate.

renal hematuria *n.* Hematuria resulting from extravasation of blood into the glomerular spaces, tubules, or pelvises of the kidneys.

renal hypertension *n.* Hypertension that is secondary to renal disease.

renal hypoplasia *n.* An abnormally small kidney that is morphologically normal but has either a reduced number of nephrons or smaller nephrons.

renal osteodystrophy *n.* A bone disease characterized by softening and fibrous degeneration of bone and the formation of cysts in bone tissue, caused by chronic renal failure.

renal papilla *n.* The apex of a renal pyramid, projecting into a calix.

renal pelvis *n.* A hollow flattened funnel-shaped expansion of the upper end of the ureter into which urine is discharged before entering the ureter.

renal pyramid *n.* Any of various pyramidal masses that are seen upon longitudinal section of the kidney and that contain part of the secreting tubules and the collecting tubules. Also called *malpighian pyramid, medullary pyramid.*

renal rickets *n.* A form of rickets occurring in children in association with, and apparently as a result of renal disease with hyperphosphatemia. Also called *pseudorickets.*

renal sinus *n.* The cavity of the kidney, containing the calices and the pelvis.

renal tubular acidosis *n.* A syndrome characterized by the inability to excrete acidic urine and by low plasma bicarbonate and high plasma chloride concentrations, often with hypokalemia.

renal tubule *n.* A tubule of the kidney, such as a collecting or convoluted tubule.

renal vein *n.* Any of the veins that accompany the renal arteries and open at right angles into the vena cava at the level of the second lumbar vertebra.

Ren·du-Os·ler-Web·er disease (rŏn-dōō′ŏs′lər-wĕb′ər, räN-dü′-, ŏz′-) *n.* See **hereditary hemorrhagic telangiectasia.**

Rendu-Osler-Weber syndrome *n.* See **hereditary hemorrhagic telangiectasia.**

ren·i·form (rĕn′ə-fôrm′, rē′nə-) *adj.* Kidney-shaped.

re·nin (rē′nĭn, rĕn′ĭn) *n.* A protein-digesting enzyme that is released by the kidneys and that catalyzes the hydrolysis of angiotensinogen to angiotensin I. Also called *angiotensinogenase.*

ren·i·por·tal (rĕn′ə-pôr′tl, rē′nə-) *adj.* **1.** Relating to the hilum of the kidney. **2.** Relating to the portal or venous capillary circulation in the kidney.

ren·nin (rĕn′ĭn) *n.* A milk-coagulating enzyme found especially in the gastric juice of the fourth stomach of young ruminants, used in making cheeses and junkets. Also called *chymosin.*

ren·nin·o·gen (rĕ-nĭn′ə-jən) *or* **ren·no·gen** (rĕn′ə-jən, -jĕn′) *n.* See **prochymosin.**

reno– *or* **reni–** *pref.* Kidney: *renogram.*

re·no·gen·ic (rē′nə-jĕn′ĭk) *adj.* Originating in or derived from the kidney.

re·no·gram (rē′nə-grăm′) *n.* **1.** A graphic record of the renal excretion of a radioactive tracer that has been injected into the renal system. **2.** A radiograph of a kidney.

re·nog·ra·phy (rē-nŏg′rə-fē) *n.* Radiography of the kidney.

re·no·meg·a·ly (rē′nō-mĕg′ə-lē) *n.* Enlargement of the kidney.

re·nop·a·thy (rē-nŏp′ə-thē) *n.* See **nephropathy.**

re·no·pri·val (rē′nō-prī′vəl) *adj.* Of, characterized by, or resulting from loss of kidney function or surgical removal of all functioning renal tissue.

re·no·troph·ic (rē′nō-trŏf′ĭk, -trō′fĭk) *or* **re·no·trop·ic** (-trŏp′ĭk, -trō′pĭk) *adj.* Influencing the growth or nutrition of the kidney.

Re·no·va (rĭ-nō′və) A trademark for the drug tretinoin.

re·no·vas·cu·lar (rē′nō-văs′kyə-lər) *adj.* Relating to the blood vessels of the kidney.

renovascular hypertension *n.* Hypertension produced by renal arterial obstruction.

Re·o·Pro (rē′ō-prō′) A trademark for the drug abciximab.

Re·o·vir·i·dae (rē′ō-vîr′ĭ-dē′) *n.* A family of double-stranded ether-resistant RNA viruses.

re·o·vi·rus (rē′ō-vī′rəs) *n.* Any member of the genus *Reovirus.*

Reovirus *n.* A genus of viruses that contain double-stranded RNA and are associated with various diseases in animals, including human respiratory and gastrointestinal infections.

rep (rĕp) *n.* Roentgen-equivalent-physical; a unit of absorbed radiation dose, equal to the amount of ionizing radiation that will transfer 93 ergs of energy to 1 gram of water or living tissue.

re·pair (rĭ-pâr′) *v.* To restore to a healthy or functioning condition after damage or injury. —*n.* Restoration of diseased or damaged tissues naturally or by surgical means.

re·par·a·tive dentin (rĭ-păr′ə-tĭv) *n.* See **tertiary dentin.**

re·pel·lent (rĭ-pĕl′ənt) *adj.* Capable of driving off or repelling. —*n.* A substance used to drive off or keep away insects.

re·per·fu·sion (rē′pər-fyoo′zhən) *n.* The restoration of blood flow to an organ or tissue that has had its blood supply cut off, as after a heart attack.

rep·e·ti·tion-com·pul·sion (rĕp′ĭ-tĭsh′ən-kəm-pŭl′shən) *n.* In psychoanalysis, the tendency to repeat earlier experiences or actions in an unconscious effort to achieve belated mastery over them.

re·pet·i·tive strain injury (rĭ-pĕt′ĭ-tĭv) *n. Abbr.* **RSI** Damage to tendons, nerves, and other soft tissues caused by the repeated performance of a limited number of physical movements and characterized by numbness, pain, and a wasting and weakening of muscle.

re·place·ment therapy (rĭ-plās′mənt) *n.* Therapy designed to compensate for a lack or deficiency arising from inadequate nutrition, from certain dysfunctions, or from losses, as by the administration of natural or synthetic substances.

re·plant (rē-plănt′) *v.* To reattach an organ, limb, or other body part surgically to the original site. —*n.* (rē′plănt′) An organ, limb, or body part that has been replanted.

re·plan·ta·tion (rē′plăn-tā′shən) *n.* Replanting of an organ or part and the reestablishment of circulation. Also called *reimplantation.*

re·ple·tion (rĭ-plē′shən) *n.* **1.** The condition of being fully supplied or completely filled. **2.** A state of excessive fullness.

rep·li·case (rĕp′lĭ-kās′, -kāz′) *n.* An enzyme that promotes the synthesis of a complementary RNA molecule from an RNA template.

rep·li·cate (rĕp′lĭ-kāt′) *v.* **1.** To duplicate, copy, reproduce, or repeat. **2.** To reproduce or make an exact copy or copies of genetic material, a cell, or an organism. —*n.* A repetition of an experiment or a procedure.

rep·li·ca·tion (rĕp′lĭ-kā′shən) *n.* **1.** The act or process of duplicating or reproducing something. **2.** Autoreproduction.

rep·li·ca·tor (rĕp′lĭ-kā′tər) *n.* The site on a bacterial genome where replication begins.

rep·li·con (rĕp′lĭ-kŏn′) *n.* A genetic element that undergoes replication as an autonomous unit.

rep·li·some (rĕp′lĭ-sōm′) *n.* Any of the sites on the matrix of a cell nucleus that contains a series of enzyme complexes in which DNA replication is considered to occur.

re·po·lar·i·za·tion (rē-pō′lər-ĭ-zā′shən) *n.* The restoration of a polarized state across a membrane.

re·port·a·ble disease (rĭ-pôr′tə-bəl) *n.* See **notifiable disease.**

re·pos·i·tor (rĭ-pŏz′ĭ-tər) *n.* An instrument used to reposition a displaced organ.

re·press (rĭ-prĕs′) *v.* **1.** To hold back by an act of volition. **2.** To exclude something from the conscious mind.

re·pressed (rĭ-prĕst′) *adj.* Being subjected to or characterized by repression.

re·press·i·ble enzyme (rĭ-prĕs′ə-bəl) *n.* An enzyme whose production is generally continuous but can be halted if a particular substance is present in concentrations greater than normal.

re·pres·sion (rĭ-prĕsh′ən) *n.* **1.** The act of repressing or the state of being repressed. **2.** The unconscious exclusion of painful impulses, desires, or fears from the conscious mind.

re·pres·sive (rĭ-prĕs′ĭv) *adj.* Causing or inclined to cause repression.

re·pres·sor (rĭ-prĕs′ər) *n.* **1.** One that represses. **2.** A protein, especially either of two proteins produced by regulatory genes, that blocks transcription of an operon.

repressor gene *n.* A gene that prevents transcription of a nonallele.

re·pro·duce (rē′prə-doos′, -dyoos′) *v.* **1.** To produce a counterpart, an image, or a copy of something. **2.** To bring something to mind again. **3.** To generate offspring by sexual or asexual means.

re·pro·duc·tion (rē′prə-dŭk′shən) *n.* **1.** The act of reproducing or the condition or process of being reproduced. **2.** Recall of a memory. **3.** The sexual or asexual process by which organisms generate others of the same kind.

re·pro·duc·tive (rē′prə-dŭk′tĭv) *adj.* **1.** Of or relating to reproduction. **2.** Tending to reproduce.

reproductive cloning *n.* The genetic duplication of an existing organism especially by transferring the nucleus of a somatic cell of the organism into an enucleated oocyte.

reproductive cycle *n.* The cycle of physiological changes that begins with conception and extends through gestation and parturition.

reproductive system *n.* The complex of male or female gonads, associated ducts, and external genitalia concerned with sexual reproduction.

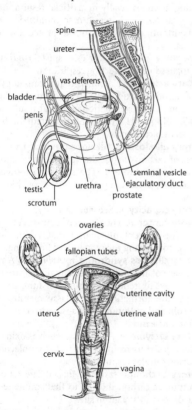

reproductive system
Top: *cross section of male reproductive system*
Bottom: *anterior view of female reproductive system*

re·pul·sion (rĭ-pŭl′shən) *n.* **1.** The act of repelling or driving apart. **2.** A feeling of extreme dislike. **3.** The tendency of particles or bodies of the same electric charge or magnetic polarity to separate.

RES *abbr.* reticuloendothelial system

Re·scrip·tor (rĭ-skrĭp′tər) A trademark for the drug delavirdine.

re·sect (rĭ-sĕkt′) *v.* To perform a resection on a part of the body.

re·sect·a·ble (rĭ-sĕk′tə-bəl) *adj.* Suitable for resection.

re·sec·tion (rĭ-sĕk′shən) *n.* **1.** Surgical removal of part of an organ or a structure. **2.** Removal of the articular ends of one or both bones forming a joint.

re·sec·to·scope (rĭ-sĕk′tə-skōp′) *n.* A surgical instrument for performing a resection without an opening or incision other than that made by the instrument.

re·serve (rĭ-zûrv′) *v.* **1.** To keep back, as for future use or for a special purpose. **2.** To set or cause to be set apart for a particular person or use. —*n.* Something kept back or saved for future use or a special purpose. —*adj.* **1.** Held back, set aside, or saved. **2.** Forming a reserve.

reserve air *n.* See **expiratory reserve volume.**

reserve force *n.* The energy residing in an organ or in any of its parts above that required for its normal functioning.

res·er·voir (rĕz′ər-vwär′, -vwôr′, -vôr′) *n.* **1.** A fluid-containing sac or cavity. **2.** An organism or a population that directly or indirectly transmits a pathogen while being virtually immune to its effects. **3.** A large or extra supply; a reserve.

reservoir bag *n.* See **breathing bag.**

reservoir host *n.* A host that serves as a source of infection and potential reinfection of humans and as a means of sustaining a parasite when it is not infecting humans.

reservoir of spermatozoa *n.* The distal portion of the tail of the epididymis and the beginning of the vas deferens, where spermatozoa are stored.

res·i·dence (rĕz′ĭ-dəns) *n.* A medical residency.

res·i·den·cy (rĕz′ĭ-dən-sē) *n.* The period during which a physician gets specialized clinical training.

res·i·dent (rĕz′ĭ-dənt) *n.* A physician during residency.

re·sid·u·al (rĭ-zĭj′ōō-əl) *adj.* **1.** Of, relating to, or characteristic of a residue. **2.** Remaining as a residue.

residual abscess *n.* An abscess recurring at the site of a former abscess as a result of the persistence of microbes and pus.

residual air *n.* See **residual volume.**

residual capacity *n.* See **residual volume.**

residual schizophrenia *n.* A condition occurring in individuals with a history of schizophrenic episodes, characterized by blunted or inappropriate emotion, social withdrawal, eccentric behavior, and the making of loose associations, and lacking in prominent psychotic symptoms.

residual urine *n.* Urine remaining in the bladder at the end of micturition, as in cases of prostatic obstruction or bladder atony.

residual volume *n. Abbr.* **RV** The volume of air remaining in the lungs after a maximal expiratory effort. Also called *residual air, residual capacity.*

res·i·due (rĕz′ĭ-dōō′) *n.* The remainder of something after removal of parts or a part.

re·sid·u·um (rĭ-zĭj′ōō-əm) *n., pl.* **–u·a** (-ōō-ə) Something remaining after removal of a part; a residue.

res·in (rĕz′ĭn) *n.* **1.** Any of numerous clear to translucent yellow or brown, solid or semisolid, viscous substances of plant origin, such as copal, rosin, and amber. **2.** Any of numerous physically similar polymerized synthetics or chemically modified natural resins including thermoplastic materials and thermosetting materials. **3.** Rosin. **4.** A precipitate formed by the addition of water to certain tinctures.

res·in·ous (rĕz′ə-nəs) *adj.* Of, relating to, or derived from a resin.

re·sis·tance (rĭ-zĭs′təns) *n.* **1.** The capacity of an organism to defend itself against a disease. **2.** The capacity of an organism, a tissue, or a cell to withstand the effects of a harmful physical or environmental agent. **3.** The opposition of a body or substance to current passing through it, resulting in a change of electrical energy into heat or another form of energy. **4.** In psychoanalysis, a process in which the ego opposes the conscious recall of repressed unpleasant experiences.

resistance plasmid *n.* Any of the conjugative or nonconjugative plasmids carrying genes responsible for antibiotic or antibacterial drug resistance among bacteria. Also called *resistance factor, R factor, R plasmid.*

resistance thermometer *n.* A device measuring temperature by the change of the electrical resistance of a metal wire.

resistance transfer factor *n.* The transfer gene of a conjugative resistance plasmid.

res·o·lu·tion (rĕz′ə-lōō′shən) *n.* **1.** The subsiding or termination of an abnormal condition, such as a fever or an inflammation. **2.** The act or process of separating or reducing something into its constituent parts. **3.** The fineness of detail that can be distinguished in an image, as on a video display terminal.

re·solve (rĭ-zŏlv′) *v.* **1.** To cause resolution of an abnormal condition. **2.** To separate an optically inactive compound or mixture into its optically active constituents. **3.** To render parts of an image visible and distinct.

re·sol·vent (rĭ-zŏl′vənt) *adj.* Causing or able to cause separation into constituents; solvent. —*n.* A resolvent substance, especially a medicine that reduces inflammation or swelling.

re·solv·ing power (rĭ-zŏl′vĭng) *n.* The ability of a lens to distinguish small objects in close proximity.

res·o·nance (rĕz′ə-nəns) *n.* **1.** The sound produced by diagnostic percussion of the normal chest. **2.** Intensification of vocal tones during articulation, as by the air cavities of the mouth and nasal passages. **3.** Intensification and prolongation of sound produced by sympathetic vibration. **4.** The property of a compound having simultaneously the characteristics of two or more structural forms that differ only in the distribution of electrons.

re·sorb (rē-zôrb′) *v.* **1.** To absorb again. **2.** To dissolve and assimilate such things as bone tissue.

res·or·cin·ol (rĭ-zôr′sə-nôl′, -nōl′) *or* **res·or·cin** (-sĭn) *n.* A white crystalline compound used primarily as an antiseptic in skin diseases such as psoriasis or eczema, but also used in the treatment of nausea, asthma, whooping cough, and diarrhea.

re·sorp·tion (rē-sôrp′shən, -zôrp′-) *n.* The act or process of resorbing.

resorption lacuna *n.* See **Howship's lacuna.**

res·pi·ra·ble (rĕs′pər-ə-bəl, rĭ-spīr′-) *adj.* **1.** Fit for breathing, as air. **2.** Capable of undergoing respiration, as certain organisms.

res·pi·ra·tion (rĕs′pə-rā′shən) *n. Abbr.* **R 1.** The act or process of inhaling and exhaling; breathing. Also called *ventilation.* **2.** The act or process by which an organism without lungs, such as a fish or plant, exchanges gases with its environment. **3.** The oxidative process occurring within living cells by which the chemical energy of organic molecules is released in a series of metabolic steps involving the consumption of oxygen and the liberation of carbon dioxide and water. **4.** Any of various analogous metabolic processes by which organisms, such as fungi, obtain energy from organic molecules.

respiration rate *n.* Frequency of breathing, expressed as the number of breaths per minute.

res·pi·ra·tor (rĕs′pə-rā′tər) *n.* **1.** A device that supplies oxygen or a mixture of oxygen and carbon dioxide for breathing, used especially in artificial respiration. Also called *inhalator, ventilator.* **2.** A screenlike device worn over the mouth or nose or both to protect the respiratory tract.

res·pi·ra·to·ry (rĕs′pər-ə-tôr′ē, rĭ-spīr′ə-) *adj.* Of, relating to, used in, or affecting respiration.

respiratory acidosis *n.* Acidosis that is caused by retention of carbon dioxide, due to inadequate pulmonary ventilation or hypoventilation, and that results in a decrease in blood pH unless compensated for by renal retention of bicarbonate.

respiratory alkalosis *n.* Alkalosis resulting from abnormal loss of carbon dioxide due to hyperventilation.

respiratory bronchiole *n.* The smallest subdivision of a bronchiole, connecting a terminal bronchiole to an alveolar duct.

respiratory capacity *n.* See **vital capacity.**

respiratory center *n.* The region of neurons in the brain that receives afferent information that is then translated to signals controlling the sequence of breathing.

respiratory distress syndrome *n. Abbr.* **RDS** A respiratory disease of newborns, especially premature infants, characterized by reduced amounts of lung surfactant, cyanosis, the formation of a glassy membrane over the alveoli, and pulmonary collapse. Also called *hyaline membrane disease.*

respiratory enzyme *n.* An enzyme, such as oxidase, that transfers electrons from its substrate to molecular oxygen during cellular respiration.

respiratory exchange ratio *n. Abbr.* **R** The ratio of the net output of carbon dioxide to the simultaneous net uptake of oxygen at a given site.

respiratory failure *n.* An acute or chronic condition in which pulmonary function is markedly impaired, usually characterized by elevated carbon dioxide or decreased oxygen (or both) in the arterial blood. Patients in respiratory failure often require ventilators to breathe.

respiratory lobule *n.* See **primary pulmonary lobule.**

respiratory minute volume *n.* The product of tidal volume and the respiratory frequency.

respiratory pause *n.* Cessation of air flow during respiration for less than ten seconds.

respiratory pigment *n.* Any of the oxygen-carrying substances in the blood and tissues, such as hemoglobin and myoglobin.

respiratory quotient *n. Abbr.* **RQ** The ratio of carbon dioxide produced by tissue metabolism to oxygen consumed in the same metabolism.

respiratory scleroma *n.* Rhinoscleroma in which the lesion involves the mucous membrane of much or all of the upper respiratory tract.

respiratory syncytial virus *n. Abbr.* **RSV** An RNA-containing virus that causes minor respiratory infections in adults and bronchitis and bronchopneumonia in children.

respiratory system *n.* The integrated system of organs involved in the intake and exchange of oxygen and carbon dioxide between the body and the environment and including the nasal passages, larynx, trachea, bronchial tubes, and lungs.

respiratory therapy *n. Abbr.* **RT** The treatment or management of acute and chronic breathing disorders, as through the use of respirators or the administration of medication in aerosol form.

respiratory tract *n.* The air passages from the nose to the pulmonary alveoli, including the pharynx, larynx, trachea, and bronchi.

re·spire (rĭ-spīr′) *v.* **1.** To breathe in and out; inhale and exhale. **2.** To undergo the metabolic process of respiration. **3.** To breathe easily again, as after a period of exertion.

res·pi·rom·e·ter (rĕs′pə-rŏm′ĭ-tər) *n.* An instrument for measuring the degree and nature of respiration.

re·sponse (rĭ-spŏns′) *n.* A reaction, as that of an organism or any of its parts, to a specific stimulus.

rest (rĕst) *n.* **1.** Cessation of work, exertion, or activity. **2.** Peace, ease, or refreshment resulting from sleep or the cessation of an activity. **3.** Sleep or quiet relaxation. **4.** Mental or emotional tranquillity. **5.** A device used as a support, as for the back. **6.** A group of embryonic cells or a portion of fetal tissue that has become displaced during development. **7.** An extension from a prosthesis that gives vertical support to a dental restoration. —*v.* **1.** To cease motion, work, or activity. **2.** To lie down, especially to sleep. **3.** To be supported or based; lie, lean, or sit.

re·ste·no·sis (rē′stə-nō′sĭs) *n.* Recurrence of stenosis after corrective surgery on a heart valve.

rest home *n.* An establishment where elderly or disabled persons are housed and cared for.

res·ti·form (rĕs′tə-fôrm′) *adj.* Having the shape of a rope; ropelike.

restiform body *n.* See **inferior cerebellar peduncle.**

rest·ing cell (rĕs′tĭng) *n.* A cell that is not actively in the process of dividing.

resting tidal volume *n.* The tidal volume under normal resting conditions.

res·ti·tu·tion (rĕs′tĭ-tōo′shən) *n.* A return to or restoration of a previous state or position, especially the return of the rotated head of a fetus to its natural alignment with the body after delivery.

rest·less legs syndrome (rĕst′lĭs) *n.* Discomfort or twitching in the legs that occurs after going to bed and often leads to insomnia.

rest mass *n.* The physical mass of a body when it is regarded as being at rest.

res·to·ra·tion (rĕs′tə-rā′shən) *n.* **1.** Any of various dental fittings, such as an inlay, crown, bridge, or denture,

that restore or replace lost tooth structure, teeth, or oral tissues. **2.** A substance used to restore the missing portion of a tooth.

re·stor·a·tive (rĭ-stôr′ə-tĭv) *adj.* **1.** Of or relating to restoration. **2.** Tending or having the power to restore. —*n.* A medicine or other agent that helps to restore health, strength, or consciousness.

restorative dentistry *n.* The branch of dentistry that deals with the restoration of diseased, injured, or abnormal teeth to normal function, as by crowns.

Res·to·ril (rĕs′tə-rĭl′) A trademark for the drug temazepam.

re·straint (rĭ-strānt′) *n.* **1.** An instrument or a means of restraint to prevent the infliction of harm to self or others, such as a straightjacket. **2.** Control or repression of feelings; constraint.

re·stric·tion enzyme (rĭ-strĭk′shən) *n.* Any of a group of enzymes that cleave DNA at specific sites to produce discrete fragments, used especially in gene-splicing. Also called *restriction endonuclease.*

restriction fragment length polymorphism *n. Abbr.* **RFLP** Intraspecies variations in the length of DNA fragments generated by the action of restriction enzymes and caused by mutations that alter the sites at which these enzymes act, changing the length, number, or production of fragments.

restriction site *n.* A site in a DNA segment in which the bordering bases are vulnerable to restriction enzymes. Also called *cleavage site.*

restriction-site polymorphism *n.* DNA polymorphism in which one of the two nucleotide sequences contains a recognition site for a particular endonuclease but the second lacks such a site.

re·sus·ci·tate (rĭ-sŭs′ĭ-tāt′) *v.* To restore consciousness, vigor, or life to.

re·sus·ci·ta·tion (rĭ-sŭs′ĭ-tā′shən) *n.* The act of resuscitating or the state of being resuscitated.

re·sus·ci·ta·tor (rĭ-sŭs′ĭ-tā′tər) *n.* One that resuscitates, as an apparatus that forces oxygen or a mixture of oxygen and carbon dioxide into the lungs of a person who has undergone partial asphyxiation.

res·ver·a·trol (rĕz-vîr′ĭ-trôl′, -trŏl′, -trōl′) *n.* A natural compound found in grapes, mulberries, peanuts, and other plants or food products, especially red wine, that may protect against cancer and cardiovascular disease by acting as an antioxidant, antimutagen, and anti-inflammatory.

re·tained menstruation (rĭ-tānd′) *n.* See **hematocolpos.**

retained testis *n.* See **undescended testis.**

re·tain·er (rĭ-tā′nər) *n.* **1.** One that retains, as a device, frame, or groove that restrains or guides, especially for a prosthesis. **2.** An appliance used to hold teeth in position after orthodontic treatment.

re·tar·date (rĭ-tär′dāt′, -dĭt) *n.* A mentally retarded person.

re·tar·da·tion (rē′tär-dā′shən) *n.* **1.** The condition of being relatively slow in mental, emotional, or physical development. **2.** The extent to which something is held back or delayed. **3.** Mental retardation.

re·tard·ed dentition (rĭ-tär′dĭd) *n.* Dentition in which processes such as calcification, growth, and eruption occur later than normal as a result of some systemic metabolic dysfunction.

retch (rĕch) *v.* To try to vomit.

re·te (rē′tē) *n., pl.* **re·ti·a** (rē′tē-ə, rē′shə) An anatomical mesh, network, or structure, as of veins, arteries, or nerves. —**re′ti·al** (-tē-əl, -shəl) *adj.*

rete ar·te·ri·o·sum (är-tîr′ē-ō′səm) *n.* A vascular network of anastomoses between minute arteries.

rete ar·tic·u·lar·e (är-tĭk′yə-lâr′ē) *n.* A vascular network near a joint.

rete cu·ta·ne·um co·ri·i (kyōō-tā′nē-əm côr′ē-ī′) *n.* A vascular network parallel to the skin surface and lying between the dermis and the superficial fascia.

rete mi·ra·bi·le (mĭ-rä′bĭ-lē) *n.* A vascular network interrupting the continuity of an artery or vein, as in the glomeruli of the kidney or in the liver.

re·ten·tion (rĭ-tĕn′shən) *n.* **1.** Involuntary withholding by the body of wastes or secretions that are normally eliminated. **2.** The holding by the body of what normally belongs in it, such as food in the stomach. **3.** An ability to recall or recognize what has been learned or experienced; memory. **4.** In dentistry, a period following orthodontic treatment when a patient wears an appliance or appliances to stabilize the teeth in their new position.

retention cyst *n.* A cyst caused by an obstruction to the excretory duct of a gland.

retention jaundice *n.* Jaundice caused by an inability of the liver to secrete enough bile pigment or by an overproduction of bile pigment.

retention suture *n.* A heavy reinforcing suture placed deeply within the muscles and fasciae of the abdominal wall to relieve tension on the primary suture line and avoid postsurgical wound disruption. Also called *tension suture.*

retention vomiting *n.* Vomiting due to mechanical obstruction, usually hours after ingestion of a meal.

rete o·var·i·i (ō-vâr′ē-ī′) *n.* A transient network of cells in the developing ovary.

rete ridge *n.* Epidermal thickenings that extend downward between dermal papillae.

rete sub·pap·il·lar·e (sŭb′păp-ə-lâr′ē) *n.* A vascular network between the papillary and reticular strata of the dermis.

rete tes·tis (tĕs′tĭs) *n.* The network of canals at the termination of the semiferous tubules.

rete ve·no·sum (vē-nō′səm) *n.* A venous network.

reticul– *pref.* Variant of **reticulo–**.

re·tic·u·lar (rĭ-tĭk′yə-lər) *or* **re·tic·u·lat·ed** (-lā′tĭd) *adj.* Resembling a net in form; netlike. —**re·tic′u·la′tion** *n.*

reticular activating system *n. Abbr.* **RAS** The part of the reticular formation in the brainstem that plays a central role in bodily and behavioral alertness; its ascending connections affect the function of the cerebral cortex and its descending connections affect bodily posture and reflex mechanisms.

reticular cell *n.* Any of the cells forming the stroma of bone marrow and lymphatic tissues whose processes make contact with those of similar cells to form a network.

reticular degeneration *n.* Severe epidermal edema re-

sulting in the occurrence of bullae that contain numerous small spaces.

reticular dystrophy of cornea *n.* A bilateral progressive superficial degeneration of the corneal epithelium and the adjacent Bowman's membrane.

reticular fiber *n.* Any of the small, branching, argyrophilic, intercellular fiber elements that may be continuous with collagen fibers.

reticular formation *n.* A massive but vaguely delimited neural apparatus composed of closely intermingled gray and white matter, extending the length of the spinal cord and into the diencephalon, and having a dominant role in the central control of autonomic and endocrine functions, bodily posture, skeletomuscular reflex activity, and general behavioral states. Also called *reticular substance.*

reticular membrane *n.* The membrane formed by cuticular plates of the cells of the spiral organ.

reticular substance *n.* **1.** A filamentous plasmatic material beaded with granules that is visible upon vital staining in the immature red blood cells. **2.** See **reticular formation.**

reticular tissue *n.* Connective tissue in which reticular fibers form a branching network usually having a network of reticular cells associated with the fibers. Also called *retiform tissue.*

re·tic·u·lat·ed bone (rĭ-tĭk′yə-lā′tĭd) *n.* See **woven bone.**

re·tic·u·lin (rĭ-tĭk′yə-lĭn) *n.* A scleroprotein present in the connective tissue framework of the lymphatic tissues.

reticulo– *or* **reticul–** *pref.* Net; network; netlike: *reticulocyte.*

re·tic·u·lo·cyte (rĭ-tĭk′yə-lō-sīt′) *n.* An immature red blood cell containing a network of basophilic filaments and occurring during blood regeneration.

re·tic·u·lo·cy·to·pe·ni·a (rĭ-tĭk′yə-lō-sī′tə-pē′nē-ə) *n.* An abnormal decrease in the number of reticulocytes in the blood. Also called *reticulopenia.*

re·tic·u·lo·cy·to·sis (rĭ-tĭk′yə-lō-sī-tō′sĭs) *n.* An increase in the number of reticulocytes in the blood.

re·tic·u·lo·en·do·the·li·al (rĭ-tĭk′yə-lō-ĕn′dō-thē′lē-əl) *adj.* Of, relating to, or being the widely diffused bodily system constituting all phagocytic cells except certain white blood cells.

reticuloendothelial system *n. Abbr.* **RES** The diffuse system constituting all phagocytic cells of the body except granulocytes including the cells lining the sinusoids of the spleen, lymph nodes, and bone marrow along with the fibroblastic reticular cells of hematopoietic tissues.

re·tic·u·lo·en·do·the·li·o·ma (rĭ-tĭk′yə-lō-ĕn′dō-thē′-lē-ō′mə) *n.* A neoplasm derived from reticuloendothelial tissue.

re·tic·u·lo·en·do·the·li·o·sis (rĭ-tĭk′yə-lō-ĕn′dō-thē′-lē-ō′sĭs) *n.* Proliferation of the reticuloendothelium in any organ or tissue.

re·tic·u·lo·en·do·the·li·um (rĭ-tĭk′yə-lō-ĕn′dō-thē′-lē-əm) *n.* The cells and tissues making up the reticuloendothelial system.

re·tic·u·lo·his·ti·o·cy·to·ma (rĭ-tĭk′yə-lō-hĭs′tē-ō-sī-tō′mə) *n.* A solitary skin nodule that is composed of glycolipid-containing, multinucleated, large histiocytes.

re·tic·u·lo·pe·ni·a (rǐ-tǐk′yə-lō-pē′nē-ə) *n.* See **reticulocytopenia.**

re·tic·u·lo·sis (rǐ-tǐk′yə-lō′sǐs) *n.* An increase in histiocytes or other reticuloendothelial elements.

re·tic·u·lo·spi·nal tract (rǐ-tǐk′yə-lō-spī′nəl) *n.* Any of several fiber tracts descending to the spinal cord from the reticular formation of the pons and medulla oblongata. Some fibers conduct impulses from the neural mechanisms regulating cardiovascular and respiratory functions to the spinal cord; others form links in extrapyramidal motor mechanisms affecting muscle tonus and somatic movement.

re·tic·u·lum (rǐ-tǐk′yə-ləm) *n., pl.* **-la** (-lə) **1.** A fine network formed by cells, by certain structures within cells, or by connective-tissue fibers between cells. **2.** See **neuroglia. 3.** The second compartment of the stomach of ruminant mammals, lined with a membrane having honeycombed ridges.

reticulum cell sarcoma *n.* A malignant tumor of reticular tissue that is composed primarily of neoplastic histocytes.

re·ti·form (rē′tə-fôrm′, rĕt′ə-) *adj.* Arranged like a net; reticulate.

retiform tissue *n.* See **reticular tissue.**

retin– *pref.* Variant of **retino–.**

ret·i·na (rĕt′n-ə) *n., pl.* **ret·i·nas** or **ret·i·nae** (rĕt′n-ē′) The delicate multilayered light-sensitive membrane lining the inner posterior chamber of the eyeball containing the rods and cones and connected by the optic nerve to the brain. —**ret′i·nal** *adj.*

Ret·in-A (rĕt′n-ā′) A trademark for a preparation of retinoic acid.

ret·i·nac·u·lum (rĕt′n-ăk′yə-ləm) *n., pl.* **-la** (-lə) A band or bandlike structure that holds an organ or a part in place. —**ret′i·nac′u·lar** (-lər) *adj.*

retinaculum of fibular muscles *n.* See **retinaculum of peroneal muscles.**

retinaculum of flexor muscles *n.* A wide band that passes from the medial malleolus to the calcaneus and to the plantar surface as far as the navicular bone and holds in place the tendons of the posterior tibial muscle, the long flexor muscle of the toes, and the long flexor muscle of the big toe.

retinaculum of peroneal muscles *n.* Any of the superior and inferior fibrous bands retaining the tendons of the long and short peroneal muscles in position as they cross the lateral side of the ankle. Also called *retinaculum of fibular muscles.*

retinaculum of skin *n.* Any of the numerous small fibrous strands that attach the dermis to the underlying superficial fascia and are particularly well developed over the breast.

retinaculum ten·di·num (tĕn′də-nəm) *n.* The annular ligament of the ankle or wrist.

ret·i·nal (rĕt′n-ăl′, -ôl′) *n.* See **retinaldehyde.**

retinal adaptation *n.* Adjustment of the eye to the degree of illumination.

retinal cone *n.* See **cone cell.**

ret·i·nal·de·hyde (rĕt′n-ăl′də-hīd′) *n.* A yellow to orange aldehyde that is a derivative of vitamin A and acts

in the retina to form the visual pigments of the rods and cones. Also called *retinal, retinene₁.*

retinaldehyde isomerase *n.* See **retinal isomerase.**

retinal detachment *n.* See **detachment of retina.**

retinal isomerase *n.* An enzyme that catalyzes the conversion of the *trans* form of retinaldehyde to 11-*cis* retinal, a reaction that is important to the regeneration of the visual pigments. Also called *retinaldehyde isomerase.*

ret·i·nene (rĕt′n-ēn′) *n.* Either of two yellow to red retinal pigments, formed by oxidation of vitamin A alcohols.

retinene₁ *n.* See **retinaldehyde.**

retinene₂ *n.* See **dehydroretinaldehyde.**

ret·i·ni·tis (rĕt′n-ī′tǐs) *n.* Inflammation of the retina.

retinitis pig·men·to·sa (pǐg′mən-tō′sə) *n.* A hereditary degenerative disease of the retina, producing conditions such as night blindness, pigmentation changes in the retina, narrowing of the visual field, and the eventual loss of vision. Also called *pigmentary retinopathy, tapetoretinal retinopathy.*

retinitis pro·lif·er·ans (prə-lǐf′ə-rănz′) *n.* See **proliferative retinopathy.**

retinitis sclo·pe·tar·i·a (sklō′pǐ-târ′ē-ə) *n.* A retinal lesion resulting from severe contusion.

retino– or **retin–** *pref.* Retina: *retinoscopy.*

ret·i·no·blas·to·ma (rĕt′n-ō-blă-stō′mə) *n., pl.* **-mas** or **-ma·ta** (-mə-tə) A hereditary malignant tumor of the retina, transmitted as a dominant trait and occurring chiefly among infants.

ret·i·no·cer·e·bral angiomatosis (rĕt′n-ō-sĕr′ə-brəl, -sə-rē′-) *n.* See **Lindau's disease.**

ret·i·no·cho·roid (rĕt′n-ō-kôr′oid′) *adj.* Relating to the choroid coat of the eye and to the retina.

ret·i·no·cho·roid·i·tis (rĕt′n-ō-kôr′oi-dī′tǐs) *n.* See **chorioretinitis.**

retinochoroiditis jux·ta·pap·il·lar·is (jŭk′stə-păp′ə-lâr′ĭs) *n.* Inflammation of the retina and choroid close to the optic nerve. Also called *Jensen's disease.*

ret·i·no·di·al·y·sis (rĕt′n-ō-dī-ăl′ĭ-sĭs) *n.* Detachment of the retina.

ret·i·no·ic acid (rĕt′n-ō′ĭk) *n.* An acid formed in the oxidation of retinaldehyde and used as a topical treatment for acne. Also called *vitamin A acid.*

ret·i·noid (rĕt′n-oid′) *n.* Any of a class of keratolytic drugs derived from retinoic acid and used in the treatment of severe acne and psoriasis.

ret·i·nol (rĕt′n-ôl′, -ōl′) *n.* See **vitamin A.**

retinol dehydrogenase *n.* An enzyme that catalyzes interconversion of retinaldehyde and retinol.

ret·i·no·pap·il·li·tis (rĕt′n-ō-păp′ə-lī′tǐs) *n.* See **papilloretinitis.**

ret·i·nop·a·thy (rĕt′n-ŏp′ə-thē) *n.* A noninflammatory degenerative disease of the retina.

retinopathy of prematurity *n.* Abnormal replacement of the sensory retina by fibrous tissue and blood vessels, occurring mainly in premature infants who are placed in a high-oxygen environment. Also called *retrolental fibroplasia, Terry's syndrome.*

ret·i·no·pex·y (rĕt′n-ō-pĕk′sē) *n.* Surgical correction of a detachment of the retina by forming chorioretinal adhesions around the torn part of the retina.

ret·i·nos·chi·sis (rĕt′n-ŏs′kĭ-sĭs) *n.* Degeneration of the retina causing splitting and the formation of cysts between retinal layers.

ret·i·no·scope (rĕt′n-ə-skōp′) *n.* An optical instrument for examining refraction of light in the eye.

ret·i·nos·co·py (rĕt′n-ŏs′kə-pē) *n.* A method of detecting errors of refraction of the eye by illuminating the retina and noting the direction of movement of the light on the retinal surface. Also called *pupilloscopy, shadow test, skiascopy.* —**ret′i·no·scop′ic** (-ə-skŏp′ĭk) *adj.*

re·tort (rĭ-tôrt′, rē′tôrt′) *n.* A closed laboratory vessel with an outlet tube, used for distillation, sublimation, or decomposition by heat.

re·trac·tile (rĭ-trăk′tĭl, -tīl′) *adj.* That can be drawn back or in, as the claws of a cat.

re·trac·tion (rĭ-trăk′shən) *n.* **1.** The act of drawing back or in; shrinking. **2.** The act of pulling apart, usually as part of a surgical procedure. **3.** The posterior movement of teeth, usually with the aid of an orthodontic appliance.

retraction nystagmus *n.* An irregular jerky nystagmus, either horizontal, vertical, or rotatory, with drawing of the eye backward into the orbit when an attempt is made to look one way or the other.

re·trac·tor (rĭ-trăk′tər) *n.* **1.** A surgical instrument used to hold back organs or the edges of an incision. **2.** A muscle, such as a flexor, that retracts an organ or a part.

re·treat from reality (rĭ-trēt′) *n.* The substitution of the imaginary for the real.

re·trench·ment (rĭ-trĕnch′mənt) *n.* The cutting away of superfluous tissue.

re·triev·al (rĭ-trē′vəl) *n.* The third stage in the memory process, after encoding and storage, involving mental processes associated with bringing stored information back into consciousness.

retro– *pref.* **1.** Backward; back: *retroposition.* **2.** Situated behind: *retroperitoneum.*

ret·ro·bul·bar anesthesia (rĕt′rō-bŭl′bər, -bär′) *n.* Injection of a local anesthetic behind the eye to produce sensory denervation of the eye.

retrobulbar neuritis *n.* See **optic neuritis.**

ret·ro·cal·ca·ne·o·bur·si·tis (rĕt′rō-kăl-kā′nē-ō-bər-sī′tĭs) *n.* See **achillobursitis.**

ret·ro·ce·dent gout (rĕt′rō-sēd′nt) *n.* The occurrence of severe gastric, cardiac, or cerebral symptoms during an attack of gout, especially when the joint symptoms suddenly subside at the same time.

ret·ro·ces·sion (rĕt′rō-sĕsh′ən) *n.* **1.** A relapse, as of a disease. **2.** Cessation of the external symptoms of a disease, followed by signs of involvement of an internal organ or part. **3.** Backward displacement of the uterus or other organ.

ret·ro·clu·sion (rĕt′rō-klōō′zhən) *n.* A form of acupressure used to halt bleeding.

ret·ro·col·lic spasm (rĕt′rō-kŏl′ĭk) *n.* Torticollis in which the spasm affects the posterior neck muscles. Also called *retrocollis.*

ret·ro·con·duc·tion (rĕt′rō-kən-dŭk′shən) *n.* Conduction backward from the ventricles or from the atrioventricular node into and through the atria.

ret·ro·cur·sive (rĕt′rō-kûr′sĭv) *adj.* Characterized by running backward.

ret·ro·cus·pid papilla (rĕt′rō-kŭs′pĭd) *n.* A small tag of tissue on the mandibular gums, lingual to the cuspid teeth, usually bilateral and is considered a normal anatomic structure.

ret·ro·de·vi·a·tion (rĕt′rō-dē′vē-ā′shən) *n.* A backward bending or inclining.

ret·ro·dis·place·ment (rĕt′rō-dĭs-plās′mənt) *n.* A backward displacement, such as retroflexion.

ret·ro·flex·ion (rĕt′rō-flĕk′shən) *n.* A backward bending, especially of the body of the uterus toward the cervix.

ret·ro·gnath·ism (rĕt′rō-năth′ĭz′əm) *n.* A condition of facial disharmony in which one or both jaws are posterior to their normal positions. —**ret′ro·gnath′ic** *adj.*

ret·ro·grade (rĕt′rə-grād′) *adj.* **1.** Moving or tending backward. **2.** Opposite to the usual order; inverted or reversed. **3.** Reverting to an earlier or inferior condition. —*v.* **1.** To move or seem to move backward; recede. **2.** To decline to an inferior state; degenerate.

retrograde amnesia *n.* A condition in which events that occurred before the onset of amnesia cannot be recalled.

retrograde beat *n.* A beat occurring as a contraction of a portion of a heart chamber cephalad to the chamber of origin.

retrograde block *n.* Impaired conduction of an impulse backward from the ventricles or atrioventricular node into the atria.

retrograde ejaculation *n.* Ejaculation in which the discharged seminal fluid travels up toward the bladder instead of outside the body through the urethra.

retrograde embolism *n.* The obstruction of a vein by a mass carried in a direction opposite to that of the normal blood current.

retrograde hernia *n.* A hernia of two loops of intestine, with the portion of intestine between the loops lying in the abdominal cavity.

retrograde menstruation *n.* A flow of menstrual blood into the fallopian tubes.

retrograde urography *n.* X-ray examination of the urinary tract following the injection of a contrast agent directly into the bladder, ureter, or renal pelvis. Also called *cystoscopic urography.*

ret·ro·gres·sion (rĕt′rə-grĕsh′ən) *n.* **1.** The act or process of deteriorating or declining. **2.** A return to a less complex biological state or stage.

ret·ro·hy·oid bursa (rĕt′rō-hī′oid′) *n.* A bursa between the posterior surface of the body of the hyoid bone and the thyrohyoid membrane. Also called *Boyer's bursa.*

ret·ro·jec·tion (rĕt′rə-jĕk′shən) *n.* The washing out of a cavity using the backward flow of an injected fluid.

ret·ro·len·tal (rĕt′rō-lĕn′tl) *adj.* Of, related to, or being posterior to the lens of the eye.

retrolental fibroplasia *n.* See **retinopathy of prematurity.**

ret·ro·man·dib·u·lar vein (rĕt′rō-măn-dĭb′yə-lər) *n.* A vein formed by union of the temporal veins in front of the ear, running behind the ramus of the mandible through the parotid gland, and uniting with the facial vein. Also called *posterior facial vein.*

ret·ro·mo·lar pad (rĕt′rō-mō′lər) *n.* A cushioned mass of tissue, frequently pear-shaped, located on the alveolar process of the mandible behind the area of the last natural molar tooth.

ret·ro·oc·u·lar (rĕt′rō-ŏk′yə-lər) *adj.* Situated behind the eye.

ret·ro·per·i·to·ne·al (rĕt′rō-pĕr′ĭ-tn-ē′əl) *adj.* Situated behind the peritoneum.

retroperitoneal space *n.* The space between the parietal peritoneum and the muscles and bones of the posterior abdominal wall.

ret·ro·per·i·to·ne·um (rĕt′rō-pĕr′ĭ-tn-ē′əm) *n.* The retroperitoneal space.

ret·ro·per·i·to·ni·tis (rĕt′rō-pĕr′ĭ-tn-ī′tĭs) *n.* Inflammation of the cellular tissue behind the peritoneum.

ret·ro·pha·ryn·geal (rĕt′rō-fə-rĭn′jəl, -făr′ĭn-jē′əl) *adj.* Situated or occurring behind the pharynx.

ret·ro·phar·ynx (rĕt′rō-făr′ĭngks) *n.* The posterior part of the pharynx.

ret·ro·pla·sia (rĕt′rō-plā′zhə) *n.* A decreased state of activity of a cell or tissue that is usually associated with retrogressive changes.

ret·ro·posed (rĕt′rə-pōzd′) *adj.* Displaced backward.

ret·ro·po·si·tion (rĕt′rō-pə-zĭsh′ən) *n.* A simple backward displacement of a structure or organ, such as the uterus, without retroversion or retroflexion.

ret·ro·po·son (rĕt′rō-pō′sən) *n.* A transposition of DNA sequences that does not occur in DNA itself but rather when mRNA is transcribed back into the genomic DNA.

ret·ro·pu·bic space (rĕt′rō-pyōō′bĭk) *n.* The area of loose pubic connective tissue between the bladder and the pubic bone and anterior abdominal wall.

ret·ro·pul·sion (rĕt′rō-pŭl′shən) *n.* **1.** An involuntary backward walking or running, as seen in Parkinsonism. **2.** A pushing back of a part or organ.

ret·ro·spec·tive falsification (rĕt′rə-spĕk′tĭv) *n.* The unconscious distortion of past experience to conform to present psychological needs.

ret·ro·spon·dy·lo·lis·the·sis (rĕt′rō-spŏn′də-lō-lĭs-thē′sĭs) *n.* Backward slippage of the body of a vertebra that moves it out of alignment with adjacent vertebrae.

ret·ro·ver·sio·flex·ion (rĕt′rō-vûr′sē-ō-flĕk′shən, -vûr′zhō-) *n.* Retroversion and retroflexion of the uterus.

ret·ro·ver·sion (rĕt′rō-vûr′zhən) *n.* **1.** A turning or tilting backward, as of the uterus. **2.** The state of being turned or tilted back. **3.** A condition in which the teeth are located in a position posterior to normal. **—ret′ro·vert′ed** *adj.*

Ret·ro·vir (rĕt′rō-vîr) A trademark for the drug zidovudine.

Ret·ro·vir·i·dae (rĕt′rō-vîr′ĭ-dē′) *n.* A family of viruses, many of which produce tumors, that contain RNA and reverse transcriptase, including the virus that causes AIDS.

ret·ro·vi·rus (rĕt′rō-vī′rəs, rĕt′rə-vī′-) *n.*, *pl.* **–rus·es** A virus of the family Retroviridae.

re·tru·sion (rĭ-trōō′zhən) *n.* Retraction from any given point, especially the backward movement of the mandible.

re·tru·sive occlusion (rĭ-trōō′sĭv) *n.* Occlusion in which the lower jaw is forcefully or habitually placed toward the back from its centric position.

Rett's syndrome (rĕts) *n.* A progressive brain disorder occurring principally in girls, characterized by autism, dementia, ataxia, and purposeless hand movements, and associated with abnormally high levels of ammonia in the blood.

re·turn extrasystole (rĭ-tûrn′) *n.* A form of reciprocal rhythm in which the impulse, having arisen in the ventricle, ascends toward the atria but before reaching the atria is reflected back to the ventricles to produce a second ventricular contraction.

re·up·take (rē-ŭp′tāk′) *n.* The reabsorption of a neurotransmitter, such as serotonin or norepinephrine, by a neuron following impulse transmission across a synapse.

re·vac·ci·na·tion (rē′văk-sə-nā′shən) *n.* Vaccination of a person previously vaccinated.

re·vas·cu·lar·i·za·tion (rē-văs′kyə-lər-ĭ-zā′shən) *n.* Re-establishment of blood supply to a part or organ.

re·ver·sal (rĭ-vûr′səl) *n.* **1.** A change to an opposite condition, direction, or position. **2.** A condition in which an individual has difficulty distinguishing the lowercase printed or written characters of particular letters: *p* from *q; g* or *b* from *d;* or *s* from *z.* **3.** The change of an emotion into its opposite, as from love into hate.

re·verse Colles' fracture (rĭ-vûrs′) *n.* See **Smith's fracture.**

re·versed coarctation (rĭ-vûrst′) *n.* Aortic arch syndrome in which blood pressure in the arms is lower than that in the legs.

reversed peristalsis *n.* A wave of intestinal contraction in a direction the reverse of normal, by which the contents of the tube are forced backward. Also called *antiperistalsis.*

reversed Prausnitz-Küstner reaction *n.* The reaction at the site of injection when serum containing reaginic antibody is injected into the skin of someone in whom the antigen is already present.

reverse Eck fistula *n.* Side-to-side anastomosis of the portal vein with the inferior vena cava, and ligation of the vena cava above the anastomosis but below the hepatic veins, thus directing the blood from the lower body through the hepatic circulation.

reverse osmosis *n.* The movement of a solvent in the opposite direction from osmosis in such a manner that the solvent moves from a solution of greater concentration through a membrane to a solution of lesser concentration.

reverse passive hemagglutination *n.* A diagnostic technique for virus infection using agglutination by viruses of red blood cells that previously have been coated with antibody specific to the virus.

reverse transcriptase *n.* A polymerase that catalyzes the formation of DNA on an RNA template, found in oncogenic viruses containing RNA, especially the retroviruses.

reverse transcription *n.* The process by which DNA is synthesized from an RNA template.

re·vers·i·ble calcinosis (rĭ-vûr′sə-bəl) *n.* Calcinosis that occasionally occurs in persons who ingest large quantities of milk and alkaline medicines.

re·ver·sion (rĭ-vûr′zhən) *n.* **1.** The return of a trait or characteristic peculiar to a remote ancestor, especially one that has been suppressed for one or more generations. **2.** A return to the normal phenotype, usually by a second mutation.

re·vert (rĭ-vûrt′) *v.* **1.** To return to a former condition, practice, subject, or belief. **2.** To undergo genetic reversion.

re·ver·tant (rĭ-vûr′tnt) *adj.* Having reverted to the normal phenotype, usually by a second mutation. —*n.* A revertant organism, cell, or strain.

re·vive (rĭ-vīv′) *v.* **1.** To bring back to life or consciousness; resuscitate. **2.** To regain health, vigor, or good spirits.

re·viv·i·fi·ca·tion (rē-vĭv′ə-fĭ-kā′shən) *n.* Refreshening the edges of a wound by paring or scraping to promote healing. Also called *vivification.*

re·vul·sion (rĭ-vŭl′shən) *n.* **1.** A sudden, strong change or reaction in feeling, especially a feeling of violent disgust or loathing. **2.** Counterirritation used to reduce inflammation or increase the blood supply to an affected area.

re·ward (rĭ-wôrd′) *n.* The return for the performance of a behavior that is desired; a positive reinforcement. —**re·ward′** *v.*

Reye's syndrome (rīz, rāz) *n.* An acute encephalopathy characterized by fever, vomiting, fatty infiltration of the liver, disorientation, and coma, occurring mainly in children and usually following a viral infection, such as chicken pox or influenza.

Rf The symbol for the element **rutherfordium.**

RF *abbr.* releasing factor; rheumatoid factor; rheumatic fever

R factor *n.* See **resistance plasmid.**

RFLP *abbr.* restriction fragment length polymorphism

Rh[1] (är′āch′) *adj.* Of or relating to the Rh factor.

Rh[2] The symbol for the element **rhodium.**

Rh₀(D) immune globulin *n.* A specific globulin fraction derived from serum of human blood donors immunized to produce antibodies against the Rh₀ antigen (D antigen), the most common antigen of the Rh blood group, used to prevent Rh-sensitization of an Rh-negative woman after delivery of a fetus that is Rh positive.

Rhab·di·tis (răb-dī′tĭs) *n.* A genus of small nematodes, some of which are parasitic on plants and animals.

rhabdo– *or* **rhabd–** *pref.* Rod; rodlike: *rhabdomyoma.*

rhab·doid (răb′doid′) *adj.* Rod-shaped.

rhab·do·my·o·blast (răb′dō-mī′ə-blăst′) *n.* A large spindle-shaped or strap-shaped cell found in some rhabdomyosarcomas.

rhab·do·my·ol·y·sis (răb′dō-mī-ŏl′ĭ-sĭs) *n.* An acute, fulminant, potentially fatal disease that destroys skeletal muscle and is often accompanied by the excretion of myoglobin in the urine.

rhab·do·my·o·ma (răb′dō-mī-ō′mə) *n.* A benign tumor derived from striated muscle.

rhab·do·my·o·sar·co·ma (răb′dō-mī′ō-sär-kō′mə) *n.* A malignant tumor derived from skeletal muscle, characterized in adults by poorly differentiated cells with large hyperchromatic nuclei. Also called *rhabdosarcoma.*

Rhab·do·vir·i·dae (răb′dō-vîr′ĭ-dē′) *n.* A family of rod- or bullet-shaped RNA viruses of vertebrates, insects, and plants, including the rabies virus.

rhab·do·vi·rus (răb′dō-vī′rəs) *n., pl.* **–rus·es** A virus of the family Rhabdoviridae.

rhag·a·des (răg′ə-dēz′) *pl.n.* Chips, cracks, or fissures occurring especially around the mouth and at other mucocutaneous junctions, seen in vitamin deficiency diseases and in congenital syphilis.

Rha·zes (rā′zēz) *or* **Ra·zi** (rä′zē) 865?–925? Persian physician whose medical writings were a major influence during the Middle Ages.

RH disease *n.* See **erythroblastosis fetalis.**

rheg·ma (rĕg′mə) *n.* A rent or fissure.

rheg·ma·tog·e·nous (rĕg′mə-tŏj′ə-nəs) *adj.* Arising from a rupture or a fracture.

rhe·ni·um (rē′nē-əm) *n. Symbol* **Re** A rare dense metallic element with a high melting point, used in plating medical instruments. Atomic number 75.

rheo– *pref.* Current; flow: *rheotaxis.*

rhe·o·base (rē′ō-bās′) *n.* The minimal strength of an electrical stimulus that is able to cause excitation of a tissue. —**rhe′o·ba′sic** *adj.*

rhe·ol·o·gy (rē-ŏl′ə-jē) *n.* The study of the deformation and flow of matter. —**rhe′o·log′i·cal** (rē′ə-lŏj′ĭ-kəl) *adj.* —**rhe′o·log′i·cal·ly** *adv.*

rhe·om·e·ter (rē-ŏm′ĭ-tər) *n.* An instrument for measuring the flow of viscous liquids, such as blood.

rhe·om·e·try (rē-ŏm′ĭ-trē) *n.* **1.** The measurement of electrical current. **2.** The measurement of blood flow.

rhe·os·to·sis (rē′ŏs-tō′sĭs) *n.* A hypertrophying and condensing osteitis which tends to run in longitudinal streaks or columns, like wax drippings on a candle, and involves a number of the long bones.

rhe·o·tax·is (rē′ə-tăk′sĭs) *n.* Movement of an organism in response to a current of fluid or air.

rhe·ot·ro·pism (rē-ŏt′rə-pĭz′əm) *n.* Growth or movement of a part of an organism in response to the motion of a current.

rhes·to·cy·the·mi·a (rĕs′tō-sī-thē′mē-ə) *n.* The presence of broken down red blood cells in the peripheral circulation.

Rhe·sus factor (rē′səs) *n.* Rh factor.

rheum (rro͞om) *n.* A watery or thin mucous discharge from the eyes or nose.

rheu·ma·tal·gia (ro͞o′mə-tăl′jə) *n.* Rheumatic pain.

rheu·mat·ic (ro͞o-măt′ĭk) *adj.* Relating to or characterized by rheumatism. —*n.* One who is affected by rheumatism.

rheumatic arteritis *n.* Arteritis due to rheumatic fever.

rheumatic endocarditis *n.* Endocarditis resulting from acute rheumatic fever, recognized clinically by valvular involvement.

rheumatic fever *n. Abbr.* **RF** An acute inflammatory disease occurring during recovery from infection with group A streptococci, having an onset marked by fever and joint pain. It is associated with polyarthritis, Sydenham's chorea, and endocarditis, and is frequently followed by scarring of the heart valves.

rheumatic heart disease *n.* Permanent damage to the valves of the heart usually caused by repeated attacks of rheumatic fever.

rheumatic pneumonia *n.* A pneumonia, occurring in severe acute rheumatic fever, in which consolidation occurs and nodules may be present in the fibrous septa of the lungs; it is usually fatal.

rheu·ma·tid (rōo′mə-tĭd′) *n.* A rheumatoid nodule or other eruption accompanying rheumatism.

rheu·ma·tism (rōo′mə-tĭz′əm) *n.* **1.** Any of several pathological conditions of the muscles, tendons, joints, bones, or nerves, characterized by discomfort and disability. **2.** Rheumatoid arthritis.

rheu·ma·toid (rōo′mə-toid′) *adj.* **1.** Of or resembling rheumatism. **2.** Suffering from rheumatism.

rheumatoid arthritis *n. Abbr.* **RA** A chronic, inflammatory arthritis, commonly involving the hands and feet, characterized by joint pain, stiffness, and weakness that can lead to deformity and disability. Also called *arthritis deformans.*

rheumatoid factor *n. Abbr.* **RF** Any of the immunoglobulins found in the serum of individuals with rheumatoid arthritis that enhance the agglutination of suspended particles that are coated with pooled human gamma globulin and that are used to diagnose the disease.

rheumatoid nodule *n.* A subcutaneous nodule occurring most commonly over bony prominences in some patients with rheumatoid arthritis.

rheumatoid spondylitis *n.* See **ankylosing spondylitis.**

rheu·ma·tol·o·gist (rōo′mə-tŏl′ə-jĭst) *n.* A specialist in the diagnosis and treatment of rheumatic disorders.

rheu·ma·tol·o·gy (rōo′mə-tŏl′ə-jē) *n.* The medical science that deals with the study and treatment of rheumatic diseases.

rhex·is (rĕk′sĭs) *n.,* *pl.* **rhex·es** (rĕk′sēz) Bursting or rupture of an organ or vessel.

Rh factor *n.* Any of several substances on the surface of red blood cells that induce a strong antigenic response in individuals lacking the substance.

rhi·nal (rī′nəl) *adj.* Nasal.

rhi·nal·gia (rī-nǎl′jə) *n.* Pain in the nose. Also called *rhinodynia.*

rhinal sulcus *n.* The shallow sulcus that delimits the anterior part of the parahippocampal gyrus from the fusiform gyrus and marks the border between the neocortex and the areas medial to it.

rhi·ne·de·ma (rī′nĭ-dē′mə) *n.* Swelling of the nasal mucous membrane.

rhi·nen·ceph·a·lon (rī′nĕn-sĕf′ə-lŏn′, -lən) *n.,* *pl.* **–la** (-lə) The olfactory region of the brain, located in the cerebrum. —**rhi′nen·ce·phal′ic** (-sə-fǎl′ĭk) *adj.*

rhi·ni·tis (rī-nī′tĭs) *n.* Inflammation of the nasal mucous membranes.

rhino– *or* **rhin–** *pref.* Nose; nasal: *rhinitis.*

rhi·no·an·tri·tis (rī′nō-ăn-trī′tĭs) *n.* Inflammation of the nasal cavities and one or both maxillary sinuses.

rhi·no·can·thec·to·my (rī′nō-kăn-thĕk′tə-mē) *n.* Excision of the inner canthus of the eye.

rhi·no·cele (rī′nə-sēl′) *n.* The cavity or ventricle of the rhinencephalon or primitive olfactory part of the telencephalon.

rhi·no·ceph·a·ly (rī′nō-sĕf′ə-lē) *n.* A form of cyclopia in which the nose is represented by a fleshy proboscis-like protuberance above the slitlike orbits.

rhi·no·chei·lo·plas·ty *or* **rhi·no·chi·lo·plas·ty** (rī′nō-kī′lə-plăs′tē) *n.* Plastic or reparative surgery of the nose and upper lip.

Rhi·no·clad·i·el·la (rī′nō-klăd′ē-ĕl′ə) *n.* A genus of dark-colored fungi that cause chromomycosis.

rhi·no·clei·sis (rī′nə-klī′sĭs) *n.* See **rhinostenosis.**

Rhi·no·cort (rī′nə-kôrt′) A trademark for the drug budesonide.

rhi·no·dac·ry·o·lith (rī′nō-dăk′rē-ə-lĭth′) *n.* A calculus in the nasolacrimal duct.

rhi·no·dyn·i·a (rī′nə-dĭn′ē-ə) *n.* See **rhinalgia.**

rhi·nog·e·nous (rī-nŏj′ə-nəs) *adj.* Originating in the nose.

rhi·no·ky·phec·to·my (rī′nō-kī-fĕk′tə-mē) *n.* Plastic surgery to correct rhinokyphosis.

rhi·no·ky·pho·sis (rī′nō-kī-fō′sĭs) *n.* A humpback deformity of the nose.

rhi·no·la·li·a (rī′nə-lā′lē-ə) *n.* A nasal tone in speech. Also called *rhinophonia.*

rhi·no·lar·yn·gi·tis (rī′nō-lăr′ĭn-jī′tĭs) *n.* Inflammation of the nasal and laryngeal mucous membranes.

rhi·no·lar·yn·gol·o·gy (rī′nō-lăr′ĭn-gŏl′ə-jē) *n.* The anatomy, physiology, and pathology of the nose and larynx.

rhi·no·lith (rī′nə-lĭth′) *n.* A calculus present in the nasal cavity.

rhi·no·li·thi·a·sis (rī′nō-lĭ-thī′ə-sĭs) *n.* The presence of calculi in the nasal cavity.

rhi·nol·o·gy (rī-nŏl′ə-jē) *n.* The anatomy, physiology, and pathology of the nose. —**rhi·nol′o·gist** *n.*

rhi·no·ma·nom·e·ter (rī′nō-mă-nŏm′ĭ-tər) *n.* A manometer used to determine the presence and amount of nasal obstruction.

rhi·no·ma·nom·e·try (rī′nō-mă-nŏm′ĭ-trē) *n.* **1.** The study and measurement of nasal airflow and pressures. **2.** The use of a rhinomanometer.

rhi·no·mu·cor·my·co·sis (rī′nō-myōo′kôr-mī-kō′sĭs, -kər-) *n.* Mucormycosis involving the nose, paranasal sinuses, the eyes, and sometimes the cranial cavity. Also called *rhinophycomycosis.*

rhi·no·my·co·sis (rī′nō-mī-kō′sĭs) *n.* Fungal infection of the nasal mucous membranes.

rhi·no·ne·cro·sis (rī′nō-nə-krō′sĭs) *n.* Necrosis of the bones of the nose.

rhi·nop·a·thy (rī-nŏp′ə-thē) *n.* Disease of the nose.

rhi·no·pho·ni·a (rī′nə-fō′nē-ə) *n.* See **rhinolalia.**

rhi·no·phy·co·my·co·sis (rī′nō-fī′kō-mī-kō′sĭs) *n.* See **rhinomucormycosis.**

rhi·no·phy·ma (rī′nō-fī′mə) *n.* Hypertrophy of the nose with follicular dilation resulting from hyperplasia of sebaceous glands accompanied by fibrosis and increased vascularity.

rhi·no·plas·ty (rī′nō-plăs′tē, -nə-) *n.* Plastic surgery of the nose.

rhi·nor·rha·gia (rī′nə-rā′jə) *n.* Nosebleed, especially one in which bleeding is profuse.

rhi·nor·rhe·a (rī′nə-rē′ə) *n.* A discharge from the nasal mucous membrane, especially if excessive.

rhi·no·sal·pin·gi·tis (rī′nō-săl′pĭn-jī′tĭs) *n.* Inflammation of the mucous membrane of the nose and of the eustachian tube.

rhi·no·scle·ro·ma (rī′nō-sklə-rō′mə) *n.* A chronic granulomatous condition involving the nose, upper lip, mouth, and upper air passages that is possibly caused by a bacterium.

rhi·nos·co·py (rī-nŏs′kə-pē) *n.* Examination of the nasal passages. —**rhi′no·scope′** (rī′nə-skōp′) *n.* —**rhi′-no·scop′ic** (-skŏp′ĭk) *adj.*

rhi·no·spo·rid·i·o·sis (rī′nō-spə-rĭd′ē-ō′sĭs) *n.* A chronic granulomatous disease of the mucous membranes of the nasal cavity characterized by polyps or other forms of hyperplasia and caused by a yeastlike microorganism *Rhinosporidium seeberi.*

rhi·no·ste·no·sis (rī′nō-stə-nō′sĭs) *n.* Obstruction of the nasal passages. Also called *rhinocleisis.*

rhi·not·o·my (rī-nŏt′ə-mē) *n.* Incision into the nose, especially incision along one side to allow viewing of the nasal passages for radical sinus operations.

rhi·no·vi·rus (rī′nō-vī′rəs) *n.* Any of a group of picornaviruses that are causative agents of disorders of the respiratory tract, such as the common cold. Also called *coryzavirus.*

Rhi·pi·ceph·a·lus (rī′pĭ-sĕf′ə-ləs, rĭp′ĭ-) *n.* A genus of ixodids including species that are vectors of various diseases in humans and domestic animals, such as Rocky Mountain spotted fever.

rhizo– *or* **rhiz–** *pref.* Root: *rhizoid.*

rhi·zoid (rī′zoid′) *adj.* **1.** Rootlike. **2.** Having irregular branching. Used of a form of bacterial growth. —*n.* **1.** A slender rootlike filament by which mosses, liverworts, and fern gametophytes attach to the substratum and absorb nourishment. **2.** A rootlike extension of the thallus of a fungus.

rhi·zo·me·li·a (rī′zə-mē′lē-ə, -mēl′yə) *n.* A disproportion in the length of the upper arms and thighs. —**rhi′-zo·me′lic** (-mē′lĭk, -mĕl′ĭk) *adj.*

rhi·zo·me·nin·go·my·e·li·tis (rī′zō-mə-nĭng′gō-mī′-ə-lī′tĭs) *n.* An inflammation that involves the nerve roots, the meninges, and the spinal cord. Also called *radiculomeningomyelitis.*

Rhi·zo·po·de·a (rī′zə-pō′dē-ə) *or* **Rhi·zop·o·da** (rī-zŏp′ə-də) *n.* A phylum of microorganisms that includes protozoa such as the ameba that move and take in nourishment by means of pseudopods.

Rhi·zo·pus (rī′zə-pəs, rī-zō′pəs) *n.* A genus of rot-causing fungi that includes the common bread mold; some species cause mucormycosis in humans.

rhi·zot·o·my (rī-zŏt′ə-mē) *n.* Surgical severance of spinal nerve roots, as for the relief of pain. Also called *radicotomy, radiculotomy.*

Rh-negative *adj.* Lacking an Rh factor.

Rh null syndrome *n.* A syndrome that is characterized by a lack of all Rh antigens, hemolytic anemia that has been compensated for by the body, and stomatocytosis.

rho *n. Symbol* ρ The 17th letter of the Greek alphabet.

Rho·de·sian trypanosomiasis (rō-dē′zhən) *n.* An acute type of African trypanosomiasis that progresses rapidly and is caused by *Trypanosoma brucei rhodesiense,* transmitted by tsetse flies. Also called *acute African sleeping sickness, acute trypanosomiasis.*

rho·di·um (rō′dē-əm) *n. Symbol* **Rh** A hard durable metallic element. Atomic number 45.

rhodo– *or* **rhod–** *pref.* Rose; rosy; red: *rhodopsin.*

rho·do·gen·e·sis (rō′də-jĕn′ĭ-sĭs) *n.* The regeneration of rhodopsin by the combination of 11-*cis*-retinal and opsin, occurring in darkness.

rho·do·phy·lax·is (rō′dō-fə-lăk′sĭs) *n.* The action of the pigment cells of the choroid of the eye in preserving or facilitating the regeneration of rhodopsin. —**rho′-do·phy·lac′tic** (-lăk′tĭk) *adj.*

rho·dop·sin (rō-dŏp′sĭn) *n.* A thermolabile protein that is sensitive to red light and is found in the external segments of the rods of the retina of the eye. Also called *visual purple.*

rhom·ben·ce·phal·ic isthmus (rŏm′bĕn-sə-făl′ĭk) *n.* **1.** A narrow portion in the embryonic neural tube delineating the mesencephalon from the rhombencephalon. **2.** The anterior portion of the rhombencephalon that connects with the mesencephalon.

rhom·ben·ceph·a·lon (rŏm′bĕn-sĕf′ə-lŏn′, -lən) *n.* The portion of the embryonic brain from which the metencephalon and myelencephalon develop, including the pons, cerebellum, and the medulla oblongata. Also called *hindbrain.*

rhom·bic (rŏm′bĭk) *adj.* **1.** Relating to the rhombencephalon. **2.** Rhomboid.

rhombo– *or* **rhomb–** *pref.* Rhombus: *rhomboid.*

rhom·bo·cele (rŏm′bə-sēl′) *n.* See **rhomboidal sinus.**

rhom·boid (rŏm′boid′) *or* **rhom·boi·dal** (rŏm-boid′l) *adj.* Resembling a parallelogram having unequal adjacent sides.

rhomboidal sinus *n.* A dilation of the central canal of the spinal cord in the lumbar region. Also called *rhombocele.*

rhomboid fossa *n.* The floor of the fourth ventricle of the brain, formed by the ventricular surface of the rhombencephalon.

rhomboid ligament *n.* See **costoclavicular ligament.**

rhonchal fremitus *n.* The vibration in the chest produced by the passage of air through bronchial tubes that are partially obstructed by mucous secretions.

rhon·chus (rŏng′kəs) *n., pl.* **–chi** (-kī) A coarse rattling sound somewhat like snoring, usually caused by secretion in a bronchial tube. —**rhon′chal** (-kəl) *adj.*

Rh-positive *adj.* Containing an Rh factor.

Rhus (rōōs, rŭs) *n.* A genus of vines and shrubs including several species, especially poison ivy, poison oak, and poison sumac.

rhythm (rĭth′əm) *n.* Movement or variation characterized by the regular recurrence or alternation of different quantities or conditions, as in the heartbeat.

rhythm method *n.* A birth control method dependent on abstinence during the period of ovulation.

rhyt·i·dec·tomy (rĭt′ĭ-dĕk′tə-mē) *n.* See **face-lift.**

rhyt·i·do·plas·ty (rĭt′ĭ-dō-plăs′tē) *n.* See **face-lift.**

rhyt·i·do·sis (rĭt′ĭ-dō′sĭs) *n.* **1.** A condition in which the face wrinkles to a degree disproportionate to age. **2.** A condition in which the cornea of the eye becomes lax and wrinkled. Also called *rutidosis.*

RIA *abbr.* radioimmunoassay

rib (rĭb) *n.* One of a series of long curved bones occurring in 12 pairs in humans and extending from the spine to or toward the sternum.

ri·ba·vi·rin (rī′bə-vī′rĭn) *n.* A synthetic antiviral ribonucleoside that inhibits DNA and RNA replication.

rib cage *n.* The enclosing structure formed by the ribs and the bones to which they are attached.

ribo– *pref.* **1.** A five-carbon sugar: *ribose.* **2.** A monosaccharide that has three carbohydrate groups arranged in the manner of ribose: *D-ribo-pentose.*

ri·bo·fla·vin (rī′bō-flā′vĭn, -bə-) *n.* An orange-yellow crystalline compound that is the principal growth-promoting factor in the vitamin B complex, naturally occurring in milk, leafy vegetables, fresh meat, and egg yolks. Also called *lactoflavin, vitamin B$_2$.*

riboflavin kinase *n.* An enzyme that catalyzes the formation of flavin mononucleotide from riboflavin, using ATP or ADP as a phosphorylating agent.

ri·bo·nu·cle·ase (rī′bō-nōō′klē-ās′, -āz′) *n.* Any of various enzymes that catalyze the hydrolysis of RNA. Also called *RNase.*

ri·bo·nu·cle·ic acid (rī′bō-nōō-klē′ĭk, -klā′-) *n.* RNA.

ri·bo·nu·cle·o·pro·tein (rī′bō-nōō′klē-ō-prō′tēn) *n.* *Abbr.* **RNP** A nucleoprotein that contains RNA.

ri·bo·nu·cle·o·side (rī′bō-nōō′klē-ə-sīd′) *n.* A nucleoside that contains ribose as its sugar component; as in uridine.

ri·bo·nu·cle·o·tide (rī′bō-nōō′klē-ə-tīd′) *n.* A nucleotide that contains ribose as its sugar and usually occurs as a component of RNA.

ri·bose (rī′bōs′) *n.* A pentose sugar occurring as a component of riboflavin, nucleotides, and nucleic acids.

ribose 5-phosphate isomerase *n.* An enzyme that plays an important role in ribose metabolism. Also called *phosphoriboisomerase.*

ribosomal RNA *n.* See **rRNA.**

ri·bo·some (rī′bə-sōm′) *n.* A minute round cytoplasmic particle composed of RNA and protein that is the site of protein synthesis as directed by mRNA.

ri·bo·su·ri·a (rī′bō-sōōr′ē-ə) *n.* Excretion of an excessive amount of ribose in the urine, usually a manifestation of muscular dystrophy.

ri·bo·syl (rī′bō-sĭl′) *n.* The radical $C_5H_9O_4$ formed from ribose.

ri·bo·zyme (rī′bə-zīm′) *n.* A strand of RNA that attaches to specific sites on other RNA strands and lyses the strands.

Rich·ards (rĭch′ərdz), **Dickinson Woodruff** 1895–1973. American physician. He shared a 1956 Nobel Prize for developing cardiac catheterization.

Ri·chet (rĭ-shā′, rē-shĕ′), **Charles Robert** 1850–1935. French physiologist. He won a 1913 Nobel Prize for the discovery of anaphylaxis.

Rich·ter's hernia (rĭk′tərz, rĭкн′-) *n.* See **parietal hernia.**

ri·cin (rī′sĭn, rĭs′ĭn) *n.* A poisonous protein that is extracted from the castor bean and is used as a biochemical reagent.

rick·ets (rĭk′ĭts) *n.* A bone disease resulting in defective skeletal growth in children, analogous to osteomalacia in adults, characterized by bone demineralization caused by deficiency or impaired metabolism of vitamin D or phosphates. Also called *infantile osteomalacia, juvenile osteomalacia, rachitis.*

Rick·etts (rĭk′ĭtz), **Howard Taylor** 1871–1910. American pathologist who discovered bacteria of the genus *Rickettsia* and determined the cause and methods of transmission of Rocky Mountain spotted fever and typhus.

Rick·ett·si·a (rĭ-kĕt′sē-ə) *n.* A genus of gram-negative bacteria that are carried as parasites by many ticks, fleas, and lice and cause diseases such as typhus, scrub typhus, and Rocky Mountain spotted fever.

Rickettsia ak·a·ri (ăk′ə-rī′) *n.* A bacterium that causes rickettsialpox in humans.

Rickettsia aus·tra·lis (ô-strā′lĭs) *n.* A bacterium causing a spotted fever that elicits the production of an antibody that is different from the one that reacts with other rickettsial species.

Rickettsia co·no·ri·i (kŏ-nôr′ē-ī′) *n.* A bacterium that causes boutonneuse fever in humans.

rick·ett·si·al (rĭ-kĕt′sē-əl) *adj.* Relating to, or caused by a member of the genus *Rickettsia.*

rick·ett·si·al·pox (rĭ-kĕt′sē-əl-pŏks′) *n.* An acute nonfatal disease caused by *Rickettsia akari* and transmitted by mites; it is characterized by a papule in the skin and symptoms that develop about a week after the appearance of the papule, consisting of fever, chills, headache, backache, sweating, and local adenitis. Also called *Kew garden fever.*

Rickettsia pro·wa·zek·i·i (prō′və-zĕk′ē-ī′) *n.* A bacterium that causes epidemic typhus fever.

Rickettsia rick·ett·si·i (rĭ-kĕt′sē-ī′) *n.* A bacterium that causes a variety of spotted fevers throughout the world including Rocky Mountain spotted fever.

Rickettsia tsu·tsu·ga·mu·shi (tsōō′tsə-gə-mōō′shē) *n.* A bacterium that causes scrub typhus.

rick·ett·si·o·sis (rĭ-kĕt′sē-ō′sĭs) *n.* Infection with Rickettsia bacteria.

Rid·au·ra (rĭd-ô′rə) A trademark for the drug auranofin.

Rid·e·al-Wal·ker coefficient (rĭd′ē-əl-wô′kər) *n.* A figure expressing the disinfecting power of a substance by relating it to the disinfecting power of phenol. Also called *phenol coefficient.*

rid·er's bone (rī′dərz) *n.* Ossification of the tendon of the long adductor muscle of the leg from strain in horseback riding.

ridge (rĭj) *n.* A long, narrow, or crested part of the body, as on the nose.

Rie·del's lobe (rēd′lz) *n.* A tonguelike process occasionally extending downward from the right lobe of the liver laterally to the gallbladder.

Riedel's struma *n.* A rare fibrous hardening of the thyroid, with adhesion to adjacent structures, that may cause tracheal compression.

Rie·der cell (rē′dər) *n.* An anaplastic cell, probably a type of white blood cell or granulocyte, that occurs in acute leukemia.

Rieder cell leukemia *n.* A form of acute granulocytic leukemia that is characterized by abnormal numbers of Rieder cells in the blood and tissues.

Rie·gel's pulse (rē′gəlz) *n.* A pulse that diminishes in volume during exhalation.

Rif·a·din (rĭf′ə-dĭn′) A trademark for the drug rifampin.

ri·fam·pin (rĭ-făm′pĭn) *or* **ri·fam·pi·cin** (-pĭ-sĭn) *n.* A semisynthetic antibiotic, derived from a form of rifamycin, that interferes with the synthesis of RNA and is used to treat bacterial and viral diseases.

rif·a·my·cin (rĭf′ə-mī′sĭn) *n.* Any of a group of antibiotics originally isolated from a strain of the soil microorganism *Streptomyces mediterranei*, used in the treatment of leprosy, tuberculosis, and other bacterial diseases.

Riggs' disease (rĭgz) *n.* Inflammation of the tissues surrounding and supporting the teeth.

right atrioventricular valve (rīt) *n.* See **tricuspid valve**.

right brachiocephalic vein *n.* A vein that receives the right vertebral and internal thoracic veins, and the right lymphatic duct.

right brain *n.* The cerebral hemisphere to the right of the corpus callosum, controlling the left side of the body.

right-brained *adj.* **1.** Having the right brain dominant. **2.** Of or relating to the thought processes involved in creativity and imagination, generally associated with the right brain. **3.** Of or relating to a person whose behavior is dominated by emotion, creativity, intuition, nonverbal communication, and global reasoning rather than logic and analysis.

right colic flexure *n.* The bend of the colon at the juncture of its ascending and transverse portions. Also called *hepatic flexure*.

right colic vein *n.* A vein that parallels the right colic artery and drains blood from the ascending colon and right flexure.

right-eyed *adj.* Tending to use the right eye instead of the left when using an instrument that permits the use of one eye only.

right-footed *adj.* Using the right leg more skillfully or easily than the left.

right gastric vein *n.* See **pyloric vein**.

right gastro-omental vein *n.* A tributary of the superior mesenteric vein that parallels the right gastroomental artery along the greater curvature of the stomach. Also called *right gastroepiploic vein*.

right-handed *adj.* Using the right hand more skillfully or easily than the left.

right heart *n.* The right atrium and right ventricle.

right hepatic duct *n.* The duct that conveys bile to the common hepatic duct from the right half of the liver.

right inferior pulmonary vein *n.* The vein returning blood from the inferior lobe of the right lung to the left atrium.

right·ing reflex (rī′tĭng) *n.* Any of various reflexes that tend to bring the body into normal position in space and resist forces acting to displace it out of normal position. Also called *static reflex*.

right lobe of liver *n.* The largest lobe of the liver, separated from the left lobe above and in front by the falciform ligament, and separated from the caudate and quadrate lobes by the sulcus for the vena cava and by the fossa for the gallbladder.

right lymphatic duct *n.* One of the two terminal lymphatic vessels, formed by the union of the right jugular lymphatic vessel and vessels from the lymph nodes of the right upper extremity, thoracic wall, and both lungs;

lying on the right side of the root of the neck and emptying into the right brachiocephalic vein. Also called *right thoracic duct*.

right ovarian vein *n.* A vein that begins at the pampiniform plexus at the hilum of the ovary and opens into the inferior vena cava.

right suprarenal vein *n.* A short vein that passes from the hilum of the right adrenal gland to the inferior vena cava.

right testicular vein *n.* A vein that passes upward from the pampiniform plexus to join the inferior vena cava.

right thoracic duct *n.* See **right lymphatic duct**.

right-to-die *adj.* Advocating or expressing, as in a living will, a person's right to refuse extraordinary life-sustaining measures intended to prolong life artificially when the person is deemed by his or her physicians to be terminally or incurably ill.

right-to-left shunt *n.* **1.** The passage of blood from the right side of the heart into the left, as through a septal defect. **2.** The passage of blood from the pulmonary artery into the aorta, as through a patent ductus arteriosus.

right ventricle *n.* The chamber on the right side of the heart that receives venous blood from the right atrium and forces it into the pulmonary artery.

right ventricular failure *n.* Congestive heart failure manifested by distention of the neck veins, enlargement of the liver, and dependent edema.

right ventricular opening *n.* An opening that leads from the right atrium into the right ventricle of the heart. Also called *tricuspid orifice*.

ri·gid·i·ty (rĭ-jĭd′ĭ-tē) *n.* **1.** The quality or state of stiffness or inflexibility. Also called *rigor*. **2.** An aspect of the personality characterized by resistance to change.

rig·or (rĭg′ər) *n.* **1.** See **rigidity** (sense 1). **2.** Shivering or trembling, as caused by a chill. **3.** A state of rigidity in living tissues or organs that prevents response to stimuli.

rigor mor·tis (môr′tĭs) *n.* Muscular stiffening following death. Also called *postmortem rigidity*.

Ri·ley-Day syndrome (rī′lē-dā′) *n.* See **familial dysautonomia**.

rim (rĭm) *n.* The border, edge, or margin of an organ or a part.

ri·ma (rī′mə) *n., pl.* **–mae** (-mē) A slit, fissure, or narrow elongated opening between two symmetrical parts.

rima glot·ti·dis (glŏt′ĭ-dĭs) *n.* The narrow opening between the vocal cords.

rima o·ris (ôr′ĭs) *n.* The opening of the mouth.

rima pu·den·di (pyoo-dĕn′dī) *n.* The cleft between the labia majora.

rima ves·tib·u·li (vĕ-stĭb′yə-lī′) *n.* The opening between the vestibular folds.

ri·mose (rī′mōs′, rī-mōs′) *adj.* Full of chinks, cracks, or crevices.

rim·u·la (rĭm′yə-lə) *n., pl.* **–lae** (-lē′) A minute slit or fissure.

ring (rĭng) *n.* **1.** A circular object, form, or arrangement with a vacant circular center. **2.** The area between two concentric circles; annulus. **3.** A group of atoms linked by bonds that may be represented graphically in circular or triangular form.

ring abscess *n.* An acute purulent inflammation of the cornea which often progresses to panophthalmia.

ring chromosome *n.* A chromosome with ends joined to form a circular structure.

Ring·er's injection (rĭng′ərz) *n.* A sterile solution of sodium chloride, potassium chloride, and calcium chloride, given intravenously as a fluid and electrolyte replenisher.

Ringer's solution *n.* **1.** A solution resembling blood serum in its salt constituents, containing sodium chloride, potassium chloride, and calcium chloride in water, used topically for burns and wounds. **2.** A salt solution usually used in combination with naturally occurring body substances or with more complex chemically defined nutritive solutions for culturing animal cells. **3.** Ringer's injection.

ring finger *n.* The third finger of the left hand.

ring-knife *n.* A circular or oval ring with an internal cutting edge used to shave off tumors in the nasal and other cavities.

ring scotoma *n.* An annular area of blindness in the visual field surrounding the point of fixation, associated with glaucoma and pigmentary degeneration of the retina.

ring syringe *n.* See **control syringe.**

ring·worm (rĭng′wûrm′) *n.* See **tinea.**

Rin·ne's test (rĭn′ēz, -əz) *n.* A hearing test in which a vibrating tuning fork is held against the mastoid process until the sound is lost and then brought close to the auditory orifice.

Ri·o·lan's anastomosis (rē′ō-länz′) *n.* A surgical connection of superior and inferior mesenteric arteries.

risk (rĭsk) *n.* **1.** The possibility of suffering a harmful event. **2.** A factor or course involving uncertain danger, as with smoking or exposure to radiation.

risk factor *n.* A characteristic, condition, or behavior that increases the possibility of disease or injury. High blood pressure, high serum cholesterol, and smoking are risk factors for heart disease.

ri·so·ri·us muscle (rĭ-sôr′ē-əs, -zôr′-) *n.* A muscle with origin from the masseter muscle, with insertion into the orbicular muscle of the mouth, with nerve supply from the facial nerve, and whose action draws out the angle of the mouth.

Ris·per·dal (rĭs′pər-dăl′) A trademark for the drug risperidone.

ris·per·i·done (rĭ-spâr′ə-dōn′) *n.* A dopamine and serotonin antagonist used to treat the hallucinations, delusions, and thought disturbances of schizophrenia and other psychoses.

ri·sus ca·ni·nus (rī′səs kā-nī′nəs) *n.* The semblance of a grin caused by facial spasm, as in tetanus. Also called *canine spasm, cynic spasm, sardonic grin.*

Rit·a·lin (rĭt′l-ĭn) A trademark for the drug methylphenidate.

rite of passage (rīt) *n.* A ritual or ceremony signifying an event in a person's life indicative of a transition from one stage to another, as from adolescence to adulthood.

ri·ton·a·vir (rĭ-tŏn′ə-vîr′) *n.* A protease-inhibiting drug usually used in combination with other drugs to suppress the replication of HIV.

Rit·ter's disease (rĭt′ərz) *n.* **1.** See **staphylococcal scalded skin syndrome. 2.** See **jaundice of newborn.**

rit·u·al (rĭch′ōō-əl) *n.* A detailed act or series of acts carried out by an individual to relieve anxiety or to forestall the development of anxiety.

Ri·tux·an (rĭ-tŭk′sən) A trademark for the drug rituximab.

ri·tux·i·mab (rĭ-tŭk′sĭ-măb′) *n.* A monoclonal antibody used to treat certain types of non-Hodgkin's lymphoma.

ri·val·ry (rī′vəl-rē) *n.* The state or condition of competition or antagonism.

riv·er blindness (rĭv′ər) *n.* See **onchocerciasis.**

Ri·vi·nus gland (rĭ-vē′nəs, rē-vē′nŏōs) *n.* See **sublingual gland.**

Rivinus incisure *n.* See **tympanic notch.**

riz·i·form (rĭz′ə-fôrm′) *adj.* Resembling grains of rice.

RLL *abbr.* right lower lobe (of the lung)

RLQ *abbr.* right lower quadrant (of the abdomen)

RMSF *abbr.* Rocky Mountain spotted fever

Rn The symbol for the element **radon.**

RN *abbr.* registered nurse

RNA (är′ĕn-ā′) *n.* Ribonucleic acid; a polymeric constituent of all living cells and many viruses, consisting of a long, usually single-stranded chain of alternating phosphate and ribose units with the bases adenine, guanine, cytosine, and uracil bonded to the ribose. The structure and base sequence of RNA are determinants of protein synthesis and the transmission of genetic information.

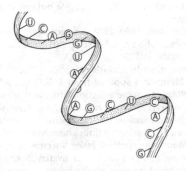

RNA

single-strand molecule containing nucleotide bases of adenine (A), guanine (G), cytosine (C), and uracil (U)

RNA interference *n.* A process in which the introduction of double-stranded RNA into a cell inhibits the expression of genes.

RNA polymerase *n.* A polymerase that catalyzes the synthesis of RNA from a DNA or RNA template.

RN·ase (är′ĕn-ās′, -āz′) *or* **RNA·ase** (är′ĕn-ā′ās′, -āz′) *n.* See **ribonuclease.**

RNA splicing *n.* See **splicing** (sense 2).

RNA tumor virus *n.* An RNA-containing virus of the subfamily Oncovirinae; oncornavirus.

RNA virus *n.* Any of a group of viruses whose nucleic acid core is composed of RNA, including the picornaviruses, retroviruses, and paramyxoviruses.

RNP *abbr.* ribonucleoprotein

Rob·bins (rŏb′ĭnz), **Frederick Chapman** 1916–2003. American microbiologist. He shared a 1954 Nobel Prize for work on the cultivation of the polio virus.

rob·ert·son·i·an translocation (rŏb′ərt-sō′nē-ən) *n.* A breakage in the short arms of two acrocentric chromosomes and the subsequent fusion of the long arms into a single chromosome. Also called *centric fusion.*

Ro·bert's pelvis (rō′bĕrts′) *n.* A pelvis that is narrowed transversely due to the almost entire absence of the alae of the sacrum.

Rob·in·son index (rŏb′ĭn-sən) *n.* An index used to calculate the work load of the heart.

Ro·bi·tus·sin (rō′bĭ-tŭs′ĭn) A trademark for the drug guaifenesin, sometimes combined with cough suppressants or decongestants.

ro·bot (rō′bŏt′) *n.* **1.** A mechanical device that sometimes resembles a human and is capable of performing a variety of often complex human tasks on command or by being programmed in advance. **2.** A machine or device that operates automatically or by remote control. **3.** A person who works mechanically without original thought, especially one who responds automatically to the commands of others.

ro·bot·ic (rō-bŏt′ĭk) *adj.* Relating to, characteristic of, or employing robots.

Ro·ceph·in (rə-sĕf′ĭn) A trademark for the drug ceftriaxone.

Ro·cha·li·mae·a (rō′chə-lī-mē′ə) *n.* A genus of bacteria, closely resembling *Rickettsia* in staining properties, morphology, and mode of transmission between hosts.

Ro·chelle salt (rə-shĕl′, rō-) *n.* See **potassium sodium tartrate.**

Rock (rŏk), **John** 1890–1984. American gynecologist and obstetrician who helped develop the first effective oral contraceptive in 1954.

Rock fever *n.* See **brucellosis.**

Rock·y Moun·tain spotted fever (rŏk′ē moun′tən) *n. Abbr.* **RMSF** An acute infectious disease that is caused by the bacteria *Rickettsia rickettsii* and is transmitted by ticks, characterized by muscular pain, high fever, and a skin rash, and is endemic throughout North America.

Rocky Mountain spotted fever vaccine *n.* A vaccine containing a suspension of inactivated *Rickettsia rickettsii* prepared by growing the microorganisms in the yolk sac of fowl eggs, used to immunize against Rocky Mountain spotted fever.

rod (rŏd) *n.* **1.** A straight slender cylindrical formation. **2.** A rod cell. **3.** An elongated bacterium; a bacillus.

rod cell *n.* Any of various cylindrically-shaped cells in the retina that respond to dim light.

ro·den·ti·cide (rō-dĕn′tĭ-sīd′) *n.* A chemical substance used to kill rodents.

ro·dent ulcer (rōd′nt) *n.* A slowly enlarging ulcerated basal cell carcinoma, usually on the face.

rod granule *n.* The nucleus of a retinal cell connecting with one of the rods.

roent·gen *or* **rönt·gen** (rĕnt′gən, -jən, rŭnt′-) *n. Abbr.* **R, r** A unit of radiation exposure that is equal to the quantity of ionizing radiation that will produce one electrostatic unit of electricity in one cubic centimeter of dry air at 0°C and standard atmospheric pressure.

Roent·gen (rĕnt′gən, -jən, rŭnt′-) *or* **Rönt·gen** (rœnt′gən) **Wilhelm Konrad** 1845–1923. German physicist who discovered x-rays and developed x-ray photography, revolutionizing medical diagnosis. He won a 1901 Nobel Prize.

roent·ge·nism (rĕnt′gə-nĭz′əm, -jə-, rŭnt′-) *n.* **1.** The use of x-rays in the diagnosis and treatment of disease. **2.** A damaging effect of x-rays on tissues.

roent·gen·o·gram (rĕnt′gə-nə-grăm′, -jə-, rŭnt′-) *n.* A photograph made with x-rays. Also called *roentgenograph.*

roent·gen·og·ra·phy (rĕnt′gə-nŏg′rə-fē, -jə-, rŭnt′-) *n.* Photography with the use of x-rays. —**roent′gen·o·graph′ic** (-gə-nə-grăf′ĭk, -jə-) *adj.*

roent·gen·ol·o·gy (rĕnt′gə-nŏl′ə-jē, -jə-, rŭnt′-) *n.* Radiology using x-rays. —**roent′gen·ol′o·gist** *n.*

roentgen ray *n.* See **x-ray** (sense 1, 2).

ro·fe·cox·ib (rō′fə-kŏk′sĭb) *n.* A nonsteroidal anti-inflammatory drug that selectively inhibits the formation of prostaglandins and was formerly used to treat pain, especially in osteoarthritis.

Ro·gaine (rō′gān′) A trademark for the drug minoxidil.

Rog·ers (rŏj′ərz), **Carl Ransom** 1902–1987. American psychologist who founded humanistic psychology.

Ro·ger's disease (rō-zhāz′) *n.* A congenital defect in the septum that separates the ventricles of the heart.

Roger's murmur *n.* A loud pansystolic murmur heard at the left sternal border, caused by a small ventricular septal defect.

Ro·hyp·nol (rō-hĭp′nôl′, -nōl′) A trademark for the drug flunitrazepam.

Ro·ki·tan·sky (rō′kĭ-tăn′skē), **Baron von Karl** 1804–1878. Austrian physician who was one of the founders of modern pathological anatomy. He performed more than 30,000 autopsies and published numerous studies on diseases of the heart and arteries based on his observations.

Rokitansky-Küs·ter-Hau·ser syndrome (-küs′tər-hou′zər) *n.* See **Mayer-Rokitansky-Küster-Hauser syndrome.**

Ro·ki·tan·sky's disease (rō′kĭ-tăn′skēz) *n.* **1.** See **acute yellow atrophy of liver. 2.** See **Chiari's syndrome.**

Rokitansky's pelvis *n.* See **spondylolisthetic pelvis.**

ro·lan·dic epilepsy (rō-lăn′dĭk) *n.* An inherited form of epilepsy occurring in children and characterized by arrested speech and muscular contractions of the side of the face and arm.

Ro·lan·do's area (rō-lăn′dōz) *n.* See **motor cortex.**

Rolando's fissure *n.* Variant of **fissure of Rolando.**

Rolando's gelatinous substance *n.* See **substantia gelatinosa.**

role *or* **rôle** (rōl) *n.* The characteristic and expected social behavior of an individual.

role model *n.* A person who serves as a model in a particular behavioral or social role for another person to emulate.

role-play (rōl′plā′) *v.* To assume deliberately the part or role of; act out. —*n.* Role-playing.

role-play·ing (rōl′plā′ĭng) *n.* A psychotherapeutic technique, designed to reduce the conflict inherent in various social situations, in which participants act out particular behavioral roles in order to expand their awareness of differing points of view.

Rolf·ing (rôl′fĭng) A service mark used for a technique of deep muscular manipulation and massage for the relief of bodily and emotional tension.

roll·er bandage (rō′lər) *n.* A strip of material, of variable width, rolled into a compact cylinder to facilitate application.

ROM *abbr.* range of motion

Rom·berg's sign (rŏm′bərgz) *n.* A sign indicating loss of proprioceptive control in which increased unsteadiness occurs when standing with the eyes closed compared with standing with the eyes open. Also called *rombergism.*

ron·geur (rôn-zhœr′, rôn-) *n.* A heavy-duty forceps for removing small pieces of bone.

rönt·gen (rĕnt′gən, -jən, rŭnt′-) *n.* Variant of **roentgen**.

roof (rōof, rŏof) *n.* The upper surface of an anatomical structure, especially one having a vaulted inner structure.

roof·ie (rōō′fē) *n.* A tablet of the sedative flunitrazepam.

roof of fourth ventricle *n.* The roof of the fourth ventricle formed by the inferior and the superior medullary vela.

roof of tympanum *n.* The roof of the middle ear, formed by the thinned anterior surface of the petrous portion of the temporal bone.

roof plate *or* **roofplate** *n.* The thin layer of the embryonic neural tube that connects the lateral plates dorsally.

root (rōot, rŏot) *n.* **1.** The embedded part of an organ or structure, such as a hair, tooth, or nerve, serving as a base or support. **2.** A primary source; an origin; radix.

root amputation *n.* Surgical removal of one or more roots of a multirooted tooth. Also called *radectomy.*

root canal *n.* **1.** The chamber of the dental pulp lying within the root portion of a tooth. Also called *pulp canal.* **2.** A treatment in which diseased tissue from this part of the tooth is removed and the resulting cavity is filled with an inert material.

root caries index *n.* The ratio of the number of teeth with carious lesions of the root and restorations of the root to the number of teeth with exposed root surfaces.

root filament *n.* Any of the small individual fiber fascicles into which the roots of each spinal nerve and several of the cranial nerves divide in a fanlike fashion before entering or leaving the spinal cord or brainstem. Also called *nerve rootlet.*

root·ing reflex (rōō′tĭng, rŏot′ĭng) *n.* A reflex in infants in which rubbing or scratching about the mouth causes the infant to turn its head toward the stimulus.

root of lung *n.* All the structures entering or leaving the lung at the hilum.

root of nail *n.* The proximal end of the nail, concealed under a fold of skin.

root of penis *n.* The proximal attached part of the penis, including the two crura and the bulb.

root of tongue *n.* The rear attached portion of the tongue.

root of tooth *n.* The part of a tooth below the neck of the tooth, covered by cementum rather than enamel and attached by the periodontal ligament to the alveolar bone.

root resection *n.* See **apicoectomy**.

root sheath *n.* Either of two epidermic layers of the hair follicle.

ro·pin·i·role (rō-pĭn′ə-rōl′) *n.* A dopamine agonist used to treat Parkinson's disease.

Ror·schach (rôr′shäk′, -shäкн′), **Hermann** 1884–1922. Swiss psychiatrist. His inkblot test, introduced in 1921, has become a standard clinical diagnostic tool in psychiatry.

ro·sa·ce·a (rō-zā′shē-ə) *n.* A chronic dermatitis of the face, especially of the nose and cheeks, characterized by a red or rosy coloration with deep-seated papules and pustules and caused by dilation of capillaries. Also called *acne erythematosa, acne rosacea.*

ros·an·i·line *or* **ros·an·i·lin** (rō-zăn′ə-lĭn) *n.* A brownish-red crystalline organic compound derived from aniline and used in the manufacture of dyes and in Schiff's reagent.

ro·sa·ry (rō′zə-rē) *n.* An arrangement or structure that is beadlike in appearance.

rose ben·gal (rōz′ bĕn-gôl′, bĕng-, bĕn′gəl, bĕng′-) *n.* A bluish-red dye used as a stain for bacteria, as a stain in the diagnosis of keratitis sicca, and in tests of liver function.

rose fever *n.* A spring or early summer hay fever. Also called *rose cold.*

ro·se·o·la (rō-zē′ə-lə, rō′zē-ō′lə) *n.* A rose-colored skin rash, sometimes occurring with diseases such as measles, syphilis, or scarlet fever.

roseola in·fan·tum (ĭn-făn′təm) *n.* See **exanthema subitum**.

Rose's position (rō′zĭz) *n.* A supine position with the head over the end of a table, used for operations within the mouth or the fauces.

rose spots *pl.n.* The characteristic rose-colored spots of typhoid fever.

ro·sette (rō-zĕt′) *n.* **1.** The segmented or mature phase of *Plasmodium malariae.* **2.** A grouping of cells characteristic of neoplasms of neuroblastic or neuroectodermal origin, in which a number of nuclei form a ring from which neurofibrils extend to interlace in the center.

ros·in (rŏz′ĭn) *n.* A translucent yellowish to dark brown resin derived from the stumps or sap of various pine trees and used as an adhesive in plasters and as a stimulant in ointments.

Ross (rôs), **Sir Ronald** 1857–1932. British physician. He won a 1902 Nobel Prize for proving that malaria is transmitted to humans by the bite of the mosquito.

Ros·so·li·mo's reflex (rŏs′ə-lē′mōz) *n.* **1.** Flexion of the toes in response to flicking the tips of the underside of the toes, indicative of lesions of the pyramidal tracts. **2.** Flexion of the fingers in response to tapping the tips of the fingers on their volar surfaces. Also called *Rossolimo's sign.*

Ross River virus *n.* A mosquito-borne alphavirus that causes epidemic polyarthritis.

ros·tel·lum (rŏ-stĕl′əm) *n.,* pl. **ros·tel·la** (rŏ-stĕl′ə) A small beaklike part, such as the hooked projection on the head of a tapeworm.

ros·trad (rŏs′trăd′) *adv.* In a direction toward the rostrum or snout end of an organism. —*adj.* Situated nearer the rostrum of an organism when compared with the position of something else.

ros·trate (rŏs′trāt′, -trĭt) *adj.* Having a beaklike part.

ros·trum (rŏs′trəm) *n.,* pl. **–trums** or **–tra** (-trə) A beaklike or snoutlike projection. —**ros′tral** (-trəl) *adj.*

ro·su·va·stat·in calcium (rŏ-sŏŏ′və-stăt′n) *n.* A statin drug used to treat hyperlipidemia.

ro·ta·ry joint (rō′tə-rē) *or* **ro·ta·to·ry joint** (rō′tə-tôr′ē) *n.* See **trochoid joint.**

ro·ta·tion (rō-tā′shən) *n.* **1.** The act or process of turning around a center or an axis. **2.** Regular and uniform variation in a sequence or series, as in the recurrence of symptoms of a disease.

ro·ta·tion·al nystagmus (rō-tā′shə-nəl) *n.* A jerky nystagmus arising from stimulation of the labyrinth of the ear by rotation of the head around any axis and induced by change of motion.

rotation flap *n.* A pedicle flap rotated from the donor site to an adjacent recipient area, usually as a direct flap.

ro·ta·tor (rō′tā′tər) *n.* A muscle that serves to rotate a part of the body.

rotator cuff *n.* A set of muscles and tendons that secures the arm to the shoulder joint and permits rotation of the arm. Also called *musculotendinous cuff.*

rotator muscle *n.* Any of a number of short transversospinal muscles chiefly developed in cervical, lumbar, and thoracic regions, arising from the transverse process of one vertebra and inserted into the root of the spinous process of the next two or three vertebrae above, with nerve supply from the dorsal branches of the spinal nerve, and whose actions rotate the vertebral column.

ro·ta·to·ry (rō′tə-tôr′ē) *adj.* **1.** Of, relating to, causing, or characterized by rotation. **2.** Occurring or proceeding in alternation or succession.

ro·ta·to·ry nystagmus (rō′tə-tôr′ē) *n.* A slight movement of the eyes around the visual axis.

ro·ta·vi·rus (rō′tə-vī′rəs) *n.,* pl. **–rus·es** Any of a group of wheel-shaped RNA viruses of the family Reoviridae, including the human gastroenteritis viruses that cause infant diarrhea. Also called *gastroenteritis virus type B.*

rote learning (rōt) *n.* Learning or memorization by repetition, often without an understanding of the reasoning or relationships involved in the material that is learned.

Roth·mund's syndrome (rôth′məndz, rōt′mŏŏnts) *n.* An inherited syndrome characterized by atrophy, pigmentation, and telangiectasia of the skin, and usually accompanied by juvenile cataract, saddle nose, congenital bone defects, disturbance of hair growth, and hypogonadism.

Roth's spots (rōts) *pl.n.* Round white spots surrounded by hemorrhage, observed in the retina in some cases of bacterial endocarditis.

ro·to·sco·li·o·sis (rō′tō-skō′lē-ō′sĭs, -skŏl′ē-) *n.* Curvature of the vertebral column resulting from the column turning on its axis.

ro·to·tome (rō′tə-tōm′) *n.* A rotating cutting instrument used in arthroscopic surgery.

Rou·get cell (rŏŏ-zhā′) *n.* Any of numerous branching contractile cells on an external capillary wall.

rough·age (rŭf′ĭj) *n.* See **fiber** (sense 5).

rou·leaux formation (rŏŏ-lō′) *n.* A stacklike arrangement of red blood cells in blood or in diluted suspensions of blood in which their biconcave surfaces are next to each other.

round atelectasis (round) *n.* See **folded lung syndrome.**

round foramen *n.* An opening in the greater wing of the sphenoid bone, transmitting the maxillary nerve.

round ligament of femur *n.* See **ligament of head of femur.**

round ligament of liver *n.* The fibrous cord that remains after the fetal umbilical vein is obliterated.

round ligament of uterus *n.* A fibromuscular band attached to the uterus on either side in front of and below the opening of the fallopian tube and passing through the inguinal canal to the labia majora.

round pronator muscle *n.* A muscle whose superficial head has origin from the humerus and whose deep head has origin from the ulna, with insertion into the radius, with nerve supply from the median nerve, and whose action pronates the forearm.

round-shouldered *adj.* Having the shoulders and upper back rounded.

round window *n.* An opening on the medial wall of the middle ear that leads into the cochlea and is covered by the secondary tympanic membrane. Also called *fenestra of cochlea.*

round·worm (round′wûrm′) *n.* See **nematode.**

Rous (rous), **Francis Peyton** 1879–1970. American pathologist. He shared a 1966 Nobel Prize for his discovery of tumor-producing viruses.

Rous-associated virus *n. Abbr.* **RAV** A helper virus that mixes phenotypically with a defective noninfectious strain of Rous sarcoma virus.

Rous sarcoma virus *n.* An avian retrovirus that causes Rous sarcoma.

Roux (rŏŏ), **Pierre Paul Émile** 1853–1933. French bacteriologist. His work with the diphtheria bacillus led to the development of antitoxins to neutralize pathogenic toxins.

Roux, Wilhelm 1850–1924. German anatomist who is noted for his research on embryonic development.

Roux-en-Y gastric bypass (rŏŏ′ĕn-wī′) *n.* A Y-shaped surgical connection that divides the small intestine and connects one end to the stomach, bile duct, or other structure and connects the opposite end to the small intestine at a point below the first connection. Also called *Roux-en-Y anastomosis.*

Row·a·sa (rō-ā′sə) A trademark for the drug mesalamine.

RPh *abbr.* Registered Pharmacist

R plasmid *n.* See **resistance plasmid.**

rpm *abbr.* revolutions per minute

RPR test *n.* See **rapid plasma reagin test.**

RQ *abbr.* respiratory quotient

–rrhagia *suff.* An abnormal or excessive flow or discharge: *menorrhagia.*

–rrhaphy *suff.* Surgical suture: *aneurysmorrhaphy.*

–rrhea *suff.* Flow; discharge: *seborrhea.*

rRNA (är′är′ĕn-ā′) *n.* The RNA that is a permanent structural part of a ribosome. Also called *ribosomal RNA.*

RSI *abbr.* repetitive strain injury

RSV *abbr.* respiratory syncytial virus

RT *abbr.* respiratory therapy

Ru The symbol for the element **ruthenium.**

RU 486 (är′yо̄о̄ fôr′ā-tē-sĭks′) *n.* A drug that chemically terminates a pregnancy. Also called *mifepristone.*

rub (rŭb) *n.* **1.** The application of friction and pressure. **2.** Such a procedure applied to the body.

rub·ber-bulb syringe (rŭb′ər-bŭlb′) *n.* A syringe with a hollow rubber bulb and a cannula provided with a check valve, used to obtain a jet of air or water.

rub·bing alcohol (rŭb′ĭng) *n.* A mixture usually consisting of 70 percent isopropyl or absolute alcohol, applied externally to relieve muscle and joint pain.

ru·be·do (rо̄о̄-bē′dō) *n.* A temporary redness of the skin.

ru·be·fa·cient (rо̄о̄′bə-fā′shənt) *adj.* Producing redness, as of the skin. —*n.* A substance that irritates the skin, causing redness. —**ru′be·fac′tion** (-făk′shən) *n.*

ru·bel·la (rо̄о̄-bĕl′ə) *n.* A mild contagious eruptive disease that is caused by the rubella virus and is capable of producing congenital defects in infants born to mothers infected during the first three months of pregnancy. Also called *epidemic roseola, German measles, three-day measles.*

rubella HI test *n.* A hemagglutination inhibition test for rubella in which the presence of hemagglutination inhibition titer in the absence of disease indicates previous infection and therefore immunity to reinfection.

rubella virus *n.* An RNA virus of the genus *Rubivirus* that causes rubella. Also called *German measles virus.*

rubella virus vaccine *n.* A vaccine containing live attenuated rubella virus prepared in duck embryo or human diploid cell culture and administered as a single subcutaneous injection to immunize against rubella.

ru·be·o·la (rо̄о̄-bē′ə-lə, rо̄о̄′bē-ō′lə) *n.* See **measles** (sense 1). —**ru·be′o·lar** *adj.*

rubeola virus *n.* See **measles virus.**

ru·be·o·sis (rо̄о̄′bē-ō′sĭs) *n.* A condition characterized by reddish discoloration, as of the skin.

rubeosis i·ri·dis di·a·bet·i·ca (ī′rĭ-dĭs dī′ə-bĕt′ĭ-kə) *n.* Neovascularization of the anterior surface of the iris of the eye, seen in chronic severe diabetes.

ru·bes·cent (rо̄о̄-bĕs′ənt) *adj.* Turning red; reddening.

ru·bid·i·um (rо̄о̄-bĭd′ē-əm) *n.* *Symbol* **Rb** A soft metallic element of the alkali group. Atomic number 37.

Ru·bin test (rо̄о̄′bĭn) *n.* A test of patency of the fallopian tubes using carbon dioxide gas passed through a cannula into the cervix.

Ru·bi·vi·rus (rо̄о̄′bə-vī′rəs) *n.* A virus genus of the family Togaviridae that includes the rubella virus.

ru·bor (rо̄о̄′bôr′) *n.* Redness, especially as a sign of inflammation.

ru·bre·dox·in (rо̄о̄′brĭ-dok′sĭn) *n.* A protein that displays electron-carrier abilities and is associated with oxidation-reduction reactions in certain bacteria and cells.

ru·bri·blast (rо̄о̄′brə-blăst′) *n.* See **pronormoblast.**

ru·bri·cyte (rо̄о̄′brĭ-sīt′) *n.* A normoblast having a polychromatic appearance.

ru·bro·spi·nal decussation (rо̄о̄′brō-spī′nəl) *n.* See **tegmental decussation** (sense 2).

ru·di·ment (rо̄о̄′də-mənt) *n.* **1.** An imperfectly or incompletely developed organ or part. **2.** Something in an incipient or undeveloped form. Often used in the plural.

ru·di·men·ta·ry (rо̄о̄′də-mĕn′tə-rē, -mĕn′trē) *adj.* **1.** Being imperfectly or incompletely developed; embryonic. **2.** Being in the earliest stages of development; incipient.

Ruf·fi·ni's corpuscle (rə-fē′nēz, rо̄о̄-) *n.* Any of numerous sensory end organs in the subcutaneous connective tissues of the fingers, consisting of an ovoid capsule within which the sensory fiber ends with numerous collateral knobs.

ru·fous (rо̄о̄′fəs) *adj.* Strong yellowish pink to moderate orange; reddish.

ru·ga (rо̄о̄′gə) *n., pl.* **–gae** (-gē′, -gī′) A fold, crease, or wrinkle, as in the lining of the stomach. Often used in the plural. —**ru′gate′** (-gāt′) *adj.*

ru·gine (rо̄о̄-zhēn′) *n.* See **raspatory.**

ru·gose (rо̄о̄′gōs′) *or* **ru·gous** (-gəs) *adj.* Having many wrinkles or creases; ridged or wrinkled.

ru·gos·i·ty (rо̄о̄-gŏs′ĭ-tē) *n.* The state or condition of being rugose.

RUL *abbr.* right upper lobe (of the lung)

rule (rо̄о̄l) *n.* **1.** A usual, customary, or generalized course of action or behavior. **2.** A generalized statement that describes what is true in most or all cases; a standard.

rule of bigeminy *n.* A rule stating that a ventricular premature heartbeat will follow the heartbeat that terminates a long cardiac cycle.

rule of outlet *n.* A rule for determining whether the pelvic outlet will allow the passage of a normal-sized fetus by calculating whether the sum of the posterior sagittal diameter and the transverse diameter of the outlet equal at least 15 centimeters.

ru·mi·nant (rо̄о̄′mə-nənt) *n.* Any of various hoofed, even-toed, usually horned mammals of the suborder Ruminantia, such as cattle, sheep, goats, deer, and giraffes, characteristically having a stomach divided into four compartments and chewing a cud consisting of regurgitated, partially digested food.

ru·pi·a (rо̄о̄′pē-ə) *pl.n.* **1.** Ulcers that develop in late secondary syphilis and are covered with yellowish or brown crusts. **2.** See **yaws.** —**ru′pi·al** *adj.*

rup·ture (rŭp′chər) *n.* **1.** The process of breaking open or bursting. **2.** A hernia, especially of the groin or intestines. **3.** A tear in an organ or a tissue. —*v.* To break open; burst.

rup·tured disk (rŭp′chərd) *n.* See **herniated disk.**

RUQ *abbr.* right upper quadrant (of the abdomen)

ru·ral leishmaniasis (rŏŏr′əl) *n.* See **zoonotic cutaneous leishmaniasis.**

Rush (rŭsh), **Benjamin** 1745–1813. American physician, politician, and educator. A signer of the Declaration of Independence, he promoted the humane treatment of the mentally ill.

Rus·sell body (rŭs′əl) *n.* A small spherical intracytoplasmic hyaline body common in plasma cells in chronic inflammation.

Rus·sell's sign (rŭs′əlz) *n.* An indication of bulimia in which abrasions and scars occur on the back of the hands as a result of manual attempts to induce vomiting.

Russell's syndrome *n.* Failure of infants and young children to thrive due to brain lesions in the region above the sella turcica, characterized by emaciation and loss of body fat.

Russell's viper venom *n.* A venom used as a coagulant in the arrest of hemorrhage from accessible sites in hemophilia.

rust (rŭst) *n.* Any of a group of parasitic fungi of the order Uredinales that are plant pathogens, especially of cereal grains, and that can produce allergy in humans when inhaled in large numbers.

rust·y sputum (rŭs′tē) *n.* A reddish-brown, bloodstained expectoration found in lobar pneumonia.

ru·the·ni·um (rōō-thē′nē-əm) *n. Symbol* **Ru** A hard acid-resistant metallic element that is found in platinum ores. Atomic number 44.

ruth·er·ford (rŭth′ər-fərd) *n.* A unit expressing the rate of decay of radioactive material, equal to one million disintegrations per second.

Ruth·er·ford (rŭth′ər-fərd, rŭth′-), **Ernest** First Baron Rutherford of Nelson. 1871–1937. New Zealand-born British physicist who classified radiation into alpha, beta, and gamma types and discovered the atomic nucleus. He won the 1908 Nobel Prize in chemistry.

ruth·er·for·di·um (rŭth′ər-fər′dē-əm) *n. Symbol* **Rf** A radioactive synthetic element whose longest-lived isotopes haved mass numbers of 253, 255, 257, and 259 with half-lives of 1.8, 1.6, 4.7, and 3.4 seconds. Atomic number 104.

ru·ti·do·sis (rōō′tĭ-dō′sĭs) *n.* See **rhytidosis** (sense 2).

Ruysch's membrane (roi′sĭz) *n.* See **choriocapillary layer.**

Ruysch's muscle *n.* The muscular tissue of the fundus of the uterus.

RV *abbr.* residual volume

RVH *abbr.* right ventricular hypertrophy

R wave *n.* The initial positive or upward deflection of the QRS complex in the electrocardiogram.

Rx The symbol for prescription or treatment.

S

σ **1.** The Greek letter *sigma*. Entries beginning with this character are alphabetized under **sigma. 2.** The symbol for **reflection coefficient. 3.** The symbol for **standard deviation.**

s *abbr. Latin* semis (half); *Latin* sinister (left)

S The symbol for the element **sulfur.**

S-A *abbr.* sinoatrial

sa·ber shin (sā′bər) *n.* A sharp-edged anteriorly convex tibia characteristic of congenital syphilis.

saber tibia *n.* Deformity of the tibia occurring in tertiary syphilis or yaws, characterized by a marked forward convexity as a result of gumma formation and periostitis.

Sa·bi·a virus (sā′bē-ə) *n.* An arbovirus having an incubation period of about 12 days and causing fever, rashes, and other infectionlike symptoms as well as hemorrhagic bleeding from internal organs, mouth, nose, and other mucous membranes.

Sa·bin (sā′bĭn), **Albert Bruce** 1906–1993. American microbiologist and physician who developed a live-virus vaccine against polio (1957), replacing the killed-virus vaccine invented by Jonas Salk.

Sabin, Florence Rena 1871–1953. American pioneer anatomist noted for her investigations of the lymphatic system. She was the first woman elected to the National Academy of Sciences (1925).

Sabin vaccine *n.* An oral vaccine that contains live attenuated polioviruses and is used to confer immunity against poliomyelitis.

sab·u·lous (săb′yə-ləs) *or* **sab·u·lose** (-lōs′) *adj.* Gritty; sandy.

sac (săk) *n.* **1.** A pouch or bursa. **2.** An encysted abscess at the root of a tooth. **3.** The capsule of a tumor or the envelope of a cyst.

sac·cade (să-käd′, sə-) *n.* A rapid intermittent eye movement, as that which occurs when the eyes fix on one point after another in the visual field. —**sac·cad′ic** (-kä′dĭk) *adj.*

sac·cate (săk′āt′) *adj.* **1.** Shaped like a pouch or sac. **2.** Having a pouch or sac.

sac·cha·rase (săk′ə-rās′, -rāz′) *n.* See **invertase.**

sac·char·ic acid (sə-kăr′ĭk) *n.* A white crystalline acid that is formed by the oxidation of glucose, sucrose, or starch.

sac·cha·ride (săk′ə-rīd′) *n.* Any of a series of compounds of carbon, hydrogen, and oxygen in which the atoms of the latter two elements are in the ratio of 2:1.

sac·cha·rif·er·ous (săk′ə-rĭf′ər-əs) *adj.* Producing sugar.

sac·cha·rin (săk′ər-ĭn) *n.* A white crystalline powder having a taste about 500 times sweeter than cane sugar, used as a calorie-free sweetener. Also called *benzosulfimide.*

sac·cha·rine (săk′ər-ĭn, -ə-rēn′, -ə-rīn′) *adj.* Of, relating to, or characteristic of sugar or saccharin; sweet.

saccharo– *or* **sacchar–** *pref.* Sugar: *saccharide.*

sac·cha·ro·lyt·ic (săk′ə-rō-lĭt′ĭk) *adj.* Capable of hydrolyzing or otherwise metabolizing a sugar molecule resulting in the production of energy.

sac·cha·ro·me·tab·o·lism (săk′ə-rō-mǐ-tăb′ə-lĭz′əm) *n.* The cellular process by which sugar is metabolized. —**sac′cha·ro·met′a·bol′ic** (-mĕt′ə-bŏl′ĭk) *adj.*

sac·cha·rum (săk′ə-rəm) *n.* Sucrose.

sac·ci·form (săk′sə-fôrm′) *adj.* Sacculate.

saccular aneurysm *or* **sacculated aneurysm** *n.* A saclike bulging on one side of an artery.

saccular gland *n.* An alveolar gland.

saccular nerve *n.* A branch of the vestibular nerve that innervates the sensory receptor in the wall of the saccule.

sac·cu·late (săk′yə-lāt′) *or* **sac·cu·lat·ed** (-lā′tĭd) *or* **sac·cu·lar** (-lər) *adj.* Formed of or divided into a series of saclike dilations or pouches.

sac·cu·la·tion (săk′yə-lā′shən) *n.* **1.** A structure formed by a group of sacs. **2.** The formation of a sac or pouch.

sac·cule (săk′yōōl) *or* **sac·cu·lus** (-yə-ləs) *n., pl.* **sac·cules** *or* **sac·cu·li** (săk′yə-lī′) **1.** A small sac. **2.** The smaller of two membranous sacs in the vestibule of the inner ear.

saccule of larynx *n.* A small pouch extending upward from the laryngeal cavity between the vestibular fold and the lamina of the thyroid cartilage.

sac·cu·lo·coch·le·ar (săk′yə-lō-kŏk′lē-ər, -kō′klē-) *adj.* Relating to the sacculus and the membranous cochlea.

sac·cus (săk′əs) *n., pl.* **sac·ci** (săk′ī, săk′sī) A sac.

sacr– *pref.* Variant of **sacro–.**

sa·crad (sā′krăd) *adv.* Toward the sacrum.

sa·cral (sā′krəl) *adj.* In the region of or relating to the sacrum.

sacral artery *n.* **1.** An artery that is one of two arteries that arise from the internal iliac artery and supplies the muscles and skin in that area and sends branches into the sacral canal; lateral sacral artery. **2.** An artery with origin in the back of the abdominal aorta, with distribution to the lower lumbar vertebrae, sacrum, and coccyx; and with anastomoses to the lateral sacral, superior and middle rectal arteries; median sacral artery.

sacral canal *n.* The continuation of the vertebral canal in the sacrum.

sacral crest *n.* Any of five rough irregular ridges on the posterior surface of the sacrum.

sacral flexure *n.* See **caudal flexure.**

sacral foramen *n.* Any of the openings between the fused vertebrae of the sacrum transmitting the sacral nerves.

sacral ganglion *n.* Any of three or four ganglions on either side that constitute the pelvic portion of the sympathetic trunk with the coccygeal ganglion and the connecting cords.

sa·cral·gia (sā-krăl′jə) *n.* Pain in the sacral region. Also called *sacrodynia.*

sa·cral·i·za·tion (sā′krə-lĭ-zā′shən) *n.* A developmental abnormality in which the first sacral vertebra becomes fused with the fifth lumbar veterbra.

sacral nerve *n.* Any of five nerves emerging from the sacral foramina: the first three enter into the formation of the sacral plexus, and the second two into the coccygeal plexus.

sacral plexus *n.* A plexus formed by the fourth and fifth lumbar nerves and by the first, second, and third sacral nerves, lying on the posterior wall of the pelvis and supplying the lower limbs.

sacral splanchnic nerve *n.* Any of the branches from the sacral sympathetic trunk that pass to the inferior hypogastric plexus.

sa·crec·to·my (sā-krĕk′tə-mē) *n.* Resection of a portion of the sacrum.

sacro– *or* **sacr–** *pref.* Sacrum: *sacroiliac.*

sac·ro·an·te·ri·or position (săk′rō-ăn-tîr′ē-ər, sā′krō-) *n.* A breech presentation of the fetus with the sacrum directed toward either the left or right front quarter of the mother's pelvis.

sac·ro·coc·cyg·e·al (săk′rō-kŏk-sĭj′ē-əl, sā′krō-) *adj.* Of, relating to, or affecting the sacrum and coccyx.

sacrococcygeal muscle *n.* An inconstant and poorly developed muscle on the dorsal and ventral surfaces of the sacrum and the coccyx.

sa·cro·dyn·i·a (sā′krō-dĭn′ē-ə, săk′rō-) *n.* See **sacralgia.**

sac·ro·il·i·ac (săk′rō-ĭl′ē-ăk′, sā′krō-) *adj.* Of, relating to, or affecting the sacrum and ilium and their articulation or associated ligaments. —*n.* The sacroiliac region or cartilage.

sac·ro·lum·bar (săk′rō-lŭm′bər, -bär′, sā′krō-) *adj.* Lumbosacral.

sac·ro·pos·te·ri·or position (săk′rō-pŏ-stîr′ē-ər, -pō-, sā′krō-) *n.* A breech presentation of the fetus with the sacrum directed toward either the left or right rear quarter of the mother's pelvis.

sac·ro·sci·at·ic (săk′rō-sī-ăt′ĭk, sā′krō-) *adj.* Of, relating to, or affecting the sacrum and ischium.

sac·ro·spi·nal (săk′rō-spī′nəl, sā′krō-) *adj.* Of, relating to, or affecting the sacrum and the spinal column above it.

sac·ro·trans·verse position (săk′rō-trănz-vûrs′, -trăns-, -trănz′vûrs′, -trăns′-, sā′krō-) *n.* A breech presentation with the fetal sacrum pointing to the right or left iliac fossa of the mother's pelvis.

sac·ro·ver·te·bral (săk′rō-vûr′tə-brəl, -vər-tē′brəl, sā′-krō-) *adj.* Of, relating to, or affecting the sacrum and the vertebrae above it.

sa·crum (sā′krəm, săk′rəm) *n., pl.* **sa·cra** (sā′krə, săk′-rə) The triangular segment of the spinal column that forms part of the pelvis and closes in the pelvic girdle posteriorly, is formed between the ages of 16 and 25 by the fusion of five originally separate sacral vertebrae, and articulates with the last lumbar vertebra, the coccyx, and the hipbone on either side.

SAD *abbr.* seasonal affective disorder

sad·dle (săd′l) *n.* A structure shaped like a saddle.

saddle back *n.* See **lordosis.**

saddle block anesthesia *n.* A form of spinal anesthesia limited in area to the buttocks, perineum, and inner surfaces of the thighs.

saddle embolus *n.* A large embolism that straddles the arterial bifurcation and thus blocks both branches.

saddle head *n.* See **clinocephaly.**

saddle joint *n.* A biaxial joint in which the double motion is effected by the opposition of two surfaces, each of which is concave in one direction and convex in the other, as in the carpometacarpal articulation of the thumb.

saddle nose *n.* A nose having a markedly depressed bridge.

sa·dism (sā′dĭz′əm, săd′ĭz′-) *n.* **1.** The act or an instance of deriving sexual gratification from infliction of pain on others. **2.** A psychosexual disorder in which sexual gratification is derived from infliction of pain on others. —**sa′dist** *n.* —**sa·dis′tic** (sə-dĭs′tĭk) *adj.*

sa·do·mas·o·chism (sā′dō-măs′ə-kĭz′əm, săd′ō-) *n.* A psychosexual disorder in which sexual gratification is obtained by engaging in sadistic and masochistic interactions. —**sa′do·mas′o·chist** *n.* —**sa′do·mas′o·chis′-tic** *adj.*

Sae·misch's operation (sā′mĭsh′ĭz) *n.* Incision of the cornea to evacuate pus.

Saemisch's section *n.* A treatment for hypopyon in which the cornea is transfixed beneath an ulcer and then cut from within outward through the base.

Saeng·er's sign (zĕng′ərz) *n.* An indication of cerebral syphilis in which the loss of the light reflex of the pupil returns after a short time in the dark.

safe period (sāf) *n.* The period in the menstrual cycle when conception is least likely, typically from ten days before to ten days after the onset of menstruation.

safe sex *n.* Sexual activity in which safeguards, such as the use of a condom, are taken to avoid acquiring or spreading a sexually transmitted disease.

safe·ty lens (sāf′tē) *n.* A lens that meets government specifications for impact resistance.

saf·ra·nine (săf′rə-nēn′, -nĭn) *or* **saf·ra·nin** (-nĭn) *n.* Any of a family of dyes based on phenazine, used in the textile industry and as a biological stain.

sag·it·tal (săj′ĭ-tl) *adj.* **1.** Of or relating to the suture uniting the two parietal bones of the skull. **2.** Of or relating to the sagittal plane.

sagittal axis *n.* **1.** The optic axis. **2.** The line around which the working condyle rotates in the frontal plane during mandibular movement.

sagittal plane *n.* A longitudinal plane that divides the body of a bilaterally symmetrical animal into right and left sections.

sagittal suture *n.* A line of union between the two parietal bones. Also called *interparietal suture.*

sa·go spleen (sā′gō) *n.* Amyloidosis in the spleen affecting chiefly the malpighian bodies.

Saint An·tho·ny's fire (sānt ăn′thə-nēz) *n.* See **erysipelas.**

Saint John's wort (jŏnz) *n.* Any of various herbs or shrubs of the genus *Hypericum,* having yellow flowers and used in alternative medicine as a treatment for mild depression.

Saint Lou·is encephalitis (lōō′ĭs) *n.* A viral encephalitis occurring in parts of North America and transmitted by a mosquito of the genus *Culex.*

Saint Louis encephalitis virus *n.* An arbovirus that causes Saint Louis encephalitis and is transmitted by a mosquito.

Saint's triad (sānts) *n.* The concurrence of hiatal hernia, diverticulosis, and cholelithiasis.

Saint Vi·tus' dance *or* **Saint Vi·tus's dance** (vī′təs, -tə-sīz) *n.* See **Sydenham's chorea**.

sal (săl) *n.* Salt.

sa·laam convulsion (sə-läm′) *n.* See **nodding spasm** (sense 2).

sal·bu·ta·mol (săl-byōō′tə-môl′, -mōl′) *n.* A sympathomimetic agent used as a bronchodilator, especially in the treatment of asthma.

sali– *pref.* Salt: *salicylate.*

sal·i·cyl·a·mide (săl′ĭ-sĭl′ə-mīd′) *n.* The amide of salicylic acid, similar in action to aspirin, and used as an analgesic, antipyretic, and antiarthritic.

sa·lic·y·late (sə-lĭs′ə-lāt′, -lĭt, săl′ĭ-sĭl′ĭt) *n.* A salt or ester of salicylic acid.

sal·i·cyl·ic acid (săl′ĭ-sĭl′ĭk) *n.* A white crystalline acid used in making aspirin and in the topical treatment of skin conditions such as eczema.

sal·i·cyl·ism (săl′ĭ-sə-lĭz′əm) *n.* A toxic syndrome caused by excessive doses of salicylic acid or any of the salicylates.

sal·i·fi·a·ble (săl′ə-fī′ə-bəl) *adj.* Capable of being made into a salt. Used of a base that combines with acids to make salts.

sa·line (sā′lēn′, -līn′) *adj.* **1.** Of, relating to, or containing salt; salty. **2.** Of or relating to chemical salts. —*n.* **1.** A salt of magnesium or of the alkalis, used in medicine as a cathartic. **2.** A saline solution, especially one that is isotonic to blood.

saline agglutinin *n.* An antibody that causes agglutination of Rh-positive red blood cells when they are suspended either in saline or in a protein medium. Also called *complete antibody.*

saline solution *n.* A solution of any salt, usually an isotonic sodium chloride solution. Also called *salt solution.*

sa·li·va (sə-lī′və) *n.* The watery mixture of secretions from the salivary and oral mucous glands that lubricates chewed food, moistens the oral walls, and contains ptyalin.

sal·i·vant (săl′ə-vănt′, -vənt) *adj.* Causing or producing a flow of saliva. —*n.* An agent that increases the flow of saliva.

sal·i·var·y (săl′ə-vĕr′ē) *adj.* **1.** Of, relating to, or producing saliva. **2.** Of or relating to a salivary gland.

salivary digestion *n.* Conversion of starch into sugar by the action of salivary amylase.

salivary duct *n.* An intralobular duct found in salivary glands and involved in the production and transport of their secretions. Also called *secretory duct.*

salivary fistula *n.* An opening between a salivary duct or gland and the skin surface or the oral cavity.

salivary gland *n.* A exocrine gland that secretes saliva, especially any of major salivary glands or minor salivary glands.

sal·i·vate (săl′ə-vāt′) *v.* **1.** To secrete or produce saliva. **2.** To produce excessive salivation in.

sal·i·va·tion (săl′ə-vā′shən) *n.* **1.** The act or process of secreting saliva. **2.** See **ptyalism.**

sal·i·va·tor (săl′ə-vā′tər) *n.* An agent that increases the flow of saliva.

Salk (sôlk), **Jonas** 1914–1995. American microbiologist who developed (1954) the first effective killed-virus vaccine against polio.

Salk vaccine *n.* A vaccine containing inactivated polioviruses, used to immunize against poliomyelitis.

sal·low (săl′ō) *adj.* Of a sickly yellowish hue or complexion. —*v.* To make sallow.

sal·me·ter·ol xi·naf·o·ate (săl-mē′tə-rôl′ zĭ-năf′ō-āt′) *n.* An inhalant powder used to treat and prevent bronchospasm in patients with asthma.

sal·mo·nel·la (săl′mə-nĕl′ə) *n., pl.* **–nel·lae** (-nĕl′ē) *or* **–nel·las** *or* **salmonella** Any of various gram-negative, rod-shaped bacteria of the genus *Salmonella,* many of which are pathogenic, causing food poisoning, typhoid, and paratyphoid fever in humans and other infectious diseases in domestic animals.

Salmonella *n.* A genus of aerobic to facultatively anaerobic gram-negative bacteria that are pathogenic in humans and animals.

Salmonella chol·er·ae·su·is (kŏl′ə-rē-sōō′ĭs) *n.* A bacterium occurring in pigs and occasionally causing acute gastroenteritis and enteric fever in humans.

Salmonella en·ter·it·i·dis (ĕn′tə-rĭt′ĭ-dĭs) *n.* Gärtner's bacillus.

Salmonella hirsch·feld·i·i (hərsh-fĕl′dē-ī′) *n.* A bacterium that causes enteric fever in humans.

Salmonella par·a·ty·phi (păr′ə-tī′fī) *n.* A bacterium that causes gastroenteritis and enteric fever.

Salmonella poisoning *n.* Gastroenteritis that is caused by food contaminated with bacteria of the genus *Salmonella* which multiply freely in the gastrointestinal tract but do not produce septicemia. Symptoms include fever, headache, nausea, vomiting, diarrhea, and abdominal pain.

Salmonella schott·mül·ler·i (shôt-myōō′lə-rī′) *n.* A bacterium that causes enteric fever in humans.

Salmonella ty·phi (tī′fī) *n.* Typhoid bacillus.

Salmonella ty·phi·mu·ri·um (tī′fə-myōōr′ē-əm) *n.* A bacterium that causes food poisoning.

Salmonella ty·pho·sa (tī-fō′sə) *n.* Typhoid bacillus.

sal·mo·nel·lo·sis (săl′mə-nĕ-lō′sĭs) *n.* Infection with bacteria of the genus *Salmonella,* characterized by gastroenteritis and fever, and caused especially by eating improperly stored or undercooked foods.

sal·ol (săl′ôl′, -ōl′) *n.* A white crystalline powder derived from salicylic acid and used as an analgesic and antipyretic.

sal·pin·gec·to·my (săl′pĭn-jĕk′tə-mē) *n.* Surgical removal of the fallopian tube. Also called *tubectomy.*

sal·pin·gem·phrax·is (săl′pĭn-jĕm-frăk′sĭs) *n.* Obstruction of a eustachian tube or fallopian tube.

sal·pin·gi·an (săl-pĭn′jē-ən) *adj.* Relating to a fallopian tube or a eustachian tube.

sal·pin·gi·tis (săl′pĭn-jī′tĭs) *n.* Inflammation of a fallopian tube or eustachian tube. —**sal′pin·git′ic** (-jĭt′ĭk) *adj.*

salpingitis isth·mi·ca no·do·sa (ĭs′mĭ-kə nō-dō′sə) *n.* See **adenosalpingitis.**

salpingo– *or* **salping–** *pref.* Salpinx: *salpingitis.*

sal·pin·go·cele (săl-pĭng′gə-sēl′) *n.* Hernia of a fallopian tube.

sal·pin·gog·ra·phy (săl′pĭng-gŏg′rə-fē) *n.* Radiographic visualization of the fallopian tubes after injection of a radiopaque substance.

sal·pin·gol·y·sis (săl′pĭng-gŏl′ĭ-sĭs) *n.* A surgical procedure for freeing a fallopian tube from adhesions.

sal·pin·go-o·o·pho·rec·to·my (săl-pĭng′gō-ō′ə-fə-rĕk′tə-mē) *n.* Surgical removal of an ovary and its fallopian tube.

sal·pin·go-o·o·pho·ri·tis (săl-pĭng′gō-ō′ə-fə-rī′tĭs) *n.* Inflammation of a fallopian tube and its ovary.

sal·pin·go-o·oph·o·ro·cele (săl-pĭng′gō-ō-ŏf′ə-rō-sēl′) *n.* Hernia of an ovary and its fallopian tube.

sal·pin·go·per·i·to·ni·tis (săl-pĭng′gō-pĕr′ĭ-tn-ī′tĭs) *n.* Inflammation of a fallopian tube, the perisalpinx, and the peritoneum.

sal·pin·go·pex·y (săl-pĭng′gə-pĕk′sē) *n.* Surgical fixation of an oviduct.

sal·pin·go·pha·ryn·geal muscle (săl-pĭng′gō-fə-rĭn′-jəl, -făr′ĭn-jē′əl) *n.* A muscle with origin from the medial lamina of the cartilaginous part of the eustachian tube, with insertion into the muscular layer of the pharynx, with nerve supply from the pharyngeal plexus, and whose action assists in elevating the pharynx and in opening the eustachian tube during swallowing.

sal·pin·go·plas·ty (săl-pĭng′gə-plăs′tē) *n.* Plastic surgery on a fallopian tube. Also called *tuboplasty.*

sal·pin·gor·rha·phy (săl′pĭng-gôr′ə-fē) *n.* Suture of a fallopian tube.

sal·pin·gos·to·my (săl′pĭng-gŏs′tə-mē) *n.* Surgical formation of an opening in a fallopian tube whose fimbriated extremity has been closed as a result of inflammation.

sal·pin·got·o·my (săl′pĭng-gŏt′ə-mē) *n.* Incision of a fallopian tube.

sal·pinx (săl′pĭngks) *n.*, *pl.* **sal·pin·ges** (săl-pĭn′jēz) **1.** See **fallopian tube. 2.** See **eustachian tube.**

salt (sôlt) *n.* **1.** A colorless or white crystalline solid, chiefly sodium chloride, used extensively as a food seasoning and preservative. **2.** A chemical compound replacing all or part of the hydrogen ions of an acid with metal ions or electropositive radicals. **3. salts** Any of various mineral salts, such as magnesium sulfate, sodium sulfate, or potassium sodium tartrate, used as laxatives or cathartics. **4. salts** Smelling salts. **5. salts** Epsom salts.

sal·ta·tion (săl-tā′shən, sôl-) *n.* **1.** The act of leaping, jumping, or dancing. **2.** Discontinuous movement, transition, or development; advancement by leaps as of a disease or physiologic function. **3.** A single mutation that drastically alters the phenotype.

sal·ta·to·ry (săl′tə-tôr′ē, sôl′-) *adj.* **1.** Of, relating to, or adapted for leaping or dancing. **2.** Proceeding by leaps rather than by smooth, gradual transitions.

saltatory conduction *n.* A form of nerve impulse conduction in which the impulse jumps from one Ranvier's node to the next, rather than traveling the entire length of the nerve fiber.

saltatory evolution *n.* The theory that the evolution of a new species from an older one may occur as a large jump, such as a major repatterning of chromosomes, rather than by gradual accumulation of small steps or mutations.

saltatory spasm *n.* A spasmodic affliction of the muscles of the lower extremities that causes a person to appear to jump when standing. Also called *static convulsion.*

Sal·ter-Harris classification (sôl′tər-) *n.* The classification of epiphysial fractures into five groups (I to V), according to different prognoses regarding the effects of the injury on subsequent growth and subsequent deformity of the epiphysis.

salt·ing out (sôl′tĭng) *n.* Precipitation, separation, or coagulation of a protein from its solution by saturation or partial saturation with a neutral salt such as sodium chloride or ammonium sulfate.

salt-losing nephritis *n.* A rare disorder that results from renal tubular damage of unknown etiology, and is characterized by abnormal renal loss of sodium chloride.

salt solution *n.* See **saline solution.**

salt substitute *n.* A low-sodium food additive that tastes like salt, such as potassium chloride, and is used as a dietary alternative to salt.

salt wasting *n.* A condition in which there is an inappropriately large renal excretion of salt despite the body's apparent need to retain it.

sa·lu·bri·ous (sə-lōō′brē-əs) *adj.* Conducive or favorable to health or well-being.

sal·u·re·sis (săl′yə-rē′sĭs) *n.* The presence of sodium in the urine.

sal·u·ret·ic (săl′yə-rĕt′ĭk) *adj.* Relating to or causing excretion of salt. —*n.* A drug that promotes excretion of salt in the urine.

sal·u·tar·y (săl′yə-tĕr′ē) *adj.* Favorable to health; wholesome.

Sal·var·san (săl′vər-săn′) A trademark for the drug arsphenamine.

salve (săv, säv) *n.* An analgesic or medicinal ointment. —**salve** *v.*

sa·mar·i·um (sə-mâr′ē-əm, -măr′-) *n. Symbol* **Sm** A metallic rare-earth element used in alloys, in infrared absorbing glass, and as a neutron absorber in certain nuclear reactors. Atomic number 62.

Sam·u·els·son (săm′yōō-əl-sən), **Bengt Ingemar** Born 1934. Swedish physician and biochemist. He shared a 1982 Noble Prize for research on prostaglandins.

SAN *abbr.* sinoatrial node

san·a·tive (săn′ə-tĭv) *adj.* Having the power to cure; healing or restorative.

san·a·to·ri·um (săn′ə-tôr′ē-əm) *or* **san·a·tar·i·um** (-târ′ē-əm) *n.*, *pl.* **–to·ri·ums** *or* **–to·ri·a** (-tôr′ē-ə) *or* **–tar·i·ums** *or* **–tar·i·a** (-târ′ē-ə) **1.** An institution for the treatment of chronic diseases or for medically supervised recuperation. **2.** A resort for improvement or maintenance of health, especially for convalescents. Also called *sanitarium.*

san·a·to·ry (săn′ə-tôr′ē) *adj.* Causing or producing health; curative.

sand (sănd) *n.* Small, loose grains of worn or disintegrated rock.

sand flea *n.* See **chigoe.**

sand fly *n.* Any of various small biting flies of the genus *Phlebotomus* of tropical areas, some of which transmit diseases.

sand·fly fever (sănd′flī′) *n.* See **phlebotomus fever.**

Sand·hoff's disease (sănd′hôfs′) *n.* A form of G_{M2} gangliosidosis that resembles Tay-Sachs disease except that it does not affect persons of Jewish descent, characterized by a defect in the production of two forms of hexosaminidase.

San·dim·mune (săn′dĭ-myoōn′) A trademark for the drug cyclosporine.

sand tumor *n.* See **psammomatous meningioma.**

sane (sān) *adj.* Of sound mind; mentally healthy. —**sane′ness** *n.*

San·fi·lip·po's syndrome (săn′fə-lĭp′ōz) *n.* An inherited disorder of mucopolysaccharide metabolism, characterized by the presence of heparitin sulfate in the urine, enlargement of the liver, severe mental retardation, and, sometimes, skeletal abnormalities. Also called *type III mucopolysaccharidosis.*

Sang·er (săng′ər), **Frederick** Born 1918. British biochemist. He won a 1958 Nobel Prize for determining the order of amino acids in the insulin molecule and shared a 1980 Nobel Prize for developing methods for mapping DNA structure and function.

Sanger, Margaret Higgins 1883–1966. American nurse who campaigned widely for birth control and founded (1929) the organization that became the Planned Parenthood Federation (1942).

san·guic·o·lous (săng-gwĭk′ə-ləs) *adj.* Living in the blood, as certain parasites.

san·gui·fa·ci·ent (săng′gwə-fā′shənt) *adj.* Of or relating to the formation of red blood cells.

san·guif·er·ous (săng-gwĭf′ər-əs) *adj.* Conveying blood.

san·gui·fi·ca·tion (săng′gwə-fĭ-kā′shən) *n.* See **hematopoiesis.**

san·guin·a·rine (săng-gwĭn′ə-rēn′, -rĭn) *n.* An alkaloid obtained from the bloodroot plant, *Sanguinaria canadensis,* used to treat and remove dental plaque.

san·guine (săng′gwĭn) *adj.* **1.** Of a healthy, reddish color; ruddy. **2.** Cheerfully confident; optimistic. **3.** *Archaic* Having blood as the dominant humor in terms of medieval physiology. **4.** *Archaic* Having the temperament and ruddy complexion that was formerly thought to be characteristic of a person dominated by this humor; passionate.

san·guin·e·ous (săng-gwĭn′ē-əs) *adj.* Of or relating to blood; bloody.

sanguino– or **sangui–** or **sanguin–** *pref.* Blood; bloody: *sanguinolent.*

san·guin·o·lent (săng-gwĭn′ə-lənt) *adj.* Mixed or tinged with blood.

san·gui·no·pu·ru·lent (săng′gwə-nō-pyoōr′ə-lənt) *adj.* Containing blood and pus.

san·guiv·o·rous (săng-gwĭv′ər-əs) *adj.* Feeding on blood, as certain bats, leeches, and insects.

sa·ni·es (sā′nē-ēz′) *n., pl.* **sanies** A thin, fetid, blood-tinged fluid consisting of serum and pus discharged from a wound, an ulcer, or a fistula.

sa·ni·o·pu·ru·lent (sā′nē-ō-pyoōr′ə-lənt, -pyoōr′yə-) *adj.* Characterized by bloody pus.

sa·ni·o·se·rous (sā′nē-ō-sîr′əs) *adj.* Characterized by blood-tinged serum.

sa·ni·ous (sā′nē-əs) *adj.* Of or relating to sanies.

san·i·tar·i·an (săn′ĭ-târ′ē-ən) *n.* A public health or sanitation expert.

san·i·tar·i·um (săn′ĭ-târ′ē-əm) *n.* See **sanatorium.**

san·i·tar·y (săn′ĭ-tĕr′ē) *adj.* **1.** Of or relating to health. **2.** Free from elements, such as filth or pathogens, that endanger health; hygienic.

sanitary napkin *n.* A disposable pad of absorbent material worn to absorb menstrual flow.

san·i·ta·tion (săn′ĭ-tā′shən) *n.* **1.** Formulation and application of measures designed to protect public health. **2.** Disposal of sewage.

san·i·ti·za·tion (săn′ĭ-tĭ-zā′shən) *n.* The process of making something sanitary, as by cleaning or disinfecting. —**san′i·tize′** (-tīz′) *v.*

san·i·ty (săn′ĭ-tē) *n.* **1.** The quality or condition of being sane; soundness of mind. **2.** Soundness of judgment or reason.

S-A node *n.* The sinoatrial node.

san·to·nin (săn′tə-nĭn) *n.* A colorless crystalline compound obtained from species of wormwood and used as an anthelmintic.

San·to·ri·ni (săn′tə-rē′nē, sän′tō-), **Giovanni Domenico** 1681–1737. Italian physician and anatomist whose works, especially *Observationes Anatomicae* (1724) are noted for their thorough descriptions and detailed illustrations.

San·to·ri·ni's duct (săn′tə-rē′nēz, sän′-) *n.* See **accessory pancreatic duct.**

sa·phe·na (sə-fē′nə) *n., pl.* **–nae** (-nē′) A saphenous vein.

sa·phe·nous nerve (sə-fē′nəs) *n.* A branch of the femoral nerve that supplies cutaneous branches to the skin of the leg and foot by way of the infrapatellar and medial crural branches.

saphenous vein *n.* Either of two main superficial veins of the leg, one larger than the other, that begin at the foot.

sapo– or **sapon–** *pref.* Soap; soapy: *saponaceous.*

sap·o·na·ceous (săp′ə-nā′shəs) *adj.* Having the qualities of soap.

sa·pon·i·fi·ca·tion (sə-pŏn′ə-fĭ-kā′shən) *n.* A reaction in which an ester is heated with an alkali, such as sodium hydroxide, producing a free alcohol and an acid salt, especially alkaline hydrolysis of a fat or oil to make soap.

sa·pon·i·fy (sə-pŏn′ə-fī′) *v.* To undergo saponification.

sap·o·nin (săp′ə-nĭn, sə-pō′-) *n.* Any of various plant glucosides that form soapy lathers when mixed and agitated with water, used in detergents, foaming agents, and emulsifiers.

sap·phism (săf′ĭz′əm) *n.* Lesbianism.

sa·pre·mi·a or **sa·prae·mi·a** (sə-prē′mē-ə) *n.* Blood poisoning resulting from the absorption of the products of putrefaction.

sapro– or **sapr–** *pref.* **1.** Decay; putrefaction; decomposition: *saprogenic.* **2.** Dead or decaying organic material: *saprophyte.*

sap·robe (săp′rōb′) *n.* An organism that derives its nourishment from nonliving or decaying organic matter. —**sap·ro′bi·al** (să-prō′bē-əl), **sap·ro′bic** (-bĭk) *adj.*

sap·ro·gen (săp′rə-jən, -jĕn′) *n.* An organism that lives on dead organic matter and causes its decay.

sap·ro·gen·ic (săp′rə-jĕn′ĭk) *or* **sa·prog·e·nous** (sə-prŏj′ə-nəs) *adj.* Of, producing, or resulting from putrefaction. —**sap′ro·ge·nic′i·ty** (-jə-nĭs′ĭ-tē) *n.*

sap·ro·phyte (săp′rə-fīt′) *n.* An organism, especially a fungus or bacterium, that grows on and derives its nourishment from dead or decaying organic matter. —**sap′ro·phyt′ic** (-fĭt′ĭk) *adj.*

sap·ro·zo·ic (săp′rə-zō′ĭk) *adj.* **1.** Obtaining nourishment by absorption of dissolved organic and inorganic materials, as occurs in certain protozoa and some fungi. **2.** Feeding on dead or on decaying animal matter.

sap·ro·zo·on·o·sis (săp′rə-zō-ŏn′ə-sĭs, -zō′ə-nō′-) *n.* A zoonosis whose causative agent requires both a vertebrate host and a nonanimal reservoir or developmental site for completion of its life cycle.

sa·quin·a·vir (sə-kwĭn′ə-vîr) *n.* A protease-inhibiting drug usually used in combination with other drugs to suppress the replication of HIV.

sar·al·a·sin acetate (sär-ăl′ə-sĭn) *n.* An angiotensin II derivative that is used in the treatment of essential hypertension.

Sar·ci·na (sär′sə-nə) *n.* A genus of anaerobic grampositive bacteria including both saprophytic and facultatively parasitic species.

sarco– *or* **sarc–** *pref.* **1.** Flesh: *sarcocele.* **2.** Striated muscle: *sarcolemma.*

sar·co·blast (sär′kə-blăst′) *n.* See **myoblast.**

sar·co·car·ci·no·ma (sär′kō-kär′sə-nō′mə) *n.* See **carcinosarcoma.**

sar·co·cele (sär′kə-sēl′) *n.* A fleshy tumor or sarcoma of the testis.

Sar·co·cys·tis (sär′kə-sĭs′tĭs) *n.* A genus of protozoan parasites, related to the sporozoan genera *Eimeria, Isospora,* and *Toxoplasma.*

Sarcocystis hom·i·nis (hŏm′ə-nĭs) *n.* A protozoan that is parasitic in human intestines and is transmitted by eating beef from cattle that have been infected by contact with contaminated human feces.

Sarcocystis su·i·hom·i·nis (soō′ē-hŏm′ə-nĭs) *n.* A widespread protozoan that causes intestinal infections in humans who have eaten pork from pigs that have become infected by contact with contaminated human feces.

Sar·co·di·na (sär′kō-dī′nə, -dē′-) *n.* A superclass of protozoans that includes the rhizopods.

sar·co·din·i·an (sär′kə-dĭn′ē-ən) *adj.* Of or belonging to the superclass Sarcodina.

sar·coid (sär′koid′) *adj.* Of or resembling flesh. —*n.* **1.** A tumor resembling a sarcoma. **2.** See **sarcoidosis.**

sar·coi·dal granuloma (sär-koid′l) *n.* An epithelioid cell granuloma similar to those seen in sarcoidosis, but not causing necrosis.

sar·coid·o·sis (sär′koi-dō′sĭs) *n., pl.* **-ses** (-sēz) A disease of unknown origin marked by formation of granulomatous lesions that appear especially in the liver, lungs, skin, and lymph nodes. Also called *Besnier-Boeck-Schaumann disease, Boeck's disease, Boeck's sarcoid, sarcoid, Schaumann's syndrome.*

sar·co·lac·tic acid (sär′kə-lăk′tĭk) *n.* An isomeric form of lactic acid produced by muscle tissue during the anaerobic metabolism of glucose.

sar·co·lem·ma (sär′kə-lĕm′ə) *n.* A thin membrane enclosing a striated muscle fiber. —**sar′co·lem′mal** *adj.*

sar·co·ma (sär-kō′mə) *n., pl.* **-mas** *or* **-ma·ta** (-mə-tə) A malignant tumor arising from connective tissues. —**sar·co′ma·toid′** (-mə-toid′), **sar·co′ma·tous** (-təs) *adj.*

sar·co·ma·to·sis (sär-kō′mə-tō′sĭs) *n.* Formation of numerous sarcomas in various parts of the body.

sar·co·mere (sär′kə-mîr′) *n.* One of the segments into which a fibril of striated muscle is divided.

sar·co·plasm (sär′kə-plăz′əm) *n.* The cytoplasm of a striated muscle fiber. —**sar′co·plas·mat′ic** (-plăz-măt′ĭk), **sar′co·plas′mic** (-mĭk) *adj.*

sarcoplasmic reticulum *n.* The endoplasmic reticulum found in striated muscle fibers.

sar·co·poi·et·ic (sär′kō-poi-ĕt′ĭk) *adj.* Forming or producing muscle.

Sar·cop·tes (sär-kŏp′tēz) *n.* A genus of acarids that includes the itch mite.

Sarcoptes sca·bi·e·i (skā′bē-ē′ī) *n.* The itch mite, varieties of which affect humans and various animals and cause scabies and mange.

sar·cop·tic (sär-kŏp′tĭk) *adj.* Of, relating to, or caused by mites of the family Sarcoptidae.

sar·cop·tid (sär-kŏp′tĭd) *n.* A mite of the family Sarcoptidae that includes species that are parasitic on the skin of humans and animals.

Sar·cop·ti·dae (sär-kŏp′tĭ-dē) *n.* A family of mites that includes the genus Sarcoptes.

sar·co·sine (sär′kə-sēn′, -sĭn) *n.* An amino acid made synthetically or formed naturally during the decomposition of creatine.

sar·co·si·ne·mi·a (sär′kə-sə-nē′mē-ə) *n.* A hereditary disorder of amino acid metabolism due to deficiency of an enzyme and characterized by elevated levels of sarcosine in blood plasma and excretion of sarcosine in the urine, failure to thrive, irritability, muscle tremors, and retarded motor and mental development. Also called *hypersarcosinemia.*

sar·co·sis (sär-kō′sĭs) *n.* **1.** An abnormal increase of body tissue. **2.** A growth of fleshy tumors. **3.** A diffuse sarcoma involving an entire organ.

sar·co·some (sär′kə-sōm′) *n.* A large specialized mitochondrion found in striated muscle.

sar·cos·to·sis (sär′kŏ-stō′sĭs) *n.* Ossification of muscular tissue.

sar·co·style (sär′kə-stīl′) *n.* See **myofibril.**

sar·cot·ic (sär-kŏt′ĭk) *adj.* **1.** Of or relating to sarcosis. **2.** Causing an increase of body tissue.

sar·co·tu·bules (sär′kō-toō′byoōlz) *pl.n.* Membranous tubules that constitute a continuous system in striated muscle and correspond to the smooth endoplasmic reticulum of other cells.

sar·cous (sär′kəs) *adj.* Of, relating to, or consisting of flesh or muscle tissue.

sar·don·ic grin (sär-dŏn′ĭk) *n.* See **risus caninus.**

SARS *abbr.* severe acute respiratory syndrome

sar·to·ri·us muscle (sär-tôr′ē-əs) *n.* A muscle with origin from the anterior superior spine of the ilium, with insertion into the medial border of the tuberosity of the tibia, with nerve supply from the femoral nerve, and whose action flexes the thigh and leg and rotates the leg medially and the thigh laterally. Also called *tailor's muscle.*

sat. *abbr.* saturate; saturation

sat·el·lite (săt′l-īt′) *n.* **1.** A minor structure accompanying a more important or larger one. **2.** A short segment of a chromosome separated from the rest by a constriction, typically associated with the formation of a nucleolus. **3.** A colony of microorganisms whose growth in culture medium is enhanced by certain substances produced by another colony in its proximity.

satellite abscess *n.* A secondary abscess formed near the primary abscess.

satellite cell *n.* Any of the cells that envelop the bodies of neurons in the peripheral nervous system.

satellite DNA *n.* A portion of DNA in animal cells whose density differs from that of the other DNA, consisting of short, repeating sequences of nucleotide pairs near the region of the centromere.

sat·el·li·to·sis (săt′l-ī-tō′sĭs) *n.* A condition characterized by an accumulation of neuroglia around the neurons of the central nervous system, often followed by neuronophagia.

sa·ti·a·tion (sā′shē-ā′shən) *n.* The state produced by having had a specific need, such as hunger or thirst, fulfilled. —**sa′ti·ate′** *v.*

sat·is·fac·tion (săt′ĭs-făk′shən) *n.* **1.** The fulfillment or gratification of a desire, a need, or an appetite. **2.** The pleasure or contentment that is derived from such gratification.

sat·u·rate (săch′ə-rāt′) *v. Abbr.* **sat. 1.** To imbue or impregnate thoroughly. **2.** To soak, fill, or load to capacity. **3.** To cause a substance to unite with the greatest possible amount of another substance. **4.** To satisfy all the chemical affinities of a substance; neutralize. **5.** To dissolve a substance up to that concentration beyond which the addition of more results in a second phase. —**sat′u·ra·ble** (săch′ər-ə-bəl) *adj.* —**sat′u·ra′tor** *n.*

sat·u·rat·ed (săch′ə-rā′tĭd) *adj.* **1.** Unable to hold or contain more; full. **2.** Soaked with moisture; drenched. **3.** Combined with or containing all the solute that can normally be dissolved at a given temperature. **4.** Having all available valence bonds filled. Used especially of organic compounds.

saturated compound *n.* An organic compound in which all the carbon atoms are connected by single bonds.

saturated fat *n.* A fat, most often of animal origin, having chains of saturated fatty acids. An excess of these fats in the diet is thought to raise the cholesterol level in the bloodstream.

saturated fatty acid *n.* A fatty acid, such as stearic acid, whose carbon chain contains no unsaturated linkages between carbon atoms and hence cannot incorporate any more hydrogen atoms.

sat·u·ra·tion (săch′ə-rā′shən) *n. Abbr.* **sat. 1.** The act or process of saturating. **2.** The condition of being saturated. **3.** The condition of being full to or beyond satisfaction; satiety. **4.** Filling of all the available sites on an enzyme molecule by its substrate, or on a hemoglobin molecule by molecular oxygen or carbon monoxide.

5. In optics, the degree which colors of the same wavelength are differentiated from one another on the basis of purity which correlates with the amount of white present, such as red from pink.

saturation index *n.* An index representing the relative concentration of hemoglobin in the red blood cells.

sat·ur·nine (săt′ər-nīn′) *adj.* **1.** Melancholy or sullen. **2.** Produced by absorption of lead.

sat·urn·ism (săt′ər-nĭz′əm) *n.* See **lead poisoning.**

sa·ty·ri·a·sis (sā′tə-rī′ə-sĭs, săt′ə-) *n.* Excessive, often uncontrollable sexual desire in a man.

sau·cer·i·za·tion (sô′sər-ĭ-zā′shən) *n.* Surgical excavation of tissue to form a shallow depression to facilitate drainage from infected areas of a wound.

Saund·by's test (sônd′bēz) *n.* A test for blood in the stool in which hydrogen peroxide solution is added to a mixture of a saturated benzidine solution and a small quantity of feces in a test tube; a persistent dark-blue color indicates the presence of blood.

sau·sage poisoning (sô′sĭj) *n.* See **allantiasis.**

saw pal·met·to (sô păl-mĕt′ō) *n.* A small creeping palm (*Serenoa repens*) of the southeast United States, whose black, one-seeded fruit is available in dried form as a nonprescription herbal remedy that is supposedly beneficial for disorders of the prostate gland.

sax·i·tox·in (săk′sĭ-tŏk′sĭn) *n.* A potent neurotoxin produced by certain dinoflagellates that accumulates in shellfish feeding on these organisms and consequently causes food poisoning in humans who eat the shellfish.

Sb The symbol for the element **antimony.**

SBE *abbr.* subacute bacterial endocarditis

Sc The symbol for the element **scandium.**

s.c. *abbr. Latin* sub cutem, sub cute; subcutaneous

scab (skăb) *n.* **1.** A crust formed from and covering a healing wound. **2.** Scabies or mange in domestic animals or livestock, especially sheep.

scab·by (skăb′ē) *adj.* **1.** Having, consisting of, or covered with scabs. **2.** Affected with scab or scabies.

sca·bi·cide (skā′bĭ-sīd′) *n.* An agent that kills itch mites. —**sca′bi·cid′al** (-sīd′l) *adj.*

sca·bies (skā′bēz) *n.* **1.** A contagious skin disease caused by *Sarcoptes scabiei* and characterized by intense itching. **2.** A similar disease in animals.

sca·bi·et·ic (skā′bē-ĕt′ĭk) *adj.* Relating to or affected with scabies.

sca·la (skā′lə) *n., pl.* **–lae** (-lē) Any of the spiral cavities of the cochlea winding around the modiolus of the ear.

scala tym·pa·ni (tĭm′pə-nī′) *n.* The division of the spiral canal of the cochlea below the spiral lamina.

scala ves·tib·u·li (vĕ-stĭb′yə-lī′) *n.* The division of the spiral canal of the cochlea above the spiral lamina in the inner ear.

scald (skôld) *v.* To burn with a hot liquid or steam. —*n.* A body injury caused by scalding.

scale¹ (skāl) *n.* **1.** A dry, thin flake of epidermis shed from the skin. **2.** One of the many small, platelike dermal or epidermal structures that characteristically form the external covering of fishes, reptiles, and certain mammals. —*v.* **1.** To come off in scales or layers; flake. **2.** To become encrusted. **3.** To remove tartar from tooth surfaces with a pointed instrument.

scale² (skāl) *n.* **1.** A system of ordered marks at fixed intervals used as a reference standard in measurement. **2.** An instrument or device bearing such marks. **3.** A proportion used in determining the dimensional relationship of a representation to that which it represents. **4.** A standard of measurement or judgment; a criterion.

scale³ (skāl) *n.* **1.** An instrument or a machine that is used for weighing. **2.** Either of the pans, trays, or dishes of a balance.

sca·le·nec·to·my (skā′lə-nĕk′tə-mē) *n.* Resection of the scalene muscles.

sca·lene muscle (skā′lēn′, skā-lēn′) *n.* Any of three muscles on each side of the neck that serve to bend and rotate the neck and that assist breathing by raising or fixing the first two ribs.

sca·le·not·o·my (skā′lə-nŏt′ə-mē) *n.* Surgical division or section of the anterior scalene muscle.

sca·le·nus anterior syndrome (skā-lē′nəs) *n.* A disorder characterized by pain and tingling in the forearm and hand similar to that occurring in cervical rib syndrome, caused by compression of the brachial plexus and subclavian artery against the first thoracic rib by a hypertonic anterior scalene muscle. Also called *scalenus anticus syndrome, Naffziger syndrome.*

scall (skôl, skäl) *or* **scald** (skôld, skäld) *n.* A scaly eruption of the skin or scalp.

scal·lop·ing (skŏl′ə-pĭng, skăl′-) *n.* A series of indentations or erosions on a normally smooth margin of a structure.

scalp (skălp) *n.* The skin covering the top of the head.

scal·pel (skăl′pəl) *n.* A small straight knife with a thin sharp blade used in surgery and dissection.

scal·prum (skăl′prəm) *n.* **1.** A large strong scalpel. **2.** See **raspatory.**

scal·y (skā′lē) *adj.* **1.** Covered or partially covered with scales. **2.** Shedding scales or flakes; flaking.

scan (skăn) *v.* **1.** To move a finely focused beam of light or electrons in a systematic pattern over a surface in order to reproduce or sense and subsequently transmit an image. **2.** To examine a body or a body part with a CAT scanner or similar scanning apparatus. **3.** To search stored computer data automatically for specific data. —*n.* **1.** The act or an instance of scanning. **2.** Examination of a body or body part by a CAT scanner or similar scanning apparatus. **3.** A picture or an image that is produced by this means. —**scan′na·ble** *adj.* —**scan′ner** *n.*

scan·di·um (skăn′dē-əm) *n. Symbol* **Sc** A highly reactive metallic element found in various rare minerals and separated as a byproduct in the processing of certain uranium ores. Atomic number 21.

scan·ning electron microscope (skăn′ĭng) *n. Abbr.* **SEM** An electron microscope that forms a three-dimensional image on a cathode-ray tube by moving a beam of focused electrons across an object and reading both the electrons scattered by the object and the secondary electrons produced by it.

Scan·zo·ni's maneuver (skăn-zō′nēz, skän-tsō′-) *n.* A method of applying an obstetrical forceps to rotate a fetus.

scaph·a (skăf′ə, skā′fə) *n.* **1.** A boat-shaped anatomical structure. **2.** The longitudinal furrow between the helix and the anthelix of the auricle of the ear.

scapho– *pref.* Boat; boat-shaped: *scaphocephalic.*

scaph·o·ce·phal·ic (skăf′ō-sə-făl′ĭk) *or* **scaph·o·ceph·a·lous** (-sĕf′ə-ləs) *adj.* Having an abnormally long, narrow skull.

scaph·oid (skăf′oid′) *adj.* Shaped like a boat; hollow. —*n.* See **navicular.**

scaphoid abdomen *n.* See **navicular abdomen.**

scaphoid scapula *n.* A scapula in which the vertebral border below the level of the spine is concave instead of convex.

scap·u·la (skăp′yə-lə) *n., pl.* **–las** *or* **–lae** (-lē′) Either of two large, flat, triangular bones forming the back part of the shoulder. Also called *shoulder blade.*

scapula a·la·ta (ā-lā′tə) *n.* See **winged scapula.**

scap·u·lar (skăp′yə-lər) *or* **scap·u·lar·y** (-lĕr′ē) *adj.* Of or relating to the shoulder or scapula.

scap·u·lec·to·my (skăp′yə-lĕk′tə-mē) *n.* Surgical removal of the scapula.

scapulo– *pref.* Shoulder: *scapulopexy.*

scap·u·lo·cla·vic·u·lar (skăp′yə-lō-klə-vĭk′yə-lər) *adj.* **1.** Acromioclavicular. **2.** Coracoclavicular.

scap·u·lo·cos·tal syndrome (skăp′yə-lō-kŏs′təl) *n.* Pain in the upper or posterior part of the shoulder radiating into the neck, head, arm, or chest, caused by an abnormal relationship between the scapula and the posterior wall of the thorax.

scap·u·lo·hu·mer·al (skăp′yə-lō-hyōō′mər-əl) *adj.* Of, characterizing, or affecting the scapula and the humerus.

scap·u·lo·pex·y (skăp′yə-lō-pĕk′sē) *n.* Surgical fixation of the scapula to the chest wall or to the spinous process of the vertebrae.

sca·pus (skā′pəs) *n., pl.* **–pi** (-pī) A shaft or stem.

scar (skär) *n.* The fibrous tissue that replaces normal tissue destroyed by injury or disease. —*v.* **1.** To mark with a scar or become marked with a scar. **2.** To form scar.

scar carcinoma *n.* Adenocarcinoma of the lung due to a peripheral lung scar or interstitial fibrosis.

scarf·skin (skärf′skĭn′) *n.* The outermost layer of skin, especially that which forms the cuticle.

scar·i·fi·ca·tion (skăr′ə-fĭ-kā′shən) *n.* The act of making shallow cuts in the skin.

scar·i·fi·ca·tor (skăr′ə-fĭ-kā′tər) *n.* A surgical instrument with several spring-operated lancets, used to scarify the skin.

scar·i·fy (skăr′ə-fī′) *v.* To make shallow cuts in the skin, as when vaccinating.

scar·la·ti·na (skär′lə-tē′nə) *n.* See **scarlet fever.** —**scar′la·ti′nal** *adj.*

scarlatina hem·or·rhag·i·ca (hĕm′ə-răj′ĭ-kə) *n.* Scarlet fever in which blood hemorrhages into the skin and mucous membranes and produces a dusky hue in the eruption.

scar·la·ti·nel·la (skär′lə-tə-nĕl′ə) *n.* See **fourth disease.**

scar·la·ti·ni·form (skär′lə-tē′nə-fôrm, -tĭn′ə-) *adj.* Resembling scarlet fever or its rash.

scar·la·ti·noid (skär′lə-tē′noid′, skär-lăt′n-oid′) *adj.* Scarlatiniform.

scar·let fever (skär′lĭt) *n.* An acute contagious disease caused by a hemolytic streptococcus, occurring predominantly among children and characterized by a scarlet skin eruption and high fever. Also called *scarlatina*.

scarlet fever antitoxin *n.* The antitoxin for the toxins produced by the bacteria that cause scarlet fever.

scarlet red *n.* An azo dye used as an agent to promote the healing of wounds and as a histological stain.

Scar·pa (skär′pə), **Antonio** 1752–1832. Italian anatomist and surgeon known for his studies of the ear and nerves and for his description of atherosclerosis.

Scar·pa's fascia (skär′pəz) *n.* The deeper, membranous or lamellar part of the subcutaneous tissue of the lower abdominal wall.

Scarpa's fluid *n.* See **endolymph.**

Scarpa's foramen *n.* Either of two foramina, designated anterior and posterior, located in the line of the intermaxillary suture, and that transmit the nasopalatine nerves.

Scarpa's membrane *n.* See **secondary tympanic membrane.**

Scarpa's triangle *n.* See **femoral triangle.**

scar tissue *n.* Dense, fibrous connective tissue that forms over a healed wound or cut.

sca·te·mi·a (skă-tē′mē-ə) *n.* Toxemia resulting from the absorption of toxins in the intestines.

scato– *pref.* Excrement: *scatology.*

sca·tol·o·gy (skă-tŏl′ə-jē) *n.* **1.** The study and analysis of feces for physiological and diagnostic purposes. Also called *coprology.* **2.** An obsession with excrement or excretory functions. **3.** The psychiatric study of such an obsession. —**scat′o·log′i·cal** (skăt′l-ŏj′ĭ-kəl), **scat′o·log′ic** (-ĭk) *adj.*

sca·toph·a·gy (skă-tŏf′ə-jē) *n.* The eating of excrement. Also called *coprophagy.*

sca·tos·co·py (skă-tŏs′kə-pē) *n.* Examination of the feces for diagnostic purposes.

scat·ter (skăt′ər) *v.* **1.** To cause to separate and go in different directions. **2.** To separate and go in different directions; disperse. **3.** To deflect radiation or particles. —*n.* The act of scattering or the condition of being scattered.

Sce·do·spor·i·um a·pi·os·per·mum (sē′dō-spôr′ē-əm ā′pē-ŏs′pər-məm) *n.* The imperfect state of the fungus *Pseudallescheria boydii,* one of 16 species of fungi that may cause mycetoma in humans.

Schal·ly (shăl′ē), **Andrew Victor** Born 1926. Polish-born American physiologist. He shared a 1977 Nobel Prize for discovering and synthesizing the hormones that control anterior pituitary hormone secretion.

Scham·berg's disease (shăm′bûrgz′) *n.* See **progressive pigmentary dermatosis.**

Schau·mann's syndrome (shou′mänz′, -mənz) *n.* See **sarcoidosis.**

Scheie's syndrome (shīz) *n.* An inherited syndrome that is a form of Hurler's syndrome and is characterized by corneal clouding and deformity of the hands; stature and intelligence usually remain normal. Also called *type IS mucopolysaccharidosis.*

sche·ma (skē′mə) *n.,* *pl.* **sche·mas** or **sche·ma·ta** (skē-mä′tə, skĭ-măt′ə) **1.** A diagrammatic representation; an outline or a model. **2.** A pattern imposed on complex reality or experience to assist in explaining it, mediate perception, or guide response.

Scheu·er·mann's disease (shoi′ər-mänz′) *n.* Epiphysial aseptic necrosis of vertebral bodies. Also called *osteochondritis deformans juvenilis dorsi.*

Schick test (shĭk) *n.* An intracutaneous test for detecting immunity or susceptibility to diphtheria.

Schick test toxin *n.* The inoculated dose of the toxin produced by *Corynebacterium diphtheriae* and used in the Schick test. Also called *diagnostic diphtheria toxin.*

Schiff's reagent (shĭfs) *n.* A solution of rosaniline and sulfurous acid used to test for aldehydes.

Schil·der's disease (shĭl′dərz) *n.* A degenerative fatal brain disease that is most common in children, characterized by the destruction of myelin in the white matter, progressive dementia, convulsions, failure of hearing, spastic paralysis, and blindness. Also called *encephalitis periaxialis diffusa.*

Schil·ler's test (shĭl′ərz) *n.* A test for cancer of the cervix, in which the cervix is stained with a solution of iodine and potassium iodide and turns dark brown in all noncancerous areas.

Schil·ling's blood count (shĭl′ĭngz) *n.* A method of counting blood cells in which the polymorphonuclear neutrophils are separated into four groups according to the number and the arrangement of the nuclear masses in each cell. Also called *Schilling's index.*

Schil·ling test (shĭl′ĭng) *n.* A test for determining the amount of vitamin B_{12} excreted in the urine, in which vitamin B_{12} tagged with a radioisotope is taken orally and quantified in urine samples.

schin·dy·le·sis (skĭn′də-lē′sĭs) *n.* A fibrous joint in which the sharp edge of one bone is received into a cleft in the edge of the other, as in the articulation of the vomer with the rostrum of the sphenoid. Also called *wedge-and-groove joint, wedge-and-groove suture.*

Schiötz tonometer (shē′ĕts, shyœts) *n.* An instrument that measures ocular tension by indicating the ease with which the cornea is indented.

schisto– *pref.* Split; cleft: *schistocyte.*

schis·to·ce·li·a (shĭs′tə-sē′lē-ə, skĭs′-) *n.* A congenital fissure of the abdominal wall.

schis·to·cor·mi·a (shĭs′tə-kôr′mē-ə, skĭs′-) *n.* A congenital cleft of the trunk, usually accompanied by imperfectly developed lower extremities. Also called *schistosomia.*

schis·to·cyte (shĭs′tə-sīt′, skĭs′-) *n.* A red blood cell having an abnormal shape as a result of fragmentation that occurs as the cell flows through damaged small vessels.

schis·to·cy·to·sis (shĭs′tə-sī-tō′sĭs, skĭs′-) *n.* **1.** The presence or accumulation of schistocytes in the blood. **2.** Fragmentation of a red blood cell.

schis·to·glos·si·a (shĭs′tə-glô′sē-ə, skĭs′-) *n.* A congenital fissure or cleft of the tongue.

Schis·to·so·ma (shĭs′tə-sō′mə, skĭs′-) *n.* A genus of digenetic trematodes that includes the blood flukes of humans and domestic animals that cause schistosomiasis. Also called *Bilharzia.*

Schistosoma hae·ma·to·bi·um (hē′mə-tō′bē-əm) *n.* A parasitic trematode found in the portal system, bladder, and rectum and common throughout Africa and parts of the Middle East. It causes schistosomiasis haematobium.

Schistosoma ja·pon·i·cum (jă-pŏn′ĭ-kəm) *n.* A trematode that causes schistosomiasis japonicum and is found throughout eastern Asia.

Schistosoma man·so·ni (măn-sō′nī) *n.* A trematode that is common in Africa, parts of the Middle East, the West Indies, South America, and certain Caribbean islands and causes schistosomiasis mansoni.

Schistosoma me·kong·i (mā-kông′ī, -kông′gī) *n.* A trematode found in the Mekong delta near Khong Island in southern Laos and northern Cambodia that causes schistosomiasis mekongi.

schis·to·some (shĭs′tə-sōm′, skĭs′-) *n.* Any of several chiefly tropical trematodes of the genus *Schistosoma,* many of which are parasitic in the blood of humans and other mammals. Also called *blood fluke.*

schistosome dermatitis *n.* An itching inflammation of the skin caused by parasitic larvae of certain schistosomes that penetrates the skin of persons who bathe in infested water. Also called *swimmer's itch.*

schis·to·so·mi·a (shĭs′tə-sō′mē-ə, skĭs′-) *n.* See **schistocormia.**

schis·to·so·mi·a·sis (shĭs′tə-sə-mī′ə-sĭs, skĭs′-) *n., pl.* **–ses** (-sēz′) Any of various generally tropical diseases that is caused by infestation with schistosomes, is widespread in rural areas of Africa, Asia, and Latin America through use of contaminated water, and is characterized by infection and gradual destruction of the tissues of the kidneys, liver, and other organs. Also called *bilharziasis.*

schistosomiasis hae·ma·to·bi·um (hē′mə-tō′bē-əm) *n.* Infestation of the urinary tract with eggs of *Schistosoma haematobium,* characterized by inflammation of the bladder and the passage of blood in the urine. Also called *endemic hematuria.*

schistosomiasis ja·pon·i·cum (jă-pŏn′ĭ-kəm) *n.* Infection with *Schistosoma japonicum,* characterized by dysenteric symptoms, painful enlargement of the liver and spleen, dropsy, urticaria, and progressive anemia. Also called *Asiatic schistosomiasis, Katayama disease, Katayama syndrome, urticarial fever, Yangtze Valley fever.*

schistosomiasis man·so·ni (măn-sō′nī) *n.* Infection of the liver and large intestine with *Schistosoma mansoni,* characterized by irritation, inflammation, and ultimately formation of fibrous tissue. Also called *Manson's disease.*

schistosomiasis me·kong·i (mā-kông′ī, -kông′gī) *n.* Infection with *Schistosoma mekongi,* producing symptoms similar to schistosomiasis japonica and chiefly affecting children in the Mekong delta.

schis·to·tho·rax (shĭs′tə-thôr′ăks′, skĭs′-) *n.* A congenital cleft of the chest wall.

schiz·am·ni·on (skĭz-ăm′nē-ən, -ŏn′) *n.* An amnion developing by the formation of a cavity within the inner cell mass, as in human development.

schiz·ax·on (skĭz-ăk′sŏn′) *n.* An axon that is divided into two branches.

schizo– or **schiz–** *pref.* **1.** Split; cleft: *schizotrichia.* **2.** Cleavage; fission: *schizogenesis.* **3.** Schizophrenia: *schizoid.*

schiz·o·af·fec·tive (skĭt′sō-ə-fĕk′tĭv) *adj.* Showing symptoms suggestive of both schizophrenia and mood disorders.

schizoaffective psychosis *n.* A psychotic disturbance in which there is a mixture of schizophrenic and manic-depressive symptoms.

schiz·o·gen·e·sis (skĭz′ō-jĕn′ĭ-sĭs, skĭt′sō-) *n.* Reproduction by fission. Also called *fissiparity.*

schi·zog·e·nous (skĭ-zŏj′ə-nəs, skĭt-sŏj′-) *adj.* **1.** Relating to or characterized by schizogenesis. **2.** Relating to or characterized by schizogony.

schi·zog·o·ny (skĭ-zŏg′ə-nē, skĭt-sŏg′-) *n.* Multiple fission in which the nucleus divides first, and then the cell divides into as many parts as there are nuclei. Also called *merogony.*

schiz·o·gy·ri·a (skĭz′ə-jī′rē-ə) *n.* A deformity of the cerebral convolutions that appears as occasional interruptions of continuity.

schiz·oid (skĭt′soid′) *adj.* **1.** Of, relating to, or having a personality marked by extreme shyness, seclusiveness, and an inability to form close friendships or social relationships. **2.** Schizophrenic. No longer in scientific use. —*n.* A schizoid or schizophrenic person.

schizoid personality *n.* A personality disorder characterized by long-term emotional coldness, indifference to praise, criticism, or the feelings of others, and an inability to form close friendships with more than one or two people.

schiz·o·my·cete (skĭz′ō-mī-sēt′) *n.* A member of the Schizomycetes; a bacterium.

Schiz·o·my·ce·tes (skĭz′ō-mī-sē′tēz) *n.* A class of unicellular or noncellular organisms that lack chlorophyll, comprise all the bacteria, and are prokaryotes, although formerly classified as fungi. Also called *fission fungi.*

schiz·ont (skĭz′ŏnt′, skĭt′sŏnt′) *n.* A sporozoan cell that reproduces by schizogony, producing a varied number of daughter trophozoites or merozoites.

schiz·o·nych·i·a (skĭz′ə-nĭk′ē-ə) *n.* A condition marked by irregular splitting of the nails.

schiz·o·pha·sia (skĭt′sə-fā′zhə) *n.* The characteristic disordered speech of a schizophrenic person. Also called *word salad.*

schiz·o·phre·ni·a (skĭt′sə-frē′nē-ə, -frĕn′ē-ə) *n.* Any of a group of psychotic disorders usually characterized by withdrawal from reality, illogical patterns of thinking, delusions, and hallucinations, and accompanied in varying degrees by other emotional, behavioral, or intellectual disturbances. Schizophrenia is often associated with dopamine imbalances in the brain and defects of the frontal lobe and may have an underlying genetic cause.

schiz·o·phren·ic (skĭt′sə-frĕn′ĭk) *adj.* Of, relating to, or affected by schizophrenia. —*n.* One who is affected with schizophrenia.

schiz·o·trich·i·a (skĭz′ə-trĭk′ē-ə) *n.* A splitting of the hairs at the ends.

schiz·o·typ·i·cal personality (skĭt′sə-tĭp′ĭ-kəl) *n.* A personality disorder characterized by eccentricities of thought, appearance, behavior, and speech, although the eccentricities are not severe enough to be considered psychotic.

Schlat·ter-Osgood disease (shlăt′ər-) *or* **Schlat·ter's disease** (-ərz) *n.* See **Osgood-Schlatter disease.**

Schlemm's canal (shlĕmz) *n.* See **venous sinus of sclera.**

Schmidt-Lanterman incisure (shmĭt′-) *n.* Any of the funnel-shaped breaks in the myelin sheath of nerve fibers, each corresponding to strands of cytoplasm that separate the two membranes composing the myelin sheath. Also called *Lanterman's incisure.*

Schön·lein (shœn′līn′), **Johann Lukas** 1793–1864. German physician. A noted teacher and microscopist, he described (1837) a form of purpura and discovered (1839) the fungus causing favus.

Schönlein-Henoch purpura *n.* See **Henoch-Schönlein purpura.**

Schön·lein's disease (shœn′līnz′) *n.* See **Henoch-Schönlein purpura.**

school phobia (skōol) *n.* The sudden aversion to or fear of attending school that occurs in young children, considered a manifestation of separation anxiety.

Schüff·ner's dot (shōof′nərz, shüf′-) *n.* Any of the fine, round, uniformly red or red-yellow staining dots occurring in red blood cells infected with *Plasmodium vivax* or *P. ovale.* Also called *Schüffner's granule.*

Schül·ler's disease *or* **Schül·ler's syndrome** (shōo′lərz, shü′-) *n.* See **Hand-Schüller-Christian disease.**

Schultz-Charl·ton reaction (shōolts′chärl′tən) *n.* The specific blanching of a scarlatinal rash at the site of an intracutaneous injection of scarlatina antiserum.

Schütz rule (shüts) *n.* A rule for determining the activity of an enzyme, especially of pepsin, by calculating the rate of the enzyme's reaction as proportional to the square root of the enzyme's concentration.

Schwach·man syndrome (shwăch′mən, shwäch′-) *n.* An inherited disorder characterized by sinusitis and bronchiectasis accompanied by pancreatic insufficiency and resulting in malnutrition; it is associated with neutropenia and a defect in neutrophile chemotaxis, short stature, and bone abnormalities.

Schwal·be's ring (shväl′bəz) *n.* 1. See **anterior limiting ring. 2.** See **posterior limiting ring.**

Schwann (shvän), **Theodor** 1810–1882. German physiologist and pioneer histologist who described (1839) the cell as the basic structure of animal tissue. He isolated pepsin in 1836, and in 1838 he described the myelin sheath.

Schwann cell (shwän, shvän) *n.* Any of the cells that cover the nerve fibers in the peripheral nervous system and form the myelin sheath. Also called *neurilemma, neurilemma cell.*

schwan·no·ma (shwä-nō′mə) *n.* 1. See **neurofibroma. 2.** See **neurilemoma.**

schwan·no·sis (shwä-nō′sĭs) *n.* A non-neoplastic proliferation of Schwann cells in the spaces around the blood vessels of the spinal cord.

Schweit·zer (shwīt′sər, shvīt′-), **Albert** 1875–1965. French philosopher, physician, and musician who founded (1913) and spent much of his life at a missionary hospital in present-day Gabon. He won the 1952 Nobel Peace Prize.

sci·age (sē-äzh′) *n.* In massage, a to-and-fro sawlike movement of the hand.

sci·at·ic (sī-ăt′ĭk) *adj.* 1. Of or relating to the ischium or

to the region of the hipbone in which it is located. **2.** Of or relating to sciatica.

sci·at·i·ca (sī-ăt′ĭ-kə) *n.* Pain along the sciatic nerve that radiates from the lower back to the buttocks and back of the thigh and is usually caused by a herniated disk of the lumbar region of the spine.

sciatic foramen *n.* Either of two foramina, designated greater and lesser, formed by the sacrospinous and sacrotuberous ligaments crossing the sciatic notches of the hipbone.

sciatic hernia *n.* Protrusion of intestine through the great sacrosciatic foramen. Also called *ischiocele.*

sciatic nerve *n.* A nerve that arises from the sacral plexus and passes through the greater sciatic foramen to about the middle of the thigh where it divides into the common peroneal and tibial nerves.

sciatic spine *n.* A pointed process from the posterior border of the ischium on a level with the lower border of the acetabulum. Also called *ischiadic spine.*

SCID *abbr.* severe combined immunodeficiency

sci·ence (sī′əns) *n.* 1. The observation, identification, description, experimental investigation, and theoretical explanation of phenomena. **2.** Such activities restricted to explaining a limited class of natural phenomena. **3.** Such activities applied to an object of inquiry or study.

sci·en·tif·ic method (sī′ən-tĭf′ĭk) *n.* The principles and empirical processes of discovery and demonstration considered characteristic of or necessary for scientific investigation, generally involving the observation of phenomena, the formulation of a hypothesis concerning the phenomena, experimentation to demonstrate the truth or falseness of the hypothesis, and a conclusion that validates or modifies the hypothesis.

scim·i·tar sign (sĭm′ĭ-tər, -tär′) *n.* A radiologic indication of anomalous pulmonary venous drainage in which a curvilinear structure is seen in the base of the lung.

scin·ti·cis·ter·nog·ra·phy (sĭn′tĭ-sĭs′tər-nŏg′rə-fē) *n.* Cisternography performed with a radiopharmaceutical and recorded with a stationary imaging device.

scin·ti·gram (sĭn′tĭ-grăm′) *n.* A two-dimensional record of the distribution of a radioactive tracer in a tissue or organ. Also called *photoscan, scintigraph, scintiscan.*

scin·ti·graph (sĭn′tĭ-grăf′) *n.* 1. A device for producing a scintigram; a scintiscanner. **2.** See **scintigram. —scin′-ti·graph′ic** *adj.*

scin·tig·ra·phy (sĭn-tĭg′rə-fē) *n.* See **scintiphotography.**

scin·til·la·scope (sĭn-tĭl′ə-skōp′) *n.* See **scintillation counter.**

scin·til·lat·ing scotoma (sĭn′tl-ā′tĭng) *n.* A localized area of blindness that may follow the appearance of brilliantly colored shimmering lights and is associated with the aura of migraine.

scin·til·la·tion (sĭn′tl-ā′shən) *n.* 1. A spark; a flash. **2.** A flash of light produced in a phosphor by absorption of an ionizing particle or photon.

scintillation counter *n.* A device for detecting and counting scintillations produced by ionizing radiation. Also called *scintillascope.*

scin·til·la·tor (sĭn′tl-ā′tər) *n.* A substance that glows when hit by high-energy particles or photons.

scin·ti·pho·tog·ra·phy (sĭn′tə-fə-tŏg′rə-fē) *n.* The process of or procedure for obtaining a scintigram. Also called *scintigraphy.*

scin·ti·scan (sĭn′tĭ-skăn′) *n.* See **scintigram.**

scin·ti·scan·ner (sĭn′tĭ-skăn′ər) *n.* The apparatus used to make a scintigram.

scir·rhous (skĭr′əs, sĭr′-) *adj.* Hardened; indurated.

scirrhous carcinoma *n.* See **fibrocarcinoma.**

scir·rhus (skĭr′əs, sĭr′-) *n., pl.* **scir·rhus·es** *or* **scir·rhi** (skĭr′ī, sĭr′ī) A hard, dense cancerous growth usually arising from connective tissue.

scis·sion (sĭzh′ən, sĭsh′-) *n.* **1.** A separation, division, or splitting, as in fission. **2.** See **cleavage** (sense 2).

scis·su·ra (sĭ-sŏŏr′ə) *n., pl.* **scis·su·rae** (sĭ-sŏŏr′ē) A cleft or fissure.

scis·sure (sĭzh′ər, sĭsh′-) *n.* A split or opening in an organ or part.

scler– *pref.* Variant of **sclero–.**

scle·ra (sklîr′ə) *n., pl.* **scle·ras** *or* **scle·rae** (sklîr′ē) The tough fibrous tunic forming the outer envelope of the eye and covering all of the eyeball except the cornea; the white of the eye. Also called *sclerotic.* —**scle′ral** *adj.*

scler·ad·e·ni·tis (sklîr′ăd-n-ī′tĭs) *n.* Inflammatory induration of a gland.

scleral staphyloma *n.* See **equatorial staphyloma.**

scleral vein *n.* Any of the tributaries to the anterior ciliary veins, draining the sclera.

scler·ec·ta·sia (sklîr′ĕk-tā′zhə) *n.* Localized bulging of the sclera lined with uveal tissue.

scle·rec·to·ir·i·dec·to·my (sklə-rĕk′tō-ĭr′ĭ-dĕk′tə-mē, -ī′rĭ-) *n.* Excision of a portion of the sclera and the iris in the treatment of glaucoma.

scle·rec·to·ir·i·do·di·al·y·sis (sklə-rĕk′tō-ĭr′ĭ-dō-dī-ăl′ĭ-sĭs, -ī′rĭ-) *n.* A surgical procedure used in treating glaucoma that combines sclerectomy and iridodialysis.

scle·rec·to·my (sklə-rĕk′tə-mē) *n.* **1.** Excision of a portion of the sclera. **2.** Surgical removal of the fibrous adhesions formed in chronic otitis media.

scler·e·de·ma (sklîr′ĭ-dē′mə) *n.* A hard nonpitting edema of the skin, having a waxy appearance with no sharp demarcation and occurring mainly in females with diabetes mellitus.

scleredema ad·ul·to·rum (ăd′ŭl-tôr′əm) *n.* A benign spreading induration of the skin and subcutaneous tissue, possibly streptococcal in origin.

scle·re·ma (sklə-rē′mə) *n.* **1.** Induration of the subcutaneous fat. **2.** Sclerema neonatorum.

sclerema ne·o·na·to·rum (nē′ō-nā-tôr′əm) *n.* Necrosis of subcutaneous fat appearing at birth or in early infancy as sharply demarcated indurated plaques, usually affecting the cheeks, buttocks, shoulders, and calves. Also called *adiponecrosis neonatorum, subcutaneous fat necrosis of newborn.*

scler·i·rit·o·my (sklîr′ī-rĭt′ə-mē) *n.* Incision of the iris and sclera.

scle·ri·tis (sklə-rī′tĭs) *n.* Inflammation of the sclera.

sclero– *or* **scler–** *pref.* **1.** Hard: *scleredema.* **2.** Hardness: *sclerogenous.* **3.** Sclera: *scleritis.*

scle·ro·at·ro·phy (sklîr′ō-ăt′rə-fē) *n.* See **sclerotylosis.**

scle·ro·blas·te·ma (sklîr′ō-blă-stē′mə) *n.* The embryonic tissue that forms bones.

scle·ro·cho·roid·i·tis (sklîr′ō-kôr′oi-dī′tĭs) *n.* Inflammation of the scleral and choroid coats of the eye.

scle·ro·con·junc·ti·val (sklîr′ō-kŏn′jŭngk-tī′vəl) *n.* Of or relating to the sclera and the conjunctiva.

scle·ro·cor·ne·a (sklîr′ō-kôr′nē-ə) *n.* **1.** The cornea and sclera regarded as forming together the hard outer coat of the eye. **2.** A congenital anomaly in which all or part of the cornea is opaque and resembles the sclera.

scle·ro·cor·ne·al junction (sklîr′ō-kôr′nē-əl) *n.* See **corneal margin.**

scle·ro·dac·ty·ly (sklîr′ō-dăk′tə-lē) *n.* See **acrosclerosis.**

scle·ro·der·ma (sklîr′ə-dûr′mə) *n.* **1.** A collagen disease characterized by the deposition of fibrous tissue into the skin and often other organs, causing tissue hardening and thickening. Also called *dermatosclerosis.* **2.** See **progressive systemic sclerosis.** —**scle′ro·der′ma·tous** (-mə-təs) *adj.*

scle·rog·e·nous (sklə-rŏj′ə-nəs) *or* **scle·ro·gen·ic** (sklîr′ə-jĕn′ĭk) *adj.* Producing hard, sclerotic tissue; causing sclerosis.

scle·roid (sklîr′oid′) *adj.* Hard or hardened.

scle·ro·i·ri·tis (sklîr′ō-ī-rī′tĭs) *n.* Inflammation of the sclera and the iris.

scle·ro·ker·a·ti·tis (sklîr′ō-kĕr′ə-tī′tĭs) *n.* Inflammatory cellular infiltration of the sclera and cornea.

scle·ro·ker·a·to·i·ri·tis (sklîr′ō-kĕr′ə-tō-ī-rī′tĭs) *n.* Inflammation of the sclera, cornea, and iris.

scle·ro·ma (sklə-rō′mə) *n., pl.* **–mas** *or* **–ma·ta** (-mə-tə) An indurated patch of body tissue especially in the upper respiratory tract.

scle·ro·ma·la·cia (sklîr′ō-mə-lā′shə) *n.* Degenerative thinning of the sclera, occurring in persons with rheumatoid arthritis and other collagen disorders.

scle·ro·mere (sklîr′ə-mîr′) *n.* A section of the skeleton, such as a vertebral segment.

scle·ro·myx·e·de·ma (sklîr′ō-mĭk′sĭ-dē′mə) *n.* Lichen myxedematosus with diffuse thickening of the skin underlying the papules.

scle·ro·nych·i·a (sklîr′ō-nĭk′ē-ə) *n.* Induration and thickening of the nails.

scle·ro·o·o·pho·ri·tis (sklîr′ō-ō′ə-fə-rī′tĭs) *n.* Inflammatory induration of the ovary.

scle·roph·thal·mi·a (sklîr′ŏf-thăl′mē-ə, ŏp-) *n.* A congenital condition in which the opacity of the sclera has advanced over the edge of the cornea so that only a small central area of the cornea remains transparent.

scle·ro·pro·tein (sklîr′ō-prō′tēn′) *n.* Any of a class of generally insoluble proteins found in skeletal and connective tissue. Also called *albuminoid.*

scle·ro·sal (sklə-rō′səl, -zəl) *adj.* Scleroid.

scle·ro·sant (sklə-rō′sənt, -zənt) *n.* An injectable irritant that is used in the treatment of varicose veins and that causes inflammation and subsequent fibrosis, thus obliterating the lumen of the vein.

scle·rose (sklə-rōz′, -rōs′) *v.* To harden; undergo sclerosis.

scle·ros·ing adenosis (sklə-rō′sĭng, -zĭng) *n.* A benign nodular breast lesion occurring most frequently in young women and consisting of hyperplastic distorted lobules of acinar tissue that exhibit increased collagenous stroma. Also called *adenofibrosis, fibrosing adenosis.*

sclerosing hemangioma *n.* See **dermatofibroma.**

sclerosing keratitis *n.* Inflammation of the cornea as a complication of scleritis, characterized by opacification of the corneal stroma.

sclerosing osteitis *n.* A fusiform thickening or increased density of bones. Also called *condensing osteitis, Garré's disease.*

scle·ro·sis (sklə-rō′sĭs) *n., pl.* **-ses** (-sēz) **1.** The hardening of a tissue or part due to chronic inflammation. **2.** A thickening or hardening of a body part or system especially from excessive formation of fibrous interstitial or glial tissue. **3.** Any of various diseases characterized by thickening or hardening, such as arteriosclerosis.

scle·ro·ste·no·sis (sklĭr′ō-stə-nō′sĭs) *n.* Induration and contraction of the tissues, as around an orifice.

scle·ros·to·my (sklə-rŏs′tə-mē) *n.* Surgical perforation of the sclera, as in the treatment of glaucoma.

scle·ro·ther·a·py (sklĭr′ō-thĕr′ə-pē) *n.* Treatment, as for varicose veins, involving the injection of a sclerosing solution into vessels or tissues.

scle·rot·ic (sklə-rŏt′ĭk) *adj.* **1.** Affected or marked by sclerosis. **2.** Of or relating to the sclera of the eye. —*n.* or **scle·rot·i·ca** (-rŏt′ĭ-kə) See **sclera.**

sclerotic body *n.* A vegetative rounded muriform cell of dematiaceous fungi, characteristic of the causative agent of chromomycosis in tissue. Also called *copper penny.*

sclerotic dentin *n.* Dentin that has become translucent due to calcification of the dentinal tubules as a result of injury or normal aging. Also called *transparent dentin.*

scle·ro·tome (sklĭr′ə-tōm′) *n.* **1.** A knife used in sclerotomy. **2.** A group of mesenchymal cells emerging from the ventromedial part of a mesodermic somite and migrating toward the notochord.

scle·rot·o·my (sklə-rŏt′ə-mē) *n.* Incision through the sclera of the eye.

scle·ro·ty·lo·sis (sklĭr′ō-tī-lō′sĭs) *n.* An inherited disorder associated with gastrointestinal cancer and marked by atrophic fibrosis of the skin, hypoplasia of the nails, and palmoplantar keratoderma. Also called *scleroatrophy.*

scle·rous (sklĭr′əs, sklĕr′-) *adj.* Scleroid.

sco·lex (skō′lĕks′) *n., pl.* **-lex·es** or **-li·ces** or **-le·ces** (-lĭ-sēz′) The knoblike anterior end of a tapeworm, having suckers or hooklike parts that in the adult stage serve as organs of attachment to the host.

sco·li·o·ky·pho·sis (skō′lē-ō-kī-fō′sĭs) *n.* A combination of lateral and posterior curvature of the spine.

sco·li·o·sis (skō′lē-ō′sĭs, skŏl′ē-) *n.* A condition of lateral curvature of the spine, which may have just one curve or primary and secondary compensatory curves and be fixed or mobile.

sco·li·ot·ic (skō′lē-ŏt′ĭk) *adj.* Of, relating to, or affected by scoliosis.

scoliotic pelvis *n.* A deformed pelvis associated with lateral curvature of the spine.

scom·broid poisoning (skŏm′broid′) *n.* Poisoning from ingestion of heat-stable toxins produced by bacterial action on inadequately preserved dark-meat fish of the order Scombroidea, including tuna, bonito, mackerel, albacore, skipjack. It is characterized by epigastric pain, nausea and vomiting, headache, thirst, difficulty in swallowing, and urticaria.

–scope *suff.* An instrument for viewing or observing: *bronchoscope.*

sco·pol·a·mine (skə-pŏl′ə-mēn′, -mĭn) *n.* A thick, syrupy, colorless alkaloid extracted from plants such as henbane and used as a mydriatic, sedative, antiemetic, and treatment for motion sickness. Also called *hyoscine.*

sco·po·phil·i·a (skō′pə-fĭl′ē-ə) *n.* See **voyeurism.**

sco·po·pho·bi·a (skō′pə-fō′bē-ə) *n.* An abnormal fear of being looked at or seen.

–scopy *suff.* Viewing; seeing; observation: *microscopy.*

scor·bu·tic (skôr-byoō′tĭk) or **scor·bu·ti·cal** (-tĭ-kəl) *adj.* Of, relating to, resembling, or affected by scurvy.

scor·bu·ti·gen·ic (skôr-byoō′tĭ-jĕn′ĭk) *adj.* Producing scurvy.

scor·di·ne·ma (skôr′də-nē′mə) *n.* An early symptom of an infectious disease marked by heaviness of the head with yawning and stretching.

scoto– *pref.* Darkness: *scotophobia.*

sco·to·ma (skə-tō′mə) *n., pl.* **-mas** or **-ma·ta** (-mə-tə) **1.** An area of diminished vision within the visual field. **2.** See **blind spot** (sense 3).

sco·tom·e·try (skə-tŏm′ĭ-trē) *n.* The plotting and measuring of a scotoma. —**sco·tom′e·ter** *n.*

sco·to·phil·i·a (skō′tə-fĭl′ē-ə) *n.* See **nyctophilia.**

sco·to·pho·bi·a (skō′tə-fō′bē-ə) *n.* See **nyctophobia.**

sco·to·pi·a (skə-tō′pē-ə) *n.* See **scotopic vision.**

sco·to·pic (skə-tō′pĭk, -tŏp′ĭk) *adj.* **1.** Of or relating to low illumination to which the eye is dark-adapted. **2.** Of or relating to scotopia.

scotopic adaptation *n.* See **dark adaptation.**

scotopic eye *n.* See **dark-adapted eye.**

scotopic vision *n.* Vision that occurs when the eye is dark-adapted. Also called *scotopia.*

sco·top·sin (skə-tŏp′sĭn) *n.* The protein component of the pigment in the rods of the retina.

Scott operation (skŏt) *n.* A jejunoileal bypass for treating morbid obesity in which the upper jejunum is joined to the terminal ileum, with the bypassed intestine closed proximally and anastomosed distally to the colon.

scra·pie (skrā′pē, skrăp′ē) *n.* A usually fatal infectious disease of sheep and goats, marked by chronic itching, loss of muscular coordination, and progressive deterioration of the central nervous system, thought to be caused by a prion.

scratch test (skrăch) *n.* A test for allergy performed by scratching the skin and applying an allergen to the wound.

screen (skrēn) *n.* **1.** One that serves to protect, conceal, or divide. **2.** The white or silver surface on which a picture is projected for viewing. **3.** A screen memory. —*v.* **1.** To process a group of people in order to select or separate certain individuals from it. **2.** To test or examine for the presence of disease or infection.

screen·ing (skrē′nĭng) *n.* **1.** The examination of a group of usually asymptomatic individuals to detect those with a high probability of having or developing a given disease. **2.** The initial evaluation of an individual, intended to determine suitability for a particular treatment modality.

screening test *n.* A test designed to identify and eliminate those who are not affected by a disease.

screen memory *n.* In psychoanalysis, the memory of an unacceptable but tolerable experience that unconsciously serves the purpose of concealing the memory of an associated experience that is more significant but emotionally more difficult to recall.

scro·bic·u·late (skrō-bĭk′yə-lĭt, -lāt′) *adj.* Marked with many shallow depressions, grooves, or pits.

scrof·u·la (skrŏf′yə-lə) *n.* A form of tuberculosis affecting the lymph nodes, especially of the neck, that is most common in children and is usually spread by unpasteurized milk from infected cows. Also called *struma*.

scrof·u·lo·der·ma (skrŏf′yə-lō-dûr′mə) *n.* See **cutaneous tuberculosis**.

scrof·u·lous (skrŏf′yə-ləs) *adj.* Relating to, affected with, or resembling scrofula.

scroll bone (skrōl) *n.* Any of the turbinate bones.

scrotal hernia *n.* A complete inguinal hernia that is located in the scrotum. Also called *oscheohydrocele, scrotocele*.

scrotal septum *n.* An incomplete wall of connective tissue and nonstriated muscle dividing the scrotum into two sacs, each containing a testis.

scrotal tongue *n.* See **furrowed tongue**.

scro·tec·to·my (skrō-tĕk′tə-mē) *n.* Surgical removal of part of the scrotum.

scro·ti·tis (skrō-tī′tĭs) *n.* Inflammation of the scrotum.

scro·to·cele (skrō′tə-sēl′) *n.* See **scrotal hernia**.

scro·to·plas·ty (skrō′tə-plăs′tē) *n.* Reparative or plastic surgery of the scrotum. Also called *oscheoplasty*.

scro·tum (skrō′təm) *n., pl.* **–tums** *or* **-ta** (-tə) The musculocutaneous sac that encloses the testes and is formed of skin, a network of nonstriated muscular fibers, cremasteric fascia, the cremaster muscle, and the serous coverings of the testes and epididymides. —**scro′tal** (skrōt′l) *adj.*

scrub nurse (skrŭb) *n.* A nurse who assists the surgeon in the operating room.

scrub suit *n.* A two-piece garment of lightweight cotton, worn by hospital staff especially when participating in surgery.

scrub typhus *n.* An acute infectious disease common in Asia caused by *Rickettsia tsutsugamushi* and transmitted by mites; it is characterized by sudden fever, painful swelling of the lymph glands, skin lesions, and skin rash. Also called *akamushi disease, Japanese river fever, mite typhus, tropical typhus, tsutsugamushi disease.*

scru·ple (skrōō′pəl) *n.* **1.** An uneasy feeling arising from conscience or principle that tends to hinder action. **2.** A unit of apothecary weight that is equal to about 1.3 grams, or 20 grains. **3.** A minute part or amount.

Scul·te·tus bandage (skəl-tē′təs) *n.* See **many-tailed bandage**.

scurf (skûrf) *n.* Scaly or shredded dry skin, such as that which occurs as dandruff.

scur·vy (skûr′vē) *n.* A disease caused by deficiency of vitamin C and characterized by spongy bleeding gums, bleeding under the skin, and weakness.

scute (skyōōt) *n.* A thin platelike structure.

scu·ti·form (skyōō′tə-fôrm′) *adj.* Having the shape of a shield.

scu·tu·lar (skyōō′chə-lər) *adj.* Of, relating to, or characterized by a scutulum.

scu·tu·lum (skyōō′chə-ləm) *n., pl.* **-la** (-lə) The characteristic lesion of favus, appearing as a yellow saucer-shaped crust made up of hyphae and spores.

scyb·a·lous (sĭb′ə-ləs) *adj.* Of, relating to, or characterized by a scybalum.

scyb·a·lum (sĭb′ə-ləm) *n., pl.* **-la** (-lə) A hard round mass of inspissated feces.

scy·phoid (sī′foid′) *adj.* Having the shape of a cup.

SD *abbr.* streptodornase

SDA *abbr.* specific dynamic action

Se The symbol for the element **selenium**.

sea·bor·gi·um (sē-bôr′gē-əm) *n. Symbol* **Sg** A radioactive synthetic element whose longest-lived isotopes have mass numbers of 259, 261, 263, 265, and 266 with half-lives of 0.9, 0.23, 0.8, 16, and 20 seconds. Atomic number 106.

Sea·bright ban·tam syndrome (sē′brīt′ băn′təm) *n.* See **pseudohypoparathyroidism**.

search·er (sûr′chər) *n.* A sounding instrument used to determine the presence of a calculus in the bladder.

sea·sick·ness (sē′sĭk′nĭs) *n.* Motion sickness resulting from the pitching and rolling of a ship or boat in water, especially at sea. Also called *mal de mer*.

sea·son·al affective disorder (sē′zə-nəl) *n. Abbr.* **SAD** A mood disorder occurring during seasons when sunlight is limited, characterized by symptoms of depression.

Sea·so·nale (sē′zə-nāl′) A trademark for an oral contraceptive that contains ethinyl estradiol and levonorgestrol and that results in quarterly rather than monthly menstrual cycles.

seat·worm (sēt′wûrm′) *n.* See **pinworm**.

se·ba·ceous (sĭ-bā′shəs) *adj.* **1.** Of, resembling, or characterized by fat or sebum; fatty. **2.** Secreting or producing fat or sebum.

sebaceous adenoma *n.* A benign tumor of sebaceous tissue, that has a more progressive growth and less mature structure than that exhibited in sebaceous gland hyperplasia.

sebaceous cyst *n.* A harmless cyst, especially on the scalp or face, containing the fatty secretion of a sebaceous gland. Also called *pilar cyst, steatocystoma, wen*.

sebaceous epithelioma *n.* A benign tumor of the epithelium of the sebaceous gland containing primarily basal or germinal cells.

sebaceous gland *n.* Any of the numerous holocrine glands in the dermis that empty into a hair follicle and produce and secrete sebum. Also called *sebaceous follicle*.

se·bif·er·ous (sĭ-bĭf′ər-əs) *or* **se·bip·a·rous** (-bĭp′ər-əs) *adj.* Producing or secreting fatty, oily, or waxy matter; sebaceous.

sebo– *or* **sebi–** *pref.* Sebum; sebaceous: *sebiferous*.

seb·o·lith (sĕb′ə-lĭth′) *n.* A concretion in a sebaceous gland.

seb·or·rhe·a *or* **seb·or·rhoe·a** (sĕb′ə-rē′ə) *n.* Overactivity of the sebaceous glands characterized by excessive secretion of sebum or an alteration in its quality, resulting in an oily coating, crusts, or scales on the skin.

seborrhea ad·i·po·sa (ăd′ə-pō′sə) *n.* See **seborrhea oleosa**.

seborrhea fa·ci·e·i (fā′sē-ē′ī′) *n.* See **seborrhea oleosa**.

seborrhea fur·fu·ra·ce·a (fûr′fə-rā′sē-ə, -shē-ə) *n.* See **seborrhea sicca** (sense 1).

seborrhea o·le·o·sa (ō′lē-ō′sə) *n.* Seborrhea especially of the nose and forehead with oily secretions. Also called *seborrhea adiposa, seborrhea faciei.*

seborrhea sic·ca (sĭkʹə) *n.* **1.** An accumulation of dry scales on the skin, especially on the scalp. Also called *seborrhea furfuracea.* **2.** Dandruff.

seb·or·rhe·ic (sĕbʹə-rēʹĭk) *adj.* Of, relating to, or affected by seborrhea.

seborrheic blepharitis *n.* A common type of chronic inflammation of the margins of the eyelids with adherence of dry scales and often associated with seborrheic dermatitis of the scalp and face.

seborrheic dermatitis *n.* A chronic form of dermatitis characterized by oily scales, crusty yellow patches, and itching, and occurring primarily on the scalp and face. Also called *dyssebacia, pityriasis alba, seborrheic dermatosis.*

seborrheic keratosis *n.* A superficial, benign, verrucose lesion consisting of proliferating epidermal cells enclosing horn cysts, usually appearing on the face, trunk, or extremities in adulthood.

se·bum (sēʹbəm) *n.* The semifluid secretion of the sebaceous glands, consisting chiefly of fat, keratin, and cellular material.

Se·cer·nen·tas·i·da (sēʹsər-nĕn-tăsʹĭ-də) *n.* A class of nematodes characterized by the presence of phasmids; it includes several parasitic to humans.

Se·che·nov (sĕchʹə-nôfʹ, syĕʹchə-nəf), **Ivan Mikhaylovich** 1829–1905. Russian psychologist. A teacher of Pavlov, he developed the theory that all conscious and unconscious acts are reflexes.

Seck·el syndrome (sĕkʹəl) *n.* An inherited disorder characterized by low birth weight, dwarfism, microcephaly, large eyes, beaked nose, receding chin, and mental retardation. Also called *Seckel dwarfism.*

sec·o·bar·bi·tal (sĕkʹō-bärʹbĭ-tôlʹ, -tălʹ) *n.* A white, odorless barbiturate used in the form of its sodium salt as a sedative and hypnotic.

Sec·o·nal (sĕkʹə-nôlʹ, -nălʹ, -nəl) A trademark for the drug secobarbital.

sec·ond (sĕkʹənd) *adj.* **1.** Coming next after the first in order, place, rank, time, or quality. **2.** Being the next closest to the innermost digit, especially on the foot. —**secʹond** *n.*

sec·ond·ar·y (sĕkʹən-dĕrʹē) *adj.* **1.** Of the second rank; not primary. **2.** Inferior. **3.** Minor; lesser. **4.** Derived from what is primary or original. **5.** Of or relating to a chemical compound characterized or formed by replacement of two atoms or radicals within a molecule. **6.** Of, relating to, or being a degree of health care intermediate between that offered in a physician's office and that available at a research hospital, as the care typically offered at a clinic or community hospital. —**secʹond·arʹi·ly** (-dârʹə-lē) *adv.*

secondary abdominal pregnancy *n.* A condition in which the embryo or fetus continues to grow in the abdominal cavity after its expulsion from the tube or other site of its primary development. Also called *abdominocyesis.*

secondary adhesion *n.* See **healing by second intention.**

secondary adrenocortical insufficiency *n.* Adrenocortical insufficiency caused by failure of ACTH secretion

resulting from anterior pituitary disease or by ACTH inhibition resulting from exogenous steroid therapy.

secondary alcohol *n.* An alcohol containing the bivalent organic radical CHOH.

secondary aldosteronism *n.* Aldosteronism due not to a defect in the adrenal cortex but to stimulation of secretion caused by extra-adrenal disorders.

secondary amenorrhea *n.* Amenorrhea in which menstruation begins at puberty but then is subsequently suppressed.

secondary amyloidosis *n.* Amyloidosis that occurs in association with another chronic disease and is characterized by the deposition of amyloid in fibrous connective tissue, especially in the spleen, liver, kidneys, adrenal glands, and arterioles.

secondary anesthetic *n.* The compound that contributes to, but is not primarily responsible for, loss of sensation when two or more anesthetics are simultaneously administered.

secondary atelectasis *n.* Pulmonary collapse, particularly of a newborn, due to hyaline membrane disease or elastic recoil of the lungs while the infant is actually dying from other causes.

secondary axis *n.* Any of several hypothetical lines passing through the optical center of a lens.

secondary cartilage *n.* Cartilage, as in certain joints, that changes directly into bone.

secondary cataract *n.* **1.** A cataract that accompanies or follows some other eye disease such as glaucoma. **2.** A cataract occurring in the remains of the lens or capsule after a cataract extraction.

secondary degeneration *n.* See **wallerian degeneration.**

secondary dentin *n.* Dentin that forms normally after a root end has formed completely.

secondary dentition *n.* **1.** The set of 32 permanent teeth whose eruptions begin from the fifth to the seventh year, lasting until the 17th to the 23rd year, when the last of the wisdom teeth appear. **2.** The eruption of the permanent teeth. Also called *permanent dentition.*

secondary deviation *n.* The deviation of the healthy eye when an eye with a paralyzed muscle focuses on an object.

secondary digestion *n.* Digestion of nutrients by the cells of the body, especially through metabolic activity, as opposed to the breakdown of nutrients by primary digestion.

secondary disease *n.* **1.** A disease that follows and results from an earlier disease, injury, or event. **2.** A wasting disorder that follows the successful transplantation of bone marrow into a patient whose immune system has been destroyed by radiation, usually accompanied by fever, diarrhea, and dermatitis.

secondary drive *n.* A drive not directly related to a biological need. Also called *acquired drive.*

secondary dysmenorrhea *n.* Dysmenorrhea due to inflammation, infection, tumor, or anatomical factors.

secondary encephalitis *n.* A usually demyelinating form of encephalitis contracted following vaccination for smallpox or during convalescence from measles, mumps, varicella, and certain other infectious diseases.

secondary follicle *n.* See **Graafian follicle.**

secondary gain *n.* Interpersonal or social advantages gained indirectly from organic illness, such as an increase in attention from others.

secondary glaucoma *n.* Glaucoma occurring as a sequel to preexisting ocular disease or injury.

secondary gout *n.* A disorder having the symptoms of gout and resulting from increased levels of uric acid in the blood brought about by a previously acquired disease of the blood or bone marrow, by lead poisoning, or by renal failure.

secondary hemochromatosis *n.* An increased intake and accumulation of iron that is secondary to a known cause, such as oral iron therapy or multiple blood transfusions.

secondary hemorrhage *n.* A hemorrhage that occurs after a period of time following an injury or an operation.

secondary lysosome *n.* A lysosome formed by the combination of a primary lysosome and a phagosome or pinosome and in which lysis takes place through the activity of hydrolytic enzymes.

secondary nondisjunction *n.* Nondisjunction occurring in an aneuploid cell that was itself the result of a primary nondisjunction.

secondary oocyte *n.* An oocyte in which the first meiotic division is completed. The second meiotic division usually stops short of completion unless fertilization occurs.

secondary process *n.* In psychoanalysis, the mental process directly related to the functions of the ego and characteristic of conscious and preconscious mental activities, marked by logical thinking and by the tendency to delay gratification by regulation of actions based on instinctual demands.

secondary saturation *n.* A technique of nitrous oxide anesthesia consisting of an abrupt curtailment of the oxygen in the inhaled mixture to produce deep anesthesia, with oxygen afterwards administered to correct overdosage and relax the muscles.

secondary sensory nucleus *n.* See **terminal nucleus**.

secondary sex characteristic *n.* Any of various characteristics specific to females or males but not directly concerned with reproduction.

secondary spermatocyte *n.* The spermatocyte derived from a primary spermatocyte by the first meiotic division and giving rise by the second meiotic division to two spermatids.

secondary syphilis *n.* The second stage of syphilis, beginning with the appearance of the dermatologic eruption, slight fever, and various constitutional symptoms.

secondary tuberculosis *n.* Tuberculosis occurring in adults and characterized by lesions near the apex of an upper lobe of the lung that may cavitate or heal with scarring; it may result from reinfection with the tubercle bacillus or from reactivation of a dormant endogenous infection.

secondary tympanic membrane *n.* The membrane closing the fenestra of the cochlea of the ear. Also called *Scarpa's membrane*.

secondary union *n.* See **healing by second intention**.

sec·ond cranial nerve (sĕk′ənd) *n.* See **optic nerve**.

second cuneiform bone *n.* See **intermediate cuneiform bone**.

second-degree burn *n.* A burn that blisters the skin and is more severe than a first-degree burn.

sec·ond·hand smoke (sĕk′ənd-hănd′) *n.* Cigarette, cigar, or pipe smoke that is inhaled unintentionally by nonsmokers and may be injurious to their health if inhaled regularly over a long period. Also called *passive smoke.*

second heart sound *n.* The heart sound that signifies the beginning of diastole and is caused by closure of the semilunar valves.

second molar *n.* The seventh permanent or fifth deciduous tooth located in the upper and lower jaw on either side.

second tooth *n.* See **permanent tooth**.

se·cre·ta (sĭ-krē′tə) *n.* Substances secreted by a cell, a tissue, or an organ; the products of secretion.

se·cre·ta·gogue (sĭ-krē′tə-gôg′) *n.* A hormone or another agent that causes or stimulates secretion.

Se·cré·tan's syndrome (sĕ-krā-tănz′, -tänz′) *n.* Factitious, traumatic, recurrent edema or hemorrhage of the back of the hand.

se·crete (sĭ-krēt′) *v.* To generate and separate a substance from cells or bodily fluids.

se·cre·tin (sĭ-krēt′n) *n.* A polypeptide hormone produced in the duodenum, especially on contact with acid, that stimulates secretion of pancreatic juice.

se·cre·tion (sĭ-krē′shən) *n.* **1.** The process of secreting a substance from a cell or gland. **2.** A substance, such as saliva, mucus, tears, bile, or a hormone, that is secreted.

se·cre·to·in·hib·i·to·ry (sĭ-krē′tō-ĭn-hĭb′ĭ-tôr′ē) *adj.* Acting to restrain or curb secretion.

se·cre·to·mo·tor (sĭ-krē′tō-mō′tər) *or* **se·cre·to·mo·to·ry** (-mō′tə-rē) *adj.* Acting to stimulate secretion.

se·cre·tor (sĭ-krē′tər) *n.* **1.** A cell, a tissue, or an organ that produces a secretion. **2.** A person whose saliva and other body fluids contain ABO antigens.

se·cre·to·ry (sĭ-krē′tə-rē) *adj.* Relating to or performing secretion.

secretory carcinoma *n.* Carcinoma of the breast composed of cells that are highly secretory; it occurs primarily in children.

secretory duct *n.* See **salivary duct**.

secretory nerve *n.* A nerve conveying impulses that excite functional activity in a gland.

secretory otitis media *n.* Inflammation of the mucosa of the middle ear, often the result of obstruction of the eustachian tube and accompanied by an accumulation of fluid. Also called *serous otitis.*

sec·tion (sĕk′shən) *n.* **1.** A cut or division. **2.** The act or process of separating or cutting, especially the surgical cutting or dividing of tissue. **3.** A thin slice, as of tissue, suitable for microscopic examination. —*v.* **1.** To separate or divide into parts. **2.** To cut or divide tissue surgically.

sec·tor·a·no·pi·a (sĕk′tər-ə-nō′pē-ə) *n.* Loss of vision in a sector of the visual field.

se·cun·di·grav·i·da (sĭ-kŭn′dĭ-grăv′ĭ-də) *n.* A woman in her second pregnancy.

se·cun·dines (sē-kŭn′dīnz′, sĕk′ən-dīnz′) *pl.n.* See **afterbirth**.

se·cun·dip·a·ra (sĕk′ən-dĭp′ər-ə) *n.* A woman who has given birth twice.

se·date (sĭ-dāt′) *v.* To administer a sedative to; calm or relieve by means of a sedative drug.

se·da·tion (sĭ-dā′shən) *n.* **1.** Reduction of anxiety, stress, irritability, or excitement by administration of a sedative agent or drug. **2.** The state or condition induced by a sedative.

sed·a·tive (sĕd′ə-tĭv) *adj.* Having a soothing, calming, or tranquilizing effect; reducing or relieving anxiety, stress, irritability, or excitement. —*n.* An agent or a drug that produces a soothing, calming, or tranquilizing effect.

sed·i·ment (sĕd′ə-mənt) *n.* Insoluble material that sinks to the bottom of a liquid, as in hypostasis.

sed·i·men·ta·tion (sĕd′ə-mən-tā′shən) *n.* The act or process of depositing or forming a sediment.

sedimentation constant *n.* A unit of time, usually between 1×10^{-13} and 200×10^{-13} per second, used in calculating the molecular weight of proteins as a function of their rate of movement during centrifugation.

sedimentation rate *n.* The degree of rapidity with which red blood cells sink in a specimen of drawn blood, which when elevated may indicate anemia or inflammation. Also called *erythrocyte sedimentation rate, sed rate.*

sedimentation test *n.* A radiographic procedure for viewing the stomach, in which a mixture of a contrast salt, such as barium or bismuth, and water is used to coat the stomach wall, thus allowing visualization of the shape and movement of the organ as well as lesions on the anterior or posterior wall.

sed·i·men·ta·tor (sĕd′ə-mən-tā′tər) *n.* A centrifuge.

sed·i·men·tom·e·ter (sĕd′ə-mən-tŏm′ĭ-tər) *n.* A photographic apparatus for the automatic recording of the blood sedimentation rate.

sed rate (sĕd) *n.* See **sedimentation rate.**

seed (sēd) *n.* **1.** A ripened plant ovule that contains an embryo. **2.** A propagative part of a plant, such as a tuber or a spore. **3.** Sperm; semen. **4.** A pellet filled with a radioactive isotope that is implanted at the site of a cancerous tumor to provide localized administration of radiation. —*v.* To inoculate a culture medium with microorganisms.

seg·ment (sĕg′mənt) *n.* **1.** A clearly differentiated subdivision of an organism or part, such as a metamere. **2.** A part of an organ having independent function, supply, or drainage. **3.** See **zona** (sense 1).

seg·men·tal anesthesia (sĕg-mĕn′tl) *n.* Loss of sensation limited to an area supplied by one or more spinal nerve roots.

segmental neuritis *n.* Inflammation occurring at several points along the course of a nerve.

segmental neuropathy *n.* Neuropathy characterized by demyelination of scattered internodal segments of peripheral nerves without affecting the axons, seen in diabetes, arsenic poisoning, lead poisoning, diphtheria, and leprosy.

seg·men·ta·tion (sĕg′mən-tā′shən) *n.* See **cleavage** (sense 1).

segmentation cavity *n.* See **blastocoel.**

seg·men·tec·to·my (sĕg′mən-tĕk′tə-mē) *n.* Excision of a segment of an organ or a gland.

seg·ment·ed cell (sĕg′mĕn′tĭd, sĕg-mĕn′-) *n.* A cell having a nucleus that is divided into lobes connected by a fine filament.

seg·re·ga·tion (sĕg′rĭ-gā′shən) *n.* **1.** The removal of certain parts or segments from a whole or mass. **2.** The separation of paired alleles especially during meiosis, so that the members of each pair of alleles appear in different gametes.

segregation analysis *n.* The determination of the number of progeny that have inherited distinct and mutually exclusive phenotypes.

segregation ratio *n.* The proportion of offspring that can be expected to be of a particular genotype or phenotype.

seg·re·ga·tor (sĕg′rĭ-gā′tər) *n.* An apparatus for obtaining urine from each kidney separately.

Seid·litz powder *or* **Seid·litz powders** (sĕd′lĭts) *n.* A mixture of tartaric acid, sodium bicarbonate, and potassium sodium tartrate, used as a mild cathartic by dissolving in water and drinking.

Sei·gnette's salt (sĕn-yĕts′) *n.* See **potassium sodium tartrate.**

seize (sēz) *v.* To exhibit symptoms of seizure activity, usually with convulsions.

sei·zure (sē′zhər) *n.* **1.** A paroxysmal episode, caused by abnormal electrical conduction in the brain, resulting in the abrupt onset of transient neurologic symptoms such as involuntary muscle movements, sensory disturbances and altered consciousness. Also called *convulsion.* **2.** A sudden attack, as of a disease.

seizure disorder *n.* See **epilepsy.**

se·lec·tion (sĭ-lĕk′shən) *n.* A natural or artificial process that favors or induces survival and perpetuation of one kind of organism over others that die or fail to produce offspring.

se·lec·tive estrogen receptor modulator (sĭ-lĕk′tĭv) *n. Abbr.* **SERM** A nonsteroidal compound, such as raloxifene or tamoxifen, designed to mimic the effect of estrogen on a specific tissue or body part by binding only to that part's estrogen receptors.

selective inhibition *n.* See **competitive inhibition.**

selective serotonin reuptake inhibitor *n.* SSRI.

selective stain *n.* A stain that colors one portion of a tissue or cell exclusively or more deeply than the remaining portions.

se·leg·i·line hydrochloride (sə-lĕj′ə-lēn′) *n.* A drug that is an irreversible inhibitor of a specific type of monoamine oxidase, used in conjunction with levodopa and carbidopa to treat patients with Parkinson's disease.

se·le·ni·um (sĭ-lē′nē-əm) *n. Symbol* **Se** A nonmetallic essential trace element used in its disulfide form as an antiseborrheic and as a radioisotope to image the pancreas and parathyroid glands. Atomic number 34.

self (sĕlf) *n., pl.* **selves** (sĕlz) **1.** The total, essential, or particular being of a person; the individual. **2.** One's consciousness of one's own being or identity; the ego. **3.** That which the immune system identifies as belonging to the body.

self-abuse *n.* **1.** Abuse of oneself or one's abilities. **2.** Masturbation.

self-analysis *n.* An independent methodical attempt by one to study and comprehend one's own personality or emotions.

self-awareness *n.* Realization of oneself as an individual entity or personality.

self-care *n.* The care of oneself without medical, professional, or other assistance or oversight.

self-concept *n.* An individual's assessment of his or her status on a single trait or on many human dimensions using societal or personal norms as criteria.

self-control *n.* Control of one's emotions, desires, or actions by one's own will.

self-curing resin *n.* See **autopolymer resin.**

self-diagnosis *n.* Diagnosis of one's own illness or disease without professional medical consultation.

self-examination *n.* **1.** An introspective consideration of one's own thoughts or emotions. **2.** Examination of one's own body for medical reasons.

self-identity *n.* **1.** The oneness of a thing with itself. **2.** An awareness of and identification with oneself as a separate individual.

self-image *n.* The conception that one has of oneself, including an assessment of qualities and personal worth.

self-limited *adj.* Running a definite course within a specific period; little modified by treatment. Used of a disease.

self-love *n.* The instinct or desire to promote one's own well-being; regard for or love of one's self.

self-medication *n.* Medication of oneself without professional supervision so as to alleviate an illness or a condition.

self-registering thermometer *n.* A thermometer that registers the maximum or minimum temperature during a period of observation.

self-replicating *adj.* Replicating oneself or itself.

self-retaining catheter *n.* A catheter constructed to remain in the urethra and bladder.

self-treatment *n.* Treatment of oneself without professional supervision so as to alleviate an illness or a condition.

sel·la (sĕl′ə) *n., pl.* **sel·lae** (sĕl′ē) A saddle-shaped anatomical structure; saddle.

sel·lar (sĕl′ər, -är′) *adj.* Of, relating to, or characterized by the sella turcica.

sella tur·ci·ca (tûr′sĭ-kə) *n.* A saddlelike prominence on the upper surface of the sphenoid bone of the skull, situated in the middle cranial fossa and dividing it into two halves.

Sel·lick's maneuver (sĕl′ĭks) *n.* A method of preventing regurgitation of an anesthetized patient during endotracheal intubation by applying pressure to the cricoid cartilage.

Sel·sun (sĕl′sŭn′) A trademark for a preparation of selenium disulfide.

Sel·ye (sĕl′yĕ, zĕl′-), **Hans Hugo Bruno** 1907–1982. Austrian-born Canadian physician who studied the physiological and biochemical results of stress and anxiety. He developed the general-adaptation syndrome as a means of expressing the reactions of the body to systemic stress.

SEM *abbr.* scanning electron microscope

se·man·tics (sĭ-măn′tĭks) *n.* **1.** The study or science of meaning in language forms. **2.** The study of the relationships between various signs and symbols and what they represent.

sem·el·in·ci·dent (sĕm′əl-ĭn′sĭ-dənt) *adj.* Occurring once only. Used of an infectious disease, one attack of which confers permanent immunity

se·men (sē′mən) *n.* A viscous whitish secretion of the male reproductive organs, containing spermatozoa and consisting of secretions of the testes, seminal vesicles, prostate, and bulbourethral glands.

se·me·nu·ri·a (sē′mə-no͝or′ē-ə) *n.* Excretion of urine containing semen. Also called *seminuria, spermaturia.*

semi– *pref.* **1.** Half: *semicanal.* **2.** Partial; partially: *semiconscious.* **3.** Resembling or having some of the characteristics of: *semilunar.*

sem·i·ca·nal (sĕm′ē-kə-năl′, sĕm′ī-) *n.* A deep groove on the edge of a bone that forms a complete canal when united with a similar groove or part of an adjoining bone; a half canal.

sem·i·cir·cu·lar canal (sĕm′ĭ-sûr′kyə-lər) *n.* Any of three bony tubes in the labyrinth of the ear within which the semicircular ducts are located.

semicircular duct *n.* Any of three small membranous tubes that lie within the bony labyrinth of the inner ear, form loops in planes at right angles to one another, and open into the vestibule.

semi-closed anesthesia (sĕm′ē-klōzd′, sĕm′ī-) *n.* Inhalation anesthesia using a circuit in which a portion of the exhaled air is exhausted from the circuit and a portion is rebreathed following removal of carbon dioxide by the anesthetic apparatus.

sem·i·co·ma (sĕm′ē-kō′mə, sĕm′ī-) *n.* A partial or mild comatose state; a coma from which a person may be roused by various stimuli. —**sem′i·co′ma·tose′** (-kō′mə-tōs′, -kŏm′ə-) *adj.*

sem·i·con·scious (sĕm′ē-kŏn′shəs, sĕm′ī-) *adj.* Not completely aware of sensations; partially conscious.

sem·i·flex·ion (sĕm′ē-flĕk′shən, sĕm′ī-) *n.* The position of a limb or muscle halfway between flexion and extension.

sem·i·lu·nar (sĕm′ē-lo͞o′nər, sĕm′ī-) *or* **sem·i·lu·nate** (-lo͞o′nāt′) *adj.* Shaped like a half-moon; crescent-shaped; lunar.

semilunar bone *n.* See **lunate bone.**

semilunar cartilage *n.* Any of the articular menisci of the knee joint.

semilunar conjunctival fold *n.* The crescent-shaped fold formed by the palpebral conjunctiva at the medial angle of the eye.

semilunar ganglion *n.* **1.** See **trigeminal ganglion. 2.** See **celiac ganglion.**

semilunar line *n.* The slight groove in the external abdominal wall parallel to the lateral edge of the rectus sheath. Also called *Spigelius line.*

semilunar valve *n.* One of three semilunar segments serving as the cusps of a valve preventing regurgitation, as in the aortic valve and the pulmonary valve.

sem·i·mem·bra·no·sus (sĕm′ē-mĕm′brə-nō′səs, sĕm′ī-) *n.* A muscle with origin from the tuberosity of the ischium, with insertion into the medial condyle of the tibia and by membrane to the tibial collateral ligament of the knee joint, the popliteal fascia, and the lateral condyle of the femur, with nerve supply from the tibial nerve, and whose action flexes the leg, rotates it medially, and makes the capsule of the knee joint tense.

sem·i·mem·bra·nous (sĕm′ē-mĕm′brə-nəs, sĕm′ī-) *adj.* Partly membranous, as a hamstring muscle.

sem·i·nal (sĕm′ə-nəl) *adj.* Of, relating to, containing, or conveying semen or seed.

seminal colliculus *n.* An elevated portion of the urethral crest upon which the two ejaculatory ducts and the prostatic utricle open.

seminal duct *n.* Any of the ducts conveying semen outward from the epididymis to the urethra, the vas deferens, the duct of the seminal vesicles, or the ejaculatory duct. Also called *gonaduct.*

seminal fluid *n.* Semen, especially its fluid component without spermatozoa.

seminal gland *n.* See **seminal vesicle.**

seminal granule *n.* One of the minute granular bodies present in the spermatic fluid.

seminal lake *n.* The vaginal vault after insemination.

seminal vesicle *n.* Either of a pair of pouchlike glands situated on each side of the male urinary bladder that secrete seminal fluid and nourish and promote the movement of spermatozoa through the urethra. Also called *gonecyst, seminal gland.*

sem·i·na·tion (sĕm′ə-nā′shən) *n.* Insemination.

sem·i·nif·er·ous (sĕm′ə-nĭf′ər-əs) *adj.* Conveying, containing, or producing semen.

seminiferous epithelium *n.* Epithelium that lines the seminiferous tubules of the testis.

seminiferous tubule *n.* One of two or three twisted curved tubules in each lobule of the testis in which spermatogenesis occurs.

seminiferous tubule dysgenesis *n.* A disorder in which the seminiferous tubules exhibit an abnormal cellular architecture, the testes are small, and few spermatozoa are formed.

sem·i·no·ma (sĕm′ə-nō′mə) *n., pl.* **–mas** *or* **–ma·ta** (-mə-tə) A malignant tumor of the testis arising from sperm-forming tissue.

sem·i·nu·ri·a (sē′mə-nōŏr′ē-ə) *n.* See **semenuria.**

sem·i·o·pen anesthesia (sĕm′ē-ō′pən, sĕm′ī-) *n.* Inhalation anesthesia in which a portion of inhaled gases is derived from an anesthesia circuit while the remainder consists of room air.

sem·i·per·me·a·ble (sĕm′ē-pûr′mē-ə-bəl, sĕm′ī-) *adj.* **1.** Partially permeable. **2.** Allowing passage of certain, especially small, molecules or ions but acting as a barrier to others. Used of biological and synthetic membranes.

sem·i·po·lar bond (sĕm′ē-pō′lər, sĕm′ī-) *n.* See **coordinate bond.**

sem·i·spi·nal muscle of head (sĕm′ē-spī′nəl, sĕm′ī-) *n.* A muscle with origin from the five or six upper thoracic vertebrae and the four lower cervical vertebrae, with insertion into the occipital bone, with nerve supply from the dorsal branches of the cervical nerve, and whose action rotates the head and draws it backward.

semispinal muscle of neck *n.* A muscle continuous with the semispinal muscle of the thorax, with origin from the second to the fifth thoracic vertebrae, with insertion into the axis and the third to the fifth cervical vertebrae, with nerve supply from the dorsal branches of the cervical and thoracic nerves, and whose action extends the cervical spine.

semispinal muscle of thorax *n.* A muscle with origin from the fifth to the eleventh thoracic vertebrae, with insertion into the first four thoracic vertebrae and the

fifth and seventh cervical vertebrae, with nerve supply from the dorsal branches of the cervical and the thoracic nerves, and whose action extends the vertebral column.

sem·i·sul·cus (sĕm′ē-sŭl′kəs, sĕm′ī-) *n.* A slight groove on the edge of a bone or other structure that forms a complete sulcus when united with a similar groove on the corresponding adjoining structure.

sem·i·syn·thet·ic (sĕm′ē-sĭn-thĕt′ĭk, sĕm′ī-) *adj.* **1.** Prepared by chemical synthesis from natural materials, as of a pharmaceutical. **2.** Consisting of a mixture of natural and synthetic substances.

sem·i·sys·tem·at·ic name (sĕm′ē-sĭs′tə-măt′ĭk, sĕm′-ī-) *n.* A name of a chemical compound that contains both systematic and trivial components, as for many generic or nonproprietary names of drugs. Also called *semitrivial name.*

sem·i·ten·di·nous muscle (sĕm′ē-tĕn′də-nəs, sĕm′ī-) *n.* A muscle with origin from the ischial tuberosity, with insertion into the medial surface of the upper quarter of the shaft of the tibia, with nerve supply from the tibial nerve, and whose action extends the thigh, flexes the leg, and rotates it medially.

sem·i·triv·i·al name (sĕm′ē-trĭv′ē-əl, sĕm′ī-) *n.* See **semisystematic name.**

Sem·mel·weis (zĕm′əl-vīs′), **Ignaz Philipp** 1818–1865. Hungarian physician who pioneered the use of antiseptics in obstetrics as the result of his discovery that puerperal fever is a form of septicemia. His methods reduced mortalities but were not widely adopted until after his death.

Sen·dai virus (sĕn-dī′) *n.* A paramyxovirus used in research laboratories for its tendency to induce genetically different cells or nuclei to fuse, the resulting hybrid cells having useful properties such as the ability to synthesize specific antibodies.

Sen·e·ca snakeroot (sĕn′ĭ-kə) *n.* An eastern North American plant having a terminal cluster of small white flowers and roots that are used medicinally.

sen·e·ga (sĕn′ĭ-gə) *n.* The dried roots of the Seneca snakeroot, used medicinally as an expectorant.

se·nes·cence (sĭ-nĕs′əns) *n.* The process of growing old; aging.

se·nes·cent (sĭ-nĕs′ənt) *adj.* Growing old; aging.

Sengs·ta·ken-Blake·more tube (sĕngz′tā′kən-blāk′-môr′) *n.* A triple-lumen tube of which one lumen is used to drain the stomach and two lumen are used to inflate attached gastric and esophageal balloons; used for treatment of bleeding esophageal varices.

se·nile (sē′nīl′, sĕn′īl′) *adj.* **1.** Relating to, characteristic of, or resulting from old age. **2.** Exhibiting the symptoms of senility, as impaired memory or the inability to perform certain mental tasks.

senile amyloidosis *n.* Amyloidosis commonly occurring with old age, usually in a mild form with amyloid deposits limited to the heart.

senile arteriosclerosis *n.* Arteriosclerosis as a result of advanced age.

senile cataract *n.* A cataract occurring spontaneously in old age and marked by increased opacity of the lens followed by its softening and shrinkage.

senile dementia *n.* A progressive, abnormally accelerated deterioration of mental faculties and emotional stability in old age, occurring especially in Alzheimer's disease.

senile elastosis *n.* Elastosis in the sun-exposed skin of old people.

senile hemangioma *n.* A red dome-shaped lesion usually occurring on the trunk and formed as a result of the weakening of the capillary wall. Also called *cherry angioma.*

senile keratosis *n.* See **actinic keratosis.**

senile lentigo *n.* See **age spot.**

senile melanoderma *n.* Pigmentation of the skin occurring with age. Also called *melasma universale.*

senile plaque *n.* A spherical mass of amyloid fibrils surrounded by distorted interwoven neuronal processes, found in the cerebral cortex in Alzheimer's disease. Also called *neuritic plaque.*

senile pruritus *n.* Itching associated with degenerative changes that occur in aging skin.

senile psychosis *n.* A mental disturbance of old age and related to degenerative cerebral processes.

senile retinoschisis *n.* Retinoschisis occurring most often in individuals over the age of 40, and affecting the outer plexiform layer of the retina.

senile tremor *n.* A tremor occurring in old people.

senile vaginitis *n.* Atrophic vaginitis occurring after menopause, often resembling adhesive vaginitis.

se·nil·ism (sē′nə-lĭz′əm) *n.* Premature senility.

se·nil·i·ty (sĭ-nĭl′ĭ-tē) *n.* **1.** The state of being senile. **2.** The mental and physical deterioration characteristic of old age.

sen·na (sĕn′ə) *n.* A plant of the genus *Cassia,* used as a laxative.

Sen·o·kot (sĕn′ə-kŏt′) An over-the-counter laxative containing senna.

se·no·pi·a (sĭ-nō′pē-ə) *n.* Improvement of near vision sometimes occurring with aging because of swelling of the crystalline lens in incipient cataract.

sen·sate (sĕn′sāt′) *or* **sen·sat·ed** (-sā′tĭd) *adj.* **1.** Perceived by a sense or the senses. **2.** Having physical sensation.

sen·sa·tion (sĕn-sā′shən) *n.* **1.** A perception associated with stimulation of a sense organ or with a specific body condition. **2.** The faculty to feel or perceive; physical sensibility. **3.** An indefinite, generalized body feeling.

sense (sĕns) *n.* **1.** Any of the faculties by which stimuli from outside or inside the body are received and felt, as the faculties of hearing, sight, smell, touch, taste, and equilibrium. **2.** A perception or feeling that is produced by a stimulus; sensation, as of hunger. —*v.* To become aware of; perceive.

sense datum *n.* A basic, unanalyzable sensation, such as color, sound, or smell, experienced upon stimulation of a sense organ or receptor.

sense of equilibrium *n.* The sense that makes it possible to maintain a normal upright posture.

sense organ *n.* A specialized organ or structure, such as the eye, ear, tongue, nose, or skin, where sensory neurons are concentrated and which functions as a receptor. Also called *sensor.*

sen·si·bil·i·ty (sĕn′sə-bĭl′ĭ-tē) *n.* **1.** The ability to perceive stimuli. **2.** Mental or emotional responsiveness

toward something, such as the feelings of another. **3.** Receptiveness to impression, whether pleasant or unpleasant; acuteness of feeling. **4.** The quality of being affected by changes in the environment.

sen·si·ble (sĕn′sə-bəl) *adj.* **1.** Perceptible by the senses or by the mind. **2.** Having the faculty of sensation; able to feel or perceive. **3.** Having a perception of something; cognizant.

sensible perspiration *n.* Perspiration excreted in sufficient quantity to appear as moisture on the skin.

sen·si·tive (sĕn′sĭ-tĭv) *adj.* **1.** Capable of perceiving with a sense or senses. **2.** Responsive to a stimulus. **3.** Susceptible to the attitudes, feelings, or circumstances of others. **4.** Easily irritated or inflamed, especially due to previous exposure to an antigen. **5.** Relating to, or characterizing a sensitized antigen.

sen·si·tiv·i·ty (sĕn′sĭ-tĭv′ĭ-tē) *n.* **1.** The quality or condition of being sensitive. **2.** The capacity of an organ or organism to respond to a stimulus. **3.** The proportion of individuals in a population that will be correctly identified when administered a test designed to detect a particular disease, calculated as the number of true positive results divided by the number of true positive and false negative results.

sensitivity training *n.* Training in small groups in which people learn how to interact with each other by developing a sensitive awareness and understanding of themselves and of their relationships with others.

sen·si·ti·za·tion (sĕn′sĭ-tĭ-zā′shən) *n.* The act or process of inducing an acquired sensitivity or allergy.

sen·si·tize (sĕn′sĭ-tīz′) *v.* To make hypersensitive or reactive to an antigen, such as pollen, especially by repeated exposure.

sen·si·tized antigen (sĕn′sĭ-tīzd′) *n.* The complex formed when antigen combines with specific antibody.

sensitized cell *n.* **1.** A cell or bacterium that has combined with specific antibody to form a complex capable of reacting with component. **2.** A small cell derived by division and differentiation from a lymphocyte.

sen·sor (sĕn′sər, -sôr′) *n.* **1.** A device, such as a photoelectric cell, that receives and responds to a signal or stimulus. **2.** See **sense organ.**

Sen·sor·caine (sĕn′sər-kān′) A trademark for the drug bupivacaine.

sensori– *pref.* Sensory: *sensorimotor.*

sen·so·ri·al (sĕn-sôr′ē-əl) *adj.* Of or relating to sensations or sensory impressions.

sen·so·ri·mo·tor (sĕn′sə-rē-mō′tər) *adj.* Of, relating to, or combining the functions of the sensory and motor activities.

sensorimotor area *n.* The precentral and postcentral gyri of the cerebral cortex.

sen·so·ri·neu·ral (sĕn′sə-rē-nŏŏr′əl) *adj.* Of, relating to, or involving the sensory nerves, especially as they affect the hearing.

sensorineural deafness *n.* Hearing loss or impairment due to a lesion or defect of the cochlea or the acoustic nerve.

sensorineural hearing impairment *n.* Hearing impairment caused by dysfunction of the neural elements involved in the conduction or interpretation of nerve impulses originating in the cochlea.

sen·so·ri·um (sĕn-sôr′ē-əm) *n.*, *pl.* **–so·ri·ums** *or* **–so·ri·a** (-sôr′ē-ə) **1.** The part of the brain that receives and coordinates all the stimuli conveyed to various sensory centers. **2.** The sensory system of the body.

sen·so·ry (sĕn′sə-rē) *adj.* **1.** Of or relating to the senses or sensation. **2.** Transmitting impulses from sense organs to nerve centers; afferent.

sensory aphasia *n.* Aphasia in which the ability to comprehend written or spoken words is lost. Also called *impressive aphasia, receptive aphasia.*

sensory cortex *n.* The somatic sensory, auditory, visual, and olfactory regions of the cerebral cortex considered as a group.

sensory deprivation *n.* The reduction or absence of usual external stimuli or perceptual opportunities, commonly resulting in psychological distress and sometimes in unpleasant hallucinations.

sensory epilepsy *n.* A form of focal epilepsy in which various disturbances of sensation occur in paroxysms that may or may not cause seizures.

sensory ganglion *n.* A cluster of primary sensory neurons forming a swelling in the course of a peripheral nerve or its dorsal root and establishing the sole afferent neural connection between the sensory periphery and the central nervous system.

sensory image *n.* An image based on one or more types of sensation.

sensory integration *n.* The coordinated organization and processing of input from somatic sense receptors by the central nervous system.

sensory integration dysfunction *n.* A neurological disorder characterized by disruption in the processing and organization of sensory information by the central nervous system, characterized by impaired sensitivity to sensory input, motor control problems, unusually high or low activity levels, and emotional instability.

sensory nerve *n.* An afferent nerve conveying impulses that are processed by the central nervous system to become part of the organism's perception of itself and of its environment.

sensory neuronopathy *n.* Neuronopathy confined to the dorsal root ganglion of the spinal cord and the trigeminal ganglion in the skull.

sensory paralysis *n.* Loss of sensation.

sensory speech center *n.* See **Wernicke's center.**

sensory urgency *n.* Urgent desire to empty the urinary bladder due to vesicourethral hypersensitivity.

sen·su·al (sĕn′shoo-əl) *adj.* **1.** Relating to or affecting any of the senses or a sense organ; sensory. **2.** Of, relating to, given to, or providing gratification of the physical and especially the sexual appetites.

sen·tient (sĕn′shənt, -shē-ənt) *adj.* **1.** Having sense perception; conscious. **2.** Experiencing sensation or feeling.

sen·ti·nel gland (sĕn′tə-nəl) *n.* A single, enlarged lymph node in the omentum that may indicate an ulcer opposite to it in the greater or lesser curvature of the stomach.

sentinel pile *n.* A thickening of the mucous membrane at the lower end of a fissure of the anus.

sentinel tag *n.* A piece of projecting edematous skin at the lower end of an anal fissure.

sep·a·ra·tion anxiety (sĕp′ə-rā′shən) *n.* A child's apprehension or fear associated with his or her separation from a parent or other significant person.

sep·sis (sĕp′sĭs) *n.*, *pl.* **–ses** (-sēz) **1.** The presence of pathogenic organisms or their toxins in the blood or tissues. **2.** The poisoned condition resulting from the presence of pathogens or their toxins.

sept– *pref.* Variant of **septo–.**

sep·tal (sĕp′təl) *adj.* Of or relating to a septum or septa.

sep·tate (sĕp′tāt′) *adj.* Divided by a septum or septa.

septate uterus *n.* A uterus that is divided into two cavities by an anteroposterior septum.

sep·tec·to·my (sĕp-tĕk′tə-mē) *n.* Excision of a septum or part of a septum.

septi– *pref.* Seven.

sep·tic (sĕp′tĭk) *adj.* **1.** Of, relating to, having the nature of, or affected by sepsis. **2.** Causing or producing sepsis; putrefactive.

septic– *pref.* Variant of **septico–.**

septic abortion *n.* Abortion complicated by fever, endometritis, and parametritis, often leading to sepsis.

sep·ti·ce·mi·a (sĕp′tĭ-sē′mē-ə) *n.* A systemic disease caused by the multiplication of microorganisms in the blood. Also called *blood poisoning, septic fever.* **—sep′ti·ce′mic** (-mĭk) *adj.*

septicemic abscess *n.* See **pyemic abscess.**

septicemic plague *n.* A usually fatal form of bubonic plague in which the bacilli are present in the bloodstream and cause toxemia.

septic fever *n.* See **septicemia.**

septic infarct *n.* An area of necrosis resulting from vascular obstruction caused by emboli consisting of clumps of bacteria or infected material.

septico– *pref.* Sepsis; septic: *septicopyemia.*

sep·ti·co·py·e·mi·a (sĕp′tĭ-kō-pī-ē′mē-ə) *n.* Pyemia and septicemia occurring together. **—sep′ti·co·py·e′mic** *adj.*

septic phlebitis *n.* Inflammation of a vein resulting from bacterial infection.

septic shock *n.* **1.** Shock associated with sepsis, usually associated with abdominal and pelvic infection resulting from trauma or surgery. **2.** Shock associated with septicemia caused by gram-negative bacteria.

septic sore throat *n.* An infection of the throat caused by hemolytic streptococci and marked by fever and inflammation of the tonsils. Also called *strep throat.*

septo– *or* **sept–** *pref.* Septum: *septotomy.*

sep·to·mar·gi·nal (sĕp′tō-mär′jə-nəl) *adj.* **1.** Of or relating to the margin of a septum. **2.** Of or relating to a margin and a septum.

sep·to·na·sal (sĕp′tō-nā′zəl) *adj.* Of or relating to the nasal septum.

sep·to-op·tic dysplasia (sĕp′tō-ŏp′tĭk) *n.* A congenital hypoplasia of the optic nerve resulting from the defective development of the retinal ganglia cells and their axons.

sep·to·plas·ty (sĕp′tə-plăs′tē) *n.* A surgical operation to correct defects or deformities of the nasal septum, often by altering or partially removing supporting structures.

sep·to·rhi·no·plas·ty (sĕp′tō-rī′nō-plăs′tē, -nə-) *n.* A surgical procedure performed to repair defects or deformities of both the nasal septum and the external nasal pyramid.

sep·tos·to·my (sĕp-tŏs′tə-mē) *n.* The surgical creation of an opening in a septum.

sep·tot·o·my (sĕp-tŏt′ə-mē) *n.* Incision of the nasal septum.

Sep·tra (sĕp′trə) A trademark for a combination of the drugs trimethoprim and sulfamethoxazole.

sep·tu·lum (sĕp′chə-ləm) *n., pl.* **-la** (-lə) A tiny or minute septum.

sep·tum (sĕp′təm) *n., pl.* **-ta** (-tə) **1.** A thin partition or membrane dividing two cavities or soft masses of tissue in an organism. **2.** The septum pellucidum.

septum pel·lu·ci·dum (pə-lōō′sĭ-dəm) *n., pl.* **septa pel·lu·ci·da** (-də) A thin membrane of nervous tissue that forms the medial wall of the lateral ventricles in the brain. Also called *septum lucidum.*

septum penis *n.* The portion of the tunica albuginea separating the two cavernous bodies of the penis.

se·quel·a (sĭ-kwĕl′ə) *n., pl.* **-quel·ae** (-kwĕl′ē) A pathological condition resulting from a disease.

se·quence (sē′kwəns, -kwĕns′) *n.* **1.** A following of one thing after another; succession. **2.** An order of succession; an arrangement. **3.** A related or continuous series. **4.** The order of constituents in a polymer, especially the order of nucleotides in a nucleic acid or of the amino acids in a protein. —*v.* **1.** To organize or arrange in a sequence. **2.** To determine the order of constituents in a polymer, such as a nucleic acid.

sequence ladder *n.* The array of bands that have been electrophoretically separated and that correspond to the nucleotide sequence of a DNA molecule that has been fragmented by endonucleases.

se·ques·tral (sĭ-kwĕs′trəl) *adj.* Of, relating to, or characterized by a sequestrum.

se·ques·tra·tion (sē′kwĭ-strā′shən, sĕk′wĭ-) *n.* **1.** The formation of a sequestrum. **2.** Loss of blood or of its fluid content into spaces within the body, so that the circulating volume diminishes. **3.** The inhibition or prevention of normal ion behavior by combination with added materials, especially the prevention of metallic ion precipitation from solution.

se·ques·trec·to·my (sē′kwĭ-strĕk′tə-mē) *n.* Surgical removal of a sequestrum.

se·ques·trum (sĭ-kwĕs′trəm) *n., pl.* **-tra** (-trə) A fragment of dead tissue, usually bone, that has separated from healthy tissue as a result of injury or disease.

se·quoi·o·sis (sē′kwoi-ō′sĭs) *n.* Extrinsic allergic alveolitis caused by inhalation of redwood sawdust containing spores of various fungi.

Ser *abbr.* serine

ser·al·bu·min (sîr′ăl-byōō′mĭn) *n.* A protein fraction of serum involved in maintaining osmotic pressure of the blood and used as a substitute for plasma in the treatment of shock. Also called *blood albumin, serum albumin.*

Ser·ax (sĕr′ăks) A trademark for the drug oxazepam.

Ser·e·vent (sĕr′ə-vĕnt′) A trademark for the drug salmeterol xinafoate.

se·ri·al extraction (sîr′ē-əl) *n.* Selective extraction of certain teeth during the early years of dental devel-

opment, usually with the eventual extraction of the first premolars to encourage autonomous adjustment of crowding of the anterior teeth.

serial radiography *n.* The making of sequential x-ray exposures of a region under study over a period of time.

serial section *n.* One of a number of consecutive histological sections.

se·ries (sîr′ēz) *n., pl.* **series 1.** A number of objects or events arranged or coming one after the other in succession. **2.** A group of objects related by linearly varying successive differences in form or configuration, as in a radioactive decay series.

ser·ine (sĕr′ēn′) *n. Abbr.* **Ser** An amino acid that is a common constituent of many proteins.

se·ri·ous (sîr′ē-əs) *adj.* Being of such import as to cause anxiety, as of a physical condition.

SERM *abbr.* selective estrogen receptor modulator

sero– *pref.* Serum: *serotherapy.*

se·ro·co·li·tis (sîr′ō-kə-lī′tĭs) *n.* See **pericolitis.**

se·ro·con·ver·sion (sîr′ō-kən-vûr′zhən, -shən) *n.* Development of antibodies in blood serum as a result of infection or immunization.

se·ro·di·ag·no·sis (sîr′ō-dī′əg-nō′sĭs) *n., pl.* **-ses** (-sēz) Diagnosis of disease based on reactions in the blood serum.

se·ro·en·ter·i·tis (sîr′ō-ĕn′tə-rī′tĭs) *n.* See **perienteritis.**

se·ro·ep·i·de·mi·ol·o·gy (sîr′ō-ĕp′ĭ-dē′mē-ŏl′ə-jē, -dĕm′ē-) *n.* Epidemiologic study through the use of serological testing to detect infection.

se·ro·fi·brin·ous (sîr′ō-fī′brə-nəs) *adj.* Of, relating to, or characterized by an exudate composed of serum and fibrin.

serofibrinous pleurisy *n.* Pleurisy characterized by a fibrinous exudate on the surface of the pleura and by an extensive effusion of serous fluid into the pleural cavity.

se·ro·fi·brous (sîr′ō-fī′brəs) *adj.* Of, relating to, or characterized by a serous membrane and a fibrous tissue.

se·rol·o·gy (sĭ-rŏl′ə-jē) *n.* **1.** The science that deals with the properties and reactions of serums, especially blood serum. **2.** The characteristics of a disease or an organism shown by study of blood serums. —**se′ro·log′ic, se′ro·log′i·cal** *adj.*

se·ro·ma (sĭ-rō′mə) *n.* A mass or swelling caused by the localized accumulation of serum within a tissue or organ.

se·ro·mem·bra·nous (sîr′ō-mĕm′brə-nəs) *adj.* Of or relating to a serous membrane.

se·ro·mu·coid (sîr′ō-myōō′koid′) *n.* A glycoprotein of serum.

se·ro·mu·cous (sîr′ō-myōō′kəs) *adj.* Of, relating to, or being a mixture of watery and mucinous material such as that of certain glands.

seromucous gland *n.* A gland containing both serous and mucous secretory cells.

se·ro·neg·a·tive (sîr′ō-nĕg′ə-tĭv) *adj.* Having a negative reaction to a serological test for a disease, especially to a test for syphilis or AIDS.

se·ro·pos·i·tive (sîr′ō-pŏz′ĭ-tĭv) *adj.* Having a positive reaction to a serological test for a disease; exhibiting seroconversion.

se·ro·pu·ru·lent (sĭr′ō-pyo͝or′ə-lənt) *adj.* Consisting of serum and pus.

se·ro·pus (sĭr′ō-pŭs′) *n.* Pus diluted with serum.

Ser·o·quel (sĕr′ə-kwĕl′) A trademark for the drug quetiapine fumarate.

se·ro·sa (sĭ-rō′sə, -zə) *n., pl.* **–sas** or **–sae** (-sē, -zē) **1.** See **serous membrane. 2.** The chorion of a bird or reptile embryo.

se·ro·san·guin·e·ous (sĭr′ō-săng-gwĭn′ē-əs) *adj.* Consisting of serum and blood.

se·ro·se·rous (sĭr′ō-sĭr′əs) *adj.* **1.** Of or relating to two serous surfaces. **2.** Of, relating to, or being a suture, as of the intestine, in which the edges of the wound are folded in a manner that brings two serous surfaces into apposition.

se·ro·si·tis (sĭr′ō-sī′tĭs) *n.* Inflammation of a serous membrane.

se·ros·i·ty (sĭ-rŏs′ĭ-tē) *n.* **1.** A serous fluid or a serum. **2.** The condition of being serous. **3.** The serous quality of a liquid.

se·ro·syn·o·vi·tis (sĭr′ō-sĭn′ə-vī′tĭs, -sī′nə-) *n.* Synovitis characterized by an increase of serous fluid.

se·ro·ther·a·py (sĭr′ō-thĕr′ə-pē) *n.* Treatment of disease by administration of a serum obtained from an immunized animal. Also called *serum therapy.*

se·ro·to·ner·gic (sĕr′ə-tn-ûr′jĭk) *or* **se·ro·to·ni·ner·gic** (-tō′nə-nûr′jĭk) *adj.* Activated by or capable of liberating serotonin, especially in transmitting nerve impulses.

se·ro·to·nin (sĕr′ə-tō′nĭn, sîr′-) *n.* An organic compound formed from tryptophan and found in animal and human tissue, especially the brain, blood serum, and gastric mucous membranes, and active in vasoconstriction, stimulation of the smooth muscles, transmission of impulses between nerve cells, and regulation of cyclic body processes. Also called *5-hydroxytryptamine.*

se·ro·type (sîr′ə-tīp′, sĕr′-) *n.* See **serovar.** —*v.* To classify according to serovar; assign to a particular serovar.

se·rous (sîr′əs) *adj.* Containing, secreting, or resembling serum.

serous cell *n.* A cell, especially of the salivary gland, that secretes a watery albuminlike fluid.

serous cyst *n.* A cyst, such as a hygroma, containing clear serous fluid.

serous fluid *n.* Any of various body fluids resembling serum, especially lymph.

serous gland *n.* A gland secreting a watery substance that may or may not contain an enzyme.

serous inflammation *n.* A form of exudative inflammation in which the exudate is predominantly fluid.

serous ligament *n.* Any of a number of peritoneal folds attaching certain of the viscera to the abdominal wall or to one another.

serous membrane *n.* A thin, two-part membrane that secretes a serous fluid and lines a closed body cavity, covering the organs that lie within that cavity. Also called *serosa, serous tunic.*

serous meningitis *n.* Acute meningitis with secondary external hydrocephalus.

serous otitis *n.* See **secretory otitis media.**

serous pleurisy *n.* Pleurisy with serous effusion.

serous synovitis *n.* Synovitis with a large effusion of nonpurulent fluid.

serous tunic *n.* See **serous membrane.**

se·ro·vac·ci·na·tion (sîr′ō-văk′sə-nā′shən) *n.* A process for producing mixed immunity by administering an injection of a serum as well as a vaccine of a modified or killed culture.

se·ro·var (sîr′ō-vâr′) *n.* A group of closely related microorganisms distinguished by a characteristic set of antigens. Also called *serotype.*

ser·pig·i·nous (sər-pĭj′ə-nəs) *adj.* Relating to or being a cutaneous lesion, such as an ulcer, having an arciform border and a wavy margin.

ser·pi·go (sər-pī′gō) *n.* Any creeping or serpiginous eruption.

ser·rate (sĕr′āt′) *or* **ser·rat·ed** (-ā′tĭd) *adj.* **1.** Having or forming a row of small, sharp, projections resembling the teeth of a saw. **2.** Having a saw-toothed edge or margin notched with toothlike projections.

serrate suture *n.* A suture whose opposing margins resemble deep sawlike indentations. Also called *dentate suture.*

ser·ra·tion (sə-rā′shən, sĕ-) *n.* **1.** The state of being serrate. **2.** A series or set of teeth or notches. **3.** A single tooth or notch in a serrate edge.

ser·ra·tus posterior inferior (sə-rā′təs) *n.* A muscle with origin from the two lower thoracic and two upper lumbar vertebrae, with insertion into the last four ribs, with nerve supply from the ninth to the twelfth intercostal nerves, and whose action draws the lower ribs backward and downward.

serratus posterior superior *n.* A muscle with origin in the spinous processes of the two lower cervical and two upper thoracic vertebrae, with insertion into the second to the fifth ribs, and with nerve supply from the first to the fourth intercostals, and whose action is to elevate the upper ribs.

serre·fine (sâr-fēn′, sĕr-) *n.* A small spring forceps used for approximating the edges of a wound, or for temporarily closing an artery during surgery.

Ser·to·li cell (sər-tō′lē, sĕr′tō-) *n.* Any of the elongated striated cells in the seminiferous tubules to which spermatids attach during spermiogenesis.

Sertoli cell-only syndrome *n.* Congenital absence of germinal epithelium from the seminiferous tubules, which contain only Sertoli cells, resulting in sterility due to the absence of living sperm cells in the semen. Also called *Del Castillo syndrome.*

Sertoli cell tumor *n.* See **androblastoma** (sense 1).

ser·tra·line (sər′trə-lēn′) *n.* A serotonin reuptake inhibitor used as an oral antidepressant.

se·rum (sîr′əm) *n., pl.* **se·rums** or **se·ra** (sîr′ə) **1.** A watery fluid, especially one that moistens the surface of serous membranes or that is exuded by such membranes when they become inflamed. **2.** The clear yellowish fluid obtained upon separating whole blood into its solid and liquid components. **3.** Such fluid from the tissues of immunized animals, containing antibodies and used to transfer immunity to another individual.

serum accelerator *n.* See **factor VII.**

serum accelerator globulin *or* **accelerator globulin** *n.* See **factor VII.**

serum agglutinin *n.* An antibody that coats bacteria or Rh-positive red blood cells, preventing them from agglutinating when suspended in saline. Also called *incomplete antibody.*

se·rum·al (sîr′ə-məl) *adj.* Relating to or derived from serum.

serum albumin *n.* See **seralbumin.**

serum disease *n.* See **serum sickness.**

serum-fast *adj.* Relating to a serum showing little or no change in its antibody titer, even under conditions of treatment or immunologic stimulation.

serum globulin *n.* A protein fraction of serum composed chiefly of antibodies.

serum hepatitis *n. Abbr.* **SH** See **hepatitis B.**

serum nephritis *n.* Glomerulonephritis occurring in serum sickness or in animals injected with foreign serum protein.

serum prothrombin conversion accelerator *n. Abbr.* **SPCA** See **factor VII.**

serum reaction *n.* See **serum sickness.**

serum shock *n.* Anaphylactic or anaphylactoid shock caused by the injection of antitoxic or other foreign serum into a sensitized individual.

serum sickness *n.* A hypersensitive reaction to the administration of a foreign serum, marked by fever, swelling, skin rash, and lymph node enlargement. Also called *serum disease, serum reaction.*

serum therapy *n.* See **serotherapy.**

ser·vice animal (sûr′vĭs) *n.* An animal, such as a dog, that has been specially trained to assist a disabled person with certain daily tasks.

Ser·zone (sûr′zōn′) A trademark for the drug nefazodone.

ses·a·moid (sĕs′ə-moid′) *adj.* **1.** Resembling a sesame seed in size or shape. **2.** Of or relating to a sesamoid bone. —*n.* A sesamoid bone or cartilage.

ses·qui·hy·drate (sĕs′kwĭ-hī′drāt′) *n.* Any of various compounds that crystallize with 1.5 molecules of water.

ses·sile (sĕs′īl′, -əl) *adj.* Permanently attached or fixed; not free-moving.

set (sĕt) *v.* **1.** To put in a specified position; place. **2.** To put into a specified state. **3.** To put into a stable position. **4.** To fix firmly or in an immobile manner. **5.** To become fixed or hardened; coagulate. **6.** To bring the bones of a fracture back into a normal position or alignment. —*n.* **1.** The act or process of setting. **2.** The condition resulting from setting. **3.** A permanent firming or hardening of a substance. **4.** The carriage or bearing of a part of the body. **5.** A particular psychological state, usually of anticipation or preparedness.

se·ta (sē′tə) *n., pl.* **–tae** (-tē) A stiff hair, bristle, or bristlelike process or part.

se·ta·ceous (sĭ-tā′shəs) *adj.* **1.** Having or consisting of bristles; bristly. **2.** Resembling bristles or a bristle.

se·ton (sēt′n) *n.* Material such as thread, wire, or gauze that is passed through subcutaneous tissues or through a cyst in order to form a sinus or fistula.

7-de·hy·dro·cho·les·ter·ol (-dē-hī′drō-kə-lĕs′tə-rôl′, -rōl′) *n.* A provitamin present in the skin of humans as well as the milk of mammals that becomes vitamin D_3 when exposed to ultraviolet light.

17-al·pha-hy·drox·y·pro·ges·ter·one (-ăl′fə-hī-drŏk′sē-prō-jĕs′tə-rōn′) *n.* A compound produced by the adrenal glands and often used therapeutically as a progestogen when such a steroid is needed for parenteral administration.

17-hy·drox·y·cor·ti·co·ste·roid test (-hī-drŏk′sē-kôr′tĭ-kō-stîr′oid′, -stĕr′-) *n.* A test employing a reaction of adrenocorticosteroid and phenylhydrazine, performed on urine and used to measure adrenocortical function, as in the diagnosis of Addison's disease and Cushing's syndrome.

17-ke·to·ste·roid (-kē′tō-stîr′oid′, -stĕr′-) *n.* A steroid having a ketone group attached to its 17th carbon atom, especially any of those produced by the adrenal cortex and gonads and occurring normally in the urine. Also called *17-oxosteroid.*

17-ox·o·ste·roid (-ŏk′sə-stîr′oid′, -stĕr′-) *n.* See **17-ketosteroid.**

sev·enth cranial nerve (sĕv′ənth) *n.* See **facial nerve.**

se·vere acute respiratory syndrome (sə-vîr′) *n. Abbr.* **SARS** A viral pneumonia that can progress to respiratory failure and is often characterized by high fever, malaise, dry cough, and shortness of breath.

severe combined immunodeficiency *n. Abbr.* **SCID** A usually fatal congenital immune system disorder in which the body is unable to produce enough B cells and T cells to resist infection.

sex (sĕks) *n.* **1.** The property or quality by which organisms are classified as female or male on the basis of their reproductive organs and functions. **2.** Either of the two divisions, designated female and male, of this classification. **3.** Females or males considered as a group. **4.** The condition or character of being female or male; the physiological, functional, and psychological differences that distinguish the female and the male. **5.** The sexual urge or instinct as it manifests itself in behavior. **6.** Sexual intercourse.

sex cell *n.* See **germ cell.**

sex change *n.* The modification of biological sex characteristics, by surgery and hormone treatment, to approximate those of the opposite sex.

sex chromatin *n.* See **Barr body.**

sex chromosome *n.* Either of a pair of chromosomes, usually designated X or Y, that combine to determine the sex and sex-linked characteristics of an individual, with XX resulting in a female and XY in a male.

sex chromosome imbalance *n.* An abnormal pattern of sex chromosomes, as occurs in men with seminiferous tubule dysgenesis or in women with Turner's syndrome.

sex determination *n.* The determination of the sex of a fetus by identifying sex chromatin in amniotic fluid obtained by amniocentesis.

sex·duc·tion (sĕks-dŭk′shən) *n.* The process by which chromosomal fragments are transferred between bacteria by means of a specific plasmid.

sex gland *n.* A testis or an ovary; a gonad.

sex hormone *n.* Any of various steroid hormones, such

as estrogen and androgen, affecting the growth or function of the reproductive organs and the development of secondary sex characteristics.

sex hygiene *n.* The branch of hygiene that is concerned with healthy sexual practices.

sex-influenced *adj.* Relating to a genetic disorder in which the same genotype has differing manifestations in the two sexes.

sex-influenced inheritance *n.* Inheritance that is autosomal but has a different intensity of expression in the two sexes, as that manifested in male pattern baldness.

sex-limited *adj.* **1.** Occurring or appearing only in one sex. Used of a genetic character or phenotype. **2.** Having a sex-limited character or phenotype.

sex-limited inheritance *n.* Inheritance in which a trait or phenotype is expressed in one sex only, as in hemophilia A.

sex linkage *n.* The condition in which a gene responsible for a specific trait is located on a sex chromosome, resulting in sex-linked inheritance of the trait.

sex-linked *adj.* **1.** Carried by a sex chromosome, especially an X-chromosome. Used of genes. **2.** Sexually determined. Used especially of inherited traits.

sex-linked character *n.* An inherited character determined by a sex-linked gene.

sex-linked gene *n.* A gene located on a sex chromosome, usually the X-chromosome.

sex-linked inheritance *n.* Inheritance that may result from a mutant gene located on either the X- or Y-chromosome.

sex·ol·o·gy (sĕk-sŏl′ə-jē) *n.* The study of human sexual behavior. —**sex·ol′o·gist** *n.*

sex ratio *n.* **1.** The proportion of males to females in a given population, usually expressed as the number of males per 100 females at a specific stage in life, especially at conception, birth, and a given stage between birth and death. **2.** The ratio of the numbers of males to females affected by a particular disease or trait.

sex reversal *n.* A process that changes the sexual identity of an individual from one sex to the other, often through a combination of surgical, pharmacologic, and psychiatric procedures.

sex role *n.* Any of the various attitudinal patterns of daily behavior that are associated with masculinity and femininity in a particular society.

sex test *n.* A method of determining genetic sex by examination of stained smears of buccal mucosal squamous epithelial cells for Barr bodies; normal females have one per cell nucleus and normal males have none.

sex·u·al (sĕk′shoo-əl) *adj.* **1.** Of, relating to, involving, or characteristic of sex, sexuality, the sexes, or the sex organs and their functions. **2.** Implying or symbolizing erotic desires or activity. **3.** Of, relating to, or involving the union of male and female gametes. —**sex′u·al·ly** *adv.*

sexual dimorphism *n.* The physical differences between male and female individuals that arise as a consequence of sexual maturation, including the secondary sex characteristics.

sexual dwarf *n.* A dwarf who exhibits normal sexual development.

sexual generation *n.* Reproduction through the union

of individuals, or the union of male and female germ cells.

sexual infantilism *n.* Failure to develop secondary sexual characteristics after the normal time of puberty.

sexual intercourse *n.* **1.** Coitus between humans. **2.** Sexual union between humans involving genital contact other than vaginal penetration by the penis.

sex·u·al·i·ty (sĕk′shoo-ăl′ĭ-tē) *n.* **1.** The condition of being characterized and distinguished by sex. **2.** Concern with or interest in sexual activity. **3.** Sexual character or potency.

sexually transmitted disease *n. Abbr.* **STD** Any of various diseases, including chancroid, chlamydia, gonorrhea, and syphilis, that are usually contracted through sexual intercourse or other intimate sexual contact.

sexual orientation *n.* The direction of one's sexual interest toward members of the same, opposite, or both sexes, especially a direction seen to be dictated by physiologic rather than sociologic forces. Replaces *sexual preference* in most contemporary uses.

sexual reproduction *n.* Reproduction by the union of male and female gametes to form a zygote. Also called *syngenesis.*

sexual selection *n.* Selection that is driven by the competition for mates and that is considered an adjunct to natural selection.

Sé·za·ry cell (sā′zə-rē, sā-zä-rē′) *n.* Any of the large mononuclear T cells occurring in the blood in Sézary syndrome.

Sézary syndrome *n.* Exfoliative dermatitis characterized by intense itching and caused by the infiltration of atypical mononuclear cells into the skin and the peripheral blood.

sg *abbr.* specific gravity

Sg The symbol for the element **seaborgium.**

SGA *abbr.* small for gestational age

SGOT (ĕs′jē′ō′tē′) *n.* Serum glutamic aminotransferase; an enzyme that catalyzes the transfer of the amino group from glutamic acid to oxaloacetic acid forming alpha-ketoglutaric acid and aspartic acid, used to measure liver function. Also called *aspartate transaminase, AST, GOT, glutamic-oxaloacetic transaminase.*

SGPT (ĕs′jē′pē′tē′) *n.* Serum pyruvate aminotransferase; an enzyme in serum and body tissues that catalyzes the transfer of amino acid groups from L-alanine to 2-ketoglutarate or the reverse, thus allowing nitrogen to be excreted or incorporated into other compounds, used to measure liver function. Also called *alanine aminotransferase, ALT, glutamic-pyruvic transaminase, GPT.*

SH *abbr.* serum hepatitis

shad·ow test (shăd′ō) *n.* See **retinoscopy.**

shaft (shăft) *n.* **1.** An elongated rodlike structure, such as the midsection of a long bone. **2.** The section of a hair projecting from the surface of the body.

sha·green skin (shə-grēn′) *n.* An oval patch of thickened, smooth or crinkled, sometimes pigmented skin appearing on the trunk or lower back in early childhood in association with tuberous sclerosis.

shak·en baby syndrome (shā′kən) *n.* A syndrome in infants in which brain injury is caused by shaking of such violence that the child's brain rebounds against the skull, resulting in bruising, swelling, and bleeding of the brain and often leading to permanent, severe brain damage or death.

shal·low breathing (shăl′ō) *n.* Breathing with abnormally low tidal volume.

shank (shăngk) *n.* The part of the human leg between the knee and ankle.

shap·ing (shā′pĭng) *n.* A technique that is used in operant conditioning in which the behavior is modified by stepwise reinforcement of behaviors that produce progressively closer approximations of the desired behavior.

Shar·pey-Scha·fer (shär′pē-shā′fər), Sir **Edward** 1850–1935. British physiologist known for his research on endocrinology, particularly for discovering (1894) the effects of the hormone epinephrine.

shave biopsy (shāv) *n.* A biopsy technique performed with a surgical blade or a razor blade and used for lesions that are elevated above the skin level or confined to the epidermis and upper dermis.

sheath (shēth) *n., pl.* **sheaths** (shē*th*z, shēths) An enveloping tubular structure, such as the tissue that encloses a muscle or nerve fiber.

sheath of eyeball *n.* A condensation of connective tissue on the outer aspect of the sclera, from which it is separated by a narrow cleftlike space. Also called *Tenon's capsule.*

sheath of Schwann *n.* See **neurilemma.**

Shee·han's syndrome (shē′ənz) *n.* Hypopituitarism arising from a severe circulatory collapse during the postpartum period, resulting in pituitary necrosis. Also called *postpartum pituitary necrosis syndrome.*

shell shock *n.* See **combat fatigue.**

Shen·ton's line (shĕn′tənz) *n.* A curved line formed by the top of the obturator foramen and the inner side of the neck of the femur, seen in a radiograph of the normal hip joint.

Sher·ring·ton (shĕr′ĭng-tən), Sir **Charles Scott** 1857–1952. British neurologist. He shared a 1932 Nobel Prize for advances in the understanding of the function of the neuron.

shi·at·su (shē-ät′so͞o) *n.* A form of therapeutic massage in which pressure is applied with the thumbs and palms to those areas of the body used in acupuncture. Also called *acupressure.*

shield (shēld) *n.* A protective device or structure, such as a lead sheet to protect an individual from x-rays.

shift (shĭft) *v.* **1.** To move or transfer from one place or position to another. **2.** To alter position or place. **3.** To exchange one thing for another of the same type or class. —*n.* **1.** A change from one person or configuration to another; a substitution. **2.** A change in position.

shift to left *n.* An increase in the percentage of immature myeloid cells in the blood.

shift to right *n.* The absence of young and immature white blood cells in a differential count of white blood cells in the blood.

Shi·ga-Kruse bacillus (shē′gə-kro͞oz′, -kro͞o′zə) *n.* A gram-negative bacterium *Shigella dysenteriae* that causes dysentery in humans and monkeys.

Shi·gel·la (shĭ-gĕl′ə) *n.* A genus of gram-negative,

aerobic, nonmotile, rod-shaped bacteria that includes some species that cause dysentery in humans.

Shigella boy·di·i (boi′dē-ī′) *n.* A bacterium present in a low proportion of cases of bacillary dysentery.

Shigella dys·en·ter·i·ae (dĭs′ən-tĕr′ē-ē′) *n.* Shiga-Kruse bacillus.

Shigella flex·ner·i (flĕks-nĕr′ī) *n.* Flexner's bacillus.

Shigella son·ne·i (sŏn′ē-ī′) *n.* Sonne bacillus.

shig·el·lo·sis (shĭg′ə-lō′sĭs) *n., pl.* **-ses** (-sēz) Dysentery caused by any of various species of *Shigella,* occurring most frequently in areas where poor sanitation and malnutrition are prevalent and commonly affecting children and infants.

shin (shĭn) *n.* **1.** The front part of the leg located below the knee and above the ankle. **2.** The tibia.

shin·bone (shĭn′bōn′) *n.* See **tibia.**

shin·gles (shĭng′gəlz) *n.* An acute infection caused by a herpesvirus and characterized by inflammation of the sensory ganglia of certain spinal or cranial nerves and the eruption of vesicles along the affected nerve path. It usually strikes only one side of the body and is often accompanied by severe neuralgia. Also called *herpes zoster, zona, zoster.*

shin splints *or* **shin·splints** (shĭn′splĭnts′) *n.* A painful condition of the shins that is caused by inflammation of the surrounding muscles, frequently occurring among runners.

shirt-stud abscess (shûrt′stŭd′) *n.* Two abscesses connected by a narrow channel, usually formed by rupture through an overlying fascia. Also called *collar-button abscess.*

shock (shŏk) *n.* **1.** Something that jars the mind or emotions as if with a violent, unexpected blow. **2.** The disturbance of function, equilibrium, or mental faculties caused by such a blow; violent agitation. **3.** A generally temporary massive physiological reaction to severe physical or emotional trauma, usually characterized by marked loss of blood pressure and depression of vital processes. **4.** The sensation and muscular spasm caused by an electric current passing through the body or a body part. **5.** The abnormally palpable impact of an accentuated heartbeat felt by a hand on the chest wall. —*v.* **1.** To induce a state of physical shock in a person. **2.** To subject a person to an electric shock.

shock lung *n.* The development of edema, impaired perfusion, and reduction in alveolar space so that the alveoli collapse, occurring during shock. Also called *pump lung.*

shock therapy *n.* Any of various treatments for mental disorders, such as major depression or schizophrenia, in which a convulsion or brief coma is induced by administering a drug or passing an electric current through the brain. Also called *shock treatment.*

Shope (shōp), **Richard** 1901–1966. American pathologist and virologist who was the first to isolate an influenza virus.

short bone (shôrt) *n.* A bone whose dimensions are approximately equal, consisting of a layer of cortical substance enclosing the spongy substance and marrow.

short ciliary nerve *n.* Any of a number of branches of the ciliary ganglion, supplying the ciliary muscles, the iris, and the tunics of the eyeball.

short elevator muscle of rib *n.* Any of the muscles that arise from the transverse processes of the last cervical vertebra and the eleven thoracic vertebrae and are inserted into the next rib below.

short gastric vein *n.* Any of the veins in the wall of the stomach that empty into the splenic vein.

short gyrus of insula *n.* Any of several short radiating gyri converging toward the base of the insula of the brain, composing the anterior two thirds of the insular cortex.

short palmar muscle *n.* A muscle with origin from the palmar aponeurosis, with insertion into the skin of the ulnar side of the hand, with nerve supply from the ulnar nerve, and whose action wrinkles the skin on the medial side of the palm.

short radial extensor muscle of wrist *n.* A muscle with origin from the lateral epicondyle of the humerus, with insertion to the base of the third metacarpal bone, with nerve supply from the radial nerve, and whose action extends and abducts the wrist toward the radius.

short·sight·ed (shôrt′sī′tĭd) *adj.* **1.** Nearsighted; myopic. **2.** Lacking foresight. —**short′sight′ed·ly** *adv.*

short·sight·ed·ness (shôrt′sī′tĭd-nĭs) *n.* Myopia.

short-term exposure limit *n.* The maximum concentration of a chemical to which workers may be exposed continuously for up to 15 minutes without danger to health or work efficiency and safety.

short-term memory *n.* *Abbr.* **STM** The phase of the memory process in which stimuli that have been recognized and registered are stored briefly.

short·wave diathermy (shôrt′wāv′) *n.* The therapeutic elevation of temperature in the tissues by means of an oscillating electric current of extremely high frequency.

short-winded *adj.* **1.** Breathing with quick, labored breaths. **2.** Likely to have difficulty in breathing, especially from exertion.

shot (shŏt) *n.* **1.** A hypodermic injection. **2.** A small amount given or applied at one time.

shot-silk retina *n.* The appearance in the retina of numerous, wavelike, opalescent reflexes similar to the light reflections appearing on certain types of silk; most commonly seen in children under the age of 10 and sometimes in teenagers.

shoul·der (shōl′dər) *n.* **1.** The joint connecting the arm with the torso. **2.** The part of the human body between the neck and upper arm.

shoulder blade *n.* See **scapula**.

shoulder girdle *n.* The pectoral girdle, especially of a human.

shoulder-girdle syndrome *n.* See **brachial plexus neuropathy**.

shoulder-hand syndrome *n.* See **brachial plexus neuropathy**.

shoulder joint *n.* A ball-and-socket joint between the head of the humerus and the glenoid cavity of the scapula.

shoulder presentation *n.* Presentation during birth in which the fetus lies with its long axis transverse to the long axis of the mother's body and with the shoulder as the presenting part.

show (shō) *n.* **1.** The first discharge of blood in menstruation. **2.** The discharge of bloody mucus from the vagina indicating the start of labor.

shunt (shŭnt) *n.* A passage between two natural body channels, such as blood vessels, especially one created surgically to divert or permit flow from one pathway or region to another; a bypass.

shut-in (shŭt′ĭn′) *n.* A person confined indoors by illness or disability. —*adj.* **1.** Confined to a home or hospital, as by illness. **2.** Disposed to avoid social contact; excessively withdrawn or introverted.

Shy-Dra·ger syndrome (shī′drā′gər) *n.* A progressive disorder of the brain and spinal cord affecting the autonomic nervous system and characterized by low blood pressure, atrophy of the iris, incontinence, the absence of sweating, impotence in males, tremor, and muscle wasting.

Si The symbol for the element **silicon**.

SI *abbr.* Système International (d'Unités) (International System of Units)

sial– *pref.* Variant of **sialo–**.

si·a·lad·en·i·tis (sī′ə-lăd′n-ī′tĭs) *or* **si·a·lo·ad·e·ni·tis** (sī′ə-lō-ăd′n-) *n.* Inflammation of a salivary gland.

si·a·lad·e·no·sis (sī′ə-lăd′n-ō′sĭs) *n.* Enlargement of the salivary glands, usually the parotids, often seen in conditions such as alcoholism and malnutrition.

si·al·a·gogue *or* **si·al·o·gogue** (sī-ăl′ə-gôg′) *n.* A drug or other agent that increases the flow of saliva. Also called *ptyalagogue*.

si·a·lec·ta·sis (sī′ə-lĕk′tə-sĭs) *n.* Dilation of a salivary duct. Also called *ptyalectasis*.

si·a·lem·e·sis (sī′ə-lĕm′ĭ-sĭs) *or* **si·a·le·me·si·a** (-lə-mē′zē-ə) *n.* **1.** Vomiting due to or accompanying excessive secretion of saliva. **2.** Vomiting of saliva.

si·al·ic (sī-ăl′ĭk) *adj.* Having or having the characteristics of saliva.

sialic acid *n.* Any of a group of amino carbohydrates that are components of mucoproteins and glycoproteins, especially in animal tissue and blood cells.

si·al·i·dase (sī-ăl′ĭ-dās′, -dāz′) *n.* See **neuraminidase**.

si·al·i·do·sis (sī-ăl′ĭ-dō′sĭs) *n.* See **cherry-red spot myoclonus syndrome**.

si·a·line (sī′ə-lēn′, -lĭn′) *adj.* Sialic.

si·a·lism (sī′ə-lĭz′əm) *n.* See **ptyalism**.

si·a·lis·mus (sī′ə-lĭz′məs) *n.* See **ptyalism**.

sialo– *or* **sial–** *pref.* Saliva; salivary glands: *sialadenitis*.

si·a·lo·ad·e·nec·to·my (sī′ə-lō-ăd′n-ĕk′tə-mē) *n.* Excision of a salivary gland.

si·a·lo·ad·e·ni·tis (sī′ə-lō-ăd′n-ī′tĭs) *n.* Variant of **sialadenitis**.

si·a·lo·ad·e·not·o·my (sī′ə-lō-ăd′n-ŏt′ə-mē) *n.* Incision into a salivary gland.

si·a·lo·an·gi·ec·ta·sis (sī′ə-lō-ăn′jē-ĕk′tə-sĭs) *n.* Dilation of salivary ducts.

si·a·lo·an·gi·i·tis (sī′ə-lō-ăn′jē-ī′tĭs) *n.* Inflammation of a salivary duct. Also called *sialodochitis*.

si·a·lo·cele (sī′ə-lō-sēl′) *n.* See **ranula**.

si·a·lo·do·chi·tis (sī′ə-lō-dō-kī′tĭs) *n.* See **sialoangiitis**.

si·a·lo·do·cho·plas·ty (sī′ə-lō-dō′kə-plăs′tē) *n.* Surgical repair of a salivary duct.

si·a·log·e·nous (sī′ə-lŏj′ə-nəs) *adj.* Producing saliva.

si·al·o·gogue (sī-ăl′ə-gôg′) *n.* Variant of **sialagogue**.

si·al·o·gram (sī-ăl′ə-grăm′) *n.* A radiograph of one or more of the salivary ducts.

si·a·log·ra·phy (sī′ə-lŏg′rə-fē) *n.* Radiographic examination of the salivary glands and ducts after the introduction of a radiopaque material into the ducts.

si·a·lo·lith (sī′ə-lō-lĭth′, sī-ăl′ə-) *n.* A calculus occurring in a salivary gland or duct.

si·a·lo·li·thi·a·sis (sī′ə-lō-lĭ-thī′ə-sĭs) *n.* Formation or presence of a salivary calculus.

si·a·lo·li·thot·o·my (sī′ə-lō-lĭ-thŏt′ə-mē) *n.* Incision into a salivary duct or gland to remove a calculus.

si·a·lo·met·a·pla·sia (sī′ə-lō-mĕt′ə-plā′zhə) *n.* Squamous cell metaplasia in the salivary ducts.

si·a·lor·rhe·a *or* **si·a·lor·rhoe·a** (sī′ə-lō-rē′ə, sī-ăl′ə-) *n.* See **ptyalism.**

si·a·los·che·sis (sī′ə-lŏs′kĭ-sĭs) *n.* Suppression of the secretion of saliva.

si·a·lo·sis (sī′ə-lō′sĭs) *n.* See **ptyalism.**

si·a·lo·ste·no·sis (sī′ə-lō-stə-nō′sĭs) *n.* Stricture of a salivary duct.

si·a·lo·syr·inx (sī′ə-lō-sîr′ĭngks) *n.* A salivary fistula passing from the salivary gland or duct to the exterior of the body, usually through the skin or oral tissues.

Si·a·mese twin (sī′ə-mēz′) *n.* Either of a pair of conjoined twins. No longer in technical use.

sib (sĭb) *n.* **1.** A blood relation; a relative. **2.** A person's relatives when considered as a group; kinfolk. **3.** A brother or sister; a sibling. —*adj.* Related by blood; kindred.

sib·i·lant (sĭb′ə-lənt) *adj.* Of, characterized by, or producing a hissing sound like that of (s) or (sh).

sibilant rale *n.* A whistling sound heard on auscultation and caused by the presence of a viscid secretion narrowing the lumen of a bronchus.

sib·ling (sĭb′lĭng) *n.* One of two or more individuals having one or both parents in common; a brother or sister.

sib·ship (sĭb′shĭp′) *n.* The children produced by one pair of parents.

si·bu·tra·mine (sə-byōō′trə-mĭn, -mēn′) *n.* A drug that suppresses appetite by inhibiting the reuptake of norepinephrine and serotonin, used in the management of obesity.

sic·ca complex (sĭk′ə) *n.* Dryness of the mucous membranes, as of the eyes and mouth, in the absence of a connective tissue disease.

sic·cant (sĭk′ənt) *adj.* Having the capability to make dry; drying.

sicca syndrome *n.* See **Sjögren's syndrome.**

sic·ca·tive (sĭk′ə-tĭv) *n.* A substance added to some medicines to promote drying; a drier.

sick (sĭk) *adj.* **1.** Suffering from or affected with a disease or disorder. **2.** Of or for sick persons. **3.** Nauseated. **4.** Mentally ill or disturbed. **5.** Constituting an unhealthy environment for those working or residing within, as of a building.

sick·bay (sĭk′bā′) *n.* **1.** The hospital and dispensary of a ship. **2.** A place in which the sick or injured are treated.

sick·bed (sĭk′bĕd′) *n.* A sick person's bed.

sick building syndrome *n.* An illness affecting workers in office buildings, characterized by skin irritations, headache, and respiratory problems, and thought to be caused by indoor pollutants, microorganisms, or inadequate ventilation.

sick headache *n.* See **migraine.**

sick·le (sĭk′əl) *v.* **1.** To cut with a sickle. **2.** To deform a red blood cell into an abnormal crescent shape. **3.** To assume an abnormal crescent shape. Used of red blood cells.

sick leave *n.* Paid absence from work allowed an employee because of sickness.

sickle cell *n.* An abnormal, crescent-shaped red blood cell that results from a single change in the amino acid sequence of the cell's hemoglobin, which causes the cell to contort, especially under low-oxygen conditions. Also called *drepanocyte, meniscocyte.*

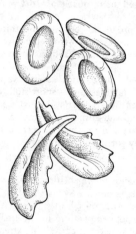

sickle cell
Top: *normal red blood cells*
Bottom: *sickle-shaped red blood cells*

sickle cell anemia *n.* A chronic, usually fatal inherited form of anemia marked by crescent-shaped red blood cells, occurring almost exclusively in Blacks, and characterized by fever, leg ulcers, jaundice, and episodic pain in the joints. Also called *crescent cell anemia, drepanocytic anemia, drepanocytosis, meniscocytosis, sickle cell disease, sickle cell syndrome.*

sickle cell C disease *n.* A hereditary blood disease caused by sickle-shaped red blood cells that contain hemoglobin S and hemoglobin C, characterized by anemia, blocked blood vessels, chronic leg ulcers, and bone deformities.

sickle cell disease *n.* See **sickle cell anemia.**

sickle cell hemoglobin *n.* See **hemoglobin S.**

sickle cell retinopathy *n.* A condition characterized by dilation and tortuosity of retinal veins, microaneurysms, and retinal hemorrhages, with advanced cases manifesting neovascularization, detachment of the retina, or vitreous hemorrhage.

sickle cell syndrome *n.* See **sickle cell anemia.**

sickle-cell test *n.* A method of determining the percentage of red blood cells containing hemoglobin S.

sickle cell-thalassemia disease *n.* See **microdrepanocytic anemia.**

sickle cell trait *n.* A hereditary condition, usually harmless and without symptoms, in which an individual carries only one gene for sickle cell anemia.

sick·le·mi·a (sĭk′ə-lē′mē-ə) *n.* The presence of sickle-shaped red blood cells in the peripheral blood, as in sickle cell trait and sickle cell anemia.

sick·ling (sĭk′lĭng) *n.* The production of sickle-shaped red blood cells, as in sickle cell anemia.

sick·ness (sĭk′nĭs) *n.* **1.** The condition of being sick; illness. **2.** A disease or an illness.

sick role *n.* The protective role given an individual who is physically or mentally ill or injured; it may be assumed by the individual or it may be imposed as a part of social custom.

sick·room (sĭk′room′, -room′) *n.* A room occupied by a sick person.

sick sinus syndrome *n.* *Abbr.* **SSS** Chaotic atrial activity characterized by an abnormally slow heartbeat punctuated by recurring ectopic beats and periods of an abnormally rapid heartbeat.

side chain (sīd) *n.* A linear group of atoms linked to a benzene ring or to any cyclic chain compound.

side effect *n.* A peripheral or secondary effect, especially an undesirable secondary effect of a drug or therapeutic regimen.

sidero– or **sider–** *pref.* Iron: *sideropenia.*

sid·er·o·blast (sĭd′ər-ə-blăst′) *n.* An erythroblast containing granules of ferritin.

sid·er·o·blas·tic anemia (sĭd′ər-ə-blăs′tĭk) *n.* Refractory anemia marked by sideroblasts in the bone marrow. Also called *sideroachrestic anemia.*

sid·er·o·cyte (sĭd′ər-ə-sīt′) *n.* A red blood cell containing granules of iron that are not part of the cell's hemoglobin.

sid·er·o·der·ma (sĭd′ə-rō-dûr′mə) *n.* A brownish discoloration of the skin on the legs caused by hemosiderin deposits.

sid·er·o·fi·bro·sis (sĭd′ə-rō-fī-brō′sĭs) *n.* Fibrosis associated with small foci in which iron is deposited.

sid·er·o·pe·ni·a (sĭd′ər-ə-pē′nē-ə) *n.* An abnormally low level of iron in the blood serum. —**sid′er·o·pe′-nic** (-nĭk) *adj.*

sid·er·o·phage (sĭd′ər-ə-fāj′) *n.* See **siderophore.**

sid·er·o·phil (sĭd′ər-ə-fĭl) or **sid·er·o·phile** (-fīl′) *adj.* Absorbing iron. —*n.* A cell or tissue that contains iron.

sid·er·oph·i·lin (sĭd′ə-rŏf′ə-lĭn, -rə-fīl′ĭn) *n.* See **transferrin.**

sid·er·oph·i·lous (sĭd′ə-rŏf′ə-ləs) *adj.* Siderophil.

sid·er·o·phore (sĭd′ər-ə-fôr′) *n.* A large, extravasated, mononuclear phagocyte containing a granule of hemosiderin. Also called *siderophage.*

sid·er·o·sil·i·co·sis (sĭd′ə-rō-sĭl′ĭ-kō′sĭs) *n.* Silicosis due to inhalation of dust containing iron and silica. Also called *silicosiderosis.*

sid·er·o·sis (sĭd′ə-rō′sĭs) *n.* **1.** Chronic inflammation of the lungs caused by excessive inhalation of dust containing iron salts or particles. **2.** Discoloration of an organ or a tissue by an iron pigment. **3.** An excess of iron in the blood.

sid·er·ot·ic (sĭd′ə-rŏt′ĭk) *n.* **1.** Pigmented by iron. **2.** Containing an excess of iron.

siderotic nodules *n.* See **Gamna-Gandy bodies.**

SIDS *abbr.* sudden infant death syndrome

sie·mens (sē′mənz) *n.,* *pl.* **siemens** A unit of electrical conductance in the International System of Units, equal to one ampere per volt.

sieve graft (sĭv) *n.* A full-thickness skin graft taken after cutting multiple holes in it with a circular punch, thus leaving islands of skin to heal the donor area.

sie·vert (sē′vərt) *n.* *Abbr.* **Sv** A unit of ionizing radiation absorbed dose equivalent in the International System of Units, obtained as a product of the absorbed dose measure in grays and a dimensionless factor, stipulated by the International Commission on Radiological Protection, and indicating the biological effectiveness of the radiation.

sig. *abbr.* *Latin* signa (sign; label); *Latin* signetur (let it be labeled; let it be signed)

sight (sīt) *n.* **1.** The ability to see. **2.** Field of vision.

sig·ma (sĭg′mə) *n.* *Symbol* **σ** The 18th letter of the Greek alphabet.

sigma factor *n.* A protein component of RNA polymerase that determines the specific site on DNA where transcription begins.

sig·moid (sĭg′moid′) or **sig·moi·dal** (sĭg-moid′l) *adj.* **1.** Having the shape of the letter S. **2.** Of or relating to the sigmoid flexure of the colon.

sigmoid artery *n.* Any of the arteries with their origin in the inferior mesenteric artery, with distribution to the descending colon and sigmoid flexure, and with anastomoses to the left colic and superior rectal arteries.

sigmoid colon *n.* See **sigmoid flexure.**

sig·moid·ec·to·my (sĭg′moi-dĕk′tə-mē) *n.* Excision of the sigmoid colon.

sigmoid flexure *n.* The S-shaped section of the colon between the pelvic brim and the third sacral segment, continuous with the rectum. Also called *sigmoid colon.*

sig·moid·i·tis (sĭg′moi-dī′tĭs) *n.* Inflammation of the sigmoid colon.

sigmoido– or **sigmoid–** *pref.* Sigmoid; sigmoid colon: *sigmoidopexy.*

sig·moi·do·pex·y (sĭg-moi′də-pĕk′sē) *n.* Surgical attachment of the sigmoid colon to a firm structure to correct rectal prolapse.

sig·moi·do·proc·tos·to·my (sĭg-moi′dō-prŏk-tŏs′tə-mē) *n.* Establishment of an artificial anus by surgically creating an opening at the junction of the sigmoid colon and the rectum. Also called *sigmoidorectostomy.*

sig·moi·do·rec·tos·to·my (sĭg-moi′dō-rĕk-tŏs′tə-mē) *n.* See **sigmoidoproctostomy.**

sig·moid·o·scope (sĭg-moi′də-skōp′) *n.* A tubular instrument for visual examination of the sigmoid flexure. —**sig′moid·os′co·py** (sĭg′moi-dŏs′kə-pē) *adj.*

sig·moid·os·to·my (sĭg′moi-dŏs′tə-mē) *n.* Establishment of an artificial anus by surgically creating an opening into the sigmoid colon.

sig·moid·ot·o·my (sĭg′moi-dŏt′ə-mē) *n.* The surgical opening of the sigmoid colon.

sigmoid sinus *n.* The S-shaped dural sinus lying on the mastoid process of the temporal bone and the jugular process of the occipital bone.

sigmoid vein *n.* Any of the tributaries of the inferior mesenteric vein that drain the sigmoid colon.

sign (sīn) *n.* An objective finding, usually detected on physical examination, from a laboratory test, or on an x-ray, that indicates the presence of abnormality or disease.

sig·nal node (sĭg′nəl) *n.* A firm, palpable, supraclavicular lymph node, usually on the left side, whose tumorous condition is usually secondary to primary carcinoma in one of the viscera. Also called *jugular gland, Virchow's node.*

sig·na·ture (sĭg′nə-chər) *n.* The part of a physician's prescription containing directions to the patient.

sig·net-ring cell (sĭg′nĭt-rĭng′) *n.* A cell with a large cytoplasmic vacuole containing mucin that compresses the nucleus to one side of the cell.

signet-ring cell carcinoma *n.* A poorly differentiated adenocarcinoma that occurs most frequently in the stomach and occasionally in the large bowel.

sign language *n.* A language that uses a system of manual, facial, and other body movements as the means of communication, especially among deaf people.

sil·ane (sĭl′ān′) *n.* Any of a group of highly reactive hydrocarbons containing tetravalent silicon instead of carbon.

sil·den·a·fil citrate (sĭl-dĕn′ə-fĭl′) *n.* A drug of the phosphodiesterase inhibitor class, used to treat erectile dysfunction by increasing the level of cyclic GMP, which increases blood flow to the erectile tissues.

si·lent (sī′lənt) *adj.* Producing no detectable signs or symptoms. Used of certain diseases or pathological processes.

silent area *n.* An area of the cerebral or cerebellar surface on which lesions cause no sensory or motor symptoms.

sil·i·ca (sĭl′ĭ-kə) *n.* A crystalline compound occurring abundantly as quartz, sand, and many other minerals and used to manufacture a variety of materials, especially glass and concrete.

sil·i·cate (sĭl′ĭ-kāt′, -kĭt) *n.* Any of numerous compounds containing silicon, oxygen, and one or more metals; a salt of silicic acid.

sil·i·ca·to·sis (sĭl′ĭ-kə-tō′sĭs) *n.* See **silicosis.**

sil·i·con (sĭl′ĭ-kən, -kŏn′) *n. Symbol* **Si** A nonmetallic element occurring extensively in the earth's crust in silica and silicates, having both an amorphous and a crystalline allotrope and used in glass and semiconducting devices and in surgical implants. Atomic number 14.

silicon dioxide *n.* Silica.

sil·i·cone (sĭl′ĭ-kōn′) *n.* Any of a group of silicon compounds in solid, liquid, or gel form, characterized by wide-range thermal stability, high lubricity, extreme water repellence, and physiological inertness and used in many medical products, including surgical implants and dental impression materials.

sil·i·co·pro·tein·o·sis (sĭl′ĭ-kō-prō′tē-nō′sĭs) *n.* An acute, usually fatal pulmonary disorder, similar to pulmonary alveolar proteinosis, resulting from exposure to high concentrations of silica dust.

sil·i·co·sid·er·o·sis (sĭl′ĭ-kō-sĭd′ə-rō′sĭs) *n.* See **siderosilicosis.**

sil·i·co·sis (sĭl′ĭ-kō′sĭs) *n.* A disease of the lungs caused by continued inhalation of the dust of minerals that contain silica and characterized by progressive fibrosis and a chronic shortness of breath. Also called *silicatosis.* —**sil′i·cot′ic** (-kŏt′ĭk) *adj.*

sil·i·co·tu·ber·cu·lo·sis (sĭl′ĭ-kō-tŏo-bûr′kyə-lō′sĭs) *n.* Silicosis associated with tuberculous pulmonary lesions.

si·lic·u·lose cataract (sə-lĭk′yə-lōs′) *n.* Calcareous degeneration of the lens capsule.

sil·i·quose (sĭl′ĭ-kwōs′) *adj.* Resembling a long slender pod. Used of a cataract resulting in shriveling of the lens and calcareous deposits in the capsule.

siliquose cataract *n.* Siliculose cataract.

sil·ver (sĭl′vər) *n. Symbol* **Ag** A lustrous ductile malleable metallic element having the highest thermal and electrical conductivity of the metals and used in dental alloys and in pharmaceuticals. Atomic number 47.

silver-fork deformity *n.* A deformity seen in Colles' fracture in which the wrist or forearm has a curve like that of the back of a fork.

silver-fork fracture *n.* A Colles' fracture of the wrist causing a silver-fork deformity.

silver iodide *n.* A pale yellow, odorless, tasteless powder that darkens when exposed to light and that is used as an antiseptic.

silver nitrate *n.* A poisonous crystalline compound with antiseptic and astringent properties, used in the prevention of ophthalmia neonatorum and in the special staining of nervous tissue, spirochetes, and reticular fibers.

silver protein *n.* A colloidal preparation of silver oxide and protein, usually gelatin or albumin, used as an antibacterial agent.

silver protein stain *n.* A silver protein complex used in staining nerve fibers, nerve endings, and flagellate protozoa.

si·meth·i·cone (sĭ-mĕth′ĭ-kōn′) *n.* A mixture of dimethyl polysiloxanes and silica gel that is used as an antiflatulent.

sim·i·an virus (sĭm′ē-ən) *n.* Any of a number of viruses of variable taxonomic classification isolated from monkeys and from cultures of monkey cells.

si·mil·i·a si·mil·i·bus cu·ran·tur (sĭ-mĭl′ē-ə sĭ-mĭl′ə-bŭs′ kyə-răn′tər) *n.* The homeopathic axiom expressing the law of similars or the doctrine that any drug capable of producing detrimental symptoms in healthy individuals will relieve similar symptoms occurring as an expression of disease.

Sim·monds disease (sĭm′əndz) *n.* Extreme and progressive emaciation, loss of body hair, and premature aging caused by atrophy or destruction of the anterior lobe of the pituitary. Also called *hypophysial cachexia, pituitary cachexia.*

sim·ple absence (sĭm′pəl) *n.* A brief loss or impairment of consciousness accompanied by the abrupt onset of spasms or twitchings of cephalic muscles that produce a 3 per second pattern of spikes and waves on an electroencephalogram. Also called *pure absence.*

simple dislocation *n.* See **closed dislocation.**

simple epithelium *n.* Epithelium made up of one layer of cells.

simple fission *n.* Division of the nucleus and then the cell body into two parts.

simple fracture *n*. See **closed fracture**.

simple glaucoma *n*. See **open-angle glaucoma**.

simple goiter *n*. Thyroid enlargement unaccompanied by constitutional effects, commonly caused by inadequate dietary intake of iodine.

simple joint *n*. A joint composed of two bones only.

simple mastectomy *n*. Surgical removal of the breast, including the nipple, areola, and most of the overlying skin.

simple microscope *n*. A microscope having one lens or lens system, such as a magnifying glass.

simple protein *n*. A protein, such as a globulin, that yields only alpha-amino acids upon hydrolysis.

simple squamous epithelium *n*. Epithelium made up of a single layer of flattened scalelike cells.

simple sugar *n*. See **monosaccharide**.

Simp·son (sĭmp′sən), Sir **James Young** 1811–1870. British obstetrician and a founder of gynecology. He is also known for introducing the use of chloroform as an anesthetic.

Sims′ position (sĭmz) *n*. A position in which the patient lies on one side with the under arm behind the back and the upper thigh flexed, used to facilitate vaginal examination. Also called *lateral recumbent position*.

sim·u·la·tion (sĭm′yə-lā′shən) *n*. **1.** Close resemblance or imitation, as of one symptom or disease by another. **2.** Assumption of a false appearance. **3.** Reproduction or representation, as of a potential situation or in experimental testing. —**sim′u·late′** (-lāt′) *v*. —**sim′u·la′·tor** (-lā′tər) *n*.

Si·mu·li·um (sĭ-myōō′lē-əm) *n*. A genus of biting gnats or midges of the family Simuliidae that includes various species that transmit the causative agent of human onchocerciasis.

si·mul·tan·ag·no·sia (sī′məl-tăn′ăg-nō′zhə) *n*. Inability to recognize multiple elements in a simultaneously displayed visual presentation; the ability to appreciate elements of a scene but not the display as a whole.

SIMV *abbr*. spontaneous intermittent mandatory ventilation

sim·va·stat·in (sĭm′və-stăt′n) *n*. A statin drug derived from the mold *Aspergillus terreus*, used to treat hyperlipidemia.

sincipital presentation *n*. Head presentation of the fetus during birth in which the large fontanel is the presenting part.

sin·ci·put (sĭn′sə-pət) *n*., *pl*. **sin·ci·puts** or **sin·cip·i·ta** (sĭn-sĭp′ĭ-tə) **1.** The upper half of the cranium, especially the anterior portion above and including the forehead. **2.** The forehead. —**sin·cip′i·tal** (-sĭp′ĭ-tl) *adj*.

Sind·bis fever (sĭnd′bĭs) *n*. A febrile illness of humans in Africa, Australia, and other countries, characterized by arthralgia, rash, and malaise. It is caused by the Sindbis virus and transmitted by culicine mosquitoes.

Sindbis virus *n*. An alphavirus that is the causative agent of Sindbis fever.

Sin·e·met (sĭn′ə-mĕt′) A trademark for the drug combination of carbidopa and L-dopa.

Sin·e·quan (sĭn′ə-kwăn′) A trademark for the drug doxepin hydrochloride.

sin·ew (sĭn′yōō) *n*. **1.** A tendon. **2.** Vigorous strength; muscular power.

sing·er′s nodes (sĭng′ərz) *pl.n*. See **vocal cord nodules**.

sin·gle blind (sĭng′gəl) *n*. A testing procedure in which the administrators do not tell the subjects if they are being given a test treatment or a control treatment, used in an effort to avoid accidental bias in the results. —**sin′gle-blind′** *adj*.

single bond *n*. A covalent bond in which one electron pair is shared by two atoms.

single photon emission computed tomography *n*. *Abbr*. **SPECT** Tomographic imaging of local metabolic and physiological functions in tissues. The image is formed by a computer synthesis of data that is transmitted by single gamma photons emitted by radionuclides administered to the patient.

sin·gle·ton (sĭng′gəl-tən) *n*. An offspring born alone.

sin·is·ter (sĭn′ĭ-stər) *adj*. On the left side; left.

sin·is·trad (sĭn′ĭ-străd′, sĭ-nĭs′trăd′) *adv*. Toward the left side.

sin·is·tral (sĭn′ĭ-strəl, sĭ-nĭs′trəl) *adj*. **1.** Of, facing, or located on the left side; left. **2.** Left-handed.

sin·is·tral·i·ty (sĭn′ĭ-străl′ĭ-tē) *n*. Preference for the left hand in performing manual tasks; left-handedness.

sinistro– or **sinistr–** *pref*. **1.** Left: *sinistral*. **2.** Levorotatory: *sinistrotorsion*.

sin·is·tro·car·di·a (sĭn′ĭ-strō-kär′dē-ə) *n*. The displacement of the heart to the left.

sin·is·tro·cer·e·bral (sĭn′ĭ-strō-sĕr′ə-brəl, -sə-rē′-) *adj*. Of or relating to the left cerebral hemisphere.

sin·is·troc·u·lar (sĭn′ĭ-strŏk′yə-lər) *adj*. Left-eyed.

sin·is·tro·gy·ra·tion (sĭn′ĭ-strō-jī-rā′shən) *n*. A twisting to the left, as of a plane of polarized light.

sin·is·tro·man·u·al (sĭn′ĭ-strō-măn′yōō-əl) *adj*. Left-handed.

sin·is·trop·e·dal (sĭn′ĭ-strŏp′ĭ-dl, sĭn′ĭ-strō-pĕd′l, -pēd′l) *adj*. Left-footed.

sin·is·tro·tor·sion (sĭn′ĭ-strō-tôr′shən) *n*. A twisting to the left. Also called *levotorsion*.

si·no·a·tri·al (sī′nō-ā′trē-əl) or **si·nu·a·tri·al** (sī′nōō-ā′trē-əl, sĭn′yōō-) *adj*. *Abbr*. **S-A** Relating to the venous sinus and the right atrium of the heart.

sinoatrial block *n*. Failure of an impulse to leave the sinoatrial node. Also called *sinoauricular block, sinus block*.

sinoatrial node *n*. *Abbr*. **SAN** A small mass of specialized cardiac muscle fibers located in the posterior wall of the right atrium of the heart that acts as a pacemaker of the cardiac conduction system by generating at regular intervals the electric impulses of the heartbeat. Also called *sinoauricular node, sinus node*.

si·no·au·ric·u·lar (sī′nō-ô-rĭk′yə-lər) *adj*. Sinoatrial.

sinoauricular block *n*. See **sinoatrial block**.

sinoauricular node *n*. See **sinoatrial node**.

si·no·pul·mo·nar·y (sī′nō-pŏŏl′mə-nĕr′ē, -pŭl′-) *adj*. Of or relating to the paranasal sinuses and the pulmonary airway.

si·nus (sī′nəs) *n*. **1.** A depression or cavity formed by a bending or curving. **2.** A channel for the passage of blood or lymph, without the coats of an ordinary vessel, such as the blood passages in the gravid uterus or in the cerebral meninges. **3.** Any of various air-filled cavities in the bones of the skull, especially one communicating with the nostrils. **4.** A dilatation in a blood vessel. **5.** A fistula or tract leading to a pus-filled cavity.

sinus arrest *n.* A pause or cessation of cardiac sinus pacemaker activity.

sinus arrhythmia *n.* Irregularity of the heartbeat due to a variation in the sinus rhythm.

sinus block *n.* See sinoatrial block.

sinus histiocytosis with massive lymphadenopathy *n.* A chronic disease that occurs in children and is characterized by massive painless cervical lymphadenopathy that is the result of distension of the lymphatic sinuses by macrophages containing ingested lymphocytes.

si·nus·i·tis (sī′nə-sī′tĭs) *n.* Inflammation of the mucous membrane of a sinus, especially of the paranasal sinuses.

sinus node *n.* See sinoatrial node.

sinus of dura mater *n.* Any of the various venous channels located in the dura mater and lined with epithelial cells. Also called *cerebral sinus, dural sinus.*

sinus of vena cava *n.* The portion of the cavity of the right atrium of the heart that receives the blood from the venae cavae and is separated from the rest of the atrium by the terminal crest.

si·nu·soid (sī′nə-soid′, -nyə-) *n.* Any of the venous cavities through which blood passes in various glands and organs, such as the adrenal gland and the liver. —*adj.* Resembling a sinus. —**si′nu·soi′dal** (-soid′l) *adj.*

si·nus·ot·o·my (sī′nə-sŏt′ə-mē, -nyə-) *n.* Incision into a sinus.

sinus pause *n.* A spontaneous interruption in the regular sinus rhythm lasting for a period that is not an exact multiple of the sinus cycle.

sinus rhythm *n.* A normal cardiac rhythm proceeding from the sinoatrial node.

si·phon (sī′fən) *n.* A tube bent into an inverted U shape of unequal lengths, used to remove fluid by means of atmospheric pressure from a cavity or reservoir at one end of the tube over a barrier and out the other end. —*v.* **1.** To draw off or convey through a siphon. **2.** To pass through a siphon.

si·phon·age (sī′fə-nĭj) *n.* The emptying of a cavity, such as the stomach, by means of a siphon.

Sip·ple's syndrome (sĭp′əlz) *n.* An inherited disorder characterized by pheochromocytoma, medullary thyroid carcinoma, and neural tumors.

si·re·no·me·li·a (sī′rə-nō-mē′lē-ə, -mēl′yə) *n.* Congenital union of the legs with partial or complete fusion of the feet.

si·ro·li·mus (sə-rō′lə-məs) *n.* An immunosuppressive drug produced by the actinomycete *Streptomyces hygroscopicus,* used in combination with cyclosporine and corticosteroids to prevent rejection of transplanted tissues or organs.

sis·o·mi·cin sulfate (sĭs′ə-mī′sĭn) *n.* An antibiotic having a spectrum of activity that is similar to that of gentamicin.

Sis·ter Jo·seph's nodule (sĭs′tər jō′səfs) *n.* A nodule in the umbilical region associated with a malignant metastatic intra-abdominal tumor.

Sister Ken·ny's treatment (kĕn′ēz) *n.* Treatment of poliomyelitis by wrapping affected parts with warm moist cloth, and later passively exercising the paralyzed muscles.

site (sīt) *n.* A place; a location. —*v.* To locate or situate at a site.

sito– *pref.* Grain; food: *sitotoxin.*

si·to·ma·ni·a (sī′tə-mā′nē-ə, -mān′yə) *n.* An abnormal craving for food.

si·to·pho·bi·a (sī′tə-fō′bē-ə) *n.* An abnormal aversion to food.

si·tos·ter·ol (sī-tŏs′tə-rôl′, -rōl′, sĭ-) *n.* Any of a group of sterols that occur in high concentrations in certain plants, such as yams, and are used in the synthesis of steroid hormones.

si·to·tax·is (sī′tə-tăk′sĭs) *n.* See sitotropism.

si·to·tox·in (sī′tə-tŏk′sĭn) *n.* A food poison, especially one developing in grain.

si·tot·ro·pism (sī-tŏt′rə-pĭz′əm) *n.* The turning of living cells toward or away from a food source. Also called *sitotaxis.*

sit·u·a·tion·al psychosis (sĭch′ōō-ā′shə-nəl) *n.* A severe, transitory emotional disorder caused by an extremely distressing event or situation.

si·tus (sī′təs) *n., pl.* **situs** Position, especially normal or original position, as of a body organ or part.

situs in·ver·sus (ĭn-vûr′səs) *n.* A congenital condition in which the organs of the viscera are transposed through the sagittal plane so that the heart, for example, is on the right side of the body. Also called *visceral inversion.*

sitz bath (sĭts, zĭts) *n.* **1.** A device shaped like a chair in which one bathes in a sitting position, immersing only the hips and buttocks. **2.** A bath taken in such a device especially for therapeutic reasons.

sixth cranial nerve (sĭksth) *n.* See abducent nerve.

sixth disease *n.* See exanthema subitum.

sixth venereal disease *n.* See venereal lymphogranuloma.

sixth-year molar *n.* The first permanent molar tooth.

siz·er (sī′zər) *n.* A cylinder of variable diameter, with rounded ends, used to measure the internal diameter of the bowel in preparation for stapling.

Sjö·gren's syndrome (shœ′grĕnz) *n.* A syndrome occurring most frequently in older women, characterized by keratoconjunctivitis sicca, dryness of mucous membranes, telangiectasias or purpuric spots on the face, and bilateral parotid enlargement; it is often associated with rheumatoid arthritis, Raynaud's phenomenon, and dental caries. Also called *sicca syndrome.*

SK *abbr.* streptokinase

skat·ole (skăt′ōl, -ôl) *n.* A crystalline organic compound that is formed in the intestine by the bacterial decomposition of tryptophan and that has a strong fecal odor, found naturally in feces, beets, and coal tar.

ska·tox·yl (skă-tŏk′sĭl) *n.* An oxidation product of skatole formed in the intestine and excreted in the urine in cases of intestinal disease.

skel·e·tal extension (skĕl′ĭ-tl) *n.* See skeletal traction.

skeletal muscle *n.* A muscle that is connected at either or both extremities with a bone and consists of elongated, multinucleated, transversely striated, skeletal muscle fibers, together with connective tissues, blood vessels, and nerves.

skeletal system *n.* The bodily system that consists of the bones, their associated cartilages, and the joints. It supports and protects the body, produces blood cells, and stores minerals.

skeletal traction *n.* Traction on a bone structure by means of a pin or wire surgically inserted into the bone. Also called *skeletal extension.*

skel·e·ton (skĕl′ĭ-tn) *n.* **1.** The internal structure composed of bone and cartilage that protects and supports the soft organs, tissues, and other parts of a vertebrate organism; endoskeleton. **2.** All the bones of the body taken collectively. **3.** The exoskeleton.

skia– *pref.* Shadow: *skiascopy.*

ski·as·co·py (skī-ăs′kə-pē) *n.* See **retinoscopy.** **—ski′a·scope′** (skī′ə-skōp′) *n.*

skilled nursing facility (skĭld) *n.* *Abbr.* **SNF** An establishment that houses chronically ill, usually elderly patients, and provides long-term nursing care, rehabilitation, and other services. Also called *long-term care facility, nursing home.*

skim milk (skĭm) *n.* The milk from which the cream has been removed.

skin (skĭn) *n.* The membranous tissue forming an external protective covering or integument of an animal and consisting of the epidermis and dermis. **—v.** To bruise, cut, or injure the skin of. **—skin′less** *adj.*

skin dose *n.* The quantity of radiation delivered to the skin surface or absorbed in the skin.

skin patch *n.* See **transdermal patch.**

Skin·ner (skĭn′ər), **B(urrhus) F(rederick)** 1904–1990. American psychologist. A leading behaviorist, Skinner influenced the fields of psychology and education with his theories of stimulus-response behavior.

skin ridge *n.* See **epidermal ridge.**

skin tag *n.* An outgrowth of epidermal and dermal fibrovascular tissue. Also called *acrochordon, soft wart.*

skin test *n.* A test for detection of an allergy or infectious disease, performed by means of a patch test, a scratch test, or an intracutaneous injection of an allergen or extract of a disease-causing organism.

skin traction *n.* Traction on an extremity by means of adhesive tape or another type of strapping applied to the limb.

sko·da·ic resonance (skō-dā′ĭk) *n.* A high-pitched sound elicited by percussing just above the site of a pleuritic effusion.

skull (skŭl) *n.* The bony or cartilaginous framework of the head, made up of the bones of the braincase and face; cranium.

skull and crossbones *n., pl.* **skulls and crossbones** A representation of a human skull above two long crossed bones, a symbol of death used as a warning label on poisons.

skull·cap (skŭl′kăp′) *n.* See **calvaria.**

SL *abbr.* sublingual

slant culture (slănt) *n.* A culture made on the slanting surface of a solidified medium in a test tube that has

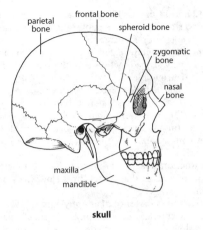

skull

been tilted to provide a greater area for growth. Also called *slope culture.*

SLE *abbr.* systemic lupus erythematosus

sleep (slēp) *n.* A natural periodic state of rest for the mind and body, in which the eyes usually close and consciousness is completely or partially lost, so that there is a decrease in bodily movement and responsiveness to external stimuli. During sleep the brain in humans and other mammals undergoes a characteristic cycle of brain-wave activity that includes intervals of dreaming. **—v.** To be in the state of sleep.

sleep apnea *n.* Apnea caused by upper airway obstruction during sleep, associated with frequent awakening and often with daytime sleepiness.

sleep-induced apnea *n.* Apnea resulting from failure of the respiratory center to stimulate adequate respiration during sleep.

sleep·ing sickness (slē′pĭng) *n.* See **encephalitis lethargica.**

sleep paralysis *n.* A condition in which, upon waking, a person is aware of the surroundings but is unable to move.

sleep·walk·ing (slēp′wô′kĭng) *n.* The act of walking or performing another activity associated with wakefulness while asleep or in a sleeplike state. Also called *noctambulism, somnambulism.* **—sleep′walk′** *v.*

slide (slīd) *n.* A small glass plate for mounting specimens to be examined under a microscope.

slid·ing flap (slī′dĭng) *n.* A rectangular flap raised in an elastic area with its free end adjacent to a defect that is covered by stretching the flap longitudinally until the end comes over it. Also called *advancement flap.*

sliding hernia *n.* A hernia in which an abdominal viscus forms part of the hernial sac. Also called *extrasaccular hernia, slipped hernia.*

sling (slĭng) *n.* A supporting bandage or suspensory device, especially a loop suspended from the neck and supporting the flexed forearm.

slipped disk (slĭpt) *n.* Protrusion of a part of an intervertebral disk through the fibrocartilage, occurring usually in the lower lumbar region and often causing back pain or sciatica.

slipped hernia *n.* See **sliding hernia.**

slip·ping rib (slĭp′ĭng) *n.* A subluxation of a rib cartilage with costochondral separation.

slipping rib cartilage *n.* Subluxation of the costal cartilage, usually at the junction with the sternum, causing pain and an audible click.

slit·lamp (slĭt′lămp′) *n.* See **biomicroscope.**

slope culture (slōp) *n.* See **slant culture.**

slough (slŭf) *n.* A layer or mass of dead tissue separated from surrounding living tissue, as in a wound, a sore, or an inflammation. —*v.* To separate from surrounding living tissue. Used of dead tissue.

slow infection (slō) *n.* An infection having a long incubation period, as that caused by a slow virus or by a prion.

slow-reacting substance of anaphylaxis *n. Abbr.* **SRS-A** A substance released in anaphylactic shock that produces slower and more prolonged contraction of muscle than does histamine. Also called *slow-reacting factor of anaphylaxis.*

slow-twitch *adj.* Of or relating to skeletal muscle that is composed of weak, slowly contracting fibers, adapted for low-intensity, high-endurance activities.

slow virus *n.* Any of a group of viruses that cause various diseases with a long, latent period and a slow progressive course, as subacute sclerosing panencephalitis. Also called *lentivirus.*

slow virus disease *n.* A disease caused by a slow virus.

Sm The symbol for the element **samarium.**

smack (smăk) *n.* Heroin.

small bowel (smōl) *n.* See **small intestine.**

small calorie *n. Abbr.* **c, cal** See **calorie** (sense 3).

small cardiac vein *n.* An inconstant vessel that accompanies the right coronary artery in the coronary sulcus from the right ventricle and empties into the coronary sinus or the middle cardiac vein.

small cell carcinoma *n.* See **oat cell carcinoma.**

small·er muscle of helix (smô′lər) *n.* A band of oblique muscular fibers that cover the ridge that runs from the helix backward and that divide the concha auriculae.

smaller posterior rectus muscle of head *n.* A muscle with origin from the posterior tubercle of the atlas, with insertion into the medial third of the occipital bone, with nerve supply from the first cervical nerve, and whose action rotates the head and draws it backward.

smaller psoas muscle *n.* An inconstant muscle with origin from the twelfth thoracic and the first lumbar vertebrae and the disk between them, with insertion into the iliopubic eminence, with nerve supply from the lumbar plexus, and whose action assists in the flexion of the lumbar spine. Also called *psoas minor.*

small·est cardiac vein (smô′lĭst) *n.* Any of the numerous small venous channels that open directly into the chambers of the heart from the capillary bed in the cardiac wall.

smallest scalene muscle *n.* An occasional independent muscular fasciculus between the anterior scalene and the middle scalene muscles, having the same action and innervation.

small increment sensitivity index *n. Abbr.* **SISI** A test for cochlear damage in which a tone above the hearing threshold is followed by a series of progressively louder tones and damage is indicated by the ability to hear the louder tones.

small intestine *n.* The narrow, winding, upper part of the intestine where digestion is completed and nutrients are absorbed by the blood. It extends from the pylorus to the cecum and consists of the duodenum, the jejunum, and the ileum. Also called *small bowel.*

small pelvis *n.* The cavity of the pelvis below the brim or below the superior aperture. Also called *pelvis minor, true pelvis.*

small·pox (smôl′pŏks′) *n.* An acute, highly infectious, often fatal disease caused by a poxvirus and characterized by high fever and aches with subsequent widespread eruption of papules that blister, produce pus, and form scabs that leave permanent pockmarks. Also called *variola.*

smallpox vaccine *n.* A vaccine containing vaccinia virus suspensions that is inoculated subcutaneously to immunize against smallpox.

smallpox virus *n.* See **variola virus.**

small pudendal lips *pl.n.* The labia minora.

small saphenous vein *n.* A vein that arises from the union of the dorsal vein of the little toe with the dorsal venous arch and ascends through the middle of the calf to the lower portion of the popliteal space where it empties into the popliteal vein.

smear (smîr) *n.* A sample, as of blood or bacterial cells, spread thinly on a slide and usually stained for microscopic examination or applied to the surface of a culture medium.

smear culture *n.* A culture made by spreading material presumed to be infected on the surface of a solidified medium.

smeg·ma (smĕg′mə) *n.* A sebaceous secretion, especially the whitish cheesy secretion that collects under the prepuce of the penis or around the clitoris.

smeg·ma·lith (smĕg′mə-lĭth′) *n.* A calcareous concretion in the smegma.

smell (smĕl) *v.* To perceive the scent of something by means of the olfactory nerves. —*n.* The sense by which odors are perceived; the olfactory sense.

smell·ing salts (smĕl′ĭng) *pl.n.* Any of various preparations of ammonium carbonate and perfume, sniffed as a restorative or stimulant especially to relieve faintness and headache.

Smith (smĭth), **Hamilton Othanel** Born 1931. American microbiologist. He shared a 1978 Nobel Prize for the discovery of restriction enzymes and their application to molecular genetics.

Smith's fracture (smĭths) *n.* A fracture of the radius of the wrist in which the lower fragment is displaced forward. Also called *reverse Colles' fracture.*

Smith's operation *n.* A surgical technique for removing a cataract within its capsule.

smog (smŏg) *n.* **1.** Fog that has become mixed and polluted with smoke. **2.** A form of air pollution produced when sunlight causes hydrocarbons and nitrogen oxides from automotive emissions to combine in a photochemical reaction.

smok·er's cough (smō′kərz) *n.* A rough, dry cough caused by excessive smoking of tobacco.

smoker's patch *n.* See **leukoplakia.**

smoker's tongue *n.* See **leukoplakia.**

smooth diet (smoōth) *n.* A diet that contains little roughage.

smooth muscle *n.* Muscle tissue that contracts without voluntary control, having fine myofibrils but lacking transverse striations and found in the walls of internal organs, blood vessels, and hair follicles.

Sn The symbol for the element **tin.**

snap (snăp) *n.* A short sharp sound; a click. Used especially of cardiac sounds.

snare (snâr) *n.* A surgical instrument with a wire loop controlled by a mechanism in the handle, used to remove growths, such as tumors and polyps.

sneeze (snēz) *v.* To expel air forcibly from the mouth and nose in an explosive, spasmodic involuntary action resulting chiefly from irritation of the nasal mucous membrane. —*n.* The act or an instance of sneezing.

Snell (snĕl), **George** 1903–1996. American geneticist. He shared a 1980 Nobel Prize for discoveries concerning cell structure that enhanced understanding of the immunological system, resulting in higher success rates in organ transplantation.

Snel·len chart (snĕl′ən) *n.* A chart for testing visual acuity, usually consisting of letters, numbers, or pictures printed in lines of decreasing size which a patient is asked to read or identify at a fixed distance.

Snel·len's test types (snĕl′ənz) *pl.n.* Letters used in testing the acuity of distant vision.

Snellen test *n.* A test for visual acuity using a Snellen chart.

SNF *abbr.* skilled nursing facility

snore (snôr) *v.* To breathe during sleep with harsh, snorting noises caused by vibration of the soft palate. —*n.* The act or an instance of snoring.

snot (snŏt) *n.* Nasal mucus; phlegm.

snout reflex (snout) *n.* A pouting or pursing of the lips that is caused by light tapping of the closed lips near the midline, seen in defective pyramidal innervation of facial musculature.

snow blindness (snō) *n.* A usually temporary loss of vision and inflammation of the conjunctiva and cornea caused by exposure to bright sunlight and ultraviolet rays reflected from snow or ice. —**snow′-blind′, snow′-blind′ed** *adj.*

snow·shoe hare virus (snō′shoo′) *n.* An arbovirus that is most commonly found in North America and that causes fever, headache, and nausea in humans.

snuff (snŭf) *v.* To inhale something audibly through the nose; sniff. —*n.* **1.** A preparation of finely pulverized tobacco that can be drawn up into the nostrils by inhaling. **2.** A medicated powder inhaled through or blown into the nose.

snuf·fle (snŭf′əl) *v.* To breathe noisily, as through a blocked nose. —*n.* **1.** The act of snuffling. **2. snuffles** Obstructed nasal respiration, especially in a newborn, sometimes due to congenital syphilis.

soap (sōp) *n.* **1.** A cleansing agent that is made from a mixture of the sodium salts of various fatty acids of natural oils and fats. **2.** A metallic salt of a fatty acid, as of aluminum or iron. —**soap** *v.*

Soa·ve operation (swä′vā, -vĕ) *n.* Endorectal pull-through for treatment of congenital megacolon.

SOB *abbr.* shortness of breath

so·cial anxiety disorder (sō′shəl) *n.* See **social phobia.**

social disease *n.* A sexually transmitted disease; a venereal disease.

so·cial·i·za·tion (sō′shə-lĭ-zā′shən) *n.* The process of learning interpersonal and interactional skills that are in conformity with the values of one's society. —**so′cial·ize′** (-shə-līz′) *v.*

so·cial·ized medicine (sō′shə-līzd′) *n.* A system for providing medical and hospital care for all at a nominal cost by means of government regulation of health services and subsidies derived from taxation.

social phobia *n.* A psychiatric disorder characterized by anxiety about being in public or social gatherings. Also called *social anxiety disorder.*

social psychiatry *n.* The branch of psychiatry that deals with the relationship between social environment and mental illness.

social psychology *n.* The branch of human psychology that deals with the behavior of groups and the influence of social factors on the individual.

socio– *pref.* **1.** Society: *sociocentric.* **2.** Social: *sociogenic.*

so·ci·o·cen·tric (sō′sē-ō-sĕn′trĭk, -shē-) *adj.* **1.** Oriented toward society; outgoing. **2.** Regarding one's own social group as superior to that of others.

so·ci·o·gen·e·sis (sō′sē-ō-jĕn′ĭ-sĭs, -shē-) *n.* The origin of social behavior that derives from past interpersonal experiences.

so·ci·o·path (sō′sē-ə-păth′, -shē-) *n.* A person affected with an antisocial personality disorder. —**so′ci·o·path′ic** *adj.*

so·ci·op·a·thy (sō′sē-ŏp′ə-thē, -shē-) *n.* The behavioral pattern exhibited by sociopaths.

sock·et (sŏk′ĭt) *n.* **1.** The concave part of a joint that receives the articular end of a bone. **2.** A hollow or concavity into which a part, such as an eye fits.

so·da (sō′də) *n.* **1.** Any of various forms of sodium carbonate. **2.** Chemically combined sodium.

soda lime *n.* A mixture of calcium hydroxide and sodium hydroxide used to absorb carbon dioxide in rebreathing apparatus and in anesthesia circuits.

so·di·um (sō′dē-əm) *n. Symbol* **Na** A soft, light, highly reactive metallic element that is naturally abundant, especially in common salt. Atomic number 11.

sodium barbital *n.* A white powder, the soluble sodium salt of barbital, used as a hypnotic and sedative.

sodium benzoate *n.* The sodium salt of benzoic acid, used as a food preservative, an antiseptic, and in the production of pharmaceuticals.

sodium bicarbonate *n.* See **baking soda.**

sodium borate *n.* A crystalline compound that is the sodium salt of boric acid and is used as an alkalizing agent and as a mild astringent in lotions, gargles, and mouthwashes.

sodium chloride *n.* Common or table salt, used as a food preservative and seasoning.

sodium cyclamate *n.* An artificially prepared salt of cyclamic acid, formerly used as a low-calorie sweetener but now banned because of the possible carcinogenic effects of its metabolic products.

sodium fluoride *n.* A colorless crystalline salt used in fluoridation of water, in treatment of tooth decay, and as an insecticide and a disinfectant.

sodium hydroxide *n.* A strongly alkaline compound used externally. Also called *caustic soda.*

sodium hypochlorite *n.* An unstable salt usually stored in solution and used as a fungicide and an oxidizing bleach.

sodium nitrite *n.* A white crystalline compound used to lower systemic blood pressure, to relieve local vasomotor spasms, to relax bronchial and intestinal spasms, and as an antidote for cyanide poisoning.

sodium nitroprusside *n.* A compound used as a reagent for the detection of organic compounds in the urine and as a potent agent for inducing hypotension through intravenous infusion.

sodium per·bo·rate (pər-bôr′āt′) *n.* A white odorless crystalline compound used as a mild alkaline oxidizing agent in dentifrices and as a topical antiseptic and deodorant.

sodium peroxide *n.* A yellowish-white powder used as a germicide, an antiseptic, and a disinfectant.

sodium-potassium pump *n.* The enzyme-based mechanism that maintains correct cellular concentrations of sodium and potassium ions by removing excess ions from inside a cell and replacing them with ions from outside the cell.

sodium pump *n.* A biologic mechanism that uses metabolic energy stored in ATP to achieve active transport of sodium ions across a membrane, such as the cell membrane or the multicellular membranes that make up the walls of renal tubules.

sodium sulfate *n.* A white crystalline compound used as a mild natural laxative and in larger doses as a hydragogue cathartic.

sodium thiosulfate *n.* A translucent crystalline compound used in conjunction with sodium nitrite as an antidote in cyanide poisoning, as a fungicide in swimming pools and baths, and as a means to measure the extracellular fluid volume of the body.

sod·om·y (sŏd′ə-mē) *n.* **1.** Anal copulation of one male with another. **2.** Anal or oral copulation with a member of the opposite sex. **3.** Copulation with an animal. —**sod′om·ite′** (-mīt′) *n.* —**sod′om·ize′** (-mīz′) *v.*

Soem·mer·ing (zœ′mər-ĭng), **Samuel Thomas von** 1755–1830. German anatomist noted for describing and naming the cranial nerves.

Soem·mer·ing's spot (sĕm′ər-ĭngz, sœ′mər-) *n.* See **macula lutea.**

soft corn (sŏft) *n.* A corn formed by pressure between two toes, with a surface softened by moisture. Also called *heloma molle.*

soft diet *n.* A normal diet limited to soft, easily digestible foods.

soft drug *n.* A drug considered to be nonaddictive and less damaging to the health than a hard drug.

soft palate *n.* The movable fold, consisting of muscular fibers enclosed in mucous membrane, that is suspended from the rear of the hard palate and closes off the nasal cavity from the oral cavity during swallowing or sucking.

soft rays *pl.n.* Radiation of relatively long wavelength and slight penetrability.

soft spot *n.* See **fontanel.**

soft tubercle *n.* A tubercle showing caseous necrosis.

soft ulcer *n.* See **chancroid.**

soft wart *n.* See **skin tag.**

sol (sôl, sōl) *n.* A colloidal dispersion of a solid in a liquid.

sol. *abbr.* solution

so·lar cheilitis (sō′lər) *n.* Mucosal atrophy, crusting, and fissuring of the border of the lips in old individuals, resulting from chronic exposure to sunlight. Also called *actinic cheilitis.*

solar elastosis *n.* Elastosis in the sun-exposed skin of old persons or in those who have chronic actinic damage.

solar ganglion *n.* See **celiac ganglion.**

solar plexus *n.* See **celiac plexus** (sense 1).

solar urticaria *n.* Urticaria resulting from exposure to sunlight.

sol·a·tion (sō-lā′shən) *n.* Transformation of a gel into a sol, as by melting gelatin.

sol·dier's heart (sōl′jərz) *n.* See **neurocirculatory asthenia.**

sole (sōl) *n.* The underside of the foot.

so·le·us (sō′lē-əs) *n.* A muscle with origin from the head and shaft of the fibula, the medial margin of the tibia, and the tendinous arch passing between the tibia and fibula, with insertion into the tuberosity of the calcaneus, with nerve supply from the tibial nerve, and whose action causes plantar flexion of the foot.

sol·id (sŏl′ĭd) *adj.* **1.** Of definite shape and volume; not liquid or gaseous. **2.** Firm or compact in substance. **3.** Having no internal cavity or hollow. —*n.* **1.** A solid substance, body, or tissue. **2.** Food that is relatively firm in substance or that must be chewed before swallowing.

sol·i·tar·y bone cyst (sŏl′ĭ-tĕr′ē) *n.* A unilocular cyst containing serous fluid and lined with a thin layer of connective tissue, usually occurring in the shaft of a long bone in growing children. Also called *osteocystoma, unicameral bone cyst.*

solitary follicle *n.* Any of the minute collections of lymphoid tissue in the mucosa of the small and large intestines, especially numerous in the cecum and in the appendix. Also called *solitary gland.*

solitary tract *n.* A slender compact bundle of primary sensory fibers that accompany the vagus, glossopharyngeal, and facial nerves and convey information from stretch receptors and chemoreceptors in the walls of the cardiovascular, respiratory, and intestinal tracts and impulses generated by the receptor cells of the taste buds in the tongue.

soln. *abbr.* solution

sol·u·bil·i·ty (sŏl′yə-bĭl′ĭ-tē) *n.* **1.** The quality or condition of being soluble. **2.** The amount of a substance that can be dissolved in a given amount of solvent.

solubility test *n.* A screening test to detect sickle-cell hemoglobin, in which blood with sickle-cell hemoglobin causes a solution to turn opaque.

sol·u·bi·lize (sŏl′yə-bə-līz′) *v.* To make substances such as fats soluble in water by the action of a detergent or similar agent.

sol·u·ble (sŏl′yə-bəl) *adj.* Capable of being dissolved, especially easily dissolved.

soluble glass *n.* A silicate of potassium or sodium, soluble in hot water but solid at ordinary temperatures, used for fixed dressings. Also called *water glass.*

sol·ute (sŏl′yo͞ot, sō′lo͞ot) *n.* A substance dissolved in another substance, usually the component of a solution present in the lesser amount.

so·lu·tion (sə-lo͞o′shən) *n. Abbr.* **sol., soln. 1.** A homogeneous mixture of two or more substances, which may be solids, liquids, gases, or a combination of these. **2.** The state of being dissolved. **3.** In pharmacology, a liquid preparation containing a solute, especially an aqueous solution of a nonvolatile substance. **4.** Termination of a disease by a crisis. **5.** A break, cut, or laceration of the solid tissues.

solution of contiguity *n.* A dislocation or displacement of two normally contiguous parts.

solution of continuity *n.* A division of bones or of soft parts that are normally continuous, as by a fracture, a laceration, or an incision. Also called *dieresis.*

sol·vent (sŏl′vənt) *adj.* Capable of dissolving another substance. —*n.* **1.** A substance in which another substance is dissolved, forming a solution. **2.** A substance capable of dissolving another substance.

so·ma (sō′mə) *n., pl.* **–mas** *or* **–ma·ta** (-mə-tə) **1.** The entire body of an organism, exclusive of the germ cells. **2.** The axial part of a body, including the head, neck, trunk, and tail. **3.** The body of a person as contrasted with the mind or psyche. **4.** See **cell body.**

somat– *pref.* Variant of **somato–.**

so·ma·tag·no·sia (sō′mə-tăg-nō′zhə) *n.* Inability to correctly identify or orient the parts of one's body or the body of another.

so·ma·tal·gia (sō′mə-tăl′jə) *n.* Pain in the body due to organic causes.

so·ma·tas·the·ni·a (sō′mə-tăs-thē′nē-ə) *or* **so·mas·the·ni·a** (sō′măs-) *n.* A condition of chronic physical weakness and fatigue.

so·ma·tes·the·sia (sō′mə-tĭs-thē′zhə) *or* **so·mes·the·sia** (sō′mĭs-) *n.* Consciousness of one's body; awareness of body sensation. —**so′ma·tes·thet′ic** (-thĕt′ĭk) *adj.*

so·mat·ic (sō-măt′ĭk) *adj.* **1.** Of, relating to, or affecting the body, especially as distinguished from a body part, the mind, or the environment; corporeal or physical. **2.** Of or relating to the wall of the body cavity, especially as distinguished from the head, limbs, or viscera. **3.** Relating to the vegetative, as distinguished from the generative, functions. **4.** Of or relating to a somatic cell or the somatoplasm. —**so·mat′i·cal·ly** *adv.*

somatic antigen *n.* An antigen located in the body of a bacterium.

somatic cell *n.* Any cell of a plant or an animal other than a germ cell.

somatic death *n.* Death of the entire body.

somatic delusion *n.* A delusion that a part of one's body has been injured or altered in some manner.

somatic motor neuron *n.* A motor neuron forming a direct synapse with striated muscle fibers via a motor end plate.

somatic motor nucleus *n.* Any of the motor nuclei innervating the tongue and external eye muscles.

somatic mutation *n.* Mutation occurring in the somatic cells as opposed to the germ cells.

somatic mutation theory of cancer *n.* The theory that cancer is caused by a mutation or mutations in the body cells, rather than germ cells, especially by nonlethal mutations associated with increased proliferation of the mutant cells.

somatic nerve *n.* Any of the nerves associated with sensation or motion.

somatic reproduction *n.* Asexual reproduction by fission or budding of somatic cells.

somatic sensory cortex *or* **somatosensory cortex** *n.* The region of the cerebral cortex receiving the somatic sensory data from the ventrobasal nucleus of the thalamus.

somatic swallow *n.* An adult or mature swallowing pattern, marked by muscular contractions that appear to be under control at a subconscious level.

so·ma·ti·za·tion (sō′mə-tĭ-zā′shən) *n.* In psychiatry, the conversion of anxiety into physical symptoms.

somatization disorder *n.* A disorder characterized by an individual's seeking help for and acquiring a complicated medical history of multiple physical symptoms referring to a variety of organ systems, but for whose complaints there is no detectable organic disorder or injury.

somato– *or* **somat–** *pref.* **1.** Body: *somatopathic.* **2.** Soma: *somatoplasm.*

so·mat·o·chrome (sō-măt′ə-krōm′, sō′mə-tə-) *n.* A nerve cell in which there is an abundance of cytoplasm completely surrounding the nucleus.

so·mat·o·form disorder (sō-măt′ə-fôrm′, sō′mə-tə-) *n.* Any of a group of disorders characterized by physical symptoms representing specific disorders for which there is no organic basis or known physiological cause, but for which there is presumed to be a psychological basis.

so·mat·o·gen·ic (sō-măt′ə-jĕn′ĭk, sō′mə-tə-) *or* **so·mat·o·ge·net·ic** (-jə-nĕt′ĭk) *adj.* **1.** Originating in the body under the influence of external forces. **2.** Having origin in body cells.

so·mat·o·lib·er·in (sō-măt′ə-lĭb′ər-ĭn, sō′mə-tə-) *n.* A decapeptide that is released by the hypothalamus and induces the release of somatotropin. Also called *growth hormone-releasing factor, somatotropin-releasing factor.*

so·mat·o·mam·mo·tro·pin (sō-măt′ə-măm′ə-trō′pĭn, sō′mə-tə-) *n.* A peptide hormone biologically related to growth hormone but produced by the normal placenta and by certain neoplasms.

so·mat·o·me·din (sō-măt′ə-mēd′n, sō′mə-tə-) *n.* A peptide synthesized in the liver, capable of stimulating certain anabolic processes in bone and cartilage, and whose secretion and biological activity are dependent on somatotropin. Also called *insulinlike growth factor.*

so·ma·to·path·ic (sō′mə-tə-păth′ĭk) *adj.* Relating to bodily or organic illness.

so·ma·top·a·thy (sō′mə-tŏp′ə-thē) *n.* Disease of the body.

so·mat·o·plasm (sō-măt′ə-plăz′əm, sō′mə-tə-) *n.* **1.** The entirety of specialized protoplasm, other than germ plasm, constituting the body. **2.** The protoplasm of a somatic cell. —**so′ma·to·plas′tic** (sō′mə-tə-plăs′tĭk) *adj.*

so·mat·o·pleure (sō-măt′ə-plŏŏr′, sō′mə-tə-) *n.* A complex sheet of embryonic cells formed by association of part of the mesoderm with the ectoderm and developing as the internal body wall. —**so·mat′o·pleu′ral** (-plŏŏr′əl), **so·mat′o·pleu′ric** (-plŏŏr′ĭk) *adj.*

so·mat·o·psy·chic (sō-măt′ə-sī′kĭk, sō′mə-tə-) *adj.* **1.** Relating to the relationship between the body and the mind. **2.** Relating to the study of the effects of the body upon the mind.

so·mat·o·psy·cho·sis (sō-măt′ə-sī-kō′sĭs, sō′mə-tə-) *n.* An emotional disorder associated with an organic disease.

so·mat·o·sen·so·ry (sə-măt′ə-sĕn′sə-rē, sō′mə-tə-) *adj.* Of or relating to the perception of sensory stimuli from the skin and internal organs.

somatosensory cortex *n.* Variant of **somatic sensory cortex.**

so·mat·o·sex·u·al (sō-măt′ə-sĕk′shŏŏ-əl, sō′mə-tə-) *adj.* Relating to the physical or physiological aspects of sexuality.

so·mat·o·stat·in (sō-măt′ə-stăt′n, sō′mə-tə-) *n.* A tetradecapeptide capable of inhibiting the release of somatotropin by the pituitary gland. Also called *somatotropin release-inhibiting factor.*

so·mat·o·stat·i·no·ma (sō-măt′ə-stăt′n-ō′mə, sō′mə-tə-) *n.* A somatostatin-secreting tumor of the pancreatic islets.

so·mat·o·ther·a·py (sō-măt′ə-thĕr′ə-pē, sō′mə-tə-) *n.* **1.** Therapy directed at bodily or physical disorders. **2.** Therapy employing chemical or physical methods, especially the treatment of mental illness by such means as drugs, shock therapy, and lobotomy.

so·mat·o·top·ag·no·sis (sō-măt′tə-tŏp′ăg-nō′sĭs, sō′-mə-tə-) *n.* Somatagnosia.

so·ma·tot·o·py (sō′mə-tŏt′ə-pē) *n.* The correspondence of receptors in regions or parts of the body via respective nerve fibers to specific functional areas of the cerebral cortex. —**so·mat′o·top′ic** (sə-măt′ə-tŏp′-ĭk, sō′mə-tə-) *adj.*

so·mat·o·troph (sō-măt′ə-trŏf′, -trōf′, sō′mə-tə-) *n.* A cell of the anterior lobe of the pituitary gland that produces somatotropin.

so·mat·o·trop·ic (sō-măt′ə-trŏp′ĭk, -trō′pĭk, sō′mə-tə-) *or* **so·mat·o·troph·ic** (-trŏf′ĭk, -trō′fĭk) *adj.* Having a stimulating effect on body growth.

so·mat·o·tro·pin (sə-măt′ə-trō′pĭn, sō′mə-tə-) *or* **so·mat·o·tro·phin** (-trō′fĭn) *n.* See **growth hormone.**

somatotropin release-inhibiting factor *n. Abbr.* **SRIF** See **somatostatin.**

somatotropin-releasing factor *n. Abbr.* **SRF** See **somatoliberin.**

so·mat·o·type (sō-măt′ə-tīp′, sō′mə-tə-) *n.* The structure or build of a person, especially to the extent to which it exhibits the characteristics of an ectomorph,

an endomorph, or a mesomorph. —**so·mat′o·typ′ic** (-tĭp′ĭk) *adj.*

–some *suff.* **1.** Body: *centrosome.* **2.** Chromosome: *autosome.*

so·mes·the·sia (sō′mĭs-thē′zhə) *n.* Variant of **somatesthesia.** —**so′mes·thet′ic** (-thĕt′ĭk) *adj.*

Som·i·nex (sŏm′ĭ-nĕks′) A trademark for the drug diphenhydramine.

so·mite (sō′mīt′) *n.* **1.** A segmental mass of mesoderm in the vertebrate embryo, occurring in pairs along the notochord and developing into muscles and vertebrae. **2.** See **metamere.**

som·nam·bu·lism (sŏm-năm′byə-lĭz′əm) *n.* See **sleepwalking.** —**som·nam′bu·lis′tic** *adj.*

somni– *or* **somn–** *pref.* Sleep: *somnambulism.*

som·ni·fa·cient (sŏm′nə-fā′shənt) *adj.* Tending to produce sleep; soporific. —**som′ni·fa′cient** *n.*

som·nif·er·ous (sŏm-nĭf′ər-əs) *adj.* Inducing sleep; soporific.

som·nil·o·quy (sŏm-nĭl′ə-kwē) *or* **som·nil·o·quism** (-kwĭz′əm) *n.* The act or habit of talking in one's sleep. —**som·nil′o·quist** *n.*

som·nip·a·thy (sŏm-nĭp′ə-thē) *n.* A disorder of sleep.

som·no·cin·e·ma·tog·ra·phy (sŏm′nō-sĭn′ə-mə-tŏg′-rə-fē) *n.* The process or technique of recording movements during sleep.

som·no·lence (sŏm′nə-ləns) *n.* **1.** A state of drowsiness; sleepiness. **2.** A condition of semiconsciousness approaching coma.

som·no·lent (sŏm′nə-lənt) *adj.* **1.** Drowsy; sleepy. **2.** Inducing or tending to induce sleep; soporific. **3.** In a condition of incomplete sleep; semicomatose.

som·no·les·cent (sŏm′nə-lĕs′ənt) *adj.* **1.** Somnolent; drowsy. **2.** Inducing sleep.

So·mo·gyi effect (sō′mō-jē′) *n.* In diabetes, the occurrence of reactive hyperglycemia following hypoglycemia. Also called *posthypoglycemic hyperglycemia, Somogyi phenomenon.*

Somogyi unit *n.* A measure of the level of activity of amylase in blood serum.

son·co·gene (sŏng′kə-jēn) *n.* One of a number of genes on specific chromosomes that can suppress the action of oncogenes.

son·ic (sŏn′ĭk) *adj.* Of, relating to, or determined by audible sound.

son·i·ca·tion (sŏn′ĭ-kā′shən) *n.* The process of dispersing, disrupting, or inactivating biological materials, such as viruses, by use of sound-wave energy.

son·i·fi·ca·tion (sŏn′ə-fĭ-kā′shən) *n.* The production of sound.

Son·ne bacillus (sŏn′ə) *n.* A gram-negative bacterium *Shigella sonnei* that causes a mild form of dysentery in adults and children.

son·o·gram (sŏn′ə-grăm′, sō′nə-) *n.* An image, as of an unborn fetus, produced by ultrasonography. Also called *echogram, sonograph, ultrasonogram.*

son·o·graph (sŏn′ə-grăf′, sō′nə-) *n.* **1.** See **ultrasonograph. 2.** See **sonogram.** —**son′o·graph′ic** *adj.*

so·nog·ra·phy (sə-nŏg′rə-fē) *n.* See **ultrasonography.**

son·o·rous rale (sŏn′ər′əs, sə-nôr′-) *n.* A cooing or snoring sound heard on auscultation, often produced by the vibration of a projecting mass of viscid secretion in a large bronchus.

so·por (sō′pər, -pôr′) *n.* A deep, lethargic, or unnatural sleep.

sop·o·rif·ic (sŏp′ə-rĭf′ĭk, sō′pə-) *adj.* **1.** Inducing or tending to induce sleep. **2.** Sleepy; drowsy.

sop·o·rous (sŏp′ər-əs, sō′pər-) *adj.* Relating to or causing sopor.

So·ra·nus (sô-rā′nəs) fl. second century AD. Greek physician. A leader of the school of physicians known as methodists, he wrote important works on midwifery and women's diseases.

sor·be·fa·cient (sôr′bə-fā′shənt) *adj.* Promoting absorption. Used of a medicine or an agent. —**sor′be·fa′cient** *n.*

sor·bic acid (sôr′bĭk) *n.* A white crystalline solid found in the berries of the mountain ash and also synthesized, used as a fungicide.

sor·bi·tol (sôr′bĭ-tôl′, -tōl′) *n.* A white, sweetish, crystalline alcohol occurring naturally or prepared synthetically, used as a sugar substitute for people with diabetes.

sor·des (sôr′dēz) *n.* A dark brown or blackish crustlike deposit on the lips, teeth, and gums of a person with dehydration resulting from a chronic debilitating disease.

sore (sôr) *n.* An open skin lesion, wound, or ulcer. —*adj.* Painful to the touch; tender. —**sore′ness** *n.*

sore throat *n.* Any of various inflammations of the tonsils, pharynx, or larynx characterized by pain in swallowing.

sorp·tion (sôrp′shən) *n.* Adsorption or absorption.

s.o.s. *abbr. Latin* si opus sit (if needed)

souf·fle (soo′fəl, soo′flə) *n.* A soft blowing sound heard on auscultation.

sound¹ (sound) *n.* **1.** Vibrations transmitted through an elastic material or a solid, liquid, or gas, with frequencies in the range of 20 to 20,000 hertz, capable of being detected by human organs of hearing. **2.** Transmitted vibrations of any frequency. **3.** A distinctive noise. —*v.* To auscultate.

sound² (sound) *adj.* **1.** Free from defect, decay, or damage; in good condition. **2.** Free from disease or injury.

sound³ (sound) *n.* An instrument used to examine or explore body cavities, as for foreign bodies or other abnormalities, or to dilate strictures in them. —*v.* To probe a body cavity with a sound.

source amnesia (sôrs) *n.* Memory loss that makes it impossible to recall the origin of the memory of a given event.

South African tick-bite fever (south) *n.* A typhuslike fever of South Africa caused by *Rickettsia rickettsii*, and usually characterized by primary eschar and regional adenitis, stiffness, and maculopapular rash on the fifth day, often with severe symptoms of the central nervous system.

South American blastomycosis *n.* See **paracoccidioidomycosis.**

South American trypanosomiasis *n.* A form of trypanosomiasis caused by *Trypanosoma cruzi* and transmitted by certain species of assassin bugs. In its acute form it causes swelling of the skin at the site of entry, with regional lymph node enlargement; in its chronic form it causes various conditions, commonly cardiomyopathy. Also called *Chagas disease, Cruz trypanosomiasis.*

South·ern blot analysis (sŭth′ərn) *n.* An electrophoretic procedure used to separate and identify DNA sequences.

space (spās) *n.* A particular area, extent, or cavity of the body.

space medicine *n.* The medical science that is concerned with the biological, physiological, and psychological effects of space flight on humans.

space sickness *n.* Motion sickness caused by sustained weightlessness during space flight, usually accompanied by disturbance of the inner ear. —**space′sick′** (spās′sĭk′) *adj.*

spa·cial formula (spā′shəl) *n.* See **stereochemical formula.**

Spal·lan·za·ni (spăl′ən-zä′nē, späl′länt-sä′nē), Lazzaro 1729–1799. Italian physiologist who disproved the theory that microorganisms generate spontaneously. He is also noted for his research on circulation and digestion.

spal·la·tion (spô-lā′shən) *n.* **1.** A nuclear reaction in which nuclei are bombarded by high-energy particles, causing the liberation of protons and alpha particles. **2.** Fragmentation.

spallation product *n.* Any of the subatomic particles produced from the spallation of an atom.

Span·ish influenza (spăn′ĭsh) *n.* Influenza that caused several waves of pandemic in 1918–1919, resulting in over 20 million deaths worldwide.

spar·ga·no·ma (spär′gə-nō′mə) *n.* A localized mass resulting from sparganosis.

spar·ga·no·sis (spär′gə-nō′sĭs) *n., pl.* **–ses** (-sēz) Infection with the plerocercoid of certain tapeworms, usually in a dermal sore resulting from direct contact with the flesh of an infected host.

spar·ing action (spâr′ĭng) *n.* The manner in which the presence of a nonessential nutritive component in the diet lowers an organism's requirement for an essential component.

spasm (spăz′əm) *n.* **1.** A sudden involuntary contraction of a muscle or group of muscles. **2.** A muscle spasm.

spasmo– *pref.* Spasm: *spasmolysis.*

spas·mod·ic (spăz-mŏd′ĭk) *adj.* **1.** Relating to, affected by, or having the character of a spasm; convulsive. **2.** Happening intermittently; fitful. **3.** Given to sudden outbursts of energy or of feeling; excitable. —**spas·mod′i·cal·ly** *adv.*

spasmodic dysmenorrhea *n.* Dysmenorrhea accompanied by painful contractions of the uterus.

spas·mol·y·sis (spăz-mŏl′ĭ-sĭs) *n.* Arrest of a spasm or convulsion.

spas·mo·lyt·ic (spăz′mə-lĭt′ĭk) *adj.* Causing arrest of a spasm; antispasmodic. —*n.* Antispasmodic.

spas·mus nu·tans (spăz′məs noo′tănz′) *n.* **1.** Nodding spasm. **2.** Nystagmus with head-nodding movements.

spas·tic (spăs′tĭk) *adj.* **1.** Relating to or affected by spasm. **2.** Relating to spastic paralysis.

spastic abasia *n.* Abasia due to spastic contraction of the leg muscles.

spastic colon *n.* See **irritable bowel syndrome.**

spastic gait *n.* A gait characterized by stiffness of legs, feet, and toes.

spastic hemiplegia *n.* Hemiplegia accompanied by spasms of the muscles of the affected side.

spastic ileus *n.* See **dynamic ileus.**

spas·tic·i·ty (spă-stĭs′ĭ-tē) *n.* **1.** A spastic state or condition. **2.** Spastic paralysis.

spastic paralysis *n.* A chronic pathological condition in which the muscles are affected by persistent spasms and exaggerated tendon reflexes because of damage to the central nervous system.

spa·tial *or* **spa·cial** (spā′shəl) *adj.* Relating to space or a space. —**spa′ti·al′i·ty** (spā′shē-ăl′ĭ-tē) *n.* —**spa′tial·ly** *adv.*

spat·u·late (spăch′ə-lĭt) *adj.* Having a broad flat end.

spay (spā) *v.* To surgically remove the ovaries of an animal.

SPCA *abbr.* serum prothrombin conversion accelerator

spe·cial anatomy (spĕsh′əl) *n.* The study of organs or organ systems that perform special physiological functions.

spe·cial·ist (spĕsh′ə-lĭst) *n.* A physician whose practice is limited to a particular branch of medicine or surgery, especially one who is certified by a board of physicians.

spe·cial·i·za·tion (spĕsh′ə-lĭ-zā′shən) *n.* **1.** The act of specializing. **2.** A specialty. **3.** Adaptation, as of an organ or organism, to a specific function or environment. **4.** See **differentiation** (sense 1).

spe·cial·ize (spĕsh′ə-līz′) *v.* **1.** To limit one's profession to a particular specialty or subject area for study, research, or treatment. **2.** To adapt to a particular function or environment.

special-needs *or* **special needs** *adj.* Of or relating to people who have specific needs, as those associated with a disability.

special sense *n.* Any of the five senses related to the organs of sight, hearing, smell, taste, and touch.

spe·cial·ty (spĕsh′əl-tē) *n.* A branch of medicine or surgery in which a physician specializes; the field or practice of a specialist.

spe·ci·a·tion (spē′shē-ā′shən, -sē-) *n.* The evolutionary formation of new biological species, usually by the division of a single species into two or more genetically distinct ones.

spe·cies (spē′shēz, -sēz) *n.*, *pl.* **species 1.** A fundamental category of taxonomic classification, ranking below a genus or subgenus and consisting of related organisms capable of interbreeding. **2.** An organism belonging to such a category, represented in binomial nomenclature by an uncapitalized Latin adjective or noun following a capitalized genus name, as in the bacterium *Escherichia coli.* **3.** A class of pharmaceutical preparations consisting of a mixture of dried plants in sufficiently fine division to be used in making boiled extracts or infusions. **4.** A specific type of atomic nucleus, atom, ion, or molecule.

species-specific *adj.* **1.** Limited to or found only in one species. **2.** Of or being a serum that acts only upon a member of the same species as that from which the original antigen was obtained.

species-specific antigen *n.* An antigen that is common to members of a single species and that provides a means by which that species can be immunologically distinguished.

spe·cif·ic (spĭ-sĭf′ĭk) *adj.* **1.** Relating to, characterizing, or distinguishing a species. **2.** Intended for, applying to, or acting on a specified thing. **3.** Designating a disease produced by a particular microorganism or condition. **4.** Having a remedial influence or effect on a particular disease. **5.** In immunology, having an affinity limited to a particular antibody or antigen. —*n.* A remedy intended for a particular ailment or disorder. —**spe·cif′i·cal·ly** *adv.*

specific action *n.* The action of a drug or treatment that has a direct, curative effect upon a disease.

specific activity *n.* Radioactivity per unit mass of a stated element or compound.

specific dynamic action *n.* *Abbr.* **SDA** An increase in the production of heat caused by the ingestion of food, especially proteins.

specific gravity *n.* *Abbr.* **sg, sp gr** The ratio of the mass of a solid or liquid to the mass of an equal volume of distilled water at 4°C (39°F) or of a gas to an equal volume of air or hydrogen under prescribed conditions of temperature and pressure.

specific immune globulin *n.* The globulin fraction of pooled sera or plasma from human donors having a normally high titer of antibodies specific for a particular antigen or a high titer of specific antibodies as a result of immunization.

specific immunity *n.* Immunity against a specific antigen or disease.

spec·i·fic·i·ty (spĕs′ə-fĭs′ĭ-tē) *n.* **1.** The condition or state of being specific. **2.** The statistical probability that an individual who does not have the particular disease being tested for will be correctly identified as negative, expressed as the proportion of true negative results to the total of true negative and false positive results.

specific opsonin *n.* Opsonin formed in response to stimulation by a specific antigen.

specific parasite *n.* A parasite that habitually lives in its present host and is particularly adapted for the host species.

specific reaction *n.* A phenomenon produced by an agent identical with or immunologically related to an agent that has altered the capacity of a certain tissue to react.

specific rotation *n.* *Symbol* α The arc of rotation, expressed in angular degrees, through which the plane of polarized light moves when it is in a light path one decimeter in length passing through a solution containing one gram of a compound per one milliliter water.

specific urethritis *n.* Urethritis caused by gonococci.

spec·i·men (spĕs′ə-mən) *n.* A sample, as of tissue, blood, or urine, used for analysis and diagnosis.

SPECT *abbr.* single photon emission computed tomography

spec·ta·cles (spĕk′tə-kəlz) *n.* See **glass** (sense 3).

Spec·ta·zole (spĕk′tə-zōl′) A trademark for the drug econazole.

Spec·tra·cef (spĕk′trə-sĕf′) A trademark for the drug cefditoren pivoxil.

spec·tral (spĕk′trəl) *adj.* Of, relating to, or produced by a spectrum. —**spec·tral′i·ty** (-trăl′ĭ-tē), **spec′tral·ness** (-trəl-nĭs) *n.*

spec·trin (spĕk′trĭn) *n.* A contractile protein of high molecular weight that is a component of a network in the membrane of red blood cells, giving the cells flexibility.

spectro– *pref.* Spectrum: *spectroscope.*

spec·trom·e·ter (spĕk-trŏm′ĭ-tər) *n.* A spectroscope equipped with scales for measuring wavelengths or indexes of refraction. —**spec′tro·met′ric** (-trə-mĕt′rĭk) *adj.*

spec·trom·e·try (spĕk-trŏm′ĭ-trē) *n.* The observation and measurement of wavelengths of light or other electromagnetic radiation.

spec·tro·pho·tom·e·ter (spĕk′trō-fō-tŏm′ĭ-tər) *n.* An instrument for measuring the intensity of light of a definite wavelength transmitted by a substance or a solution, thus providing a measure of the amount of material in the solution absorbing the light. —**spec′-tro·pho′to·met′ric** (-fō′tə-mĕt′rĭk) *adj.*

spectrophotometric analysis *n.* The determination of the structure or quantity of substances by measuring their capacity to absorb light of various wavelengths. Also called *spectrophotometry.*

spec·tro·scope (spĕk′trə-skōp′) *n.* An instrument for producing and observing spectra. —**spec′tro·scop′ic** (-skŏp′ĭk), **spec′tro·scop′i·cal** (-ĭ-kəl) *adj.*

spec·tros·co·py (spĕk-trŏs′kə-pē) *n.* The study of spectra, especially experimental observation of optical spectra. —**spec·tros′co·pist** *n.*

spec·trum (spĕk′trəm) *n., pl.* **–trums** *or* **–tra** (-trə) **1.** The distribution of a characteristic of a physical system or phenomenon, especially the distribution of energy emitted by a radiant source arranged in order of wavelengths. **2.** The color image presented when white light is resolved into its constituent colors: red, orange, yellow, green, blue, indigo, violet. **3.** The plot of intensity as opposed to wavelength of light emitted or absorbed by a substance, usually characteristic of the substance and used in qualitative and quantitative analysis. **4.** The distribution of atomic or subatomic particles in a system, as in a magnetically resolved molecular beam, arranged in order of masses. **5.** The group of pathogenic organisms against which an antibiotic or other antibacterial agent is effective.

spec·u·lum (spĕk′yə-ləm) *n., pl.* **–lums** *or* **–la** (-lə) **1.** A mirror or polished metal plate that is used as a reflector in optical instruments. **2.** An instrument that is used to dilate the opening of a body cavity for medical examination.

speculum forceps *n.* A type of tubular forceps for use through a speculum.

speech (spēch) *n.* **1.** The faculty or act of expressing thoughts, feelings, or perceptions by the articulation of words. **2.** Vocal communication; conversation.

speech bulb *n.* A prosthetic speech aid used to close a cleft or other opening in the hard or soft palate, or to

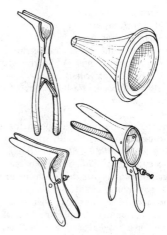

speculum
Top left to right: *nasal and ear specula*
Bottom left to right: *rectal and vaginal specula*

replace absent tissue necessary for the production of good speech.

speech pathology *n.* The science concerned with the diagnosis and treatment of functional and organic speech defects and disorders. Also called *speech-language pathology.*

speech therapy *n.* Treatment of speech defects and disorders, especially through use of exercises and audiovisual aids that develop new speech habits.

speed·ball (spēd′bôl′) *n.* An intravenous dose of cocaine mixed with heroin or an amphetamine.

Spe·mann (shpā′män′), **Hans** 1869–1941. German zoologist and physiologist. He won a 1935 Nobel Prize for his discovery of the organizer effect in embryonic development.

Spens' syndrome (spĕnz) *n.* See **Adams-Stokes syndrome.**

sperm (spûrm) *n., pl* **sperm** *or* **sperms 1.** A male gamete or reproductive cell; a spermatozoon. **2.** Semen.

sperm– *pref.* Variant of **spermi–.**

sperma– *pref.* Variant of **spermi–.**

sper·ma·cyt·ic seminoma (spûr′mə-sĭt′ĭk) *n.* A relatively slow-growing, locally invasive type of testicular seminoma that does not metastasize.

sperm-aster *n.* A centrosome with astral rays in the cytoplasm of an inseminated ovum; it is brought in by the penetrating spermatozoon and gives rise to the mitotic spindle of the first-cleavage division.

sper·mat·ic (spər-măt′ĭk) *adj.* **1.** Of, relating to, or resembling sperm. **2.** Containing, conveying, or producing sperm.

spermatic artery *n.* **1.** The cremasteric artery. **2.** The testicular artery.

spermatic cord *n.* A cordlike structure, consisting of the vas deferens and its accompanying arteries, veins, nerves, and lymphatic vessels, that passes from the abdominal cavity through the inguinal canal down into the scrotum to the back of the testicle. Also called *testicular cord.*

spermatic duct *n.* See **vas deferens.**

sper·ma·tid (spûr′mə-tĭd) *n.* Any of the four haploid cells formed by meiosis in a male organism that develop into spermatozoa without further division.

spermato– *or* **spermat–** *pref.* **1.** Sperm: *spermatic.* **2.** Spermatozoon: *spermatogenesis.*

sper·mat·o·blast (spər-măt′ə-blăst′, spûr′mə-tə-) *n.* See **spermatogonium.**

sper·mat·o·cele (spər-măt′ə-sēl′, spûr′mə-tə-) *n.* A cyst of the epididymis containing spermatozoa.

sper·mat·o·cide (spər-măt′ə-sīd′, spûr′mə-tə-) *n.* See **spermicide. —sper·mat′o·cid′al** (-sīd′l) *adj.*

sper·mat·o·cyte (spər-măt′ə-sīt′, spûr′mə-tə-) *n.* A diploid cell that undergoes meiosis to form four spermatids. **—sper·mat′o·cyt′al** (-sīt′l) *adj.*

sper·mat·o·gen·e·sis (spər-măt′ə-jĕn′ĭ-sĭs, spûr′mə-tə-) *n.* Formation and development of spermatozoa by meiosis and spermiogenesis. Also called *spermatocytogenesis.* **—sper·mat′o·ge·net′ic** (-jə-nĕt′ĭk), **sper·mat′o·gen′ic** (-jĕn′ĭk) *adj.*

sper·mat·o·go·ni·um (spər-măt′ə-gō′nē-əm, spûr′mə-tə-) *n.*, *pl.* **–ni·a** (-nē-ə) Any of the cells of the gonads in male organisms that are the progenitors of spermatocytes. Also called *spermatoblast.*

sper·ma·toid (spûr′mə-toid′) *adj.* Resembling a sperm or the whiplike tail of a sperm.

sper·ma·tol·y·sis (spûr′mə-tŏl′ĭ-sĭs) *n.* The destructive dissolution of spermatozoa.

sper·mat·o·poi·et·ic (spər-măt′ə-poi-ĕt′ĭk, spûr′mə-tə-) *adj.* **1.** Producing sperm. **2.** Secreting semen.

sper·mat·or·rhe·a *or* **sper·mat·or·rhoe·a** (spər-măt′ə-rē′ə, spûr′mə-tə-) *n.* Involuntary discharge of semen without orgasm.

sper·mat·o·zo·on (spər-măt′ə-zō′ŏn′, -ən, spûr′mə-tə-) *n.*, *pl.* **–zo·a** (-zō′ə) The mature male gamete or sex cell that consists of a cylindrical nucleated cell with a short neck and a thin motile tail, contains genetic information to be transmitted by the male, exhibits autokinesia, and is able to effect zygosis with an ovum; sperm. **—sper·mat′o·zo′al** (-zō′əl), **sper·mat′o·zo′an** (-zō′ən), **sper·mat′o·zo′ic** (-zō′ĭk) *adj.*

sper·ma·tu·ri·a (spûr′mə-tŏŏr′ē-ə) *n.* See **semenuria.**

spermi– *or* **sperma–** *or* **spermo–** *or* **sperm–** *pref.* Sperm; semen: *spermatocide.*

sper·mi·cide (spûr′mĭ-sīd′) *n.* An agent that kills spermatozoa, especially as a contraceptive. Also called *spermatocide.* **—sper′mi·cid′al** (-sīd′l) *adj.*

sper·mi·dine (spûr′mĭ-dēn′) *n.* A polyamine compound found in ribosomes and living tissues and having various metabolic functions. It was originally isolated from semen.

sper·mi·duct (spûr′mĭ-dŭkt′) *n.* **1.** See **vas deferens. 2.** See **ejaculatory duct.**

sper·mi·o·gen·e·sis (spür′mē-ō-jĕn′ĭ-sĭs) *n.* The stage of spermatogenesis during which spermatids are transformed into spermatozoa.

sper·mo·lith (spûr′mə-lĭth′) *n.* A concretion in the vas deferens.

sperm washing *n.* A procedure for separating sperm cells from the seminal fluid, used especially in the treatment of male infertility.

Sper·ry (spĕr′ē), **Roger Wolcott** 1913–1994. American neurobiologist. He shared a 1981 Nobel Prize for studies of the organization and functioning of the brain.

SPF *abbr.* sun protection factor

sp gr *abbr.* specific gravity

sph *abbr.* spherical lens

sphac·e·late (sfăs′ə-lāt′) *v.* To develop or produce gangrenous or necrotic tissue. **—sphac′e·la′tion** *n.*

sphac·e·lism (sfăs′ə-lĭz′əm) *n.* The condition manifested by a sphacelus.

sphac·e·lo·der·ma (sfăs′ə-lō-dûr′mə) *n.* Gangrene of the skin.

sphac·e·lous (sfăs′ə-ləs) *adj.* Sloughing, gangrenous, or necrotic.

sphac·e·lus (sfăs′ə-ləs) *n.* A mass of sloughing, gangrenous, or necrotic matter.

S phase *n.* The phase of the mitotic cycle during which DNA synthesis occurs.

sphe·ni·on (sfē′nē-ŏn′) *n.* The tip of the sphenoidal angle of the parietal bone, used as a craniometric point.

spheno– *or* **sphen–** *pref.* Wedge; wedge-shaped: *sphenocephaly.*

sphe·no·ceph·a·ly (sfē′nō-sĕf′ə-lē) *n.* The condition of having a wedge-shaped head.

sphe·no·eth·moi·dal suture (sfē′nō-ĕth-moid′l) *n.* The line of union between the crest of the sphenoid bone and the perpendicular and cribriform plates of the ethmoid bone.

sphe·noid (sfē′noid′) *n.* The sphenoid bone. **—adj. 1.** Of or relating to the sphenoid bone. **2.** Wedge-shaped. **—sphe·noi′dal** (-noid′l) *adj.*

sphenoidal sinus *n.* Either of a pair of cavities in the body of the sphenoid bone that communicate with the nasal cavity.

sphenoidal spine *n.* A rearward and downward projection from either of the greater wings of the sphenoid bone. Also called *alar spine, spinous process.*

sphenoid bone *n.* A compound bone with winglike processes, situated at the base of the skull.

sphenoid crest *n.* A vertical ridge in the midline of the anterior surface of the sphenoid bone.

sphe·noid·i·tis (sfē′noi-dī′tĭs) *n.* **1.** Inflammation of the sphenoidal sinus. **2.** Necrosis of the sphenoid bone.

sphe·noid·ot·o·my (sfē′noi-dŏt′ə-mē) *n.* Surgical creation of an opening in the anterior wall of the sphenoidal sinus.

sphe·no·pal·a·tine artery (sfē′nō-păl′ə-tīn′) *n.* An artery with origin in the maxillary artery, with distribution to the nasal wall and septum, and with anastomoses to the branches of the descending palatine, superior labial, and infraorbital arteries.

sphenopalatine foramen *n.* The opening formed from the sphenopalatine notch of the palatine bone in articulation with the sphenoid bone.

sphenopalatine ganglion *n.* See **pterygopalatine ganglion.**

sphe·no·pa·ri·e·tal sinus (sfē′nō-pə-rī′ĭ-təl) *n.* A paired sinus of the dura mater that begins on the parietal bone and empties into the cavernous sinus.

sphe·nor·bit·al (sfē-nôr′bĭ-tl) *adj.* Of or being the portions of the sphenoid bone contributing to the orbital cavities.

sphe·not·ic (sfē-nŏt′ĭk) *adj.* Relating to the sphenoid bone and the bony case of the ear.

sphere (sfîr) *n.* A ball-shaped or a globular body. —**spher′al** (sfîr′əl) *adj.*

spher·i·cal (sfîr′ĭ-kəl, sfĕr′-) *adj.* Having the shape of or approximating a sphere; globular.

spherical aberration *n.* A blurred image that occurs when light from the margin of a lens or mirror with a spherical surface comes to a shorter focus than light from the central portion. Also called *dioptric aberration.*

spherical lens *n. Abbr.* **sph** A lens in which all refracting surfaces are spherical.

sphero– or **spher–** *pref.* Sphere; spherical: *spherocyte.*

spher·o·cyte (sfîr′ə-sīt′, sfĕr′-) *n.* A small spherical red blood cell, characteristic of hereditary spherocytosis and of certain hemolytic anemias. —**spher′o·cyt′ic** (-sĭt′ĭk) *adj.*

spherocytic anemia *n.* See **hereditary spherocytosis.**

spher·o·cy·to·sis (sfîr′ō-sī-tō′sĭs, sfĕr′-) *n.* The presence of spherocytes in the blood.

spher·oid (sfîr′oid′, sfĕr′-) or **sphe·roi·dal** (sfī-roid′l) *adj.* Having a generally spherical shape. —**spher′oid′** *n.*

spher·o·pha·ki·a (sfîr′ə-fā′kē-ə, sfĕr′ə-) *n.* A congenital bilateral anomaly in which the lenses of the eye are small, spherical, and prone to subluxation. Also called *microphakia.*

sphinc·ter (sfĭngk′tər) *n.* A ringlike muscle that normally maintains constriction of a body passage or orifice and that relaxes as required by normal physiological functioning. Also called *anatomical sphincter.* —**sphinc′ter·al, sphinc·ter′ic** (-tĕr′ĭk) *adj.*

sphinc·ter·al·gia (sfĭngk′tə-răl′jə) *n.* Pain in the muscles of the anal sphincter.

sphinc·ter·ec·to·my (sfĭngk′tə-rĕk′tə-mē) *n.* **1.** Excision of a portion of the pupillary border of the iris. **2.** Excision of a sphincter muscle.

sphinc·ter·is·mus (sfĭngk′tə-rĭz′məs) *n.* Spasmodic contraction of the muscles of the anal sphincter.

sphinc·ter·i·tis (sfĭngk′tə-rī′tĭs) *n.* Inflammation of a sphincter.

sphincter muscle of common bile duct *n.* A smooth muscle sphincter at the terminal end of the common bile duct.

sphincter muscle of pancreatic duct *n.* A smooth muscle sphincter of the main pancreatic duct within the duodenal papilla.

sphincter muscle of pupil *n.* A ring of smooth muscle fibers surrounding the pupillary border of the iris.

sphincter muscle of pylorus *n.* See **pyloric sphincter.**

sphincter muscle of urethra *n.* A muscle with origin from the ramus of the pubis, with insertion with its fellow muscle in the median raphe behind and in front of the urethra, with nerve supply from the pudendal nerve, and whose action constricts the membranous urethra.

sphincter muscle of urinary bladder *n.* A vesical sphincter made up of a thickening of the middle muscular layer of the bladder around the urethral opening.

sphinc·ter·ol·y·sis (sfĭngk′tə-rŏl′ĭ-sĭs) *n.* An operation to correct anterior synechia.

sphinc·ter·o·plas·ty (sfĭngk′tər-ə-plăs′tē) *n.* Reparative or plastic surgery of a sphincter muscle.

sphinc·ter·ot·o·my (sfĭngk′tə-rŏt′ə-mē) *n.* Incision into a sphincter muscle.

sphin·go·lip·id (sfĭng′gō-lĭp′ĭd, -lī′pĭd) *n.* Any of a group of lipids, such as sphingomyelins or cerebrosides, that yield sphingosine or its derivatives upon hydrolysis.

sphin·go·lip·i·do·sis (sfĭng′gō-lĭp′ĭ-dō′sĭs) *n.* Any of various diseases, such as gangliosidosis or Gaucher's disease, characterized by abnormal sphingolipid metabolism. Also called *sphingolipodystrophy.*

sphin·go·my·e·lin (sfĭng′gō-mī′ə-lĭn) *n.* Any of a group of phospholipids that are found especially in nerve tissue and yield sphingosine, choline, a fatty acid, and phosphoric acid upon hydrolysis.

sphingomyelin lipidosis *n.* See **Niemann-Pick disease.**

sphingomyelin phosphodiesterase *n.* An enzyme that catalyzes the hydrolysis of sphingomyelin to ceramide and phosphocholine.

sphin·go·sine (sfĭng′gə-sēn′) *n.* A basic, long-chain, unsaturated amino alcohol, found combined with lipids in the brain and in nerve tissue.

sphyg·mic (sfĭg′mĭk) *adj.* Of or relating to the pulse.

sphygmic interval *n.* The period in the cardiac cycle when the semilunar valves are open and blood is ejected from the ventricles into the arterial system. Also called *ejection period, sphygmic period.*

sphygmo– or **sphygm–** *pref.* Pulse: *sphygmograph.*

sphyg·mo·chron·o·graph (sfĭg′mō-krŏn′ə-grăf′, -krō′nə-) *n.* A modified sphygmograph that graphically represents the time relations between the beat of the heart and the pulse.

sphyg·mo·gram (sfĭg′mə-grăm′) *n.* The record or tracing produced by a sphygmograph.

sphyg·mo·graph (sfĭg′mə-grăf′) *n.* An instrument for graphically recording the form, strength, and variations of the arterial pulse. —**sphyg′mo·graph′ic** *adj.* —**sphyg·mog′ra·phy** (-mŏg′rə-fē) *n.*

sphyg·moid (sfĭg′moid′) *adj.* Resembling a pulse.

sphyg·mo·ma·nom·e·ter (sfĭg′mō-mă-nŏm′ĭ-tər) or **sphyg·mom·e·ter** (sfĭg-mŏm′ĭ-tər) *n.* An instrument for measuring blood pressure in the arteries, especially one consisting of a pressure gauge and a rubber cuff that wraps around the upper arm and inflates to constrict the arteries. —**sphyg′mo·man′o·met′ric** (-măn′ə-mĕt′rĭk) *adj.*

sphyg·mos·co·py (sfĭg-mŏs′kə-pē) *n.* Examination of the pulse.

sphy·rec·to·my (sfī-rĕk′tə-mē) *n.* Surgical removal of the malleus.

sphy·rot·o·my (sfī-rŏt′ə-mē) *n.* Surgical section of a part of the malleus.

spi·ca bandage (spī′kə) *n.* Successive strips of material applied to the body and the first part of a limb, or to the hand and a finger, that overlap slightly so as to resemble an ear of wheat.

spic·ule (spĭk′yōol) or **spic·u·la** (-yə-lə) *n.,* *pl.* **–ules** or **–u·lae** (-yə-lē) A needlelike structure or part. —**spic′u·lar** (-yə-lər), **spic′u·late** (-yə-lĭt, -lāt′) *adj.*

spi·der (spī′dər) *n.* **1.** Any of numerous arachnids of the order Araneae, having a body divided into a cephalothorax bearing eight legs, two poison fangs, and two feelers and an unsegmented abdomen bearing several spinnerets that produce the silk used to make nests, cocoons, or webs for trapping insects. **2.** An arterial spider.

spider-burst *n.* Radiating dull-red capillary lines on the skin of the leg, usually without any visible or palpable varicose veins, due to deep-seated venous dilation.

spider nevus *n.* See **arterial spider.**

spider telangiectasia *n.* See **arterial spider.**

Spiel·mey·er-Vogt disease (shpēl′mī′ər-) *n.* The late juvenile type of cerebral sphingolipidosis. Also called *Batten-Mayou disease, ceroid lipofuscinosis, Vogt-Spielmeyer disease.*

spi·ge·li·an (spī-jē′lē-ən) *n.* Relating to or described by Flemish botanist and anatomist Adrian van der Spieghel (1578-1625).

Spi·ge·li·us′ line (spī-jē′lē-ə-sĭz, -jēl′yə-sĭz) *n.* See **semilunar line.**

Spigelius′ lobe *n.* See **caudate lobe.**

spike (spīk) *n.* A brief electrical event of 3 to 25 milliseconds that gives the appearance in the electroencephalogram of a rising and falling vertical line.

spike potential *n.* The main wave in the action potential of a nerve that is followed by negative and positive afterpotentials.

spi·na (spī′nə) *n., pl.* **–nae** (-nē) A spine-shaped or sharp thornlike anatomical process.

spina bif·i·da (bĭf′ĭ-də) *n.* A congenital defect in which the spinal column is imperfectly closed so that part of the meninges or spinal cord may protrude, often resulting in neurological disorders. Also called *hydrocele spinalis.*

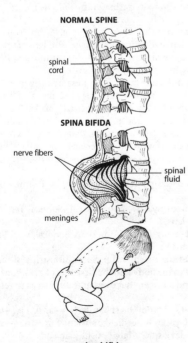

spina bifida
Top: *normal spinal cord*
Center: *myelomeningocele spina bifida*
Bottom: *showing the protrusion*

spina bifida a·per·ta (ə-pûr′tə) *n.* See **spina bifida manifesta.**

spina bifida cys·ti·ca (sĭs′tĭ-kə) *n.* Spina bifida with protrusion of the meninges or spinal cord.

spina bifida man·i·fes·ta (măn′ə-fĕs′tə) *n.* Spina bifida in which the vertebral defect is apparent and may be associated with a meningeal or spinal cord anomaly. Also called *spina bifida aperta.*

spina bifida oc·cul·ta (ə-kŭl′tə) *n.* Spina bifida with no protrusion of the meninges or spinal cord. Also called *cryptomerorrhachischis.*

spi·nal (spī′nəl) *adj.* **1.** Relating to or situated near the spinal column or spinal cord. **2.** Relating to any spine or spinous process.

spinal analgesia *n.* The deactivation of sensory nerves by injecting a local anesthetic into the subarachnoid space of the spine.

spinal anesthesia *n.* **1.** Anesthesia produced by injection of a local anesthetic solution into the spinal subarachnoid space. **2.** Loss of sensation produced by disease of the spinal cord.

spinal artery *n.* **1.** An artery with origin in the vertebral artery, with distribution to the spinal cord and the pia mater, and with anastomoses to the branches of the intercostal and lumbar arteries; anterior spinal artery. **2.** An artery with origin in the vertebral artery, with distribution to the medulla, spinal cord, and pia mater; and with anastomoses to the spinal branches of the intercostal arteries; posterior spinal artery.

spinal atrophy *n.* See **tabes dorsalis.**

spinal block *n.* **1.** Pathological obstruction of the flow of cerebrospinal fluid in the spinal subarachnoid space. **2.** Spinal anesthesia. Not in technical use.

spinal canal *n.* See **vertebral canal.**

spinal column *n.* The series of articulated vertebrae, separated by intervertebral disks and held together by muscles and tendons, that extends from the cranium to the coccyx, encasing the spinal cord and forming the supporting axis of the body. Also called *backbone, rachis, spine, vertebral column.*

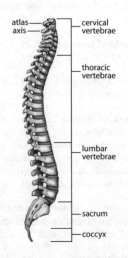

spinal column
right lateral view of an adult human spinal column

spinal concussion *n.* Sudden transient loss of function of the spinal cord due to trauma.

spinal cord *n.* The thick, whitish cord of nerve tissue that extends from the medulla oblongata down through the spinal column and from which the spinal nerves branch off to various parts of the body. Also called *spinal marrow.*

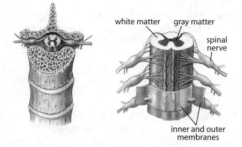

white matter   gray matter

spinal nerve

inner and outer membranes

spinal cord
Left: *cross section of vertebral column showing the spinal cord within the column*
Right: *segment of spinal cord with nerve fibers arising from it*

spinal curvature *n.* Any of several deformities characterized by abnormal curvature of the spine, such as kyphosis or scoliosis.

spinal decompression *n.* The relief of pressure upon the spinal cord as caused by a tumor, cyst, hematoma, or bone, through surgery.

spinal fluid *n.* See **cerebrospinal fluid.**

spinal fusion *n.* A surgical procedure in which vertebrae are joined. Also called *spondylosyndesis.*

spinal ganglion *n.* The ganglion of the posterior root of each spinal segmental nerve, containing the cell bodies of the unipolar primary sensory neurons. Also called *dorsal root ganglion.*

spinal headache *n.* A headache that is brought on by sitting or assuming an upright posture following spinal anesthesia; it is usually relieved by lying down.

spinal marrow *n.* See **spinal cord.**

spinal meningitis *n.* Inflammation of the membranes enclosing the spinal cord, especially a usually fatal form that affects infants and young children and is caused by a strain of gram-negative bacteria (*Hemophilus influenzae*).

spinal muscle of head *n.* An inconstant extension of the spinal muscle of the neck to the occipital bone, sometimes fusing with the semispinal muscle of the head.

spinal muscle of neck *n.* An inconstant or rudimentary muscle with origin from the sixth and seventh cervical vertebrae, with insertion into the axis and third cervical vertebra, with nerve supply from the dorsal branches of the cervical nerve, and whose action extends the cervical spine.

spinal muscle of thorax *n.* A muscle with origin from the upper lumbar and two lower thoracic vertebrae, with insertion into the middle and upper thoracic vertebrae, with nerve supply from the dorsal branches of the thoracic and the upper lumbar nerves, and whose action supports and extends the vertebral column.

spinal nerve *n.* Any of 31 pairs of nerves emerging from the spinal cord, each attached to the cord by two roots, anterior or ventral and posterior or dorsal, the latter provided with a spinal ganglion. The two roots unite in the intervertebral foramen but divide again into ventral and dorsal rami, or anterior and posterior primary divisions, the former supplying the foreparts of the body and limbs, the latter the muscles and skin of the back.

spinal paralysis *n.* Loss of motor power due to a lesion of the spinal cord.

spinal puncture *n.* See **lumbar puncture.**

spinal reflex *n.* A reflex arc involving the spinal cord.

spinal root *n.* Any of the roots of the accessory nerve that arise from the ventrolateral part of the first five segments of the spinal cord.

spinal tap *n.* See **lumbar puncture.**

spinal vein *n.* Any of the veins that drain the spinal cord and form a plexus on the surface of the cord from which veins pass along the spinal roots to the internal vertebral venous plexus.

spi·nate (spī′nāt′) *adj.* Having spines; spined.

spin·dle (spĭn′dl) *n.* **1.** A fusiform structure, usually composed of microtubules. **2.** Mitotic spindle.

spindle cell *n.* A spindle-shaped cell characteristic of certain tumors.

spindle cell carcinoma *n.* A carcinoma composed of elongated cells, frequently a poorly differentiated squamous cell carcinoma.

spindle cell lipoma *n.* A microscopically distinctive form of lipoma in which adipose tissue is infiltrated by fibroblasts and collagen.

spindle fiber *n.* One of a network of achromatic filaments that extend inward from the poles of a dividing cell, forming a spindle-shaped figure.

spine (spīn) *n.* **1.** See **spinal column. 2.** Any of various short pointed projections, processes, or appendages of bone.

spine of scapula *n.* The prominent triangular ridge on the dorsal aspect of the scapula.

spinn·bar·keit (spĭn′bär′kīt, shpĭn′-) *n.* The stringy, elastic character of cervical mucus during the ovulatory period.

spino– *pref.* Spine; spinous: *spinocerebellar.*

spi·no·bul·bar (spī′nō-bŭl′bər, -bär′) *adj.* Relating to the medulla oblongata and the spinal cord.

spi·no·cer·e·bel·lum (spī′nō-sĕr′ə-bĕl′əm) *n.* See **paleocerebellum.**

spi·no·tha·lam·ic tract (spī′nō-thə-lăm′ĭk) *n.* A large ascending bundle of fibers in the ventral half of the lateral funiculus of the spinal cord, arising in the posterior horn at all levels of the cord and continuing into the brainstem. It is composed in the spinal cord of a lateral part that conveys impulses associated with pain and temperature sensation and of an anterior part that is involved in tactile sensation.

spi·nous (spī′nəs) *adj.* Relating to, shaped like, or having a spine or spines.

spinous layer *n.* See **prickle cell layer.**

spinous process *n.* **1.** See **sphenoidal spine. 2.** The dorsal projection from the center of a vertebral arch.

spin·y-head·ed worm (spī′nē-hĕd′ĭd) *n.* See **Acanthocephala.**

spir– *pref.* Variant of **spiro–**.

spi·rad·e·no·ma (spī-răd′n-ō′mə) *n.* A benign tumor of the sweat glands.

spi·ral (spī′rəl) *adj.* Coiling or developing around an axis in a constantly changing series of planes; helical. —*n.* A structure in the shape of a coil. —*v.* To take the form or course of a spiral.

spiral bandage *n.* A bandage encircling a limb, with successive turns overlapping the preceding ones.

spiral canal of cochlea *n.* The winding tube located in the bony labyrinth of the ear. Also called *cochlear canal.*

spiral canal of modiolus *n.* The space in the modiolus containing the spiral ganglion of the cochlea.

spiral crest *n.* The thickened periosteal lining of the bony cochlea forming the outer wall of the cochlear duct to which the basal lamina attaches. Also called *spiral ligament of cochlea.*

spiral fold of cystic duct *n.* A series of crescent-shaped folds of mucous membrane in the upper part of the cystic duct, arranged in a somewhat spiral manner. Also called *spiral valve.*

spiral fracture *n.* A fracture in which the bone has been twisted apart and the line of break is helical.

spiral ganglion of cochlea *n.* An elongated ganglion of bipolar sensory nerve cell bodies on the cochlear part of the vestibulocochlear nerve in the spiral canal of the modiolus. Also called *Corti's ganglion.*

spiral joint *n.* See **cochlear joint.**

spiral lamina of cochlea *n.* A spiral bony shelf extending from the modiolus across the spiral canal of the cochlea, forming the division between the scala vestibuli and scala tympani in the inner ear.

spiral ligament of cochlea *n.* See **spiral crest.**

spiral line *n.* See **intertrochanteric line.**

spiral organ *n.* See **organ of Corti.**

spiral valve *n.* See **spiral fold of cystic duct.**

spiral vein of modiolus *n.* A vein in the modiolus of the cochlea that is a tributary to the labyrinthine vein and the vein of the cochlear canal.

spi·ril·lar (spī-rĭl′ər) *adj.* S-shaped. Used of a bacterial cell.

spi·ril·lum (spī-rĭl′əm) *n., pl.* **–ril·la** (-rĭl′ə) **1.** A member of the genus *Spirillum.* **2.** Any of various other spiral-shaped microorganisms.

Spirillum *n.* A genus of large, aerobic, gram-negative bacteria having an elongated spiral form and a tuft of flagella.

Spirillum mi·nus (mī′nəs) *n.* A bacterium that causes a rat-bite fever.

spir·it (spĭr′ĭt) *n.* **1. spirits** An alcohol solution of an essential or volatile substance. **2. spirits** An alcoholic beverage, especially distilled liquor. **3.** A liquid that has been distilled.

spirit lamp *n.* A lamp that burns alcohol or other liquid fuel and is used mainly for heating in laboratory work.

spiro– or **spir–** *pref.* **1.** Spiral; coil; coil-shaped: *spirillar.* **2.** Breath; breathing; *spirograph.*

Spi·ro·chae·ta (spī′rə-kē′tə) *n.* A genus of motile bacteria that are flexible, undulating, spiral-shaped rods having flagellalike, tapering ends.

spi·ro·chete (spī′rə-kēt′) *n.* Any of various slender, spiral, motile bacteria of the order Spirochaetales, many of which are pathogenic, causing syphilis, relapsing fever, yaws, and other diseases.

spi·ro·che·te·mi·a (spī′rə-kē-tē′mē-ə) *n.* The presence of spirochetes in the blood.

spi·ro·che·to·sis (spī′rə-kē-tō′sĭs) *n., pl.* **–ses** (-sēz) Any of various diseases, such as syphilis, caused by infection with spirochetes.

spi·ro·gram (spī′rə-grăm′) *n.* The tracing made by the spirograph.

spi·ro·graph (spī′rə-grăf′) *n.* An instrument for registering the depth and rapidity of respiratory movements. —**spi′ro·graph′ic** *adj.* —**spi·rog′ra·phy** (spī-rŏg′rə-fē) *n.*

spi·rom·e·ter (spī-rŏm′ĭ-tər) *n.* An instrument for measuring the volume of air entering and leaving the lungs. —**spi′ro·met′ric** (-rə-mĕt′rĭk) *adj.* —**spi·rom′e·try** *n.*

spi·ro·no·lac·tone (spī′rə-nō-lăk′tōn, spī-rō′-) *n.* An aldosterone antagonist and antiandrogen that promotes diuresis and is used to treat conditions characterized by hypertension and fluid retention as well as androgenic syndromes in women.

spi·ru·roid (spī′rə-roid′) *n.* A member of the superfamily Spiruroidea. —**spi′ru·oid′** *adj.*

Spi·ru·roi·de·a (spī′rə-roi′dē-ə) *n.* A superfamily of arthropod-borne, frequently pathogenic nematode parasites of the alimentary tract, the respiratory system, or the orbital, nasal, or oral cavities of vertebrates.

spis·si·tude (spĭs′ĭ-tōōd′) *n.* The condition of a fluid thickened almost to a solid by inspissation.

spit·tle (spĭt′l) *n.* Spit; saliva.

splanch·na·poph·y·sis (splăngk′nə-pŏf′ĭ-sĭs) *n.* An apophysis of a vertebra, lying on the side that is opposite the neural apophysis and enclosing a viscus.

splanch·nec·to·pi·a (splăngk′nĕk-tō′pē-ə) *n.* Displacement of any of the parts of the viscera. Also called *splanchnodiastasis.*

splanch·nes·the·sia (splăngk′nĭs-thē′zhə) *n.* See **visceral sense.**

splanch·nes·thet·ic sensibility (splăngk′nĭs-thĕt′ĭk) *n.* See **visceral sense.**

splanch·nic (splăngk′nĭk) *adj.* Of or relating to the viscera; visceral.

splanchnic anesthesia *n.* Loss of sensation in areas of the visceral peritoneum innervated by the splanchnic nerves. Also called *visceral anesthesia.*

splanch·ni·cec·to·my (splăngk′nĭ-sĕk′tə-mē) *n.* Surgical resection of the splanchnic nerves and usually of the celiac ganglion.

splanchnic ganglion *n.* A small sympathetic ganglion often present with the greater splanchnic nerve.

splanch·ni·cot·o·my (splăngk′nĭ-kŏt′ə-mē) *n.* Surgical section of a splanchnic nerve or nerves.

splanchnic wall *n.* The wall of one of the viscera or the splanchnopleure from which it is formed.

splanchno– or **splanchni–** *pref.* Viscera; visceral: *splanchnopathy.*

splanch·no·cele (splăngk′nə-sēl′) *n.* **1.** The primitive body cavity in the embryo. **2.** Hernia of any of the abdominal viscera.

splanch·no·di·as·ta·sis (splăngk′nō-dī-ăs′tə-sĭs) *n.* See **splanchnectopia.**

splanch·no·lith (splăngk′nə-lĭth′) *n.* A calculus that occurs in the intestine.

splanch·no·meg·a·ly (splăngk′nō-mĕg′ə-lē) *n.* See **visceromegaly.**

splanch·nop·a·thy (splăngk-nŏp′ə-thē) *n.* Disease of the abdominal viscera.

splanch·no·pleure (splăngk′nə-ploŏr′) *n.* A layer of embryonic cells formed by association of part of the mesoderm with the endoderm and developing into the wall of the viscera. —**splanch′no·pleur′ic** *adj.*

splanch·nop·to·sis (splăngk′nŏp-tō′sĭs, -nō-tō′-) *n.* See **visceroptosis.**

splanch·no·scle·ro·sis (splăngk′nō-sklə-rō′sĭs) *n.* Hardening of any of the viscera through connective tissue overgrowth.

splanch·no·skel·e·tal (splănk′nō-skĕl′ĭ-tl) *adj.* Relating to the visceroskeleton.

splanch·no·skel·e·ton (splăngk′nō-skĕl′ĭ-tn) *n.* See **visceroskeleton** (sense 2).

splanch·no·tribe (splăngk′nə-trīb′) *n.* An instrument used for occluding the intestine temporarily prior to resection.

splay·foot (splā′foŏt′) *n.* See **flatfoot.**

spleen (splēn) *n.* A large, highly vascular lymphoid organ, lying to the left of the stomach below the diaphragm and serving to store blood, disintegrate old blood cells, filter foreign substances from the blood, and to produce lymphocytes.

splen– *pref.* Variant of **spleno–.**

sple·nal·gia (splĭ-năl′jə) *n.* Pain in the spleen. Also called *splenodynia.*

sple·nec·to·my (splĭ-nĕk′tə-mē) *n.* Surgical removal of the spleen.

splen·ec·to·pi·a (splĕn′ĭk-tō′pē-ə, splē′nĭk-) *or* **sple·nec·to·py** (splĭ-nĕk′tə-pē) *n.* **1.** Displacement of the spleen. **2.** Presence of deposits of splenic tissue, usually in the region of the spleen.

splen·ic (splĕn′ĭk) *adj.* Of, in, near, or relating to the spleen.

splenic anemia *n.* See **Banti's syndrome.**

splenic artery *n.* See **lienal artery.**

splenic flexure *n.* See **left colic flexure.**

splenic lymph follicle *n.* See **malpighian corpuscle** (sense 2).

splenic pulp *n.* The soft, reddish brown substance that fills the sinuses of the spleen. Also called *red pulp.*

splenic sinus *n.* An elongated venous channel in the spleen, lined by rod-shaped cells.

splenic vein *n.* A vein that arises by the union of several small veins at the hilum on the anterior surface of the spleen, passes to the left kidney, and runs to the neck of the pancreas where it joins the superior mesenteric vein to form the portal vein.

sple·ni·tis (splĭ-nī′tĭs) *n.* Inflammation of the spleen.

sple·ni·um (splē′nē-əm) *n.,* *pl.* **–ni·a** (-nē-ə) **1.** A compress or bandage. **2.** An anatomical structure resembling a bandaged part.

splenium cor·po·ris cal·lo·si (kôr′pər-ĭs kə-lō′sī) *n.* The thickened extremity located in the posterior portion of the corpus callosum.

sple·ni·us muscle of head (splē′nē-əs) *n.* A muscle with origin from the nuchal ligament of the last four cervical vertebrae and from the supraspinous ligament

of the first and second thoracic vertebrae, with insertion into the mastoid process, with nerve supply from the dorsal branches of the second to the sixth cervical nerves, and whose action rotates the head and extends the neck.

splenius muscle of neck *n.* A muscle with origin from the supraspinous ligament and the spinous processes of the third to fifth thoracic vertebrae, with insertion into the first and second cervical vertebrae, with nerve supply from the dorsal branches of the fourth to the eighth cervical nerves, and whose action rotates and extends the neck.

spleno– *or* **splen–** *pref.* Spleen: *splenomegaly.*

sple·no·cele (splē′nə-sēl′) *n.* A splenic hernia.

sple·no·dyn·i·a (splē′nō-dĭn′ē-ə) *n.* See **splenalgia.**

sple·nog·ra·phy (splĭ-nŏg′rə-fē) *n.* Radiographic examination of the spleen after injection of contrast material.

sple·no·hep·a·to·meg·a·ly (splē′nō-hĕp′ə-tə-mĕg′ə-lē, -hĭ-păt′ə-) *n.* Enlargement of the spleen and the liver.

sple·noid (splē′noid′) *adj.* Resembling the spleen.

sple·no·ma (splĭ-nō′mə) *n.* An enlarged spleen.

sple·no·ma·la·cia (splē′nō-mə-lā′shə) *n.* Softening of the spleen.

sple·no·med·ul·lar·y (splē′nō-mĕd′l-ĕr′ē, -mə-dŭl′ə-rē) *adj.* Splenomyelogenous.

sple·no·meg·a·ly (splē′nō-mĕg′ə-lē, splĕn′ō-) *n.* Enlargement of the spleen. Also called *megalosplenia.*

sple·no·my·e·log·e·nous (splē′nō-mī-ə-lŏj′ə-nəs) *adj.* Originating in the spleen and the bone marrow; splenomedullary.

sple·no·my·e·lo·ma·la·cia (splē′nō-mī′ə-lō-mə-lā′shə) *n.* Pathological softening of the spleen and the bone marrow.

sple·nop·a·thy (splĭ-nŏp′ə-thē) *n.* Disease of the spleen.

sple·no·pex·y (splē′nə-pĕk′sē) *n.* The process of surgically fixing an ectopic or floating spleen. Also called *splenorrhaphy.*

sple·no·por·tog·ra·phy (splē′nō-pôr-tŏg′rə-fē) *n.* X-ray visualization of the portal circulation that uses radiopaque material introduced into the spleen. —**sple′-no·por′to·gram′** (-pôr′tə-grăm′) *n.*

sple·nop·to·sis (splē′nŏp-tō′sĭs) *n.* Downward displacement of the spleen.

sple·no·re·nal ligament (splē′nō-rē′nəl, splĕn′ō-) *n.* The portion of the greater omentum extending from spleen to diaphragm near the left kidney.

splenorenal shunt *n.* Anastomosis of the splenic vein to the left renal vein, usually end-to-side, for control of portal hypertension.

sple·nor·rha·gia (splē′nə-rā′jə) *n.* Hemorrhage from a ruptured spleen.

sple·nor·rha·phy (splĭ-nôr′ə-fē) *n.* **1.** Suture of a ruptured spleen. **2.** See **splenopexy.**

sple·not·o·my (splĭ-nŏt′ə-mē) *n.* Incision into the spleen.

sple·no·tox·in (splē′nō-tŏk′sĭn) *n.* A cytotoxin specific for cells of the spleen.

splic·ing (splī′sĭng) *n.* **1.** Gene-splicing. **2.** The removal of introns and the joining of exons from mRNA precursors. Also called *RNA splicing.*

splint (splĭnt) *n.* **1.** A rigid device used to prevent motion of a joint or of the ends of a fractured bone. **2.** A dental appliance put on the teeth to protect them from grinding or from moving out of place. —*v.* To support or restrict with a splint.

split (splĭt) *v.* **1.** To divide from end to end or along the grain by or as if by a sharp blow; tear. **2.** To break, burst, or rip apart with force; rend. **3.** To separate; disunite. **4.** To break apart or divide a chemical compound into simpler constituents.

split-brain *adj.* Of, relating to, or subjected to surgical separation of the hemispheres of the brain by severing the corpus callosum.

split hand *n.* See **cleft hand.**

split pelvis *n.* A pelvis in which the symphysis pubis is absent and the pelvic bones are separated, usually associated with exstrophy of the bladder.

split personality *n.* Multiple personality. No longer in scientific use.

split renal-function test *n.* See **differential ureteral-catheterization test.**

split-skin graft *n.* See **split-thickness graft.**

split-thickness flap *n.* A surgical flap that consists of the mucosa and submucosa but does not include periosteum. Also called *partial-thickness flap.*

split-thickness graft *n.* A skin graft of the epidermis and part of the dermis. Also called *partial-thickness graft, split-skin graft.*

split·ting (splĭt′ĭng) *n.* The chemical change in which a covalent bond in a molecule is cleaved, producing two or more simpler fragments.

spm *abbr.* suppression and mutation (used of a gene that leads to unstable mutants)

spo·dog·e·nous (spō-dŏj′ə-nəs) *adj.* Of or caused by waste material in an organ.

spon·dee (spŏn′dē′) *n.* A word or metrical foot having two equally stressed syllables, used in testing speech and hearing.

spon·dy·lal·gia (spŏn′dl-ăl′jə) *n.* Pain occurring in the spine.

spon·dyl·ar·thri·tis (spŏn′dl-är-thrī′tĭs) *n.* Inflammation of the intervertebral articulations.

spon·dy·li·tis (spŏn′dl-ī′tĭs) *n.* Inflammation of one or more vertebrae. —**spon′dy·lyt′ic** (-ĭt′ĭk) *adj.*

spondylitis de·for·mans (dē-fôr′mănz′) *n.* Arthritis and osteitis deformans involving the spinal column, marked by nodular deposits at the edges of the intervertebral disks, by ossification of the ligaments, and by bony ankylosis of the intervertebral articulations, resulting in a rounded kyphosis with rigidity. Also called *Bechterew's disease, Strümpell's disease.*

spondylo– or **spondyl–** *pref.* Vertebra; vertebrae: *spondylolysis.*

spon·dy·lo·ep·i·phys·i·al dysplasia (spŏn′dl-ō-ĕp′ə-fĭz′ē-əl) *n.* A complex of conditions, possibly genetic in cause, characterized by insufficient growth of the vertebral column and flattened vertebrae, and often involving the epiphyses at the hip and shoulder, resulting in a type of dwarfism.

spon·dy·lo·lis·the·sis (spŏn′dl-ō-lĭs-thē′sĭs) *n.* Forward displacement of one of the lower lumbar vertebrae over the vertebra below it or over the sacrum. —**spon′dy·lo·lis·thet′ic** (-thĕt′ĭk) *adj.*

spondylolisthetic pelvis *n.* A pelvis whose brim is occluded to a greater or lesser degree by a forward dislocation of the body of the lower lumbar vertebra. Also called *Prague pelvis, Rokitansky's pelvis.*

spon·dy·lol·y·sis (spŏn′dl-ŏl′ĭ-sĭs) *n.* Degeneration of the articulating part of a vertebra.

spon·dy·lop·a·thy (spŏn′dl-ŏp′ə-thē) *n.* Disease of the vertebrae or of the spinal column.

spon·dy·lo·py·o·sis (spŏn′dl-ō-pī-ō′sĭs) *n.* Suppurative inflammation of a vertebral body.

spon·dy·los·chi·sis (spŏn′dl-ŏs′kĭ-sĭs) *n.* Congenital fissure of one or more of the vertebral arches. Also called *rachischisis, cleft spine.*

spon·dy·lo·sis (spŏn′dl-ō′sĭs) *n.* **1.** Ankylosis of the vertebral bones. **2.** A degenerative disease of the spinal column, especially one leading to fusion and immobilization of the vertebral bones.

spon·dy·lo·syn·de·sis (spŏn′dl-ō-sĭn-dē′sĭs) *n.* See **spinal fusion.**

sponge (spŭnj) *n.* **1.** Any of numerous aquatic invertebrate animals of the phylum Porifera. **2.** The light, fibrous, absorbent skeleton of certain of these organisms. **3.** A piece of absorbent porous material, such as cellulose, plastic, or rubber, used especially for washing and cleaning. **4.** A gauze pad used to absorb blood and other fluids, as in surgery or in dressing a wound. **5.** A contraceptive sponge. —*v.* To wash, moisten, or absorb with a sponge.

sponge bath *n.* A bath in which a wet sponge or washcloth is used without immersing the body in water.

spon·gi·form (spŭn′jə-fôrm′) *adj.* Resembling a sponge, as in appearance or porosity.

spongiform encephalopathy *n.* Encephalopathy characterized by progressive diffuse vacuolation of the cerebral cortex.

spongio– *pref.* Sponge; spongelike: *spongiocyte.*

spon·gi·o·blast (spŭn′jē-ō-blăst′) *n.* An embryonic epithelial cell that gives rise to the neuroglia.

spon·gi·o·blas·to·ma (spŭn′jē-ō-blă-stō′mə) *n.* A glioma derived from spongioblasts.

spon·gi·o·cyte (spŭn′jē-ə-sīt′) *n.* **1.** Any of the cells of the neuroglia. **2.** A cell in the zona fasciculata of the adrenal cortex containing lipid droplets that show pronounced vacuolization.

spon·gi·oid (spŭn′jē-oid′) *adj.* Having a spongelike appearance or texture.

spon·gi·ose (spŭn′jē-ōs′) *adj.* Porous; spongy.

spon·gi·o·sis (spŭn′jē-ō′sĭs) *n.* Intercellular edema of the epidermis.

spon·gi·o·si·tis (spŭn′jē-ə-sī′tĭs) *n.* Inflammation of the spongy tissue between the cavernous bodies of the penis.

spong·y (spŭn′jē) *adj.* Resembling a sponge in appearance, elasticity, or porosity. —**spong′i·ness** *n.*

spongy bone *n.* **1.** Bone in which the spicules form a latticework, with interstices filled with embryonic connective tissue or bone marrow. Also called *cancellous bone, spongy substance, trabecular bone.* **2.** Any of the turbinate bones.

spongy degeneration *n.* A rare, inherited, fatal brain disease of infancy that is characterized by the widespread loss of myelin from nerve sheaths and the presence of round empty spaces in the brain, giving it a spongelike appearance, and resulting in progressive paralysis, blindness, and megalencephaly. Also called *Canavan's disease.*

spongy substance *n.* See **spongy bone** (sense 1).

spon·ta·ne·ous abortion (spŏn-tā′nē-əs) *n.* A naturally occurring termination of a pregnancy. Also called *miscarriage.*

spontaneous amputation *n.* **1.** Congenital amputation. **2.** Amputation resulting from a pathological process rather than from trauma.

spontaneous gangrene of newborn *n.* Gangrene due to vascular occlusion of unknown cause, usually in marasmic or dehydrated infants.

spontaneous intermittent mandatory ventilation *n. Abbr.* **SIMV** Intermittent mandatory ventilation spontaneously initiated by the patient to increase tidal volume, and subsequently synchronized with the patient's respiratory cycle.

spontaneous mutation *n.* A mutation that arises naturally and not as a result of exposure to mutagens. Also called *natural mutation.*

spontaneous pneumothorax *n.* A pneumothorax occurring secondary to parenchymal lung disease.

spontaneous version *n.* A turning of the fetus resulting from the unaided contraction of the uterine muscle.

spoon nail (spo̅o̅n) *n.* See **koilonychia.**

spo·rad·ic (spə-răd′ĭk, spô-) *or* **spo·rad·i·cal** (-ĭ-kəl) *adj.* **1.** Occurring at irregular intervals. **2.** Occurring singly; not grouped.

spo·ran·gi·um (spə-răn′jē-əm) *n., pl.* **-gi·a** (-jē-ə) A cell within a fungus in which asexual spores are produced by progressive cleavage. —**spo·ran′gi·al** (-jē-əl) *adj.*

Sporanox (spôr′ə-nŏks′) A trademark for the drug itraconazole.

spore (spôr) *n.* **1.** A small, usually single-celled asexual or sexual reproductive body that is highly resistant to desiccation and heat and is capable of growing into a new organism, produced especially by certain bacteria, fungi, algae, and nonflowering plants. **2.** A dormant, nonreproductive body formed by certain bacteria in response to adverse environmental conditions. —**spo·ra′ceous** (spə-rā′shəs, spô-) *adj.*

spo·ri·cide (spôr′ĭ-sīd′) *n.* An agent that kills spores. —**spo′ri·cid′al** (-sīd′l) *adj.*

spo·rid·i·um (spə-rĭd′ē-əm, spô-) *n., pl.* **-i·a** (-ē-ə) **1.** A protozoan spore. **2.** A protozoan organism in its embryonic stage.

sporo– *or* **spori–** *or* **spor–** *pref.* Spore: *sporocyte.*

spo·ro·ag·glu·ti·na·tion (spôr′ō-ə-glo̅o̅t′n-ā′shən) *n.* A method for diagnosing various mycoses based on the fact that the blood serum in diseases caused by fungi contains specific agglutinins that cause clumping of the spores of these organisms.

spo·ro·blast (spôr′ə-blăst′) *n.* An early stage in the development of a sporocyst, prior to differentiation of the sporozoites.

spo·ro·cyst (spôr′ə-sĭst′) *n.* **1.** A larval form in many trematode flatworms that develops in the body of its molluscan intermediate host. **2.** A secondary cyst that develops from a sporoblast and produces within itself one or several sporozoites.

spo·ro·gen·e·sis (spôr′ə-jĕn′ĭ-sĭs) *n.* **1.** Reproduction by means of spores. **2.** Production or formation of spores. —**spo′ro·gen′ic** (-jĕn′ĭk), **spo·rog′e·nous** (spə-rŏj′ə-nəs, spô-) *adj.*

spo·rog·o·ny (spə-rŏg′ə-nē, spô-) *n.* Reproduction by asexual division of a spore or zygote, characteristic of many sporozoans. Sporogony results in the production of sporozoites. —**spo′ro·gon′ic** (spôr′ə-gŏn′ĭk), **spo·rog′o·nous** (spə-rŏg′ə-nəs, spô-) *adj.*

spo·ront (spôr′ŏnt) *n.* An organism or a cell produced by sporogony.

Spo·ro·thrix (spôr′ə-thrĭks′) *n.* A genus of dimorphic imperfect fungi, including the species *S. schenckii,* the causative agent of sporotrichosis.

spo·ro·tri·cho·sis (spôr′ō-trĭ-kō′sĭs) *n.* A chronic infectious disease of domestic mammals and humans characterized by nodules or ulcers in the lymph nodes and skin and caused by a saprophytic or parasitic fungus of the genus *Sporothrix,* especially *S. schenckii,* commonly found in soil and wood.

Spo·ro·zo·a (spôr′ə-zō′ə) *or* **Spo·ro·zo·e·a** (-zō′ē-ə) *n.* A large class of parasitic protozoa, most of which reproduce sexually and asexually in alternate generations by means of spores. They are frequently transmitted by bloodsucking insects to different hosts, where they cause many serious diseases, such as malaria and coccidiosis.

spo·ro·zo·an (spôr′ə-zō′ən) *or* **spo·ro·zo·on** (-ŏn′, -ən) *n.* An organism of the class Sporozoa. —**spo′ro·zo′an** *adj.*

spo·ro·zo·ite (spôr′ə-zō′īt′) *n.* Any of the minute undeveloped sporozoans produced by multiple fission of a zygote or spore, especially at the stage just before it infects a new host cell.

sports medicine (spôrts) *n.* The branch of medicine that deals with injuries or illnesses resulting from participation in sports and athletic activities.

spor·u·lar (spôr′yə-lər) *adj.* Relating to a spore or sporule.

spor·u·late (spôr′yə-lāt′) *v.* To produce or release spores.

spor·u·la·tion (spôr′yə-lā′shən) *n.* The production or release of spores.

spor·ule (spôr′yo̅o̅l) *n.* A small spore.

spot (spŏt) *n.* **1.** A mark on a surface differing sharply in color from its surroundings. **2.** A stain or blot. —*v.* To lose a slight amount of blood through the vagina.

spot·ted fever (spŏt′ĭd) *n.* A tick typhus caused by *Rickettsia rickettsii,* such as Rocky Mountain spotted fever.

spot test for infectious mononucleosis *n.* A test used for the diagnosis of infectious mononucleosis.

sprain (sprān) *n.* An injury to a ligament when the joint is carried through a range of motion greater than its normal range without dislocation or fracture. —*v.* To cause a sprain to a joint or ligament.

sprain fracture *n.* An avulsion fracture in which a small portion of bone has been pulled or pushed off, often occurring in the ankle.

spray (sprā) *n.* A fine jet of liquid discharged from a pressurized container. —*v.* To disperse a liquid in a jet of droplets.

spring conjunctivitis (sprĭng) *n.* See **vernal conjunctivitis.**

spring ligament *n.* A dense fibroelastic ligament in the foot extending from the calcaneus to the navicular bone and supporting the head of the talus.

sprue (sprōō) *n.* **1.** A chronic disease that is characterized by diarrhea, steatorrhea, emaciation, and anemia, caused by defective absorption of nutrients from the intestinal tract. Also called *psilosis*. **2.** Wax or metal used to form the pathway for forcing molten metal into a mold in the making of a dental casting.

spud (spŭd) *n.* A blunt triangular knife used for removing foreign bodies from the cornea.

spur (spûr) *n.* A spine or projection from a bone.

spu·ri·ous (spyŏŏr′ē-əs) *adj.* Similar in appearance or symptoms but unrelated in morphology or pathology; false.

spurious ankylosis *n.* See **extracapsular ankylosis.**

spu·tum (spyŏŏ′təm) *n., pl.* **–ta** (-tə) Matter coughed up and usually expelled from the mouth, especially mucus or mucopurulent matter expectorated in diseases of the air passages.

SQ *abbr.* subcutaneous

squa·ma (skwā′mə, skwä′-) *n., pl.* **–mae** (-mē′) **1.** A thin platelike mass, as of bone. **2.** A scale or scalelike structure. —**squa′mate′** (-māt′) *adj.*

squamo– *pref.* Scale; scaly: *squamosal.*

squa·mo·sa (skwā-mō′sə) *n., pl.* **–sae** (-sē) The squama of the temporal bone or of the frontal and occipital bones.

squa·mo·sal (skwə-mō′səl) *adj.* Of or relating to the thin, platelike part of the temporal bone. —*n.* A squamosal bone.

squa·mous (skwā′məs, skwä′-) *or* **squa·mose** (-mōs′) *adj.* **1.** Covered with or formed of scales; scaly. **2.** Resembling a scale or scales; thin and flat. **3.** Squamosal.

squamous cell *n.* A flat, scalelike epithelial cell.

squamous cell carcinoma *n.* A carcinoma that arises from squamous epithelium and is the most common form of skin cancer. Also called *cancroid, epidermoid carcinoma.*

squamous epithelium *n.* Epithelium consisting of one or more cell layers, the most superficial of which is composed of flat, scalelike or platelike cells.

squamous metaplasia *n.* See **epidermalization.**

squamous metaplasia of amnion *n.* See **amnion nodosum.**

squamous odontogenic tumor *n.* A benign epithelial odontogenic tumor that appears radiologically as a lesion closely associated with the tooth root and that is composed of islands of squamous epithelium enclosed by a peripheral layer of flattened cells.

squamous suture *n.* A suture whose opposing margins are scalelike and overlapping.

squa·mo·zy·go·mat·ic (skwā′mō-zī′gə-mät′ĭk, -zĭg′ə-) *adj.* Of or relating to the squama and the zygomatic process of the temporal bone.

squint (skwĭnt) *n.* See **strabismus.**

Sr The symbol for the element **strontium.**

SRF *abbr.* somatotropin-releasing factor

SRIF *abbr.* somatotropin release-inhibiting factor

SRS-A *abbr.* slow-reacting substance of anaphylaxis

SSPE *abbr.* subacute sclerosing panencephalitis

SSRI *n.* Selective serotonin reuptake inhibitor; a class of drugs that inhibit the reuptake of serotonin in the central nervous system, used to treat depression and other psychiatric disorders.

SSS *abbr.* sick sinus syndrome

stab cell (stăb) *n.* See **band cell.**

stab culture *n.* A culture made by inserting an inoculating needle with inoculum down the center of a solid medium contained in a test tube.

stab drain *n.* A drain passed into a cavity through a puncture made adjacent to a surgical wound to prevent the wound from becoming infected.

sta·bi·late (stā′bə-lāt′) *n.* A population of organisms similar to but more stable than a strain and maintained in viable condition for a particular purpose.

sta·bile (stā′bĭl, -bəl, -bīl′, -bēl′) *adj.* Resistant to change; stable; steady.

sta·bil·i·ty (stə-bĭl′ĭ-tē) *n.* The condition of being stable or resistant to change.

sta·bi·lize (stā′bə-līz′) *v.* To bring to or reach a stable or steadfast state. —**sta′bi·li·za′tion** (-lĭ-zā′shən) *n.*

sta·ble (stā′bəl) *adj.* **1.** Resistant to change of position or condition. **2.** Not subject to mental illness or irrationality. **3.** Having no known mode of decay; indefinitely long-lived. Used of atomic particles. **4.** Not easily decomposed or otherwise modified chemically.

stable isotope *n.* An isotope of an element that shows no tendency to undergo radioactive breakdown.

stac·ca·to speech (stə-kä′tō) *n.* Abrupt speech in which each syllable is produced separately, associated with multiple sclerosis.

staff (stăf) *n.* **1.** A specific group of workers. **2.** See **director.** —*v.* **1.** To provide with a staff of workers or assistants. **2.** To serve on the staff of.

staff cell *n.* See **band cell.**

staff of Aes·cu·la·pi·us (ĕs′kyə-lā′pē-əs) *n.* A rod with a single serpent twining around it, used as the symbol of medicine.

stage (stāj) *n.* **1.** A period in the course of a disease. **2.** The platform on a microscope that supports a slide for viewing. **3.** A particular step, phase, or position in a developmental process. —*v.* To determine the extent or progression of.

stag-horn calculus (stăg′hôrn′) *n.* A renal calculus that branches into the infundibula and calices. Also called *coral calculus, dendritic calculus.*

stag·ing (stā′jĭng) *n.* The classification of neoplasms according to the extent of the tumor.

stag·nant anoxia (stăg′nənt) *n.* See **ischemic hypoxia.**

stag·na·tion (stăg-nā′shən) *n.* **1.** The retardation or cessation of the flow of blood in the blood vessels, as in passive congestion. **2.** The accumulation of a normally circulating fluid in a part or an organ.

stain (stān) *n.* **1.** A reagent or dye that is used for staining microscopic specimens. **2.** A procedure in which a dye or a combination of dyes and reagents is used to color the constituents of cells and tissues. —*v.* To treat specimens for the microscope with a reagent or dye that makes visible certain structures without affecting others.

stain·ing (stā′nĭng) *n.* **1.** The act of applying a stain. **2.** Modification of the color of the tooth or of the denture base to give a more realistic appearance.

stair·case (stâr′kās′) *n*. A series of reactions or responses that follow one another in progressively increasing or decreasing intensity, so that a chart shows a continuous rise or fall.

staircase phenomenon *n*. See **treppe**.

stal·ag·mom·e·ter (stăl′ăg-mŏm′ĭ-tər) *n*. An instrument for determining exactly the number of drops in a given quantity of liquid, used as a measure of the surface tension of a fluid.

stalk (stôk) *n*. A slender or elongated support or structure, as one that connects or supports an organ.

stam·mer (stăm′ər) *n*. A speech disorder characterized by hesitation and repetition of sounds, or by mispronunciation or transposition of certain consonants, especially *l*, *r*, and *s*. —*v*. To speak with a stammer.

stan·dard (stăn′dərd) *n*. **1.** An acknowledged measure of comparison for quantitative or qualitative value; a criterion. **2.** An object that under specified conditions defines, represents, or records the magnitude of a unit. —*adj*. **1.** Serving as or conforming to a standard of measurement or value. **2.** Widely recognized as a model of authority or excellence.

standard bicarbonate *n*. The plasma bicarbonate concentration of a sample of blood; abnormally high or low values indicate metabolic alkalosis or acidosis, respectively.

standard deviation *n*. *Symbol* σ A statistic used as a measure of the dispersion or variation in a distribution, equal to the square root of the arithmetic mean of the squares of the deviations from the arithmetic mean.

standard error of difference *n*. A statistical index of the probability that a difference between the statistical means of two samples is greater than zero.

stan·dard·i·za·tion (stăn′dər-dĭ-zā′shən) *n*. **1.** The making of a solution of definite strength so that it may be used for comparison and in tests. **2.** The making of a drug or other preparation so that it conforms to the type or standard.

stan·dard·ize (stăn′dər-dīz′) *v*. **1.** To cause to conform to a standard. **2.** To evaluate by comparing with a standard.

standard lead (lēd) *n*. **1.** Any of three standard bipolar limb leads of an electrocardiograph, designated I, II and III. Lead I records potential difference between the right and left arms; lead II, the difference between right arm and left leg; lead III, the difference between left arm and left leg. **2.** A record obtained from such a lead.

standard solution *n*. A solution of known concentration, used as a standard of comparison or analysis.

standard temperature *n*. A temperature of 0°C or 273 Kelvin.

standard volume *n*. The volume of an ideal gas at standard temperature and pressure: 22.414 liters.

stand·still (stănd′stĭl′) *n*. Complete cessation of activity or progress.

Stan·ford-Binet test (stăn′fərd-) *n*. A standardized intelligence test adapted from the Binet-Simon scale for use in the United States, especially in the assessment of children. Also called *Stanford-Binet intelligence scale*.

Stan·ley (stăn′lē), **Wendell Meredith** 1904–1971. American biochemist. He shared a 1946 Nobel Prize for discovering methods of producing pure enzymes and virus proteins.

stan·nic (stăn′ĭk) *adj*. Of, relating to, or containing tin, especially with valence 4.

stan·nous (stăn′əs) *adj*. Of, relating to, or containing tin, especially with valence 2.

stannous fluoride *n*. A preparation of stannous tin and fluoride used to fluoridate toothpaste and other dental preparations.

stan·num (stăn′əm) *n*. The element tin.

stan·o·lone (stăn′ə-lōn′) *n*. See **dihydrotestosterone**.

sta·pe·dec·to·my (stā′pĭ-dĕk′tə-mē, -pē-) *n*. Surgical removal of all or part of the stapes of the middle ear, followed by replacement with a prosthesis.

sta·pe·di·al (stā-pē′dē-əl) *adj*. Relating to the stapes.

sta·pe·di·o·te·not·o·my (stā-pē′dē-ō-tĕ-nŏt′ə-mē) *n*. Division of the tendon of the stapedius muscle.

sta·pe·di·us (stā-pē′dē-əs) *n*. A muscle with origin from the internal walls of the pyramidal eminence in the tympanic cavity of the ear, with insertion into the neck of the stapes, with nerve supply from the facial nerve, and whose action draws the head of the stapes backward.

sta·pes (stā′pēz) *n*., *pl*. **stapes** *or* **sta·pe·des** (stā′pĭ-dēz′) The smallest of the three auditory ossicles, whose base fits into the oval window and whose head is articulated with the lenticular process of the long limb of the incus. Also called *stirrup*.

stapes-mobilization operation *n*. An operation involving the fracture of tissue that has immobilized the stapes; it is performed to restore hearing, especially in patients with otosclerosis.

staph (stăf) *n*. Staphylococcus. —**staph** *adj*.

Staph·cil·lin (stăf-sĭl′ĭn) A trademark for the drug methicillin.

staph·y·lec·to·my (stăf′ə-lĕk′tə-mē) *n*. See **uvulectomy**.

staph·yl·e·de·ma (stăf′ə-lĭ-dē′mə) *n*. Edema of the uvula.

staph·y·line (stăf′ə-līn′, -lēn′) *adj*. **1.** Shaped like a bunch of grapes; botryoid. **2.** Relating to the uvula.

sta·phyl·i·on (stā-fĭl′ē-ŏn′) *n*. The midpoint of the posterior edge of the hard palate.

staphylo– *or* **staphyl–** *pref*. **1.** Cluster; resembling a cluster: *staphylococcus*. **2.** The uvula: *staphyledema*.

staphylococcal scalded skin syndrome *n*. A disease affecting infants in which large areas of skin peel off in the manner of a second-degree burn, caused by upper respiratory staphylococcal infection. Also called *Lyell's disease, Ritter's disease*.

staph·y·lo·coc·ce·mi·a (stăf′ə-lō-kŏk-sē′mē-ə) *n*. The presence of staphylococci in the blood.

staph·y·lo·coc·co·sis (stăf′ə-lō-kŏ-kō′sĭs) *n*., *pl*. **–ses** (-sēz) Infection by a species of *Staphylococcus*.

staph·y·lo·coc·cus (stăf′ə-lō-kŏk′əs) *n*., *pl*. **–coc·ci** (-kŏk′sī, -kŏk′ī) A spherical gram-positive parasitic bacterium of the genus *Staphylococcus*, usually occurring in clusters and causing boils, septicemia, and other infections. —**staph′y·lo·coc′cal** (-kŏk′əl), **staph′y·lo·coc′·cic** (-kŏk′sĭk, -kŏk′ĭk) *adj*.

staphylococcus antitoxin *n.* A preparation containing antitoxin globulins or their derivatives that act to neutralize a lethal toxin produced by *Staphylococcus aureus*.

Staphylococcus au·re·us (ô′rē-əs) *n.* A bacterium that causes furunculosis, pyemia, osteomyelitis, suppuration of wounds, and food poisoning.

Staphylococcus py·og·e·nes al·bus (pī-ŏj′ə-nēz ăl′-bəs) *n.* A strain of *Staphylococcus aureus* that forms white colonies.

staph·y·lo·der·ma (stăf′ə-lō-dûr′mə) *n.* Pyoderma due to staphylococci.

staph·y·lo·der·ma·ti·tis (stăf′ə-lō-dûr′mə-tī′tĭs) *n.* Inflammation of the skin caused by staphylococci.

staph·y·lo·di·al·y·sis (stăf′ə-lō-dī-ăl′ĭ-sĭs) *n.* See **uvuloptosis.**

staph·y·lo·ki·nase (stăf′ə-lō-kī′nās′, -năz′, -kĭn′ās′, -āz′) *n.* A enzyme from *Staphylococcus aureus* that catalyzes the conversion of plasminogen to plasmin.

staph·y·lol·y·sin (stăf′ə-lŏl′ĭ-sĭn) *n.* **1.** A hemolysin produced by a staphylococcus. **2.** An antibody causing lysis of staphylococci.

staph·y·lo·ma (stăf′ə-lō′mə) *n.* A bulging of the cornea or sclera due to inflammatory softening.

staph·y·lom·a·tous (stăf′ə-lŏm′ə-təs) *adj.* Relating to or marked by staphyloma.

staph·y·lon·cus (stăf′ə-lŏng′kəs) *n.* A tumor or swelling of the uvula.

staph·y·lo·phar·yn·gor·rha·phy (stăf′ə-lō-făr′ĭng-gôr′ə-fē) *n.* Surgical repair of defects in the uvula or soft palate and the pharynx. Also called *palatopharyngorrhaphy.*

staph·y·lo·plas·ty (stăf′ə-lō-plăs′tē) *n.* Plastic surgery of the uvula and the soft palate.

staph·y·lop·to·sis (stăf′ə-lŏp-tō′sĭs) *n.* See **uvuloptosis.**

staph·y·lor·rha·phy (stăf′ə-lôr′ə-fē) *n.* See **palatorrhaphy.**

staph·y·los·chi·sis (stăf′ə-lŏs′kĭ-sĭs) *n.* A bifid uvula, with or without cleft of the soft palate.

staph·y·lot·o·my (stăf′ə-lŏt′ə-mē) *n.* **1.** See **uvulotomy. 2.** Surgical division of a staphyloma.

staph·y·lo·tox·in (stăf′ə-lō-tŏk′sĭn) *n.* The toxin produced by a *Staphylococcus* species.

sta·pling (stā′plĭng) *n.* The fastening together of two tissues with a staple or staples.

starch (stärch) *n.* **1.** A naturally abundant nutrient carbohydrate found chiefly in the seeds, fruits, tubers, roots, and stem pith of plants, and commonly prepared as a white, amorphous, tasteless powder used in powders, ointments, and pastes. Also called *amylum.* **2.** A food having a high content of starch, such as rice, bread, and potatoes.

Star·ling (stär′lĭng), Sir **Ernest** 1866–1927. British physiologist. With Sir William Bayliss he discovered (1902) the hormone secretin.

Star·ling's curve (stär′lĭngz) *n.* A curve that indicates the ratio of cardiac output to atrial pressure. Also called *Frank-Starling curve.*

Starling's hypothesis *n.* The hypothesis that fluid filtration through capillary membranes is dependent on the balance between the pressure the blood places on the membranes and the osmotic pressure of the membranes.

Starling's law *n.* See **law of heart.**

star·tle epilepsy (stär′tl) *n.* Reflex epilepsy in which seizures are provoked by hearing a sudden noise.

startle reflex *n.* **1.** The reflex response of an infant in which the limb and neck muscles contract when the infant is allowed to drop a short distance or is startled by a sudden noise or jolt. Also called *Moro's reflex, parachute reflex.* **2.** See **cochleopalpebral reflex.**

star·va·tion (stär-vā′shən) *n.* **1.** The act or process of starving. **2.** The condition of being starved.

starve (stärv) *v.* **1.** To suffer or die from extreme or prolonged lack of food. **2.** To deprive of food so as to cause suffering or death.

sta·sis (stā′sĭs, stăs′ĭs) *n., pl.* **sta·ses** (stā′sēz, stăs′ēz) Stoppage of the normal flow of a body substance, as of blood through an artery or of intestinal contents through the bowels.

–stasis *suff.* **1.** Slowing; stoppage: *cytostasis.* **2.** Stable state: *homeostasis.*

stasis dermatitis *n.* Inflammation and scaling of the legs due to impaired venous circulation.

stasis eczema *n.* Eczematous eruption on the legs due to or aggravated by vascular stasis.

stat (stăt) *adv.* With no delay. —*adj.* Immediate.

–stat *suff.* **1.** Something that stabilizes: *barostat.* **2.** Something that inhibits: *hemostat.*

state (stāt) *n.* A condition or situation; status.

state-dependent learning *n.* Learning associated with a specific state of sleep or wakefulness or with a chemically altered state, such that the learned information cannot be recalled or used unless the subject is restored to the state that existed when learning first occurred.

stat·ic convulsion (stăt′ĭk) *n.* See **saltatory spasm.**

static reflex *n.* See **righting reflex.**

stat·in (stăt′n) *n.* Any of a class of drugs that inhibit a key enzyme involved in the synthesis of cholesterol and promote receptor binding of LDL cholesterol, resulting in decreased levels of serum cholesterol.

stato– *pref.* Equilibrium; balance: *statoacoustic.*

stat·o·a·cous·tic (stăt′ō-ə-kōō′stĭk) *adj.* Relating to equilibrium and hearing.

stat·o·co·ni·um (stăt′ə-kō′nē-əm) *n., pl.* **–ni·a** (-nē-ə) Any of the crystalline particles of calcium carbonate and a protein adhering to the gelatinous membrane of the maculae of the utricle and saccule. Also called *statolith, otoconium.*

stat·o·ki·net·ic reflex (stăt′ō-kĭ-nĕt′ĭk, -kī-) *n.* A reflex that, through stimulation of the receptors in the neck muscles and semicircular canals, brings about movements of the limbs and eyes appropriate to a given movement of the head.

stat·o·lith (stăt′l-ĭth′) *n.* **1.** A small, movable concretion of calcium carbonate found in statocysts; an otolith. **2.** See **statoconium.**

stat·o·ton·ic reflexes (stăt′ə-tŏn′ĭk) *pl.n.* Reflexes that control the tone of the limb muscles to maintain or regain a desired body position.

stat·ure (stăch′ər) *n.* The height of a person.

sta·tus (stā′təs, stăt′əs) *n.* A state or condition.

status asth·mat·i·cus (ăz-măt′ĭ-kəs, ăs-) *n.* A condition of severe, prolonged asthma.

status ep·i·lep·ti·cus (ĕp′ə-lĕp′tĭ-kəs) *n.* A condition in which one major attack of epilepsy succeeds another with little or no intermission.

stau·ri·on (stôr′ē-ŏn′) *n.* A craniometric point at the intersection of the median and transverse palatine sutures.

stau·ro·ple·gia (stôr′ə-plē′jə) *n.* See **alternating hemiplegia**.

stav·u·dine (stăv′yōō-dēn′) *n.* A nucleoside analog antiviral drug used to treat infection with HIV by inhibiting replication of the virus.

STD *abbr.* sexually transmitted disease

stead·y state (stĕd′ē) *n.* **1.** A state obtained in moderate muscular exercise when the removal of lactic acid by oxidation keeps pace with its production. **2.** A condition in which the formation of substances keeps pace with their destruction so that all volumes, concentrations, pressures, and flows remain constant. **3.** A stable condition that does not change over time or in which change in one direction is continually balanced by change in another.

steal (stēl) *n.* The diversion of blood flow from its normal course.

ste·ap·sin (stē-ăp′sĭn) *n.* A digestive enzyme of pancreatic juice that catalyzes the hydrolysis of fats to fatty acids and glycerol. Also called *triacylglycerol lipase*.

ste·a·rate (stē′ə-rāt′, stîr′āt′) *n.* A salt or ester of stearic acid.

ste·ar·ic acid (stē-ăr′ĭk, stîr′ĭk) *n.* A colorless, odorless, waxlike fatty acid occurring naturally in animal and vegetable fats and used in pharmaceutical preparations, ointments, soaps, and suppositories.

Stearns alcoholic amentia (stûrnz) *n.* A temporary mental disorder resulting from alcohol abuse, similar to delirium tremens but longer lasting.

stearo– *or* **stear–** *pref.* Fat: *stearate*.

ste·a·ti·tis (stē′ə-tī′tĭs) *n.* An inflammation of adipose tissue.

steato– *or* **steat–** *pref.* Fat: *steatolytic*.

ste·a·to·cys·to·ma (stē′ə-tō-sĭ-stō′mə) *n.* **1.** A cyst with cells of a sebaceous gland in its wall. **2.** See **sebaceous cyst**.

steatocystoma mul·ti·plex (mŭl′tə-plĕks′) *n.* Widespread, multiple, thin-walled cysts of the skin, lined by squamous epithelium, and including lobules of sebaceous cells.

ste·a·tol·y·sis (stē′ə-tŏl′ĭ-sĭs) *n.* Hydrolysis or emulsion of fat in the digestive process. —**ste′a·to·lyt′ic** (-tə-lĭt′ĭk) *adj.*

ste·a·to·ne·cro·sis (stē′ə-tō-nə-krō′sĭs) *n.* See **fat necrosis**.

ste·at·o·pyg·i·a (stē-ăt′ə-pĭj′ē-ə, -pī′jē-ə) *or* **ste·a·to·py·ga** (stē′ə-tō-pī′gə, stē-ăt′ə-) *n.* Excessive accumulation of fat on the buttocks. —**ste′a·to·pyg′ic** (-pĭj′ĭk, -pī′jĭk), **ste′a·to·py′gous** (-pī′gəs) *adj.*

ste·a·tor·rhe·a *or* **ste·a·tor·rhoe·a** (stē′ə-tə-rē′ə, stē-ăt′ə-) *n.* Excessive discharge of fat in the feces, as occurring in pancreatic disease and in malabsorption syndromes.

ste·a·to·sis (stē′ə-tō′sĭs) *n.* See **fatty degeneration**.

steg·no·sis (stĕg-nō′sĭs) *n.* **1.** A stoppage of a secretion. **2.** A constriction or stenosis.

steg·not·ic (stĕg-nŏt′ĭk) *adj.* Astringent or constipating. —*n.* An agent that is astringent or constipating.

Stein (stīn), **William Howard** 1911–1980. American biochemist. He shared a 1972 Nobel Prize for pioneering studies of ribonuclease.

Stein·berg thumb sign (stīn′bərg) *n.* An indication of Marfan's syndrome in which the thumb projects well beyond the ulnar surface of the hand when it is held across the palm of the same hand.

Stei·nert's disease (stī′nərts, shtī′-) *n.* See **myotonic dystrophy**.

Stein-Lev·en·thal syndrome (-lĕv′ən-thôl) *n.* See **polycystic ovary disease**.

stel·la (stĕl′ə) *n.,* *pl.* **stel·lae** (stĕl′ē) A star or star-shaped figure.

stel·late (stĕl′āt′) *or* **stel·lat·ed** (-ā′tĭd) *adj.* Arranged or shaped like a star; radiating from a center.

stellate abscess *n.* A star-shaped necrosis surrounded by epithelioid cells, as in swollen inguinal lymph nodes in lymphogranuloma venereum.

stellate block *n.* Injection of local anesthetic solution in the vicinity of the stellate ganglion.

stellate cell *n.* A star-shaped cell, such as an astrocyte or Kupffer cell, that has many filaments extending radially.

stellate fracture *n.* A bone fracture in which the lines of break radiate from a point, usually from the site of an injury.

stellate ganglion *n.* See **cervicothoracic ganglion**.

stellate hair *n.* A hair that is split into several strands at the free end.

stellate ligament *n.* See **radiate ligament of rib**.

stellate reticulum *n.* A network of stellate epithelial cells in the center of the enamel organ between the outer and inner enamel epithelium.

stellate vein *n.* A stellate venule.

stellate venule *n.* Any of a number of venules in the renal cortex gathered in star-shaped groups.

stel·lu·la (stĕl′yə-lə) *n.,* *pl.* **–lae** (-lē′) A small star or star-shaped figure.

Stell·wag's sign (stĕl′wăgz′, shtĕl′väks′) *n.* An indication of Graves disease in which there is infrequent and incomplete blinking of the eye.

stem (stĕm) *n.* A supporting structure resembling the stalk of a plant.

stem cell *n.* An unspecialized cell that gives rise to a specific specialized cell, such as a blood cell.

stem cell factor *n.* A cytokine that promotes the differentiation and growth of hematopoietic stem cells into other types of cells.

stem cell leukemia *n.* A form of leukemia characterized by abnormal cells that are very poorly differentiated but that are considered to be precursors of lymphoblasts, myeloblasts, or monoblasts. Also called *embryonal leukemia*.

sten·i·on (stĕn′ē-ŏn′) *n.* The termination in either temporal fossa of the shortest transverse diameter of the skull.

steno– *pref.* Narrow; small: *stenothorax.*

sten·o·car·di·a (stĕn′ə-kär′dē-ə) *n.* See **angina pectoris.**

sten·o·ceph·a·ly (stĕn′ō-sĕf′ə-lē) *n.* Marked narrowness of the head. —**sten′o·ce·phal′ic** (-sə-făl′ĭk), **sten′o·ceph′a·lous** (-sĕf′ə-ləs) *adj.*

sten·o·cho·ri·a (stĕn′ə-kôr′ē-ə) *n.* Abnormal contraction of a canal or orifice.

sten·o·pe·ic (stĕn′ə-pē′ĭk) *adj.* Having a narrow opening or slit.

ste·no·sal murmur (stə-nō′səl) *n.* An arterial murmur due to a narrowing of the vessel from pressure or organic change.

Ste·no's duct (stē′nōz, stā′-) *n.* See **parotid duct.**

ste·nosed (stə-nōzd′, -nōst′) *adj.* Marked by or showing stenosis; narrowed; strictured.

ste·no·sis (stə-nō′sĭs) *n., pl.* **–ses** (-sēz) A constriction or narrowing of a duct or passage; a stricture.

sten·o·sto·mi·a (stĕn′ə-stō′mē-ə) *n.* Narrowness of the oral cavity.

sten·o·ther·mal (stĕn′ə-thûr′məl) *or* **sten·o·ther·mic** (-mĭk) *or* **sten·o·ther·mous** (-məs) *adj.* Capable of living or growing only within a limited range of temperature. Used of bacteria. —**sten′o·therm′** *n.*

sten·o·tho·rax (stĕn′ō-thôr′ăks′) *n.* A narrow, contracted chest.

ste·not·ic (stə-nŏt′ĭk) *adj.* Of or affected with stenosis.

sten·ox·e·nous (stə-nŏk′sə-nəs) *adj.* Of or relating to a parasite having a narrow range of potential hosts.

Sten·sen's duct (stĕn′sənz, stän′-) *n.* See **parotid duct.**

stent (stĕnt) *n.* **1.** A device that is used to maintain a bodily orifice or cavity during skin grafting, or to immobilize a skin graft following placement. **2.** A slender thread, rod, or catheter placed within the lumen of tubular structures, such as a blood vessel, to provide support during or after anastomosis.

ste·pha·ni·on (stə-fā′nē-ŏn′) *n.* A point on the cranium where the coronal suture intersects the inferior temporal line. —**ste·pha′ni·al** *adj.*

step·page (stĕp′ĭj) *n.* The peculiar gait seen in neuritis of the peroneal nerve and in tabes dorsalis, characterized by high stepping to allow the drooping foot and toes to clear the ground.

sterco– *pref.* Feces; fecal: *stercoraceous.*

ster·co·bi·lin (stûr′kō-bī′lĭn, -bĭl′ĭn) *n.* A brown degradation product of hemoglobin present in feces.

ster·co·lith (stûr′kə-lĭth′) *n.* See **coprolith.**

ster·co·ra·ceous (stûr′kə-rā′shəs) *or* **ster·co·ral** (stûr′-kər-əl) *or* **ster·co·rous** (-kər-əs) *adj.* Relating to or containing feces.

stercoraceous vomiting *n.* See **fecal vomiting.**

stercoral abscess *n.* An abscess containing pus and feces. Also called *fecal abscess.*

stercoral fistula *n.* See **intestinal fistula.**

stercoral ulcer *n.* An ulcer of the colon due to pressure and irritation from retained fecal masses.

ster·co·ro·ma (stûr′kə-rō′mə) *n.* See **coproma.**

ster·cus (stûr′kəs) *n.* See **feces.**

stere (stîr) *n.* A unit of volume equal to one cubic meter.

stereo– *pref.* **1.** Solid; solid body: *stereotropism.* **2.** Three-dimensional: *stereochemistry.*

ster·e·o·ar·throl·y·sis (stĕr′ē-ō-är-thrŏl′ĭ-sĭs) *n.* The surgical formation of a new movable joint in cases of bony ankylosis.

ster·e·o·cam·pim·e·ter (stĕr′ē-ō-kăm-pĭm′ĭ-tər) *n.* An apparatus for studying the central visual fields.

stereochemical formula *n.* A chemical formula that indicates the spatial arrangement of atoms or atomic groupings in a molecule. Also called *spacial formula.*

ster·e·o·chem·is·try (stĕr′ē-ō-kĕm′ĭ-strē) *n.* The branch of chemistry that deals with the spatial arrangement of atoms in molecules and the effects such arrangements have on the chemical and physical properties of the molecules, especially where asymmetric centers of substitution lead to optical rotation. —**ster′-e·o·chem′i·cal** (-ĭ-kəl) *adj.*

ster·e·o·cin·e·fluo·rog·ra·phy (stĕr′ē-ō-sĭn′ē-floŏ-rŏg′rə-fē, -flô-) *n.* The motion-picture recording of three-dimensional radiographic images obtained by stereoscopic fluoroscopy.

ster·e·o·e·lec·tro·en·ceph·a·log·ra·phy (stĕr′ē-ō-ĭ-lĕk′trō-ĕn-sĕf′ə-lŏg′rə-fē) *n.* The recording of electrical activity in three planes of the brain by means of surface and depth electrodes.

ster·e·o·en·ceph·a·lom·e·try (stĕr′ē-ō-ĕn-sĕf′ə-lŏm′-ĭ-trē) *n.* The localization of brain structures by use of three-dimensional coordinates.

ster·e·o·en·ceph·a·lot·o·my (stĕr′ē-ō-ĕn-sĕf′ə-lŏt′ə-mē) *n.* The use of stereotaxis in surgery of the brain.

ster·e·og·no·sis (stĕr′ē-ŏg-nō′sĭs) *n.* The perception of the form of an object by means of touch. —**ster′e·og·nos′tic** (-nŏs′tĭk) *adj.*

ster·e·o·i·so·mer (stĕr′ē-ō-ī′sə-mər) *n.* A molecule containing the same number and kind of atomic groupings as another but having a different spatial arrangement, thus exhibiting different properties.

ster·e·o·i·som·er·ism (stĕr′ē-ō-ī-sŏm′ə-rĭz′əm) *n.* Isomerism created by differences in the spatial arrangement of atoms in a molecule.

ster·e·om·e·try (stĕr′ē-ŏm′ĭ-trē) *n.* **1.** The measurement of a solid object or of the cubic capacity of a vessel. **2.** The determination of the specific gravity of a liquid.

ster·e·op·a·thy (stĕr′ē-ŏp′ə-thē) *n.* Persistent stereotyped thinking.

ster·e·o·ra·di·og·ra·phy (stĕr′ē-ō-rā′dē-ŏg′rə-fē) *n.* The method of taking radiographs from two slightly different positions so as to obtain a stereoscopic effect.

ster·e·o·scope (stĕr′ē-ə-skōp′) *n.* An optical instrument with two eyepieces used to impart a three-dimensional effect to two photographs of the same scene taken at slightly different angles.

ster·e·o·scop·ic (stĕr′ē-ə-skŏp′ĭk) *n.* **1.** Of, relating to, or characterized by stereoscopy. **2.** Of or relating to a stereoscope.

stereoscopic microscope *n.* A microscope having double eyepieces and objectives and independent light paths, producing a three-dimensional image.

stereoscopic vision *n.* The single perception of a slightly different image from each eye, resulting in depth perception.

ster·e·os·co·py (stĕr′ē-ŏs′kə-pē) *n.* An optical technique by which two images of the same object are blended into one, giving a three-dimensional appearance to the single image.

stereotactic instrument *n.* An apparatus attached to the head, used to localize precisely an area in the brain by means of coordinates related to intracerebral structures.

stereotactic radiosurgery *n.* Stereotaxis in which tissue destruction is produced by ionizing radiation rather than by surgical incision.

ster·e·o·tax·is (stĕr′ē-ə-tăk′sĭs) *or* **ster·e·o·tax·y** (stĕr′-ē-ə-tăk′sē) *n.* **1.** A surgical technique that uses medical imaging to locate precisely in three dimensions an anatomical site to which a surgical instrument or a beam of radiation is directed. Also called *stereotactic surgery.* **2.** Movement of an organism in response to contact with a solid body. Also called *thigmotaxis.* —**ster′e·o·tac′tic** (-tăk′tĭk), **ster′e·o·tax′ic** (-tăk′sĭk), **ster′e·o·tac′ti·cal** (-tăk′tĭ-kəl), **ster′e·o·tax′i·cal** (-tăk′-sĭ-kəl) *adj.*

ster·e·ot·ro·pism (stĕr′ē-ŏt′rə-pĭz′əm) *n.* See **thigmotropism.** —**ster′e·o·trop′ic** (-ē-ə-trŏp′ĭk) *adj.*

ster·e·o·ty·py (stĕr′ē-ə-tī′pē) *n.* **1.** The maintenance of one attitude for a long period. **2.** The constant repetition of certain meaningless gestures or movements.

ster·ic (stĕr′ĭk) *or* **ster·i·cal** (-ĭ-kəl) *n.* Of or relating to the spatial arrangement of atoms in a molecule; stereochemical. —**ster′i·cal·ly** *adv.*

ster·ile (stĕr′əl, -īl′) *adj.* **1.** Not producing or incapable of producing offspring. **2.** Free from all live bacteria or other microorganisms and their spores. —**ster′ile·ness, ste·ril′i·ty** (stə-rĭl′ĭ-tē) *n.*

sterile cyst *n.* A hydatid cyst that has no brood capsules or viable scolexes.

ster·il·i·za·tion (stĕr′ə-lĭ-zā′shən) *n.* **1.** The act or procedure of sterilizing. **2.** The condition of being sterile or sterilized.

ster·il·ize (stĕr′ə-līz′) *v.* **1.** To make free from live bacteria or other microorganisms. **2.** To deprive a person or animal of the ability to produce offspring, as by removing the reproductive organs.

ster·il·iz·er (stĕr′ə-lī′zər) *n.* An apparatus for rendering objects aseptic.

ster·nal (stûr′nəl) *adj.* Of, relating to, or occurring near the sternum.

sternal angle *n.* The angle between the upper part of the sternum and the body of the sternum.

ster·nal·gia (stər-năl′jə) *n.* Pain in the sternum or in the sternal region. Also called *sternodynia.*

sternal line *n.* A vertical line corresponding to the lateral margin of the sternum.

sternal muscle *n.* An inconstant muscle running parallel to the sternum across the costosternal origin of the greater pectoral muscle and usually connected with the sternocleidomastoid muscle and the rectus muscle of the abdomen.

sternal plane *n.* A plane along the front surface of the sternum.

sternal puncture *n.* Removal of bone marrow from the manubrium of the sternum with a needle.

Stern·berg (stûrn′bûrg′), **George Miller** 1838–1915.

American army physician who was US surgeon general (1893–1902) and organized (1900) the Yellow Fever Commission.

Stern·berg-Reed cell (stûrn′bûrg′-, shtĕrn′bĕrk′-) *n.* See **Reed-Sternberg cell.**

ster·ne·bra (stûr′nə-brə) *n., pl.* **–brae** (-brē) One of the four segments of the primordial sternum of the embryo, the fusion of which forms the body of the adult sternum.

sterno– *or* **stern–** *pref.* Sternum: *sternocostal.*

ster·no·cla·vic·u·lar (stûr′nō-klə-vĭk′yə-lər) *adj.* Of, relating to, or connecting the sternum and clavicle.

sternoclavicular angle *n.* The angle formed by the junction of the clavicle with the sternum.

ster·no·clei·do·mas·toid (stûr′nō-klī′də-măs′toid) *adj.* Relating to or characterizing the sternum, the clavicle, and the mastoid process. —*n.* A muscle with origin from the anterior surface of the episternum and from the sternal end of the clavicle, with insertion into the mastoid process and the superior nuchal line, with nerve supply from the accessory nerve, and whose action turns the head obliquely to the opposite side and flexes the neck and extends the head when both sides act together. Also called *sternomastoid.*

sternocleidomastoid vein *n.* A vein that arises in the sternocleidomastoid muscle and drains into the internal jugular vein.

ster·no·cos·tal (stûr′nō-kŏs′təl) *adj.* Of or relating to both the sternum and the ribs.

sternocostal ligament *n.* Either of two sets of ligaments connecting the rib cartilages and the sternum.

ster·no·dyn·i·a (stûr′nō-dĭn′ē-ə) *n.* See **sternalgia.**

ster·no·hy·oid (stûr′nō-hī′oid′) *n.* A muscle with origin from the episternum and the first costal cartilage, with insertion into the hyoid bone, with nerve supply from the upper cervical nerve through the cervical ansa, and whose action depresses the hyoid bone.

ster·noid (stûr′noid′) *adj.* Resembling the sternum.

ster·no·mas·toid (stûr′nō-măs′toid′) *n.* See **sternocleidomastoid** .

ster·no·pa·gia (stûr′nō-pā′jə) *n.* The condition of conjoined twins united at the sternum or at the ventral walls of the chest.

ster·no·per·i·car·di·al (stûr′nō-pĕr′ĭ-kär′dē-əl) *adj.* Relating to the sternum and the pericardium.

ster·nos·chi·sis (stər-nŏs′kĭ-sĭs) *n.* Congenital cleft of the sternum.

ster·no·thy·roid (stûr′nō-thī′roid′) *n.* A muscle with origin from the episternum and the first or second costal cartilage, with insertion into the thyroid cartilage, with nerve supply from the upper cervical nerve through the cervical ansa, and whose action depresses the larynx.

ster·not·o·my (stər-nŏt′ə-mē) *n.* An incision into or through the sternum.

ster·no·ver·te·bral (stûr′nō-vûr′tə-brəl, -vər-tē′brəl) *adj.* Of or relating to the sternum and the vertebrae.

ster·num (stûr′nəm) *n., pl.* **–nums** *or* **–na** (-nə) A long flat bone, articulating with the cartilages of the first seven ribs and with the clavicle, forming the middle part of the anterior wall of the thorax, and consisting of the corpus, manubrium, and xiphoid process. Also called *breastbone.*

ster·nu·ta·tion (stûr′nyə-tā′shən) *n.* **1.** The act of sneezing. **2.** A sneeze.

ster·nu·ta·to·ry (stûr-nyo͞o′tə-tôr′ē, -no͞o′-) *adj.* Causing or producing sneezing. —*n.* A sternutatory substance, such as pepper.

ster·oid (stĕr′oid′, stîr′-) *n.* Any of numerous naturally occurring or synthetic fat-soluble organic compounds having as a basis 17 carbon atoms arranged in four rings and including the sterols and bile acids, adrenocortical and sex hormones, certain natural drugs such as digitalis compounds, and the precursors of certain vitamins. Also called *steroid hormone.* —*adj.* or **ste·roid·al** (stĭ-roid′l, stĕ-) Relating to or characteristic of steroids or steroid hormones.

steroid acne *n.* Acne similar to acne vulgaris but resulting from administration of steroids.

steroid hormone *n.* See **steroid.**

ste·roid·o·gen·e·sis (stĭ-roi′də-jĕn′ĭ-sĭs, stîr′oi-, stĕr′-) *n.* The biological synthesis of steroids. —**ste·roid′o·gen′ic** (-jĕn′ĭk) *adj.*

steroid ulcer *n.* An ulcer, usually on the leg or foot, developing from a wound in patients undergoing long-term steroid therapy, due to the inhibitory effects of steroids on wound healing.

ster·ol (stĕr′ôl′, -ōl′, stîr′-) *n.* Any of a group of predominantly unsaturated solid alcohols of the steroid group, such as cholesterol and ergosterol, present in the fatty tissues of plants and animals.

ster·tor (stûr′tər) *n.* A heavy snoring inspiratory sound occurring in coma or deep sleep, sometimes due to obstruction of the larynx or upper airways. —**ster′to·rous** *adj.* —**ster′to·rous·ly** *adv.*

ste·thal·gia (stĕ-thăl′jə) *n.* Pain in the chest.

stetho– or **steth–** *pref.* Chest: *stethalgia.*

steth·o·go·ni·om·e·ter (stĕth′ō-gō′nē-ŏm′ĭ-tər) *n.* An apparatus used in the measurement of the curvatures of the thorax.

steth·o·scope (stĕth′ə-skōp′) *n.* Any of various instruments used for listening to sounds produced within the body. —**steth′o·scop′ic** (-skŏp′ĭk) *adj.* —**ste·thos′co·py** (stĕ-thŏs′kə-pē) *n.*

steth·o·spasm (stĕth′ə-spăz′əm) *n.* A spasm of the chest.

Ste·vens-John·son syndrome (stē′vənz-jŏn′sən) *n.* A severe inflammatory eruption of the skin and mucous membranes, usually occurring in children and young adults following a respiratory infection or as an allergic reaction to drugs or other substances.

Stew·art-Holmes sign (sto͞o′ərt-) *n.* A sign that occurs in conditions of cerebellar deficit in which the individual is unable to check a movement when passive resistance is suddenly released. Also called *rebound phenomenon.*

Stewart-Treves syndrome (-trēvz′) *n.* Lymphangiosarcoma arising in an arm affected by postmastectomy lymphedema.

sthe·ni·a (sthē′nē-ə) *n.* A condition of bodily strength, vigor, or vitality.

sthen·ic (sthĕn′ĭk) *adj.* Strong; active.

stib·i·a·lism (stĭb′ē-ə-lĭz′əm) *n.* Chronic poisoning with antimony.

Stick·ler syndrome (stĭk′lər) *n.* See **hereditary progressive arthro-ophthalmopathy.**

stiff-man syndrome (stĭf′măn′) *n.* A chronic, progressive but variable disorder of the central nervous system having no known cause and associated with fluctuating muscle spasms and stiffness.

stig·ma (stĭg′mə) *n.,* *pl.* **stig·mas** or **stig·ma·ta** (stĭg-mä′tə, -măt′ə, stĭg′mə-) **1.** Visible evidence of a disease. **2.** A spot or blemish on the skin. **3.** A bleeding spot on the skin considered as a manifestation of conversion disorder. **4.** The orange pigmented eyespot of certain chlorophyll-bearing protozoa, such as *Euglena viridis.* It serves as a light filter by absorbing certain wavelengths. **5.** A mark of shame or discredit. **6.** Follicular stigma.

stig·mat·ic (stĭg-măt′ĭk) *adj.* Relating to or marked by a stigma.

stig·ma·tism (stĭg′mə-tĭz′əm) *n.* The condition of having stigmas.

stig·ma·ti·za·tion (stĭg′mə-tĭ-zā′shən) *n.* The production of stigmas, especially of hysterical origin.

stil·bene (stĭl′bēn′) *n.* A colorless or yellowish unsaturated crystalline hydrocarbon compound that is the chemical basis for diethylstilbestrol and other synthetic estrogenic compounds.

stil·bes·trol (stĭl-bĕs′trôl′, -trōl′) *n.* DES.

still·birth (stĭl′bûrth′) *n.* **1.** The birth of a dead child or fetus. **2.** A child or fetus dead at birth.

still·born (stĭl′bôrn′) *adj.* Dead at birth.

still layer (stĭl) *n.* The layer of the bloodstream next to the wall in the capillary vessels; it flows slowly and transports the white blood cells. Also called *Poiseuille's space.*

Still's disease (stĭlz) *n.* See **juvenile rheumatoid arthritis.**

Still's murmur *n.* A murmur whose sound resembles the noise produced by a twanging string.

stim·u·lant (stĭm′yə-lənt) *n.* An agent that arouses organic activity, strengthens the action of the heart, increases vitality, and promotes a sense of well-being. —*adj.* Serving as or being a stimulant.

stim·u·late (stĭm′yə-lāt′) *v.* To arouse a body or a responsive structure to increased functional activity.

stim·u·la·tion (stĭm′yə-lā′shən) *n.* **1.** Arousal of the body or of individual organs or other parts to increased functional activity. **2.** The condition of being stimulated. **3.** The application of a stimulus to a responsive structure, such as a nerve or muscle, regardless of whether the strength of the stimulus is sufficient to produce excitation.

stim·u·la·tor (stĭm′yə-lā′tər) *n.* Someone or something that stimulates.

stim·u·lus (stĭm′yə-ləs) *n.,* *pl.* **-li** (-lī′) **1.** A stimulant. **2.** That which can elicit or evoke an action or response in a cell, an excitable tissue, or an organism.

stimulus sensitive myoclonus *n.* Myoclonus induced by a variety of stimuli, such as talking, loud noises, or tapping.

sting (stĭng) *v.* **1.** To pierce or wound painfully with or as if with a sharp-pointed structure or organ, as that of certain insects. **2.** To introduce venom by stinging. **3.** To cause to feel a sharp smarting pain by or as if by pricking with a sharp point. —*n.* **1.** The act of stinging. **2.** The wound or pain caused by or as if by stinging. **3.** The venom apparatus of a stinging organism.

stip·pled epiphysis (stĭp′əld) *n.* A congenital abnormality of the epiphyses marked by multiple ossification centers that severely deform the long bone and give it a stippled appearance and a thickened shaft. Also called *dysplasia epiphysialis punctata.*

stip·pling (stĭp′lĭng) *n.* **1.** A speckling of a blood cell or other structure with fine dots when exposed to a basic stain as a result of the presence of free basophil granules in the cell protoplasm. **2.** The orange-peel appearance of normal gums.

stir·rup (stûr′əp, stĭr′-) *n.* See **stapes**.

stitch (stĭch) *n.* **1.** A sudden sharp pain, especially in the side. **2.** A single suture. —*v.* To suture.

stitch abscess *n.* An abscess around a stitch or suture.

STM *abbr.* short-term memory

stock culture (stŏk) *n.* A culture of a microorganism maintained solely to keep it viable for subculture into fresh medium.

Stock·holm syndrome (stŏk′hōlm′, -hōm′) *n.* A phenomenon in which a hostage begins to identify with and grow sympathetic to his or her captor.

stock·ing anesthesia (stŏk′ĭng) *n.* Loss of sensation in an area that would be covered by a stocking.

stock vaccine *n.* A vaccine made from a stock microbial strain.

stoi·chi·om·e·try (stoi′kē-ŏm′ĭ-trē) *n.* **1.** Calculation of the quantities of reactants and products in a chemical reaction. **2.** The quantitative relationship between reactants and products in a chemical reaction. —**stoi′chi·o·met′ric** (-ə-mĕt′rĭk) *adj.* —**stoi′chi·o·met′ri·cal·ly** *adv.*

stoke (stōk) *n.* A unit of kinematic viscosity equal to that of a fluid with a viscosity of one poise and a density of one gram per milliliter.

Stokes (stōks), **William** 1804–1878. British physician. Known especially for his studies of diseases of the chest and heart, he expanded on the observations of John Cheyne in describing the breathing irregularity now known as Cheyne-Stokes respiration.

Stokes-Adams disease *n.* See **Adams-Stokes syndrome**.

Stokes-Adams syndrome *n.* See **Adams-Stokes syndrome**.

Stokes' amputation (stōks) *n.* See **Gritti-Stokes amputation**.

sto·ma (stō′mə) *n.*, *pl.* **–mas** *or* **–ma·ta** (-mə-tə) **1.** A minute opening or pore, as in the surface of a membrane. **2.** A mouthlike opening, such as the oral cavity of a nematode. **3.** A surgically constructed opening, especially one made in the abdominal wall to permit the passage of waste. —**sto′mal** *adj.*

stom·ach (stŭm′ək) *n.* The enlarged saclike portion of the digestive tract between the esophagus and small intestine, lying just beneath the diaphragm.

stom·ach·ache (stŭm′ək-āk′) *n.* Pain in the stomach or abdomen.

stom·ach·al (stŭm′ə-kəl) *adj.* Of or relating to the stomach.

sto·mach·ic (stə-măk′ĭk) *n.* An agent that improves appetite and digestion. —*adj.* **1.** Of or relating to the stomach. **2.** Beneficial to or stimulating digestion in the stomach.

stomach pump *n.* An apparatus for removing the contents of the stomach by means of suction.

stomach tube *n.* A flexible tube inserted into the stomach through which liquid food is passed.

sto·mal ulcer (stō′məl) *n.* A mucosal ulcer in the jejunum mucosa near the opening between the stomach and jejunum, occurring after gastrojejunostomy.

sto·ma·tal·gia (stō′mə-tăl′jə) *n.* Pain in the mouth. Also called **stomatodynia**.

sto·ma·ti·tis (stō′mə-tī′tĭs) *n.* Inflammation of the mucous membrane of the mouth.

stomatitis med·i·ca·men·to·sa (mĕd′ĭ-kə-mən-tō′sə) *n.* Allergic inflammatory changes in the oral soft tissues associated with the use of drugs or medicaments, usually those taken systemically.

stomato– *or* **stomat–** *pref.* Mouth; stoma: *stomatitis.*

sto·ma·to·cy·to·sis (stō′mə-tō-sī-tō′sĭs) *n.* A hereditary deformation of red blood cells, which are swollen and cup-shaped. It causes congenital hemolytic anemia.

sto·ma·to·dyn·i·a (stō′mə-tə-dĭn′ē-ə) *n.* See **stomatalgia**.

sto·ma·tog·nath·ic system (stō′mə-tŏg-năth′ĭk, -tō-năth′-) *n.* The structures involved in speech and in the receiving, chewing, and swallowing of food.

sto·ma·to·ma·la·cia (stō′mə-tō-mə-lā′shə) *n.* Pathological softening of any of the structures of the mouth.

sto·ma·to·my·co·sis (stō′mə-tō-mī-kō′sĭs) *n.* A fungal disease of the mouth.

sto·ma·to·ne·cro·sis (stō′mə-tō-nə-krō′sĭs) *n.* See **noma**.

sto·ma·top·a·thy (stō′mə-tŏp′ə-thē) *n.* A disease of the mouth.

sto·ma·to·plas·ty (stō′mə-tə-plăs′tē) *n.* Reconstructive or plastic surgery of the mouth. —**sto′ma·to·plas′tic** (-plăs′tĭk) *adj.*

sto·ma·tor·rha·gia (stō′mə-tə-rā′jə) *n.* Bleeding from any part of the oral cavity.

sto·mo·de·um (stō′mə-dē′əm) *n.* A midline ectodermal depression ventral to the embryonic brain and surrounded by the mandibular arch. It becomes continuous with the foregut and forms the mouth. —**sto′mo·de′al** *adj.*

–stomy *suff.* A surgical operation in which an artificial opening is made into an organ or part: *colostomy.*

stone (stōn) *n.* See **calculus** (sense 1).

stone heart *n.* See **ischemic contracture of left ventricle**.

Stook·ey-Scarff operation (stŏŏk′ē-skärf′) *n.* See **third ventriculostomy** (sense 1).

stool (stōŏl) *n.* Evacuated fecal matter.

Stopes (stōps), **Marie Carmichael** 1880–1958. British social reformer who opened England's first birth control clinic (1924) in London and later promoted family planning in east Asia.

stor·age (stôr′ĭj) *n.* The second of three stages in the memory process, involving mental processes associated with retention of stimuli that have been registered and modified by encoding.

storage disease *n.* Any of various metabolic disorders usually caused by a congenital enzyme deficiency and characterized by the accumulation of a specific substance, such as a lipid or protein, within tissues.

sto·ri·form (stôr′ə-fôrm′) *adj.* Having a cartwheel pattern, such as spindle cells having elongated nuclei radiating from a center.

storm (stôrm) *n.* An exacerbation of symptoms or a crisis in the course of a disease.

STP (ĕs′tē-pē′) *n.* See **DOM.**

stra·bis·mom·e·ter (străb′ĭz-mŏm′ĭ-tər, strā′bĭz-) *n.* A calibrated plate with the upper margin curved to conform with the lower eyelid, used to measure strabismus.

stra·bis·mus (strə-bĭz′məs) *n.* A visual defect in which one eye cannot focus with the other on an objective because of imbalance of the eye muscles. Also called *heterotropia, squint, tropia.* —**stra·bis′mal** (-məl), **stra·bis′mic** (-mĭk) *adj.*

stra·bot·o·my (strə-bŏt′ə-mē) *n.* Surgical division of one or more of the ocular muscles or their tendons for the correction of strabismus.

straight gyrus (strāt) *n.* A gyrus running along the medial part of the orbital surface of the frontal lobe of the cerebral hemisphere and bounded laterally by the olfactory sulcus.

straight muscle *n.* Any of the rectus muscles.

straight sinus *n.* An unpaired sinus of the dura mater in the posterior part of the falx cerebri. Also called *tentorial sinus.*

strain¹ (strān) *v.* **1.** To pull, draw, or stretch tight. **2.** To stretch or exert one's muscles or nerves to the utmost. **3.** To injure or impair by overuse or overexertion; wrench. **4.** To filter, trickle, percolate, or ooze. **5.** To pass a liquid through a filtering agent such as a strainer. **6.** To draw off or remove by filtration. —*n.* **1.** The act of straining. **2.** The state of being strained. **3.** Extreme or laborious effort. **4.** A great or excessive pressure, demand, or stress on one's body, mind, or resources. **5.** A wrench, twist, or other physical injury resulting from excessive tension, effort, or use.

strain² (strān) *n.* **1.** The collective descendants of a common ancestor; a race, stock, line, or breed. **2.** Any of the various lines of ancestry united in an individual or a family; ancestry or lineage. **3.** A group of organisms of the same species, having distinctive characteristics but not usually considered a separate breed or variety. **4.** An artificial variety of a domestic animal or cultivated plant.

strain fracture *n.* A fracture in which a piece of bone attached to a tendon, ligament, or capsule is torn away by an internal or an external force.

strait (strāt) *n.* A narrow passage, such as the upper or lower opening of the pelvic canal.

strait·jack·et *or* **straight·jack·et** (strāt′jăk′ĭt) *n.* A long-sleeved jacketlike garment used to bind the arms tightly against the body as a means of restraining a violent person.

stran·gle (străng′gəl) *v.* To compress the trachea so as to prevent sufficient passage of air; suffocate.

stran·gu·late (străng′gyə-lāt′) *v.* **1.** To strangle. **2.** To compress, constrict, or obstruct a body part so as to cut off the flow of blood or other fluid. **3.** To be or become strangled, compressed, constricted, or obstructed.

stran·gu·lat·ed hernia (străng′gyə-lā′tĭd) *n.* An irreducible hernia in which normal blood supply is arrested.

stran·gu·la·tion (străng′gyə-lā′shən) *n.* **1.** The act of strangling or strangulating. **2.** The state of being strangled or strangulated. **3.** Constriction of a body part so as to cut off the flow of blood or another fluid.

stran·gu·ry (străng′gyə-rē) *n.* Slow, painful urination, in which the urine is passed drop by drop.

strap (străp) *n.* A strip or piece of adhesive plaster. —*v.* To support or bind a part, especially with overlapping strips of adhesive plaster.

strap cell *n.* An elongated tumor cell of uniform width that may show cross-striations.

strat·i·fi·ca·tion (străt′ə-fĭ-kā′shən) *n.* An arrangement in layers or strata.

strat·i·fied (străt′ə-fīd′) *adj.* Arranged in the form of layers or strata.

stratified epithelium *n.* Epithelium made up of a series of layers, the cells of each varying in size and shape. Also called *laminated epithelium.*

stra·tig·ra·phy (strə-tĭg′rə-fē) *n.* See **tomography.** —**strat′i·graph′ic** (străt′ĭ-grăf′ĭk) *adj.*

stra·tum (strā′təm, străt′əm) *n., pl.* **–tums** *or* **-ta** (-tə) **1.** A horizontal layer of material, especially one of several parallel layers arranged one on top of another. **2.** Any of the layers of differentiated tissue forming an anatomical structure. —**stra′tal** (-təl) *adj.*

stratum com·pac·tum (kəm-păk′təm) *n.* The superficial layer of decidual tissue in the pregnant uterus.

stratum cor·ne·um (kôr′nē-əm) *n.* The horny outer layer of the epidermis, consisting of several layers of flat, keratinized, nonnucleated, dead or peeling cells. Also called *corneal layer, horny layer.*

stratum func·tion·a·le (fŭngk′shə-nā′lē) *n.* The endometrium except for the basal layer.

stratum lu·ci·dum (lōō′sĭ-dəm) *n.* See **clear layer of epidermis.**

stratum spon·gi·o·sum (spŏn′jē-ō′səm) *n.* The middle layer of the endometrium, formed chiefly of dilated glandular structures and flanked by the stratum compactum on the luminal side and by the basal layer on the myometrial side.

straw·ber·ry mark (strô′bĕr′ē) *n.* A raised, shiny, red nevus or birthmark, occurring usually on the face or scalp and resembling a strawberry. Also called *strawberry nevus.*

strawberry tongue *n.* The presence of a whitish coat on the tongue through which the enlarged papillae project as red points, characteristic of scarlet fever.

streak (strēk) *n.* A line, stripe, smear, or band differentiated by color or texture from its surroundings.

streak culture *n.* A culture made by lightly stroking an inoculating needle or a loop bearing inoculum over the surface of a solid medium.

stream·ing (strē′mĭng) *n.* Streaming movement.

streaming movement *n.* Movement characteristic of the protoplasm of white blood cells, amebas, and other unicellular organisms, involving massing of the protoplasm, its extrusion in the form of a pseudopod, and a flow of the protoplasmic mass into the pseudopod.

street virus (strēt) *n.* The virulent rabies virus from a rabid domestic animal that has contracted the disease from a bite or scratch of another animal.

strep (strĕp) *adj.* Streptococcal. —*n.* Streptococcus.

streph·o·sym·bo·li·a (strĕf′ō-sĭm-bō′lē-ə) *n.* The perception of objects reversed as if in a mirror; specifically, difficulty in distinguishing written or printed letters that extend in opposite directions but are otherwise similar, such as *b* and *d.*

strep throat *n.* See **septic sore throat.**

strep·ti·ce·mi·a (strĕp′tĭ-sē′mē-ə) *n.* See **streptococcemia.**

strepto– *pref.* **1.** Twisted; twisted chain: *streptococcus.* **2.** Streptococcus: *streptolysin.*

Strep·to·ba·cil·lus (strĕp′tō-bə-sĭl′əs) *n.* A genus of gram-negative, rod-shaped, often pathogenic bacteria that typically occurs in chains, including a species that causes a type of rat-bite fever.

strep·to·cer·ci·a·sis (strĕp′tō-sər-kī′ə-sĭs) *n.* Infection with the nematode *Dipetalonema streptocerca.*

strep·to·coc·ce·mi·a (strĕp′tə-kŏk-sē′mē-ə) *n.* The presence of streptococci in the blood. Also called *strepticemia, streptosepticemia.*

strep·to·coc·cus (strĕp′tə-kŏk′əs) *n., pl.* **–coc·ci** (-kŏk′sī, -kŏk′ī) A bacterium of the genus *Streptococcus.* —**strep′to·coc′cal, strep′to·coc′cic** *adj.*

Streptococcus *n.* A genus of gram-positive, anaerobic, often pathogenic bacteria having an ovoid or spherical appearance and occurring in pairs or chains, including many erythrocytolytic and pathogenic species that cause erysipelas, scarlet fever, and septic sore throat in humans.

streptococcus erythrogenic toxin *n.* A culture filtrate of the endotoxin that is produced by strains of beta-hemolytic streptococci and that produces an erythematous reaction at inoculation sites on the skin of susceptible persons. Also called *Dick test toxin, erythrogenic toxin.*

Streptococcus mu·tans (myōō′tănz′) *n.* A species of *Streptococcus* associated with the production of dental caries.

Streptococcus pneu·mo·ni·ae (nōō-mō′nē-ē) *n.* Pneumococcus.

Streptococcus py·og·e·nes (pī-ŏj′ə-nēz) *n.* A bacterium that causes the formation of pus or of fatal septicemias.

Streptococcus vir·i·dans (vîr′ĭ-dănz′) *n.* Any of the alpha-hemolytic streptococci.

strep·to·dor·nase (strĕp′tō-dôr′nās, -nāz) *n. Abbr.* **SD** An enzyme produced by hemolytic streptococci that is used medicinally, often in combination with streptokinase, to dissolve purulent or fibrinous secretions from infections.

strep·to·kin·ase (strĕp′tō-kĭn′ās, -āz, -kī′nās, -nāz) *n. Abbr.* **SK** A proteolytic enzyme produced by hemolytic streptococci, capable of dissolving fibrin and used medically to dissolve blood clots.

streptokinase-streptodornase *n.* A purified mixture containing streptokinase, streptodornase, and other proteolytic enzymes. It is used by topical application, or by injection into body cavities, to remove clotted blood and fibrinous and purulent accumulations of exudate.

strep·tol·y·sin (strĕp-tŏl′ĭ-sĭn, strĕp′tə-lī′sĭn) *n.* A hemolysin produced by streptococci.

Strep·to·my·ces (strĕp′tə-mī′sēz) *n.* A genus of actinomycetes that are chiefly saprophytic soil forms, including several strains that produce antibiotics.

strep·to·my·cin *or* **strep·to·my·cin A** (strĕp′tə-mī′sĭn) *n.* An antibiotic obtained from *Streptomyces griseus* and used against the tubercle bacillus and other bacteria.

strep·to·ni·grin (strĕp′tə-nī′grĭn) *n.* A highly toxic antibiotic produced by a species of the genus *Streptomyces* and active against various tumors.

strep·to·sep·ti·ce·mi·a (strĕp′tō-sĕp′tĭ-sē′mē-ə) *n.* See **streptococcemia.**

strep·to·zo·cin (strĕp′tə-zō′sĭn) *or* **strep·to·zot·o·cin** (-zŏt′ə-sĭn) *n.* An antineoplastic agent produced by an actinomycete and active against tumors but damaging to insulin-producing cells and now regarded as a carcinogen.

stress (strĕs) *n.* **1.** An applied force or system of forces that tends to strain or deform a body. **2.** The resisting force set up in a body as a result of an externally applied force. **3.** A physical or psychological stimulus that can produce mental tension or physiological reactions that may lead to illness.

stress fracture *n.* A fatigue fracture of bone caused by repeated application of a heavy load, such as the constant pounding on a surface by runners, gymnasts, and dancers.

stress incontinence *n.* A sudden, involuntary release of urine caused by muscular strain accompanying laughing, sneezing, coughing, or exercise, seen primarily in older women with weakened pelvic musculature. Also called *stress urinary incontinence.*

stress reaction *n.* An acute emotional reaction to physical or psychological stress. Also called *acute situational reaction.*

stress shielding *n.* Osteopenia occurring in bone as the result of removal of normal stress from the bone by an implant.

stress test *n.* A graded test to measure an individual's heart rate and oxygen intake while undergoing strenuous physical exercise, as on a treadmill.

stress ulcers *pl.n.* Acute peptic ulcers occurring in association with various other pathologic conditions, including burns, cor pulmonale, intracranial lesions, and surgical operations.

stress urinary incontinence *n.* See **stress incontinence.**

stretch·er (strĕch′ər) *n.* A litter, usually of canvas stretched over a frame, used to transport the sick, wounded, or dead.

stretch mark (strĕch) *n.* A shiny line on the skin of the abdomen, breasts, thighs, or buttocks caused by the prolonged stretching of the skin and weakening of elastic tissues, as in pregnancy or obesity.

stretch receptor *n.* A sensory receptor in a muscle that responds to the stretching of tissue.

stretch reflex *n.* See **myotatic reflex.**

stri·a (strī′ə) *n., pl.* **stri·ae** (strī′ē) **1.** A thin, narrow groove or channel. **2.** A thin line or band, especially one of several that are parallel or close together. **3.** A thin line, band, stripe, or streak distinguished from the tissue in which it is found; a striation.

striae a·tro·phi·cae (ə-trō′fĭ-kē′, ə-trŏf′ĭ-) *pl.n.* Stretch marks.

striae grav·i·dar·um (grăv′ĭ-dâr′əm) *pl.n.* Stretch marks resulting from pregnancy.

stri·ate (strī′āt′) *v.* To mark with striae or striations. —*adj. also* **stri·at·ed** (-ā′tĭd) **1.** Marked with striae; striped, grooved, or ridged. **2.** Consisting of a stria or striae.

striate body *n.* The caudate and lentiform nuclei considered as one structure, having a striated appearance on section due to its slender fascicles of myelinated fibers.

striated border *n.* The free surface of the columnar absorptive cells of the intestine formed by microvilli.

striated muscle *n.* Skeletal, voluntary, and cardiac muscle, distinguished from smooth muscle by transverse striations of the fibers.

striate vein *n.* Either of the thalamostriate veins: inferior thalamostriate and superior thalamostriate.

stri·a·tion (strī-ā′shən) *n.* **1.** The state of being striated or having striae. **2.** A stria.

stri·a·to·ni·gral (strī-ā′tə-nī′grəl) *adj.* Of or relating to the efferent connection of the striatum with the substantia nigra.

stri·a·tum (strī-ā′təm) *n., pl.* **-ta** (-tə) A collective term for the caudate nucleus, the putamen, and the globus pallidus, which form the corpus striatum.

stric·ture (strĭk′chər) *n.* A circumscribed narrowing of a hollow structure.

stric·tur·ot·o·my (strĭk′chə-rŏt′ə-mē) *n.* The surgical opening or division of a stricture.

stri·dor (strī′dər, -dôr′) *n.* A high-pitched noisy sound occurring during inhalation or exhalation, a sign of respiratory obstruction.

strid·u·lous (strĭj′ə-ləs) *adj.* **1.** Characterized by or making a shrill grating sound or noise. **2.** Relating to or characterized by stridor.

strip (strĭp) *v.* **1.** To press out or drain off by milking. **2.** To make a subcutaneous excision of a vein in its longitudinal axis, usually of a leg vein.

stro·bi·la (strō-bī′lə) *n., pl.* **-lae** (-lē) The segmented main body part of the adult tapeworm.

stro·bo·scop·ic microscope (strō′bə-skŏp′ĭk) *n.* A microscope having a light source that flashes at a constant rate so that the motility of an object may be analyzed.

stroke (strōk) *n.* **1.** A sudden severe attack, as of paralysis or sunstroke. **2.** A sudden loss of brain function caused by a blockage or rupture of a blood vessel to the brain, resulting in necrosis of brain tissue and characterized by loss of muscular control, diminution or loss of sensation or consciousness, dizziness, slurred speech, or other symptoms that vary with the extent and severity of brain damage. Also called *cerebral accident, cerebral infarction, cerebrovascular accident.*

stroke volume *n.* The volume of blood pumped out of one ventricle of the heart in a single beat.

stroke work index *n.* A measure of the work done by the heart with each contraction and equal to the stroke volume of the heart multiplied by the arterial pressure and divided by the body surface area.

stro·ma (strō′mə) *n., pl.* **-ma·ta** (-mə-tə) **1.** The connective tissue framework of an organ, a gland, or other structure, as distinguished from the tissues performing the special function of the organ or part. **2.** The spongy and colorless framework of a cell. —**stro′mal** *adj.* —**stro·mat′ic** (-măt′ĭk) *adj.*

stro·muhr (strō′mōōr′) *n.* An instrument for measuring the quantity of blood that flows per unit of time through a blood vessel.

Stron·gy·loi·des (strŏn′jə-loi′dēz) *n.* A genus of small nematode intestinal parasites that includes the species that causes strongyloidiasis in humans.

stron·gy·loi·di·a·sis (strŏn′jə-loi-dī′ə-sĭs) *or* **stron·gy·loi·do·sis** (-dō′sĭs) *n.* Infection with the nematode *Strongyloides stercoralis.*

stron·ti·um (strŏn′chē-əm, -tē-əm, -shəm) *n. Symbol* **Sr** A soft, easily oxidized metallic element that ignites spontaneously in air when finely divided, used in pharmaceuticals and in radioisotope form for bone imaging. Atomic number 38.

stroph·u·lus (strŏf′yə-ləs) *n.* See **heat rash.**

struc·tur·al formula (strŭk′chər-əl) *n.* A chemical formula that shows the number and kinds of atoms in a molecule and how the atoms and bonds in the molecule are arranged.

structural gene *n.* A gene that determines the amino acid sequence of a specific protein or peptide.

structural isomerism *n.* Isomerism involving the same atoms in different arrangements.

struc·ture (strŭk′chər) *n.* **1.** The arrangement or formation of the tissues, organs, or other parts of an organism. **2.** A tissue, an organ, or other formation made up of different but related parts.

stru·ma (strōō′mə) *n., pl.* **-mas** *or* **-mae** (-mē) **1.** Goiter. **2.** See **scrofula. 3.** Enlargement of a tissue. No longer in technical use. —**stru·mat′ic** (-măt′ĭk), **stru′mose′** (-mōs′), **stru′mous** (-məs) *adj.*

struma lym·pho·ma·to·sa (lĭm-fō′mə-tō′sə) *n.* See **Hashimoto's disease.**

struma o·var·i·i (ō-vâr′ē-ī′) *n.* A rare ovarian tumor composed mostly of thyroid tissue.

stru·mec·to·my (strōō-mĕk′tə-mē) *n.* Surgical removal of all or a portion of a goitrous tumor.

stru·mi·form (strōō′mə-fôrm′) *adj.* Resembling goiter.

stru·mi·tis (strōō-mī′tĭs) *n.* Inflammation of the thyroid gland.

Strüm·pell-Marie disease (strōōm′pəl-, shtrüm′-) *n.* See **ankylosing spondylitis.**

Strüm·pell's disease (strōōm′pəlz, shtrüm′-) *n.* **1.** See **spondylitis deformans. 2.** See **acute epidemic leukoencephalitis.**

Strümpell-Westphal disease *n.* See **pseudosclerosis.**

strych·nine (strĭk′nīn′, -nĭn, -nēn′) *n.* An extremely poisonous white crystalline alkaloid used as a poison for rodents and formerly used topically as a central nervous system stimulant.

strych·nin·ism (strĭk′nī-nĭz′əm, -nĭ-, -nē-) *n.* Chronic strychnine poisoning, characterized by tremors and twitching, progressing to severe convulsions and respiratory arrest.

Stry·ker frame (strī′kər) *n.* A frame that allows an individual to be turned in various planes as a single unit without moving parts of the body separately.

STS *abbr.* serologic test for syphilis

S-T segment *n.* The part of an electrocardiogram immediately following the QRS complex and merging into the T wave.

Stu·art factor (stoō′ərt) *or* **Stuart-Prow·er factor** (-prou′ər) *n.* See **prothrombinase.**

stud·y (stŭd′ē) *n.* Research, detailed examination, or analysis of an organism, object, or phenomenon. —*v.* To research, examine, or analyze something.

stump (stŭmp) *n.* **1.** The extremity of a limb left after amputation. **2.** The pedicle remaining after removal of the tumor to which it was attached.

stump cancer *n.* A carcinoma of the stomach developing after gastroenterostomy or gastric resection for benign disease.

stu·por (stoō′pər) *n.* A state of impaired consciousness characterized by a marked diminution in the capacity to react to environmental stimuli. —**stu′por·ous** *adj.*

Sturge-Web·er syndrome (stûrj′wĕb′ər) *n.* A congenital syndrome characterized by a port-wine stain nevus in the distribution of the trigeminal nerve, homolateral meningeal angioma with intracranial calcification and neurologic signs, and angioma of the choroid, often with secondary glaucoma. Also called *angiophacomatosis, encephalofacial angiomatosis, encephalotrigeminal angiomatosis, Sturge's disease, Sturge-Weber disease.*

stut·ter (stŭt′ər) *n.* A phonatory or articulatory disorder characterized by difficult enunciation of words with frequent halting and repetition of the initial consonant or syllable. —*v.* To utter with spasmodic repetition or prolongation of sounds.

sty *or* **stye** (stī) *n., pl.* **sties** *or* **styes** (stīz) Inflammation of one or more sebaceous glands of an eyelid. Also called *hordeolum.*

styl– *pref.* Variant of **stylo–.**

sty·let (stī-lĕt′, stī′lĭt) *n.* **1.** A fine wire that is run through a catheter, cannula, or hollow needle to keep it stiff or clear of debris. **2.** A slender surgical probe. Also called *stylus.*

stylo– *or* **styl–** *pref.* Styloid; styloid process: *stylohyal.*

sty·lo·glos·sus (stī′lō-glô′səs) *n.* A muscle with origin from the lower end of the styloid process, with insertion into the side and undersurface of the tongue, with nerve supply from the hypoglossal nerve, and whose action retracts the tongue.

sty·lo·hy·al (stī′lō-hī′əl) *adj.* Stylohyoid.

sty·lo·hy·oid (stī′lō-hī′oid′) *adj.* Relating to the styloid process of the temporal bone and to the hyoid bone. —*n.* A muscle with origin from the styloid process of the temporal bone, with insertion into the hyoid bone by two slips on either side of the intermediate tendon of the digastric muscle, with nerve supply from the facial nerve, and whose action elevates the hyoid bone.

sty·loid (stī′loid′) *n.* Of or relating to any of several slender pointed bone processes, especially the spine that projects from the base of the temporal bone.

sty·loid·i·tis (stī′loi-dī′tĭs) *n.* Inflammation of a styloid process.

styloid process of radius *n.* A thick, pointed projection on the lateral side of the distal extremity of the radius.

styloid process of temporal bone *n.* A slender, pointed projection from the petrous portion of the temporal bone where it joins the tympanic portion, giving attachment to the styloglossus, stylohyoid, and stylopharyngeus muscles and to the stylohyoid and stylomandibular ligaments.

styloid process of ulna *n.* A cylindrical, pointed projection from the medial and posterior aspect of the head of the ulna, to the tip of which is attached the ulnar collateral ligament of the wrist.

sty·lo·mas·toid artery (stī′lō-măs′toid′) *n.* An artery with origin in the posterior auricular artery, with distribution to the external ear, mastoid cells, semicircular canals, stapedius muscle, and vestibule, and with anastomoses to the tympanic branches of the internal carotid and the ascending pharyngeal arteries, and to the auditory branch of the basilar artery.

stylomastoid foramen *n.* An opening on the lower surface of the temporal bone, between the styloid and mastoid processes, that transmits the facial nerve and the stylomastoid artery.

stylomastoid vein *n.* A vein that drains the tympanic cavity and empties into the retromandibular vein.

sty·lo·pha·ryn·geal muscle (stī′lō-fə-rĭn′jəl, -făr′ĭn-jē′əl) *n.* A muscle with origin from the root of the styloid process, with insertion into the thyroid cartilage and the wall of the pharynx, with nerve supply from the glossopharyngeal nerve, and whose action elevates the pharynx and the larynx.

sty·lus (stī′ləs) *n., pl.* **–lus·es** *or* **–li** (-lī) **1.** A pencil-shaped structure. **2.** A pencil-shaped medicinal preparation for external application; as a medicated bougie. **3.** See **stylet** (sense 2).

stype (stīp) *n.* A tampon.

styp·tic (stĭp′tĭk) *adj.* **1.** Contracting the tissues or blood vessels; astringent. **2.** Tending to check bleeding by contracting the tissues or the blood vessels; hemostatic. —*n.* A styptic drug or substance. —**styp·tic′i·ty** (-tĭs′ĭ-tē) *n.*

styptic pencil *n.* A short medicated stick, often of alum, applied to a cut to check bleeding.

sty·rene (stī′rēn′) *n.* A colorless oily liquid from which polystyrenes, plastics, and synthetic rubber are produced. Also called *vinylbenzene.*

sub– *pref.* **1.** Below; under; beneath: *subcutaneous.* **2.** Subordinate; secondary: *subinfection.* **3.** Subdivision: *subkingdom.* **4.** Less than completely or normally; nearly; almost: *subfertility.*

sub·ab·dom·i·nal (sŭb′ăb-dŏm′ə-nəl) *adj.* Located or occurring below the abdomen.

sub·a·cro·mi·al bursa (sŭb′ə-krō′mē-əl) *n.* The bursa between the acromial process and the capsule of the shoulder joint.

sub·a·cute (sŭb′ə-kyoōt′) *adj.* Between acute and chronic. —**sub′a·cute′ly** *adv.*

subacute bacterial endocarditis *n. Abbr.* **SBE** A subacute bacterial infection of the endocardium or heart valves, most frequently seen in patients with congenital or acquired valvular or cardiac defects, characterized by a heart murmur and septicemia.

subacute combined degeneration of spinal cord *n.* The degeneration of the posterior and lateral columns of the spinal cord caused by a deficiency of vitamin B$_{12}$ and usually associated with pernicious anemia, resulting in a prickling or burning sensation of the skin and a loss of coordination. Also called *Putnam-Dana syndrome, vitamin B$_{12}$ neuropathy.*

subacute inflammation *n.* Inflammation that lasts longer than acute inflammation but is not chronic.

subacute mi·gra·to·ry panniculitis (mī′grə-tôr′ē) *n.* A condition characterized by the development of tender nodular lesions of changing configuration on the lateral aspect of one or both legs that may persist for many months.

subacute necrotizing myelitis *n.* A disorder of the lower spinal cord in adult males resulting in progressive paraplegia.

subacute sclerosing panencephalitis *n. Abbr.* **SSPE** An often fatal degenerative disease of the central nervous system occurring chiefly in young people, caused by slow infection with a measles virus and characterized by progressive loss of mental and motor functions ending in dementia and paralysis.

subacute spongiform encephalopathy *n.* A form of spongiform encephalopathy, such as Creutzfeldt-Jakob disease, kuru, or Gerstmann-Sträussler syndrome, that is associated with a slow virus, is transmissible, and has a rapidly progressive, fatal course. Also called *transmissible encephalopathy.*

sub·a·or·tic stenosis (sŭb′ā-ôr′tĭk) *n.* Narrowing of the outflow tract of the left ventricle caused by an obstruction shortly below the aortic valve.

sub·ap·i·cal (sŭb-ăp′ĭ-kəl, -ā′pĭ-) *adj.* Located below the apex of a part. **—sub·ap′i·cal·ly** *adv.*

sub·a·rach·noid space (sŭb′ə-răk′noid′) *n.* The space between the arachnoid membrane and pia mater that is filled with cerebrospinal fluid and contains the large blood vessels that supply the brain and spinal cord.

sub·ar·cu·ate fossa (sŭb-är′kyoŏ-ĭt, -āt′) *n.* An irregular depression on the rear surface of the petrous portion of the temporal bone, above and a little to the side of the internal ear.

sub·a·tom·ic (sŭb′ə-tŏm′ĭk) *adj.* **1.** Of or relating to the constituents of the atom. **2.** Having dimensions or participating in reactions characteristic of the constituents of the atom.

subatomic particle *n.* Any of various units of matter below the size of an atom, including the elementary particles and hadrons.

sub·ax·i·al (sŭb-ăk′sē-əl) *adj.* Located below the axis of the body or a body part.

sub·ax·il·lary (sŭb-ăk′sə-lĕr′ē) *adj.* Situated beneath the axilla or armpit.

sub·cal·lo·sal gyrus (sŭb′kə-lō′səl) *n.* A slender vertical whitish band immediately anterior to the anterior commissure of the brain. Also called *paraterminal gyrus, peduncle of corpus callosum.*

sub·cap·su·lar cataract (sŭb-kăp′sə-lər) *n.* A cataract in which the opacities are concentrated beneath or within the capsule of the lens.

sub·car·ti·lag·i·nous (sŭb′kär-tl-ăj′ə-nəs) *adj.* **1.** Partly cartilaginous. **2.** Located beneath a cartilage.

sub·cho·ri·al space (sŭb-kôr′ē-əl) *n.* The placental part adjacent to and beneath the chorion. Also called *subchorial lake.*

sub·class (sŭb′klăs′) *n.* A taxonomic category of ranking between a class and an order.

sub·cla·vi·an ansa (sŭb-klā′vē-ən) *n.* The cord that connects the middle and cervical stellate sympathetic ganglions and forms a loop around the subclavian artery.

subclavian artery *n.* An artery originating on the left from the aortic arch and on the right from the brachiocephalic artery with branches to the vertebral artery, the thyrocervical trunk, the internal thoracic artery, the costocervical trunk, and the descending scapular artery, and directly continuous with the axillary artery.

subclavian muscle *n.* A muscle with origin from the first costal cartilage, with insertion into the inferior surface of the acromial end of the clavicle, with nerve supply from the subclavian nerve, and whose action steadies the clavicle or elevates the first rib.

subclavian nerve *n.* A branch arising from the superior trunk of the brachial plexus and supplying the subclavius muscle.

subclavian steal *n.* Obstruction of the subclavian artery proximal to the origin of the vertebral artery. Blood flow through the vertebral artery is reversed, causing symptoms of cerebrovascular insufficiency.

subclavian steal syndrome *n.* Cerebrovascular insufficiency resulting from subclavian steal.

subclavian triangle *n.* The triangle bounded by the clavicle, by the omohyoid muscle, and by the sternocleidomastoid muscle, containing the subclavian artery and vein. Also called *omoclavicular triangle.*

subclavian vein *n.* A continuation of the axillary vein at the lateral border of the first rib, passing medially to join the internal jugular vein and forming the brachiocephalic vein on each side.

sub·clin·i·cal (sŭb-klĭn′ĭ-kəl) *adj.* Not manifesting characteristic clinical symptoms. Used of a disease or condition.

subclinical absence *n.* Transient impairment of thinking without overt manifestations, demonstrable only by psychological testing, and accompanied by an outburst of spike and wave complexes appearing at a rate of 3 per second on an electroencephalogram.

subclinical diabetes *n.* A form of diabetes mellitus that is clinically evident only under certain circumstances, such as pregnancy or extreme stress.

sub·con·scious (sŭb-kŏn′shəs) *adj.* Not wholly conscious; partially or imperfectly conscious. **—n.** The part of the mind below the level of conscious perception. **—sub·con′scious·ly** *adv.*

sub·con·scious·ness (sŭb-kŏn′shəs-nĭs) *n.* The state in which mental processes take place without the conscious perception of the individual.

sub·cor·ne·al pustular dermatosis (sŭb-kôr′nē-əl) *n.* A chronic skin disorder characterized by the eruption of sterile vesicles and pustules beneath the horny layer of the epidermis.

sub·cor·tex (sŭb-kôr′tĕks) *n., pl.* **-ti·ces** (-tĭ-sēz′) The portion of the brain immediately below the cerebral cortex. **—sub·cor′ti·cal** (-tĭ-kəl) *adj.*

sub·cos·tal artery (sŭb-kŏs′təl) *n.* An artery with its origin in the thoracic aorta, with distribution from the inferior to the twelfth rib.

subcostal muscle *n.* Any of a number of inconstant muscles having the same direction as the internal intercostal muscles but passing deep to one or more ribs.

subcostal nerve *n.* The ventral branch of the 12th thoracic nerve, supplying parts of the abdominal muscles and giving off cutaneous branches to the skin of the lower abdominal wall and to the gluteal region.

subcostal plane *n.* A horizontal plane passing through the lower limits of the tenth costal cartilages, marking the boundary between the hypochondriac and epigastric regions and between the lateral and umbilical regions.

sub·crep·i·tant (sŭb-krĕp′ĭ-tənt) *adj.* Nearly or faintly crepitant. Used of a rale.

sub·cul·ture (sŭb′kŭl′chər) *n.* A culture made by transferring to a fresh medium microorganisms from a previous culture.

sub·cu·ta·ne·ous (sŭb′kyōō-tā′nē-əs) *adj. Abbr.* **s.c.,** **SQ** Located, found, or placed just beneath the skin; hypodermic. —**sub′cu·ta′ne·ous·ly** *adv.*

subcutaneous emphysema *n.* The presence of air or gas in subcutaneous tissues. Also called *aerodermectasia, pneumoderma.*

subcutaneous fat necrosis of newborn *n.* See **sclerema neonatorum.**

subcutaneous flap *n.* A pedicle flap in which the pedicle is denuded of epithelium and buried in the subcutaneous tissue of the recipient area.

subcutaneous mastectomy *n.* Surgical removal of the breast tissues, with preservation of the skin, nipple, and areola, usually followed by the implantation of a prosthesis.

subcutaneous operation *n.* An operation, as for the division of a tendon, performed without incising the skin beyond a minute opening.

subcutaneous ring *n.* See **superficial inguinal ring.**

subcutaneous tenotomy *n.* Division of a tendon by means of a small pointed knife introduced through skin and subcutaneous tissue without an incision.

subcutaneous tissue *n.* A layer of loose, irregular connective tissue immediately beneath the skin; it contains fat cells except in the auricles, eyelids, penis, and scrotum.

subcutaneous vein of abdomen *n.* Any of a network of superficial veins of the abdominal wall that empty into the thoracoepigastric, superficial epigastric, or superior epigastric veins.

sub·cu·tic·u·lar (sŭb′kyōō-tĭk′yə-lər) *adj.* Located or occurring beneath the cuticle or epidermis.

sub·cu·tis (sŭb-kyōō′tĭs) *n.* See **tela subcutanea.**

sub·del·toid bursa (sŭb-dĕl′toid′) *n.* The bursa between the deltoid and the capsule of the shoulder joint.

sub·der·mal (sŭb-dûr′məl) *adj.* Located or placed beneath the skin; subcutaneous.

sub·di·gas·tric node (sŭb′dī-gǎs′trĭk) *n.* See **jugulodigastric node.**

sub·duct (səb-dŭkt′) *v.* To pull or draw downward.

sub·dur·al (səb-dōōr′əl) *adj.* Located or occurring beneath the dura mater.

subdural hemorrhage *n.* Extravasation of blood between the dural and arachnoidal membranes. Also called *subdural hematoma.*

subdural space *n.* The narrow space between the dura mater and the arachnoid membrane.

sub·en·do·car·di·al layer (sŭb′ĕn-dō-kär′dē-əl) *n.* The layer of loose connective tissue that joins the endocardium and myocardium.

sub·en·do·the·li·al layer (sŭb′ĕn-dō-thē′lē-əl) *n.* The thin layer of connective tissue lying between the endothelium and elastic lamina in the intima of blood vessels.

sub·en·do·the·li·um (sŭb′ĕn-dō-thē′lē-əm) *n.* The connective tissue between the endothelium and the inner elastic membrane in the intima of arteries.

sub·ep·en·dy·mo·ma (sŭb′ĭ-pĕn′də-mō′mə) *n.* An ependymoma in which there are discrete, lobulated nodules in the walls of the anterior third or posterior fourth ventricles of the brain.

sub·fam·i·ly (sŭb′fǎm′ə-lē) *n.* A taxonomic category ranking between a family and a genus.

sub·fer·til·i·ty (sŭb′fər-tĭl′ĭ-tē) *n.* A less than normal capacity for reproduction.

sub·ge·nus (sŭb′jē′nəs) *n., pl.* **–gen·e·ra** (-jĕn′ər-ə) A taxonomic category ranking between a genus and a species. —**sub′ge·ner′ic** (-jə-nĕr′ĭk) *adj.*

sub·gin·gi·val curettage (sŭb-jĭn′jə-vəl, -jĭn-jī′-) *n.* The removal of subgingival calculus or ulcerated epithelial and granulomatous tissues from periodontal pockets with a curette.

subgingival space *n.* See **gingival sulcus.**

sub·glos·sal (sŭb-glô′səl) *adj.* Below or beneath the tongue; hypoglossal.

sub·grun·da·tion (sŭb′grŭn-dā′shən) *n.* Depression of one fragment of a broken cranial bone below the other.

sub·hy·oid (sŭb-hī′oid′) *adj.* Beneath the hyoid bone.

su·bic·u·lum (sə-bĭk′yə-ləm, sōō-) *n., pl.* **–la** (-lə) An underlying supporting structure.

sub·il·i·um (sŭb-ĭl′ē-əm) *n.* The portion of the ilium contributing to the acetabulum. —**sub·il′i·ac′** (-ǎk′) *adj.*

sub·in·fec·tion (sŭb′ĭn-fĕk′shən) *n.* A secondary infection occurring in a person exposed to and successfully resisting another infectious disease.

sub·in·vo·lu·tion (sŭb′ĭn-və-lōō′shən) *n.* Failure of the uterus to return to its normal size following childbirth.

sub·ja·cent (sŭb-jā′sənt) *adj.* Below or beneath another part. —**sub·ja′cen·cy** *n.*

sub·jec·tive (səb-jĕk′tĭv) *adj.* **1.** Of, relating to, or designating a symptom or condition perceived by the patient and not by the examiner. **2.** Existing only in the mind; illusory.

subjective sensation *n.* A sensation that cannot be readily linked to a verifiable external stimulus.

subjective symptom *n.* A symptom apparent to the individual afflicted but not observable by others.

sub·king·dom (sŭb′kĭng′dəm) *n.* A taxonomic category constituting a major division of a kingdom.

sub·la·tion (sŭb-lā′shən) *n.* The detachment, elevation, or removal of a part.

sub·le·thal (sŭb-lē′thəl) *adj.* Not sufficient to cause death. —**sub·le′thal·ly** *adv.*

sub·leu·ke·mic leukemia (sŭb′lōō-kē′mĭk) *n.* Leukemia that is characterized by the presence of abnormal white blood cells in the peripheral blood but in which the total number of white blood cells is normal.

sub·li·mate (sŭb′lə-māt′) *v.* **1.** To transform directly from the solid to the gaseous state or from the gaseous to the solid state without becoming a liquid. **2.** To modify the natural expression of an instinctual impulse, especially a sexual one, in a socially acceptable manner.

sub·li·ma·tion (sŭb′lə-mā′shən) *n.* **1.** The act or process of sublimating. **2.** Something that has been sublimated. **3.** An unconscious defense mechanism in which unacceptable instinctual drives and wishes are modified into more personally and socially acceptable channels.

sub·lim·i·nal (sub-lĭm′ə-nəl) *adj.* **1.** Below the threshold of conscious perception. Used of stimuli. **2.** Inadequate to produce conscious awareness but able to evoke a response.

sub·lin·gual (sub-lĭng′gwəl) *adj. Abbr.* **SL** Below or beneath the tongue; hypoglossal.

sublingual artery *n.* An artery with origin in the lingual artery, with distribution to the extrinsic muscles of the tongue, the sublingual gland, and the mucosa of the region, and with anastomoses to the artery of the opposite side and the submental artery.

sublingual caruncle *n.* A papilla on each side of the frenulum of the tongue marking the opening of the submandibular duct.

sublingual cyst *n.* See **ranula.**

sublingual duct *n.* Any of the ducts of the sublingual salivary glands, including Bartholin's duct and the ducts of Rivinus.

sublingual gland *n.* Either of two salivary glands situated in the mucus membrane on the floor of the mouth beneath the tongue. Also called *Rivinus gland.*

sublingual nerve *n.* A branch of the lingual nerve supplying parasympathetic fibers to the sublingual gland and sensory fibers to the mucous membrane of the floor of the mouth.

sublingual pit *n.* A shallow depression lodging the sublingual gland, located on either side of the mental spine on the inner surface of the body of the mandible above the mylohyoid line.

sublingual vein *n.* A tributary of the lingual vein.

sub·lux·a·tion (sŭb′lŭk-sā′shən) *n.* Incomplete or partial dislocation, as of a bone in a joint.

sub·mam·ma·ry mastitis (sub-măm′ə-rē) *n.* Inflammation of the tissues around the mammary gland. Also called *paramastitis.*

sub·man·dib·u·lar duct (sub′măn-dĭb′yə-lər) *n.* The duct of the submandibular gland, which opens beneath the tongue. Also called *submaxillary duct, Wharton's duct.*

submandibular fovea *n.* The depression in which the submandibular gland is lodged, located on the medial surface of the body of the mandible below the mylohyoid line.

submandibular ganglion *n.* A small parasympathetic ganglion suspended from the lingual nerve, with its postganglionic branches going to the submandibular

and sublingual glands and its preganglionic fibers coming from the salivary nucleus. Also called *submaxillary ganglion.*

submandibular gland *n.* Either of two major salivary glands situated in the neck near the lower edge of each side of the mandible and emptying into the submandibular duct. Also called *maxillary gland, submaxillary gland.*

submandibular triangle *n.* The triangle of the neck bounded by the mandible and the two bellies of the digastric muscle, containing the submandibular gland. Also called *digastric triangle, gastric triangle, submaxillary triangle.*

sub·max·il·la (sŭb′măk-sĭl′ə) *n.* See **mandible.**

sub·max·il·lar·i·tis (sŭb′măk-sĭl′ə-rī′tĭs) *n.* Inflammation of the submandibular salivary gland, usually due to the mumps virus.

sub·max·il·lar·y (sub-măk′sə-lĕr′ē) *adj.* **1.** Of or relating to the lower jaw; mandibular. **2.** Situated beneath the maxilla. —*n.* An anatomical part, such as a gland or nerve, situated beneath the maxilla.

submaxillary duct *n.* See **submandibular duct.**

submaxillary ganglion *n.* See **submandibular ganglion.**

submaxillary gland *n.* See **submandibular gland.**

submaxillary triangle *n.* See **submandibular triangle.**

sub·men·tal artery (sub-mĕn′tl) *n.* An artery with origin in the facial artery, with distribution to the mylohyoid muscle, the submandibular and sublingual glands, and the structures of the lower lip, and with anastomoses to the inferior labial and a branch of the inferior dental and sublingual arteries.

submental vein *n.* A vein that is situated below the chin, anastomoses with the sublingual vein, connects with the anterior jugular vein, and empties into the facial vein.

sub·met·a·cen·tric (sŭb′mĕt-ə-sĕn′trĭk) *adj.* Having the centromere near the center but not in the middle, so that one arm is shorter than the other. Used of a chromosome.

sub·mi·cro·scop·ic (sŭb′mī-krə-skŏp′ĭk) *adj.* Too small to be visible under the most powerful optical microscope.

sub·mu·co·sa (sŭb′myōō-kō′sə) *n.* A layer of loose connective tissue beneath a mucous membrane.

sub·mu·co·sal plexus (sŭb′myōō-kō′səl) *n.* A gangliated plexus of unmyelinated nerve fibers, derived chiefly from the superior mesenteric plexus, and ramifying in the intestinal submucosa.

sub·na·si·on (sub-nā′zī-ŏn′) *n.* The point of the angle between the septum of the nose and the surface of the upper lip.

sub·nu·cle·us (sŭb′nōō′klē-əs) *n.* A secondary nucleus into which a large nerve nucleus may be divided.

sub·oc·cip·i·tal muscle (sŭb′ŏk-sĭp′ĭ-tl) *n.* Any of a group of muscles located immediately below the occipital bone.

suboccipital nerve *n.* The dorsal branch of the first cervical nerve, sending branches to the greater and the lesser posterior rectus muscles of the head, to the superior and inferior oblique muscles of the head, to the lateral rectus muscle of the head, and to the semispinal muscle of the head.

sub·oc·cip·i·to·breg·mat·ic diameter (sŭb'ŏk-sĭp'ĭ-tō-brĕg-măt'ĭk) *n.* The diameter of the fetal head from the lowest posterior point of the occipital bone to the center of the anterior fontanel.

sub·or·bit·al (sŭb-ôr'bĭ-tl) *adj.* Situated on or below the floor of the orbit of the eye. —*n.* A suborbital part, such as a bone, nerve, or cartilage.

sub·or·der (sŭb'ôr'dər) *n.* A taxonomic category ranking between an order and a family.

sub·pap·u·lar (sŭb-păp'yə-lər) *adj.* Relating to the eruption of few and scattered papules, in which the lesions are very slightly elevated.

sub·per·i·os·te·al amputation (sŭb'pĕr-ē-ŏs'tē-əl) *n.* Amputation in which the periosteum is stripped back from the bone that is to be amputated and replaced afterward to form a periosteal flap over the cut end. Also called *periosteoplastic amputation.*

sub·per·i·to·ne·al fascia (sŭb'pĕr-ĭ-tn-ē'əl) *n.* The thin layer of fascia and adipose tissue between the peritoneum and the transverse fascia. Also called *extraperitoneal fascia.*

sub·phy·lum (sŭb'fī'ləm) *n.,* *pl.* **–la** (-lə) A taxonomic category ranking between a phylum and a class.

sub·pu·bic angle (sŭb-pyoō'bĭk) *n.* The angle formed by the inferior rami of the pubic bones. Also called *pubic angle.*

sub·scap·u·lar artery (sŭb-skăp'yə-lər) *n.* An artery with origin in the axillary artery, with branches to the circumflex scapular and thoracodorsal arteries, with distribution to the muscles of the shoulder and scapular region, and with anastomoses to the branches of the transverse cervical, suprascapular, lateral thoracic, and intercostal arteries.

subscapular muscle *n.* A muscle with origin from the subscapular fossa, with insertion into the humerus, with nerve supply from the upper and lower subscapular nerves from the fifth and sixth cervical nerves, and whose action rotates the arm medially.

subscapular nerve *n.* A branch of the posterior cord of the brachial plexus that supplies the subscapular muscle.

sub·scrip·tion (səb-skrĭp'shən) *n.* The part of a prescription giving the directions to the pharmacist.

sub·se·rous (sŭb-sîr'əs) *adj.* Located beneath a serous membrane.

subserous plexus *n.* The subserous part of the enteric plexus of autonomic nerves.

sub·si·dence (səb-sīd'ns, sŭb'sĭ-dns) *n.* Sinking or settling in a bone, as of a prosthetic component of a total joint implant.

sub·sid·i·ar·y atrial pacemaker (səb-sĭd'ē-ĕr'ē) *n.* A secondary source for rhythmic control of the heart, available for controlling cardiac activity if the sinoatrial pacemaker fails.

sub·spi·na·le (sŭb'spī-nā'lē) *n.* The most posterior midline point on the premaxilla between the anterior nasal spine and prosthion. Also called *point A.*

sub·stance (sŭb'stəns) *n.* **1.** That which has mass and occupies space; matter. **2.** A material of a particular kind or constitution.

substance abuse *n.* Excessive use of a potentially addictive substance, especially one that may modify body functions, such as alcohol and drugs. Also called *chemical abuse.* —**substance abuser** *n.*

substance abuse disorder *n.* Any of a category of disorders in which pathological behavioral changes are associated with the regular use of substances that affect the central nervous system.

substance P *n.* A short-chain polypeptide that functions as a neurotransmitter especially in the transmission of pain impulses from peripheral receptors to the central nervous system.

sub·stan·ti·a (sŭb-stăn'shē-ə) *n.,* *pl.* **-ti·ae** (-shē-ē') Substance.

substantia al·ba (ăl'bə) *n.* See **white matter.**

substantia ge·lat·i·no·sa (jə-lăt'n-ō'sə, jĕl'ə-tn-ō'sə) *n.* The apical part of the posterior horn of the gray matter of the spinal cord, composed largely of very small nerve cells and whose gelatinous appearance is due to its very low content of myelinated nerve fibers. It functions in the integration of sensory stimuli that give rise to the sensations of heat and pain. Also called *Rolando's gelatinous substance.*

substantia gris·e·a (grĭs'ē-ə, grĭz'-) *n.* See **gray matter.**

substantia med·ul·lar·is (mĕd'l-âr'ĭs) *n.* **1.** Medulla. **2.** Medullary substance.

substantia ni·gra (nī'grə, nĭg'rə) *n.* A layer of large pigmented nerve cells in the mesencephalon that produce dopamine and whose destruction is associated with Parkinson's disease. Also called *nigra.*

sub·ster·nal goiter (sŭb-stûr'nəl) *n.* Goiter, chiefly of the lower part of the isthmus of the thyroid gland, that is not easily palpable.

sub·sti·tu·tion (sŭb'stĭ-toō'shən) *n.* **1.** The replacement of an atom or a group of atoms in a compound by another atom or group of atoms. **2.** An unconscious defense mechanism by which the unacceptable or unattainable is replaced by something more acceptable or attainable.

substitution product *n.* A product obtained by replacing one atom or group in a molecule with another atom or group.

substitution therapy *n.* Replacement therapy in which a substitute substance is used.

substitution transfusion *n.* See **exchange transfusion.**

sub·strate (sŭb'strāt') *n.* **1.** The material or substance on which an enzyme acts. **2.** A surface on which an organism grows or is attached.

sub·struc·ture (sŭb'strŭk'chər) *n.* A tissue or structure wholly or partly beneath the surface. —**sub·struc'tur·al** *adj.*

subthalamic nucleus *n.* A circumscript nucleus that is located in the ventral part of the subthalamus, receives a massive projection from the lateral segment of the globus pallidus, and projects to both pallidal segments and to the mesencephalic tegmentum.

sub·thal·a·mus (sŭb-thăl'ə-məs) *n.* The part of the diencephalon that is wedged ventrally between the thalamus on the dorsal side and the cerebral peduncle, is lateral to the dorsal half of the hypothalamus, and is caudally continuous with the mesencephalic tegmentum. —**sub'tha·lam'ic** (-thə-lăm'ĭk) *adj.*

sub·thresh·old stimulus (sŭb-thrĕsh'ōld', -hōld') *n.* See **inadequate stimulus.**

subtotal hysterectomy *n.* See **supracervical hysterectomy.**

sub·un·gual (sŭb-ŭng′gwəl) *or* **sub·un·gui·al** (-gwē-əl) *adj.* Beneath a fingernail or toenail.

sub·u·nit vaccine (sŭb′yōō′nĭt) *n.* A vaccine containing viral antigens made free of viral nucleic acid by chemical extraction and containing only minimal amounts of nonviral antigens derived from the culture medium; it is less likely to cause adverse reactions than a vaccine containing the whole virion.

sub·vag·i·nal (sŭb-văj′ə-nəl) *adj.* **1.** Located below the vagina. **2.** Located on the inner side of any sheath.

sub·vi·rus (sŭb-vī′rəs) *n.,* *pl.* **-rus·es** A viral protein or other substance smaller than a virus and having some viral properties. **—sub·vi′ral** (-rəl) *adj.*

sub·vo·cal speech (sŭb-vō′kəl) *n.* Slight movements of the speech muscles, related to thinking but producing no sound.

sub·vo·lu·tion (sŭb′və-loō′shən) *n.* The surgical reversal of a flap of mucous membrane to prevent adhesion, as in the operation for pterygium.

suc·ci·nate (sŭk′sə-nāt′) *n.* A salt or ester of succinic acid.

suc·cin·ic acid (sək-sĭn′ĭk) *n.* A colorless crystalline dicarboxylic acid important in the Krebs cycle.

suc·ci·nyl·cho·line (sŭk′sə-nĭl-kō′lēn′) *n.* A crystalline compound formed by esterification of succinic acid with choline and used medically to produce brief but complete muscular relaxation during surgical anesthesia.

suc·ci·nyl·co·en·zyme A (sŭk′sə-nĭl-kō-ĕn′zīm′) *n.* The condensation product of succinic acid and coenzyme A that is one of the intermediates in the Krebs cycle. Also called *succinyl-CoA.*

suc·cor·rhe·a (sŭk′ə-rē′ə) *n.* An abnormal increase in the secretion of a gastric juice.

suc·cus (sŭk′əs) *n.,* *pl.* **suc·ci** (sŭk′ī, -sī) A fluid, such as gastric juice or vegetable juice, contained in or secreted by living tissue. No longer in technical use.

suck·ing reflex (sŭk′ĭng) *n.* Sucking movements of an infant's lips elicited by touching them or the adjacent skin.

sucking wound *n.* See **open pneumothorax.**

su·cral·fate (soō-krăl′fāt′) *n.* A polysaccharide with antipeptic activity used to treat duodenal ulcers.

su·crase (soō′krās′, -krāz′) *n.* See **invertase.**

su·crose (soō′krōs′) *n.* A nonreducing crystalline disaccharide made up of glucose and fructose, found in many plants but extracted as ordinary sugar mainly from sugar cane and sugar beets, and widely used as a sweetener or preservative.

su·cro·se·mi·a (soō′krō-sē′mē-ə) *n.* The presence of sucrose in the blood.

sucrose pol·y·es·ter (pŏl′ē-ĕs′tər) *n.* A complex synthetic compound of sucrose and fatty acids that the body is unable to digest or absorb, produced commercially as a partial substitute for fats in cooking oils, shortening, butter, and other high-calorie or high-cholesterol foods.

su·cro·su·ria (soō′krō-soōr′ē-ə) *n.* Excretion of sucrose in the urine.

suc·tion curettage (sŭk′shən) *n.* See **vacuum aspiration.**

suction drainage *n.* The closed drainage of a cavity using a suction apparatus attached to a drainage tube.

suc·to·ri·al (sŭk-tôr′ē-əl) *adj.* Relating to or adapted for sucking.

Su·da·fed (soō′də-fĕd′) A trademark for the drug pseudoephedrine.

su·da·men (soō-dā′mən) *n.,* *pl.* **-dam·i·na** (-dăm′ə-nə) A small vesicle caused by retention of fluid in a sweat follicle or in the epidermis. **—su·dam′i·nal** (-dăm′ə-nəl) *adj.*

Su·dan dye (soō-dăn′) *n.* Any of several fat-soluble aromatic dyes used as biological stains.

su·dan·o·phil·ic (soō-dăn′ə-fĭl′ĭk) *adj.* Staining easily with Sudan dyes.

su·dan·o·pho·bic (soō-dăn′ə-fō′bĭk) *adj.* Failing to stain with a Sudan dye.

Sudan yellow *n.* A yellow stain for fats.

su·da·tion (soō-dā′shən) *n.* Perspiration.

sud·den infant death syndrome (sŭd′n) *n. Abbr.* **SIDS** A fatal syndrome affecting apparently healthy sleeping infants under a year old and that is characterized by a sudden cessation of breathing. Also called *crib death.*

Su·deck's atrophy (soō′dĕks, zoō′-) *n.* Acute atrophy of a bone, usually one of the carpal or tarsal bones, following a slight injury such as a sprain.

su·do·mo·tor (soō′də-mō′tər) *adj.* Relating to the nerves that stimulate the sweat glands to activity.

sudomotor fiber *n.* Any of the postganglionic sympathetic nerve fibers innervating the sweat glands.

su·dor (soō′dər, -dôr′) *n.* Sweat.

sudor– *pref.* Perspiration; sweat: *sudoresis.*

su·dor·al (soō′dər-əl, -dôr′əl) *adj.* Relating to perspiration.

su·do·re·sis (soō′də-rē′sĭs) *n.* Profuse sweating.

su·dor·if·er·ous (soō′də-rĭf′ər-əs) *adj.* Carrying or producing sweat.

sudoriferous gland *n.* See **sweat gland.**

su·dor·if·ic (soō′də-rĭf′ĭk) *adj.* Causing or increasing sweat.

su·dor·ip·a·rous (soō′də-rĭp′ər-əs) *adj.* Secreting sweat.

su·fen·ta·nil citrate (soō-fĕn′tə-nĭl) *n.* An injectable general anesthetic with narcotic action.

suf·fo·cate (sŭf′ə-kāt′) *v.* **1.** To impair the respiration of; asphyxiate. **2.** To suffer from lack of oxygen; to be unable to breathe. **—suf′fo·ca′tion** *n.*

suf·fo·ca·tive goiter (sŭf′ə-kā′tĭv) *n.* A goiter that causes extreme dyspnea by pressure on the trachea.

suf·fu·sion (sə-fyoō′zhən) *n.* **1.** The act of pouring a fluid over the body. **2.** The condition of being wet with a fluid. **3.** A spreading out of a body fluid from a vessel into the surrounding tissues. **4.** The reddening of a surface. **—suf·fuse′** (-fyoōz′) *v.*

sug·ar (shoŏg′ər) *n.* **1.** A crystalline or powdered substance consisting of sucrose obtained mainly from sugar cane and sugar beets and used in many medicines to improve their taste. **2.** Any of a class of water-soluble crystalline carbohydrates, including sucrose and lactose, having a characteristically sweet taste and classified as monosaccharides, disaccharides, and trisaccharides.

sugar diabetes *n.* Insulin-dependent diabetes; diabetes mellitus.

sug·gest·i·bil·i·ty (səg-jĕs′tə-bĭl′ĭ-tē, sə-jĕs′-) *n.* Responsiveness or susceptibility to suggestion.

sug·gest·i·ble (səg-jĕs′tə-bəl, sə-jĕs′-) *adj.* Readily influenced by suggestion.

sug·ges·tion (səg-jĕs′chən, sə-jĕs′-) *n.* Implanting of an idea in the mind of another by a word or act so as to influence conduct or physical condition.

sug·gil·la·tion (sŭg′jə-lā′shən, sŭj′ə-) *n.* **1.** A black-and-blue mark. **2.** See **livedo.**

su·i·cid·al (soo′ĭ-sīd′l) *adj.* **1.** Of or relating to suicide. **2.** Likely to attempt suicide.

su·i·cide (soo′ĭ-sīd′) *n.* **1.** The act or an instance of intentionally killing oneself. **2.** One who commits suicide.

sul·cate (sŭl′kāt′) *adj.* Having narrow, deep grooves.

sul·cus (sŭl′kəs) *n.,* *pl.* **–ci** (-kī, -sī) **1.** Any of the grooves on the brain surface, bounding the gyri; a fissure. **2.** A long narrow groove or depression, as in an organ or a tissue. —**sul′cal** *adj.*

sulcus of sclera *n.* A slight groove on the external surface of the eyeball, indicating the line of union of the sclera and the cornea.

sul·fa (sŭl′fə) *adj.* Of, relating to, or containing sulfanilamide or any sulfa drug.

sul·fa·di·a·zine (sŭl′fə-dī′ə-zēn′) *n.* A sulfa drug that is used in the treatment of meningitis and other infections.

sulfa drug *n.* Any of a group of synthetic organic compounds, derived chiefly from sulfanilamide, chemically similar to PABA and capable of inhibiting bacterial growth and activity by interfering with the metabolic processes in bacteria that require PABA. Also called *sulfonamide.*

sul·fa·me·thox·a·zole (sŭl′fə-mə-thŏk′sə-zōl) *n.* A sulfonamide antibiotic that is used especially in combination with trimethoprim to treat bacterial urinary tract infections and other infectious conditions, such as malaria.

sul·fa·nil·a·mide (sŭl′fə-nĭl′ə-mīd′, -mĭd) *n.* A white, odorless crystalline sulfonamide used in the treatment of various bacterial infections.

sul·fa·tase (sŭl′fə-tās′) *n.* Any of a group of enzymes that catalyze the hydrolysis of sulfuric acid esters and are found in animal tissues and bacteria.

sul·fate (sŭl′fāt′) *n.* **1.** A salt or ester of sulfuric acid. **2.** The bivalent group SO_4. **3.** A chemical compound containing such a group. —*v.* **1.** To treat or react with sulfuric acid or a sulfate. **2.** To become sulfated.

sul·fa·ti·date (sŭl′fə-tī′dāt′) *or* **sul·fa·tide** (sŭl′fə-tīd′) *n.* Any of the cerebroside sulfuric esters containing sulfate groups in the sugar portion of the molecule.

sul·fa·tion (sŭl-fā′shən) *n.* The addition of sulfate groups as esters to molecules.

sulf·he·mo·glo·bi·ne·mi·a (sŭlf-hē′mə-glō′bə-nē′mē-ə) *n.* Presence of sulfmethemoglobin in the blood.

sulf·hy·dryl (sŭlf-hī′drəl) *n.* The univalent radical group, SH, present in many biologically active molecules such as coenzymes and certain proteins.

sul·fide (sŭl′fīd′) *n.* A compound of bivalent sulfur with an electropositive element or group, especially a binary compound of sulfur with a metal.

sul·fi·nyl (sŭl′fə-nĭl′) *n.* The bivalent group SO.

sul·fite (sŭl′fīt′) *n.* A salt or ester of sulfurous acid. —**sul·fit′ic** (-fīt′ĭk) *adj.*

sulfite oxidase *n.* An enzyme present in the liver that catalyzes the oxidation of inorganic sulfate ion with molecular oxygen.

sulf·met·he·mo·glo·bin (sŭlf′mĕt-hē′mə-glō′bĭn) *or* **sulf·he·mo·glo·bin** (sŭlf-hē′mə-) *n.* The complex formed by the reaction of a sulfide and hemoglobin in the presence of oxygen.

sulfo– *or* **sulf–** *pref.* Sulfur: *sulfate.*

sulfon– *pref.* **1.** Sulfonic: *sulfonamide.* **2.** Sulfonyl: *sulfonmethane.*

sul·fon·a·mide (sŭl-fŏn′ə-mīd′, -mĭd) *n.* **1.** Any of a group of organic sulfur compounds that includes the sulfa drugs. **2.** See **sulfa drug.**

sul·fo·nate (sŭl′fə-nāt′) *n.* A salt or ester of sulfonic acid. —*v.* **1.** To introduce one or more sulfonic acid groups into an organic compound. **2.** To treat with sulfonic acid. —**sul′fo·na′tion** *n.*

sul·fone (sŭl′fōn′) *n.* Any of various organic sulfur compounds having a sulfonyl group attached to two carbon atoms, especially such a compound formerly used as a drug to treat leprosy or tuberculosis.

sul·fon·ic (sŭl-fŏn′ĭk) *adj.* Of or relating to the chemical group SO_2OH.

sulfonic acid *n.* Any of several organic acids containing one or more sulfonic groups.

sul·fon·meth·ane (sŭl′fŏn-mĕth′ān′, -fŏn-) *n.* A colorless crystalline or powdered compound used medicinally as a hypnotic.

sul·fo·nyl (sŭl′fə-nĭl′) *n.* The bivalent radical SO_2. Also called *sulfuryl.*

sul·fo·nyl·u·re·a (sŭl′fə-nĭl-yoo-rē′ə) *n.* Any of a group of hypoglycemic drugs, such as tolbutamide, that act on the beta cells of the pancreas to increase the secretion of insulin.

sul·fo·sal·i·cyl·ic acid (sŭl′fō-săl′ĭ-sĭl′ĭk) *n.* An acid that precipitates protein in solution.

sulfosalicylic acid turbidity test *n.* A test for measuring protein in urine, in which sulfosalicylic acid is added to urine; turbidity of precipitation is approximately proportional to protein concentration.

sul·fo·trans·fer·ase (sŭl′fō-trăns′fə-rās′, -rāz′) *n.* An enzyme that catalyzes the transfer of a sulfate group from one compound to the hydroxyl group of another.

sulf·ox·ide (sŭl-fŏk′sīd′) *n.* Any of various compounds that contain a sulfinyl group.

sul·fur *or* **sul·phur** (sŭl′fər) *n. Symbol* **S** A yellow nonmetallic element occurring widely in nature in several free and combined allotropic forms and used in the manufacture of pharmaceuticals and many sulfur compounds, especially sulfuric acid. Atomic number 16.

sulfur-35 *n.* A radioisotope of sulfur that is a beta emitter with half-life of 87.2 days, used as a tracer in metabolic studies.

sul·fu·ric acid (sŭl-fyŏŏr′ĭk) *n.* A colorless, nearly odorless, corrosive liquid that is used occasionally as a caustic. Also called *vitriol.*

sulfuric ether *n.* See **diethyl ether.**

sul·fur·ous (sŭl′fər-əs, -fyər-, sŭl-fyŏŏr′əs) *adj.* **1.** Of, relating to, derived from, or containing sulfur, especially with valence 4. **2.** Characteristic of or emanating from burning sulfur.

sul·fur·yl (sŭl′fə-rĭl′, -fyə-) *n.* See **sulfonyl.**

su·lin·dac (sə-lĭn′dăk) *n.* An anti-inflammatory nonsteroid agent with analgesic and antipyretic actions.

su·mac *or* **su·mach** (sŏŏ′măk, shŏŏ′-) *n.* Any of various shrubs or small trees of the genus *Rhus,* having compound leaves, clusters of small greenish flowers, and usually red, hairy fruit. Some species, such as poison ivy, cause an acute itching rash on contact.

su·ma·trip·tan (sŏŏ′mə-trĭp′tn) *n.* A drug of the triptan class given as a nasal spray, and orally or by injection in its succinate form, used to treat migraine headaches.

sum·ma·tion (sə-mā′shən) *n.* The process by which multiple or repeated stimuli can produce a response in a nerve, muscle, or other part that one stimulus alone cannot produce.

summation gallop *n.* A gallop characterized by the superimposition of abnormal third and fourth heart sounds, usually indicative of myocardial disease.

sum·mer diarrhea (sŭm′ər) *n.* Diarrhea affecting infants or young children in hot weather, usually caused by acute gastroenteritis due to bacterial infection. Also called *choleraic diarrhea.*

Sum·ner (sŭm′nər), **James Batcheller** 1887–1955. American biochemist. He shared a 1946 Nobel Prize for his pioneering work on crystallizing enzymes.

sump drain (sŭmp) *n.* A drain consisting of a smaller tube within a larger tube through which fluid passes as a result of suction.

sump syndrome *n.* A complication of side-to-side choledochoduodenostomy in which the lower end of the common bile duct occasionally acts as a diverticulum and traps food particles, a process that may result in infection.

sun block (sŭn) *n.* A preparation, as of PABA, that prevents sunburn by filtering out the sun's ultraviolet rays, usually offering more protection than a sunscreen.

sun·burn (sŭn′bûrn′) *n.* Inflammation and erythema of the skin, often with blistering, caused by overexposure to the ultraviolet rays of direct sunlight. —**sun′burn′** *v.*

sun protection factor *n. Abbr.* **SPF** The ratio of the minimal ultraviolet dose required to produce erythema with and without a sunscreen; a measure of the degree to which a sunscreen protects the skin from ultraviolet radiation, the higher the number the greater degree of protection.

sun·screen (sŭn′skrēn′) *n.* A preparation, often in the form of a cream or lotion, used to protect the skin from the ultraviolet rays of the sun.

sun·stroke *or* **sun stroke** (sŭn′strōk′) *n.* Heatstroke that results from undue exposure to the sun's rays and is marked by prostration and collapse, but not by fever.

super– *pref.* **1.** Above; over; upon: *superstructure.* **2.** Superior in size, quality, number, or degree: *supersonic.* **3.** Exceeding a norm: *supersaturate.* **4.** Excessive in degree or intensity: *superexcitation.* **5.** Containing a specified ingredient in an unusually high proportion: *superoxide.*

su·per·a·cute (sŏŏ′pər-ə-kyŏŏt′) *adj.* Marked by great severity of symptoms and rapid progress; extremely acute. Used of the course of a disease.

su·per·al·i·men·ta·tion (sŏŏ′pər-ăl′ə-měn-tā′shən) *n.* The administration or consumption of nutrients beyond normal.

su·per·bug (sŏŏ′pər-bŭg′) *n.* Any of various disease-causing bacteria that develop a resistance to drugs normally used to control or eradicate them.

su·per·cil·i·ar·y (sŏŏ′pər-sĭl′ē-ĕr′ē) *adj.* Of, relating to, or being in the area of the eyebrow.

superciliary arch *n.* A smooth elevation extending laterally from the glabella on either side, above the orbital margin of the frontal bone.

su·per·cil·i·um (sŏŏ′pər-sĭl′ē-əm) *n., pl.* **–i·a** (-ē-ə) **1.** The eyebrow. **2.** An individual hair of the eyebrow.

su·per·class (sŏŏ′pər-klăs′) *n.* A taxonomic category ranking below a phylum and above a class.

su·per·duct (sŏŏ′pər-dŭkt′) *v.* To elevate or draw upward.

su·per·e·go (sŏŏ′pər-ē′gō, -ĕg′ō) *n., pl.* **–gos** In psychoanalytic theory, the division of the psyche that censors and restrains the ego and has identified itself unconsciously with important persons from early life. It results from incorporating the values and wishes of these persons into one's own standards.

su·per·ex·ci·ta·tion (sŏŏ′pər-ĕk′sī-tā′shən) *n.* **1.** The act of exciting or stimulating unduly. **2.** A condition of extreme excitement or overstimulation.

su·per·fi·cial (sŏŏ′pər-fĭsh′əl) *adj.* **1.** Of, affecting, or being on or near the surface. **2.** Not thorough.

superficial dorsal veins of clitoris *pl.n.* Any of the paired tributaries to the external pudendal vein on either side.

superficial dorsal veins of penis *pl.n.* Any of the paired tributaries of the external pudendal veins on each side, superficial to the fascia.

superficial epigastric vein *n.* A vein that drains the lower and medial part of the anterior abdominal wall and empties into the great saphenous vein.

superficial fascia *n.* See **tela subcutanea.**

superficial fascia of perineum *n.* The membranous layer of the subcutaneous tissue in the urogenital region attaching posteriorly to the border of the urogenital diaphragm, at the sides to the ischiopubic rami, and continuing anteriorly to the abdominal wall. Also called *Colles' fascia.*

superficial flexor muscle of fingers *n.* A muscle with origin from the medial epicondyle of the humerus, the medial border of the coronoid process, and a tendinous arch between these points, and from the middle third of the radius, with insertion to the sides of the middle phalanx of each finger, with nerve supply from the median nerve, and whose action flexes the middle phalanges of the fingers.

superficial inguinal ring *n.* The opening in the aponeurosis of the external oblique muscle of the abdominal wall through which the male spermatic cord or the female round ligament emerges from the inguinal canal. Also called *subcutaneous ring*.

superficial lingual muscle *n.* An intrinsic muscle of the tongue, running beneath the mucous membrane from base to tip on the back of the tongue.

superficial perineal space *n.* The space bounded above by the perineal membrane and below by the superficial perineal fascia and containing the root structure of the penis or clitoris

superficial peroneal nerve *n.* A branch of the common peroneal nerve that passes downward in front of the fibula to supply the long and short peroneal muscles and terminates in the skin of the dorsum of the foot and of the toes.

superficial reflex *n.* A reflex elicited by stimulation of the skin.

superficial temporal vein *n.* Any of the veins that pass from the temporal region to join the retromandibular vein.

superficial transverse muscle of perineum *n.* An inconstant muscle with origin from the ramus of the ischium, with insertion into the central tendon of the perineum, with nerve supply from the pudendal nerve, and whose action draws back and fixes the central tendon of the perineum.

su·per·fi·cies (soo′pər-fĭsh′ēz, -fĭsh′ē-ēz′) *n., pl.* **superficies 1.** The outer surface of an area or a body. **2.** External appearance or aspect.

su·per·in·duce (soo′pər-ĭn-doos′) *v.* To introduce as an addition to something already existing.

su·per·in·fect (soo′pər-ĭn-fĕkt′) *v.* To cause to be further infected with a microorganism; infect a second time or more.

su·per·in·fec·tion (soo′pər-ĭn-fĕk′shən) *n.* **1.** The act or process of superinfecting a cell or an organism. **2.** An infection following a previous infection, especially when caused by microorganisms that have become resistant to the antibiotics used earlier.

su·per·in·vo·lu·tion (soo′pər-ĭn′və-loo′shən) *n.* A reduction in the size of the uterus after childbirth to below its normal size. Also called *hyperinvolution*.

su·pe·ri·or (soo-pîr′ē-ər) *adj.* **1.** Higher than another in rank, station, or authority. **2.** Situated above or directed upward. **3.** Situated nearer the top of the head.

superior alveolar nerve *n.* Any of three branches of the maxillary nerve, designated posterior, middle, and anterior, that enter the maxilla to supply the upper teeth and the gingiva.

superior anastomotic vein *n.* A large communicating vein between the superficial middle cerebral vein and the superior sagittal sinus, passing upward from the lateral sulcus and often following the line of the central sulcus.

superior artery of knee *n.* **1.** An artery with origin in the popliteal artery, with distribution to the knee joint, and with anastomoses to the circumflex femoral, tibial, and lateral inferior genicular arteries; lateral superior artery of knee. **2.** An artery with origin in the popliteal artery, with distribution to the knee joint, and with anastomoses to the descending genicular and superior genicular arteries; medial superior artery of knee.

superior basal vein *n.* A tributary to the common basal vein, draining the lateral and anterior part of the inferior lobe of each lung.

superior cerebellar peduncle *n.* A large bundle of nerve fibers that originates from the dentate nucleus of the cerebellum and emerges from the cerebellum along the lateral wall of the fourth ventricle.

superior cerebral vein *n.* Any of the veins that drain the dorsal convexity of the cerebrum and empty into the superior sagittal sinus.

superior cervical cardiac nerve *n.* A nerve that arises from the lower part of the superior cervical ganglion of the sympathetic trunk and that passes down to form, with branches of the vagus nerve; the cardiac plexus.

superior choroid vein *n.* A vein that follows the choroid plexus of the lateral ventricle and unites with the superior thalamostriate vein and the anterior vein of the septum pellucidum to form the internal cerebral vein.

superior cluneal nerve *n.* Any of the terminal branches of the dorsal rami of the lumbar nerves, supplying the skin of the upper half of the gluteal region.

superior constrictor muscle of pharynx *n.* A muscle with origin in the medial pterygoid plate, pterygomandibular raphe, mylohyoid line of the mandible, and the floor of the mouth and the side of the tongue, with insertion to the posterior wall of the pharynx, with nerve supply from the pharyngeal plexus, and whose action narrows the pharynx.

superior dental plexus *n.* A plexus that is formed by branches of the infraorbital nerve and gives off dental and gingival branches.

superior epigastric vein *n.* Any of the accompanying veins of the superior epigastric artery that are tributaries of the internal thoracic vein.

superior ganglion of glossopharyngeal nerve *n.* See **jugular ganglion** (sense 1).

superior ganglion of vagus *n.* See **jugular ganglion** (sense 2).

superior ge·mel·lus muscle (jə-mĕl′əs) *n.* A muscle with origin in the ischial spine and the lesser sciatic notch, with insertion to the tendon of the internal obturator muscle, with nerve supply from the sacral plexus, and whose action rotates the thigh laterally.

superior gluteal nerve *n.* A nerve that arises from the fourth and fifth lumbar nerves and the first sacral nerve and supplies the gluteus medius and minimus muscles and tensor muscle of the broad fascia.

superior gluteal vein *n.* Either of the veins that accompany the gluteal artery, unite in the pelvis, and empty into the internal iliac vein.

superior intercostal vein *n.* **1.** A tributary of the azygos vein, formed by union of the right second, third, and fourth posterior intercostal veins; right superior intercostal vein. **2.** A vein that is formed by the union of the left second, third and fourth intercostal veins, passes across the arch of the aorta, empties into the left brachiocephalic vein, and frequently communicates with the accessory hemiazygos vein; left superior intercostal vein.

su·pe·ri·or·i·ty complex (soo-pîr′ē-ôr′ĭ-tē) *n.* **1.** An exaggerated feeling of being superior to others. **2.** A psychological defense mechanism in which a person's feelings of superiority counter or conceal his or her feelings of inferiority.

superior labial vein *n.* A vein that drains the upper lip and empties into the facial vein.

superior laryngeal nerve *n.* A branch of the vagus nerve at the inferior ganglion. At the thyroid cartilage, it divides into two branches, the internal, which supplies the mucous membrane of the larynx above the vocal cords; and the external, which supplies the inferior pharyngeal constrictor and the cricothyroid muscles.

superior laryngeal vein *n.* A vein that accompanies the superior laryngeal artery and empties into the superior thyroid vein.

superior lateral cutaneous nerve of arm *n.* A branch of the axillary nerve supplying the skin over the lower portion of the deltoid muscle.

superior limb *n.* See upper extremity.

superior limbic keratoconjunctivitis *n.* Inflammatory edema of the central area of the superior corneoscleral limbus of the eye, usually in both eyes, and marked by spontaneous healing and recurrence.

superior longitudinal fasciculus *n.* A bundle of long association fibers in the lateral portion of the medullary center of the cerebral hemisphere, connecting the frontal, occipital, and temporal lobes.

superior medullary velum *n.* The thin layer of white matter stretching between the two superior cerebellar peduncles, forming part of the roof of the fourth ventricle.

superior mesenteric lymph node *n.* Any of numerous nodes located in the mesentery along the superior mesenteric artery and its branches to the jejunum and the ileum, from which they receive lymph.

superior mesenteric plexus *n.* An autonomic plexus that is a continuation or part of the celiac plexus, sends nerves to the intestines, and with the vagus forms the subserous, myenteric, and submucous plexuses.

superior mesenteric vein *n.* A vein that begins at the ileum in the right iliac fossa, ascends in the root of the mesentery, and unites behind the pancreas with the splenic vein to form the portal vein.

superior oblique muscle *n.* A muscle with origin above the medial margin of the optic canal, with insertion by a tendon passing through the trochlea to the sclera between the superior rectus and lateral rectus muscles, with nerve supply from the trochlear nerve, and whose action directs the pupil of the eye downward and outward.

superior oblique muscle of head *n.* A muscle with origin from the transverse process of the atlas, with insertion into the lateral third of the inferior nuchal line, with nerve supply from the suboccipital nerve, and whose action rotates the head.

superior ophthalmic vein *n.* A vein that begins from the nasofrontal vein, passes along the medial wall of the eye socket and through the orbital fissure, and empties into the cavernous sinus.

superior orbital fissure *n.* A cleft between the greater and the lesser wing of the sphenoid, through which pass the oculomotor and trochlear nerves, the ophthalmic division of the trigeminal nerve, the abducens nerve, and the ophthalmic veins.

superior petrosal sinus *n.* A paired sinus of the dura mater in the groove on the superior margin of the petrous part of the temporal bone, connecting the cavernous sinus with the transverse sinus.

superior phrenic vein *n.* Any of the small veins that are tributaries to the azygos and hemiazygos veins and drain the upper surface of the diaphragm.

superior pulmonary vein *n.* **1.** A vein that returns blood from the left superior lobe of the lung to the left atrium; left superior pulmonary vein. **2.** A vein that returns blood from the superior and middle lobes of the right lung to the left atrium; right superior pulmonary vein.

superior rectal vein *n.* A vein that drains the greater part of the rectal venous plexus and ascends between layers of the mesorectum to the brim of the pelvis to become the inferior mesenteric vein.

superior rectus muscle *n.* A muscle with origin from the superior part of the common tendinous ring, with insertion into the superior part of the sclera of the eye, with nerve supply from the oculomotor nerve, and whose action directs the pupil upward and medialward.

superior retinaculum of extensor muscles *n.* The ligament that binds down the extensor tendons proximal to the ankle joint and is continuous above with the deep fascia of the leg.

superior sagittal sinus *n.* An unpaired dural sinus in the sagittal groove.

superior salivary nucleus *n.* A group of preganglionic parasympathetic motor neurons situated near the inferior salivary nucleus and governing secretion of the lacrimal, sublingual, and submaxillary glands by way of the facial nerve and the sphenopalatine and submandibular ganglia.

superior tarsal muscle *n.* A layer of smooth muscle that extends from the aponeurosis of the elevator muscle of the upper eyelid to the superior tarsus, is innervated by sympathetic nerves, and acts to hold the upper lid in an elevated position.

superior temporal line *n.* The upper of two curved lines on the parietal bone, to which the temporal fascia is attached.

superior temporal sulcus *n.* The longitudinal sulcus separating the superior and middle temporal gyri.

superior thal·a·mo·stri·ate vein (thăl′ə-mō-strī′āt′) *n.* A long vein that passes forward in the groove between the thalamus and caudate nucleus and joins the choroid vein and the veins of the septum pellucidum to form the internal cerebral veins.

superior thyroid vein *n.* A vein that receives blood from the upper part of the thyroid gland and the larynx, accompanies the superior thyroid artery, and empties into the internal jugular vein.

superior vein of cerebellar hemisphere *n.* Any of several veins draining the superior part of the cerebellar hemispheres and terminating in the superior petrosal sinus or in the petrosal vein.

superior vein of eyelid *n.* Any of the veins draining the upper eyelid into the angular vain.

superior vein of vermis *n.* A vein on the upper surface of the vermis, that ends in the internal cerebral vein and drains part of the upper cerebellum.

superior vena cava *n. Abbr.* **SVC** A large vein formed by the union of the two brachiocephalic veins and the azygos vein that receives blood from the head, neck, upper limbs, and chest, and empties into the right atrium of the heart. Also called *precava*.

su·per·mo·til·i·ty (so͞o′pər-mō-tĭl′ĭ-tē) *n.* Excessive motility.

su·per·nu·mer·ar·y (so͞o′pər-no͞o′mə-rĕr′ē) *adj.* Exceeding the normal or usual number; extra.

su·per·o·lat·er·al (so͞o′pə-rō-lăt′ər-əl) *adj.* At the side and above.

su·per·o·vu·late (so͞o′pər-ō′vyə-lāt′, -ŏv′yə-) *v.* **1.** To produce mature ova at an accelerated rate or in a large number at one time. **2.** To cause to superovulate. —**su′per·o′vu·la′tion** *n.*

su·per·ox·ide (so͞o′pər-ŏk′sīd′) *n.* A compound containing a univalent anionic oxygen molecule or the univalent anion itself.

superoxide dismutase *n.* An enzyme that catalyzes the decomposition of a superoxide into hydrogen peroxide and oxygen.

su·per·sat·u·rate (so͞o′pər-săch′ə-rāt′) *v.* To cause a chemical solution to be more highly concentrated than is normally possible under certain conditions of temperature and pressure. —**su′per·sat′u·ra′tion** *n.*

su·per·scrip·tion (so͞o′pər-skrĭp′shən) *n.* The part of a prescription that bears the Latin word *recipe* represented by ℞.

su·per·son·ic (so͞o′pər-sŏn′ĭk) *adj.* **1.** Having, caused by, or relating to a speed greater than the speed of sound in a given medium, especially air. **2.** Of or relating to sound waves beyond human audibility. —**su′per·son′i·cal·ly** *adv.*

su·per·struc·ture (so͞o′pər-strŭk′chər) *n.* A structure above the surface.

su·pi·nate (so͞o′pə-nāt′) *v.* To assume, or to be placed in, a supine position. —**su′pi·na′tion** *n.*

su·pi·na·tor muscle (so͞o′pə-nā′tər) *n.* A muscle with origin from the humerus and the ulna, with insertion into the radius, with nerve supply from the radial nerve, and whose action supinates the forearm.

su·pine (so͞o-pīn′, so͞o′pīn′) *adj.* **1.** Lying on the back; having the face upward. **2.** Having the palm of the hand or sole of the foot upward.

sup·ple·men·tal air (sŭp′lə-měn′tl) *n.* See **expiratory reserve volume.**

sup·port (sə-pôrt′) *v.* **1.** To bear the weight of, especially from below. **2.** To hold in position so as to keep from falling, sinking, or slipping. **3.** To be capable of bearing; withstand. **4.** To keep from weakening or failing; strengthen. **5.** To provide for or maintain, by supplying with money or necessities. **6.** To endure; tolerate. —*n.* **1.** The act of supporting. **2.** The state of being supported. **3.** One that supports or maintains. **4.** Maintenance, as of a family, with the necessities of life.

sup·pos·i·to·ry (sə-pŏz′ĭ-tôr′ē) *n.* A small plug of medication designed to melt at body temperature within a body cavity other than the mouth, especially the rectum or vagina.

sup·press (sə-prĕs′) *v.* **1.** To curtail or inhibit the activity of something, such as the immune system. **2.** To deliberately exclude unacceptable desires or thoughts

from the mind. **3.** To reduce the incidence or severity of a condition or symptom, such as a hemorrhage.

sup·pres·sion (sə-prĕsh′ən) *n.* **1.** The act of suppressing or the state of being suppressed. **2.** Conscious exclusion of unacceptable desires, thoughts, or memories from the mind. **3.** The sudden arrest of the secretion of a fluid, such as urine or bile. **4.** The checking or curtailing of an abnormal flow or discharge. **5.** The effect of a second genetic mutation that reverses a phenotypic change that had been caused by a previous mutation at a different location on the chromosome.

sup·pres·sor mutation (sə-prĕs′ər) *n.* A mutation that alters the anticodon in a tRNA so that it is complementary to a termination codon, thus suppressing termination of the amino acid chain.

suppressor T cell *n.* A T cell that reduces or suppresses the immune response of B cells or of other T cells to an antigen.

sup·pu·rant (sŭp′yə-rənt) *adj.* Causing or inducing suppuration. —*n.* An agent that promotes the suppuration process.

sup·pu·rate (sŭp′yə-rāt′) *v.* To form or discharge pus.

sup·pu·ra·tion (sŭp′yə-rā′shən) *n.* The formation or discharge of pus. Also called *pyesis, pyopoiesis, pyosis*. —**sup′pu·ra′tive** *adj.*

suppurative arthritis *n.* Acute inflammation of the synovial membranes accompanied by purulent effusion into a joint and caused by bacterial infection. Also called *purulent synovitis, pyarthrosis*.

suppurative gingivitis *n.* Gingivitis in which the gums exude pus.

suppurative hyalitis *n.* Purulent inflammation of the vitreous humor of the eye resulting from exudation from adjacent structures.

suppurative inflammation *n.* See **purulent inflammation.**

suppurative nephritis *n.* Focal glomerulonephritis with abscess formation in the kidney.

supra– *pref.* **1.** Above; over; on top of: *supracostal*. **2.** Greater than; transcending: *supraliminal*.

su·pra·bulge (so͞o′prə-bŭlj′) *n.* The portion of the crown of a tooth that converges toward the occlusal surface of the tooth.

su·pra·cal·lo·sal gyrus (so͞o′prə-kə-lō′səl) *n.* A thin layer of gray matter on the dorsal surface of the corpus callosum.

su·pra·cer·vi·cal hysterectomy (so͞o′prə-sûr′vĭ-kəl) *n.* Fundusectomy of the uterus, leaving the cervix in place. Also called *subtotal hysterectomy*.

su·pra·cho·roid (so͞o′prə-kôr′oid′) *adj.* On the outer side of the choroid of the eye.

su·pra·cli·noid aneurysm (so͞o′prə-klī′noid′) *n.* An intracranial aneurysm of the internal carotid artery that occurs above the clinoid bone.

su·pra·cos·tal (so͞o′prə-kŏs′təl) *adj.* Located above the ribs.

su·pra·cris·tal (so͞o′prə-krĭs′təl) *adj.* Above a crest.

su·pra·duc·tion (so͞o′prə-dŭk′shən) *n.* The moving upward of one eye independently of the other. Also called *sursumduction*.

su·pra·ep·i·con·dy·lar process (so͞o′prə-ĕp′ĭ-kŏn′dl-ər) *n.* An inconstant spine projecting from the anteromedial surface of the humerus above the medial epicondyle to which it is joined by a fibrous band, forming the supracondylar foramen that transmits the brachial artery and median nerve.

su·pra·lim·i·nal (soō'prə-lĭm'ə-nəl) *adj.* Being above the threshold of consciousness or of sensation. Used of stimuli.

su·pra·mar·gi·nal gyrus (soō'prə-mär'jə-nəl) *n.* A folded convolution capping the posterior extremity of the lateral sulcus.

su·pra·mas·toid crest (soō'prə-măs'toid') *n.* The ridge that forms the posterior root of the zygomatic process of the temporal bone.

su·pra·max·il·la (soō'prə-măk-sĭl'ə) *n.,* pl. **–max·il·lae** (-măk-sĭl'ē) The upper jaw or jawbone.

su·pra·max·il·lar·y (soō'prə-măk'sə-lĕr'ē) *adj.* **1.** Of or relating to the upper jaw. **2.** Located above the upper jaw.

su·pra·me·a·tal triangle (soō'prə-mē-āt'l) *n.* A triangle formed by the root of the zygomatic arch, the posterior wall of the bony external acoustic meatus, and a line connecting the extremities of the first two. It is used as a guide in mastoid operations. Also called *Macewen's triangle.*

su·pra·men·ta·le (soō'prə-měn-tā'lē) *n.* The most posterior midline point, above the chin and on the mandible between the infradentale and the pogonion. Also called *point B.*

su·pra·nu·cle·ar (soō'prə-noō'klē-ər) *adj.* **1.** Located above the level of the motor neurons of the spinal or cranial nerves. Used to indicate disorders of movement caused by destruction or functional impairment of brain structures, such as the motor cortex, pyramidal tract, or corpus striatum. **2.** Of or relating to the part of a cell between the nucleus and the distal border.

supranuclear paralysis *n.* Paralysis that is due to lesions above the primary motor neurons.

su·pra·oc·clu·sion (soō'prə-ə-kloō'zhən) *n.* A condition in which a tooth extends beyond the occlusal plane.

su·pra·op·tic commissure (soō'prə-ŏp'tĭk) *n.* Any of the commissural fibers that lie above and behind the optic chiasm.

supraoptic nucleus of hypothalamus *n.* A large-celled, neurosecretory nucleus in the hypothalamus, located over the lateral border of the optic tract, whose neurons produce vasopressin that is released into the general circulation from the axon terminals in the supraopticohypophysial tract.

su·pra·or·bit·al (soō'prə-ôr'bĭ-tl) *adj.* Located above the orbit of the eye.

supraorbital arch *n.* See **supraorbital ridge.**

supraorbital artery *n.* An artery with origin in the ophthalmic artery, with distribution to the scalp and the scalp muscle, and with anastomoses to the branches of the superficial temporal and the supratrochlear arteries.

supraorbital foramen *n.* An opening in the supraorbital margin of the frontal bone at the junction of the medial and intermediate thirds.

supraorbital nerve *n.* A branch of the frontal nerve, that itself branches to the forehead, scalp, upper eyelid, and frontal sinus.

supraorbital ridge *n.* The curved upper border of the entrance to the eye socket. Also called *supraorbital arch.*

supraorbital vein *n.* A vein that drains the front of the scalp and unites with the supratrochlear vein to form the angular vein.

su·pra·or·bi·to·me·a·tal plane (soō'prə-ôr'bĭ-tō-mē-āt'l) *n.* A plane that passes the superior orbital margins as well as the superior margins of the external acoustic meatuses.

su·pra·pa·tel·lar bursa (soō'prə-pə-tĕl'ər) *n.* A large bursa between the lower part of the thigh and the tendon of the quadriceps muscle, usually communicating with the cavity of the knee joint.

su·pra·phys·i·o·log·ic (soō'prə-fĭz'ē-ə-lŏj'ĭk) *or* **su·pra·phys·i·o·log·i·cal** (-ĭ-kəl) *adj.* **1.** Indicating a dose that is larger or more potent than would occur naturally, as of a chemical agent that mimics a hormone. **2.** Of or relating to the physiological effects of such a dose.

su·pra·pu·bic cystotomy (soō'prə-pyoō'bĭk) *n.* Incision above the pubic symphysis and into the bladder. Also called *epicystotomy.*

su·pra·re·nal (soō'prə-rē'nəl) *adj.* Located on or above the kidney. —*n.* A suprarenal part, especially an adrenal gland.

suprarenal artery *n.* **1.** An artery with origin in the renal artery, with distribution to an adrenal gland; inferior suprarenal artery. **2.** An artery with origin in the aorta, with distribution to an adrenal gland, and with anastomoses to the superior and inferior suprarenal arteries; middle suprarenal artery. **3.** An artery with origin in the inferior phrenic artery, with distribution to an adrenal gland; superior suprarenal artery.

su·pra·re·nal·ec·to·my (soō'prə-rē'nə-lĕk'tə-mē) *n.* See **adrenalectomy.**

suprarenal gland *n.* See **adrenal gland.**

su·pra·scap·u·lar (soō'prə-skăp'yə-lər) *adj.* Located above the scapula, as an artery or a nerve.

suprascapular artery *n.* An artery with its origin in the thyrocervical trunk, with distribution to the clavicle, scapula, muscles of the shoulder, and shoulder joint; and with anastomoses to the transverse cervical circumflex scapular artery. Also called *transverse scapular artery.*

suprascapular nerve *n.* A nerve that arises from the fifth and sixth cervical nerves, supplies the supraspinatus and infraspinatus muscles, and sends branches to the shoulder joint.

suprascapular vein *n.* A vein that accompanies the suprascapular artery and empties into the external jugular vein.

su·pra·scle·ral (soō'prə-sklîr'əl) *adj.* Located on the outer side of the sclera.

su·pra·spi·na·tus (soō'prə-spī-nā'təs) *n.* A muscle with origin from the supraspinous fossa of the scapula, with insertion into the humerus, with nerve supply from the suprascapular nerve, and whose action abducts the arm.

su·pra·spi·nous ligament (soō'prə-spī'nəs) *n.* A fibrous band attached to the tips of the spinous processes from the seventh cervical vertebra to the sacrum.

su·pra·troch·le·ar artery (soō'prə-trŏk'lē-ər) *n.* See **frontal artery.**

supratrochlear nerve *n.* A branch of the frontal nerve supplying the medial part of the upper eyelid, the central part of the skin of the forehead, and the root of the nose.

supratrochlear vein *n.* Any of the veins that drain the front part of the scalp and unite with the supraorbital vein to form the angular vein.

su·pra·val·var stenosis (sōō′prə-văl′vər) *n.* Narrowing of the aorta above the aortic valve, usually by a constricting ring.

su·pra·ven·tric·u·lar (sōō′prə-věn-trĭk′yə-lər) *adj.* Located or occurring above the ventricles.

supraventricular crest *n.* The internal muscular ridge that separates the arterial cone from the rest of the cavity of the right ventricle of the heart.

supraventricular tachycardia *n.* *Abbr.* **SVT** A tachycardia that originates above the ventricles of the heart, as in the atria or the atrioventricular node.

su·pra·ver·gence (sōō′prə-vûr′jəns) *n.* The upward rotation of one eye while the other eye remains stationary. Also called *sursumvergence.*

su·pra·ver·sion (sōō′prə-vûr′zhən) *n.* **1.** The act or an instance of turning upward. **2.** The condition in which a tooth is out of the line of occlusion in an occlusal direction, resulting in a deep overbite. **3.** The act or process of moving the eyes upwards. Also called *sursumversion.*

su·pra·vi·tal (sōō′prə-vīt′l) *adj.* Relating to or capable of staining living cells after their removal from a living or recently dead organism.

supravital stain *n.* A procedure in which living tissue is removed from the body and cells are placed in a nontoxic dye solution so that their vital processes may be studied.

su·ra (sōōr′ə) *n.,* *pl.* **su·rae** (sōōr′ē) The calf of the leg. —**su′ral** *adj.*

sural artery *n.* Any of four or five arteries arising from the popliteal artery, with distribution to the muscles and integument of the calf, and with anastomoses to the posterior tibial, medial and lateral inferior genicular arteries.

sural nerve *n.* A nerve that is formed by the union of the medial sural cutaneous nerve and a branch of the common peroneal nerve and accompanies the small saphenous vein around the lateral malleolus to the dorsum of the foot.

sur·face (sûr′fəs) *n.* The outer or topmost part of a solid structure.

surface-active *adj.* Of, relating to, or being a substance capable of reducing the surface tension of a liquid in which it is dissolved. Used especially of detergents.

surface analgesia *n.* See **topical anesthesia.**

surface anatomy *n.* The study of the configuration of the surface of the body, especially in relation to its internal parts.

surface epithelium *n.* Epithelium covering the embryonic genital ridges and the gonads that develop from them. Also called *germinal epithelium.*

surface tension *n.* A property of liquids arising from unbalanced molecular cohesive forces at or near the surface, as a result of which the surface tends to contract and exhibit properties resembling those of a stretched elastic membrane.

surface-tension theory of narcosis *n.* The theory that substances that lower the surface tension of water pass more readily into a cell and cause narcosis by decreasing metabolism.

sur·fac·tant (sər-făk′tənt, sûr′făk′-) *n.* **1.** A surface-active substance. **2.** A substance composed of lipoprotein that is secreted by the alveolar cells of the lung and serves to maintain the stability of pulmonary tissue by reducing the surface tension of fluids that coat the lung.

surf·er's knobs (sûr′fərz) *pl.n.* Tumorlike skin nodules just below the knees, on the tops of the feet, and often on the toes, common among surfers who paddle in a kneeling position.

sur·geon (sûr′jən) *n.* A physician who specializes in surgery.

Surgeon General *n.,* *pl.* **Surgeons General 1.** The chief general officer in the medical departments of the US Army, Navy, or Air Force. **2.** The chief medical officer in the US Public Health Service or in a state public health service.

sur·geon's knot (sûr′jənz) *n.,* *pl.* **surgeons' knots** Any of several knots, especially one similar to a square knot, used in surgery for tying ligatures or stitching incisions.

sur·ger·y (sûr′jə-rē) *n.* **1.** The branch of medicine that deals with the diagnosis and treatment of injury, deformity, and disease by manual and instrumental means. **2.** A surgical operation or procedure, especially one involving the removal or replacement of a diseased organ or tissue. **3.** An operating room or a laboratory of a surgeon or of a hospital's surgical staff. **4.** The skill or work of a surgeon.

sur·gi·cal (sûr′jĭ-kəl) *adj.* **1.** Of, relating to, or characteristic of surgeons or surgery. **2.** Used in surgery. **3.** Resulting from or occurring after surgery.

surgical abdomen *n.* See **acute abdomen.**

surgical anatomy *n.* The application of anatomical knowledge to surgical diagnosis and treatment.

surgical anesthesia *n.* **1.** Anesthesia administered so that a surgical procedure can be performed. **2.** Loss of sensation with muscle relaxation adequate for surgery.

surgical diathermy *n.* The use of electrocautery for coagulation or cauterization, as for sealing a blood vessel, resulting in local tissue destruction.

surgical emphysema *n.* Subcutaneous emphysema from air trapped in the tissues during a surgical operation or by injury.

surgical microscope *n.* A binocular microscope used to visualize fine structures within the area of a surgical procedure. Also called *operating microscope.*

surgical pathology *n.* A field in anatomical pathology concerned with examination of surgical specimens of tissues removed from living patients for the purpose of diagnosis of disease and guidance in the care of patients.

surgical prosthesis *n.* An appliance serving as an aid to or as a part of a surgical procedure, such as a heart valve or cranial plate.

surgical splint *n.* Any of various devices used to maintain tissues in a new position following surgery.

sur·gi·cen·ter (sûr′jĭ-sĕn′tər) *n.* A surgical facility for operations that do not require hospitalization.

sur·ro·gate (sûr′ə-gĭt, -gāt′) *n.* **1.** One that takes the place of another; a substitute. **2.** A person or an animal that functions as a substitute for another, as in a social or family role. **3.** A figure of authority who takes the place of the father or mother in a person's unconscious or emotional life. **4.** A surrogate mother.

surrogate mother *n.* A woman who agrees to bear a child for another woman, either through artificial insemination by the other woman's husband or partner or by carrying until birth the other woman's surgically implanted fertilized egg. —**surrogate motherhood** *n.*

sur·sum·duc·tion (sûr′səm-dŭk′shən) *n.* See **supraduction.**

sur·sum·ver·gence (sûr′səm-vûr′jəns) *n.* See **supravergence.**

sur·sum·ver·sion (sûr′səm-vûr′zhən) *n.* See **supraversion** (sense 3).

sur·veil·lance (sər-vā′ləns) *n.* **1.** Close observation of a person or group, especially one under suspicion. **2.** The act of observing or the condition of being observed. **3.** The collection, collation, analysis, and dissemination of data. **4.** A type of observational study that involves continuous monitoring of disease occurrence within a population.

sus·cep·ti·ble (sə-sĕp′tə-bəl) *adj.* **1.** Likely to be affected with a disease, infection, or condition. **2.** Especially sensitive; highly impressionable. —**sus·cep·ti·bil′i·ty** (sə-sĕp′tə-bĭl′ĭ-tē) *n.*

sus·pend·ed animation (sə-spĕn′dĭd) *n.* A temporary interruption of the vital functions resembling death.

sus·pen·sion (sə-spĕn′shən) *n.* **1.** A noncolloidal dispersion of solid particles in a liquid, often used for pharmaceutical preparations. **2.** The fixation of an organ to other tissue for support, as the uterus. **3.** The hanging of a part from a support, such as a plaster-encased limb.

sus·pen·soid (sə-spĕn′soid′) *n.* A colloid solution in which the disperse particles are solid and remain sharply demarcated from the fluid in which they are suspended.

sus·pen·so·ry (sə-spĕn′sə-rē) *adj.* Of or relating to a ligament, muscle, or other structure that supports or suspends an organ or another part. —*n.* **1.** A support or truss. **2.** An athletic supporter.

suspensory bandage *n.* An expandable bag used to support the scrotum and its contents.

suspensory ligament of axilla *n.* A downward extension of the clavipectoral fascia that attaches to the axillary fascia, forming the armpit hollow.

suspensory ligament of breast *n.* Any of the numerous, well-developed fibrous bands of the skin that extend from the overlying skin to the fibrous stroma of the mammary gland.

suspensory ligament of eyeball *n.* A thickening of the inferior part of the bulbar sheath that supports the eye within its orbit.

suspensory ligament of lens *n.* See **ciliary zonule.**

suspensory ligament of ovary *n.* A band of peritoneum that extends upward from the upper pole of the ovary and contains the ovarian vessels and the ovarian plexus of nerves.

suspensory muscle of duodenum *n.* A broad flat band

of smooth muscle and fibrous tissue attached to the right crus of the diaphragm and to the duodenum at its junction with the jejunum.

sus·tained-ac·tion tablet (sə-stānd′ăk′shən) *n.* A tablet that releases its active ingredient in specified doses at timed intervals. Also called *sustained-release tablets.*

sus·ten·tac·u·lar (sŭs′tən-tăk′yə-lər) *adj.* Serving to support.

sustentacular cell *n.* One of the supporting cells of an epithelial membrane or tissue.

sus·ten·tac·u·lum (sŭs′tən-tăk′yə-ləm) *n.,* *pl.* **–la** (-lə) An anatomical structure that supports another anatomical structure.

Sus·ti·va (sə-stē′və) A trademark for the drug efavirenz.

Suth·er·land (sŭth′ər-lənd), **Earl Wilbur, Jr** 1915–1974. American physiologist. He won a 1971 Nobel Prize for showing that cyclic AMP within the cell is the agent that moderates the action of hormones.

Sut·ton (sŭt′n), **Walter Stanborough** 1877–1916. American physician and geneticist who described the behavior of chromosomes in cell division and provided evidence that chromosomes contain units of inheritance.

Sut·ton's disease (sŭt′nz) *n.* **1.** See **periadenitis mucosa necrotica recurrens. 2.** See **halo nevus.**

su·tu·ra (soo-toor′ə) *n.,* *pl.* **–tu·rae** (-toor′ē) An anatomical suture.

sutural bone *n.* Any of several irregular bones that are located along the sutures of the cranium, particularly those bones related to the parietal bone. Also called *wormian bone.*

sutural ligament *n.* A delicate membrane binding skull bones together at the cranial sutures.

su·ture (soo′chər) *n.* **1.** The line of junction or an immovable joint between two bones, especially of the skull. **2.** The process of joining two surfaces or edges together along a line by or as if by sewing. **3.** The surgical method used to close a wound or join tissues. **4.** The fine thread or other material used surgically to close a wound or join tissues. **5.** The line so formed. —*v.* To join by means of sutures or a suture. —**su′tur·al** *adj.*

su·tur·ec·to·my (soo′chə-rĕk′tə-mē) *n.* The surgical removal of a cranial suture.

SV40 (ĕs′vē-fôr′tē) *n.* A virus that causes cancers in monkeys and that is used widely in genetic and medical research.

SVC *abbr.* superior vena cava

Sved·berg unit (svĕd′bərg, -bĕr′ē) *n.* A sedimentation constant of 1×10^{-13} seconds.

SVT *abbr.* supraventricular tachycardia

swab (swŏb) *n.* **1.** A small piece of absorbent material attached to the end of a stick or wire and used for cleansing or applying medicine. **2.** A specimen of mucus or other material removed with a swab.

swal·low (swŏl′ō) *v.* To pass something, as food or drink, through the mouth and throat into the stomach.

swal·low·ing reflex (swŏl′ō-ĭng) *n.* Swallowing caused by stimulation of the palate, fauces, or posterior pharyngeal wall. Also called *pharyngeal reflex.*

swamp fever (swŏmp) *n.* See **malaria.**

Swan-Ganz catheter (swŏn′gănz′) *n.* A soft catheter

with an expandable balloon tip that is used for measuring blood pressure in the pulmonary artery.

S wave *n.* A downward deflection of the QRS complex in an electrocardiogram following an R wave.

sweat (swĕt) *v.* To excrete perspiration through the pores in the skin; perspire. —*n.* **1.** The colorless saline moisture excreted by the sweat glands; perspiration. **2.** The process of sweating.

sweat gland *n.* Any of the small, tubular glands that are found nearly everywhere in the skin of humans, that secrete perspiration externally through pores, and that comprise the apocrine sweat and eccrine glands. Also called *sudoriferous gland.*

sweat gland carcinoma *n.* A sporatically growing tumor that is nodular and fixed to the skin and underlying structure.

Swed·ish massage (swē′dĭsh) *n.* A system of therapeutic massage and exercise for the muscles and joints, developed in Sweden in the 19th century.

swell·ing (swĕl′ĭng) *n.* **1.** Something swollen, especially an abnormally swollen body part or area. **2.** A primordial elevation that develops into a fold, ridge, or process.

Swift's disease (swĭfts) *n.* See **acrodynia** (sense 1).

swim·mer's itch (swĭm′ərz) *n.* See **schistosome dermatitis.**

swim·ming pool conjunctivitis (swĭm′ĭng pōol′) *n.* See **inclusion conjunctivitis.**

swimming pool granuloma *n.* A chronic, low-grade, wartlike lesion most commonly seen on the knee and caused by mycobacterial infection of a cut or scrape sustained in a swimming pool.

swine influenza (swīn) *n.* A highly contagious form of human influenza caused by a filterable virus identical or related to a virus formerly isolated from infected swine. Also called *swine flu.*

switch·ing site (swĭch′ĭng) *n.* Any of the break points in a DNA sequence at which a gene segment unites with another gene segment and causes genetic rearrangement of the sequence, as in the production of the immunoglobulins.

Swy·er-James syndrome (swī′ər-) *n.* Decrease in size of one lung due to obliterating bronchiolitis or some other disorder and resulting in compensatory overinflation of the normal lung.

sx *abbr.* symptoms

sy·co·ma (sī-kō′mə) *n.* A pendulous figlike growth or wart.

sy·co·si·form (sī-kō′sə-fôrm′) *adj.* Resembling sycosis.

sy·co·sis (sī-kō′sĭs) *n.* A chronic inflammation of the hair follicles, especially of the beard, characterized by the eruption of pimples and nodules. Also called *ficosis.*

Syd·en·ham (sĭd′n-əm), **Thomas** 1624–1689. English physician who advocated the Hippocratic ideals of observation and experience in medicine, and recorded detailed firsthand accounts of numerous maladies, including gout, malarial fever, measles, dysentery, hysteria, and Sydenham's chorea.

Syd·en·ham's chorea (sĭd′n-əmz) *n.* An acute toxic or infective disorder of the nervous system, usually associated with acute rheumatic fever, occurring in young persons and characterized by involuntary, irregular,

jerky movement of the muscles of the face, neck, and limbs. Also called *Saint Vitus' dance.*

syl·vi·an (sĭl′vē-ən) *adj.* Relating to or described by Franciscus Sylvius (Franz de la Boö; 1614–1672), German-born Dutch physician and anatomist, or Jacobus Sylvius (Jaques Dubois; 1478–1555), French anatomist.

sylvian aqueduct *n.* See **cerebral aqueduct.**

sylvian fissure *n.* Variant of **fissure of Sylvius.**

sym– *pref.* Variant of **syn–.**

sym·bal·lo·phone (sĭm-băl′ə-fōn′) *n.* A stethoscope fitted with two chest pieces, allowing a lateral comparison of sounds.

sym·bi·on (sĭm′bē-ŏn′, -bī-) *or* **sym·bi·ote** (-ōt′) *or* **sym·bi·ont** (-ŏnt′) *n.* An organism associated with another in symbiosis. Also called *mutualist.*

sym·bi·o·sis (sĭm′bē-ō′sĭs, -bī-) *n.,* *pl.* **–ses** (-sēz) **1.** A close, prolonged association between two or more different organisms of different species that may, but does not necessarily, benefit each member. **2.** A relationship of mutual benefit or dependence.

sym·bi·ot·ic (sĭm′bē-ŏt′ĭk, -bī-) *adj.* Of, resembling, or relating to symbiosis.

sym·bleph·a·ron (sĭm-blĕf′ə-rŏn′) *n.* The adhesion of one or both eyelids to the eyeball.

sym·bleph·a·ro·pte·ryg·i·um (sĭm-blĕf′ə-rō-tə-rĭj′ē-əm) *n.* The union of eyelid to eyeball by a cicatricial band of membrane similar to a pterygium.

sym·bol (sĭm′bəl) *n.* **1.** Something that represents something else by association, resemblance, or convention, especially a material object used to represent something invisible. **2.** A printed or written sign used to represent an operation, an element, a quantity, or a relation, as in mathematics or chemistry. **3.** A conventional sign.

sym·bol·ism (sĭm′bə-lĭz′əm) *n.* **1.** A mental state in which everything that happens is regarded by the individual as symbolic of his or her own thoughts. **2.** The disguised representation in conscious thought of unconscious or repressed contents or events.

sym·bol·i·za·tion (sĭm′bə-lĭ-zā′shən) *n.* An unconscious mental mechanism whereby one object or idea is represented by another and is not consciously recognized as such.

sym·brach·y·dac·ty·ly (sĭm-brăk′ē-dăk′tə-lē) *n.* A condition in which abnormally short fingers or toes are joined or webbed in their proximal portions.

Sym·me·trel (sĭm′ə-trĕl′) A trademark for the drug amantadine hydrochloride.

sym·met·ri·cal gangrene (sĭ-mĕt′rĭ-kəl) *n.* Gangrene affecting the extremities of both sides of the body; seen especially in severe arteriosclerosis, myocardial infarction, and ball-valve thrombus.

sym·me·try (sĭm′ĭ-trē) *n.* Exact correspondence of form and constituent configuration on opposite sides of a dividing line or plane or about a center or an axis.

sympath– *pref.* Variant of **sympatho–.**

sym·pa·thec·to·my (sĭm′pə-thĕk′tə-mē) *or* **sym·pa·the·tec·to·my** (sĭm′pə-thē-tĕk′tə-mē) *n.* Surgical removal of a part of the sympathetic nervous system.

sym·pa·thet·ic (sĭm′pə-thĕt′ĭk) *adj.* Of, relating to, or acting on the sympathetic nervous system.

sympathetic amine *n.* See **sympathomimetic amine.**

sympathetic ganglia *n.* Any of the ganglia of the autonomic nervous system composed of adrenergic neurons receiving afferent fibers originating from preganglionic visceral motor neurons in the lateral horn of the thoracic and upper lumbar segments of the spinal cord.

sympathetic imbalance *n.* See **vagotonia.**

sympathetic nerve *n.* One of the nerves of the sympathetic nervous system.

sympathetic nervous system *n.* The part of the autonomic nervous system originating in the thoracic and lumbar regions of the spinal cord that in general inhibits or opposes the physiological effects of the parasympathetic nervous system, as in tending to reduce digestive secretions or speed up the heart.

sympathetic ophthalmia *n.* A swelling of the uvea in an uninjured eye caused by a wound of the uvea of the other eye. It may eventually lead to bilateral blindness.

sympathetic trunk *n.* Either of two long ganglionated nerve strands along the vertebral column that are connected to each spinal nerve by gray matter rami and that receive fibers from the spinal cord through white matter rami connecting with the thoracic and upper lumbar spinal nerves.

sympathetic uveitis *n.* Inflammation of the uveal tract of the uninjured eye due to a perforating wound of the uveal tract of the other eye.

sym·pa·thet·o·blast (sĭm′pə-thĕt′ə-blăst′) *n.* See **sympathoblast.**

sym·pa·thet·o·blas·to·ma (sĭm′pə-thĕt′ō-blă-stō′mə) *n.* See **sympathoblastoma.**

sympathico– *pref.* Sympathetic nervous system: *sympathicotonia.*

sym·path·i·co·blast (sĭm-păth′ĭ-kō-blăst′) *n.* See **sympathoblast.**

sym·path·i·co·blas·to·ma (sĭm-păth′ĭ-kō-blă-stō′mə) *n.* See **sympathoblastoma.**

sym·path·i·co·go·ni·o·ma (sĭm-păth′ĭ-kō-gō′nē-ō′-mə) *n.* See **sympathoblastoma.**

sym·path·i·co·lyt·ic (sĭm-păth′ĭ-kō-lĭt′ĭk) *adj.* Having sympatholytic activity.

sym·path·i·co·mi·met·ic (sĭm-păth′ĭ-kō-mĭ-mĕt′ĭk, -mī-) *adj.* Sympathomimetic.

sym·path·i·co·to·ni·a (sĭm-păth′ĭ-kō-tō′nē-ə) *n.* A condition in which there is increased tonicity of the sympathetic nervous system, marked by vascular spasm and high blood pressure.

sym·path·i·co·ton·ic (sĭm-păth′ĭ-kō-tŏn′ĭk) *adj.* Of, relating to, or characterized by sympathicotonia.

sym·path·i·co·trip·sy (sĭm-păth′ĭ-kō-trĭp′sē) *n.* Surgical crushing of the sympathetic ganglion.

sym·path·i·co·tro·pic (sĭm-păth′ĭ-kō-trŏp′ĭk) *adj.* Having a specific affinity for the sympathetic nervous system.

sym·pa·thin (sĭm′pə-thĭn) *n.* A substance, such as norepinephrine, that diffuses into the circulation from the terminals of active sympathetic nerves and serves as a chemical mediator.

sympatho– *or* **sympath–** *pref.* Sympathetic nervous system: *sympathoadrenal.*

sym·pa·tho·blast (sĭm′pə-thō-blăst′) *n.* A primitive cell derived from neuroglia of the neural crest that develops into a cell of the adrenal medulla. Also called *sympathetoblast, sympathicoblast.*

sym·pa·tho·blas·to·ma (sĭm′pə-thō-blă-stō′mə) *n.* A completely undifferentiated malignant tumor made up of sympathoblasts and originating from embryonal cells of the sympathetic nervous system. Also called *sympathetoblastoma, sympathicoblastoma, sympathicogonioma, sympathogonioma.*

sym·pa·tho·go·ni·a (sĭm′pə-thō-gō′nē-ə) *pl.n.* The completely undifferentiated cells that develop into cells of the sympathetic nervous system.

sym·pa·tho·go·ni·o·ma (sĭm′pə-thō-gō′nē-ō′mə) *n.* See **sympathoblastoma.**

sym·pa·tho·lyt·ic (sĭm′pə-thō-lĭt′ĭk) *adj.* Opposing the physiological effects caused by stimulation of the sympathetic nervous system.

sym·pa·tho·mi·met·ic (sĭm′pə-thō-mĭ-mĕt′ĭk, -mī-) *adj.* Producing physiological effects resembling those caused by the action of the sympathetic nervous system. —**sym′pa·tho·mi·met′ic** *n.*

sympathomimetic amine *n.* An agent that elicits physiological responses similar to those produced during adrenergic nerve activity. Also called *adrenergic amine, adrenomimetic amine, sympathetic amine.*

sym·pa·thy (sĭm′pə-thē) *n.* **1.** A relation between parts or organs by which a disease or disorder in one induces an effect in the other. **2.** Mental contagion, as in yawning induced by seeing another person yawn. **3.** Mutual understanding or affection arising from a relationship or an affinity, in which whatever affects one correspondingly affects the other.

sym·phal·an·gism (sĭm-făl′ən-jĭz′əm) *n.* **1.** See **syndactyly. 2.** Ankylosis of the finger or toe joints.

sym·phys·i·al (sĭm-fĭz′ē-əl) *or* **sym·phy·se·al** (sĭm′fĭ-sē′əl, sĭm-fĭz′ē-əl) *adj.* Of, relating to, or characterized by a symphysis.

sym·phys·i·on (sĭm-fĭz′ē-ŏn′) *n.* The most anterior point of the alveolar process of the mandible.

sym·phys·i·ot·o·my (sĭm-fĭz′ē-ŏt′ə-mē, sĭm′fə-zē-) *n.* Surgical division of the pubic symphysis, especially to permit the passage of a fetus during delivery. Also called *pelviotomy, synchondrotomy.*

sym·phy·sis (sĭm′fĭ-sĭs) *n., pl.* **–ses** (-sēz′) **1.** A form of cartilaginous joint in which union between two bones is effected by fibrocartilage without a synovial membrane. **2.** A union, meeting point, or commissure of two structures. **3.** A growing together of bones originally separate, as of the two pubic bones. **4.** A line or junction thus formed. **5.** A pathological adhesion or growing together.

sym·po·di·a (sĭm-pō′dē-ə) *n.* Fusion of the feet, as in sirenomelia.

sym·port (sĭm′pôrt′) *n.* The transport of two different molecules or ions in the same direction through a membrane using a common carrier mechanism.

symp·tom (sĭm′təm, sĭmp′-) *n.* A subjective indication of a disorder or disease, such as pain, nausea, or weakness.

symp·to·mat·ic (sĭm′tə-măt′ĭk, sĭmp′-) *adj.* **1.** Of, relating to, or based on symptoms. **2.** Constituting a symptom, as of a disease.

symptomatic porphyria *n.* See **porphyria cutanea tarda.**

symptomatic pruritus *n.* Itching occurring as a symptom of some systemic illness.

symptomatic reaction *n.* An allergic response to a test for or a therapeutic dose of an allergen or atopen that resembles the original allergic response.

symp·to·ma·tol·o·gy (sĭm′tə-mə-tŏl′ə-jē, sĭmp′-) *n.* **1.** The medical science of symptoms. **2.** The combined symptoms of a disease.

symp·to·mat·o·lyt·ic (sĭm′tə-măt′ə-lĭt′ĭk, sĭmp′tə-) *or* **symp·to·mo·lyt·ic** (-tə-mə-lĭt′ĭk) *adj.* Serving to eradicate symptoms.

symptom complex *n.* A group of symptoms that occur together and are characteristic of a certain disease, disorder, or condition.

symptom formation *n.* The process of developing a physical or behavioral substitute for an unconscious impulse or a conflict that causes anxiety, such as avoiding crowds. Also called *symptom substitution.*

symp·to·sis (sĭm-tō′sĭs, sĭmp-) *n.* A localized or general wasting of the body.

syn– *or* **sym–** *pref.* **1.** Together; with: *synclonus.* **2.** United: *syncephaly.* **3.** Same; similar: *synteny.* **4.** At the same time: *synesthesia.*

syn·apse (sĭn′ăps′, sĭ-năps′) *n.* The junction across which a nerve impulse passes from an axon terminal to a neuron, a muscle cell, or a gland cell.

syn·ap·sis (sĭ-năp′sĭs) *n.,* *pl.* **–ses** (-sēz) The side-by-side association of homologous paternal and maternal chromosomes during early meiotic prophase.

syn·ap·tic (sĭ-năp′tĭk) *adj.* Of or relating to synapsis or a synapse.

synaptic cleft *n.* See **synaptic gap.**

synaptic conduction *n.* The conduction of a nerve impulse across a synapse.

synaptic gap *n.* The minute space between the cell membrane of an axon terminal and of the target cell with which it synapses. Also called *synaptic cleft.*

synaptic vesicle *n.* Any of several small, intracellular, membrane-bound vesicles at a synaptic junction of neurons that contain the neurotransmitter.

syn·ap·ti·ne·mal complex (sĭ-năp′tə-nē′məl) *n.* A submicroscopic structure interposed between the homologous chromosome pairs during synapsis.

syn·ap·to·some (sĭ-năp′tə-sōm′) *n.* A saclike structure containing synaptic vesicles and mitochondria, which breaks away from axon terminals when brain tissue is homogenized under controlled conditions.

syn·ar·thro·di·a (sĭn′ăr-thrō′dē-ə) *n.,* *pl.* **–di·ae** (-dē-ē′) See **immovable joint.**

syn·ar·thro·di·al (sĭn′ăr-thrō′dē-əl) *adj.* Of or relating to synarthrosis.

synarthrodial joint *n.* **1.** See **immovable joint.** **2.** See **movable joint** (sense 2).

syn·ar·thro·phy·sis (sĭn-är′thrō-fī′sĭs) *n.* The process or condition of ankylosis.

syn·ar·thro·sis (sĭn′ăr-thrō′sĭs) *n.,* *pl.* **–ses** (-sēz) **1.** See **immovable joint.** **2.** See **movable joint** (sense 1, 2).

syn·can·thus (sĭn-kăn′thəs) *n.* Adhesion of the eyeball to the orbital structures.

syn·ceph·a·lus (sĭn-sĕf′ə-ləs) *n.* Conjoined twins having a single head.

syn·chei·li·a *or* **syn·chi·li·a** (sĭn-kī′lē-ə) *n.* Congenital adhesion of the lips.

syn·chei·ri·a *or* **syn·chi·ri·a** (sĭn-kī′rē-ə) *n.* A form of dyscheiria in which a stimulus applied to one side of the body is referred to both sides.

syn·chon·dro·di·al joint (sĭng′kŏn-drō′dē-əl, sĭn′-) *n.* See **synchondrosis.**

syn·chon·dro·se·ot·o·my (sĭn′kŏn-drō′sē-ŏt′ə-mē) *n.* A procedure for cutting through a synchondrosis, especially cutting through the sacroiliac ligaments and forcibly closing the arch of the pubes in the treatment of exstrophy of the bladder.

syn·chon·dro·sis (sĭng′kŏn-drō′sĭs, sĭn′-) *n.,* *pl.* **–ses** (-sēz) A rigid union between two bones formed either by hyaline cartilage or by fibrocartilage. Also called *synchondrodial joint.*

syn·chon·drot·o·my (sĭn′kŏn-drŏt′ə-mē) *n.* See **symphysiotomy.**

syn·chro·ni·a (sĭn-krō′nē-ə, sĭng-) *n.* **1.** See **synchronism.** **2.** The origination, development, involution, or functioning of tissues or organs at the usual time.

syn·chron·ic study (sĭn-krŏn′ĭk, sĭng-) *n.* A study of the structure of a population at one point in time. Also called *cross-sectional study.*

syn·chro·nism (sĭng′krə-nĭz′əm, sĭn′-) *n.* Coincidence in time; simultaneousness. Also called *synchronia.*

syn·chro·nous (sĭng′krə-nəs, sĭn′-) *adj.* Occurring or existing at the same time.

syn·chy·sis (sĭn′kĭ-sĭs, sĭng′-) *n.* The collapse of the collagenous framework of the vitreous humor with liquefaction of the vitreous body.

synchysis scin·til·lans (sĭn′tə-lănz′) *n.* An accumulation of cholesterol crystals in the vitreous humor, having the appearance of glistening spots in the eye.

syn·clit·ic (sĭn-klĭt′ĭk, sĭng-) *adj.* Of, relating to, or marked by synclitism.

syn·cli·tism (sĭn′klĭ-tĭz′əm, sĭng′-) *n.* The condition of parallelism between the plane of the pelvis and that of the fetal head.

syn·clo·nus (sĭn′klō′nəs) *n.* **1.** Clonic spasm or tremor of several muscles at the same time. **2.** A disease characterized by such spasms or tremors.

syn·co·pal (sĭng′kə-pəl, sĭn′-) *adj.* Of or relating to syncope.

syn·co·pe (sĭng′kə-pē, sĭn′-) *n.* A brief loss of consciousness caused by a sudden fall of blood pressure or failure of the cardiac systole, resulting in cerebral anemia.

syn·cop·ic (sĭn-kŏp′ĭk) *adj.* Syncopal.

syncytial knot *n.* A localized aggregation of syncytiotrophoblastic nuclei in the villi of the placenta during early pregnancy. Also called *syncytial bud.*

syn·cy·ti·o·tro·pho·blast (sĭn-sĭsh′ē-ō-trō′fə-blăst′) *n.* The syncytial outer layer of the trophoblast. Also called *syntrophoblast.*

syn·cy·ti·um (sĭn-sĭsh′ē-əm) *n.,* *pl.* **–cy·ti·a** (-sĭsh′ē-ə) A mass of cytoplasm having many nuclei but no internal cell boundaries. —**syn·cy′ti·al** *adj.*

syn·dac·tyl·i·a (sĭn′dăk-tĭl′ē-ə) *n.* See **syndactyly.**

syn·dac·tyl·ism (sĭn-dăk′tə-lĭz′əm) *n.* See **syndactyly.**

syn·dac·ty·lous (sĭn-dăk′tə-ləs) *adj.* Having fused or webbed fingers or toes.

syn·dac·ty·ly (sĭn-dăk′tə-lē) *n.* Webbing or fusion of the fingers or toes, involving soft parts only or including bone structure. Also called *symphalangism, syndactylia, syndactylism, zygodactyly.*

syn·de·sis (sĭn′dĭ-sĭs, sĭn-dē′-) *n.* See **arthrodesis.**

syn·des·mec·to·my (sĭn′dĕz-mĕk′tə-mē) *n.* The cutting away of a section of a ligament.

syn·des·mec·to·pi·a (sĭn-dĕz′mĕk-tō′pē-ə) *n.* Displacement of a ligament.

syn·des·mi·tis (sĭn′dĕz-mī′tĭs) *n.* Inflammation of a ligament.

syndesmo– or **syndesm–** *pref.* Ligament; ligamentous: *syndesmosis.*

syn·des·mo·di·al (sĭn′dĕz-mō′dē-əl) *adj.* Relating to syndesmosis.

syndesmodial joint *n.* See **syndesmosis.**

syn·des·mo·pex·y (sĭn-dĕz′mə-pĕk′sē) *n.* The surgical joining of two ligaments or the attachment of a ligament in a new place.

syn·des·mo·phyte (sĭn-dĕz′mə-fīt′) *n.* An osseous excrescence attached to a ligament.

syn·des·mo·plas·ty (sĭn-dĕz′mə-plăs′tē) *n.* Plastic surgery on a ligament.

syn·des·mor·rha·phy (sĭn′dĕz-môr′ə-fē) *n.* The suturing or repair of ligaments.

syn·des·mo·sis (sĭn′dĕz-mō′sĭs) *n., pl.* **–ses** (-sēz) A form of fibrous joint in which opposing surfaces that are relatively far apart are united by ligaments. Also called *syndesmodial joint.* —**syn′des·mot′ic** (-mŏt′ĭk) *adj.*

syn·des·mot·o·my (sĭn′dĕz-mŏt′ə-mē) *n.* Surgical division of a ligament.

syn·drome (sĭn′drōm′) *n.* A group of symptoms that collectively indicate or characterize a disease, a psychological disorder, or another abnormal condition. —**syn·drom′ic** (-drō′mĭk, -drŏm′ĭk) *adj.*

syndrome X *n.* A cluster of metabolic abnormalities, including insulin resistance, high blood levels of triglycerides, low blood levels of HDL-cholesterol, and obesity, that increase the risk of chronic diseases such as hypertension, coronary artery disease, and diabetes. Also called *metabolic syndrome.*

syn·ech·i·a (sĭ-nĕk′ē-ə, -nē′kē-ə) *n., pl.* **syn·ech·i·ae** (sĭ-nĕk′ē-ē′, -nē′kē-ē′) **1.** An adhesion of parts, especially involving the iris. **2.** Anterior synechia. **3.** Posterior synechia.

syn·ech·i·ot·o·my (sĭ-nĕk′ē-ŏt′ə-mē) *n.* Surgical division of a synechia.

syn·en·ceph·a·lo·cele (sĭn′ĕn-sĕf′ə-lō-sēl′) *n.* Protrusion of brain substance through a defect in the skull together with adhesions preventing restoration.

syn·er·e·sis (sĭ-nĕr′ĭ-sĭs) *n., pl.* **–ses** (-sēz′) The contraction of a gel, as a blood clot, and the exudation of part of its liquid component.

syn·er·get·ic (sĭn′ər-jĕt′ĭk) *adj.* Synergistic.

syn·er·gic (sĭ-nûr′jĭk) *adj.* Synergistic.

syn·er·gism (sĭn′ər-jĭz′əm) *n.* Synergy.

syn·er·gist (sĭn′ər-jĭst) *n.* A synergistic organ, drug, or agent.

syn·er·gis·tic (sĭn′ər-jĭs′tĭk) *adj.* **1.** Of or relating to synergy or a synergist. **2.** Producing or capable of producing synergy.

synergistic muscles *pl.n.* Muscles having similar and mutually helpful functions or actions.

syn·er·gy (sĭn′ər-jē) *n.* The interaction of two or more agents or forces so that their combined effect is greater than the sum of their individual effects.

syn·es·the·sia (sĭn′ĭs-thē′zhə) *n.* **1.** A condition in which one type of stimulation evokes the sensation of another, as when the hearing of a sound produces the visualization of a color. **2.** A sensation felt in one part of the body as a result of stimulus that is applied to another, as in referred pain. —**syn′es·thet′ic** (-thĕt′ĭk) *adj.*

syn·es·the·si·al·gia (sĭn′ĭs-thē′zē-ăl′jə) *n.* Painful synesthesia.

syn·ga·my (sĭng′gə-mē) *n.* The fusion of two gametes in fertilization. —**syn·gam′ic** (sĭn-găm′ĭk), **syn′ga·mous** (sĭng′gə-məs) *adj.*

syn·ge·ne·ic (sĭn′jə-nē′ĭk) *adj.* Genetically identical or closely related, so as to allow tissue transplant; immunologically compatible.

syngeneic graft *n.* See **syngraft.**

syngeneic homograft *n.* See **syngraft.**

syn·gen·e·sis (sĭn-jĕn′ĭ-sĭs) *n.* See **sexual reproduction.** —**syn′ge·net′ic** (-jə-nĕt′ĭk) *adj.*

syn·graft (sĭn′grăft′) *n.* A graft of tissue that is obtained from a donor who is genetically identical to the recipient. Also called *isogeneic graft, isogeneic homograft, isograft, isologous graft, isoplastic graft, syngeneic graft, syngeneic homograft.*

syn·i·ze·sis (sĭn′ĭ-zē′sĭs) *n.* **1.** Closure or obliteration of the pupil of the eye. **2.** The phase of meiosis in some species in which the chromatin contracts into a mass at one side of the nucleus.

syn·kar·y·on (sĭn-kăr′ē-ŏn′, -ē-ən) *n.* The nucleus of a fertilized egg immediately after the male and female nuclei have fused.

syn·ki·ne·sis (sĭn′kə-nē′sĭs, -kĭ-, sĭng′-) *n.* Involuntary movement of muscles or limbs accompanying a voluntary movement. —**syn′ki·net′ic** (-nĕt′ĭk) *adj.*

syn·o·nych·i·a (sĭn′ə-nĭk′ē-ə) *n.* Fusion of two or more nails of the digits, as in syndactyly.

syn·oph·thal·mi·a (sĭn′ŏf-thăl′mē-ə, -ŏp-) or **syn·oph·thal·mus** (-məs) *n.* See **cyclopia.**

syn·or·chi·dism (sĭn-ôr′kĭ-dĭz′əm) or **syn·or·chism** (sĭn-ôr′kĭz′əm) *n.* Congenital fusion of the testes in the abdominal cavity.

syn·os·che·os (sĭn-ŏs′kē-ŏs′) *n.* Partial or complete adhesion of the penis and scrotum.

syn·os·te·ot·o·my (sĭn-ŏs′tē-ŏt′ə-mē) *n.* See **arthrotomy.**

syn·os·to·sis (sĭn′ŏ-stō′sĭs) *n., pl.* **–ses** (-sēz) Fusion of normally separate bones. Also called *bony ankylosis, true ankylosis.* —**syn′os·tot′ic** (-tŏt′ĭk) *adj.*

syn·o·ti·a (sĭ-nō′shē-ə, -shə) *n.* Fusion or close approach of the lobes of the ears in otocephaly.

syn·o·vec·to·my (sĭn′ō-vĕk′tə-mē) *n.* Excision of part or all of the synovial membrane of a joint. Also called *villusectomy.*

syn·o·vi·a (sĭ-nō′vē-ə) *n.* A clear, thixotropic lubricating fluid secreted by membranes in joint cavities, tendon sheaths, and bursae. Also called *synovial fluid.* —syn·o′vi·al *adj.*

synovial bursa *n.* A sac containing synovial fluid at sites of friction, as between a tendon and a bone over which it moves, or subcutaneously over a bony prominence.

synovial crypt *n.* A diverticulum of the synovial membrane of a joint.

synovial cyst *n.* See **ganglion** (sense 2).

synovial fluid *n.* See **synovia.**

synovial frenulum *n.* See **vinculum of tendons.**

synovial hernia *n.* The protrusion of an inner synovial membrane through an opening in the stratum fibrosum of a joint capsule.

synovial joint *n.* See **movable joint** (sense 1).

synovial ligament *n.* One of the large synovial folds in a joint.

synovial membrane *n.* The connective-tissue membrane that lines the cavity of a synovial joint and produces the synovial fluid. Also called *synovium.*

synovial sheath *n.* The membrane lining the cavity of bone through which a tendon moves.

syn·o·vi·o·ma (sĭ-nō′vē-ō′mə) *n.* A tumor of synovial origin, involving a joint or tendon sheath.

syn·o·vi·tis (sĭn′ə-vī′tĭs, sī′nə-) *n.* Inflammation of a synovial membrane.

synovitis sic·ca (sĭk′ə) *n.* See **dry synovitis.**

syn·o·vi·um (sĭ-nō′vē-əm) *n.* See **synovial membrane.**

syn·pol·y·dac·ty·ly (sĭn′pŏl-ē-dăk′tə-lē) *n.* Syndactyly associated with polydactyly.

syn·te·ny (sĭn′tə-nē) *n.* The condition of two or more genes being on the same chromosome whether or not there is demonstrable linkage between them. —**syn·ten′ic** (-tĕn′ĭk) *adj.*

syn·thase (sĭn′thās′, -thāz′) *n.* Any of various enzymes that catalyze the synthesis of a substance without the use of a high-energy source such as cleavage of a phosphate bond in ATP.

syn·the·sis (sĭn′thĭ-sĭs) *n.,* *pl.* **-ses** (-sēz′) **1.** The combining of separate elements or substances to form a coherent whole. **2.** Formation of a chemical compound from simpler compounds or elements. **3.** A period in the cell cycle.

syn·the·size (sĭn′thĭ-sīz′) *v.* **1.** To combine so as to form a new, complex product. **2.** To form or produce by chemical synthesis.

syn·the·tase (sĭn′thĭ-tās′, -tāz′) *n.* See **ligase.**

syn·thet·ic (sĭn-thĕt′ĭk) *adj.* **1.** Relating to or involving synthesis. **2.** Produced by chemical synthesis, especially not of natural origin. —*n.* A synthetic chemical compound or material.

synthetic dye *n.* Any of the organic dyes originally derived from coal-tar derivatives, but currently synthesized from benzene and its derivatives.

Syn·throid (sĭn′throid′) A trademark for the drug levothyroxine sodium.

syn·ton·ic (sĭn-tŏn′ĭk) *adj.* Characterized by a normal emotional responsiveness to the environment.

syn·tro·pho·blast (sĭn-trō′fə-blăst′) *n.* See **syncytiotrophoblast.**

syn·tro·py (sĭn′trə-pē) *n.* **1.** The occasional tendency of two diseases to coalesce into one. **2.** The psychological state of wholesome association with others. **3.** A

number of similar structures inclined in one general direction, such as the ribs.

syph·i·lid (sĭf′ə-lĭd) *n.* Any of the cutaneous and mucous membrane lesions characteristic of secondary and tertiary syphilis.

syph·i·lis (sĭf′ə-lĭs) *n.* A chronic infectious disease caused by *Treponema pallidum,* either transmitted by direct contact, usually in sexual intercourse, or passed from mother to child in utero, and progressing through three stages characterized respectively by local formation of chancres, ulcerous skin eruptions, and systemic infection that leads to general paresis.

syph·i·lit·ic (sĭf′ə-lĭt′ĭk) *adj.* Of, relating to, or affected with syphilis. —*n.* A person with syphilis.

syphilitic abscess *n.* See **gummatous abscess.**

syphilitic aneurysm *n.* An aneurysm, usually involving the thoracic aorta, resulting from tertiary syphilitic aortitis.

syphilitic leukoderma *n.* A fading of the roseola that occurs with secondary syphilis, leaving reticulated depigmented and hyperpigmented areas located primarily on the sides of the neck. Also called *melanoleukoderma colli.*

syphilitic roseola *n.* Roseola marking the first eruption of syphilis, occurring 6 to 12 weeks after the initial lesion.

syphilo– *or* **syphil–** *or* **syphili–** *pref.* Syphilis; syphilitic: *syphilid.*

syph·i·lo·ma (sĭf′ə-lō′mə) *n.,* *pl.* **–mas** *or* **–ma·ta** (-mə-tə) See **gumma.**

Syr·ette (sĭ-rĕt′) A trademark for a collapsible tube having an attached hypodermic needle containing a single dose of medicine.

syr·ing·ad·e·no·ma (sĭr′ĭng-ăd′n-ō′mə, -găd′-) *or* **sy·rin·go·ad·e·no·ma** (sə-rĭng′gō-) *n.* A benign sweat gland tumor showing the glandular differentiation typical of secretory cells.

sy·ringe (sə-rĭnj′, sîr′ĭnj) *n.* **1.** An instrument used to inject fluids into the body or draw them from it. **2.** A hypodermic syringe.

sy·rin·ge·al (sə-rĭn′jē-əl) *adj.* Of, relating to, or resembling a syrinx.

syr·in·gec·to·my (sĭr′ĭn-jĕk′tə-mē) *n.* See **fistulectomy.**

syr·in·gi·tis (sĭr′ĭn-jī′tĭs) *n.* Inflammation of the eustachian tube.

syringo– *or* **syring–** *pref.* **1.** Fistula: *syringotomy.* **2.** Syrinx: *syringomyelocele.*

sy·rin·go·bul·bi·a (sə-rĭng′gō-bŭl′bē-ə) *n.* The abnormal presence of a fluid-filled cavity in the brainstem, analogous to syringomyelia.

sy·rin·go·car·ci·no·ma (sə-rĭng′gō-kär′sə-nō′mə) *n.* A malignant epithelial tumor that has undergone cystic change.

sy·rin·go·cele (sə-rĭng′gə-sēl′) *n.* A meningomyelocele in which there is a cavity in the protruding spinal cord.

sy·rin·go·cyst·ad·e·no·ma (sə-rĭng′gō-sĭ-stăd′n-ō′mə) *n.* A benign cystic tumor of the sweat glands.

sy·rin·go·cys·to·ma (sə-rĭng′gō-sĭ-stō′mə) *n.* See **hidrocystoma.**

syr·in·go·ma (sĭr′ĭng-gō′mə) *n.* A benign, often multiple, tumor of the sweat glands composed of very small round cysts.

sy·rin·go·me·nin·go·cele (sə-rĭng′gō-mə-nĭng′gə-sēl′) *n.* Spina bifida in which the dorsal sac consists chiefly of membranes enclosing a cavity that communicates with a syringomyelic cavity.

sy·rin·go·my·e·li·a (sə-rĭng′gō-mī-ē′lē-ə) *n.* A chronic disease of the spinal cord characterized by the presence of fluid-filled cavities and leading to spasticity and sensory disturbances. Also called *hydrosyringomyelia, Morvan's disease.* —**sy·rin′go·my·el′ic** (-ĕl′ĭk) *adj.*

sy·rin·go·my·e·lo·cele (sə-rĭng′gō-mī′ə-lə-sēl′) *n.* A form of spina bifida in which the fluid of the syrinx in the spinal cord is increased, expanding the cord tissue into a thin-walled sac that in turn expands through the vertebral defect.

syr·in·got·o·my (sĭr′ĭng-gŏt′ə-mē) *n.* See **fistulotomy.**

syr·inx (sîr′ĭngks) *n.,* *pl.* **syr·inx·es** *or* **sy·rin·ges** (sə-rĭn′jēz, -rĭng′gēz) A pathological tube-shaped cavity in the brain or spinal cord.

syr·up (sĭr′əp, sûr′-) *n.* A concentrated solution of sugar in water, often used as a vehicle for medicine.

sys·sar·co·sis (sĭs′är-kō′sĭs) *n.,* *pl* **−ses** (-sēz) The union or attachment of bones, such as the hyoid bone and lower jaw, by muscle.

sys·tal·tic (sĭ-stôl′tĭk, -stăl′-) *adj.* Alternately contracting and dilating, as the heart; pulsating.

sys·tem (sĭs′təm) *n.* **1.** A group of interacting, interrelated, or interdependent elements forming a complex whole. **2.** An organism or body considered as a whole, especially with regard to its vital processes or functions. **3.** A group of physiologically or anatomically complementary organs or parts.

sys·te·ma (sĭ-stē′mə) *n.* A complex of anatomical structures functionally related; a system.

sys·tem·at·ic name (sĭs′tə-măt′ĭk) *n.* A name composed of words or symbols that precisely describe chemical structure, thus allowing the structure of a chemical to be derived from its name.

sys·tem·a·tized delusion (sĭs′tə-mə-tīzd′) *n.* Any of various delusions that are logically founded upon false premises and form part of an organized group of related delusions.

Sys·tème In·ter·na·tion·al d′U·ni·tés (sē-stĕm′ ăn-tĕr-nä-syôN-näl′ dü-nē-tā′) *n.* International System of Units.

sys·tem·ic (sĭ-stĕm′ĭk) *adj.* **1.** Of or relating to a system. **2.** Of, relating to, or affecting the entire body or an entire organism. **3.** Relating to or affecting a particular body system, especially the nervous system. **4.** Relating to systemic circulation.

systemic anaphylaxis *n.* See **generalized anaphylaxis.**

systemic circulation *n.* Circulation of blood throughout the body through the arteries, capillaries, and veins, which carry oxygenated blood from the left ventricle to various tissues and return venous blood to the right atrium.

systemic lupus er·y·the·ma·to·sus (ĕr′ə-thē′mə-tō′səs, -thĕm′ə-) *n. Abbr.* **SLE** A chronic multisystemic inflammatory disease with variable features, frequently including fever, weakness and fatigability, joint pains or arthritis, skin lesions on the face, neck, or upper extremities, and often affecting the kidneys, spleen, and various other organs. Also called *disseminated lupus erythematosus.*

systemic vascular resistance *n.* An index of arteriolar constriction throughout the body, calculated by dividing the blood pressure by the cardiac output.

sys·to·le (sĭs′tə-lē) *n.* The rhythmic contraction of the heart, especially of the ventricles, by which blood is driven through the aorta and pulmonary artery after each dilation or diastole. Also called *miocardia.* —**sys·tol′ic** (sĭ-stŏl′ĭk) *adj.*

systolic gallop *n.* A triple cadence to the heart sounds in which the extra sound occurs during systole, usually in the form of a systolic click.

systolic murmur *n.* A murmur heard during ventricular systole.

systolic pressure *n.* The highest arterial blood pressure reached during any given ventricular cycle.

systolic thrill *n.* A thrill felt during ventricular systole over the precordium or over a blood vessel.

sys·trem·ma (sĭ-strĕm′ə) *n.* A muscular cramp in the calf of the leg in which the contracted muscles form a hard ball.

syz·y·gy (sĭz′ə-jē) *n.* **1.** The association of gregarine protozoa end-to-end or in lateral pairing without sexual fusion. **2.** The pairing of chromosomes in meiosis. —**sy·zyg′i·al** (sĭ-zĭj′ē-əl) *adj.*

Szent–Györ·gyi (sänt-jôr′jē, sĕnt-dyœr′dyĭ), **Albert** 1893–1986. Hungarian-born American biochemist who was the first to isolate vitamin C. He won a 1937 Nobel Prize for discoveries relating to biological combustion.

T

θ The Greek letter *theta*. Entries beginning with this character are alphabetized under **theta**.

τ The Greek letter *tau*. Entries beginning with this character are alphabetized under **tau**.

t *abbr.* temperature

T¹ The symbol for the isotope **tritium**.

T² *abbr.* tablespoon; absolute temperature; tesla; tetanus toxoids vaccine; tetanus vaccine

T-3 *abbr.* 3,5,3'-triiodothyronine

T4 *abbr.* thyroxine

Ta The symbol for the element **tantalum**.

ta·ba·nid (tə-bā′nĭd, -băn′ĭd) *n.* Any of various blood-sucking dipterous flies of the family Tabanidae, including the horseflies, that are involved in the transmission of several blood-borne parasites.

ta·bes (tā′bēz) *n., pl.* **tabes** 1. Progressive bodily wasting or emaciation. 2. Tabes dorsalis. —**ta·bes′cence** (tə-bĕs′əns) *n.* —**ta·bes′cent** *adj.* —**ta·bet·ic** (tə-bĕt′-ĭk) *adj.*

tabes dor·sa·lis (dôr-sā′lĭs, -săl′ĭs) *n.* A late form of syphilis resulting in hardening of the dorsal columns of the spinal cord and characterized by shooting pains, emaciation, loss of muscular coordination, and disturbances of sensation and digestion. Also called *Duchenne's disease, locomotor ataxia, spinal atrophy.*

tabes mes·en·ter·i·ca (mĕz′ĕn-tĕr′ĭ-kə) *n.* Tuberculosis of the mesenteric and retroperitoneal lymph nodes.

tabetic arthropathy *n.* A neuropathic joint commonly associated with tabes dorsalis or diabetic neuropathy. Also called *Charcot's joint.*

ta·bet·i·form (tə-bĕt′ə-fôrm′) *adj.* Resembling tabes.

tab·la·ture (tăb′lə-chŏor′, -chər) *n.* 1. An engraved tablet or surface. 2. The cranial bones considered as two laminae separated by the diploe.

ta·ble (tā′bəl) *n.* 1. An article of furniture supported by one or more vertical legs and having a flat horizontal surface. 2. An orderly arrangement of data, especially one in which the data are arranged in columns and rows in an essentially rectangular form. 3. An abbreviated list, as of contents; a synopsis. 4. The inner or outer flat layer of bones of the skull separated by the diploe.

ta·ble·spoon (tā′bəl-spŏon′) *n. Abbr.* **T, tbsp.** A measure of about 3 teaspoons or 15 milliliters.

tab·let (tăb′lĭt) *n.* A small flat pellet of medication to be taken orally.

ta·boo *or* **ta·bu** (tə-bōo′, tă-) *n., pl.* **–boos** *or* **–bus** A ban or an inhibition resulting from social custom or emotional aversion. —*adj.* Excluded or forbidden from use, approach, or mention.

ta·bo·pa·re·sis (tā′bō-pə-rē′sĭs, -păr′ĭ-sĭs) *n.* A condition in which the symptoms of tabes dorsalis and general paresis occur together.

tab·u·lar (tăb′yə-lər) *adj.* 1. Having a plane surface; flat. 2. Organized as a table or list. 3. Calculated by means of a table.

tache (tăsh, täsh) *n.* A circumscribed discoloration of the skin or mucous membrane, as a freckle.

tache noir (nwär′) *n.* A necrotic area covered with a black crust that characteristically appears at the site of the bite in certain tick-borne diseases.

ta·chet·ic (tə-kĕt′ĭk, tă-) *adj.* Of, relating to, or marked by bluish or brownish spots.

ta·chis·to·scope (tă-kĭs′tə-skōp′) *n.* An apparatus that projects a series of images onto a screen at rapid speed to test visual perception, memory, and learning. —**ta·chis′to·scop′ic** (-skŏp′ĭk) *adj.*

ta·chom·e·ter (tă-kŏm′ĭ-tər) *n.* An instrument used to measure the rotations per minute of a rotating shaft.

tachy– *pref.* Rapid; accelerated: *tachycardia.*

tach·y·ar·rhyth·mi·a (tăk′ē-ə-rĭth′mē-ə) *n.* An excessively rapid heartbeat accompanied by arrhythmia.

tach·y·car·di·a (tăk′ĭ-kär′dē-ə) *n.* A rapid heart rate, especially one above 100 beats per minute in an adult. Also called *tachyrhythmia.*

tachycardia-bradycardia syndrome *n.* A syndrome characterized by alternating periods of slow and rapid heartbeat.

tach·y·car·di·ac (tăk′ĭ-kär′dē-ăk′) *adj.* Of, relating to, or affected by tachycardia.

tachycardia window *n.* In paroxysmal tachycardia, the period of time between the earliest and latest premature activation that can excite the paroxysm.

tach·y·pha·gia (tăk′ə-fā′jə) *n.* Rapid eating; bolting of food.

tach·y·phy·lax·is (tăk′ə-fĭ-lăk′sĭs) *n.* 1. Rapid desensitization to a pharmacologically or physiologically active substance, produced by inoculation with a series of small doses. 2. A rapidly decreasing response to a drug following its initial administration.

tach·yp·ne·a (tăk′ĭp-nē′ə, tăk′ĭ-nē′ə) *n.* Rapid breathing. Also called *polypnea.*

tach·y·rhyth·mi·a (tăk′ə-rĭth′mē-ə) *n.* See **tachycardia**.

ta·chys·ter·ol (tə-kĭs′tə-rôl′, -rōl′) *n.* An isomer of ergosterol that forms vitamin D_2 when irradiated with ultraviolet light.

tac·rine hydrochloride (tăk′rēn′, -rĭn) *n.* An acetylcholinesterase inhibitor drug that is used to treat mild-to-moderate dementia in patients with Alzheimer's disease.

ta·cro·li·mus (tə-krō′lə-məs) *n.* An immunosuppressive drug produced by the actinomycete *Streptomyces tsukubaensis,* used in combination with corticosteroids to prevent rejection of organ transplants.

tac·tile (tăk′təl, -tīl′) *adj.* 1. Perceptible to the sense of touch; tangible. 2. Used for feeling. 3. Of, relating to, or proceeding from the sense of touch; tactual.

tactile anesthesia *n.* Loss or impairment of the sense of touch.

tactile corpuscle *n.* Any of numerous minute oval end organs of touch in sensitive skin, as in the palms, fingertips, and soles of the feet. Also called *Meissner's corpuscle.*

tactile disk *n.* A cup-shaped tactile nerve ending that is in contact with a single modified epithelial cell. Also called *Merkel's corpuscle, tactile meniscus.*

tactile fremitus *n.* The vibration felt by a hand placed on a chest during vocal fremitus.

tactile image *n.* An image of an object as perceived by the sense of touch.

tactile meniscus *n.* See **tactile disk.**

tactile papilla *n.* Any of the papillae of the skin containing a tactile cell or corpuscle.

tac·tom·e·ter (tăk-tŏm′ĭ-tər) *n.* See **aesthesiometer.**

tac·to·re·cep·tor (tăk′tō-rĭ-sĕp′tər) *n.* A receptor that responds to touch.

tac·tu·al (tăk′chōō-əl) *adj.* Tactile.

TAD *abbr.* transient acantholytic dermatosis

ta·da·la·fil (tə-dä′lə-fĭl′) *n.* A phosphodiesterase inhibitor drug used to treat erectile dysfunction for up to several days by increasing the level of cyclic GMP, which increases blood flow to the erectile tissues.

tae·ni·a *or* **te·ni·a** (tē′nē-ə) *n., pl* **–ni·as** *or* **–ni·ae** (-nē-ē′) **1.** A ribbonlike band of tissue or muscle. **2.** A flatworm of the genus *Taenia,* which includes many tapeworms. Not in technical use.

Tae·ni·a (tē′nē-ə) *n.* A genus of cestodes that formerly included most of the tapeworms but is now restricted to those species infecting carnivores with a cysticercus.

tae·ni·a·cide *or* **te·ni·a·cide** (tē′nē-ə-sīd′) *n.* An agent that kills tapeworms.

tae·ni·a·fuge *or* **te·ni·a·fuge** (tē′nē-ə-fyōōj′) *n.* An agent that expels tapeworms from the body.

Taenia sag·i·na·ta (săj′ə-nā′tə) *n.* A tapeworm that is parasitic in humans and is acquired by eating infected beef that is insufficiently cooked.

tae·ni·a·sis *or* **te·ni·a·sis** (tē-nī′ə-sĭs) *n.* Infestation with tapeworms.

Taenia so·li·um (sō′lē-əm) *n.* A tapeworm that is parasitic in humans and is acquired by eating infected pork that is insufficiently cooked.

tae·ni·id (tē′nē-ĭd) *n.* A member of the parasitic cestode family Taeniidae, which includes the genera *Taenia, Multiceps,* and *Echinococcus.*

tae·ni·oid (tē′nē-oid′) *adj.* Of or relating to cestodes of the genus *Taenia.*

TAF *abbr.* tumor angiogenic factor

tag (tăg) *n.* **1.** A strip of leather, paper, metal, or plastic attached to something or hung from a wearer's neck to identify, classify, or label. **2.** A small outgrowth or polyp. —*v.* **1.** To label, identify, or recognize with or as if with a tag. **2.** To incorporate into a compound a readily detected substance making the compound detectable so that its metabolic or chemical history may be followed.

Tag·a·met (tăg′ə-mĕt′) A trademark for the drug cimetidine.

TAH *abbr.* total abdominal hysterectomy

TAH-BSO *abbr.* total abdominal hysterectomy with bilateral salpingo-oopherectomy

tail (tāl) *n.* The posterior part of an animal, especially when elongated and extending beyond the trunk or main part of the body.

tail·bone (tāl′bōn′) *n.* See **coccyx.**

tail bud *n.* The rapidly proliferating mass of cells at the caudal extremity of the embryo. Also called *end bud.*

tail fold *n.* The ventral folding of the caudal extremity of the embryonic disk.

tai·lor's muscle (tā′lərz) *n.* See **sartorius muscle.**

Ta·ka·ha·ra's disease (tăk′ə-här′əz, tä′kə-hä′rəz) *n.* See **acatalasemia.**

Ta·ka·ya·su's disease (tăk′ə-yăs′ōōz, tä′kə-yä′sōōz) *n.* See **pulseless disease.**

Takayasu's syndrome *n.* See **pulseless disease.**

talc (tălk) *n.* A fine-grained white, greenish, or gray mineral, having a soft soapy feel and used in talcum and face powder. Also called *talcum.*

tal·co·sis (tăl-kō′sĭs) *n., pl.* **–ses** (-sēz) A form of pneumoconiosis caused by the inhalation of talc mixed with silicates.

tal·cum (tăl′kəm) *n.* See **talc.**

tal·i·ped (tăl′ə-pĕd′) *adj.* Having a clubfoot; clubfooted. —*n.* A person with a clubfoot.

tal·i·ped·ic (tăl′ə-pĕd′ĭk, -pē′dĭc) *adj.* Having a clubfoot or clubfeet.

tal·i·pes (tăl′ə-pēz′) *n.* See **clubfoot.**

talipes cal·ca·ne·o·val·gus (kăl-kā′nē-ō-văl′gəs) *n.* A congenital deformity that is a combination of talipes calcaneus and talipes valgus, marked by a dorsiflexed, everted, and abducted foot.

talipes cal·ca·ne·o·var·us (kăl-kā′nē-ō-vâr′əs) *n.* A congenital deformity that is a combination of talipes calcaneus and talipes varus, marked by a dorsiflexed, inverted, and adducted foot.

talipes cal·ca·ne·us (kăl-kā′nē-əs) *n.* A deformity due to weakness or absence of the calf muscles in which the axis of the calcaneus becomes vertically oriented.

talipes ca·vus (kā′vəs) *n.* A deformity of the foot in which the normal arch is exaggerated.

talipes e·qui·no·val·gus (ĭ-kwī′nō-văl′gəs, ĕk′wə-) *n.* A deformity that is a combination of talipes equinus and talipes valgus, marked by a plantar-flexed, everted, and abducted foot.

talipes e·qui·no·var·us (ĭ-kwī′nō-vâr′əs, ĕk′wə-) *n.* A deformity that is a combination of talipes equinus and talipes varus, marked by a plantar-flexed, inverted, and adducted foot.

talipes e·qui·nus (ĭ-kwī′nəs) *n.* A deformity resulting in permanent extension of the foot so that only the ball rests on the ground.

talipes pla·nus (plā′nəs) *n.* See **flatfoot.**

talipes val·gus (văl′gəs) *n.* A deformity resulting in permanent eversion of the foot so that only the inner side of the sole rests on the ground.

talipes var·us (vâr′əs) *n.* A deformity resulting in inversion of the foot so that only the outer side of the sole rests on the ground. Also called *pes varus.*

tal·i·pom·a·nus (tăl′ə-pŏm′ə-nəs, -pō-mā′nəs, -măn′əs) *n.* A congenital or acquired deformity of the hand. Also called *clubhand.*

talo– *pref.* Talus: talocrural.

ta·lo·cal·ca·ne·o·na·vic·u·lar joint (tā′lō-kăl-kā′nē-ō-nə-vĭk′yə-lər) *n.* A ball-and-socket joint, part of the transverse tarsal joint, formed by the head of the talus articulating with the navicular bone and the anterior part of the calcaneus.

ta·lo·cru·ral (tā′lō-kroŏr′əl) *adj.* Of or relating to the talus and the bones of the leg.

talocrural joint *n.* See **ankle joint.**

ta·lus (tā′ləs) *n., pl.* **–li** (-lī′) **1.** The bone of the ankle that articulates with the tibia and fibula to form the ankle joint. Also called *anklebone, astragalus.* **2.** The ankle. —**ta′ler** (-lər) *adj.*

Tal·win (tăl′wĭn) A trademark for the drug pentazocine hydrochloride.

Tam·bo·cor (tăm′bə-kôr′) A trademark for the drug flecainide acetate.

tam·bour sound (tăm′boŏr′, tăm-boŏr′) *n.* A heart sound, usually the aortic- or pulmonic-valve closure sound when it has a booming and ringing quality like that of a drum.

Tamm-Hors·fall mucoprotein (tăm′hôrs′fôl) *n.* A substance derived from the secretion of renal tubular cells and is a normal constituent of urine.

ta·mox·i·fen (tə-mŏk′sə-fĕn) *n.* A nonsteroidal estrogen antagonist used in the treatment of advanced breast cancer in women whose tumors are estrogen-dependent and also used prophylactically by some women at risk for breast cancer.

tam·pon (tăm′pŏn′) *n.* A plug of absorbent material inserted into a body cavity or wound to check a flow of blood or to absorb secretions, especially one designed for insertion into the vagina during menstruation. —*v.* To plug or stop with a tampon.

tam·pon·ade (tăm′pə-nād′) *or* **tam·pon·age** (tăm′pə-nĭj) *n.* The insertion or use of a tampon.

tan·gen·ti·al·i·ty (tăn-jĕn′shē-ăl′ĭ-tē) *n.* A disturbance in the associative thought process in which one tends to digress readily from one topic under discussion to other topics that arise through association.

Tan·gier disease (tăn-jîr′) *n.* An inheritable disorder of lipid metabolism that is characterized by almost complete absence from plasma of high-density lipoproteins, by the storage of cholesterol esters in foam cells, and by the enlargement of the liver, spleen, and lymph nodes. Also called *familial high-density lipoprotein disease.*

tan·go·re·cep·tor (tăng′gō-rĭ-sĕp′tər) *n.* A cutaneous receptor that responds to touch and pressure.

tan·nate (tăn′āt′) *n.* A salt or ester of tannic acid.

Tan·ner growth chart (tăn′ər) *n.* A series of charts for measuring different aspects of the physical development of children according to sex, age, and stages of puberty.

Tanner stage *n.* A stage of puberty in the Tanner growth chart, based on the growth of pubic hair in both sexes, the development of the genitalia in boys, and the development of the breasts in girls.

tan·nic (tăn′ĭk) *adj.* Of, relating to, or obtained from tannin.

tannic acid *n.* **1.** A white or yellowish astringent powder used as a denaturant and in tanning and textiles. **2.** A lustrous yellowish to light brown amorphous, powdered, flaked, or spongy mass derived from the bark and fruit of many plants and used as a mordant and to clarify wine and beer.

tan·ta·lum (tăn′tə-ləm) *n. Symbol* **Ta** A hard heavy metallic element that is exceptionally resistant to chemical attack below 150°C and is used to make electronic components and surgical instruments. Atomic number 73.

T antigen *n.* See **tumor antigen.**

tan·trum (tăn′trəm) *n.* A fit of bad temper.

tap (tăp) *n.* The removal of fluid from a body cavity. —*v.* **1.** To withdraw fluid from a body cavity, as with a trocar and cannula, hollow needle, or catheter. **2.** To strike lightly with the finger or a hammerlike instrument, as in percussion or to elicit a tendon reflex.

Tap·a·zole (tăp′ə-zōl′) A trademark for the drug methimazole.

ta·pe·to·ret·i·nal (tə-pē′tō-rĕt′n-əl) *adj.* Of or relating to the tapetum and the retina.

tapetoretinal retinopathy *n.* See **retinitis pigmentosa.**

ta·pe·tum (tə-pē′təm) *n., pl.* **–ta** (-tə) **1.** A membranous layer or region, especially the iridescent membrane of the choroid of certain mammals. **2.** A layer of fibers of the corpus callosum forming the roof of part of the lateral ventricle of the brain.

tape·worm (tāp′wûrm′) *n.* Any of various ribbonlike, often very long flatworms of the class Cestoda, that lack an alimentary canal and are intestinal parasites in humans.

ta·pir mouth (tā′pər) *n.* Protrusion of the lips due to weakness of the oral muscle in certain forms of juvenile muscular dystrophy.

ta·pote·ment (tə-pōt′mənt, tä-pôt-mäɴ′) *n.* A striking with the side of the hand, usually with partly flexed fingers, used in massage.

ta·ran·tu·la (tə-răn′chə-lə) *n., pl.* **–las** *or* **–lae** (-lē′) Any of various large, hairy, chiefly tropical spiders of the family Theraphosidae, capable of inflicting a painful but not seriously poisonous bite.

tar·dive (tär′dĭv) *adj.* Having symptoms that develop slowly or that appear long after inception. Used of a disease.

tardive cyanosis *n.* See **cyanose tardive.**

tardive dyskinesia *n.* A chronic disorder of the nervous system characterized by involuntary jerky movements of the face, tongue, jaws, trunk, and limbs, usually developing as a late side effect of prolonged treatment with antipsychotic drugs. Also called *tardive oral dyskinesia.*

tar·get (tär′gĭt) *n.* **1.** One to be influenced or changed by an action or event. **2.** A desired goal. **3.** A usually metal part in an x-ray tube on which a beam of electrons is focused and from which x-rays are emitted. **4.** A target organ.

target cell *n.* **1.** A red blood cell having a dark center surrounded by a light band that is itself encircled by a darker ring, and occurring in certain anemias and after splenectomy. **2.** A cell selectively affected by a particular agent, such as a virus, drug, or hormone.

target gland *n.* An endocrine gland directly affected by the hormone of another gland.

target heart rate *n.* A heart rate that is attained during aerobic exercise and represents the minimum level of exertion at which cardiovascular fitness can increase for an individual in a given age group.

target organ *n.* A tissue or organ that is affected by a specific hormone.

target response *n.* See **operant.**

tar·ry cyst (tär′ē) *n.* A cyst or collection of old blood that has a black appearance and is usually caused by endometriosis.

tars– *pref.* Variant of **tarso–.**

tars·ad·e·ni·tis (tär′săd-n-ī′tĭs) *n.* Inflammation of the tarsal borders of the eyelids and Meibomian glands.

tar·sal (tär′səl) *adj.* **1.** Of, relating to, or situated near the tarsus of the foot. **2.** Of or relating to the tarsus of the eyelid.

tarsal artery *n.* **1.** An artery with its origin in the dorsal artery of the foot, with distribution to the tarsal joints and the short extensor muscle of the toes, and with anastomoses to the arcuate, peroneal, lateral plantar, and anterior lateral malleolar arteries; lateral tarsal artery. **2.** An artery that is one of two small branches of the dorsal artery of the foot, with distribution to the medial malleolar network; medial tarsal artery.

tarsal bone *n.* Any of the seven bones of the tarsus.

tarsal canal *n.* See **tarsal sinus.**

tarsal cyst *n.* Chronic, inflammatory granuloma of the Meibomian gland.

tar·sa·le (tär-sā′lē) *n., pl.* **–sa·li·a** (-sā′lē-ə) Any of the tarsal bones.

tar·sal·gia (tär-săl′jə) *n.* See **podalgia.**

tarsal gland *n.* See **Meibomian gland.**

tarsal joint *n.* Any of the joints that unite the tarsal bones. Also called *intertarsal joint.*

tarsal plate *n.* See **tarsus** (sense 2).

tarsal sinus *n.* A hollow or canal formed by the groove of the talus and the groove of the calcaneus. Also called *tarsal canal.*

tarsal tunnel syndrome *n.* A syndrome characterized by pain and numbness in the sole, caused by entrapment neuropathy of the posterior tibial nerve.

tar·sec·to·my (tär-sĕk′tə-mē) *n.* **1.** Excision of the tarsus of the foot. **2.** Excision of a segment of the tarsus of an eyelid.

tar·si·tis (tär-sī′tĭs) *n.* **1.** Inflammation of the tarsus of the foot. **2.** Inflammation of the tarsal border of an eyelid.

tarso– *or* **tars–** *pref.* Tarsus; tarsal: *tarsoclasia.*

tar·so·chei·lo·plas·ty (tär′sō-kī′lə-plăs′tē) *n.* Plastic surgery on the edge of the eyelid.

tar·soc·la·sis (tär-sŏk′lə-sĭs) *or* **tar·so·cla·sia** (tär′sō-klā′zhə) *n.* The surgical fracture of the tarsus as a treatment for clubfoot.

tar·so·ma·la·cia (tär′sō-mə-lā′shə) *n.* Softening of the tarsal cartilages of the eyelids.

tar·so·meg·a·ly (tär′sō-mĕg′ə-lē) *n.* Congenital maldevelopment and overgrowth of a tarsal bone.

tar·so·met·a·tar·sal (tär′sō-mĕt′ə-tär′səl) *adj.* Of or relating to the tarsal and metatarsal bones.

tarsometatarsal joint *n.* Any of the three joints between the tarsal and metatarsal bones: a medial joint between the first cuneiform and first metatarsal, an intermediate joint between the second and third cuneiforms and corresponding metatarsals, and a lateral joint between the cuboid and fourth and fifth metatarsals. Also called *Lisfranc's joint.*

tar·so·pha·lan·ge·al (tär′sō-fə-lăn′jē-əl, -fā-) *adj.* Of or relating to the tarsus and the phalanges.

tar·so·phy·ma (tär′sō-fī′mə) *n.* A growth or tumor of the tarsus of the eyelid.

tar·so·plas·ty (tär′sə-plăs′tē) *n.* See **blepharoplasty.**

tar·sor·rha·phy (tär-sôr′ə-fē) *n.* A partial or complete suture of the eyelid margins performed to shorten the palpebral fissure or to protect the cornea. Also called *blepharorrhaphy.*

tar·so·tar·sal (tär′sō-tär′səl) *adj.* Mediotarsal.

tar·sot·o·my (tär-sŏt′ə-mē) *n.* **1.** Incision of the tarsus of an eyelid. **2.** An operation on the tarsus of the foot.

tar·sus (tär′səs) *n., pl.* **–si** (-sī) **1.** The area of articulation between the foot and the leg, comprising the seven bones of the instep: the talus, calcaneus, navicular, three cuneiform, and cuboid bones. **2.** The fibrous plate that supports and shapes the edges of the eyelids. Also called *tarsal plate.*

TAR syndrome (tär, tē′ā-är′) *n.* See **thrombocytopenia-absent radius syndrome.**

tar·tar (tär′tər) *n.* A hard, yellowish deposit on the teeth, consisting of organic secretions and food particles deposited in various salts, such as calcium carbonate. Also called *dental calculus.*

tartar emetic *n.* A poisonous crystalline compound used in medicine as an expectorant and in the treatment of parasitic infections, such as schistosomiasis.

tart cell *n.* **1.** A granulocyte that has engulfed the nucleus of another cell, the structure of which is still well preserved. **2.** This type of ingested nucleus, especially as found as an artifact in lupus erythematosus cell preparations.

tar·trate (tär′trāt′) *n.* A salt or ester of tartaric acid.

taste (tāst) *n.* **1.** The sense that distinguishes the sweet, sour, salty, and bitter qualities of dissolved substances in contact with the taste buds on the tongue. **2.** This sense in combination with the senses of smell and touch, which together receive a sensation of a substance in the mouth. **3.** The sensation of sweet, sour, salty, or bitter qualities produced by or as if by a substance placed in the mouth. **4.** The unified sensation produced by any of these qualities plus a distinct smell and texture; flavor. —*v.* **1.** To distinguish the flavor of something by taking it into the mouth. **2.** To eat or drink a small quantity of something. **3.** To distinguish flavors in the mouth. **4.** To have a distinct flavor.

taste bud *n.* One of a number of flask-shaped receptor cell nests located in the epithelium of the papillae of the tongue and in the soft palate, epiglottis, and pharynx that mediate the sense of taste.

taste cell *n.* A darkly staining neuroepithelial cell in a taste bud that makes synaptic contact with sensory nerve fibers thus serving as receptors for taste. Also called *gustatory cell.*

taste hair *n.* Any of the hairlike projections of the gustatory cells of taste buds.

TAT *abbr.* Thematic Apperception Test

tat·too (tă-tōo′) *n., pl.* **–toos** A permanent mark or design made on the skin by a process of pricking and ingraining an indelible pigment or by raising scars. —*v.* **1.** To mark the skin with a tattoo. **2.** To form a tattoo on the skin.

Ta·tum (tā′təm), **Edward Lawrie** 1909–1975. American biochemist. Through his genetic research with bacteria, he showed how genes transmit hereditary characteristics and shared a 1958 Nobel Prize for his discoveries.

tau *n. Symbol* τ The 19th letter of the Greek alphabet.

tau·rine (tôr′ēn′) *n.* A colorless crystalline substance formed by the hydrolysis of taurocholic acid and found in the fluids of the muscles and lungs of many animals.

tau·ro·cho·late (tôr′ō-kō′lāt′) *n.* A salt of taurocholic acid.

tau·ro·cho·lic acid (tôr′ō-kō′lĭk, -kŏl′ĭk) *n.* A crystalline acid involved in the emulsification of fats and occurring as a sodium salt in the bile of humans and other mammals. Also called *cholaic acid.*

Taus·sig (tou′sĭg), **Helen** 1898–1986. American pediatrician and embryologist noted for her work on congenital defects of the heart. With Alfred Blalock she developed the pulmonary bypass operation for the treatment of blue babies.

Taussig-Bing syndrome (-bĭng′) *n.* A rare malformation of the heart characterized by transposition of the aorta, which arises from the right ventricle, and by ventricular septal defect, hypertrophy of the right ventricle, and a pulmonary artery that is situated behind the aorta.

tauto– *or* **taut–** *pref.* Same; identical: *tautomeric.*

tautomeric fiber *n.* Any of the nerve fibers of the spinal cord that do not extend beyond the limits of the spinal cord segment in which they originate.

tau·tom·er·ism (tô-tŏm′ə-rĭz′əm) *n.* Chemical isomerism in which the isomeric forms differ little, usually only in the position of a hydrogen atom, and are able to exist in equilibrium and react with each other. —**tau′to·mer′ic** (tô′tə-mĕr′ĭk) *adj.*

tax·is (tăk′sĭs) *n., pl.* **tax·es** (tăk′sēz) **1.** The responsive movement of a free-moving organism or cell toward or away from an external stimulus, such as light. **2.** The moving of a body part by manipulation into normal position, as after a dislocation.

–taxis *suff.* **1.** Order; arrangement: *stereotaxis.* **2.** Responsive movement; taxis: *chemotaxis.*

Tax·ol (tăk′sôl′) A trademark for the drug paclitaxel.

tax·on (tăk′sŏn′) *n., pl.* **tax·a** (tăk′sə) A taxonomic category or group, such as a phylum, order, family, genus, or species.

tax·on·o·my (tăk-sŏn′ə-mē) *n.* **1.** The classification of organisms in an ordered system that indicates natural relationships. **2.** The science, laws, or principles of classification; systematics. —**tax′o·nom′ic** (-sə-nŏm′ĭk), **tax′o·nom′i·cal** (-ĭ-kəl) *adj.*

Tay-Sachs disease (tā′săks′) *n.* A lyposomal storage disease that is the infantile type of cerebral sphingolipidosis. Also called G_{M2} *gangliosidosis.*

Tb The symbol for the element **terbium.**

TB *abbr.* tuberculosis

TBG *abbr.* thyroid-binding globulin

T-binder *n.* Two strips of cloth positioned at right angles and used for retaining a dressing. Also called *T-bandage.*

tbsp. *abbr.* tablespoon

TBV *abbr.* total blood volume

Tc The symbol for the element **technetium.**

T cell *n.* A principal type of white blood cell that completes maturation in the thymus and that has various roles in the immune system, including the identification of specific foreign antigens in the body and the activation and deactivation of other immune cells. Also called *T lymphocyte.*

Td *abbr.* tetanus-diphtheria toxoids vaccine

Te The symbol for the element **tellurium.**

teach·ing hospital (tē′chĭng) *n.* A hospital closely associated with a medical school and serving as a practical educational site for medical students, interns, residents, and allied health personnel.

Teale's amputation (tēlz) *n.* **1.** Amputation of the thigh or the lower half of the forearm with the construction of a long posterior rectangular flap and a short anterior one. **2.** Amputation of the leg with the construction of a long anterior rectangular flap and a short posterior one.

tear¹ (târ) *n.* A rip or rent in a material or structure.

tear² (tîr) *n.* A drop of the clear salty liquid that is secreted by the lacrimal gland of the eye to lubricate the surface between the eyeball and eyelid and to wash away irritants.

tear·drop (tîr′drŏp′) *n.* **1.** A single tear. **2.** An object shaped like a tear.

tear gas (tîr) *n.* A gas that causes irritation of the eyes and profuse tearing.

tear·ing (tîr′ĭng) *n.* Epiphora.

tear sac (tîr) *n.* See **lacrimal sac.**

tear stone (tîr) *n.* See **dacryolith.**

tease (tēz) *v.* To separate the structural parts of a tissue, as with a needle, in order to prepare it for microscopic examination.

tea·spoon (tē′spōōn′) *n. Abbr.* **tsp., tsp** A measure of about 1 fluid dram or 5 milliliters.

teat (tēt, tĭt) *n.* **1.** See **nipple. 2.** The female breast; mamma. **3.** A papilla.

tech·ne·ti·um (tĕk-nē′shē-əm, -shəm) *n. Symbol* **Tc** A radioactive metal, the first synthetically produced element, used as a tracer and in diagnostic imaging. Atomic number 43.

tech·ni·cian (tĕk-nĭsh′ən) *n.* One whose occupation requires training in a specific technical process. Also called *technologist.*

tech·nique (tĕk-nēk′) *or* **tech·nic** (tĕk′nĭk) *n.* The skill and procedure with which a surgical operation or experiment, for example, is carried out.

tech·nol·o·gist (tĕk-nŏl′ə-jĭst) *n.* See **technician.**

tec·ton·ic keratoplasty (tĕk-tŏn′ĭk) *n.* The surgical grafting of corneal material in an area where corneal tissue has been lost.

tec·to·ri·al (tĕk-tôr′ē-əl) *adj.* Of, relating to, or characteristic of a tectorium.

tectorial membrane of cochlear duct *n.* A gelatinous membrane that overlies the spiral organ in the inner ear. Also called *Corti's membrane, tectorium.*

tec·to·spi·nal (tĕk′tō-spī′nəl) *adj.* Of or relating to nerve fibers that pass from the tectum mesencephali to the spinal cord.

tec·tum (tĕk′təm) *n., pl.* **–ta** (-tə) A rooflike structure of the body, especially the dorsal part of the mesencephalon. —**tec′tal** (-təl) *adj.*

tectum mes·en·ceph·a·li (mĕs'ĕn-sĕf'ə-lī') *n.* See **lamina tecti mesencephali.**

teeth (tēth) *n.* Plural of **tooth.**

teeth·ing (tē'thĭng) *n.* The eruption or cutting of the teeth.

teeth·ridge (tēth'rĭj') *n.* The ridge of gum behind the upper front teeth.

tef·lu·rane (tĕf'lə-rān') *n.* A general anesthetic having moderate potency, administered by inhalation.

teg·men (tĕg'mən) *n.*, *pl.* **–mi·na** (-mə-nə) A covering or an integument of a part. Also called *tegmentum.*

tegmen mas·toi·de·um (mă-stoi'dē-əm) *n.* The lamina of bone that roofs over the mastoid cells.

tegmental decussation *n.* **1.** The dorsal tegmental decussation of the left and right tectospinal and tectobulbar tracts, located in the mesencephalon. Also called *fountain decussation, Meynert's decussation.* **2.** The ventral tegmental decussation of left and right tracts that control flexor muscle tone, located in the mesencephalon. Also called *Forel's decussation, rubrospinal decussation.*

tegmental nucleus *n.* Either of two small round cell groups in the caudal part of the midbrain, associated with the mamillary body via the mamillary peduncle and mamillotegmental tract.

tegmental syndrome *n.* A syndrome characterized by hemiplegia and paresis or paraylsis of the eye muscles and caused by a lesion in the tegmentum of the mesencephalon.

teg·men·tum (tĕg-mĕn'təm) *n.*, *pl.* **–ta** (-tə) **1.** See **tegmen. 2.** The mesencephalic tegmentum. —**teg·men'tal** *adj.*

tegmentum of rhombencephalon *n.* The portion of the pons and the medulla oblongata continuous with the mesencephalic tegmentum.

Teg·re·tol (tĕg'rə-tōl', -tôl') A trademark for the drug carbamazepine.

teg·u·ment (tĕg'yə-mənt) *n.* A natural outer covering; an integument.

teg·u·men·tal (tĕg'yə-mĕn'tl) *or* **teg·u·men·ta·ry** (-mĕn'tə-rē) *adj.* Of or relating to the integument.

tei·cho·ic acid (tī-kō'ĭk) *n.* One of two types of polymers present in gram-positive bacteria, especially in the cell walls.

tei·chop·si·a (tī-kŏp'sē-ə) *n.* A transient visual sensation of bright shimmering colors, as that preceding scintillating scotoma in migraine.

tel-¹ *pref.* Variant of **tele-.**

tel-² *pref.* Variant of **telo-.**

te·la (tē'lə) *n.*, *pl.* **–lae** (-lē) **1.** A thin weblike structure. **2.** A tissue, especially of delicate formation.

tel·an·gi·ec·ta·sia (tĕl-ăn'jē-ĕk-tā'zhə) *or* **tel·an·gi·ec·ta·sis** (-ĕk'tə-sĭs) *n.* Chronic dilation of groups of capillaries causing elevated dark red blotches on the skin. —**tel·an'gi·ec·tat'ic** (-tăt'ĭk) *adj.*

telangiectatic angioma *n.* An angioma composed of dilated blood vessels.

telangiectatic fibroma *n.* A benign neoplasm of fibrous tissue having numerous, frequently dilated, vascular channels. Also called *angiofibroma.*

telangiectatic osteogenic sarcoma *n.* A cystic form of osteogenic sarcoma in which aneurysmal blood-filled spaces are lined with sarcoma cells that produce osteoid.

telangiectatic wart *n.* See **angiokeratoma.**

tel·an·gi·o·sis (tĕl-ăn'jē-ō'sĭs) *n.* Disease of the capillaries and terminal arterioles.

tela sub·cu·ta·ne·a (sŭb'kyōō-tā'nē-ə) *n.* A loose fibrous envelope beneath the skin, containing the cutaneous vessels and nerves. Also called *hypodermis, subcutis, superficial fascia.*

tela sub·mu·co·sa (sŭb'myōō-kō'sə) *n.* The layer of connective tissue beneath the mucous membrane. Also called *tunica submucosa.*

tele- *or* **tel–** *pref.* Distance; distant: *teletherapy.*

tel·e·can·thus (tĕl'ĭ-kăn'thəs) *n.* An abnormally increased distance between the medial canthi of the eyelids.

tel·e·di·ag·no·sis (tĕl'ĭ-dī'əg-nō'sĭs) *n.* A diagnosis that is made at a remote location and is based on the evaluation of data transmitted from instruments that monitor the patient and a transfer link to a diagnostic center.

tel·e·med·i·cine (tĕl'ĭ-mĕd'ĭ-sĭn) *n.* The use of telecommunications technology to provide, enhance, or expedite health care services, as by accessing off-site databases or transmitting diagnostic images for examination at another site.

te·lem·e·try (tə-lĕm'ĭ-trē) *n.* The science and technology of automatic measurement and transmission of data by radio or other means from remote sources to receiving stations for recording and analysis.

telencephalic flexure *n.* A flexure appearing in the embryonic forebrain region.

tel·en·ceph·a·lon (tĕl'ĕn-sĕf'ə-lŏn', -lən) *n.* The anterior portion of the prosencephalon, constituting the cerebral hemispheres and composing with the diencephalon the prosencephalon. Also called *endbrain.* —**tel'en·ce·phal'ic** (-sə-făl'ĭk) *adj.*

tel·e·o·mi·to·sis (tĕl'ē-ō-mī-tō'sĭs) *n.* A completed mitosis.

tel·e·op·si·a (tĕl'ē-ŏp'sē-ə) *n.* A vision disorder characterized by errors in judging the distance of objects and arising from lesions in the parietal temporal region of the brain.

tel·e·or·gan·ic (tĕl'ē-ôr-găn'ĭk) *adj.* Necessary to maintain life.

te·lep·a·thy (tə-lĕp'ə-thē) *n.* Communication by means other than through the normal senses.

tel·e·ra·di·og·ra·phy (tĕl'ə-rā'dē-ŏg'rə-fē) *n.* Radiography performed with the tube held about six feet from the body. Also called *teleroentgenography.*

tel·er·gy (tĕl'ər-jē) *n.* See **automatism** (sense 4).

tel·e·roent·gen·og·ra·phy (tĕl'ə-rĕnt'gə-nŏg'rə-fē, -jə-, -rŭnt'-) *n.* See **teleradiography.**

tel·e·ther·a·py (tĕl'ə-thĕr'ə-pē) *n.* Radiation therapy that is administered at a distance from the body.

tel·lu·ric (tĕ-lŏŏr'ĭk) *adj.* **1.** Of or relating to Earth; terrestrial. **2.** Derived from or containing tellurium, especially with valence 6.

tel·lu·ri·um (tĕ-lŏŏr'ē-əm) *n. Symbol* **Te** A brittle metallic element usually found in combination with gold and other metals, used to alloy stainless steel and lead, and in thermoelectric devices. Atomic number 52.

telo– or **tel–** pref. End: telophase.

tel·o·cen·tric (tĕl′ə-sĕn′trĭk, tē′lə-) adj. Of or relating to a chromosome having the centromere in a terminal position.

tel·o·den·dron (tĕl′ə-dĕn′drən, -drŏn′) n. The terminal arborization of an axon.

tel·o·gen (tĕl′ə-jĕn′, tē′lə-) n. The resting phase of the follicle in the hair cycle.

tel·o·lec·i·thal (tĕl′ə-lĕs′ə-thəl, tē′lə-) adj. Having a yolk that is concentrated at one end.

te·lom·er·ase (tə-lŏm′ə-rās′, -rāz′) n. An enzyme found in the telomeres of certain chromosomes that is active in cell division and may have a role in the proliferation of cancer cells.

tel·o·mere (tĕl′ə-mîr′, tē′lə-) n. Either end of a chromosome; a terminal chromosome.

tel·o·phase (tĕl′ə-fāz′, tē′lə-) n. The final stage of mitosis or meiosis during which the chromosomes of daughter cells are grouped in new nuclei. —**tel′o·phas′ic** adj.

te·maz·e·pam (tə-măz′ə-păm′) n. A benzodiazepine sedative primarily used to relieve insomnia.

Tem·in (tĕm′ĭn), **Howard Martin** 1934–1994. American oncologist. He shared a 1975 Nobel Prize for research on the interaction of tumor viruses and genetic material.

temp. abbr. temperature; temporal

tem·per (tĕm′pər) n. **1.** A state of mind or emotions; mood. **2.** A tendency to become easily angry or irritable. **3.** An outburst of rage.

tem·per·a·ment (tĕm′prə-mənt, tĕm′pər-ə-) n. **1.** The manner of thinking, behaving, or reacting characteristic of a specific person. **2.** Disposition; temper.

tem·per·ance (tĕm′pər-əns, tĕm′prəns) n. **1.** Moderation and self-restraint, as in behavior or expression. **2.** Restraint in the use of or abstinence from alcoholic liquors.

tem·per·ate (tĕm′pər-ĭt, tĕm′prĭt) adj. Exercising moderation and self-restraint.

temperate bacteriophage n. A bacteriophage whose genome incorporates with and replicates with that of the host bacterium.

tem·per·a·ture (tĕm′pər-ə-choŏr′, -chər, tĕm′prə-) n. Abbr. **T, t, temp. 1.** The degree of hotness or coldness of a body or an environment. **2.** A specific degree of hotness or coldness as indicated on or referred to a standard scale. **3.** The degree of heat in the body of a living organism, usually about 37.0°C (98.6°F) in humans. **4.** An abnormally high condition of body heat caused by illness; a fever.

tem·plate or **tem·plet** (tĕm′plĭt) n. **1.** A pattern or gauge, such as a thin metal plate with a cut pattern, used as a guide in making something accurately, as in woodworking. **2.** A molecule, such as DNA, that serves as a pattern for the synthesis of a macromolecule, as of RNA.

tem·ple (tĕm′pəl) n. **1.** The flat region on either side of the forehead. **2.** Either of the sidepieces of a frame for eyeglasses that extends along the temple and over the ear.

tem·po·la·bile (tĕm′pō-lā′bĭl′, -bəl) adj. Subject to change or destruction with the passage of time.

tem·po·ral (tĕm′pər-əl, tĕm′prəl) adj. Abbr. **temp.** Of, relating to, or near the temples of the skull.

temporal arteritis n. Arteritis that occurs in older persons and that is characterized by severe bitemporal headache, sudden loss of vision, and the presence of multinucleated giant cells in temporal, retinal, or intracerebral arteries. Also called cranial arteritis, giant cell arteritis.

temporal artery n. **1.** An artery with origin in the superficial temporal artery, with distribution to the temporal fascia and muscle, and with anastomoses to the branches of the maxillary artery; middle temporal artery. **2.** Either of two arteries with their origin in the maxillary artery, with distribution to the temporal muscle, and with anastomoses to the branches of the temporal, lacrimal, and meningeal arteries; deep temporal artery. **3.** An artery with origin in the external carotid artery, with branches to the transverse facial, middle temporal, orbital, parotid, anterior auricular, frontal, and parietal arteries; superficial temporal artery.

temporal bone n. Either of a pair of compound bones forming the sides and base of the skull.

temporal fossa n. The space on the side of the cranium bounded by the temporal lines and terminating below at the level of the zygomatic arch.

temporal gyrus n. **1.** A sagittal convolution on the inferolateral border of the temporal lobe of the cerebrum, separated from the middle temporal gyrus by the inferior temporal sulcus and including the fusiform gyrus; inferior temporal gyrus. **2.** A longitudinal gyrus on the lateral surface of the temporal lobe of the brain, between the superior and inferior temporal sulci; middle temporal gyrus. **3.** A longitudinal gyrus on the lateral surface of the temporal lobe between the lateral fissure and the superior temporal sulcus; superior temporal gyrus.

temporal lobe n. The lowest of the major subdivisions of the cortical mantle of the brain, containing the sensory center for hearing and forming the rear two thirds of the ventral surface of the cerebral hemisphere. It is separated from the frontal and parietal lobes above it by the fissure of Sylvius.

temporal lobe epilepsy n. See **psychomotor epilepsy.**

temporal muscle n. A muscle with origin from the temporal fossa, with insertion into the anterior border of the ramus and the mandible, with nerve supply from the deep temporal branches of the mandibular division of the trigeminal nerve, and whose action closes the jaw.

temporal plane n. A slightly depressed area on the side of the cranium, formed by the temporal and parietal bones, the greater wing of the sphenoid, and a part of the frontal bone.

temporal pole n. The most prominent anterior part of the temporal lobes of the brain.

temporal process n. The posterior projection of the zygomatic bone articulating with the zygomatic process of the temporal bone to form the zygomatic arch.

temporal ridge n. Temporal line, designated inferior and superior.

tem·po·rar·y cartilage (tĕm′pə-rĕr′ē) *n.* Cartilage that normally becomes converted to bone to form a part of the skeleton. Also called *precursory cartilage.*

temporary denture *n.* See **interim denture.**

temporary parasite *n.* An organism accidentally ingested that survives briefly in the intestine.

temporary tooth *n.* See **deciduous tooth.**

temporo– *pref.* Temporal: *temporomandibular.*

tem·po·ro·man·dib·u·lar (tĕm′pə-rō-măn-dĭb′yə-lər) *adj.* Of, relating to, or formed by the temporal bone and the mandible.

temporomandibular joint *n.* See **mandibular joint.**

temporomandibular joint dysfunction *n.* Impaired functioning of the temporomandibular articulation of the jaw.

temporomandibular joint syndrome *n. Abbr.* **TMJ** A disorder that is caused by faulty articulation of the temporomandibular joint and is characterized by facial pain, headache, ringing ears, dizziness, and stiffness of the neck. Also called *myofacial pain-dysfunction syndrome.*

temporomandibular nerve *n.* See **zygomatic nerve.**

tem·po·ro·max·il·lar·y (tĕm′pə-rō-măk′sə-lĕr′ē) *adj.* Of, relating to, or formed by the temporal bone and the maxillary bones.

tem·po·ro·pa·ri·e·tal muscle (tĕm′pə-rō-pə-rī′ĭ-təl) *n.* The part of the epicranial muscle with origin from the galea aponeurotica and with insertion into the cartilage of the auricle of the ear.

tem·po·sta·bile (tĕm′pō-stā′bĭl, -bəl, -bīl′, -bēl′) *adj.* Not subject to change or destruction with the passage of time.

TEN *abbr.* toxic epidermal necrolysis

te·na·cious (tə-nā′shəs) *adj.* **1.** Clinging to another object or surface; adhesive. **2.** Holding together firmly; cohesive.

te·nac·u·lum (tə-năk′yə-ləm) *n., pl.* **-la** (-lə) A long-handled, slender, hooked instrument for lifting and holding parts, such as blood vessels, during surgery.

tenaculum forceps *n.* A forceps with jaws ending in sharp inward-pointing hooks.

te·nal·gia (tĕ-năl′jə) *n.* Pain in a tendon. Also called *tenodynia, tenontodynia.*

ten·der (tĕn′dər) *adj.* **1.** Easily crushed or bruised; fragile. **2.** Easily hurt; sensitive. **3.** Painful; sore.

ten·der·ness (tĕn′dər-nĭs) *n.* The condition of being tender or sore to the touch.

ten·di·ni·tis *or* **ten·do·ni·tis** (tĕn′də-nī′tĭs) *n.* Inflammation of a tendon.

ten·di·no·plas·ty (tĕn′də-nə-plăs′tē) *n.* See **tenontoplasty.**

ten·di·no·su·ture (tĕn′də-nō-sōō′chər) *n.* See **tenorrhaphy.**

ten·di·nous (tĕn′də-nəs) *adj.* Of, having, or resembling a tendon.

tendinous arch *n.* A fibrous band arching over a vessel or nerve as it passes through a muscle, protecting it from compression.

tendinous arch of pelvic fascia *n.* A linear thickening of the superior fascia of the pelvic diaphragm extending posteriorly from the body of the pubis alongside the bladder and vagina in the female, and providing attachment to the supporting ligaments of the pelvic viscera.

tendinous cord *n.* Any of the tendinous strands running from the papillary muscles to the atrioventricular valves.

tendinous synovitis *n.* See **tenosynovitis.**

tendo– *pref.* Tendon: *tendosynovitis.*

ten·dol·y·sis (tĕn-dŏl′ĭ-sĭs) *or* **te·nol·y·sis** (tĕ-nŏl′lĭ-sĭs) *n.* The release of a tendon from adhesions, usually by surgery.

ten·don (tĕn′dən) *n.* A band of tough, inelastic fibrous tissue that connects a muscle with its bony attachment and consists of rows of elongated cells, minimal ground substance, and densely arranged, almost parallel, bundles of collageneous fibers.

tendon cell *n.* Any of various elongated fibroblastic cells arranged in rows between the collagenous tendon fibers.

ten·do·ni·tis (tĕn′də-nī′tĭs) *n.* Variant of **tendinitis.**

tendon reflex *n.* A myotatic or deep reflex in which the muscle stretch receptors are stimulated by percussing the tendon of a muscle.

tendon sheath syndrome *n.* Limitation of passive movement on attempted elevation of the eye when looking toward the nose, due to fascial interference with the superior oblique muscle on the same side as the affected eye.

ten·do·plas·ty (tĕn′də-plăs′tē) *n.* See **tenontoplasty.**

ten·do·syn·o·vi·tis (tĕn′dō-sĭn′ə-vī′tĭs, -sī′nə-) *n.* Variant of **tenosynovitis.**

ten·dot·o·my (tĕn-dŏt′ə-mē) *n.* See **tenotomy.**

ten·do·vag·i·nal (tĕn′dō-văj′ə-nəl) *adj.* Relating to a tendon and its sheath.

ten·do·vag·i·ni·tis (tĕn′dō-văj′ə-nī′tĭs) *n.* Variant of **tenovaginitis.**

te·nec·to·my (tĕ-nĕk′tə-mē) *n.* The surgical resection of part of a tendon. Also called *tenonectomy.*

te·nes·mic (tə-nĕz′mĭk) *adj.* Relating to, marked by, or affected with tenesmus.

te·nes·mus (tə-nĕz′məs) *n.* A painful spasm of the anal sphincter accompanied by an urgent desire to evacuate the bowel or bladder and involuntary straining that results in the passing of little or no matter.

te·ni·a (tē′nē-ə) *n.* Variant of **taenia.**

tenia cho·roi·de·a (kô-roi′dē-ə) *n.* The somewhat thickened line along which a choroid membrane is attached to the rim of a ventricle of the brain.

te·ni·a·cide (tē′nē-ə-sīd′) *n.* Variant of **taeniacide.**

tenia co·li (kō′lī) *n.* Any of the three bands in which the longitudinal muscular fibers of the large intestine, except the rectum, are collected: the mesocolic band, located at the place corresponding to the mesenteric attachment; the free band, located opposite the mesocolic band; and the omental band, located at the place corresponding to the site of adhesion of the greater omentum to the transverse colon.

te·ni·a·fuge (tē′nē-ə-fyōōj′) *n.* Variant of **taeniafuge.**

te·ni·al (tē′nē-əl) *adj.* **1.** Of or relating to a tapeworm or tapeworms. **2.** Of or relating to a taenia.

te·ni·a·sis (tē-nī′ə-sĭs) *n.* Variant of **taeniasis.**

ten·nis elbow (tĕn′ĭs) *n.* A painful inflammation of the tissue surrounding the elbow, caused by strain from playing tennis and other sports. Also called *lateral humeral epicondylitis.*

tennis thumb *n.* Tendonitis with calcification in the tendon of the long flexor of the thumb, caused by exercise in which the thumb is subject to pressure or strain.

teno– *or* **tenon–** *pref.* Tendon: *tenotomy.*

te·nod·e·sis (tə-nŏd′ĭ-sĭs, tĕn′ə-dē′sĭs) *n.* The surgical anchoring of a tendon, as to a bone.

ten·o·dyn·i·a (tĕn′ə-dĭn′ē-ə) *n.* See **tenalgia.**

te·nol·y·sis (tĕ-nŏl′ĭ-sĭs) *n.* Variant of **tendolysis.**

ten·o·my·o·plas·ty (tĕn′ō-mī′ə-plăs′tē) *n.* See **tenontomyoplasty.**

ten·o·my·ot·o·my (tĕn′ō-mī-ŏt′ə-mē) *n.* See **myotenotomy.**

ten·o·nec·to·my (tĕn′ə-nĕk′tə-mē) *n.* See **tenectomy.**

ten·o·ni·tis (tĕn′ə-nī′tĭs) *n.* **1.** Inflammation of Tenon's capsule or the connective tissue within Tenon's space. **2.** Tendinitis.

ten·o·nom·e·ter (tĕn′ə-nŏm′ĭ-tər) *n.* A tonometer.

Te·non's capsule (tē′nənz, tə-nôNz) *n.* See **sheath of eyeball.**

Tenon's space *n.* See **episcleral space.**

ten·on·ti·tis (tĕn′ən-tī′tĭs) *n.* Tendinitis.

tenonto– *or* **tenont–** *pref.* Tendon: *tenontomyoplasty.*

te·non·to·dyn·i·a (tə-nŏn′tə-dĭn′ē-ə, tĕn′ən-tō-) *n.* See **tenalgia.**

te·non·to·my·o·plas·ty (tə-nŏn′tō-mī′ə-plăs′tē) *n.* A surgical procudure used in the radical correction of hernia that combines tenontoplasty and myoplasty. Also called *tenomyoplasty.*

te·non·to·plas·ty (tə-nŏn′tə-plăs′tē) *n.* Reparative or plastic surgery of the tendons. Also called *tendinoplasty, tendoplasty, tenoplasty.*

ten·o·phyte (tĕn′ə-fīt′) *n.* A bony or a cartilaginous growth in or on a tendon.

ten·o·plas·ty (tĕn′ə-plăs′tē) *n.* See **tenontoplasty.**

ten·o·re·cep·tor (tĕn′ō-rĭ-sĕp′tər) *n.* A receptor in a tendon, activated by increased tension.

te·nor·rha·phy (tĕ-nôr′ə-fē) *n.* The surgical suture of the divided ends of a tendon. Also called *tendinosuture, tenosuture.*

ten·o·si·tis (tĕn′ə-sī′tĭs) *n.* Tendinitis.

ten·os·to·sis (tĕn′ŏ-stō′sĭs) *n.* The ossification of a tendon.

ten·o·sus·pen·sion (tĕn′ō-sə-spĕn′shən) *n.* The use of a tendon as a suspensory ligament.

ten·o·su·ture (tĕn′ō-sōō′chər) *n.* See **tenorrhaphy.**

ten·o·syn·o·vec·to·my (tĕn′ō-sĭn′ō-vĕk′tə-mē) *n.* Excision of a tendon sheath.

ten·o·syn·o·vi·tis (tĕn′ō-sĭn′ə-vī′tĭs, -sī′nə-) *or* **ten·do·syn·o·vi·tis** (tĕn′dō-) *n.* Inflammation of a tendon and its enveloping sheath. Also called *tendinous synovitis, tenovaginitis.*

te·not·o·my (tĕ-nŏt′ə-mē) *n.* The surgical division of a tendon to correct a deformity caused by congenital or acquired shortening of a muscle, as for the correction of strabismus. Also called *tendotomy.*

ten·o·vag·i·ni·tis (tĕn′ō-văj′ə-nī′tĭs) *or* **ten·do·vag·i·ni·tis** (tĕn′dō-) *n.* See **tenosynovitis.**

TENS (tĕnz) *n.* Transcutaneous electrical nerve stimulation; a technique used to relieve pain in an injured or diseased part of the body in which electrodes applied to the skin deliver intermittent stimulation to surface nerves and block the transmission of pain signals.

ten·sion (tĕn′shən) *n. Abbr.* **T 1.** The act or process of stretching something tight. **2.** The condition of so being stretched. **3.** A force tending to stretch or elongate something. **4.** The partial pressure of a gas, especially dissolved in a liquid such as blood. **5.** Mental, emotional, or nervous strain. **6.** Barely controlled hostility or a strained relationship between people or groups.

tension cavity *n.* A cavity in the lung in which the air pressure is greater than that of the atmosphere.

tension curve *n.* A line tracing the direction of the trabeculae in cancellous bone tissue, indicating the direction of tension placed on the bone.

tension headache *n.* A headache associated with nervous tension, anxiety, or stress, often related to chronic contraction of the scalp muscles.

tension suture *n.* See **retention suture.**

ten·sor (tĕn′sər, -sôr′) *n.* A muscle that stretches or tightens a body part.

tensor muscle of broad fascia *n.* A muscle with origin from the anterior superior spine and the adjacent lateral surface of the ilium, with insertion into the iliotibial band of the broad fascia, with nerve supply from the superior gluteal nerve, and whose action tenses the broad fascia and flexes, abducts, and medially rotates the thigh.

tensor muscle of soft palate *n.* A muscle with origin from the sphenoid bone and the eustachian tube, with insertion into the hard and soft palate, with nerve supply from the branches of the trigeminal nerve through the otic ganglion, and whose action tenses the soft palate and opens the eustachian tube.

tensor muscle of tympanic membrane *n.* A muscle with origin from the eustachian tube, with insertion into the handle of the malleus, with nerve supply from the branches of the trigeminal nerve through the otic ganglion, and whose action draws the handle of the malleus medialward and tenses the tympanic membrane.

tent[1] (tĕnt) *n.* A canopy used in various types of inhalation therapy to control the humidity and oxygen concentration of inspired air.

tent[2] (tĕnt) *n.* A small, cylindrical plug of lint or gauze used to keep open or probe a wound or an orifice. *—v.* To keep a wound or an orifice open with such a plug.

ten·ta·cle (tĕn′tə-kəl) *n.* An elongated, flexible, unsegmented extension, as one of those surrounding the mouth or oral cavity of the squid, used for feeling, grasping, or locomotion.

tenth cranial nerve (tĕnth) *n.* See **vagus nerve.**

ten·to·ri·al (tĕn-tôr′ē-əl) *adj.* Relating to a tentorium.

tentorial sinus *n.* See **straight sinus.**

ten·to·ri·um (tĕn-tôr′ē-əm) *n., pl.* **–to·ri·a** (-tôr′ē-ə) A membranous cover or horizontal partition.

tentorium cer·e·bel·li (sĕr′ə-bĕl′ī) *n.* A fold of dura mater forming a roof over the posterior cranial fossa, except for an anterior median opening through which the mesencephalon passes, and separating the cerebellum from the basal surface of the occipital and temporal lobes of the cerebral cortex.

TEPP (tē′ē-pē′pē) *n.* Tetraethyl pyrophosphate; a crystalline organophosphorus compound that inhibits the action of acetylcholinesterase and is used as a stimulant of the parasympathetic nervous system.

tera– *pref.* One trillion (10^{12}): *terahertz.*

ter·as (tĕr′əs) *n., pl.* **ter·a·ta** (tĕr′ə-tə) A malformed fetus with deficient, redundant, misplaced, or misshapen parts. —**te·rat′ic** (tə-răt′ĭk) *adj.*

ter·a·tism (tĕr′ə-tĭz′əm) *n.* A congenital malformation or monster.

terato– *pref.* Teras: *teratogen.*

ter·a·to·blas·to·ma (tĕr′ə-tō-blă-stō′mə) *n.* See **teratoma.**

ter·a·to·car·ci·no·ma (tĕr′ə-tō-kär′sə-nō′mə) *n.* 1. A malignant teratoma occurring most commonly in the testis. 2. A malignant epithelioma arising in a teratoma.

te·rat·o·gen (tə-răt′ə-jən, tĕr′ə-tə-) *n.* An agent, such as a virus, a drug, or radiation, that can cause malformations or functional damage to an embryo or a fetus.

ter·a·to·gen·e·sis (tĕr′ə-tə-jĕn′ĭ-sĭs) *n.* Development of malformed organisms or growths. Also called *teratogeny.*

ter·a·to·gen·ic (tĕr′ə-tə-jĕn′ĭk) *adj.* Of, relating to, or causing malformations of an embryo or a fetus.

ter·a·to·ge·nic·i·ty (tĕr′ə-tō-jə-nĭs′ĭ-tē) *n.* The capability of producing fetal malformation.

ter·a·tog·e·ny (tĕr′ə-tŏj′ə-nē) *n.* See **teratogenesis.**

ter·a·toid (tĕr′ə-toid′) *adj.* Resembling a teras; grotesquely deformed.

teratoid tumor *n.* See **teratoma.**

ter·a·tol·o·gy (tĕr′ə-tŏl′ə-jē) *n.* The biological study of malformations and monstrosities. —**ter′a·to·log′ic** (-tl-ŏj′ĭk) *adj.*

ter·a·to·ma (tĕr′ə-tō′mə) *n., pl.* **–mas** *or* **–ma·ta** (-mə-tə) A tumor consisting of different types of tissue, as of skin, hair, and muscle, that is caused by the development of independent germ cells. Also called *teratoblastoma, teratoid tumor.* —**ter′a·to′ma·tous** (-tō′mə-təs) *adj.*

ter·a·to·sis (tĕr′ə-tō′sĭs) *n.* Teratism.

te·ra·zo·sin hydrochloride (tə-rā′zə-sĭn) *n.* A crystalline compound that blocks adrenergic receptors and is used to treat hypertension.

ter·bi·um (tûr′bē-əm) *n. Symbol* **Tb** A soft metallic rare-earth element that is used in x-ray tubes. Atomic number 65.

te·res (tîr′ēz, tĕr′-) *adj.* Being round and long. Used of certain muscles and ligaments.

teres major *n.* A muscle with origin from the lower third of the border of the scapula, with insertion into the medial border of the humerus, with nerve supply from the lower subscapular nerve from the fifth and the sixth cervical nerves, and whose action adducts and extends the arm and rotates it medially.

teres minor *n.* A muscle with origin from the lateral border of the scapula, with insertion into the great tuberosity of the humerus, with nerve supply from the axillary nerve from the fifth and the sixth cervical nerves, and whose action adducts the arm and rotates it laterally.

term (tûrm) *n.* 1. A limited period of time. 2. The end of a normal gestation period.

Ter·man (tûr′mən), **Lewis Madison** 1877–1956. American psychologist who developed the intelligence quotient (IQ) as a measure of intelligence and created an English version of the tests used in the Binet-Simon scale.

ter·mi·nal (tûr′mə-nəl) *adj.* 1. Of, relating to, situated at, or forming a limit, a boundary, an extremity, or an end. 2. Of, relating to, occurring at, or being the end of a section or series; final. 3. Causing, ending in, or approaching death; fatal.

terminal artery *n.* See **end artery.**

terminal bar *n.* The zones where epithelial cells contact each other.

terminal boutons *pl.n.* See **axon terminals.**

terminal bronchiole *n.* The last portion of the nonrespiratory conducting airway, which subdivides into respiratory bronchioles.

terminal filum *n.* A long slender strand of connective tissue extending from the end of the medullary cone to the termination of the vertebral canal.

terminal hair *n.* A mature hair.

terminal ileitis *n.* See **Crohn's disease.**

terminal infection *n.* An acute infection, commonly pneumonic or septic, that occurs toward the end of a disease and often causes death.

terminal line *n.* An oblique ridge located on the inner surface of the ilium, continuing on the pubis and separating the small from the large pelvis. Also called *iliopectineal line.*

terminal nerve *n.* Any of the plexiform nerve strands passing parallel and medial to the olfactory tracts, distributing with the olfactory nerves and passing centrally into the anterior perforated substance.

terminal nucleus *n.* Any of the groups of nerve cells in the rhombencephalon and spinal cord in which the afferent fibers of the spinal and cranial nerves terminate. Also called *secondary sensory nucleus.*

terminal stria *n.* A slender, compact bundle of fibers connecting the amygdala with the hypothalamus and other basal forebrain regions.

terminal sulcus *n.* A V-shaped groove on the surface of the tongue, marking the separation between the oral and pharyngeal parts.

ter·mi·na·ti·o (tûr′mə-nā′shē-ō) *n., pl.* **–na·ti·o·nes** (-nā′shē-ō′nēz) A termination or ending, especially a nerve ending.

term infant *n.* An infant that is born between the end of the 37th week and the end of the 42nd week of gestation.

ter·mi·no·ter·mi·nal anastomosis (tûr′mə-nō-tûr′-mə-nəl) *n.* A surgical connection of the central end of an artery with the peripheral end of the corresponding vein, and between the peripheral end of the artery with the central end of the vein.

ter·na·ry (tûr′nə-rē) *adj.* Composed of three or arranged in threes, as a chemical compound containing three elements. —*n.* A group of three.

ter·pene (tûr′pēn′) *n.* Any of various unsaturated hydrocarbons in essential oils and certain resins of plants and used in organic syntheses.

ter·race (tĕr′ĭs) *v.* To suture in several rows, as when closing a wound through a considerable thickness of tissue.

Ter·ra·my·cin (tĕr′ə-mī′sĭn) A trademark for the drug oxytetracycline.

ter·ri·to·ri·al·i·ty (tĕr′ĭ-tôr′ē-ăl′ĭ-tē) *n.* **1.** A behavior pattern in animals consisting of the occupation and defense of a territory. **2.** A similar behavior pattern in humans consisting of the tendency to defend a particular domain or sphere of influence or interest.

ter·ri·to·ri·al matrix (tĕr′ĭ-tôr′ē-əl) *n.* Basophilic material surrounding isogenous groups of cartilage cells.

Ter·ry's syndrome (tĕr′ēz) *n.* See **retinopathy of prematurity.**

ter·tian (tûr′shən) *adj.* Recurring every other day or, when considered inclusively, every third day. Used of a fever. —*n.* A tertian fever.

tertian malaria *n.* See **vivax malaria.**

ter·ti·ar·y (tûr′shē-ĕr′ē) *adj.* **1.** Third in place, order, degree, or rank. **2.** Of or relating to salts of acids containing three replaceable hydrogen atoms. **3.** Of or relating to organic compounds in which a group is bound to three nonelementary radicals.

tertiary alcohol *n.* An alcohol containing the trivalent organic radical COH.

tertiary dentin *n.* Morphologically irregular dentin formed in response to an irritant, such as caries, disease, or drilling to prepare a cavity for filling. Also called *irregular dentin, reparative dentin.*

tertiary syphilis *n.* The final stage of syphilis, marked by gumma formation, cellular infiltration, and cardiovascular and central nervous system lesions.

tes·la (tĕs′lə) *n. Abbr.* **T** A unit of magnetic field intensity in the International System of Units equal to the magnitude of the magnetic field vector necessary to produce a force of one newton on a charge of one coulomb moving perpendicular to the direction of the magnetic field vector with a velocity of one meter per second.

tes·sel·lat·ed (tĕs′ə-lā′tĭd) *adj.* Composed of or patterned in small squares. —**tes′sel·la′tion** *n.*

tessellated fundus *n.* A normal retina having a deeply pigmented choroid that gives it the appearance of having dark polygonal areas between the choroidal vessels. Also called *leopard retina.*

test (tĕst) *n.* **1.** A procedure for critical evaluation; a means of determining the presence, quality, or truth of something; an examination, or experiment. **2.** A physical or chemical change by which a substance may be detected or its properties ascertained. **3.** A reagent used to cause or promote such a change. —*v.* **1.** To subject to a test; try. **2.** To determine the presence or properties of a substance. **3.** To administer a test. **4.** To exhibit a given characteristic when subjected to a test.

tes·tal·gia (tĕs-tăl′jə) *n.* See **orchialgia.**

tes·tec·to·my (tĕs-tĕk′tə-mē) *n.* See **orchiectomy.**

tes·ti·cle (tĕs′tĭ-kəl) *n.* A testis, especially one contained within the scrotum.

tes·tic·u·lar (tĕ-stĭk′yə-lər) *adj.* Of or relating to a testicle or testis.

testicular artery *n.* An artery with origin in the aorta, with branches to the ureteral, cremasteric, and epididymal arteries, with distribution to the testicle, and with anastomoses to the branches of the renal, inferior epigastric, and deferential arteries. Also called *internal spermatic artery.*

testicular cord *n.* See **spermatic cord.**

testicular feminization syndrome *n.* A type of familial male pseudohermaphroditism characterized by female external genitalia, an incompletely developed vagina often with a rudimentary uterus and fallopian tubes, testes present within the abdomen, inguinal canals, or labia majora, and amenorrhea and scant or absent pubic and axillary hair at puberty.

tes·tis (tĕs′tĭs) *n., pl.* **–tes** (-tēz) The male reproductive gland, the source of spermatozoa and the androgens, normally occurring paired in an external scrotum. Also called *didymus, orchis.*

tes·ti·tis (tĕ-stī′tĭs) *n.* See **orchitis.**

test meal *n.* Bland food given to stimulate gastric secretion before analysis of gastric contents.

tes·tos·ter·one (tĕs-tŏs′tə-rōn′) *n.* A steroid hormone and the most potent naturally occurring androgen that is formed by the interstitial cells of the testes, and possibly by the ovary and adrenal cortex, may be produced in nonglandular tissues from precursors such as androstenedione, and is used in the treatment of hypogonadism, cryptorchism, carcinomas, and menorrhagia.

test profile *n.* An array of laboratory tests usually conducted using automated methods and equipment and designed to gather biochemical and other information on the organ systems of individuals admitted to a hospital or clinic.

test solution *n.* A solution of a reagent in a specified strength, used in chemical analysis or testing.

test tube *n.* A clear, cylindrical glass tube usually open at one end and rounded at the other, used in laboratory experimentation.

test-tube *adj.* **1.** Produced or cultivated in a test tube. **2.** Conceived by or developed from fertilization in laboratory apparatus or by artificial insemination.

test-tube baby *n.* A baby developed from an egg that was fertilized outside the body and then implanted in the uterus.

test types *pl.n.* Letters printed in various sizes used to test the acuity of vision.

te·tan·ic (tĕ-tăn′ĭk) *adj.* **1.** Of or causing tetanus or tetany. **2.** Marked by sustained muscular contractions. —*n.* An agent that in poisonous doses produces tonic muscular spasm.

te·tan·i·form (tĕ-tăn′ə-fôrm′) *adj.* Resembling tetanus; tetanoid.

tet·a·nig·e·nous (tĕt′n-ĭj′ə-nəs) *adj.* Causing tetanus or tetanoid spasms.

tet·a·nism (tĕt′n-ĭz′əm) *n.* See **neonatal tetany.**

tet·a·nize (tĕt′n-īz′) *v.* To affect with tetanic convulsions; produce or induce tetanus in. —**tet′a·ni·za′tion** (tĕt′n-ĭ-zā′shən) *n.*

tetano– *or* **tetan–** *pref.* Tetanus; tetany: *tetanigenous.*

tet·a·node (tĕt′n-ōd′) *n.* The quiet interval between the recurrent tonic spasms in tetanus.

tet·a·noid (tĕt′n-oid′) *adj.* **1.** Resembling tetanus. **2.** Resembling tetany.

tet·a·no·spas·min (tĕt′n-ō-spăz′mĭn) *n.* The neurotoxin of *Clostridium tetani* that causes the characteristic signs and symptoms of tetanus.

tet·a·nus (tĕt′n-əs) *n.* **1.** An acute, often fatal disease that is characterized by spasmodic contraction of voluntary muscles, especially one occurring in the neck and jaw, and that is caused by the bacterium *Clostridium tetani,* which usually enters the body through an infected wound and produces a neurotoxin. Also called *lockjaw.* **2.** A state of continuous muscular contraction, especially when induced artificially by rapidly repeated stimuli.

tetanus and gas gangrene antitoxin *n.* A solution of tetanus and gas gangrene antitoxins.

tetanus antitoxin *n.* The antitoxin specific for the neurotoxin produced by *Clostridium tetani.*

tetanus-diphtheria toxoids vaccine *n. Abbr.* **Td** One of the forms of the diphtheria, tetanus toxoids, and pertussis vaccine, containing tetanus and diphtheria toxoids and used to immunize against tetanus and diphtheria.

tetanus immune globulin *n.* A sterile solution of globulins that are derived from the blood plasma of adult human donors who exhibit a high titer of antibodies specific for tetanus because of immunization with tetanus toxoid, used as a passive immunizing agent.

tet·a·nus ne·o·na·to·rum (nē′ō-nă-tôr′əm) *n.* Tetanus affecting newborns, usually due to infection of the severed umbilical cord.

tetanus toxin *n.* The neurotropic exotoxin of *Clostridium tetani* that causes tetanus.

tetanus toxoids vaccine *n. Abbr.* **T** One of the forms of the diphtheria, tetanus toxoids, and pertussis vaccine, containing tetanus toxoids and used to immunize against tetanus.

tetanus vaccine *n. Abbr.* **T** Tetanus toxoids vaccine.

tet·a·ny (tĕt′n-ē) *n.* An abnormal condition that is characterized by periodic painful muscular spasms and tremors, is caused by faulty calcium metabolism, and is associated with diminished function of the parathyroid glands. Also called *intermittent cramp, intermittent tetanus.*

te·tar·ta·nop·si·a (tĕ-tär′tə-nŏp′sē-ə) *n.* A homonymous form of quadrantic hemianopsia. Also called *tetartanopia.*

teth·ered cord syndrome (tĕth′ərd) *n.* Sacral retention of the spinal cord by the terminal filum, causing incontinence and progressive motor and sensory impairment in the legs.

tetra– *or* **tetr–** *pref.* **1.** Four: *tetradactyl.* **2.** Composed of or containing four atoms, molecules, or groups: *tetrasaccharide.*

tet·ra·caine hydrochloride (tĕt′rə-kān′) *n.* A crystalline compound related to procaine and used as a local anesthetic.

tet·ra·chlo·ride (tĕt′rə-klôr′īd′) *n.* A chemical compound containing four chlorine atoms per molecule.

tet·ra·chlo·ro·eth·ane (tĕt′rə-klôr′ō-ĕth′ān′) *n.* A toxic, nonflammable solvent used in the manufacture of paint and varnish removers, photographic films, lacquers, and insecticides.

tet·ra·chlo·ro·meth·ane (tĕt′rə-klôr′ō-mĕth′ān′) *n.* See **carbon tetrachloride.**

tet·ra·co·sac·tide (tĕt′rə-kō-săk′tīd′) *n.* See **cosyntropin.**

tet·ra·crot·ic (tĕt′rə-krŏt′ĭk) *adj.* Of or relating to a pulse curve with four upstrokes in the cycle.

tet·ra·cy·clic antidepressant (tĕt′rə-sī′klĭk, -sĭk′lĭk) *n.* Any of a class of antidepressants whose chemical structure includes four benzene rings.

tet·ra·cy·cline (tĕt′rə-sī′klēn′, -klĭn) *n.* **1.** A yellow crystalline compound synthesized or derived from certain actinomycetes of the genus *Streptomyces* and used as a broad-spectrum antibiotic. **2.** An antibiotic, such as oxytetracycline, having the same basic structure.

tet·rad (tĕt′răd′) *n.* **1.** A group or set of four. **2.** A tetravalent atom, radical, or element. **3.** A group of four chromatids formed from each of a pair of homologous chromosomes that split longitudinally during the prophase of meiosis.

tet·ra·dac·tyl (tĕt′rə-dăk′təl) *or* **tet·ra·dac·ty·lous** (-tə-ləs) *adj.* Having only four fingers or toes on a hand or foot.

tet·ra·eth·yl lead *or* **tet·ra·eth·yl·lead** (tĕt′rə-ĕth′əl-lĕd′) *n.* A colorless, poisonous, oily liquid used in gasoline for internal-combustion engines as an antiknock agent.

tetraethyl pyrophosphate *n.* TEPP.

tetrahydro– *pref.* Containing four hydrogen atoms: *tetrahydrocannabinol.*

tet·ra·hy·dro·can·nab·i·nol (tĕt′rə-hī′drə-kə-năb′ə-nôl′, -nōl′) *n.* THC.

te·tral·o·gy (tĕ-trăl′ə-jē, -trŏl′-) *n.* A complex of four symptoms.

tetralogy of Fallot *n.* See **Fallot's tetralogy.**

tet·ra·mer (tĕt′rə-mər) *n.* A polymer consisting of four identical monomers. —**tet·ra·mer·ic** (-mĕr′ĭk) *adj.*

tet·ra·pa·re·sis (tĕt′rə-pə-rē′sĭs, -păr′ĭ-sĭs) *n.* Weakness of all four limbs. Also called *quadriparesis.*

tet·ra·pep·tide (tĕt′rə-pĕp′tīd′) *n.* A peptide composed of four amino acids.

tet·ra·ple·gia (tĕt′rə-plē′jə) *n.* See **quadriplegia.**

tet·ra·ploid (tĕt′rə-ploid′) *adj.* Having four times the haploid number of chromosomes in the cell nucleus. —*n.* A tetraploid individual.

tet·ra·sac·cha·ride (tĕt′rə-săk′ə-rīd′) *n.* A sugar containing four monosaccharide molecules.

tet·ra·so·mic (tĕt′rə-sō′mĭk) *adj.* Relating to a cell nucleus in which one chromosome occurs four times, while all others are present in the normal number.

tet·ra·va·lent (tĕt′rə-vā′lənt) *adj.* Having a valence of four; quadrivalent.

te·tro·do·tox·in (tĕ-trō′də-tŏk′sĭn) *n.* A potent neurotoxin, found in many puffer fish and certain newts.

tet·rose (tĕt′rōs′, -rōz′) *n.* A monosaccharide containing no more than four carbon atoms in its primary chain.

tet·ter (tĕt′ər) *n.* Any of various skin diseases, such as eczema, psoriasis, or herpes, characterized by eruptions and itching.

text blindness *n.* See **alexia.**

tex·ti·form (tĕk′stə-fôrm′) *adj.* Resembling a web.

tex·tur·al (tĕks′chər-əl) *adj.* Relating to the texture of the tissues.

tex·ture (tĕks′chər) *n.* The composition or structure of a tissue or organ. —**tex′tured** *adj.*

Tev·e·ten (tĕv′ĭ-tn) A trademark for the drug eprosartan mesylate.

Th The symbol for the element **thorium.**

thal·a·men·ceph·a·lon (thăl′ə-mĕn-sĕf′ə-lŏn′) *n.* The

part of the diencephalon comprising the thalamus and its associated structures.

thalamo– *or* **thalam–** *pref.* Thalamus: *thalamotomy.*

thal·a·mo·cor·ti·cal (thăl′ə-mō-kôr′tĭ-kəl) *adj.* Relating to the thalamus and the cerebral cortex.

thal·a·mot·o·my (thăl′ə-mŏt′ə-mē) *n.* Destruction of a portion of the thalamus by stereotaxis to relieve tremor.

thal·a·mus (thăl′ə-məs) *n., pl.* **–mi** (-mī′) A large ovoid mass of gray matter that forms the larger dorsal subdivision of the diencephalon and is located medial to the internal capsule and to the body and tail of the caudate nucleus. It functions in the relay of sensory impulses to the cerebral cortex. —**tha·lam·ic** (thə-lăm′ĭk) *adj.*

thal·as·se·mi·a (thăl′ə-sē′mē-ə) *n.* Any of a group of inherited forms of anemia occurring chiefly among people of Mediterranean descent, caused by faulty synthesis of part of the hemoglobin molecule. Also called *Mediterranean anemia.*

thalassemia ma·jor (mā′jər) *n.* A usually fatal form of thalassemia appearing in infancy or childhood in which normal hemoglobin is absent, characterized by severe anemia, enlargement of the heart, liver, and spleen, and skeletal deformation. Also called *Cooley's anemia.*

tha·lid·o·mide (thə-lĭd′ə-mīd′) *n.* A sedative and hypnotic drug that was withdrawn from sale after it was found to cause severe birth defects when taken during pregnancy.

thal·lic (thăl′lĭk) *adj.* **1.** Of or relating to conidia produced with no enlargement or growth after delimitation by septa in the hypha. **2.** Of, relating to, or containing thallium, especially with valence 3.

thal·li·um (thăl′ē-əm) *n. Symbol* **Tl** A soft, malleable, highly toxic metallic element whose radioisotopes are used in diagnostic imaging. Atomic number 81.

thal·lus (thăl′əs) *n., pl.* **–lus·es** *or* **thal·li** (thăl′ī) A plant body or fungus undifferentiated into stem, root, or leaf.

thanato– *pref.* Death: *thanatology.*

than·a·to·bi·o·log·ic (thăn′ə-tō-bī′ə-lŏj′ĭk) *adj.* Of or relating to the processes concerned in life and death.

than·a·to·gno·mon·ic (thăn′ə-tō-nō-mŏn′ĭk, -tŏg′-nō-) *adj.* Indicating the approach of death.

than·a·toid (thăn′ə-toid′) *adj.* **1.** Resembling death. **2.** Mortal; deadly.

than·a·tol·o·gy (thăn′ə-tŏl′ə-jē) *n.* The study of death and dying, especially of their psychological and social aspects.

Than·a·tos *or* **than·a·tos** (thăn′ə-tōs′) *n.* See **death instinct.**

THC (tē′ăch-sē′) *n.* Tetrahydrocannabinol; a compound that is obtained from cannabis or is made synthetically; it is the primary intoxicant in the illegal drugs marijuana and hashish.

the·ba·ine (thē′bə-ēn′, thĭ-bā′ĭn) *n.* A poisonous crystalline alkaloid obtained from opium. Also called *paramorphine.*

the·ca (thē′kə) *n., pl.* **–cae** (-sē′, -kē′) A case, covering, or sheath, such as the outer covering of the cocoon of certain insects.

theca-cell tumor *n.* See **thecoma.**

theca cor·dis (kôr′dĭs) *n.* See **pericardium.**

theca fol·lic·u·li (fə-lĭk′yə-lī′) *n.* The wall of a vesicular ovarian follicle.

the·cal (thē′kəl) *adj.* Of or relating to a sheath, especially a tendon sheath.

the·ci·tis (thē-sī′tĭs) *n.* Inflammation of the sheath of a tendon.

the·co·ma (thē-kō′mə) *n.* A tumor derived from ovarian mesenchyme and consisting chiefly of spindle-shaped cells that frequently contain small droplets of fat; it may form considerable quantities of estrogens, causing development of secondary sexual features in prepubertal girls or endometrial hyperplasia in older individuals. Also called *theca-cell tumor.*

the·co·steg·no·sis (thē′kō-stĕg-nō′sĭs) *n.* Constriction of a tendon sheath.

thee·lin (thē′lĭn) *n.* See **estrone.**

thee·lol (thē′lôl′, -lŏl′) *n.* See **estriol.**

Thei·ler (tī′lər), **Max** 1899–1972. South African-born American microbiologist. He won a 1951 Nobel Prize for developing a vaccine for yellow fever.

the·lar·che (thē-lär′kē) *n.* The beginning of development of the breasts in the female.

The·la·zi·a (thə-lā′zē-ə) *n.* A genus of spiruroid nematodes that inhabit the lacrimal ducts and surface of the eyes of various domestic and wild animals but rarely of humans.

the·la·zi·a·sis (thē′lə-zī′ə-sĭs, thĕl′ə-) *n.* Infection with nematodes of the genus *Thelazia.*

the·le·plas·ty (thē′lə-plăs′tē) *n.* See **mammillaplasty.**

the·li·um (thē′lē-əm) *n., pl.* **–li·a** (-lē-ə) **1.** A papilla. **2.** A cellular layer. See **nipple.**

thelo– *or* **thel–** *pref.* Nipple: *thelarche.*

the·lor·rha·gia (thē′lə-rā′jə) *n.* Bleeding from the nipple.

T-helper cell *n.* Immune system cells that produce lymphokines that regulate the activities of other immune system cells, such as T cells, B cells, and monocytes, that are necessary for the differentiating of B cells into antibody-producing cells, and that often decrease in concentration following HIV infection.

The·mat·ic Apperception Test (thĭ-măt′ĭk) *n. Abbr.* **TAT** A psychological test in which the subject is asked to tell a story about a set of standard pictures showing everyday situations, thereby revealing his or her own attitudes and feelings.

the·nal·dine (thē-năl′dēn′) *n.* An antihistaminic and antipruritic agent.

the·nar (thē′när′, -nər) *n.* The fleshy mass on the palm at the base of the thumb. Also called *thenar prominence.* —*adj.* Of or relating to the thenar.

the·o·bro·mine (thē′ō-brō′mēn′) *n.* A bitter, colorless alkaloid found in chocolate products and used as a diuretic, vasodilator, and myocardial stimulant.

the·oph·yl·line (thē-ŏf′ə-lĭn, thē′ō-fĭl′ēn′) *n.* A colorless crystalline alkaloid derived from tea leaves or made synthetically, used as a cardiac stimulant and diuretic.

The·o·rell (tā′ə-rĕl′), **Axel Hugo Theodor** 1903–1982. Swedish biochemist. He won a 1955 Nobel Prize for research on the oxidation of enzymes.

the·o·rem (thē′ər-əm, thîr′əm) *n.* **1.** An idea that is demonstrably true or is assumed to be so. **2.** A mathematical proposition that has been or is to be proved on the basis of explicit assumptions.

the·o·ret·i·cal (thē′ə-rĕt′ĭ-kəl) *adj.* **1.** Of, relating to, or based on theory. **2.** Restricted to theory; not practical.

the·o·ry (thē′ə-rē, thîr′ē) *n.* **1.** A systematically organized body of knowledge applicable in a relatively wide variety of circumstances, especially a system of assumptions, accepted principles, and rules of procedure devised to analyze, predict, or otherwise explain the nature or behavior of a specified set of phenomena. **2.** Abstract reasoning; speculation.

thèque (tĕk) *n.* An aggregation of nevus cells or other cells in the epidermis.

ther·a·peu·tic (thĕr′ə-pyoo′tĭk) *or* **ther·a·peu·ti·cal** (-tĭ-kəl) *adj.* **1.** Having or exhibiting healing powers. **2.** Of or relating to therapeutics.

therapeutic abortion *n.* Induced abortion.

therapeutic cloning *n.* A procedure in which damaged tissues or organs are repaired or replaced with genetically identical cells that originate from undifferentiated stem cells.

therapeutic crisis *n.* A turning point in psychiatric treatment leading to positive or negative change.

therapeutic index *n.* The ratio between the toxic dose and the therapeutic dose of a drug, used as a measure of the relative safety of the drug for a particular treatment.

therapeutic ratio *n.* The ratio of the maximally tolerated dose of a drug to the minimally curative or effective dose.

ther·a·peu·tics (thĕr′ə-pyoo′tĭks) *n.* Medical treatment of disease; the art or science of healing. **—ther′a·peu′tist** *n.*

ther·a·pist (thĕr′ə-pĭst) *n.* One who specializes in the provision of a particular therapy.

ther·a·py (thĕr′ə-pē) *n.* **1.** The treatment of illness or disability. **2.** Psychotherapy. **3.** A healing power or quality.

therm– *pref.* Variant of **thermo–**.

–therm *suff.* An organism having a specified kind of body temperature: *exotherm.*

ther·ma·co·gen·e·sis (thûr′mə-kō-jĕn′ĭ-sĭs) *n.* Elevation of body temperature by the use of a drug.

ther·mal (thûr′məl) *adj.* **1.** Of, relating to, using, producing, or caused by heat. **2.** Intended or designed in such a way as to help retain body heat.

thermal anesthesia *or* **ther·mic anesthesia** (thûr′mĭk) *n.* Loss of the ability to sense temperature.

thermal capacity *n.* See **heat capacity**.

therm·al·ge·si·a (thûr′məl-jē′zē-ə, -zhə) *n.* Extreme sensitivity to warmth or heat.

ther·mal·gia (thər-măl′jə) *n.* Burning pain.

therm·an·al·ge·si·a (thûrm′ăn-əl-jē′zē-ə, -zhə) *n.* See **thermoanesthesia**.

therm·an·es·the·sia (thûrm′ăn-ĭs-thē′zhə) *n.* See **thermoanesthesia**.

therm·es·the·sia (thûrm′ĭs-thē′zhə) *n.* See **thermoesthesia**.

therm·es·the·si·om·e·ter (thûrm′ĭs-thē′zē-ŏm′ĭ-tər) *n.* See **thermoesthesiometer**.

thermo– *or* **therm–** *pref.* Heat: *thermogenesis.*

ther·mo·an·es·the·sia (thûr′mō-ăn′ĭs-thē′zhə) *n.* Loss of the ability to distinguish between heat and cold. Also

called *thermanalgesia, thermanesthesia, thermoanalgesia.*

ther·mo·cau·ter·y (thûr′mō-kô′tə-rē) *n.* Cauterization using heat, as with a heated wire.

ther·mo·chem·is·try (thûr′mō-kĕm′ĭ-strē) *n.* The study of the chemistry of heat and heat-associated chemical phenomena.

ther·mo·co·ag·u·la·tion (thûr′mō-kō-ăg′yə-lā′shən) *n.* The use of heat produced by high-frequency electric current to bring about localized destruction of tissues.

ther·mo·cou·ple (thûr′mə-kŭp′əl) *n.* A thermoelectric device used to measure temperatures accurately, especially one consisting of two dissimilar metals joined so that a potential difference generated between the points of contact is a measure of the temperature difference between the points.

ther·mo·dif·fu·sion (thûr′mō-dĭ-fyoo′zhən) *n.* The diffusion of fluids, either gaseous or liquid, as influenced by their temperature.

ther·mo·du·ric (thûr′mō-door′ĭk) *adj.* Capable of surviving high temperatures, especially those of pasteurization. Used of a microorganism.

ther·mo·dy·nam·ic (thûr′mō-dī-năm′ĭk) *adj.* **1.** Characteristic of or resulting from the conversion of heat into other forms of energy. **2.** Of or relating to thermodynamics.

ther·mo·dy·nam·ics (thûr′mō-dī-năm′ĭks) *n.* **1.** Physics that deals with the relationships between heat and other forms of energy. **2.** Thermodynamic phenomena and processes.

thermodynamic theory of narcosis *n.* The theory that interposition of narcotic molecules in the nonaqueous cellular phase causes changes that interfere with ionic exchange.

ther·mo·es·the·sia (thûr′mō-ĭs-thē′zhə) *n.* Ability to feel hot or cold; sensitivity to variations in temperature. Also called *thermesthesia.*

ther·mo·es·the·si·om·e·ter (thûr′mō-ĭs-thē′zē-ŏm′ĭ-tər) *n.* An instrument for testing sensitivity to temperature variations. Also called *thermesthesiometer.*

ther·mo·ex·ci·to·ry (thûr′mō-ĭk-sī′tə-rē, -ĕk′sĭ-tôr′ē) *adj.* Stimulating the production of heat.

ther·mo·gen·e·sis (thûr′mō-jĕn′ĭ-sĭs, -mə-) *n.* Generation or production of heat, especially by physiological processes. **—ther′mo·ge·net′ic** (-jə-nĕt′ĭk), **ther′mo·gen′ic** (-jĕn′ĭk) *adj.*

ther·mo·gram (thûr′mə-grăm′) *n.* A regional temperature map of the surface of a part of the body made by a thermograph.

ther·mo·graph (thûr′mə-grăf′) *n.* **1.** A thermometer that records the temperature it indicates. **2.** The apparatus used in diagnostic thermography.

ther·mog·ra·phy (thər-mŏg′rə-fē) *n.* A diagnostic technique in which an infrared camera is used to measure temperature variations on the surface of the body, producing images that reveal sites of abnormal tissue growth.

ther·mo·in·hib·i·to·ry (thûr′mō-ĭn-hĭb′ĭ-tôr′ē) *adj.* Inhibiting or arresting thermogenesis.

ther·mo·la·bile (thûr′mō-lā′bĭl, -bīl′) *adj.* Subject to destruction, decomposition, or great change by moderate heating. Used especially of biochemical substances. **—ther′mo·la·bil′i·ty** (-bĭl′ĭ-tē) *n.*

ther·mol·y·sis (thər-mŏl′ĭ-sĭs) *n.* **1.** Dissipation of heat from the body, as by evaporation. **2.** Dissociation or decomposition of chemical compounds by heat. —**ther′mo·lyt′ic** (thûr′mə-lĭt′ĭk) *adj.*

ther·mo·mas·sage (thûr′mō-mə-säzh′) *n.* Physical therapy using both heat and massage.

ther·mom·e·ter (thər-mŏm′ĭ-tər) *n.* An instrument for measuring temperature.

ther·mom·e·try (thər-mŏm′ĭ-trē) *n.* **1.** Measurement of temperature. **2.** The technology of temperature measurement. —**ther′mo·met′ric** (thûr′mō-mĕt′rĭk) *adj.*

ther·mo·phile (thûr′mə-fīl′) *or* **ther·mo·phil** (-fĭl) *n.* An organism that thrives at a temperature of 50°C or higher.

ther·mo·phil·ic (thûr′mə-fĭl′ĭk) *adj.* Requiring high temperatures for normal development, as certain bacteria.

ther·mo·phore (thûr′mə-fôr′) *n.* A device for applying heat to a body part.

ther·mo·phy·lic (thûr′mə-fī′lĭk) *adj.* Capable of surviving at high temperatures. Used of a microorganism.

ther·mo·plac·en·tog·ra·phy (thûr′mə-plăs′ən-tŏg′rə-fē) *n.* A determination of placental position by infrared detection of the blood flowing through the placenta.

ther·mo·ple·gia (thûr′mə-plē′jə) *n.* Sunstroke.

ther·mo·re·cep·tor (thûr′mō-rĭ-sĕp′tər) *n.* A sensory receptor that responds to heat and cold.

ther·mo·reg·u·late (thûr′mō-rĕg′yə-lāt′) *v.* To regulate body temperature.

ther·mo·reg·u·la·tion (thûr′mō-rĕg′yə-lā′shən) *n.* Maintenance of a constant internal body temperature independent of the environmental temperature. —**ther′mo·reg′u·la·to·ry** (-rĕg′yə-lə-tôr′ē) *adj.*

ther·mo·scope (thûr′mə-skōp′) *n.* An instrument that indicates slight differences of temperature but does not record them.

ther·mo·sta·ble (thûr′mō-stā′bəl) *or* **ther·mo·sta·bile** (-bəl, -bīl′) *adj.* Unaffected by relatively high temperatures, as certain ferments or toxins.

ther·mo·ste·re·sis (thûr′mō-stə-rē′sĭs) *n.* Deprivation of heat.

ther·mo·sys·tal·tic (thûr′mō-sĭ-stôl′tĭk, -stăl′-) *adj.* Causing contraction, as of the muscles, by the influence of heat.

ther·mo·tax·is (thûr′mə-tăk′sĭs) *n.,* *pl.* **-tax·es** (-tăk′sēz) **1.** Movement of a living organism in response to changes in temperature. **2.** Normal regulation or adjustment of body temperature. —**ther′mo·tac′tic** (-tăk′tĭk), **ther′mo·tax′ic** (-tăk′sĭk) *adj.*

ther·mo·ther·a·py (thûr′mō-thĕr′ə-pē) *n.* Medical therapy involving the application of heat.

ther·mo·to·nom·e·ter (thûr′mō-tō-nŏm′ĭ-tər) *n.* An instrument for measuring the degree of muscular contraction under the influence of heat.

ther·mot·ro·pism (thər-mŏt′rə-pĭz′əm) *n.* The tendency of plants or other organisms to bend toward or away from heat. —**ther′mo·trop′ic** (thûr′mə-trŏp′ĭk) *adj.*

–thermy *suff.* Heat: *diathermy.*

the·ta (thā′tə, thē′-) *n.* *Symbol* θ The eighth letter of the Greek alphabet.

theta wave *n.* A waveform on an electroencephalogram having a frequency of 4 to 8 hertz, recorded chiefly in the hippocampus of carnivorous mammals when they are alert or aroused. Also called *theta rhythm.*

thi– *pref.* Variant of *thio–.*

thi·a·ben·da·zole (thī′ə-bĕn′də-zōl′) *n.* A white compound used as an antifungal agent and as an anthelmintic; it is effective against a broad spectrum of infectious agents.

thi·a·mine (thī′ə-mĭn, -mēn′) *or* **thi·a·min** (-mĭn) *n.* A vitamin of the vitamin B complex, found in meat, yeast, and the bran coat of grains, and necessary for carbohydrate metabolism and normal neural activity. Also called *vitamin B₁.*

thi·a·zide (thī′ə-zīd′, -zĭd) *n.* See benzothiadiazide.

thi·a·zine (thī′ə-zēn′) *or* **thi·a·zin** (-zĭn) *n.* Any of a class of organic chemical compounds containing a ring composed of one sulfur atom, one nitrogen atom, and four carbon atoms, used in making dyes.

thi·a·zo·li·dine·di·one (thī′ə-zō′lĭ-dīn′dī-ōn′, -dē-ōn′) *n.* *Abbr.* **TZD** A class of drugs used to treat type 2 diabetes mellitus by decreasing insulin resistance.

thick (thĭk) *adj.* **1.** Relatively great in extent from one surface to the opposite, usually in the smallest solid dimension; not thin. **2.** Measuring a specified number of units in this dimension. **3.** Heavy in form, build, or stature; thickset. **4.** Having component parts in a close, crowded state or arrangement; dense. **5.** Having or suggesting a heavy or viscous consistency. **6.** Having a great number; abounding. **7.** Impenetrable by the eyes. **8.** Not easy to hear or understand; indistinctly articulated. **9.** Noticeably affecting sound; conspicuous. **10.** Producing indistinctly articulated sounds.

thick·ness (thĭk′nĭs) *n.* **1.** The quality or condition of being thick. **2.** The dimension between two surfaces of an object, usually the one of smallest measure. **3.** A layer or stratum.

thi·e·mi·a (thī-ē′mē-ə) *n.* The presence of sulfur in the blood.

thi·e·nyl·al·a·nine (thī′ə-nĭl-ăl′ə-nēn′) *n.* A compound that is structurally similar to phenylalanine and inhibits the growth of *Escherichia coli.*

thi·eth·yl·per·a·zine maleate (thī-ĕth′əl-pĕr′ə-zēn′) *n.* A drug used to control nausea and vomiting.

thigh (thī) *n.* The part of the leg between the hip and the knee. Also called *femur.*

thigh·bone (thī′bōn′) *n.* See femur.

thig·mes·the·sia (thĭg′mĭs-thē′zhə) *n.* Sensibility to touch.

thig·mo·tax·is (thĭg′mə-tăk′sĭs) *n.* See stereotaxis (sense ?). —**thig′mo·tac′tic** (-tăk′tĭk) *adj.*

thig·mot·ro·pism (thĭg-mŏt′rə-pĭz′əm) *n.* The turning or bending response of an organism or part of an organism upon direct contact with a solid surface or object. Also called *stereotropism.* —**thig′mo·trop′ic** (thĭg′-mə-trŏp′ĭk, -trō′pĭk) *adj.*

thi·mer·o·sal (thī-mĕr′ə-săl′) *n.* A mercury-based crystalline powder with antibacterial and antifungal properties, used as a local antiseptic and preservative in vaccines and other drugs.

think (thĭngk) *v.* **1.** To exercise the power of reason, as by conceiving ideas, drawing inferences, and using judgment. **2.** To weigh or consider an idea. **3.** To bring a thought to mind by imagination or invention. **4.** To recall a thought or an image to mind.

think·ing (thĭng′kĭng) *n*. The act or practice of a person who thinks; thought. —*adj*. Characterized by thought or thoughtfulness; rational.

thinking through *n*. The psychological process of understanding one's own behavior.

thin-layer chromatography *n*. *Abbr*. **TLC** Chromatography through a thin layer of cellulose or similar inert material supported on a glass or plastic plate.

thin section (thĭn) *n*. A section of tissue less than 0.1 micrometer in thickness, fixed and embedded in a plastic resin for examination by electron microscope. Also called *ultrathin section*.

thio– or **thi–** *pref*. Containing sulfur, used especially of a compound in which oxygen has been replaced by a divalent sulfur: *thioacid*.

thi·o·ac·id (thī′ō-ăs′ĭd) *n*. An organic acid in which one or more of the oxygen atoms have been replaced by sulfur atoms.

thi·o·bar·bi·tu·rate (thī′ō-bär-bĭch′ər-ĭt, -ə-rāt′, -bär′- bĭ-tŏŏr′ĭt, -āt′) *n*. Any of the hypnotics of the barbiturate group in which a particular oxygen atom is replaced by a sulfur atom.

thi·o·di·phen·yl·a·mine (thī′ō-dī-fĕn′əl-ə-mēn′, -ăm′- ĭn, -fē′nəl-) *n*. See **phenothiazine** (sense 1).

thi·o·ki·nase (thī′ō-kī′nās′, -nāz′, -kĭn′ās′, -āz′) *n*. See **acyl-CoA synthetase**.

thi·ol (thī′ôl′, -ōl′) *n*. **1**. See **mercaptan**. **2**. A mixture of sulfurated and sulfonated petroleum oils that is purified with ammonia and is used in the treatment of skin diseases.

thion– *pref*. Sulfur: *thionic*.

thi·on·ic (thī-ŏn′ĭk) *adj*. Of, relating to, containing, or derived from sulfur.

thi·o·nine (thī′ə-nēn′, -nĭn) *n*. A dark-green powder that turns water purple when mixed in solution, used as a basic stain in histology for chromatin and mucin because of its metachromatic properties.

thi·o·pen·tal sodium (thī′ō-pĕn′tăl′, -tôl′) *n*. A yellowish-white hygroscopic powder injected intravenously as a general anesthetic and used in psychotherapy to induce a relaxed state.

thi·o·rid·a·zine (thī′ə-rĭd′ə-zēn′) *n*. A white or yellow powder, a derivative of phenothiazine, that is used orally as a tranquilizer to treat various psychotic conditions.

thi·o·sul·fate (thī′ō-sŭl′fāt′) *n*. A salt or ester of thiosulfuric acid.

thi·o·sul·fu·ric acid (thī′ō-sŭl-fyŏŏr′ĭk) *n*. An acid formed by replacement of an oxygen atom by a sulfur atom in sulfuric acid, known only in solution or by its salts and esters.

thi·o·thix·ene (thī′ō-thĭk′sēn′) *n*. An antipsychotic drug that is given orally and intramuscularly, used primarily in the treatment of schizophrenia.

thi·o·u·ra·cil (thī′ō-yŏŏr′ə-sĭl′) *n*. A white crystalline compound that interferes with the synthesis of thyroxine, used to reduce thyroid gland activity, especially in the treatment of hyperthyroidism.

thi·o·xan·thene (thī′ō-zăn′thēn) *n*. A class of tricyclic compounds resembling phenothiazine and having antipsychotic and antiemetic properties.

third (thûrd) *adj*. **1**. Coming next after second, as in order, rank, or time. **2**. Being the digit that is adjacent to and is on the outermost side of the second digit, as on a foot. —**third** *n*.

third cranial nerve *n*. See **oculomotor nerve**.

third cuneiform bone *n*. See **lateral cuneiform bone**.

third-degree burn *n*. A severe burn in which the skin and underlying tissues are destroyed and nerve endings are exposed.

third fibular muscle *n*. See **third peroneal muscle**.

third heart sound *n*. The heart sound that occurs in early diastole and corresponds with the first phase of rapid ventricular filling.

third molar *n*. The eighth permanent tooth in the upper and lower jaw on either side.

third occipital nerve *n*. The mediodorsal branch of the third cervical nerve, usually joined with the greater occipital nerve but also existing as an independent nerve having cutaneous branches to the scalp and the nape.

third peroneal muscle *n*. A muscle with origin in common with the long extensor muscle of the toes, with insertion into the base of the fifth metatarsal bone, with nerve supply from a branch of the peroneal nerve, and whose action assists in the dorsal flexion of the foot. Also called *third fibular muscle*.

third ventricle *n*. A narrow, vertically oriented cavity in the midplane below the corpus callosum that communicates with each of the lateral ventricles through the interventricular foramen.

third ventriculostomy *n*. **1**. A ventriculostomy from the third ventricle to the prechiasmal and interpeduncular cisterns. Also called *Stookey-Scarff operation*. **2**. A ventriculostomy from the third ventricle to the interpeduncular cistern. Also called *Dandy operation*.

thirst (thûrst) *n*. **1**. A sensation of dryness in the mouth and throat related to a need or desire to drink. **2**. The desire or need to drink. —*v*. To feel a need to drink.

thix·o·la·bile (thĭk′sō-lā′bĭl′, -bəl) *adj*. Susceptible to thixotropy.

thix·ot·ro·py (thĭk-sŏt′rə-pē) *n*. The property exhibited by certain gels of becoming fluid when stirred or shaken and returning to the semisolid state upon standing. —**thix′o·trop′ic** (thĭk′sə-trŏp′ĭk) *adj*.

Thom·as (tŏm′əs), **E(dward) Donnall** Born 1920. American physician. He shared a 1990 Nobel Prize for developing techniques of transplanting bone marrow.

Tho·ma's ampulla (tō′məz) *n*. A dilation of the arterial capillary beyond the sheathed splenic artery.

Thomas splint *n*. A long leg splint that extends from a ring at the hip to beyond the foot, allowing traction to a fractured leg, and is used in emergencies and for transportation.

Thomp·son's test (tŏmp′sənz, tŏm′-) *n*. A test for determining the extent of gonorrhea in which an infected patient urinates first into one glass and then into another; if gonococci and gonorrheal threads are found only in the first glass, the probability is that the infection is limited to the anterior urethra. Also called *two-glass test*.

Thom·sen's disease (tŏm′sənz) *n*. See **myotonia congenita**.

thorac– *pref*. Variant of **thoraco–**.

tho·ra·cal·gia (thôr′ə-kăl′jə) *n*. Pain in the chest. Also called *thoracodynia*.

tho·ra·cec·to·my (thôr′ə-sĕk′tə-mē) *n*. Surgical resection of a portion of a rib.

tho·ra·cen·te·sis (thôr′ə-sĕn-tē′sĭs) *n*. Paracentesis of the pleural cavity. Also called *pleurocentesis, thoracocentesis*.

tho·rac·ic (thə-răs′ĭk) *adj*. Of, relating to, or situated in or near the thorax.

thoracic artery *n*. **1.** The internal mammary artery, with origin in the subclavian artery and bifurcations to the musculophrenic and superior epigastric arteries; internal thoracic artery. **2.** The external mammary artery, with origin in the axillary artery and distribution to the muscles of the chest and mammary gland; lateral thoracic artery. **3.** An artery with origin in the axillary artery, with distribution to the muscles of the chest, and with anastomoses to the branches of the suprascapular, internal thoracic, and thoracoacromial arteries; superior thoracic artery.

thoracic cage *n*. The part of the skeleton enclosing the thorax, consisting of the thoracic vertebrae, ribs, costal cartilages, and sternum.

thoracic cardiac nerve *n*. Any of the branches from the second to the fifth segments of the thoracic sympathetic trunk that pass forward to enter the cardiac plexus.

thoracic cavity *n*. The space within the walls of the chest, bounded below by the diaphragm and above by the neck, and containing the heart and the lungs.

thoracic duct *n*. The largest lymph vessel in the body, which collects lymph from the left side of the body above the diaphragm and from all parts below the diaphragm. Also called *left lymphatic duct*.

thoracic ganglion *n*. Any of 11 or 12 ganglions at the level of the head of each rib on either side that with the connecting nerve cords constitute the thoracic portion of the sympathetic trunk.

thoracic iliocostal muscle *n*. A muscle with origin from the medial side of the angles of the lower six ribs, with insertion to the angles of the upper six ribs, with nerve supply from the dorsal branches of the thoracic nerves, and whose action extends, abducts, and rotates the thoracic vertebrae.

thoracic limb *n*. See **upper extremity**.

thoracic longissimus muscle *n*. A muscle with origin from the transverse processes of the lower thoracic vertebrae, with insertion into the ribs between the angles and tubercles, and into the transverse processes of the upper lumbar vertebrae, by medial slips into the accessory processes of the upper lumbar vertebrae and into the transverse processes of the thoracic vertebrae, with nerve supply from the dorsal branches of the thoracic and the lumbar nerves, and whose action extends the vertebral column.

thoracic nerve *n*. Any of 12 mixed motor and sensory nerves on each side of the spine, supplying muscles and skin of the thoracic and the abdominal walls.

thoracic nucleus *n*. A column of large neurons located in the base of the posterior gray column of the spinal cord, extending from the first thoracic through the second lumbar segment, and giving rise to the dorsal spinocerebellar tract of the same side. Also called *dorsal nucleus*.

thoracic outlet syndrome *n*. Compression of the brachial plexus and subclavian artery by attached muscles in the region of the first rib and the clavicle, characterized by pain in the arm, numbness in the fingers, and weakness in the hand muscles.

thoracic wall *n*. See **chest wall**.

thoraco– *or* **thorac–** *pref*. Thorax: *thoracoscope*.

tho·ra·co·a·cro·mi·al (thôr′ə-kō-ə-krō′mē-əl) *adj*. Acromiothoracic.

thoracoacromial artery *n*. An artery with origin in the axillary artery, with distribution to the muscles and skin of the shoulder and upper chest, and with anastomoses to the branches of the superior, internal, and lateral thoracic, posterior and anterior circumflex humeral, and suprascapular arteries. Also called *acromiothoracic artery*.

thoracoacromial vein *n*. The vein corresponding to the thoracocromial artery and emptying into the axillary vein.

tho·ra·co·ce·los·chi·sis (thôr′ə-kō-sē-lŏs′kĭ-sĭs) *n*. A congenital fissure of the thoracic and the abdominal cavities. Also called *thoracogastroschisis*.

tho·ra·co·cen·te·sis (thôr′ə-kō-sĕn-tē′sĭs) *n*. See **thoracentesis**.

tho·ra·co·cyl·lo·sis (thôr′ə-kō-sə-lō′sĭs) *n*. Deformity of the chest.

tho·ra·co·cyr·to·sis (thôr′ə-kō-sîr-tō′sĭs, -sər-) *n*. Abnormally wide curvature of the chest wall.

tho·ra·co·dor·sal artery (thôr′ə-kō-dôr′səl) *n*. An artery with origin in the subscapular artery, with distribution to the muscles of the upper part of the back, and with anastomoses to the branches of the lateral thoracic artery.

thoracodorsal nerve *n*. A nerve that arises from the posterior cord of the brachial plexus, contains fibers from the sixth, seventh, and eighth cervical nerves, and supplies the latissimus dorsi muscle.

tho·ra·co·dyn·i·a (thôr′ə-kō-dĭn′ē-ə) *n*. See **thoracalgia**.

tho·ra·co·ep·i·gas·tric vein (thôr′ə-kō-ĕp′ĭ-găs′trĭk) *n*. Either of two veins, sometimes a single vein, arising from the region of the superficial epigastric vein and opening into the axillary vein or the lateral thoracic vein.

tho·ra·co·gas·tros·chi·sis (thôr′ə-kō-gă-strŏs′kĭ-sĭs) *n*. See **thoracoceloschisis**.

tho·ra·co·lum·bar (thôr′ə-kō-lŭm′bər, -bär) *adj*. **1.** Of or relating to the thoracic and lumbar parts of the spinal column. **2.** Of or relating to the thoracic and lumbar nerves. **3.** Of or relating to the sympathetic division of the autonomic nervous system.

thoracolumbar fascia *n*. The fascia covering the deep muscles of the back.

tho·ra·col·y·sis (thôr′ə-kŏl′ĭ-sĭs) *n*. The loosening of adhesions of the lung to the chest wall.

tho·ra·com·e·ter (thôr′ə-kŏm′ĭ-tər) *n*. An instrument for measuring the varying circumference of the chest in respiration.

tho·ra·co·my·o·dyn·i·a (thôr′ə-kō-mī′ō-dĭn′ē-ə) *n*. Pain in the muscles of the chest wall.

tho·ra·cop·a·thy (thôr'ə-kŏp'ə-thē) *n.* A disease of the thoracic organs or tissues.

tho·ra·co·plas·ty (thôr'ə-kō-plăs'tē) *n.* **1.** Reparative or plastic surgery performed on the thorax. **2.** Conventional thoracoplasty.

tho·ra·cos·chi·sis (thôr'ə-kŏs'kĭ-sĭs) *n.* Congenital fissure of the chest wall.

tho·ra·co·scope (thə-rā'kə-skōp', -răk'ə-) *n.* An endoscope for examination of the chest cavity.

tho·ra·cos·co·py (thôr'ə-kŏs'kə-pē) *n.* Endoscopic examination of the chest cavity.

tho·ra·co·ste·no·sis (thôr'ə-kō-stə-nō'sĭs) *n.* Abnormal narrowness of the chest wall.

tho·ra·cos·to·my (thôr'ə-kŏs'tə-mē) *n.* The surgical formation of an opening into the chest cavity.

tho·ra·cot·o·my (thôr'ə-kŏt'ə-mē) *n.* Incision into the chest wall. Also called *pleurotomy.*

tho·rax (thôr'ăks') *n., pl.* **tho·rax·es** *or* **tho·ra·ces** (thôr'ə-sēz') **1.** The part of the human body between the neck and the diaphragm, partially encased by the ribs and containing the heart and lungs; the chest. **2.** A part in other vertebrates that corresponds to the human thorax. **3.** The second or middle region of the body of an arthropod, between the head and the abdomen, in insects bearing the legs and wings.

Tho·ra·zine (thôr'ə-zēn') A trademark for the drug chlorpromazine.

tho·ri·um (thôr'ē-əm) *n. Symbol* **Th** A radioactive metallic element that is used in magnesium alloys; its longest-lived isotope, Th 232, has a half-life of 1.41 × 10^{10} years. Atomic number 90.

Thorn·dike (thôrn'dīk'), **Edward Lee** 1874–1949. American educational psychologist noted for his study of animal intelligence and for his methods of measuring intelligence.

thought (thôt) *n.* **1.** The act or the process of thinking; cogitation. **2.** A product of thinking, such as an idea. **3.** The faculty of thinking or reasoning.

Thr *abbr.* threonine

thread·worm (thrĕd'wûrm') *n.* **1.** A nematode of the genus *Strongyloides,* parasitic in the small intestine of mammals. **2.** See **pinworm.**

thread·y pulse (thrĕd'ē) *n.* A small fine pulse that feels like a small cord or thread under the finger.

3,5,3'-tri·i·o·do·thy·ro·nine (-trī'ī-ō'dō-thī'rə-nēn', -nĭn) *n. Abbr.* **T-3** A thyroid hormone found in plasma and the thyroid gland that is similar to thyroxine in biological action, used in the treatment of hypothyroidism.

3',5'-cyclic AMP synthetase *n.* See **adenylate cyclase.**

three-day measles *n.* See **rubella.**

three-glass test *n.* A test to determine the location of an infection affecting the male urinary system.

3-hy·drox·y·ty·ra·mine (-hī-drŏk'sē-tī'rə-mēn') *n.* See **dopamine.**

thre·o·nine (thrē'ə-nēn', -nĭn) *n. Abbr.* **Thr** A colorless crystalline amino acid that is derived from the hydrolysis of protein and is an essential component of human nutrition.

thresh·old (thrĕsh'ōld', -hōld') *n.* **1.** The place or point of beginning; the outset. **2.** The lowest point at which a stimulus begins to produce a sensation. **3.** The minimal stimulus that produces excitation of any structure, eliciting a motor response.

threshold limit value *n. Abbr.* **TLV** The maximum concentration of a chemical allowable for repeated exposure without producing adverse health effects.

threshold stimulus *n.* A stimulus that is just strong enough to evoke a response.

threshold substance *n.* A material excreted in the urine only when its concentration in the plasma exceeds a certain value.

thrill (thrĭl) *n.* The vibration accompanying a cardiac or vascular murmur, detectible on palpation.

thrix (thrĭks) *n.* Hair; a hair.

throat (thrōt) *n.* **1.** The portion of the digestive tract that lies between the rear of the mouth and the esophagus and includes the fauces and the pharynx. **2.** The anterior portion of the neck.

throat·wash (thrōt'wŏsh') *n.* See **gargle.**

throb (thrŏb) *v.* To beat rapidly or perceptibly, such as occurs in the heart or a constricted blood vessel. —*n.* A strong or rapid beat; a pulsation.

throm·base (thrŏm'bās', -bāz') *n.* See **thrombin.**

throm·bas·the·ni·a (thrŏm'băs-thē'nē-ə) *or* **throm·bo·as·the·ni·a** (thrŏm'bō-ăs-) *n.* An abnormality of blood platelets, as in Glanzmann's thrombasthenia.

throm·bec·to·my (thrŏm-bĕk'tə-mē) *n.* Excision of a thrombus.

throm·bin (thrŏm'bĭn) *n.* An enzyme in blood formed from prothrombin that facilitates blood clotting by reacting with fibrinogen to form fibrin. Also called *thrombase.*

thrombo– *or* **thromb–** *pref.* Blood clot; blood clotting: *thromboplastin.*

throm·bo·an·gi·i·tis (thrŏm'bō-ăn'jē-ī'tĭs) *n.* Inflammation of the intima of a blood vessel together with thrombosis.

thromboangiitis o·blit·er·ans (ə-blĭt'ə-rănz') *n.* Inflammation of the medium-sized arteries and veins, especially of the legs, that is associated with thrombotic occlusion and that commonly results in ischemia and gangrene. Also called *Buerger's disease, Winiwarter-Buerger disease.*

throm·bo·ar·te·ri·tis (thrŏm'bō-är'tə-rī'tĭs) *n.* Arterial inflammation with thrombus formation.

throm·boc·la·sis (thrŏm-bŏk'lə-sĭs) *n.* See **thrombolysis.** —**throm·bo·clas·tic** (thrŏm'bō-klăs'tĭk) *adj.*

throm·bo·cyst (thrŏm'bə-sĭst') *or* **throm·bo·cys·tis** (thrŏm'bə-sĭs'tĭs) *n.* A membranous sac enclosing a thrombus.

throm·bo·cy·tas·the·ni·a (thrŏm'bō-sī'tăs-thē'nē-ə) *n.* A group of hemorrhagic disorders in which the platelets may be within or only slightly below the normal numerical range but are morphologically abnormal or are lacking in factors that are effective in the coagulation of blood.

throm·bo·cyte (thrŏm'bə-sīt') *n.* See **platelet.** —**throm·bo·cyt·ic** (-sĭt'ĭk) *adj.*

throm·bo·cy·the·mi·a (thrŏm'bō-sī-thē'mē-ə) *n.* See **thrombocytosis.**

thrombocytic series *n.* The cells that are in various stages of thrombocytopoietic development in the bone marrow.

throm·bo·cy·top·a·thy (thrŏm′bō-sī-tŏp′ə-thē) *n.* A disorder of the blood coagulating mechanism that results from dysfunction of the platelets.

throm·bo·cy·to·pe·ni·a (thrŏm′bō-sī′tə-pē′nē-ə) *n.* An abnormal decrease in the number of platelets in the blood. Also called *thrombopenia.* —**throm′bo·cy′-to·pe′nic** (-pē′nĭk) *adj.*

thrombocytopenia-absent radius syndrome *n.* Congenital absence of the radius accompanied by thrombocytopenia and sometimes by congenital heart disease and renal anomalies. Also called *TAR syndrome.*

thrombocytopenic purpura *n.* See **idiopathic thrombocytopenic purpura.**

throm·bo·cy·to·poi·e·sis (thrŏm′bō-sī′tə-poi-ē′sĭs) *n.* The process of formation of thrombocytes, usually in the bone marrow. —**throm′bo·cy′to·poi·et′ic** (-ĕt′ĭk) *adj.*

throm·bo·cy·to·sis (thrŏm′bō-sī-tō′sĭs) *n.* An increase in the number of platelets in the blood. Also called *thrombocythemia.*

throm·bo·e·las·to·gram (thrŏm′bō-ĭ-lăs′tə-grăm′) *n.* A recording of the coagulation process made by a thromboelastograph.

throm·bo·e·las·to·graph (thrŏm′bō-ĭ-lăs′tə-grăf′) *n.* An apparatus for recording elastic variations of a thrombus during the process of coagulation.

throm·bo·em·bo·lism (thrŏm′bō-ĕm′bə-lĭz′əm) *n.* Occlusion of a blood vessel due to a thrombus.

throm·bo·end·ar·ter·ec·to·my (thrŏm′bō-ĕn′där-tə-rĕk′tə-mē) *n.* An operation to remove a thrombus along with the intima and atheromatous material from an occluded artery.

throm·bo·gen·ic (thrŏm′bə-jĕn′ĭk) *adj.* Causing or resulting in thrombosis or coagulation of the blood.

throm·boid (thrŏm′boid′) *adj.* Of or resembling a thrombus.

throm·bo·ki·nase (thrŏm′bō-kī′nās, -nāz) *n.* See **thromboplastin.**

throm·bo·lym·phan·gi·tis (thrŏm′bō-lĭm′făn-jī′tĭs) *n.* Inflammation of a lymphatic vessel with the formation of a lymph clot.

throm·bol·y·sis (thrŏm-bŏl′ĭ-sĭs) *n.,* *pl.* **-ses** (-sēz) Dissolution or destruction of a thrombus. Also called *thromboclasis.* —**throm′bo·lyt′ic** (-bə-lĭt′ĭk) *adj.*

throm·bon (thrŏm′bŏn′, -bən) *n.* The total mass of circulating blood platelets and their precursors.

throm·bop·a·thy (thrŏm-bŏp′ə-thē) *n.* A disorder of blood platelets resulting in defective thromboplastin, without obvious change in the appearance or number of platelets.

throm·bo·pe·ni·a (thrŏm′bə-pē′nē-ə) *n.* See **thrombocytopenia.**

throm·bo·phil·i·a (thrŏm′bə-fĭl′ē-ə) *n.* A disorder of the hemopoietic system in which there is an increased tendency for thrombosis.

throm·bo·phle·bi·tis (thrŏm′bō-flĭ-bī′tĭs) *n.* Inflammation of a vein caused by or associated with the formation of a blood clot.

thrombophlebitis mi·grans (mī′grănz′) *n.* Slowly advancing thrombophlebitis, appearing in one vein and then another.

throm·bo·plas·tic (thrŏm′bō-plăs′tĭk) *adj.* **1.** Causing or promoting blood clotting. **2.** Of or relating to thromboplastin.

throm·bo·plas·tid (thrŏm′bō-plăs′tĭd) *n.* A platelet.

throm·bo·plas·tin (thrŏm′bō-plăs′tĭk) *n.* A plasma protein present in tissues, platelets, and white blood cells necessary for the coagulation of blood and, in the presence of calcium ions, necessary for the conversion of prothrombin to thrombin. Also called *factor III, platelet tissue factor, thrombokinase.*

throm·bo·poi·e·sis (thrŏm′bō-poi-ē′sĭs) *n.* **1.** The process of blood clot formation. **2.** The formation of blood platelets.

throm·bosed (thrŏm′bōst, -bōzd) *adj.* **1.** Clotted. **2.** Of, being, or characterizing a blood vessel that is the seat of thrombosis.

throm·bose par ef·fort (trôn-bōz′ pär ĕ-fôr′) *n.* Thrombosis caused by stress or spontaneous thrombosis of the subclavian or axillary vein. Also called *Paget-von Schrötter syndrome.*

throm·bo·sis (thrŏm-bō′sĭs) *n.,* *pl.* **-ses** (-sēz) Formation or presence of a thrombus.

throm·bo·sta·sis (thrŏm′bō-stā′sĭs, thrŏm-bŏs′tə-sĭs) *n.* Local arrest of the circulation by thrombosis.

throm·bo·sthe·nin (thrŏm′bō-sthē′nĭn) *n.* A contractile protein in platelets that is active in the formation of blood clots.

throm·bot·ic (thrŏm-bŏt′ĭk) *adj.* Relating to, caused by, or characterized by thrombosis.

thrombotic thrombocytopenic purpura *n.* A disease of unknown origin, characterized by abnormally low levels of platelets in the blood, the formation of blood clots in the arterioles and capillaries of many organs, and neurological damage.

throm·box·ane (thrŏm-bŏk′sān) *n.* Any of several compounds, originally derived from prostaglandin precursors in platelets, that stimulate aggregation of platelets and constriction of blood vessels.

throm·bus (thrŏm′bəs) *n.,* *pl.* **-bi** (-bī) A fibrinous clot formed in a blood vessel or in a chamber of the heart.

through drainage (thrōō) *n.* The passage of an open-ended perforated tube through a cavity to drain or irrigate the cavity.

thrush (thrŭsh) *n.* A contagious disease caused by a fungus, *Candida albicans,* that occurs most often in infants and children, characterized by small whitish eruptions on the mouth, throat, and tongue, and usually accompanied by fever, colic, and diarrhea.

thu·li·um (thōō′lē-əm) *n. Symbol* **Tm** A rare-earth element having an x-ray emitting isotope that is used in small portable medical x-ray units. Atomic number 69.

thumb (thŭm) *n.* The short thick digit of the human hand, next to the index finger and opposable to each of the other four digits.

thumb forceps *n.* A forceps operated by compression with thumb and forefinger.

thym– *pref.* Variant of **thymo–.**

thy·mec·to·my (thī-mĕk′tə-mē) *n.* Surgical removal of the thymus gland.

thy·mel·co·sis (thī′mĕl-kō′sĭs) *n.* Suppuration of the thymus gland.

thymi– *pref.* Variant of **thymo–.**

–thymia *suff.* State or condition of mind: *dysthymia.*

thy·mic (thī′mĭk) *adj.* Of or relating to the thymus.

thymic abscesses *pl.n.* See **Dubois abscesses.**

thymic alymphoplasia *n.* Thymic hypoplasia that includes an absence of Hassall's concentric corpuscles and a deficiency of lymphocytes in the thymus and usually in the lymph nodes, spleen, and gastrointestinal tract.

thymic corpuscle *n.* Any of numerous small spherical bodies found in the medulla of the lobules of the thymus, composed of keratinized, usually squamous, epithelial cells arranged around clusters of degenerating lymphocytes, eosinophils, and macrophages. Also called *Hassall's concentric corpuscle.*

thy·mi·co·lym·phat·ic (thī′mĭ-kō-lĭm-făt′ĭk) *adj.* Relating to the thymus and the lymphatic system.

thymic vein *n.* Any of the small veins from the thymus that empty into the left brachiocephalic vein.

thy·mi·dine (thī′mĭ-dēn′) *n.* A nucleoside composed of thymine and deoxyribose.

thymidine triphosphate *n.* The immediate precursor of thymidylic acid in DNA.

thy·mi·dyl·ic acid (thī′mĭ-dĭl′ĭk) *n.* A nucleotide component of DNA that yields thymine, ribose, and phosphoric acid when hydrolyzed.

thy·mine (thī′mēn′) *n.* A pyrimidine base that is an essential constituent of DNA.

thy·mi·tis (thī-mī′tĭs) *n.* Inflammation of the thymus gland.

thymo– *or* **thymi–** *or* **thym–** *pref.* Thymus: *thymokinetic.*

thy·mo·cyte (thī′mə-sīt′) *n.* A lymphocyte that develops in the thymus and is the precursor of a T cell.

thy·mo·ki·net·ic (thī′mō-kĭ-nĕt′ĭk, -kī-) *adj.* Activating the thymus gland.

thy·mol (thī′môl′, -mōl′) *n.* A white crystalline aromatic compound derived from thyme oil and other oils or made synthetically and used as an antiseptic, a fungicide, and a preservative.

thy·mo·ma (thī-mō′mə) *n.* A usually benign tumor of the thymus.

thy·mo·pri·val (thī′mə-prī′vəl) *or* **thy·mo·priv·ic** (-prĭv′ĭk) *or* **thy·mo·pri·vous** (-prī′vəs) *adj.* Marked by premature atrophy or removal of the thymus.

thy·mo·sin (thī′mə-sĭn) *n.* A hormone secreted by the thymus that stimulates development of T cells.

thy·mus (thī′məs) *n., pl.* **–mus·es** A lymphoid organ that is located in the superior mediastinum and lower part of the neck and is necessary in early life for the normal development of immunological function.

thymus corpuscle *n.* Variant of **thymic corpuscle.**

thyro– *or* **thyr–** *pref.* Thyroid: *thyroxine.*

thy·ro·ac·tive (thī′rō-ăk′tĭv) *adj.* Stimulating activity of the thyroid gland.

thy·ro·ad·e·ni·tis (thī′rō-ăd′n-ī′tĭs) *n.* See **thyroiditis.**

thy·ro·a·pla·sia (thī′rō-ə-plā′zhə) *n.* Defective development of the thyroid gland and deficiency of its secretion.

thy·ro·ar·y·te·noid (thī′rō-ăr′ĭ-tē′noid′, -ə-rĭt′n-oid′) *adj.* Relating to the thyroid and arytenoid cartilages.

thyroarytenoid muscle *n.* A muscle with origin from the inner surface of the thyroid cartilage, that inserts into the muscular process and the outer surface of the arytenoid muscle, supplied by the recurrent laryngeal nerve, whose action shortens the vocal cords.

thy·ro·cal·ci·to·nin (thī′rō-kăl′sĭ-tō′nĭn) *n.* See **calcitonin.**

thy·ro·car·di·ac disease (thī′rō-kär′dē-ăk′) *n.* Heart disease resulting from hyperthyroidism.

thy·ro·cele (thī′rə-sēl′) *n.* Enlargement of the thyroid gland.

thy·ro·cer·vi·cal trunk (thī′rō-sûr′vĭ-kəl) *n.* A short arterial trunk arising from the subclavian artery and dividing generally into three branches.

thy·ro·cri·co·to·my (thī′rō-krī-kŏt′ə-mē) *n.* Surgical division of the cricothyroid membrane.

thy·ro·ep·i·glot·tic (thī′rō-ĕp′ĭ-glŏt′ĭk) *adj.* Relating to the thyroid cartilage and the epiglottis.

thyroepiglottic muscle *n.* A muscle with origin from the inner surface of the thyroid cartilage, in common with the thyroarytenoid muscle, insertion into the epiglottis, supplied by the recurrent laryngeal nerve, whose action depresses the base of the epiglottis.

thy·ro·gen·ic (thī′rə-jĕn′ĭk) *or* **thy·rog·e·nous** (thī-rŏj′ə-nəs) *adj.* Originating in the thyroid gland.

thy·ro·glob·u·lin (thī′rō-glŏb′yə-lĭn) *n.* **1.** A thyroid protein that is the precursor to iodine-containing hormones and is typically present in the colloid of thyroid gland follicles. **2.** A substance extracted from the thyroid glands of hogs, formerly used as a thyroid hormone supplement to treat hypothyroidism.

thy·ro·glos·sal (thī′rō-glô′səl) *adj.* Relating to the thyroid gland and the tongue.

thy·ro·hy·al (thī′rō-hī′əl) *n.* The greater horn of the hyoid bone.

thy·ro·hy·oid (thī′ō-hī′oid′) *adj.* Of or relating to the thyroid cartilage and the hyoid bone. —*n.* A continuation of the sternothyroid muscle, with origin from the oblique line of the thyroid cartilage, with insertion into the body of the hyoid bone, with nerve supply from the upper cervical nerve, and whose action moves the hyoid bone closer to the larynx.

thyrohyoid membrane *n.* A thin, fibrous, membranous sheet filling the gap between the hyoid bone and the thyroid cartilage.

thy·roid (thī′roid′) *n.* **1.** The thyroid gland. **2.** The thyroid cartilage. **3.** A powdered preparation of the thyroid gland of certain domestic animals, used in the treatment of cretinism and myxedema, in certain cases of obesity, and in skin disorders. —**thy′roid′** *adj.* —**thy·roi′dal** *adj.*

thyroid artery *n.* **1.** An artery with origin in the aortic arch or the brachiocephalic artery and distribution to the thyroid gland; lowest thyroid artery. **2.** An artery with origin in the thyrocervical trunk and branches to the ascending cervical, inferior laryngeal, muscular, esophageal, and tracheal arteries; inferior thyroid artery. **3.** An artery with origin in the external carotid artery and branches to the infrahyoid, superior laryngeal, sternocleidomastoid, and cricothyroid arteries; superior thyroid artery.

thyroid-binding globulin *n.* A glycoprotein to which thyroid hormone binds in the blood and from which it is released into tissue cells.

thyroid bruit *n.* A vascular murmur heard over a hyperactive thyroid gland.

thyroid cartilage *n.* The largest cartilage of the larynx, having two broad processes that join anteriorly to form the Adam's apple.

thyroid crisis *n.* See **thyrotoxic crisis.**

thy·roid·ec·to·my (thī′roi-děk′tə-mē) *n.* Surgical removal of the thyroid gland. —**thy′roid·ec′to·mize′** *v.*

thyroid gland *n.* A two-lobed endocrine gland located in front of and on either side of the trachea and producing various hormones, such as calcitonin.

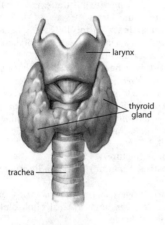

thyroid gland
anterior view of thyroid gland

thyroid hormone *n.* A hormone, especially thyroxine or triiodothyronine, produced by the thyroid gland.

thy·roid·i·tis (thī′roi-dī′tĭs) *n.* Inflammation of the thyroid gland. Also called *thyroadenitis.*

thyroid-stimulating hormone *n. Abbr.* **TSH** See **thyrotropin.**

thyroid-stimulating hormone stimulation test *n.* A test that measures the uptake of I¹³¹ in the thyroid gland before and after the administration of thyroid-stimulating hormone, used to distinguish primary hyperthyroidism from secondary or tertiary hyperthyroidism.

thyroid storm *n.* See **thyrotoxic crisis.**

thyroid suppression test *n.* A test of thyroid function used to diagnose difficult cases of hyperthyroidism in which triiodothyronine is administered for a period of 7 to 10 days.

thy·ro·lib·er·in (thī′rō-lĭb′ər-ĭn) *n.* See **thyrotropin-releasing hormone.**

thy·ro·meg·a·ly (thī′rō-měg′ə-lē) *n.* Enlargement of the thyroid gland.

thy·ro·nine (thī′rə-nēn′, -nĭn) *n.* An amino acid that occurs in proteins only in the form of iodinated derivatives such as thyroxine.

thy·ro·par·a·thy·roid·ec·to·my (thī′rō-păr′ə-thī′roi-děk′tə-mē) *n.* Surgical removal of the thyroid and parathyroid glands.

thy·ro·pri·val (thī′rə-prī′vəl) *or* **thy·ro·priv·ic** (-prĭv′ĭk) *adj.* Relating to hypothyroidism produced by disease or by thyroidectomy.

thy·ro·priv·i·a (thī′rə-prĭv′ē-ə) *n.* A state characterized by reduced activity of the thyroid.

thy·rop·to·sis (thī′rŏp-tō′sĭs) *n.* Downward placement of the thyroid gland.

thy·rot·o·my (thī-rŏt′ə-mē) *n.* **1.** Incision of the thyroid gland. **2.** See **laryngofissure.**

thy·ro·tox·ic (thī′rō-tŏk′sĭk) *adj.* Characterizing the state that is produced by excessive quantities of thyroid hormone.

thyrotoxic crisis *n.* A sudden worsening of thyrotoxicosis following shock, injury, or thyroidectomy. Also called *thyroid crisis, thyroid storm.*

thy·ro·tox·i·co·sis (thī′rō-tŏk′sĭ-kō′sĭs) *n.* A toxic condition resulting from excessive amounts of thyroid hormones in the body, as that occurring in hyperthyroidism.

thy·ro·troph (thī′rə-trŏf′, -trōf′) *n.* A cell that is located in the anterior lobe of the pituitary gland and that produces thyrotropin.

thy·ro·trop·ic (thī′rə-trŏp′ĭk, -trō′pĭk) *or* **thy·ro·troph·ic** (-trŏf′ĭk, -trō′fĭk) *adj.* Stimulating or nurturing the thyroid gland.

thy·ro·tro·pin (thī′rə-trō′pĭn, thī-rŏt′rə-) *or* **thy·ro·tro·phin** (-fĭn) *n.* A glycoprotein hormone secreted by the anterior lobe of the pituitary gland that stimulates and regulates activity of the thyroid gland. Also called *thyroid-stimulating hormone, thyrotropic hormone.*

thyrotropin-releasing hormone *n. Abbr.* **TRH** A tripeptide hormone secreted by the hypothalamus that stimulates the release of thyrotropin. Also called *thyroliberin.*

thyrotropin-releasing hormone stimulation test *n.* A test used primarily to distinguish pituitary from hypothalamic causes of thyroid disorders.

thy·rox·ine (thī-rŏk′sēn′, -sĭn) *or* **thy·rox·in** (-rŏk′sĭn) *n. Abbr.* **T4** An iodine-containing hormone that is produced by the thyroid gland, increases the rate of cell metabolism, regulates growth, and is made synthetically for treatment of thyroid disorders.

Ti The symbol for the element **titanium.**

TIA *abbr.* transient ischemic attack

tib·i·a (tĭb′ē-ə) *n., pl.* **–i·as** *or* **–i·ae** (-ē-ē′) The inner and larger of the two bones of the lower leg, extending from the knee to the ankle, and articulating with the femur, fibula, and talus. Also called *shinbone.* —**tib′i·al** *adj.*

tibial artery *n.* **1.** An artery with origin in the popliteal artery, with branches to the posterior and anterior tibial recurrent, lateral and medial anterior malleolar arteries, the dorsal artery of the foot, the lateral tarsal, medial tarsal, arcuate, dorsal metatarsal, and dorsal digital arteries; anterior tibial artery. **2.** An artery with origin in the popliteal artery, with branches to the peroneal artery, the nutrient artery of the fibula, the lateral and medial posterior malleolar arteries, the nutrient artery of the tibia, and the medial and lateral plantar arteries; posterior tibial artery.

tibial nerve *n.* One of two major divisions of the sciatic nerve, supplying the hamstring muscles, the muscles of the back of the leg, the muscles of the plantar aspect of the foot, and the skin on the back of the leg and on the sole of the foot.

tibia val·ga (văl′gə) *n.* Knock-knee.

tibia var·a (vâr′ə) *n.* Bowleg.

tib·i·o·fib·u·lar (tĭb′ē-ō-fĭb′yə-lər) *adj.* Of, relating to, or involving both the tibia and the fibula.

tic (tĭk) *n.* A habitual spasmodic muscular movement or contraction, usually of the face or extremities. Also called *habit spasm.*

ti·car·cil·lin disodium (tī′kär-sĭl′ĭn) *n.* The disodium salt of a semisynthetic bactericide used in the treatment of *Pseudomonas aeruginosa* infections.

tic dou·lou·reux (dōō′lə-rōō′) *n.* See **trigeminal neuralgia.**

tick (tĭk) *n.* **1.** Any of numerous small bloodsucking parasitic arachnids of the families Ixodidae and Argasidae, many of which transmit febrile diseases, such as Rocky Mountain spotted fever and Lyme disease. **2.** Any of various usually wingless, louselike insects of the family Hippobosciddae that are parasitic on sheep, goats, and other animals.

tick-borne *adj.* Carried or transmitted by ticks, as certain diseases.

tick-borne encephalitis virus *n.* An arbovirus of the genus *Flavivirus* that occurs in two subtypes, Central European and Eastern, causing two forms of encephalitis; it is transmitted by ticks.

tick fever *n.* Any of various febrile diseases transmitted by ticks, such as Rocky Mountain spotted fever and Texas fever.

tick paralysis *n.* Ascending paralysis caused by the attachment of certain ticks, especially of the genera *Dermacentor* and *Ixodes.* Removal of the tick usually results in rapid recovery.

tick typhus *n.* Any of various tick-borne rickettsial diseases identified by their immunological reactions and, in some cases, by their pathogenicity.

Ti·clid (tī′klĭd) A trademark for the drug ticlopidine hydrochloride.

ti·clo·pi·dine hydrochloride (tī-klō′pə-dēn′) *n.* A drug that blocks platelet aggregation, used to prevent stroke and to treat intermittent claudication.

t.i.d. *abbr. Latin* ter in die (three times a day)

tid·al (tīd′l) *adj.* Resembling the tides; alternately rising and falling.

tidal air *n.* See **tidal volume.**

tidal drainage *n.* The use of an apparatus that can be intermittently filled and emptied to drain the urinary bladder.

tidal volume *n.* The volume of air inspired or expired in a single breath during regular breathing. Also called *tidal air.*

tide (tīd) *n.* An alternate increase and decrease, as of levels of a substance in the blood or digestive tract.

tier·fell·nae·vus (tîr′fĕl-nē′vəs, -nĕv′əs) *n.* See **bathing trunk nevus.**

Tie·tze's syndrome (tē′tsēz) *n.* Inflammation of the cartilage of the rib cage, causing pain in the chest similar to angina pectoris.

tight junction (tīt) *n.* An intercellular junction between epithelial cells in which the outer layers of the cell membranes fuse, reducing the ability of larger molecules and water to pass between the cells.

Ti·lade (tī′lād′) A trademark for the drug nedocromil sodium.

tilt-ta·ble (tĭlt′tā′-bəl) *n.* An examining table that can be tilted to a nearly upright position for assessment of a patient's circulatory response to gravitational change.

time (tīm) *n.* **1.** A duration or relation of events expressed in terms of past, present, and future, and measured in units such as minutes, hours, days, months, or years. **2.** A certain period during which something is done.

timed-release *or* **time-release** *adj.* Releasing ingredients gradually to produce a sustained effect.

Ti·men·tin (tī′mĕn′tn) A trademark for the drug ticarcillin disodium.

ti·mo·lol maleate (tī′mō-lōl′) *n.* A beta-blocker drug used primarily in the treatment of hypertension and after myocardial infarction.

tim·o·thy hay bacillus (tĭm′ə-thē hā′) *n.* An aerobic, gram-negative, nonmotile bacterium, *Mycobacterium phlei,* that is found in soil and dust and on plants.

tim·pa·num (tĭm′pə-nəm) *n.* Variant of **tympanum.**

tin (tĭn) *n. Symbol* **Sn** A malleable metallic element used to coat other metals to prevent corrosion. Atomic number 50.

tinct *abbr.* tincture

tinc·to·ri·al (tĭngk-tôr′ē-əl) *adj.* Relating to coloring or staining.

tinc·ture (tĭngk′chər) *n.* **1.** A coloring or dyeing substance. **2.** *Abbr.* **tinct, tr** An alcohol solution of a nonvolatile medicine.

tine (tīn) *n.* **1.** The slender pointed end of an instrument, such as an explorer used in dentistry. **2.** An instrument usually containing several individual prongs and used to introduce antigen, such as tuberculin, into the skin.

tin·e·a (tĭn′ē-ə) *n.* Any of various fungal infections of the skin, hair, or nails that are caused chiefly by species of the genera *Microsporum, Trichophyton,* and *Epidermophyton.* Also called *ringworm.* **—tin′e·al** *adj.*

tinea bar·bae (bär′bē) *n.* See **barber's itch.**

tinea cap·i·tis (kăp′ĭ-tĭs) *n.* A fungal infection of the scalp, characterized by patches of apparent baldness, scaling, black dots, and occasionally erythema and pyoderma.

tinea cor·po·ris (kôr′pər-ĭs) *n.* A fungal infection of the body, characterized by a scaling macular eruption that frequently forms annular lesions on nonhairy parts of the body.

tinea cru·ris (krŏŏr′ĭs) *n.* A fungal infection of the skin of the groin, occurring especially in males. Also called *eczema marginatum, jock itch.*

tinea im·bri·ca·ta (ĭm′brĭ-kā′tə) *n.* An eruption of concentric rings of overlapping scales that form papulosquamous patches on the skin, caused by the fungus *Trichophyton concentricum.*

tinea kerion *n.* An inflammatory pustular fungus infection of the scalp and beard with infiltration of the surrounding parts, commonly caused by *Microsporum audouinii.*

tinea ped·is (pĕd′ĭs) *n.* See **athlete's foot.**

tinea sycosis *n.* See **barber's itch.**

tinea un·gui·um (ŭng′gwē-əm) *n.* See **onychomycosis.**

tinea ver·si·col·or (vûr′sĭ-kŭl′ər) *n.* An eruption of tan or brown, branny patches on the skin of the trunk, caused by the fungus *Pityrosporum furfur* and often appearing white in contrast with hyperpigmented skin after exposure to intense sunlight. Also called *pityriasis versicolor.*

Ti·nel's sign (tĭ-nĕlz′, tē-) *n.* A sensation of tingling felt in the distal extremity of a limb when percussion is made over the site of an injured nerve, indicating a partial lesion or early regeneration in the nerve.

tine test *n.* A tuberculin test in which the antigen is introduced into the skin by means of tines.

tin·ni·tus (tĭ-nī′təs, tĭn′ĭ-) *n., pl.* **–tus·es** A sound in one ear or both ears, such as buzzing, ringing, or whistling, occurring without an external stimulus and usually caused by a specific condition, such as an ear infection, the use of certain drugs, a blocked auditory tube or canal, or a head injury.

tir·ing (tīr′ĭng) *n.* See **cerclage** (sense 1).

Ti·se·li·us (tē-sā′lē-əs), **Arne Wilhelm Kaurin** 1902–1971. Swedish biochemist. He won a 1948 Nobel Prize for his study of serum proteins.

tis·sue (tĭsh′o͞o) *n.* An aggregation of morphologically similar cells and associated intercellular matter acting together to perform specific functions in the body. There are four basic types of tissue: muscle, nerve, epithelial, and connective.

tissue culture *n.* **1.** The technique or process of keeping tissue viable in a culture medium. **2.** A culture of tissue grown by this technique or process.

tissue lymph *n.* Lymph derived chiefly from fluid in tissue spaces rather than from the blood.

tissue plasminogen activator *n. Abbr.* **TPA 1.** An enzyme that catalyzes the conversion of plasminogen to plasmin, used to dissolve blood clots rapidly and selectively, especially in the treatment of heart attacks. **2.** A preparation of this enzyme that is produced by genetic engineering and used to dissolve clots blocking coronary arteries in heart attack and cranial arteries in certain cases of stroke.

tissue respiration *n.* The interchange of gases that occurs between the blood and the tissues. Also called *internal respiration.*

tissue-specific antigen *n.* See **organ-specific antigen.**

tissue tension *n.* A theoretical condition of equilibrium between the tissues and cells, whereby overaction of a part is restrained by the pull of the mass.

ti·ta·ni·um (tī-tā′nē-əm, tĭ-) *n. Symbol* **Ti** A strong, low-density, highly corrosion-resistant metallic element, used in ultraviolet sunscreens and as a surgical aid to repair fractures. Atomic number 22.

ti·ter *or* **ti·tre** (tī′tər) *n.* **1.** The concentration of a substance in solution or the strength of such a substance determined by titration. **2.** The minimum volume needed to cause a particular result in titration. **3.** The dilution of a serum containing a specific antibody at which the solution retains the minimum level of activity needed to neutralize or precipitate an antigen.

ti·trate (tī′trāt′) *v.* To determine the concentration of a solution by titration or perform the operation of titration. —**ti′trat·a·ble** *adj.* —**ti′tra′tor** *n.*

ti·tra·tion (tī-trā′shən) *n.* The process, operation, or method of determining the concentration of a sub-

stance in a solution to which the addition of a reagent having a known concentration is made in carefully measured amounts until a reaction of definite and known proportion is completed, as shown by a color change or by electrical measurement, and then calculating the unknown concentration.

tit·u·ba·tion (tĭch′ə-bā′shən) *n.* The staggering or stumbling gait that is characteristic of certain nervous disorders.

Tl The symbol for the element **thallium.**

TLC *abbr.* thin-layer chromatography; total lung capacity

TLV *abbr.* threshold limit value

T lymphocyte *n.* See **T cell.**

tm *abbr.* temperature midpoint (on the Celsius scale)

Tm¹ The symbol for the element **thulium.**

Tm² *abbr.* transport maximum; tubular maximum

TMJ *abbr.* temporomandibular joint syndrome

T-mycoplasma *n.* See **Ureaplasma.**

Tn *abbr.* intraocular tension

TNF *abbr.* tumor necrosis factor

TNM staging (tē′ĕn-ĕm′) *n.* A system of evaluation of tumors, based on three variables: primary tumor (T), regional nodes (N), and metastasis (M).

to·bac·co heart (tə-băk′ō) *n.* A rapid, irregular heart rate resulting from excessive use of tobacco.

tobacco mosaic virus *n.* A retrovirus that causes a disease in tobacco and some other plants and is widely used in the study of viruses and viral diseases.

toco– *pref.* Childbirth; labor: *tocolytic.*

to·co·dy·na·graph (tō′kō-dī′nə-grăf′, tŏk′ō-) *n.* The recording made by a tocodynamometer.

to·co·dy·na·mom·e·ter (tō′kō-dī′nə-mŏm′ĭ-tər, tŏk′-ō-) *n.* An instrument for measuring the force of uterine contractions.

to·cog·ra·phy (tō-kŏg′rə-fē) *n.* The process of recording uterine contractions.

to·col (tō′kôl) *n.* A colorless viscous oil synthesized through condensation of hydroquinone and phytol and used as an antioxidant.

to·col·o·gy *or* **to·kol·o·gy** (tō-kŏl′ə-jē) *n.* The science of childbirth; midwifery or obstetrics.

to·co·lyt·ic (tō′kə-lĭt′ĭk) *adj.* Of or being an agent that arrests uterine contractions in labor.

to·coph·er·ol (tō-kŏf′ə-rôl′, -rōl′) *n.* Any of a group of closely related, fat-soluble alcohols that behave similarly to vitamin E and are present in milk, lettuce, and wheat germ oil and certain other vegetable oils.

Todd (tŏd), Sir **Alexander Robertus** 1907–1997. British chemist. He won a 1957 Nobel Prize for his study of nucleic acids and nucleotide structures.

Todd's paralysis (tŏdz) *n.* Temporary paralysis that occurs in the limb or limbs involved in the jacksonian convulsions of epilepsy after the attack is over.

toe (tō) *n.* Any of the digits of a foot.

toe-drop *n.* A drooping of the toes and front part of the foot due to paralysis of the muscles that flex the foot back.

toe-nail (tō′nāl′) *n.* The thin, horny, transparent plate covering the upper surface of the end of a toe.

toe reflex *n.* **1.** A reflex in which strong passive flexion of the great toe excites contraction of the flexor muscles in the leg. **2.** See **Babinski's reflex.**

To·fra·nil (tō-frā′nĭl) A trademark for the drug imipramine pamoate.

To·ga·vir·i·dae (tō′gə-vîr′ĭ-dē) *n.* A family of RNA viruses that includes the causative agents of encephalitis, rubella, yellow fever, and dengue.

to·ga·vi·rus (tō′gə-vī′rəs) *n.* A virus of the family Togaviridae.

tol·bu·ta·mide (tŏl-byōō′tə-mīd′) *n.* An orally active hypoglycemic agent used in the treatment of adult-onset diabetes mellitus.

tolbutamide test *n.* A test to detect insulin-producing tumors in which plasma insulin and glucose are measured at intervals after an intravenous dose of tolbutamide.

tol·er·ance (tŏl′ər-əns) *n.* **1.** Decreased responsiveness to a stimulus, especially over a period of continued exposure. **2.** The capacity to absorb a drug continuously or in large doses without adverse effect; diminution in the response to a drug after prolonged use. **3.** Physiological resistance to a poison. **4.** Acceptance of a tissue graft or transplant without immunological rejection. **5.** Unresponsiveness to an antigen that normally produces an immunological reaction. **6.** The ability of an organism to resist or survive infection by a parasitic or pathogenic organism. —**tol′er·ant** *adj.*

tolerance dose *n.* The largest quantity of a substance, radiologic or pharmacologic, that an organism can endure without exhibiting unfavorable or injurious effects.

tol·er·ate (tŏl′ə-rāt′) *v.* **1.** To allow without prohibiting or opposing; permit. **2.** To put up with; endure. **3.** To have tolerance for a substance or pathogen.

tol·er·o·gen·ic (tŏl′ər-ə-jĕn′ĭk) *adj.* Producing immunological tolerance.

To·lo·sa-Hunt syndrome (tə-lō′sə-) *n.* Cavernous sinus syndrome caused by an idiopathic granuloma.

to·lu·i·dine blue O (tō-lōō′ĭ-dēn′, -dĭn, tə-) *n.* A blue basic dye used as a heparin antagonist, an antibacterial agent, a nuclear and metachromatic stain, and a stain for electrophoretic analysis of RNA, RNase, and mucopolysaccharides.

–tome *suff.* **1.** Part; area; segment: *dermatome.* **2.** Cutting instrument: *microtome.*

to·men·tum (tō-mĕn′təm) *n., pl.* **-ta** (-tə) A network of extremely small blood vessels passing between the pia mater and the cerebral cortex.

to·mo·gram (tō′mə-grăm′) *n.* An x-ray image produced by tomography.

to·mo·graph (tō′mə-grăf′) *n.* The radiographic equipment used in tomography.

to·mog·ra·phy (tō-mŏg′rə-fē) *n.* Any of several techniques for making detailed x-rays of a plane section of a solid object, such as the body, while blurring out the images of other planes. Also called *laminagraphy, planigraphy, planography, stratigraphy.* —**to′mo·graph′ic** (tō′mə-grăf′ĭk) *adj.*

–tomy *suff.* Act of cutting; incision: *gastrotomy.*

tone (tōn) *n.* **1.** The quality or character of sound. **2.** The character of voice expressing an emotion. **3.** The normal state of elastic tension or partial contraction in resting muscles. **4.** Normal firmness of a tissue or an organ. —*v.* To give tone or firmness to.

To·ne·ga·wa (tô-nĕ′gä-wä), **Susumu** Born 1939. Japanese molecular biologist. He won a 1987 Nobel Prize for discovering how certain cells of the immune system can genetically rearrange themselves to produce diverse antibodies.

tongue (tŭng) *n.* A mobile mass of muscular tissue that is covered with mucous membrane, occupies much of the cavity of the mouth, forms part of its floor, bears the organ of taste, and assists in chewing, swallowing, and speech.

tongue crib *n.* An appliance used to control visceral swallowing and tongue thrusting in infants and to encourage somatic tongue posture and function.

tongue depressor *n.* A thin blade for pressing down the tongue during a medical examination of the mouth and throat; a spatula.

tongue-swallowing *n.* A slipping back of the tongue against the pharynx, causing choking.

tongue thrust *n.* The infantile pattern of the suckle-swallow movement in which the tongue is placed between the incisor teeth or between the alveolar ridges during the initial stage of swallowing.

tongue-tie *n.* Restricted mobility of the tongue resulting from abnormal shortness of the frenum. Also called *ankyloglossia.*

–tonia *suff.* Degree or state of tonicity: *myotonia.*

ton·ic (tŏn′ĭk) *adj.* **1.** Of or producing tone or tonicity in muscles or tissue. **2.** Characterized by continuous tension or contraction of muscles, as a convulsion or spasm. **3.** Producing or stimulating physical, mental, or emotional vigor. —*n.* An agent, such as a medication, that restores or increases body tone.

tonic-clonic *adj.* Both tonic and clonic. Used of a convulsion or muscular spasms.

tonic contraction *n.* The sustained contraction of a muscle, as is necessary for maintaining posture.

tonic convulsion *n.* A convulsion in which muscle contraction is prolonged.

tonic epilepsy *n.* A convulsive seizure during which the body is rigid.

to·nic·i·ty (tō-nĭs′ĭ-tē) *n.* **1.** Normal firmness or functional readiness in body tissues or organs. **2.** The sustained partial contraction of resting or relaxed muscles. **3.** The osmotic pressure or tension of a solution, usually relative to that of blood.

ton·i·co·clon·ic (tŏn′ĭ-kō-klŏn′ĭk) *adj.* Tonic-clonic.

tonic pupil *n.* A usually enlarged pupil that responds very slowly to changes in focal length and exposure to light. Also called *Piltz sign, Westphal-Piltz pupil.*

tonic spasm *n.* A continuous involuntary muscular contraction. Also called *entasia.*

tono– *pref.* Tone; tension; pressure: *tonography.*

ton·o·clon·ic (tŏn′ō-klŏn′ĭk) *adj.* Tonic-clonic.

tonoclonic spasm *n.* The convulsive contraction of muscles.

ton·o·fi·bril (tŏn′ō-fī′brəl, -fĭb′rəl) *n.* One of a system of fibers found in the cytoplasm of epithelial cells.

ton·o·fil·a·ment (tŏn′ō-fĭl′ə-mənt) *n.* A structural cytoplasmic protein, bundles of which together form a tonofibril.

ton·o·graph (tŏn′ə-grăf′, tō′nə-) *n.* A tonometer equipped to make a graphic recording.

to·nog·ra·phy (tō-nŏg′rə-fē) *n.* Continuous measurement of intraocular pressure to determine the facility of aqueous outflow, used to determine the presence of glaucoma.

to·nom·e·ter (tō-nŏm′ĭ-tər) *n.* Any of various instruments for measuring pressure or tension, especially one used in tonography. —**to′no·met′ric** (tō′nə-mĕt′rĭk) *adj.* —**to·nom′e·try** *n.*

to·no·plast (tō′nə-plăst′) *n.* An intracellular structure or vacuole.

to·no·top·ic (tō′nə-tŏp′ĭk) *adj.* Of or being a structural arrangement, as in the auditory pathway, such that different tone frequencies are transmitted separately along specific parts of the structure.

to·no·trop·ic (tō′nə-trŏp′ĭk, -trō′pĭk) *adj.* Relating to the shortening of the resting length of a muscle.

ton·sil (tŏn′səl) *n.* **1.** A collection of lymphoid tissue. **2.** A small oral mass of lymphoid tissue, especially either of two such masses embedded in the lateral walls of the opening between the mouth and the pharynx, of uncertain function, but believed to help protect the body from respiratory infections. Also called *faucial tonsil, palatine tonsil.*

ton·sil·la (tŏn-sĭl′ə) *n., pl.* **-sil·lae** (-sĭl′ē) A tonsil.

ton·sil·lar (tŏn′sə-lər) *or* **ton·sil·lar·y** (tŏn′sə-lĕr′ē) *adj.* Of or relating to a tonsil, especially the palatine tonsil.

tonsillar crypt *n.* One of the deep recesses that extend into the palatine and pharyngeal tonsils.

tonsillar fossa *n.* The depression between the palatoglossal and palatopharyngeal arches occupied by the palatine tonsil. Also called *amygdaloid fossa.*

ton·sil·lec·to·my (tŏn′sə-lĕk′tə-mē) *n.* Surgical removal of tonsils or a tonsil.

ton·sil·li·tis (tŏn′sə-lī′tĭs) *n.* Inflammation of a tonsil, especially the palatine tonsil. —**ton′sil·lit′ic** (-lĭt′ĭk) *adj.*

tonsillo– *or* **tonsill–** *pref.* Tonsil: *tonsillectomy.*

ton·sil·lo·lith (tŏn-sĭl′ə-lĭth′) *n.* A calcareous concretion in a tonsil.

ton·sil·lot·o·my (tŏn′sə-lŏt′ə-mē) *n.* The cutting away of a portion of a hypertrophied palatine tonsil.

to·nus (tō′nəs) *n.* Body or muscular tone; tonicity.

tooth (tōōth) *n., pl.* **teeth** (tēth) One of a set of hard, bonelike structures rooted in sockets in the jaws of vertebrates, typically composed of a core of soft pulp surrounded by a layer of hard dentin that is coated with cement or enamel at the crown and used chiefly for biting or chewing food or as a means of attack or defense.

tooth·ache (tōōth′āk′) *n.* An aching pain in or near a tooth. Also called *dentalgia, odontalgia.*

tooth bud *n.* The primordial structures from which a tooth is formed.

tooth germ *n.* A mass of tissue, including the enamel organ and dentinal papilla, that has the potential of developing into a tooth; tooth bud.

tooth pulp *n.* See **dental pulp**.

top·ag·no·sis (tŏp′ăg-nō′sĭs) *n.* Inability to recognize or determine the location of tactile sensations. Also called *topoanesthesia.*

to·pal·gia (tə-păl′jə) *n.* Pain localized in one spot without evident organic basis.

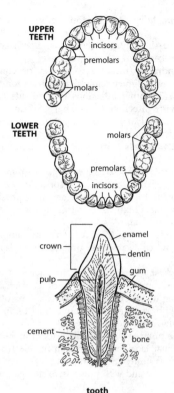

tooth
Top: *adult permanent teeth*
Bottom: *cross section of an incisor*

to·pec·to·my (tə-pĕk′tə-mē) *n.* Surgical removal of specific areas of the frontal lobe of the cerebral cortex as a treatment for certain mental disorders. Also called *corticectomy.*

top·es·the·sia (tŏp′ĭs-thē′zhə) *n.* Ability to recognize the location of tactile sensations.

to·pha·ceous (tə-fā′shəs) *adj.* **1.** Of or characteristic of a tophus. **2.** Sandy; gritty.

tophaceous gout *n.* Gout in which deposits of uric acid and urates occur as tophi.

to·phus (tō′fəs) *n., pl.* **–phi** (-fī) **1.** A deposit of urates in the skin and tissue around a joint or in the external ear. **2.** Dental calculus; tartar.

top·i·cal (tŏp′ĭ-kəl) *adj.* Of or applied to a definite or localized area of the body. —**top′i·cal·ly** *adv.*

topical anesthesia *n.* Superficial loss of sensation in mucous membranes or skin, produced by direct application of local anesthetic solutions, ointments, or jellies. Also called *surface analgesia.*

Top·i·cort (tŏp′ĭ-kôrt′) A trademark for the drug desoximetasone.

topo– *or* **top–** *pref.* Place; area: *topoanesthesia.*

top·o·an·es·the·sia (tŏp′ō-ăn′ĭs-thē′zhə) *n.* See **topagnosis**.

topographic anatomy *n.* See **regional anatomy**.

to·pog·ra·phy (tə-pŏg′rə-fē) *n.* The description of the regions of the body or of a body part, especially the regions of a definite and limited area of the surface.

—**top·o·graph·ic** (-grăf′ĭk), **top·o·graph·i·cal** (-ĭ-kəl) *adj.*

top·o·nar·co·sis (tŏp′ō-när-kō′sĭs) *n.* Localized cutaneous anesthesia.

TORCH syndrome (tôrch) *n.* A group of congenital infections with similar clinical manifestations: toxoplasmosis (T), other infections (O), rubella (R), cytomegalovirus infection (C), and herpes simplex (H).

Tor·e·can (tôr′ə-kăn′) A trademark for the drug thiethylperazine maleate.

Torn·waldt's abscess (tôrn′välts) *n.* Chronic infection of the pharyngeal bursa.

tor·pid (tôr′pĭd) *adj.* **1.** Deprived of power of motion or feeling. **2.** Lethargic; apathetic. —**tor·pid′i·ty** *n.*

tor·por (tôr′pər) *n.* **1.** A state of mental or physical inactivity or insensibility. **2.** Lethargy; apathy. —**tor′po·rif′ic** (-pə-rĭf′ĭk) *adj.*

torpor ret·i·nae (rĕt′n-ē′) *n.* A form of nyctalopia characterized by retinal response only to strong luminous stimuli.

torque (tôrk) *n.* A turning or twisting force.

Tor·re's syndrome (tôr′āz) *n.* A disorder characterized by multiple tumors of the sebaceous glands often accompanied by malignant gastrointestinal tumors. Also called *Muir-Torre syndrome.*

tor·sade de pointes (tôr-säd′ də pwănt′) *n.* Paroxysms of ventricular tachycardia in which the electrocardiogram shows a steady undulation in the QRS axis in runs of 5 to 20 beats and with progressive changes in direction.

tor·si (tôr′sē) *n.* A plural of torso.

tor·sion (tôr′shən) *n.* **1.** A twisting or rotation of a part on its long axis. **2.** Twisting of the cut end of an artery to arrest hemorrhage. **3.** Ocular rotation around the anteroposterior axis. —**tor′sion·al** *adj.*

torsional deformity *n.* A deformity caused by rotation of a portion of an extremity in relationship to the long axis of the entire extremity.

torsion forceps *n.* A forceps used for applying torsion on an artery to arrest hemorrhage.

torsion fracture *n.* A bone fracture resulting from the twisting of a limb.

torsion spasm *n.* A spasmodic twisting of the body and pelvis.

tor·si·ver·sion (tôr′sə-vûr′shən) *n.* A malposition of a tooth in which it is rotated on its long axis. Also called *torsoclusion.*

tor·so (tôr′sō) *n., pl.* **-sos** *or* **-si** (-sē) The human body excluding the head and limbs; trunk.

tor·so·clu·sion (tôr′sə-klōō′zhən) *n.* **1.** Acupressure performed by entering a needle in the tissues parallel with an artery, turning it so that it crosses the artery transversely, and then passing it into the tissues on the opposite side of the vessel. **2.** See torsiversion.

tor·ti·col·lis (tôr′tĭ-kŏl′ĭs) *n.* A contracted state of the neck muscles producing an unnatural position of the head. Also called *wryneck.* —**tor′ti·col′lar** (-kŏl′ər) *adj.*

tortuosity (tôr′chōō-ŏs′ĭ-tē) *n.* **1.** The quality or condition of being tortuous; twistedness or crookedness. **2.** A bent or twisted part, passage, or thing.

tor·tu·ous (tôr′chōō-əs) *adj.* Having many turns; winding or twisting.

tor·u·lop·so·sis (tôr′yə-lŏp-sō′sĭs) *n.* An opportunistic infection in humans caused by the yeast *Torulopsis glabrata* and usually seen in patients treated with antibiotics, corticosteroids, or immunosuppressive agents.

tor·u·lus (tôr′yə-ləs) *n., pl.* **-li** (-lī) A minute elevation in the skin.

to·rus (tôr′əs) *n., pl.* **to·ri** (tôr′ī) A bulging or rounded projection or swelling, such as is caused by a bone or muscle.

torus fracture *n.* A deformity in children caused by the longitudinal compression of the soft bone in either the radius or ulna, or both, and characterized by localized bulging.

to·tal abdominal hysterectomy (tōt′l) *n. Abbr.* **TAH** An abdominal hysterectomy in which the uterus and cervix are removed.

total aphasia *n.* See global aphasia.

total body hypothermia *n.* Deliberate reduction of total body temperature to reduce the general metabolism of the tissues.

total hyperopia *n. Abbr.* **Ht** The total amount of hyperopia, comprising both latent and manifest hyperopia, which can be determined only after complete paralysis of accommodation with a mydriatic drug.

total joint arthroplasty *n.* Arthroplasty in which both joint surfaces are replaced with artificial materials, usually metal and high-density plastic.

total lung capacity *n. Abbr.* **TLC** The volume of gas that is contained in the lungs at the end of maximal inspiration.

total ophthalmoplegia *n.* Paralysis of both the extrinsic and intrinsic ocular muscles.

total parenteral nutrition *n. Abbr.* **TPN** Nutrition maintained entirely by intravenous injection or by some other nongastrointestinal route.

total transfusion *n.* See exchange transfusion.

to·tip·o·ten·cy (tō-tĭp′ə-tən-sē, tō′tĭ-pōt′n-sē) *or* **to·tip·o·tence** (tō-tĭp′ə-təns, tō′tĭ-pōt′ns) *n.* The ability of a cell, such as an egg, to give rise to unlike cells and to develop into or generate a new organism or part. —**to·tip′o·tent** *adj.*

touch (tŭch) *n.* **1.** The physiological sense by which external objects or forces are perceived through contact with the body. **2.** Digital examination. —**touch·a·ble** *adj.*

Tou·rette's syndrome (tōō-rĕts′) *or* **Tou·rette syndrome** (-rĕt′) *n.* A severe neurological disorder characterized by multiple facial and other body tics, usually beginning in childhood or adolescence and often accompanied by grunts and compulsive utterances, as of interjections and obscenities. Also called *Gilles de la Tourette's disease.*

tour·ni·quet (tōōr′nĭ-kĭt, tûr′-) *n.* A device, typically a tightly encircling bandage, used to check bleeding by temporarily stopping the flow of blood through a large artery in a limb.

Tou·ton giant cell (tōōt′n) *n.* A lipid-laden histiocyte in which multiple nuclei are grouped around a small island of cytoplasm.

To·vell tube (tə-vĕl′) *n.* An endotracheal tube that has a wire spiral embedded in its wall to prevent obstruction of the lumen when the tube is compressed and to prevent kinking when the tube is bent at a sharp angle.

tox– *pref.* Variant of **toxi–**.

tox·e·mi·a (tŏk-sē′mē-ə) *n.* A condition in which the blood contains bacterial toxins disseminated from a local source of infection or metabolic toxins resulting from organ failure or other disease. Also called *blood poisoning.* —**tox·e′mic** *adj.*

toxemia of pregnancy *n.* See **preeclampsia**.

toxi– *or* **toxo–** *or* **tox–** *pref.* Poison; poisonous: *toxemia; toxoplasmosis.*

tox·ic (tŏk′sĭk) *adj.* **1.** Of, relating to, or caused by a toxin or other poison. **2.** Capable of causing injury or death, especially by chemical means; poisonous. —*n.* A toxic chemical or other substance.

tox·i·cant (tŏk′sĭ-kənt) *n.* **1.** A poison or poisonous agent. **2.** An intoxicant. —*adj.* Poisonous; toxic.

toxic cirrhosis *n.* Cirrhosis of the liver resulting from chronic poisoning.

toxic epidermal necrolysis *n. Abbr.* **TEN** A life-threatening, exfoliative mucocutaneous disease in which much of the skin becomes intensely red, blisters, and peels off in the manner of a second-degree burn. Toxic epidermal necrolysis is thought to be an idiosyncratic reaction to a drug or other chemical agent.

toxic goiter *n.* Goiter that forms an excessive secretion, causing signs and symptoms of hyperthyroidism.

toxic hemoglobinuria *n.* Hemoglobinuria occurring after the ingestion of various poisons, in certain blood diseases, and in certain infections.

tox·ic·i·ty (tŏk-sĭs′ĭ-tē) *n.* **1.** The quality or condition of being toxic. **2.** The degree to which a substance is toxic.

toxic megacolon *n.* Acute dilation of the colon, seen in ulcerative colitis.

toxic nephrosis *n.* Necrosis due to chemical poisons, septicemia, or bacterial toxemia.

toxic neuritis *n.* Neuritis due to the action of a poison, such as alcohol, lead, or arsenic.

toxico– *or* **toxic–** *pref.* Poison: *toxicosis.*

Tox·i·co·den·dron (tŏk′sĭ-kō-děn′drŏn′) *n.* An alternative genus for six species of poison ivies and poison oaks within the genus *Rhus.*

tox·i·co·gen·ic (tŏk′sĭ-kō-jěn′ĭk) *adj.* **1.** Producing poison or toxic substances. **2.** Derived from or containing toxic matter.

tox·i·coid (tŏk′sĭ-koid′) *adj.* Having an action like that of a poison.

tox·i·col·o·gy (tŏk′sĭ-kŏl′ə-jē) *n.* The study of the nature, effects, and detection of poisons and the treatment of poisoning. —**tox′i·co·log′i·cal** (-kə-lŏj′ĭ-kəl), **tox′i·co·log′ic** (-ĭk) *adj.* —**tox′i·col′o·gist** *n.*

tox·i·co·path·ic (tŏk′sĭ-kō-păth′ĭk) *adj.* Of or being a pathological state caused by the action of a poison.

tox·i·co·sis (tŏk′sĭ-kō′sĭs) *n., pl.* **-ses** (-sēz) **1.** Systemic poisoning. **2.** A diseased condition resulting from poisoning.

toxic shock syndrome *n. Abbr.* **TSS** An acute infection characterized by high fever, a sunburnlike rash, vomiting, and diarrhea, followed in severe cases by shock, that is caused by a toxin-producing strain of *Staphy-*

lococcus aureus, occurring chiefly among young menstruating women who use vaginal tampons. Also called *toxic shock.*

toxic tetanus *n.* See **drug tetanus**.

tox·i·gen·ic (tŏk′sə-jěn′ĭk) *adj.* Producing a poison; toxicogenic. —**tox′i·ge·nic′i·ty** (-jə-nĭs′ĭ-tē) *n.*

tox·in (tŏk′sĭn) *n.* A poisonous substance, especially a protein, that is produced by living cells or organisms and is capable of causing disease when introduced into the body tissues but is often also capable of inducing neutralizing antibodies or antitoxins.

toxin-antitoxin *n.* A mixture of a toxin and its antitoxin with a slight excess of toxin, formerly used as a vaccine.

tox·in·ic (tŏk-sĭn′ĭk) *adj.* Of or relating to a toxin.

tox·i·no·gen·ic (tŏk′sə-nə-jěn′ĭk) *adj.* Producing a toxin; toxicogenic.

tox·i·path·ic (tŏk′sə-păth′ĭk) *adj.* Relating to a diseased state caused by a poison.

toxo– *pref.* Variant of **toxi–**.

tox·o·ca·ri·a·sis (tŏk′sō-kă-rī′ə-sĭs) *n.* Infection with nematodes of the genus *Toxocara.*

tox·oid (tŏk′soid′) *n.* A substance that has been treated to destroy its toxic properties but that retains the capacity to stimulate production of antitoxins, used in immunization.

tox·o·phil (tŏk′sə-fĭl) *or* **tox·o·phile** (-fīl′) *adj.* Susceptible to the action of a poison.

tox·o·phore (tŏk′sə-fôr′) *n.* The chemical group of a toxin that produces the poisonous effect. —**tox·oph′o·rous** (tŏk-sŏf′ər-əs) *adj.*

Tox·o·plas·ma gon·di·i (tŏk′sə-plăz′mə gŏn′dē-ī′) *n.* A sporozoan species that is an intracellular parasite in a variety of vertebrates and is the causative agent of toxoplasmosis.

tox·o·plas·mo·sis (tŏk′sō-plăz-mō′sĭs) *n., pl.* **-mo·ses** (-mō′sēz) An infectious disease caused by the protozoan *Toxoplasma gondii.* The congenital form, resulting from parasites in the infected mother being transmitted to the fetus, is characterized by lesions of the central nervous system that can cause blindness and brain damage. Acquired toxoplasmosis is characterized by fever, swollen lymph nodes, and lesions in the liver, heart, lungs, and brain.

tox·o·py·rim·i·dine (tŏk′sō-pī-rĭm′ĭ-dēn′, -pĭ-) *n.* A metabolite resulting from the hydrolysis of thiamine and appearing in the urine. Also called *pyramine.*

TPA *abbr.* tissue plasminogen activator

TPI test (tē′pē-ī′) *n.* See **Treponema pallidum immobilization test**.

TPN *abbr.* total parenteral nutrition

tr *abbr.* tincture

tra·bec·u·la (trə-běk′yə-lə) *n., pl.* **-lae** (-lē′) **1.** Any of the supporting strands of connective tissue projecting into an organ and constituting part of the framework of that organ. **2.** Any of the fine spicules forming a network in cancellous bone. —**tra·bec′u·lar** *adj.*

trabecular bone *n.* See **spongy bone** (sense ?).

trabecular reticulum *n.* A network of fibers involved in the drainage of the aqueous humor of the eye and located at the iridocorneal angle between the anterior chamber of the eye and the venous sinus of the sclera.

tra·bec·u·lo·plas·ty (trə-běk′yə-lə-plăs′tē) *n.* Photocoagulation of the trabecular meshwork of the eye by means of a laser. It is used in the treatment of glaucoma.

tra·bec·u·lot·o·my (trə-běk′yə-lŏt′ə-mē) *n.* Surgical opening of the canal of Schlemm to treat glaucoma.

trace element (trās) *n.* **1.** A chemical element required in minute quantities by an organism to maintain proper physical functioning. **2.** A minute quantity or amount, as of a chemical compound.

trac·er (trā′sər) *n.* **1.** A substance, such as a dye or a radioactive isotope, that is introduced into and followed through a biological or chemical process, by virtue of its radioactive signature, color, or other distinguishing physical property, thus providing information on the course of the process or on the components or events involved. **2.** An instrument used in dissecting nerves and blood vessels.

trache– *pref.* Variant of **tracheo–**.

tra·che·a (trā′kē-ə) *n., pl.* **–che·as** *or* **–che·ae** (-kē-ē′) The airway that extends from the larynx into the thorax where it divides into the right and left bronchi. It is composed of thin incomplete rings of hyaline cartilage connected by a membrane called the annular ligament. Also called *windpipe.* **—tra′che·al** *adj.*

tracheal cartilage *n.* Any of the incomplete rings of hyaline cartilage forming the wall of the trachea. Also called *tracheal ring.*

tracheal muscle *n.* The band of smooth muscular fibers in the membrane of the trachea, connecting posteriorly the ends of the tracheal cartilage.

tracheal ring *n.* See **tracheal cartilage.**

tracheal tube *n.* See **endotracheal tube.**

tracheal tugging *n.* **1.** A downward pull of the trachea symptomatic of aneurysm of the aortic arch. **2.** A jerky type of inspiration seen when the intercostal muscles and the sternocostal parts of the diaphragm are paralyzed by deep general anesthesia or by muscle relaxants.

tracheal vein *n.* Any of several small venous trunks from the trachea that empty into the brachiocephalic vein or into the superior vena cava.

tra·che·i·tis (trā′kē-ī′tĭs) *or* **tra·chi·tis** (trə-kī′tĭs) *n.* Inflammation of the trachea.

trach·e·lec·to·my (trăk′ə-lěk′tə-mē) *n.* See **cervicectomy.**

trach·e·le·ma·to·ma (trăk′ə-lē′mə-tō′mə, -lěm′ə-) *n.* A hematoma of the neck.

trach·e·lism (trăk′ə-lĭz′əm) *or* **trach·e·lis·mus** (trăk′ə-lĭz′məs) *n.* A spasmodic bending backward of the neck, as that preceding an epileptic attack.

trach·e·li·tis (trăk′ə-lī′tĭs) *n.* See **cervicitis.**

trachelo– *or* **trachel–** *pref.* Neck; cervix; cervical: *trachelocystitis.*

trach·e·lo·breg·mat·ic diameter (trăk′ə-lō-brěg-măt′ĭk) *n.* The diameter of the fetal head from the middle of the anterior fontanelle to the neck.

trach·e·lo·cys·ti·tis (trăk′ə-lō-sĭ-stī′tĭs) *n.* Inflammation of the neck of the bladder.

trach·e·lo·dyn·i·a (trăk′ə-lō-dĭn′ē-ə) *n.* See **cervicodynia.**

trach·e·lo·pex·y (trăk′ə-lō-pěk′sē) *n.* Surgical fixation of the uterine cervix.

trach·e·lo·plas·ty (trăk′ə-lō-plăs′tē) *n.* Surgical repair of the uterine cervix.

trach·e·lor·rha·phy (trăk′ə-lôr′ə-fē) *n.* Suture of a laceration of the uterine cervix.

trach·e·lot·o·my (trăk′ə-lŏt′ə-mē) *n.* See **cervicotomy.**

tracheo– *or* **trache–** *pref.* Trachea: *tracheid.*

tra·che·o·aer·o·cele (trā′kē-ō-âr′ō-sēl′) *n.* An air cyst in the neck, due to the distention of a tracheocele.

tra·che·o·bron·chi·al (trā′kē-ō-brŏng′kē-əl) *adj.* Of or relating to the trachea and the bronchi.

tra·che·o·bron·chi·tis (trā′kē-ō-brŏn-kī′tĭs, -brŏng-) *n.* Inflammation of the mucous membrane of the trachea and bronchi.

tra·che·o·bron·chos·co·py (trā′kē-ō-brŏng-kŏs′kə-pē) *n.* Endoscopic examination of the interior of the trachea and the bronchi.

tra·che·o·cele (trā′kē-ə-sēl′) *n.* A protrusion of the mucous membrane through a defect in the wall of the trachea.

tra·che·o·e·soph·a·ge·al (trā′kē-ō′ĭ-sŏf′ə-jē′əl) *adj.* Of or relating to the trachea and the esophagus.

tra·che·o·la·ryn·geal (trā′kē-ō-lə-rĭn′jəl, -lăr′ĭn-jē′əl) *adj.* Of or relating to the trachea and the larynx.

tra·che·o·ma·la·cia (trā′kē-ō-mə-lā′shə) *n.* Degeneration of the elastic and connective tissue of the trachea.

tra·che·o·meg·a·ly (trā′kē-ō-měg′ə-lē) *n.* An abnormally dilated trachea, which may result from infection or prolonged positive pressure ventilation.

tra·che·o·path·i·a (trā′kē-ə-păth′ē-ə) *or* **tra·che·op·a·thy** (-ŏp′ă-thē) *n.* Disease of the trachea.

tra·che·o·pha·ryn·geal (trā′kē-ō-fə-rĭn′jəl, -făr′ĭn-jē′əl) *adj.* Relating to the trachea and the pharynx.

tra·che·oph·o·ny (trā′kē-ŏf′ə-nē) *n.* The hollow voice sound heard on auscultation over the trachea.

tra·che·o·plas·ty (trā′kē-ə-plăs′tē) *n.* Reparative or plastic surgery of the trachea.

tra·che·o·py·o·sis (trā′kē-ō-pī-ō′sĭs) *n.* Suppurative inflammation of the trachea.

tra·che·or·rha·gia (trā′kē-ə-rā′jə) *n.* Hemorrhage from the mucous membrane of the trachea.

tra·che·os·chi·sis (trā′kē-ŏs′kĭ-sĭs) *n.* A congenital fissure of the trachea.

tra·che·os·co·py (trā′kē-ŏs′kə-pē) *n.* Examination of the interior of the trachea, as with a laryngoscope. **—tra′che·o·scop′ic** (-ə-skŏp′ĭk) *adj.*

tra·che·o·ste·no·sis (trā′kē-ō-stə-nō′sĭs) *n.* Abnormal narrowing of the lumen of the trachea.

tra·che·os·to·my (trā′kē-ŏs′tə-mē) *n.* **1.** Surgical construction of a respiratory opening in the trachea. **2.** The opening so made. **3.** A tracheotomy performed in order to insert a catheter or tube into the trachea, especially to facilitate breathing.

tra·che·ot·o·my (trā′kē-ŏt′ə-mē) *n.* Incision into the trachea through the neck.

tracheotomy tube *n.* A curved tube used to keep the stoma unobstructed after tracheotomy.

tra·chi·tis (trə-kī′tĭs) *n.* Variant of **tracheitis.**

tra·cho·ma (trə-kō′mə) *n.* A contagious disease of the conjunctiva and cornea, caused by the bacterium *Chlamydia trachomatis* and marked by inflammation, hypertrophy, and formation of granules of adenoid tissue. It is a major cause of blindness in Asia and Africa. Also called *contagious granular conjunctivitis,*

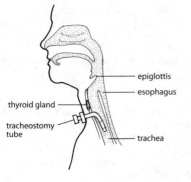

tracheostomy

Egyptian ophthalmia, granular conjunctivitis, granular ophthalmia.

trachoma body *n.* An intracytoplasmic body found in the conjunctival epithelial cells in acute trachoma.

tra·cho·ma·tous (trə-kō′mə-təs) *adj.* Relating to or suffering from trachoma.

trachomatous keratitis *n.* Vascular keratitis that occurs at the upper limbus of the cornea resulting in formation of a pannus.

trachomatous panniculus *n.* A panniculus of the superior cornea of the eye associated with trachoma.

trac·ing (trā′sĭng) *n.* A graphic record of mechanical or electrical events that is recorded by a pointed instrument.

tract (trăkt) *n.* **1.** An elongated assembly of tissue or organs having a common origin, function, and termination, or a serial arrangement having a common function. **2.** A bundle of nerve fibers having a common origin, termination, and function.

trac·tion (trăk′shən) *n.* **1.** The act of drawing or pulling. **2.** A pulling force. **3.** A sustained pull applied mechanically, especially to the arm, leg, or neck, to correct fractured or dislocated bones, to overcome muscle spasms, or to relieve pressure.

traction alopecia *n.* Loss of hair due to from prolonged pulling on the hair, usually associated with certain hairstyles or a habit of twisting the hair.

traction diverticulum *n.* A diverticulum formed by the pulling force of contracting bands of adhesion and occurring mainly in the esophagus.

traction epiphysis *n.* A secondary center of ossification forming at the attachment site of a tendon.

trac·tot·o·my (trăk-tŏt′ə-mē) *n.* Incision of a nerve tract in the brainstem or spinal cord, usually for the relief of pain.

tra·gus (trā′gəs) *n.,* *pl.* **–gi** (-gī, -jī) **1.** The tonguelike projection of skin-covered cartilage in front of the external acoustic meatus. Also called *hircus.* **2.** Any of the hairs growing at the entrance to the external acoustic meatus. Also called *hircus.* —**tra′gal** *adj.*

train·ing group (trā′nĭng) *n.* A group that participates in sensitivity training.

trait (trāt) *n.* **1.** A genetically determined structure, attribute, or function. **2.** A distinct pattern of behavior.

trance (trăns) *n.* An altered state of consciousness as in hypnosis, catalepsy, or ecstasy.

Tran·date (trăn′dāt′) A trademark for the drug labetalol hydrochloride.

tran·ex·am·ic acid (trăn′ĭk-săm′ĭk) *n.* A competitive inhibitor of plasminogen activation and of plasmin. It is used in hemophilia to reduce or to prevent the occurence of hemorrhage.

tran·quil·ize *or* **tran·quil·lize** (trăng′kwə-līz′, trăn′-) *v.* **1.** To make tranquil; pacify. **2.** To sedate or relieve of anxiety or tension by the administration of a drug. **3.** To become tranquil; relax. **4.** To have a calming or soothing effect. —**tran′quil·i·za′tion** (-kwə-lĭ-zā′shən) *n.*

tran·quil·iz·er (trăng′kwə-līz′ər, trăn′-) *n.* Any of various drugs used to reduce tension or anxiety; an antianxiety agent.

trans (trăns, trănz) *adj.* Having two genes, each carrying a mutation, located on opposite chromosomes of a homologous pair.

trans– *pref.* **1.** Across; on the other side; beyond: *transilient.* **2.** Through: *transpiration.* **3.** Change; transfer: *transketolation.* **4.** Having a pair of identical atoms on opposite sides of two atoms linked by a double bond. Used of a geometric isomer. Usually in italic: *trans-butene.*

trans·a·cet·y·lase (trăns′ə-sĕt′l-ās′, -āz′, trănz′-) *n.* See **acetyltransferase.**

trans·a·cet·y·la·tion (trăns′ə-sĕt′l-ā′shən, trănz′-) *n.* The transfer of an acetyl group from one compound to another.

trans·ac·tion·al analysis (trăn-săk′shə-nəl, -zăk′-) *n.* A system of psychotherapy that analyzes personal relationships and interactions in terms of conflicting or complementary ego states that correspond to the roles of parent, child, and adult.

trans·ac·yl·ase (trăns-ăs′ə-lās′, -lāz′, trănz′-) *n.* See **acyltransferase.**

trans·al·do·la·tion (trăns-ăl′də-lā′shən, trănz-) *n.* A reaction involving the transfer of an aldol group from one compound to another.

trans·am·i·di·na·tion (trăns-ăm′ĭ-də-nā′shən, trănz-) *n.* A reaction involving the transfer of an amidine group from one compound to another.

trans·am·i·nase (trăns-ăm′ə-nās′, -nāz′, trănz-) *n.* See **aminotransferase.**

trans·am·i·na·tion (trăns-ăm′ə-nā′shən, trănz-) *n.* **1.** Transfer of an amino group from one chemical compound to another. **2.** Transposition of an amino group within a chemical compound.

trans·ca·lent (trăn-skā′lənt) *adj.* Diathermanous.

trans·car·bam·yl·ase (trăns′kär-băm′ə-lās′, -lāz′) *or* **trans·car·bam·o·yl·ase** (trăns′kär-băm′ō-ə-lās′, -lāz′) *n.* Any of various enzymes that catalyze the transfer of carbamyl groups from one molecule to another. Also called *carbamyltransferase.*

trans·car·box·yl·ase (trăns′kär-bŏk′sə-lās′, -lāz′) *n.* See **carboxyltransferase.**

trans·cel·lu·lar fluid (trăn-sĕl′yə-lər) *n.* A body fluid that is not inside cells but is separated from plasma and interstitial fluid by cellular barriers.

trans·co·bal·a·min (trăns′kō-băl′ə-mĭn) *n.* Any of a family of cobalamin-binding proteins, deficiencies of which have been associated with low serum cobalamin levels.

trans·cor·ti·cal (trăns-kôr′tĭ-kəl) *adj.* **1.** Across or through the cortex of an organ. **2.** From one part of the cerebral cortex to another.

transcortical apraxia *n.* See **ideokinetic apraxia.**

trans·cor·tin (trăns-kôr′tn) *n.* A plasma globulin that binds hydrocortisone and related corticosteroids. Also called *corticosteroid-binding globulin.*

tran·scrip·tase (trăn-skrĭp′tās, -tāz) *n.* **1.** A polymerase that catalyzes the formation of RNA from a DNA template in the process of transcription. **2.** Reverse transcriptase.

tran·scrip·tion (trăn-skrĭp′shən) *n.* **1.** The act or process of transcribing. **2.** Something that has been transcribed. **3.** The process by which mRNA is synthesized from a DNA template resulting in the transfer of genetic information from the DNA molecule to mRNA.

trans·cu·ta·ne·ous (trăns′kyōō-tā′nē-əs) *adj.* Transdermal.

transcutaneous electrical nerve stimulation *n.* TENS.

trans·cy·to·sis (trăns′sī-tō′sĭs, trănz′-) *n.* A mechanism for transcellular transport in which a cell encloses extracellular material in an invagination of the cell membrane to form a vesicle, then moves the vesicle across the cell to eject the material through the opposite cell membrane by the reverse process. Also called *vesicular transport.*

trans·der·mal (trăns-dûr′məl, trănz-) *adj.* Through or by way of the skin.

transdermal patch *n.* A medicated adhesive pad that is placed on the skin to deliver a timed-release dose of medication through the skin into the bloodstream. Also called *skin patch.*

trans·duce (trăns-dōōs′, trănz-) *v.* **1.** To convert energy from one form to another. **2.** To transfer genetic material or characteristics from one bacterial cell to another. Used of a bacteriophage or plasmid.

trans·duc·er cell (trăns-dōō′sər, trănz-) *n.* Any of various cells that respond to a mechanical, thermal, photic, or chemical stimulus by generating an electrical impulse that is synaptically transmitted to a sensory neuron in contact with the cell.

trans·duc·tion (trăns-dŭk′shən, trănz-) *n.* Transfer of genetic material or characteristics from one bacterial cell to another by a bacteriophage or plasmid.

tran·sec·tion (trăn-sĕk′shən) *n.* **1.** A cross section along a long axis. **2.** Division by cutting across.

trans·fec·tion (trăns-fĕk′shən) *n.* Infection of a bacterium or cell with DNA or RNA isolated from a bacteriophage or from an animal or a plant virus, resulting in replication of the complete virus.

trans·fer (trăns′fər) *n.* **1.** The conveyance or removal of something from one place to another. **2.** A condition in which learning in one situation influences learning in another situation. It may be positive, as when learning one behavior facilitates the learning of something else, or negative, as when one habit interferes with the acquisition of a later one. —**trans·fer′** (trăns-fûr′, trănz′fər) *v.*

trans·fer·ase (trăns′fə-rās′, -rāz′) *n.* Any of various enzymes that catalyze the transfer of a chemical group, such as a phosphate or an amine, from one molecule to another.

trans·fer·ence (trăns-fûr′əns, trăns′fər-əns) *n.* In psychoanalysis, the process by which emotions associated with one person, such as a parent, unconsciously shift to another, especially to the analyst.

transfer factor *n.* **1.** The transfer gene of a conjugative plasmid, especially of the resistance plasmid. **2.** A substance free of nucleic acid and antibody, that is obtained from the white blood cells of a person with a delayed-type sensitivity and will transfer the specific sensitivity to the recipient after injection into the skin of a nonsensitive person.

trans·fer·rin (trăns-fĕr′ĭn) *n.* A beta globulin in blood serum that combines with and transports iron. Also called *siderophilin.*

transfer RNA *n.* See **tRNA.**

trans·fix·ion (trăns-fĭk′shən) *n.* In amputation, passing the knife from side to side through tissues close to the bone and dividing muscles from within outward.

transfixion suture *n.* **1.** A crisscross stitch placed so as to control bleeding from a tissue surface or small vessel when it is tied. **2.** A suture used to fix the columella to the nasal septum.

trans·for·ma·tion (trăns′fər-mā′shən) *n.* **1.** See **metamorphosis** (sense 1). **2.** The genetic alteration of a bacterial cell by introduction of DNA from another cell or from a virus.

trans·form·ing factor (trăns-fôr′mĭng) *n.* The DNA responsible for bacterial transformation.

trans·fuse (trăns-fyōōz′) *v.* To administer a transfusion of or to. —**trans·fus′a·ble** *adj.*

trans·fu·sion (trăns-fyōō′zhən) *n.* **1.** The transfer of whole blood or blood products from one individual to another. **2.** The intravascular injection of physiological saline solution.

transfusion nephritis *n.* The renal failure and tubular damage that results from the transfusion of incompatible blood; the hemoglobin of the hemolyzed red cells is deposited as casts in the renal tubules.

trans·gen·der (trăns-jĕn′dər, trănz-) *or* **trans·gendered** (-dərd) *adj.* Transsexual.

trans·gen·e·sis (trăns-jĕn′ĭ-sĭs, trănz-) *n.* The transfer of cloned genetic material from one species or breed to another.

trans·gen·ic (trăns-jĕn′ĭk, trănz-) *adj.* **1.** Of, relating to, or being an organism whose genome has been altered by the transfer of a gene or genes from another species or breed: *transgenic mice.* **2.** Of or relating to the study of transgenic organisms.

trans·hi·a·tal (trăns′hī-āt′l, trănz′-) *adj.* Across or through a hiatus.

transhiatal esophagectomy *n.* Resection of the esophagus by blunt dissection from a cervical incision from above and transhiatal approach through an abdominal incision.

tran·si·ent acantholytic dermatosis (trăn′shənt, -zhənt, -zē-ənt) *n. Abbr.* **TAD** A papular eruption that occurs chiefly on the chest and back in which the tissues are affected with acantholysis, lasting from a few weeks to several months and occurring predominantly in males over the age of 40.

transient hypogammaglobulinemia of infancy *n.* A temporary form of primary immunodeficiency that occurs in infants usually within the first six months following birth and is associated with an increased susceptibility to bacterial infection.

transient ischemic attack *n. Abbr.* **TIA** A temporary blockage of the blood supply to the brain, typically caused by an embolus and usually lasting ten minutes or less, during which dizziness, blurring of vision, numbness on one side of the body, and other symptoms of a stroke may occur. Also called *ministroke.*

transient synovitis *n.* A painful hip condition of children, usually of boys and generally affecting only one hip, having an unknown cause and producing symptoms similar to those of osteochondritis deformans juvenilis. Also called *pseudocoxalgia.*

tran·sil·ient (trăn-sĭl′yənt, -zĭl′-) *adj.* Jumping across; passing over. Used especially of the cortical association fibers in the brain that pass between nonadjacent convolutions.

tran·si·tion (trăn-zĭsh′ən) *n.* **1.** A period during childbirth that precedes the expulsive phase of labor, characterized by strong uterine contractions and nearly complete cervical dilation. **2.** A point mutation in a polynucleic acid, in which a pyrimidine is replaced by another pyrimidine, or a purine is replaced by another purine.

tran·si·tion·al cell carcinoma (trăn-zĭsh′ə-nəl) *n.* A malignant neoplasm derived from transitional epithelium and occurring primarily in the urinary bladder, ureters, or renal pelvises.

transitional denture *n.* A partial denture that serves as a temporary prosthesis and allows for the addition of more teeth as more natural teeth are lost and that will be replaced once the tissue changes that follow the extraction of natural teeth have occurred.

transitional epithelium *n.* Stratified epithelium in which the individual layers are formed by a transformation of the cells from the layer below.

transitional zone *n.* **1.** The region of the lens of the eye where cells from the anterior epithelial capsule become transformed into the fibers that compose the lens substance. **2.** The portion of a scleral contact lens that joins the corneal and scleral sections.

tran·si·tion gyrus (trăn-zĭsh′ən) *n.* A small convolution connecting two lobes or two main gyri in the depth of a sulcus. Also called *annectent gyrus.*

transition mutation *n.* A point mutation involving substitution of one base pair for another by replacement of one purine by another purine and of one pyrimidine by another pyrimidine but without change in the purine-pyrimidine orientation.

trans·ke·to·la·tion (trăns′kē-tə-lā′shən) *n.* A reaction involving the transfer of a ketol group from one compound to another.

trans·late (trăns-lāt′, trănz-, trăns′lāt′, trănz′-) *v.* **1.** To render in another language. **2.** To put into simpler terms; explain or interpret. **3.** To subject mRNA to translation. —**trans·lat′a·bil′i·ty** *n.* —**trans·lat′a·ble** *adj.*

trans·la·tion (trăns-lā′shən, trănz-) *n.* **1.** The act or process of translating, especially from one language into another. **2.** The state of being translated. **3.** A translated version of a text. **4.** The process by which mRNA, tRNA, and ribosomes effect the production of a protein

molecule from amino acids, the specificity of synthesis being controlled by the base sequences of the mRNA. **5.** Movement of a tooth through alveolar bone without change in axial inclination. —**trans·la′tion·al** *adj.*

trans·lo·cate (trăns-lō′kāt′, trănz-) *v.* **1.** To change from one place or one position to another; to displace. **2.** To transfer a chromosomal segment to a new position; to cause to undergo translocation.

trans·lo·ca·tion (trăns′lō-kā′shən, trănz′-) *n.* Transposition of two segments between nonhomologous chromosomes as a result of abnormal breakage and refusion of reciprocal segments.

translocation Down syndrome *n.* A condition in which, as a result of translocation of a large segment of chromosome 21 to another chromosome, an individual has virtually the genetic equivalent of three chromosomes 21 and thus has the phenotype of Down syndrome but with the normal number of chromosomes.

trans·lu·min·al (trăns-lōō′mə-nəl, trănz-) *adj.* Passing or occurring across a lumen.

trans·mem·brane (trăns-mĕm′brān, trănz-) *adj.* Passing or occurring across a membrane.

trans·meth·yl·ase (trăns-mĕth′ə-lās′, -lāz′, trănz-) *n.* See **methyltransferase.**

trans·meth·yl·a·tion (trăns-mĕth′ə-lā′shən, trănz-) *n.* The transfer of a methyl group from one compound to another.

trans·mi·gra·tion (trăns′mī-grā′shən, trănz′-) *n.* Movement from one site to another, which may entail the crossing of some usually limiting membrane or barrier, as in diapedesis.

trans·mis·si·ble (trăns-mĭs′ə-bəl, trănz-) *adj.* Capable of being conveyed from one person to another.

transmissible encephalopathy *n.* See **subacute spongiform encephalopathy.**

trans·mis·sion (trăns-mĭsh′ən, trănz-) *n.* **1.** The conveyance of disease from one person to another. **2.** The passage of a nerve impulse across synapses or at myoneural junctions.

trans·mit (trăns-mĭt′, trănz-) *v.* **1.** To send from one person, thing, or place to another; convey. **2.** To cause to spread; pass on. **3.** To impart or convey to others by heredity or inheritance; hand down. —**trans·mit′ta·ble** *adj.*

trans·mu·ral (trăns-myŏŏr′əl, trănz-) *adj.* Passing through a wall, as of the body or of a cyst or any hollow structure.

trans·mu·ta·tion (trăns′myŏŏ-tā′shən, trănz′-) *n.* **1.** A change; transformation. **2.** In physics, the transformation of one element into another by one or a series of nuclear reactions.

trans·par·ent dentin (trăns-pâr′ənt) *n.* See **sclerotic dentin.**

trans·pep·ti·dase (trăns-pĕp′tĭ-dās′, -dāz′) *n.* An enzyme that catalyzes a transpeptidation.

trans·pep·ti·da·tion (trăns-pĕp′tĭ-dā′shən) *n.* A reaction involving the transfer of one or more amino acids from one peptide chain to another.

trans·phos·pha·tase (trăns-fŏs′fə-tās′, -tāz′) *n.* See **phosphotransferase.**

trans·phos·pho·ryl·a·tion (trăns-fŏs′fər-ə-lā′shən) *n.* A reaction involving transfer of a phosphoric group from one compound to another.

tran·spi·ra·tion (trăn′spə-rā′shən) *n.* The passage of watery vapor through the skin or through any membrane or pore.

trans·pla·cen·tal (trăns′plə-sĕn′tl) *adj.* Relating to or involving passage through or across the placenta. —**trans′pla·cen′tal·ly** *adv.*

trans·plant (trăns-plănt′) *v.* To transfer a tissue or an organ from one body or body part to another. —*n.* (trăns′plănt′) **1.** The act or process of transplanting. **2.** The tissue or organ so used.

trans·plan·ta·tion (trăns′plăn-tā′shən) *n.* The act or process of transplanting a tissue or an organ from one body or body part to another.

trans·port (trăns′pôrt′) *n.* The movement or transference of biochemical substances that occurs in biological systems.

transport maximum *n. Abbr.* **Tm** The maximal rate of secretion or reabsorption of a substance by the renal tubules. Also called *tubular maximum.*

transport medium *n.* A medium for transporting clinical specimens to the laboratory for examination.

trans·pos·ase (trăns-pō′zās, -zāz′) *n.* An enzyme required for transposition of DNA segments.

trans·pose (trăns-pōz′) *v.* To transfer one tissue, organ, or part to the place of another.

trans·po·si·tion (trăns′pə-zĭsh′ən) *n.* **1.** Removal from one place to another. **2.** The state of being transposed or of being on the wrong side of the body. **3.** Transfer of a segment of DNA to a new position on the same or another chromosome, plasmid, or cell.

transposition of great vessels *n.* A congenital cardiovascular malformation in which the aorta arises from the right ventricle while the pulmonary artery arises from the left ventricle.

trans·po·son (trăns-pō′zŏn) *n.* A segment of DNA having a repeat of an insertion sequence element at each end as well as genes specific to some other activity such as resistance to antibiotics; it is capable of migrating to a new position within the same or another chromosome, plasmid, or cell and thereby transferring genetic properties.

trans·py·lor·ic plane (trăns′pī-lôr′ĭk, -pĭ-) *n.* An Addison's clinical plane passing horizontally midway between the upper margins of the sternum and the pubic symphysis, corresponding to the disk between the first and second lumbar vertebrae.

trans·sex·u·al (trăns-sĕk′shōō-əl) *n.* **1.** A person who strongly identifies with the opposite gender and who chooses to live as a member of the opposite gender or to become one by surgery. —*adj.* **1.** Of or relating to such a person. **2.** Relating to medical and surgical procedures designed to alter a person's external sexual characteristics so they resemble those of the opposite gender.

trans·sex·u·al·ism (trăns-sĕk′shōō-ə-lĭz′əm) *n.* **1.** The state of being a transsexual. **2.** The desire to change one's anatomic sexual characteristics to conform physically with one's perception of self as a member of the opposite sex.

trans·syn·ap·tic degeneration (trăns′sĭ-năp′tĭk) *n.* The atrophy of nerve cells following damage to the axons that make synaptic connections with them.

trans·tho·rac·ic (trăns′thə-răs′ĭk) *adj.* Across or through the thoracic cavity or chest wall. —**trans′tho·rac′i·cal·ly** *adv.*

transthoracic esophagectomy *n.* The resection of the esophagus through a thoracotomy incision.

transthoracic plane *n.* An Addison's clinical plane passing across the thorax above the lower border of the body of the sternum.

tran·su·date (trăn-sōō′dāt′, trăn′sōō-dāt′) *or* **tran·su·da·tion** (trăn′sōō-dā′shən) *n.* **1.** A product of the process of passing through a membrane, pore, or interstice. **2.** A substance that transudes.

tran·sude (trăn-sōōd′, -zōōd′) *v.* To pass through pores or interstices in the manner of perspiration. —**tran·su′da·to·ry** (trăn-sōō′də-tôr′ē) *adj.*

trans·u·re·ter·o·u·re·ter·os·to·my (trăns′yōō-rē′tə-rō-yōō-rē′tə-rŏs′tə-mē, trănz′-) *n.* The suture of the transected end of one ureter into the intact opposite ureter.

trans·u·re·thral resection (trăns′yōō-rē′thrəl, trănz′-) *n.* Surgical removal of the prostate gland or bladder lesions by means of an endoscope inserted through the urethra, usually for the relief of prostatic obstruction or for treatment of bladder malignancies.

trans·vec·tor (trăns-vĕk′tər, -tôr′, trănz-) *n.* An animal that transmits a toxic substance that it does not produce but that has accumulated in its body from other sources.

trans·verse (trăns-vûrs′, trănz-, trăns′vûrs′, trănz′-) *adj.* Lying across the long axis of the body or of a part.

transverse amputation *n.* Amputation in which the incision through the extremity is at right angles to the long axis.

transverse cervical artery *n.* An artery with origin in the thyrocervical trunk, with superficial cervical and descending scapular branches. Also called *transverse artery of neck.*

transverse colon *n.* The part of the colon that lies across the upper part of the abdominal cavity.

trans·ver·sec·to·my (trăns′vər-sĕk′tə-mē, trănz′-) *n.* Excision of the transverse process of a vertebra.

transverse diameter *n.* The diameter of the pelvic inlet measured between the two most widely separated points.

transverse facial artery *n.* An artery with origin in the superficial temporal artery, with distribution to the parotid gland, parotid duct, masseter muscle, and overlying skin; and with anastomoses to the infraorbital and buccal branches of the maxillary artery, and the buccal and masseteric branches of the facial artery.

transverse facial fracture *n.* See **craniofacial disjunction fracture.**

transverse fascia *n.* The fascia lining the abdominal cavity, between the inner surfaces of the abdominal musculature and the peritoneum.

transverse fissure of cerebrum *n.* The space between the corpus callosum and the fornix above, and the dorsal surface of the thalamus below.

transverse fold of rectum *n.* Any of three or four horizontal crescentic folds in the rectal mucous membrane above the anus.

transverse foramen *n.* An opening in the transverse process of a cervical vertebra for the passage of the vertebral artery and vein and the sympathetic nerve plexus. Also called *vertebroarterial foramen.*

transverse fracture *n.* A fracture in which the line of break forms a right angle with the axis of the bone.

transverse hermaphroditism *n.* Pseudohermaphroditism in which the external genital organs are characteristic of one sex and the gonads are characteristic of the other sex.

transverse horizontal axis *n.* The hypothetical line around which the mandible may rotate through the horizontal plane.

transverse lie *n.* An anatomical relationship in which the long axis of the fetus lies at right angles to the long axis of the mother.

transverse ligament of elbow *n.* A bundle of fibers running from the olecranon to the coronoid process of the elbow in association with the ulnar collateral ligament. Also called *Cooper's ligament.*

transverse ligament of knee *n.* A transverse band that passes between the lateral and medial menisci in the front part of the knee joint.

transverse ligament of perineum *n.* The thickened front border of the urogenital diaphragm, formed by the fusion of its two fascial layers.

transverse muscle of abdomen *n.* A muscle with origin from the seventh to the twelfth costal cartilages, lumbar fascia, iliac crest, and inguinal ligament; with insertion into the xiphoid cartilage, linea alba, and the pubic tubercle and pecten, with nerve supply from the lower thoracic nerve, and whose action compresses the abdominal contents.

transverse muscle of chin *n.* Inconstant fibers of the depressor muscle of the angle of the mouth that continue into the neck and cross to the opposite side below the chin.

transverse muscle of nape *n.* An occasional muscle passing between the tendons of the trapezius and the sternocleidomastoid muscles.

transverse muscle of tongue *n.* An intrinsic muscle of the tongue, whose fibers arise from the septum and radiate to the dorsum and the sides.

transverse nerve of neck *n.* A branch of the cervical plexus that supplies the skin over the anterior triangle of the neck.

transverse plane *n.* See **horizontal plane.**

transverse presentation *n.* An abnormal presentation during birth, neither head nor breech, in which the fetus is positioned transversely in the uterus across the axis of the birth canal.

transverse process *n.* A process projecting on either side of the arch of a vertebra.

transverse rhombencephalic flexure *n.* See **pontine flexure.**

transverse scapular artery *n.* See **suprascapular artery.**

transverse sinus *n.* A paired dural sinus that begins at the confluence of the sinuses and terminates in the sigmoid sinus.

transverse sinus of pericardium *n.* A passage in the pericardium between the origins of the great vessels and the atria.

transverse tarsal joint *n.* The joint between the talus and calcaneus posteriorly and the navicular and cuboid bones anteriorly. Also called *Chopart's joint.*

transverse temporal gyrus *n.* Either of two or any of three convolutions that run transversely on the surface of the temporal lobe, border on the lateral fissure, and are separated by the transverse temporal sulci. Also called *Heschl's gyrus.*

transverse vein of face *n.* A tributary of the retromandibular vein, anastomosing with the facial vein.

transverse vein of neck *n.* Any of the veins that accompany the transverse arteries of the neck and empty into the external jugular vein or sometimes into the subclavian vein.

trans·ver·sion (trăns-vûr′zhən, trănz-) *n.* Eruption of a tooth in a position normally occupied by another.

transversion mutation *n.* A point mutation involving base substitution in which the orientation of purine and pyrimidine is reversed.

trans·ver·so·spi·nal·es (trănz-vûr′sō-spī′nə-lēs′) *pl.n.* The muscles that originate from the transverse processes of the vertebrae, pass to the spinous processes of higher vertebrae, acting as rotators, and include the semispinal and the rotator muscles.

trans·ves·tism (trăns-vĕs′tĭz′əm, trănz-) *or* **trans·ves·ti·tism** (-tĭ-tĭz′əm) *n.* The practice of dressing in clothes traditionally associated with the opposite gender.

trans·ves·tite (trăns-vĕs′tīt′, trănz-) *n.* One who practices transvestism.

Tran·tas dot (trăn′təs, trän′täs) *n.* Any of the pale, grayish-red gelatinous nodules occurring on the edge of the conjunctiva in vernal conjunctivitis.

tra·pe·zi·al (trə-pē′zē-əl) *adj.* Relating to a trapezium or to the trapezius muscle.

tra·pe·zi·form (trə-pē′zə-fôrm′) *adj.* Shaped or having a form like a trapezium.

tra·pe·zi·um (trə-pē′zē-əm) *n.,* pl. **-zi·ums** *or* **-zi·a** (-zē-ə) **1.** A quadrilateral having no parallel sides. **2.** A bone in the wrist at the base of the thumb, articulating with the first and second metacarpal, scaphoid, and trapezoid bones.

tra·pe·zi·us (trə-pē′zē-əs) *n.* A muscle with origin from the superior nuchal line, the external occipital protuberance, the nuchal ligament, the spinous processes of the seventh cervical and thoracic vertebrae, with insertion into the lateral third of the posterior surface of the clavicle, the medial side of the acromion, and the upper border of the spine of the scapula, with nerve supply from the accessory nerve and the cervical plexus, and whose action draws the head to one side or backward and rotates the scapula.

trap·e·zoid (trăp′ĭ-zoid′) *n.* **1.** A quadrilateral having two parallel sides. **2.** A small bone in the wrist that is situated near the base of the index finger and that articulates with the second metacarpal, trapezium, capitate, and scaphoid bones. —**trap′e·zoid′, trap′e·zoi′dal** (-zoid′l) *adj.*

trapezoid ligament *n.* The lateral part of the coracoclavicular ligament that attaches to the trapezoid line of the clavicle.

trapezoid line *n.* The area on the lower sueface of the clavicle near its lateral extremity, to which the trapezoid ligament is attached. Also called *trapezoid ridge.*

tras·tu·zu·mab (trăs-tōō′zə-măb′) *n.* A monoclonal IgG antibody derived from recombinant DNA, used intravenously to treat metastatic breast cancer.

Trau·be-Her·ing curves (trou′bə-hĕr′ĭng) *pl.n.* Curved lines representing slow oscillations in blood pressure usually extending over several respiratory cycles. Also called *Traube-Hering waves.*

traum– *pref.* Wound; injury: *traumasthenia.*

trau·ma (trô′mə, trou′-) *n., pl.* **–mas** *or* **–ma·ta** (-mə-tə) **1.** A serious bodily injury or shock, as from violence or an accident. **2.** A severely disturbing experience that leads to lasting psychological or emotional impairment. **—trau·mat′ic** (-măt′ĭk) *adj.*

trauma center *n.* A medical facility that is designated to treat severe physical trauma as a result of the specialized training of its staff and the availability of appropriate diagnostic and treatment tools.

traumat– *pref.* Variant of **traumato–**.

traumatic amenorrhea *n.* Absence of menstruation because of endometrial scarring or cervical stenosis.

traumatic amputation *n.* Amputation resulting from an accidental injury.

traumatic anesthesia *n.* Loss of sensation resulting from nerve injury.

traumatic asphyxia *n.* Asphyxia produced by a sudden increase in venous pressure, common in those who have been hanged and occurring occasionally in crush injuries.

traumatic discopathy *n.* An injury characterized by fissuration, laceration, or fragmentation of a disk or surrounding ligaments, with or without displacement of fragments against the spinal cord, nerve roots, or ligaments.

traumatic neuritis *n.* Inflammation of a nerve following an injury.

traumatic neuroma *n.* A proliferation of Schwann cells and axons that may develop at the proximal end of a severed or injured nerve. Also called *amputation neuroma, false neuroma.*

traumatic occlusion *n.* See **traumatogenic occlusion**.

traumatic tetanus *n.* Tetanus following infection of a wound.

trau·ma·tism (trô′mə-tĭz′əm, trou′-) *n.* **1.** The physical or psychological condition produced by a trauma. **2.** A wound or an injury.

traumato– *or* **traumat–** *pref.* Wound; injury: *traumatopnea.*

trau·ma·to·gen·ic occlusion (trô′mə-tə-jĕn′ĭk, trou′-) *n.* A malocclusion capable of producing injury to the teeth or associated structures. Also called *traumatic occlusion.*

trau·ma·tol·o·gy (trô′mə-tŏl′ə-jē, trou′-) *n.* The branch of medicine that deals with the treatment of serious wounds and injuries. **—trau′ma·tol′o·gi·cal** *adj.* **—trau′ma·tol′o·gist** *n.*

trau·ma·top·ne·a (trô′mə-tŏp-nē′ə, trou′-) *n.* Passage of air in and out through a wound of the chest wall.

trav·el·ers′ diarrhea *or* **trav·el·er′s diarrhea** (trăv′əl-ərz, trăv′lərz) *n.* Diarrhea and abdominal cramps occurring among travelers to regions where sanitation is poor, commonly caused by a toxin-producing strain of the bacterium *Escherichia coli.*

tra·zo·done hydrochloride (trā′zə-dōn′) *n.* A triazolopyridine antidepressant drug.

treat (trēt) *v.* **1.** To give medical aid to someone. **2.** To give medical aid to counteract a disease or condition.

treat·ment (trēt′mənt) *n.* Administration or application of remedies to a patient or for a disease or an injury; medicinal or surgical management; therapy.

Trem·a·to·da (trĕm′ə-tō′də) *n.* A class of flatworms of the phylum Platyhelminthes, including both external and internal parasites of animal hosts, that have a thick outer cuticle and one or more suckers or hooks for attaching to host tissue; the flukes.

trem·a·tode (trĕm′ə-tōd′) *n.* Any of numerous flatworms of the class Trematoda. Also called *fluke.*

trem·a·to·di·a·sis (trĕm′ə-tō-dī′ə-sĭs) *n.* Infestation or infection with trematodes, often caused by ingestion of inadequately cooked food.

trem·or (trĕm′ər) *n.* **1.** An involuntary trembling movement. **2.** Minute ocular movement occurring during fixation on an object.

trem·u·lous (trĕm′yə-ləs) *adj.* Characterized by tremor. **—trem′u·lous·ness** *n.*

trench fever (trĕnch) *n.* An acute infectious disease characterized by chills and fever, caused by the microorganism *Rickettsia quintana,* and transmitted by the louse *Pediculus humanus.*

trench foot *n.* A condition of the foot resembling frostbite, caused by prolonged exposure to cold and dampness and often affecting soldiers in trenches. Also called *immersion foot.*

trench mouth *n.* An acute, sometimes recurrent lesion of the mouth, gums, and throat often associated with fusiform bacilli and spirochetes, marked by ulceration and necrosis of the gum margin, destruction of the interdental papillae, and foul breath. Also called *acute necrotizing ulcerative gingivitis, fusospirillary gingivitis, fusospirochetal gingivitis, necrotizing ulcerative gingivitis, ulceromembranous gingivitis, Vincent's angina, Vincent's disease.*

Tren·de·len·burg position (trĕn′dl-ən-bûrg′) *n.* A supine position with the patient inclined at an angle of 45 degrees; so that the pelvis is higher than the head, used during and after operations in the pelvis or for shock.

Tren·de·len·burg's sign (trĕn′dl-ən-bûrgz′) *n.* An indication of congenital dislocation of the hip or of hip abductor weakness in which the pelvis on the side opposite to the dislocation will sag when the hip and knee of the normal side are flexed.

Trendelenburg's test *n.* A test of the valvular competence of the leg veins in which the leg is raised above the level of the heart until the veins are empty and then the leg is rapidly lowered.

Tren·tal (trĕn′tăl′) A trademark for the drug pentoxifylline.

tre·pan (trĭ-păn′) *n.* A trephine. **—**v. To trephine.

treph·i·na·tion (trĕf′ə-nā′shən) *n.* Removal of a circular piece of bone, especially of the skull, by a trephine. Also called *trepanation.*

tre·phine (trĭ-fīn′) *n.* A cylindrical or crown saw for the removal of a disk of bone, especially from the skull, or removal of other firm tissue such as that of the cornea. **—**v. To operate on with a trephine.

trep·i·dant (trĕp′ĭ-dənt) *adj.* Relating to or characterized by trepidation.

trep·i·da·ti·o cor·dis (trĕp′ĭ-dā′shē-ō kôr′dĭs) *n.* Palpitation of the heart.

trep·i·da·tion (trĕp′ĭ-dā′shən) *n.* **1.** An involuntary trembling or quivering. **2.** A state of anxious fear; apprehension.

Trep·o·ne·ma (trĕp′ə-nē′mə) *n.* A genus of anaerobic spirochetes including species that cause syphilis, pinta, and yaws.

trep·o·ne·mal (trĕp′ə-nē′məl) *adj.* Relating to *Treponema*.

Treponema pal·li·dum (păl′ĭ-dəm) *n.* A spirochete that causes syphilis in humans.

Treponema pallidum hemagglutination test *n.* A test for the serologic diagnosis of syphilis in which tanned sheep red blood cells are coated with the antigen of *Treponema pallidum* and combined with nonspecific serum antibody of an individual.

Treponema pallidum immobilization test *n.* A test for syphilis in which an antibody other than Wassermann antibody is present in the serum of a syphilitic patient; in the presence of complement, the patient's serum causes the immobilization of actively motile *Treponema pallidum* obtained from testes of a rabbit infected with syphilis. Also called *TPI test*.

Treponema per·ten·u·e (pər-tĕn′yoo-ē′) *n.* A spirochete that causes yaws.

trep·o·ne·ma·to·sis (trĕp′ə-nē′mə-tō′sĭs) *n., pl.* **-ses** (-sēz) See **treponemiasis**.

trep·o·neme (trĕp′ə-nēm′) *n.* A member of the genus *Treponema*.

trep·o·ne·mi·a·sis (trĕp′ə-nē-mī′ə-sĭs) *n.* Infection caused by a spirochete of the genus *Treponema*. Also called *treponematosis*.

trep·o·ne·mi·cid·al (trĕp′ə-nē′mĭ-sīd′l) *n.* An agent destructive to any species of *Treponema*. Also called *antitreponemal*. —**trep′o·ne′mi·cid′al** *adj.*

trep·pe (trĕp′ə) *n.* The occurrence of a successive increase in amplitude of the first few contractions of cardiac muscle that has received a number of stimuli of the same intensity following a quiescent period. Also called *staircase phenomenon*.

tre·sis (trē′sĭs) *n.* Perforation.

tret·i·noin (trĕt′n-oin′) *n.* An isomer of retinoic acid, used in the treatment of acne.

TRH *abbr.* thyrotropin-releasing hormone

tri– *pref.* **1.** Three: *tricuspid.* **2.** Containing three atoms, molecules, or groups: *triacetic acid.*

tri·a·ce·tic acid (trī′ə-sē′tĭk) *n.* An acid formed during the synthesis of fatty acids.

tri·ac·yl·glyc·er·ol (trī-ăs′əl-glĭs′ə-rôl′, -rōl′) *n.* A naturally occurring ester of three fatty acids and glycerol that is the chief constituent of fats and oils. Also called *triglyceride*.

triacylglycerol lipase *n.* See **steapsln**.

tri·ad (trī′ăd′, -əd) *n.* **1.** A collection of three things or symptoms having something in common. **2.** The transverse tubule, and the terminal cisternae on each side of it, in a skeletal muscle fiber.

triad syndrome *n.* See **abdominal muscle deficiency syndrome**.

tri·age (trē-äzh′, trē′äzh′) *n.* A process for sorting injured people into groups based on their need for or likely benefit from immediate medical treatment. Triage is used on the battlefield, at disaster sites, and in hospital emergency rooms when limited medical resources must be allocated.

tri·al denture (trī′əl, trīl) *n.* A setup of artificial teeth made for placement in a person's mouth before a denture is completed.

trial frame *n.* An adjustable frame that holds trial lenses used during retinoscopy or refraction tests on the eye.

trial lens *n.* Any of a set of cylindrical and spherical lenses used in testing vision.

tri·am·cin·o·lone (trī′ăm-sĭn′ə-lōn′) *n.* A synthetic glucocorticoid used as an anti-inflammatory drug in the treatment of allergic and respiratory disorders.

tri·am·te·rene (trī′ăm′tə-rēn′) *n.* A diuretic agent that allows potassium to be retained rather than eliminated, often used in conjunction with hydrochlorothiazide.

tri·an·gle (trī′ăng′gəl) *n.* A three-sided area, space, or structure.

triangle of auscultation *n.* The space bounded by the lower border of the trapezius, the latissimus dorsi, and the medial margin of the scapula.

triangle of safety *n.* The area at the lower left sternal border where the pericardium is not covered by lung.

tri·an·gu·lar bandage (trī-ăng′gyə-lər) *n.* A piece of cloth cut in the shape of a right-angled triangle and used as a sling.

triangular bone *n.* An independent ossicle sometimes present in the tarsus and usually forming part of the talus.

triangular muscle *n.* See **depressor muscle of angle of mouth**.

Tri·at·o·ma (trī-ăt′ə-mə) *n.* A genus of insects that includes important vectors of *Trypanosoma cruzi.*

tri·a·zo·lam (trī-ā′zə-lăm) *n.* A benzodiazepine derivative used as a sedative and hypnotic.

tri·az·o·lo·pyr·i·dine antidepressant (trī-ăz′ə-lō-pĭr′ĭ-dēn′, -ā′zə-, -ə-zō′lō-) *n.* Any of a class of antidepressants, such as trazodone, structurally and pharmacologically unrelated to other antidepressants, whose clinical effectiveness is similar to that of tricyclic antidepressants but with fewer anticholinergic side effects.

tri·ba·sic (trī-bā′sĭk) *adj.* **1.** Relating to an acid containing three replaceable hydrogen atoms per molecule. **2.** Relating to a base or salt containing three univalent basic atoms or radicals per molecule.

tribe (trīb) *n.* An occasional taxonomic category placed between a subfamily and a genus or between a suborder and a family and usually containing several genera.

tri·bra·chi·a (trī-brā′kē-ə) *n.* A condition seen in conjoined twins when the fusion has merged the adjacent arms to form a single one, so that there are only three arms for the two bodies.

tri·bro·mo·eth·a·nol (trī-brō′mō-ĕth′ə-nôl′, -nōl′) *n.* A crystalline compound having a slight aromatic odor and taste and used as a basal anesthetic.

tri·car·box·yl·ic acid cycle (trī′kär-bŏk-sĭl′ĭk) *n.* See **Krebs cycle.**

tri·ceps (trī′sĕps′) *n., pl.* **–ceps·es** (-sĕp′sĭz) or **triceps** **1.** A three-headed muscle of the upper arm, whose long or scapular head has origin from the lateral border of the scapula, the lateral head, origin from the lateral and posterior surface of the humerus, and the medial head from the posterior surface of the humerus; with insertion into the olecranon of the ulna, with nerve supply from the radial nerve, and whose action extends the forearm; the triceps brachii. **2.** The gastrocnemius and soleus muscles of the calf considered as one muscle; the triceps surae.

triceps reflex *n.* A sudden contraction of the triceps muscle caused by a firm tap on its tendon when the forearm hangs loosely at a right angle with the upper arm.

triceps su·rae reflex (sŏŏr′ē) *n.* See **Achilles reflex.**

trich– *pref.* Variant of **tricho–.**

tri·chi·a·sis (trĭ-kī′ə-sĭs) *n.* A condition in which the hair adjacent to a natural opening turns inward and causes irritation, as in the inward turning of the eyelashes upon the eye.

trich·i·lem·mo·ma (trĭk′ə-lĕ-mō′mə) *n.* A benign tumor derived from the outer root sheath epithelium of a hair follicle.

tri·chi·na (trĭ-kī′nə) *n., pl.* **–nae** (-nē) A small, slender parasitic nematode (*Trichinella spiralis*) that infests the intestines of various mammals and whose larvae move through the bloodstream, becoming encysted in muscles.

Trich·i·nel·la (trĭk′ə-nĕl′ə) *n.* A genus of parasitic nematodes, including the species *Trichinella spiralis,* which causes trichinosis.

trich·i·no·sis (trĭk′ə-nō′sĭs) *n.* A disease caused by eating undercooked meat, usually pork, that is infested with trichinae that develop as adults in the intestines and as larvae in the muscles and cause intestinal pain, fever, nausea, muscular pain, and edema.

trich·i·nous (trĭk′ə-nəs, trĭ-kī′-) *adj.* **1.** Containing trichina. **2.** Of or relating to trichinae or trichinosis.

tri·chi·tis (trĭ-kī′tĭs) *n.* Inflammation of the hair bulbs.

tri·chlo·ride (trī-klôr′īd′) *or* **tri·chlo·rid** (-klôr′ĭd) *n.* A compound containing three chlorine atoms per molecule.

tri·chlor·meth·yl chloroformate (trī′klôr-mĕth′əl) *n.* See **diphosgene.**

tri·chlo·ro·a·ce·tic acid (trī-klôr′ō-ə-sē′tĭk) *n.* A colorless, deliquescent, corrosive, crystalline compound used topically as an astringent and antiseptic.

tri·chlo·ro·eth·yl·ene (trī-klôr′ō-ĕth′ə-lēn′) *n.* An analgesic and inhalation anesthetic used in minor surgical operations and in obstetrics.

tri·chlo·ro·meth·ane (trī-klôr′ō-mĕth′ān′) *n.* Chloroform.

tricho– *or* **trich–** *pref.* Hair; thread; filament: *trichonocardiosis.*

trich·o·be·zoar (trĭk′ō-bē′zôr′) *n.* See **hairball.**

trich·o·cla·sia (trĭk′ō-klā′zhə) *or* **tri·choc·la·sis** (trī-kŏk′lə-sĭs) *n.* See **trichorrhexis nodosa.**

trich·o·dis·co·ma (trĭk′ō-dĭ-skō′mə) *n.* See **haarscheibe tumor.**

trich·o·ep·i·the·li·o·ma (trĭk′ō-ĕp′ə-thē′lē-ō′mə) *n.* One of multiple small, benign nodules, occurring mostly on the skin of the face, derived from basal cells of hair follicles enclosing keratin pearls. Also called *epithelioma adenoides cysticum.*

trich·o·glos·si·a (trĭk′ō-glô′sē-ə) *n.* See **hairy tongue.**

trich·oid (trĭk′oid′, trī′koid′) *adj.* Resembling hair.

trich·o·lith (trĭk′ə-lĭth′) *n.* A small mass of hair; a hairball.

trich·o·lo·gia (trĭk′ə-lō′jə) *n.* A nervous habit of plucking at the hair.

trich·o·meg·a·ly (trĭk′ə-mĕg′ə-lē) *n.* A congenital condition in which the eyelashes are abnormally long.

trich·o·mo·na·cide (trĭk′ə-mō′nə-sīd′) *n.* An agent that is destructive to a trichomonad.

trich·o·mo·nad (trĭk′ə-mō′năd′) *n.* Any of various flagellate protozoa of the genus *Trichomonas.*

Trich·o·mon·as (trĭk′ə-mō′nəs) *n.* A genus of parasitic protozoan flagellates that cause trichomoniasis.

Trichomonas te·nax (tē′năks′) *n.* A protozoan that lives as a commensal in the mouth; it is found especially in tartar around the teeth or in defects of carious teeth.

Trichomonas vag·i·na·lis (văj′ə-nā′lĭs) *n.* A protozoan found in the vagina and urethra of women and in the urethra and prostate gland of men.

trich·o·mo·ni·a·sis (trĭk′ə-mə-nī′ə-sĭs) *n., pl.* **–ses** (-sēz′) **1.** A vaginal inflammation caused by a trichomonad (*Trichomonas vaginalis*) and resulting in a refractory discharge and itching. **2.** An infection that is caused by trichomonads, as a disease of cattle that commonly results in infertility or abortion in infected cows.

trichomoniasis vaginitis *n.* Acute or subacute vaginitis or urethritis caused by infection with the trichomonads *Trichomonas vaginalis.* Infection may be venereal or may be caused by other forms of contact.

trich·o·my·co·sis (trĭk′ō-mī-kō′sĭs) *n.* **1.** A disease of hair caused by infection with fungus. No longer in technical use. **2.** Trichonocardiosis. **3.** Trichomycosis axillaris.

trichomycosis ax·il·lar·is (ăk′sə-lâr′ĭs) *n.* Infection of the axillary and pubic hairs with the development of yellow, black, or red concretions around the hair shafts. Also called *lepothrix, trichonodosis.*

trich·o·no·car·di·o·sis (trĭk′ə-nō-kär′dē-ō′sĭs) *n.* An infection of hair shafts, especially of the axillary and pubic regions, with microorganisms of the genus *Nocardia.* Yellow, red, or black concretions develop around the infected hair shafts.

trich·o·no·do·sis (trĭk′ə-nō-dō′sĭs) *n.* See **trichomycosis axillaris.**

tri·chop·a·thy (trĭ-kŏp′ə-thē) *n.* Disease of the hair. Also called *trichonosis, trichosis.* —**trich′o·path′ic** (trĭk′ə-păth′ĭk) *adj.*

tri·choph·a·gy (trĭ-kŏf′ə-jē) *n.* Habitual biting of the hair.

trich·o·phyt·ic (trĭk′ə-fĭt′ĭk) *adj.* Relating to trichophytosis.

trich·o·phy·tid (trĭk′ə-fī′tĭd, trĭ-kŏf′ĭ-) *n.* An eruption caused by an allergic reaction to infection with a trichophyton.

trich·o·phy·to·be·zoar (trĭk′ə-fī′tō-bē′zôr′) *n.* An indigestible mass of hair and vegetable fibers found usually in the stomach of ruminant animals or occasionally in the stomach of humans.

trich·o·phy·ton (trĭk′ə-fī′tŏn′, trĭ-kŏf′ĭ-) *n.* A member of the genus *Trichophyton.*

Trich·o·phy·ton (trĭk′ə-fī′tŏn′, trī-kŏf′ĭ-) *n.* A genus of pathogenic fungi causing dermatophytosis in the hair, skin, and nails of humans.

Trichophyton con·cen·tri·cum (kən-sĕn′trĭ-kəm) *n.* The fungal parasite that causes tinea imbricata.

Trichophyton men·tag·ro·phy·tes (mĕn-tăg′rō-fī′tēz) *n.* A zoophilic small-spored fungal parasite that causes infection of hair, skin, and nails.

Trichophyton ru·brum (roo′brəm) *n.* A fungal parasite that causes persistent infections in the nails.

Trichophyton schoen·lein·i·i (shœn-lī′nē-ī′) *n.* The fungal parasite that causes favus.

Trichophyton ton·su·rans (tŏn′syə-rănz′, -shə-) *n.* The fungal parasite that is the causative agent of epidemic dermatophytosis.

Trichophyton vi·o·la·ce·um (vī′ə-lā′sē-əm) *n.* The fungal parasite that causes favus infection of the scalp.

trich·o·phy·to·sis (trĭk′ə-fī-tō′sĭs) *n.* A superficial fungus infection caused by a trichophyton.

tri·chop·ti·lo·sis (trĭ-kŏp′tə-lō′sĭs, trĭk′ə-tə-) *n.* A splitting of the shaft of the hair, giving it a feathery appearance.

trich·or·rhex·is (trĭk′ə-rĕk′sĭs) *n.* A condition in which the hairs readily break or split. Also called *trichoschisis.*

trichorrhexis in·vag·i·na·ta (ĭn-văj′ə-nā′tə) *n.* See **bamboo hair.**

trichorrhexis no·do·sa (nō-dō′sə) *n.* A condition in which minute nodes are formed in the hair shafts, weakening the hair and causing splitting and breaking. Also called *clastothrix, trichoclasia.*

tri·chos·chi·sis (trĭ-kŏs′kĭ-sĭs) *n.* See **trichorrhexis.**

tri·cho·sis (trĭ-kō′sĭs) *n.* See **trichopathy.**

Trich·o·spo·ron (trĭk′ə-spôr′ŏn′, trĭ-kŏs′pə-rŏn′) *n.* A genus of imperfect fungi that are part of the normal flora of the intestinal tract of humans and that includes the causative agent of trichosporosis.

trich·o·spo·ro·sis (trĭk′ə-spə-rō′sĭs, -spô-) *n.* A superficial mycotic infection of the hair in which nodular masses of fungi become attached to the hair shafts.

tri·chos·ta·sis spi·nu·lo·sa (trĭ-kŏs′tə-sĭs spī′nyə-lō′sə, spĭn′yə-, trĭk′ə-stā′sĭs) *n.* A condition in which hair follicles are blocked with a keratin plug containing lanugo hairs.

trich·o·thi·o·dys·tro·phy (trĭk′ə-thī′ō-dĭs′trə-fē) *n.* An abnormality of the hair shaft, probably inherited, characterized by fine brittle hairs with abnormally low sulfur content.

trich·o·til·lo·ma·ni·a (trĭk′ō-tĭl′ə-mā′nē-ə, -mān′yə) *n.* A compulsion to pull out one's own hair.

–trichous *suff.* Having a specified kind of hair or hairlike part: *peritrichous.*

tri·chro·mat·ic (trī′krō-măt′ĭk) *or* **tri·chrome** (trī′krōm′) *or* **tri·chro·mic** (trī-krō′mĭk) *adj.* **1.** Having or relating to the three primary colors, red, blue, and green. **2.** Having perception of the three primary colors, as in normal vision.

tri·chro·ma·top·si·a (trī′krō-mə-tŏp′sē-ə) *n.* Normal color vision; the ability to perceive the three primary colors.

trichrome stain *n.* A staining method utilizing a combination of three different dyes to identify different cell or tissue elements.

trich·u·ri·a·sis (trĭk′yə-rī′ə-sĭs) *n., pl.* **–ses** (-sēz) Infection with a nematode. It is usually asymptomatic and not associated with peripheral eosinophilia, but in massive infections it frequently causes diarrhea or rectal prolapse.

Trich·u·ris (trī-kyoor′ĭs) *n.* A genus of aphasmid nematodes related to the trichina worm and parasitic in the intestines of mammals. Also called *whipworm.*

tri·cip·i·tal (trī-sĭp′ĭ-tl) *adj.* Having three heads, as a triceps muscle.

tri·cor·nute (trī-kôr′noot′) *adj.* Having three cornua or horns.

tri·crot·ic (trī-krŏt′ĭk) *adj.* Marked by three waves in the arterial pulse tracing.

tri·cus·pid (trī-kŭs′pĭd) *n.* An organ or a part, especially a tooth, having three cusps. —*adj.* also **tri·cus·pi·dal** (-pĭ-dəl) *or* **tri·cus·pi·date** (-pĭ-dāt′) **1.** Having three points, prongs, or cusps. **2.** Of or relating to the tricuspid valve.

tricuspid atresia *n.* The congenital absence of the normal tricuspid orifice.

tricuspid insufficiency *n.* Valvular insufficiency involving the tricuspid valve.

tricuspid murmur *n.* A murmur produced at the tricuspid orifice.

tricuspid orifice *n.* See **right ventricular opening.**

tricuspid stenosis *n.* Pathological narrowing of the orifice of the tricuspid valve.

tricuspid valve *n.* The three-segmented valve of the heart that keeps blood in the right ventricle from flowing back into the right atrium. Also called *right atrioventricular valve.*

tri·cy·clic antidepressant (trī-sī′klĭk, -sĭk′lĭk) *n.* Any of a class of antidepressants, such as amitriptyline, that are structurally related to the phenothiazine antipsychotics.

tri·den·tate (trī-dĕn′tāt′) *adj.* Three-toothed; three-pronged.

tri·der·mic (trī-dûr′mĭk) *adj.* Relating to or derived from the three primary germ layers of the embryo.

tri·fa·cial (trī-fā′shəl) *adj.* Trigeminal.

trifacial neuralgia *n.* See **trigeminal neuralgia.**

tri·fid (trī′fĭd′) *adj.* Divided into three narrow parts or lobes.

tri·fo·cal lens (trī-fō′kəl, trī′fō′-) *n.* A lens having one section that corrects for distant vision, a second section that corrects for intermediate vision, and a third that corrects for near vision.

tri·fur·ca·tion (trī′fər-kā′shən) *n.* A division into three branches. —**tri·fur′cate** *v.*

tri·gas·tric (trī-găs′trĭk) *adj.* Having three bellies. Used of a muscle with two tendinous interruptions.

tri·gem·i·nal (trī-jĕm′ə-nəl) *adj.* Of or relating to the trigeminal nerves.

trigeminal cavity *n.* See **Meckel's cavity.**

trigeminal ganglion *n.* The large, flattened, sensory ganglion of the trigeminal nerve, lying close to the cavernous sinus along the medial part of the middle cranial fossa. Also called *gasserian ganglion, semilunar ganglion.*

trigeminal nerve *n.* The chief sensory nerve of the face and the motor nerve of the muscles of chewing. The nuclei of the nerve are in the mesencephalon and in the pons and extend down into the cervical portion of the spinal cord. The nerve emerges by two sensory and motor roots from the pons and enters a cavity of the dura mater at the temporal bone, where its sensory root expands to form the trigeminal ganglion that forms three branches that are designated ophthalmic, maxillary, and mandibular. Also called *fifth cranial nerve, trigeminus.*

trigeminal neuralgia *n.* Paroxysmal shooting pains of the facial area around one or more branches of the trigeminal nerve, of unknown cause, but often precipitated by touching specific areas in or about the mouth. Also called *Fothergill's disease, Fothergill's neuralgia, prosopalgia, prosoponeuralgia, tic douloureux, trifacial neuralgia.*

trigeminal pulse *n.* A pulse in which the beats occur in threes, with a pause after every third beat.

trigeminal rhizotomy *n.* Division or section of a sensory root of the fifth cranial nerve.

trigeminal rhythm *n.* A cardiac dysrhythmia in which heartbeats occur in groups of threes, usually composed of a sinus beat followed by two extrasystolic beats. Also called *trigeminy.*

tri·gem·i·nus (trī-jĕm′ə-nəs) *n.* See **trigeminal nerve.**

tri·gem·i·ny (trī-jĕm′ə-nē) *n.* See **trigeminal rhythm.**

trig·ger area (trĭg′ər) *n.* A point or circumscribed area that when irritated or stimulated will give rise to physiological or pathological change elsewhere.

trig·gered activity (trĭg′ərd) *n.* One or a series of spontaneously generated heartbeats originating from an action potential that produces an after-depolarization that reaches activation threshold.

trigger point *n.* A specific point on the body at which touch or pressure will elicit pain.

trigger zone *n.* A specific area that, when stimulated by touch, pain, or pressure, excites an attack of neurologic pain.

tri·glyc·er·ide (trī-glĭs′ə-rīd′) *n.* See **triacylglycerol.**

tri·gone (trī′gōn′) *n.* 1. A triangle or trigonum. 2. The first three dominant cusps of an upper molar tooth.

trigone of bladder *n.* See **vesical triangle.**

tri·go·nid (trī′gə-nĭd, trī-gŏn′ĭd) *n.* The first three dominant cusps of a lower molar tooth.

tri·go·ni·tis (trī′gə-nī′tĭs) *n.* Inflammation of the urinary bladder, localized in the mucous membrane at the trigonum vesicae.

trig·o·no·ceph·a·ly (trĭg′ə-nō-sĕf′ə-lē, trī-gō′nō-) *n.* A malformation characterized by a triangular configuration of the skull, due in part to premature synostosis of the cranial bones with accompanying compression of the cerebral hemispheres.

tri·go·num (trī-gō′nəm) *n.*, *pl.* **-na** (-nə) A triangular anatomical area.

tri·hy·dric alcohol (trī-hī′drĭk) *n.* An alcohol containing three hydroxyl groups, such as glycerol.

tri·i·o·do·thy·ro·nine (trī′ī-ō′dō-thī′rə-nēn′,-nĭn) *n.* See **3,5,3′-triiodothyronine.**

tri·labe (trī′lāb′) *n.* A three-pronged forceps for removal of foreign bodies from the bladder.

Tri·la·fon (trī′lə-fŏn′) A trademark for the drug perphenazine.

tri·lam·i·nar (trī-lăm′ə-nər) *adj.* Having three layers.

tri·lo·bate (trī-lō′bāt′) *or* **tri·lo·bat·ed** (-bā′tĭd) *or* **tri·lobed** (trī′lōbd′) *adj.* Having three lobes.

tri·loc·u·lar (trī-lŏk′yə-lər) *adj.* Having three cavities or cells.

tril·o·gy of Fallot (trĭl′ə-jē) *n.* An atrial septal defect associated with pulmonic stenosis and right ventricular hypertrophy.

tri·mes·ter (trī-mĕs′tər, trī′mĕs′-) *n.* A period of three months.

tri·meth·a·di·one (trī-mĕth′ə-dī′ōn′) *n.* A white crystalline substance used as an anticonvulsant in the treatment of epilepsy.

tri·meth·o·prim (trī-mĕth′ə-prĭm) *n.* An antibiotic usually used to treat urinary tract infections, often in combination with sulfamethoxazole.

tri·meth·yl·a·mine (trī-mĕth′ə-lə-mēn′, -lăm′ēn, -mə-thĭl′ə-mēn′) *n.* A degradation product of nitrogenous plant and animal substances.

tri·meth·yl·am·i·nu·ri·a (trī-mĕth′ə-lăm′ə-noŏr′ē-ə) *n.* Increased excretion of trimethylamine in urine and sweat, with a characteristic fishy body odor.

tri·ni·tro·cel·lu·lose (trī′nī-trō-sĕl′yə-lōs′, -lōz′) *n.* See **pyroxylin.**

tri·nu·cle·o·tide (trī-noō′klē-ə-tīd′) *n.* A triplet of nucleotides; a codon.

tri·ose (trī′ōs′) *n.* A monosaccharide that contains three carbon atoms.

tri·ose·phos·phate isomerase (trī′ōs-fŏs′fāt′) *n.* An enzyme that catalyzes the interconversion of two isomeric three-carbon phosphorylated sugars during glycolysis. Also called *phosphotriose isomerase.*

tri·ox·ide (trī-ŏk′sīd′) *or* **tri·ox·id** (-ŏk′sĭd) *n.* An oxide containing three oxygen atoms per molecule.

tri·phen·yl·meth·ane dye (trī-fĕn′əl-mĕth′ān′, -fē′-nəl-) *n.* Any of a group of dyes used as nuclear, cytoplasmic, and connective tissue stains.

tri·phos·phate (trī-fŏs′fāt′) *n.* A salt or ester containing three phosphate groups.

tri·ple bond (trĭp′əl) *n.* A covalent bond in which three electron pairs are shared between two atoms.

tri·ple·gia (trī-plē′jə) *n.* 1. Paralysis of an upper and a lower extremity and of the face. 2. Paralysis of both extremities on one side and one extremity on the opposite side.

triple point *n.* The temperature and pressure at which three different phases, such as gaseous, liquid, and solid phases, of a particular substance can coexist in equilibrium.

triple response *n.* The triphasic response to the firm stroking of the skin characterized by sharply demarcated erythema, a brief blanching of the skin, and release of histamine from the mast cells, followed by arteriolar dilation causing an intense red flare that extends beyond the margins of the line of pressure, and ending with the appearance of a line wheal having the configuration of the original stroking.

trip·let (trĭp′lĭt) *n.* 1. Any of three children delivered at the same birth. 2. A set of three similar objects, such as a compound lens in a microscope formed of three planoconvex lenses. 3. A unit of three successive nucleotides in a DNA or RNA molecule that codes for a specific amino acid; a codon or anticodon.

triple vision *n.* See **triplopia.**

trip·loid (trĭp′loid′) *adj.* Having three times the haploid number of chromosomes in the cell nucleus. —*n.* A triploid organism or cell. —**trip′loi·dy** *n.*

trip·lo·pi·a (trĭp-lō′pē-ə) *n.* A visual defect in which three images are seen of the same object. Also called *triple vision.*

–tripsy *suff.* A crushing: *lithotripsy.*

trip·tan (trĭp′tn) *n.* Any of a class of drugs that act as agonists of serotonin, result in cranial vasoconstriction, and are used for the prophylaxis and treatment of migraine headaches.

tri·que·trum (trī-kwē′trəm) *n.* A bone of the wrist in the proximal row of the carpus, articulating with the lunate, pisiform, and hamate bones. Also called *cuneiform bone, pyramidal bone.*

tris– *pref.* Three: *trisplanchnic.*

tris·mus (trĭz′məs) *n.* A firm closing of the jaw due to tonic spasm of the muscles of mastication from disease of the motor branch of the trigeminal nerve. It is usually associated with general tetanus. Also called *lockjaw.*

tri·so·my (trī-sō′mē, trī′sō′-) *n.* The condition of having three copies of a given chromosome or chromosome segment in each somatic cell rather than the normal number of two. —**tri·so′mic** *adj.*

trisomy 13 *n.* A syndrome characterized by mental retardation and defects to the central nervous system and heart, caused by having three copies of chromosome 13.

trisomy 21 *n.* See **Down syndrome.**

trisomy 21 syndrome *n.* See **Down syndrome.**

tri·splanch·nic (trī-splăngk′nĭk) *adj.* Of, characterized by, or having three visceral cavities: skull, thorax, and abdomen.

tri·stich·i·a (trī-stĭk′ē-ə) *n.* The presence of three rows of eyelashes.

tri·sul·cate (trī-sŭl′kāt′) *adj.* Having or characterized by three grooves.

tri·ta·nom·a·ly (trī′tə-nŏm′ə-lē) *n.* Partial color blindness resulting from a deficiency of a blue-sensitive retinal pigment.

tri·tan·o·pi·a (trī′tə-nō′pē-ə) *n.* A deficiency in color preception characterized by an inability to discern blue and yellow due to an absence of blue-sensitive pigment in the retina.

trit·i·um (trĭt′ē-əm, trĭsh′ē-) *n. Symbol* **T** A rare radioactive hydrogen isotope with atomic mass 3 and half-life 12.5 years, prepared artificially for use as a tracer and as a constituent of hydrogen bombs. Also called *hydrogen-3.*

tri·ton tumor (trī′tŏn′) *n.* A peripheral nerve tumor with striated muscle differentiation, often seen in neurofibromatosis.

trit·u·rate (trĭch′ə-rāt′) *v.* To rub, crush, grind, or pound into fine particles or a powder. —*n.* A triturated substance, especially a powdered drug. —**trit′u·ra·ble** (-ər-ə-bəl) *adj.*

trit·u·ra·tion (trĭch′ə-rā′shən) *n.* The process of reducing a substance to a fine powder.

tri·va·lent (trī-vā′lənt) *adj.* Having valence 3. —**tri·va′lence, tri·va′len·cy** *n.*

triv·i·al name (trĭv′ē-əl) *n.* **1.** A common, historic, or convenient name for a substance, derived often from the source in which the substance was discovered, but unsystematic and not used in modern official nomenclature, as *aspirin* for *salicylic acid.* **2.** A common or vernacular name as distinguished from a specific name, as *human* for *Homo sapiens.*

tRNA (tē′är-ĕn-ā′) *n.* One of a class of RNA molecules that transports amino acids to ribosomes for incorporation into a polypeptide undergoing synthesis. Also called *transfer RNA.*

tro·car (trō′kär′) *n.* A sharp-pointed surgical instrument, used with a cannula to puncture a body cavity for fluid aspiration.

tro·chan·ter (trō-kăn′tər) *n.* Any of several bony processes on the upper part of the femur.

tro·chan·ter·i·an (trō′kən-tĕr′ē-ən, -kăn-) *or* **tro·chan·ter·ic** (-tĕr′ĭk) *adj.* Of or relating to a trochanter, especially the greater trochanter.

tro·che (trō′kē) *n.* A small, circular medicinal lozenge; a pastille.

troch·le·a (trŏk′lē-ə) *n., pl.* **–le·ae** (-lē-ē′) **1.** An anatomical structure that resembles a pulley, especially the part of the distal end of the humerus that articulates with the ulna. **2.** A fibrous loop in the eye socket near the nasal process of the frontal bone, through which the tendon of the superior oblique muscle of the eye passes.

troch·le·ar (trŏk′lē-ər) *adj.* **1.** Of, resembling, or situated near a trochlea. **2.** Of or relating to the trochlear nerve.

trochlear nerve *n.* A nerve that originates in the mesencephalon below the cerebral aqueduct and supplies the superior oblique muscle of the eyeball. Also called *fourth cranial nerve.*

trochlear spine *n.* A spicule of bone arising from the edge of the trochlear pit of the eye, giving attachment to the pulley of the superior oblique muscle of the eyeball.

tro·choid (trō′koid′, trŏk′oid′) *or* **tro·choi·dal** (trō-koid′l, trŏk-oid′l) *adj.* **1.** Capable of or exhibiting rotation about a central axis. **2.** Permitting rotation, as a pivot.

trochoid joint *n.* A joint in which a section of a cylinder of one bone fits into a corresponding cavity on the other, as in the proximal articulation between the radius and ulna. Also called *pivot joint, rotary joint.*

Trog·lo·tre·ma sal·min·co·la (trŏg′lə-trē′mə săl-mĭng′kə-lə, -mĭn′-) *n.* See **Nanophyetus salmincola.**

Tro·land (trō′lənd), **Leonard Thompson** 1889–1932. American psychologist noted for his experiments with human vision.

Trom·bic·u·la (trŏm-bĭk′yə-lə) *n.* A genus of mites whose larvae are pests of humans and other animals and that includes species that are agents of transmission for tsutsugamushi disease.

trom·bic·u·li·a·sis (trŏm-bĭk′yə-lī′ə-sĭs) *or* **trom·bic·u·lo·sis** (-lō′sĭs) *n.* Infestation with chiggers.

trom·bic·u·lid (trŏm-bĭk′yə-lĭd) *n.* A member of the family Trombiculidae. —**trom·bic′u·lid** *adj.*

Trom·bic·u·li·dae (trŏm-bĭk′yə-lī′dē) *n.* A family of mites whose larvae are parasitic to vertebrates and whose nymphs and adults are bright red and live on insect eggs or on microorganisms in the soil.

tro·meth·a·mine (trō-mĕth′ə-mēn′) *n.* A weakly basic compound used as an alkalizing agent and as a buffer in enzymatic reactions.

trop– *pref.* Variant of tropo–.

troph·ec·to·derm (trŏf-ĕk'tə-dûrm', trō-fĕk'-) *n.* The cell layer from which the trophoblast differentiates.

troph·e·de·ma (trŏf'ĭ-dē'mə, trō'fĭ-) *n.* See **hereditary lymphedema.**

troph·e·sy (trŏf'ĭ-sē) *n.* A disorder of the trophic nerves. —**tro·phe'sic** (trə-fē'zĭk) *adj.*

troph·ic (trŏf'ĭk, trō'fĭk) *adj.* Of, relating to, or characterized by nutrition.

–trophic *suff.* Of, relating to, or characterized by a specified kind of nutrition: *organotrophic.*

trophic ulcer *n.* An ulcer due to impaired nutrition of the part.

tropho– or **troph–** *pref.* Nutrition; nutritive: *trophoblast.*

tro·pho·blast (trō'fə-blăst') *n.* The outermost layer of cells of the blastocyst that attaches the fertilized ovum to the uterine wall and serves as a nutritive pathway for the embryo. Also called *trophoderm.* —**tro'pho·blas'tic** *adj.*

trophoblastic lacuna *n.* One of the spaces in the chorion that becomes an intervillous space after the chorionic villi are formed.

tro·pho·blas·to·ma (trō'fō-blă-stō'mə) *n.* See **choriocarcinoma.**

tro·pho·derm (trō'fə-dûrm') *n.* See **trophoblast.**

tro·pho·der·ma·to·neu·ro·sis (trō'fō-dûr'mə-tō-nŏŏ-rō'sĭs) *n.* Trophic changes to the skin due to neural inflammation.

tro·pho·neu·ro·sis (trō'fō-nŏŏ-rō'sĭs, -trŏf'ō-) *n.* A trophic disorder of a part or region resulting from disease or injury to nerves enervating the area. —**tro'pho·neu·rot'ic** (-rŏt'ĭk) *adj.*

trophoneurotic anemia *n.* Anemia believed to be the result of a profound nervous shock.

trophoneurotic leprosy *n.* See **anesthetic leprosy.**

tro·pho·plast (trō'fə-plăst') *n.* See **plastid** (sense 1).

tro·phot·ro·pism (trō-fŏt'rə-pĭz'əm) *n.* Movement of living cells toward or away from nutritive material. Also called *trophotaxis.* —**tro'pho·trop'ic** (trō'fə-trŏp'-ĭk) *adj.*

tro·pho·zo·ite (trō'fə-zō'īt') *n.* The asexual form of certain sporozoans, such as the schizont of the plasmodia of malaria and related parasites.

–trophy *suff.* Nutrition; growth: *hypertrophy.*

tro·pi·a (trō'pē-ə) *n.* 1. Abnormal deviation of the eye. 2. See **strabismus.**

–tropic *suff.* Affecting or attracted to something specified: *gonadotropic.*

trop·i·cal abscess (trŏp'ĭ-kəl) *n.* See **amebic abscess.**

tropical acne *n.* Severe acne occurring in hot humid climates and covering the entire trunk, shoulders, upper arms, buttocks, and thighs.

tropical anemia *n.* Any of various anemic conditions occurring in persons in tropical climates, usually resulting from nutritional deficiencies or hookworm infestation.

tropical bubo *n.* See **venereal lymphogranuloma.**

tropical diarrhea *n.* See **tropical sprue.**

tropical eosinophilia *n.* Eosinophilia characterized by cough, asthmatic attacks, and enlarged spleen, and believed to be caused by filarial infection; it occurs most frequently in India and southeast Asia.

tropical lichen *n.* See **heat rash.**

tropical medicine *n.* The branch of medicine that deals with diseases occurring in tropical countries.

tropical sore *n.* The lesion that occurs in cutaneous leishmaniasis.

tropical splenomegaly syndrome *n.* See **hyperreactive malarious splenomegaly.**

tropical sprue *n.* Sprue occurring in the tropics, associated with enteric infection and nutritional deficiency, and often complicated by anemia due to folic acid deficiency. Also called *tropical diarrhea.*

tropical typhus *n.* See **scrub typhus.**

tro·pine (trō'pēn', -pĭn) or **tro·pin** (-pĭn) *n.* A white, crystalline, poisonous alkaloid obtained chiefly by hydrolysis of atropine.

tro·pism (trō'pĭz'əm) *n.* The turning or bending movement of a living organism or part toward or away from an external stimulus, such as light, heat, or gravity. —**tro'pic, tro·pis'tic** *adj.*

–tropism *suff.* Tropism: *stereotropism.*

tropo– or **trop–** *pref.* Tropism: *tropocollagen.*

tro·po·col·la·gen (trō'pə-kŏl'ə-jən, trŏp'ə-) *n.* The molecular component of a collagen fiber, consisting of three polypeptide chains coiled around each other.

tro·po·my·o·sin (trō'pə-mī'ə-sĭn, trŏp'ə-) *n.* Any of a group of muscle proteins that bind to molecules of actin and troponin to regulate the interaction of actin and myosin.

tro·po·nin (trō'pə-nĭn, trŏp'ə-) *n.* A calcium-regulated protein in muscle tissue occurring in three subunits with tropomyosin.

troponin I (ī) *n.* A subunit of troponin found in muscle and cartilage that inhibits the formation of blood vessels and is under investigation as a potential cancer therapy.

–tropy *suff.* The state of turning in a specified way or from a specified stimulus: *thixotropy.*

Trous·seau's sign (trŏŏ-sōz') *n.* An indication of latent tetany in which carpal spasm occurs when the upper arm is compressed, as by a tourniquet or a blood pressure cuff.

Trousseau's syndrome *n.* **1.** The occurrence of thrombophlebitis migrans with visceral cancer. **2.** See **gastric vertigo.**

true ankylosis (trŏŏ) *n.* See **synostosis.**

true conjugate *n.* See **conjugate.**

true diverticulum *n.* A diverticulum that includes all the layers of the wall from which it protrudes.

true hermaphrodite *n.* An individual having both ovarian and testicular tissues.

true knot *n.* An intertwining of a segment of umbilical cord, usually without obstructing circulation, commonly formed by the fetus slipping through a loop of the cord.

true pelvis *n.* See **small pelvis.**

true rib *n.* Any of the seven upper pairs of ribs attached to the sternum by costal cartilage.

true vocal cord *n.* See **vocal cord.**

trun·cal (trŭng'kəl) *adj.* **1.** Of or relating to the trunk of the body. **2.** Of or relating to an arterial or nerve trunk.

trun·cate (trŭng'kāt') *v.* To shorten by or as if by

cutting off, especially by cutting across at right angles to the long axis.

trunk (trŭngk) *n.* **1.** The body excluding the head and limbs. **2.** The main stem of a blood vessel or nerve apart from the branches. **3.** A large collecting lymphatic vessel.

truss (trŭs) *n.* A supportive device, usually consisting of a pad with a belt, worn to prevent enlargement of a hernia or the return of a reduced hernia. —*v.* To support or brace with a truss.

truth serum (trōōth) *n.* Any of various hypnotic or anesthetic drugs, such as scopolamine or thiopental sodium, used to induce a subject under questioning to talk without inhibition.

Try *abbr.* tryptophan

try·pan blue (trī′pən, trĭp′ən) *n.* An acid dye used for staining of the reticuloendothelial system, the kidney tubules, and cells in tissue culture.

try·pan·o·cide (trĭ-păn′ə-sīd′) *n.* An agent that kills trypanosomes. Also called *trypanosomicide.* —**try·pan′-o·cid′al** (-sīd′l) *adj.*

Try·pan·o·so·ma (trĭ-păn′ə-sō′mə) *n.* A genus of parasitic flagellate protozoa of the family Trypanosomatidae, transmitted to the vertebrate bloodstream, lymph, and spinal fluid by certain insects and often causing diseases such as sleeping sickness in humans and various other diseases in domesticated animals.

Trypanosoma bru·ce·i gam·bi·en·se (brōō′sē-ī′ găm′bē-ĕn′sē) *n.* A protozoan that is the causative agent of Gambian trypanosomiasis.

Trypanosoma brucei rho·de·si·en·se (rō-dē′zē-ĕn′sē) *n.* A protozoan that is the causative agent of Rhodesian trypanosomiasis.

Trypanosoma cru·zi (krōō′zī) *n.* A protozoan that is the causative agent of South American trypanosomiasis.

Trypanosoma gam·bi·en·se (găm′bē-ĕn′sē) *n. Trypanosoma brucei gambiense.*

Trypanosoma rho·de·si·en·se (rō-dē′zē-ĕn′sē) *n. Trypanosoma brucei rhodesiense.*

try·pan·o·some (trĭ-păn′ə-sōm′) *n.* A member of the genus *Trypanosoma* or of the family Trypanosomatidae. —**try·pan′o·so′mal, try·pan′o·som′ic** (-sŏm′ĭk) *adj.*

try·pan·o·so·mi·a·sis (trĭ-păn′ə-sō-mī′ə-sĭs) *n., pl.* **-ses** (-sēz′) A disease or an infection caused by a trypanosome.

try·pan·o·so·mi·cide (trĭ-păn′ə-sō′mĭ-sīd′) *n.* See **trypanocide.** —**try·pan′o·so′mi·cid′al** (-sīd′l) *adj.*

try·pan·o·so·mid (trĭ-păn′ə-sō′mĭd) *n.* A skin lesion resulting from trypanosomiasis.

try·pars·a·mide (trĭ-pär′sə-mīd′) *n.* A crystalline powder used in the treatment of trypanosomiasis.

tryp·sin (trĭp′sĭn) *n.* An enzyme of pancreatic juice that hydrolyzes proteins into smaller polypeptide units.

tryp·sin·o·gen (trĭp-sĭn′ə-jən) *or* **tryp·so·gen** (trĭp′sə-jən) *n.* The inactive precursor of trypsin, produced by the pancreas and converted to trypsin in the small intestine by enterokinase.

tryp·ta·mine (trĭp′tə-mēn′) *n.* A crystalline substance that is formed in plant and animal tissues from tryptophan and is an intermediate in various metabolic processes.

tryp·tic (trĭp′tĭk) *adj.* Relating to or resulting from trypsin.

tryp·to·phan (trĭp′tə-făn′) *or* **tryp·to·phane** (-fān′) *n. Abbr.* **Try** An essential amino acid formed from proteins during the digestive process by the action of proteolytic enzymes.

tryptophan 2,3-dioxygenase *n.* An oxidoreductase whose concentration is regulated by hormones produced in the adrenal glands; it is present in the liver. Also called *tryptophanase.*

tryp·to·pha·nase (trĭp′tə-fə-nās′, -nāz′, trĭp-tŏf′ə-) *n.* **1.** An enzyme that catalyzes the cleavage of tryptophan to indole, pyruvic acid, and ammonia and that is commonly found in bacteria. **2.** See **tryptophan 2,3-dioxygenase.**

tryp·to·pha·nu·ri·a (trĭp′tə-fə-nōōr′ē-ə) *n.* Increased urinary excretion of tryptophan.

tset·se fly *or* **tzet·ze fly** (tsĕt′sē, tsē′tsē) *n.* Any of several two-winged bloodsucking African flies of the genus *Glossina,* often carrying and transmitting pathogenic trypanosomes to humans and livestock.

TSH *abbr.* thyroid-stimulating hormone

tsp *or* **tsp.** *abbr.* teaspoon

TSS *abbr.* toxic shock syndrome

TSTA *abbr.* tumor-specific transplantation antigen

tsu·tsu·ga·mu·shi disease (tsōō′tsə-gə-mōō′shē) *n.* See **scrub typhus.**

T tubule *n.* The tubule that passes in a transverse manner from the sarcolemma across a myofibril of striated muscle.

TU *abbr.* toxic unit

tu·bal (tōō′bəl) *adj.* Of, relating to, or occurring in a tube, such as the fallopian tube or the eustachian tube.

tubal ligation *n.* A method of female sterilization in which the fallopian tubes are surgically tied.

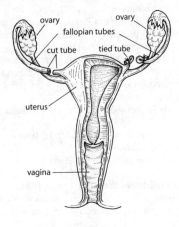

ovary   ovary
fallopian tubes
cut tube   tied tube
uterus
vagina

tubal ligation

tubal pregnancy *n.* An ectopic pregnancy developing in the fallopian tube.

tube (tōōb) *n.* **1.** A hollow cylinder, especially one that conveys a fluid or functions as a passage. **2.** An anatomical structure or organ having the shape or function of a tube; a duct.

tu·bec·to·my (tōō-bĕk′tə-mē) *n.* See **salpingectomy.**

tubed flap *n.* A surgical flap in which the sides of the pedicle are sutured together to create a tube, with the entire surface covered by skin. Also called *Filatov flap.*

tu·ber (tōō′bər) *n., pl.* **tubers** *or* **–ber·a** (-bər-ə) A localized rounded projection or swelling; a knob, tuberosity, or eminence.

tuber ci·ne·re·um (sə-nîr′ē-əm) *n.* A prominence of the base of the hypothalamus, extending ventrally into the infundibulum and pituitary stalk.

tu·ber·cle (tōō′bər-kəl) *n.* **1.** An anatomical nodule. Also called *tuberculum.* **2.** A small elevation on the surface of a tooth. **3.** A nodule or swelling, especially a mass of lymphocytes and epithelioid cells forming the characteristic granulomatous lesion of tuberculosis.

tubercle bacillus *n.* The rod-shaped, gram-negative, aerobic bacterium *Mycobacterium tuberculosis* that causes tuberculosis. Also called *Koch's bacillus.*

tubercle of rib *n.* The knob on which a rib articulates with the transverse process of a vertebra.

tubercle of trapezium *n.* A prominent ridge on the trapezium that forms the lateral border of the groove holding the radial carpal tendon of the hand.

tubercula do·lo·ro·sa (dō′lə-rō′sə) *pl.n.* Multiple cutaneous myomas or neuromas that are painful when pressure is applied.

tu·ber·cu·lar (tōō-bûr′kyə-lər) *adj.* **1.** Of, relating to, or covered with tubercles; tuberculate. **2.** Of, relating to, or affected with tuberculosis. —*n.* A person having tuberculosis.

tu·ber·cu·late (tōō-bûr′kyə-lĭt) *or* **tu·ber·cu·lat·ed** (-lā′tĭd) *adj.* **1.** Having or affected with tubercles. **2.** Tubercular.

tu·ber·cu·lid (tōō-bûr′kyə-lĭd) *n.* A lesion of the skin or of mucous membrane resulting from sensitization to the tubercle bacillus.

tu·ber·cu·lin (tōō-bûr′kyə-lĭn) *n.* A sterile liquid culture containing proteins of tubercle bacilli used chiefly in diagnostic tests for tuberculosis.

tuberculin test *n.* Any of various skin tests used to determine infection with *Mycobacterium tuberculosis,* in which tuberculin or its purified protein is introduced into the skin by injection or tines.

tu·ber·cu·li·tis (tōō-bûr′kyə-lī′tĭs) *n.* Inflammation of a tubercle.

tuberculo– *or* **tubercul–** *pref.* Tubercle; tuberculous; tuberculosis: *tuberculoma.*

tu·ber·cu·lo·cele (tōō-bûr′kyə-lə-sēl′) *n.* Tuberculosis of the testes.

tu·ber·cu·lo·fi·broid (tōō-bûr′kyə-lō-fī′broid′) *n.* An encapsulated nodule formed in a focus of tuberculous granulomatous inflammation during the healing process.

tu·ber·cu·loid (tōō-bûr′kyə-loid′) *adj.* **1.** Resembling tuberculosis. **2.** Resembling a tubercle.

tuberculoid leprosy *n.* A benign, stable, and resistant form of leprosy in which the lepromin reaction is strongly positive but which shows little or no *Mycobacterium leprae* present in the tissues, and in which the lesions are inflamed, red, well-defined plaques that infiltrate the nervous tissue causing a loss of skin sensation as well as sensorimotor damage to nerves serving the area. Also called *cutaneous leprosy, nodular leprosy.*

tu·ber·cu·lo·ma (tōō-bûr′kyə-lō′mə) *n.* A non-neoplastic mass, usually in the lungs or brain, caused by a localized tuberculous infection.

tu·ber·cu·lo·sis (tōō-bûr′kyə-lō′sĭs) *n. Abbr.* **TB 1.** An infectious disease of humans and animals caused by the tubercle bacillus and characterized by the formation of tubercles on the lungs and other tissues of the body, often developing long after the initial infection. **2.** Tuberculosis of the lungs, characterized by the coughing up of mucus and sputum, fever, weight loss, and chest pain.

tuberculosis cu·tis in·du·ra·ti·va (kyōō′tĭs ĭn-door′ə-tī′və) *n.* See **erythema induratum.**

tuberculosis cutis ver·ru·co·sa (vĕr′ə-kō′sə) *n.* A tuberculous skin lesion having a warty surface and a chronically inflamed base. Also called *tuberculous wart.*

tuberculosis vaccine *n.* See **BCG vaccine.**

tu·ber·cu·lo·stat·ic (tōō-bûr′kyə-lō-stăt′ĭk) *adj.* Of, relating to, or being an agent that inhibits the growth of tubercle bacilli.

tu·ber·cu·lous (tōō-bûr′kyə-ləs) *adj.* **1.** Of, relating to, or having tuberculosis. **2.** Of, affected with, or caused by tubercles.

tuberculous abscess *n.* An abscess caused by the tubercle bacillus.

tuberculous meningitis *n.* See **basilar meningitis.**

tuberculous spondylitis *n.* A spinal infection associated with tuberculosis and characterized by a sharp angulation of the spine where tubercle lesions are present. Also called *Pott's disease.*

tuberculous wart *n.* See **tuberculosis cutis verrucosa.**

tu·ber·cu·lum (tōō-bûr′kyə-ləm) *n., pl.* **-la** (-lə) **1.** See **tubercle** (sense 1). **2.** A circumscribed, rounded, solid elevation on the skin, mucous membrane, or surface of an organ. **3.** A slight elevation from the surface of a bone giving attachment to a muscle or ligament.

tuberculum ar·thrit·i·cum (är-thrĭt′ĭ-kəm) *n.* A gouty concretion in or around a joint.

tu·ber·os·i·ty (tōō′bə-rŏs′ĭ-tē) *n.* **1.** The quality or condition of being tuberous. **2.** A projection or protuberance, especially one at the end of a bone for the attachment of a muscle or tendon.

tu·ber·ous (tōō′bər-əs) *or* **tu·ber·ose** (-bə-rōs′) *adj.* **1.** Producing or bearing tubers. **2.** Being or resembling a knot; nodular; lumpy.

tuberous sclerosis *n.* An inherited disease characterized by hamartomas of the brain, retina, and viscera, as well as epileptic seizures, mental retardation, and skin nodules of the face. Also called *Bourneville's disease.*

tubo– *pref.* Tube; tubular: *tubotorsion.*

tu·bo·ab·dom·i·nal pregnancy (tōō′bō-ăb-dŏm′ə-nəl) *n.* Development of an ectopic pregnancy partly in the fallopian tube and partly in the abdominal cavity.

tu·bo·cu·ra·rine chloride (tōō′bō-kyōō-rä′rēn′, -rĭn) *n.* An alkaloid that competes with acetylcholine for myoneural receptors, blocks ganglionic transmission, and releases histamine; it is used to relax skeletal muscles during surgical operations.

tu·bo·o·var·i·an (tōō′bō-ō-vâr′ē-ən) *adj.* Of or relating to the fallopian tube and ovary.

tubo-ovarian pregnancy *n.* An ectopic pregnancy developing at the fimbriated extremity of the fallopian tube and involving the ovary.

tu·bo·plas·ty (tōō′bō-plăs′tē) *n.* See **salpingoplasty**.

tu·bo·tor·sion (tōō′bō-tôr′shən) *n.* The twisting of a tubular structure, such as a fallopian tube.

tu·bo·tym·pan·ic (tōō′bō-tĭm-păn′ĭk) *or* **tu·bo·tym·pa·nal** (-tĭm′pə-nəl) *adj.* Of or relating to the eustachia tube and the tympanic cavity of the ear.

tu·bo·u·ter·ine (tōō′bō-yōō′tər-ĭn, -tə-rīn′) *adj.* Of or relating to a fallopian tube and to the uterus.

tu·bu·lar carcinoma (tōō′byə-lər) *n.* A well-differentiated form of breast carcinoma characterized by invasion of the stroma by small epithelial tubules.

tubular cyst *n.* See **tubulocyst**.

tubular forceps *n.* A long slender forceps intended for use through a cannula or other tubular instrument.

tubular gland *n.* A gland composed of one or more tubules ending in a blind extremity.

tubular maximum *n. Abbr.* **Tm** See **transport maximum**.

tu·bule (tōō′byōol) *n.* A very small tube or tubular structure; tubulus.

tu·bu·lin (tōō′byə-lĭn) *n.* A globular protein that is the structural constituent of microtubules.

tu·bu·lo·ac·i·nar gland (tōō′byə-lō-ăs′ĭ-nər, -när′) *n.* A gland having branching tubules each of which ends in a secretory acini. Also called *acinotubular gland*.

tu·bu·lo·al·ve·o·lar gland (tōō′byə-lō-ăl-vē′ə-lər) *n.* A gland whose secretory portions end in tubular and alveolar configurations.

tu·bu·lo·cyst (tōō′byə-lə-sĭst′) *n.* A cyst formed by the dilation of a blocked canal or tube. Also called *tubular cyst*.

tu·bu·lo·in·ter·sti·tial nephritis (tōō′byə-lō-ĭn′tər-stĭsh′əl) *n.* Nephritis affecting the renal tubules and interstitial tissue that is characterized by infiltration by plasma cells and mononuclear cells and is seen in lupus nephritis, allograft rejection, and methicillin sensitization.

tu·bu·lor·rhex·is (tōō′byə-lə-rĕk′sĭs) *n.* Localized necrosis of the epithelial lining in renal tubules, with focal rupture or loss of basement membrane.

tu·bus (tōō′bəs) *n., pl.* **-bi** (-bī) A tube or a canal.

tuff·stone body (tŭf′stōn′) *n.* A granule found primarily in Schwann cells of individuals affected with metachromatic leukodystrophy.

tuft·ed cell (tŭf′tĭd) *n.* A cell present in the olfactory bulb that transmits sensory impulses in a manner comparable to mitral cells, but is smaller and located more superficially than such cells.

tu·la·re·mi·a (tōō′lə-rē′mē-ə) *n.* An infectious disease caused by the bacterium *Francisella tularensis* that chiefly affects rodents but can also be transmitted to humans, in whom it causes intermittent fever and swelling of lymph nodes.

tu·me·fa·cient (tōō′mə-fā′shənt) *adj.* Producing or tending to produce tumefaction.

tu·me·fac·tion (tōō′mə-făk′shən) *n.* **1.** The act or process of puffing or swelling. **2.** A swollen condition. **3.** A puffy or swollen part; tumescence.

tu·me·fy (tōō′mə-fī′) *v.* To swell or cause to swell.

tu·mes·cence (tōō-mĕs′əns) *n.* **1.** A swelling or an enlargement. **2.** A swollen condition. **3.** A swollen part or organ.

tu·mes·cent (tōō-mĕs′ənt) *adj.* **1.** Somewhat tumid. **2.** Becoming swollen; swelling.

tu·mid (tōō′mĭd) *adj.* **1.** Swollen; distended. Used of a body part or organ. **2.** Of a bulging shape; protuberant.

tum·my tuck (tŭm′ē) *n.* Abdominoplasty. Used informally.

tu·mor (tōō′mər) *n.* **1.** An abnormal growth of tissue resulting from uncontrolled, progressive multiplication of cells and serving no physiological function; a neoplasm. **2.** A swollen part; a swelling.

tumor angiogenic factor *n. Abbr.* **TAF** A substance released by solid tumors that induces formation of new blood vessels to supply the tumor.

tumor antigen *n.* Any of several antigens present in tumors induced by certain types of adenoviruses and papovaviruses or in cells transformed in vitro by those viruses. Also called *neoantigen, T antigen*.

tumor burden *n.* The total mass of tumor tissue carried by an individual with cancer.

tu·mor·i·cid·al (tōō′mər-ə-sīd′l) *adj.* Of or being destructive to tumor cells.

tu·mor·i·gen·e·sis (tōō′mər-ə-jĕn′ĭ-sĭs) *n.* Formation or production of tumors.

tu·mor·i·gen·ic (tōō′mər-ə-jĕn′ĭk) *adj.* Capable of causing tumors.

tumor lysis syndrome *n.* A syndrome characterized by abnormally high levels of phosphates, potassium, and uric acid and by abnormally low levels of calcium in the blood following induction chemotherapy of malignant tumors, possibly caused by the release of intracellular products by cell lysis.

tumor marker *n.* A substance, released into the circulation by tumor tissue, whose detection in the serum indicates the presence of a specific type of tumor.

tumor necrosis factor *n. Abbr.* **TNF** A protein that is produced in the presence of an endotoxin, especially by monocytes and macrophages, is able to attack and destroy tumor cells, and exacerbates chronic inflammatory diseases.

tumor-specific transplantation antigen *n. Abbr.* **TSTA** Any of several surface antigens of virus-transformed tumor cells, which elicit an immune rejection of the virus-free cells when transplanted into an individual that has been immunized against the specific cell-transforming virus.

tumor suppressor gene *n.* A gene that suppresses cellular proliferation. When inherited in a mutated state, it is associated with the development of various cancers, including most familial cancers. Also called *antioncogene*.

tumor stage *n.* The extent of the spread of a malignant tumor from its site of origin.

tumor virus *n.* See **oncogenic virus**.

Tums (tŭmz) A trademark for an over-the-counter preparation of calcium carbonate.

Tun·ga pen·e·trans (tŭng′gə pĕn′ĭ-trănz′) n. Chigoe.

tung·sten (tŭng′stən) n. *Symbol* **W** A hard brittle corrosion-resistant metallic element that has the highest melting point of any metal and that is used in high-temperature structural materials and in electrical elements, notably lamp filaments. Atomic number 74. Also called *wolfram*.

tu·nic (tōō′nĭk) n. A coat or layer enveloping an organ or a part; tunica.

tu·ni·ca (tōō′nĭ-kə) n., pl. **-cae** (-kē′, -sē′) An enclosing or enveloping membrane or layer of tissues, as of a blood vessel or other tubular structure.

tunica ad·ven·ti·ti·a (ăd′vĕn-tĭsh′ē-ə) n. The outermost fibrous coat of a vessel or of an organ that is derived from the surrounding connective tissue. Also called *membrana adventitia*.

tunica al·bu·gin·e·a (ăl′bōō-jĭn′ē-ə, -byōō-) n. A dense collagenous sheath surrounding a structure.

tunica con·junc·ti·va (kŏn′jŭngk-tī′və) n. The conjunctiva.

tunica ex·ter·na (ĭk-stûr′nə) n. The outer of two or more enveloping layers of any structure, especially the fibroelastic coat of a blood or lymph vessel.

tunica fi·bro·sa (fī-brō′sə) n. A fibrous envelope surrounding an anatomical part.

tunica in·ti·ma (ĭn′tə-mə) n. The innermost membrane of a blood or lymph vessel.

tunica me·di·a (mē′dē-ə) n. The middle, usually muscular, coat of a blood or lymph vessel.

tunica mu·co·sa (myōō-kō′sə) n. A mucous membrane.

tunica mus·cu·lar·is (mŭs′kyə-lâr′ĭs) n. The muscular, usually middle, layer or coat of a tubular anatomical structure.

tunica pro·pri·a (prō′prē-ə) n. The particular envelope of a part, as distinguished from the peritoneal or other envelope common to several parts.

tunica re·flex·a (rĭ-flĕk′sə) n. The reflected layer of the vascular layer of testis that lines the scrotum.

tunica sub·mu·co·sa (sŭb′myōō-kō′sə) n. See **tela submucosa**.

tunica vag·i·na·lis tes·tis (văj′ə-nā′lĭs tĕs′tĭs) n. The serous sheath of the testis and epididymis, derived from the peritoneum, and consisting of an outer and inner serous layer.

tunica vas·cu·lo·sa (văs′kyə-lō′sə) n. A histological layer supplied with blood vessels.

tun·nel (tŭn′əl) n. A passage located through or under a barrier.

tunnel disease n. See **ancylostomiasis**.

tunnel vision n. Vision in which the visual field is severely constricted.

tur·bid (tûr′bĭd) adj. Having sediment or foreign particles stirred up or suspended; muddy; cloudy. —**tur·bid′i·ty** n.

tur·bi·dim·e·try (tûr′bĭ-dĭm′ĭ-trē) n. A method for determining the concentration of a substance in a solution by measuring the loss in intensity of a light beam through a solution that contains suspended particulate matter.

tur·bi·nate (tûr′bə-nĭt, -nāt′) or **tur·bi·nat·ed** (-nā′tĭd) adj. **1.** Shaped like a top. **2.** Of or relating to a turbinate bone.

turbinate bone n. A small curved bone that extends horizontally along the lateral wall of the nasal passage in humans and other animals.

tur·bi·nec·to·my (tûr′bə-nĕk′tə-mē) n. Surgical removal of a turbinate bone.

tur·bi·not·o·my (tûr′bə-nŏt′ə-mē) n. Incision into or excision of a turbinate bone.

Tur·cot syndrome (tər-kō′) n. An inherited syndrome marked by polyps of the colon and brain tumors.

tur·ges·cence (tûr-jĕs′əns) n. **1.** The condition of being swollen; tumescence. **2.** The process of swelling.

tur·ges·cent (tûr-jĕs′ənt) adj. Tumescent.

tur·gid (tûr′jĭd) adj. Swollen or distended, as from a fluid; bloated; tumid.

tur·gor (tûr′gər, -gôr′) n. **1.** The state of being turgid. **2.** The normal fullness or tension produced by the fluid content of blood vessels, capillaries, and cells.

tu·ris·ta (tōō-rē′stə) n. Diarrhea occurring in travelers as a result of a change in food and water. Not in technical use.

Tur·ner's syndrome (tûr′nərz) n. A congenital condition of females associated with a defect or an absence of an X-chromosome, characterized by short stature, webbed neck, outward-turning elbows, shield-shaped chest, sexual underdevelopment, and amenorrhea. Also called *XO syndrome*.

Turner's tooth n. Hypoplasia of the enamel involving a single permanent tooth.

turn·o·ver flap (tûrn′ō′vər) n. A hinged flap that is turned over 180°, usually to receive a second flap.

TURP abbr. transurethral resection of the prostate

tus·sal (tŭs′əl) adj. Tussive.

tus·sis (tŭs′ĭs) n., pl. **-ses** (-sēz) A cough.

tus·sive (tŭs′ĭv) adj. Of or relating to a cough.

tussive fremitus n. The vibration felt by a hand placed on the chest of an individual who is coughing.

T wave n. The first deflection in the electrocardiogram following the QRS complex, representing ventricular repolarization.

twelfth cranial nerve n. See **hypoglossal nerve**.

twelfth-year molar n. The second permanent molar tooth.

25-hy·drox·y·cho·le·cal·cif·er·ol (-hī-drŏk′sē-kō′lĭ-kăl-sĭf′ə-rôl′, -rōl′) n. A metabolite of vitamin D_3 that is produced primarily in the liver and is the circulating form of vitamin D in the body. It promotes intestinal absorption of calcium and is used in the treatment of rickets.

21-hy·drox·y·pro·ges·ter·one (-hī-drŏk′sē-prō-jĕs′tə-rōn′) n. See **deoxycorticosterone**.

twi·light sleep (twī′līt′) n. An amnesic condition characterized by insensibility to pain without loss of consciousness, induced by an injection of morphine and scopolamine, formerly used to relieve the pain of childbirth.

twilight state n. A condition of disordered consciousness during which actions may be performed without conscious volition and without any remembrance afterward.

twin (twĭn) *n.* One of two offspring born at the same birth. —*adj.* **1.** Being two or one of two offspring born at the same birth. **2.** Consisting of two identical or similar parts; double.

twinge (twĭnj) *n.* A sharp, sudden physical pain. —*v.* To cause to feel a sharp pain.

twin·ning (twĭn′ĭng) *n.* **1.** The bearing of twins. **2.** A pairing or union of two similar or identical objects.

twin-twin transfusion *n.* Direct vascular anastomosis between the placental circulation of twins.

twist·ed hairs (twĭs′tĭd) *pl.n.* A condition in which the hair shafts are twisted as a result of distortion of the follicles, as from a scarring inflammatory process or mechanical stress. Also called *pili torti.*

twitch (twĭch) *v.* **1.** To draw, pull, or move suddenly and sharply; jerk. **2.** To move jerkily or spasmodically. **3.** To ache sharply from time to time; twinge. —*n.* A sudden involuntary or spasmodic muscular movement.

2,3-di·phos·pho·glyc·er·ate (dī-fŏs′fō-glĭs′ə-rāt′) *n.* An isomer of 1,3-diphosphoglycerate that occurs in red blood cells and is essential to the normal functioning of hemoglobin.

2,4,5-T *n.* (2,4,5-Trichlorophenoxy)acetic acid; a herbicide that is the principal constituent of the defoliant Agent Orange.

2,5-di·me·thox·y-4-meth·yl·am·phet·a·mine (dī′mə-thŏk′sē- -mĕth′əl-ăm-fĕt′ə-mēn, -mĭn) *n.* DOM.

two-carbon fragment *n.* The acetyl radical carried by coenzyme A during transacetylation.

two-glass test *n.* See **Thompson's test.**

2-phe·nox·y·eth·a·nol (-fĭ-nŏk′sē-ĕth′ə-nôl′, -nōl′) *n.* An antibacterial agent effective against gram-negative bacteria that are resistant to other antiseptics and used as a topical treatment for wound infections.

Twort (twôrt), **Frederick William** 1877–1950. British bacteriologist who discovered bacteriophages, the large viruses that attack and destroy bacteria.

two-step exercise test *n.* A test for coronary insufficiency in which an individual ascends and descends two, nine-inch high steps while an electrocardiograph records cardiac activity during the exercise and at intervals afterwards. Also called *Master's test, Master's two-step exercise test.*

two-way catheter *n.* See **double-channel catheter.**

tx *abbr.* treatment

ty·lec·to·my (tī-lĕk′tə-mē) *n.* Surgical removal of a tumor from the breast. Also called *lumpectomy.*

Ty·le·nol (tī′lə-nôl′) A trademark for the drug acetaminophen.

ty·lo·ma (tī-lō′mə) *n.* See **callosity.**

ty·lo·sis (tī-lō′-sĭs) *n., pl.* **–ses** (-sēz) **1.** Inflammation of the eyelids, characterized by thickening and hardening of the edges. **2.** A thickening of the horny layer of the skin as a result of chronic pressure or friction.

tympan– *pref.* Variant of **tympano–.**

tym·pa·nec·to·my (tĭm′pə-nĕk′tə-mē) *n.* Surgical excision of the tympanic membrane of the ear.

tympani– *pref.* Variant of **tympano–.**

tym·pan·ic (tĭm-păn′ĭk) *adj.* **1.** Relating to or resembling a drum of the ear. **2.** *or* **tym·pa·nal** (tĭm′pə-nəl) Of or relating to the tympanic cavity or membrane. **3.** Resonant. **4.** Tympanitic.

tympanic antrum *n.* See **mastoid antrum.**

tympanic artery *n.* **1.** An artery with origin in the maxillary artery, with distribution to the middle ear, and with anastomoses to the tympanic branches of the internal carotid and ascending pharyngeal stylomastoid arteries; anterior tympanic artery. **2.** An artery with origin in the pharyngeal artery, with distribution to the middle ear, and with anastomoses to tympanic branches of other arteries; inferior tympanic artery. **3.** An artery with origin in the stylomastoid artery, with distribution to the middle ear, and with anastomoses to the other tympanic arteries; posterior tympanic artery. **4.** An artery with origin in the middle meningeal artery, with distribution to the middle ear, and with anastomoses to the other tympanic arteries; superior tympanic artery.

tympanic bone *n.* The bony ring in the fetus that develops after birth into the tympanic part of the temporal bone of the skull, partially enclosing the middle ear and supporting the eardrum. Also called *tympanic ring.*

tympanic canal *n.* A minute canal that passes from the petrous portion of the temporal bone between the jugular fossa and carotid canal to the floor of the tympanic cavity and transmits the tympanic branch of the glossopharyngeal nerve. Also called *tympanic canaliculus.*

tympanic cavity *n.* See **middle ear.**

tympanic ganglion *n.* A small ganglion on the tympanic nerve during its passage through the petrous portion of the temporal bone.

tympanic incisure *n.* See **tympanic notch.**

tympanic membrane *n.* See **eardrum.**

tympanic nerve *n.* A nerve from the inferior ganglion of the glossopharyngeal nerve, passing to the tympanic cavity and forming the tympanic plexus that supplies the mucous membrane of the tympanic cavity, the mastoid cells, and the eustachian tube.

tympanic notch *n.* The notch in the superior part of the tympanic ring, bridged by the flaccid part of the tympanic membrane. Also called *Rivinus incisure, tympanic incisure.*

tympanic opening of auditory tube *n.* An opening located in the front part of the tympanic cavity below the canal for the tensor muscle of the tympanic membrane.

tympanic plate *n.* The bony plate between the anterior wall of the external acoustic meatus and the posterior wall of the mandibular fossa.

tympanic plexus *n.* A plexus that is located on the promontory of the labyrinthine wall of the tympanic cavity, is formed by the tympanic nerve, by an anastomotic branch of the facial nerve, and by sympathetic branches coming from the internal carotid plexus, supplies the mucosa of the middle ear, the mastoid cells, and the auditory tube, and gives off the lesser petrosal nerve to the otic ganglion.

tympanic ring *n.* See **tympanic bone.**

tympanic sinus *n.* A depression in the tympanic cavity behind the tympanic promontory.

tympanic vein *n.* Any of the veins that exit from the tympanic cavity and empty into the retromandibular vein.

tym·pa·ni·tes (tĭm′pə-nī′tēz) *n.* A distention of the abdomen resulting from the accumulation of gas or air in the intestine or peritoneal cavity. Also called *meteorism, tympany.* —**tym′pa·nism** *n.*

tym·pa·nit·ic (tĭm′pə-nĭt′ĭk) *adj.* **1.** Of or relating to tympanites. **2.** Of or relating to the quality of sound elicited by percussing over the inflated intestine or over a large pulmonary cavity; tympanic.

tympanitic resonance *n.* A drumlike resonance obtained by percussing over a large space filled with air, such as the stomach, intestine, or large pulmonary cavity.

tym·pa·ni·tis (tĭm′pə-nī′tĭs) *n.* See **myringitis.**

tympano– *or* **tympani–** *or* **tympan–** *pref.* **1.** Tympanum; tympanic: *tympanoplasty.* **2.** Tympanites: *tympanism.*

tym·pa·no·cen·te·sis (tĭm′pə-nō-sĕn-tē′sĭs) *n.* Puncture of the tympanic membrane with a needle to aspirate fluid from the middle ear.

tym·pa·no·mas·toid fissure (tĭm′pə-nō-măs′toid′) *n.* A fissure that separates the tympanic portion from the mastoid portion of the temporal bone and transmits the auricular branch of the vagus nerve. Also called *auricular fissure.*

tym·pa·no·mas·toid·i·tis (tĭm′pə-nō-măs′toi-dī′tĭs) *n.* Inflammation of the middle ear and the mastoid cells.

tym·pa·no·plas·ty (tĭm′pə-nə-plăs′tē, -nō-) *n.* Surgical repair or reconstruction of the middle ear.

tym·pa·nos·to·my (tĭm′pə-nŏs′tə-mē) *n.* See **myringotomy.**

tympanostomy tube *n.* A small tube inserted through the tympanic membrane after myringotomy to aerate the middle ear; often used in the treatment of secretory otitis media.

tym·pa·not·o·my (tĭm′pə-nŏt′ə-mē) *n.* See **myringotomy.**

tym·pa·nous (tĭm′pə-nəs) *adj.* Of or relating to tympanites; tympanitic.

tym·pa·num *or* **tim·pa·num** (tĭm′pə-nəm) *n., pl.* **–nums** *or* **–na** (-nə) **1.** See **middle ear. 2.** See **eardrum.**

tym·pa·ny (tĭm′pə-nē) *n.* **1.** A low-pitched, resonant, drumlike note obtained by percussing the surface of a large air-containing space. **2.** See **tympanites.**

Tyn·dall phenomenon (tĭn′dl) *n.* The occurrence of visible floating particles in gases or liquids that are illuminated by a ray of sunlight and are viewed at right angles to the illuminating ray.

type (tīp) *n.* **1.** A number of people or things having in common traits or characteristics that distinguish them as a group or class. **2.** The general character or structure held in common by a number of people or things considered as a group or class. **3.** A person or thing having the features of a group or class. **4.** An example or a model having the ideal features of a group or class. **5.** A taxonomic group, especially a genus or species, chosen as the representative example in characterizing the larger taxonomic group to which it belongs. **6.** The specimen on which the original description and naming of a taxon is based. —*v.* To determine the antigenic characteristics of a blood or tissue sample.

type 1 diabetes *n.* See **diabetes mellitus** (sense 1).

type 2 diabetes *n.* See **diabetes mellitus** (sense 2).

type 1 glycogenosis *n.* Glycogenosis caused by glucose 6-phosphatase deficiency and resulting in the accumulation of excessive amounts of glycogen, particularly in liver and kidney tissues. Also called *Gierke's disease, von Gierke's disease.*

type 2 glycogenosis *n.* Glycogenosis caused by a deficiency of acid maltase, resulting in the accumulation of glycogen in all organs and marked by cardiorespiratory failure and death, usually before age 2. Also called *generalized glycogenosis, Pompe's disease.*

type 3 glycogenosis *n.* Glycogenosis due to a deficiency of amylo-1,6-glucosidase, resulting in the accumulation of abnormal glycogen in liver and muscle tissues and characterized by symptoms that are similar to but milder than those of type 1 glycogenosis. Also called *Cori's disease, debrancher deficiency limit dextrinosis, Forbes disease.*

type 4 glycogenosis *n.* Glycogenosis due to brancher enzyme deficiency, resulting in the accumulation of abnormal glycogen in liver, kidney, muscle, and other tissues and characterized by progressive cirrhosis of the liver, leading to liver failure and death, usually before age 2. Also called *Andersen's disease, brancher deficiency amylopectinosis.*

type 5 glycogenosis *n.* Glycogenosis due to a phosphorylase deficiency resulting in the accumulation of glycogen in muscle and characterized by muscle cramping that limits the ability to perform strenuous exercise. Also called *McArdle-Schmid-Pearson disease, McArdle's disease.*

type 6 glycogenosis *n.* Glycogenosis due to a phosphorylase deficiency resulting in an accumulation of glycogen in the liver and characterized by symptoms similar to but milder than those of type 1 glycogenosis. Also called *Hers disease.*

type I acrocephalosyndactyly *n.* Acrocephalosyndactyly with the second through fifth digits fused into one mass with a common nail, often accompanied by moderately severe acne vulgaris on the forearms. Also called *Apert's syndrome.*

type I familial hyperlipoproteinemia *n.* Familial hyperlipoproteinemia marked by the increased serum concentrations of chylomicrons and triglycerides, which decrease if the diet becomes fat free, decreased concentrations of high- and low-density lipoproteins, which increase if the diet is fat free, and decreased tissue lipoprotein lipase activity. It is marked by paroxysms of abdominal pain, enlargement of the spleen and liver, and eruptive xanthomas. Also called *familial fat-induced hyperlipemia, familial hyperchylomicronemia, familial hypertriglyceridemia.*

type I mucopolysaccharidosis *n.* See **Hurler's syndrome.**

type IS mucopolysaccharidosis *n.* See **Scheie's syndrome.**

type II acrocephalosyndactyly *n.* Acrocephalosyndactyly with the facial characteristics of Crouzon disease and a hypoplastic maxilla. Also called *Apert-Crouzon syndrome.*

type II familial hyperlipoproteinemia *n.* The most common form of familial hyperlipoproteinemia, characterized by normal concentrations of serum triglycerides and by increased serum concentrations of cholesterol, phospholipids, and low-density lipoproteins. It is marked by generalized xanthomatosis and coronary atherosclerosis. Also called *familial broad-beta hyperlipoproteinemia, familial hyperbetalipoproteinemia, familial hypercholesterolemia.*

type II mucopolysaccharidosis *n.* See **Hunter's syndrome.**

type III acrocephalosyndactyly *n.* Mild acrocephalosyndactyly with asymmetry of the skull and soft tissue syndactyly of the second and third fingers and toes. Also called *Chotzen syndrome.*

type III familial hyperlipoproteinemia *n.* Familial hyperlipoproteinemia marked by an abnormal tolerance of glucose and by an increase in serum concentrations of low-density lipoproteins, pre-low-density lipoproteins, cholesterol, and phospholipids as well as an endogenous increase in serum triglycerides induced by a high-carbohydrate diet. It is marked by eruptive xanthomas and atherosclerosis. Also called *carbohydrate-induced hyperlipemia, familial broad-beta hyperlipoproteinemia, familial hyperbetalipoproteinemia and hyperprebetalipoproteinemia, familial hypercholesterolemia with hyperlipemia.*

type III mucopolysaccharidosis *n.* See **Sanfilippo's syndrome.**

type IV familial hyperlipoproteinemia *n.* Familial hyperlipoproteinemia characterized by increased serum concentrations of pre-low-density lipoproteins and triglycerides on a normal diet but normal concentrations of low-density lipoproteins, cholesterol, and phospholipids. It is marked by paroxysms of abdominal pain, abnormal glucose tolerance, and susceptibility to ischemic heart disease. Also called *carbohydrate-induced hyperlipemia, endogenous hyperglyceridemia, familial hyperprebetalipoproteinemia, familial hypertriglyceridemia.*

type IV mucopolysaccharidosis *n.* See **Morquio's syndrome.**

type V acrocephalosyndactyly *n.* Acrocephalosyndactyly with broad short thumbs and great toes, often with duplication of the great toes and syndactyly of other digits. Also called *Pfeiffer syndrome.*

type V familial hyperlipoproteinemia *n.* Familial hyperlipoproteinemia characterized by increased serum concentrations of chylomicrons, pre-low-density lipoproteins, and triglycerides that are considered to be the result of a combination of fat and carbohydrate-induced hyperlipemia. It is marked by atherosclerosis, paroxysms of abdominal pain, enlargement of the spleen and liver, and abnormal glucose tolerance. Also called *combined fat and carbohydrate-induced hyperlipemia, familial hyperchylomicronemia with hyperprebetalipoproteinemia.*

type V mucopolysaccharidosis *n.* Scheie's syndrome. No longer in technical use.

type VI mucopolysaccharidosis *n.* See **Maroteaux-Lamy syndrome.**

type VII mucopolysaccharidosis *n.* Mucopolysaccharidosis due to beta-glucuronidase deficiency.

type A behavior *n.* A behavior pattern that is characterized by tenseness, impatience, and aggressiveness, often resulting in stress-related symptoms such as insomnia and indigestion and possibly increasing the risk of heart disease. Also called *type A personality.*

type B behavior *n.* A behavior pattern characterized by a relaxed manner, patience, and friendliness that possibly decreases one's risk of heart disease. Also called *type B personality.*

typh·lec·ta·sis (tĭf-lĕk′tə-sĭs) *n.* Dilation of the intestinal cecum.

typh·lec·to·my (tĭf-lĕk′tə-mē) *n.* See **cecectomy.**

typh·len·ter·i·tis (tĭf-lĕn′tə-rī′tĭs) *or* **typh·lo·en·ter·i·tis** (tĭf′lō-ĕn′-) *n.* See **cecitis.**

typh·li·tis (tĭf-lī′tĭs) *n.* See **cecitis.**

typhlo– *or* **typhl–** *pref.* **1.** Cecum: *typhlitis.* **2.** Blindness: *typhlosis.*

typh·lo·dic·li·di·tis (tĭf′lō-dĭk′lĭ-dī′tĭs) *n.* Inflammation of the ileocecal valve of the intestine.

typh·lo·li·thi·a·sis (tĭf′lō-lĭ-thī′ə-sĭs) *n.* The condition of having fecal concretions in the cecum.

typh·lo·pex·y (tĭf′lə-pĕk′sē) *n.* See **cecopexy.**

typh·lor·rha·phy (tĭf-lôr′ə-fē) *n.* See **cecorrhaphy.**

typh·lo·sis (tĭf-lō′sĭs) *n.* Blindness.

typh·los·to·my (tĭf-lŏs′tə-mē) *n.* See **cecostomy.**

typh·lot·o·my (tĭf-lŏt′ə-mē) *n.* See **cecotomy.**

ty·phoid (tī′foid′) *n.* Typhoid fever. —*adj.* **ty·phoidal** (tī-foid′l) Of, relating to, or resembling typhoid fever.

typhoid bacillus *n.* An aerobic, gram-negative, rod-shaped bacterium, *Salmonella typhi,* that causes typhoid fever.

typhoid fever *n.* An acute infectious disease caused by *Salmonella typhi* and characterized by a continued fever, physical and mental depression, an eruption of rose-colored spots on the chest and abdomen, tympanites, and diarrhea. Also called *enteric fever.*

ty·phoi·din (tī-foi′dĭn) *n.* A culture of typhoid bacilli, used to test for the presence of typhoid fever.

typhoid vaccine *n.* A vaccine containing a suspension of inactivated *Salmonella typhi,* used to immunize against typhoid fever.

ty·phus (tī′fəs) *n.* Any of several forms of infectious disease caused by Rickettsia, especially those transmitted by fleas, lice, or mites, and characterized generally by severe headache, sustained high fever, depression, delirium, and the eruption of red rashes on the skin. Also called *camp fever, prison fever.* —**ty′phous** (-fəs) *adj.*

typhus vaccine *n.* A vaccine containing a suspension of inactivated *Rickettsia prowazekii* that has been grown in embryonate eggs, used to immunize against epidemic typhus.

typ·ing (tī′pĭng) *n.* The process of classifying organisms or things according to type.

Tyr *abbr.* tyrosine

ty·ra·mine (tī′rə-mēn′) *n.* A colorless crystalline amine found in mistletoe, putrefied animal tissue, certain cheeses, and ergot, or produced synthetically, used as a sympathomimetic agent.

ty·ro·ci·dine *or* **ty·ro·ci·din** (tī′rə-sīd′n) *n.* A polypeptide antibiotic, produced by the soil microorganism *Bacillus brevis,* which is a major constituent of tyrothricin.

ty·ro·ke·to·nu·ri·a (tī′rō-kē′tə-no͞or′ē-ə) *n.* Urinary excretion of ketonic metabolites of tyrosine.

ty·ro·ma (tī-rō′mə) *n.* A caseous tumor.

ty·ro·sine (tī′rə-sēn′) *n. Abbr.* **Tyr** A white crystalline amino acid that is derived from the hydrolysis of proteins such as casein and is a precursor of epinephrine, thyroxine, and melanin.

ty·ro·si·ne·mi·a (tī′rə-sĭ-nē′mē-ə) *n.* An inherited disorder of tyrosine metabolism marked by an increase in the concentration of tyrosine in the blood, an increase in urinary excretion of tyrosine and related compounds, hepatosplenomegaly, nodular cirrhosis of the liver, multiple renal tubular reabsorptive defects, and vitamin D-resistant rickets.

ty·ro·si·no·sis (tī′rə-sĭ-nō′sĭs) *n.* A rare, possibly inherited disorder of tyrosine metabolism characterized by enhanced urinary excretion of certain metabolites upon ingestion of tyrosine.

ty·ro·si·nu·ri·a (tī′rə-sĭ-no͞or′ē-ə) *n.* Excretion of tyrosine in the urine.

ty·ro·syl·u·ri·a (tī′rə-sĭ-lo͞or′ē-ə) *n.* Enhanced urinary excretion of metabolites of tyrosine, as that occurring in certain diseases including tyrosinosis, scurvy, and pernicious anemia.

ty·ro·thri·cin (tī′rō-thrī′sĭn) *n.* A gray-brown mixture consisting mainly of tryocidine and gramicidin, used as a topical antibiotic in treating infections caused by gram-positive bacteria.

TZD *abbr.* thiazolidinedione

tzet·ze fly (tsĕt′sē, tsē′tsē) *n.* Variant of **tsetse fly**.

U

υ The Greek letter *upsilon*. Entries beginning with this character are alphabetized under **upsilon**.

U The symbol for the element **uranium**.

U/A *abbr.* urinalysis

u·bi·qui·nol (yōo′bĭ-kwī′nôl, yōo-bĭk′wə-nôl) *n.* A compound formed in the reduction of ubiquinone.

u·bi·qui·none (yōo′bĭ-kwĭ-nōn′, yōo-bĭk′wə-nōn′) *n.* A quinone compound that serves as an electron carrier between various flavoproteins and in cellular respiration.

u·biq·ui·tin (yōo-bĭk′wĭ-tĭn) *n.* A polypeptide found in all eukaryotic cells, including plant cells, that participates in a variety of cellular functions including protein degradation.

UDP *abbr.* uridine diphosphate

UGI *abbr.* upper gastrointestinal (as in series)

Uht·hoff sign (ōot′hŏf) *n.* An indication of multiple sclerosis in which vasodilation from exposure to heat or from exertion may cause transient visual impairment or weakness.

ul·cer (ŭl′sər) *n.* A lesion of the skin or of a mucous membrane, such as the one lining the stomach or duodenum, that is accompanied by formation of pus and necrosis of surrounding tissue, usually resulting from inflammation or ischemia.

ul·cer·ate (ŭl′sə-rāt′) *v.* To develop an ulcer; become ulcerous. —**ul′cer·a′tive** (-sə-rā′tĭv, -sər-ə-tĭv) *adj.*

ul·cer·a·tion (ŭl′sə-rā′shən) *n.* **1.** Development of an ulcer. **2.** An ulcer or an ulcerous condition.

ulcerative colitis *n.* A chronic disease of unknown cause, characterized by ulceration of the colon and rectum with bleeding, mucosal crypt abscesses, and inflammatory pseudopolyps, often causing anemia, hypoproteinemia, and electrolyte imbalance.

ulcerative stomatitis *n.* See **canker sore.**

ul·cer·o·gen·ic (ŭl′sə-rō-jĕn′ĭk) *adj.* Tending to cause an ulcer.

ul·cer·o·mem·bra·nous gingivitis (ŭl′sə-rō-mĕm′brə-nəs) *n.* See **trench mouth.**

ul·cer·ous (ŭl′sər-əs) *adj.* **1.** Of the nature of ulcers or an ulcer. **2.** Having ulcers or an ulcer.

ule– *pref.* Variant of **ulo–**.

u·ler·y·the·ma (yōo-lĕr′ə-thē′mə) *n.* An erythema marked by scarring of skin tissue.

ulerythema sy·co·si·for·me (sī-kō′sə-fôr′mē) *n.* See **lupoid sycosis.**

ul·na (ŭl′nə) *n.,* *pl.* **–nas** *or* **–nae** (-nē) The larger bone of the two bones of the forearm, extending from elbow to wrist on the side opposite the thumb. Also called *cubitus, elbow bone.* —**ul′nar** *adj.*

ul·nad (ŭl′năd′) *adj.* In a direction toward the ulna.

ulnar artery *n.* An artery with its origin in the brachial artery, with branches to the recurrent ulnar, interosseous, dorsal and palmar carpal, and deep palmar arteries and the superficial palmar arch with its digital branches.

ulnar collateral artery *n.* **1.** An artery with origin in the brachial artery, with distribution to the arm muscles at the back of the elbow; inferior ulnar collateral artery. **2.** An artery with origin in the brachial artery, with distribution to the elbow joint; superior ulnar collateral artery.

ulnar extensor muscle of wrist *n.* A muscle with origin from the humerus and the ulna, with insertion to the base of the fifth metacarpal bone, with nerve supply from the radial nerve, and whose action extends and abducts the wrist toward the ulna.

ulnar flexor muscle of wrist *n.* A muscle with its origin from the humeral head and from the ulnar head, with insertion to the pisiform bone, with nerve supply from the ulnar nerve, and whose action flexes and abducts the wrist toward the ulna.

ulnar nerve *n.* A nerve that arises from the medial cord of the brachial plexus and gives off numerous muscular and cutaneous branches in the forearm, and supplies the intrinsic muscles of the hand and the skin of the medial side of the hand. Also called *cubital nerve.*

ulnar vein *n.* Any of the veins that accompany the ulnar artery.

ulo– *or* **ule–** *pref.* Scar; scarring: *ulodermatitis.*

u·lo·der·ma·ti·tis (yōo′lō-dûr′mə-tī′tĭs) *n.* Inflammation of the skin resulting in destruction of tissue and the formation of scars.

u·loid (yōo′loid′) *adj.* Resembling a scar. —*n.* A scarlike lesion due to a degenerative process in deeper layers of skin.

ultra– *pref.* **1.** Beyond; on the other side of: *ultraviolet.* **2.** Beyond the range, scope, or limit of: *ultrasonic.*

ul·tra·cen·tri·fuge (ŭl′trə-sĕn′trə-fyōoj′) *n.* A centrifuge that uses high-velocity rotations to achieve the separation of colloidal or submicroscopic particles. —**ul′tra·cen·trif′u·gal** (-trĭf′yə-gəl, -trĭf′ə-gəl) *adj.* —**ul′tra·cen′tri·fu·ga′tion** (-fyōo-gā′shən) *n.*

ul·tra·di·an (ŭl-trā′dē-ən) *adj.* Relating to or exhibiting periodic physiological activity that occurs more than once every 24 hours.

ul·tra·fil·tra·tion (ŭl′trə-fĭl-trā′shən) *n.* The filtration of a colloidal substance through a semipermeable medium that allows only small molecules through.

ul·tra·li·ga·tion (ŭl′trə-lī-gā′shən) *n.* Ligation of a blood vessel beyond the point where a branch is given off.

ul·tra·mi·cro·scope (ŭl′trə-mī′krə-skōp′) *n.* A microscope with high-intensity illumination used to study very minute objects.

ul·tra·mi·cro·scop·ic (ŭl′trə-mī′krə-skŏp′ĭk) *adj.* **1.** Too minute to be seen with an ordinary microscope. **2.** Of or relating to an ultramicroscope.

ul·tra·son·ic (ŭl′trə-sŏn′ĭk) *adj.* **1.** Of or relating to acoustic frequencies above the range audible to the human ear, or above approximately 20,000 hertz. **2.** Of, relating to, or involving ultrasound.

ul·tra·son·ics (ŭl′trə-sŏn′ĭks) *n.* **1.** The acoustics of ultrasonic sound. **2.** The science and technology that deals with ultrasound.

ul·tra·son·o·gram (ŭl′trə-sŏn′ə-grăm′, -sō′nə-) *n.* See **sonogram.**

ul·tra·son·o·graph (ŭl′trə-sŏn′ə-grăf′, -sō′nə-) *n.* An apparatus for producing images obtained by ultrasonography. Also called *sonograph.*

ul·tra·so·nog·ra·phy (ŭl′trə-sə-nŏg′rə-fē) *n.* Diagnostic imaging in which ultrasound is used to visualize an internal body structure or a developing fetus. Also called *echography, sonography.* —**ul′tra·so·nog′ra·pher** *n.* —**ul′tra·son′o·graph′ic** (-sŏn′ə-grăf′ĭk, -sō′-nə-) *adj.*

ul·tra·sound (ŭl′trə-sound′) *n. Abbr.* **U/S 1.** Ultrasonic sound. **2.** The use of ultrasonic waves for diagnostic or therapeutic purposes, specifically to visualize an internal body structure, monitor a developing fetus, or generate localized deep heat to the tissues.

ultrasound cardiography *n.* See **echocardiography.**

ul·tra·struc·tur·al anatomy (ŭl′trə-strŭk′chər-əl) *n.* The study of structures of the body too small to be seen with a light microscope.

ul·tra·thin section (ŭl′trə-thĭn′) *n.* See **thin section.**

ul·tra·vi·o·let (ŭl′trə-vī′ə-lĭt) *adj. Abbr.* **UV** Of or relating to the range of invisible radiation wavelengths from about 4 nanometers, on the border of the x-ray region, to about 380 nanometers, just beyond the violet in the visible spectrum. —*n.* Ultraviolet light or the ultraviolet part of the spectrum.

ultraviolet keratoconjunctivitis *n.* Acute keratoconjunctivitis caused by exposure to intense ultraviolet radiation.

ultraviolet lamp *n.* A lamp, especially a mercury-vapor lamp, that produces ultraviolet rays.

ultraviolet microscope *n.* A microscope having a quartz and fluorite optical system that allows the transmission of light waves shorter than those of the visible spectrum.

ul·tra·vi·rus (ŭl′trə-vī′rəs) *n.* A filterable virus.

um·bil·i·cal (ŭm-bĭl′ĭ-kəl) *adj.* **1.** Of or relating to the navel. **2.** Relating to the umbilical region of the abdomen. —**um·bil′i·cal·ly** *adv.*

umbilical artery *n.* Either of two arteries that before birth is a continuation of the common iliac artery and after birth partly forms the medial umbilical ligament and partly is reduced in size and gives off the superior vesical artery.

umbilical cord *n.* The flexible cordlike structure connecting a fetus at the navel with the placenta and containing two umbilical arteries and one vein that transport nourishment to the fetus and remove its wastes. Also called *funis.*

umbilical hernia *n.* A hernia in which part of the intestine protrudes through the abdominal wall under the skin at the umbilicus. Also called *exomphalos.*

umbilical ligament *n.* **1.** The obliterated umbilical artery that persists as a fibrous cord passing upward alongside the bladder to the umbilicus; medial umbilical ligament. **2.** The remnant of the urachus that persists as a midline fibrous cord located between the apex of the bladder and the umbilicus; middle umbilical ligament.

umbilical region *n.* The middle region of the abdomen centered around the navel.

umbilical ring *n.* An opening in the abdominal wall through which the umbilical cord passes and meets the fetus.

umbilical vein *n.* The left umbilical vein.

umbilical vesicle *n.* See **yolk sac.**

um·bil·i·cate (ŭm-bĭl′ĭ-kĭt) *or* **um·bil·i·cat·ed** (-kā′tĭd) *adj.* **1.** Having a central mark or depression resembling a navel. **2.** Having a navel.

um·bil·i·ca·tion (ŭm-bĭl′ĭ-kā′shən) *n.* **1.** A pit or navel-like depression. **2.** Formation of a depression at the apex of a papule, vesicle, or pustule.

um·bil·i·cus (ŭm-bĭl′ĭ-kəs, ŭm′bə-lī′kəs) *n., pl* **–ci** (-sī′) See **navel.**

um·bo (ŭm′bō) *n., pl.* **um·bos** *or* **um·bo·nes** (ŭm-bō′nēz) A small anatomical projection on a surface, such as that on the inner surface of the tympanic membrane at the end of the manubrium of the malleus, corresponding to the most depressed point of the membrane. —**um′bo·nal** (ŭm′bə-nəl, ŭm-bō′nəl), **um·bon′ic** (ŭm-bŏn′ĭk) *adj.*

UMP *abbr.* uridine phosphate

un– *pref.* Not: *unmyelinated.*

un·bal·anced translocation (ŭn-băl′ənst) *n.* A condition, resulting from fertilization of a gamete containing a translocation chromosome by a normal gamete, in which a segment of the translocation chromosome is represented three times in each cell and a trisomic state exists even though the individual has 46 chromosomes.

un·cal (ŭng′kəl) *adj.* Of or relating to the uncus.

un·ci·form (ŭn′sə-fôrm′) *adj.* Shaped like a hook.

unciform bone *n.* See **hamate.**

Un·ci·nar·i·a (ŭn′sə-nâr′ē-ə) *n.* A genus of nematode hookworms including species that infect various carnivorous mammals, formerly including species now classified under the genera *Ancylostoma* and *Necator.*

un·ci·na·ri·a·sis (ŭn′sə-nə-rī′ə-sĭs) *n.* See **ancylostomiasis.**

un·ci·nate (ŭn′sə-nāt′, -nĭt) *adj.* Unciform.

uncinate epilepsy *n.* A form of psychomotor epilepsy initiated by a dreamy state and by hallucinations of smell and taste, usually caused by a medial temporal lesion. Also called *uncinate fit.*

uncinate fasciculus *n.* A band of long association fibers connecting the frontal and temporal lobes of the cerebrum.

uncinate fit *n.* See **uncinate epilepsy.**

uncinate gyrus *n.* See **uncus** (sense 2).

un·com·pen·sat·ed alkalosis (ŭn-kŏm′pən-sā′tĭd) *n.* A rise in the alkalinity of body fluids without any compensating physiological action to lower the pH.

un·con·di·tioned reflex (ŭn′kən-dĭsh′ənd) *n.* An instinctive reflex not dependent on previous learning or experience.

unconditioned response *n.* A natural, usually unvarying response evoked by a stimulus in the absence of learning or conditioning.

unconditioned stimulus *n.* A stimulus that elicits an

unconditioned response; for example, food is an unconditioned stimulus for a hungry animal, and salivation is the unconditioned response.

un·con·scious (ŭn-kŏn′shəs) *adj.* **1.** Of or in a state of unconsciousness; not conscious. **2.** Occurring in the absence of conscious awareness or thought, as an emotion or motive. **3.** Without conscious control; involuntary or unintended. —*n.* In psychoanalytic theory, the division of the mind containing elements of psychic makeup, such as memories or repressed desires, that are not subject to conscious perception or control but that often affect conscious thoughts and behavior. —**un·con′scious·ly** *adv.*

un·con·scious·ness (ŭn-kŏn′shəs-nĭs) *n.* A state of impaired consciousness in which one shows no responsiveness to environmental stimuli but may respond to deep pain with involuntary movements.

unc·tion (ŭngk′shən) *n.* The action of applying or rubbing with an ointment or oil.

unc·tu·ous (ŭngk′cho̅o̅-əs) *adj.* Containing or composed of oil or fat.

un·cus (ŭng′kəs) *n.,* *pl.* **un·ci** (ŭn′sī) **1.** A hook-shaped part or process. **2.** The anterior hooked extremity of the parahippocampal gyrus on the basomedial surface of the temporal lobe. Also called *uncinate gyrus.*

un·der·arm (ŭn′dər-ärm′) *adj.* Located, placed, or used under the arm. —*n.* The armpit.

un·der·bite (ŭn′dər-bīt′) *n.* Malocclusion in which the lower teeth overlap the upper teeth.

un·der·de·vel·oped (ŭn′dər-dĭ-vĕl′əpt) *adj.* Not adequately or normally developed; immature.

un·der·min·ing ulcer (ŭn′dər-mī′nĭng) *n.* A chronic skin ulcer having overhanging margins, caused by bacterial infection.

un·der·sexed (ŭn′dər-sĕkst′) *adj.* Having low sexual desire or potency.

un·der·shoot (ŭn′dər-sho̅o̅t′) *n.* A temporary decrease below the final steady-state value that may occur immediately following the removal of an influence that had been raising that value.

un·der·weight (ŭn′dər-wāt′) *adj.* Weighing less than is normal, healthy, or required. —*n.* Insufficiency of weight.

un·de·scend·ed testicle (ŭn′dĭ-sĕn′dĭd) *n.* An undescended testis.

undescended testis *n.* A testis that has remained in the abdomen or inguinal canal and not descended into the scrotum. Also called *retained testis.*

un·de·ter·mined nitrogen (ŭn′dĭ-tûr′mĭnd) *n.* The concentration of nitrogen in blood or urine, for example, that can be directly estimated, excluding the nitrogen in such substances as urea, uric acid, or amino acids.

un·dif·fer·en·ti·at·ed (ŭn′dĭf-ə-rĕn′shē-ā′tĭd) *adj.* Having no special structure or function; primitive; embryonic.

undifferentiated type fever *n.* Any of a group of illnesses resulting from infection by any of the arboviruses pathogenic to humans, in which the only constant manifestation is fever.

un·du·lant fever (ŭn′jə-lənt, -də-) *n.* See **brucellosis**.

un·du·lat·ing membrane (ŭn′jə-lā′tĭng, -də-) *n.* An organelle of locomotion in certain flagellate parasites consisting of a finlike extension of the cytoplasmic membrane with the flagellar sheath.

undulating pulse *n.* A pulse in which there is a succession of waves.

ung. *abbr. Latin* unguentum (unguent; ointment)

un·gual (ŭng′gwəl) *adj.* Of or relating to fingernails or toenails.

un·guent (ŭng′gwənt) *n.* A soothing or medicinal salve. —**un′guen·tar′y** (-tĕr′ē) *adj.*

un·gui·nal (ŭng′gwə-nəl) *adj.* Ungual.

un·guis (ŭng′gwĭs) *n., pl.* **–gues** (-gwēz) Any of the thin horny translucent plates covering the upper surface at the end of each finger and toe, consisting of a visible body and a root concealed under a fold of skin; a fingernail or toenail. Also called *onyx.*

uni– *pref.* Single; one: *univalent.*

u·ni·ax·i·al joint (yo̅o̅′nē-ăk′sē-əl) *n.* A joint that permits movement around one axis only.

u·ni·cam·er·al (yo̅o̅′nĭ-kăm′ər-əl) *adj.* Monolocular.

unicameral bone cyst *n.* See **solitary bone cyst**.

unicameral cyst *n.* See **unilocular cyst**.

u·ni·cel·lu·lar (yo̅o̅′nĭ-sĕl′yə-lər) *adj.* Having or consisting of a single cell, as the protozoans; one-celled. —**u′ni·cel′lu·lar′i·ty** (-lăr′ĭ-tē) *n.*

unicellular gland *n.* A single secretory cell.

u·ni·cor·nous (yo̅o̅′nĭ-kôr′nəs) *adj.* Having a single horn or cornu.

u·ni·corn uterus (yo̅o̅′nĭ-kôrn′) *n.* A uterus with one lateral half undeveloped or absent.

u·ni·glan·du·lar (yo̅o̅′nĭ-glăn′jə-lər) *adj.* Having or involving a single gland.

u·ni·lat·er·al (yo̅o̅′nə-lăt′ər-əl) *adj.* On, having, or confined to only one side. —**u′ni·lat′er·al·ly** *adv.*

unilateral anesthesia *n.* See **hemianesthesia**.

unilateral hemianopsia *n.* A condition in which vision is lost in half the visual field of one eye. Also called *uniocular hemianopsia.*

unilateral hermaphroditism *n.* Hermaphroditism in which there is gonadal tissue typical of both sexes on one side of the body and either an ovary or testis on the other.

u·ni·lo·bar (yo̅o̅′nə-lō′bər, -bär′) *adj.* One-lobed.

u·ni·lo·cal (yo̅o̅′nə-lō′kəl) *adj.* Of or being a trait in which the genetic component is contributed predominantly by one locus.

u·ni·loc·u·lar (yo̅o̅′nə-lŏk′yə-lər) *adj.* Having a single compartment or cavity; monolocular.

unilocular cyst *n.* A cyst having a single sac. Also called *unicameral cyst.*

unilocular joint *n.* A joint having only one cavity.

un·in·hib·it·ed neurogenic bladder (ŭn′ĭn-hĭb′ĭ-tĭd) *n.* An abnormal condition, either congenital or acquired, of urinary bladder function in which normal inhibitory control of the function of the detrusor muscle by the central nervous system is impaired or underdeveloped, resulting in precipitant or uncontrolled urination or anuresis or both.

un·in·ter·rupt·ed suture (ŭn′ĭn-tə-rŭp′tĭd) *n.* See **continuous suture**.

u·ni·oc·u·lar hemianopsia (yōō′nē-ŏk′yə-lər) *n.* See unilateral hemianopsia.

un·ion (yōōn′yən) *n.* **1.** The joining or amalgamation of two or more bodies. **2.** The structural adhesion of the edges of a wound.

u·ni·o·vu·lar (yōō′nē-ō′vyə-lər, -ŏv′yə-) *adj.* Relating to or formed from a single ovum.

U·ni·pen (yōō′nə-pĕn′) A trademark for the drug nafcillin sodium.

u·ni·pen·nate (yōō′nə-pĕn′āt′) *adj.* Of or being a muscle whose fibers are attached obliquely to one side of a lateral tendon.

u·ni·po·lar (yōō′nĭ-pō′lər) *n.* **1.** Having a single fibrous process. Used of a neuron. **2.** Situated at only one extremity of a cell. —**u′ni·po·lar′i·ty** (-pō-lăr′ĭ-tē, -pə-) *n.*

unipolar lead (lēd) *n.* **1.** A lead of an electrocardiograph in which one electrode is placed on the chest in the vicinity of the heart or on one of the limbs, while the other is placed at an area of zero potential. **2.** A record obtained from such a lead.

unipolar neuron *n.* A neuron whose cell body emits a single axonal process resulting from the fusion of two polar processes during development, one branch of the process serving as a sensory nerve fiber and a second branch entering into synaptic contact with neurons in the spinal cord or brainstem.

u·ni·port (yōō′nə-pôrt′) *n.* Transport of a molecule or ion through a membrane by a carrier mechanism without known coupling to the transport of any other molecule or ion.

u·nit (yōō′nĭt) *n.* **1.** An entity regarded as an elementary structural or functional constituent of a whole. **2.** A precisely specified quantity in terms of which the magnitudes of other quantities of the same kind can be stated. **3.** The quantity of a serum, drug, or other agent necessary to produce a specific effect.

United States Pharmacopeia *n. Abbr.* **USP** A book that is the officially recognized authority and standard on the description of drugs, chemicals, and medicinal preparations in the United States.

unit membrane *n.* A trilaminar structure of the cell membrane as seen in cross section through an electron microscope.

u·ni·va·lent (yōō′nĭ-vā′lənt) *adj.* **1.** Having valence 1. **2.** Having only one valence. **3.** Of or relating to a chromosome that is not paired or united with its homologous chromosome during synapsis. —*n.* A univalent chromosome. —**u′ni·va′lence, u′ni·va′len·cy** *n.*

u·ni·ver·sal donor (yōō′nə-vûr′səl) *n.* A person whose red blood cells do not contain agglutinogen A or B and are therefore not agglutinated by plasma containing either of the ordinary isoagglutinins, alpha or beta; a person who has group O blood.

universal recipient *n.* A person who has group AB blood and is therefore able to receive blood from any other group in the ABO system.

un·my·e·lin·at·ed (ŭn-mī′ə-lĭ-nā′tĭd) *adj.* Lacking a myelin sheath. Used of a nerve fiber.

unmyelinated fiber *n.* Any of the nerve fibers that lack a fatty sheath but that are enveloped by a sheath of Schwann cells as are other nerve fibers. Also called *gray fiber, nonmedullated fiber.*

Un·na boot (ōō′nə) *n.* A compression dressing consisting of a paste, primarily made of zinc oxide, that is applied both under and over a gauze bandage, used on the lower leg for venous ulcers, phlebitis, sprains, and other disorders.

un·of·fi·cial (ŭn′ə-fĭsh′əl) *adj.* Of or being a drug that is not listed in the *United States Pharmacopeia* or the *National Formulary.*

un·phys·i·o·log·ic (ŭn′fĭz-ē-ə-lŏj′ĭk) *adj.* Relating to conditions in an organism that are abnormal.

un·san·i·tar·y (ŭn-săn′ĭ-tĕr′ē) *adj.* Not sanitary.

un·sat·u·rat·ed (ŭn-săch′ə-rā′tĭd) *adj.* **1.** Of or relating to a solution in which the solvent is capable of dissolving still more of the solute; not saturated. **2.** Of or relating to a chemical compound in which all the affinities are not satisfied, so that still other atoms or radicals may be added to it. **3.** Of or relating to chemical compounds containing double and triple bonds.

unsaturated fat *n.* A fat having chains of unsaturated fatty acids.

unsaturated fatty acid *n.* A fatty acid, such as oleic acid, whose carbon chain possesses one or more double or triple bonds and hence can incorporate additional hydrogen atoms.

un·sta·ble angina (ŭn-stā′bəl) *n.* Angina pectoris characterized by pain of coronary origin that occurs in response to less exercise or other stimuli than usually required to produce pain.

un·stri·at·ed (ŭn-strī′ā′tĭd) *adj.* Lacking striations; smooth-textured. Used of muscles.

un·sys·tem·a·tized delusion (ŭn-sĭs′tə-mə-tīzd′) *n.* One of a group of apparently discrete, disconnected delusions.

up·per airway (ŭp′ər) *n.* The portion of the respiratory tract that extends from the nostrils or mouth through the larynx.

upper extremity *n.* The shoulder, arm, forearm, wrist, or hand. Also called *superior limb, thoracic limb.*

upper GI series *n.* A radiologic study in which barium sulfate is swallowed, providing an image of the upper gastrointestinal tract including the esophagus, stomach, and duodenum. Also called *barium swallow.*

upper motor neuron *n.* A motor neuron whose cell body is located in the motor area of the cerebral cortex and whose processes connect with motor nuclei in the brainstem or the anterior horn of the spinal cord.

upper uterine segment *n.* The main portion of the body of the gravid uterus, the contraction of which furnishes the chief force of expulsion in labor.

UPPP *abbr.* uvulopalatopharyngoplasty

up·take (ŭp′tāk′) *n.* The absorption by a tissue of a substance, such as a nutrient, and its permanent or temporary retention.

ur– *pref.* Variant of **uro–.**

u·ra·chus (yōōr′ə-kəs) *n.* The portion of the reduced allantoic stalk between the apex of the bladder and the umbilicus. —**u′ra·chal** *adj.*

u·ra·cil (yōōr′ə-sĭl) *n.* A pyrimidine base that is an essential constituent of RNA.

u·ra·ni·um (yŏŏ-rā′nē-əm) *n. Symbol* **U** An easily oxidized radioactive toxic metallic element having 16 known isotopes, of which U 238 is the most naturally abundant. Atomic number 92.

urano– *pref.* Hard palate: *uranoplasty.*

u·ra·no·plas·ty (yŏŏr′ə-nə-plăs′tē) *n.* See **palatoplasty.**

u·ra·nor·rha·phy (yŏŏr′ə-nôr′ə-fē) *n.* See **palatorrhaphy.**

u·ra·nos·chi·sis (yŏŏr′ə-nŏs′kĭ-sĭs) *n.* Cleft of the hard palate.

u·ra·no·staph·y·los·chi·sis (yŏŏr′ə-nō-stăf′ə-lŏs′kĭ-sĭs) *n.* Cleft of the soft and hard palates.

u·ra·nyl (yŏŏr′ə-nĭl, yŏŏ-rā′nəl) *n.* The divalent radical $UO_2{}^{2+}$.

u·rar·thri·tis (yŏŏr′är-thrī′tĭs) *n.* Gouty inflammation of a joint.

u·rase (yŏŏr′ās′, -āz′) *n.* Variant of **urease.**

u·rate (yŏŏr′āt′) *n.* A salt of uric acid.

u·ra·te·mi·a (yŏŏr′ə-tē′mē-ə) *n.* Presence of urates, especially sodium urate, in the blood.

urate oxidase *n.* An enzyme that catalyzes the oxidation of uric acid. Also called *uricase.*

u·ra·to·sis (yŏŏr′ə-tō′sĭs) *n.* A pathological condition due to the presence of urates in the blood or tissues.

u·ra·tu·ri·a (yŏŏr′ə-tŏŏr′ē-ə) *n.* Presence of an increased amount of urates in the urine.

u·re·a (yŏŏ-rē′ə) *n.* A water-soluble compound that is the major nitrogenous end product of protein metabolism and is the chief nitrogenous component of the urine in mammals and other organisms. Also called *carbamide.*

urea– *pref.* Urea; urine: *ureapoiesis.*

urea clearance *n.* The volume of plasma or blood that would be completely cleared of urea by one minute's excretion of urine.

urea cycle *n.* The sequence of chemical reactions that takes place in the liver and that results in the production of urea. The key reaction is the hydrolysis of arginine by arginase to ornithine and urea. Also called *Krebs-Henseleit cycle, Krebs ornithine cycle, Krebs urea cycle.*

urea frost *n.* Minute flakes of urea sometimes observed on the skin in patients with uremia.

u·re·a·gen·e·sis (yŏŏ-rē′ə-jĕn′ĭ-sĭs) *n.* Formation of urea, especially the metabolism of amino acids to urea. Also called *ureapoiesis.*

urea nitrogen *n.* The concentration of nitrogen in blood or urine, for example, derived from urea.

U·re·a·plas·ma (yŏŏ-rē′ə-plăz′mə) *n.* A genus of nonmotile gram-negative bacteria that require urea and cholesterol for growth and are associated with nongonococcal urethritis and prostatitis in males and with genitourinary tract infections and reproductive failure in females. Also called *T-mycoplasma.*

u·re·a·poi·e·sis (yŏŏ-rē′ə-poi ē′sĭs) *n.* See **ureagenesis.**

u·re·ase (yŏŏr′ē-ās′, -āz′) *or* **u·rase** (yŏŏr′ās′, -āz′) *n.* An enzyme that cataylzes the hydrolysis of urea to form ammonium carbonate.

u·rec·chy·sis (yŏŏ-rĕk′ĭ-sĭs) *n.* Extravasation of urine into the tissues.

u·re·de·ma (yŏŏr′ĭ-dē′mə) *or* **u·ro·e·de·ma** (yŏŏr′ō-) *n.* Edema due to infiltration of urine into the subcutaneous tissues.

u·rel·co·sis (yŏŏr′ĕl-kō′sĭs) *n.* Ulceration of the urinary tract.

u·re·mi·a *or* **u·rae·mi·a** (yŏŏ-rē′mē-ə) *n.* **1.** The accumulation of urinary waste products in the blood. Also called *azotemia.* **2.** A toxic condition caused by uremia. —**u·re′mic** *adj.*

uremic frost *n.* Powdery deposits of urea and uric acid salts on the skin, especially the face, usually the result of severe uremia.

u·re·mi·gen·ic (yŏŏ-rē′mə-jĕn′ĭk) *adj.* **1.** Caused by uremia. **2.** Causing or resulting in uremia.

u·re·si·es·the·sia (yŏŏ-rē′sē-ĕs-thē′zhə) *n.* The normal urge to urinate.

u·re·sis (yŏŏ-rē′sĭs) *n.* See **urination.**

u·re·ter (yŏŏ-rē′tər, yŏŏr′ĭ-tər) *n.* The long narrow duct that conveys urine from the kidney to the urinary bladder. —**u·re′ter·al, u′re·ter′ic** (yŏŏr′ĭ-tĕr′ĭk) *adj.*

u·re·ter·al·gia (yŏŏ-rē′tə-răl′jə) *n.* Pain in the ureter.

ureteral meatus *n.* The opening of either ureter into the bladder, situated at either angle of the trigone. Also called *ureteral opening.*

u·re·ter·cys·to·scope (yŏŏ-rē′tər-sĭs′tə-skōp′, yŏŏr′ĭ-tər-) *or* **u·re·ter·o·cys·to·scope** (yŏŏ-rē′tə-rō-) *n.* A cystoscope with an attachment for catheterization of the ureters.

u·re·ter·ec·ta·sia (yŏŏ-rē′tə-rĕk-tā′zhə, -yŏŏr′ĭ-tə-) *n.* Dilation of a ureter.

u·re·ter·ec·to·my (yŏŏ-rē′tə-rĕk′tə-mē) *n.* Excision of all or part of a ureter.

u·re·ter·i·tis (yŏŏ-rē′tə-rī′tĭs, -yŏŏr′ĭ-tə-) *n.* Inflammation of a ureter.

uretero– *pref.* Ureter; urethral: *ureteropathy.*

u·re·ter·o·cele (yŏŏ-rē′tə-rō-sēl′) *n.* Saccular dilation of the terminal portion of the ureter at the entrance into the urinary bladder, due to a congenital stricture of the ureteral meatus.

u·re·ter·o·ce·lor·ra·phy (yŏŏ-rē′tə-rō′sē-lôr′ə-fē, -sĭ-) *n.* Excision and suturing of a ureterocele through an open cystotomy incision.

u·re·ter·o·co·los·to·my (yŏŏ-rē′tə-rō-kə-lŏs′tə-mē) *n.* Surgical implantation of the ureter into the colon.

u·re·ter·o·cys·tos·to·my (yŏŏ-rē′tə-rō-sĭ-stŏs′tə-mē) *n.* See **ureteroneocystostomy.**

u·re·ter·o·di·al·y·sis (yŏŏ-rē′tə-rō-dī-ăl′ĭ-sĭs) *n.* See **ureterolysis** (sense 1).

u·re·ter·o·en·ter·os·to·my (yŏŏ-rē′tə-rō-ĕn′tə-rŏs′tə-mē) *n.* Surgical formation of an opening between a ureter and the intestine.

u·re·ter·og·ra·phy (yŏŏ-rē′tə-rŏg′rə-fē) *n.* X-ray examination of the ureter after injection of a contrast medium.

u·re·ter·o·il·e·o·ne·o·cys·tos·to·my (yŏŏ-rē′tə-rō-ĭl′ē-ō-nē′ō-sĭ-stŏs′tə-mē) *n.* Surgical restoration of the continuity of the urinary tract by anastomosis of the upper segment of a partially destroyed ureter to a segment of the ileum, the lower end of which is then implanted into the bladder.

u·re·ter·o·il·e·os·to·my (yŏŏ-rē′tə-rō-ĭl′ē-ŏs′tə-mē) *n.* Surgical implantation of a ureter into an isolated segment of the ileum which drains through an abdominal stoma.

u·re·ter·o·lith (yŏŏ-rē′tə-rō-lĭth′) *n.* A calculus in the ureter.

u·re·ter·o·li·thi·a·sis (yŏŏ-rē′tə-rō-lĭ-thī′ə-sĭs) *n.* Formation or presence of a calculus or calculi in one or both ureters.

u·re·ter·o·li·thot·o·my (yŏŏ-rē′tə-rō-lĭ-thŏt′ə-mē) *n.* Surgical removal of a calculus lodged in a ureter.

u·re·ter·ol·y·sis (yŏŏ-rē′tə-rŏl′ĭ-sĭs) *n.* **1.** Rupture of a ureter. Also called *ureterodialysis.* **2.** Paralysis of the ureter. **3.** Surgical freeing of the ureter from surrounding disease or adhesions.

u·re·ter·o·ne·o·cys·tos·to·my (yŏŏ-rē′tə-rō-nē′ō-sĭ-stŏs′tə-mē) *n.* An operation to implant the upper end of a transected ureter into the bladder. Also called *ureterocystostomy.*

u·re·ter·o·ne·o·py·e·los·to·my (yŏŏ-rē′tə-rō-nē′ō-pī′ə-lŏs′tə-mē) *n.* Surgical reimplantation of the ureter into the pelvis of the kidney. Also called *ureteropyeloneostomy.*

u·re·ter·o·ne·phrec·to·my (yŏŏ-rē′tə-rō-nə-frĕk′tə-mē) *n.* Surgical removal of a kidney with its ureter.

u·re·ter·op·a·thy (yŏŏ-rē′tə-rŏp′ə-thē) *n.* Disease of the ureter.

u·re·ter·o·plas·ty (yŏŏ-rē′tə-rō-plăs′tē) *n.* Reparative or plastic surgery of either or both ureters.

u·re·ter·o·py·e·li·tis (yŏŏ-rē′tə-rō-pī′ə-lī′tĭs) *n.* Inflammation of the pelvis of a kidney and its ureter. Also called *ureteropyelonephritis.*

u·re·ter·o·py·e·log·ra·phy (yŏŏ-rē′tə-rō-pī′ə-lŏg′rə-fē) *n.* See **pyelography.**

u·re·ter·o·py·e·lo·ne·os·to·my (yŏŏ-rē′tə-rō-pī′ə-lō-nē-ŏs′tə-mē) *n.* See **ureteroneopyelostomy.**

u·re·ter·o·py·e·lo·ne·phri·tis (yŏŏ-rē′tə-rō-pī′ə-lō-nə-frī′tĭs) *n.* See **ureteropyelitis.**

u·re·ter·o·py·e·lo·plas·ty (yŏŏ-rē′tə-rō-pī′ə-lə-plăs′tē) *n.* Plastic surgery of the ureter and of the pelvis of the kidney.

u·re·ter·o·py·e·los·to·my (yŏŏ-rē′tə-rō-pī′ə-lŏs′tə-mē) *n.* Surgical formation of a junction of the ureter and the renal pelvis.

u·re·ter·o·py·o·sis (yŏŏ-rē′tə-rō-pī-ō′sĭs) *n.* Accumulation of pus in a ureter.

u·re·ter·o·re·nal reflux (yŏŏ-rē′tə-rō-rē′nəl) *n.* Reflux of urine from the ureter into the pelvis of the kidney.

u·re·ter·or·rha·gia (yŏŏ-rē′tə-rō-rā′jə) *n.* Hemorrhage from a ureter.

u·re·ter·or·rha·phy (yŏŏ-rē′tə-rôr′ə-fē) *n.* Suture of a ureter.

u·re·ter·o·sig·moid·os·to·my (yŏŏ-rē′tə-rō-sĭg′moi-dŏs′tə-mē) *n.* Surgical implantation of a ureter into the sigmoid colon.

u·re·ter·os·to·my (yŏŏ-rē′tə-rŏs′tə-mē) *n.* Surgical establishment of an external opening into the ureter.

u·re·ter·ot·o·my (yŏŏ-rē′tə-rŏt′ə-mē) *n.* Incision of a ureter.

u·re·ter·o·u·re·ter·os·to·my (yŏŏ-rē′tə-rō-yŏŏ-rē′tə-rŏs′tə-mē) *n.* The establishment of an anastomosis between the two ureters or between two segments of the same ureter.

u·re·ter·o·ves·i·cos·to·my (yŏŏ-rē′tə-rō-vĕs′ĭ-kŏs′tə-mē) *n.* Surgical joining of a ureter to the bladder.

urethr– *pref.* Variant of **urethro–.**

u·re·thra (yŏŏ-rē′thrə) *n., pl.* **–thras** *or* **–thrae** (-thrē) The canal through which urine is discharged from the bladder in most mammals and through which semen is discharged in the male. Also called *urogenital canal.* **—u·re′thral** *adj.*

urethral artery *n.* An artery with origin in the perineal artery, with distribution to part of the urethra.

urethral caruncle *n.* A small, fleshy, sometimes painful growth on the mucous membrane, usually occurring at the meatus of the female urethra.

urethral crest *n.* **1.** In the female, a conspicuous longitudinal fold of mucosa on the posterior wall of the urethra. **2.** In the male, a longitudinal fold on the posterior wall of the urethra extending from the uvula of the bladder through the part of the urethra that traverses the bladder.

u·re·thral·gi·a (yŏŏr′ĭ-thrăl′jə) *n.* Pain in the urethra. Also called *urethrodynia.*

urethral gland *n.* Any of the numerous mucous glands in the wall of the male or female urethra.

urethral groove *n.* The groove on the undersurface of the embryonic penis that ultimately is closed to form the penile portion of the urethra.

urethral hematuria *n.* Hematuria in which the site of bleeding is in the urethra.

urethral papilla *n.* The slight projection in the vestibule of the vagina marking the urethral orifice.

urethral valve *n.* Any of various folds in the mucous membrane of the urethra.

u·re·thra·tre·sia (yŏŏ-rē′thrə-trē′zhə) *n.* Imperforation or occlusion of the urethra.

u·re·threc·to·my (yŏŏr′ĭ-thrĕk′tə-mē) *n.* Excision of a part or all of the urethra.

u·re·threm·or·rha·gia (yŏŏ-rē′thrĕm-ə-rā′jə) *n.* The occurrence of bleeding from the urethra. Also called *urethrorrhagia.*

u·re·threm·phrax·is (yŏŏ-rē′thrĕm-frăk′sĭs, yŏŏr′ə-) *n.* Obstruction of the flow of urine through the urethra. Also called *urethrophraxis.*

u·re·thrism (yŏŏr′ə-thrĭz′əm) *or* **u·re·thris·mus** (yŏŏr′-ə-thrĭz′məs) *n.* Irritability or spasmodic stricture of the urethra. Also called *urethrospasm.*

u·re·thri·tis (yŏŏr′ĭ-thrī′tĭs) *n.* Inflammation of the urethra.

urethritis pe·trif·i·cans (pə-trĭf′ĭ-kănz′) *n.* Urethritis in which there is a deposit of calcareous matter in the wall of the urethra.

urethro– *or* **urethr–** *pref.* Urethra; urethral: *urethroscope.*

u·re·thro·bal·a·no·plas·ty (yŏŏ-rē′thrō-băl′ə-nō-plăs′tē) *n.* The surgical repair of hypospadias and epispadias.

u·re·thro·bul·bar (yŏŏ-rē′thrō-bŭl′bər, -bär′) *adj.* Bulbourethral.

u·re·thro·cele (yŏŏ-rē′thrə-sēl′) *n.* A prolapse of the female urethra.

u·re·thro·cys·ti·tis (yŏŏ-rē′thrō-sĭ-stī′tĭs) *n.* Inflammation of the urethra and the bladder.

u·re·thro·cys·tom·e·try (yŏŏ-rē′thrō-sĭ-stŏm′ĭ-trē) *n.* A procedure that simultaneously measures pressures in the urinary bladder and the urethra.

u·re·thro·dyn·i·a (yŏŏ-rē′thrō-dĭn′ē-ə) *n.* See **urethralgia.**

u·re·thro·per·i·ne·o·scro·tal (yŏŏ-rē′thrō-pĕr′ə-nē′ə-skrōt′l) *adj.* Relating to the urethra, perineum, and scrotum.

u·re·thro·pex·y (yŏŏ-rē′thrə-pĕk′sē) *n.* Surgical suspension of the urethra from the posterior surface of the pubic symphysis in order to correct urinary stress incontinence.

u·re·thro·phrax·is (yŏŏ-rē′thrə-frăk′sĭs) *n.* See **urethremphraxis.**

u·re·thro·phy·ma (yŏŏ-rē′thrə-fī′mə) *n.* A tumor or circumscribed swelling of the urethra.

u·re·thro·plas·ty (yŏŏ-rē′thrə-plăs′tē) *n.* Reparative or plastic surgery of the urethra.

u·re·thror·rha·gia (yŏŏ-rē′thrə-rā′jə) *n.* See **urethremorrhagia.**

u·re·thror·rha·phy (yŏŏr′ə-thrôr′ə-fē) *n.* Suture of the urethra.

u·re·thror·rhe·a (yŏŏ-rē′thrə-rē′ə) *n.* An abnormal discharge from the urethra.

u·re·thro·scope (yŏŏ-rē′thrə-skōp′) *n.* An instrument for examining the interior of the urethra. —**u′re′-thro·scop′ic** (-skŏp′ĭk) *adj.* —**u′re·thros′co·py** (yŏŏr′-ə-thrŏs′kə-pē) *n.*

u·re·thro·spasm (yŏŏ-rē′thrə-spăz′əm) *n.* See **urethrism.**

u·re·thro·stax·is (yŏŏ-rē′thrə-stăk′sĭs) *n.* Oozing of blood from the mucous membrane of the urethra.

u·re·thro·ste·no·sis (yŏŏ-rē′thrō-stə-nō′sĭs) *n.* Stricture of the urethra.

u·re·thros·to·my (yŏŏr′ə-thrŏs′tə-mē) *n.* **1.** Surgical construction of an artificial excretory opening from the urethra. **2.** The opening that is created by such a procedure.

u·re·throt·o·my (yŏŏr′ə-thrŏt′ə-mē) *n.* Surgical incision of a stricture of the urethra.

u·re·thro·vag·i·nal fistula (yŏŏ-rē′thrō-văj′ə-nəl) *n.* A fistula between the urethra and the vagina.

u·re·thro·ves·i·co·pex·y (yŏŏ-rē′thrō-vĕs′ĭ-kə-pĕk′sē) *n.* Surgical suspension of the urethra and the base of the bladder to correct stress incontinence.

u·ret·ic (yŏŏ-rĕt′ĭk) *adj.* Of urine; urinary.

–uretic *suff.* Urine: *diuretic.*

urge incontinence (ûrj) *n.* Leakage of urine when the desire to void is strong. Also called *urgency incontinence.*

ur·gen·cy (ûr′jən-sē) *n.* A strong desire to urinate, accompanied by a fear of leakage.

urgency incontinence *n.* See **urge incontinence.**

ur·hi·dro·sis (yŏŏr′hī-drō′sĭs, -hĭ-) *n.* Variant of **uridrosis.**

URI *abbr.* upper respiratory infection

–uria *suff.* **1.** The condition of having a specified substance in the urine: *aciduria.* **2.** The condition of having a specified kind of urine: *polyuria.*

u·ric (yŏŏr′ĭk) *adj.* Relating to, contained in, or obtained from urine.

uric acid *n.* A semisolid compound that is a nitrogenous end product of protein and purine metabolism and is a nitrogenous component of urine.

u·ri·case (yŏŏr′ĭ-kās′, -kāz′) *n.* See **urate oxidase.**

urico– or **uric–** *pref.* Uric acid: *uricolytic.*

u·ri·col·y·sis (yŏŏr′ĭ-kŏl′ĭ-sĭs) *n.* Decomposition of uric acid. —**u′ri·co·lyt′ic** (yŏŏr′ĭ-kō-lĭt′ĭk) *adj.*

u·ri·co·su·ri·a (yŏŏr′ĭ-kə-soŏr′ē-ə) *n.* The presence of excessive amounts of uric acid in the urine. —**u′ri·co·su′ric** (-soŏr′ĭk) *adj.*

u·ri·co·tel·ic (yŏŏr′ĭ-kō-tĕl′ĭk) *adj.* Excreting uric acid as the chief component of nitrogenous waste.

u·ri·dine (yŏŏr′ĭ-dēn′) *n.* A white odorless powder that is the nucleoside of uracil and is important in carbohydrate metabolism.

uridine diphosphate *n. Abbr.* **UDP** A uridine compound that serves as a glycosyl carrier in the synthesis of glycogen and starch.

uridine phosphate *n. Abbr.* **UMP** See **uridylic acid.**

uridine triphosphate *n. Abbr.* **UTP** A phosphorylated nucleoside of uridine that participates in the biosynthesis of glycogen.

u·ri·dro·sis (yŏŏr′ĭ-drō′sĭs) or **ur·hi·dro·sis** (yŏŏr′hī-) *n.* Excretion of urea or uric acid in the sweat.

u·ri·dyl·ic acid (yŏŏr′ĭ-dĭl′ĭk) *n.* A nucleoside of uridine formed in the hydrolysis of RNA. Also called *uridine phosphate.*

urin– *pref.* Variant of **urino–.**

u·ri·nal (yŏŏr′ə-nəl) *n.* A vessel into which urine is passed.

u·ri·nal·y·sis (yŏŏr′ə-năl′ĭ-sĭs) *n., pl.* **–ses** (-sēz′) *Abbr.* **U/A** Laboratory analysis of urine, used to help diagnose disease or detect a specific substance.

u·ri·nar·y (yŏŏr′ə-nĕr′ē) *adj.* **1.** Relating to urine and its production, function, or excretion. **2.** Of or relating to the organs involved in the formation and excretion of urine.

urinary bladder *n.* A musculomembranous elastic receptacle in the anterior part of the pelvic cavity serving as the temporary storage place for urine.

urinary calculus *n.* A hard mass of mineral salts in the urinary tract. Also called *cystolith, urolith, vesical calculus.*

urinary nitrogen *n.* The nitrogen that is excreted as urea, amino acids, or uric acid, as in the urine.

urinary sand *n.* Small calculous particles passed in the urine.

urinary stress incontinence *n.* Leakage of urine as a result of coughing, straining, or sudden movement.

urinary stuttering *n.* Frequent involuntary interruption occurring during the act of urination.

urinary system *n.* The organs and passages of the urinary tract.

urinary tract *n.* The passage from the pelvis of the kidney through the ureters, bladder, and urethra to the external urinary opening. See illustration on page 860.

u·ri·nate (yŏŏr′ə-nāt′) *v.* To excrete urine.

u·ri·na·tion (yŏŏr′ə-nā′shən) *n.* The passing of urine. Also called *emiction, miction, micturition, uresis.*

u·rine (yŏŏr′ĭn) *n.* The waste product secreted by the kidneys that in mammals is a fluid that is yellow to amber in color, slightly acidic, and discharged from the body through the urethra.

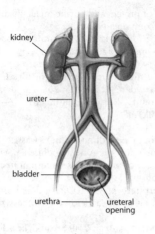

kidney

ureter

bladder

urethra — ureteral opening

urinary tract

urino– or **urin–** *pref.* Urine: *urinalysis*

u·ri·no·gen·i·tal (yŏor′ə-nō-jĕn′ĭ-tl) *adj.* Variant of **urogenital.**

u·ri·nog·e·nous (yŏor′ə-nŏj′ə-nəs) *adj.* **1.** Producing or excreting urine. **2.** Of urinary origin.

u·ri·no·ma (yŏor′ə-nō′mə) *n.*, *pl.* **–mas** or **–ma·ta** (-mə-tə) A cyst containing urine.

u·ri·nom·e·ter (yŏor′ə-nŏm′ĭ-tər) *n.* A hydrometer for measuring the specific gravity of urine.

u·ri·nom·e·try (yŏor′ə-nŏm′ĭ-trē) *n.* The determination of the specific gravity of urine.

u·ri·nos·co·py (yŏor′ə-nŏs′kə-pē) *n.* See **uroscopy.**

uro– or **ur–** *pref.* **1.** Urine: *uric.* **2.** Urinary tract: *urolithiasis.*

u·ro·bi·lin (yŏor′ō-bī′lĭn, -bĭl′ĭn) *n.* A pigment in urine that produces an orange-red color whose intensity varies with its degree of oxidation.

u·ro·bi·li·ne·mi·a (yŏor′ō-bī′lə-nē′mē-ə, -bĭl′ə-) *n.* The presence of urobilins in the blood.

u·ro·bi·lin·o·gen (yŏor′ō-bī-lĭn′ə-jən, -jĕn′) *n.* The precursor of urobilin and a product of the reduction of bilirubin.

u·ro·bi·li·nu·ri·a (yŏor′ō-bī′lə-nŏor′ē-ə) *n.* The presence of excess urobilins in the urine.

u·ro·can·ate (yŏor′ō-kăn′āt′) *n.* A salt or ester of urocanic acid.

urocanate hydratase *n.* An enzyme that catalyzes the conversion of urocanic acid in histidine catabolism.

u·ro·can·ic acid (yŏor′ə-kăn′ĭk) *n.* An acid derived from the oxidative deamination of histidine and present in dog's urine.

u·ro·cele (yŏor′ə-sēl′) *n.* Extravasation of urine into the scrotal sac. Also called *uroscheocele.*

u·ro·che·si·a (yŏor′ə-kē′zē-ə, -zhə) *n.* Passage of urine from the anus.

u·ro·chrome (yŏor′ə-krōm′) *n.* A compound of urobilin and a peptide that is the principal pigment of urine.

u·ro·cys·ti·tis (yŏor′ō-sĭ-stī′tĭs) *n.* Inflammation of the urinary bladder.

u·ro·dyn·i·a (yŏor′ə-dĭn′ē-ə) *n.* Pain on urination.

u·ro·e·de·ma (yŏor′ō-ĭ-dē′mə) *n.* Variant of **uredema.**

u·ro·fla·vin (yŏor′ə-flā′vĭn) *n.* A fluorescent product of riboflavin catabolism, found in urine and feces.

u·ro·fol·li·tro·pin (yŏor′ō-fŏl′ĭ-trō′pĭn) *n.* A preparation of gonadotropin extracted from the urine of postmenopausal women used with human chorionic gonadotropin to induce ovulation.

u·ro·gas·trone (yŏor′ə-găs′trōn′) *n.* A fluorescent pigment extracted from urine that inhibits gastric secretion and motility.

u·ro·gen·i·tal (yŏor′ō-jĕn′ĭ-tl) or **u·ri·no·gen·i·tal** (yŏor′ə-nō-) *adj.* Genitourinary.

urogenital canal *n.* See **urethra.**

urogenital diaphragm *n.* A triangular sheet of muscle between the ischiopubic rami, composed of the sphincter muscle of the urethra and the deep transverse muscles of the perineum.

urogenital mesentery *n.* See **diaphragmatic ligament of mesonephros.**

urogenital ridge *n.* One of the paired longitudinal ridges developing in the dorsal body wall of the embryo, formed at first by the growing mesonephros and later by the mesonephros and the gonad. Also called *mesonephric fold, Wolffian ridge.*

urogenital sinus *n.* The ventral part of the cloaca after its separation from the rectum, giving rise to the lower part of the bladder in both sexes, to the prostatic portion of the male urethra, and to the urethra and vestibule in the female.

urogenital system *n.* The organs involved in the formation and excretion of urine together with those involved in sexual reproduction. Also called *genitourinary system.*

u·rog·e·nous (yŏo-rŏj′ə-nəs) *adj.* **1.** Producing urine. **2.** Produced or derived from urine.

u·ro·gram (yŏor′ə-grăm′) *n.* A radiograph of the urinary tract.

u·rog·ra·phy (yŏo-rŏg′rə-fē) *n.* Radiography of the urinary tract. —**u′ro·graph′ic** (yŏor′ə-grăf′ĭk) *adj.*

u·ro·ki·nase (yŏor′ō-kī′nās, -nāz) *n.* An enzyme that catalyzes the conversion of plasminogen to plasmin and is produced in the kidney, excreted in the urine, and used to dissolve blood clots. Also called *plasminogen activator.*

u·ro·lith (yŏor′ə-lĭth′) *n.* See **urinary calculus.** —**u′ro·lith′ic** *adj.*

u·ro·li·thi·a·sis (yŏor′ō-lĭ-thī′ə-sĭs) *n.* A diseased condition resulting from the presence or formation of calculi in the urinary tract.

u·rol·o·gy (yŏo-rŏl′ə-jē) *n.* The medical specialty concerned with the study, diagnosis, and treatment of diseases of the urinary tract in females and of the genitourinary tract in males. —**ur′o·log′ic** (yŏor′ə-lŏj′ĭk), **ur′o·log′i·cal** (-ĭ-kəl) *adj.* —**u·rol′o·gist** *n.*

u·ron·cus (yŏo-rŏng′kəs, -rŏn′-) *n.* A circumscribed swelling containing extravasated urine.

u·ro·ne·phro·sis (yŏor′ō-nə-frō′sĭs) *n.* See **hydronephrosis.**

–uronic *suff.* Connected with urine: *hyaluronic acid.*

u·ron·ic acid (yŏo-rŏn′ĭk) *n.* A product of the oxidation of sugar occurring in various polysaccharides and in urine and containing both an aldehyde and a carboxyl group.

u·rop·a·thy (yŏŏ-rŏp′ə-thē) *n.* A disorder involving the urinary tract.

u·ro·phan·ic (yŏŏr′ə-făn′ĭk) *adj.* Appearing in the urine.

u·ro·pla·ni·a (yŏŏr′ə-plā′nē-ə) *n.* Extravasation of urine.

u·ro·poi·e·sis (yŏŏr′ō-poi-ē′sĭs) *n.* The production and excretion of urine. —**u′ro·poi·et′ic** (-ĕt′ĭk) *adj.*

u·ro·por·phy·rin (yŏŏr′ō-pôr′fə-rĭn) *n.* A porphyrin excreted in the urine, such as urobilin.

u·ro·por·phy·rin·o·gen (yŏŏr′ō-pôr′fə-rĭn′ə-jən, -jĕn′) *n.* Any of various porphyrins that can be converted to uroporphyrins.

u·ro·ra·di·ol·o·gy (yŏŏr′ō-rā′dē-ŏl′ə-jē) *n.* Examination of the urinary tract by radiological techniques.

u·ros·che·o·cele (yŏŏ-rŏs′kē-ə-sēl′) *n.* See urocele.

u·ros·che·sis (yŏŏ-rŏs′kĭ-sĭs) *n.* 1. The retention of urine. 2. The suppression of urine.

u·ros·co·py (yŏŏ-rŏs′kə-pē) *n.* Examination of urine for diagnostic purposes. Also called *urinoscopy.* —**u′-ro·scop′ic** (yŏŏr′ə-skŏp′ĭk) *adj.*

u·ro·sep·sis (yŏŏr′ō-sĕp′sĭs) *n.* Sepsis resulting from the decomposition of extravasated urine.

u·ros·to·my (yŏŏ-rŏs′tə-mē) *n.* Surgical construction of an artificial excretory opening from the urinary tract.

u·ro·tho·rax (yŏŏr′ō-thôr′ăks′) *n.* The presence of urine in the thoracic cavity.

u·ro·u·re·ter (yŏŏr′ō-yŏŏ-rē′tər, -yŏŏr′ĭ-tər) *n.* See hydroureter.

ur·ti·cant (ûr′tĭ-kənt) *adj.* Causing itching or stinging. —*n.* A substance that causes itching or stinging.

ur·ti·car·i·a (ûr′tĭ-kâr′ē-ə) *n.* A skin condition characterized by welts that itch intensely, caused by an allergic reaction, an infection, or a nervous condition. Also called *hives, nettle rash.*

urticaria en·dem·i·ca (ĕn-dĕm′ĭ-kə) *n.* Urticaria caused by contact with the nettling hairs of certain caterpillars.

ur·ti·car·i·al (ûr′tĭ-kâr′ē-əl) *adj.* Relating to or marked by urticaria.

urticarial fever *n.* See schistosomiasis japonicum.

urticaria med·i·ca·men·to·sa (mĕd′ĭ-kə-mən-tō′sə) *n.* Urticaria due to an allergic reaction to a drug.

urticaria pig·men·to·sa (pĭg′mən-tō′sə) *n.* Mastocytosis resulting from congenital excess of mast cells in the superficial dermis and characterized by brownish papules that urticate when stroked.

ur·ti·cate (ûr′tĭ-kāt′) *v.* To undergo urtication. —*adj.* (-kĭt, -kāt′) Characterized by the presence of urticaria.

ur·ti·ca·tion (ûr′tĭ-kā′shən) *n.* 1. The formation or development of urticaria. 2. The sensation of having been stung by nettles. 3. A lashing with nettles formerly used to treat a paralyzed part of the body.

u·ru·shi·ol (ŏŏ-rŏŏ′shē-ôl′, -ōl′) *n.* A toxic substance constituting the active allergen of the irritant oil present in poison ivy, poison oak, and poison sumac.

U/S *abbr.* ultrasound

USAN *abbr.* United States Adopted Names (used for nonproprietary names of drugs adopted by a committee of medical professionals and drug manufacturers)

Ush·er's syndrome (ŭsh′ərz) *n.* An inherited syndrome characterized by sensorineural deafness and retinitis pigmentosa.

USP *abbr.* United States Pharmacopoeia

USPHS *abbr.* United States Public Health Service

USP unit *n.* A unit as defined and adopted by the *United States Pharmacopeia.*

ut dict. *abbr. Latin* ut dictum (as directed)

uter– *pref.* Variant of utero–.

u·ter·ine (yŏŏ′tər-ĭn, -tə-rīn′) *adj.* Of, relating to, or in the region of the uterus.

uterine artery *n.* An artery with its origin in the internal iliac artery, with distribution to the uterus, the upper part of the vagina, the round ligament, and part of the uterine tube.

uterine calculus *n.* See uterolith.

uterine cavity *n.* The space within the uterus extending from the cervical canal to the openings of the uterine tubes.

uterine cycle *n.* The menstrual cycle.

uterine gland *n.* Any of the numerous branched tubular glands in the mucus membrane of the uterus.

uterine placenta *n.* See maternal placenta.

uterine sinus *n.* A small irregular vascular channel in the endometrium.

uterine souffle *n.* A blowing sound, synchronous with the cardiac systole of the mother, heard on auscultation over the pregnant uterus. Also called *placental souffle.*

uterine tube *n.* See fallopian tube.

uterine vein *n.* Either of two veins on each side that arise from the uterine plexus, pass through a part of the broad ligament and through a peritoneal fold, and empty into the hypogastric vein.

utero– *or* **uter–** *pref.* Uterus: *uteroscopy.*

u·ter·o·cys·tos·to·my (yŏŏ′tə-rō-sĭ-stŏs′tə-mē) *n.* Surgical formation of a communication between the uterus and the bladder.

u·ter·o·fix·a·tion (yŏŏ′tə-rō-fĭk-sā′shən) *n.* See hysteropexy.

u·ter·o·lith (yŏŏ′tər-ə-lĭth′) *n.* An abnormal concretion of the uterus, usually a calcified myoma. Also called *hysterolith, uterine calculus.*

u·ter·om·e·ter (yŏŏ′tə-rŏm′ĭ-tər) *n.* See hysterometer.

u·ter·o·pex·y (yŏŏ′tər-ə-pĕk′sē) *n.* See hysteropexy.

u·ter·o·pla·cen·tal sinus (yŏŏ′tə-rō-plə-sĕn′tl) *n.* Any of the irregular vascular spaces in the zone of the chorionic attachment to the decidua basalis.

u·ter·o·plas·ty (yŏŏ′tər-ə-plăs′tē) *n.* Plastic surgery of the uterus. Also called *hysteroplasty, metroplasty.*

u·ter·o·sal·pin·gog·ra·phy (yŏŏ′tə-rō-săl′pĭng-gŏg′rə-fē) *n.* See hysterosalpingography.

u·ter·o·scope (yŏŏ′tər-ə-skōp′) *n.* See hysteroscope.

u·ter·os·co·py (yŏŏ′tə-rŏs′kə-pē) *n.* See hysteroscopy.

u·ter·ot·o·my (yŏŏ′tə-rŏt′ə-mē) *n.* See hysterotomy.

u·ter·o·ton·ic (yŏŏ′tə-rō-tŏn′ĭk) *adj.* Giving tone to the uterine muscle. —*n.* An agent that overcomes relaxation of the muscular wall of the uterus.

u·ter·o·tu·bog·ra·phy (yŏŏ′tə-rō-tŏŏ-bŏg′rə-fē) *n.* See hysterosalpingography.

u·ter·us (yŏŏ′tər-əs) *n., pl.* **u·ter·us·es** *or* **u·ter·i** (yŏŏ′tə-rī′) A hollow muscular organ consisting of a body, fundus, isthmus, and cervix located in the pelvic cavity of female mammals, in which the fertilized egg implants and develops into the fetus. Also called *metra, womb.*

uterus di·del·phys (dī-dĕl′fĭs) *n.* A double uterus with double cervix and double vagina, caused by a failure of the müllerian ducts to unite.

UTI *abbr.* urinary tract infection

u·til·i·za·tion review (yōot′l-ĭ-zā′shən) *n.* A process for monitoring the use, delivery, and cost-effectiveness of services, especially those provided by medical professionals.

UTP *abbr.* uridine triphosphate

u·tri·cle[1] (yōo′trĭ-kəl) *n.* A membranous sac contained within the labyrinth of the inner ear and connected with the semicircular canals.

utricle[2] *n.* A small vestigial blind pouch of the prostate gland; the prostatic utricle.

u·tric·u·lar[1] (yōo-trĭk′yə-lər) *adj.* 1. Of, relating to, or resembling a utricle. 2. Having one or more utricles.

utricular[2] *adj.* Of the uterus.

utricular nerve *n.* A branch of the utriculoampullar nerve, supplying the macula of the utricle.

u·tric·u·li·tis (yōo-trĭk′yə-lī′tĭs) *n.* 1. Inflammation of the internal ear. 2. Inflammation of the prostatic utricle.

u·tric·u·lo·am·pul·lar nerve (yōo-trĭk′yə-lō-ăm-pŏŏl′-ər, -pŭl′-) *n.* A division of the vestibular part of the eighth cranial nerve, giving off branches to the macula of the utricle and to the ampullary crests of the anterior and lateral semicircular ducts.

u·tric·u·lo·sac·cu·lar (yōo-trĭk′yə-lō-săk′yə-lər) *adj.* Of the utricle and the saccule of the inner ear.

u·tric·u·lus (yōo-trĭk′yə-ləs) *n., pl.* **-li** (-lī′) An anatomical sac or pouch, especially the one within the inner ear; utricle.

UV *abbr.* ultraviolet

u·ve·a (yōo′vē-ə) *n.* The vascular, pigmentary, middle coat of the eye comprising the choroid, ciliary body, and iris. —**u′ve·al** *adj.*

u·ve·i·tis (yōo′vē-ī′tĭs) *n.* Inflammation of the uvea. —**u′ve·it′ic** (-ĭt′ĭk) *adj.*

u·ve·o·pa·rot·id fever (yōo′vē-ō-pə-rŏt′ĭd) *n.* A form of sarcoidosis characterized by chronic enlargement of the parotid glands, inflammation of the uveal tract, and low-grade fever. Also called *Heerfordt's disease.*

u·ve·o·scle·ri·tis (yōo′vē-ō-sklə-rī′tĭs) *n.* Inflammation of the sclera due to extension of inflammation from the uvea.

u·vi·form (yōo′və-fôrm′) *adj.* 1. Having the form of a grape. 2. Having numerous rounded protuberances resembling a bunch of grapes; botryoid.

UV index (yōo′vē′) *n.* A scale ranging from zero to ten, used in estimating the risk for sunburn that an unprotected fair-skinned person would have if exposed to the ultraviolet radiation in midday sunlight.

u·vu·la (yōo′vyə-lə) *n., pl.* **-las** *or* **-lae** (-lē) A small conical pendent fleshy mass of tissue, especially the uvula palatina.

uvula cer·e·bel·li (sĕr′ə-bĕl′ī) *n.* See **uvula vermis.**

uvula pal·a·ti·na (păl′ə-tī′nə) *n.* The uvula hanging from the the middle of the soft palate.

u·vu·lar (yōo′vyə-lər) *adj.* Of, relating to, or associated with the uvula.

uvula ver·mis (vûr′mĭs) *n.* A triangular elevation on the vermis of the cerebellum, lying between the two cerebellar tonsils in front of the cerebellar pyramid. Also called *uvula cerebelli.*

uvula ve·si·cae (vĭ-sī′kē, vĭ-sē′kē) *n.* A slight projection into the cavity of the bladder just behind the urethral opening, marking the location of the middle lobe of the prostate gland.

u·vu·lec·to·my (yōo′vyə-lĕk′tə-mē) *n.* Excision of the uvula. Also called *staphylectomy.*

u·vu·li·tis (yōo′vyə-lī′tĭs) *n.* An inflammation of the uvula.

uvulo– *or* **uvul–** *pref.* Uvula: *uvuloptosis.*

u·vu·lo·pal·a·to·pha·ryn·go·pla·sty (yōo′vyə-lō-păl′-ə-tō-fə-rĭng′gə-plăs′tē) *n. Abbr.* **UPPP** A surgical procedure for treating severe obstructive sleep apnea, in which the airway at the back of the throat is widened by the removal of excess soft tissue including the uvula, tonsils, and part of the soft palate.

u·vu·lop·to·sis (yōo′vyə-lŏp-tō′sĭs) *n.* Relaxation or elongation of the uvula. Also called *staphylodialysis, staphyloptosis.*

u·vu·lot·o·my (yōo′vyə-lŏt′ə-mē) *n.* Incision of the uvula. Also called *staphylotomy.*

U wave *n.* A positive wave following the T wave of the electrocardiogram.

V

v *abbr.* venous blood (used as a subscript)

V The symbol for the element **vanadium**.

V *Abbr.* **volt**

VA *abbr.* viral antigen

V-A *abbr.* ventriculoatrial

vac·ci·na (văk-sī′nə) *n.* Vaccinia.

vac·ci·nal (văk′sə-nəl, văk-sē′-) *adj.* 1. Of or relating to vaccination or a vaccine. 2. Induced by vaccination.

vac·ci·nate (văk′sə-nāt′) *v.* To inoculate with a vaccine in order to produce immunity to an infectious disease such as diphtheria or typhus. —**vac′ci·na′tor** *n.*

vac·ci·na·tion (văk′sə-nā′shən) *n.* 1. Inoculation with a vaccine in order to protect against a particular disease. 2. A scar left on the skin by vaccinating.

vac·cine (văk-sēn′ văk′sēn′) *n.* 1. A preparation of a weakened or killed pathogen, such as a bacterium or virus, or of a portion of the pathogen's structure that upon administration stimulates antibody production against the pathogen but is incapable of causing severe infection. 2. A vaccine prepared from the cowpox virus and inoculated against smallpox.

vac·ci·nee (văk′sə-nē′) *n.* An individual who has been vaccinated.

vaccine lymph *n.* Lymph collected from the vaccinia vesicles of infected calves and used for active immunization against smallpox.

vac·cin·i·a (văk-sĭn′ē-ə) *n.* 1. See **cowpox**. 2. An infection induced in humans by inoculation with the vaccinia virus in order to confer resistance to smallpox; it is usually limited to the site of inoculation. Also called *primary reaction*. —**vac·cin′i·al** *adj.*

vaccinia virus *n.* A virus of the genus *Orthopoxvirus* used in the immunization against smallpox.

vac·cin·i·form (văk-sĭn′ə-fôrm′) *adj.* Of or resembling vaccinia.

vac·ci·ni·za·tion (văk′sə-nĭ-zā′shən) *n.* Vaccination repeated at short intervals until the antigen produces no response.

vac·ci·nol·o·gy (văk′sə-nŏl′ə-jē) *n.* The science or methodology of vaccine development.

VACTERL syndrome (văk′tərl) *n.* A syndrome seen in embryos and fetuses characterized by abnormalities of vertebrae (V), anus (A), cardiovascular tree (C), trachea (T), esophagus (E), renal system (R), and limb buds (L), associated with the administration of sex hormones during early pregnancy.

vac·u·o·lat·ed (văk′yōō-ō-lā′tĭd) *or* **vac·u·o·late** (-lāt′, -lĭt) *adj.* Containing vacuoles or a vacuole.

vac·u·o·la·tion (văk′yōō-ō-lā′shən) *or* **vac·u·o·li·za·tion** (-lĭ-zā′shən) *n.* 1. The formation of vacuoles. 2. The condition of having vacuoles.

vac·u·ole (văk′yōō-ōl′) *n.* 1. A small cavity in the cytoplasm of a cell, bound by a single membrane and containing water, food, or metabolic waste. 2. A small space or cavity in a tissue. —**vac′u·o′lar** (-ō′lər, -lär′) *adj.*

vac·u·tome (văk′yə-tōm′) *n.* An electrodermatome that applies suction to the skin to raise it before an advancing blade, usually for taking a split-thickness skin graft.

vac·u·um (văk′yōō-əm, -yōōm, -yəm) *n., pl.* **-u·ums** *or* **-u·a** (-yōō-ə) 1. Absence of matter. 2. A space empty of matter. 3. A space relatively empty of matter. 4. A space in which the pressure is significantly lower than atmospheric pressure.

vacuum aspiration *n.* A method of abortion performed during the first trimester, in which the contents of the uterus are withdrawn through a narrow tube. Also called *suction curettage, vacuum curettage*.

vag·a·bond's disease (văg′ə-bŏndz′) *n.* See **parasitic melanoderma**.

va·gal (vā′gəl) *adj.* Of or relating to the vagus nerve.

vagal attack *n.* A paroxysmal condition marked by slow pulse, a fall in blood pressure, and sometimes by convulsions, thought to be the result of sudden stimulation of the vagus nerve mediated through receptors located in the carotid sinus, the aortic arch, or the heart. Also called *vasovagal attack, vasovagal syncope*.

vagal trunk *n.* Either of two nerve bundles into which the esophageal plexus continues as it passes through the diaphragm.

vagin– *pref.* Variant of **vagino–**.

va·gi·na (və-jī′nə) *n., pl.* **-nas** *or* **-nae** (-nē) 1. The genital canal in the female, leading from the opening of the vulva to the cervix of the uterus. 2. A sheathlike anatomical structure.

vag·i·nal (văj′ə-nəl) *adj.* 1. Of or relating to the vagina. 2. Relating to or resembling a sheath.

vaginal artery *n.* An artery with origin in the internal iliac artery, with distribution to the vagina, the base of the bladder, and the rectum, and with anastomoses to the uterine and internal pudendal arteries.

vaginal atresia *n.* Imperforation or occlusion of the vagina. Also called *colpatresia*.

vaginal celiotomy *n.* An incision into the abdomen through the vagina.

vaginal gland *n.* Any of the mucous glands in the mucous membrane of the vagina.

vaginal hysterectomy *n.* The surgical removal of the uterus through the vagina without incising the wall of the abdomen.

vaginal hysterotomy *n.* Incision into the uterus via the vagina.

vag·i·na·li·tis (văj′ə-nə-lī′tĭs) *n.* Inflammation of the tunica vaginalis testis.

vaginal nerve *n.* Any of several nerves passing from the uterovaginal plexus to the vagina.

vaginal opening *n.* The narrowest portion of the vaginal canal, located in the floor of the vestibule, behind the urethral orifice.

vag·i·nate (văj′ə-nĭt, -nāt′) *or* **vag·i·nat·ed** (-nā′tĭd) *adj.* 1. Forming or enclosed in a sheath. 2. Resembling a sheath.

vag·i·nec·to·my (văj′ə-něk′tə-mē) *n.* **1.** Surgical removal of all or part of the vagina. Also called *colpectomy.* **2.** Surgical removal of the serous membrane covering the testis and epididymis.

vag·i·nis·mus (văj′ə-nĭz′məs) *n.* A usually prolonged and painful contraction or spasm of the vagina.

vag·i·ni·tis (văj′ə-nī′tĭs) *n.* Inflammation of the vagina. Also called *colpitis.*

vaginitis em·phy·se·ma·to·sa (ěm′fĭ-sē′mə-tō′sə, -zē′-) *n.* Vaginitis characterized by the accumulation of gas in small connective tissue spaces that are lined by foreign body giant cells.

vagino– *or* **vagin–** *pref.* Vagina; vaginal: *vaginitis.*

vag·i·no·cele (văj′ə-nō-sēl′) *n.* See **colpocele** (sense 1).

vag·i·no·dyn·i·a (văj′ə-nō-dĭn′ē-ə) *n.* Vaginal pain. Also called *colpalgia, colpodynia.*

vag·i·no·fix·a·tion (văj′ə-nō-fĭk-sā′shən) *n.* Suture of a relaxed and prolapsed vagina to the abdominal wall. Also called *colpopexy, vaginopexy.*

vag·i·no·my·co·sis (văj′ə-nō-mī-kō′sĭs) *n.* Inflammation of the vagina due to infection by a fungus.

vag·i·nop·a·thy (văj′ə-nŏp′ə-thē) *n.* Any disease that affects the vagina.

vag·i·no·per·i·ne·o·plas·ty (văj′ə-nō-pěr′ə-nē′ə-plăs′tē) *n.* Plastic surgery that is performed to repair an injury to the perineum and to the vagina. Also called *colpoperineoplasty.*

vag·i·no·per·i·ne·or·rha·phy (văj′ə-nō-pěr′ə-nē-ôr′ə-fē) *n.* Surgical repair of a lacerated vagina and perineum. Also called *colpoperineorrhaphy.*

vag·i·no·per·i·ne·ot·o·my (văj′ə-nō-pěr′ə-nē-ŏt′ə-mē) *n.* Surgical division of the outlet of the vagina and of the adjacent portion of the perineum to facilitate childbirth.

vag·i·no·pex·y (văj′ə-nə-pěk′sē) *n.* See **vaginofixation.**

vag·i·no·plas·ty (văj′ə-nə-plăs′tē) *n.* Plastic surgery of the vagina. Also called *colpoplasty.*

vag·i·nos·co·py (văj′ə-nŏs′kə-pē) *n.* Examination of the vagina, usually by means of an endoscope.

vag·i·no·sis (văj′ə-nō′sĭs) *n.* A disease of the vagina, especially one caused by bacteria of the genus *Gardnerella.*

vag·i·not·o·my (văj′ə-nŏt′ə-mē) *n.* Incision of the vagina. Also called *colpotomy.*

va·gi·tus u·ter·i·nus (və-jī′təs yōō′tə-rī′nəs) *n.* Crying of the fetus while still within the uterus, occurring at times when the membranes have been ruptured and air has entered the uterine cavity.

vago– *pref.* Vagus: *vagotonia.*

va·gol·y·sis (vā-gŏl′ĭ-sĭs) *n.* Surgical destruction of the vagus nerve.

va·go·lyt·ic (vā′gə-lĭt′ĭk) *adj.* Relating to or causing inhibition of the vagus nerve. —*n.* An agent that has inhibitory effects on the vagus nerve.

va·go·mi·met·ic (vā′gō-mĭ-mět′ĭk, mī-) *adj.* Mimicking action of efferent fibers of the vagus nerve.

va·got·o·my (vā-gŏt′ə-mē) *n.* Surgical division of fibers of the vagus nerve, used to diminish acid secretion of the stomach and control a duodenal ulcer.

va·go·to·ni·a (vā′gə-tō′nē-ə) *n.* Overactivity or irritability of the vagus nerve, adversely affecting function of the blood vessels, stomach, and muscles. Also called *sympathetic imbalance.* —**va′go·ton′ic** (-tŏn′ĭk) *adj.*

va·go·trop·ic (vā′gə-trŏp′ĭk, -trō′pĭk) *adj.* Affecting or acting on the vagus nerve. Used chiefly of a drug.

va·go·va·gal (vā′gō-vā′gəl) *adj.* Relating to a process that utilizes both afferent and efferent fibers of the vagus nerve.

va·grant's disease (vā′grənts) *n.* See **parasitic melanoderma.**

va·gus (vā′gəs) *n., pl.* **-gi** (-gī, -jī) The vagus nerve.

vagus nerve *n.* Either of the tenth pair cranial nerves that originate from the medulla oblongata and supply multiple vital organs, including the lungs, heart, and gastrointestinal viscera. Also called *pneumogastric nerve, tenth cranial nerve.*

vagus pulse *n.* A slow pulse due to the inhibitory action of the vagus nerve on the heart.

Val *abbr.* valine

val·a·cy·clo·vir hydrochloride (văl′ə-sī′klō-vîr′) *n.* A purine nucleoside analog that is derived from acyclovir and used in the treatment of herpes simplex and herpes zoster infections.

va·lence (vā′ləns) *or* **va·len·cy** (-lən-sē) *n.* **1.** The combining capacity of an atom or radical that is determined by the number of electrons that it will lose, add, or share when it reacts with other atoms. **2.** A positive or negative integer used to represent this capacity. **3.** The number of components of an antigen molecule to which an antibody molecule can bind. **4.** The attraction or aversion that an individual feels toward a specific object or event.

–valent *suff.* Having a specified valence or valences: *polyvalent.*

Val·en·tine's position (văl′ən-tīnz′) *n.* A supine position on a table with double inclined plane so as to cause flexion at the hips, used to facilitate urethral irrigation.

val·e·tu·di·nar·i·an (văl′ĭ-tōōd′n-âr′ē-ən) *n.* A sickly or weak person, especially one who is constantly and morbidly concerned with his or her health. —*adj.* **1.** Chronically ailing; sickly. **2.** Constantly and morbidly concerned with one's health.

val·e·tu·di·nar·y (văl′ĭ-tōōd′n-ěr′ē) *adj.* Of, relating to, or typical of a valetudinarian. —*n.* A valetudinarian.

val·gus (văl′gəs) *adj.* Characterized by an abnormal outward turning of a bone, especially of the hip, knee, or foot; occasionally used to indicate an inward turning. —*n.* A bone of the leg or foot characterized by such an abnormality.

val·ine (văl′ēn, vā′lēn′) *n. Abbr.* **Val** An essential amino acid that is a constituent of proteins, especially fibrous proteins.

Val·i·um (văl′ē-əm) A trademark for the drug diazepam.

val·late (văl′āt) *adj.* Surrounded with a wall or elevation; cupped.

vallate papilla *n.* Any of the eight or ten projections from the dorsum of the tongue that form a row in front of and parallel with the terminal sulcus. Also called *circumvallate papilla.*

val·lec·u·la (vă-lěk′yə-lə, və-) *n., pl.* **-lae** (-lē′) An anatomical crevice or depression on any surface, such as the deep hollow on the inferior surface of the cerebellum, between the hemispheres, in which the medulla oblongata rests.

Val·leix's point (vă-lāz′) *n.* Any of various points in the course of a nerve upon which pressure is painful in cases of neuralgia.

vall·ey fever (văl′ē) *n.* See **coccidioidomycosis.**

val·pro·ate (văl-prō′āt) *n.* The sodium salt of valproic acid used orally in the treatment of epilepsy.

val·pro·ic acid (văl-prō′ĭk) *n.* An anticonvulsive drug used to treat seizure disorders.

Val·sal·va (văl-săl′və, văl-säl′vä), **Antonio Maria** 1666–1723. Italian anatomist known for his detailed studies of the ear, his innovative surgical approach to aneurysms, and the use of the Valsalva maneuver. He was also an early advocate for the compassionate treatment of the mentally ill.

Val·sal·va maneuver (văl-săl′və) *n.* **1.** Expiratory effort against a closed glottis, which increases pressure within the thoracic cavity and thereby impedes venous return of blood to the heart. The maneuver results in changes in blood pressure and heart rate and is used in conjunction with other tests to diagnose cardiac abnormalities and to treat various conditions, especially some abnormal heart rhythms. **2.** Expiratory effort when the mouth is closed and the nostrils are pinched shut, which forces air into the eustachian tubes and increases pressure on the inside of the eardrum.

val·sar·tan (văl-sär′tn) *n.* An oral drug that is an angiotensin II receptor antagonist, used to treat hypertension.

Val·trex (văl′trĕks′) A trademark for the drug valacyclovir hydrochloride.

val·ue (văl′yōō) *n.* **1.** A principle, standard, or quality considered worthwhile or desirable. **2.** An assigned or calculated numerical quantity.

val·val (văl′vəl) *or* **val·var** (-vər) *adj.* Valvular.

val·vate (văl′vāt′) *adj.* Having valves or valvelike parts.

valve (vălv) *n.* **1.** A membranous structure in a hollow organ or passage, as in an artery or vein, that folds or closes to prevent the return flow of the body fluid passing through it. **2.** Any of various devices that regulate the flow of gases, liquids, or loose materials through piping or through apertures by opening, closing, or obstructing ports or passageways. **3.** The movable control element of such a device.

val·vo·plas·ty (văl′və-plăs′tē) *n.* See **valvuloplasty.**

val·vot·o·my (văl-vŏt′ə-mē) *n.* **1.** The surgical cutting of a constricted cardiac valve to relieve obstruction. Also called *valvulotomy.* **2.** An incision into a valvular structure.

val·vu·lar (văl′vyə-lər) *adj.* Relating to, having, or operating by means of valves or valvelike parts.

valvular endocarditis *n.* Endocarditis confined to the endocardium of the heart valves.

valvular insufficiency *n.* Failure of the cardiac valves to close perfectly, thus allowing regurgitation of blood past the closed valve.

val·vule (văl′vyōōl′) *or* **val·vu·la** (-vyə-lə) *n., pl.* **–vules** *or* **–vu·lae** (-vyə-lē′) A small anatomical valve or valvelike structure.

val·vu·li·tis (văl′vyə-lī′tĭs) *n.* Inflammation of a valve, especially a cardiac valve.

val·vu·lo·plas·ty (văl′vyə-lə-plăs′tē) *n.* Plastic surgery to repair a valve, especially a cardiac valve. Also called *valvoplasty.*

val·vu·lot·o·my (văl′vyə-lŏt′ə-mē) *n.* See **valvotomy** (sense 1).

va·na·di·um (və-nā′dē-əm) *n. Symbol* **V** A soft ductile metallic element, used in rust-resistant high-speed tools, as a carbon stabilizer in some steels, and as a catalyst. Atomic number 23.

Van Bu·chem's syndrome (văn bōō′kĕmz, văn) *n.* An inherited skeletal dysplasia characterized by enlargement of the lower jaw and thickening of the long bones and the top of the skull. Also called *generalized cortical hyperostosis.*

Van·ce·nase (văn′sə-nāz′) A trademark for the drug beclomethasone dipropionate.

Van·ce·ril (văn′sə-rĭl′) A trademark for the drug beclomethasone dipropionate.

Van·co·cin (văn′kō-sĭn) A trademark for the drug vancomycin.

van·co·my·cin (văng′kə-mī′sĭn, văn′kə-) *n.* An antibiotic that is produced by the actinomycete *Streptomyces orientalis* and is effective against staphylococci and spirochetes.

van der Waals force (văn′ dər wôlz′, wälz′) *n.* A weak attractive force between atoms or nonpolar molecules caused by an instantaneous dipole moment of one atom or molecule that induces a similar temporary dipole moment in adjacent atoms or molecules.

Vane (văn), **John Robert** 1927–2004. British pharmacologist. He shared a 1982 Nobel Prize for research on prostaglandins.

va·nil·la (və-nĭl′ə) *n.* **1.** Any of various tropical American vines of the genus *Vanilla,* especially *V. planifolia,* cultivated for its long narrow seedpods from which a flavoring agent is obtained. **2.** The seedpod of this plant. Also called *vanilla bean.* **3.** A flavoring extract prepared from the cured seedpods of this plant or produced synthetically. —*adj.* Flavored with vanilla.

va·nil·lin (və-nĭl′ĭn, văn′ə-lĭn) *n.* A white or yellowish crystalline compound found in vanilla beans and certain balsams and resins and used in flavorings and pharmaceuticals.

va·nil·lism (və-nĭl′ĭz′əm) *n.* **1.** Irritation of the skin, nasal mucous membrane, and conjunctiva, sometimes seen in people who work with vanilla. **2.** Infestation of the skin by sarcoptic mites found in vanilla pods.

van·il·lyl·man·del·ic acid (văn′ə-lĭl′măn-dĕl′ĭk, və-nĭl′əl-) *n.* The major urinary metabolite of adrenal and sympathetic catecholamines.

vanillylmandelic acid test *n.* A test for catecholamine-secreting tumors performed on a 24-hour urine specimen and based on the fact that vanillylmandelic acid is the major urinary metabolite of norepinephrine and epinephrine.

van·ish·ing lung syndrome (văn′ə-shĭng) *n.* A radiologic sign of progressive decrease of the radiologic density of the lung due to a variety of pathophysiologic conditions.

Van·tin (văn′tn) A trademark for the drug cefpodoxime proxetil.

va·por (vā′pər) *n.* **1.** Barely visible or cloudy diffused matter, such as mist, fumes, or smoke, suspended in the air. **2.** The state of a substance that exists below its critical temperature and that may be liquefied by application of sufficient pressure. **3.** The gaseous state of a substance that is liquid or solid under ordinary conditions. **4.** The vaporized form of a medicinal preparation to be administered by inhalation. **5.** A mixture of a vapor and air, as an explosive mixture of gasoline and air burned in an internal-combustion engine. **6. vapors** Exhalations within an organ, especially the stomach, supposed to affect the mental or physical condition. No longer in technical use. **7. vapors** A nervous disorder such as depression or hysteria. No longer in technical use.

va·por·es·cence (vā′pə-rĕs′əns) *n.* The formation of vapor.

va·por·i·za·tion (vā′pə-rĭ-zā′shən) *n.* **1.** The conversion of a solid or liquid into a vapor. **2.** Therapeutic application of a vapor.

va·por·ize (vā′pə-rīz′) *v.* To convert or be converted into a vapor.

va·por·iz·er (vā′pə-rī′zər) *n.* A device used to vaporize medicine for inhaling.

Va·quez disease (vă-kā′, vä-) *n.* See **erythremia.**

var·den·a·fil hydrochloride (vär-dĕn′ə-fĭl) *n.* A phosphodiesterase inhibitor drug used to treat erectile dysfunction by increasing the level of cyclic GMP, which increases blood flow to the erectile tissues.

var·i·a·ble (vâr′ē-ə-bəl, vâr′-) *adj.* **1.** Likely to change or vary; subject to variation; changeable. **2.** Tending to deviate, as from a normal or recognized type; aberrant. **3.** Having no fixed quantitative value. —*n.* **1.** Something that varies or that is prone to variation. **2.** A quantity that is capable of assuming any of a set of values.

variable region *n.* The portion of the amino terminal of an immunoglobulin's heavy and light chains having a variable amino acid sequence.

var·i·ance (vâr′ē-əns, vâr′-) *n.* **1.** The state or quality of being variant or variable; a variation. **2.** The state or fact of differing or of being in conflict. **3.** The square of the standard deviation.

var·i·ant (vâr′ē-ənt, vâr′-) *adj.* **1.** Having or exhibiting variation; differing. **2.** Tending or liable to vary; variable. **3.** Deviating from a standard, usually by only a slight difference. —*n.* Something that differs in form only slightly from something else.

var·i·a·tion (vâr′ē-ā′shən, vâr′-) *n.* **1.** The act, process, or result of varying. **2.** The state or fact of being varied. **3.** The extent or degree to which something varies. **4.** Something that is slightly different from another of the same type. **5.** Marked difference or deviation from the normal or recognized form, function, or structure. **6.** An organism exhibiting such difference or deviation. **7.** A function that relates the values of one variable to those of other variables.

var·i·ca·tion (văr′ĭ-kā′shən) *n.* The formation or presence of varices.

var·i·ce·al (văr′ĭ-sē′əl) *adj.* Of, relating to, or caused by a varix or varices.

var·i·cel·la (văr′ĭ-sĕl′ə) *n.* See **chickenpox.**

varicella encephalitis *n.* Encephalitis occurring as a complication of chickenpox.

varicella-zoster virus *n.* A herpesvirus that causes chickenpox and shingles. Also called *chickenpox virus, herpes zoster virus.*

var·i·cel·li·form (văr′ĭ-sĕl′ə-fôrm′) *adj.* Resembling chickenpox.

var·i·ci·form (văr′ĭ-sə-fôrm′, və-rĭs′ə-) *adj.* Resembling a varix.

varico– *or* **varic–** *pref.* Varix; varicose: *varicocele.*

var·i·co·bleph·a·ron (văr′ĭ-kō-blĕf′ə-rŏn′) *n.* A varicosity of the eyelid.

var·i·co·cele (văr′ĭ-kō-sēl′) *n.* A varicose condition of veins of the spermatic cord or the ovaries, forming a soft tumor.

var·i·co·ce·lec·to·my (văr′ĭ-kō-sə-lĕk′tə-mē) *n.* Surgery for the relief of a varicocele by ligature and excision and by ligation of the dilated veins.

var·i·cog·ra·phy (văr′ĭ-kŏg′rə-fē) *n.* Radiography of varicose veins following injection of a radiopaque contrast medium.

var·i·coid (văr′ĭ-koid′) *adj.* Resembling a dilated vein; variciform.

var·i·com·pha·lus (văr′ĭ-kŏm′fə-ləs) *n.* A swelling formed by varicose veins at the umbilicus.

var·i·co·phle·bi·tis (văr′ĭ-kō-flĭ-bī′tĭs) *n.* Inflammation of varicose veins.

var·i·cose (văr′ĭ-kōs′) *adj.* Relating to, affected with, or characterized by varices or varicosis.

varicose aneurysm *n.* A blood-containing sac communicating with both an artery and a vein.

varicose ulcer *n.* Loss of skin surface in the drainage area of a varicose vein, usually in the leg, resulting from stasis and infection.

varicose vein *n.* **1.** An abnormally dilated or swollen vein. **2. varicose veins** The condition of having abnormally dilated or swollen veins, especially in the legs.

var·i·co·sis (văr′ĭ-kō′sĭs) *n., pl.* **–ses** (-sēz) **1.** The condition of being varicose. **2.** Formation of varices.

var·i·cos·i·ty (văr′ĭ-kŏs′ĭ-tē) *n.* **1.** Varicosis. **2.** A varicose enlargement or swelling.

var·i·cot·o·my (văr′ĭ-kŏt′ə-mē) *n.* Surgical removal of varicose veins.

va·ric·u·la (və-rĭk′yə-lə) *n., pl.* **–lae** (-lē) A varicose condition of veins of the conjunctiva. Also called *conjunctival varix.*

var·i·cule (văr′ĭ-kyōōl′) *n.* A small varicose vein ordinarily seen in the skin.

var·i·e·gate porphyria (vâr′ē-ĭ-gāt′) *n.* A hereditary disorder characterized by abdominal pain, neuropsychiatric abnormalities, dermal sensitivity to light and mechanical trauma, and increased fecal excretion of protoporphyrin and coproporphyrin.

var·i·o·la (və-rī′ə-lə, vâr′ē-ō′lə) *n.* See **smallpox.** —**va·ri′o·lar** (-lər), **va·ri′o·lous** (-ləs) *adj.*

var·i·o·late (vâr′ē-ə-lāt′) *adj.* Having pustules or pitted scars like those of smallpox. —*v.* To inoculate with smallpox virus.

variola virus *n.* A virus of the genus *Orthopoxvirus* that causes smallpox. Also called *smallpox virus.*

va·ri·o·li·form (və-rī′ə-lə-fôrm′, vâr′ē-ō′lə-) *adj.* Resembling smallpox.

var·i·o·loid (vâr′ē-ə-loid′, văr′-, və-rī′ə-loid′) *adj.* Varioliform. —*n.* A mild form of smallpox occurring in people who have been previously vaccinated or who have had the disease.

va·ri·o·lous (və-rī'ə-ləs, vâr'ē-ōl'-) *adj.* Of, relating to, or affected with smallpox.

var·ix (văr'ĭks) *n., pl.* **–i·ces** (-ĭ-sēz') An abnormally dilated or swollen vein, artery, or lymph vessel.

Var·mus (vär'məs), **Harold Eliot** Born 1939. American microbiologist. He shared a 1989 Nobel Prize for discovering a sequence of genes that can cause cancer when mutated.

var·us (vâr'əs) *adj.* Characterized by an abnormal inward turning of a bone, especially of the hip, knee, or foot; occasionally used to indicate an outward turning. —*n.* A bone of the leg or foot characterized by such an abnormality.

var·y (vâr'ē) *v.* **1.** To make or cause changes in the characteristics or attributes of; modify or alter. **2.** To undergo or show change. **3.** To be different; deviate.

vas (văs) *n., pl.* **va·sa** (vā'zə) An anatomical duct or canal conveying any liquid, such as blood, lymph, chyle, or semen.

vas– *pref.* Variant of **vaso–**.

vasa brev·i·a (brĕv'ē-ə) *pl.n.* The gastric arteries considered as a group.

va·sal (vā'səl, -zəl) *adj.* Of, relating to, or connected with a vessel or duct of the body.

vasa pre·vi·a (prē'vē-ə) *n.* The presentation of the umbilical blood vessels in advance of the fetal head during labor.

vasa rec·ta (rĕk'tə) *pl.n.* **1.** See **arteriolae rectae. 2.** The collecting tubules of the kidney.

vasa va·so·rum (vā-sôr'əm, -zôr'-) *pl.n.* Small arteries that are distributed to the outer and middle coats of the larger blood vessels and to their corresponding veins.

vas·cu·lar (văs'kyə-lər) *adj.* Of, relating to, or containing blood vessels.

vascular cataract *n.* A congenital cataract in which degenerated lens is replaced with mesodermic tissue.

vascular compartment *n.* The medial compartment located beneath the inguinal ligament for the passage to the femoral vessels and separated from the muscular lacuna by the iliopectineal arch.

vascular dementia *n.* A steplike deterioration in intellectual functions that result from multiple infarctions of the cerebral hemispheres. Also called *multi-infarct dementia.*

vascular hemophilia *n.* See **von Willebrand's disease.**

vas·cu·lar·i·ty (văs'kyə-lăr'ĭ-tē) *n.* The condition of being vascular.

vas·cu·lar·i·za·tion (văs'kyə-lər-ĭ-zā'shən) *n.* **1.** The formation of blood vessels. **2.** An abnormal or pathological formation of blood vessels.

vas·cu·lar·ize (văs'kyə-lə-rīz') *v.* To make or become vascular.

vas·cu·lar·ized graft (văs'kyə-lə-rīzd') *n.* A graft after the recipient vasculature has been connected with the vessels in the graft.

vascular keratitis *n.* Keratitis characterized by superficial cellular infiltration of the cornea and the formation of blood vessels between the limiting layer of the cornea and the epithelium.

vascular layer *n.* The outer portion of the choroid of the eye, containing the largest blood vessels. Also called *vascular layer of choroid.*

vascular leiomyoma *n.* A leiomyoma apparently arising from the smooth muscle of blood vessels. Also called *angioleiomyoma, angiomyoma.*

vascular nerve *n.* A small nerve filament that supplies the wall of a blood vessel.

vascular polyp *n.* A bulging or protruding angioma of the nasal mucous membrane.

vascular ring *n.* Anomalous arteries congenitally encircling the trachea and the esophagus that may produce pressure symptoms.

vascular spider *n.* See **arterial spider.**

vascular system *n.* See **circulatory system.**

vascular zone *n.* An area in the external auditory canal of the ear where a number of minute blood vessels enter from the mastoid bone.

vas·cu·la·ture (văs'kyə-lə-chŏŏr') *n.* Arrangement of blood vessels in the body or in an organ or body part.

vas·cu·li·tis (văs'kyə-lī'tĭs) *n.* Inflammation of a blood or lymph vessel. Also called *angiitis.*

vasculo– *pref.* Blood vessel: *vasculopathy.*

vas·cu·lo·my·e·li·nop·a·thy (văs'kyə-lō-mī'ə-lə-nŏp'-ə-thē) *n.* Vasculopathy of the small cerebral vessels followed by perivascular demyelination.

vas·cu·lop·a·thy (văs'kyə-lŏp'ə-thē) *n.* Disease of the blood vessels.

vas def·er·ens (văs' dĕf'ər-ənz, -ə-rĕnz') *n., pl.* **vasa def·er·en·ti·a** (dĕf'ə-rĕn'shē-ə) The main secretory duct of the testicle, through which semen is carried from the epididymis to the prostatic urethra, where it ends as the ejaculatory duct. Also called *deferent duct, spermatic duct, spermiduct.*

va·sec·to·mize (və-sĕk'tə-mīz') *v.* To perform a vasectomy on.

va·sec·to·my (və-sĕk'tə-mē) *n.* Surgical removal of all or part of the vas deferens, usually as a means of sterilization. Also called *deferentectomy, gonangiectomy.*

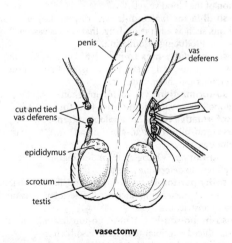

penis

vas deferens

cut and tied vas deferens

epididymus

scrotum

testis

vasectomy

vas ef·fer·ens (văs' ĕf'ər-ənz, -ə-rĕnz') *n., pl.* **vasa ef·fer·en·ti·a** (ĕf'ə-rĕn'shē-ə) Any of a number of small ducts that carry semen from the testis to the epididymis.

Vas·e·line (văs'ə-lēn', văs'ə-lēn') A trademark for a brand of petroleum jelly.

vas·i·fac·tion (văs′ə-făk′shən) *n.* See **angiopoiesis.** —**vas′i·fac′tive** *adj.*

vas·i·form (văs′ə-fôrm′) *adj.* Shaped like a vas or tubular structure.

vas·i·tis (və-sī′tĭs, vă-) *n.* See **deferentitis.**

vaso– *or* **vas–** *pref.* **1.** Blood vessel: *vasoconstriction.* **2.** Vas deferens: *vasectomy.* **3.** Vessel: *vasiform.*

va·so·ac·tive (vā′zō-ăk′tĭv) *adj.* Causing constriction or dilation of blood vessels.

vasoactive amine *n.* A substance containing amino groups, such as histamine or serotonin, that acts on the blood vessels to alter their permeability or to cause vasodilation.

vasoactive intestinal polypeptide *n. Abbr.* **VIP** A polypeptide hormone usually secreted by non-beta islet cell tumors of the pancreas, producing copious watery diarrhea and fecal electrolyte loss, resulting in hypokalemia.

va·so·con·stric·tion (vā′zō-kən-strĭk′shən) *n.* Constriction of a blood vessel, as by a nerve or drug.

va·so·con·stric·tive (vā′zō-kən-strĭk′tĭv) *adj.* Causing constriction of the blood vessels.

va·so·con·stric·tor (vā′zō-kən-strĭk′tər) *n.* Something, such as a nerve or drug, that causes vasoconstriction. —*adj.* Producing vasoconstriction.

va·so·de·pres·sion (vā′zō-dĭ-prĕsh′ən) *n.* Reduction of tone in blood vessels with vasodilation and resulting in lowered blood pressure.

va·so·de·pres·sor (vā′zō-dĭ-prĕs′ər) *n.* An agent that lowers blood pressure through reduction in peripheral resistance. —*adj.* Producing vasodepression.

va·so·di·la·tion (vā′zō-dī-lā′shən, -dĭ-) *or* **va·so·dil·a·ta·tion** (-dĭl′ə-tā′shən, -dī′lə-) *n.* Dilation of a blood vessel, as by the action of a nerve or drug. Also called *phlebarteriectasia.*

va·so·di·la·tive (vā′zō-dī-lā′tĭv, -dĭ-) *adj.* Causing dilation of the blood vessels.

va·so·di·la·tor (vā′zō-dī-lā′tər, -dĭ-, -dī′lā-) *n.* Something, such as a nerve or drug, that causes vasodilation. —*adj.* Producing vasodilation.

va·so·ep·i·did·y·mos·to·my (vā′zō-ĕp′ĭ-dĭd′ə-mŏs′tə-mē) *n.* Surgical creation of a passage between the vas deferens and the epididymis.

va·so·for·ma·tion (vā′zō-fôr-mā′shən) *n.* See **angiopoiesis.** —**va′so·form′a·tive** (-fôr′mə-tĭv) *adj.*

vasoformative cell *n.* See **angioblast** (sense 2).

va·so·gan·gli·on (vā′zō-găng′glē-ən) *n.* A mass of blood vessels.

va·sog·ra·phy (vă-zŏg′rə-fē) *n.* Radiography of the vas deferens to determine patency.

va·so·hy·per·ton·ic (vā′zō-hī′pər-tŏn′ĭk) *adj.* Relating to or characterizing increased arteriolar tension or vasoconstriction.

va·so·hy·po·ton·ic (vā′zō-hī′pō-tŏn′ĭk) *adj.* Relating to reduced arteriolar tension or vasodilation.

va·so·in·hib·i·tor (vā′zō-ĭn-hĭb′ĭ-tər) *n.* An agent that restricts or prevents the functioning of the vasomotor nerves.

va·so·in·hib·i·to·ry (vā′zō-ĭn-hĭb′ĭ-tôr′ē) *adj.* Inhibiting the action of the vasomotor nerves.

va·so·li·ga·tion (vā′zō-lī-gā′shən) *n.* Surgical ligation of the vas deferens as a means of sterilization. —**va′so·li′gate** (-lī′gāt) *v.*

va·so·mo·tion (vā′zō-mō′shən) *n.* Change in the caliber of a blood vessel. Also called *angiokinesis.*

va·so·mo·tor (vā′zō-mō′tər) *adj.* Causing or regulating dilation or constriction of the blood vessels. Also called *angiokinetic.*

vasomotor angina *n.* Angina pectoris that is caused by a vasomotor disorder and that is marked by chest pain that is comparatively light. Also called *angina pectoris vasomotoria.*

vasomotor imbalance *n.* See **autonomic imbalance.**

vasomotor nerve *n.* A motor nerve effecting dilation, such as a vasodilator nerve, or contraction, such as a vasoconstrictor nerve, of the blood vessels.

vasomotor paralysis *n.* See **vasoparesis.**

vasomotor rhinitis *n.* Congestion of nasal mucosa without infection or allergy.

va·so·neu·rop·a·thy (vā′zō-nŏŏ-rŏp′ə-thē) *n.* A disease involving the nerves and the blood vessels.

va·so·or·chi·dos·to·my (vā′zō-ôr′kĭ-dŏs′tə-mē) *n.* The surgical reestablishment of blocked seminiferous channels by uniting tubules of the epididymis or the rete testis to the divided end of the vas deferens.

va·so·pa·ral·y·sis (vā′zō-pə-răl′ĭ-sĭs) *n.* Paralysis or lack of constricting ability in blood vessels. Also called *angioparalysis.*

va·so·pa·re·sis (vā′zō-pə-rē′sĭs, -păr′ĭ-sĭs) *n.* A mild degree of vasoparalysis. Also called *angioparesis, vasomotor paralysis.*

va·so·pres·sin (vā′zō-prĕs′ĭn) *n. Abbr.* **VP** A hormone, related to oxytocin, that is secreted by the posterior lobe of the pituitary gland, constricts blood vessels, raises blood pressure, stimulates intestinal motility, and reduces the excretion of urine. Also called *antidiuretic hormone.*

va·so·pres·sor (vā′zō-prĕs′ər) *adj.* Producing constriction of the blood vessels and a consequent rise in blood pressure. —*n.* An agent that causes a rise in blood pressure.

va·so·punc·ture (vā′zō-pŭngk′chər) *n.* The puncture of a blood vessel with a needle.

va·so·re·flex (vā′zō-rē′flĕks′) *n.* A reflex that increases or decreases the caliber of blood vessels.

va·so·re·lax·a·tion (vā′zō-rē′lăk-sā′shən) *n.* Reduction in tension of the blood vessel walls.

va·so·sec·tion (vā′zō-sĕk′shən) *n.* See **vasotomy.**

va·so·sen·so·ry (vā′zō-sĕn′sə-rē) *adj.* **1.** Relating to sensation in the blood vessels. **2.** Of or relating to sensory nerve fibers that innervate blood vessels.

va·so·spasm (vā′zō-spăz′əm) *n.* A sudden constriction of a blood vessel that reduces the blood flow. Also called *angiospasm.* —**va′so·spas′tic** (-spăs′tĭk) *adj.*

va·so·stim·u·lant (vā′zō-stĭm′yə-lənt) *adj.* Exciting vasomotor action. —*n.* **1.** An agent that excites the vasomotor nerves to action. **2.** An agent that increases vascular tension.

va·sos·to·my (vă-zŏs′tə-mē) *n.* Surgical creation of an opening into the vas deferens.

Vas·o·tec (văz′ō-tĕk′) A trademark for the drug enalapril maleate.

va·sot·o·my (vă-zŏt′ə-mē) *n.* Incision into or division of the vas deferens. Also called *vasosection.*

va·so·to·ni·a (vā′zō-tō′nē-ə) *n.* The tone of blood vessels, particularly of the arterioles. Also called *angiotonia.* —**va′so·ton′ic** (-tŏn′ĭk) *adj.*

va·so·trip·sy (vā′zə-trĭp′sē) *n.* See **angiotripsy.**

va·so·troph·ic (vā′zə-trŏf′ĭk, -trō′fĭk) *adj.* Relating to the nutrition of the blood vessels or lymphatics.

va·so·trop·ic (vā′zə-trŏp′ĭk, -trō′pĭk) *adj.* Tending to act on the blood vessels.

va·so·va·gal (vā′zō-vā′gəl) *adj.* Relating to or involving blood vessels and the vagus nerve.

vasovagal attack *n.* See **vagal attack.**

vasovagal syncope *n.* See **vagal attack.**

va·so·va·sos·to·my (vā′zō-vā-zŏs′tə-mē) *n.* The surgical creation of a passage connecting the ends of a severed vas deferens, usually to restore fertility in a vasectomized man.

va·so·ve·sic·u·lec·to·my (vā′zō-vě-sĭk′yə-lěk′tə-mē) *n.* The excision of the vas deferens and seminal vesicles.

vas·tus lat·e·ra·lis (văs′təs lăt′ə-rā′lĭs, -răl′ĭs) *n.* A muscle with origin from the posterior ridge of the femur as far as the greater trochanter, with insertion into the tibia, with nerve supply from the femoral nerve, and whose action extends the leg.

vastus me·di·a·lis (mē′dē-ā′lĭs, -ăl′ĭs) *n.* A muscle with origin from the shaft of the femur, with insertion into the tibial tuberosity, with nerve supply from the femoral nerve, and whose action extends the leg.

VATER *abbr.* vertebral defects, anal atresia, tracheoesophageal fistula with esophageal atresia, renal defects, and radial dysplasia (symptom complex associated with Fanconi's anemia)

Va·ter's ampulla (fä′tərz) *n.* The dilation within the major duodenal papilla, formed by the junction of the common bile duct and the main pancreatic duct.

VBAC *abbr.* vaginal birth after cesarean

VC *abbr.* vital capacity

VD *abbr.* venereal disease

VDRL (vē′dē-är-ĕl′) *n.* A flocculation test for syphilis, using cardiolipin-lecithin-cholesterol antigen as developed by the Venereal Disease Research Laboratory, a former federal facility.

vec·tion (věk′shən) *n.* The transference of pathogens from the sick to the healthy by a vector.

vec·tor (věk′tər) *n.* **1.** An organism, such as a mosquito or tick, that carries disease-causing microorganisms from one host to another. **2.** A bacteriophage, a plasmid, or another agent that transfers genetic material from one location to another. **3.** A quantity, such as velocity, specified by a magnitude and a direction.

vec·tor·car·di·o·gram (věk′tər-kär′dē-ə-grăm′) *n.* A graphic representation of the magnitude and direction of the electrical currents of the heart's action in the form of a vector loop.

vec·tor·car·di·og·ra·phy (věk′tər-kär′dē-ŏg′rə-fē) *n.* **1.** Electrocardiography in which the heart's activation currents are represented by vector loops. **2.** The study and interpretation of vectorcardiograms.

vec·to·ri·al (věk-tôr′ē-əl) *adj.* Of, relating to, or characterized by a vector.

ve·gan (vē′gən, věj′ən) *n.* A vegetarian who eats plant products only, especially one who uses no products derived from animals, as fur or leather.

veg·e·ta·ble (věj′tə-bəl, věj′ĭ-tə-) *n.* **1.** A plant cultivated for an edible part, such as the root of the beet, the leaf of spinach, or the flower buds of broccoli or cauliflower. **2.** The edible part of such a plant. —*adj.* Of, relating to, or derived from plants or a plant.

veg·e·tal (věj′ĭ-tl) *adj.* **1.** Of, relating to, or characteristic of plants. **2.** Relating to growth rather than to sexual reproduction; vegetative.

vegetal pole *n.* The part of a telolecithal egg in which the bulk of the yolk is situated. Also called *vitelline pole.*

veg·e·tar·i·an (věj′ĭ-târ′ē-ən) *n.* One who practices vegetarianism. —*adj.* **1.** Of or relating to vegetarianism or vegetarians. **2.** Consisting primarily or wholly of vegetables and vegetable products.

veg·e·tar·i·an·ism (věj′ĭ-târ′ē-ə-nĭz′əm) *n.* The practice of subsisting on a diet composed primarily or wholly of vegetables, grains, fruits, nuts, and seeds, with or without eggs and dairy products.

veg·e·ta·tion (věj′ĭ-tā′shən) *n.* **1.** The process of growth in plants. **2.** An abnormal bodily growth or excrescence, especially a clot composed largely of fused blood platelets, fibrin, and sometimes bacteria that is adherent to a diseased heart valve. **3.** A vegetative state of impaired consciousness.

veg·e·ta·tive (věj′ĭ-tā′tĭv) *adj.* **1.** Of, relating to, or capable of growth. **2.** Of or functioning in processes such as growth or nutrition rather than sexual reproduction. **3.** Of or relating to asexual reproduction, such as fission or budding. **4.** Of or relating to the resting stage of a cell or its nucleus. **5.** Of or relating to a pathological vegetation. **6.** Of or being a state of grossly impaired consciousness, as after severe head trauma or brain disease, in which an individual is incapable of voluntary or purposeful acts and only responds reflexively to painful stimuli.

vegetative bacteriophage *n.* A stage in bacteriophage synthesis in which its nucleic acid multiplies within the host bacterium independent of the bacterial multiplication process.

vegetative endocarditis *n.* Endocarditis that is associated with the presence of fibrinous clots forming on the ulcerated surfaces of the valves. Also called *verrucous endocarditis.*

ve·hi·cle (vē′ĭ-kəl) *n.* A substance of no therapeutic value that is used to convey an active medicine for administration.

veil (vāl) *n.* **1.** See **caul. 2.** See **velum** (sense 1).

Veil·lo·nel·la (vā′yə-nĕl′ə) *n.* A genus of gram-negative bacteria that are parasitic in the mouth and in the intestinal and respiratory tracts.

vein (vān) *n.* Any of the branching blood vessels carrying blood toward the heart. All veins except the pulmonary vein carry dark unaerated blood. —*v.* To supply or fill with veins. —**vein′al** *adj.*

vein of bulb of penis *n.* A tributary of the internal pudendal vein that drains the bulb of the penis.

vein of cochlear canal *n.* A vein that drains the cochlea and the sacculus and empties into the superior bulb of the jugular vein, accompanying the cochlear aqueduct through the canal.

vein of eyelid *n.* Either of the tributaries of the superior ophthalmic vein that drain the superior eyelid, designated inferior or superior.

vein of kidney *n.* Any of the tributaries of the renal veins that parallel the arteries and that drain the kidney.

vein of knee *n.* Genicular vein.

vein of pterygoid canal *n.* A vein that accompanies the pterygoid nerve and artery through the pterygoid canal and empties into the pharyngeal vein.

vein of vestibular aqueduct *n.* A vein that accompanies the endolymphatic duct and terminates in the inferior petrosal sinus.

vein of vestibular bulb *n.* A tributary of the internal pudendal vein that drains the bulb of the vestibule.

veins of vertebral column *pl.n.* The veins of the internal and external vertebral venous plexuses, the basivertebral veins, and the anterior and posterior spinal veins.

ve·la·men (və-lā′mən) *n.,* *pl.* **–lam·i·na** (-lăm′ə-nə) See **velum** (sense 1).

vel·a·men·tous (vĕl′ə-mĕn′təs) *adj.* Resembling a veil in shape and composition.

ve·lar (vē′lər) *adj.* **1.** Of or relating to a velum. **2.** Concerning or using the soft palate.

Vel·ban (vĕl′băn′) A trademark for the drug vinblastine sulfate.

vel·lus (vĕl′əs) *n.* The fine hair present on the body before puberty.

ve·loc·i·ty (və-lŏs′ĭ-tē) *n.* Rapidity or speed of motion; specifically, the distance traveled per unit time.

ve·lo·pha·ryn·geal (vē′lō-fə-rĭn′jəl, -făr′ĭn-jē′əl) *adj.* Of or relating to the soft palate and the posterior nasopharyngeal wall.

velopharyngeal insufficiency *n.* An anatomical deficiency in the soft palate or superior constrictor muscle resulting in the inability to achieve velopharyngeal closure and often resulting in defective speech.

Vel·peau bandage (vĕl-pō′) *n.* A bandage used to support and immobilize an arm, with the forearm positioned obliquely across and upward on the front of the chest.

ve·lum (vē′ləm) *n.,* *pl.* **–la** (-lə) **1.** An anatomical structure resembling a veil or curtain. Also called *veil, velamen.* **2.** See **greater omentum. 3.** A serous membrane or membranous envelope or covering.

ve·na (vē′nə) *n.,* *pl.* **–nae** (-nē) A vein.

vena ca·va (kā′və) *n.,* *pl.* **venae ca·vae** (kā′vē) Either of the two venae cavae, designated inferior and superior. Also called *cava.*

ve·na·ca·vog·ra·phy (vē′nə-kā-vŏg′rə-fē) *n.* Angiography of a vena cava.

venae cav·er·no·sae pe·nis (kăv′ər-nō′sē pē′nĭs) *pl.n.* The cavernous venous spaces in the erectile tissue of the penis.

venae rec·tae (rĕk′tē) *n.* The ascending limbs of the arteriolae rectae in the renal medulla.

vene– *pref.* Variant of **veno–.**

ve·nec·ta·sia (vē′nĕk-tā′zhə) *n.* See **phlebectasia.**

ve·nec·to·my (vē-nĕk′tə-mē) *n.* See **phlebectomy.**

ve·neer (və-nîr′) *n.* A layer of tooth-colored material, usually porcelain or acrylic resin, attached to and covering the surface of a metal crown or natural tooth structure.

ven·e·na·tion (vĕn′ə-nā′shən) *n.* **1.** Introduction of a venom into animal tissue. **2.** The poisoned condition produced by a venom.

ve·nene (və-nēn′, vĕn′ēn) *n.* A preparation of snake venoms used in the treatment of epilepsy.

ven·e·nous (vĕn′ə-nəs) *adj.* Venomous; poisonous.

ve·ne·re·al (və-nîr′ē-əl) *adj.* **1.** Transmitted by sexual intercourse. **2.** Of or relating to a sexually transmitted disease. **3.** Of or relating to sexual intercourse. **4.** Of or relating to the genitals.

venereal bubo *n.* An enlarged gland in the groin associated with a venereal disease, especially chancroid.

venereal disease *n. Abbr.* **VD** Any of several contagious diseases, such as syphilis and gonorrhea, contracted through sexual intercourse; a sexually transmitted disease.

venereal lymphogranuloma *n.* A venereal infection usually caused by *Chlamydia* and characterized by a transient genital ulcer and inguinal adenopathy in the male; in the female, perirectal nodes are involved, and rectal stricture is a common occurrence. Also called *climatic bubo, Nicolas-Favre disease, sixth venereal disease, tropical bubo.*

venereal ulcer *n.* See **chancroid.**

venereal wart *n.* See **genital wart.**

ve·ne·re·ol·o·gy (və-nîr′ē-ŏl′ə-jē) *n.* The study of sexually transmitted diseases.

ven·e·sec·tion (vĕn′ĭ-sĕk′shən, vē′nĭ-) *n.* See **phlebotomy.**

ve·ni·punc·ture or **ve·ne·punc·ture** (vē′nĭ-pŭngk′chər, vĕn′ĭ-) *n.* Puncture of a vein, as for drawing blood, intravenous feeding, or the administration of medicine.

ven·la·fax·ine hydrochloride (vĕn′lə-făk′sēn, -sĭn) *n.* An oral antidepressant that inhibits neuronal reuptake of serotonin, norepinephrine, and dopamine in the central nervous system.

veno– or **veni–** or **vene–** *pref.* Vein; venous: *venipuncture.*

ve·no·gram (vē′nə-grăm′) *n.* **1.** A radiograph of a vein after injection of a radiopaque substance. **2.** See **phlebogram.**

ve·nog·ra·phy (vĭ-nŏg′rə-fē) *n.* **1.** Radiography of veins or a vein after injection of a radiopaque substance. **2.** See **phlebography.**

ven·om (vĕn′əm) *n.* **1.** A poisonous secretion of an animal, such as a snake, spider, or scorpion, usually transmitted by a bite or sting. **2.** A poison.

ve·no·mo·tor (vē′nō-mō′tər) *adj.* Relating to or causing change in the caliber of a vein.

ve·no·oc·clu·sive disease (vē′nō-ə-klōō′sĭv) *n.* An inflammatory condition, especially of the liver, characterized by the occlusion and destruction of tiny veins.

veno-occlusive disease of liver *n.* A disease of the liver characterized by the inflammation and destruction of minute hepatic veins, usually caused by drinking tea made from plants containing toxic substances.

ve·no·per·i·to·ne·os·to·my (vē′nō-pĕr′ĭ-tn-ē-ŏs′tə-mē) *n.* Surgical insertion of the saphenous vein into the peritoneal cavity to drain ascitic fluid.

ve·no·scle·ro·sis (vē′nō-sklə-rō′sĭs) *n.* See **phleboscle-rosis.**

ve·nose (vē′nōs′) *adj.* **1.** Having noticeable veins or veinlike markings. **2.** Venous.

ve·nos·i·ty (vē-nŏs′ĭ-tē) *n.* **1.** The quality or condition of being venous or venose. **2.** An excess of venous blood.

ve·nos·ta·sis (vē-nŏs′tə-sĭs, vē′nō-stā′sĭs) *n.* See **phle-bostasis** (sense 2).

ve·nos·to·my (vē-nŏs′tə-mē) *n.* See **cutdown.**

ve·not·o·my (vē-nŏt′ə-mē) *n.* See **phlebotomy.**

ve·nous (vē′nəs) *adj.* Of, relating to, or contained in the veins.

venous angle *n.* The angle formed by the junction of the internal jugular and subclavian veins.

venous blood *n. Abbr.* **v** Blood that has passed through the capillaries of various tissues other than the lungs, is found in the veins, in the right chambers of the heart, and in pulmonary arteries, and is usually dark red as a result of a lower content of oxygen.

venous capillary *n.* A blood capillary opening into a venule.

venous hum *n.* A humming sound, usually continuous, heard during auscultation of the veins at the base of the neck, especially in anemia.

venous hyperemia *n.* See **passive hyperemia.**

venous insufficiency *n.* Inadequate drainage of venous blood from a part, resulting in edema or dermatosis.

venous pulse *n.* The pulsation occurring in the veins, especially in the internal jugular vein.

venous return *n.* The blood returning to the heart via the inferior and superior venae cavae.

venous sinus *n.* A cavity at the caudal end of the em-bryonic cardiac tube in which veins from the intra- and extraembryonic circulatory arcs unite. In adults it de-velops into the sinuses of the venae cavae.

venous sinus of sclera *n.* A vascular structure near the anterior edge of the sclera and encircling the cornea. Also called *circular sinus, Schlemm's canal.*

venous sphygmograph *n.* See **phlebograph.**

venous star *n.* A small red nodule formed by a dilated vein in the skin. It is caused by increased venous pres-sure.

ve·no·ve·nos·to·my (vē′nō-vē-nŏs′tə-mē) *n.* The sur-gical formation of an anastomosis between two veins. Also called *phlebophlebostomy.*

vent (vĕnt) *n.* An opening into a cavity or canal, espe-cially one through which contents are discharged.

ven·ter (vĕn′tər) *n.* **1.** See **abdomen. 2.** See **belly** (sense 4). **3.** One of the large cavities of the body. **4.** A cav-ity or hollowed surface, especially of a bone. **5.** The uterus.

ven·ti·la·tion (vĕn′tl-ā′shən) *n.* **1.** The replacement of fresh air or gas for stale or noxious air or gas in a space. **2.** See **respiration** (sense 1). **3.** Aeration or oxygenation, as of blood. **4.** The verbal expression of feelings or emotions in psychotherapy. —**ven′ti·late′** *v.*

ventilation-perfusion scan *n.* A diagnostic test for pul-monary embolism in which an x-ray of the lung records the distribution and perfusion of a radionuclide that is inhaled and a second radionuclide that is administered intravenously. Also called *V/Q scan.*

ven·ti·la·tor (vĕn′tl-ā′tər) *n.* See **respirator** (sense 1).

Ven·to·lin (vĕn′tl-ĭn) A trademark for the drug albu-terol.

ventr– *pref.* Variant of **ventro–.**

ven·trad (vĕn′trăd) *adv.* Toward the ventral side or sur-face.

ven·tral (vĕn′trəl) *adj.* **1.** Relating to or situated on or close to the abdomen; abdominal. **2.** Relating to or situated on or close to the anterior aspect of the body.

ventral column of spinal cord *n.* See **anterior column of spinal cord.**

ventral horn *n.* See **anterior horn** (sense 1, 2).

ventral plate *n.* See **floor plate.**

ventral plate of neural tube *n.* See **basal lamina.**

ventral root *n.* The motor root of a spinal nerve.

ventral thalamic peduncle *n.* The massive system of fiber bundles emerging through the ventral, lateral, and anterior borders of the thalamus to join the internal capsule.

ven·tri·cle (vĕn′trĭ-kəl) *n.* A small cavity or chamber within a body or organ, especially the right or left ven-tricle of the heart or any of the interconnecting ventri-cles of the brain.

ven·tri·cose (vĕn′trĭ-kōs′) *adj.* Inflated, swollen, or dis-tended, especially on one side.

ven·tric·u·lar (vĕn-trĭk′yə-lər) *adj.* Of or relating to a ventricle or ventriculus.

ventricular artery *n.* Any of the arteries that are branches of the right and left coronary arteries dis-tributed to the muscle of the ventricles.

ventricular band of larynx *n.* See **vestibular fold.**

ventricular complex *n.* The continuous QRST wave in each beat in an electrocardiogram.

ventricular conduction *n.* See **intraventricular conduc-tion.**

ventricular escape *n.* Cardiologic escape in which a ventricular pacemaker sets the heart's beat before the sinoatrial pacemaker.

ventricular extrasystole *n.* A premature contraction of the ventricle. Also called *infranodal extrasystole.*

ventricular fibrillation *n. Abbr.* **VF** An often fatal form of arrhythmia characterized by rapid, irregular fibrillar twitching of the ventricles of the heart instead of nor-mal contractions, resulting in a loss of pulse. Also called *v-fib.*

ventricular fusion beat *n.* A fusion beat that occurs when the ventricles are activated partly by the descend-ing sinus or atrioventricular nodal impulse and partly by an ectopic ventricular impulse.

ventricular rhythm *n.* See **idioventricular rhythm.**

ventricular septal defect *n. Abbr.* **VSD** A congenital de-fect in the septum between the cardiac ventricles, usu-ally resulting from failure of the spiral septum to close the interventricular foramen.

ven·tric·u·li·tis (vĕn-trĭk′yə-lī′tĭs) *n.* Inflammation of the ventricles of the brain.

ventriculo– *pref.* Ventricle: *ventriculoatrial.*

ven·tric·u·lo·a·tri·al (vĕn-trĭk′yə-lō-ā′trē-əl) *adj. Abbr.* **V-A** Of or relating to the ventricles and atria of the heart.

ven·tric·u·lo·cis·ter·nos·to·my (vĕn-trĭk′yə-lō-sĭs′-tər-nŏs′tə-mē) *n.* The surgical formation of an opening between the ventricles of the brain and the cerebellomedullary cistern.

ven·tric·u·log·ra·phy (věn-trĭk′yə-lŏg′rə-fē) *n.* Radiography of the ventricles of the brain by injection of either a contrast medium or radiopaque agent.

ven·tric·u·lo·mas·toid·os·to·my (věn-trĭk′yə-lō-măs′-toi-dŏs′tə-mē) *n.* A surgical procedure used in treating hydrocephalus in which a communication is established between the lateral cerebral ventricle and the mastoid antrum.

ven·tric·u·lo·plas·ty (věn-trĭk′yə-lə-plăs′tē) *n.* Surgical repair of a defect in a ventricle of the heart.

ven·tric·u·lo·punc·ture (věn-trĭk′yə-lō-pŭngk′chər) *n.* The insertion of a needle into a ventricle.

ven·tric·u·los·co·py (věn-trĭk′yə-lŏs′kə-pē) *n.* Examination of a ventricle of the brain by means of an endoscope.

ven·tric·u·los·to·my (věn-trĭk′yə-lŏs′tə-mē) *n.* A surgical procedure used in the treatment of hydrocephalus in which an opening is established in a ventricle, usually from the third ventricle to the subarachnoid space.

ven·tric·u·lo·sub·a·rach·noid (věn-trĭk′yə-lō-sŭb′ə-răk′noid′) *adj.* Of or relating to the ventricles of the brain and the subarachnoid space.

ven·tric·u·lot·o·my (věn-trĭk′yə-lŏt′ə-mē) *n.* Incision into a ventricle of the brain or heart.

ven·tric·u·lus (věn-trĭk′yə-ləs) *n., pl.* **-li** (-lī′) **1.** A ventricle. **2.** The stomach.

ven·tri·duc·tion (věn-trĭ-dŭk′shən) *n.* The drawing of a part toward the abdomen or the abdominal wall.

ventro– *or* **ventr–** *pref.* Ventral: *ventriduction.*

ven·tros·co·py (věn-trŏs′kə-pē) *n.* See **peritoneoscopy.**

ven·trot·o·my (věn-trŏt′ə-mē) *n.* See **celiotomy.**

ven·ule (věn′yo͞ol, vēn′-) *n.* A small vein, especially one joining capillaries to larger veins. Also called *capillary vein.* —**ven′u·lar** (-yə-lər) *adj.*

ve·rap·a·mil (və-răp′ə-mĭl′) *n.* A vasodilator that inhibits calcium activity, used to treat hypertension, angina pectoris, and certain cardiac arrhythmias.

ver·big·er·a·tion (vər-bĭj′ə-rā′shən) *n.* Obsessive repetition of meaningless words and phrases, especially as a symptom of mental illness.

verge (vûrj) *n.* The extreme edge or margin; a border.

ver·gence (vûr′jəns) *n.* A disjunctive movement of the eyes in which the fixation axes are not parallel.

vermi– *pref.* Worm: *vermicide.*

ver·mi·cid·al (vûr′mĭ-sīd′l) *adj.* Destructive to parasitic intestinal worms.

ver·mi·cide (vûr′mĭ-sīd′) *n.* An agent used to kill parasitic intestinal worms.

ver·mic·u·lar (vər-mĭk′yə-lər) *adj.* **1.** Having the shape or motion of a worm. **2.** Caused by or relating to worms.

vermicular movement *n.* See **peristalsis.**

vermicular pulse *n.* A small rapid pulse giving a sensation of a moving worm to the finger.

ver·mic·u·la·tion (vər-mĭk′yə-lā′shən) *n.* Motion resembling that of a worm, especially the wavelike contractions of the intestine; peristalsis.

ver·mic·u·lose (vər-mĭk′yə-lōs′) *or* **ver·mic·u·lous** (-ləs) *adj.* **1.** Infested with worms or larvae. **2.** Being wormlike.

ver·mi·form (vûr′mə-fôrm′) *adj.* Resembling or having the long, thin, cylindrical shape of a worm.

vermiform appendix *n.* A wormlike intestinal diverticulum starting from the blind end of the cecum in the lower right-hand part of the abdomen and ending in a blind extremity.

ver·mif·u·gal (vər-mĭf′yə-gəl, vûr′mə-fyo͞o′gəl) *adj.* Causing expulsion of parasitic intestinal worms.

ver·mi·fuge (vûr′mə-fyo͞oj′) *n.* See **anthelmintic.**

ver·mil·ion border (vər-mĭl′yən) *n.* The exposed margin of the upper or lower lip.

ver·mil·ion·ec·to·my (vər-mĭl′yən-ĕk′tə-mē) *n.* Excision of the vermilion border of the lip.

ver·min (vûr′mĭn) *n., pl.* **vermin** Any of various small animals or insects, such as rats or cockroaches, that are destructive, annoying, or injurious to health.

ver·mi·na·tion (vûr′mə-nā′shən) *n.* **1.** The production or breeding of worms or larvae. **2.** Infestation by vermin, especially parasitic vermin.

ver·min·ous (vûr′mə-nəs) *adj.* **1.** Of, relating to, or caused by vermin. **2.** Infested with vermin.

ver·mis (vûr′mĭs) *n., pl.* **–mes** (-mēz) The narrow middle zone occurring between the two hemispheres of the cerebellum.

ver·nal conjunctivitis (vûr′nəl) *n.* A chronic form of conjunctivitis affecting both eyes, characterized by abnormal sensitivity to light and intense itching that recurs seasonally during warm weather. Also called *spring conjunctivitis.*

Ver·net′s syndrome (věr-nāz′) *n.* A syndrome characterized by paralysis of the glossopharyngeal, vagus, and accessory cranial nerves, causing paralysis of the soft palate, fauces, pharynx, and vocal cords, most commonly as the result of a head injury.

ver·nix ca·se·o·sa (vûr′nĭks kā′sē-ō′sə) *n.* The substance consisting of desquamated epithelial cells and sebaceous matter that covers the skin of the fetus.

ver·ru·ca (və-ro͞o′kə) *n., pl.* **–cae** (-kē) See **wart.**

verruca a·cu·mi·na·ta (ə-kyo͞o′mə-nā′tə) *n.* See **genital wart.**

verruca nec·ro·gen·i·ca (něk′rō-jěn′ĭ-kə) *n.* See **postmortem wart.**

verruca per·u·a·na (pěr′o͞o-ä′nə) *n.* See **Peruvian wart.**

verruca pe·ru·vi·a·na (pə-ro͞o′vē-ä′nə) *n.* See **Peruvian wart.**

verruca pla·na (plā′nə) *n.* See **flat wart.**

verruca plan·tar·is (plăn-târ′ĭs) *n.* See **plantar wart.**

verruca vul·gar·is virus (vŭl-gâr′ĭs) *n.* See **human papilloma virus.**

ver·ru·ci·form (və-ro͞o′sə-fôrm′) *adj.* Resembling or shaped like a wart.

ver·ru·cous (və-ro͞o′kəs) *or* **ver·ru·cose** (-kōs′) *adj.* Covered with warts or wartlike projections.

verrucous carcinoma *n.* A well-differentiated squamous cell carcinoma, especially of the oral cavity or penis, that rarely metastasizes.

verrucous endocarditis *n.* See **vegetative endocarditis.**

verrucous hemangioma *n.* A skin lesion appearing at birth or in early childhood on the legs, consisting of bluish-red nodules with a warty surface.

verrucous nevus *n.* A wartlike, often linear skin lesion appearing at birth or early in childhood and occurring in various sizes, groupings, and locations.

verrucous xanthoma *n.* A papilloma of the oral mucosa and skin in which squamous epithelium covers connective-tissue papillae filled with large foamy histiocytes.

ver·ru·ga (və-rōō′gə) *n.* See **wart**.

verruga per·u·a·na (pĕr′ōō-ä′nə) *n.* See **Peruvian wart**.

ver·sion (vûr′zhən, -shən) *n.* **1.** Deflection of an organ, such as the uterus, from its normal position. **2.** The changing of position of the fetus in the uterus, either spontaneously or as a result of manipulation. **3.** The conjugate rotation of the eyes in the same direction.

vertebr– *pref.* Variant of **vertebro–**.

ver·te·bra (vûr′tə-brə) *n.,* *pl.* **–bras** or **–brae** (-brā′, -brē′) Any of the bones or cartilaginous segments of the spinal column, usually 33 in number.

vertebra den·ta·ta (dĕn-tā′tə) *n.* See **axis** (sense 3).

ver·te·bral (vûr′tə-brəl, vər-tē′brəl) *adj.* **1.** Of, relating to, or of the nature of a vertebra. **2.** Having or consisting of vertebrae. **3.** Having a spinal column.

vertebral arch *n.* The posterior projection from the body of a vertebra that encloses the vertebral foramen. Also called *neural arch*.

vertebral artery *n.* The first branch of the subclavian artery, divided into four parts: the prevertebral part, before it enters the foramen of the transverse process of the sixth cervical vertebra; the transverse part, in the transverse foramina of the first six cervical vertebrae; the atlas, running along the posterior arch of the atlas; and the intracranial part, within the cranial cavity to unite with the artery from the other side to form the basilar artery.

vertebral canal *n.* The canal that contains the spinal cord, spinal meninges, and related structures and is formed by the vertebral foramina of successive vertebrae of the articulated spinal column. Also called *spinal canal*.

vertebral column *n.* See **spinal column**.

vertebral foramen *n.* The opening formed by the union of the vertebral arch with its body.

vertebral formula *n.* A formula indicating the number of vertebrae in each segment of the spinal column.

vertebral nerve *n.* A nerve that arises from the cervicothoracic ganglion, ascends along the vertebral artery to the level of the axis or atlas, and gives branches to the cervical nerves and meninges.

vertebral rib *n.* See **floating rib**.

vertebral vein *n.* Either of two veins that derive from tributaries that run through the foramina in the transverse processes of the first six cervical vertebrae and form a plexus around the vertebral artery and that empty as a single trunk into the brachiocephalic vein, designated right and left.

vertebra pla·na (plā′nə) *n.* Spondylitis with reduction of the vertebral body to a thin disk.

Ver·te·bra·ta (vûr′tə-brā′tə, -brä′-) *n.* A primary division of the phylum Chordata that includes the fishes, amphibians, reptiles, birds, and mammals, all of which are characterized by a segmented spinal column and a distinct, well-differentiated head.

ver·te·brate (vûr′tə-brĭt, -brāt′) *adj.* **1.** Having a spinal column. **2.** Of or characteristic of a vertebrate. —*n.* A member of the subphylum Vertebrata.

ver·te·brat·ed catheter (vûr′tə-brā′tĭd) *n.* A catheter made of several segments fitted together so as to be flexible.

ver·te·brec·to·my (vûr′tə-brĕk′tə-mē) *n.* Excision of a vertebra.

vertebro– or **vertebr–** *pref.* Vertebra; vertebral: *vertebrochondral*.

ver·te·bro·ar·te·ri·al foramen (vûr′tə-brō-är-tîr′ē-əl) *n.* See **transverse foramen**.

ver·te·bro·chon·dral (vûr′tə-brō-kŏn′drəl) *adj.* Of or relating to the three false ribs, designated eighth, ninth, and tenth, that are connected with the vertebrae at one extremity and with the costal cartilages at the other and do not articulate directly with the sternum.

ver·te·bro·cos·tal (vûr′tə-brō-kŏs′təl) *adj.* **1.** Costovertebral. **2.** Vertebrochondral.

vertebrocostal trigone *n.* A triangular area in the diaphragm near the lateral arcuate ligament, devoid of muscle fibers, and covered by pleura above and by peritoneum below.

ver·te·bro·ster·nal (vûr′tə-brō-stûr′nəl) *n.* See **sternovertebral**.

ver·tex (vûr′tĕks′) *n.,* *pl.* **–tex·es** or **–ti·ces** (-tĭ-sēz′) **1.** The highest point; the apex. **2.** The topmost point of the vault of the skull; the crown of the head. **3.** The portion of the fetal head bounded by the planes of the trachelobregmatic and biparietal diameters, with the posterior fontanel at the apex.

vertex presentation *n.* Head presentation of the fetus during birth in which the upper back part of the fetal head is the presenting part.

ver·ti·cal (vûr′tĭ-kəl) *adj.* **1.** Of or relating to the vertex of the head. **2.** Being or situated at right angles to the horizon; upright.

vertical banded gastroplasty *n.* A gastroplasty for the treatment of morbid obesity in which an upper gastric pouch is formed by a vertical staple line, with a cloth band applied to prevent dilation at the outlet into the main pouch.

vertical growth phase *n.* The late pattern of growth of cutaneous malignant melanoma in which tumor cells spread from the epidermis into the dermis.

vertical muscle of tongue *n.* An intrinsic muscle of the tongue, consisting of fibers that pass from the aponeurosis of the dorsum to the aponeurosis of the inferior surface.

vertical nystagmus *n.* An up-and-down oscillation of the eyes.

vertical overlap *n.* **1.** See **overbite**. **2.** The distance that teeth vertically lap over their antagonists.

vertical strabismus *n.* Strabismus in which the visual axis of one eye deviates upward or downward.

vertical transmission *n.* Transmission of a virus by means of the genetic apparatus of a cell in which the viral genome is integrated.

ver·ti·cil·late (vûr′tĭ-sĭl′ĭt, -āt′) *adj.* Arranged in or forming a whorl or whorls.

ver·tig·i·nous (vər-tĭj′ə-nəs) *adj.* **1.** Affected by vertigo; dizzy. **2.** Tending to produce vertigo.

ver·ti·go (vûr′tĭ-gō′) *n.,* *pl.* **–goes** or **–gos** A sensation of irregular or whirling motion, either of oneself or of external objects, often caused by inner ear disease.

ver·y low-density lipoprotein (vĕr′ē) *n. Abbr.* **VLDL** A lipoprotein containing a very large proportion of lipids to protein and carrying most cholesterol from the liver to the tissues.

Ve·sa·li·us (vĭ-sā′lē-əs, -zā′-), **Andreas** 1514–1564. Flemish anatomist and surgeon who is considered the founder of modern anatomy and who wrote *On the Structure of the Human Body* (1543).

vesic– *pref.* Variant of **vesico–**.

ve·si·ca (və-sī′kə, -sē′-, vĕs′ĭ-kə) *n., pl.* **–cae** (-kē, -sē) **1.** A bladder, especially the urinary bladder or the gallbladder. **2.** A hollow structure or sac containing a serous fluid. —**ves′i·cal** (vĕs′ĭ-kəl) *adj.*

vesical artery *n.* **1.** An artery with origin in the internal iliac artery, with distribution to the base of the bladder, ureter, and (in the male) to the seminal vesicles and the vas deferens, with branches to the prostate, and with anastomosis to the middle rectal artery; inferior vesical artery. **2.** An artery with its origin in the umbilical artery, with distribution to the bladder, urachus, and ureter, and with anastomoses to the other vesical branches; superior vesical artery.

vesical calculus *n.* See **urinary calculus**.

vesical diverticulum *n.* A true or false diverticulum of the bladder wall.

vesical hematuria *n.* Hematuria in which the site of bleeding is in the urinary bladder.

vesical hernia *n.* The protrusion of a segment of the bladder through the abdominal wall or into the inguinal canal.

vesical triangle *n.* A smooth triangular area at the base of the bladder between the openings of the two ureters and the opening of the urethra. Also called *trigone of bladder*.

vesical vein *n.* Any of the veins that drain the vesical plexus and join the internal iliac veins.

ves·i·cant (vĕs′ĭ-kənt) *n.* A blistering agent, especially mustard gas, used in chemical warfare. —*adj.* Causing blisters.

vesica pros·tat·i·ca (prŏ-stăt′ĭ-kə) *n.* The prostatic utricle.

ves·i·ca·tion (vĕs′ĭ-kā′shən) *n.* See **vesiculation** (sense 1).

ves·i·cle (vĕs′ĭ-kəl) *n.* **1.** A small structure resembling a bladder. **2.** A small circumscribed elevation of the skin containing serum. **3.** A small sac or cyst containing liquid or gas.

vesico– *or* **vesic–** *pref.* **1.** Bladder: *vesicoclysis.* **2.** Vesicle; blister: *vesicant.*

ves·i·co·cele (vĕs′ĭ-kō-sēl′) *n.* See **cystocele**.

ves·i·coc·ly·sis (vĕs′ĭ-kŏk′lĭ-sĭs) *n.* The washing out of the urinary bladder.

ves·i·co·fix·a·tion (vĕs′ĭ-kō-fĭk-sā′shən) *n.* The surgical fixation of the uterus to the bladder wall.

ves·i·co·pus·tu·lar (vĕs′ĭ-kō-pŭs′chə-lər) *or* **ve·sic·u·lo·pus·tu·lar** (və-sīk′yə-lō-) *adj.* Of, relating to, or consisting of a mixed eruption of vesicles and pustules.

ves·i·co·rec·tos·to·my (vĕs′ĭ-kō-rĕk-tŏs′tə-mē) *n.* Surgical formation of a passage between the rear of the bladder and the rectum to serve as an alternate route for the urine. Also called *cystoproctostomy, cystorectostomy.*

ves·i·co·sig·moid·os·to·my (vĕs′ĭ-kō-sĭg′moi-dŏs′tə-mē) *n.* Surgical formation of a communication between the bladder and the sigmoid colon.

ves·i·co·spi·nal (vĕs′ĭ-kō-spī′nəl) *adj.* Of or relating to the spinal-neural mechanisms that control retention and evacuation of urine by the bladder.

ves·i·cos·to·my (vĕs′ĭ-kŏs′tə-mē) *n.* Surgical creation of a stoma between the anterior bladder wall and the skin of the lower abdomen, for temporary or permanent lower urinary tract diversion.

ves·i·cot·o·my (vĕs′ĭ-kŏt′ə-mē) *n.* See **cystotomy**.

ves·i·co·u·re·ter·al reflux (vĕs′ĭ-kō-yoo-rē′tər-əl) *n.* Reflux of urine from the bladder into the ureter.

vesicoureteral valve *n.* A mechanism in the wall of the intravesical portion of the ureter that prevents the reflux of urine from the bladder into the ureter.

ves·i·co·u·ter·ine fistula (vĕs′ĭ-kō-yoo′tər-ĭn, -tə-rīn′) *n.* A fistula between bladder and uterus.

vesicouterine ligament *n.* A peritoneal fold extending from the uterus to the posterior part of the bladder.

vesicouterine pouch *n.* A pocket formed by the deflection of the peritoneum from the bladder to the uterus.

ve·sic·u·lar (vĕ-sīk′yə-lər) *adj.* **1.** Of or relating to vesicles. **2.** Composed of or containing vesicles. **3.** Having the form of a vesicle.

vesicular murmur *n.* See **vesicular respiration**.

vesicular ovarian follicle *n.* See **Graafian follicle**.

vesicular resonance *n.* The sound obtained by percussing over the normal lungs.

vesicular respiration *n.* The respiratory murmur heard on auscultation of the normal lung. Also called *vesicular murmur.*

vesicular transport *n.* See **transcytosis**.

ve·sic·u·late (vĕ-sīk′yə-lāt′) *v.* To make or become vesicular. —*adj.* (-lĭt, -lāt′) Full of or bearing vesicles; vesicular.

ve·sic·u·la·tion (vĕ-sīk′yə-lā′shən) *n.* **1.** The formation of vesicles. Also called *blistering, vesication.* **2.** The presence of vesicles.

ve·sic·u·lec·to·my (vĕ-sīk′yə-lĕk′tə-mē) *n.* Surgical resection of part or all of a seminal vesicle.

ve·sic·u·li·form (vĕ-sīk′yə-lə-fôrm′) *adj.* Of or resembling a vesicle.

ve·sic·u·li·tis (vĕ-sīk′yə-lī′tĭs) *n.* Inflammation of a vesicle, especially a seminal vesicle.

vesiculo– *pref.* Vesicle: *vesiculotomy.*

ve·sic·u·lo·cav·ern·ous (vĕ-sīk′yə-lō-kăv′ər-nəs) *adj.* Being both vesicular and cavernous, as of sound produced upon ausculation or the structure of certain neoplasms.

ve·sic·u·log·ra·phy (vĕ-sīk′yə-lŏg′rə-fē) *n.* Radiography of the seminal vesicles.

ve·sic·u·lo·pap·u·lar (vĕ-sīk′yə-lō-păp′yə-lər) *adj.* Of, relating to, or consisting of a combination of vesicles and papules.

ve·sic·u·lo·pros·ta·ti·tis (vĕ-sīk′yə-lō-prŏs′tə-tī′tĭs) *n.* Inflammation of bladder and prostate.

ve·sic·u·lo·pus·tu·lar (və-sīk′yə-lō-pŭs′chə-lər) *adj.* Variant of **vesicopustular**.

ve·sic·u·lot·o·my (vĕ-sīk′yə-lŏt′ə-mē) *n.* Surgical division of the seminal vesicles.

ve·sic·u·lo·tu·bu·lar (vĕ-sīk′yə-lō-too′byə-lər) *adj.* Relating to or being an auscultatory sound having a vesicular and a tubular quality.

ve·sic·u·lo·tym·pan·ic (vĕ-sĭk′yə-lō-tĭm-păn′ĭk) *adj.* Of, relating to, or being a percussion sound having a vesicular and a tympanic quality.

ve·sic·u·lo·tym·pa·nit·ic resonance (vĕ-sĭk′yə-lō-tĭm′pə-nĭt′ĭk) *n.* A sound, partly tympanitic, partly vesicular, obtained by percussing the lung cavity of an individual with pulmonary emphysema.

ve·sic·u·lous (vĕ-sĭk′yə-ləs) *adj.* Vesicular.

ves·sel (vĕs′əl) *n.* A duct, canal, or other tube that contains or conveys a body fluid such as blood or lymph.

ves·tib·u·lar (vĕ-stĭb′yə-lər) *adj.* Of, relating to, or serving as a vestibule, especially of the ear.

vestibular canal *n.* The division of the spiral canal of the cochlea lying above the spiral lamina and the vestibular membrane.

vestibular crest *n.* An oblique ridge on the inner wall of the vestibule of the labyrinth, bounding the spherical recess above and behind.

vestibular fold *n.* Either of a pair of folds of mucous membrane stretching across the laryngeal cavity from the angle of the thyroid cartilage to the arytenoid cartilage to enclose the rima vestibuli. Also called *false vocal cord, ventricular band of larynx.*

vestibular ganglion *n.* A collection of bipolar nerve-cell bodies forming a swelling on the vestibular part of the eighth nerve in the internal acoustic meatus and associated with the utriculoampullar and saccular nerves.

vestibular gland *n.* Any of the glands that open into the vestibule of the vagina.

vestibular labyrinth *n.* The portion of the membranous labyrinth located within the semicircular canals and the vestibule of the osseous labyrinth.

vestibular membrane *n.* The membrane separating the cochlear duct from the vestibular canal of the ear. Also called *Reissner's membrane.*

vestibular nerve *n.* The superior part of the vestibulocochlear nerve peripheral to the vestibulocochlear nerve root, composed of nerve processes that have their terminals on hair cells of the ampullae of the semicircular ducts and the maculas of the saccule and utricle and the bipolar neurons of the vestibular ganglion.

vestibular nucleus *n.* Any of a group of four nuclei, designated lateral, medial, superior, and inferior, that are located in the lateral region of the rhombencephalon, receive the incoming fibers of the vestibular nerve, and project via the medial longitudinal fasciculus to the abducens, trochlear, and oculomotor nuclei and to the ventral horn of the spinal cord, on both the left and the right sides.

vestibular nystagmus *n.* A nystagmus resulting from physiological stimuli to the labyrinth of the ear. Also called *labyrinthine nystagmus.*

vestibular organ *n.* The structure composed of the utricle, saccule, and the three semicircular ducts of the membranous labyrinth of the inner ear.

vestibular vein *n.* Any of the tributaries of the labyrinthine veins and of the vein that drains the saccule and utricle.

ves·ti·bule (vĕs′tə-byōōl′) *n.* A cavity, chamber, or channel that leads to or is an entrance to another cavity, especially that of the ear.

vestibule of mouth *n.* See **buccal cavity.**

vestibule of nose *n.* The anterior part of the nasal cavity, enclosed by cartilage.

vestibule of vagina *n.* The space behind the glans clitoridis, between the labia minora, containing the openings of the vagina, the urethra, and the ducts of the greater vestibular glands.

vestibulo– *pref.* Vestibule: *vestibuloplasty.*

ves·tib·u·lo·coch·le·ar (vĕ-stĭb′yə-lō-kŏk′lē-ər, -kō′-klē-) *adj.* Of or relating to the vestibule and the cochlea of the ear.

vestibulocochlear nerve *n.* A composite sensory nerve that emerges from the brainstem at the cerebellopontine angle, that innervates the receptor cells of the membranous labyrinth, and that consists of two major anatomically and functionally distinct components: the vestibular nerve and the cochlear nerve. Also called *acoustic nerve, eighth cranial nerve.*

ves·tib·u·lo·plas·ty (vĕ-stĭb′yə-lō-plăs′tē) *n.* A surgical procedure to restore alveolar ridge height by lowering muscles attaching to the buccal, labial, and lingual aspects of the jaws.

ves·tib·u·lo·spi·nal reflex (vĕ-stĭb′yə-lō-spī′nəl) *n.* Any of many reflexes that originate with vestibular stimulation and control body posture.

ves·tib·u·lot·o·my (vĕ-stĭb′yə-lŏt′ə-mē) *n.* Incision of the vestibule of the labyrinth of the ear.

ves·tib·u·lum (vĕ-stĭb′yə-ləm) *n., pl.* **-la** (-lə) A cavity, chamber, or channel; vestibule.

ves·tige (vĕs′tĭj) *n.* A rudimentary or degenerate, usually nonfunctioning structure that is the remnant of an organ or part that was fully developed or functioning in a preceding generation or an earlier stage of development.

ves·tig·i·al (vĕ-stĭj′ē-əl, -stĭj′əl) *adj.* Occurring or persisting as a rudimentary or degenerate structure.

vestigial organ *n.* A rudimentary structure in humans corresponding to a functional structure or organ in ancestral animals.

vet·er·i·nar·i·an (vĕt′ər-ə-nâr′ē-ən, vĕt′rə-) *n.* A person who practices veterinary medicine.

vet·er·i·nar·y (vĕt′ər-ə-nĕr′ē, vĕt′rə-) *adj.* Of or relating to veterinary medicine. —*n.* A veterinarian.

veterinary anatomy *n.* The study of the structures of domestic animals.

veterinary medicine *n.* The branch of medicine that deals with the causes, diagnosis, and treatment of diseases and injuries of animals, especially domestic animals.

VF *abbr.* ventricular fibrillation

V-fib (vē′fĭb′) *n.* See **ventricular fibrillation.**

VHDL *abbr.* very high density lipoprotein

vi·a·ble (vī′ə-bəl) *adj.* **1.** Capable of living, developing, or germinating under favorable conditions. **2.** Capable of living outside the uterus. Used of a fetus or newborn. —**vi′a·bil′i·ty** *n.*

Vi·ag·ra (vī-ăg′rə) A trademark for the drug sildenafil citrate.

Vi·bra·my·cin (vī-brä-mī′sĭn) A trademark for the drug doxycycline.

vi·brat·ing line (vī′brā′tĭng) *n.* The imaginary line across the posterior palate, marking the division between the movable and immovable tissues.

Vib·ri·o (vĭb′rē-ō) *n.* A genus of gram-negative, motile, S-shaped or comma-shaped bacteria some species of which are saprophytes in salt and fresh water and in soil, while others are parasites or pathogens.

Vibrio al·gi·no·lyt·i·cus (ăl′jə-nō-lĭt′ĭ-kəs) *n.* A bacterium associated with wound and ear infections and with bacteremia in immunocompromised individuals and in individuals with severe burns.

Vibrio chol·er·ae (kŏl′ə-rē) *n.* A bacterium that causes Asiatic cholera in humans; Koch's bacillus.

Vibrio fe·tus (fē′təs) *n.* A bacterium that causes infections in humans as well as abortion in sheep and cattle.

Vibrio flu·vi·a·lis (floo′vē-ā′lĭs) *n.* A bacterium associated with diarrheal disease.

Vibrio fur·nis·si·i (fər-nĭs′ē-ī) *n.* An aerogenic bacterium associated with diarrheal disease and with outbreaks of gastroenteritis.

Vibrio mim·i·cus (mĭm′ĭ-kəs) *n.* A bacterium associated with diarrheal disease and ear infections.

Vib·ri·o·na·ce·ae (vĭb′rē-ō-nā′sē-ē′) *n.* A family of gram-negative, rod-shaped, facultatively anaerobic bacteria that have flagella and are usually motile and are found in fresh or sea water and, occasionally, in fish and humans.

Vibrio par·a·hae·mo·lyt·i·cus (păr′ə-hē′mə-lĭt′ĭ-kəs) *n.* A marine bacterium that may contaminate shellfish and cause human gastroenteritis.

vib·ri·o·sis (vĭb′rē-ō′sĭs) *n., pl.* **–ses** (-sēz) Infection caused by a species of *Vibrio*, especially an infection caused by *V. parahaemolyticus* as a result of eating undercooked seafood from contaminated waters.

Vibrio vul·nif·i·cus (vŭl-nĭf′ĭ-kəs) *n.* A bacterium capable of causing septicemia in individuals with an underlying chronic disease, especially hepatic disease, as well as causing wound infections, especially to persons who handle shellfish.

vi·bris·sa (vī-brĭs′ə, və-) *n., pl.* **–bris·sae** (-brĭs′ē) **1.** Any of the hairs growing at the anterior nares. **2.** Any of the long, stiff hairs projecting from the anterior nares of most mammals, as cat whiskers.

vi·bro·car·di·o·gram (vī′brō-kär′dē-ə-grăm′) *n.* A graphic record of chest vibrations produced by hemodynamic events of the cardiac cycle.

vi·car·i·ous (vī-kâr′ē-əs, vĭ-) *adj.* **1.** Felt or undergone as if one were taking part in the experience or feelings of another. **2.** Occurring in or performed by a part of the body not normally associated with a certain function.

vicarious hypertrophy *n.* Hypertropy of an organ following failure of another organ to which it is functionally related.

vicarious menstruation *n.* Bleeding from a surface other than the mucous membrane of the uterine cavity that occurs at the time when normal menstruation should take place.

vi·cious circle (vĭsh′əs) *n.* A condition in which a disorder or disease gives rise to another that subsequently affects the first.

Vic·o·dan (vī′kə-dn) A trademark for a drug combination of hydrocodone bitartrate and acetaminophen.

Vicq d'A·zyr's bundle (vēk′ dä-zîrz′) *n.* See **mamillothalamic fascicle.**

vi·dar·a·bine (vī-där′ə-bēn′) *n.* A purine nucleoside obtained from a species of *Streptomyces* and used in the treatment of herpes simplex infections.

vig·il·am·bu·lism (vĭj′ə-lăm′byə-lĭz′əm) *n.* A condition of unconsciousness regarding one's surroundings together with automatism of motion.

vil·lo·ma (vĭ-lō′mə) *n.* See **papilloma.**

vil·lo·si·tis (vĭl′ə-sī′tĭs) *n.* Inflammation of the villous surface of the placenta.

vil·los·i·ty (vĭ-lŏs′ĭ-tē) *n.* **1.** The condition of being villous. **2.** A villous formation, surface, or coating. **3.** A villus.

vil·lous (vĭl′əs) *or* **vil·lose** (-ōs′) *adj.* Of, relating to, resembling, or covered with villi.

villous adenoma *n.* A usually solitary, often large sessile tumor of the mucosa of the large intestine composed of mucinous epithelium covering delicate vascular projections. Also called *papillary adenoma of large intestine.*

villous carcinoma *n.* A carcinoma having numerous, closely packed, papillary projections of neoplastic epithelial tissue.

villous tenosynovitis *n.* A condition in which diffuse outgrowths arise in periarticular soft tissue of a joint, usually in the hands.

vil·lus (vĭl′əs) *n., pl.* **vil·li** (vĭl′ī) **1.** A minute projection arising from a mucous membrane, especially one of the vascular projections of the small intestine. **2.** Such a projection of the chorion that contributes to placental formation in mammals.

vil·lus·ec·to·my (vĭl′ə-sĕk′tə-mē) *n.* See **synovectomy.**

vi·men·tin (vī-mĕn′tĭn) *n.* The polypeptide that copolymerizes with other subunits to form the intermediate filament cytoskeleton of mesenchymal cells.

vin·blas·tine sulfate (vĭn-blăs′tēn′) *n.* The sulfate salt of a dimeric alkaloid obtained from a plant of the genus *Vinca* and used as an antineoplastic agent in the treatment of Hodgkin's disease, choriocarcinoma, acute and chronic leukemias, and other neoplastic diseases. Also called *vincaleukoblastine.*

Vin·ca (vĭng′kə) *n.* A genus of evergreens usually found in the Eastern hemisphere.

vin·ca·leu·ko·blas·tine (vĭng′kə-loo′kə-blăs′tēn′) *n.* See **vinblastine sulfate.**

Vin·cent's angina (vĭn′sənts) *n.* See **trench mouth.**

Vincent's disease *n.* See **trench mouth.**

vin·cris·tine sulfate (vĭn-krĭs′tēn′) *n.* The sulfate salt of a dimeric alkaloid obtained from a plant of the genus *Vinca* that exhibits antineoplastic activity similar to that of vinblastine sulfate and is used especially in the treatment of lymphocytic lymphosarcoma and acute leukemia.

vin·cu·lum (vĭng′kyə-ləm) *n., pl.* **–lums** *or* **–la** (-lə) A uniting band or bandlike structure, such as a frenum or ligament.

vinculum of tendons *n.* Any of the fibrous bands that extend from the flexor tendons of the fingers and toes to the capsules of the interphalangeal joints and to the phalanges and convey small vessels to the tendons. Also called *synovial frenulum.*

vin·e·gar (vĭn′ĭ-gər) *n.* An impure dilute solution of

acetic acid obtained by fermentation beyond the alcohol stage and used as a preservative.

vi·nyl (vī′nəl) *n.* The univalent radical CH_2-CH derived from ethylene.

vi·nyl·ben·zene (vī′nəl-bĕn′zēn′, -bĕn-zēn′) *n.* See **styrene**.

vinyl chloride *n.* A flammable gas used in the plastics industry as a monomer for polyvinyl chloride and suspected of being a potent carcinogen in humans.

vinyl ether *n.* See **divinyl ether**.

vi·nyl·eth·yl ether (vī′nəl-ĕth′əl) *n.* See **ethylvinyl ether**.

vi·o·let (vī′ə-lĭt) *n.* **1.** The hue of the short-wave end of the visible spectrum, evoked in the human observer by radiant energy with wavelengths of approximately 380 to 420 nanometers. **2.** Any of a group of colors, reddish-blue in hue, that may vary in lightness and saturation.

vi·o·my·cin (vī′ə-mī′sĭn) *n.* An antibiotic produced by the actinomycete *Streptomyces puniceus,* used in the treatment of tuberculosis.

Vi·oxx (vī′ŏks′) A trademark for the drug rofecoxib.

VIP *abbr.* vasoactive intestinal polypeptide

vi·po·ma (vī-pō′mə) *n.* An endocrine tumor, usually originating in the pancreas, that produces a vasoactive intestinal polypeptide believed to cause profound cardiovascular and electrolyte changes with vasodilatory hypotension, watery diarrhea, hypokalemia, and dehydration.

vir– *pref.* Variant of **viro–**.

Vir·a·A (vîr′ə-ā′) A trademark for the drug vidarabine.

Vir·a·cept (vîr′ə-sĕpt′) A trademark for the drug nelfinavir.

vi·ral (vī′rəl) *adj.* Of, relating to, or caused by a virus.

viral antigen *n. Abbr.* **VA** An antigen with multiple antigenicities that is protein in nature, strain-specific, and closely associated with the virus particle.

viral dysentery *n.* A profuse watery diarrhea believed to be the result of viral infection.

viral envelope *n.* The outer structure that encloses the nucleocapsids of some viruses.

viral hemagglutination *n.* The agglutination of suspended red blood cells by viruses, usually by the virion itself but in some instances by products of viral growth.

viral hepatitis *n.* Any of various forms of hepatitis caused by a virus.

viral load *n.* The concentration of a virus, such as HIV, in the blood.

viral tropism *n.* The specificity of a virus for a particular host tissue, determined in part by the interaction of viral surface structures with receptors present on the surface of the host cell.

Vir·a·mune (vîr′ə-myoōn′) A trademark for the drug nevirapine.

Vir·a·zole (vîr′ə-zōl′) A trademark for the drug ribavirin.

Vir·chow (vîr′kō, fîr′кнō), **Rudolf** 1821–1902. German physician and pathologist known for his contributions to cell theory and the study of disease.

Vir·chow's cell (vîr′kōz, fîr′-) *n.* **1.** The cavities in osseous tissue containing bone cells. **2.** A bone cell. **3.** See **corneal corpuscle**.

Virchow's crystals *pl.n.* Crystals of hematoidin frequently observed in extravasated blood in tissues.

Virchow's node *n.* See **signal node**.

vi·re·mi·a (vī-rē′mē-ə) *n.* The presence of viruses in the bloodstream.

vir·gin (vûr′jĭn) *n.* A person who has not experienced sexual intercourse. —**vir′gin·al** (-jə-nəl) *adj.*

vir·gin·i·ty (vər-jĭn′ĭ-tē) *n.* The quality or condition of being a virgin.

vi·ri·cide (vī′rĭ-sīd′) *or* **vi·ru·cide** (vī′rə-) *n.* An agent that inhibits or destroys viruses. —**vi′ri·cid′al** (-sīd′l) *adj.*

–viridae *suff.* Virus family: *Orthomyxoviridae.*

vir·ile (vîr′əl, -īl′) *adj.* **1.** Of, relating to, or having the characteristics of an adult male, especially the ability to perform sexually as a male. **2.** Having or showing masculine spirit, strength, vigor, or power. **3.** Sexually potent.

vir·i·les·cence (vîr′ə-lĕs′əns) *n.* The assumption of male characteristics by a female.

vir·il·ism (vîr′ə-lĭz′əm) *n.* The presence of male secondary sexual characteristics in a female.

vi·ril·i·ty (və-rĭl′ĭ-tē) *n.* **1.** The quality or state of being virile. **2.** Masculine vigor; potency.

vir·il·i·za·tion (vîr′ə-lĭ-zā′shən) *n.* Development of male secondary sexual characteristics. —**vir′il·ize′** (-ə-līz′) *v.*

–virinae *suff.* Subfamily of viruses: *Oncovirinae.*

vi·ri·on (vī′rē-ŏn′, vîr′ē-) *n.* A complete viral particle, consisting of RNA or DNA surrounded by a protein shell and constituting the infective form of a virus.

viro– *or* **vir–** *pref.* Virus: *virology.*

vi·ro·gene (vī′rə-jēn′) *n.* A gene capable of specifying the synthesis of a virus in a cell.

vi·ro·gen·e·sis (vī′rō-jĕn′ĭ-sĭs, -rə-) *n.* Production or formation of a virus.

vi·roid (vī′roid′) *n.* An infectious particle, smaller than a virus, that consists solely of a strand of RNA and is capable of causing disease in plants.

vi·rol·o·gy (vī-rŏl′ə-jē) *n.* The study of viruses and viral diseases. —**vi′ro·log′i·cal** (vī′rə-lŏj′ĭ-kəl), **vi′ro·log′ic** (-ĭk) *adj.* —**vi·rol′o·gist** *n.*

vi·ro·sis (vī-rō′sĭs) *n., pl.* **–ses** (-sēz) A disease caused by a virus.

vir·tu·al cautery (vûr′choō-əl) *n.* See **potential cautery**.

virtual colonoscopy *n.* A screening examination of the colon in which x-rays obtained by CAT scan are used to generate computerized three-dimensional images of the colonic mucosa.

vi·ru·cid·al (vī′rə-sīd′l) *adj.* Destructive to viruses.

vi·ru·cide (vī′rə-sīd′) *n.* Variant of **viricide**.

vir·u·lence (vîr′yə-ləns, vîr′ə-) *n.* **1.** The quality of being poisonous. **2.** The capacity of a microorganism to cause disease.

vir·u·lent (vîr′yə-lənt, vîr′ə-) *adj.* **1.** Extremely infectious, malignant, or poisonous. Used of a disease or toxin. **2.** Capable of causing disease by breaking down protective mechanisms of the host. Used of a pathogen. **3.** Intensely irritating, obnoxious, or harsh.

virulent bacteriophage *n.* A bacteriophage that lyses bacteria it infects.

vir·u·lif·er·ous (vĭr'yə-lĭf'ər-əs, vĭr'ə-) *adj.* Carrying or containing a virus.

vi·ru·ri·a (vī-rŏŏr'ē-ə) *n.* Presence of living viruses in the urine.

vi·rus (vī'rəs) *n., pl.* **–rus·es 1.** Any of a large group of submicroscopic agents that act as parasites and consist of a segment of DNA or RNA surrounded by a coat of protein. Because viruses are unable to replicate without a host cell, they are not considered living organisms in conventional taxonomic systems. Nonetheless, they are described as "live" when they are capable of replicating and causing disease. **2.** A disease caused by a virus.

–virus *suff.* Genus of viruses: *Influenzavirus.*

virus-associated he·mo·phag·o·cyt·ic syndrome (hē'-mō-făg'ə-sĭt'ĭk) *n.* A syndrome that resembles malignant histiocytosis and follows infection with a herpes virus, such as Epstein-Barr virus.

virus keratoconjunctivitis *n.* See **epidemic keratoconjunctivitis.**

virus punctate keratoconjunctivitis *n.* Keratoconjunctivitis having symptoms similar to those of inclusion conjunctivitis, associated with punctate keratitis of the epithelial and subepithelial layers of the cornea.

virus shedding *n.* Excretion of virus from the infected host by any route.

virus-transformed cell *n.* A cell that has been genetically changed to a tumor cell and that passes the change to its daughter cells.

vis·cer·a (vĭs'ər-ə) *pl.n.* **1.** The soft internal organs of the body, especially those contained within the abdominal and thoracic cavities. **2.** The intestines.

vis·cer·ad (vĭs'ə-răd') *adj.* In a direction toward the viscera.

vis·cer·al (vĭs'ər-əl) *adj.* Relating to, situated in, or affecting the viscera.

visceral anesthesia *n.* See **splanchnic anesthesia.**

visceral arch *n.* See **branchial arch.**

visceral cleft *n.* A cleft between two branchial arches in the embryo.

visceral disease virus *n.* See **cytomegalovirus.**

visceral ganglion *n.* See **autonomic ganglion.**

vis·cer·al·gia (vĭs'ə-răl'jə) *n.* Pain in any part of the viscera.

visceral inversion *n.* See **situs inversus.**

visceral larva migrans *n.* A disease, chiefly of children, caused by ingestion of nematode ova, usually of *Toxocara canis,* characterized by high eosinophilia and often liver enlargement, fever, cough, and hyperglobulinemia.

visceral layer *n.* **1.** See **epicardium. 2.** The inner part of the tunica vaginalis testis, which is in direct contact with the testis and epididymis.

visceral leishmaniasis *n.* A chronic, often fatal disease occurring chiefly in Asia, caused by a protozoan parasite *(Leishmania donovani)* and characterized by irregular fever, enlargement of the spleen and liver, and emaciation. Also called *kala-azar.*

visceral node *n.* Any of the lymph nodes draining the viscera of the abdomen or the pelvis.

visceral sense *n.* The perception of the presence of the internal organs. Also called *splanchnesthesia, splanchnesthetic sensibility.*

visceral swallow *n.* An immature swallowing pattern, as of infants, marked by a thrust of the tongue and resembling the peristaltic, wavelike, muscular contractions observed in the gut.

viscero– *pref.* Viscera; visceral: *visceroptosis.*

vis·cer·o·gen·ic (vĭs'ər-ə-jĕn'ĭk) *adj.* Of, relating to, or being reflexes, such as sensory reflexes, that are visceral in origin.

vis·cer·o·in·hib·i·to·ry (vĭs'ə-rō-ĭn-hĭb'ĭ-tôr'ē) *adj.* Inhibiting or arresting the functional activity of the viscera.

vis·cer·o·meg·a·ly (vĭs'ər-ə-mĕg'ə-lē) *n.* Abnormal enlargement of the viscera. Also called *organomegaly, splanchnomegaly.*

vis·cer·o·mo·tor (vĭs'ər-ə-mō'tər) *adj.* Producing or related to movements of the viscera.

vis·cer·o·pleu·ral (vĭs'ə-rō-plŏŏr'əl) *adj.* Relating to the pleural and thoracic viscera.

vis·cer·op·to·sis (vĭs'ə-rŏp-tō'sĭs) *n.* Descent of the viscera from their normal positions. Also called *splanchnoptosis.*

vis·cer·o·sen·so·ry (vĭs'ə-rō-sĕn'sə-rē) *adj.* Of or relating to the sensory innervation of internal organs.

vis·cer·o·skel·e·ton (vĭs'ə-rō-skĕl'ĭ-tn) *n.* **1.** A bony formation in an organ, as in the heart, tongue, or penis. **2.** The part of the skeleton protecting the viscera, such as the rib cage and the pelvic bones. Also called *splanchnoskeleton.* —**vis'cer·o·skel'e·tal** (-skĕl'ĭ-tl) *adj.*

vis·cer·o·so·mat·ic (vĭs'ə-rō-sō-măt'ĭk) *adj.* Of or relating to both the viscera and the body.

vis·cer·o·troph·ic (vĭs'ə-rō-trŏf'ĭk, -trō'fĭk) *adj.* Of, relating to, or being a trophic change determined by the viscera.

vis·cer·o·trop·ic (vĭs'ə-rō-trŏp'ĭk, -trō'pĭk) *adj.* Relating to or affecting the viscera.

vis·cid (vĭs'ĭd) *adj.* **1.** Thick and adhesive. Used of a fluid. **2.** Covered with a sticky coating. —**vis·cid'i·ty, vis'cid·ness** *n.*

vis·cos·i·ty (vĭ-skŏs'ĭ-tē) *n.* **1.** The condition or property of being viscous. **2.** The degree to which a fluid resists flow under an applied force, measured by the tangential friction force per unit area divided by the velocity gradient under conditions of streamline flow; coefficient of viscosity.

vis·cous (vĭs'kəs) *adj.* **1.** Having relatively high resistance to flow. **2.** Viscid.

vis·i·ble spectrum (vĭz'ə-bəl) *n.* The part of the electromagnetic spectrum visible to the human eye, extending from extreme red, 760.6 nanometers, to extreme violet, 393.4 nanometers.

vi·sion (vĭzh'ən) *n.* **1.** The faculty of sight; eyesight. **2.** The manner in which an individual sees or conceives of something.

vis·it·ing nurse (vĭz'ĭ-tĭng) *n.* A registered nurse employed by a public health agency or hospital to promote community health and especially to visit and administer treatment to sick people in their homes.

Vis·ta·ril (vĭs'tə-rĭl') A trademark for a drug preparation of hydroxyzine.

vi·su·al (vĭzh′ōō-əl) *adj.* **1.** Of or relating to the sense of sight. **2.** Seen or able to be seen by the eye; visible. **3.** Optical.

visual acuity *n.* Sharpness of vision, especially as tested with a Snellen chart. Normal visual acuity based on the Snellen chart is 20/20.

visual allesthesia *n.* A condition in which visual images are transposed from one half of the visual field to the other, either vertically or horizontally. Also called *optical allachesthesia.*

visual angle *n.* The angle formed at the retina by the meeting of lines drawn from the periphery of the viewed object.

visual aphasia *n.* **1.** See **alexia. 2.** Anomia. Not in technical use.

visual area *n.* See **visual cortex.**

visual axis *n.* A straight line extending from the viewed object through the center of the pupil to the yellow spot of the retina.

visual cortex *n.* The region of the cerebral cortex occupying the entire surface of the occipital lobe and receiving the visual data from the lateral geniculate body of the thalamus. Also called *visual area.*

visual evoked potential *n.* The measurement that results from the recordings of an electroencephalogram from the occipital area of the scalp as the result of retinal stimulation by a light flashing at quarter-second intervals, as given by a computer that averages the electroencephalogram response of 100 consecutive flashes.

visual field *n.* The area simultaneously visible to one eye without movement.

visual pigment *n.* Any of the photopigments in the retinal cones and rods that absorb light and photochemically initiate the phenomenon of vision.

visual purple *n.* See **rhodopsin.**

visual receptor cell *n.* **1.** A rod cell. **2.** A cone cell.

visual violet *n.* See **iodopsin.**

vi·su·og·no·sis (vĭzh′ōō-ŏg-nō′sĭs) *n.* Recognition and understanding of visual impressions.

vis·u·o·mo·tor (vĭzh′ōō-ō-mō′tər) *adj.* Of or relating to motor activity dependent on or involving sight.

vi·su·o·sen·so·ry (vĭzh′ōō-ō-sĕn′sə-rē) *adj.* Of or relating to the perception of visual stimuli, especially to the portion of the brain that functions in such perception.

vis·u·o·spa·tial (vĭsh′ōō-ō-spā′shəl) *adj.* Of or relating to visual perception of spatial relationships among objects.

vi·tal (vīt′l) *adj.* **1.** Of, relating to, or characteristic of life. **2.** Necessary to the continuation of life. **3.** Used or done on a living cell or tissue, as in staining. **4.** Destructive to life; fatal, as of an injury.

vital capacity *n.* *Abbr.* **VC** The amount of air that can be forcibly expelled from the lungs following breathing in as deeply as possible. Also called *respiratory capacity.*

vital index *n.* The ratio of births to deaths within a population during a given time.

vi·tal·i·ty (vī-tăl′ĭ-tē) *n.* **1.** The capacity to live, grow, or develop. **2.** Physical or intellectual vigor; energy.

vitality test *n.* Any of a group of thermal and electrical tests used to aid in assessing the health of dental pulp. Also called *pulp test.*

vi·ta·lom·e·ter (vī′tə-lŏm′ĭ-tər) *n.* An electrical device for measuring the vitality of tooth pulp.

vital pulp *n.* Living dental pulp that responds to electric and thermal stimulation.

vital red *n.* An acid dye used as a vital stain.

vi·tals (vīt′lz) *pl.n.* **1.** The vital body organs. **2.** The parts that are essential to continued functioning, as of a system.

vital signs *pl.n.* The rates or values indicating an individual's pulse, temperature, and respiration.

vital stain *n.* A stain applied to cells or parts of cells while they are still living.

vital statistics *pl.n.* Statistics concerning the important events in human life, such as births, deaths, marriages, and migrations.

vi·ta·mer (vī′tə-mər) *n.* One of two or more related chemical substances that fulfill the same specific vitamin function.

vi·ta·min (vī′tə-mĭn) *n.* Any of various fat-soluble or water-soluble organic substances essential in minute amounts for normal growth and activity of the body and obtained naturally from plant and animal foods.

vitamin A *n.* A fat-soluble vitamin or a mixture of vitamins, especially vitamin A_1 or a mixture of vitamins A_1 and A_2, occurring principally in fish-liver oils, milk, and some yellow and dark green vegetables, and functioning in normal cell growth and development with deficiencies causing hardening and roughening of the skin, night blindness, and degeneration of mucous membranes. Also called *retinol.*

vitamin A_1 *n.* A yellow crystalline compound extracted from egg yolks, milk, and cod-liver oil.

vitamin A_2 *n.* A golden yellow oil occurring chiefly in the livers of freshwater fish and having about 40 percent of the biological activity of vitamin A_1.

vitamin A acid *n.* See **retinoic acid.**

vitamin B *n.* **1.** Vitamin B complex. **2.** A member of the vitamin B complex, especially thiamine.

vitamin B_1 *n.* See **thiamine.**

vitamin B_2 *n.* See **riboflavin.**

vitamin B_6 *n.* Pyridoxine and related compounds.

vitamin B_{12} *n.* A complex compound containing cobalt, found especially in liver and widely used to treat pernicious anemia. Also called *antipernicious anemia factor, cobalamin, cyanocobalamin, extrinsic factor.*

vitamin B_{12} neuropathy *n.* See **subacute combined degeneration of spinal cord.**

vitamin B_c *n.* See **folic acid.**

vitamin B_x *n.* See **PABA.**

vitamin B complex *n.* A group of water-soluble vitamins including thiamine, riboflavin, niacin, pantothenic acid, biotin, pyridoxine, folic acid, inositol, and vitamin B_{12} and occurring chiefly in yeast, liver, eggs, and some vegetables. Also called *B complex.*

vitamin C *n.* See **ascorbic acid.**

vitamin D *n.* A fat-soluble vitamin occurring in several forms, especially vitamin D_2 or vitamin D_3, required for normal growth of teeth and bones, and produced in general by ultraviolet irradiation of sterols found in milk, fish, and eggs.

vitamin D₂ *n.* A white crystalline compound produced by ultraviolet irradiation of ergosterol. Also called *calciferol, ergocalciferol.*

vitamin D₃ *n.* A colorless crystalline compound found in fish-liver oils, irradiated milk, and all irradiated animal foodstuffs and having biological activity similar to vitamin D₂. Also called *cholecalciferol.*

vitamin D milk *n.* Cow's milk that has had vitamin D added to it.

vitamin D-resistant rickets *n.* An inherited form of rickets characterized by high concentrations of phosphate in the blood due to defective renal tubular reabsorption of phosphate and subnormal absorption of dietary calcium. Also called *X-linked hypophosphatemic osteomalacia.*

vitamin E *n.* A fat-soluble vitamin found chiefly in plant leaves, wheat germ oil, and milk and used to treat sterility and various abnormalities of the muscles, red blood cells, liver, and brain.

vitamin G *n.* Riboflavin.

vitamin H *n.* Biotin.

vitamin K *n.* Any of several fat-soluble compounds that are found in alfalfa, hog liver, fish meal, and vegetable oils and are essential for the production of normal amounts of prothrombin. Also called *antihemorrhagic factor.*

vitamin K₁ *n.* A yellow viscous oil found in leafy green vegetables or made synthetically, used by the body to form prothrombin.

vitamin K₂ *n.* Any of various yellowish crystalline compounds isolated from putrefied fish meal or from various intestinal bacteria and used to stop hemorrhaging. Also called *menaquinone.*

vitamin P *n.* A water-soluble vitamin, found as a crystalline substance especially in citrus juices, that functions as a bioflavonoid in promoting capillary resistance to hemorrhaging. Also called *capillary permeability factor.*

vi·tel·li·form degeneration (vĭ-tĕl′ə-fôrm′, vī-) *n.* Macular degeneration in Best's disease.

vi·tel·line (vĭ-tĕl′ĭn, -ēn′, vī-) *adj.* Of, relating to, or associated with the yolk of an egg. —*n.* The yolk of an egg.

vitelline membrane *n.* **1.** The membrane enveloping the yolk of an egg. Also called *ovular membrane, yolk membrane.* **2.** The pellucid zone of a mammalian ovum. Also called *yolk membrane.*

vitelline pole *n.* See **vegetal pole.**

vitelline vessel *n.* **1.** The artery that carries blood to the yolk sac from the embryo. **2.** The vein that carries blood from the yolk sac to the embryo.

vi·tel·lo·in·tes·ti·nal cyst (vĭt′l-ō-ĭn-tĕs′tə-nəl, vĭt′-) *n.* A small tumor that is at the umbilicus of an infant and is caused by the persistence of a segment of the vitellointestinal duct.

vi·tel·lus (vĭ-tĕl′əs, vī-) *n., pl.* **-lus·es** The yolk of an egg.

vi·ti·a·tion (vĭsh′ē-ā′shən) *n.* A change in a process that impairs utility or reduces efficiency.

vit·i·lig·i·nous (vĭt′l-ĭj′ə-nəs) *adj.* Of, relating to, or characterized by vitiligo.

vit·i·li·go (vĭt′l-ī′gō, -ē′gō) *n., pl.* **-gos** *or* **vit·i·lig·i·nes** (vĭt′l-ĭj′ə-nēz) See **leukoderma.**

vit·rec·to·my (vĭ-trĕk′tə-mē) *n.* Surgical removal of the vitreous humor from the eyeball.

vit·re·i·tis (vĭt′rē-ī′tĭs) *n.* See **hyalitis.**

vitreo– *pref.* Vitreous: *vitreoretinal.*

vit·re·o·den·tin (vĭt′rē-ō-dĕn′tĭn) *n.* A variety of dentin having a particular brittle hardness.

vit·re·o·ret·i·nal (vĭt′rē-ō-rĕt′n-əl) *adj.* Of, relating to, or affecting the limit between the retina and the vitreous body.

vitreoretinal choroidopathy syndrome *n.* An inherited eye disorder that is characterized by peripheral pigmentary retinopathy, retinal vascular abnormalities, opacity of the vitreous humor, choroidal atrophy, and presenile cataracts.

vit·re·ous (vĭt′rē-əs) *adj.* **1.** Of, relating to, resembling, or having the nature of glass; glassy. **2.** Of or relating to the vitreous body. —*n.* The vitreous body.

vitreous body *n.* A transparent jellylike substance enclosing the vitreous humor and filling the interior of the eyeball behind the lens. Also called *hyaloid body, vitreum.*

vitreous chamber of eye *n.* The large space between the lens and the retina, filled with the vitreous body.

vitreous detachment *n.* The separation of the peripheral vitreous humor from the retina.

vitreous hernia *n.* Internal prolapse of the vitreous humor into the anterior chamber of the eye; it may follow removal or displacement of the lens from the lenticular space.

vitreous humor *n.* **1.** The clear gelatinous substance that fills the eyeball between the retina and the lens. **2.** The vitreous body.

vitreous membrane *n.* **1.** A condensation of fine collagen fibers in the cortex of the vitreous body. Also called *hyaloid membrane.* **2.** See **limiting layer of cornea** (sense 2). **3.** See **basal layer** (sense 2).

vit·re·um (vĭt′rē-əm) *n.* See **vitreous body.**

vit·ri·fi·ca·tion (vĭt′rə-fĭ-kā′shən) *n.* The process of using heat and fusion to convert dental porcelain to a glassy substance.

vit·ri·ol (vĭt′rē-ōl′, -əl) *n.* **1.** Any of various sulfates of metals, such as ferrous sulfate, zinc sulfate, or copper sulfate. **2.** See **sulfuric acid.**

vi·vax (vī′văks) *n.* **1.** The protozoan (*Plasmodium vivax*) that causes the most common form of malaria. **2.** Vivax malaria.

vivax malaria *n.* Malaria in which the paroxysms recur every third day, counting inclusively, and are induced by the release of merozoites and their invasion of new red blood cells. Also called *tertian malaria.*

vivi– *pref.* Living; alive: *viviparous.*

viv·i·fi·ca·tion (vĭv′ə-fĭ-kā′shən) *n.* **1.** The process of converting protein from food into the living matter of the cells. **2.** See **revivification.**

vi·vip·a·rous (vī-vĭp′ər-əs, vĭ-) *adj.* Giving birth to living offspring that develop within the mother's body as for most mammals.

viv·i·sec·tion (vĭv′ĭ-sĕk′shən, vĭv′ĭ-sĕk′-) *n.* The act or practice of cutting into or performing surgery on living animals, especially for the purpose of scientific research. —**viv′i·sec′tion·ist** n.

VLDL abbr. very low-density lipoprotein

VMD abbr. Latin Veterinariae Medicinae Doctor (Doctor of Veterinary Medicine)

VNA abbr. Visiting Nurse Association

vo·cal (vō′kəl) adj. 1. Of or relating to the voice. 2. Capable of emitting sound or speech.

vocal cord n. The sharp edge of a fold of mucous membrane stretching along either wall of the larynx from the angle between the laminae of the thyroid cartilage to the vocal process of the arytenoid cartilage. Vibrations of these cords are used in voice production. Also called *true vocal cord, vocal fold*.

vocal cord nodules pl.n. Small circumscribed beadlike enlargements on the vocal cords caused by overuse or abuse of the voice. Also called *singer's nodes*.

vocal fold n. See **vocal cord**.

vocal fremitus n. The vibration felt by a hand placed on the chest of an individual who is speaking.

vocal ligament n. The band that extends on either side from the thyroid cartilage to the vocal process of the arytenoid cartilage.

vocal muscle n. A muscle with origin from the depression between the two laminae of the thyroid cartilage, with insertion into the vocal process of the arytenoid, with nerve supply from the recurrent laryngeal nerve, and whose action shortens and relaxes the vocal cords.

vocal resonance n. Abbr. **VR** The voice sounds heard on auscultation of the chest of an individual who is vocalizing in some manner.

vocal tic n. An involuntary, abrupt, and inappropriate grunt, bark, or other exclamation or utterance, occurring especially in Tourette's syndrome.

Vogt-Spielmeyer disease (fōkt′-) n. See **Spielmeyer-Vogt disease**.

Voh·win·kel syndrome (vō-wĭng′kəl, fō-vĭng′-) n. See **mutilating keratoderma**.

voice (vois) n. The sound made by air passing out through the larynx and upper respiratory tract and produced by the vibration of the vocal organs.

void (void) v. To excrete body wastes. —adj. Containing no matter; empty.

void·ing cystogram (voi′dĭng) n. See **cystourethrogram**.

Voigt's lines (voits) n. Boundaries on a skin area innervated by a main cutaneous nerve.

Voit (foit), **Carl von** 1831–1908. German physiologist known for his studies on metabolism.

vo·la (vō′lə) n., pl **-lae** (-lē) The palm or sole. —**vo′lar** (-lər) adj.

vol·a·tile (vŏl′ə-tl, -tīl′) adj. 1. Evaporating readily at normal temperatures and pressures. 2. That can be readily vaporized. 3. Tending to violence; explosive, as of behavior.

volatile oil n. A rapidly evaporating oil of plant derivation, especially an essential oil, that is capable of distillation and that does not leave a stain. Also called *ethereal oil*.

vol·a·til·i·za·tion (vŏl′ə-tl-ĭ-zā′shən) n. See **evaporation** (sense 2).

vo·li·tion (və-lĭsh′ən) n. 1. The act or an instance of making a conscious choice or decision. 2. A conscious choice or decision. 3. The power or faculty of choosing; the will. —**vo·li′tion·al** adj.

volitional tremor n. See **intention tremor**.

Volk·mann's canal (fōlk′mənz, -mänz′) n. Any of the various canals in bone that transmit blood vessels from the periosteum into the bone.

Volkmann's contracture n. Contraction of the hand and fingers and related tissue degeneration caused by reduced blood flow, as from an injury or improper use of a tourniquet.

vol·ley (vŏl′ē) n. The bursting forth of many things together, such as a synchronous group of impulses induced simultaneously by artificial stimulation of either nerve fibers or muscle fibers.

volt (vōlt) n. Abbr. **V** A unit of electromotive force in the International System of Units that will produce a current of 1 ampere in a circuit that has resistance of 1 ohm.

volt·age (vōl′tĭj) n. Electromotive force or potential difference, usually expressed in volts.

volt·am·pere (vōlt′ăm′pîr) n. A unit of electrical power equivalent to 1 watt or one thousandth (10^{-3}) of a kilowatt.

Vol·ta·ren (vōl′tə-rĕn) A trademark for the drug diclofenac potassium.

vol·ume (vŏl′yōōm, -yəm) n. 1. The amount of space occupied by a three-dimensional object or region of space, expressed in cubic units. 2. The capacity of such a region or of a specified container, expressed in cubic units.

volume index n. An index representing the relative size of red blood cells, equal to the percentage of hematocrit that is normal divided by the percentage of red blood cells that are normal.

vol·u·met·ric (vŏl′yōō-mĕt′rĭk) adj. Of or relating to measurement by volume. —**vol′u·met′ri·cal·ly** adv.

volumetric analysis n. 1. Quantitative analysis using accurately measured titrated volumes of standard chemical solutions. 2. Analysis of a gas by volume.

volumetric solution n. Abbr. **VS** A solution made by mixing specified volumes of the components.

vol·un·tar·y (vŏl′ən-tĕr′ē) adj. 1. Arising from or acting on one's own free will. 2. Normally controlled by individual volition, as of respiration. 3. Capable of making choices; having the faculty of will.

voluntary muscle n. A muscle, such as any of the striated muscles except the heart, whose action is normally controlled by individual volition.

vo·lute (və-lōōt′) adj. Rolled up; convoluted.

vol·vu·lo·sis (vŏl′vyə-lō′sĭs) n. See **onchocerciasis**.

vol·vu·lus (vŏl′vyə-ləs) n. Abnormal twisting of the intestine causing obstruction.

vo·mer (vō′mər) n. A thin flat bone of trapezoidal shape that forms the inferior and posterior portion of the nasal septum and articulates with the sphenoid and ethmoid bones, the two maxillae, and the two palatine bones. —**vo′mer·ine′** (-mə-rīn′) adj.

vomerine cartilage n. A narrow strip of cartilage located between the lower edge of the cartilage of the nasal septum and the vomer. Also called *vomeronasal cartilage.*

vom·i·ca (vŏm′ĭ-kə) *n.* **1.** Profuse expectoration of putrid matter. **2.** An abnormal pus-containing cavity, usually in a lung, caused by deterioration of tissue. **3.** The pus contained in such a cavity.

vom·it (vŏm′ĭt) *v.* To eject part or all of the stomach contents through the mouth, usually in a series of involuntary spasmic movements. —*n.* **1.** The act or an instance of ejecting matter from the stomach through the mouth. **2.** Matter ejected from the stomach through the mouth. **3.** An emetic.

vom·it·ing of pregnancy (vŏm′ĭ-tĭng) *n.* Vomiting occurring in the early months of pregnancy, as in morning sickness.

vomiting reflex *n.* Contraction of the abdominal muscles with relaxation of the cardiac sphincter of the stomach and of the muscles of the throat elicited by a variety of stimuli, especially by a stimulus applied to the fauces. Also called *pharyngeal reflex.*

vom·i·tive (vŏm′ĭ-tĭv) *n.* An emetic. —*adj.* Relating to or causing vomiting.

vom·i·to·ry (vŏm′ĭ-tôr′ē) *adj.* Inducing vomiting; vomitive. —*n.* **1.** Something that induces vomiting. **2.** An aperture through which matter is discharged.

vom·i·tu·ri·tion (vŏm′ĭ-chə-rĭsh′ən) *n.* Forceful attempts at vomiting without bringing up the contents of the stomach; retching. Also called *dry vomiting.*

vom·i·tus (vŏm′ĭ-təs) *n.* Vomited matter.

von E·co·no·mo's disease (vŏn ĕk′ə-nō′mōz, fôn) *n.* See **encephalitis lethargica.**

von Gier·ke's disease (vŏn gîr′kəz, fôn) *n.* See **type 1 glycogenosis.**

von Grae·fe's sign (vŏn grā′fəz) *n.* Variant of **Graefe's sign.**

von Hip·pel-Lindau disease *or* **von Hippel-Lindau syndrome** (vŏn hĭp′əl-, fôn) *n.* See **Lindau's disease.**

von Reck·ling·hau·sen's disease (vŏn rĕk′lĭng-hou′zənz, fôn) *n.* See **neurofibromatosis.**

von Wil·le·brand's disease (vŏn wĭl′ə-brăndz′, fôn vĭl′ə-bränts′) *n.* A hereditary predisposition to hemorrhaging characterized by bleeding from mucous membranes and various abnormalities in the blood components responsible for clotting. Also called *angiohemophilia, vascular hemophilia.*

vor·tex (vôr′tĕks′) *n., pl.* **–tex·es** *or* **–ti·ces** (-tĭ-sēz′) A spiral motion of fluid within a limited area, especially a whirling mass of water or air that sucks everything near it toward its center.

vortex vein *n.* Any of the veins in the tunica vasculosa that are formed of branches from the posterior surface of the eye and the ciliary body and empty into the superior or the inferior ophthalmic vein. Also called *vorticose vein.*

vox·el (vŏk′səl) *n.* The basic unit of computed tomography reconstruction, represented as a pixel in a computed tomography image display.

voy·eur (voi-yûr′) *n.* **1.** A person who derives sexual gratification from observing nudity or sexual acts of others, especially from a secret vantage point. **2.** An obsessive observer of sordid or sensational subjects.

voy·eur·ism (voi-yûr′ĭz′əm) *n.* The practice of being a voyeur. Also called *scopophilia.*

VP *abbr.* vasopressin

V/Q scan (vē′kyōō′) *n.* See **ventilation-perfusion scan.**

VR *abbr.* vocal resonance

VS *abbr.* volumetric solution

VSD *abbr.* ventricular septal defect

vul·gar·is (vŭl-gâr′ĭs) *adj.* Being of the usual type; common.

vul·ner·a·ble phase (vŭl′nər-ə-bəl) *n.* A phase in the cardiac cycle during which an ectopic impulse may lead to repetitive activity, such as flutter or fibrillation, of the affected chamber.

vul·ner·ar·y (vŭl′nə-rĕr′ē) *adj.* Used in the healing or treating of wounds. —*n.* A remedy used in healing or treating wounds.

vul·sel·lum (vŭl-sĕl′əm) *n., pl.* **-la** (-lə) A forceps with a small hook or hooks at the tip of each blade.

vul·va (vŭl′və) *n., pl.* **–vae** (-vē) The external genital organs of the female, including the labia majora, labia minora, clitoris, and vestibule of the vagina. —**vul′val, vul′var** (-vər, -vär′) *adj.*

vul·vec·to·my (vŭl-vĕk′tə-mē) *n.* Surgical removal of the vulva.

vul·vi·tis (vŭl-vī′tĭs) *n.* Inflammation of the vulva.

vulvo– *or* **vulv–** *pref.* Vulva: *vulvitis.*

vul·vo·dyn·i·a (vŭl′vō-dĭn′ē-ə) *n.* Chronic vulvar pain.

vul·vo·vag·i·nal (vŭl′vō-văj′ə-nəl) *adj.* Of or relating to the vulva and the vagina.

vul·vo·vag·i·ni·tis (vŭl′vō-văj′ə-nī′tĭs) *n.* Inflammation of the vulva and the vagina, or of the vulvovaginal glands.

V wave *n.* A large pressure wave that is visible in electrocardiograms from either the atrium or the incoming veins and is normally produced by venous return.

V-Y plas·ty (vē′wī′ plăs′tē) *n.* A surgical method for lengthening tissues in one direction by cutting in the lines of a V, sliding the two segments apart, and closing in the lines of a Y.

W

W¹ The symbol for the element **tungsten**.

W² *Abbr.* **watt**

Waar·den·burg syndrome (wôr′dn-bûrg′, vär′-) *n.* An inherited syndrome marked by displacement of the medial canthi and lacrimal puncta, a broad nasal bridge, multicolored or hyperpigmented irises, cochlear deafness, and a white forelock.

Wag·ner von Jau·regg (väg′nər fôn you′rĕk′), **Julius** 1857–1940. Austrian neurologist and psychiatrist. He shared a 1927 Nobel Prize for using a malaria inoculation in the treatment of general paralysis.

waist (wāst) *n.* **1.** The part of the human trunk between the bottom of the rib cage and the pelvis. **2.** The middle section or part of an object, especially when narrower than the rest.

waist of heart *n.* The middle segment of the cardiac silhouette in a chest x-ray.

Waks·man (wăks′mən), **Selman Abraham** 1888–1973. Russian-born American microbiologist. He won a 1952 Nobel Prize for discovering the antibiotic streptomycin.

Wald (wôld), **George** 1906–1997. American biologist. He shared a 1967 Nobel Prize for research on the role of vitamin A in vision.

Wal·den·ström's macroglobulinemia (väl′dən-strĕmz′, -strœmz′) *n.* Macroglobulinemia occurring in older persons, especially women, characterized by anemia, hyperglobulinemia, and the proliferation of cells resembling white blood cells or plasma cells in the bone marrow.

Wal·dey·er's fossa (väl′dī′ərz) *n.* Either of two peritoneal recesses, the inferior and the superior, lying behind the duodenal fold.

wale (wāl) *n.* A mark raised on the skin, as by a whip; a weal or welt. —*v.* To raise marks on the skin, as by whipping.

walk (wôk) *v.* To move over a surface by taking steps with the feet at a pace slower than a run. —*n.* **1.** The gait of a human in which the feet are lifted alternately with one part of a foot always on the ground. **2.** The characteristic way in which one walks.

walk·er (wô′kər) *n.* **1.** A frame device used to support someone, such as an infant learning to walk or a convalescent learning to walk again. **2.** A shoe specially designed for walking comfortably. Often used in the plural.

walk-through angina *n.* Angina pectoris in which continuing activity, such as walking, does not increase or prolong the pain, but instead brings about relief.

wall (wôl) *n.* An investing part enclosing a cavity, chamber, or other anatomical unit.

Wal·lace (wŏl′ĭs), **Alfred Russel** 1823–1913. British naturalist who developed a concept of evolution that paralleled the work of Charles Darwin.

wal·le·ri·an degeneration (wŏ-lîr′ē-ən) *n.* The degeneration of a nerve fiber that has been separated from its nutritive center by injury or disease, characterized by segmentation of the myelin and resulting in atrophy and destruction of the axon. Also called *orthograde degeneration, secondary degeneration.*

wall·eye (wôl′ī′) *n.* **1.** Absence of color in the iris. **2.** The condition of having a dense white opacity of the cornea. **3.** See **exotropia**.

wall·eyed (wôl′īd′) *adj.* **1.** Having a walleye. **2.** Affected with walleye. **3.** Having large bulging or staring eyes. **4.** Having eyes with distended pupils.

Wal·thard's cell rest (väl′tärts) *n.* An accumulation of epithelial cells in the peritoneum of the uterine tubes or ovary.

waltzed flap (wôltst, wôlst) *n.* See **caterpillar flap**.

wan·der·ing (wŏn′dər-ĭng) *adj.* Moving about freely; not fixed; abnormally motile.

wandering abscess *n.* An abscess formed by pus burrowing along fascial planes and occurring at a distance from the primary focus of infection. Also called *migrating abscess.*

wandering cell *n.* See **ameboid cell**.

wandering goiter *n.* See **diving goiter**.

wandering kidney *n.* See **floating kidney**.

wandering pacemaker *n.* A disturbance of the normal cardiac rhythm in which the site of the controlling pacemaker shifts from beat to beat, usually between the sinoatrial and atrioventricular nodes.

Wan·gen·steen tube (wăng′gən-stēn′) *n.* A modified siphon that maintains constant negative pressure; used in the treatment of gastric and intestinal distention.

War·burg (wôr′bərg, vär′bŏŏrk′), **Otto Heinrich** 1883–1970. German biochemist. He won a 1931 Nobel Prize for research on the respiration of cells.

ward (wôrd) *n.* **1.** A room in a hospital usually holding six or more patients. **2.** A division in a hospital for the care of a particular group of patients.

war·fa·rin sodium (wôr′fər-ĭn) *n.* An anticoagulant with the same actions as dicumarol.

warm-blood·ed (wôrm′blŭd′ĭd) *adj.* Maintaining a relatively constant and warm body temperature independent of environmental temperature; homeothermic. —**warm′-blood′ed·ness** *n.*

War·ren (wôr′ən), **John Collins** 1778–1856. American surgeon who gave the first public demonstration (1846) of the use of ether as an anesthetic for a surgical procedure.

wart (wôrt) *n.* A hard, rough lump that grows on the skin and is caused by infection with certain viruses; it typically occurs on the hands or feet. Also called *verruca, verruga.*

War·thin's tumor (wôr′thĭnz) *n.* See **adenolymphoma**.

wart·y dyskeratoma (wôr′tē) *n.* A benign solitary tumor of the skin, usually of the scalp, face, or neck, that appears to arise from a hair follicle and includes extensive epithelial downgrowth.

wash (wŏsh) *v.* **1.** To cleanse, using water or other liquid, usually with soap, detergent, or bleach, by immersing, dipping, rubbing, or scrubbing. **2.** To make moist or wet. —*n.* **1.** The act or process of cleansing or washing. **2.** A solution used to cleanse or bathe a part.

Was·ser·mann (wä′sər-mən, vä′sər-män′), **August von** 1866–1925. German physician who developed the Wasserman test for the detection of syphilis.

Was·ser·mann·fast (wä′sər-mən-făst′) *adj.* Having a positive Wassermann test in spite of treatment.

Was·ser·mann reaction (wä′sər-mən) *n. Abbr.* **WR** A complement-fixing reaction in the Wassermann test.

Wassermann test *n.* A diagnostic test for syphilis involving the fixation or inactivation of a complement by an antibody in a blood serum sample.

waste (wāst) *v.* To gradually lose energy, strength, or bodily substance, as from disease. —*n.* The undigested residue of food eliminated from the body; excrement.

waste product *n.* **1.** Useless or worthless debris produced during or as a result of an activity or other process. **2.** Organic waste matter such as urine, feces, or dead cells.

wast·ing (wās′tĭng) *adj.* **1.** Gradually deteriorating; declining. **2.** Sapping the strength or substance of the body, as a disease; emaciating. —*n.* Emaciation.

wa·ter (wô′tər) *n.* **1.** A clear, colorless, odorless, and tasteless liquid essential for most plant and animal life and the most widely used of all solvents. Freezing point 0°C (32°F); boiling point 100°C (212°F); specific gravity (4°C) 1.0000; weight per gallon (15°C) 8.338 pounds (3.782 kilograms). **2.** Any of the liquids that are present in or passed out of the body, such as urine, perspiration, tears, or saliva. **3.** The fluid that surrounds a fetus in the uterus; amniotic fluid. **4.** An aqueous solution of a substance, especially a gas.

water bag *n.* The membranous sac filled with amniotic fluid that protects a fetus during pregnancy. Also called *bag of waters.*

water balance *n.* See **fluid balance.**

water blister *n.* A blister having watery contents without blood or pus.

wa·ter·fall (wô′tər-fôl′) *n.* Blood flow in vascular beds where lateral pressure greatly exceeds venous pressure and tends to collapse vessels.

water for injection *n.* Water that has been purified by distillation for the preparation of products for parenteral use.

water glass *n.* See **soluble glass.**

water-hammer pulse *n.* A pulse having a forcible impulse immediately followed by collapse, characteristic of aortic incompetency. Also called *cannonball pulse, Corrigan's pulse.*

Wa·ter·house-Frid·er·ich·sen syndrome (wô′tər-hous′frĭd′ə-rĭk′sən) *n.* Acute fulminating meningococcal septicemia occurring mainly in children under 10 years old and characterized by vomiting, diarrhea, extensive purpura, cyanosis, convulsions, and circulatory collapse, usually accompanied by meningitis and hemorrhage into the adrenal glands.

water of crystallization *n.* Water in chemical combination with a crystal, necessary for the maintenance of crystalline properties but capable of being removed by sufficient heat.

water of hydration *n.* Water chemically combined with a substance in such a way that it can be removed, as by heating, without substantially changing the chemical composition of the substance.

water of metabolism *n.* Water that is formed in the body by oxidation of the hydrogen in foods, as in the metabolism of fat.

water on the brain *n.* Hydrocephalus.

wa·ter·shed (wô′tər-shĕd′) *n.* **1.** A ridge between two areas that directs drainage to either side. **2.** The area of marginal blood flow at the extreme periphery of a vascular bed. **3.** Ridges of the lumbar vertebrae and the pelvic brim formed in the abdominal cavity, which determine the direction in which a free effusion will gravitate when the body is supine.

watershed infarction *n.* Infarction of the cerebral cortex in an area of blood supply between two major cerebral arteries.

water-trap stomach *n.* A stomach that does not empty itself properly due to a relatively high pyloric outlet.

wa·ter·y (wô′tə-rē) *adj.* **1.** Filled with, consisting of, or soaked with water; wet or soggy. **2.** Secreting or discharging water or watery fluid, especially as a symptom of disease.

Wat·son (wŏt′sən), **James Dewey** Born 1928. American biologist who with Francis Crick proposed a spiral model, the double helix, for the molecular structure of DNA. He shared a 1962 Nobel Prize for advances in the study of genetics.

Watson-Crick helix *n.* See **double helix.**

Watson-Crick model *n.* A three-dimensional model of the DNA molecule, consisting of two polynucleotide strands wound in the form of a double helix and joined in a ladderlike fashion by hydrogen bonds between purine and pyrimidine bases.

watt (wŏt) *n. Abbr.* **W** A unit of power in the International System of Units equal to one joule per second.

wave (wāv) *n.* **1.** A disturbance traveling through a medium by which energy is transferred from one particle of the medium to another without causing any permanent displacement of the medium itself. **2.** A graphic representation of the variation of such a disturbance with time. **3.** A single cycle that is representative of such a disturbance.

wave·length (wāv′lĕngkth′, -lĕngth′) *n. Symbol* **λ** The distance between one peak or crest of a wave of light, heat, or other energy and the next corresponding peak or crest.

wax (wăks) *n.* **1.** Any of various natural, oily or greasy heat-sensitive substances, consisting of hydrocarbons or esters of fatty acids that are insoluble in water but soluble in most organic solvents. **2.** Cerumen. **3.** A solid plastic or pliable liquid substance, such as paraffin, originating from petroleum and found in rock layers and often used in medicinal preparations.

wax·ing (wăk′sĭng) *or* **wax·ing-up** (wăk′sĭng-ŭp′) *n.* The shaping of the contours of a trial denture or crown in wax prior to its casting in metal.

wax·y degeneration (wăk′sē) *n.* **1.** See **amyloid degeneration. 2.** See **Zenker's degeneration.**

waxy kidney *n.* See **amyloid kidney.**

waxy spleen *n.* Amyloidosis of the spleen.

Wb *abbr.* weber

WBC *abbr.* white blood cell

WDLL *abbr.* well-differentiated lymphocytic lymphoma

weal (wēl) *n.* A ridge on the flesh raised by a blow; a welt.

wean (wēn) *v.* **1.** To deprive permanently of breast milk and begin to nourish with other food. **2.** To accustom the young of a mammal to take nourishment other than by suckling. **3.** To gradually withdraw from a life-support system.

wear-and-tear pigment (wâr′ənd-târ′) *n.* Lipofuscin that accumulates in aging or atrophic cells as a residue of lysosomal digestion.

web (wĕb) *n.* **1.** A membrane or fold of skin connecting the toes, as of certain mammals. **2.** A structure of delicate, threadlike filaments characteristically spun by spiders.

webbed fingers (wĕbd) *n.* Two or more fingers united by a common sheath of skin.

webbed neck *n.* The broad neck due to lateral folds of skin extending from the clavicle to the head, as in Turner's syndrome.

web·bing (wĕb′ĭng) *n.* A congenital condition in which adjacent structures or parts are joined by a broad band of tissue that is not normally present to such a degree.

web·er (wĕb′ər, vā′bər) *n. Abbr.* **Wb** A unit of magnetic flux in the International System of Units equal to the product of one tesla and one square meter.

We·ber (vā′bər), **Ernst Heinrich** 1795–1878. German physiologist and psychologist who studied sensory response and is considered a founder of experimental psychology.

Web·er-Christian disease (wĕb′ər-) *n.* See **nodular nonsuppurative panniculitis.**

We·ber-Fechner law (vā′bər-) *n.* The principle that the intensity of a sensation varies by a series of equal arithmetic increments as the strength of the stimulus is increased geometrically. Also called *Fechner-Weber law.*

We·ber's gland (vā′bərz) *n.* Any of the various muciparous glands on either side of the posterior border of the tongue.

We·ber's paradox (vā′bərz) *n.* The paradox stating that, if a muscle is loaded beyond its power to contract, it may elongate.

Web·er's syndrome (wĕb′ərz) *n.* A form of alternating hemiplegia caused by a lesion in the cerebral peduncle and resulting in paralysis of the oculomotor nerve on the side of the lesion and paralysis of the extremities and of the face and tongue on the opposite side.

We·ber's test (vā′bərz) *n.* A test for differentiating conductive hearing impairment from sensorineural hearing impairment. A vibrating tuning fork is applied to one of several points in the midline of the forehead; if the sound is heard better in the impaired ear, the middle-ear apparatus is at fault; if the sound is heard better in the normal ear, the hearing impairment is caused by diseased sensorineural apparatus.

web·foot (wĕb′fŏŏt′) *n.* A foot with webbed toes.

Wechs·ler adult intelligence scale (wĕks′lər) *n.* A standardized intelligence test for assessing people aged 16 and older.

Wechsler intelligence scale for children *n.* A standardized intelligence test that is used for assessing children from 5 to 15 years old.

Wechsler preschool and primary scale for intelligence *n.* A standardized intelligence test for assessing preschool children.

wedge-and-groove joint (wĕj′ənd-grŏŏv′) *n.* See **schindylesis.**

wedge-and-groove suture *n.* See **schindylesis.**

wedge bone *n.* Either of two of the cuneiform bones, the lateral or the medial.

wedge pressure *n.* The intravascular pressure reading obtained when a fine catheter is advanced until it completely occludes a small blood vessel.

wedge resection *n.* Surgical removal of a wedge-shaped portion of tissue, as of the ovary.

We·ge·ner's granulomatosis (vā′gə-nərz) *n.* A rare fatal immune disorder, occurring mainly in people in their 40's and 50's, and characterized by granulomatous vasculitis of the small vessels, progressive ulceration of the upper respiratory tract, purulent discharge from the nose, obstruction of the nasal area, and sometimes discharge from the ear, spitting of blood, pulmonary cavitation, and fever.

weight (wāt) *n. Abbr.* **wt 1.** The force with which a body is attracted to Earth or another celestial body and which is equal to the product of the object's mass and the acceleration of gravity. **2.** A measure of the heaviness of an object.

Weil-Fe·lix test (vīl′fā′lĭks) *n.* A test to determine infection with a species of *Rickettsia* in which certain strains of *Proteus vulgaris* are agglutinated when combined with the serum of infected individuals. Also called *Weil-Felix reaction.*

Weil's disease (wīlz, vīlz) *n.* A severe form of leptospirosis characterized by jaundice, fever, muscle pain, and a tendency to hemorrhage.

Weis·mann (vīs′män′), **August Friedrich Leopold** 1834–1914. German biologist who asserted that hereditary characteristics are transmitted by a germinal plasm.

Weit·brecht's foramen (vīt′brĕkts, -brĕkнts) *n.* An opening in the articular capsule of the shoulder joint, communicating with the subtendinous bursa of the subscapular muscle.

Welch (wĕlch, wĕlsh), **William Henry** 1850–1934. American pathologist and bacteriologist who discovered the bacteria that causes gas gangrene.

Well·bu·trin (wĕl′byŏŏ-trĭn) A trademark for the drug bupropion hydrochloride, used to treat depression.

well-dif·fer·en·ti·at·ed lymphocytic lymphoma (wĕl′-dĭf′ə-rĕn′shē-ā′tĭd) *n. Abbr.* **WDLL** A disease that is essentially the same as chronic lymphocytic leukemia except that lymphocytes are not increased in the peripheral blood.

Wel·ler (wĕl′ər), **Thomas Huckle** Born 1915. American microbiologist. He shared a 1954 Nobel Prize for work on the cultivation of the polio virus.

well·ness (wĕl′nĭs) *n.* The condition of good physical, mental and emotional health, especially when maintained by an appropriate diet, exercise, and other lifestyle modifications.

Wells (wĕlz), **Horace** 1815–1848. American dentist who was the first to use nitrous oxide to anesthetize patients during oral surgery.

Wells' syndrome (wĕlz) *n.* Recurrent cellulitis followed by an eruption of skin lesions that are usually brawny, filled with fluid, and heavily infiltrated by eosinophils and histiocytes. Also called *eosinophilic cellulitis.*

welt (wĕlt) *n.* **1.** A ridge or bump on the skin caused by a lash or blow or sometimes by an allergic reaction. **2.** See **wheal.**

wen (wĕn) *n.* See **sebaceous cyst.**

Wenck·e·bach period (vĕn′kə-bäk′, -bäκн′) *n.* A sequence of cycles in the electrocardiogram ending in a dropped beat due to atrioventricular block, with the preceding cycles showing progressively lengthening P-R intervals; the P-R interval following the dropped beat is again shortened.

Werl·hof's disease (wûrl′hôfs′, vĕrl′-) *n.* See **idiopathic thrombocytopenic purpura.**

Wer·ner's syndrome (vĕr′nərz) *n.* A hereditary disease of young adults characterized by short stature, early graying, cataracts, vascular disorders, and generally premature aging and death.

Wer·nick·e-Korsakoff encephalopathy (vĕr′nĭ-kē-, -kə-) *n.* Encephalopathy due to Wernicke's syndrome and Korsakoff's syndrome.

Wernicke-Korsakoff syndrome *n.* Wernicke's syndrome and Korsakoff's syndrome occurring together.

Wer·nick·e's center (vĕr′nĭ-kēz, -kəz) *n.* A large region of the parietal and temporal lobes of the left cerebral hemisphere, thought to be essential for understanding and formulating coherent, propositional speech. Also called *sensory speech center, Wernicke's area.*

Wernicke's encephalopathy *n.* See **Wernicke's syndrome.**

Wernicke's reaction *n.* A reaction seen in hemianopsia in which the pupil constricts when light is directed to the normal side of the retina, but fails to constrict when light is directed to the retina's blind side. Also called *hemiopic pupillary reaction, Wernicke's sign.*

Wernicke's syndrome *n.* A disease of the nervous system caused by a deficiency of thiamine and characterized by abnormal eye movements, a loss of muscle coordination, tremors, and confusion; it is almost always followed by amnesia and is most often seen in chronic alcoholics. Also called *Wernicke's encephalopathy.*

Wert·heim's operation (vĕrt′hīmz′) *n.* A radical hysterectomy for treatment of uterine cancer, in which as much as possible of the vagina is excised, and lymph nodes are excised throughout a broad area.

Wes·ter·gren method (wĕs′tər-grĕn′, vĕs′-) *n.* A method for estimating the sedimentation rate of red blood cells in whole blood by mixing venous blood with an aqueous solution of sodium citrate and allowing the mixture to stand in an upright standard pipet and, after one hour, reading the millimeters the cells have descended.

West·ern blot analysis (wĕs′tərn) *n.* An electrophoretic procedure for separating proteins.

Western blot test *n.* A serum electrophoretic analysis used to identify proteins.

West Nile virus (wĕst nīl) *n.* A flavivirus that is transmitted by the bite of a mosquito and that can cause mild febrile illness as well as severe, sometimes fatal encephalitis and meningitis.

West·phal-Erb sign (wĕst′fôl-, vĕst′fäl-) *n.* See **Erb-Westphal sign.**

Westphal-Piltz pupil *n.* See **tonic pupil.**

West·phal's sign (wĕst′fôlz, vĕst′fälz) *n.* See **Erb-Westphal sign.**

Westphal-Strümpell disease *n.* See **pseudosclerosis.**

wet gangrene (wĕt) *n.* Ischemic necrosis of an extremity with bacterial infection.

wet leishmaniasis *n.* See **zoonotic cutaneous leishmaniasis.**

wet lung *n.* The lung in pulmonary edema.

wet nurse *n.* A woman employed to breast-feed a child that is not her own.

wet pleurisy *n.* Pleurisy with effusion.

Whar·ton's duct (wôr′tnz) *n.* See **submandibular duct.**

Wharton's jelly *n.* The mucous connective tissue of the umbilical cord.

wheal (wēl) *n.* A small swelling on the skin, as from an insect bite, that usually itches or burns. Also called *welt.*

wheal-and-flare reaction *n.* The characteristic immediate reaction to an injected allergen in a skin test, in which an irregular blanched wheal appears, surrounded by an area of redness. Also called *wheal-and-erythema reaction.*

wheel·chair *or* **wheel chair** (wēl′châr′) *n.* A chair mounted on large wheels for the use of a sick or disabled person.

wheeze (wēz) *v.* To breathe with difficulty, producing a hoarse whistling sound. —*n.* A wheezing sound.

whelk (wĕlk) *n.* An inflamed swelling, such as a pimple or pustule.

whip·lash (wĭp′lăsh′) *n.* Whiplash injury.

whiplash injury *n.* A hyperextension-hyperflexion injury to the cervical spine caused by an abrupt jerking movement of the head, either in a backward or forward direction.

Whip·ple (wĭp′əl), **George Hoyt** 1878–1976. American pathologist. He shared a 1934 Nobel Prize for discovering that a diet of liver relieves anemia.

Whip·ple's disease (wĭp′əlz) *n.* A rare disease in which the intestinal wall is invaded by macrophages containing the remnants of bacteria and which is characterized by steatorrhea, generalized lymphadenopathy, arthritis, fever, and cough. Also called *intestinal lipodystrophy.*

Whipple's operation *n.* See **pancreatoduodenectomy.**

whip·worm (wĭp′wûrm′) *n.* See **Trichuris.**

white blood cell (wīt) *n. Abbr.* **WBC** Any of the colorless or white cells in the blood that have a nucleus and cytoplasm and help protect the body from infection and disease through specialized neutrophils, lymphocytes, and monocytes. Also called *leukocyte, white corpuscle.*

white-coat hypertension *n.* Transient hypertension that occurs during a medical examination, presumably as a result of anxiety.

white fiber *n.* See **collagen fiber.**

white gangrene *n.* Death of a body part accompanied by the formation of grayish white sloughs. Also called *leukonecrosis.*

white·head (wīt′hĕd′) *n.* **1.** A tiny epidermal cystlike mass with a narrow or obstructed opening on the skin surface, which may rupture, caused by the retention of secretions of a sebaceous gland. Also called *closed comedo.* **2.** See **milium.**

White·head's operation (wīt′hĕdz′) *n.* Excision of hemorrhoids by two circular incisions above and below involved veins, allowing normal mucosa to be pulled down and sutured to anal skin.

white infarct *n.* See **anemic infarct.**

white line *n.* See **linea alba.**

white line of anal canal *n.* A bluish pink zone located in the mucosa of the anal canal below the pectinate line at the interval between the subcutaneous part of the external sphincter and the lower border of the internal sphincter. Also called *Hilton's white line.*

white matter *n.* Whitish nerve tissue, especially of the brain and spinal cord, chiefly composed of myelinated nerve fibers and containing few or no neuronal cell bodies or dendrites. Also called *alba, substantia alba, white substance.*

white muscle *n.* A muscle in which large pale fibers predominate and mitochondria and myoglobin are sparse.

white plague *n.* Tuberculosis, especially of the lungs.

white pulp *n.* The part of the spleen that consists of lymphatic nodules and other concentrations of lymphatic tissue.

white rat *n.* A domesticated albino variety of the Norway rat, used extensively in laboratory experiments.

white sponge nevus *n.* A hereditary mucosal keratosis of the mouth characterized by a thickened white spongy fold of mucosa.

white substance *n.* See **white matter.**

whit·low (wĭt′lō′) *n.* See **felon.**

WHO *abbr.* World Health Organization

whole (hōl) *adj.* **1.** Not wounded, injured, or impaired; sound or unhurt. **2.** Having been restored; healed. —*n.* An entity or system made up of interrelated parts.

whole blood *n.* Blood from which no constituent such as plasma or platelets has been removed.

whole-body counter *n.* A device used to measure the total radiation in the body, usually containing a number of sensitive detectors and shielding to block out ambient radiation.

whole-body titration curve *n.* A graphic representation of the ionic changes in blood in response to disturbances in its acid-base balance.

whole-cell vaccine *n.* Vaccine made up of suspensions of killed bacteria.

whoop (hōōp, wōōp) *n.* The paroxysmal gasp characteristic of whooping cough.

whoop·ing cough (hōō′pĭng, wōō′-, hōōp′ĭng) *n.* A highly contagious disease of the respiratory system, usually affecting children, that is caused by *Bordetella pertussis* and is marked in its advanced stage by spasms of coughing interspersed with deep, noisy inspirations. Also called *pertussis.*

whooping cough vaccine *n.* See **pertussis vaccine.**

whorl (wôrl, wûrl) *n.* **1.** A form that coils or spirals; a curl or swirl. **2.** A turn of the cochlea or of the ethmoidal crest. **3.** An area of hair growing in a radial manner. **4.** One of the circular ridges or convolutions of a fingerprint.

whorled (wôrld, wûrld) *adj.* Having, arranged in, or forming whorls or a whorl.

Wi·dal test (vē-däl′) *n.* A test of blood serum that uses an agglutination reaction to diagnose typhoid fever.

Wie·land (vē′länt′), **Heinrich Otto** 1877–1957. German chemist. He won a 1927 Nobel Prize for his research on bile acids.

Wie·sel (vē′səl), **Torsten Nils** Born 1924. Swedish-born American physiologist. He shared a 1981 Nobel Prize for studies on the organization and function of the brain.

wild type (wīld) *n.* The typical form of an organism, strain, gene, or characteristic as it occurs in nature, as distinguished from mutant forms that may result from selective breeding.

Wil·kins (wĭl′kĭnz), **Maurice Hugh Frederick** 1916–2004. British biophysicist. He shared a 1962 Nobel Prize for his contributions to the determination of the structure of DNA.

Wil·lis (wĭl′ĭs), **Thomas** 1621–1675. English anatomist and physician known for his studies of the nervous system and the brain. He discovered the circle of Willis at the base of the brain.

Wilms' tumor (vĭlms) *n.* A malignant renal tumor occurring in young children and composed of small spindle cells and other tissue. Also called *adenomyosarcoma, embryoma of kidney, nephroblastoma, renal carcinosarcoma.*

Wil·son-Mik·i·ty syndrome (wĭl′sən-mĭk′ĭ-tē) *n.* See **pulmonary dysmaturity syndrome.**

Wil·son's disease (wĭl′sənz) *n.* An inherited disorder of copper metabolism characterized by cirrhosis, degeneration of the basal ganglia of the brain, and the deposition of green pigment in the periphery of the cornea. Also called *hepatolenticular degeneration.*

Win·daus (vĭn′dous′), **Adolf** 1876–1959. German chemist. He won a Nobel Prize (1928) for his research on sterols and their relationship to vitamins, especially vitamin D.

wind·burn (wĭnd′bûrn′) *n.* A reddened irritation of the skin caused by exposure to the wind.

win·dow (wĭn′dō) *n.* A fenestra.

wind·pipe (wĭnd′pīp′) *n.* See **trachea.**

wing (wĭng) *n.* **1.** Any of various paired movable organs of flight, such as the modified forelimb of a bird or bat or one of the membranous organs extending from the thorax of an insect. **2.** Something that resembles a wing in appearance, function, or position relative to a main body.

winged catheter (wĭngd) *n.* A soft rubber catheter with small flaps at each side of the end that serve to retain it in the bladder.

winged scapula *n.* A condition characterized by protrusion of the medial border of the scapula from the thorax as the scapula rotates out, caused by paralysis of the anterior serratus muscle. Also called *scapula alata.*

Wi·ni·war·ter-Buerger disease (wĭn′ə-wär′tər-, vĭn′ĭ-vär′tər) *n.* See **thromboangiitis obliterans.**

wink (wĭngk) *v.* **1.** To close and open the eyelid of one eye deliberately, as to convey a message, signal, or suggestion. **2.** To close and open the eyelids of both eyes; blink. —*n.* A quick closing and opening of the eyelids; a blink.

wink reflex *n.* Reflex closing of eyelids in response to a stimulus.

Win·ni·cott (wĭn′ə-kŏt′), **Donald Woods** 1896–1971. British pediatrician and child psychiatrist noted for his contributions to object relations theory, which deals with the relationship between children and familiar, inanimate objects that mitigate anxiety during times of stress.

wir·ing (wīr′ĭng) *n.* The fastening together of the ends of a broken bone with wire sutures.

Wir·sung's canal (vĭr′sŏŏngz′) *n.* See **pancreatic duct.**

wir·y (wīr′ē) *adj.* **1.** Resembling wire in form or quality, especially in stiffness. **2.** Sinewy and lean. **3.** Filiform and hard. Used of a pulse.

wiry pulse *n.* A small, fine, incompressible pulse.

wis·dom tooth (wĭz′dəm) *n.* The third molar tooth on both sides of each jaw that erupts from the 17th to the 23rd year.

wish fulfillment (wĭsh) *n.* In psychoanalytic theory, the satisfaction of a desire, need, or impulse through a dream or other exercise of the imagination.

Wis·kott-Aldrich syndrome (wĭs′kŏt-, vĭs′kôt-) *n.* An inherited immunodeficiency disorder occurring in male children, characterized by thrombocytopenia, eczema, melena, and susceptibility to recurrent bacterial infections. Also called *Aldrich syndrome.*

Wiss·ler's syndrome (wĭs′lərz, vĭs′-) *n.* A condition occurring in children and adolescents, characterized by high intermittent fever, irregularly recurring macular and maculo-papular eruption, leukocytosis, joint pain, and occasionally eosinophilia and raised red blood cell sedimentation rate.

witch hazel (wĭch) *n.* **1.** Any of several deciduous shrubs or small trees of the genus *Hamamelis,* especially *H. virginiana,* of eastern North America, having yellow flowers that bloom in late autumn or winter. **2.** An alcoholic solution containing an extract of the bark and leaves of this plant, applied externally as a mild astringent.

witch's milk (wĭch′ĭz) *n.* Milk resembling colostrum sometimes secreted from the breasts of newborns of either sex three to four days after birth and lasting no longer than two weeks, due to endocrine stimulation from the mother before birth.

with·draw·al (wĭth-drô′əl, wĭth-) *n.* **1.** Detachment, as from social or emotional involvement. **2.** Discontinuation of the use of an addictive substance. **3.** The physiological and mental readjustment that accompanies such discontinuation. **4.** A pattern of behavior, observed in schizophrenia and depression, that is characterized by a pathological retreat from interpersonal contact and social involvement and that leads to self-preoccupation. **5.** Coitus interruptus.

withdrawal symptom *n.* Any of a group of physical and psychological symptoms occurring in an individual deprived of an accustomed dose of an addicting agent.

wnl *abbr.* within normal limits

wob·ble (wŏb′əl) *n.* **1.** A movement or rotation with an uneven or rocking motion or an unsteady motion from side to side. **2.** The ability of one tRNA anticodon to recognize two mRNA codons, as in the third base of a tRNA anticodon pairing with any of a variety of bases that occupy the third position of different mRNA codons instead of pairing according to base pairing rules. —**wob′bler** *n.*

Wohl·fahr·ti·a (vōl-fär′tē-ə) *n.* A genus of flesh flies whose larvae breed in ulcerated surfaces and flesh wounds.

wohl·fahr·ti·o·sis (vōl-fär′tē-ō′sĭs) *n.* An infection of animals and humans caused by infestation with the larvae of flies of the genus Wohlfahrtia.

Wolfe graft (wŏŏlf) *n.* A full-thickness skin graft without any subcutaneous fat. Also called *Wolfe-Krause graft.*

Wolff (vôlf), **Kaspar Friedrich** 1733–1794. German anatomist noted for his pioneering work in embryology. His chief work, *Theoria Generationis* (1759), refuted the theory of preformation, which held that the embryo is a fully formed miniature adult.

Wolff·i·an *or* **wolff·i·an** (wŏŏl′fē-ən) *adj.* Relating to or described by Kaspar Friedrich Wolff.

wolffian body *n.* See **mesonephros.**

wolffian cyst *n.* A cyst arising from a mesonephric structure.

wolffian duct *n.* A duct in the embryo draining the mesonephric tubules, becoming the vas deferens in the male and forming vestigial structures in the female. Also called *mesonephric duct.*

wolffian rest *n.* Remnants of the wolffian duct in the female genital tract that give rise to cysts.

Wolffian ridge *n.* See **urogenital ridge.**

Wolff-Parkinson-White syndrome (wŏŏlf′-) *n.* An electrocardiographic pattern sometimes associated with paroxysmal tachycardia, characterized by a short P-R interval together with a prolonged QRS complex with a delta wave. Also called *preexcitation syndrome, WPW syndrome.*

Wolff's law (vôlfs) *n.* The principle that every change in the form and the function of a bone or in the function of the bone alone, leads to changes in its internal architecture and in its external form.

Wolf-Or·ton body (wŏŏlf′ôr′tn) *n.* An intranuclear inclusion body of nonviral origin found in cells of malignant neoplasms.

wolf·ram (wŏŏl′frəm) *n.* See **tungsten.**

Wol·man's disease (wôl′mənz) *n.* An inherited disorder of lipid metabolism caused by a deficiency of lysosomal acid lipase and resulting in the widespread accumulation of cholesterol esters and triglycerides in the internal organs.

womb (wŏŏm) *n.* See **uterus.**

wood alcohol (wŏŏd) *n.* See **methanol.**

Wood's lamp (wŏŏdz) *n.* An ultraviolet lamp with a nickel oxide filter that only allows light with a maximal wavelength of about 3660 angstroms to be emitted; it is used to detect hairs that are infected with *Microsporum* fungi.

Wood's light *n.* Ultraviolet light produced by Wood's lamp.

wood sugar *n.* See **xylose.**

wool·ly-hair nevus (wŏŏl′ē-hâr′) *n.* A congenital condition in which hair in a circumscribed area of the scalp is kinky or woolly. Also called *allotrichia circumscripta.*

wool-sorter's disease *n.* A pulmonary form of anthrax that results from the inhalation of spores of the bacterium *Bacillus anthracis* in the wool of contaminated sheep.

word blindness *n.* See **alexia.**

word deafness *n.* Aphasia in which the meaning of ordinary spoken words becomes incomprehensible.

word salad *n.* See **schizophasia.**

work·a·hol·ic (wûr′kə-hô′lĭk) *n.* One who has a compulsive and unrelenting need to work.

work·ers′ compensation (wûr′kərz) *n.* Payments required by law to be made to an employee who is injured or disabled in connection with work.

work·up (wûrk′ŭp′) *n. Abbr.* **w/u** A thorough medical examination for diagnostic purposes.

worm (wûrm) *n.* **1.** Any of various invertebrates, as those of the phyla Annelida, Nematoda, Nemertea, or Platyhelminthes, having a long, flexible, rounded or flattened body, often without obvious appendages. **2.** Any of various crawling insect larvae, such as a grub or caterpillar, having a soft, elongated body. **3.** Any of various unrelated animals, such as the shipworm or the slowworm, resembling a worm in habit or appearance. **4. worms** Infestation of the intestines or other parts of the body with worms or wormlike parasites; helminthiasis.

wor·mi·an (wôr′mē-ən, wûr′-) *adj.* Relating to or described by Danish physician and anatomist Ole Worm (1588–1654).

wormian bone *n.* See **sutural bone.**

wound (wo̅o̅nd) *n.* **1.** Injury to a part or tissue of the body, especially one caused by physical trauma and characterized by tearing, cutting, piercing, or breaking of the tissue. **2.** An incision. —**wound** *v.*

wound clip *n.* A metal clasp or device for bringing tissue edges together for the suture of skin incisions.

wo·ven bone (wō′vən) *n.* Bony tissue characteristic of the embryonic skeleton in which the collagen fibers of the matrix are arranged irregularly in the form of interlacing networks. Also called *nonlamellar bone, reticulated bone.*

W-plas·ty (dŭb′əl-yo̅o̅-plăs′tē, -yŏo-) *n.* A procedure to prevent the contracture of a straight-line scar in which the edges of a wound are trimmed in the shape of a W and closed in a zigzag fashion.

WPW syndrome *n.* See **Wolff-Parkinson-White syndrome.**

WR *abbr.* Wassermann reaction

Wright (rīt), Sir **Almroth Edward** 1861–1947. British physician and pathologist who developed (1896) a vaccine against typhoid fever.

Wright′s stain (rīts) *n.* A specially prepared mixture of methylene blue and eosin in methanol, used in staining blood smears.

wrist (rĭst) *n.* **1.** The joint between the hand and the forearm. **2.** See **carpus.**

wrist-drop *n.* Paralysis of the extensor muscles of the wrist and fingers causing the hand to hang down at the wrist. Also called *carpoptosis, drop hand.*

wrist joint *n.* The joint between the distal end of the radius and its articular disk and the proximal row of carpal bones, except the pisiform bone. Also called *radiocarpal joint.*

wrist sign *n.* An indication of Marfan's syndrome in which the thumb and fifth finger overlap appreciably when the wrist is gripped with the opposite hand.

writ·er′s cramp (rī′tərz) *n.* A cramp or spasm of the muscles of the fingers, hand, and forearm during writing.

writ·ing hand (rī′tĭng) *n.* A contraction of the hand muscles seen in Parkinson's disease, in which the fingers appear to be in the position of holding a pen.

wry·neck (rī′nĕk′) *n.* See **torticollis.**

wt *abbr.* weight

w/u *abbr.* workup

Wu·cher·e·ri·a (wo̅o̅′chə-rîr′ē-ə, vo̅o̅′kə-) *n.* A genus of filarial nematodes of the family Onchocercidae characterized by adult forms that live chiefly in lymphatic vessels, causing obstruction to lymph flow and producing large numbers of embryos or microfilariae that circulate in the bloodstream.

Wuchereria ban·crof·ti (băn-krôf′tī) *n.* A parasitic nematode that is transmitted to humans by mosquitoes and is the causative agent of elephantiasis.

wu·cher·e·ri·a·sis (wo̅o̅′chər-ə-rī′ə-sĭs, vo̅o̅′kər-) *n.* Infestation with worms of the genus *Wuchereria.*

Wundt (vo̅o̅nt), **Wilhelm** 1832–1920. German physiologist who founded the first experimental psychology laboratory. His *Principles of Physiological Psychology* (1873–1874) is considered a classic text.

Wy·burn-Ma·son syndrome (wī′bərn-mā′sən) *n.* Arteriovenous malformation on the cerebral cortex, retinal arteriovenous angioma, and facial nevus, usually occurring in mentally retarded individuals.

X

ξ The Greek letter *xi*. Entries beginning with this character are alphabetized under **xi**.

Xan·ax (zăn′ăks′) A trademark for the drug alprazolam.

xan·than gum (zăn′thən) *n*. A natural gum of high molecular weight produced by culture fermentation of glucose and used as a stabilizer in commercial food preparation.

xan·the·las·ma (zăn′thə-lăz′mə) *n*. Xanthoma of the eyelid.

xan·the·mi·a (zăn-thē′mē-ə) *n*. See **carotenemia**.

xan·thene (zăn′thēn′) *n*. A yellow crystalline organic compound that is soluble in ether and is used as a fungicide and in organic synthesis.

xanthene dye *n*. Any of the brilliant fluorescent yellow to pink to bluish red dyes having xanthene central to their molecular structure.

xan·thic (zăn′thĭk) *adj*. **1.** Having a yellow or yellowish color. **2.** Of or relating to xanthine.

xan·thine (zăn′thēn′, -thĭn) *n*. **1.** A yellowish-white crystalline purine base that is a precursor of uric acid and is found in blood, urine, and muscle tissue. **2.** Any of several derivatives of this compound.

xan·thi·nu·ri·a (zăn′thə-nŏŏr′ē-ə) *n*. **1.** Excretion of abnormally large amounts of xanthine in the urine. **2.** An inherited metabolic disorder resulting from defective synthesis of xanthine oxidase and characterized by urinary excretion of xanthine in place of uric acid.

xan·thism (zăn′thĭz′əm) *n*. A pigmentary anomaly of Blacks characterized by red or yellow-red hair color, copper-red skin, and often fading of the pigment of the iris.

xantho– or **xanth–** *pref*. Yellow: *xanthochromia*.

xan·tho·chroid (zăn′thə-kroid′) *adj*. Having a light complexion and light hair.

xan·tho·chro·mat·ic (zăn′thə-krō-măt′ĭk) or **xan·tho·chro·mic** (-krō′mĭk) *adj*. Yellow.

xan·tho·chro·mi·a (zăn′thə-krō′mē-ə) *n*. The occurrence of patches of yellow color in the skin resembling xanthoma but without nodules or plates. Also called *xanthoderma*.

xan·tho·der·ma (zăn′thə-dûr′mə) *n*. **1.** A yellow coloration of the skin. **2.** See **xanthochromia**.

xan·tho·gran·u·lo·ma (zăn′thə-grăn′yə-lō′mə) *n*. An infiltration of retroperitoneal tissue by lipid macrophages, usually occurring in women.

xan·tho·ma (zăn-thō′mə) *n*., *pl*. **–mas** or **–ma·ta** (-mə-tə) A yellowish-orange, lipid-filled nodule or plaque in the skin, often on an eyelid or over a joint.

xanthoma dis·sem·i·na·tum (dĭ-sĕm′ə-nā′təm) *n*. See **xanthomatosis**.

xanthoma mul·ti·plex (mŭl′tə-plĕks′) *n*. See **xanthomatosis**.

xanthoma pal·pe·brar·um (păl′pə-brâr′əm) *n*. The most common type of xanthoma consisting of soft yellow-orange plaque occurring in groups around the eyes.

xanthoma pla·num (plā′nəm) *n*. A form of xanthoma consisting of a yellow band or rectangular plate in the dermis.

xan·tho·ma·to·sis (zăn′thō-mə-tō′sĭs) *n*. A metabolic disorder characterized by excessive accumulation of lipids in the body and a resulting spread of xanthomas. Also called *lipid granulomatosis, xanthoma disseminatum, xanthoma multiplex*.

xanthomatosis bul·bi (bŭl′bī) *n*. The ulcerative fatty degeneration of the cornea after injury.

xan·tho·ma·tous (zăn-thō′mə-təs, -thŏm′ə-) *adj*. Of or relating to xanthoma.

xanthoma tu·be·ro·sum (tōō′bə-rō′səm) *n*. Xanthomatosis associated with certain types of familial hyperlipoproteinemia. Also called *xanthoma tuberosum simplex*.

xan·thop·si·a (zăn-thŏp′sē-ə) *n*. Chromatopsia in which all objects appear yellow.

xan·tho·sine (zăn′thə-sēn′, -sĭn) *n*. The deamination product of guanosine.

xan·tho·sis (zăn-thō′sĭs) *n*. A yellowish discoloration of degenerating tissues, especially seen in malignant neoplasms.

xan·thu·ren·ic acid (zăn′thə-rĕn′ĭk, zănth′yə-) *n*. A yellow crystalline phenolic acid excreted in the urine of pyridoxine-deficient test animals that have been fed a diet containing additional tryptophan.

X-chromosome *n*. The sex chromosome associated with female characteristics, occurring paired in the female and singly in the male sex-chromosome pair.

Xe The symbol for the element **xenon**.

xeno– or **xen–** *pref*. **1.** Stranger; foreigner: *xenophobia*. **2.** Strange; foreign; different: *xenophthalmia*.

xen·o·bi·ot·ic (zĕn′ə-bī-ŏt′ĭk, zē′nə-) *adj*. Foreign to the body or to living organisms. Used of chemical compounds. —*n*. A xenobiotic chemical.

xen·o·di·ag·no·sis (zĕn′ə-dī′əg-nō′sĭs, zē′nə-) *n*., *pl*. **–ses** (-sēz) Diagnosis of an infectious disease at an early stage by exposing a presumably infected individual or tissue to a clean, laboratory-bred mosquito, tick, or other vector and, following a suitable incubation period, examining the vector for the presence of the infective microorganism.

xen·o·ge·ne·ic (zĕn′ə-jə-nē′ĭk, -nā′-, zē′nə-) *adj*. Derived or obtained from an organism of a different species, as a tissue graft.

xen·o·gen·e·sis (zĕn′ə-jĕn′ĭ-sĭs, zē′nə-) *n*. **1.** The supposed production of offspring that are markedly different from either parent. **2.** See **alternation of generations**.

xen·o·gen·ic (zĕn′ə-jĕn′ĭk, zē′nə-) or **xe·nog·e·nous** (zə-nŏj′ə-nəs) *adj*. **1.** Originating outside the organism or from a foreign substance introduced into the organism. **2.** Xenogeneic.

xen·o·graft (zĕn′ə-grăft′, zē′nə-) *n*. See **heterograft**.

890

xe·non (zē′nŏn′) *n. Symbol* **Xe** A colorless, odorless, highly unreactive gaseous element found in minute quantities in the atmosphere and extracted commercially from liquefied air, used as an anesthetic and, in radioisotope form, for diagnostic imaging. Atomic number 54.

xenon-133 *n.* A radioisotope of xenon having gamma emissions and a physical half-life of 5.27 days and used in the study of pulmonary function and organ blood flow.

xen·o·par·a·site (zĕn′ə-păr′ə-sīt′, zē′nə-) *n.* An ectoparasite that becomes pathogenic when the resistance of its host weakens.

xen·o·pho·bi·a (zĕn′ə-fō′bē-ə, zē′nə-) *n.* Fear and contempt of strangers or foreign peoples.

xen·oph·thal·mi·a (zĕn′ŏf-thăl′mē-ə, zē′nŏf-) *n.* Inflammation resulting from the presence of a foreign body in the eye.

Xen·op·syl·la (zĕn′ŏp-sĭl′ə, zĕn′ə-sĭl′ə) *n.* A genus of fleas parasitic on rats and involved in the transmission of bubonic plague.

xen·o·trans·plan·ta·tion (zĕn′ə-trăns′plăn-tā′shən, zē′nə-) *n.* The surgical transfer of cells, tissues, or especially whole organs from one species to another.

xen·o·trop·ic virus (zĕn′ə-trŏp′ĭk, -trō′pĭk, zē′nə-) *n.* An oncornavirus that does not produce disease in its natural host and replicates only in tissue culture cells derived from a different species.

xero– *or* **xer–** *pref.* Dry; dryness: *xeroderma.*

xe·ro·chi·li·a (zîr′ə-kī′lē-ə) *n.* Dryness of the lips.

xe·ro·der·ma (zîr′ō-dûr′mə) *or* **xe·ro·der·mi·a** (-mē-ə) *n.* Excessive or abnormal dryness of the skin, as in ichthyosis.

xeroderma pig·men·to·sum (pĭg′mən-tō′səm, -mĕn-) *n.* A rare hereditary skin disorder caused by a defect in the enzymes that repair DNA damaged by ultraviolet light and resulting in hypersensitivity to the carcinogenic effect of ultraviolet light.

xe·rog·ra·phy (zĭ-rŏg′rə-fē) *n.* See **xeroradiography.**

xe·ro·ma (zĭ-rō′mə) *n.* See **xerophthalmia.**

xe·ro·me·ni·a (zîr′ə-mē′nē-ə) *n.* The occurrence of the usual physical manifestations at the menstrual period but without the show of blood.

xe·roph·thal·mi·a (zîr′ŏf-thăl′mē-ə) *n.* Extreme dryness of the conjunctiva resulting from disease localized in the eye or from a systemic deficiency of vitamin A. Also called *xeroma.*

xe·ro·ra·di·og·ra·phy (zîr′ə-rā′dē-ŏg′rə-fē) *n.* A dry photographic or photocopying process in which a negative image formed by a resinous powder on an electrically charged plate is electrically transferred to and thermally fixed as positive on a paper or other copying surface. Also called *xeroradiograph.* —**xe′ro·ra′di·o·graph** (-rā′dē-ō-grăf′) *n.*

xe·ro·sis (zĭ-rō′sĭs) *n., pl.* **–ses** (-sēz) **1.** Abnormal dryness, especially of the skin, eyes, or mucous membranes. **2.** The normal hardening of aging tissue.

xe·ro·sto·mi·a (zîr′ə-stō′mē-ə) *n.* Dryness of the mouth resulting from diminished or arrested salivary secretion.

xe·rot·ic (zĭ-rŏt′ĭk) *adj.* **1.** Dry. **2.** Affected with or characterized by xerosis.

xi (zī, sī, ksē) *n. Symbol* ξ The 14th letter of the Greek alphabet.

X-inactivation *n.* See **Lyonization.**

xiph·i·ster·num (zĭf′ĭ-stûr′nəm) *n.* See **xiphoid process.** —**xiph′i·ster′nal** *adj.*

xipho– *or* **xiphi–** *or* **xiph–** *pref.* Xiphoid or xiphoid process: *xiphisternum.*

xiph·oid (zĭf′oid′) *adj.* Sword-shaped.

xiph·oid·i·tis (zĭf′oi-dī′tĭs) *n.* Inflammation of the xiphoid process.

xiphoid process *n.* The cartilage at the lower end of the sternum. Also called *ensiform cartilage, ensiform process, xiphisternum, xiphoid cartilage.*

X-linked *adj.* Of, relating to, or characterized by genes situated on the X-chromosome.

X-linked gene *n.* A gene located on an X-chromosome.

X-linked hypogammaglobulinemia *or* **X-linked infantile hypogammaglobulinemia** *n.* An X-linked primary immunodeficiency characterized by a deficiency of circulating B-cells with a corresponding decrease in immunoglobulins and increased susceptibility to infection by pyogenic bacteria after the loss of maternal antibodies.

X-linked hy·po·phos·pha·te·mic osteomalacia (hī′pō-fŏs′fə-tē′mĭk) *n.* See **vitamin D-resistant rickets.**

Xo·lair (zō′lâr′) A trademark for the drug omalizumab.

XO syndrome (ĕks′sō′) *n.* See **Turner's syndrome.**

x-radiation *n.* **1.** Treatment with or exposure to x-rays. **2.** Radiation composed of x-rays.

x-ray *or* **X-ray** *n.* **1.** A relatively high-energy photon with wavelength in the approximate range from 0.01 to 10 nanometers. Also called *roentgen ray.* **2.** A stream of such photons used for their penetrating power in radiography, radiology, radiotherapy, and scientific research. Often used in the plural. Also called *roentgen ray.* **3.** A photograph taken with x-rays. —*v.* **1.** To irradiate with x-rays. **2.** To photograph with x-rays.

x-ray microscope *n.* An instrument using x-rays to render a highly magnified image.

x-ray therapy *n.* Medical treatment using controlled doses of x-ray radiation.

XXY syndrome (ĕks′ĕks-wī′) *n.* See **Klinefelter's syndrome.**

xy·li·tol (zī′lĭ-tôl′, -tōl′, -tŏl′) *n.* A sweet white crystalline alcohol derived from xylose and used especially as a sugar substitute in oral health products.

Xy·lo·caine (zī′lə-kān′) A trademark for the drug lidocaine and its hydrochloride salt.

xy·lose (zī′lōs′) *n.* A white crystalline sugar used in dyeing and tanning and in diabetic diets. Also called *wood sugar.*

xy·lu·lose (zī′lə-lōs′, zīl′yə-) *n.* A pentose sugar that is a part of carbohydrate metabolism and is found in the urine in pentosuria.

xys·ma (zĭz′mə) *n.* Shreds of membrane occasionally found in feces.

xys·ter (zĭs′tər) *n.* A surgical instrument for scraping bones.

XYY syndrome (ĕks′wī-wī′) *n.* A chromosomal anomaly that is characterized by the presence of one X-chromosome and two Y-chromosomes and thought to be associated with tallness, aggressiveness, and acne.

Y

Y The symbol for the element **yttrium**.

Ya·low (yăl′ō), **Rosalyn Sussman** Born 1921. American biophysicist who in 1959 developed the radioimmunoassay (RIA) procedure, a highly precise method of measuring minute concentrations of biological substances in the body using radioactive-labeled material.

Yang·tze Valley fever (yăng′sē′, -tsē′) *n.* See **schistosomiasis japonicum.**

yawn (yôn) *v.* To open the mouth wide with a deep inhalation, usually involuntarily from drowsiness, fatigue, or boredom. —*n.* The act of yawning.

yaws (yôz) *n.* An infectious tropical disease caused by *Treponema pertenue,* characterized by the development of crusted granulomatous ulcers on the extremities that may cause bone and joint destruction in later stages of the disease. Also called *boubas, bubas, frambesia, granuloma tropicum, pian, rupia.*

Yb The symbol for the element **ytterbium**.

Y cartilage *n.* The Y-shaped connecting cartilage in the acetabulum that joins the ilium, ischium, and pubis.

Y-chromosome *n.* The sex chromosome that is associated with male characteristics, occurring with one X-chromosome in the male sex chromosome pair.

yeast (yēst) *n.* **1.** Any of various unicellular fungi of the genus *Saccharomyces,* especially *S. cerevisiae,* reproducing by budding and from ascospores and capable of fermenting carbohydrates. **2.** Any of various similar fungi. **3.** A commercial preparation in either powdered or compressed form containing yeast cells and inert material and used especially as a leavening agent or as a dietary supplement.

yel·low atrophy of liver (yĕl′ō) *n.* See **acute yellow atrophy of liver.**

yellow bile *n.* See **choler.**

yellow body *n.* See **corpus luteum.**

yellow bone marrow *n.* Bone marrow in which the meshes of the reticular network are filled with fat.

yellow cartilage *n.* See **elastic cartilage.**

yellow enzyme *n.* Any of various flavoproteins that take part in oxidation-reduction.

yellow fever *n.* An infectious tropical disease caused by an arbovirus transmitted by mosquitoes of the genera *Aedes,* especially *A. aegypti* and *Haemogogus,* and characterized by high fever, jaundice, and vomit that is dark in color as a result of gastrointestinal hemorrhaging.

yellow fever vaccine *n.* A vaccine containing a live attenuated strain of yellow fever virus that has been grown in embryonate fowl eggs, used to immunize against yellow fever.

yellow fever virus *n.* An arbovirus of the genus *Flavivirus* that causes yellow fever and is transmitted by mosquitoes.

yellow fiber *n.* See **elastic fiber.**

yellow hepatization *n.* The final stage of hepatization of lung tissue in pneumonia, in which the exudate is becoming purulent.

yellow spot *n.* See **macula lutea.**

Yer·sin (yĕr-săN′), **Alexandre Émile John** 1863–1943. Swiss-born French bacteriologist. His work with the diphtheria bacillus led to the development of antitoxins to neutralize pathogenic toxins.

yer·sin·i·a (yər-sĭn′ē-ə) *n.* A bacterium of the genus *Yersinia.*

Yersinia *n.* A genus of gram-negative parasitic bacteria of the family Enterobacteriaceae that cause various diseases in humans and animals.

Yersinia en·ter·o·co·lit·i·ca (ĕn′tərō-kō-lĭt′ĭ-kə) *n.* A bacterium that causes yersiniosis.

Yersinia pes·tis (pĕs′tĭs) *n.* A bacterium that causes plague and is transmitted from rats to humans by the rat flea *Xenopsylla cheopis.* Also called *Pasteurella pestis.*

Yersinia pseu·do·tu·ber·cu·lo·sis (soo′dō-too-bûr′kyə-lō′sĭs) *n.* A bacterium that causes acute mesenteric lymphadenitis in humans. Also called *Pasteurella pseudotuberculosis.*

yer·sin·i·o·sis (yər-sĭn′ē-ō′sĭs) *n.* An infectious disease marked by diarrhea, enteritis, ileitis, pseudoappendicitis, erythema nodosum, and sometimes septicemia or acute arthritis.

–yl *suff.* A monovalent organic acid radical: *carbonyl.*

–ylene *suff.* A bivalent organic radical: *methylene.*

Y ligament *n.* See **iliofemoral ligament.**

Y-linked gene *n.* A gene located on a Y-chromosome. Also called *holandric gene.*

Yo·con (yō′kŏn) A trademark for the drug yohimbine hydrochloride.

yo·him·bine hydrochloride (yō-hĭm′bēn′) *n.* An alpha-blocker drug that is derived from the bark of a tree, *Corynanthe yohimbe,* and is used as a mydriatic and as a treatment for erectile dysfunction.

yoke (yōk) *n.* See **jugum** (sense 1).

yolk (yōk) *n.* The portion of the egg of an animal that consists of protein and fat from which the early embryo gets its main nourishment and of protoplasmic substances from which the embryo develops.

yolk membrane *n.* See **vitelline membrane.**

yolk sac *n.* A membranous sac attached to an embryo, enclosing food yolk. Also called *umbilical vesicle.*

yolk-sac tumor *n.* See **endodermal sinus tumor.**

yolk stalk *n.* A narrow ductlike part that connects the yolk sac to the middle of the digestive tract of an embryo. Also called *omphalomesenteric duct.*

Young (yŭng), **John** 1907–1997. British biologist whose experiments with the giant nerve cells of squid contributed to the knowledge of the anatomy and physiology of nerves.

Young, Thomas 1773–1829. British physician and physicist who in 1801 postulated the three-color theory of color vision. Young also discovered (1801) astigmatism and described accommodation.

Young-Helm·holtz theory of color vision (-hĕlm′hōlts) *n.* The theory that there are three sets of color-perceiving elements in the retina, red, green, and violet. Perception of the other colors arises from the combined stimulation of these elements.

Young's rule (yŭngz) *n.* A rule for calculating the dose of medicine correct for a child by adding 12 to the child's age, dividing the sum by the child's age, then dividing the adult dose by the figure obtained.

yp·si·lon (ŭp′sə-lŏn′, yōōp′-) *n.* Variant of **upsilon**.

Y-shaped ligament *n.* See **iliofemoral ligament.**

yt·ter·bi·um (ĭ-tûr′bē-əm) *n. Symbol* **Yb** A soft bright allotropic rare-earth element, whose radioisotope is used in diagnostic imaging of the brain. Atomic number 70.

yt·tri·um (ĭt′rē-əm) *n. Symbol* **Y** A silvery, ductile, rare-earth element used in various alloys. Atomic number 39.

yup·pie flu (yŭp′ē) *n.* Chronic fatigue syndrome. Used informally.

Z

ζ The Greek letter *zeta*. Entries beginning with this character are alphabetized under **zeta**.

za·fir·lu·kast (zə-fîr′lōō-kăst′) *n.* A leukotriene receptor antagonist that reduces inflammation and is used to treat asthma.

zal·ci·ta·bine (zăl′sĭ-tə-bīnē′) *n.* See **ddC**.

za·na·ma·vir (zə-nä′mə-vîr′) *n.* A neuraminidase inhibitor used to treat influenza.

Zantac (zăn′tăk′) A trademark for the drug ranitidine.

Z band *n.* See **Z line**.

Z-DNA *n.* A form of DNA in which the double helix twists in a left-hand direction, thus producing a zigzag appearance.

ZDV *abbr.* zidovudine

ze·a·xan·thin (zē′ə-zăn′thēn′, -thĭn) *n.* A carotenoid that is found in some fruits and vegetables and may reduce the risk of certain eye diseases.

ze·bra body (zē′brə) *n.* A granule found in Schwann cells and macrophages of individuals suffering from metachromatic leukodystrophy.

zed·o·ar·y (zĕd′ō-ĕr′ē) *n.* **1.** An Indian plant that has yellow flowers, purple bracts, and starchy tuberous rhizomes. **2.** The dried rhizomes of this plant that are used as a condiment as well as in perfumes, medicines, and cosmetics.

Zeis gland (zīs, tsīs) *n.* Any of the numerous sebaceous glands opening into the follicles of the eyelashes.

Zen·ker's degeneration (zĕng′kərz, tsĕng′) *n.* A form of severe hyaline degeneration or necrosis in skeletal muscle, occurring in severe infections. Also called *waxy degeneration, Zenker's necrosis.*

Zenker's diverticulum *n.* See **hypopharyngeal diverticulum**.

Zenker's necrosis *n.* See **Zenker's degeneration**.

Zer·it (zâr′ĭt) A trademark for the drug stavudine.

ze·ro (zîr′ō) *n., pl.* **–ros** *or* **–roes** **1.** The numerical symbol 0, indicating the absence of quantity or mass. **2.** The temperature indicated by the numeral 0 on a thermometer. —*v.* To adjust an instrument or device to zero value.

Zes·tril (zĕs′trĭl′) A trademark for the drug lisinopril.

ze·ta (zā′tə, zē′-) *n. Symbol* ζ The sixth letter of the Greek alphabet.

ze·ta·crit (zā′tə-krĭt′) *n.* Vertical centrifugation of blood in capillary tubes allowing controlled compaction and dispersion of the red blood cells.

zeta sedimentation ratio *n.* The ratio of the zetacrit to the hematocrit, used as an indicator of the red blood cell sedimentation rate.

Zet·i·a (zĕt′ē-ə) A trademark for the drug ezetimibe.

Z filament *n.* The thin zigzag strand at the Z line of striated muscle fibers to which the actin filaments attach.

zi·do·vu·dine (zĭ-dō′vyōō-dēn′) *n. Abbr.* **ZDV AZT**.

Zie·gler's operation (zē′glərz) *n.* A V-shaped iridotomy for the formation of an artificial pupil.

Zin·a·cef (zĭn′ə-sĕf′) A trademark for the drug cefuroxime.

zinc (zĭngk) *n. Symbol* **Zn** A metallic element that is brittle at room temperature but becomes malleable when heated and is used in various pharmaceuticals, including astringents and antiseptics. Atomic number 30.

zinc-65 *n.* A radioisotope of zinc with a half-life of 245 days, used as a tracer in studies of zinc metabolism.

zinc ointment *n.* A salve consisting of about 20 percent zinc oxide with beeswax or paraffin and petrolatum, used in the treatment of skin disorders.

zinc oxide *n.* An amorphous white or yellowish powder used as a pigment and in pharmaceuticals and cosmetics.

Zinn's membrane (zĭnz) *n.* The anterior layer of the iris of the eye.

Zinn's zonule *n.* See **ciliary zonule**.

Zins·ser (zĭn′sər), **Hans** 1878–1940. American bacteriologist and pioneer immunologist who first differentiated epidemic from endemic forms of typhus.

zir·co·ni·um (zûr-kō′nē-əm) *n. Symbol* **Zr** A strong ductile metallic element obtained primarily from zircon, and used in deodorants and dermatologic preparations. Atomic number 40.

zit (zĭt) *n.* A pimple.

Zith·ro·max (zĭth′rə-măks′) A trademark for the drug azithromycin dihydrate.

Z line *n.* A dark thin protein band to which actin filaments are attached in a striated muscle fiber, marking the boundaries between adjacent sarcomeres. Also called *Z band.*

Zn The symbol for the element **zinc**.

zo– *pref.* Variant of **zoo–**.

zo·ac·an·tho·sis (zō′ăk′ən-thō′sĭs) *n.* An eruption caused by piercing of the skin with the hair, bristles, or stingers of an animal.

zo·an·thro·py (zō-ăn′thrə-pē) *n.* A delusion that one is an animal.

Zo·cor (zō′kôr′) A trademark for the drug simvastatin.

–zoic *suff.* Relating to a specified manner of animal existence: *holozoic.*

Zo·la·dex (zō′lə-dĕks′) A trademark for the drug goserelin acetate.

Zol·lin·ger-El·li·son syndrome (zŏl′ĭn-jər-ĕl′ĭ-sən) *n.* A gastrointestinal disease characterized by chronic peptic ulcers, gastric hypersecretion, and gastrinomas of the pancreatic islets of Langerhans.

zol·mi·trip·tan (zŏl′mĭ-trĭp′tn) *n.* A serotonin receptor agonist used to treat migraine headaches.

Zo·loft (zō′lôft′) A trademark for the serotonin-inhibiting antidepressant sertraline hydrochloride.

zol·pi·dem tartrate (zōl′pə-dĕm′) *n.* A nonbenzodiazepine hypnotic drug used to treat insomnia.

Zo·mig (zō′mĭg′) A trademark for the drug zolmitriptan.

zo·na (zō′nə) *n., pl.* **–nae** (-nē) **1.** An encircling or beltlike anatomical structure. Also called *segment, zone.* **2.** See **shingles.**

zona fas·cic·u·la·ta (fə-sĭk′yə-lā′tə) *n.* The layer of radially arranged cell cords in the cortical portion of the suprarenal gland.

zona glo·mer·u·lo·sa (glō-mĕr′yə-lō′sə) *n.* The outer layer of the cortex of the suprarenal gland, just beneath the capsule.

zona hem·or·rhoi·da·lis (hĕm′ə-roi-dā′lĭs) *n.* The part of the anal canal that contains the rectal venous plexus. Also called *annulus hemorrhoidalis.*

zo·nal necrosis (zō′nəl) *n.* Necrosis predominantly affecting or limited to a defined anatomical area.

zona oph·thal·mi·ca (ŏf-thāl′mĭ-kə) *n.* The occurrence of herpes zoster in the region in which the ophthalmic nerve is distributed.

zona pel·lu·ci·da (pə-lōō′sĭ-də) *n.* The thick solid transparent outer membrane of a developed mammalian ovum. Also called *oolemma.*

zona re·tic·u·lar·is (rĭ-tĭk′yə-lâr′ĭs) *n.* The inner layer of the cortex of the adrenal gland in which cell cords form a network.

zona tec·ta (tĕk′tə) *n.* See **arcuate zone.**

zone (zōn) *n.* **1.** An area or a region distinguished from adjacent parts by a distinctive feature or characteristic. **2.** See **zona** (sense 1). **3.** A segment.

zo·nes·the·sia (zō′nĭs-thē′zhə) *n.* A sensation of constriction as if a cord were being drawn around the body. Also called *girdle sensation.*

zo·nif·u·gal (zō-nĭf′yə-gəl) *adj.* Passing out of or away from a region.

zon·ing (zō′nĭng) *n.* An unexpectedly strong immunologic reaction in a small amount of serum, probably the result of high antibody titer.

zo·nip·e·tal (zō-nĭp′ĭ-tl) *adj.* Passing into a region from without.

zonular band *n.* See **orbicular zone.**

zonular cataract *n.* See **lamellar cataract.**

zonular space *n.* A space between the fibers of the ciliary zonule at the equator of the lens of the eye.

zon·ule (zōn′yōōl) *n.* A small zone, as of a ligament. —**zo′nu·lar** (zōn′yə-lər) *adj.*

zo·nu·li·tis (zōn′yə-lī′tĭs) *n.* Inflammation of the ciliary zonule.

zo·nu·lol·y·sis (zōn′yə-lŏl′ĭ-sĭs) *or* **zo·nu·ly·sis** (-lī′sĭs) *n.* Enzymatic dissolution of the ciliary zonule to facilitate surgical removal of a cataract.

zoo– *or* **zo–** *pref.* Animal; animal kingdom: *zoonosis.*

zo·o·e·ras·ti·a (zō′ō-ə-răs′tē-ə) *n.* Sexual intercourse between a human and an animal.

zo·o·gen·ic (zō′ə-jĕn′ĭk) *or* **zo·og·e·nous** (zō-ŏj′ə-nəs) *adj.* Originating in or produced by animals.

zo·o·graft (zō′ə-grăft′) *n.* A graft in which tissue from an animal is transferred to a human.

zo·o·graft·ing (zō′ə-grăf′tĭng) *n.* See **zooplasty.**

zo·oid (zō′oid) *n.* **1.** An organic cell or organized body that has independent movement within a living organism, especially a motile gamete such as a spermatozoon. **2.** An independent animallike organism produced asexually, as by budding or fission. **3.** One of the dis-

tinct individuals forming a colonial animal such as a coral.

zo·o·lag·ni·a (zō′ə-lăg′nē-ə) *n.* Sexual attraction to animals.

Zo·o·mas·ti·go·pho·re·a (zō′ə-măs′tĭ-gō-fôr′ē-ə, -gŏf′ə-rē′ə) *n.* A class of flagellates having animal-like rather than plantlike characteristics, including parasites such as trypanosomes and trichomonads.

–zoon *suff.* Animal; independently moving organic unit: *spermatozoon.*

zo·on·o·sis (zō-ŏn′ə-sĭs, zō′ə-nō′-) *n., pl.* **-ses** (-sēz′) A disease of animals, such as rabies or psittacosis, that can be transmitted to humans. —**zo′o·not′ic** (zō′ə-nŏt′ĭk) *adj.*

zoonotic cutaneous leishmaniasis *n.* An acute form of cutaneous leishmaniasis occurring among people living in rural areas near infected rodents and characterized by rapidly developing skin lesions that become severely inflamed, with moist necrotizing sores that often leave disfiguring scars. Also called *rural leishmaniasis, wet leishmaniasis.*

zoonotic potential *n.* The potential for animal infections to be transmissible to humans.

zo·o·par·a·site (zō′ə-păr′ə-sīt′) *n.* An animal parasite.

zo·o·phil·i·a (zō′ə-fĭl′ē-ə) *or* **zo·oph·i·lism** (zō-ŏf′ə-lĭz′əm) *or* **zo·oph·i·ly** (-ə-lē) *n.* Attraction to or affinity for animals.

zo·o·pho·bi·a (zō′ə-fō′bē-ə) *n.* An abnormal fear of animals.

zo·o·plas·ty (zō′ə-plăs′tē) *n.* Surgical transfer of tissue from an animal to a human. Also called *zografting.*

zo·os·ter·ol (zō-ŏs′tə-rôl′, -rōl′) *n.* A sterol produced by animals rather than plants.

zo·o·tox·in (zō′ə-tŏk′sĭn) *n.* A toxin of animal origin.

zos·ter (zŏs′tər) *n.* See **shingles.**

zos·ter·i·form (zŏ-stĕr′ə-fôrm′) *or* **zos·ter·oid** (zŏs′tə-roid′) *adj.* Resembling herpes zoster.

zoster immune globulin *n.* A globulin fraction of pooled plasma from human donors who have recovered from infection by herpes zoster, used in the prevention and treatment of chickenpox.

Zo·syn (zō′sĭn) A trademark for the drug piperacillin sodium.

Zo·vi·rax (zō′və-răks′) A trademark for the drug acyclovir.

Z-plas·ty (zē′plăs′tē) *n.* A surgical procedure to elongate a contracted scar or to rotate tension 90°, in which the middle line of the Z-shaped incision is made along the line of greatest tension or contraction, and triangular flaps are raised on opposite sides of the two ends and then transposed.

Zr The symbol for the element **zirconium.**

zwit·ter hypothesis (zwĭt′ər, tsvĭt′-) *n.* The hypothesis that an ampholyteric electrode, such as an amino acid, yields equal numbers of basic and acid ions at the isoelectric point, thus becoming a zwitterion.

zwit·ter·i·on (zwĭt′ər-ī′ən, swĭt′-, tsvĭt′-) *n.* See **dipolar ion.** —**zwit′ter·i·on′ic** (-ī-ŏn′ĭk) *adj.*

Zy·ban (zī′băn) A trademark for the drug bupropion dipropionate, used to treat nicotine dependence.

zy·gal (zī′gəl) *adj.* Having a shape like a yoke or like the letter H.

zygo– *or* **zyg–** *pref.* **1.** Yoke; pair: *zygodactyly.* **2.** Union: *zygosis.*

zy·go·dac·ty·ly (zī′gə-dăk′tə-lē) *n.* See **syndactyly.**

zy·go·gen·e·sis (zī′gō-jĕn′ĭ-sĭs) *n.* Reproduction involving the formation of a zygote.

zy·go·ma (zī-gō′mə, zĭ-) *n.* **1.** See **zygomatic arch. 2.** See **zygomatic bone.**

zy·go·mat·ic (zī′gə-măt′ĭk, zĭg′ə-) *adj.* Of, relating to, or located in the area of the zygoma.

zygomatic arch *n.* The arch formed by the temporal process of the zygomatic bone and the zygomatic process of the temporal bone. Also called *zygoma.*

zygomatic bone *n.* A quadrilateral bone that forms the cheek prominence and articulates with the frontal, sphenoid, temporal, and maxillary bones. Also called *cheekbone, jugal bone, malar bone, zygoma.*

zygomatic fossa *n.* See **infratemporal fossa.**

zygomatic nerve *n.* A branch of the maxillary nerve that divides and supplies the skin of the temporal and zygomatic regions. Also called *temporomandibular nerve.*

zy·go·mat·i·co·fa·cial foramen (zī′gə-măt′ĭ-kō-fā′-shəl) *n.* The opening on the lateral surface of the zygomatic bone, transmitting the zygomaticofacial nerve.

zy·go·mat·i·co·max·il·lar·y suture (zī′gə-măt′ĭ-kō-măk′sə-lĕr′ē) *n.* The articulation of the zygomatic bone with the zygomatic process of the maxilla.

zy·go·mat·i·co-or·bit·al artery (zī′gə-măt′ĭ-kō-ôr′bĭtl) *n.* An artery with its origin usually in the superficial temporal artery, sometimes in the middle temporal artery, with distribution to the orbicular muscle of the eye and portions of the orbit, and with anastomoses to the lacrimal and palpebral branches of the ophthalmic artery.

zygomatico-orbital foramen *n.* The common opening on the orbital surface of the zygomatic bone, transmitting the zygomaticofacial and zygomaticotemporal nerves.

zy·go·mat·i·co·tem·po·ral foramen (zī′gə-măt′ĭ-kōtĕm′pər-əl, -tĕm′prəl) *n.* The opening on the temporal surface of the zygomatic bone of the canal for passage of the zygomaticotemporal nerve.

zygomatic process *n.* Any of three processes that articulate with the zygomatic bone, especially the process from the temporal bone that articulates to form the zygomatic arch.

zygomatic process of frontal bone *n.* The projection of the frontal bone that joins the zygomatic bone to form the lateral margin of the eye socket.

zygomatic process of maxilla *n.* The rough projection from the maxilla that articulates with the zygomatic bone. Also called *malar process.*

zygomatic process of temporal bone *n.* The anterior process of the temporal bone that articulates with the temporal process of the zygomatic bone to form the zygomatic arch.

zy·go·max·il·lar·e (zī′gə-măk′sə-lâr′ē) *n.* A craniometric point located externally at the lowest extent of the zygomaticomaxillary suture. Also called *zygomaxillary point.*

zy·go·mor·phic (zī′gə-môr′fĭk, zĭg′ə-) *or* **zy·go·mor·phous** (-fəs) *adj.* Bilaterally symmetrical. Used of organisms or parts.

Zy·go·my·ce·tes (zī′gō-mī-sē′tēz) *n.* A subclass of fungi characterized by sexual reproduction resulting in the formation of a large multinucleate spore formed by union of similar gametes.

zy·go·my·co·sis (zī′gō-mī-kō′sĭs) *n.* A fungus infection caused by various genera of the class Zygomycetes. Also called *mucormycosis, phycomycosis.*

zy·gon (zī′gŏn′) *n.* The short crossbar connecting the branches of a zygal fissure.

zy·go·ne·ma (zī′gə-nē′mə) *n.* See **zygotene.**

zy·go·sis (zī-gō′sĭs, zĭ-) *n., pl.* **–ses** (-sēz) The union of gametes to form a zygote; conjugation.

zy·gos·i·ty (zī-gŏs′ĭ-tē) *n.* The genetic condition of a zygote, especially with respect to its being a homozygote or a heterozygote.

zy·gote (zī′gōt′) *n.* **1.** The cell that is formed by the union of two gametes, especially a fertilized ovum before cleavage. **2.** The organism that develops from a zygote. —**zy·got′ic** (-gŏt′ĭk) *adj.*

zy·go·tene (zī′gə-tēn′) *n.* The stage of meiotic prophase during which the precise point-for-point pairing of the homologous chromosomes begins. Also called *zygonema.*

–zygous *suff.* Having a zygotic constitution of a specified kind: *heterozygous.*

Zy·lo·prim (zī′lə-prĭm′) A trademark for the drug allopurinol.

zy·mase (zī′mās′, -māz′) *n.* The enzyme complex in yeasts that catalyzes the breakdown of sugar into alcohol and carbon dioxide.

–zyme *suff.* Enzyme: *lysozyme.*

zymo– *pref.* **1.** Fermentation: *zymogenic.* **2.** Enzyme: *zymogram.*

zy·mo·deme (zī′mə-dēm′) *n.* An isozyme pattern, identified electrophoretically.

zy·mo·gen (zī′mə-jən) *n.* See **proenzyme.**

zy·mo·gen·e·sis (zī′mə-jĕn′ĭ-sĭs) *n.* The process by which a proenzyme becomes transformed into an active enzyme.

zy·mo·gen·ic (zī′mə-jĕn′ĭk) *or* **zy·mog·e·nous** (zīmŏj′ə-nəs) *adj.* **1.** Of or relating to a proenzyme. **2.** Causing fermentation. **3.** Enzyme-producing.

zy·mo·gen·ic cell (zī′mə-jĕn′ĭk) *n.* A cell that forms and secretes an enzyme, especially a secretory cell that lines the lumen of the gastric glands of the stomach or a pepsin-secreting acinar cell of the pancreas. Also called *chief cell, peptic cell.*

zy·mol·y·sis (zī-mŏl′ĭ-sĭs) *n.* Fermentation.

zy·mo·sis (zī-mō′sĭs) *n.* **1.** Fermentation. **2.** The process of infection. **3.** An infectious disease, especially one caused by a fungus.

Zy·prex·a (zī-prĕk′sə) A trademark for the drug olanzapine.

Zyr·tec (zŭr′tĕk′) A trademark for the drug cetirizine hydrochloride.

APPENDIXES

MEASUREMENTS

length

U.S. customary unit	U.S. equivalents	metric equivalents	metric unit	number of meters	U.S. equivalent
inch	$1/_{12}$ foot	2.540 centimeters	kilometer	1,000	0.621 mile
foot	$1/_3$ yard, 12 inches	0.305 meter	hectometer	100	109.361 yards
yard	3 feet, 36 inches	0.914 meter	decameter	10	32.808 feet
rod	$5^1/_2$ yards, $16^1/_2$ feet	5.029 meters	meter	1	39.370 inches
mile (statute, land)	1,760 yards, 5,280 feet	1.609 kilometers	decimeter	0.1	3.937 inches
			centimeter	0.01	0.394 inch
mile (nautical)	1.151 statute miles	1.852 kilometers	millimeter	0.001	0.039 inch

volume and capacity

U.S. customary unit	U.S. equivalents	metric equivalents	metric unit of volume	cubic meters	U.S. equivalent
cubic inch	0.00058 cubic foot	16.387 cubic centimeters	decastere	10	13.079 cubic yards
			stere	1	1.308 cubic yards
cubic foot	1,728 cubic inches	0.028 cubic meter	decistere	0.1	3.531 cubic feet
cubic yard	27 cubic feet	0.765 cubic meter	cubic centimeter	0.000001	0.061 cubic inch

U.S. customary liquid measure	U.S. equivalents	metric equivalents	metric unit of capacity	liters	U.S. equivalent
fluid ounce	8 fluid drams, 1.805 cubic inches	29.574 millimeters	hectoliter	100	26.42 gallons
			decaliter	10	2.642 gallons
pint	16 fluid ounces, 28.875 cubic inches	0.473 liter	liter	1	1.057 quarts
			deciliter	0.1	0.211 pint
quart	2 pints, 57.75 cubic inches	0.946 liter	centiliter	0.01	0.338 fluid ounce
			milliliter	0.001	0.271 fluid dram
gallon	4 quarts, 231 cubic inches	3.785 liters			

weight and mass

U.S. customary unit (avoirdupois)	U.S. equivalents	metric equivalents	metric unit	number of grams	U.S. equivalent and apothecary equivalent
grain	0.037 dram, 0.002286 ounce	64.799 milligrams	metric ton	1,000,000	1.102 tons (short)
			quintal	100,000	220.462 pounds
dram	27.344 grains	1.772 grams			267.923 pounds (apoth.)
ounce	16 drams, 437.5 grains	28.350 grams	kilogram	1,000	2.205 pounds
					2.679 pounds (apoth.)
pound	16 ounces, 7,000 grains	453.592 grams	hectogram	100	3.527 ounces
					3.215 ounces (apoth.)
ton (short)	2,000 pounds	0.907 metric ton	decagram	10	0.353 ounce
					0.322 ounce (apoth.)

apothecary unit	apothecary equivalents	metric equivalents			
grain	$1/_{20}$ scruple	64.799 milligrams	gram	1	0.035 ounce
					0.032 ounce (apoth.)
scruple	20 grains, $1/_3$ dram	1.296 grams			
dram	3 scruples, $1/_8$ ounce	3.888 grams	decigram	0.1	1.543 grains
ounce	8 drams, $1/_{12}$ pound	31.103 grams	centigram	0.01	0.154 grain
pound	12 ounces	373.2417 grams	milligram	0.001	0.015 grain

METRIC CONVERSION CHART

when you know	multiply by	to find
length		
millimeters	0.04	inches
centimeters	0.39	inches
meters	3.28	feet
meters	1.09	yards
kilometers	0.62	miles
inches	25.40	millimeters
inches	2.54	centimeters
feet	30.48	centimeters
yards	0.91	meters
miles	1.61	kilometers
speed		
miles per hour	1.61	kilometers per hour
kilometers per hour	0.62	miles per hour
volume		
milliliters	0.20	teaspoons
milliliters	0.07	tablespoons
milliliters	0.03	fluid ounces
liters	4.23	cups
liters	2.11	pints
liters	1.06	quarts
liters	0.26	gallons
cubic meters	35.31	cubic feet
cubic meters	1.31	cubic yards
teaspoons	4.93	milliliters
tablespoons	14.79	milliliters
fluid ounces	29.57	milliliters
cups	0.24	liters
pints	0.47	liters
quarts	0.95	liters
gallons	3.79	liters
cubic feet	0.03	cubic meters
cubic yards	0.76	cubic meters

when you know	multiply by	to find
mass and weight		
grams	0.035	ounce
grams	0.032	ounce (apoth.)
kilograms	2.20	pounds
kilograms	2.68	pounds (apoth.)
tons (1,000 kg)	1.10	short tons
ounces	28.35	grams
ounces (apoth.)	31.10	grams
pounds	0.45	kilograms
pounds (apoth.)	0.37	kilograms
short tons (2,000 lb)	0.91	metric tons
temperature		
degrees Fahrenheit	$(°F − 32) ÷ 1.8$	degrees Celsius
degrees Celsius	$(°C × 1.8) + 32$	degrees Fahrenheit

metric prefixes

prefix	symbol	factor		
exa-	E	10^{18}	=	1,000,000,000,000,000,000
peta-	P	10^{15}	=	1,000,000,000,000,000
tera-	T	10^{12}	=	1,000,000,000,000
giga-	G	10^{9}	=	1,000,000,000
mega-	M	10^{6}	=	1,000,000
kilo-	k	10^{3}	=	1,000
hecto-	h	10^{2}	=	100
deca-	da	10	=	10
deci-	d	10^{-1}	=	0.1
centi-	c	10^{-2}	=	0.01
milli-	m	10^{-3}	=	0.001
micro-	μ	10^{-6}	=	0.000,001
nano-	n	10^{-9}	=	0.000,000,001
pico-	p	10^{-12}	=	0.000,000,000,001
femto-	f	10^{-15}	=	0.000,000,000,000,001
atto-	a	10^{-18}	=	0.000,000,000,000,000,001

RECOMMENDED DAILY ALLOWANCES OF VITAMINS AND MINERALS[1]

category	age in years	weight in pounds[2]	height in inches[2]	protein (g)	Fat-soluble vitamins			
					vitamin A (μg RE)[3]	vitamin D (μg)[4]	vitamin E (mg alpha-TE)[5]	vitamin K (μg)
infants	to 6 months	13	24	13	375	7.5	3	5
	6 months to 1 year	20	28	14	375	10	4	10
children	1-3	29	35	16	400	10	6	15
	4-6	44	44	24	500	10	7	20
	7-10	62	52	28	700	10	7	30
males	11-14	99	62	45	1,000	10	10	45
	15-18	145	69	59	1,000	10	10	60
	19-24	160	70	58	1,000	10	10	70
	25-50	174	70	63	1,000	5	10	80
	51+	170	68	63	1,000	5	10	80
females	11-14	101	62	46	800	10	8	45
	15-18	120	64	44	800	10	8	55
	19-24	128	65	46	800	10	8	60
	25-50	138	64	50	800	5	8	65
	51+	143	63	50	800	5	8	65
pregnant				60	800	10	10	65
lactating	first 6 months			65	1,300	10	12	65
	second 6 months			62	1,200	10	11	65

[1]RDAs of the Food and Nutrition Board of the National Academy of Sciences–National Research Council, 1989 revision
[2]median weights and heights for U.S. individuals of designated ages, as reported in key reference studies
[3]retinol equivalents: 1RE = 6μg beta-carotene or 5 IU vitamin A

Water-soluble vitamins							Minerals						
vitamin C (mg)	thia-mine (mg)	ribo-flavin (mg)	niacin (mg NE)[6]	vitamin B$_6$ (mg)	folate (µg)	vitamin B$_{12}$ (µg)	calcium (mg)	phos-phorus (mg)	mag-nesium (mg)	iron (mg)	zinc (mg)	iodine (µg)	sele-nium (µg)
30	0.3	0.4	5	0.3	25	0.3	400	300	40	6	5	40	10
35	0.4	0.5	6	1.6	35	0.5	600	500	60	10	5	60	15
40	0.7	0.8	9	1.0	60	0.7	800	800	80	10	10	70	20
45	0.9	1.1	12	1.1	75	1.0	800	800	120	10	10	90	20
45	1.0	1.2	13	1.4	100	1.4	800	800	170	10	10	120	30
50	1.3	1.5	17	1.7	150	2.0	1,200	1,200	270	12	15	150	40
60	1.5	1.8	20	2.0	200	2.0	1,200	1,200	400	12	15	150	50
60	1.5	1.7	19	2.0	200	2.0	1,200	1,200	350	10	15	150	70
60	1.5	1.7	19	2.0	200	2.0	800	800	350	10	15	150	70
60	1.2	1.4	15	2.0	200	2.0	800	800	350	10	15	150	70
50	1.1	1.3	15	1.4	150	2.0	1,200	1,200	280	15	12	150	45
60	1.1	1.3	15	1.5	180	2.0	1,200	1,200	300	15	12	150	50
60	1.1	1.3	15	1.6	180	2.0	1,200	1,200	280	15	12	150	55
60	1.1	1.3	15	1.6	180	2.0	800	800	280	15	12	150	55
60	1.0	1.2	13	1.6	180	2.0	800	800	280	10	12	150	55
70	1.5	1.6	17	2.2	400	2.2	1,200	1,200	300	30	15	175	65
95	1.6	1.8	20	2.1	280	2.6	1,200	1,200	355	15	19	200	75
90	1.6	1.7	20	2.1	260	2.6	1,200	1,200	340	15	16	200	75

[4]as cholecalciferol with 10 µg cholecalciferol = 400 IU vitamin D
[5]alpha-tocopherol equivalents: 1 alpha-TE = 1 mg d-alpha-tocopherol
[6]1 niacin equivalent: 1 NE = 1 mg niacin or 60 mg dietary tryptophan

PERIODIC TABLE OF THE ELEMENTS

1
H
Hydrogen
1.00794

— atomic number
— symbol
— atomic weight (or mass number of most stable isotope if in parentheses)

The Periodic Table arranges the chemical elements in two ways. The first is by **atomic number,** starting with hydrogen (atomic number =1) in the upper left-hand corner and continuing in ascending order from left to right. The second is by the number of electrons in the outermost shell. Elements having the same number of electrons in the outermost shell are placed in the same column. Since the number of electrons in the outermost shell in large part determines the chemical nature of an element, elements in the same column have similar chemical properties.

This arrangement of the elements was devised by **Dmitri Mendeleev** in 1869,

Group 1a

Period 1	1 **H** Hydrogen 1.00794	**Group 2a**							
Period 2	3 **Li** Lithium 6.941	4 **Be** Beryllium 9.0122							
Period 3	11 **Na** Sodium 22.9898	12 **Mg** Magnesium 24.305	**Group 3b**	**Group 4b**	**Group 5b**	**Group 6b**	**Group 7b**	**Group 8**	**Group 8**
Period 4	19 **K** Potassium 39.098	20 **Ca** Calcium 40.08	21 **Sc** Scandium 44.956	22 **Ti** Titanium 47.87	23 **V** Vanadium 50.942	24 **Cr** Chromium 51.996	25 **Mn** Manganese 54.9380	26 **Fe** Iron 55.845	27 **Co** Cobalt 58.9332
Period 5	37 **Rb** Rubidium 85.47	38 **Sr** Strontium 87.62	39 **Y** Yttrium 88.906	40 **Zr** Zirconium 91.22	41 **Nb** Niobium 92.906	42 **Mo** Molybdenum 95.94	43 **Tc** Technetium (98)	44 **Ru** Ruthenium 101.07	45 **Rh** Rhodium 102.905
Period 6	55 **Cs** Cesium 132.905	56 **Ba** Barium 137.33	57–71* Lanthanides	72 **Hf** Hafnium 178.49	73 **Ta** Tantalum 180.948	74 **W** Tungsten 183.84	75 **Re** Rhenium 186.2	76 **Os** Osmium 190.2	77 **Ir** Iridium 192.2
Period 7	87 **Fr** Francium (223)	88 **Ra** Radium (226)	89–103 ** Actinides	104 **Rf** Rutherfordium (261)	105 **Db** Dubnium (262)	106 **Sg** Seaborgium (266)	107 **Bh** Bohrium (264)	108 **Hs** Hassium (265)	109 **Mt** Meitnerium (268)

*LANTHANIDES	57 **La** Lanthanum 138.91	58 **Ce** Cerium 140.12	59 **Pr** Praseodymium 140.908	60 **Nd** Neodymium 144.24	61 **Pm** Promethium (145)	62 **Sm** Samarium 150.36	63 **Eu** Europium 151.96	
**ACTINIDES	89 **Ac** Actinium (227)	90 **Th** Thorium 232.038	91 **Pa** Protactinium 231.036	92 **U** Uranium 238.03	93 **Np** Neptunium (237)	94 **Pu** Plutonium (244)	95 **Am** Americium (243)	

ALPHABETICAL TABLE OF THE ELEMENTS

Element	Symbol	Atomic Number	Element	Symbol	Atomic Number	Element	Symbol	Atomic Number	Element	Symbol	Atomic Number
Actinium	Ac	89	Cadmium	Cd	48	Einsteinium	Es	99	Helium	He	2
Aluminum	Al	13	Calcium	Ca	20	Element 111	–	111	Holmium	Ho	67
Americium	Am	95	Californium	Cf	98	Element 112	–	112	Hydrogen	H	1
Antimony	Sb	51	Carbon	C	6	Erbium	Er	68	Indium	In	49
Argon	Ar	18	Cerium	Ce	58	Europium	Eu	63	Iodine	I	53
Arsenic	As	33	Cesium	Cs	55	Fermium	Fm	100	Iridium	Ir	77
Astatine	At	85	Chlorine	Cl	17	Fluorine	F	9	Iron	Fe	26
Barium	Ba	56	Chromium	Cr	24	Francium	Fr	87	Krypton	Kr	36
Berkelium	Bk	97	Cobalt	Co	27	Gadolinium	Gd	64	Lanthanum	La	57
Beryllium	Be	4	Copper	Cu	29	Gallium	Ga	31	Lawrencium	Lr	103
Bismuth	Bi	83	Curium	Cm	96	Germanium	Ge	32	Lead	Pb	82
Bohrium	Bh	107	Darmstadtium	Ds	110	Gold	Au	79	Lithium	Li	3
Boron	B	5	Dubnium	Db	105	Hafnium	Hf	72	Lutetium	Lu	71
Bromine	Br	35	Dysprosium	Dy	66	Hassium	Hs	108	Magnesium	Mg	12

before many of the elements now known were discovered. To maintain the overall logic of the table, Mendeleev allowed space for undiscovered elements whose existence he predicted. This space has since been partly filled in, most recently by the addition of elements 104–112. Elements 111 and 112 have been isolated experimentally but not yet officially named.†

The **lanthanide** series (elements 57–71) and the **actinide** series (elements 89–103) are composed of elements with Group 3b chemical properties. They are placed below the main body of the table to make it easier to read.

| Metals | Nonmetals | Noble gases |

Group 0

| | | | | | 2 **He** Helium 4.0026 |

Group 3a	Group 4a	Group 5a	Group 6a	Group 7a	
5 **B** Boron 10.811	6 **C** Carbon 12.011	7 **N** Nitrogen 14.0067	8 **O** Oxygen 15.9994	9 **F** Fluorine 18.9984	10 **Ne** Neon 20.183

Group 8	Group 1b	Group 2b	13 **Al** Aluminum 26.9815	14 **Si** Silicon 28.086	15 **P** Phosphorus 30.9738	16 **S** Sulfur 32.066	17 **Cl** Chlorine 35.453	18 **Ar** Argon 39.948
28 **Ni** Nickel 58.69	29 **Cu** Copper 63.546	30 **Zn** Zinc 65.39	31 **Ga** Gallium 69.72	32 **Ge** Germanium 72.61	33 **As** Arsenic 74.9216	34 **Se** Selenium 78.96	35 **Br** Bromine 79.904	36 **Kr** Krypton 83.80
46 **Pd** Palladium 106.4	47 **Ag** Silver 107.868	48 **Cd** Cadmium 112.41	49 **In** Indium 114.82	50 **Sn** Tin 118.71	51 **Sb** Antimony 121.76	52 **Te** Tellurium 127.60	53 **I** Iodine 126.9045	54 **Xe** Xenon 131.29
78 **Pt** Platinum 195.08	79 **Au** Gold 196.967	80 **Hg** Mercury 200.59	81 **Tl** Thallium 204.38	82 **Pb** Lead 207.2	83 **Bi** Bismuth 208.98	84 **Po** Polonium (210)	85 **At** Astatine (210)	86 **Rn** Radon (222)
110 **Ds** Darmstadtium (269)	111† (272)	112† (277)						

† Until official names are given to new elements, names based on a Latin translation of the atomic number are used; e.g. *ununbium* (Latin *unus* '1' + *unus* '1' + *bi-* '2') for element 112.

64 **Gd** Gadolinium 157.25	65 **Tb** Terbium 158.925	66 **Dy** Dysprosium 162.50	67 **Ho** Holmium 164.930	68 **Er** Erbium 167.26	69 **Tm** Thulium 168.934	70 **Yb** Ytterbium 173.04	71 **Lu** Lutetium 174.97
96 **Cm** Curium (247)	97 **Bk** Berkelium (247)	98 **Cf** Californium (251)	99 **Es** Einsteinium (252)	100 **Fm** Fermium (257)	101 **Md** Mendelevium (258)	102 **No** Nobelium (259)	103 **Lr** Lawrencium (262)

Element	Symbol	Atomic Number	Element	Symbol	Atomic Number	Element	Symbol	Atomic Number	Element	Symbol	Atomic Number
Manganese	Mn	25	Palladium	Pd	46	Ruthenium	Ru	44	Terbium	Tb	65
Meitnerium	Mt	109	Phosphorus	P	15	Rutherfordium	Rf	104	Thallium	Tl	81
Mendelevium	Md	101	Platinum	Pt	78	Samarium	Sm	62	Thorium	Th	90
Mercury	Hg	80	Plutonium	Pu	94	Scandium	Sc	21	Thulium	Tm	69
Molybdenum	Mo	42	Polonium	Po	84	Seaborgium	Sg	106	Tin	Sn	50
Neodymium	Nd	60	Potassium	K	19	Selenium	Se	34	Titanium	Ti	22
Neon	Ne	10	Praseodymium	Pr	59	Silicon	Si	14	Tungsten	W	74
Neptunium	Np	93	Promethium	Pm	61	Silver	Ag	47	Uranium	U	92
Nickel	Ni	28	Protactinium	Pa	91	Sodium	Na	11	Vanadium	V	23
Niobium	Nb	41	Radium	Ra	88	Strontium	Sr	38	Xenon	Xe	54
Nitrogen	N	7	Radon	Rn	86	Sulfur	S	16	Ytterbium	Yb	70
Nobelium	No	102	Rhenium	Re	75	Tantalum	Ta	73	Yttrium	Y	39
Osmium	Os	76	Rhodium	Rh	45	Technetium	Tc	43	Zinc	Zn	30
Oxygen	O	8	Rubidium	Rb	37	Tellurium	Te	52	Zirconium	Zr	40

SKELETAL MUSCLES

anterior view of skeletal muscles

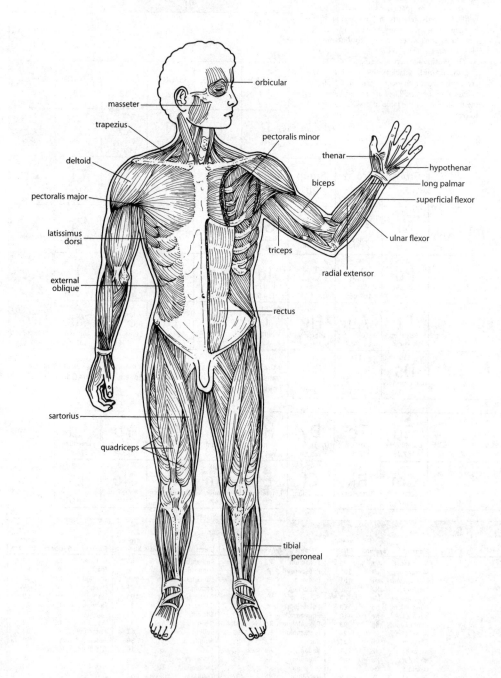

orbicular

masseter

trapezius

pectoralis minor

deltoid

thenar

biceps

hypothenar

long palmar

superficial flexor

pectoralis major

latissimus dorsi

ulnar flexor

triceps

external oblique

radial extensor

rectus

sartorius

quadriceps

tibial

peroneal

SKELETAL MUSCLES

posterior view of skeletal muscles

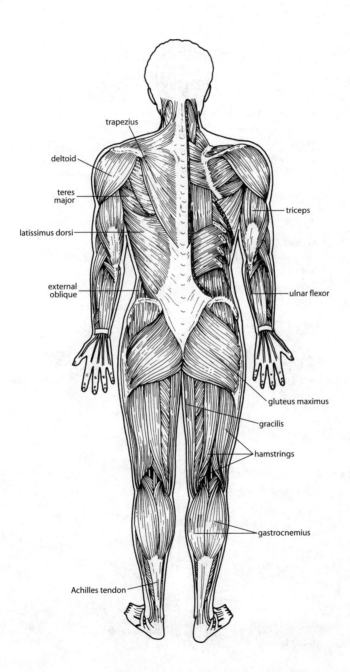

trapezius

deltoid

teres major

latissimus dorsi

external oblique

triceps

ulnar flexor

gluteus maximus

gracilis

hamstrings

gastrocnemius

Achilles tendon

SKELETON

anterior view of an adult skeleton

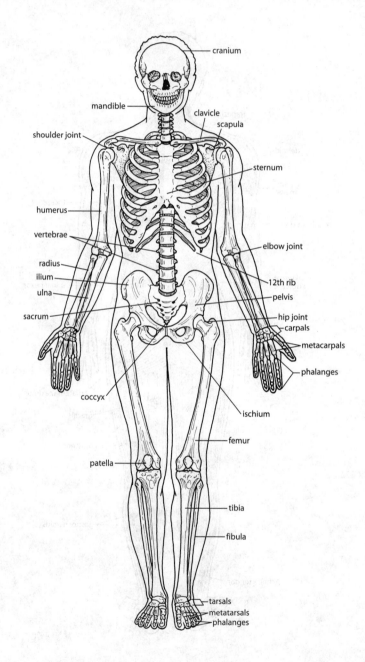

cranium

mandible

shoulder joint

clavicle

scapula

sternum

humerus

vertebrae

radius

ilium

ulna

sacrum

elbow joint

12th rib

pelvis

hip joint

carpals

metacarpals

phalanges

coccyx

ischium

femur

patella

tibia

fibula

tarsals

metatarsals

phalanges

VASCULAR SYSTEM

Anterior view with veins shown in black. For veins and arteries that occur on both sides of the body, only one is labeled; eg., the right femoral vein has a matching left femoral vein.

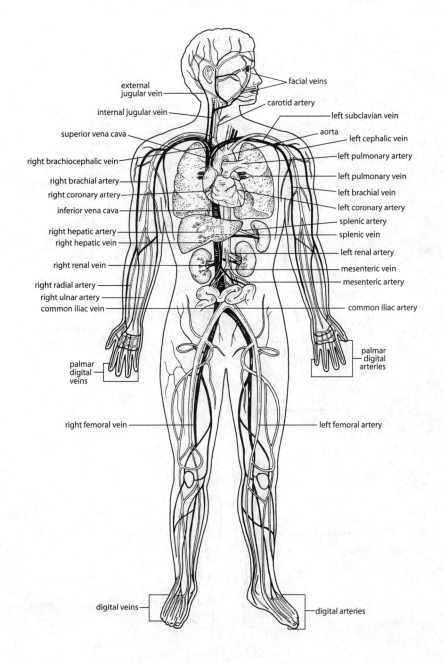

external jugular vein

internal jugular vein

superior vena cava

right brachiocephalic vein

right brachial artery

right coronary artery

inferior vena cava

right hepatic artery

right hepatic vein

right renal vein

right radial artery

right ulnar artery

common iliac vein

palmar digital veins

right femoral vein

digital veins

facial veins

carotid artery

left subclavian vein

aorta

left cephalic vein

left pulmonary artery

left pulmonary vein

left brachial vein

left coronary artery

splenic artery

splenic vein

left renal artery

mesenteric vein

mesenteric artery

common iliac artery

palmar digital arteries

left femoral artery

digital arteries

NERVOUS SYSTEM

posterior view

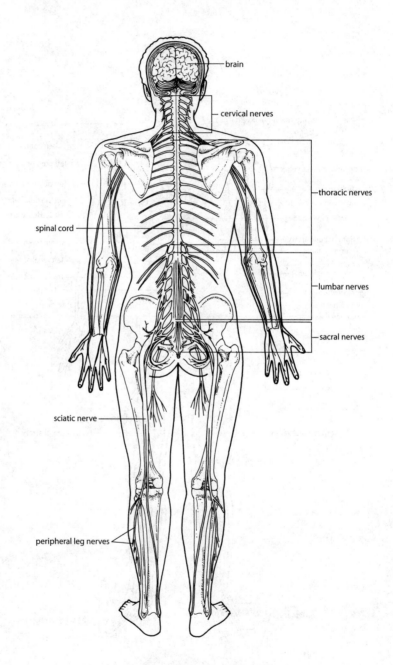

brain

cervical nerves

thoracic nerves

spinal cord

lumbar nerves

sacral nerves

sciatic nerve

peripheral leg nerves

A–Z Illustration Credits

adrenal gland Cecile Duray-Bito; **aneurysm** Laurel Cook Lhowe; **arthritis** Laurel Cook Lhowe; **asthma** Laurel Cook Lhowe; **astigmatism** Cecile Duray-Bito; **atherosclerosis** Elizabeth Morales; **balloon angioplasty** Laurel Cook Lhowe; **biopsy** Laurel Cook Lhowe; **blood cell** Laurel Cook Lhowe; **bone** Carlyn Iverson; **brain** Laurel Cook Lhowe; **cataract** Laurel Cook Lhowe; **cell** Laurel Cook Lhowe; **cerebral embolism** Laurel Cook Lhowe; **cleft lip** Laurel Cook Lhowe; **cleft palate** Laurel Cook Lhowe; **cone** Precision Graphics; **coronary bypass** Laurel Cook Lhowe; **dental caries** Laurel Cook Lhowe; **diaphragm** Laurel Cook Lhowe; **digestive system** Laurel Cook Lhowe; **diverticulum** Laurel Cook Lhowe; **DNA** Laurel Cook Lhowe; **ear** Laurel Cook Lhowe; **ectopic pregnancy** Laurel Cook Lhowe; **embryo** Laurel Cook Lhowe; **endocrine system** Laurel Cook Lhowe; **enzyme** Elizabeth Morales; **epidural hematoma** Laurel Cook Lhowe; **eye** Laurel Cook Lhowe; **floating rib** Laurel Cook Lhowe; **fontanel** Laurel Cook Lhowe; **foot** Laurel Cook Lhowe; **forceps** Laurel Cook Lhowe; **fracture** Laurel Cook Lhowe; **germ layer** Laurel Cook Lhowe; **hair** Carlyn Iverson; **hand** Laurel Cook Lhowe; **heart** Laurel Cook Lhowe; **hyperopia** Cecile Duray-Bito; **inner ear** Laurel Cook Lhowe; **intervertebral disk** Carlyn Iverson; **intestine** Laurel Cook Lhowe; **joint (ball and socket)** Carlyn Iverson; **joint (knee)** Carlyn Iverson; **karyotype** Laurel Cook Lhowe; **kidney** Carlyn Iverson; **lens** Laurel Cook Lhowe;

liver Laurel Cook Lhowe; **lung** Laurel Cook Lhowe; **meiosis** Cecile Duray-Bito; **mitochondrion** Elizabeth Morales; **mitosis** Cecile Duray-Bito; **mouth** Laurel Cook Lhowe; **muscle** Laurel Cook Lhowe; **myopia** Cecile Duray-Bito; **neuron** Laurel Cook Lhowe; **olecranon** Carlyn Iverson; **osteoporosis** Laurel Cook Lhowe; **pacemaker** Laurel Cook Lhowe; **pancreas** Laurel Cook Lhowe; **patella** Laurel Cook Lhowe; **placenta** Laurel Cook Lhowe; **polyp** Laurel Cook Lhowe; **reproductive system** Laurel Cook Lhowe **RNA** Laurel Cook Lhowe; **sickle cell** Laurel Cook Lhowe; **skull** Laurel Cook Lhowe; **speculum** Laurel Cook Lhowe; **spina bifida** Laurel Cook Lhowe; **spinal column** Carlyn Iverson; **spinal cord** Carlyn Iverson; **thyroid gland** Carlyn Iverson; **tooth** Laurel Cook Lhowe; **tracheostomy** Laurel Cook Lhowe; **tubal ligation** Laurel Cook Lhowe; **urinary tract** Carlyn Iverson; **vasectomy** Laurel Cook Lhowe

Backmatter Illustration Credits

measurements Publisher's Design & Production Services; **metric conversion chart** Publisher's Design & Production Services; **recommended daily allowances** Hans + Cassady; **periodic table of the elements** Catherine Hawkes **skeletal muscles** Laurel Cook Lhowe; **skeleton** Laurel Cook Lhowe; **vascular system** Laurel Cook Lhowe; **nervous system** Laurel Cook Lhowe